P9-CQX-268

WinkingSkull.com PLUS

Your study aid for must-know anatomy

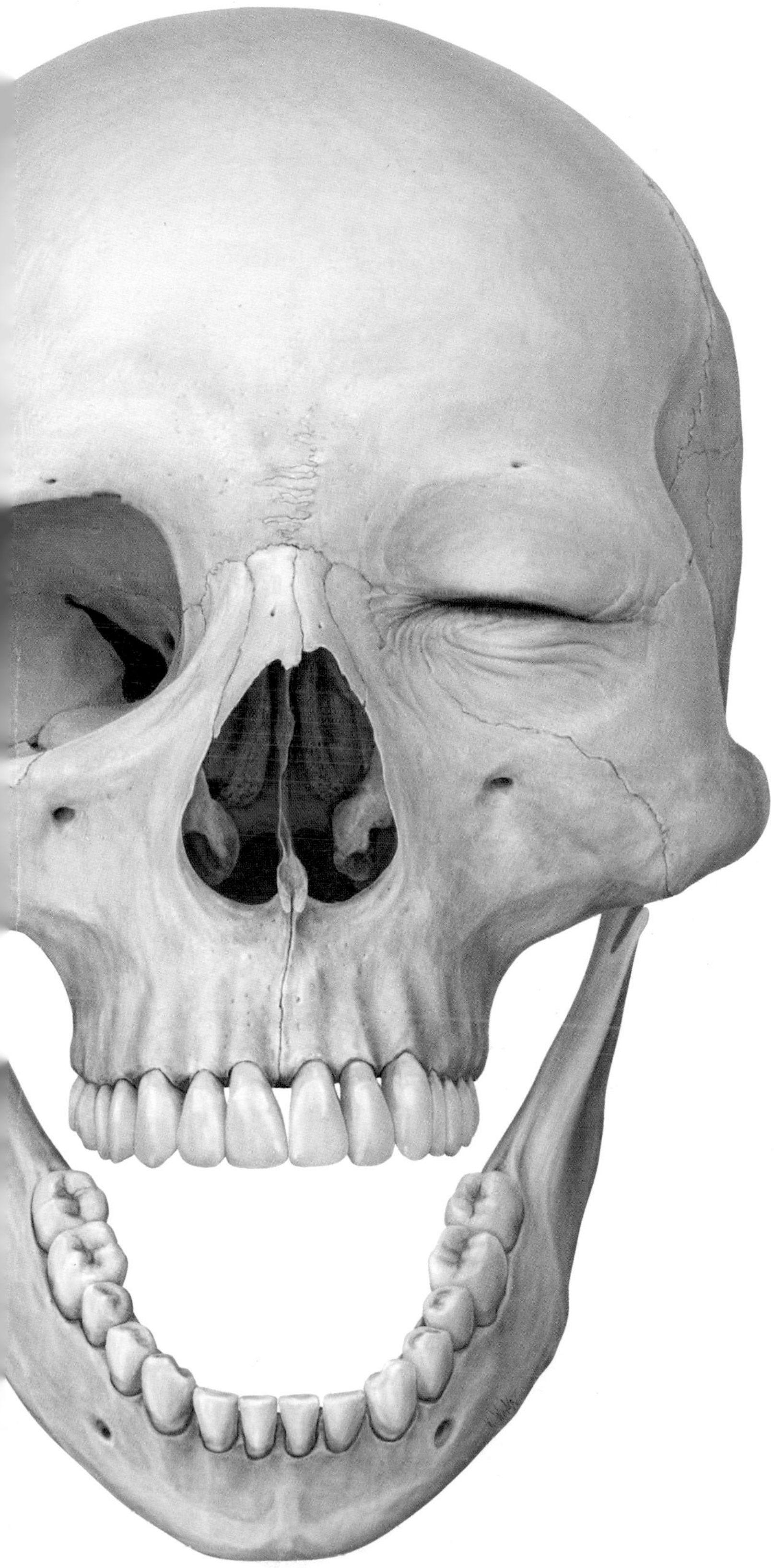

Register for WinkingSkull.com *PLUS* – master human anatomy with this unique interactive online learning tool.

Use the access code below to register for **WinkingSkull.com** *PLUS* and view over 560 full-color illustrations and radiographs from Thieme's bestselling *Atlas of Anatomy* and radiology publications. After studying this invaluable image bank, you can quiz yourself on key body structures and get your score instantly to check your progress or to compare with other users' results.

WinkingSkull.com *PLUS* has everything you need for course study and exam prep:

- More than 560 full-color anatomy illustrations
- Intuitive design that simplifies navigation
- "Labels-on, labels-off" function that makes studying easy and fun
- Timed self-tests–with instant results
- Exclusive clinical material, including MRIs and CT scans with paired explanatory schematics

Simply visit WinkingSkull.com and follow these instructions to get started today.

If you do not already have a free WinkingSkull.com account, visit www.winkingskull.com, click on "Register Now," and complete the registration form. Enter the scratch-off code below.

If you already have a WinkingSkull.com account, go to the "My Account" page and click on the "Enter WinkingSkull PLUS Access Code" link. Enter the scratch-off code below.

4PKZNT6J

This product cannot be returned if the access code panel is scratched off.

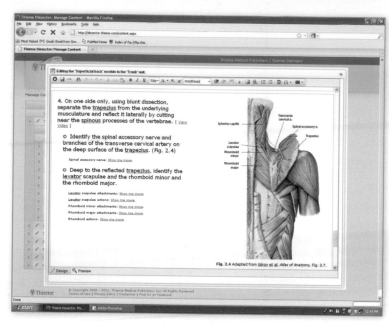

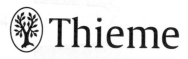

Atlas of Anatomy
Second Edition

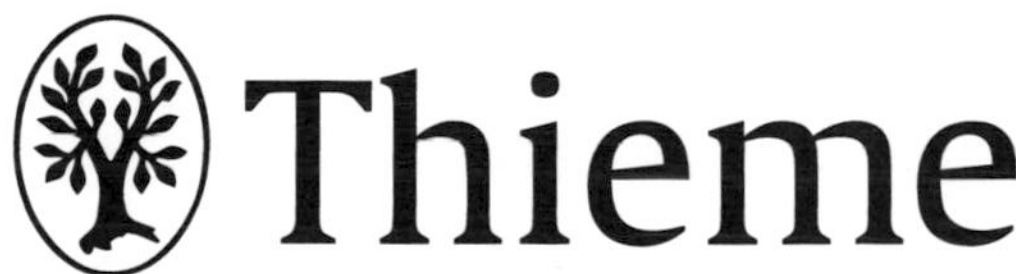
Thieme

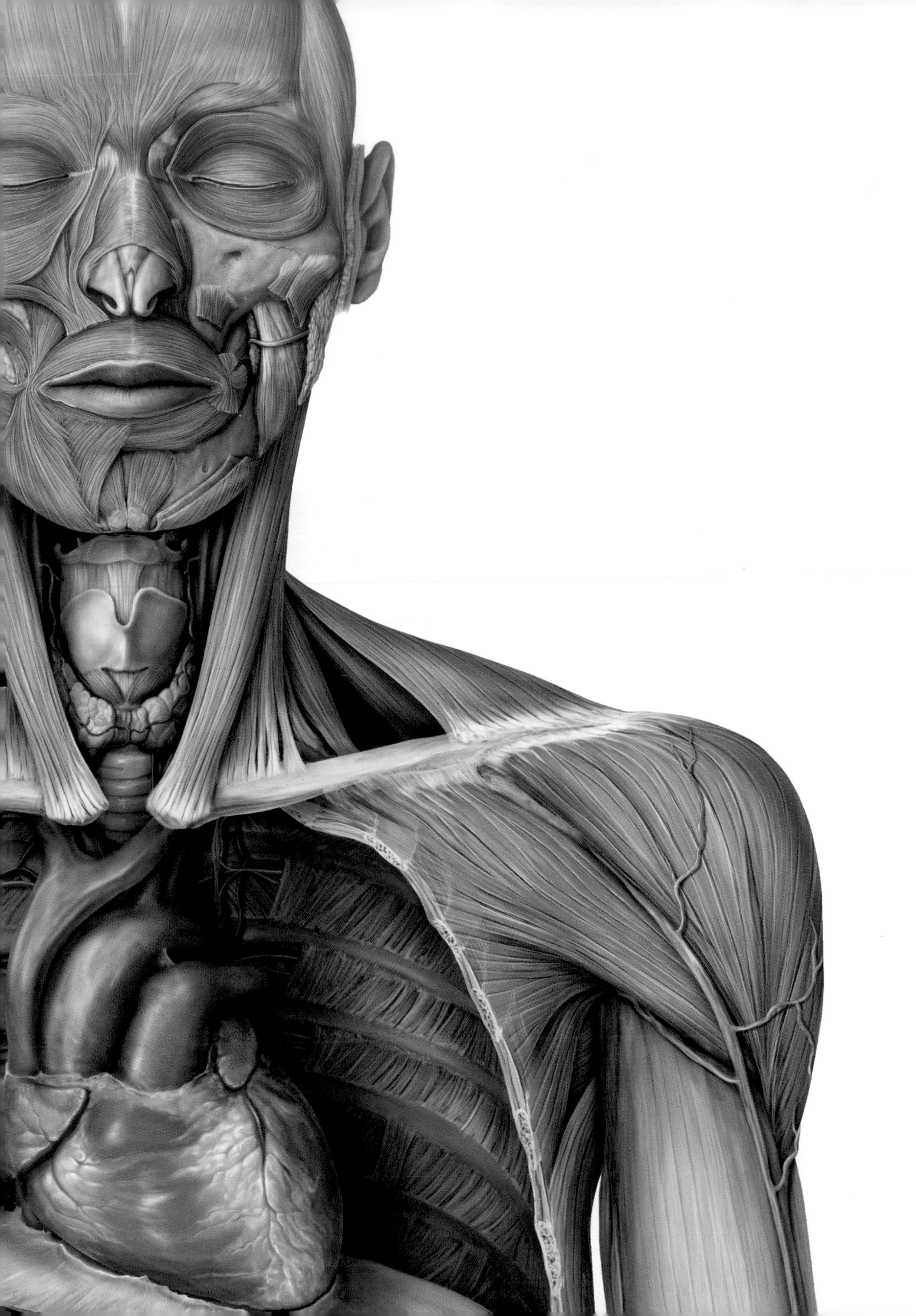

Atlas of Anatomy
Second Edition

Edited by
Anne M. Gilroy
Brian R. MacPherson
Lawrence M. Ross

Based on the work of
Michael Schuenke
Erik Schulte
Udo Schumacher

Illustrated by
Markus Voll
Karl Wesker

Thieme
Stuttgart · New York

Thieme Medical Publishers, Inc.
333 Seventh Avenue
New York, New York 10001

Anne M. Gilroy, MA
Dept. of Cell Biology and Dept. of Surgery
University of Massachusetts Medical School
55 Lake Avenue North
Worcester, MA 01655-0333

Brian R. MacPherson, PhD
Department of Anatomy and Neurobiology
University of Kentucky College of Medicine
MN225 Chandler Medical Center
Lexington, KY 40536-0298

Lawrence M. Ross, MD, PhD
Department of Neurobiology and Anatomy
University of Texas Medical School at Houston
6431 Fannin, Suite 7.046
Houston, TX 77030

Michael Schuenke, MD, PhD
Institute of Anatomy
Christian Albrecht University Kiel
Otto-Hahn-Platz 8
D-24118 Kiel

Erik Schulte, MD
Department of Functional and Clinical Anatomy
University Medicine
Johannes Gutenberg University
Saarstrasse 19-21
D-55099 Mainz

Udo Schumacher, MD, FRCPath, CBiol, FSB, DSc
Institute of Anatomy and Experimental Morphology
Center for Experimental Medicine
University Cancer Center
University Medical Center Hamburg-Eppendorf
Martinistrasse 52
D-20246 Hamburg

Editorial Assistant: Debra A. Zharnest
Production Editor: Megan Conway
Developmental Editor: Avalon Garcia
Vice President and Editorial Director, Educational Products:
Anne T. Vinnicombe
Senior Vice President, International Marketing and Sales:
Cornelia Schulze
Chief Financial Officer: Sarah Vanderbilt
President: Brian D. Scanlan

Illustrators: Markus Voll and Karl Wesker
Compositor: WEYOU Consulting KG, Leonberg, Germany
Printer: Transcontinental Interglobe, Inc.

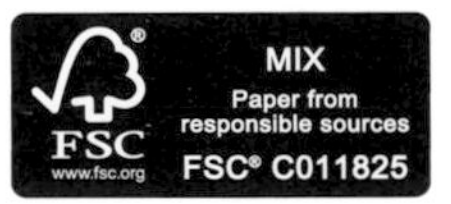
MIX
Paper from responsible sources
FSC
www.fsc.org
FSC® C011825

Library of Congress Cataloging-in-Publication Data

Atlas of anatomy / edited by Anne M. Gilroy, Brian R. MacPherson, Lawrence M. Ross ; based on the work of Michael Schuenke, Erik Schulte, Udo Schumacher ; illustrated by Markus Voll, Karl Wesker. -- 2nd ed.
p. ; cm.
Includes index.
ISBN 978-1-60406-745-3 (softcover : alk. paper) -- ISBN 978-1-60406-746-0 (electronic)
I. Gilroy, Anne M. II. MacPherson, Brian R. III. Ross, Lawrence M. IV. Schuenke, Michael. V. Schulte, Erik. VI. Schumacher, Udo.
[DNLM: 1. Anatomy--Atlases. QS 17]

611.0022'2--dc23
2012004056

Important note: Medical knowledge is ever-changing. As new research and clinical experience broaden our knowledge, changes in treatment and drug therapy may be required. The authors and editors of the material herein have consulted sources believed to be reliable in their efforts to provide information that is complete and in accord with the standards accepted at the time of publication. However, in view of the possibility of human error by the authors, editors, or publisher of the work herein or changes in medical knowledge, neither the authors, editors, nor publisher, nor any other party who has been involved in the preparation of this work, warrants that the information contained herein is in every respect accurate or complete, and they are not responsible for any errors or omissions or for the results obtained from use of such information. Readers are encouraged to confirm the information contained herein with other sources. For example, readers are advised to check the product information sheet included in the package of each drug they plan to administer to be certain that the information contained in this publication is accurate and that changes have not been made in the recommended dose or in the contraindications for administration. This recommendation is of particular importance in connection with new or infrequently used drugs.

Some of the product names, patents, and registered designs referred to in this book are in fact registered trademarks or proprietary names even though specific reference to this fact is not always made in the text. Therefore, the appearance of a name without designation as proprietary is not to be construed as a representation by the publisher that it is in the public domain.

Fig. B, Clinical Box, p. 11: With permission from J. Jallo and A.R. Vaccaro: Neurotrauma and Critical Care of the Spine, Thieme Medical Publishers, Inc., © 2009, p. 150, Fig. 10.4A.

Printed in Canada
5 4 3 2

ISBN: 978-1-60406-745-3 eISBN: 978-1-60406-746-0

Dedication

To my father, Francis Gilroy, whose dedication to medicine has been a greater inspiration to me than he has ever realized; to my students who lovingly tolerate, and sometimes share, my passion for human anatomy; and most of all, to my sons, Colin & Bryan, whose love and support I treasure beyond all else.

— A.M.G.

To my friend and mentor, Dr. Ken McFadden of the Division of Anatomy at the University of Alberta, who ensured I received the training in gross anatomy instruction required to be successful, and to the thousands of professional students who I have taught over the past 30 years, honing these skills. However, none of the success I've enjoyed during my time in academia would have been possible without the constant support, participation, and encouragement of my wife, Cynthia Long.

— B.R.M.

To my wife Irene, and to the children, Chip, Jennifer, Jocelyn & Barry, Tricia, Katie & Snapper, Trey & Alison, and to all my students who have taught me so well.

— L.M.R.

Acknowledgements

We would like to thank the authors of the original award-winning Thieme Atlas of Anatomy, three-volume series, Michael Schuenke, Erik Schulte, and Udo Schumacher, and the illustrators, Karl Wesker and Marcus Voll, for their work over the course of many years.

We thank the many instructors and students who have pointed out to us what we have done well and brought to our attention errors, ambiguities, and new information, or have suggested how we could present a topic more effectively. This input, combined with our experience teaching with the Atlas, have guided our work on this edition.

We again cordially thank the members of the first edition Advisory Board for their contributions:

- Bruce M. Carlson, MD, PhD
  University of Michigan
  Ann Arbor, Michigan
- Derek Bryant (Class of 2011)
  University of Toronto Medical School
  Burlington, Ontario
- Peter Cole, MD
  Glamorum Healing Centre
  Orangeville, Ontario
- Michael Droller, MD
  The Mount Sinai Medical Center
  New York, New York
- Anthony Firth, PhD
  Imperial College London
  London
- Mark H. Hankin, PhD
  University of Toledo, College of Medicine
  Toledo, Ohio
- Katharine Hudson (Class of 2010)
  McGill Medical School
  Montreal, Quebec
- Christopher Lee (Class of 2010)
  Harvard Medical School
  Cambridge, Massachusetts
- Francis Liuzzi, PhD
  Lake Erie College of Osteopathic Medicine
  Bradenton, Florida
- Graham Louw, PhD
  University of Cape Town Medical School
  University of Cape Town
- Estomih Mtui, MD
  Weill Cornell Medical College
  New York, New York
- Srinivas Murthy, MD
  Harvard Medical School
  Boston, Massachusetts
- Jeff Rihn, MD
  The Rothman Institute
  Philadelphia, Pennsylvania
- Lawrence Rizzolo, PhD
  Yale University
  New Haven, Connecticut
- Mikel Snow, PhD
  University of Southern California
  Los Angeles, California
- Kelly Wright (Class of 2010)
  Wayne State University School of Medicine
  Detroit, Michigan

Foreword

This Atlas of Anatomy, in my opinion, is the finest single-volume atlas of human anatomy that has ever been created. Two factors make it so: the images and the way they have been organized.

The artists, Markus Voll and Karl Wesker, have created a new standard of excellence in anatomical art. Their graceful use of transparency and their sensitive representation of light and shadow give the reader an accurate three-dimensional understanding of every structure.

The authors have organized the images so that they give just the flow of information a student needs to build up a clear mental image of the human body. Each two-page spread is a self-contained lesson that unobtrusively shows the hand of an experienced and thoughtful teacher. I wish I could have held this book in my hands when I was a student; I envy any student who does so now.

Robert B. Acland
Louisville, KY

February 2012

Preface to the First Edition

Each of the authors was amazed, and impressed with the extraordinary detail, accuracy, and beauty of the illustrations that were created for the Thieme Atlas of Anatomy. We feel these images are one of the most significant additions to anatomical education in the past 50 years. It was our intent to use these exceptional illustrations as the cornerstone of our effort in creating a concise single volume Atlas of Anatomy for the curious and eager health science student.

Our challenge was first to select from this extensive collection, those images that are most instructive and illustrative of current dissection approaches. Along the way however, we realized that creating a single volume atlas was much more than choosing images: each image has to convey a significant amount of detail while the appeal and labeling need to be clean and soothing to the eye. Therefore, hundreds of illustrations were drawn new or modified to fit the approach of this new atlas. In addition, key schematic diagrams and simplified summary-form tables were added wherever needed. Dozens of applicable radiographic images and important clinical correlates have been added where appropriate. Additionally, surface anatomy illustrations are accompanied by questions designed to direct the student's attention to anatomic detail that is most relevant in conducting the physical exam. Elements from each of these features are arranged in a regional format to facilitate common dissection approaches. Within each region, the various components are examined systemically, followed by topographical images to tie the systems together within the region. In all of this, a clinical perspective on the anatomical structures is taken. The unique two facing pages "spread" format focuses the user to the area/topic being explored.

We hope these efforts — the results of close to 100 combined years experience teaching the discipline of anatomy to bright, enthusiastic students — has resulted in a comprehensive, easy-to-use resource and reference.

We would like to thank our colleagues at Thieme Publishers who so professionally facilitated this effort. We cannot thank enough, Cathrin E. Schulz, M.D., Editorial Director Educational Products, who so graciously reminded us of deadlines, while always being available to "trouble shoot" problems. More importantly, she encouraged, helped, and complimented our efforts.

We also wish to extend very special thanks and appreciation to Bridget Queenan, Developmental Editor, who edited and developed the manuscript with an outstanding talent for visualization and intuitive flow of information. We are very grateful to her for catching many details along the way while always patiently responding to requests for artwork and labeling changes.

Cordial thanks to Elsie Starbecker, Senior Production Editor, who with great care and speed produced this atlas with its over 2.200 illustrations. Finally thanks to Rebecca McTavish, Developmental Editor, for joining the team in the correction phase. So very much of their hard work has made the Atlas of Anatomy a reality.

Anne M. Gilroy
Brian R. MacPherson
Lawrence M. Ross

March 2008,
Worcester, MA, Lexington, KY and Houston, TX

Preface to the Second Edition

We were gratified by the high praise we received from all corners of the anatomic world after publication of the first edition of Atlas of Anatomy. The generous comments of colleagues and students assured us that the atlas was a valuable addition to the learning experience, citing among other things the unparalleled artwork that extends to the level of individual muscles and muscles tables presented in an easy-to-learn summary format. We are especially indebted to those of you who reported omissions, inconsistencies, and typographical, factual, and even artistic errors that escaped the authors, editors, and reviewers. We encourage your continued input, as this motivates and helps us to make each edition of the atlas even more effective than the previous one.

Our mission in this new edition, as in the first edition, is to provide the most complete, up-to-date and effective reference for teaching and studying human anatomy. The core of this new edition remains the more than 2,400 elegant illustrations and schematics, over 150 summary tables, and the effective two-page spreads for presenting concepts. As in the first edition, the presentation is by region and within each region the content is presented in a similar order. Each unit now starts with the surface anatomy of that region and follows with bones, muscles, vasculature, nerves, through to the topographical summary of the area. Where appropriate, sectional anatomy is found at the end of each chapter. In this edition we have reorganized some chapters and spreads in an effort to more closely parallel the progression and content of a typical dissection curriculum. New artwork and expanded text now offers more comprehensive coverage of specific topics. Images that illustrate more than one organ or region are still conveniently repeated as needed. In this second edition of Atlas of Anatomy, readers will find that we have:

- reorganized the material of the combined Abdomen & Pelvis unit into two separate units, Abdomen and Pelvis & Perineum, with the addition of many new illustrations.
- moved the spreads on the spinal cord and cranial meninges from the Neuroanatomy unit into the Back and Head & Neck units, where they are more accessible to students of gross anatomy.
- expanded the surface anatomy spreads and moved them to the beginning of each unit.
- added sectional anatomy spreads to the end of each unit.
- added new and updated artwork in all sections of the atlas.

We hope that students and teaching faculty find these revisions helpful.

Our colleagues at Thieme Publishers have been the essential core of this effort and we are enormously grateful for their support. We especially thank Anne Vinnicombe, Editorial Director for Educational Products, who throughout this project has been available to advise, encourage, and at times even commiserate with each of us. Her professional vision has been a valuable contribution to this manuscript. She is the force who kept us on track and always moving forward.

We also want to thank our Developmental Editor, Avalon Garcia, who worked tirelessly, and with admirable patience, to coordinate and interpret our input.

Additional thanks go to our Production Editor, Megan Conway, who in spite of the hectic schedules of the three authors, coordinated the production of this new volume with remarkable speed with the able help of Editorial Assistant, Debra Zharnest,

Anne M. Gilroy
Brian R. MacPherson
Lawrence M. Ross

February 2012
Worcester, MA, Lexington, KY, and Houston, TX

Table of Contents

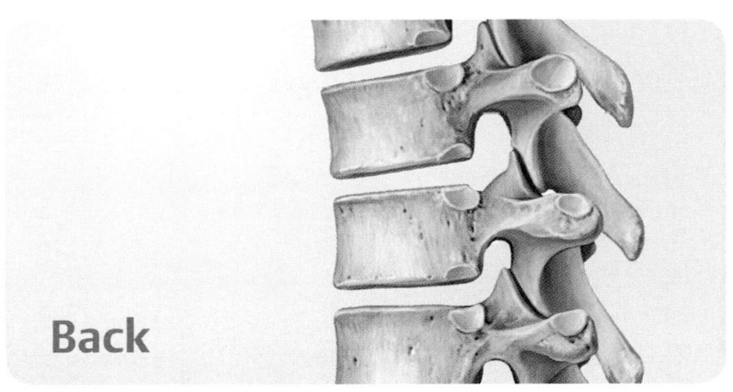
Back

1 **Surface Anatomy**

Surface Anatomy 2

2 **Bones, Ligaments & Joints**

Vertebral Column: Overview 4
Vertebral Column: Elements 6
Cervical Vertebrae 8
Thoracic & Lumbar Vertebrae 10
Sacrum & Coccyx 12
Intervertebral Disks 14
Joints of the Vertebral Column: Overview 16
Joints of the Vertebral Column: Craniovertebral Region 18
Vertebral Ligaments: Overview & Cervical Spine 20
Vertebral Ligaments: Thoracolumbar Spine 22

3 **Muscles**

Muscles of the Back: Overview 24
Intrinsic Muscles of the Cervical Spine 26
Intrinsic Muscles of the Back 28
Muscle Facts (I) 30
Muscle Facts (II) 32
Muscle Facts (III) 34

4 **Neurovasculature**

Arteries & Veins of the Back 36
Nerves of the Back 38
Spinal Cord 40
Spinal Cord Segments and Spinal Nerves 42
Arteries & Veins of the Spinal Cord 44
Neurovascular Topography of the Back 46

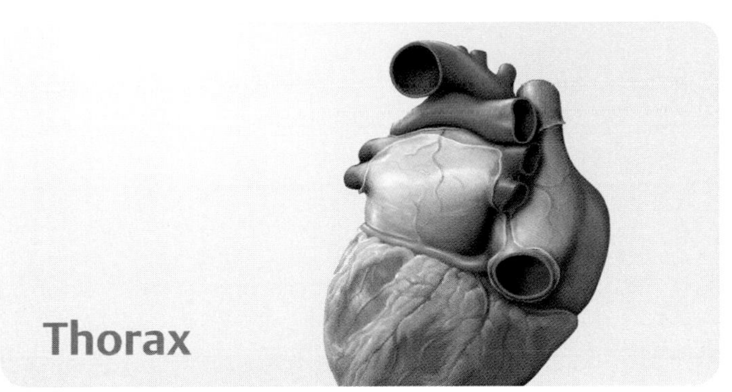
Thorax

5 **Surface Anatomy**

Surface Anatomy 50

6 **Thoracic Wall**

Thoracic Skeleton 52
Sternum & Ribs 54
Joints of the Thoracic Cage 56
Thoracic Wall Muscle Facts 58
Diaphragm 60
Neurovasculature of the Diaphragm 62
Arteries & Veins of the Thoracic Wall 64
Nerves of the Thoracic Wall 66
Neurovascular Topography of the Thoracic Wall 68
Female Breast 70
Lymphatics of the Female Breast 72

7 **Thoracic Cavity**

Divisions of the Thoracic Cavity 74
Arteries of the Thoracic Cavity 76
Veins of the Thoracic Cavity 78
Lymphatics of the Thoracic Cavity 80
Nerves of the Thoracic Cavity 82

8 **Mediastinum**

Mediastinum: Overview 84
Mediastinum: Structures 86
Heart: Functions and Relations 88
Pericardium 90
Heart: Surfaces & Chambers 92
Heart: Valves 94
Arteries & Veins of the Heart 96
Conduction & Innervation of the Heart 98
Heart: Radiology 100
Pre- & Postnatal Circulation 102
Esophagus 104
Neurovasculature of the Esophagus 106
Lymphatics of the Mediastinum 108

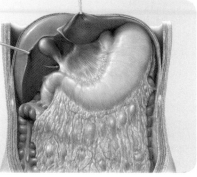

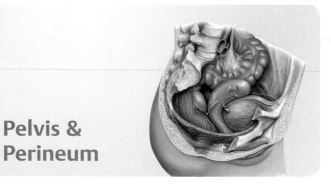

9 Pleural Cavity

Pleural Cavity Chambers 110
Pleura: Subdivisions, Recesses & Innervation 112
Lungs 114
Lung: Radiology 116
Bronchopulmonary Segments of the Lungs 118
Trachea & Bronchial Tree 120
Respiratory Mechanics 122
Pulmonary Arteries & Veins 124
Neurovasculature of the Tracheobronchial Tree 126
Lymphatics of the Pleural Cavity 128

Abdomen

10 Surface Anatomy

Surface Anatomy 132

11 Abdominal Wall

Bony Framework for the Abdominal Wall 134
Muscles of the Anterolateral Abdominal Wall 136
Muscles of the Posterior Abdominal Wall & Diaphragm . . . 138
Abdominal Wall Muscle Facts 140
Inguinal Region & Canal 142
Spermatic Cord, Scrotum & Testis 144
Anterior Abdominal Wall & Inguinal Hernias 146

12 Abdominal Cavity & Spaces

Divisions of the Abdominopelvic Cavity 148
Peritoneal Cavity & Greater Sac 150
Omental Bursa, or Lesser Sac 152
Mesenteries & Posterior Wall 154

13 Internal Organs

Stomach 156
Duodenum 158
Jejunum & Ileum 160
Cecum, Appendix & Colon 162
Liver: Overview 164
Liver: Segments & Lobes 166
Gallbladder & Bile Ducts 168
Pancreas & Spleen 170
Kidneys & Suprarenal Glands (I) 172
Kidneys & Suprarenal Glands (II) 174

14 Neurovasculature

Arteries of the Abdomen 176
Abdominal Aorta & Renal Arteries 178
Celiac Trunk 180
Superior & Inferior Mesenteric Arteries 182
Veins of the Abdomen 184
Inferior Vena Cava & Renal Veins 186
Portal Vein 188
Superior & Inferior Mesenteric Veins 190
Lymphatics of the Abdominal Organs 192
Lymph Nodes of the Posterior Abdominal Wall 194
Lymph Nodes of the Supracolic Organs 196
Lymph Nodes of the Infracolic Organs 198
Nerves of the Abdominal Wall 200
Autonomic Innervation: Overview 202
Autonomic Plexuses 204
Innervation of the Abdominal Organs 206
Innervation of the Intestines 208
Sectional Anatomy of the Abdomen 210

Pelvis & Perineum

15 Surface Anatomy

Surface Anatomy 214

16 Bones, Ligaments & Muscles

Pelvic Girdle 216
Female & Male Pelvis 218
Female & Male Pelvic Measurements 220
Pelvic Ligaments 222
Muscles of the Pelvic Floor & Perineum 224
Pelvic Floor & Perineal Muscle Facts 226

17 Spaces

Contents of the Pelvis 228
Peritoneal Relationships 230
Pelvis & Perineum 232

18 Internal Organs

Rectum & Anal Canal 234
Ureters 236
Urinary Bladder & Urethra 238
Overview of the Genital Organs 240

Uterus & Ovaries 242
Ligaments & Fascia of the Deep Pelvis 244
Vagina 246
Female External Genitalia 248
Penis, Testis & Epididymis 250
Male Accessory Sex Glands 252

19 Neurovasculature

Arteries & Veins of the Pelvis 254
Arteries & Veins of the Rectum & Genitalia 256
Lymph Nodes of the Abdomen & Pelvis 258
Lymph Nodes of the Genitalia 260
Autonomic Plexuses of the Pelvis 262
Autonomic Innervation: Urinary & Genital Organs 264
Neurovasculature of the Female Perineum & Genitalia 266
Neurovasculature of the Male Perineum & Genitalia 268
Sectional Anatomy of the Pelvis & Perineum 270

Upper Limb

20 Surface Anatomy

Surface Anatomy 274

21 Shoulder & Arm

Bones of the Upper Limb 276
Clavicle & Scapula 278
Humerus 280
Joints of the Shoulder 282
Joints of the Shoulder: Glenohumeral Joint 284
Subacromial Space & Bursae 286
Anterior Muscles of the Shoulder & Arm (I) 288
Anterior Muscles of the Shoulder & Arm (II) 290
Posterior Muscles of the Shoulder & Arm (I) 292
Posterior Muscles of the Shoulder & Arm (II) 294
Muscle Facts (I) 296
Muscle Facts (II) 298
Muscle Facts (III) 300
Muscle Facts (IV) 302

22 Elbow & Forearm

Radius & Ulna 304
Elbow Joint 306
Ligaments of the Elbow Joint 308
Radioulnar Joints 310
Muscles of the Forearm (I) 312
Muscles of the Forearm (II) 314
Muscle Facts (I) 316
Muscle Facts (II) 318
Muscle Facts (III) 320

23 Wrist & Hand

Bones of the Wrist & Hand 322
The Carpal Bones 324
Joints of the Wrist & Hand 326
Ligaments of the Hand 328
Ligaments of the Wrist 330
Ligaments of the Fingers 332
Muscles of the Hand: Superficial & Middle Layers 334
Muscles of the Hand: Middle & Deep Layers 336
Dorsum of the Hand 338
Muscle Facts (I) 340
Muscle Facts (II) 342

24 Neurovasculature

Arteries of the Upper Limb 344
Veins & Lymphatics of the Upper Limb 346
Nerves of the Brachial Plexus 348
Supraclavicular Branches & Posterior Cord 350
Posterior Cord: Axillary & Radial Nerves 352
Medial & Lateral Cords 354
Median & Ulnar Nerves 356
Superficial Veins & Nerves of the Upper Limb 358
Posterior Shoulder & Axilla 360
Anterior Shoulder 362
Topography of the Axilla 364
Topography of the Brachial & Cubital Regions 366
Topography of the Forearm 368
Topography of the Carpal Region 370
Topography of the Palm of the Hand 372
Topography of the Dorsum of the Hand 374
Sectional Anatomy of the Upper Limb 376

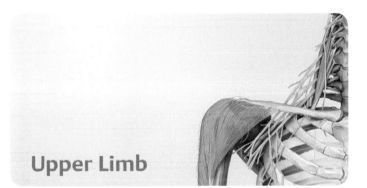

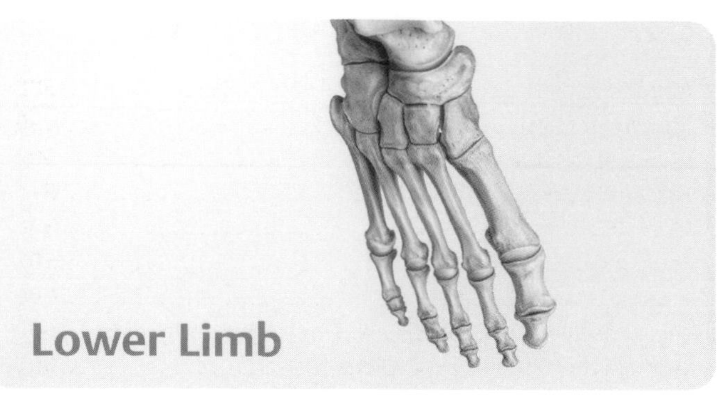

Lower Limb

25 Surface Anatomy

Surface Anatomy 380

26 Hip & Thigh

Bones of the Lower Limb 382
Femur 384
Hip Joint: Overview 386
Hip Joint: Ligaments & Capsule 388
Anterior Muscles of the Hip, Thigh & Gluteal Region (I) . . . 390
Anterior Muscles of the Hip, Thigh & Gluteal Region (II) . . . 392
Posterior Muscles of the Hip, Thigh & Gluteal Region (I) . . . 394
Posterior Muscles of the Hip, Thigh & Gluteal Region (II) . . 396
Muscle Facts (I) 398
Muscle Facts (II) 400
Muscle Facts (III) 402

27 Knee & Leg

Tibia & Fibula 404
Knee Joint: Overview 406
Knee Joint: Capsule, Ligaments & Bursae 408
Knee Joint: Ligaments & Menisci 410
Cruciate Ligaments 412
Knee Joint Cavity 414
Muscles of the Leg: Anterior & Lateral Compartments 416
Muscles of the Leg: Posterior Compartment 418
Muscle Facts (I) 420
Muscle Facts (II) 422

28 Ankle & Foot

Bones of the Foot 424
Joints of the Foot (I) 426
Joints of the Foot (II) 428
Joints of the Foot (III) 430
Ligaments of the Ankle & Foot 432
Plantar Vault & Arches of the Foot 434
Muscles of the Sole of the Foot 436
Muscles & Tendon Sheaths of the Foot 438
Muscle Facts (I) 440
Muscle Facts (II) 442

29 Neurovasculature

Arteries of the Lower Limb 444
Veins & Lymphatics of the Lower Limb 446
Lumbosacral Plexus 448
Nerves of the Lumbar Plexus 450
Nerves of the Lumbar Plexus: Obturator & Femoral Nerves 452
Nerves of the Sacral Plexus 454
Nerves of the Sacral Plexus: Sciatic Nerve 456
Superficial Nerves & Vessels of the Lower Limb 458
Topography of the Inguinal Region 460
Topography of the Gluteal Region 462
Topography of the Anterior, Medial & Posterior Thigh 464
Topography of the Posterior Compartment of the Leg & Foot 466
Topography of the Lateral & Anterior Compartments of the Leg 468
Topography of the Sole of the Foot 470
Sectional Anatomy of the Thigh & Leg 472

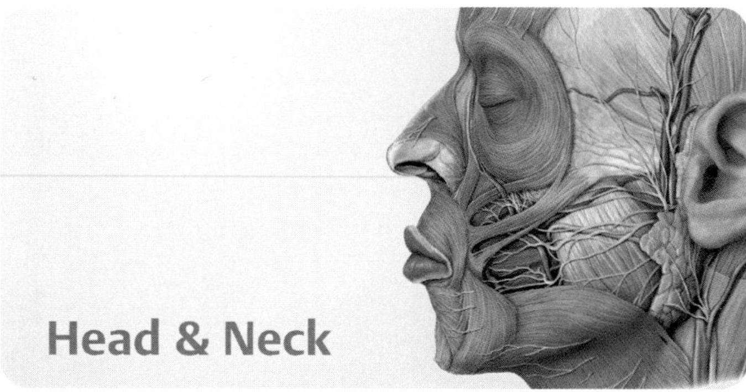

Head & Neck

30 Surface Anatomy

Surface Anatomy 476

31 Bones of the Head

Anterior & Lateral Skull 478
Posterior Skull & Calvaria 480
Base of the Skull 482
Neurovascular Pathways Exiting or Entering the Cranial Cavity 484
Ethmoid & Sphenoid Bones 486

32 Muscles of the Skull & Face

Muscles of Facial Expression & of Mastication 488
Muscle Origins & Insertions on the Skull 490
Muscle Facts (I) 492
Muscle Facts (II) 494

33 Cranial Nerves

Cranial Nerves: Overview 496
CN I & II: Olfactory & Optic Nerves 498
CN III, IV & VI: Oculomotor, Trochlear & Abducent Nerves . 500

CN V: Trigeminal Nerve 502
CN VII: Facial Nerve 504
CN VIII: Vestibulocochlear Nerve 506
CN IX: Glossopharyngeal Nerve 508
CN X: Vagus Nerve 510
CN XI & XII: Accessory & Hypoglossal Nerves 510

34 Neurovasculature of the Skull & Face

Innervation of the Face 514
Arteries of the Head & Neck 516
External Carotid Artery:
Anterior, Medial & Posterior Branches 518
External Carotid Artery: Terminal Branches 520
Veins of the Head & Neck 522
Meninges 524
Dural Sinuses 526
Topography of the Superficial Face 528
Topography of the Parotid Region & Temporal Fossa 530
Topography of the Infratemporal Fossa 532
Topography of the Pterygopalatine Fossa 534

35 Orbit & Eye

Bones of the Orbit 536
Muscles of the Orbit 538
Neurovasculature of the Orbit 540
Topography of the Orbit 542
Orbit & Eyelid 544
Eyeball 546
Cornea, Iris & Lens 548

36 Nasal Cavity & Nose

Bones of the Nasal Cavity 550
Paranasal Air Sinuses 552
Neurovasculature of the Nasal Cavity 554

37 Temporal Bone & Ear

Temporal Bone 556
External Ear & Auditory Canal 558
Middle Ear: Tympanic Cavity 560
Middle Ear: Ossicular Chain & Tympanic Membrane 562
Arteries of the Middle Ear 564
Inner Ear 566

38 Oral Cavity & Pharynx

Bones of the Oral Cavity 568
Temporomandibular Joint 570
Teeth 572
Oral Cavity Muscle Facts 574
Innervation of the Oral Cavity 576
Tongue 578
Topography of the Oral Cavity & Salivary Glands 580
Tonsils & Pharynx 582
Pharyngeal Muscles 584
Neurovasculature of the Pharynx 586

39 Neck

Muscle Facts (I) 588
Muscle Facts (II) 590
Muscle Facts (III) 592
Arteries & Veins of the Neck 594
Innervation of the Neck 596
Larynx: Cartilage & Structure 598
Larynx: Muscles & Levels 600
Neurovasculature of the Larynx, Thyroid & Parathyroids . . . 602
Topography of the Neck: Regions & Fascia 604
Topography of the Anterior Cervical Region 606
Topography of the Anterior & Lateral Cervical Regions 608
Topography of the Lateral Cervical Region 610
Topography of the Posterior Cervical Region 612
Lymphatics of the Neck 614
Coronal Sections of the Head 616
Transverse Sections of the Head & Neck 618
Sagittal Sections of the Head 620

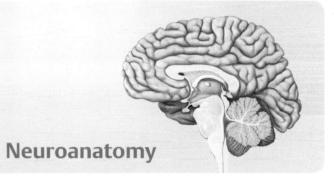

Neuroanatomy

40 Brain

Nervous System: Overview 624
Telencephalon 626
Telencephalon & Diencephalon 628
Diencephalon, Brainstem & Cerebellum 630
Ventricles & CSF Spaces 632

41 Blood Vessels of the Brain

Veins of the Brain 634
Arteries of the Brain 636

42 Functional Systems

Circuitry 638
Sensory & Motor Pathways 640
Sensory Systems (I) 642
Sensory Systems (II) 644
Sensory Systems (III) 646

43 Autonomic Nervous System

Autonomic Nervous System 648

Index 652

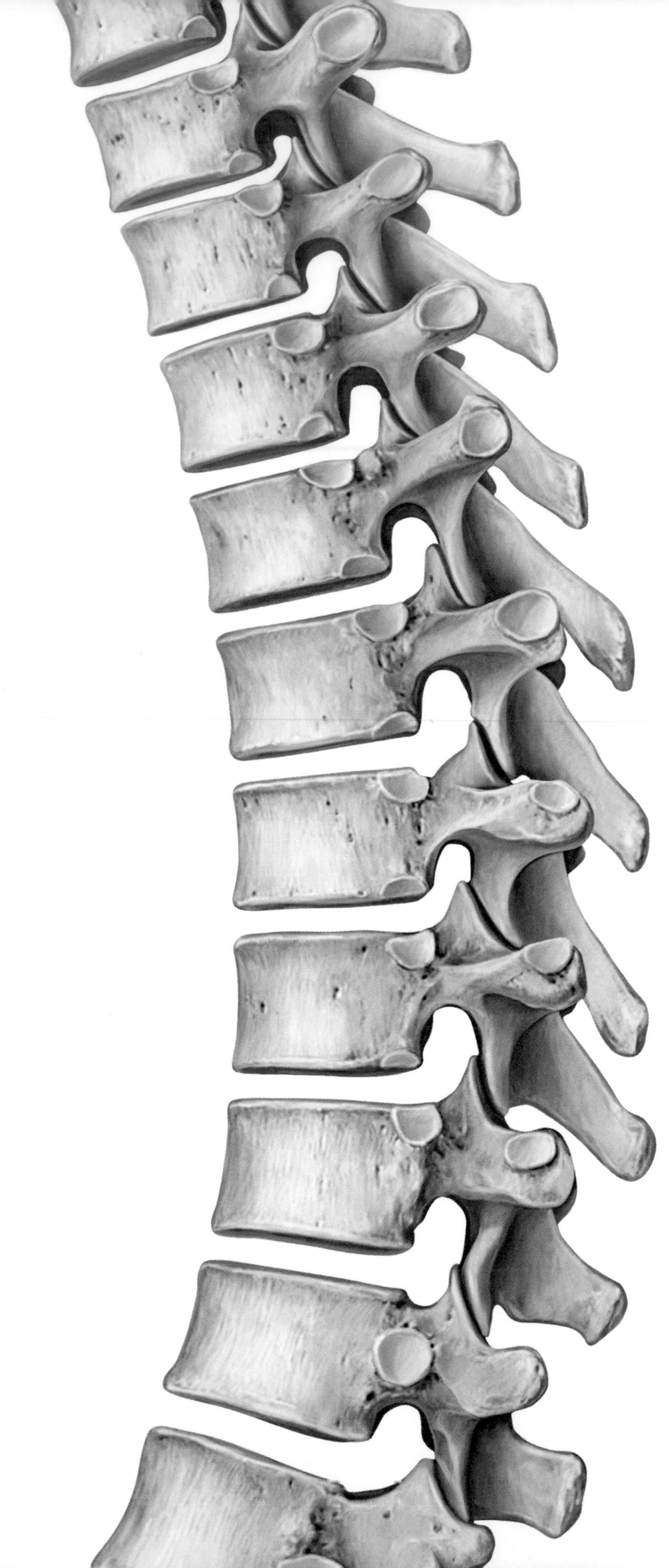

Back

1 Surface Anatomy

Surface Anatomy 2

2 Bones, Ligaments & Joints

Vertebral Column: Overview 4
Vertebral Column: Elements 6
Cervical Vertebrae 8
Thoracic & Lumbar Vertebrae 10
Sacrum & Coccyx 12
Intervertebral Disks 14
Joints of the Vertebral Column: Overview 16
Joints of the Vertebral Column: Craniovertebral Region 18
Vertebral Ligaments: Overview & Cervical Spine 20
Vertebral Ligaments: Thoracolumbar Spine 22

3 Muscles

Muscles of the Back: Overview 24
Intrinsic Muscles of the Cervical Spine 26
Intrinsic Muscles of the Back 28
Muscle Facts (I) 30
Muscle Facts (II) 32
Muscle Facts (III) 34

4 Neurovasculature

Arteries & Veins of the Back 36
Nerves of the Back 38
Spinal Cord 40
Spinal Cord Segments & Spinal Nerves 42
Arteries & Veins of the Spinal Cord 44
Neurovascular Topography of the Back 46

Surface Anatomy

Fig. 1.1 **Palpable structures of the back**
Posterior view.

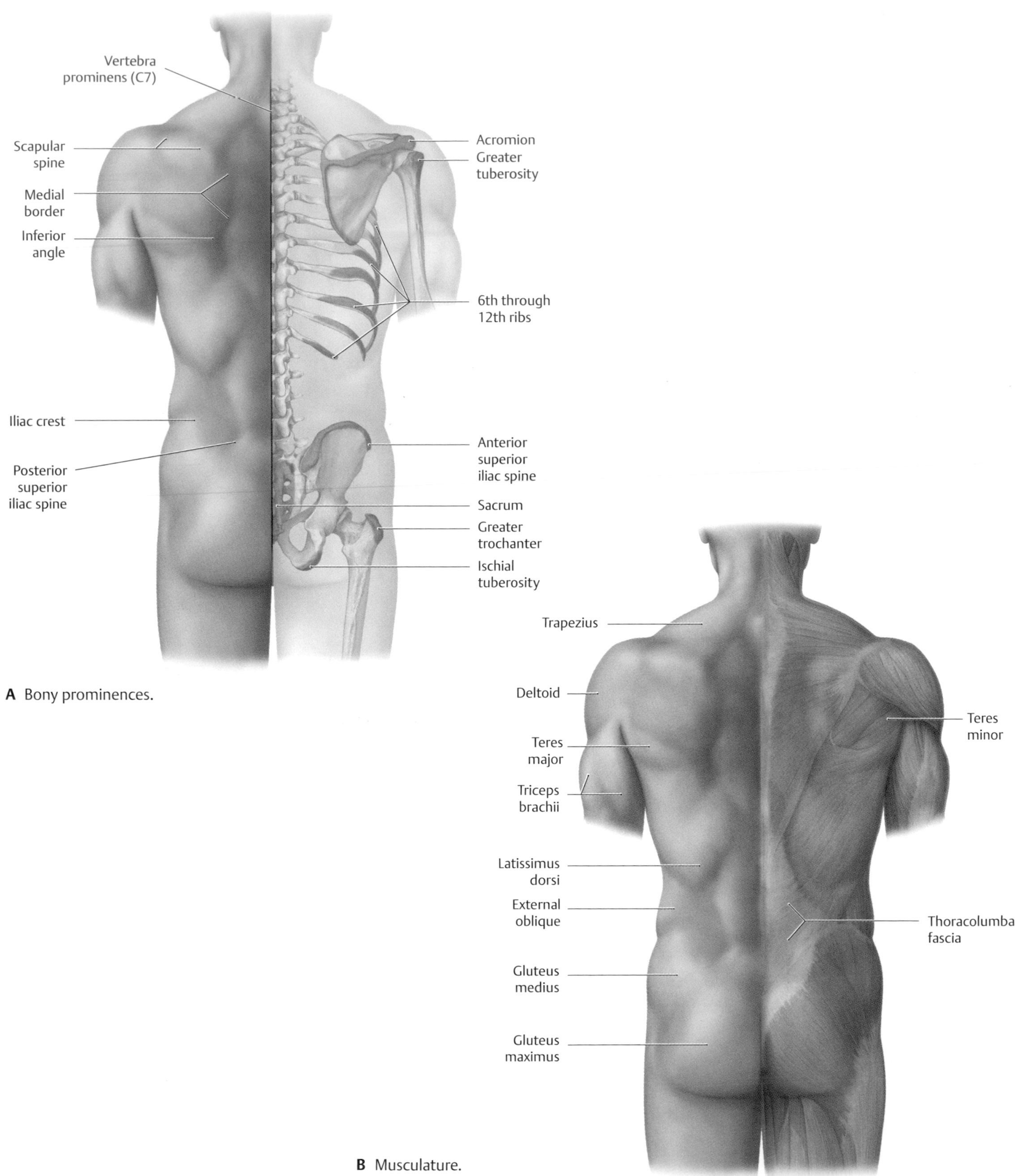
Vertebra prominens (C7)
Scapular spine
Medial border
Inferior angle
Acromion
Greater tuberosity
6th through 12th ribs
Iliac crest
Posterior superior iliac spine
Anterior superior iliac spine
Sacrum
Greater trochanter
Ischial tuberosity
Trapezius
Deltoid
Teres major
Triceps brachii
Latissimus dorsi
External oblique
Gluteus medius
Gluteus maximus
Teres minor
Thoracolumbar fascia

A Bony prominences.

B Musculature.

Fig. 1.2 **Regions of the back and buttocks**
Posterior view.

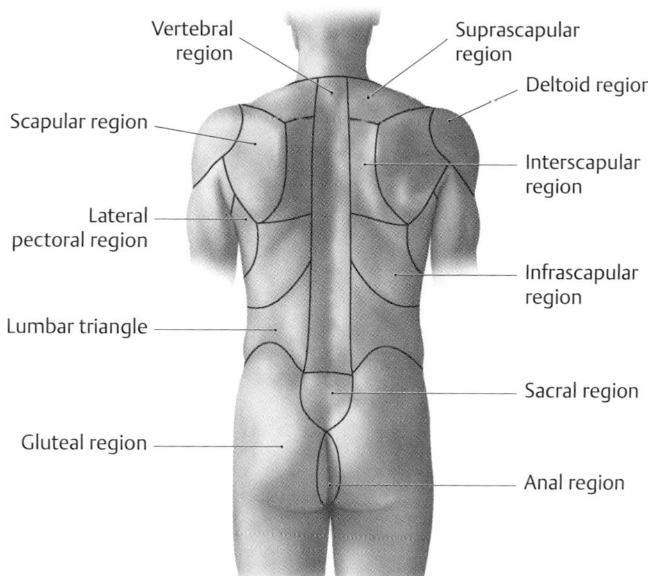
Vertebral region
Suprascapular region
Deltoid region
Scapular region
Interscapular region
Lateral pectoral region
Infrascapular region
Lumbar triangle
Sacral region
Gluteal region
Anal region

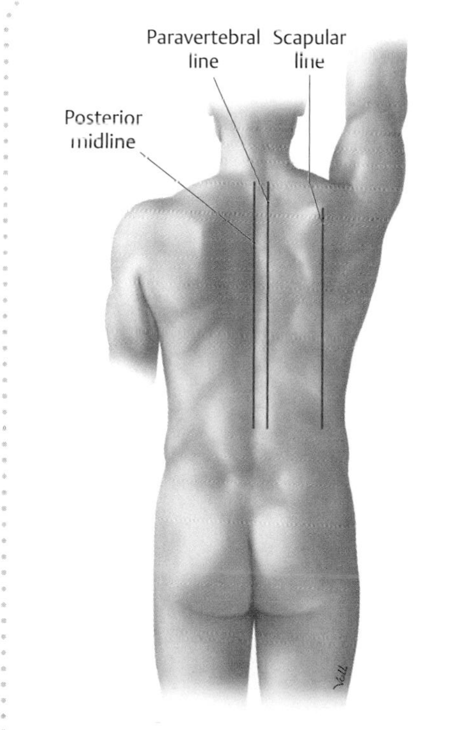
Paravertebral line
Scapular line
Posterior midline

Table 1.1	Reference lines of the back
Posterior midline	Posterior trunk midline at the level of the spinous processes
Paravertebral line	Line at the level of the transverse processes
Scapular line	Line through the inferior angle of the scapula

Fig. 1.3 **Spinous processes and landmarks of the back**
Posterior view.

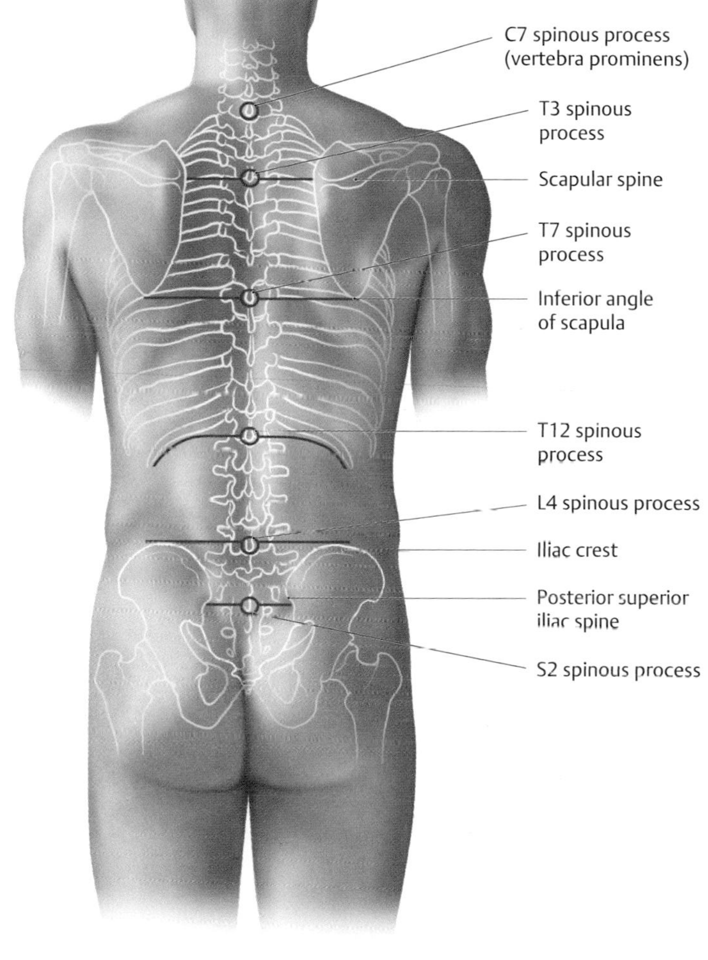
C7 spinous process (vertebra prominens)
T3 spinous process
Scapular spine
T7 spinous process
Inferior angle of scapula
T12 spinous process
L4 spinous process
Iliac crest
Posterior superior iliac spine
S2 spinous process

Table 1.2 **Spinous processes that provide useful posterior landmarks**

Vertebral spinous process	Posterior landmark
C7	Vertebra prominens (the projecting spinous process of C7 is clearly visible and palpable)
T3	The scapular spine
T7	The inferior angle of the scapula
T12	Just below the 12th rib
L4	The summit of the iliac crest
S2	The posterior superior iliac spine (recognized by small skin depressions directly over the iliac spines)

Vertebral Column: Overview

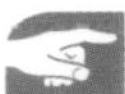

The vertebral column (spine) is divided into four regions: the cervical, thoracic, lumbar, and sacral spines. Both the cervical and lumbar spines demonstrate lordosis (inward curvature); the thoracic and sacral spines demonstrate kyphosis (outward curvature).

Fig. 2.1 **Vertebral column**
Left lateral view.

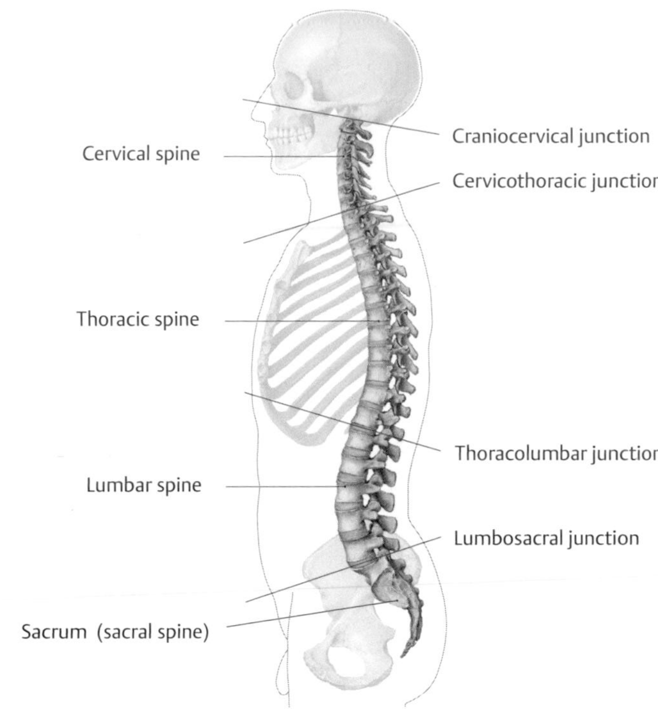
Cervical spine
Craniocervical junction
Cervicothoracic junction
Thoracic spine
Thoracolumbar junction
Lumbar spine
Lumbosacral junction
Sacrum (sacral spine)

A Regions of the spine.

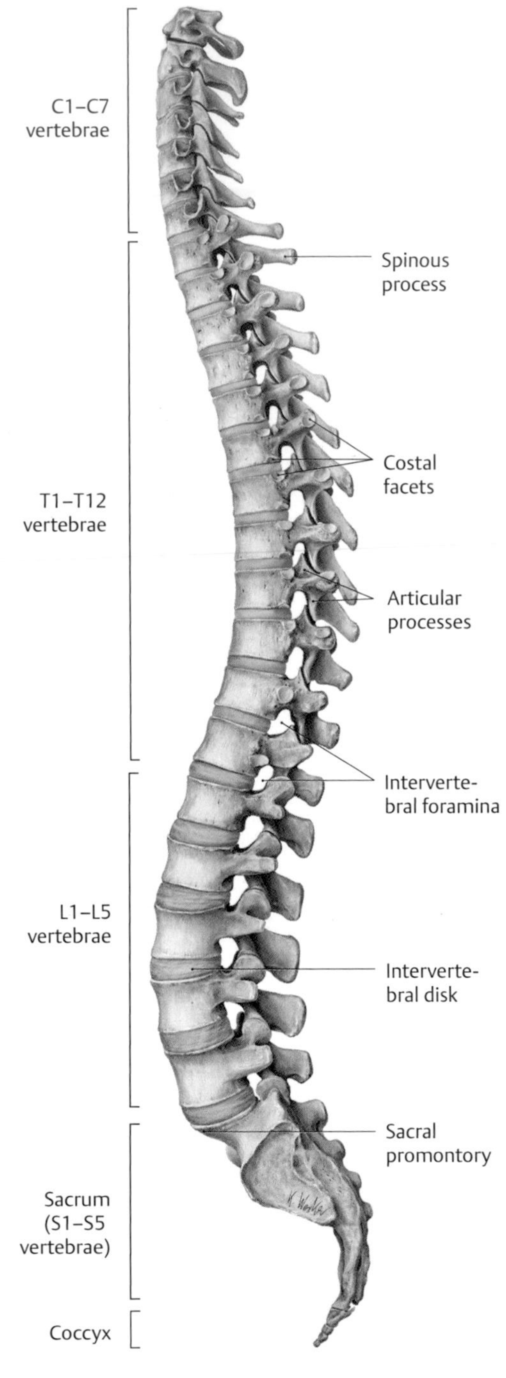
C1–C7
vertebrae
Spinous
process
Costal
facets
T1–T12
vertebrae
Articular
processes
Interverte-
bral foramina
L1–L5
vertebrae
Interverte-
bral disk
Sacral
promontory
Sacrum
(S1–S5
vertebrae)
Coccyx

B Bony vertebral column.

Clinical

Spinal development

The characteristic curvatures of the adult spine appear over the course of postnatal development, being only partially present in a newborn. The newborn has a "kyphotic" spinal curvature (**A**); lumbar lordosis develops later and becomes stable at puberty (**C**).

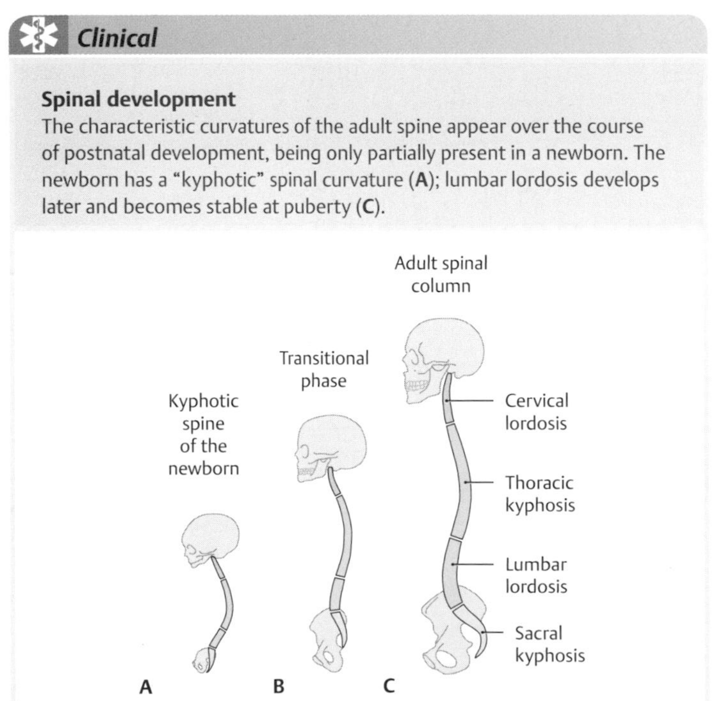
Adult spinal
column
Transitional
phase
Kyphotic
spine
of the
newborn
Cervical
lordosis
Thoracic
kyphosis
Lumbar
lordosis
Sacral
kyphosis
A
B
C

Fig. 2.2 Normal anatomical position of the spine
Left lateral view.

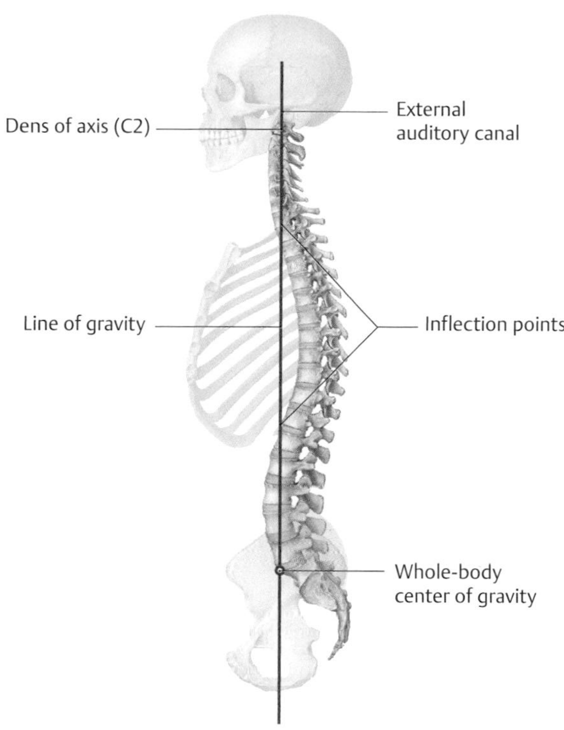

Dens of axis (C2)
External auditory canal
Line of gravity
Inflection points
Whole-body center of gravity

A Line of gravity. The line of gravity passes through certain anatomical landmarks, including the inflection points at the cervicothoracic and thoracolumbar junctions. It continues through the center of gravity (anterior to the sacral promontory) before passing through the hip joint, knee, and ankle.

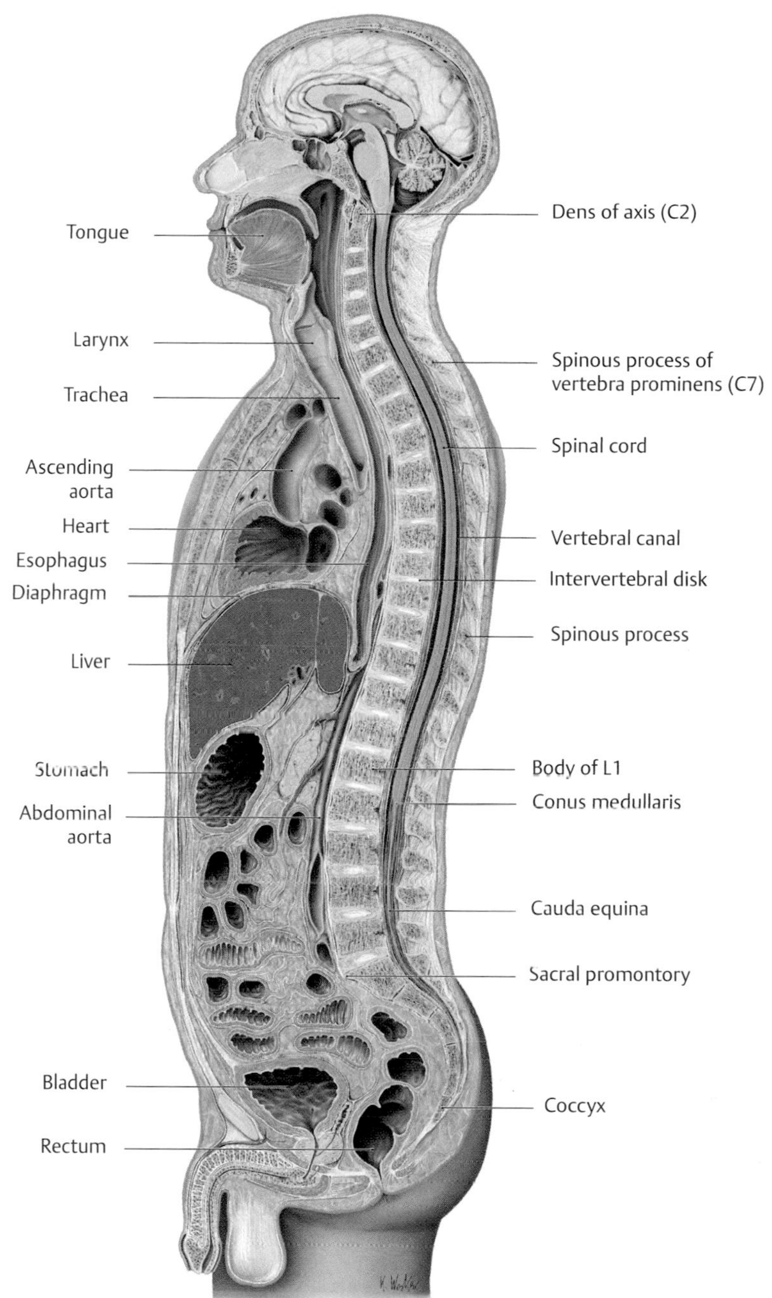

Tongue
Larynx
Trachea
Ascending aorta
Heart
Esophagus
Diaphragm
Liver
Stomach
Abdominal aorta
Bladder
Rectum
Dens of axis (C2)
Spinous process of vertebra prominens (C7)
Spinal cord
Vertebral canal
Intervertebral disk
Spinous process
Body of L1
Conus medullaris
Cauda equina
Sacral promontory
Coccyx

B Midsagittal section through an adult male.

Vertebral Column: Elements

Fig. 2.3 **Bones of the vertebral column**
The transverse processes of the lumbar vertebrae are originally rib rudiments and so are named costal processes.

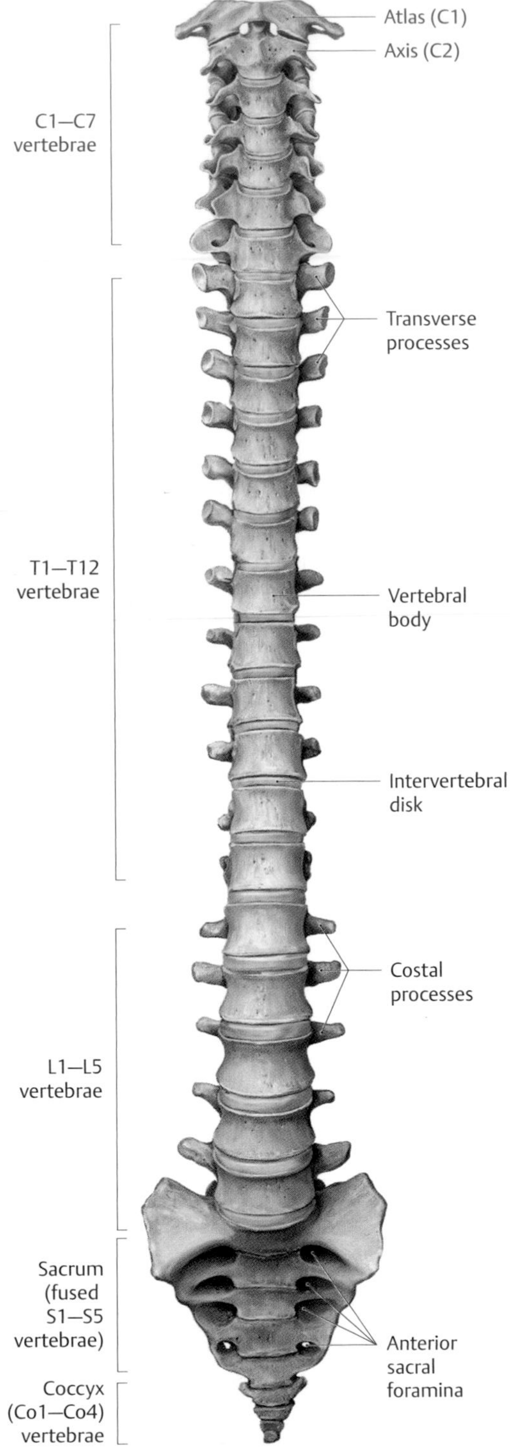

Atlas (C1)
Axis (C2)
C1—C7 vertebrae
Transverse processes
T1—T12 vertebrae
Vertebral body
Intervertebral disk
Costal processes
L1—L5 vertebrae
Sacrum (fused S1—S5 vertebrae)
Anterior sacral foramina
Coccyx (Co1—Co4) vertebrae

A Anterior view.

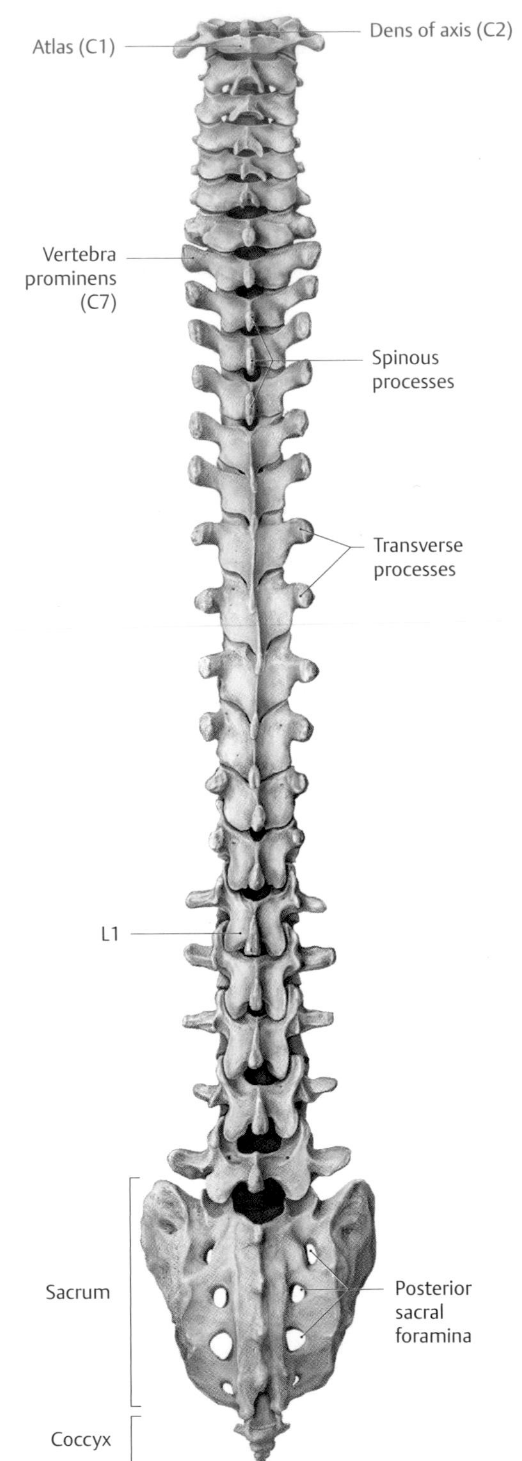

Atlas (C1)
Dens of axis (C2)
Vertebra prominens (C7)
Spinous processes
Transverse processes
L1
Sacrum
Posterior sacral foramina
Coccyx

B Posterior view.

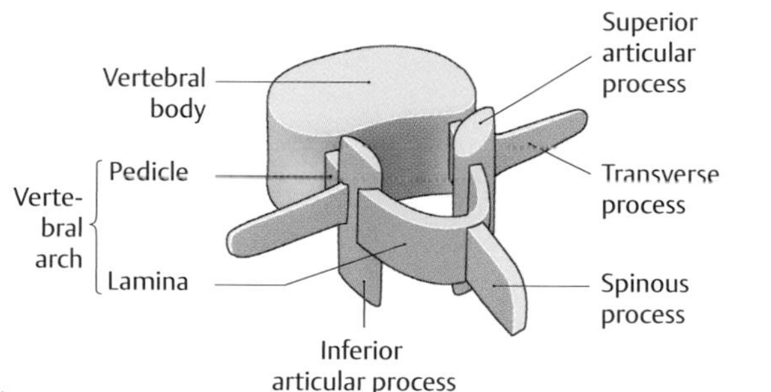
Vertebral body
Superior articular process
Pedicle
Vertebral arch
Transverse process
Lamina
Spinous process
Inferior articular process

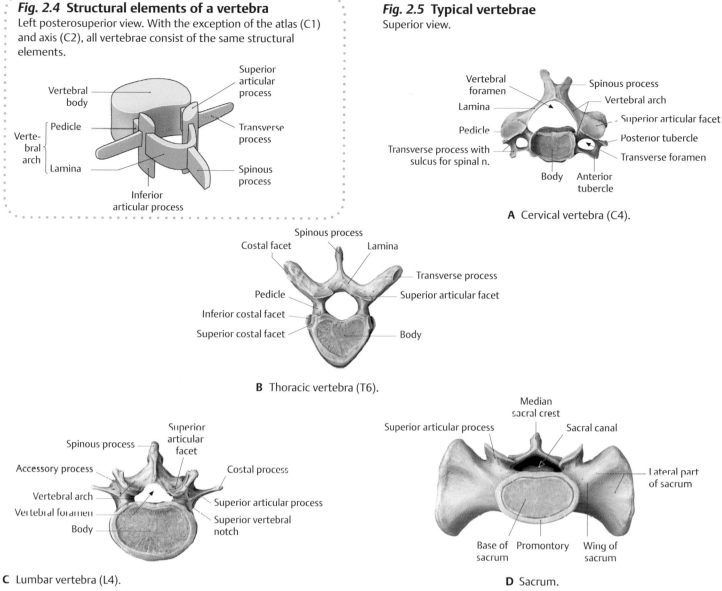

Fig. 2.4 **Structural elements of a vertebra**
Left posterosuperior view. With the exception of the atlas (C1) and axis (C2), all vertebrae consist of the same structural elements.

Fig. 2.5 **Typical vertebrae**
Superior view.

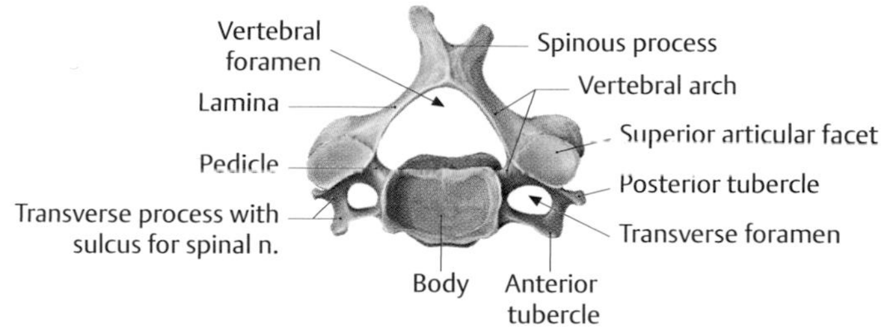
Vertebral foramen
Lamina
Pedicle
Transverse process with sulcus for spinal n.
Spinous process
Vertebral arch
Superior articular facet
Posterior tubercle
Transverse foramen
Body
Anterior tubercle

A Cervical vertebra (C4).

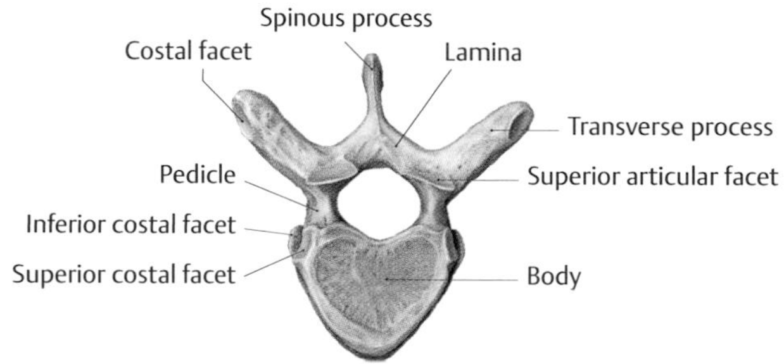
Spinous process
Costal facet
Lamina
Transverse process
Pedicle
Superior articular facet
Inferior costal facet
Superior costal facet
Body

B Thoracic vertebra (T6).

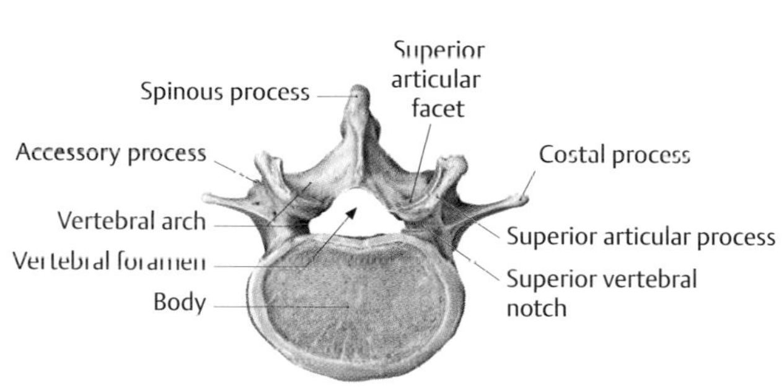
Spinous process
Superior articular facet
Accessory process
Costal process
Vertebral arch
Superior articular process
Vertebral foramen
Superior vertebral notch
Body

C Lumbar vertebra (L4).

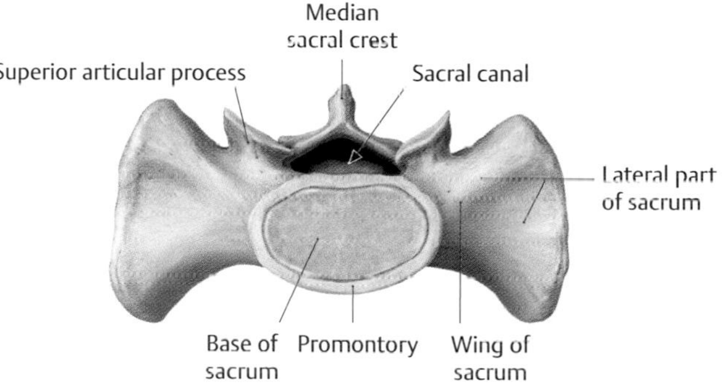
Median sacral crest
Superior articular process
Sacral canal
Lateral part of sacrum
Base of sacrum
Promontory
Wing of sacrum

D Sacrum.

Table 2.1 **Structural elements of vertebrae**

Vertebrae	Body	Vertebral foramen	Transverse processes	Articular processes	Spinous process
Cervical vertebrae C3*–C7	Small (kidney-shaped)	Large (triangular)	Small (may be absent in C7); anterior and posterior tubercles enclose transverse foramen	Superoposteriorly and inferoanteriorly; oblique facets: most nearly horizontal	Short (C3–C5); bifid (C3–C6); long (C7)
Thoracic vertebrae T1–T12	Medium (heart-shaped); includes costal facets	Small (circular)	Large and strong; length decreases T1–T12; costal facets (T1–T10)	Posteriorly (slightly laterally) and anteriorly (slightly medially); facets in coronal plane	Long, sloping postero-inferiorly; tip extends to level of vertebral body below
Lumbar vertebrae L1–L5	Large (kidney-shaped)	Medium (triangular)	Called costal processes, long and slender; accessory process on posterior surface	Posteromedially (or medially) and anterolaterally (or laterally); facets nearly in sagittal plane; mammillary process on posterior surface of each superior articular process	Short and broad
Sacral vertebrae (sacrum) S1–S5 (fused)	Decreases from base to apex	Sacral canal	Fused to rudimentary rib (ribs, see pp. 52–55)	Superoposteriorly (SI) superior surface of lateral sacrum-auricular surface	Median sacral crest

*C1 (atlas) and C2 (axis) are considered atypical (see pp. 8–9).

Cervical Vertebrae

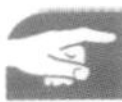

The seven vertebrae of the cervical spine differ most conspicuously from the common vertebral morphology. They are specialized to bear the weight of the head and allow the neck to move in all directions. C1 and C2 are known as the atlas and axis, respectively. C7 is called the vertebra prominens for its long, palpable spinous process.

Fig. 2.6 **Cervical spine**
Left lateral view.

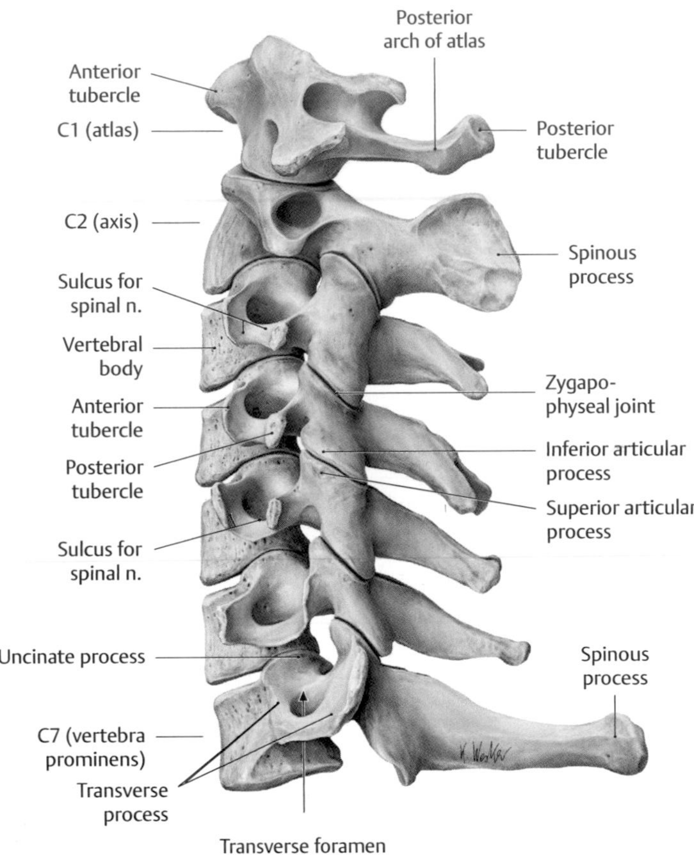
Posterior arch of atlas
Anterior tubercle
C1 (atlas)
Posterior tubercle
C2 (axis)
Spinous process
Sulcus for spinal n.
Vertebral body
Zygapophyseal joint
Anterior tubercle
Inferior articular process
Posterior tubercle
Superior articular process
Sulcus for spinal n.
Uncinate process
Spinous process
C7 (vertebra prominens)
Transverse process
Transverse foramen

A Bones of the cervical spine, left lateral view.

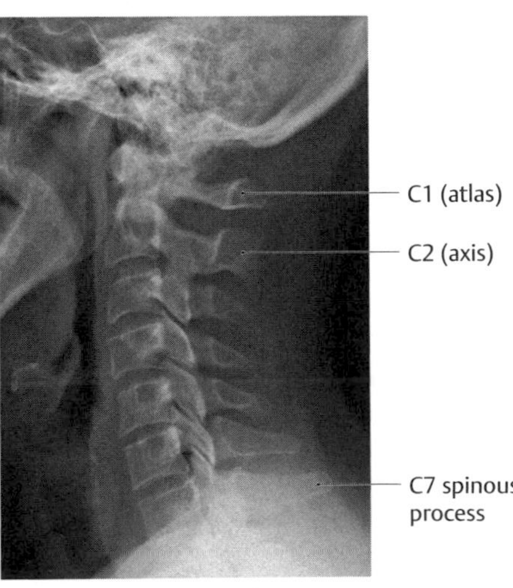
C1 (atlas)
C2 (axis)
C7 spinous process

B Radiograph of the cervical spine, left lateral view.

Fig. 2.7 **Atlas (C1)**

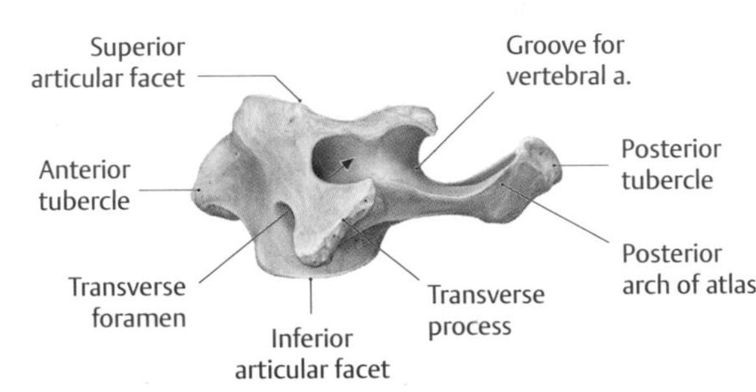
Superior articular facet
Groove for vertebral a.
Anterior tubercle
Posterior tubercle
Posterior arch of atlas
Transverse foramen
Transverse process
Inferior articular facet

A Left lateral view.

Fig. 2.8 **Axis (C2)**

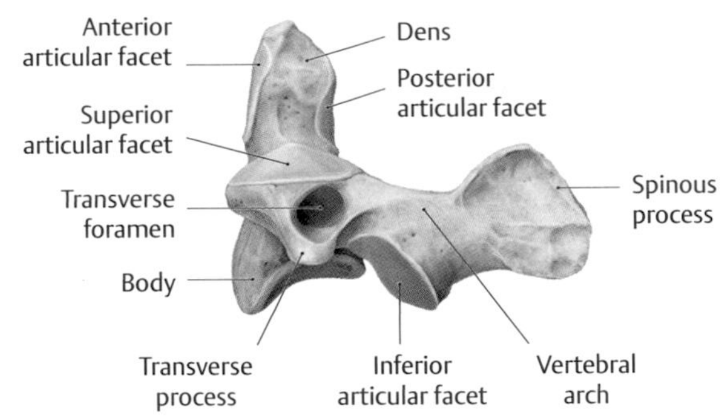
Anterior articular facet
Dens
Posterior articular facet
Superior articular facet
Spinous process
Transverse foramen
Body
Transverse process
Inferior articular facet
Vertebral arch

A Left lateral view.

Fig. 2.9 **Typical cervical vertebra (C4)**

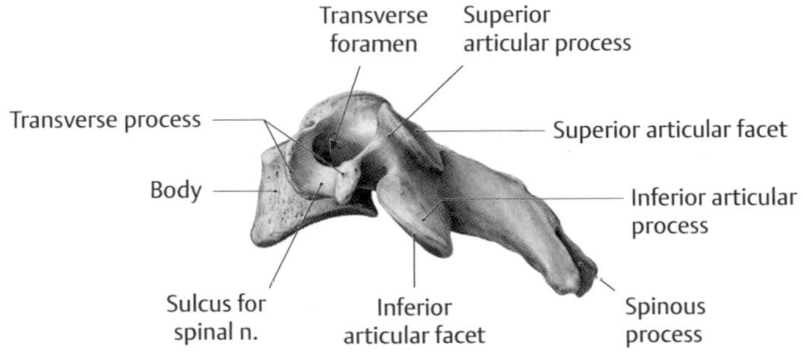
Transverse foramen
Superior articular process
Transverse process
Superior articular facet
Body
Inferior articular process
Sulcus for spinal n.
Inferior articular facet
Spinous process

A Left lateral view.

Clinical

Injuries in the cervical spine

The cervical spine is prone to hyperextension injuries, such as "whiplash," which can occur when the head extends back much farther than it normally would. The most common injuries of the cervical spine are fractures of the dens of the axis, traumatic spondylolisthesis (ventral slippage of a vertebral body), and atlas fractures. Patient prognosis is largely dependent on the spinal level of the injuries (see p. 42).

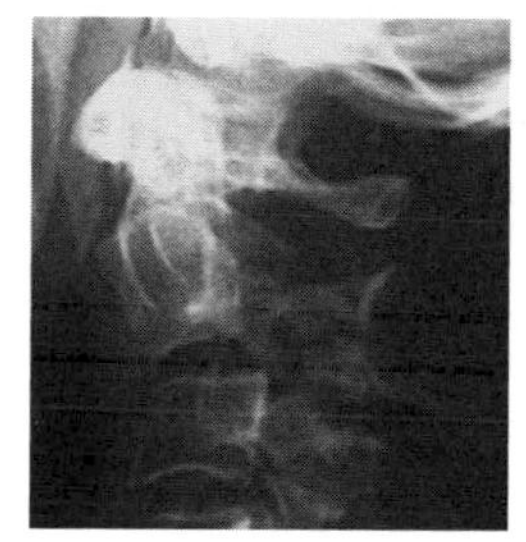

This patient hit the dashboard of his car while not wearing a seat belt. The resulting hyperextension caused the traumatic spondylolisthesis of C2 (axis) with fracture of the vertebral arch of C2, as well as tearing of the ligaments between C2 and C3. This injury is often referred to as "hangman's fracture."

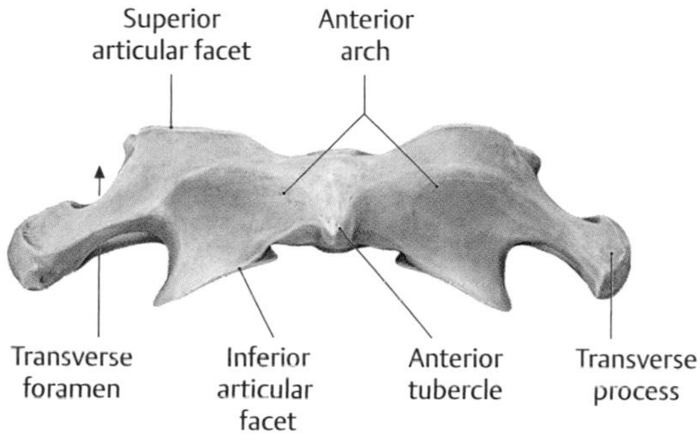
Superior articular facet
Anterior arch
Transverse foramen
Inferior articular facet
Anterior tubercle
Transverse process

B Anterior view.

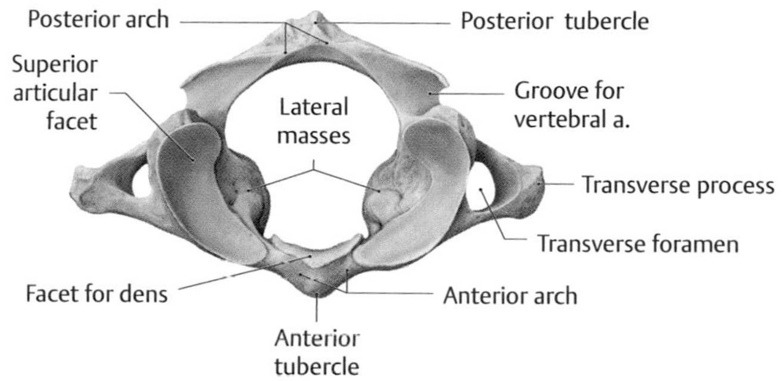
Posterior arch
Posterior tubercle
Superior articular facet
Lateral masses
Groove for vertebral a.
Transverse process
Transverse foramen
Facet for dens
Anterior arch
Anterior tubercle

C Superior view.

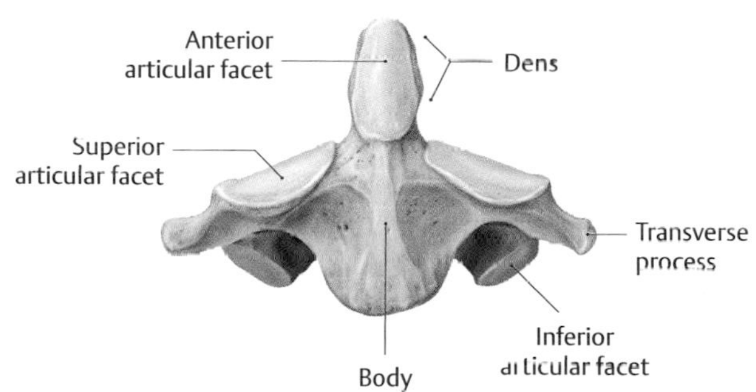
Anterior articular facet
Dens
Superior articular facet
Transverse process
Inferior articular facet
Body

B Anterior view.

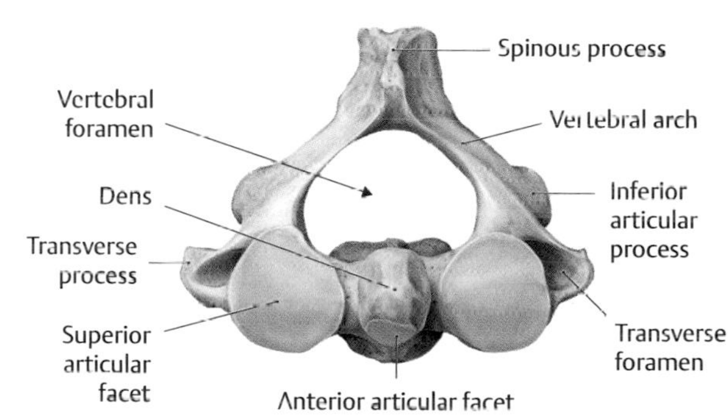
Spinous process
Vertebral foramen
Vertebral arch
Dens
Inferior articular process
Transverse process
Superior articular facet
Transverse foramen
Anterior articular facet

C Superior view.

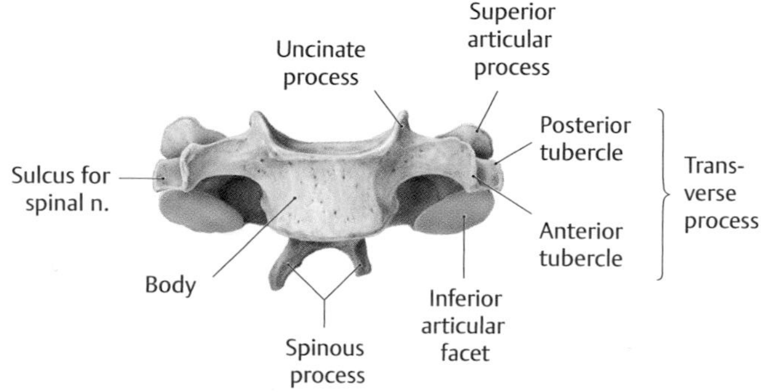
Superior articular process
Uncinate process
Posterior tubercle
Sulcus for spinal n.
Trans-verse process
Anterior tubercle
Body
Inferior articular facet
Spinous process

B Anterior view.

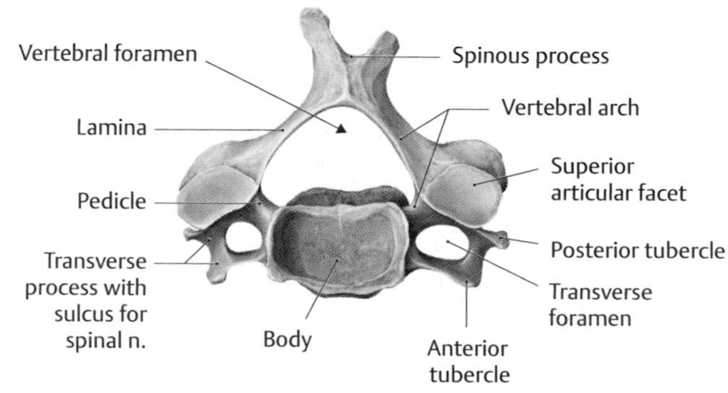
Vertebral foramen
Spinous process
Vertebral arch
Lamina
Superior articular facet
Pedicle
Posterior tubercle
Transverse process with sulcus for spinal n.
Transverse foramen
Body
Anterior tubercle

C Superior view.

Thoracic & Lumbar Vertebrae

Fig. 2.10 **Thoracic spine**
Left lateral view.

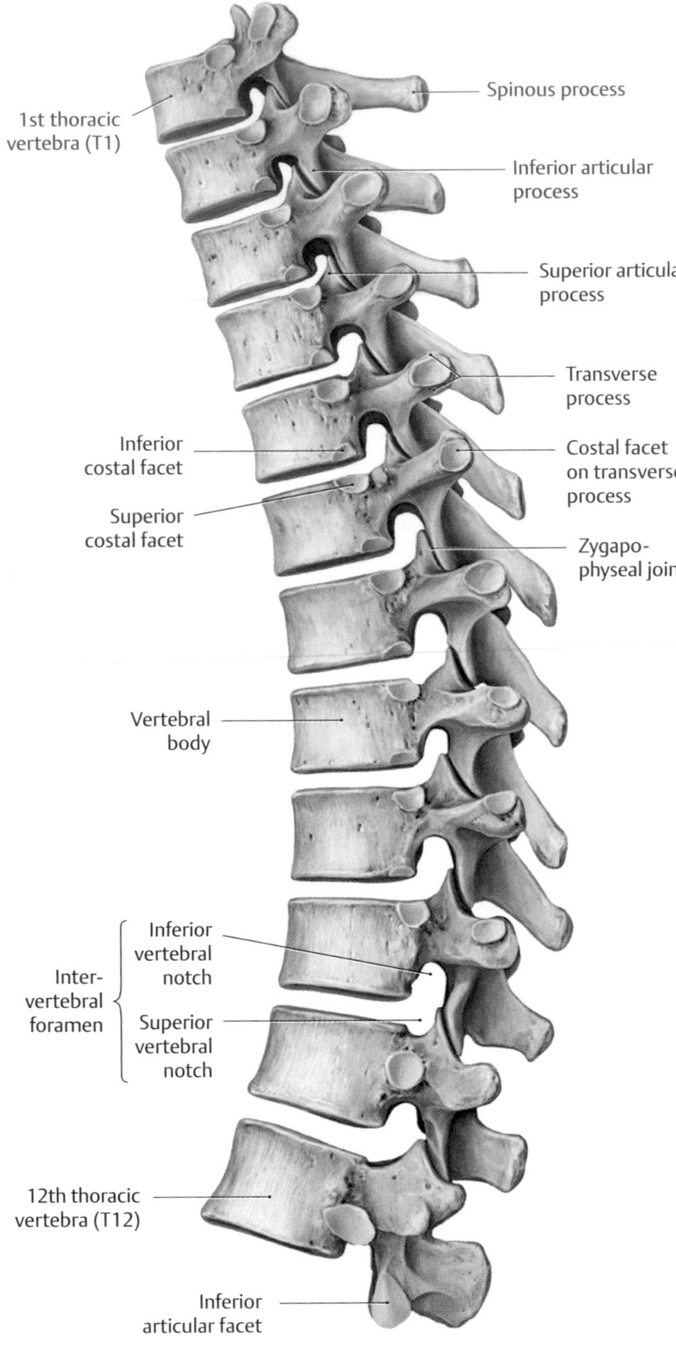

1st thoracic vertebra (T1)
Spinous process
Inferior articular process
Superior articular process
Transverse process
Inferior costal facet
Costal facet on transverse process
Superior costal facet
Zygapo-physeal joint
Vertebral body
Inter-vertebral foramen
Inferior vertebral notch
Superior vertebral notch
12th thoracic vertebra (T12)
Inferior articular facet

Fig. 2.11 **Typical thoracic vertebra (T6)**

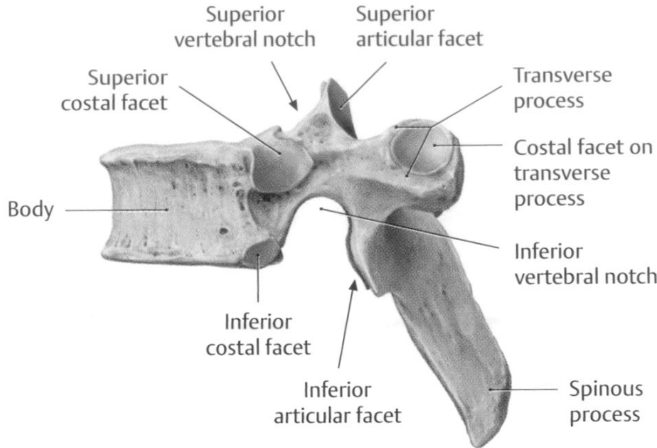

Superior vertebral notch
Superior articular facet
Superior costal facet
Transverse process
Costal facet on transverse process
Body
Inferior vertebral notch
Inferior costal facet
Inferior articular facet
Spinous process

A Left lateral view.

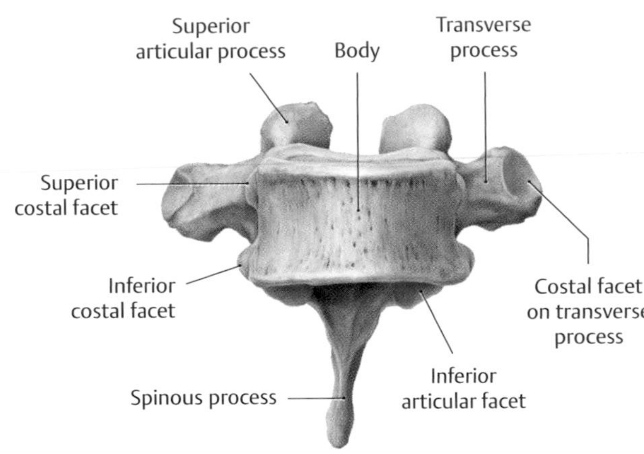

Superior articular process
Body
Transverse process
Superior costal facet
Inferior costal facet
Costal facet on transverse process
Inferior articular facet
Spinous process

B Anterior view.

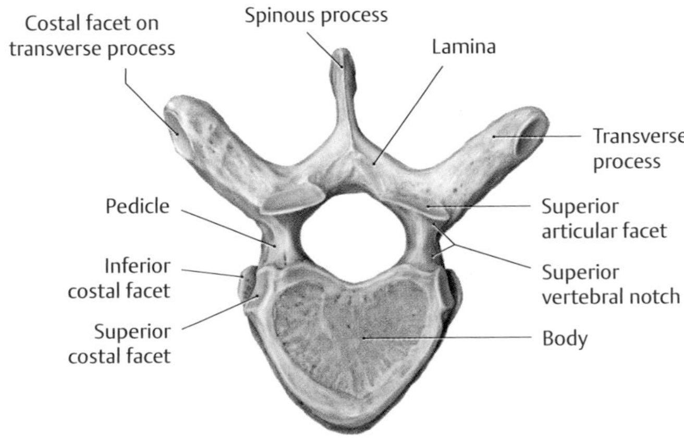

Costal facet on transverse process
Spinous process
Lamina
Transverse process
Pedicle
Superior articular facet
Inferior costal facet
Superior vertebral notch
Superior costal facet
Body

C Superior view.

Fig. 2.12 **Lumbar spine**
Left lateral view.

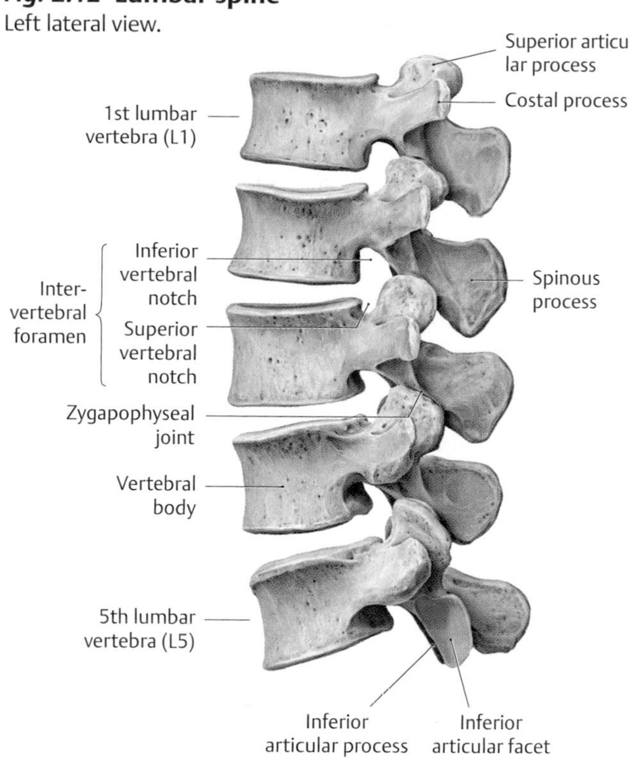
Superior articular process
Costal process
1st lumbar vertebra (L1)
Inferior vertebral notch
Inter-vertebral foramen
Superior vertebral notch
Spinous process
Zygapophyseal joint
Vertebral body
5th lumbar vertebra (L5)
Inferior articular process
Inferior articular facet

Clinical

Osteoporosis
The spine is the structure most affected by degenerative diseases of the skeleton, such as arthrosis and osteoporosis. In osteoporosis, more bone material gets reabsorbed than built up, resulting in a loss of bone mass. Symptoms include compression fractures and resulting back pain.

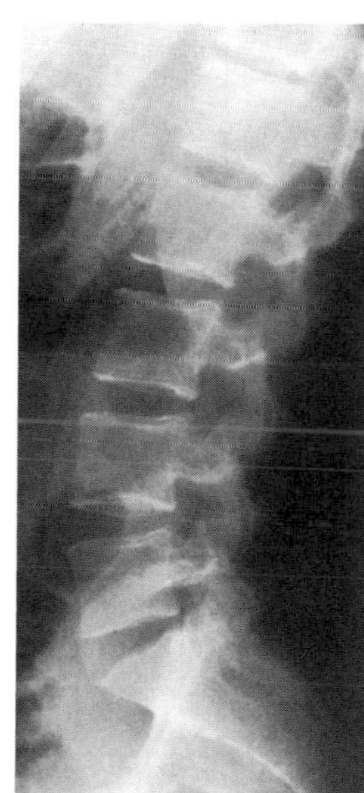

A Radiograph of a normal lumbar spine, left lateral view.

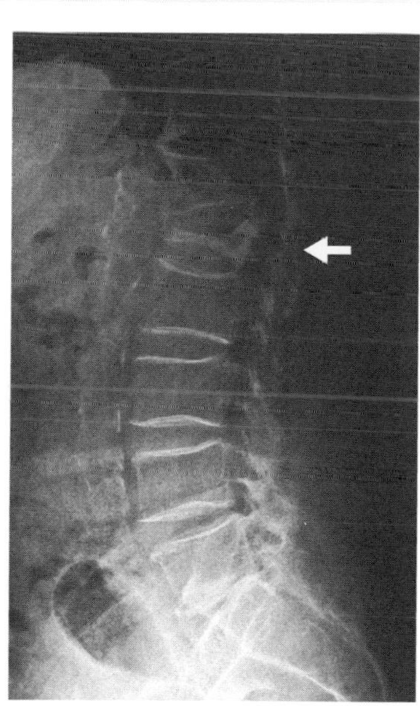

B Radiograph of an osteoporotic lumbar spine with a compression fracture at L1 (*arrow*). Note that the vertebral bodies are decreased in density, and the internal trabecular structure is coarse.

Fig. 2.13 **Typical lumbar vertebra (L4)**

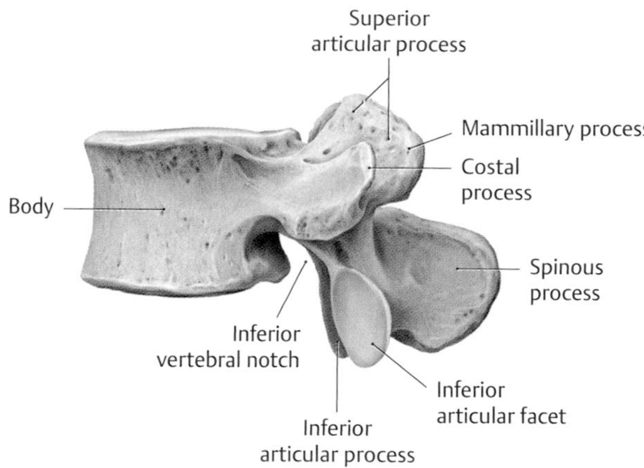
Superior articular process
Mammillary process
Costal process
Body
Spinous process
Inferior vertebral notch
Inferior articular facet
Inferior articular process

A Left lateral view.

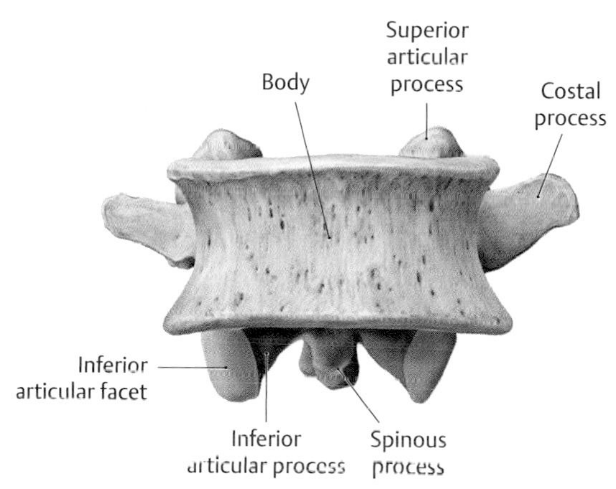
Body
Superior articular process
Costal process
Inferior articular facet
Inferior articular process
Spinous process

B Anterior view.

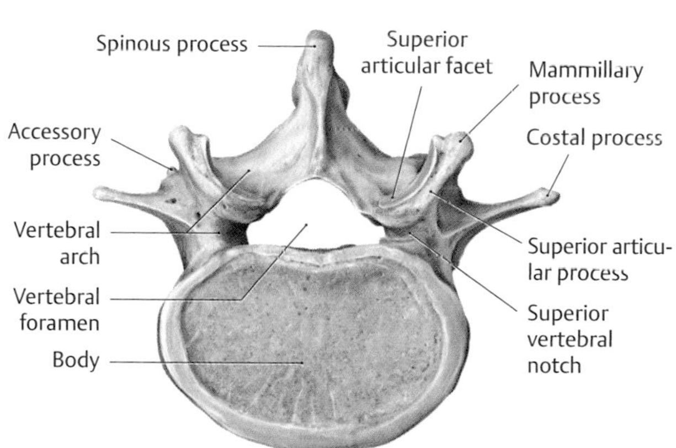
Spinous process
Superior articular facet
Mammillary process
Accessory process
Costal process
Vertebral arch
Superior articular process
Vertebral foramen
Superior vertebral notch
Body

C Superior view.

Sacrum & Coccyx

The sacrum is formed from five postnatally fused sacral vertebrae. The base of the sacrum articulates with the 5th lumbar vertebra, and the apex articulates with the coccyx, a series of three or four rudimentary vertebrae. See Fig. 16.1, p. 214, for the sacroiliac joint.

***Fig. 2.14* Sacrum and coccyx**

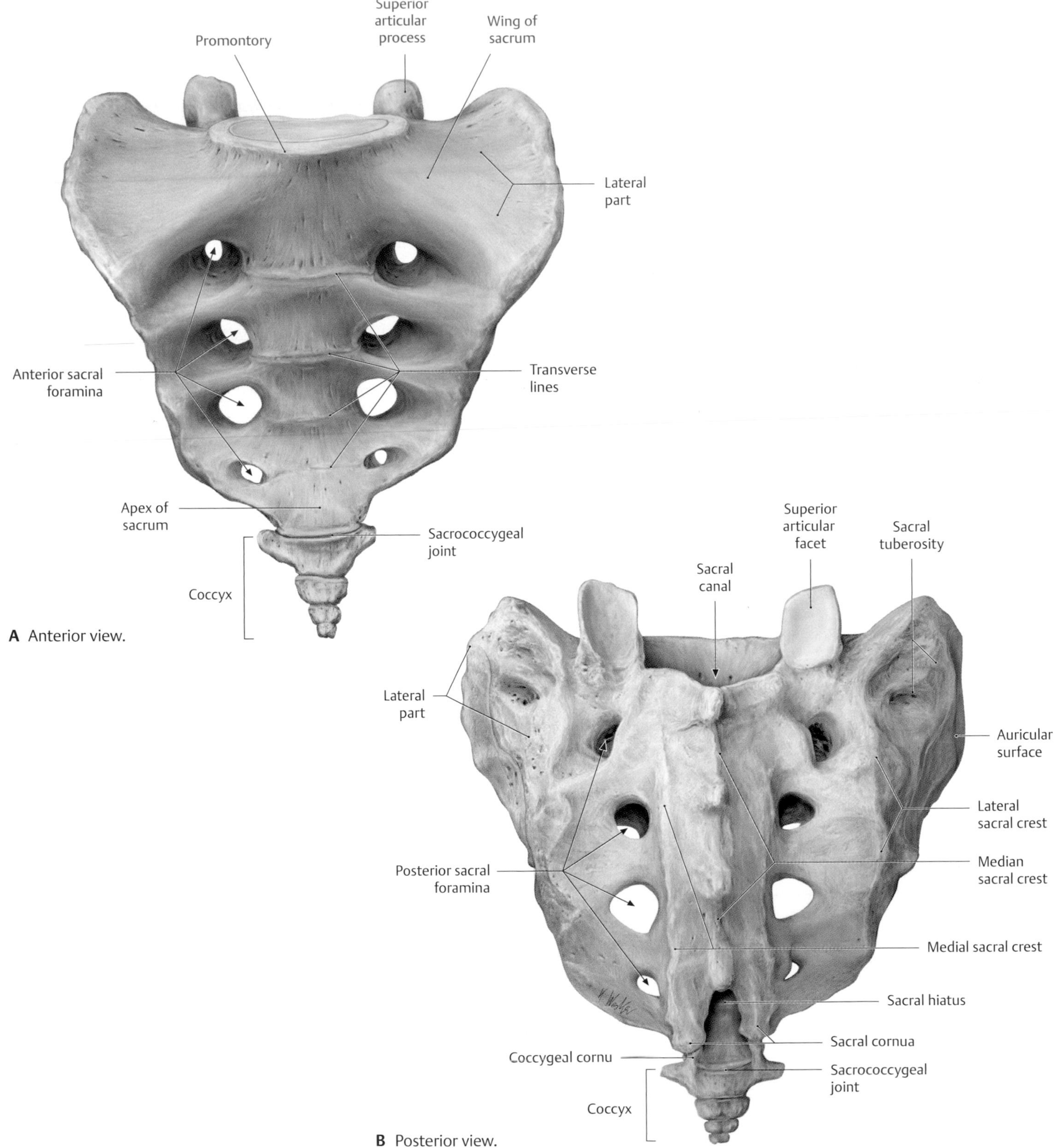

Promontory
Superior articular process
Wing of sacrum
Lateral part
Anterior sacral foramina
Transverse lines
Apex of sacrum
Sacrococcygeal joint
Coccyx
Superior articular facet
Sacral tuberosity
Sacral canal
Lateral part
Auricular surface
Lateral sacral crest
Median sacral crest
Posterior sacral foramina
Medial sacral crest
Sacral hiatus
Sacral cornua
Coccygeal cornu
Sacrococcygeal joint
Coccyx

A Anterior view.

B Posterior view.

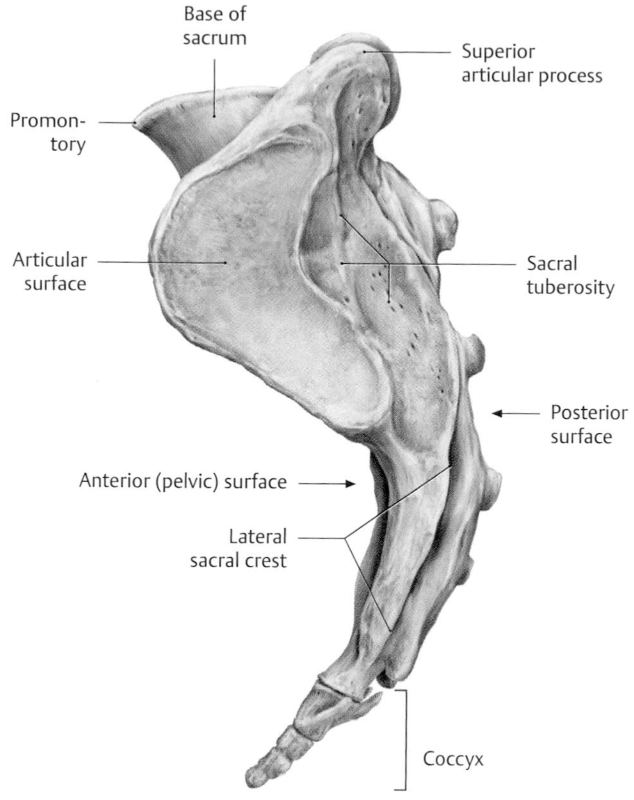
Base of
sacrum
Superior
articular process
Promon-
tory
Articular
surface
Sacral
tuberosity
Posterior
surface
Anterior (pelvic) surface
Lateral
sacral crest
Coccyx

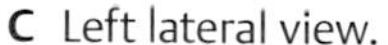
C Left lateral view.

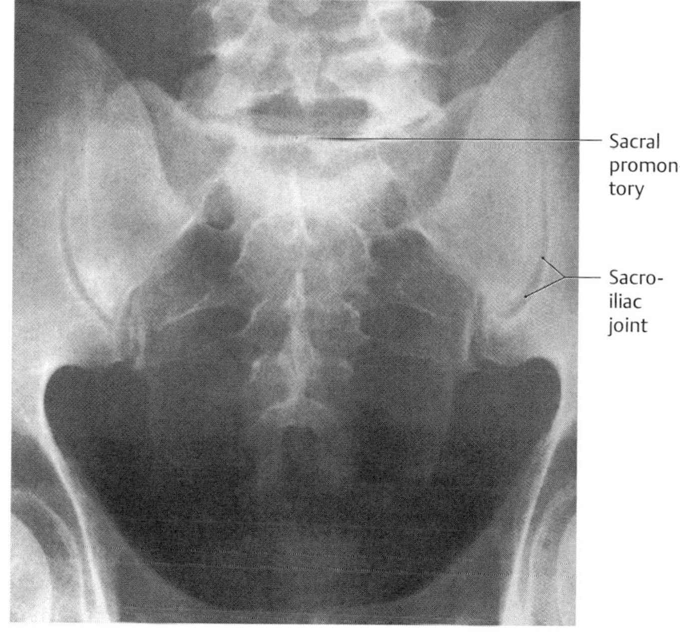
Sacral
promon-
tory
Sacro-
iliac
joint

D Radiograph of sacrum, anteroposterior view.

Fig. 2.15 Sacrum

Superior view.

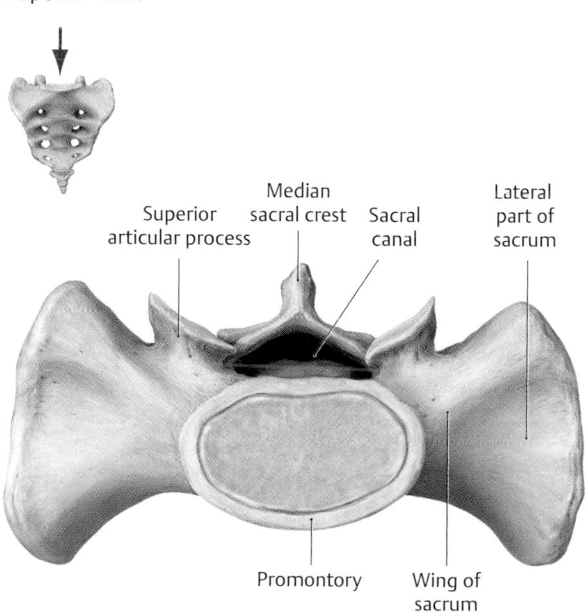
Superior
articular process
Median
sacral crest
Sacral
canal
Lateral
part of
sacrum
Promontory
Wing of
sacrum

A Base of sacrum, superior view.

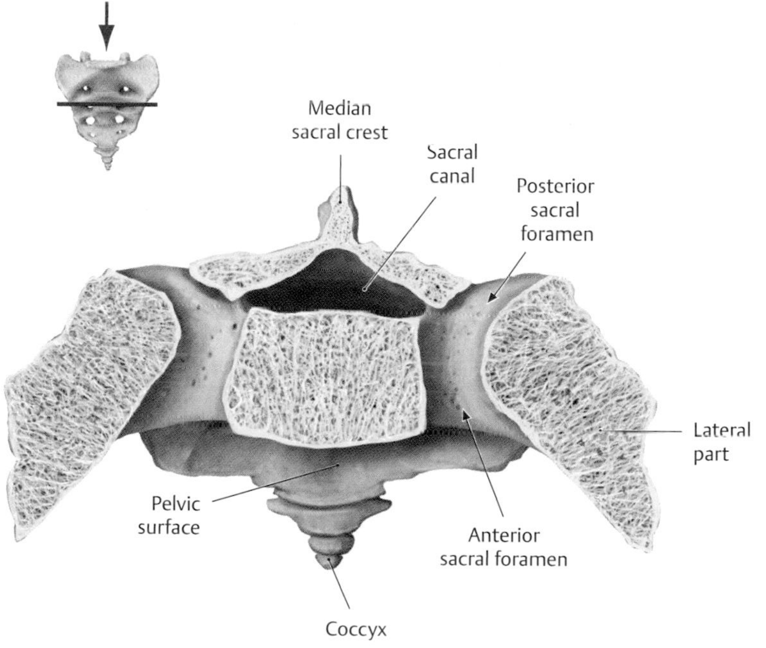
Median
sacral crest
Sacral
canal
Posterior
sacral
foramen
Lateral
part
Pelvic
surface
Anterior
sacral foramen
Coccyx

B Transverse section through second sacral vertebra demonstrating anterior and posterior sacral foramina, superior view.

Intervertebral Disks

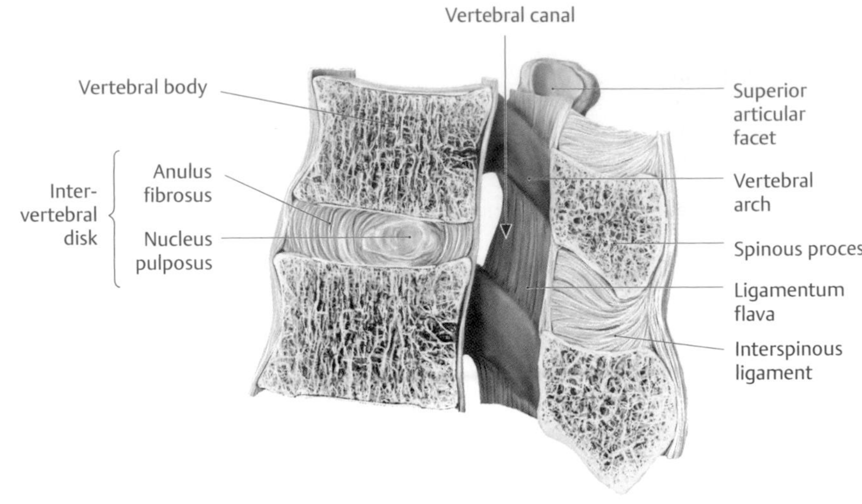
Vertebral canal
Vertebral body
Inter-
vertebral
disk
Anulus
fibrosus
Nucleus
pulposus
Superior
articular
facet
Vertebral
arch
Spinous process
Ligamentum
flava
Interspinous
ligament

Fig. 2.16 **Intervertebral disk in the vertebral column**
Sagittal section of T11–T12, left lateral view. The intervertebral disks occupy the spaces between vertebrae (intervertebral joints, see p. 16).

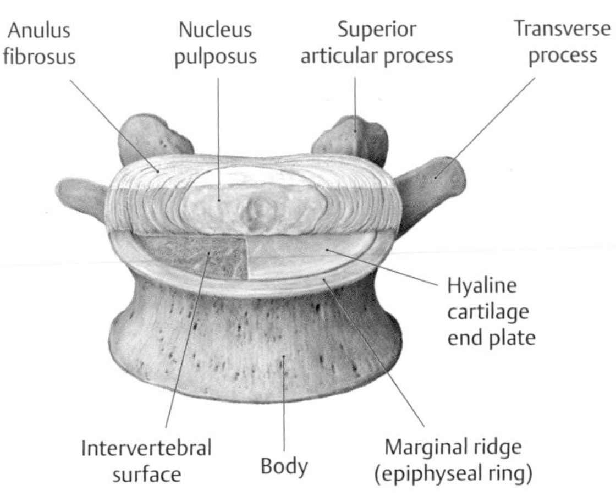
Anulus
fibrosus
Nucleus
pulposus
Superior
articular process
Transverse
process
Hyaline
cartilage
end plate
Intervertebral
surface
Body
Marginal ridge
(epiphyseal ring)

Fig. 2.17 **Structure of intervertebral disk**
Anterosuperior view with the anterior half of the disk and the right half of the end plate removed. The intervertebral disk consists of an external fibrous ring (anulus fibrosus) and a gelatinous core (nucleus pulposus).

Fig. 2.18 **Relation of intervertebral disk to vertebral canal**
Fourth lumbar vertebra, superior view.

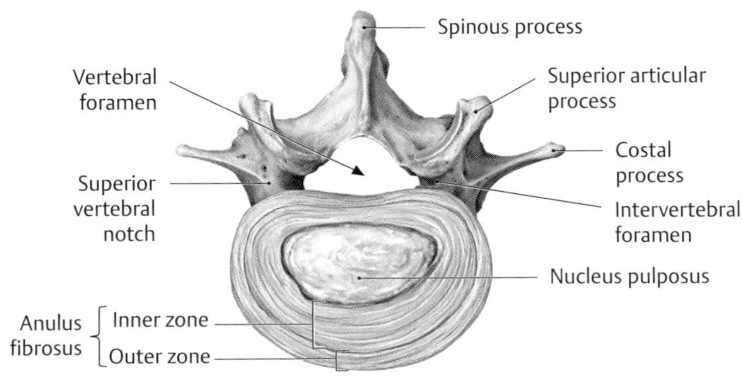
Spinous process
Vertebral
foramen
Superior articular
process
Costal
process
Superior
vertebral
notch
Intervertebral
foramen
Nucleus pulposus
Anulus
fibrosus
Inner zone
Outer zone

Fig. 2.19 **Outer zone of the anulus fibrosus**
Anterior view of L3–L4 with intervertebral disk.

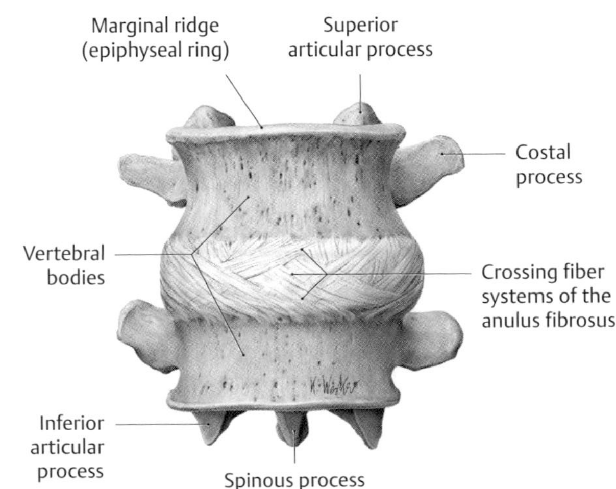
Marginal ridge
(epiphyseal ring)
Superior
articular process
Costal
process
Vertebral
bodies
Crossing fiber
systems of the
anulus fibrosus
Inferior
articular
process
Spinous process

Clinical

Disk herniation in the lumbar spine

As the stress resistance of the anulus fibrosus declines with age, the tissue of the nucleus pulposus may protrude through weak spots under loading. If the fibrous ring of the anulus ruptures completely, the herniated material may compress the contents of the intervertebral foramen (nerve roots and blood vessels). These patients often suffer from severe local back pain. Pain is also felt in the associated dermatome (see p. 42). When the motor part of the spinal nerve is affected, the muscles served by that spinal nerve will show weakening. It is an important diagnostic step to test the muscles innervated by a nerve from a certain spinal segment, as well as the sensitivity in the specific dermatome. Example: The first sacral nerve root innervates the gastrocnemius and soleus muscles; thus, standing or walking on toes can be affected (see p. 414).

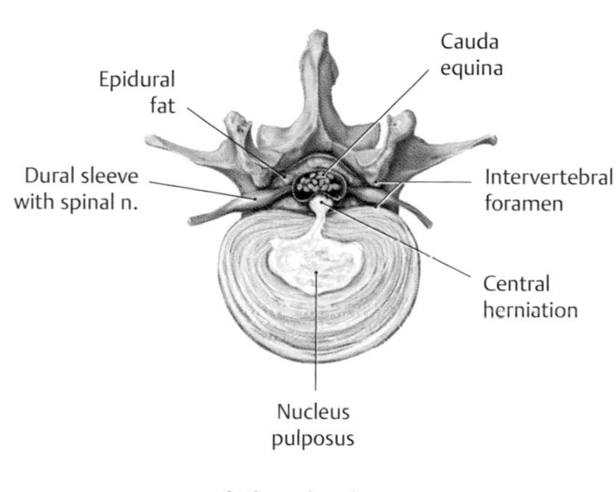
Epidural fat
Cauda equina
Dural sleeve with spinal n.
Intervertebral foramen
Central herniation
Nucleus pulposus

A Superior view.

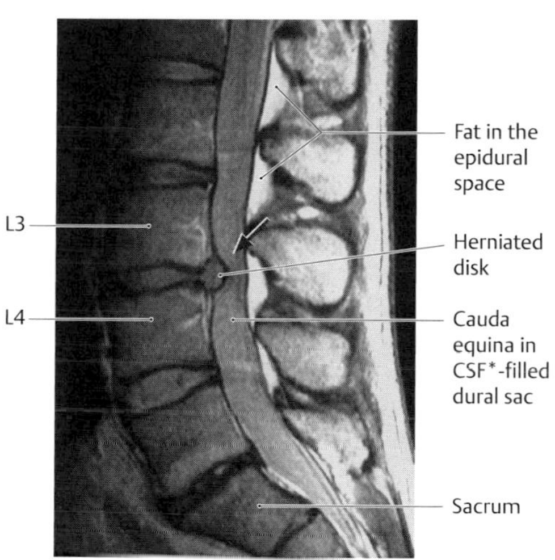
L3
L4
Fat in the epidural space
Herniated disk
Cauda equina in CSF*-filled dural sac
Sacrum

B Midsagittal T2-weighted MRI (magnetic resonance image).

Posterior herniation (A, B) In the MRI, a conspicuously herniated disk at the level of L3–L4 protrudes posteriorly (transligamentous herniation). The dural sac is deeply indented at that level. *CSF (cerebrospinal fluid).

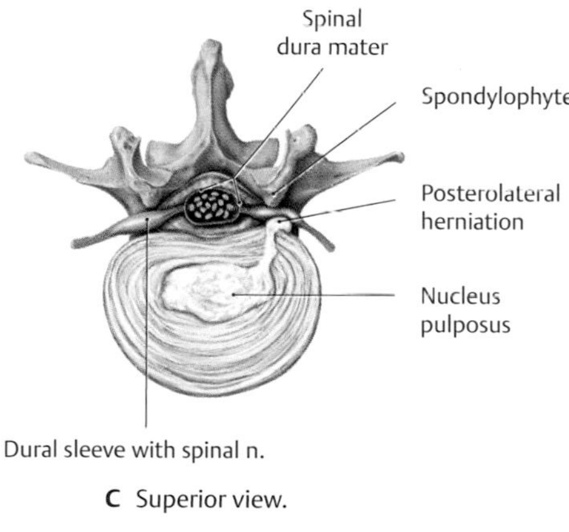
Spinal dura mater
Spondylophyte
Posterolateral herniation
Nucleus pulposus
Dural sleeve with spinal n.

C Superior view.

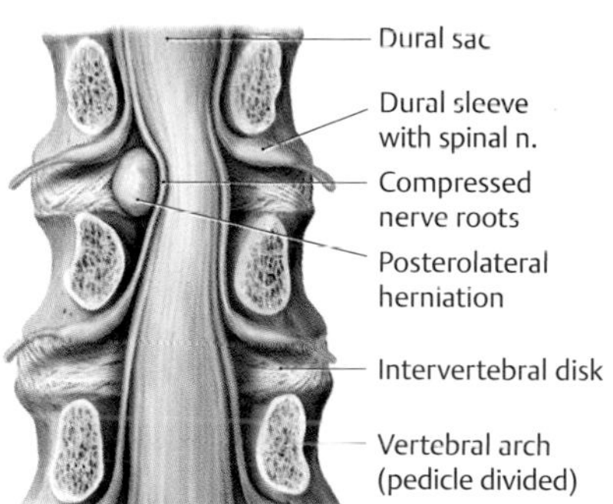
Dural sac
Dural sleeve with spinal n.
Compressed nerve roots
Posterolateral herniation
Intervertebral disk
Vertebral arch (pedicle divided)

D Posterior view, vertebral arches removed.

Posterolateral herniation (C, D) A posterolateral herniation may compress the spinal nerve as it passes through the intervertebral foramen. If more medially positioned, the herniation may spare the nerve at that level but impact nerves at inferior levels.

Joints of the Vertebral Column: Overview

Table 2.2	Joints of the vertebral column	
Craniovertebral joints		
①	Atlanto-occipital joints	Occiput–C1
②	Atlantoaxial joints	C1–C2
Joints of the vertebral bodies		
③	Uncovertebral joints	C3–C7
④	Intervertebral joints	C2–S1
Joints of the vertebral arch		
⑤	Zygapophyseal joints	C2–S1

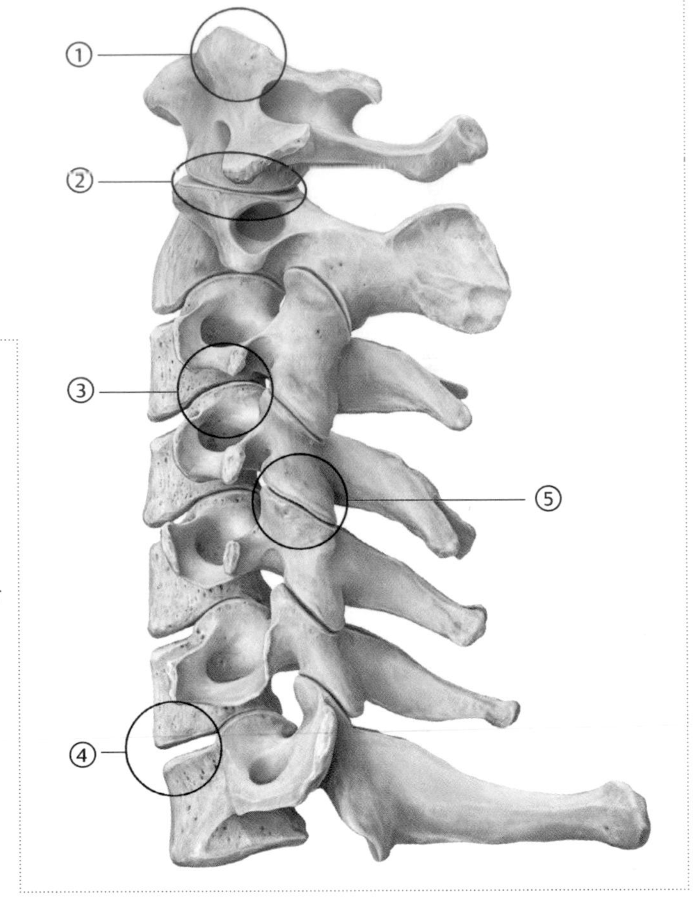
①
②
③
⑤
④

Fig. 2.20 Zygapophyseal (intervertebral facet) joints
The orientation of the zygapophyseal joints differs between the spinal regions, influencing the degree and direction of movement.

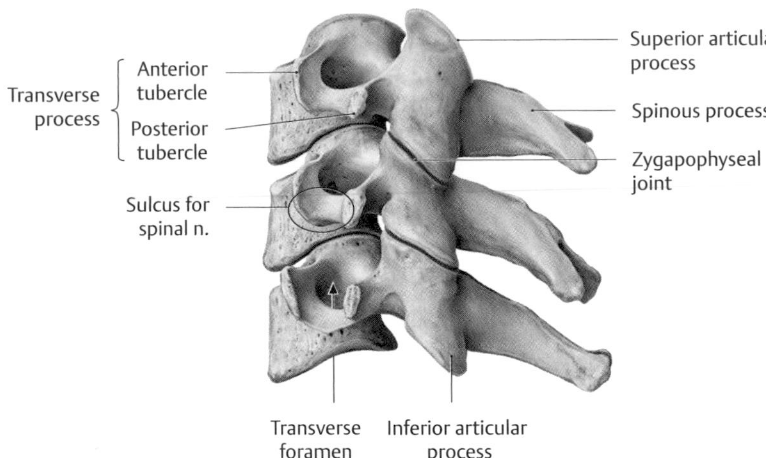
Transverse process
Anterior tubercle
Posterior tubercle
Sulcus for spinal n.
Superior articular process
Spinous process
Zygapophyseal joint
Transverse foramen
Inferior articular process

A Cervical region, left lateral view. The zygapophyseal joints lie 45 degrees from the horizontal.

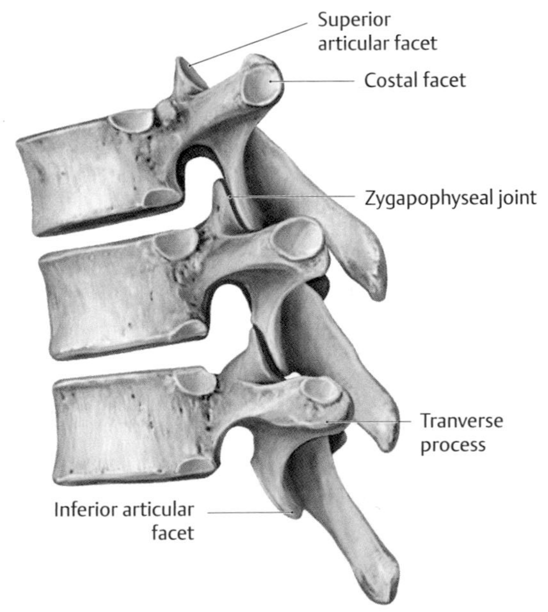
Superior articular facet
Costal facet
Zygapophyseal joint
Tranverse process
Inferior articular facet

B Thoracic region, left lateral view. The joints lie in the coronal plane.

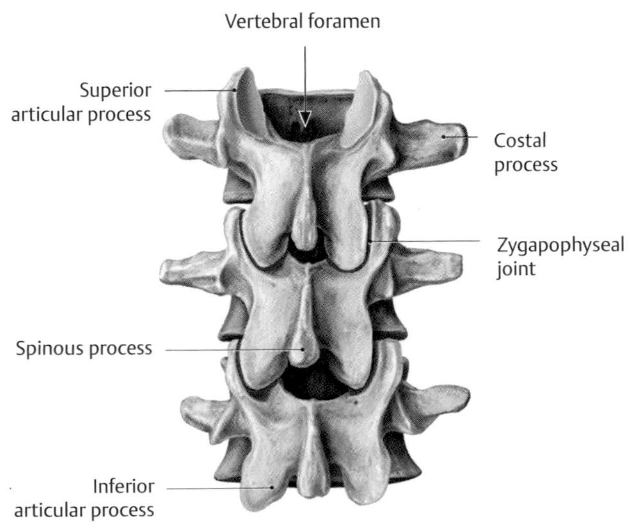
Vertebral foramen
Superior articular process
Costal process
Zygapophyseal joint
Spinous process
Inferior articular process

C Lumbar region, posterior view. The joints lie in the sagittal plane.

Fig. 2.21 Uncovertebral joints

Anterior view. Uncovertebral joints form during childhood between the uncinate processes of C3–C7 and the vertebral bodies immediately superior. The joints may result from fissures in the cartilage of the disks that assume an articular character. If the fissures become complete tears, the risk of pulposus herniation is increased (see p. 15).

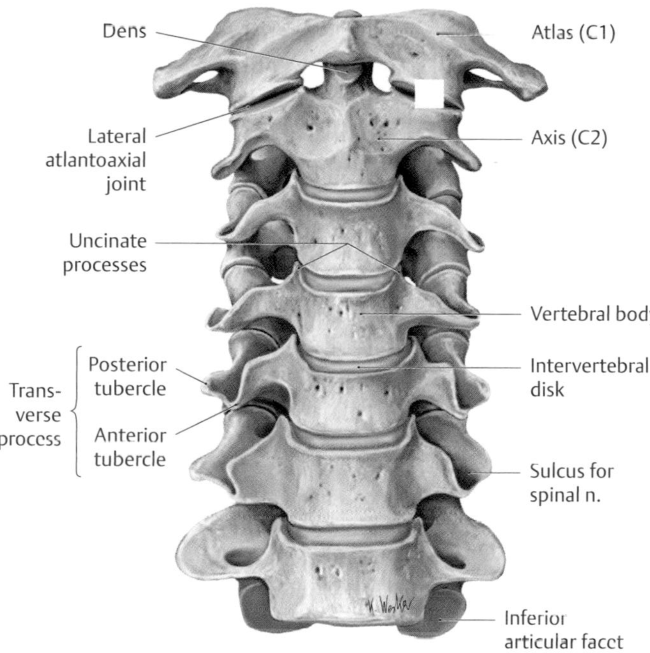
Dens
Atlas (C1)
Lateral atlantoaxial joint
Axis (C2)
Uncinate processes
Vertebral body
Trans-verse process
Posterior tubercle
Anterior tubercle
Intervertebral disk
Sulcus for spinal n.
Inferior articular facet

A Uncovertebral joints in the cervical spine of an 18-year-old man, anterior view.

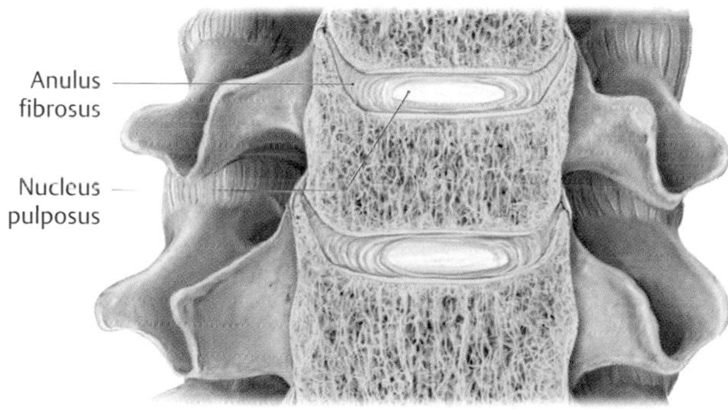
Anulus fibrosus
Nucleus pulposus

B Uncovertebral joint (enlarged), anterior view of coronal section.

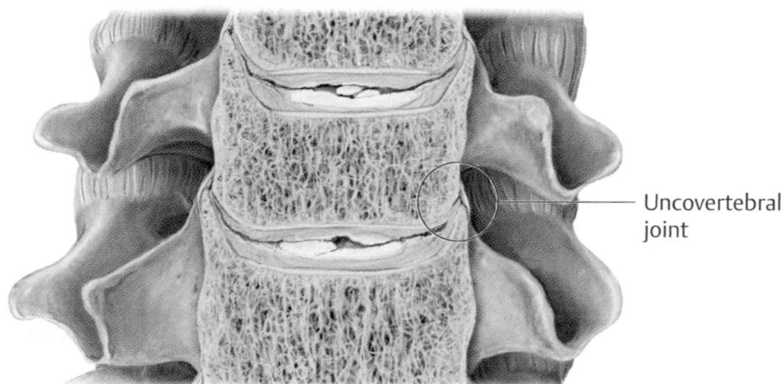
Uncovertebral joint

C Uncovertebral joints, split intervertebral disks, anterior view of coronal section.

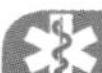 *Clinical*

Proximity of the spinal nerve and vertebral artery to the uncinate process

The spinal nerve and vertebral artery pass through the intervertebral and transverse foramina, respectively. Bony outgrowths (osteophytes) on the uncinate process resulting from uncovertebral arthrosis (degeneration) may compress both the nerve and the artery and can lead to chronic pain in the neck.

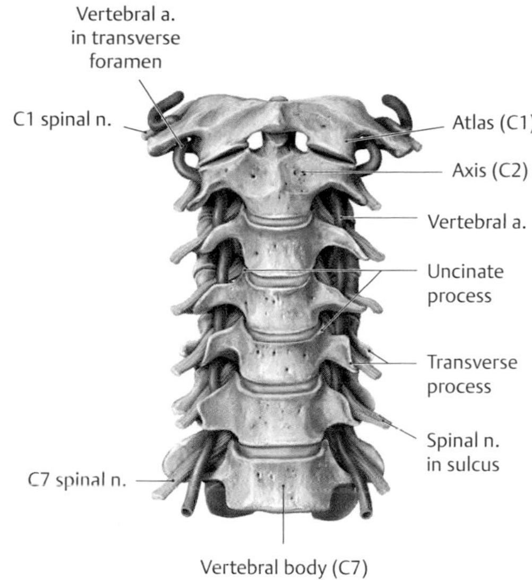
Vertebral a. in transverse foramen
C1 spinal n.
Atlas (C1)
Axis (C2)
Vertebral a.
Uncinate process
Transverse process
Spinal n. in sulcus
C7 spinal n.
Vertebral body (C7)

A Cervical spine, anterior view.

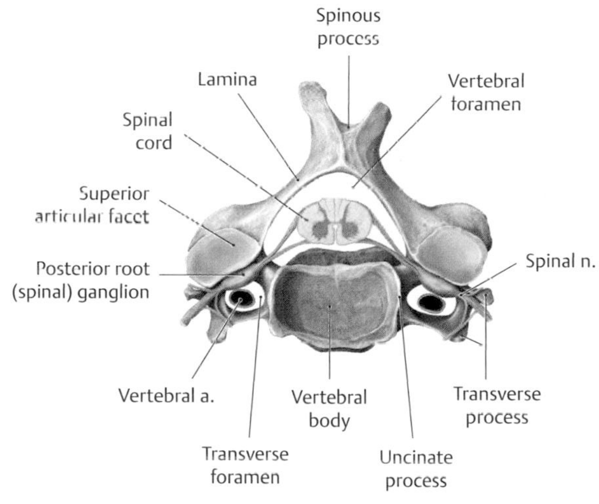
Spinous process
Lamina
Vertebral foramen
Spinal cord
Superior articular facet
Posterior root (spinal) ganglion
Spinal n.
Vertebral a.
Vertebral body
Transverse process
Transverse foramen
Uncinate process

B Fourth cervical vertebra, superior view.

Joints of the Vertebral Column: Craniovertebral Region

Fig. 2.22 Craniovertebral joints

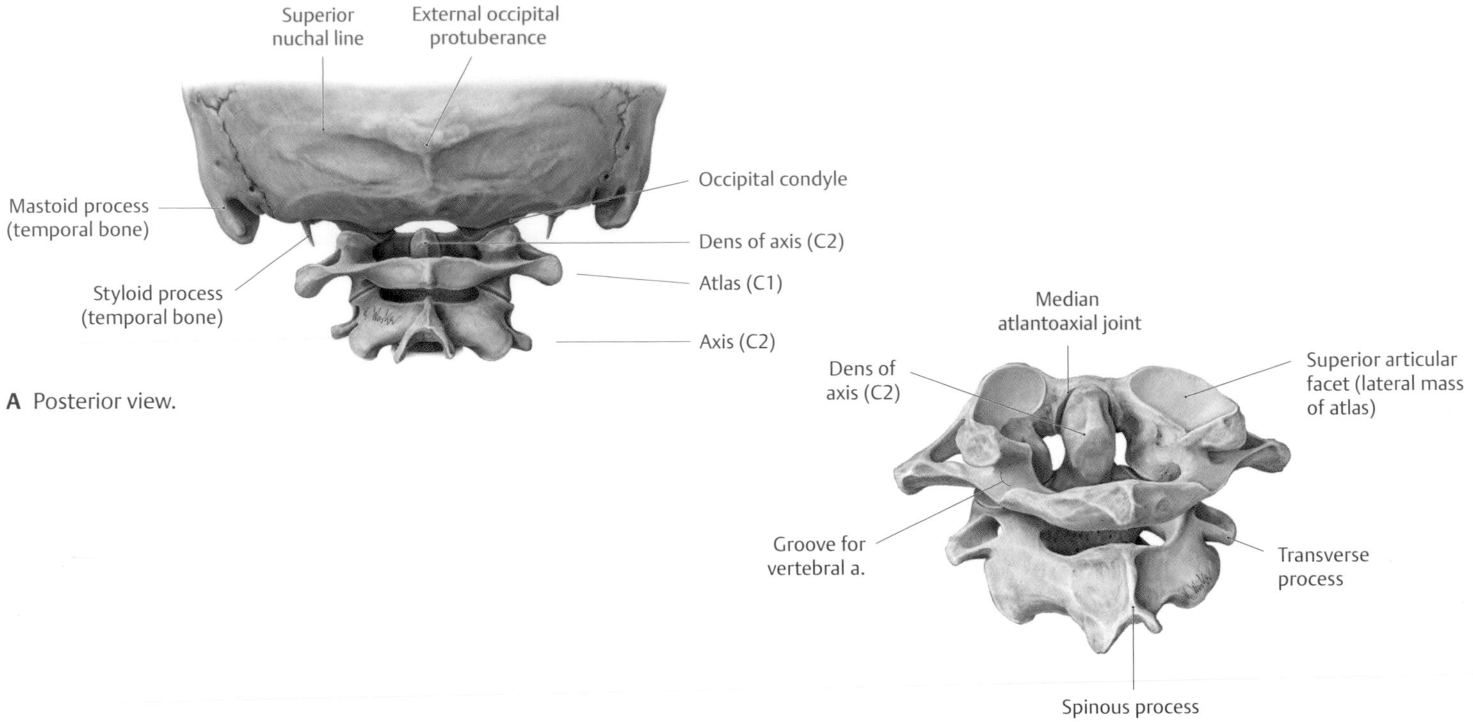

Superior nuchal line
External occipital protuberance
Mastoid process (temporal bone)
Styloid process (temporal bone)
Occipital condyle
Dens of axis (C2)
Atlas (C1)
Axis (C2)
Median atlantoaxial joint
Dens of axis (C2)
Superior articular facet (lateral mass of atlas)
Groove for vertebral a.
Transverse process
Spinous process

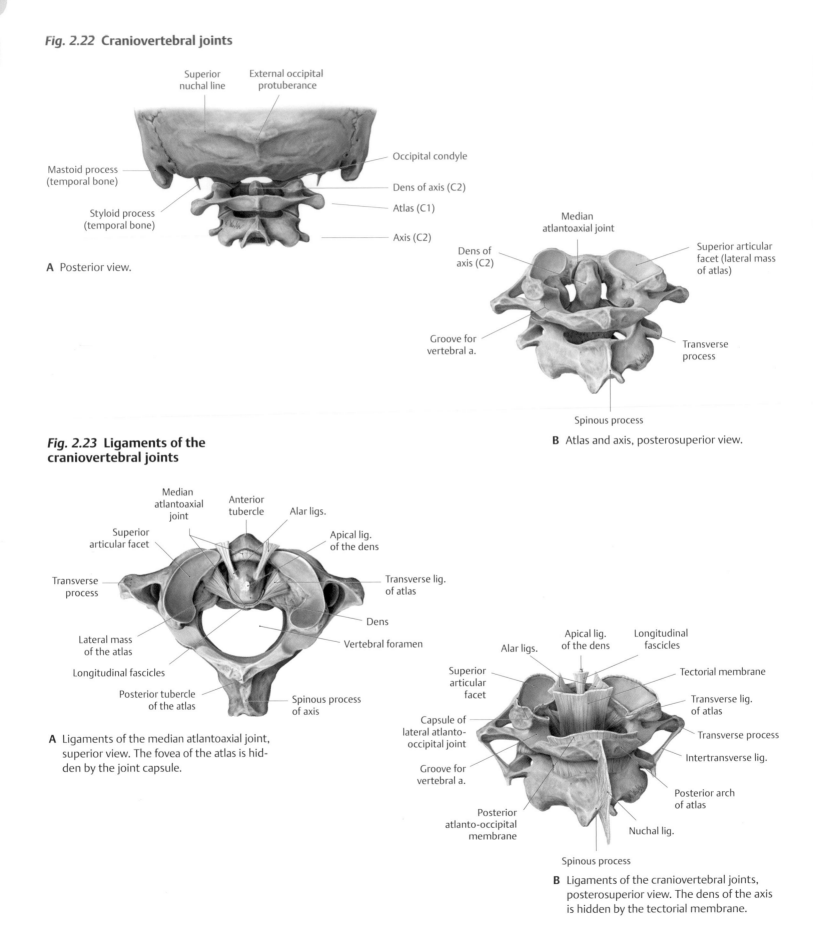

A Posterior view.

B Atlas and axis, posterosuperior view.

Fig. 2.23 Ligaments of the craniovertebral joints

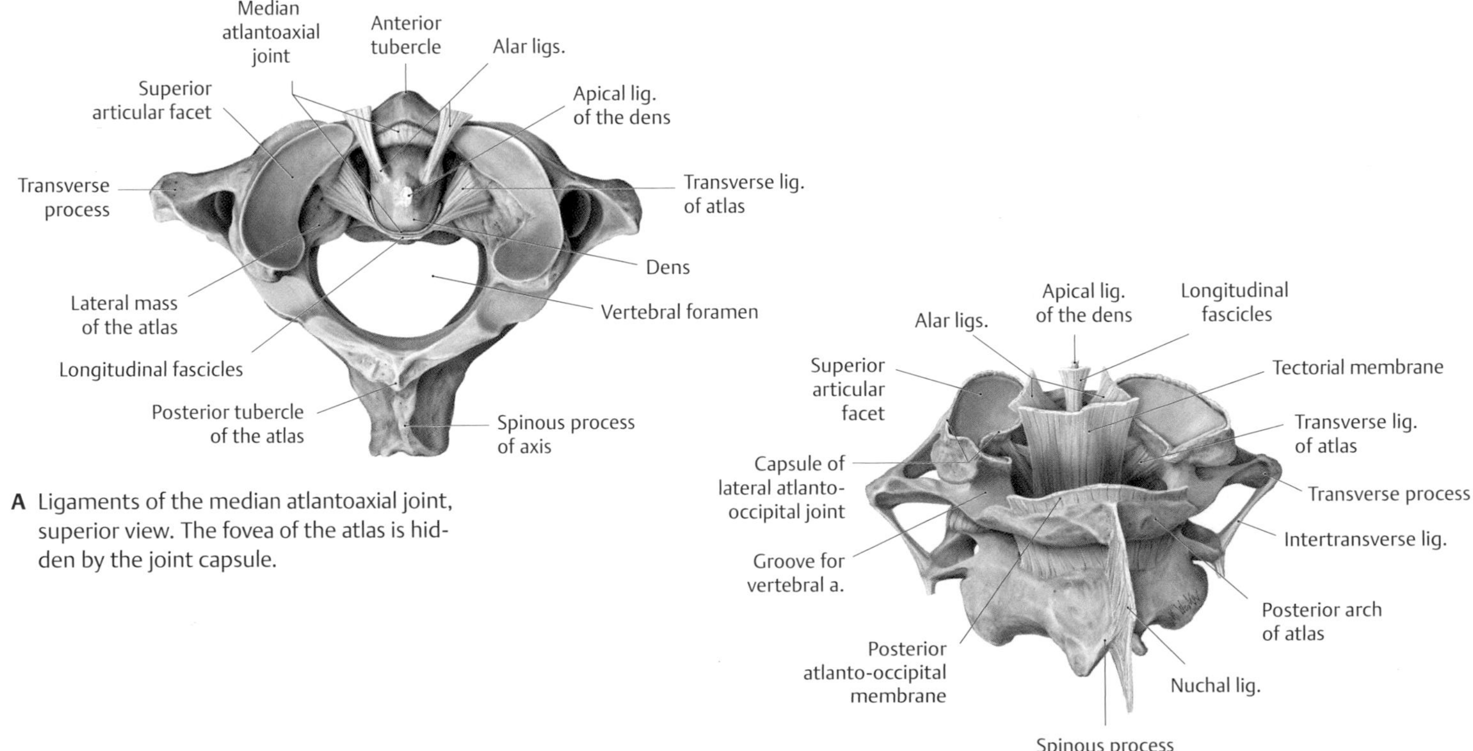

Median atlantoaxial joint
Anterior tubercle
Alar ligs.
Superior articular facet
Apical lig. of the dens
Transverse process
Transverse lig. of atlas
Dens
Lateral mass of the atlas
Vertebral foramen
Longitudinal fascicles
Posterior tubercle of the atlas
Spinous process of axis
Alar ligs.
Apical lig. of the dens
Longitudinal fascicles
Superior articular facet
Tectorial membrane
Transverse lig. of atlas
Capsule of lateral atlanto-occipital joint
Transverse process
Intertransverse lig.
Groove for vertebral a.
Posterior arch of atlas
Posterior atlanto-occipital membrane
Nuchal lig.
Spinous process

A Ligaments of the median atlantoaxial joint, superior view. The fovea of the atlas is hidden by the joint capsule.

B Ligaments of the craniovertebral joints, posterosuperior view. The dens of the axis is hidden by the tectorial membrane.

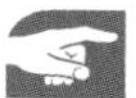

The atlanto-occipital joints are the two articulations between the convex occipital condyles of the occipital bone and the slightly concave superior articular facets of the atlas (C1). The atlanto-axial joints are the two lateral and one medial articulations between the atlas (C1) and axis (C2).

Fig. 2.24 Dissection of the craniovertebral joint ligaments

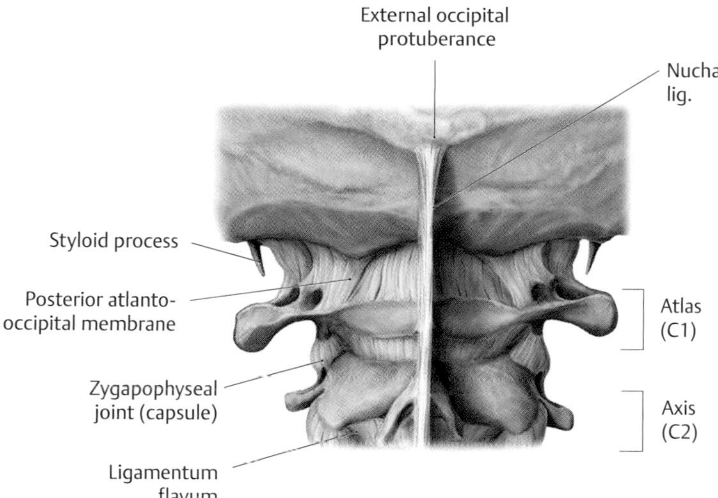
External occipital protuberance
Nuchal lig.
Styloid process
Posterior atlanto-occipital membrane
Atlas (C1)
Zygapophyseal joint (capsule)
Axis (C2)
Ligamentum flavum

A Nuchal ligament and posterior atlanto-occipital membrane.

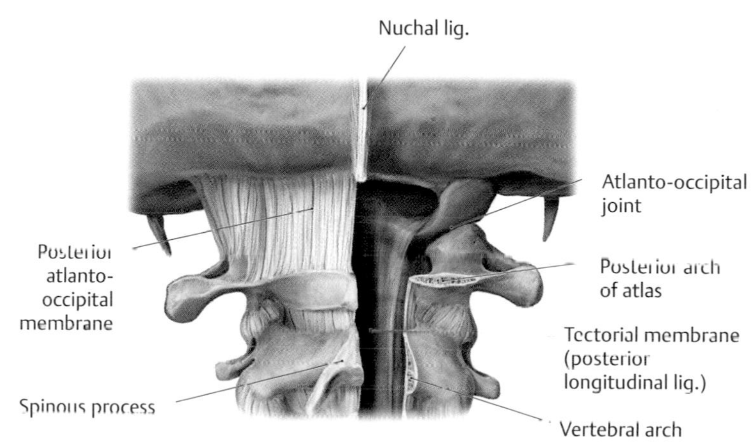
Nuchal lig.
Atlanto-occipital joint
Posterior atlanto-occipital membrane
Posterior arch of atlas
Tectorial membrane (posterior longitudinal lig.)
Spinous process
Vertebral arch

B Posterior longitudinal ligament. *Removed:* Spinal cord; vertebral canal windowed.

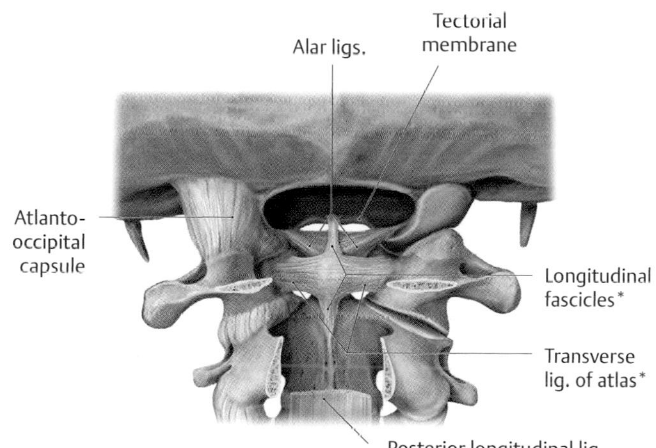
Alar ligs.
Tectorial membrane
Atlanto-occipital capsule
Longitudinal fascicles*
Transverse lig. of atlas*
Posterior longitudinal lig.

C Cruciform ligament of atlas (*). *Removed:* Tectorial membrane, posterior atlanto-occipital membrane, and vertebral arches.

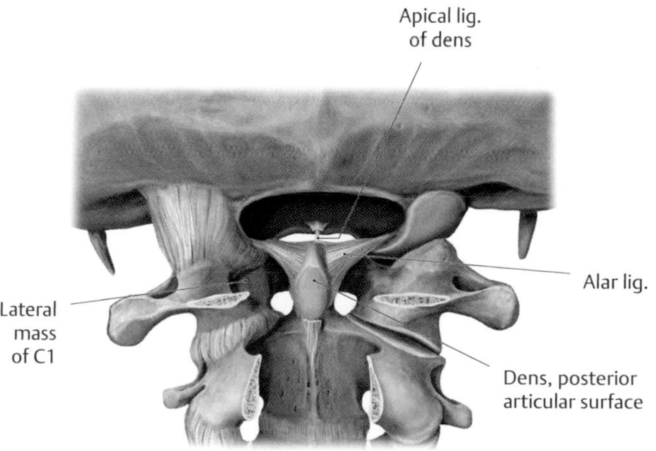
Apical lig. of dens
Alar lig.
Lateral mass of C1
Dens, posterior articular surface

D Alar and apical ligaments *Removed:* Transverse ligament of atlas.

Vertebral Ligaments: Overview & Cervical Spine

The ligaments of the spinal column bind the vertebrae and enable the spine to withstand high mechanical loads and shearing stresses and limit the range of motion. The ligaments are subdivided into vertebral body ligaments and vertebral arch ligaments.

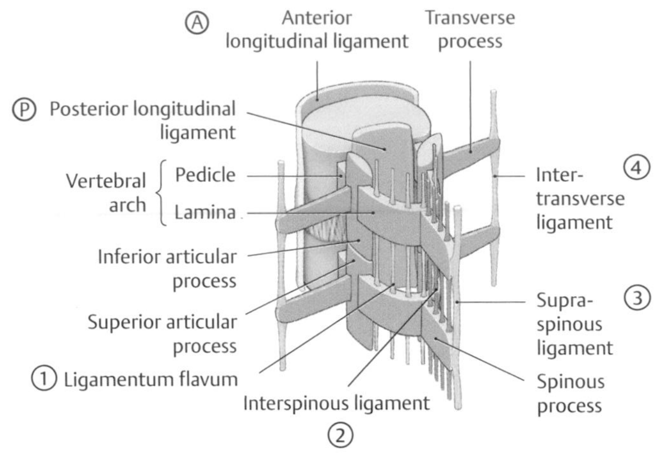

Ⓐ Anterior longitudinal ligament
Transverse process
Ⓟ Posterior longitudinal ligament
Vertebral arch
Pedicle
Lamina
Inferior articular process
Superior articular process
① Ligamentum flavum
Interspinous ligament
②
Inter-transverse ligament ④
Supra-spinous ligament ③
Spinous process

Fig. 2.25 **Vertebral ligaments**
Viewed obliquely from the left posterior view.

Table 2.3	**Vertebral ligaments**	
Ligament		**Location**
Vertebral body ligaments		
Ⓐ	Anterior longitudinal ligament	Along anterior surface of vertebral body
Ⓟ	Posterior longitudinal ligament	Along posterior surface of vertebral body
Vertebral arch ligaments		
①	Ligamenta flava	Between laminae
②	Interspinous ligaments	Between spinous process
③	Supraspinous ligaments	Along posterior ridge of spinous processes
④	Intertransverse ligaments	Between transverse processes
Nuchal ligament*		Between external occipital protuberance and spinous process of C7

*Corresponds to a supraspinous ligament that is broadened superiorly.

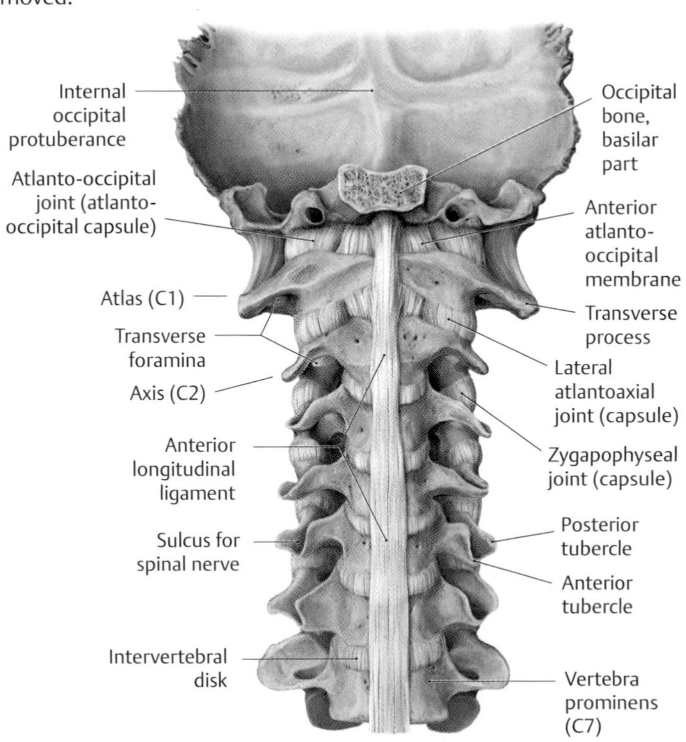

Internal occipital protuberance
Atlanto-occipital joint (atlanto-occipital capsule)
Atlas (C1)
Transverse foramina
Axis (C2)
Anterior longitudinal ligament
Sulcus for spinal nerve
Intervertebral disk
Occipital bone, basilar part
Anterior atlanto-occipital membrane
Transverse process
Lateral atlantoaxial joint (capsule)
Zygapophyseal joint (capsule)
Posterior tubercle
Anterior tubercle
Vertebra prominens (C7)

Fig. 2.26 **Anterior longitudinal ligament**
Anterior longitudinal ligament. Anterior view with base of skull removed.

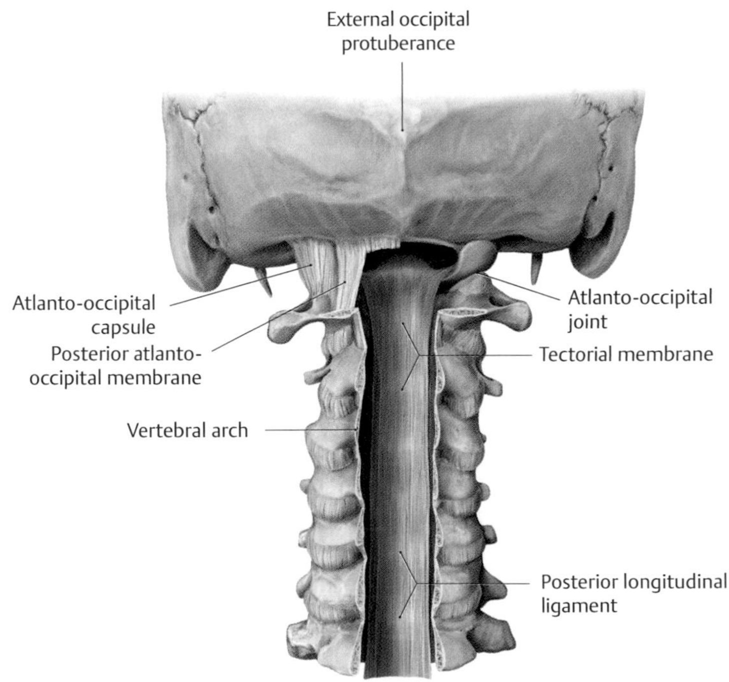

External occipital protuberance
Atlanto-occipital capsule
Posterior atlanto-occipital membrane
Vertebral arch
Atlanto-occipital joint
Tectorial membrane
Posterior longitudinal ligament

Fig. 2.27 **Posterior longitudinal ligament**
Posterior view with vertebral canal windowed and spinal cord removed. The tectorial membrane is a broadened expansion of the posterior longitudinal ligament.

Fig. 2.28 Ligaments of the cervical spine

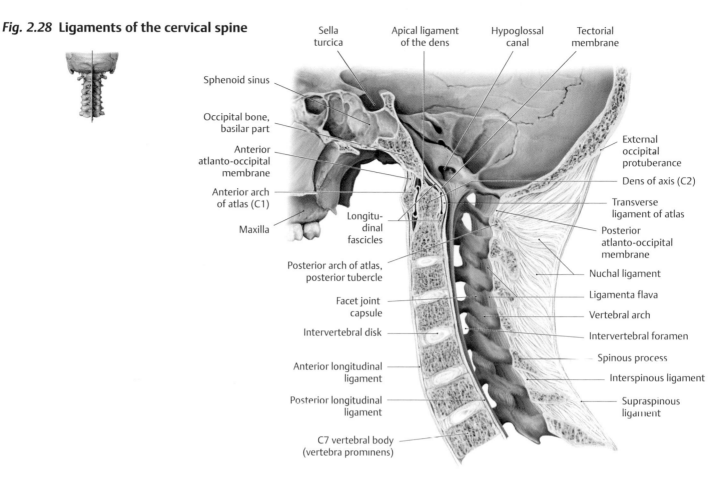

Sella turcica
Apical ligament of the dens
Hypoglossal canal
Tectorial membrane
Sphenoid sinus
Occipital bone, basilar part
Anterior atlanto-occipital membrane
Anterior arch of atlas (C1)
Maxilla
Longitudinal fascicles
Posterior arch of atlas, posterior tubercle
Facet joint capsule
Intervertebral disk
Anterior longitudinal ligament
Posterior longitudinal ligament
C7 vertebral body (vertebra prominens)
External occipital protuberance
Dens of axis (C2)
Transverse ligament of atlas
Posterior atlanto-occipital membrane
Nuchal ligament
Ligamenta flava
Vertebral arch
Intervertebral foramen
Spinous process
Interspinous ligament
Supraspinous ligament

A Midsagittal section, left lateral view. The nuchal ligament is the broadened, sagittally oriented part of the supraspinous ligament that extends from the vertebra prominens (C7) to the external occipital protuberance.

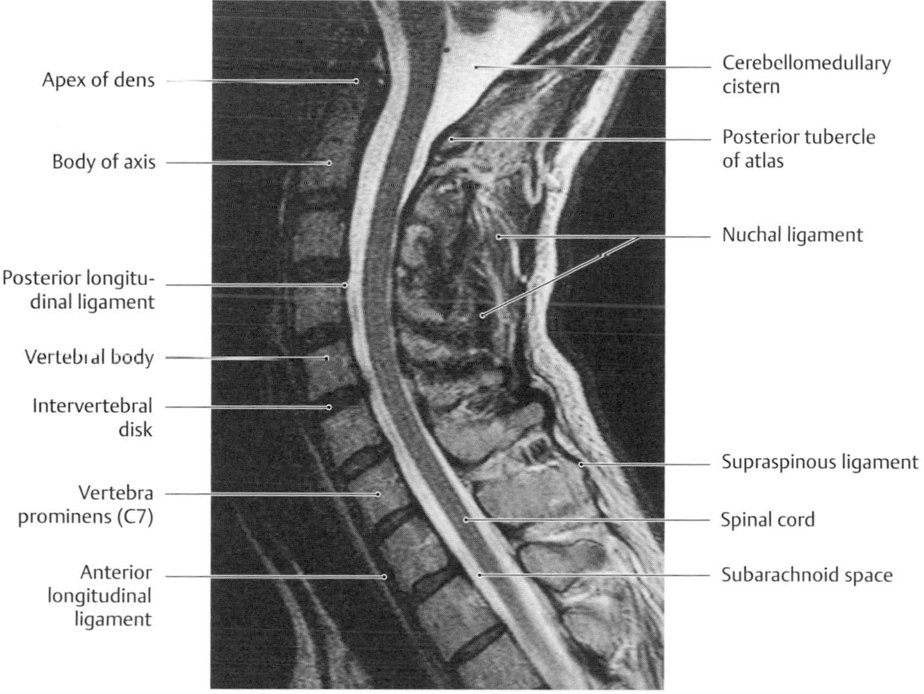
Apex of dens
Body of axis
Posterior longitudinal ligament
Vertebral body
Intervertebral disk
Vertebra prominens (C7)
Anterior longitudinal ligament
Cerebellomedullary cistern
Posterior tubercle of atlas
Nuchal ligament
Supraspinous ligament
Spinal cord
Subarachnoid space

B Midsagittal T2-weighted MRI, left lateral view.

Vertebral Ligaments: Thoracolumbar Spine

Fig. 2.29 **Ligaments of the vertebral column: Thoracolumbar junction**
Left lateral view of T11–L3, with T11–T12 sectioned in the midsagittal plane.

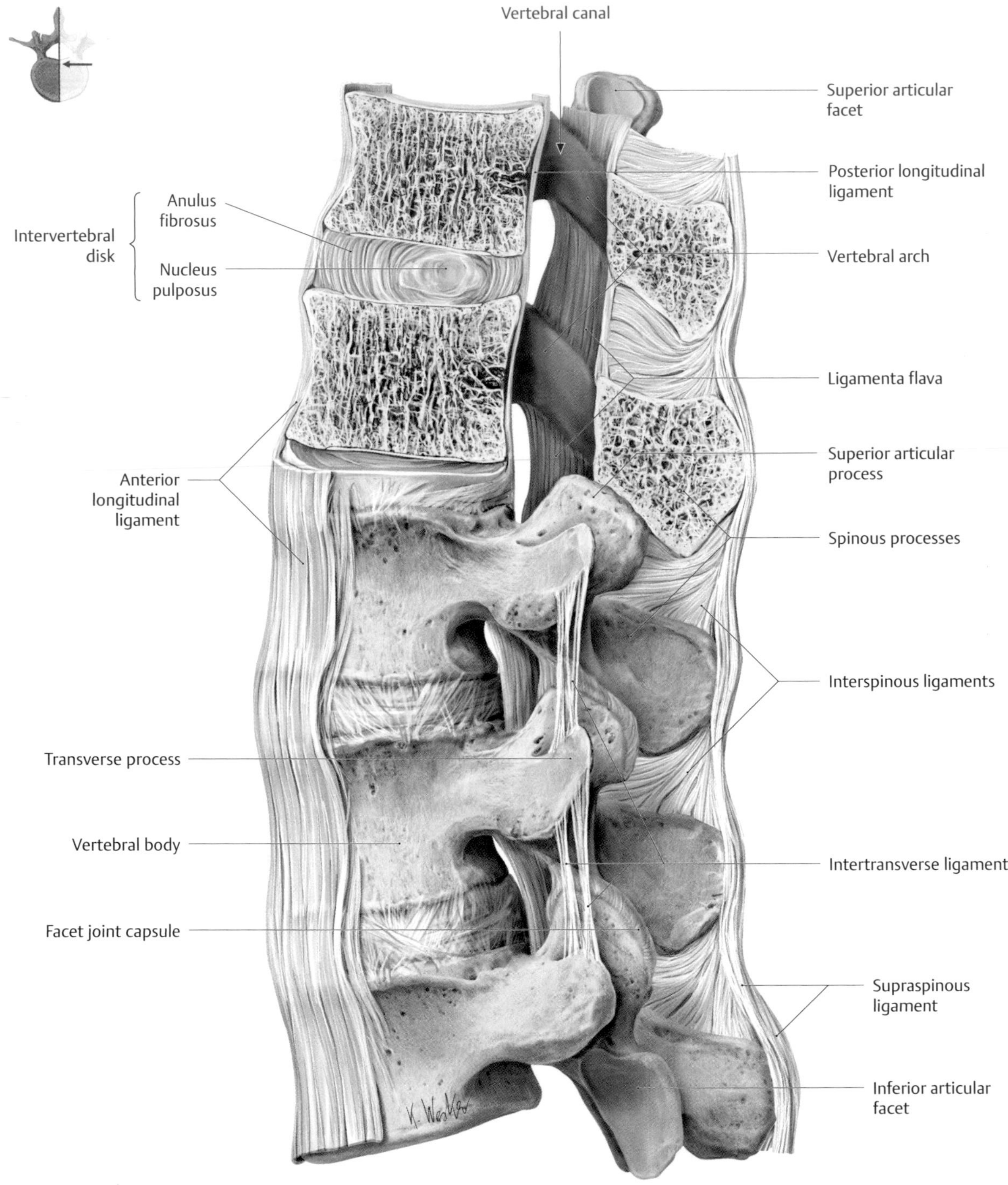
Vertebral canal
Superior articular facet
Posterior longitudinal ligament
Vertebral arch
Ligamenta flava
Superior articular process
Spinous processes
Interspinous ligaments
Intertransverse ligaments
Supraspinous ligament
Inferior articular facet
Intervertebral disk
Anulus fibrosus
Nucleus pulposus
Anterior longitudinal ligament
Transverse process
Vertebral body
Facet joint capsule

Fig. 2.30 **Anterior longitudinal ligament**
Anterior view of L3–L5.

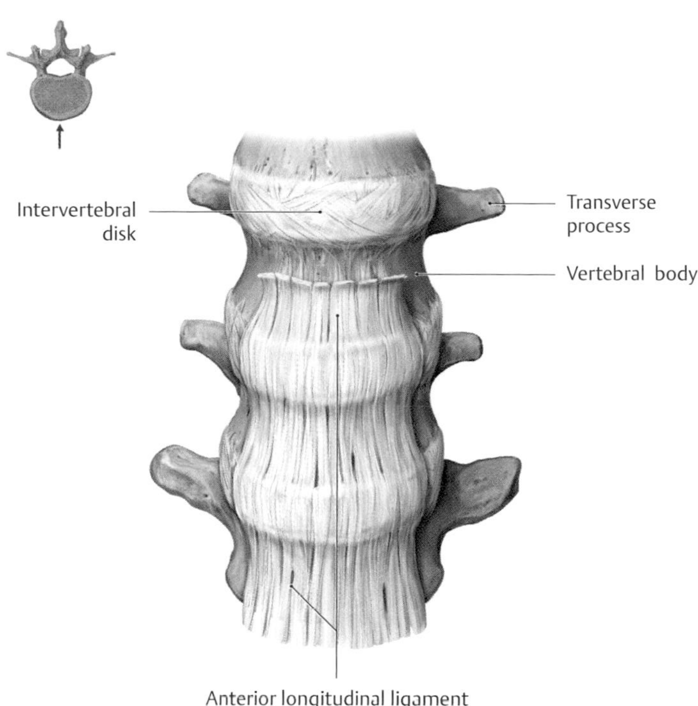
Intervertebral disk
Transverse process
Vertebral body
Anterior longitudinal ligament

Fig. 2.32 **Posterior longitudinal ligament**
Posterior view of opened vertebral canal at level of L2–L5. *Removed:* L2–L4 vertebral arches at pedicular level.

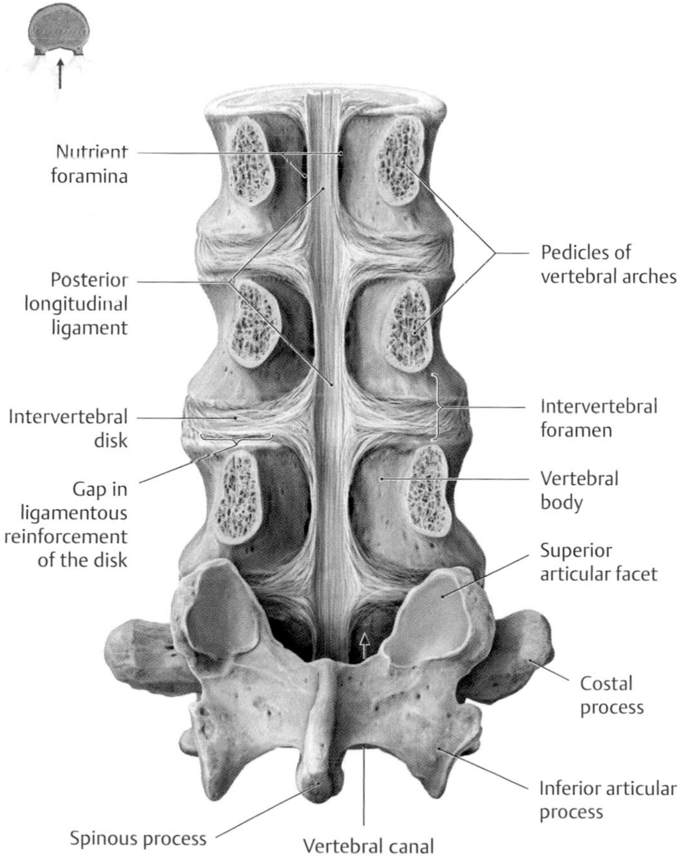
Nutrient foramina
Posterior longitudinal ligament
Intervertebral disk
Gap in ligamentous reinforcement of the disk
Pedicles of vertebral arches
Intervertebral foramen
Vertebral body
Superior articular facet
Costal process
Inferior articular process
Spinous process
Vertebral canal

Fig. 2.31 **Ligamenta flava and intertransverse ligaments**
Anterior view of opened vertebral canal at level of L2–L5. *Removed:* L2–L4 vertebral bodies.

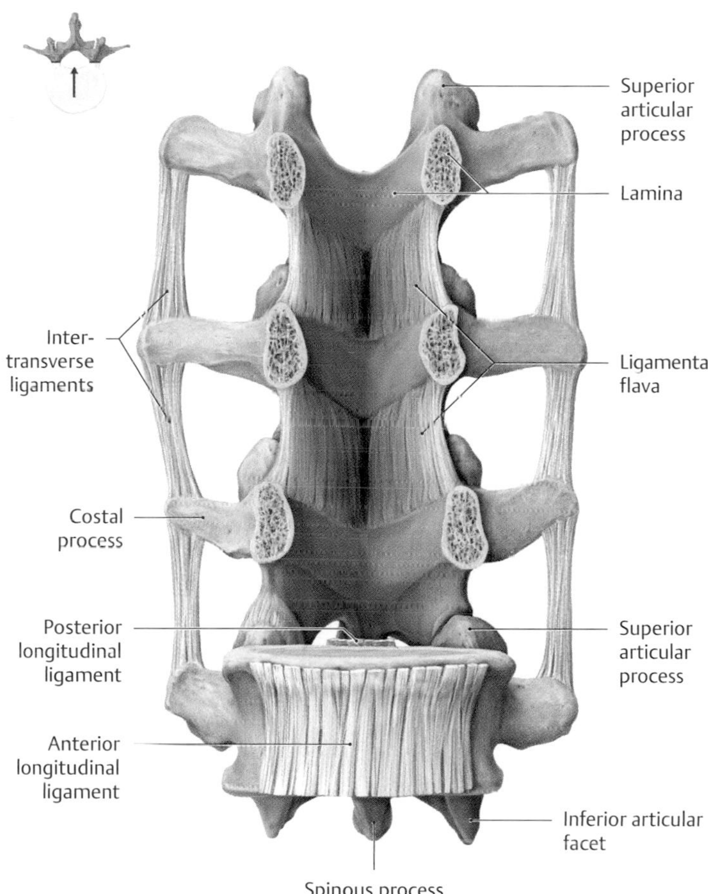
Superior articular process
Lamina
Inter-transverse ligaments
Ligamenta flava
Costal process
Posterior longitudinal ligament
Superior articular process
Anterior longitudinal ligament
Inferior articular facet
Spinous process

Muscles of the Back: Overview

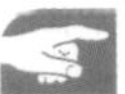

The muscles of the back are divided into two groups, the extrinsic and the intrinsic muscles, which are separated by the superficial layer of the thoracolumbar fascia. The superficial extrinsic muscles are considered muscles of the upper limb that have migrated to the back; these muscles are discussed in the Upper Limb, pp. 296–301.

Fig. 3.1 **Superficial extrinsic muscles of the back**
Posterior view. *Removed:* Trapezius and latissimus dorsi (right). *Revealed:* Thoracolumbar fascia. *Note:* The superficial layer of the thoracolumbar fascia is reinforced by the aponeurotic origin of the latissimus dorsi.

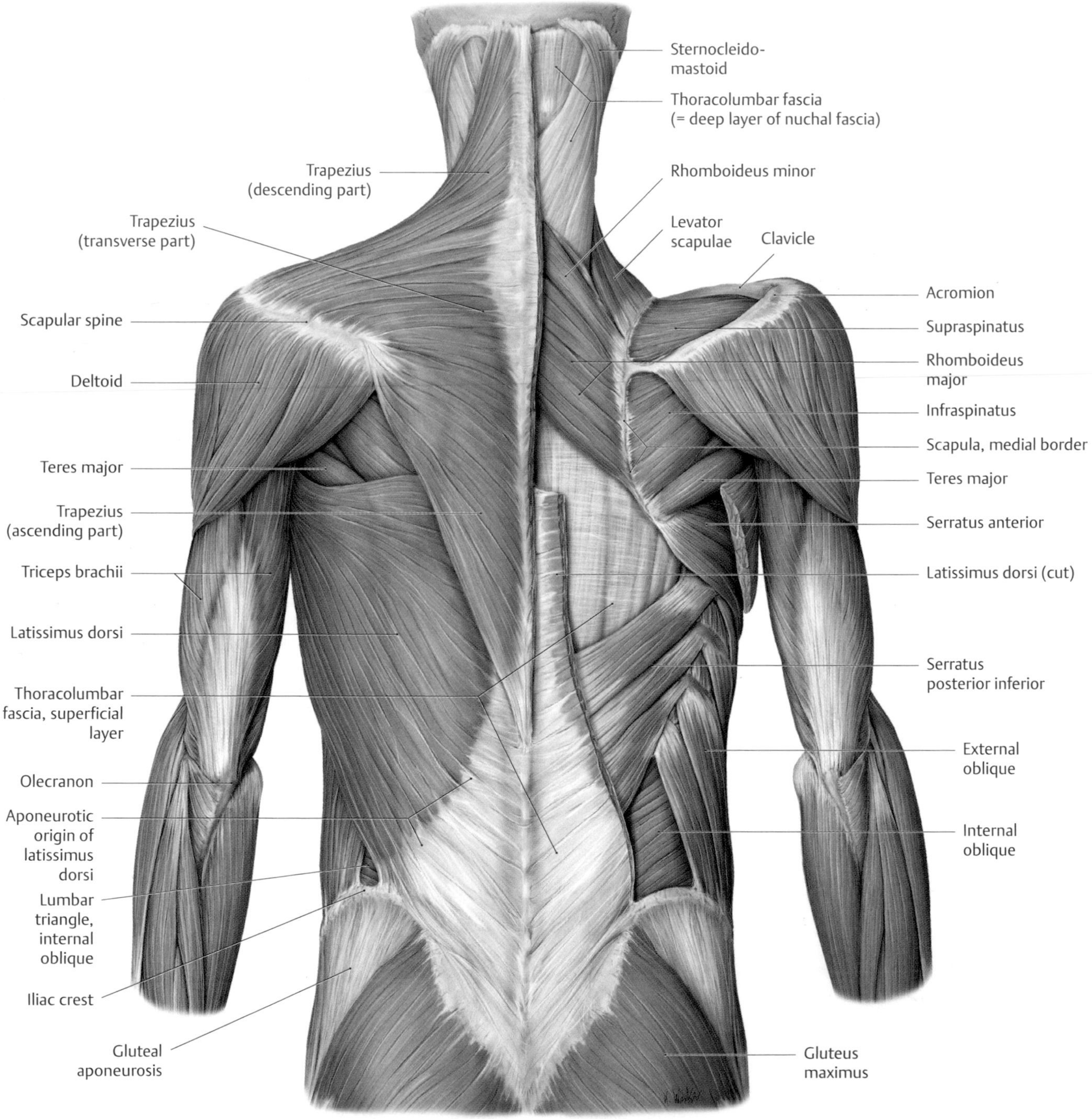

Sternocleido-mastoid
Thoracolumbar fascia (= deep layer of nuchal fascia)
Trapezius (descending part)
Rhomboideus minor
Trapezius (transverse part)
Levator scapulae
Clavicle
Acromion
Scapular spine
Supraspinatus
Rhomboideus major
Deltoid
Infraspinatus
Scapula, medial border
Teres major
Teres major
Trapezius (ascending part)
Serratus anterior
Triceps brachii
Latissimus dorsi (cut)
Latissimus dorsi
Serratus posterior inferior
Thoracolumbar fascia, superficial layer
External oblique
Olecranon
Aponeurotic origin of latissimus dorsi
Internal oblique
Lumbar triangle, internal oblique
Iliac crest
Gluteal aponeurosis
Gluteus maximus

Fig. 3.2 **Thoracolumbar fascia**

Transverse section, superior view. The intrinsic back muscles are sequestered in an osseofibrous canal, formed by the thoracolumbar fascia, the vertebral arches, and the spinous and transverse processes of associated vertebrae. The thoracolumbar fascia consists of a superficial and a deep layer that unite at the lateral margin of the intrinsic back muscles. In the neck, the superficial layer blends with the nuchal fascia (deep layer), becoming continuous with the deep cervical fascia (prevertebral layer).

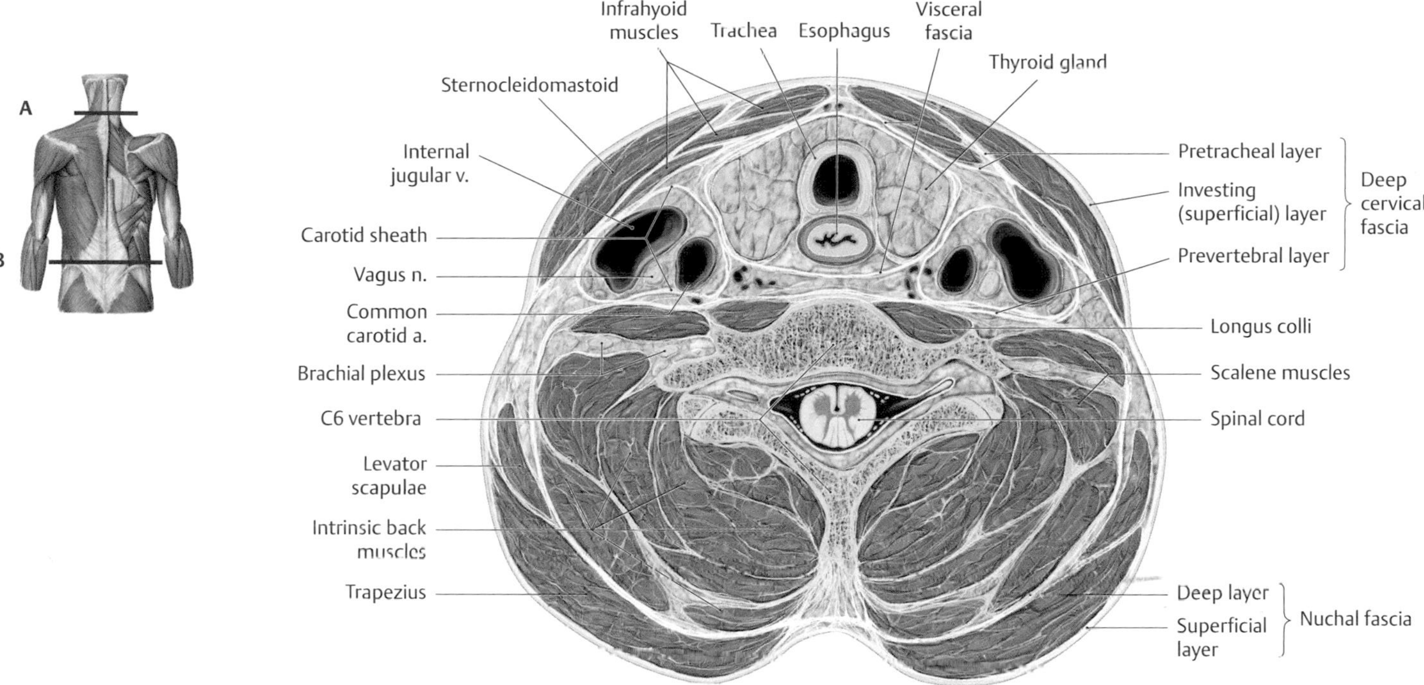
A
B
Infrahyoid muscles
Trachea
Esophagus
Visceral fascia
Thyroid gland
Sternocleidomastoid
Internal jugular v.
Carotid sheath
Vagus n.
Common carotid a.
Brachial plexus
C6 vertebra
Levator scapulae
Intrinsic back muscles
Trapezius
Pretracheal layer
Investing (superficial) layer
Prevertebral layer
Deep cervical fascia
Longus colli
Scalene muscles
Spinal cord
Deep layer
Superficial layer
Nuchal fascia

A Transverse section at level of C6 vertebra, superior view.

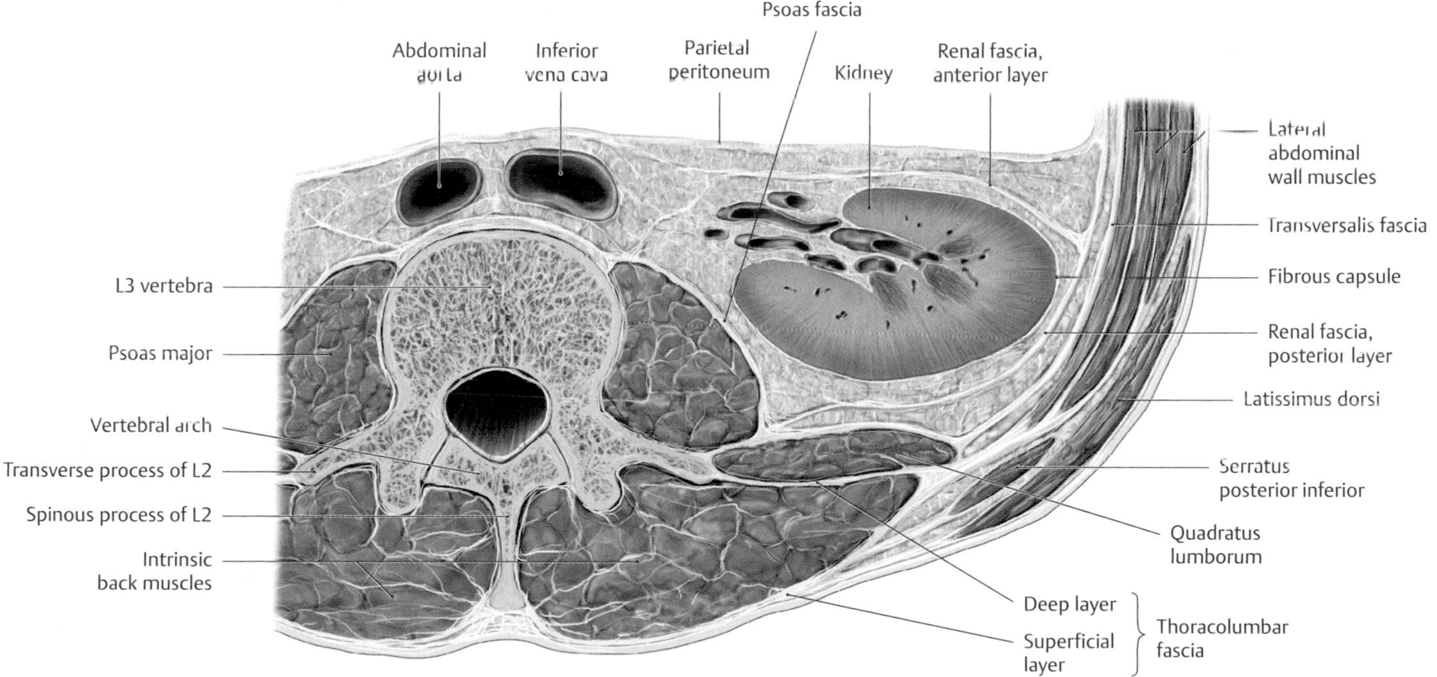
Psoas fascia
Abdominal aorta
Inferior vena cava
Parietal peritoneum
Kidney
Renal fascia, anterior layer
Lateral abdominal wall muscles
Transversalis fascia
Fibrous capsule
Renal fascia, posterior layer
Latissimus dorsi
Serratus posterior inferior
Quadratus lumborum
L3 vertebra
Psoas major
Vertebral arch
Transverse process of L2
Spinous process of L2
Intrinsic back muscles
Deep layer
Superficial layer
Thoracolumbar fascia

B Transverse section at level of L2, superior view.
Removed: Cauda equina and anterior trunk wall.

Intrinsic Muscles of the Cervical Spine

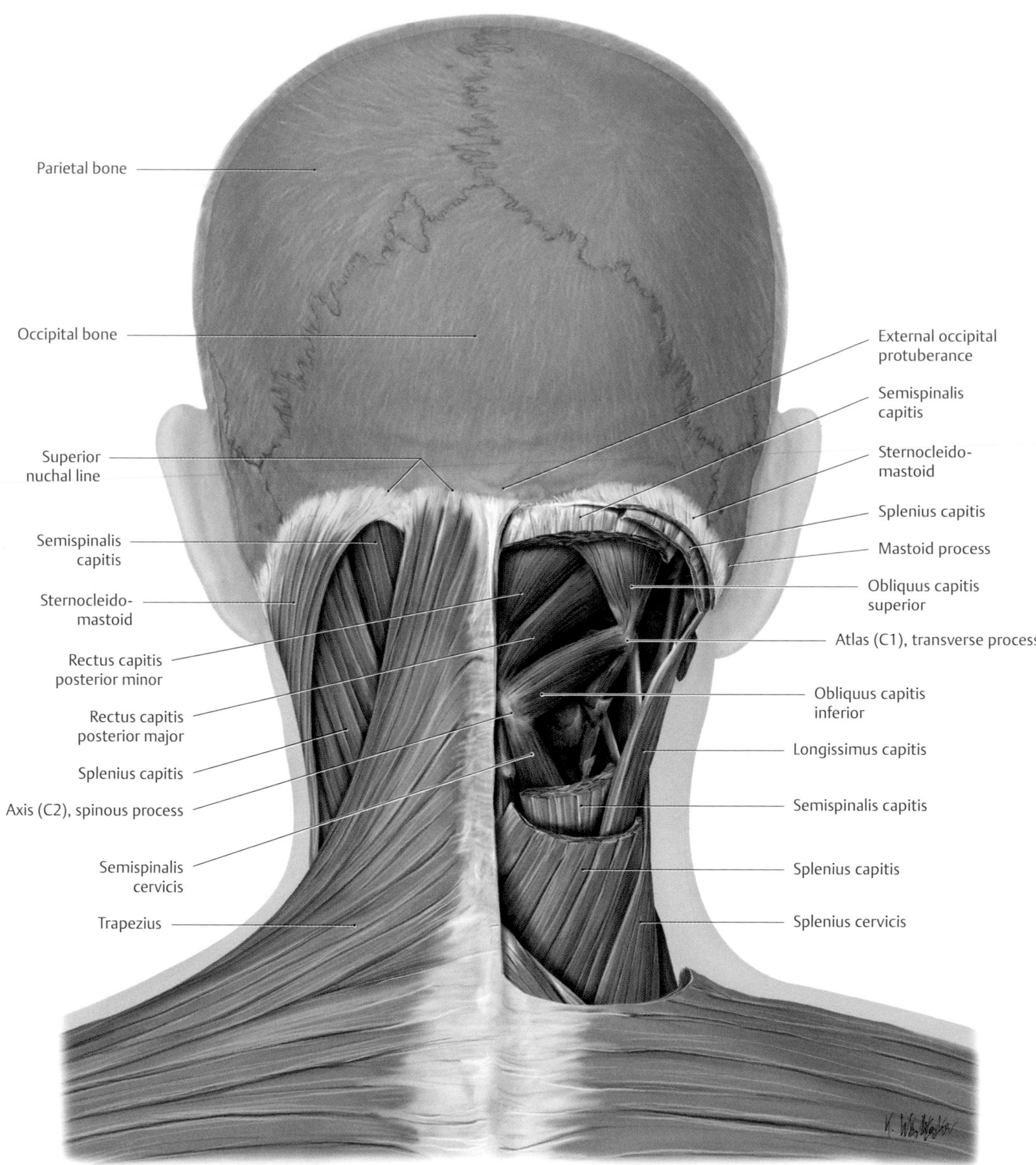
Parietal bone
Occipital bone
Superior nuchal line
Semispinalis capitis
Sternocleido-mastoid
Rectus capitis posterior minor
Rectus capitis posterior major
Splenius capitis
Axis (C2), spinous process
Semispinalis cervicis
Trapezius
External occipital protuberance
Semispinalis capitis
Sternocleido-mastoid
Splenius capitis
Mastoid process
Obliquus capitis superior
Atlas (C1), transverse process
Obliquus capitis inferior
Longissimus capitis
Semispinalis capitis
Splenius capitis
Splenius cervicis

Fig. 3.3 **Muscles in the nuchal region**
Posterior view. *Removed:* Trapezius, sternocleidomastoid, splenius, and semispinalis muscles (right). *Revealed:* Nuchal muscles (right).

Fig. 3.4 Short nuchal muscles

Posterior view. See Fig. 3.6.

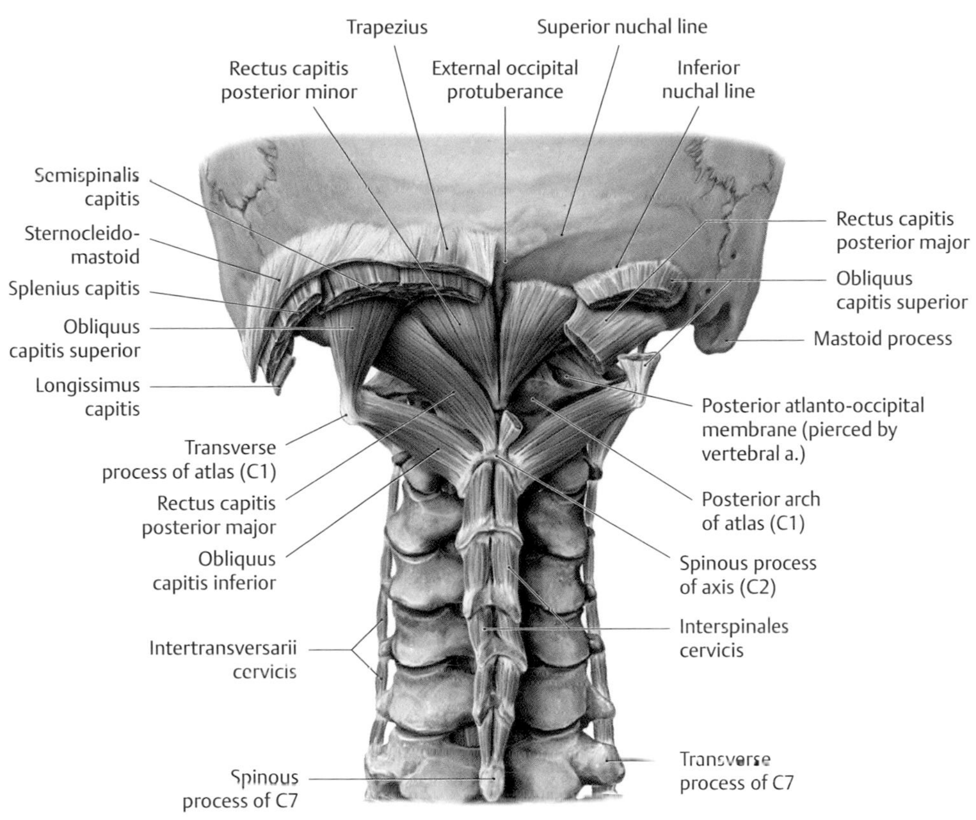
Trapezius
Superior nuchal line
Rectus capitis posterior minor
External occipital protuberance
Inferior nuchal line
Semispinalis capitis
Sternocleido-mastoid
Splenius capitis
Obliquus capitis superior
Longissimus capitis
Transverse process of atlas (C1)
Rectus capitis posterior major
Obliquus capitis inferior
Intertransversarii cervicis
Spinous process of C7
Rectus capitis posterior major
Obliquus capitis superior
Mastoid process
Posterior atlanto-occipital membrane (pierced by vertebral a.)
Posterior arch of atlas (C1)
Spinous process of axis (C2)
Interspinales cervicis
Transverse process of C7

A Course of the short nuchal muscles.

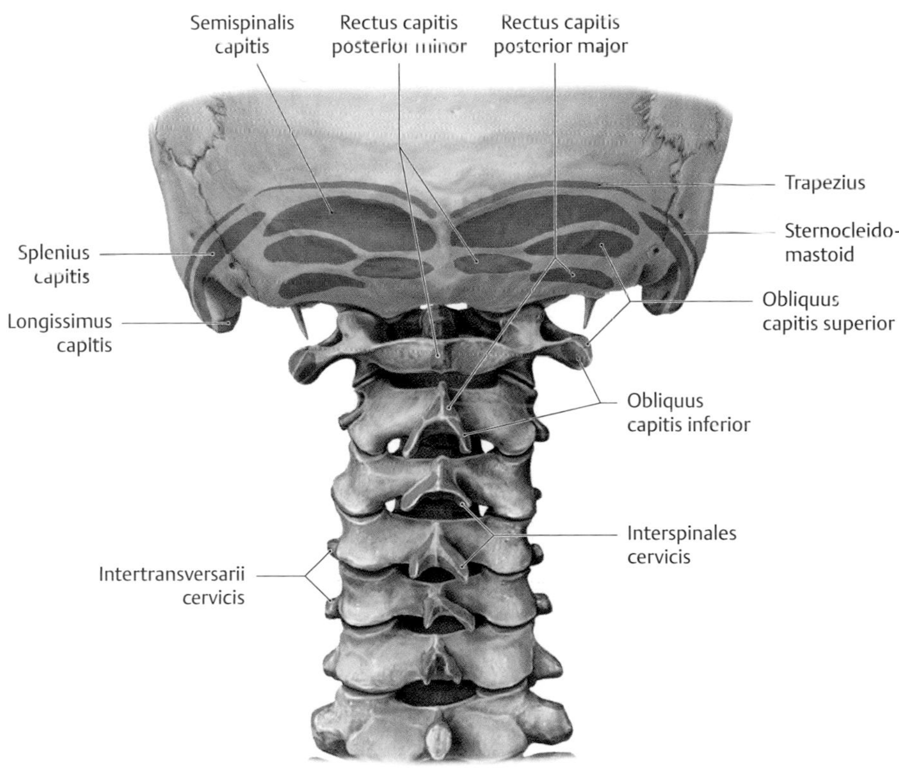
Semispinalis capitis
Rectus capitis posterior minor
Rectus capitis posterior major
Trapezius
Sternocleido-mastoid
Splenius capitis
Longissimus capitis
Obliquus capitis superior
Obliquus capitis inferior
Interspinales cervicis
Intertransversarii cervicis

B Suboccipital region. Muscle origins are shown in red, insertions in blue.

Intrinsic Muscles of the Back

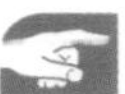

The extrinsic muscles of the back (trapezius, latissimus dorsi, levator scapulae, and rhomboids) are discussed in the Upper Limb, pp. 298-299. The serratus posterior, considered an intermediate extrinsic back muscle, has been included with the superficial intrinsic muscles in this unit.

Fig. 3.5 **Intrinsic muscles of the back**
Posterior view. Sequential dissection of the thoracolumbar fascia, superficial intrinsic muscles, intermediate intrinsic muscles, and deep intrinsic muscles of the back.

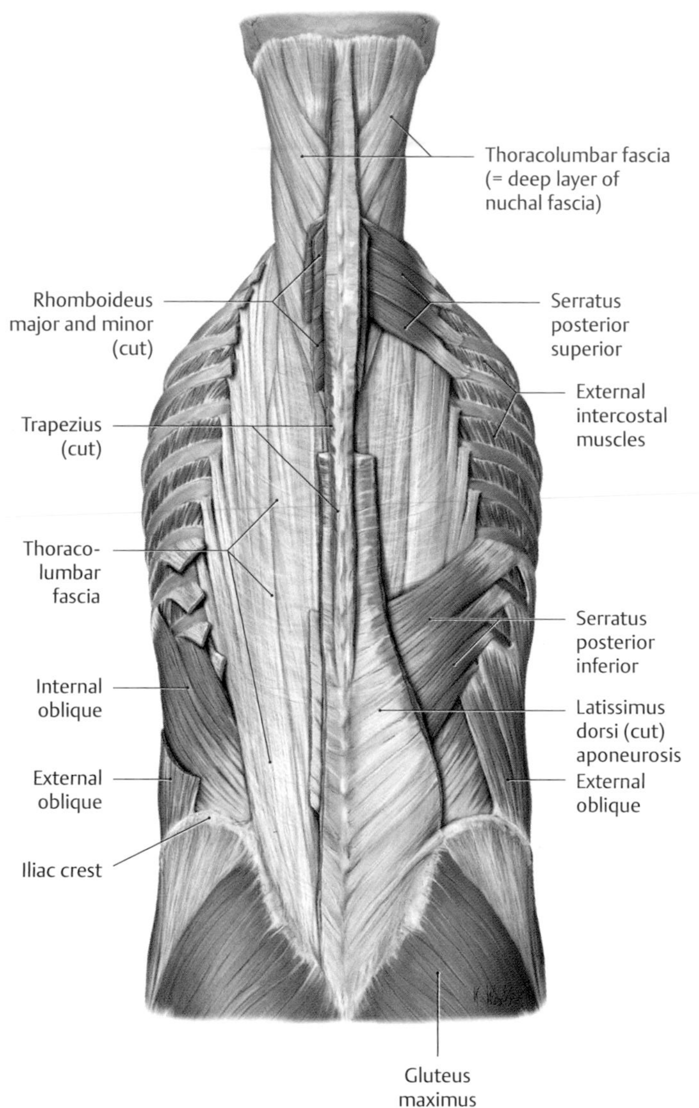
Thoracolumbar fascia (= deep layer of nuchal fascia)
Rhomboideus major and minor (cut)
Serratus posterior superior
External intercostal muscles
Trapezius (cut)
Thoraco-lumbar fascia
Serratus posterior inferior
Internal oblique
Latissimus dorsi (cut) aponeurosis
External oblique
External oblique
Iliac crest
Gluteus maximus

A Thoracolumbar fascia. *Removed:* Shoulder girdles and extrinsic back muscles (except serratus posterior and aponeurotic origin of latissimus dorsi). *Revealed:* Superficial layer of thoracolumbar fascia.

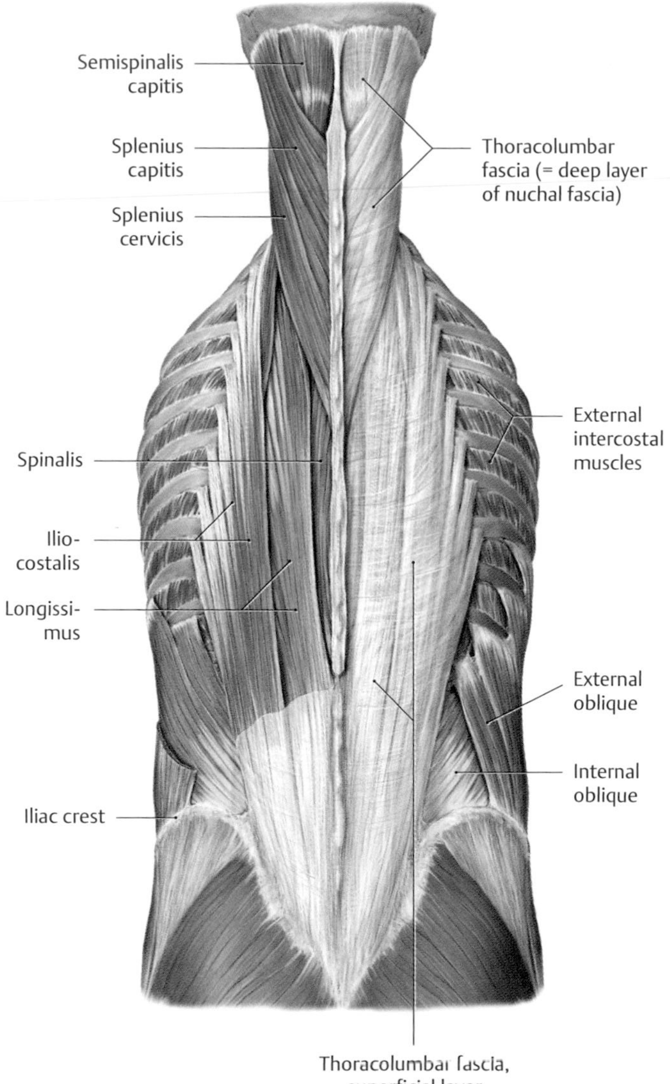
Semispinalis capitis
Splenius capitis
Splenius cervicis
Thoracolumbar fascia (= deep layer of nuchal fascia)
External intercostal muscles
Spinalis
Ilio-costalis
Longissi-mus
External oblique
Internal oblique
Iliac crest
Thoracolumbar fascia, superficial layer

B Superficial and intermediate intrinsic back muscles. *Removed:* Thoracolumbar fascia (left). *Revealed:* Erector spinae and splenius muscles.

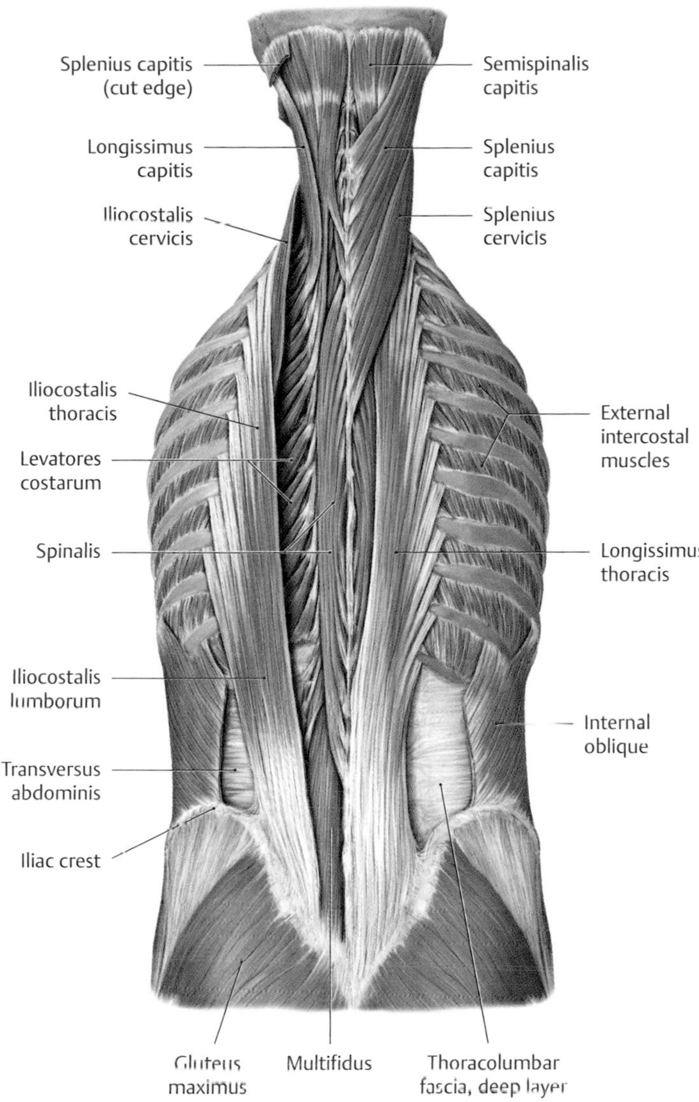
Splenius capitis (cut edge)
Semispinalis capitis
Longissimus capitis
Splenius capitis
Iliocostalis cervicis
Splenius cervicis
Iliocostalis thoracis
External intercostal muscles
Levatores costarum
Spinalis
Longissimus thoracis
Iliocostalis lumborum
Internal oblique
Transversus abdominis
Iliac crest
Gluteus maximus
Multifidus
Thoracolumbar fascia, deep layer

C Intermediate and deep intrinsic back muscles. *Removed:* Longissimus thoracis and cervicis, splenius muscles (left); iliocostalis (right). *Note:* The deep layer of the thoracolumbar fascia gives origin to the internal oblique and transversus abdominus. *Revealed:* Deep muscles of the back.

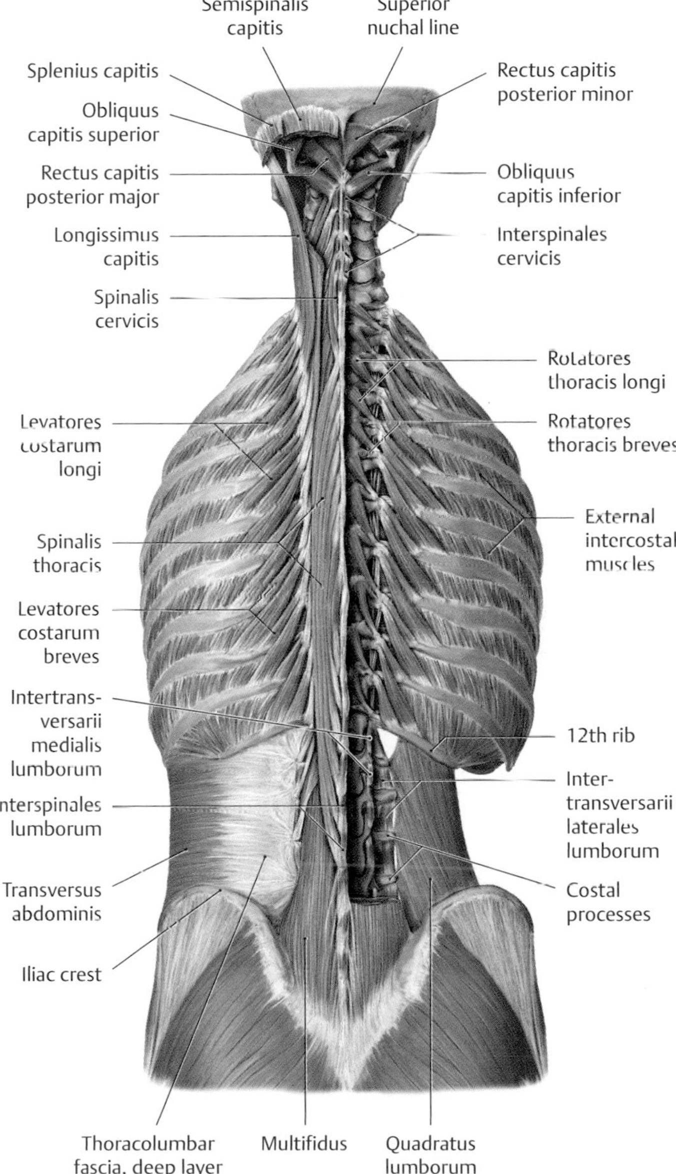
Semispinalis capitis
Superior nuchal line
Splenius capitis
Rectus capitis posterior minor
Obliquus capitis superior
Rectus capitis posterior major
Obliquus capitis inferior
Longissimus capitis
Interspinales cervicis
Spinalis cervicis
Rotatores thoracis longi
Levatores costarum longi
Rotatores thoracis breves
External intercostal muscles
Spinalis thoracis
Levatores costarum breves
Intertrans-versarii medialis lumborum
12th rib
Inter-transversarii laterales lumborum
Interspinales lumborum
Transversus abdominis
Costal processes
Iliac crest
Thoracolumbar fascia, deep layer
Multifidus
Quadratus lumborum

D Deep intrinsic back muscles. *Removed:* Superficial and intermediate intrinsic back muscles (all); deep fascial layer and multifidus (right). *Revealed:* Intertransversarii and quadratus lumborum (right).

Muscle Facts (I)

Fig. 3.6 **Short nuchal and craniovertebral joint muscles**

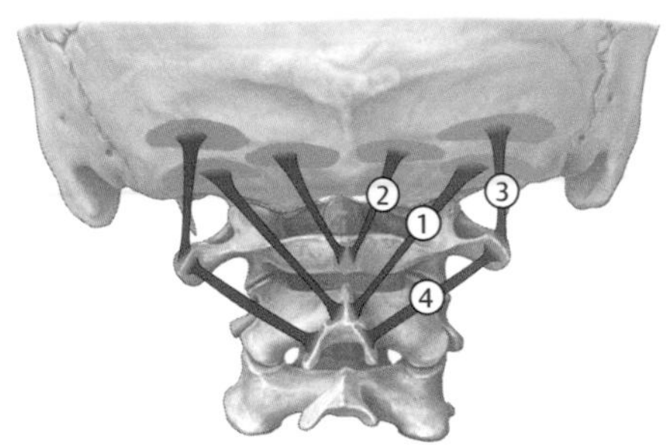

1
2
3
4

A Posterior view, schematic.

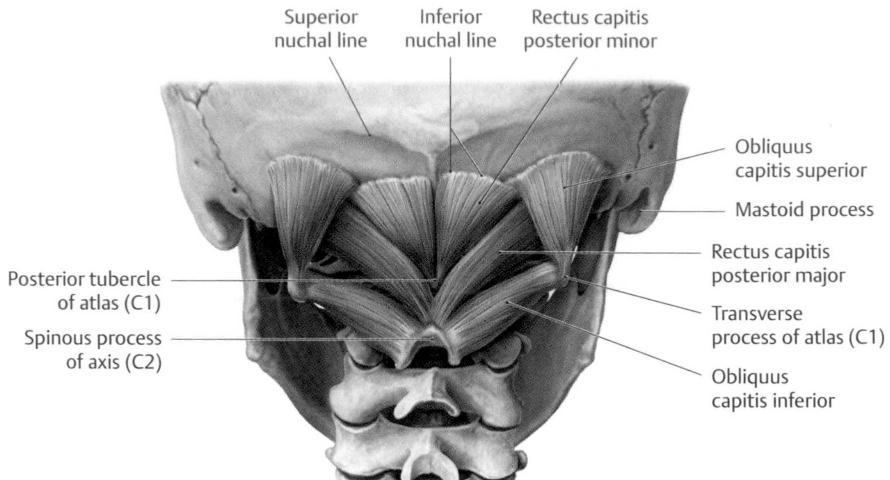

Superior nuchal line
Inferior nuchal line
Rectus capitis posterior minor
Obliquus capitis superior
Mastoid process
Rectus capitis posterior major
Posterior tubercle of atlas (C1)
Transverse process of atlas (C1)
Spinous process of axis (C2)
Obliquus capitis inferior

B Suboccipital muscles, posterior view.

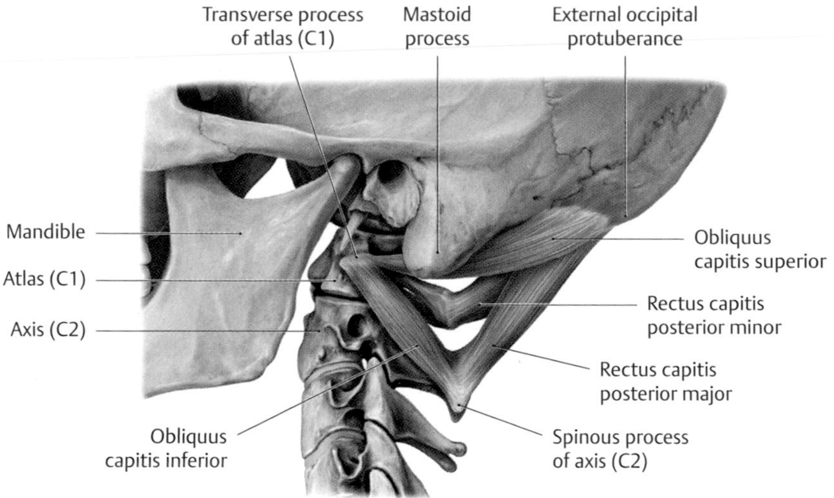

Transverse process of atlas (C1)
Mastoid process
External occipital protuberance
Mandible
Obliquus capitis superior
Atlas (C1)
Rectus capitis posterior minor
Axis (C2)
Rectus capitis posterior major
Obliquus capitis inferior
Spinous process of axis (C2)

C Suboccipital muscles, left lateral view.

Table 3.1 **Short nuchal and craniovertebral joint muscles**

Muscle		Origin	Insertion	Innervation	Action
Rectus capitis posterior	① Rectus capitis posterior major	C2 (spinous process)	Occipital bone (inferior nuchal line, middle third)	C1 (posterior ramus = suboccipital n.)	*Bilateral:* Extends head *Unilateral:* Rotates head to same side
	② Rectus capitis posterior minor	C1 (posterior tubercle)	Occipital bone (inferior nuchal line, inner third)		
Obliquus capitis	③ Obliquus capitis superior	C1 (transverse process)	Occipital bone (inferior nuchal line, middle third; above rectus capitis posterior major)		*Bilateral:* Extends head *Unilateral:* Tilts head to same side; rotates to opposite side
	④ Obliquus capitis inferior	C2 (spinous process)	C1 (transverse process)		*Bilateral:* Extends head *Unilateral:* Rotates head to same side

Fig. 3.7 Prevertebral muscles

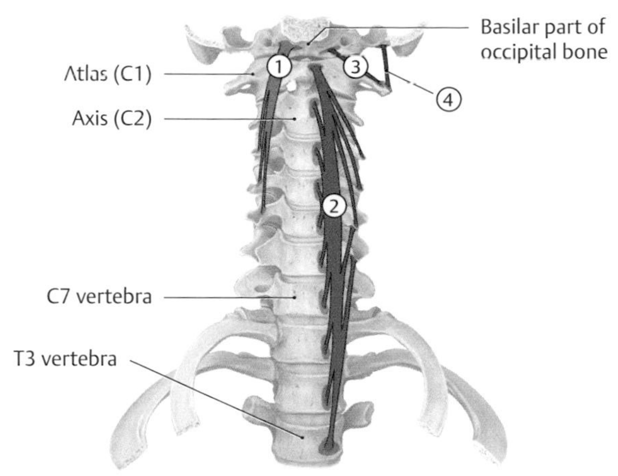
Basilar part of occipital bone
Atlas (C1)
Axis (C2)
C7 vertebra
T3 vertebra
①
②
③
④

A Anterior view, schematic.

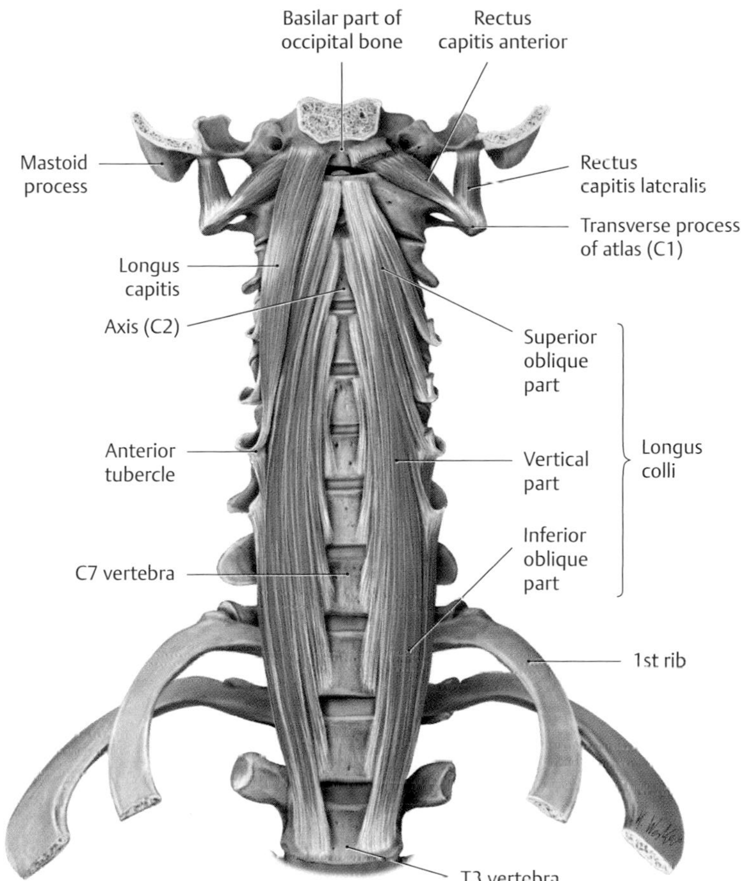
Basilar part of occipital bone
Rectus capitis anterior
Mastoid process
Rectus capitis lateralis
Transverse process of atlas (C1)
Longus capitis
Axis (C2)
Superior oblique part
Anterior tubercle
Vertical part
Longus colli
Inferior oblique part
C7 vertebra
1st rib
T3 vertebra

B Prevertebral muscles, anterior view. *Removed:* Longus capitis (left); cervical viscera.

Table 3.2 **Prevertebral muscles**

Muscle		Origin	Insertion	Innervation	Action
① Longus capitis		C3–C6 (transverse processes, anterior tubercles)	Occipital bone (basilar part)	Direct branches from cervical plexus (C1–C3)	*Bilateral:* Flexes head *Unilateral:* Tilts and slightly rotates head to same side
② Longus colli (cervicis)	Vertical (medial) part	C5–T3 (anterior sides of vertebral bodies)	C2–C4 (anterior sides of vertebral bodies)	Direct branches from cervical plexus (C2–C6)	*Bilateral:* Flexes cervical spine *Unilateral:* Tilts and rotates cervical spine to same side
	Superior oblique part	C3–C5 (transverse processes, anterior tubercles)	C1 (transverse process, anterior tubercle)		
	Inferior oblique part	T1–T3 (anterior sides of vertebral bodies)	C5–C6 (transverse processes, anterior tubercles)		
③ Rectus capitis anterior		C1 (lateral mass)	Occipital bone (basilar part)	C1 (anterior ramus)	*Bilateral:* Flexion at atlanto-occipital joint *Unilateral:* Lateral flexion at atlanto-occipital joint
④ Rectus capitis lateralis		C1 (transverse process)	Occipital bone (basilar part, lateral to occipital condyles)		

Muscle Facts (II)

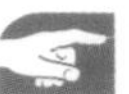

The intrinsic back muscles are divided into superficial, intermediate, and deep layers. The serratus posterior muscles are extrinsic back muscles, innervated by the anterior rami of intercostal nerves, not the posterior rami, which innervate the intrinsic back muscles. They are included here as they are encountered in dissection of the back musculature.

Table 3.3 Superficial intrinsic back muscles

Muscle		Origin	Insertion	Innervation	Action
Serratus posterior	① Serratus posterior superior	Nuchal ligament; C7–T3 (spinous processes)	2nd–4th ribs (superior borders)	Spinal nn. T2–T5 (anterior rami)	Elevates ribs
	② Serratus posterior inferior	T11–L2 (spinous processes)	8th–12th ribs (inferior borders, near angles)	Spinal nn. T9–T12 (anterior rami)	Depresses ribs
Splenius	③ Splenius capitis	Nuchal ligament; C3–C7 (spinous processes)	Occipital bone (lateral superior nuchal line; mastoid process)	Spinal nn. C1–C6 (posterior rami, lateral branches)	*Bilateral:* Extends cervical spine and head *Unilateral:* Flexes and rotates head to the same side
	④ Splenius cervicis	T3–T6 (spinous processes)	C1–C2 (transverse processes)		

Fig. 3.8 **Superficial intrinsic back muscles, schematic**
Right side, posterior view.

Fig. 3.9 **Intermediate intrinsic back muscles, schematic**
Right side, posterior view. These muscles are collectively known as the erector spinae.

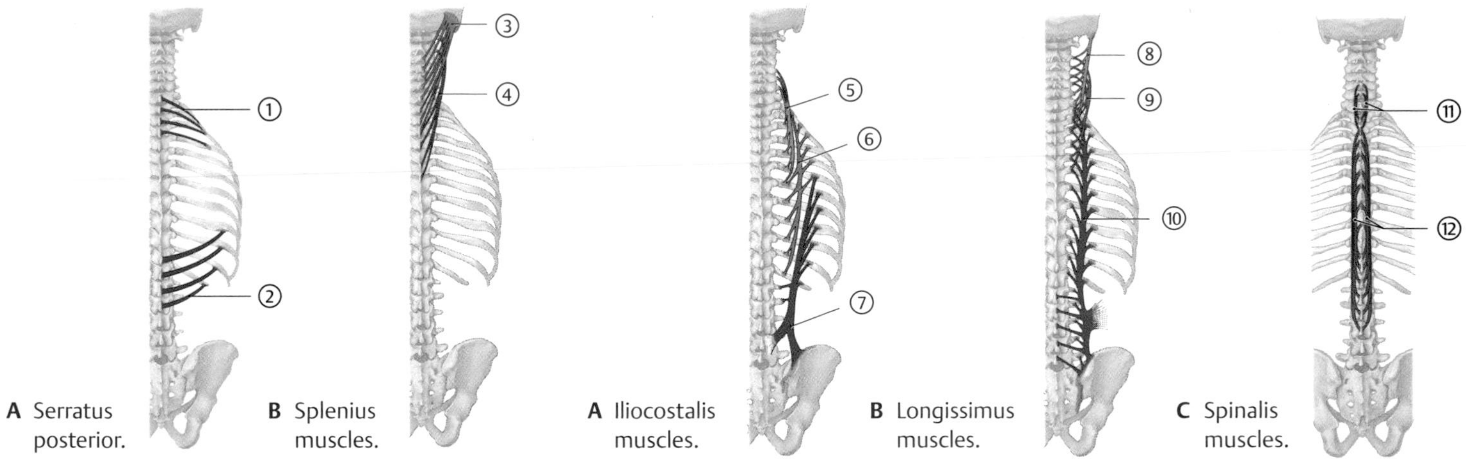

①
②
③
④
⑤
⑥
⑦
⑧
⑨
⑩
⑪
⑫

Fig. 3.8: **A** Serratus posterior. **B** Splenius muscles.

Fig. 3.9: **A** Iliocostalis muscles. **B** Longissimus muscles. **C** Spinalis muscles.

Table 3.4 Intermediate intrinsic back muscles

Muscle		Origin	Insertion	Innervation	Action
Iliocostalis	⑤ Iliocostalis cervicis	3rd–7th ribs	C4–C6 (transverse processes)	Spinal nn. C8–L1 (posterior rami, lateral branches)	*Bilateral:* Extends spine *Unilateral:* Bends spine laterally to same side
	⑥ Iliocostalis thoracis	7th–12th ribs	1st–6th ribs		
	⑦ Iliocostalis lumborum	Sacrum; iliac crest; thoracolumbar fascia	6th–12th ribs; thoracolumbar fascia (deep layer); upper lumbar vertebrae (transverse processes)		
Longissimus	⑧ Longissimus capitis	T1–T3 (transverse processes); C4-C7 (transverse and articular processes)	Temporal bone (mastoid process)	Spinal nn. C1–L5 (posterior rami, lateral branches)	*Bilateral:* Extends head *Unilateral:* Flexes and rotates head to same side
	⑨ Longissimus cervicis	T1–T6 (transverse processes)	C2–C5 (transverse processes)		*Bilateral:* Extends spine *Unilateral:* Bends spine laterally to same side
	⑩ Longissimus thoracis	Sacrum; iliac crest; lumbar vertebrae (spinous processes); lower thoracic vertebrae (transverse processes)	2nd–12th ribs; lumbar vertebrae (costal processes); thoracic vertebrae (transverse processes)		
Spinalis	⑪ Spinalis cervicis	C5–T2 (spinous processes)	C2–C5 (spinous processes)	Spinal nn. (posterior rami)	*Bilateral:* Extends cervical and thoracic spine *Unilateral:* Bends cervical and thoracic spine to same side
	⑫ Spinalis thoracis	T10–L3 (spinous processes, lateral surfaces)	T2–T8 (spinous processes, lateral surfaces)		

Fig. 3.10 Superficial and intermediate intrinsic back muscles
Posterior view.

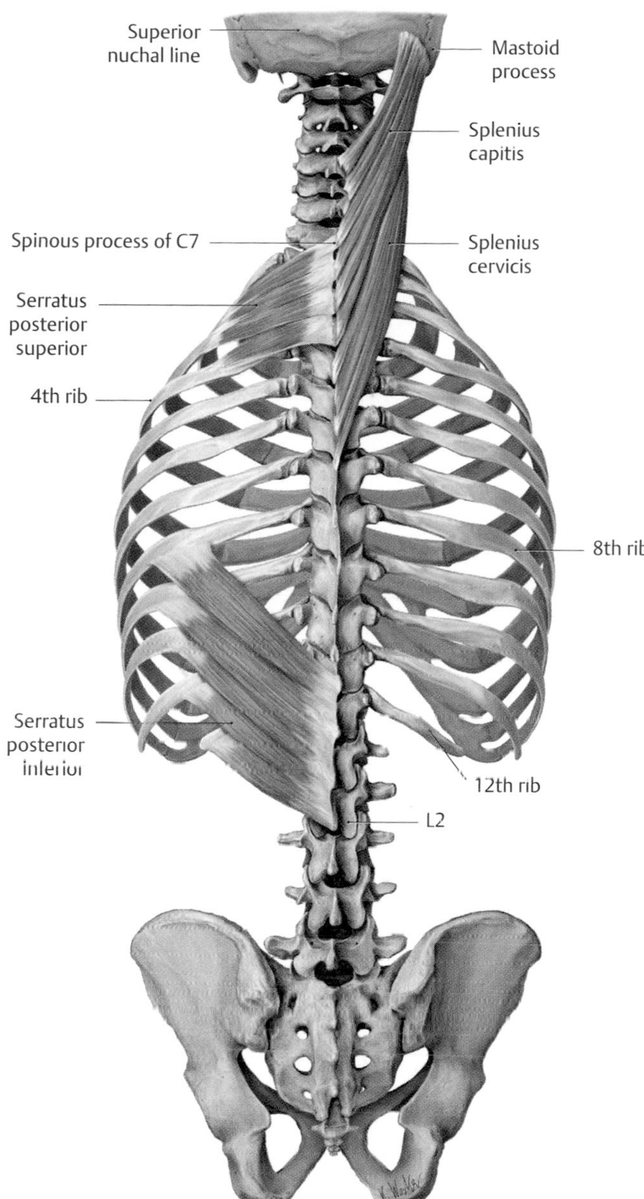
Superior nuchal line
Mastoid process
Splenius capitis
Spinous process of C7
Splenius cervicis
Serratus posterior superior
4th rib
8th rib
Serratus posterior inferior
12th rib
L2

A Superficial back muscles: Splenius and serratus posterior muscles.

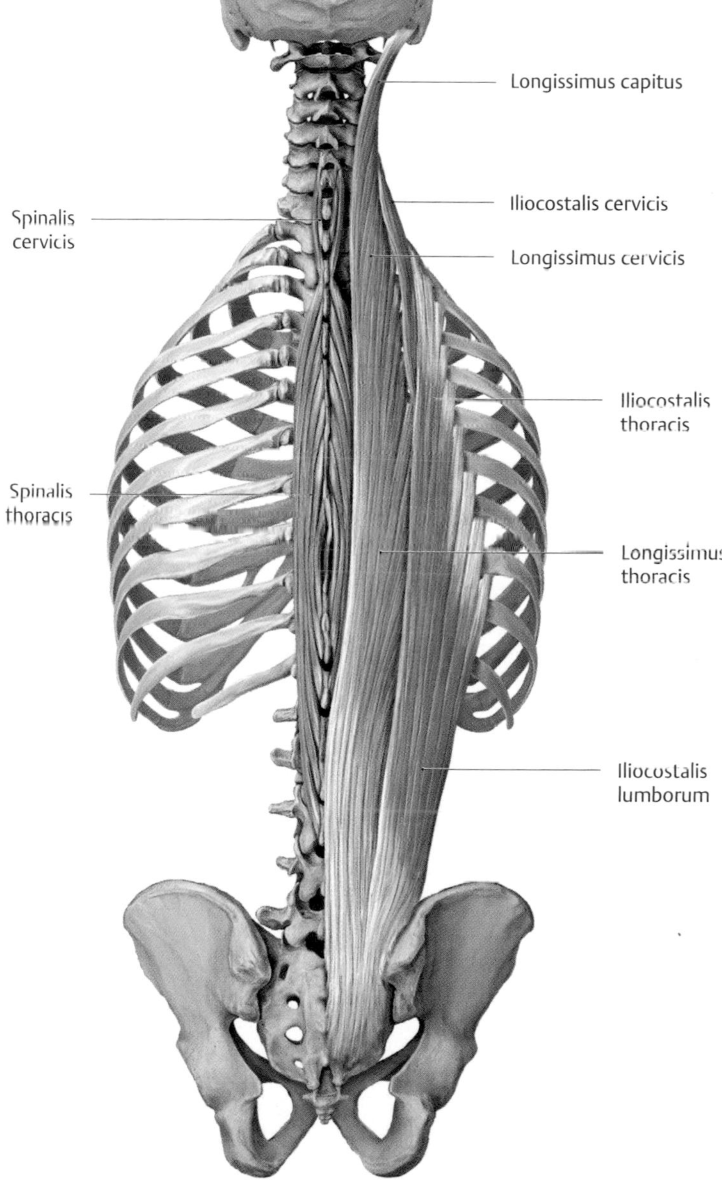
Longissimus capitus
Iliocostalis cervicis
Spinalis cervicis
Longissimus cervicis
Iliocostalis thoracis
Spinalis thoracis
Longissimus thoracis
Iliocostalis lumborum

B Intermediate intrinsic back muscles: Iliocostalis, longissimus, and spinalis muscles.

Muscle Facts (III)

The deep intrinsic back muscles are divided into two groups: transversospinal and deep segmental muscles. The transversospinalis muscles pass between the transverse and spinous processes of the vertebrae.

Table 3.5 Transversospinalis muscles

Muscle		Origin	Insertion	Innervation	Action
Rotatores	① Rotatores breves	T1–T12 (between transverse and spinous processes of adjacent vertebrae)			*Bilateral:* Extends thoracic spine *Unilateral:* Rotates spine to opposite side
	② Rotatores longi	T1–T12 (between transverse and spinous processes, skipping one vertebra)			
Multifidus ③		C2–sacrum (between transverse and spinous processes, skipping two to four vertebrae)		Spinal nn. (posterior rami)	*Bilateral:* Extends spine *Unilateral:* Flexes spine to same side, rotates to opposite side
Semispinalis	④ Semispinalis capitis	C4–T7 (transverse and articular processes)	Occipital bone (between superior and inferior nuchal lines)		*Bilateral:* Extends thoracic and cervical spines and head (stabilizes craniovertebral joints)
	⑤ Semispinalis cervicis	T1–T6 (transverse processes)	C2–C5 (spinous processes)		*Unilateral:* Bends head, cervical and thoracic spines to same side, rotates to opposite side
	⑥ Semispinalis thoracis	T6–T12 (transverse processes)	C6–T4 (spinous processes)		

Fig. 3.11 **Transversospinalis muscles**
Posterior view, schematic.

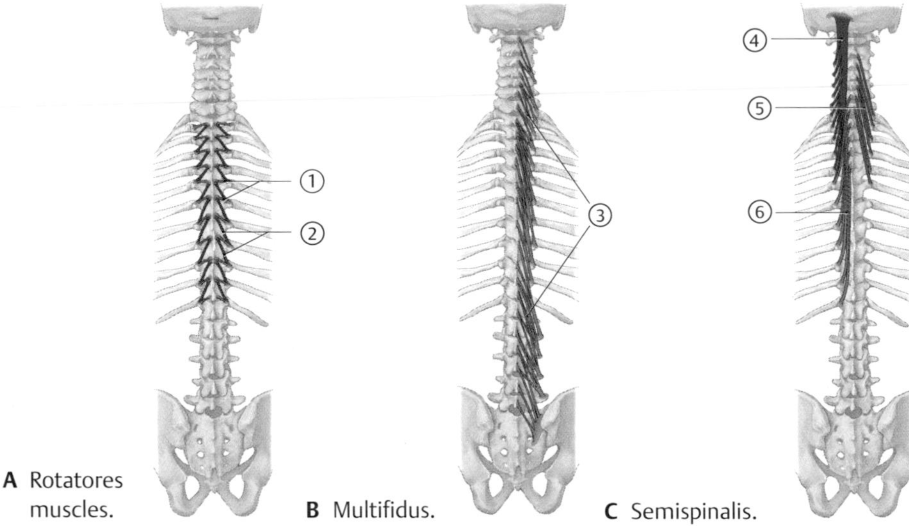

①
②
③
④
⑤
⑥

A Rotatores muscles. **B** Multifidus. **C** Semispinalis.

Fig. 3.12 **Deep segmental muscles**
Posterior view, schematic.

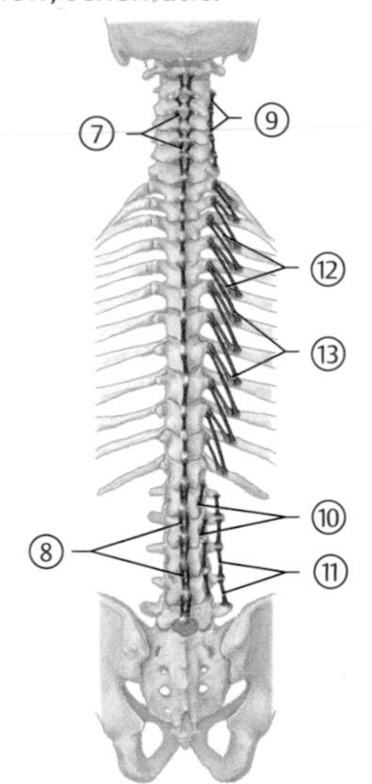

⑦
⑨
⑫
⑬
⑩
⑧
⑪

Table 3.6 Deep segmental back muscles

Muscle		Origin	Insertion	Innervation	Action
Interspinales*	⑦ Interspinales cervicis	C1–C7 (between spinous processes of adjacent vertebrae)		Spinal nn. (posterior rami)	Extends cervical and lumbar spines
	⑧ Interspinales lumborum	L1–L5 (between spinous processes of adjacent vertebrae)			
Inter-transversarii*	Intertransversarii anteriores cervicis	C2–C7 (between anterior tubercles of adjacent vertebrae)		Spinal nn. (anterior rami)	*Bilateral:* Stabilizes and extends the cervical and lumbar spines *Unilateral:* Bends the cervical and lumbar spines laterally to same side
	⑨ Intertransversarii posteriores cervicis	C2–C7 (between posterior tubercles of adjacent vertebrae)		Spinal nn. (posterior rami)	
	⑩ Intertransversarii mediales lumborum	L1–L5 (between mammillary processes of adjacent vertebrae)			
	⑪ Intertransversarii laterales lumborum	L1–L5 (between transverse processes of adjacent vertebrae)			
Levatores costarum	⑫ Levatores costarum breves	C7–T11 (transverse processes)	Costal angle of next lower rib		*Bilateral:* Extends thoracic spine *Unilateral:* Bends thoracic spine to same side, rotates to opposite side
	⑬ Levatores costarum longi		Costal angle of rib two vertebrae below		

*Both the interspinales and intertransversarii muscles traverse the entire spine; only their clinically relevant components have been included.

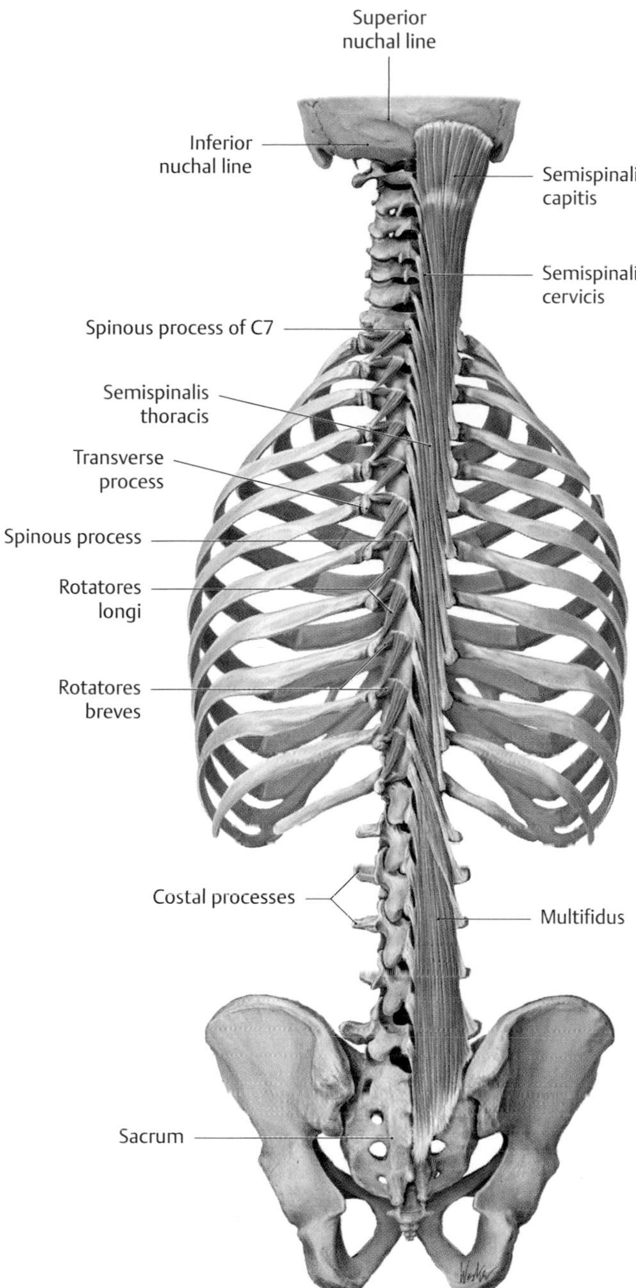

Superior nuchal line
Inferior nuchal line
Semispinalis capitis
Semispinalis cervicis
Spinous process of C7
Semispinalis thoracis
Transverse process
Spinous process
Rotatores longi
Rotatores breves
Costal processes
Multifidus
Sacrum

A Transversospinalis muscles: Rotatores, multifidus, and semispinalis.

Fig. 3.13 **Deep intrinsic back muscles**
Posterior view.

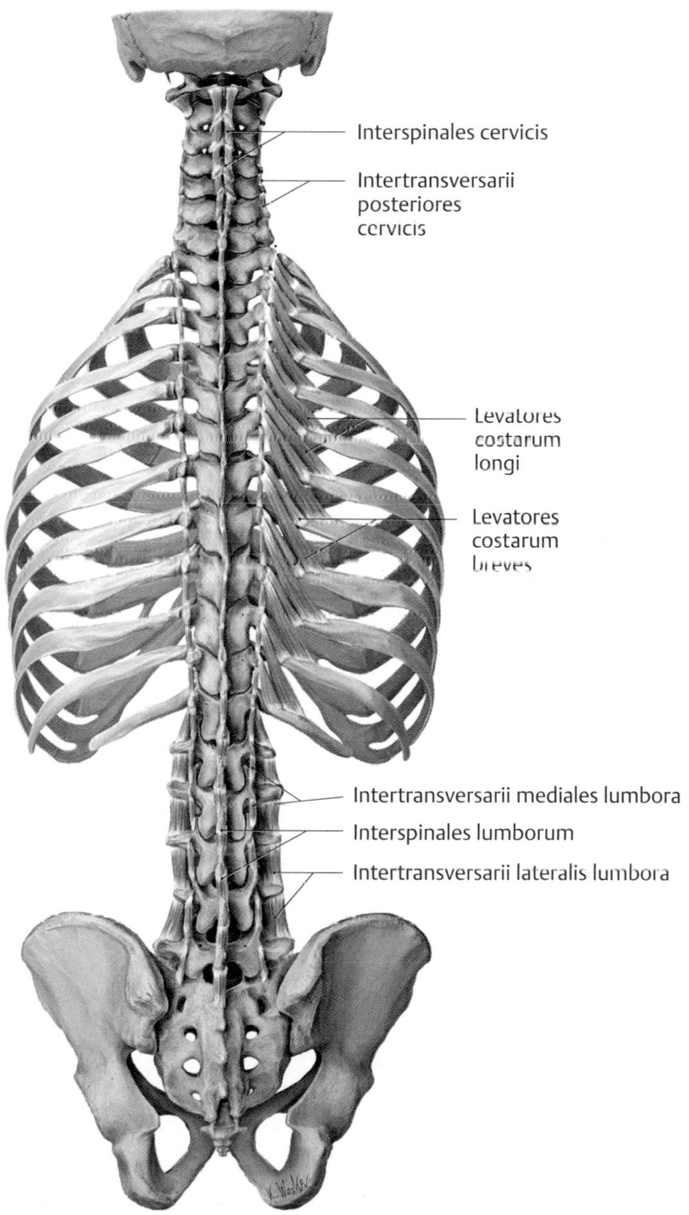

Interspinales cervicis
Intertransversarii posteriores cervicis
Levatores costarum longi
Levatores costarum breves
Intertransversarii mediales lumbora
Interspinales lumborum
Intertransversarii lateralis lumbora

B Deep segmental muscles: Interspinales, intertransversarii, and levatores costarum.

Arteries & Veins of the Back

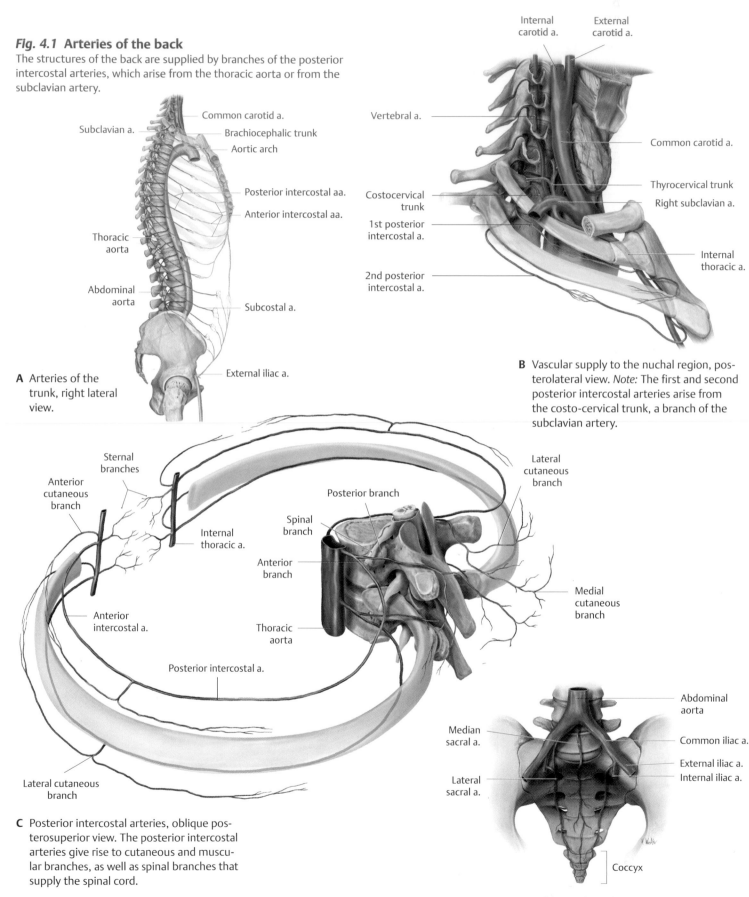

Fig. 4.1 Arteries of the back

The structures of the back are supplied by branches of the posterior intercostal arteries, which arise from the thoracic aorta or from the subclavian artery.

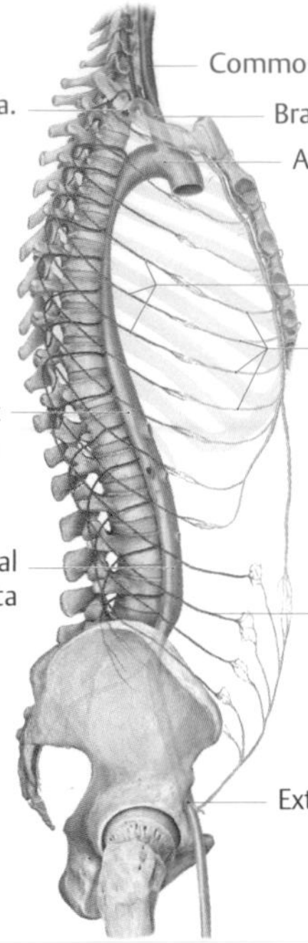

Common carotid a.
Subclavian a.
Brachiocephalic trunk
Aortic arch
Posterior intercostal aa.
Anterior intercostal aa.
Thoracic aorta
Abdominal aorta
Subcostal a.
External iliac a.

A Arteries of the trunk, right lateral view.

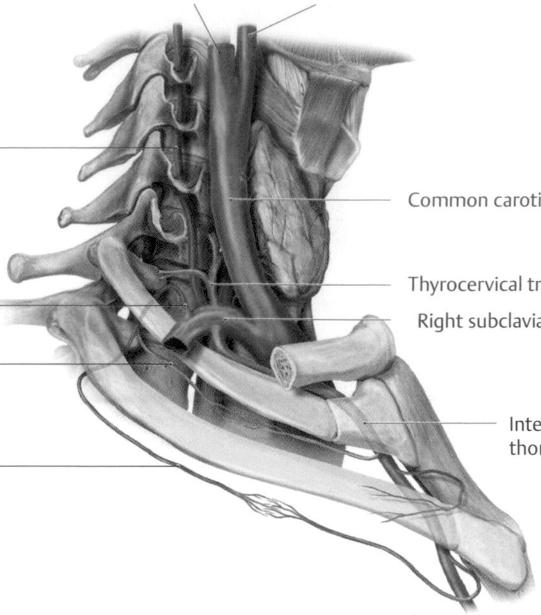

Internal carotid a.
External carotid a.
Vertebral a.
Common carotid a.
Thyrocervical trunk
Costocervical trunk
Right subclavian a.
1st posterior intercostal a.
Internal thoracic a.
2nd posterior intercostal a.

B Vascular supply to the nuchal region, posterolateral view. *Note:* The first and second posterior intercostal arteries arise from the costo-cervical trunk, a branch of the subclavian artery.

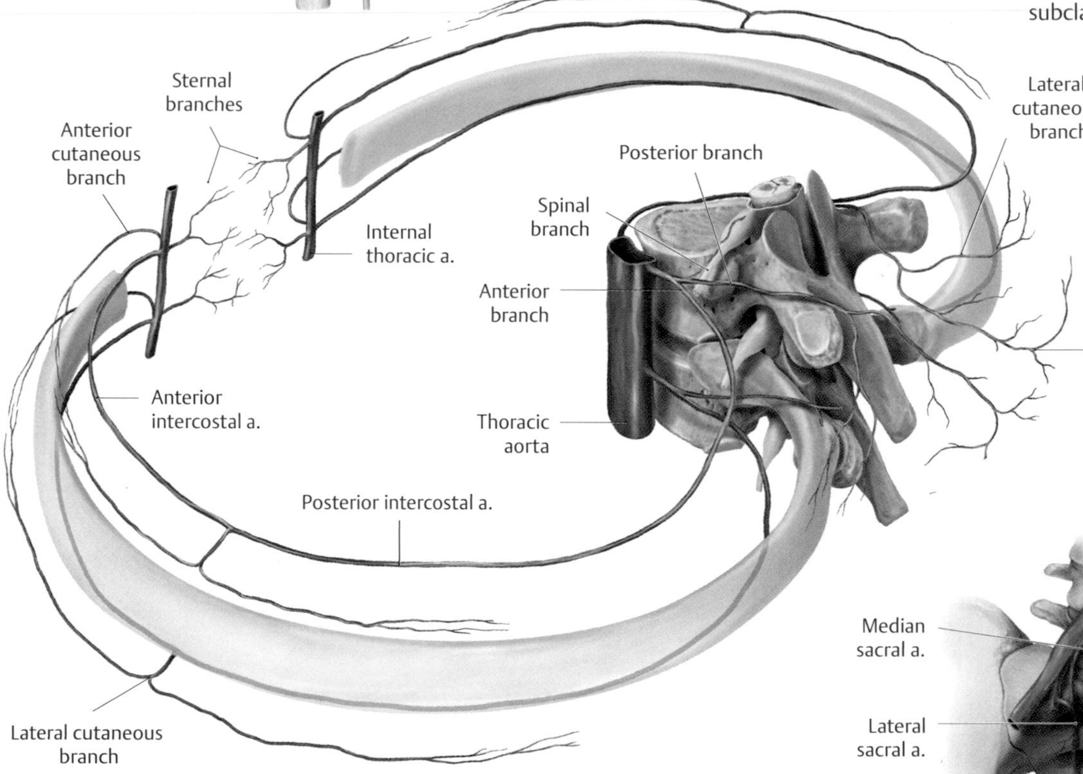

Sternal branches
Anterior cutaneous branch
Lateral cutaneous branch
Posterior branch
Spinal branch
Internal thoracic a.
Anterior branch
Medial cutaneous branch
Anterior intercostal a.
Thoracic aorta
Posterior intercostal a.
Lateral cutaneous branch

C Posterior intercostal arteries, oblique posterosuperior view. The posterior intercostal arteries give rise to cutaneous and muscular branches, as well as spinal branches that supply the spinal cord.

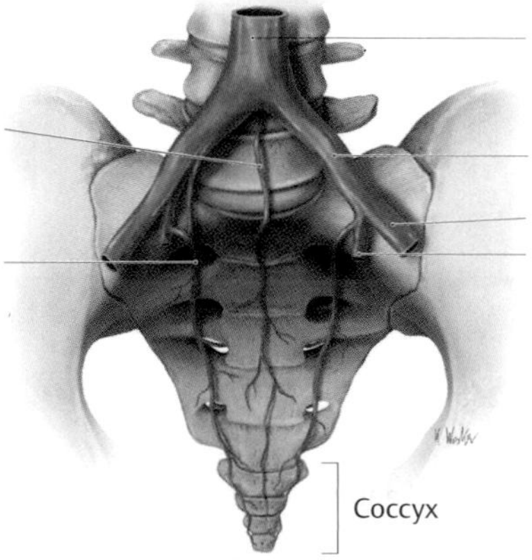

Abdominal aorta
Median sacral a.
Common iliac a.
External iliac a.
Lateral sacral a.
Internal iliac a.
Coccyx

D Vascular supply to the sacrum, anterior view.

Fig. 4.2 **Veins of the back**

The veins of the back drain into the azygos vein via the posterior intercostal veins, hemiazygos vein, and ascending lumbar veins. The interior of the spinal column is drained by the vertebral venous plexus that runs the length of the spine.

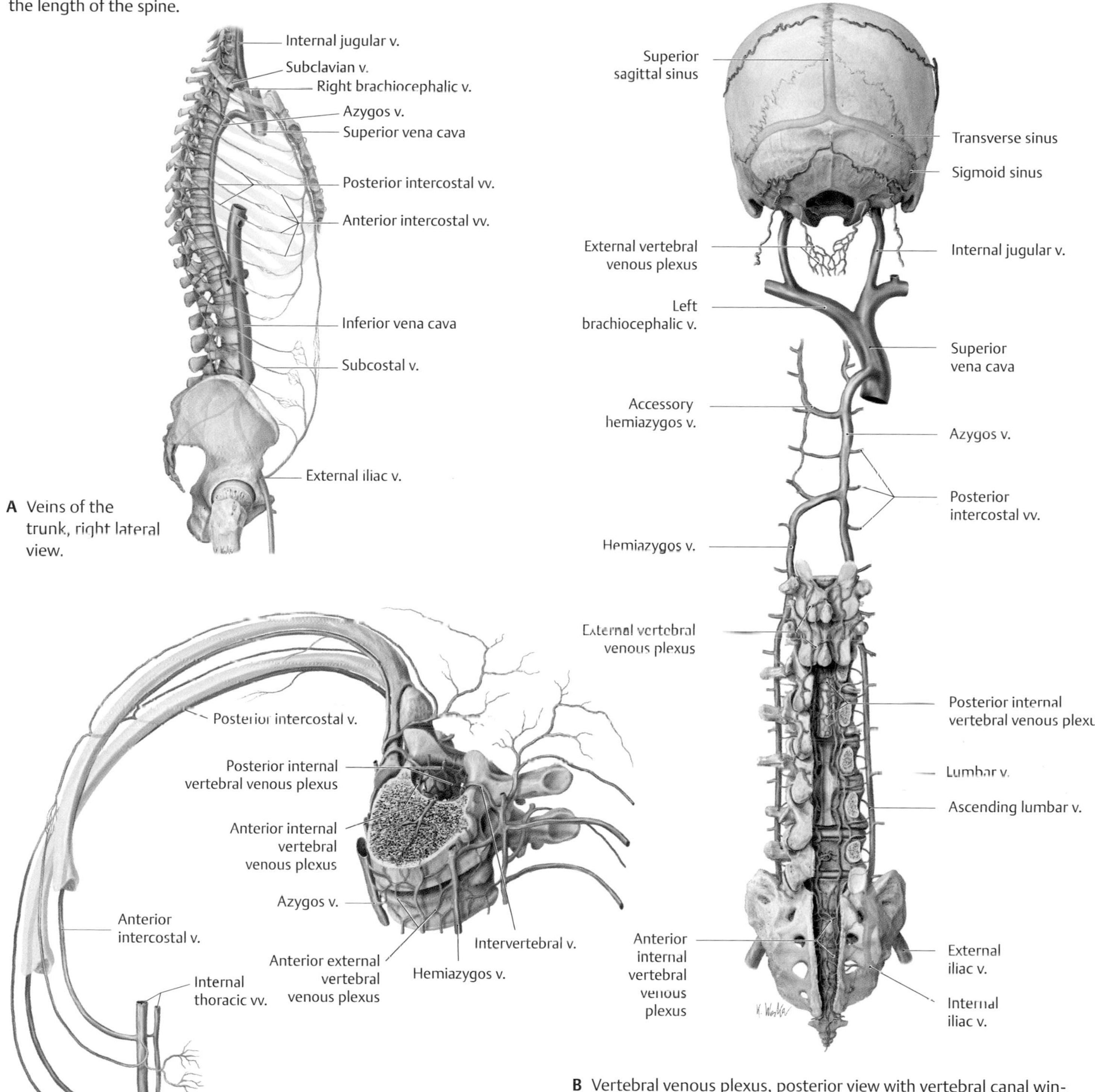

Internal jugular v.
Subclavian v.
Right brachiocephalic v.
Azygos v.
Superior vena cava
Posterior intercostal vv.
Anterior intercostal vv.
Inferior vena cava
Subcostal v.
External iliac v.
Superior sagittal sinus
Transverse sinus
Sigmoid sinus
External vertebral venous plexus
Internal jugular v.
Left brachiocephalic v.
Superior vena cava
Accessory hemiazygos v.
Azygos v.
Posterior intercostal vv.
Hemiazygos v.
External vertebral venous plexus
Posterior internal vertebral venous plexus
Lumbar v.
Ascending lumbar v.
Anterior internal vertebral venous plexus
External iliac v.
Internal iliac v.
Posterior intercostal v.
Posterior internal vertebral venous plexus
Anterior internal vertebral venous plexus
Azygos v.
Anterior intercostal v.
Intervertebral v.
Anterior external vertebral venous plexus
Hemiazygos v.
Internal thoracic vv.

A Veins of the trunk, right lateral view.

B Vertebral venous plexus, posterior view with vertebral canal windowed in the lumbar and sacral spine. The external vertebral venous plexus communicates with the sigmoid sinus through emissary veins in the skull. The *external* vertebral venous plexus is divided into an anterior and a posterior portion that run along the exterior of the spinal column. The anterior and posterior *internal* vertebral venous plexus run in the vertebral foramen and drain the spinal cord.

C Intercostal veins and anterior vertebral venous plexus, anterosuperior view. The intercostal veins follow a similar course as the intercostal nerves and arteries (see pp. 36, 38). *Note:* The anterior external vertebral venous plexus can be seen communicating with the azygos vein.

Nerves of the Back

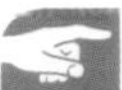

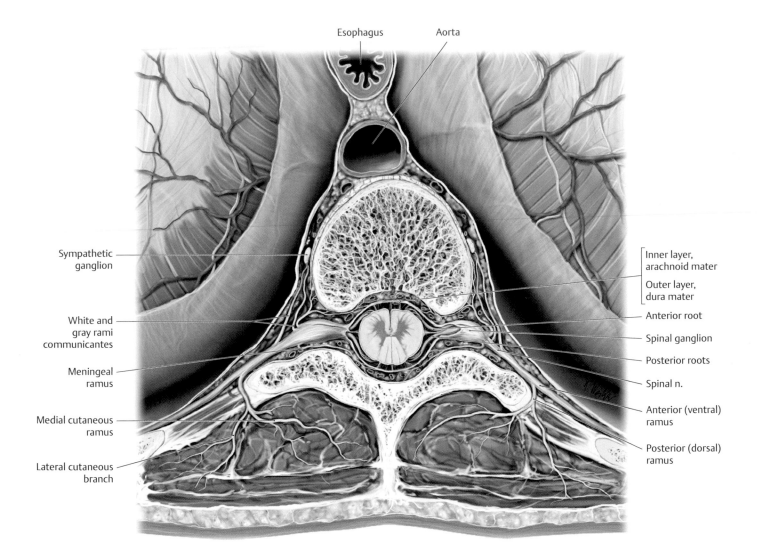

The back receives its innervation from branches of the spinal nerves. The *posterior (dorsal) rami* of the spinal nerves supply most of the intrinsic muscles of the back. The extrinsic muscles of the back are supplied by the *anterior (ventral) rami* of the spinal nerves.

Fig. 4.3 **Nerves of the back**
Cross section of the vertebral column and spinal cord with surrounding musculature, superior view.

Esophagus
Aorta
Sympathetic ganglion
White and gray rami communicantes
Meningeal ramus
Medial cutaneous ramus
Lateral cutaneous branch
Inner layer, arachnoid mater
Outer layer, dura mater
Anterior root
Spinal ganglion
Posterior roots
Spinal n.
Anterior (ventral) ramus
Posterior (dorsal) ramus

Fig. 4.4 Nerves of the nuchal region
Right side, posterior view. Like the back, the nuchal region receives most of its motor and sensory innervation from the *posterior* rami of the spinal nerves. The posterior rami of C1–C3 have specific names: suboccipital nerve (C1), greater occipital nerve (C2), and third occipital nerve (C3). The lesser occipital and great auricular nerves arise from the *anterior* rami of the C1–C4 spinal nerves and innervate the skin of the anterolateral head and neck. The anterior rami of C1–C4 also give rise to the *ansa cervicalis,* which innervates the infrahyoid muscles (see p. 590).

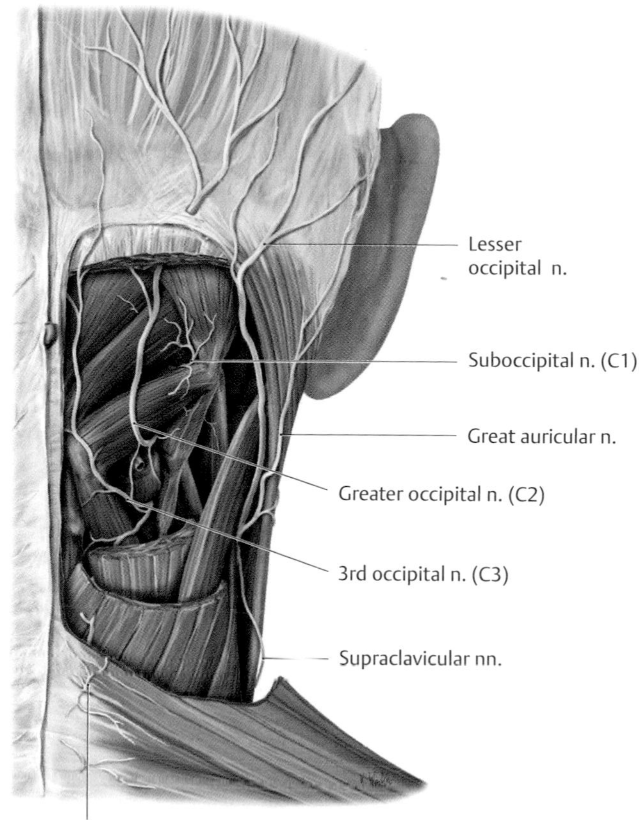
Lesser occipital n.
Suboccipital n. (C1)
Great auricular n.
Greater occipital n. (C2)
3rd occipital n. (C3)
Supraclavicular nn.
C5 spinal n., posterior ramus

Fig. 4.5 Cutaneous innervation of the back
Color denotes the skin areas innervated by (**A**) particular peripheral nerves or (**B**) particular pairs of segmental spinal nerves. Patterns of loss of cutaneous sensation can be helpful in diagnosis of nerve lesions.

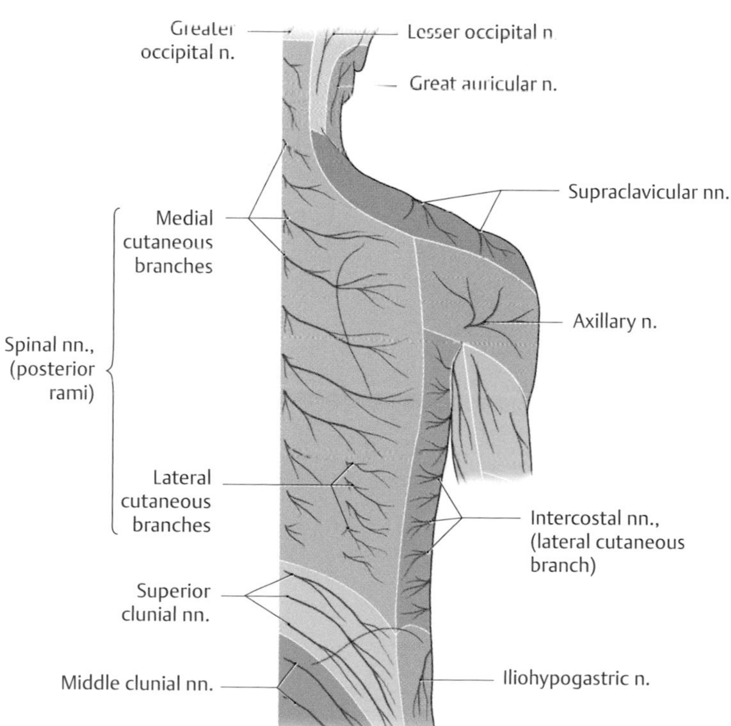
Greater occipital n.
Lesser occipital n
Great auricular n.
Supraclavicular nn.
Medial cutaneous branches
Spinal nn., (posterior rami)
Axillary n.
Lateral cutaneous branches
Intercostal nn., (lateral cutaneous branch)
Superior clunial nn.
Middle clunial nn.
Iliohypogastric n.

A Cutaneous innervation patterns of specific peripheral nerves.

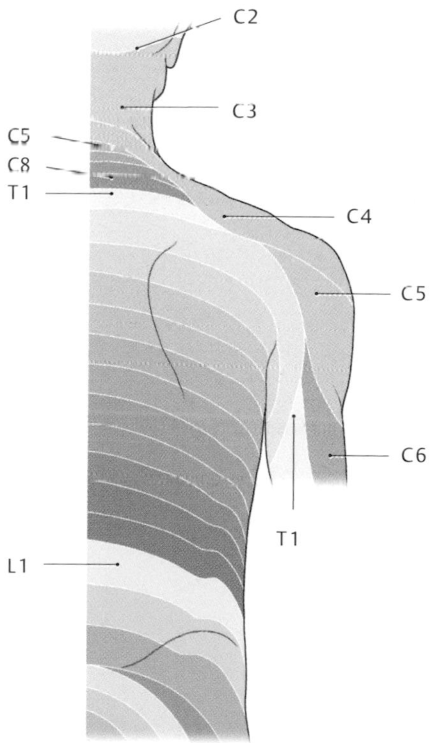
C2
C3
C5
C8
T1
C4
C5
C6
T1
L1

B Dermatomes: Dermatomes are bilateral bandlike areas of skin receiving innervation from a single pair of spinal nerves (from a single segment of the spinal cord). *Note:* Spinal nerve C1 is purely motor; consequently there is no C1 dermatome.

Spinal Cord

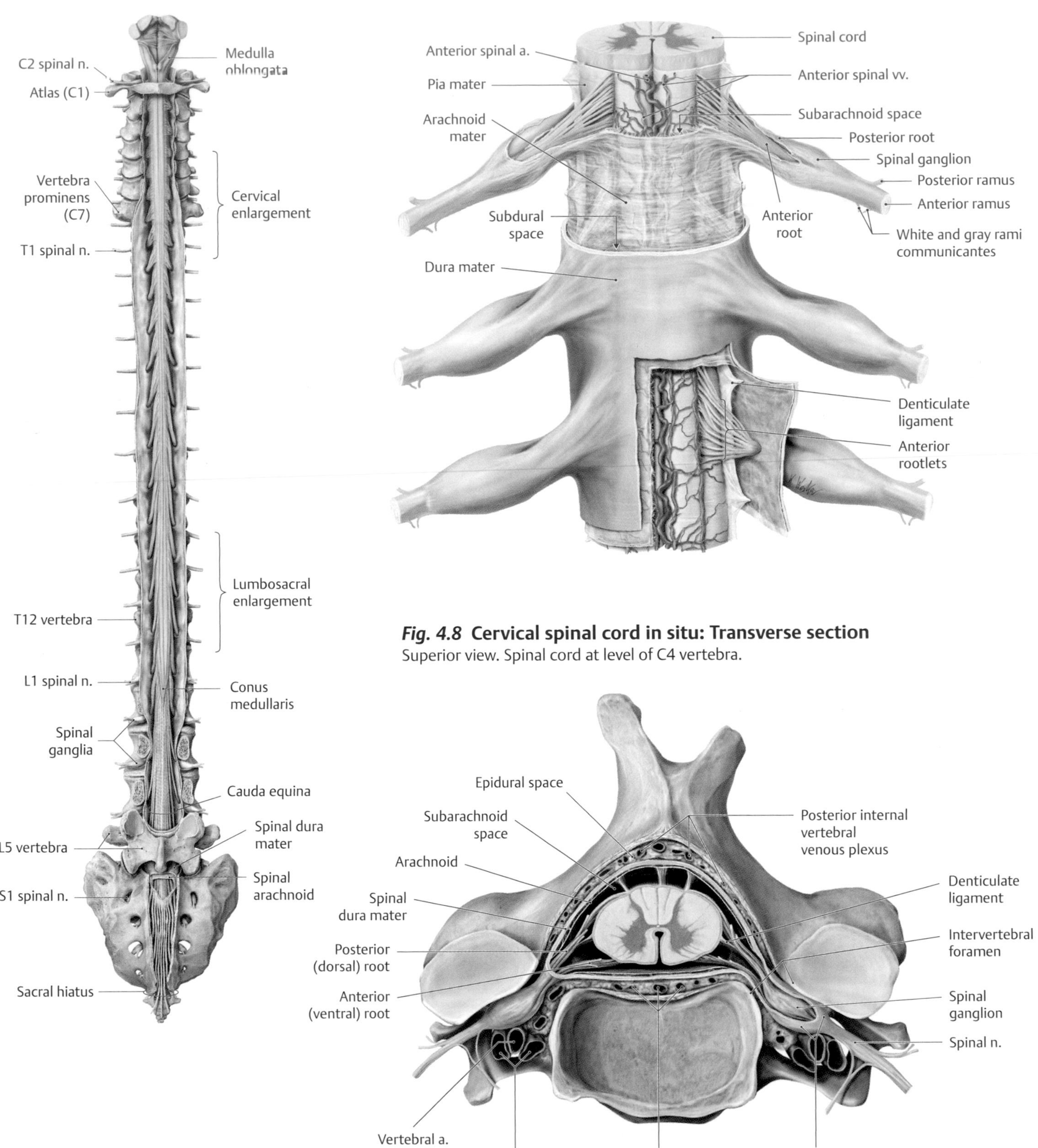
Medulla oblongata
C2 spinal n.
Atlas (C1)
Vertebra prominens (C7)
Cervical enlargement
T1 spinal n.
Lumbosacral enlargement
T12 vertebra
L1 spinal n.
Conus medullaris
Spinal ganglia
Cauda equina
Spinal dura mater
L5 vertebra
Spinal arachnoid
S1 spinal n.
Sacral hiatus
Anterior spinal a.
Spinal cord
Anterior spinal vv.
Pia mater
Arachnoid mater
Subarachnoid space
Posterior root
Spinal ganglion
Posterior ramus
Anterior ramus
Subdural space
Anterior root
White and gray rami communicantes
Dura mater
Denticulate ligament
Anterior rootlets
Epidural space
Subarachnoid space
Posterior internal vertebral venous plexus
Arachnoid
Denticulate ligament
Spinal dura mater
Intervertebral foramen
Posterior (dorsal) root
Anterior (ventral) root
Spinal ganglion
Spinal n.
Vertebral a.
Vertebral vv.
Anterior internal vertebral venous plexus
Root sleeve

Fig. 4.6 **Spinal cord in situ**
Posterior view with vertebral canal windowed.

Fig. 4.7 **Spinal cord and its meningeal layers**
Posterior view. The dura matter is opened and the arachnoid is sectioned.

Fig. 4.8 **Cervical spinal cord in situ: Transverse section**
Superior view. Spinal cord at level of C4 vertebra.

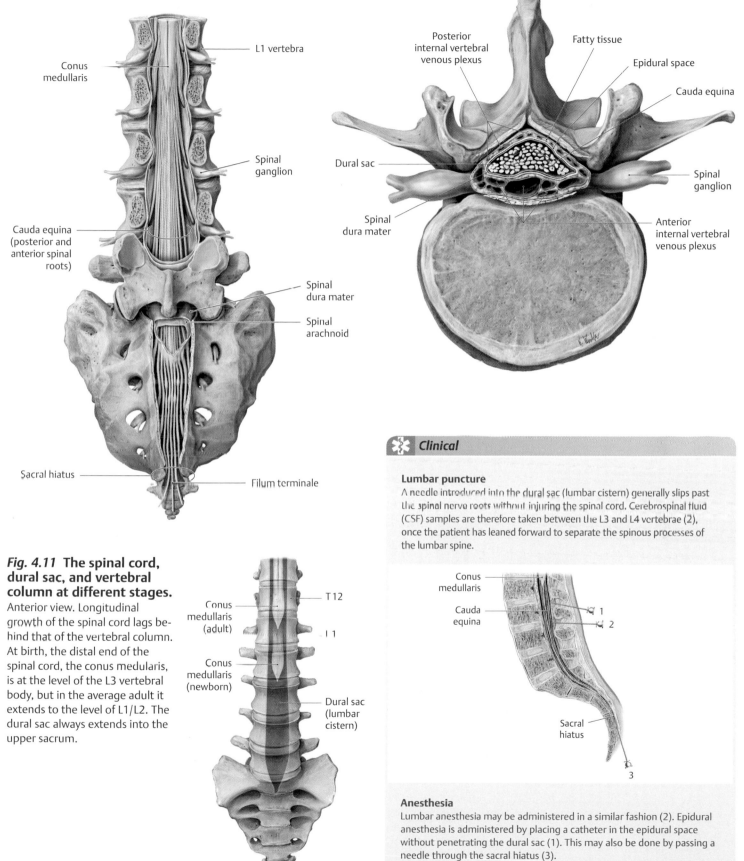

Fig. 4.9 Cauda equina in the vertebral canal

Posterior view. The lamina and posterior surface of the sacrum have been partially removed.

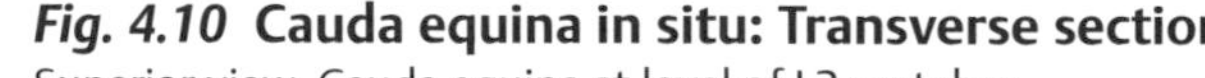

Fig. 4.10 Cauda equina in situ: Transverse section

Superior view. Cauda equina at level of L2 vertebra.

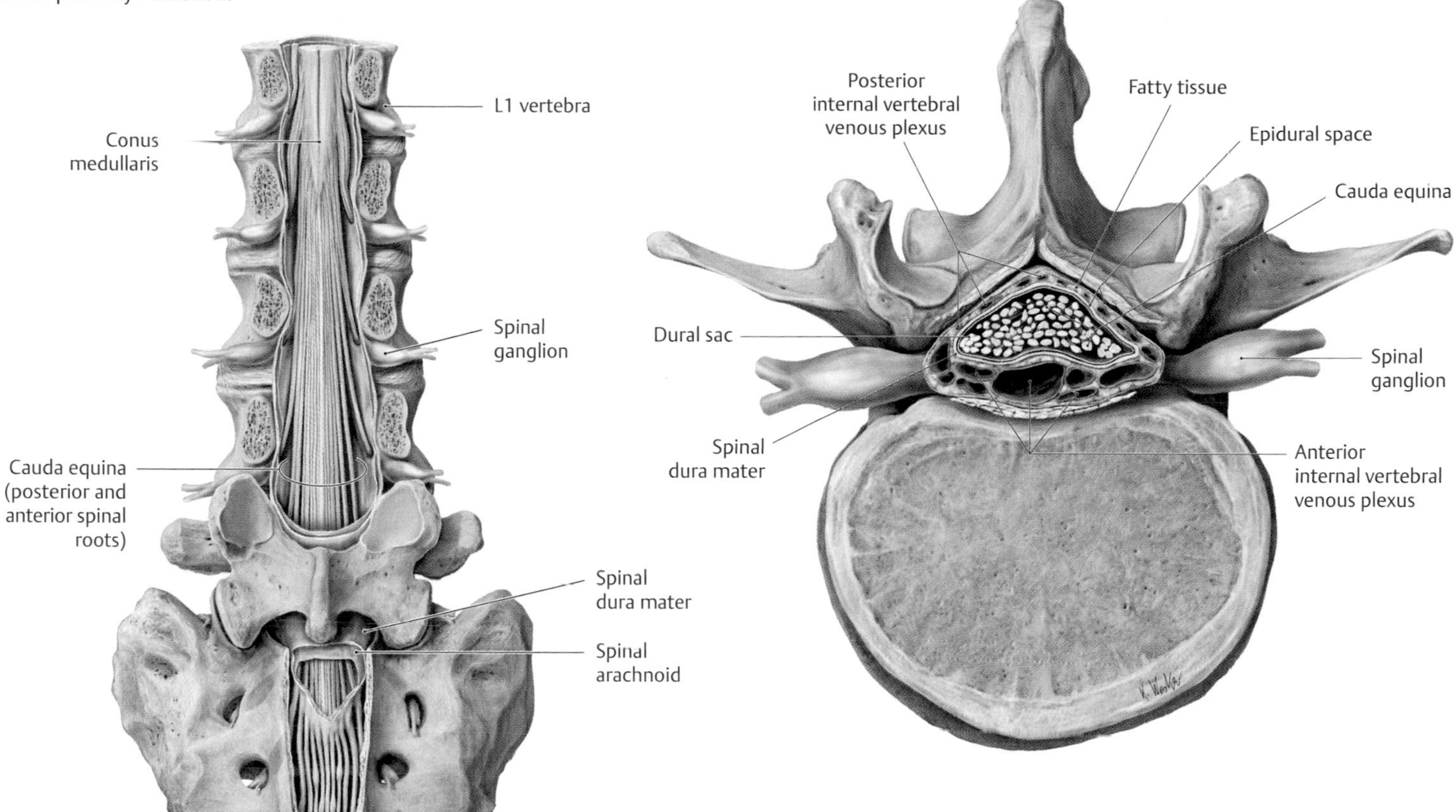
L1 vertebra
Conus medullaris
Spinal ganglion
Cauda equina (posterior and anterior spinal roots)
Spinal dura mater
Spinal arachnoid
Sacral hiatus
Filum terminale
Posterior internal vertebral venous plexus
Fatty tissue
Epidural space
Cauda equina
Dural sac
Spinal ganglion
Spinal dura mater
Anterior internal vertebral venous plexus

Fig. 4.11 The spinal cord, dural sac, and vertebral column at different stages.

Anterior view. Longitudinal growth of the spinal cord lags behind that of the vertebral column. At birth, the distal end of the spinal cord, the conus medularis, is at the level of the L3 vertebral body, but in the average adult it extends to the level of L1/L2. The dural sac always extends into the upper sacrum.

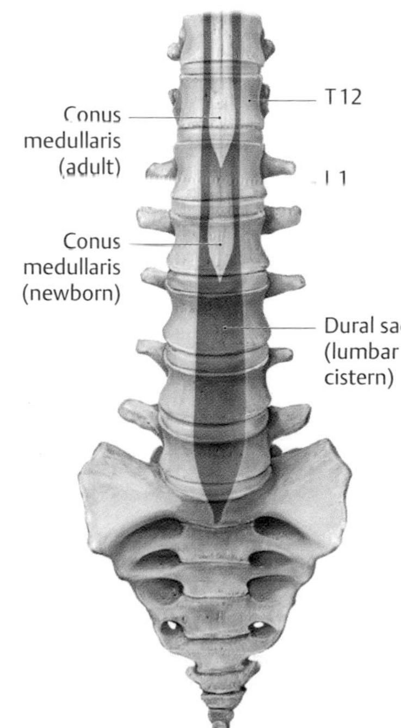
Conus medullaris (adult)
T12
L1
Conus medullaris (newborn)
Dural sac (lumbar cistern)

Clinical

Lumbar puncture

A needle introduced into the dural sac (lumbar cistern) generally slips past the spinal nerve roots without injuring the spinal cord. Cerebrospinal fluid (CSF) samples are therefore taken between the L3 and L4 vertebrae (2), once the patient has leaned forward to separate the spinous processes of the lumbar spine.

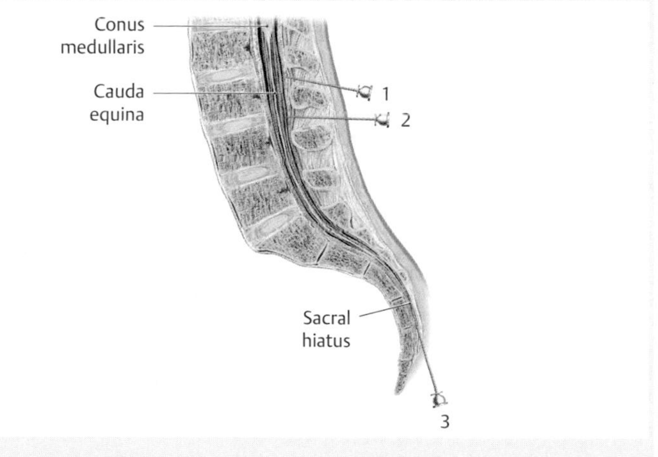
Conus medullaris
Cauda equina
1
2
Sacral hiatus
3

Anesthesia

Lumbar anesthesia may be administered in a similar fashion (2). Epidural anesthesia is administered by placing a catheter in the epidural space without penetrating the dural sac (1). This may also be done by passing a needle through the sacral hiatus (3).

Spinal Cord Segments & Spinal Nerves

Fig. 4.12 Spinal cord segment

The spinal cord consists of 31 segments, each innervating a specific area of the skin (a dermatome) of the head, trunk, or limbs. Afferent (sensory) posterior rootlets and efferent (motor) anterior rootlets form the posterior and anterior roots of the spinal nerve for that segment. The two roots fuse to form a mixed (motor and sensory) spinal nerve that exits the intervertebral foramen and immediately thereafter divides into an anterior and posterior ramus (or branch).

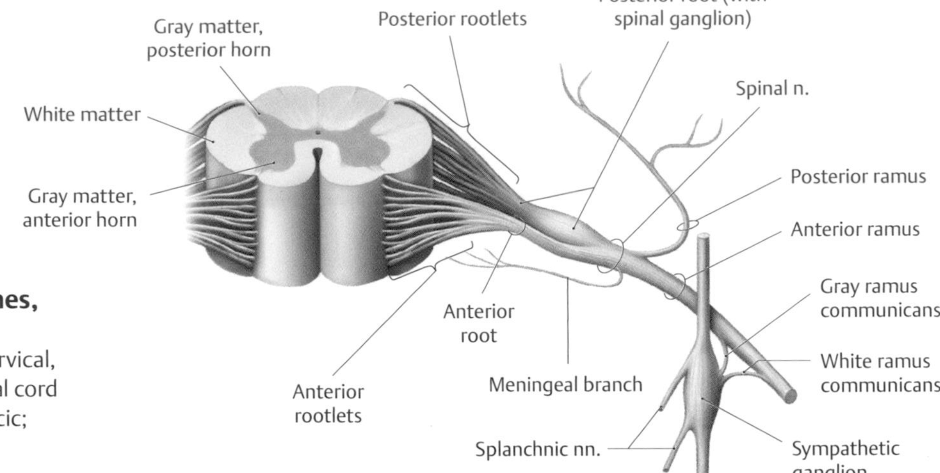
Gray matter, posterior horn
Posterior rootlets
Posterior root (with spinal ganglion)
Spinal n.
White matter
Gray matter, anterior horn
Posterior ramus
Anterior ramus
Gray ramus communicans
White ramus communicans
Anterior root
Meningeal branch
Anterior rootlets
Splanchnic nn.
Sympathetic ganglion

Fig. 4.13 Spinal cord segments, dermatomes, and effects of spinal cord lesions

The spinal cord is divided into four major regions: cervical, thoracic, lumbar, and sacral. The regions of the spinal cord are designated by colors: red, cervical; brown, thoracic; green, lumbar; blue, sacral.

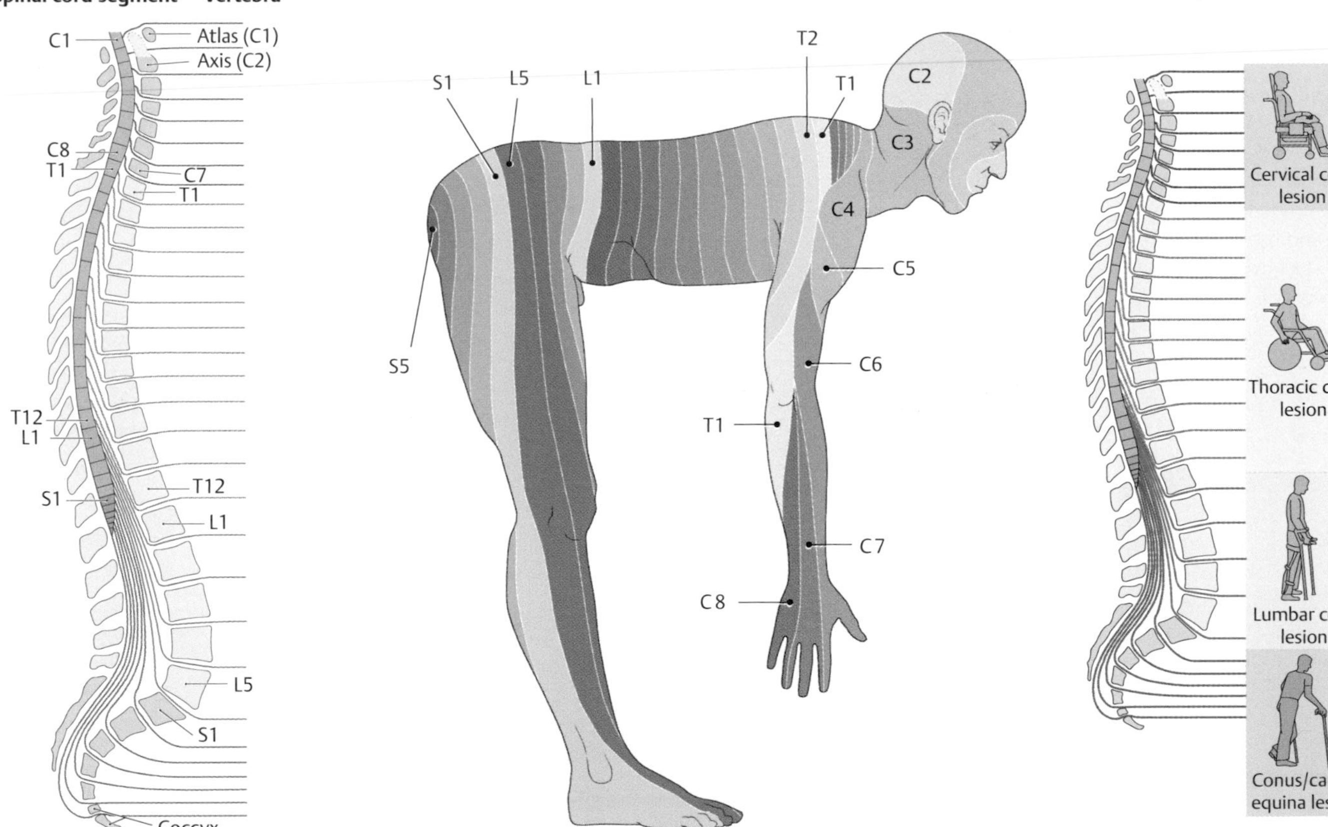
Spinal cord segment
Vertebra
C1
Atlas (C1)
Axis (C2)
C8
T1
C7
T1
T12
L1
S1
T12
L1
L5
S1
Coccyx
T2
S1
L5
L1
T1
C2
C3
C4
C5
S5
C6
T1
C7
C8
Cervical cord lesion
Thoracic cord lesion
Lumbar cord lesion
Conus/cauda equina lesion

A Spinal cord segments. Initially spinal nerves pass out above the vertebrae for which they are numbered. However, since there is an 8th cervical spinal nerve but no 8th cervical vertebrae, C8 passes out above vertebral level T1, and the spinal nerve for T1 and following pass out below the vertebral level for which they are numbered.

B Dermatomes, bandlike areas of skin receiving sensory innervation from a single pair of spinal nerves (from a single segment of the spinal cord). *Note:* Spinal nerve C1 is purely motor; consequently there is no C1 dermatome.

C Effects of lesions in each region of the spinal cord.

Fig. 4.14 Spinal nerve branches

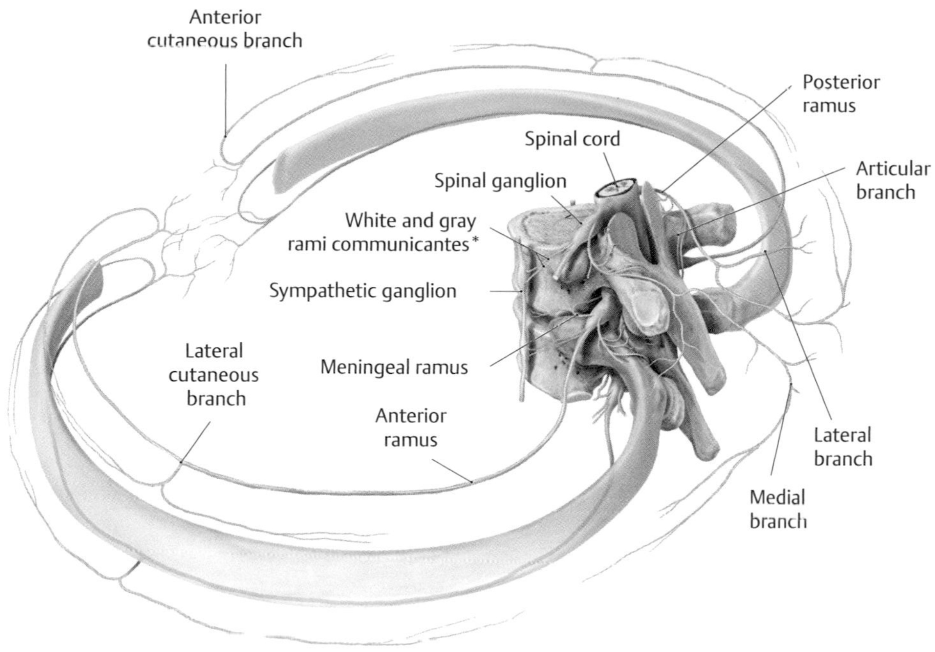
Anterior cutaneous branch
Posterior ramus
Spinal cord
Articular branch
Spinal ganglion
White and gray rami communicantes*
Sympathetic ganglion
Lateral cutaneous branch
Meningeal ramus
Anterior ramus
Lateral branch
Medial branch

A Superolateral view of a thoracic spinal nerve. The *posterior (dorsal) rami* of the spinal nerves give rise to muscular and cutaneous branches, as well as articular branches to the zygapophyseal joints. The *anterior (ventral) rami* of the spinal nerves form the cervical plexus (C1–C4), the brachial plexus (C5–T1), the lumbar plexus (T12–L4), and the sacral plexus (L4–S3). The anterior rami of spinal nerves T1–T11 produce the intercostal nerves (T12 produces the subcostal nerve).

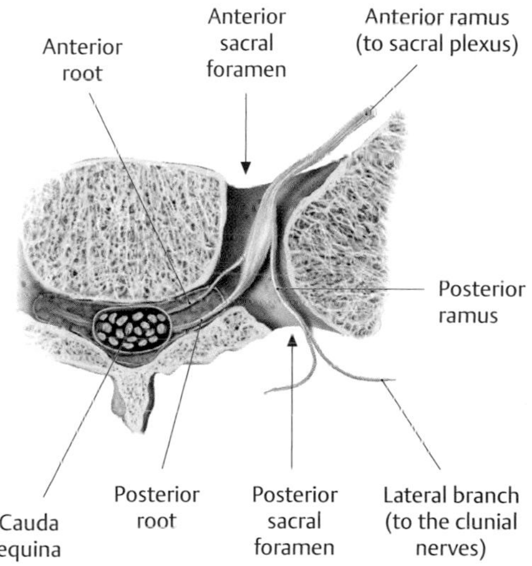
Anterior root
Anterior sacral foramen
Anterior ramus (to sacral plexus)
Posterior ramus
Cauda equina
Posterior root
Posterior sacral foramen
Lateral branch (to the clunial nerves)

B Spinal nerve branches in the sacral foramina. Superior view of transverse section through right half of sacrum.

Table 4.1 Branches of a spinal nerve

Branches			Territory
Meningeal ramus			Spinal meninges; ligaments of spinal column
Posterior (dorsal) ramus	Medial branches	Articular branch	Zygapophyseal joints
		Muscular branch	Intrinsic back muscles
		Cutaneous branch	Skin of posterior head, neck, back, and buttocks
	Lateral branches	Cutaneous branch	
		Muscular branch	Intrinsic back muscles
Anterior (ventral) ramus	Lateral cutaneous branches		Skin of lateral chest wall
	Anterior cutaneous branches		Skin of anterior chest wall

*The white and gray rami communicantes carry pre- and postganglionic fibers between the sympathetic trunk and spinal nerve. They are shown on p. 647.

Arteries & Veins of the Spinal Cord

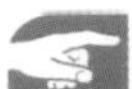

Like the spinal cord itself, the arteries and veins of the spinal cord consist of multiple horizontal systems (blood vessels of the spinal cord segments) that are integrated into a vertical system.

Fig. 4.15 **Arteries of the spinal cord**
The unpaired anterior and paired posterior spinal arteries typically arise from the vertebral arteries. As they descend within the vertebral canal, the spinal arteries are reinforced by anterior and posterior segmental medullary arteries. Depending on the spinal level, these reinforcing branches may arise from the vertebral, ascending or deep cervical, posterior intercostal, lumbar, or lateral sacral arteries.

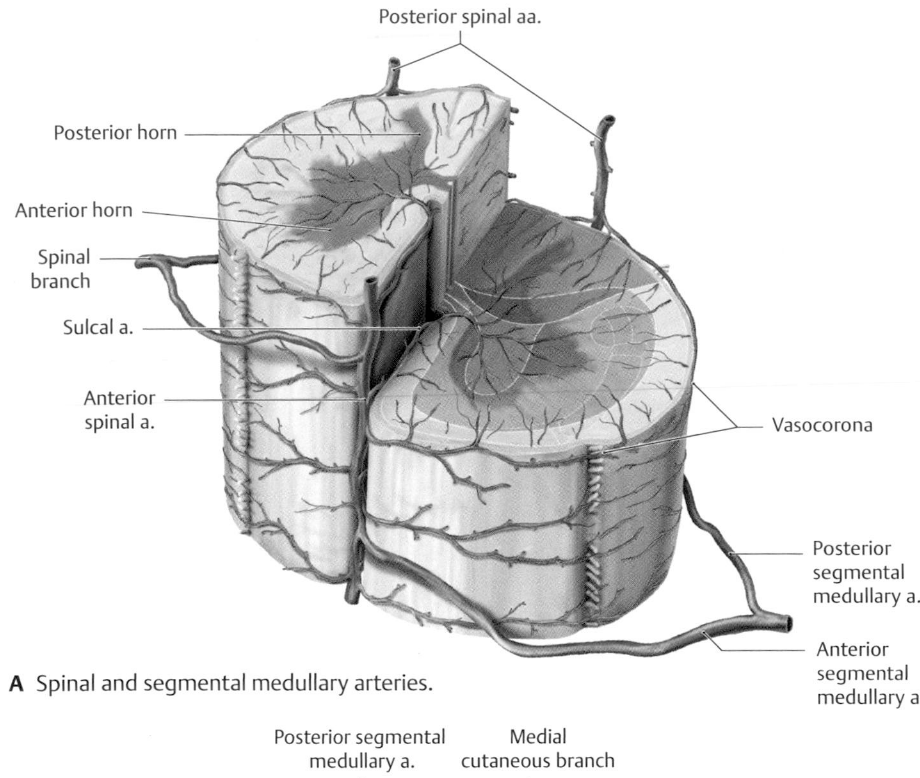
Posterior spinal aa.
Posterior horn
Anterior horn
Spinal branch
Sulcal a.
Anterior spinal a.
Vasocorona
Posterior segmental medullary a.
Anterior segmental medullary a.

A Spinal and segmental medullary arteries.

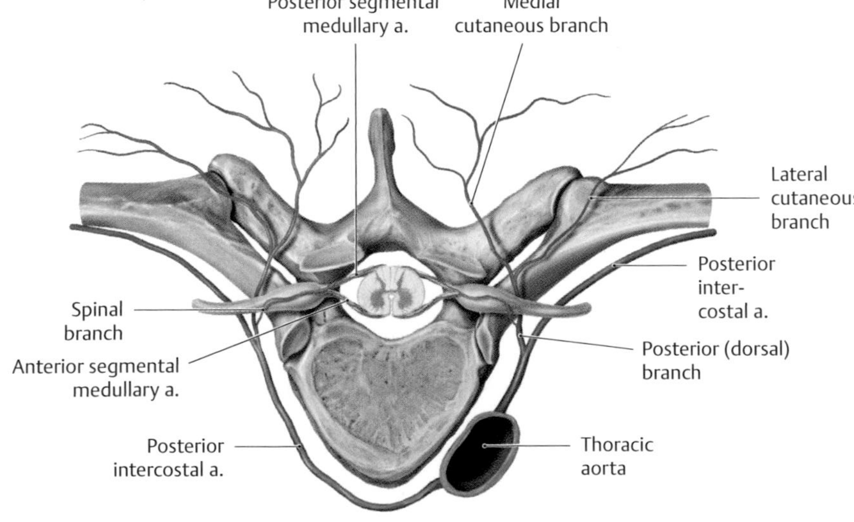
Posterior segmental medullary a.
Medial cutaneous branch
Lateral cutaneous branch
Posterior inter-costal a.
Posterior (dorsal) branch
Spinal branch
Anterior segmental medullary a.
Posterior intercostal a.
Thoracic aorta

B Origins of the segmental medullary arteries. In the thorax, the segmental medullary arteries arise from the spinal branch of the posterior intercostal arteries (see p. 36).

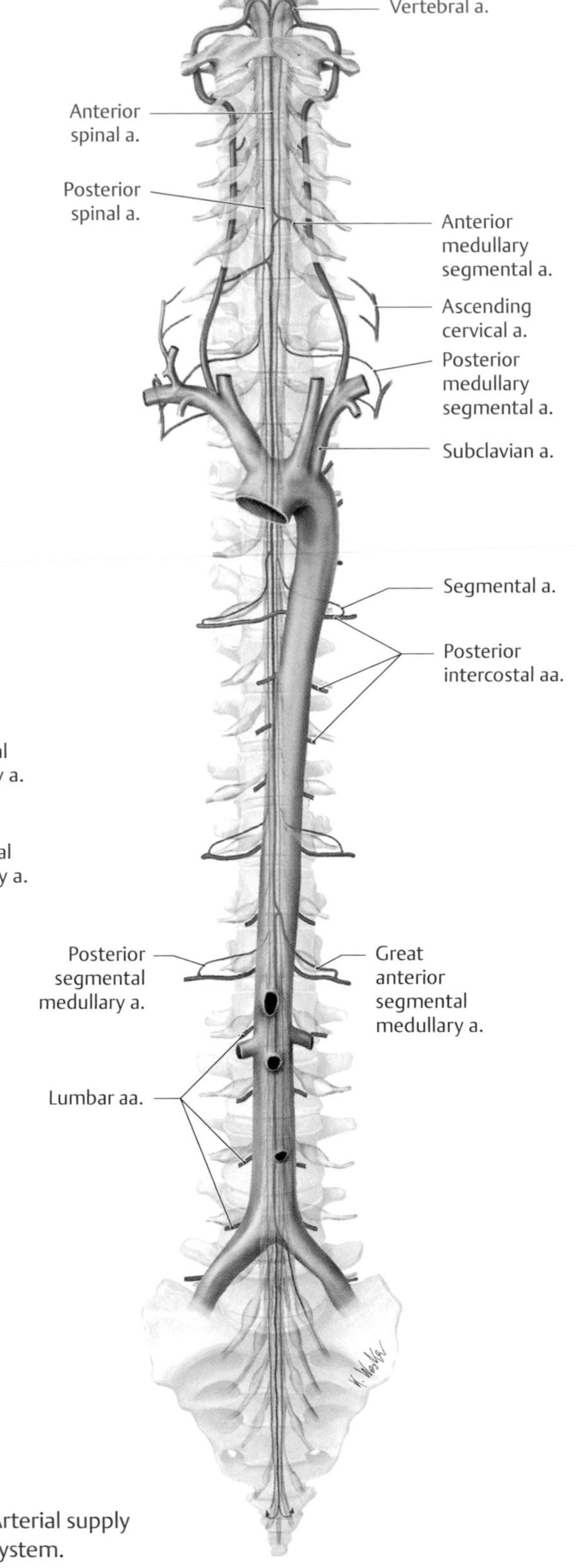
Basilar a.
Vertebral a.
Anterior spinal a.
Posterior spinal a.
Anterior medullary segmental a.
Ascending cervical a.
Posterior medullary segmental a.
Subclavian a.
Segmental a.
Posterior intercostal aa.
Posterior segmental medullary a.
Great anterior segmental medullary a.
Lumbar aa.

C Arterial supply system.

Fig. 4.16 Veins of the spinal cord
The interior of the spinal cord drains via venous plexuses into an anterior and a posterior spinal vein. The radicular and spinal veins connect the veins of the spinal cord with the internal vertebral venous plexus. The intervertebral and basivertebral veins connect the internal and external venous plexuses, which drain into the azygos system.

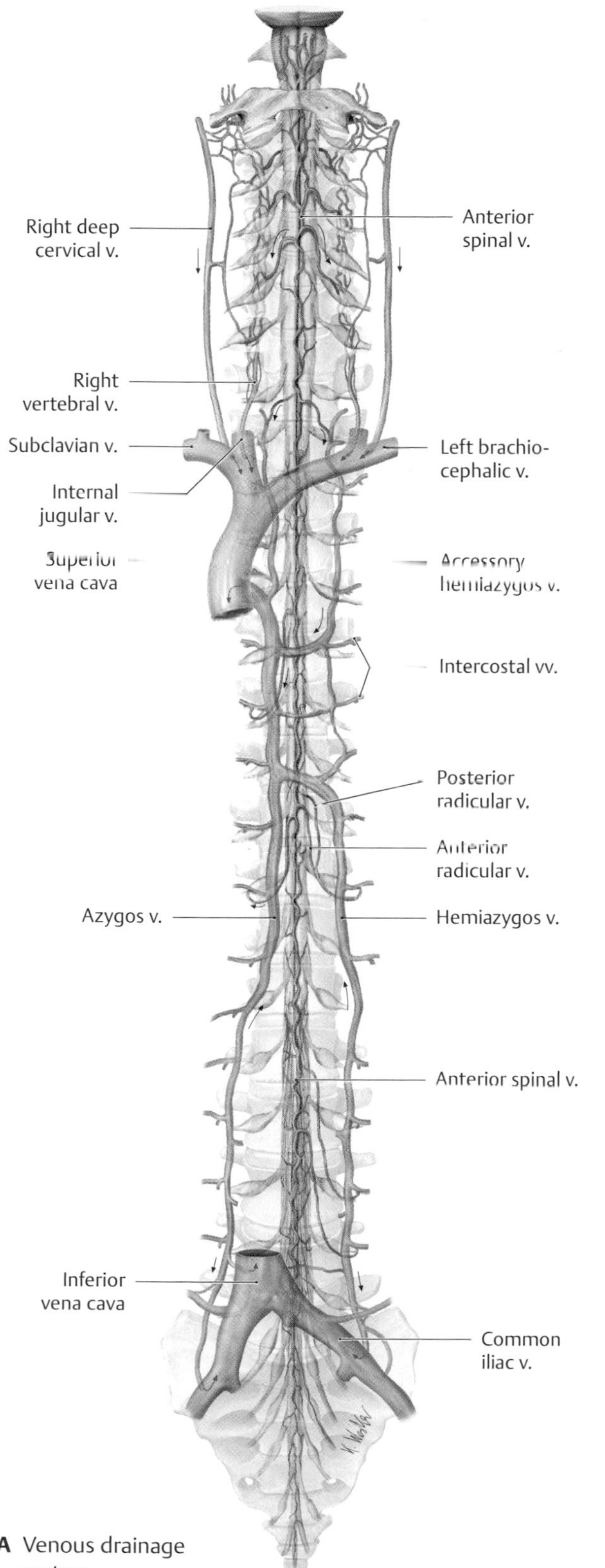
Right deep cervical v.
Anterior spinal v.
Right vertebral v.
Subclavian v.
Left brachio-cephalic v.
Internal jugular v.
Superior vena cava
Accessory hemiazygos v.
Intercostal vv.
Posterior radicular v.
Anterior radicular v.
Azygos v.
Hemiazygos v.
Anterior spinal v.
Inferior vena cava
Common iliac v.

A Venous drainage system.

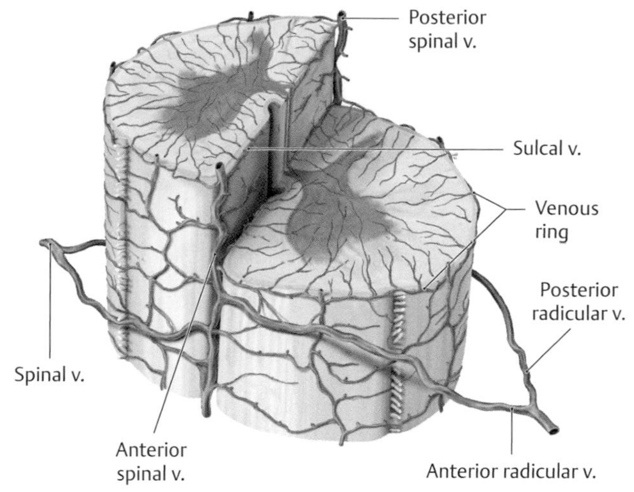
Posterior spinal v.
Sulcal v.
Venous ring
Posterior radicular v.
Spinal v.
Anterior spinal v.
Anterior radicular v.

B Spinal and radicular veins.

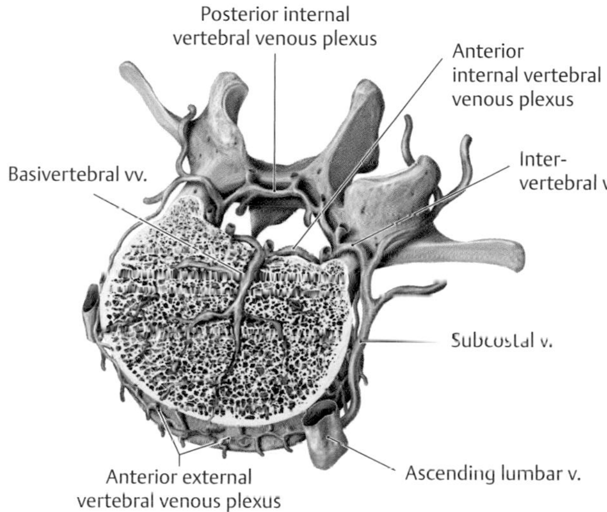
Posterior internal vertebral venous plexus
Anterior internal vertebral venous plexus
Basivertebral vv.
Inter-vertebral v.
Subcostal v.
Anterior external vertebral venous plexus
Ascending lumbar v.

C Vertebral venous plexuses.

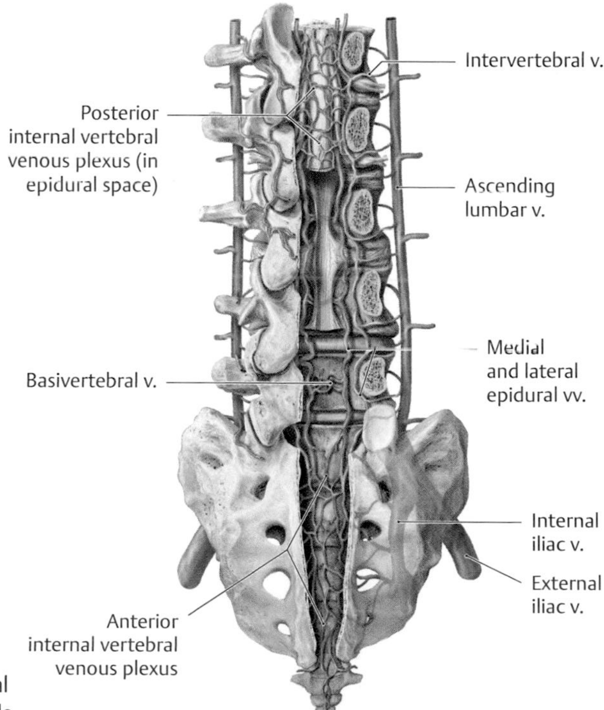
Intervertebral v.
Posterior internal vertebral venous plexus (in epidural space)
Ascending lumbar v.
Medial and lateral epidural vv.
Basivertebral v.
Internal iliac v.
External iliac v.
Anterior internal vertebral venous plexus

D Veins in the sacral and lumbar canals.

Neurovascular Topography of the Back

Fig. 4.17 **Neurovasculature of the nuchal region**
Posterior view. *Removed:* Trapezius, sternocleidomastoid, and semispinalis capitis. *Revealed:* Suboccipital region. See p. 68 for the course of the intercostal vessels.

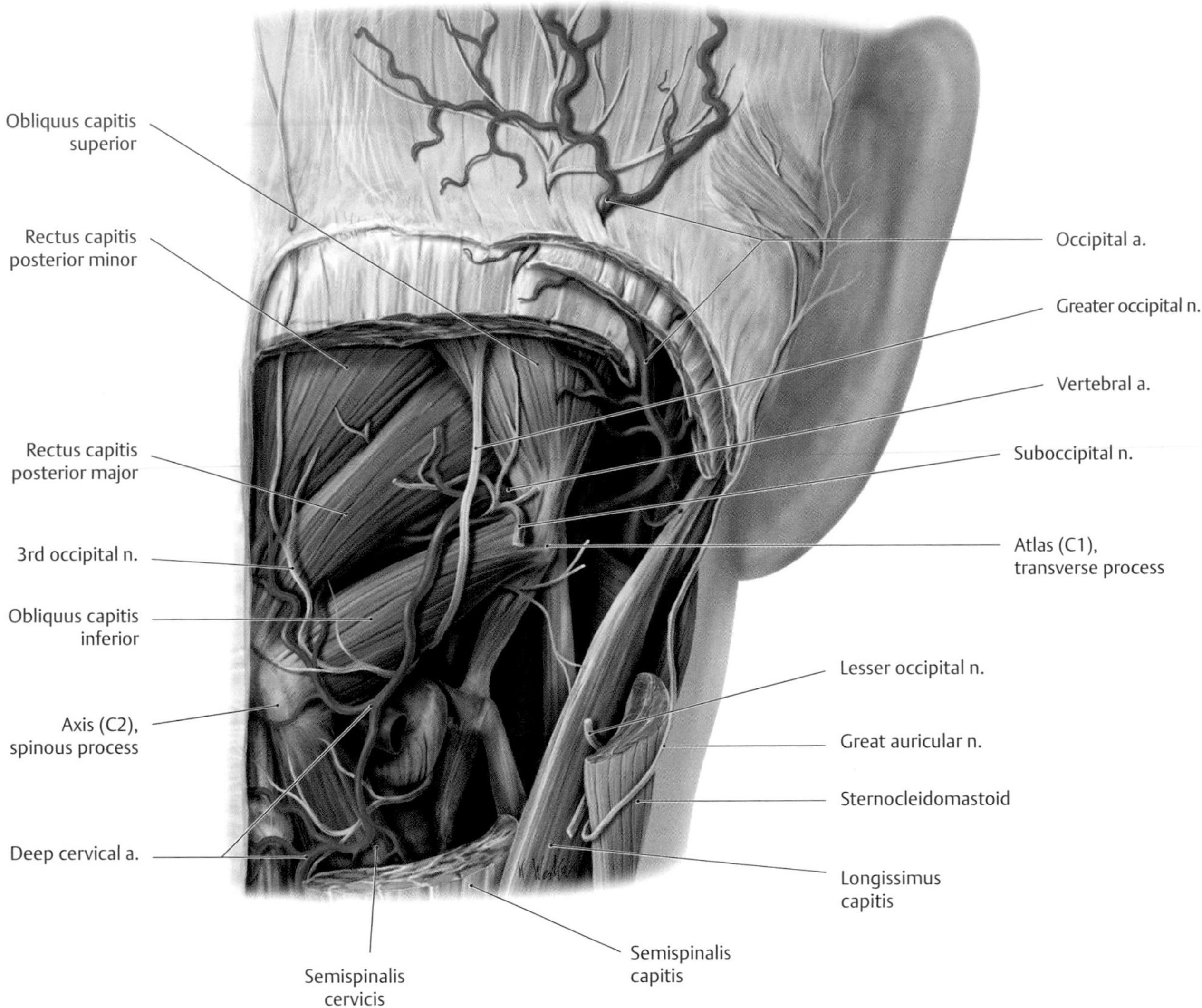
Obliquus capitis superior
Rectus capitis posterior minor
Rectus capitis posterior major
3rd occipital n.
Obliquus capitis inferior
Axis (C2), spinous process
Deep cervical a.
Semispinalis cervicis
Semispinalis capitis
Occipital a.
Greater occipital n.
Vertebral a.
Suboccipital n.
Atlas (C1), transverse process
Lesser occipital n.
Great auricular n.
Sternocleidomastoid
Longissimus capitis

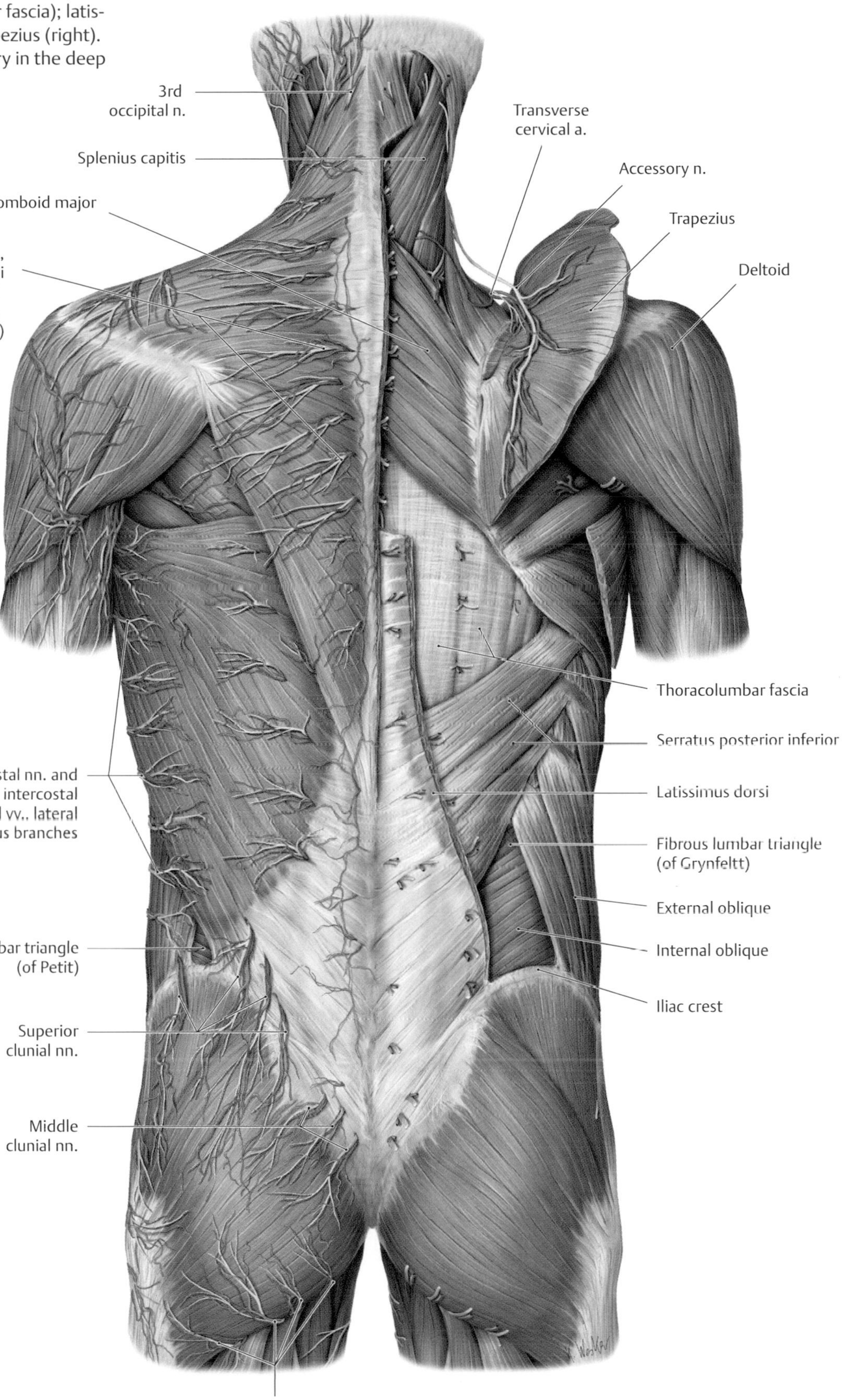

Fig. 4.18 **Neurovasculature of the back**

Posterior view. *Removed:* Muscle fascia (except superficial layer of thoracolumbar fascia); latissimus dorsi (right). *Reflected:* Trapezius (right). *Revealed:* Transverse cervical artery in the deep scapular region.

3rd occipital n.
Splenius capitis
Rhomboid major
Spinal nn., posterior rami (medial cutaneous branches)
Transverse cervical a.
Accessory n.
Trapezius
Deltoid
Thoracolumbar fascia
Serratus posterior inferior
Latissimus dorsi
Fibrous lumbar triangle (of Grynfeltt)
External oblique
Internal oblique
Iliac crest
Intercostal nn. and posterior intercostal aa. and vv., lateral cutaneous branches
Iliolumbar triangle (of Petit)
Superior clunial nn.
Middle clunial nn.
Inferior clunial nn.

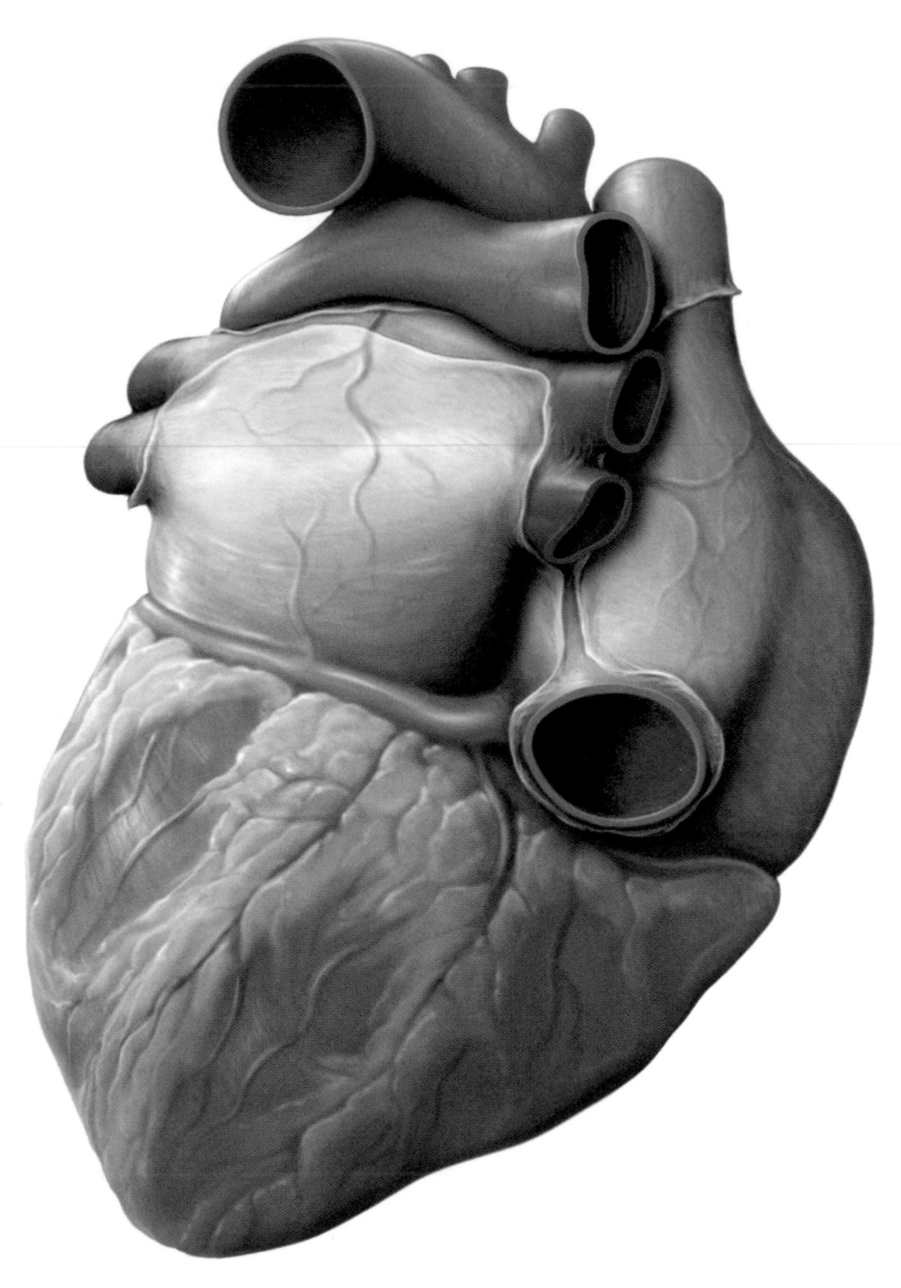

Thorax

5 Surface Anatomy

Surface Anatomy 50

6 Thoracic Wall

Thoracic Skeleton 52
Sternum & Ribs 54
Joints of the Thoracic Cage 56
Thoracic Wall Muscle Facts 58
Diaphragm 60
Neurovasculature of the Diaphragm 62
Arteries & Veins of the Thoracic Wall 64
Nerves of the Thoracic Wall 66
Neurovascular Topography of the Thoracic Wall 68
Female Breast 70
Lymphatics of the Female Breast 72

7 Thoracic Cavity

Divisions of the Thoracic Cavity 74
Arteries of the Thoracic Cavity 76
Veins of the Thoracic Cavity 78
Lymphatics of the Thoracic Cavity 80
Nerves of the Thoracic Cavity 82

8 Mediastinum

Mediastinum: Overview 84
Mediastinum: Structures 86
Heart: Functions and Relations 88
Pericardium 90
Heart: Surfaces & Chambers 92
Heart: Valves 94
Arteries & Veins of the Heart 96
Conduction & Innervation of the Heart 98
Heart: Radiology 100
Pre- & Postnatal Circulation 102
Esophagus 104
Neurovasculature of the Esophagus 106
Lymphatics of the Mediastinum 108

9 Pleural Cavity

Pleural Cavities 110
Pleura: Subdivisions, Recesses & Innervation 112
Lungs 114
Lung: Radiology 116
Bronchopulmonary Segments of the Lungs 118
Trachea & Bronchial Tree 120
Respiratory Mechanics 122
Pulmonary Arteries & Veins 124
Neurovasculature of the Tracheobronchial Tree 126
Lymphatics of the Pleural Cavity 128

Surface Anatomy

Fig. 5.1 **Regions of the thorax**
Anterior view.

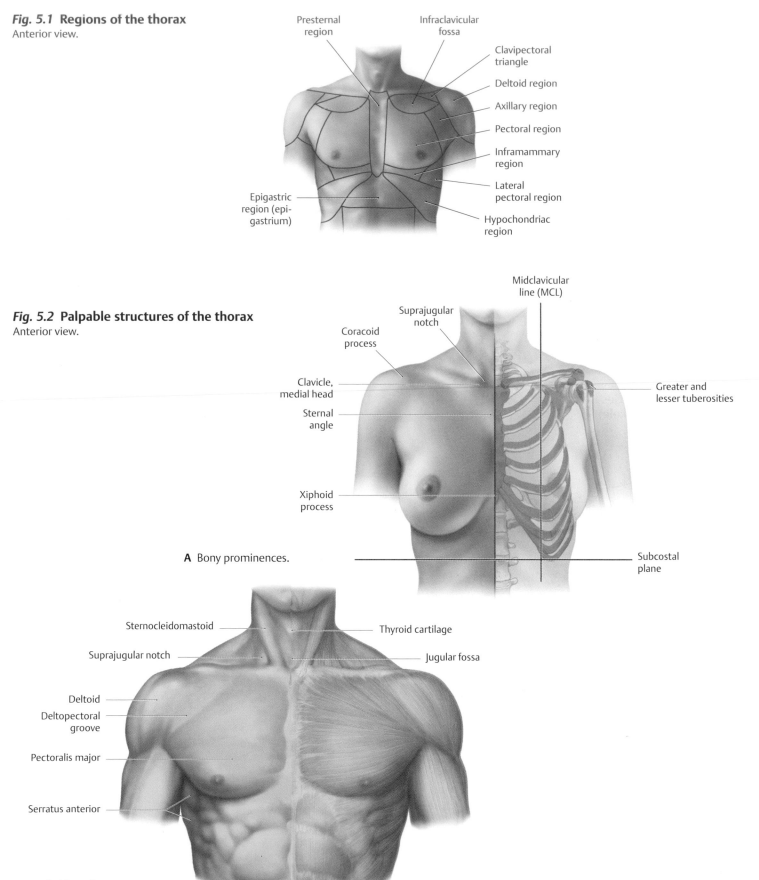

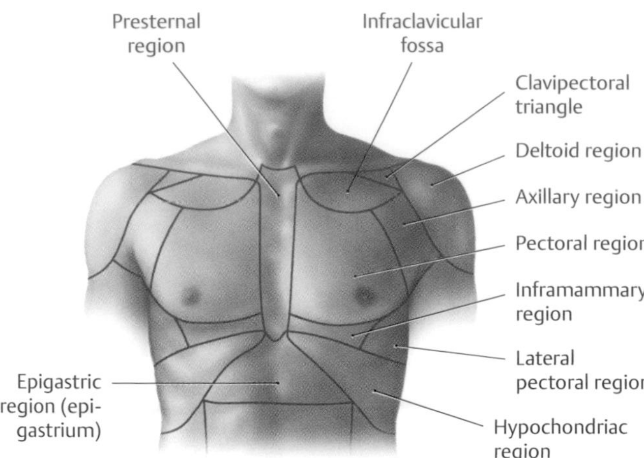
Presternal region
Infraclavicular fossa
Clavipectoral triangle
Deltoid region
Axillary region
Pectoral region
Inframammary region
Lateral pectoral region
Hypochondriac region
Epigastric region (epigastrium)

Fig. 5.2 **Palpable structures of the thorax**
Anterior view.

Midclavicular line (MCL)
Suprajugular notch
Coracoid process
Clavicle, medial head
Greater and lesser tuberosities
Sternal angle
Xiphoid process
Subcostal plane

A Bony prominences.

Sternocleidomastoid
Thyroid cartilage
Suprajugular notch
Jugular fossa
Deltoid
Deltopectoral groove
Pectoralis major
Serratus anterior

B Musculature.

Fig. 5.3 Vertical reference lines of the thorax

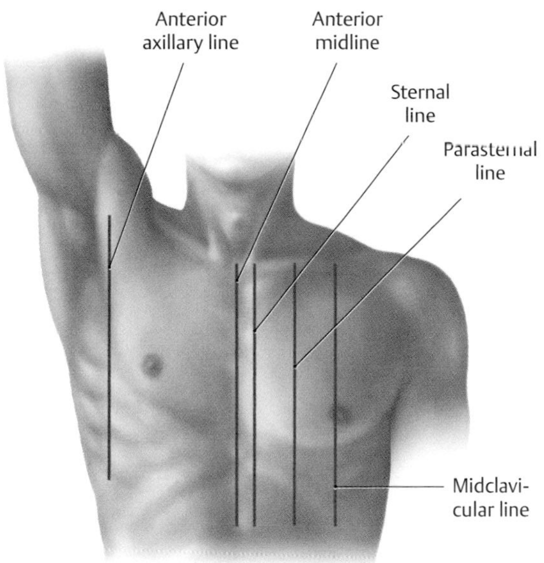
Anterior axillary line
Anterior midline
Sternal line
Parasternal line
Midclavicular line

A Anterior view.

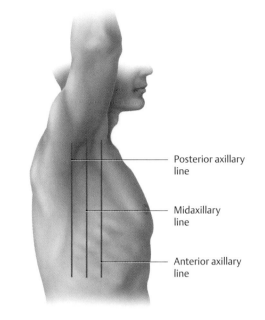

B Right lateral view.

Posterior axillary line
Midaxillary line
Anterior axillary line

Fig. 5.4 Pleural cavities and lungs projected onto the thoracic skeleton

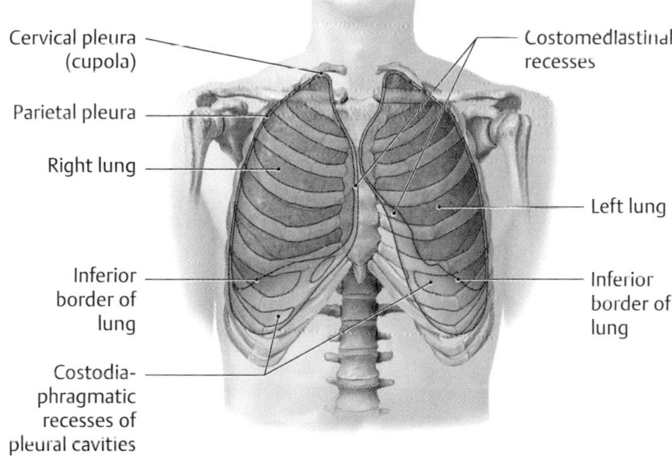
Cervical pleura (cupola)
Parietal pleura
Right lung
Inferior border of lung
Costodiaphragmatic recesses of pleural cavities
Costomediastinal recesses
Left lung
Inferior border of lung

A Anterior view.

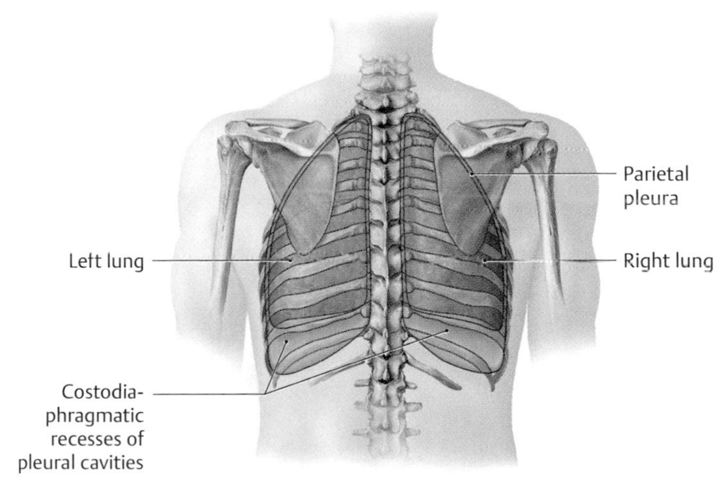
Parietal pleura
Left lung
Right lung
Costodiaphragmatic recesses of pleural cavities

B Posterior view.

Thoracic Skeleton

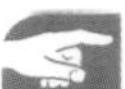

The thoracic skeleton consists of 12 thoracic vertebrae (p. 10), 12 pairs of ribs with costal cartilages, and the sternum. In addition to participating in respiratory movements, it provides a measure of protection to vital organs. The female thorax is generally narrower and shorter than the male equivalent.

Fig. 6.1 Thoracic skeleton

Clavicular notch
Superior thoracic aperture
Jugular notch
Manubrium
Sternal angle
Body
Xiphoid process
Sternum
Costal cartilage
Costal margin (arch)
Inferior thoracic aperture

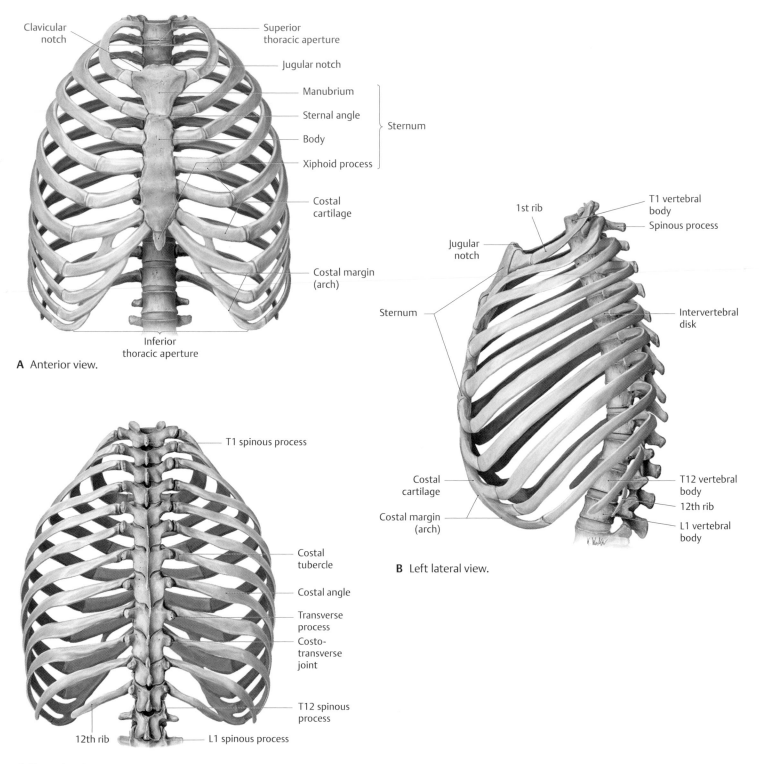

A Anterior view.

1st rib
T1 vertebral body
Spinous process
Jugular notch
Sternum
Intervertebral disk
Costal cartilage
Costal margin (arch)
T12 vertebral body
12th rib
L1 vertebral body

B Left lateral view.

T1 spinous process
Costal tubercle
Costal angle
Transverse process
Costo-transverse joint
T12 spinous process
12th rib
L1 spinous process

C Posterior view.

Fig. 6.2 Structure of a thoracic segment
Superior view of 6th rib pair.

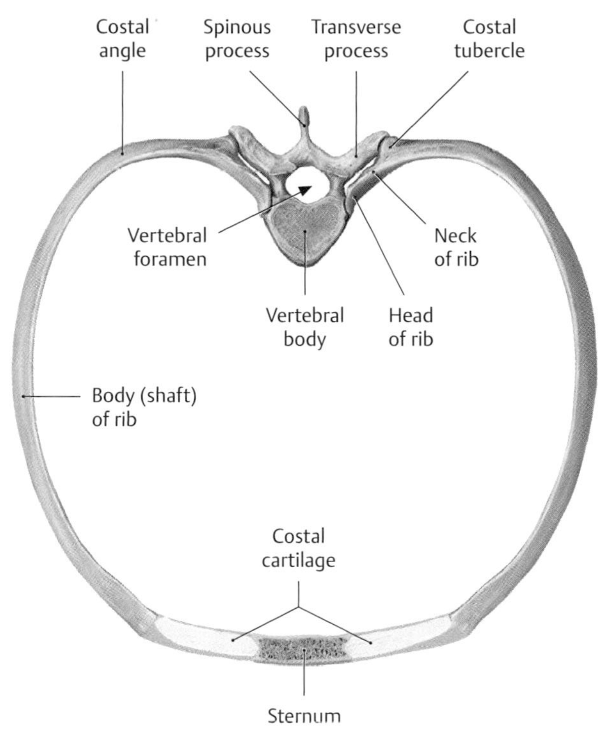
Costal angle
Spinous process
Transverse process
Costal tubercle
Vertebral foramen
Neck of rib
Vertebral body
Head of rib
Body (shaft) of rib
Costal cartilage
Sternum

Table 6.1	Elements of a thoracic segment	
Vertebra		
Rib	Bony part (costal bone)	Head
		Neck
		Costal tubercle
		Body (including costal angle)
	Costal part (costal cartilage)	
Sternum (articulates with costal cartilage of true ribs only; see Fig. 6.3)		

Fig. 6.3 Types of ribs
Left lateral view.

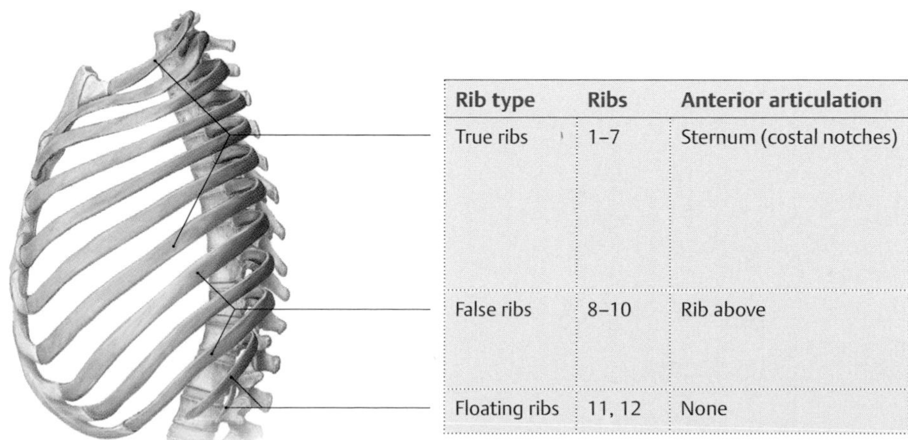

Rib type	Ribs	Anterior articulation
True ribs	1–7	Sternum (costal notches)
False ribs	8–10	Rib above
Floating ribs	11, 12	None

Sternum & Ribs

Fig. 6.4 **Sternum**

The sternum is a blade-like bone consisting of the manubrium, body, and xiphoid process. The junction of the manubrium and body (the sternal angle) is typically elevated and marks the articulation of the second rib. The sternal angle is an important landmark for internal structures.

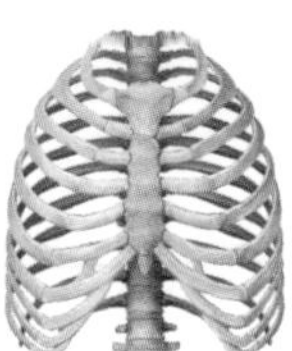

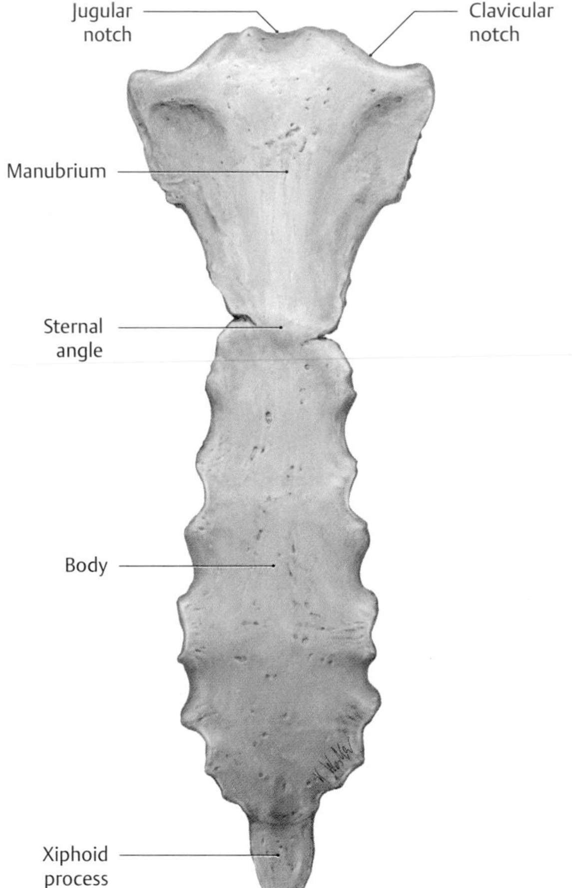
Jugular notch
Clavicular notch
Manubrium
Sternal angle
Body
Xiphoid process

A Anterior view.

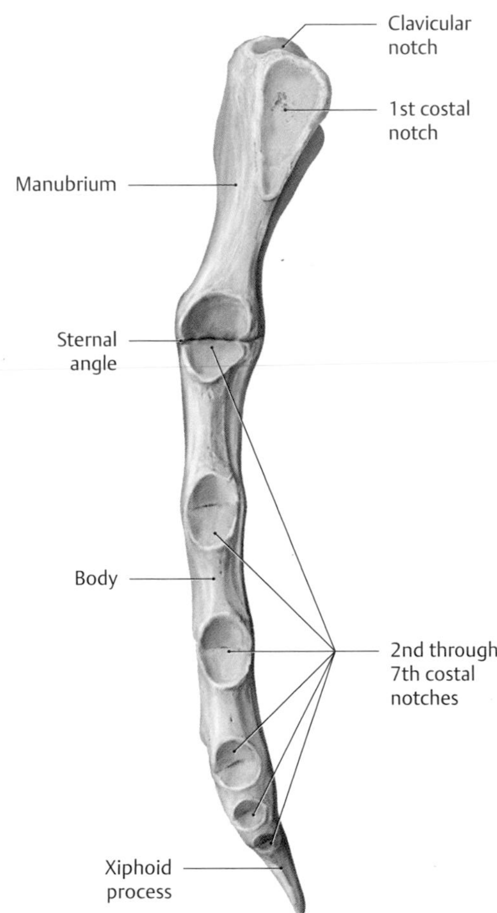
Clavicular notch
1st costal notch
Manubrium
Sternal angle
Body
2nd through 7th costal notches
Xiphoid process

B Left lateral view. The costal notches are sites of articulation with the costal cartilage of the true ribs (see Fig. 6.3).

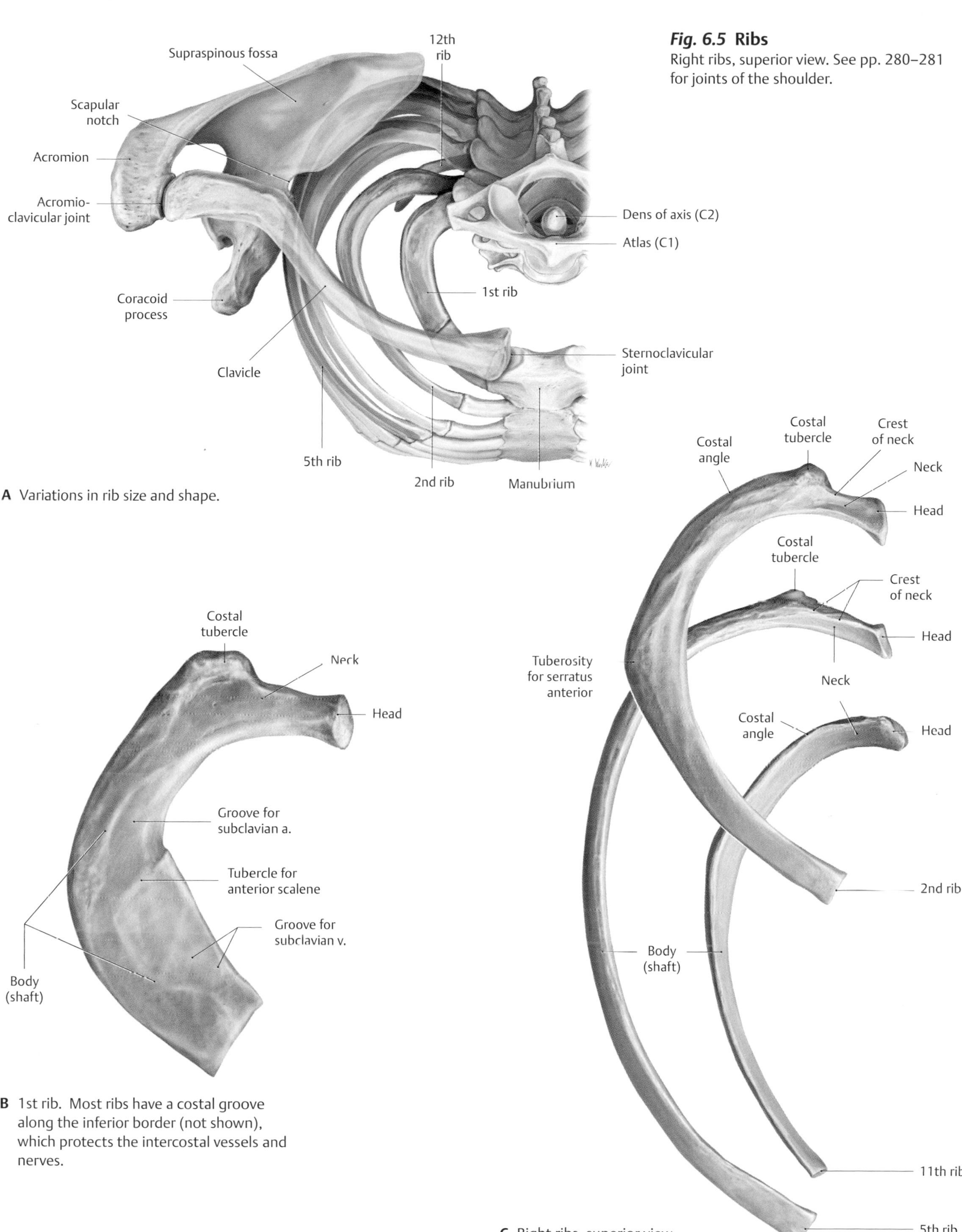

Supraspinous fossa
12th rib
Scapular notch
Acromion
Acromio-clavicular joint
Dens of axis (C2)
Atlas (C1)
1st rib
Coracoid process
Sternoclavicular joint
Clavicle
5th rib
2nd rib
Manubrium
Costal tubercle
Neck
Head
Groove for subclavian a.
Tubercle for anterior scalene
Groove for subclavian v.
Body (shaft)
Costal angle
Costal tubercle
Crest of neck
Neck
Head
Costal tubercle
Crest of neck
Head
Tuberosity for serratus anterior
Neck
Costal angle
Head
2nd rib
Body (shaft)
11th rib
5th rib

Fig. 6.5 **Ribs**
Right ribs, superior view. See pp. 280–281 for joints of the shoulder.

A Variations in rib size and shape.

B 1st rib. Most ribs have a costal groove along the inferior border (not shown), which protects the intercostal vessels and nerves.

C Right ribs, superior view.

Joints of the Thoracic Cage

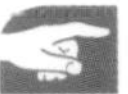

The diaphragm is the chief muscle for quiet respiration (see p. 60). The muscles of the thoracic wall (see p. 58) contribute to deep (forced) inspiration.

Fig. 6.6 **Rib cage movement**

Full inspiration (red); full expiration (blue). In deep inspiration, there is an increase in transverse and sagittal thoracic diameters, as well as the infrasternal angle. The descent of the diaphragm further increases the volume of the thoracic cavity.

Inspiration

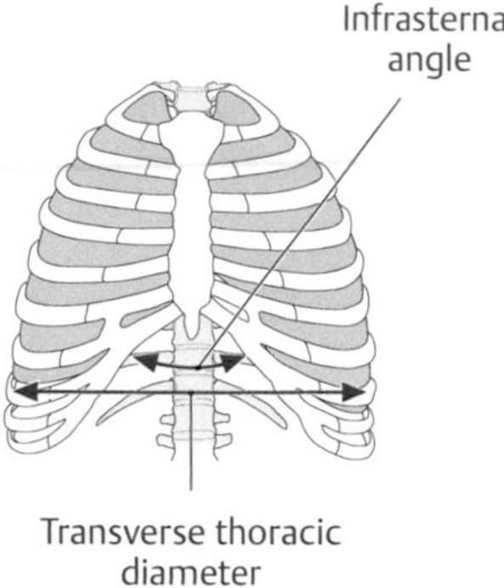
Infrasternal angle
Transverse thoracic diameter

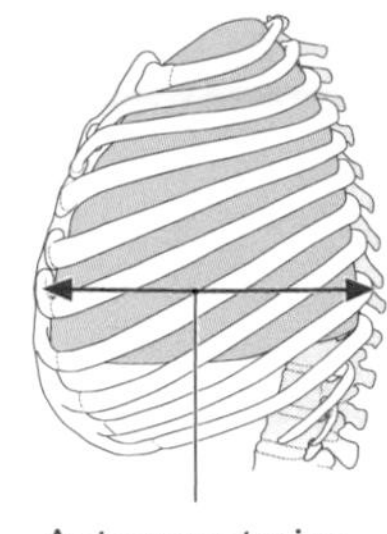
Anteroposterior thoracic diameter

Expiration

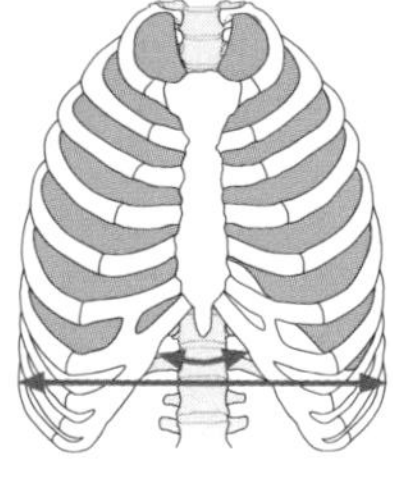

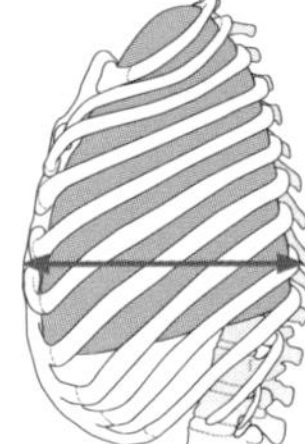

A Anterior view.

B Left lateral view.

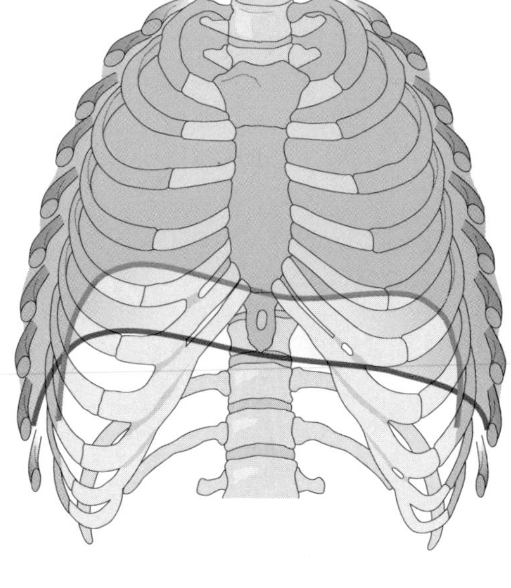

C Position of diaphragm during respiration.

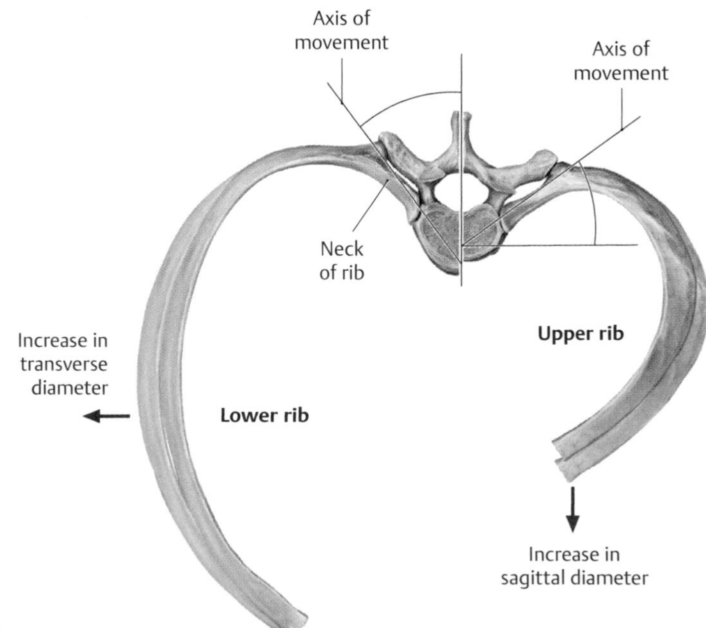
Axis of movement
Axis of movement
Neck of rib
Upper rib
Lower rib
Increase in transverse diameter
Increase in sagittal diameter

D Axes of rib movement, superior view.

Fig. 6.7 Sternocostal joints

Anterior view with right half of sternum sectioned frontally. True joints are generally found only at ribs 2 to 5; ribs 1, 6, and 7 attach to the sternum by synchondroses.

Fig. 6.8 Costovertebral joints

Two synovial joints make up the costovertebral articulation of each rib. The costal tubercle of each rib articulates with the costal facet of its accompanying vertebra (**A**). The head of most ribs articulates with the vertebra of its own number and the vertebra immediately superior. Ribs 1, 11, and 12 typically articulate only with their own vertebrae.

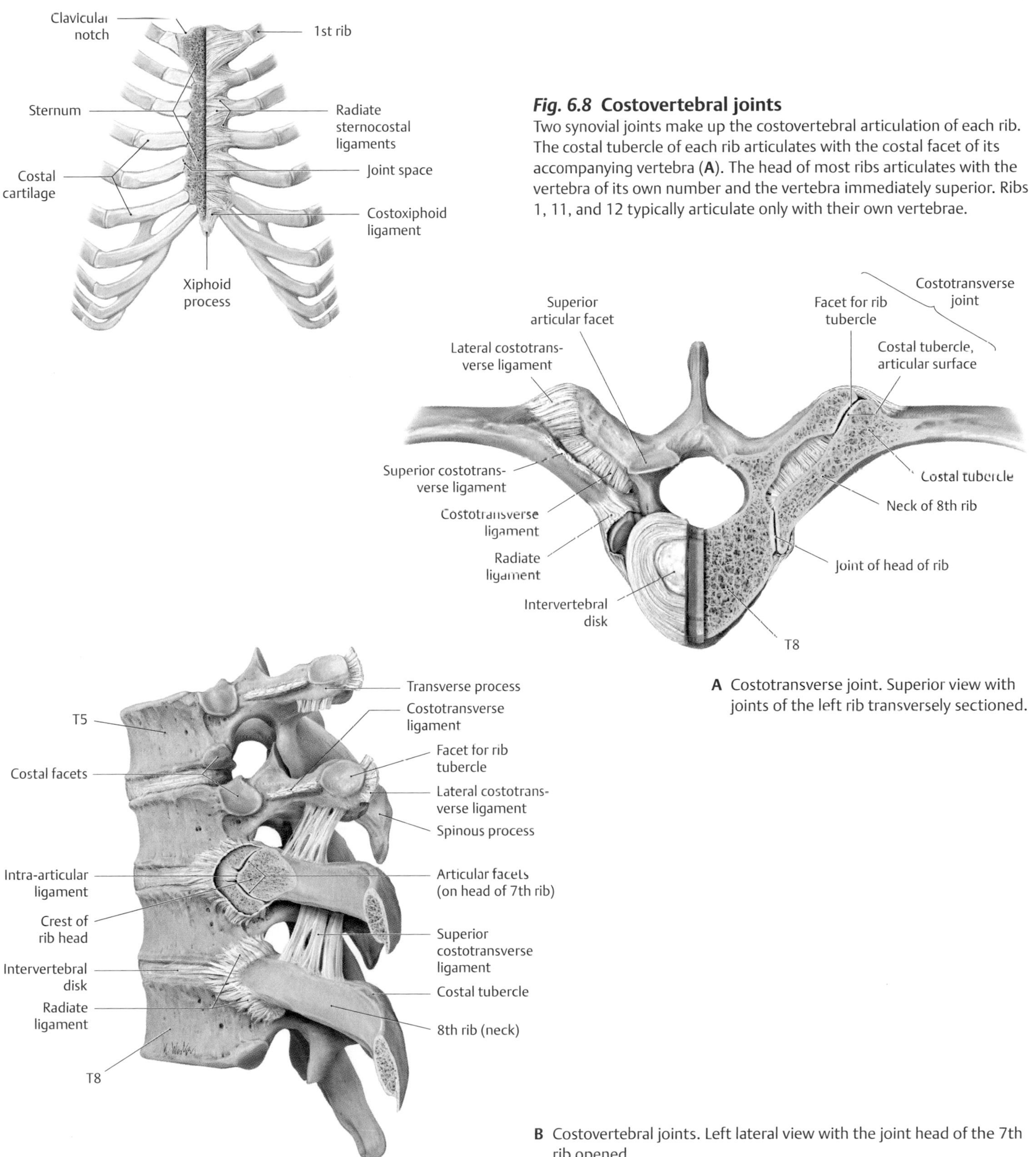

Clavicular notch
1st rib
Sternum
Radiate sternocostal ligaments
Costal cartilage
Joint space
Costoxiphoid ligament
Xiphoid process
Superior articular facet
Facet for rib tubercle
Costotransverse joint
Lateral costotransverse ligament
Costal tubercle, articular surface
Superior costotransverse ligament
Costal tubercle
Costotransverse ligament
Neck of 8th rib
Radiate ligament
Joint of head of rib
Intervertebral disk
T8
T5
Transverse process
Costotransverse ligament
Facet for rib tubercle
Costal facets
Lateral costotransverse ligament
Spinous process
Intra-articular ligament
Articular facets (on head of 7th rib)
Crest of rib head
Superior costotransverse ligament
Intervertebral disk
Costal tubercle
Radiate ligament
8th rib (neck)
T8

A Costotransverse joint. Superior view with joints of the left rib transversely sectioned.

B Costovertebral joints. Left lateral view with the joint head of the 7th rib opened.

Thoracic Wall Muscle Facts

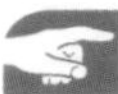

The muscles of the thoracic wall are primarily responsible for chest respiration, although other muscles aid in *deep* inspiration: the pectoralis major and serratus anterior are discussed with the shoulder (see pp. 296–297), and the serratus posterior is discussed with the back (see p. 32).

Fig. 6.9 **Muscles of the thoracic wall**

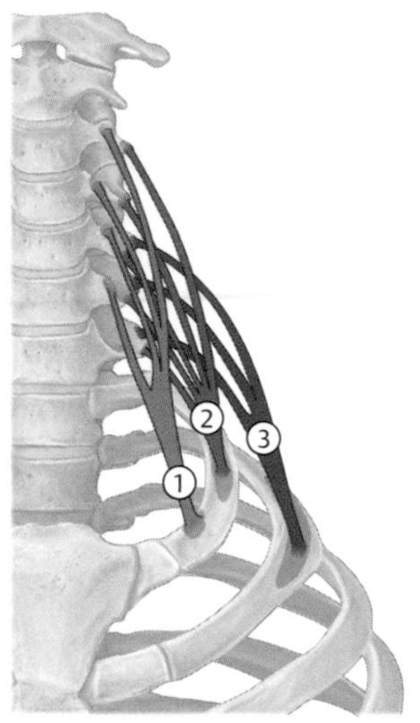
1
2
3

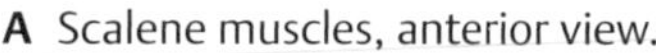

A Scalene muscles, anterior view.

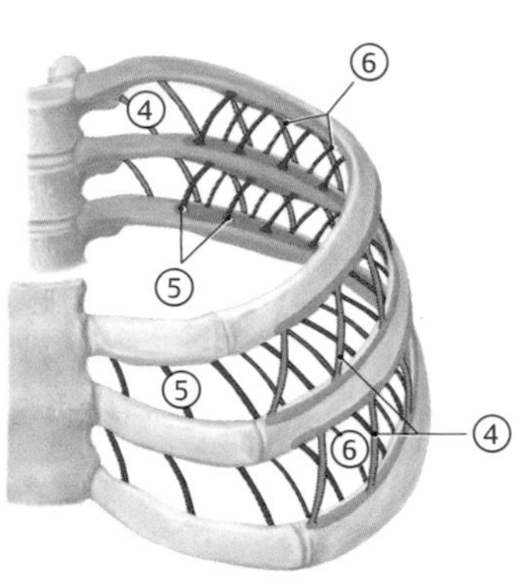
6
4
5
5
6
4

B Intercostal muscles, anterior view.

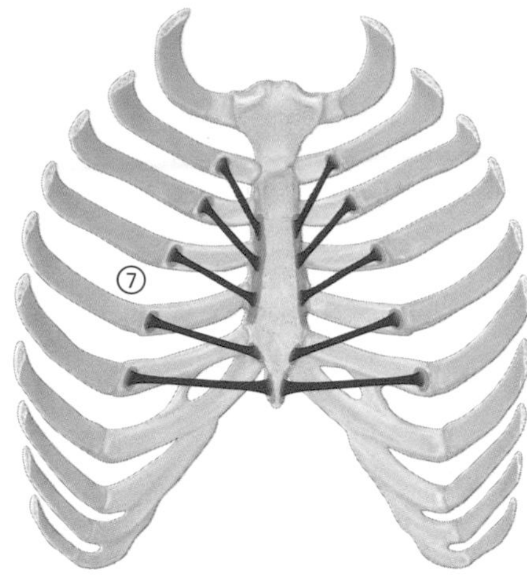
7

C Transversus thoracis, posterior view.

Table 6.2	**Muscles of the thoracic wall**				
Muscle		**Origin**	**Insertion**	**Innervation**	**Action**
Scalene mm.	① Anterior scalene m.	C3–C6 (transverse processes, anterior tubercles)	1st rib (anterior scalene tubercle)	Direct branches from cervical and brachial plexus (C3–C6)	*With ribs mobile*: Raises upper ribs (inspiration) *With ribs fixed*: Bends cervical spine to same side (unilateral); flexes neck (bilateral)
	② Middle scalene m.	C3–C7 (transverse processes, posterior tubercles)	1st rib (posterior to groove for subclavian a.)		
	③ Posterior scalene m.	C5–C7 (transverse processes, posterior tubercles)	2nd rib (outer surface)		
Intercostal mm.	④ External intercostal mm.	Lower margin of rib to upper margin of next lower rib (courses obliquely forward and downward from costal tubercle to chondro-osseous junction)		1st to 11th intercostal nn.	Raises ribs (inspiration); supports intercostal spaces; stabilizes chest wall
	⑤ Internal intercostal mm.	Lower margin of rib to upper margin of next lower rib (courses obliquely forward and upward from costal angle to sternum)			Lowers ribs (expiration); supports intercostal spaces, stabilizes chest wall
	⑥ Innermost intercostal mm.				
Subcostal mm.		Lower margin of lower ribs to inner surface of ribs two to three ribs below		Adjacent intercostal nn.	Lowers ribs (expiration)
⑦ Transversus thoracis m.		Sternum and xiphoid process (inner surface)	2nd to 6th ribs (costal cartilage, inner surface)	2nd to 6th intercostal nn.	Weakly lowers ribs (expiration)

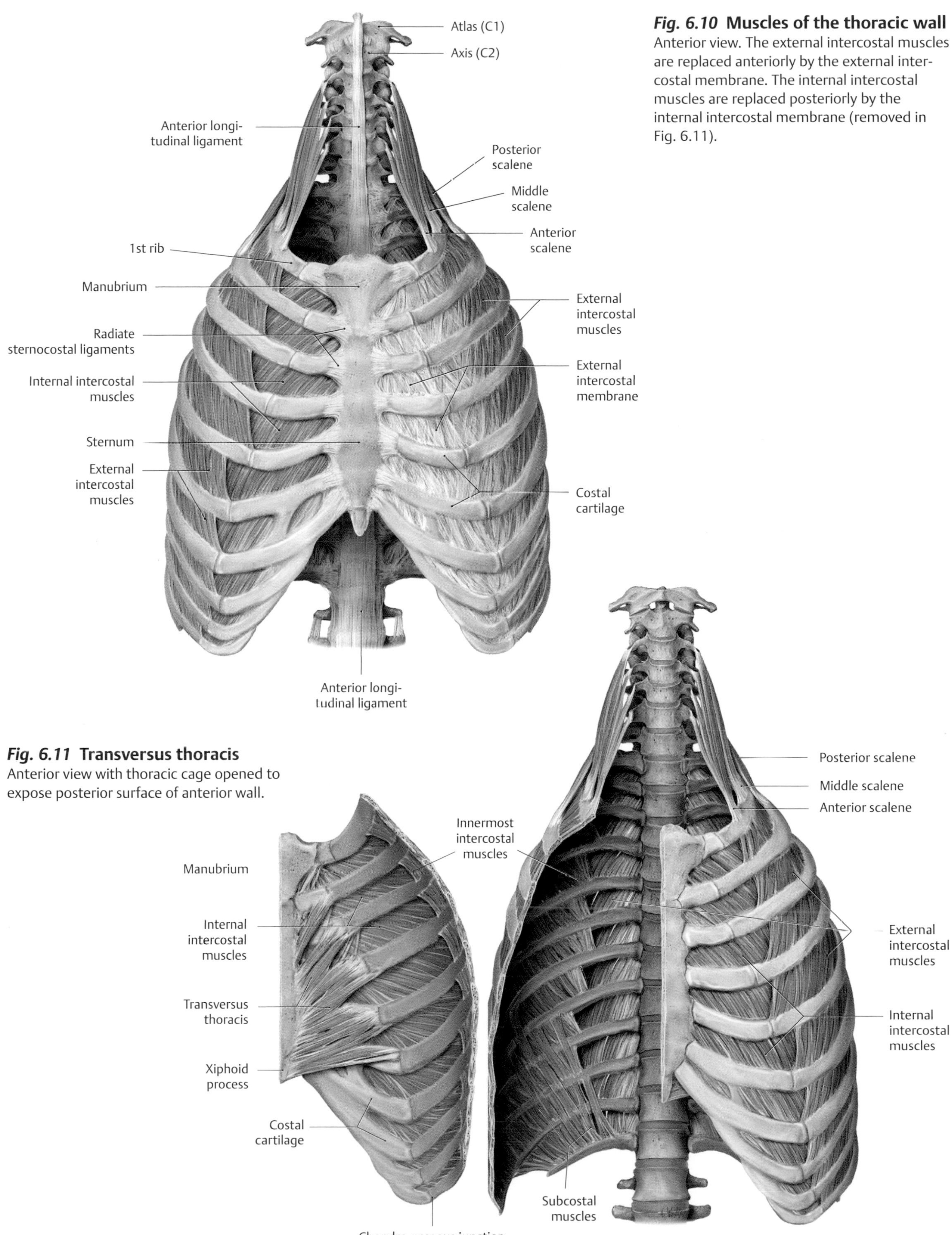

Atlas (C1)
Axis (C2)
Anterior longi-tudinal ligament
Posterior scalene
Middle scalene
Anterior scalene
1st rib
Manubrium
External intercostal muscles
Radiate sternocostal ligaments
External intercostal membrane
Internal intercostal muscles
Sternum
External intercostal muscles
Costal cartilage
Anterior longi-tudinal ligament
Posterior scalene
Middle scalene
Anterior scalene
Innermost intercostal muscles
Manubrium
Internal intercostal muscles
External intercostal muscles
Transversus thoracis
Internal intercostal muscles
Xiphoid process
Costal cartilage
Subcostal muscles
Chondro-osseous junction

Fig. 6.10 **Muscles of the thoracic wall**
Anterior view. The external intercostal muscles are replaced anteriorly by the external intercostal membrane. The internal intercostal muscles are replaced posteriorly by the internal intercostal membrane (removed in Fig. 6.11).

Fig. 6.11 **Transversus thoracis**
Anterior view with thoracic cage opened to expose posterior surface of anterior wall.

Diaphragm

Fig. 6.12 **Diaphragm**
The diaphragm, which separates the thorax from the abdomen, has two asymmetric domes and three apertures (for the aorta, vena cava, and esophagus; see Fig. 6.13B).

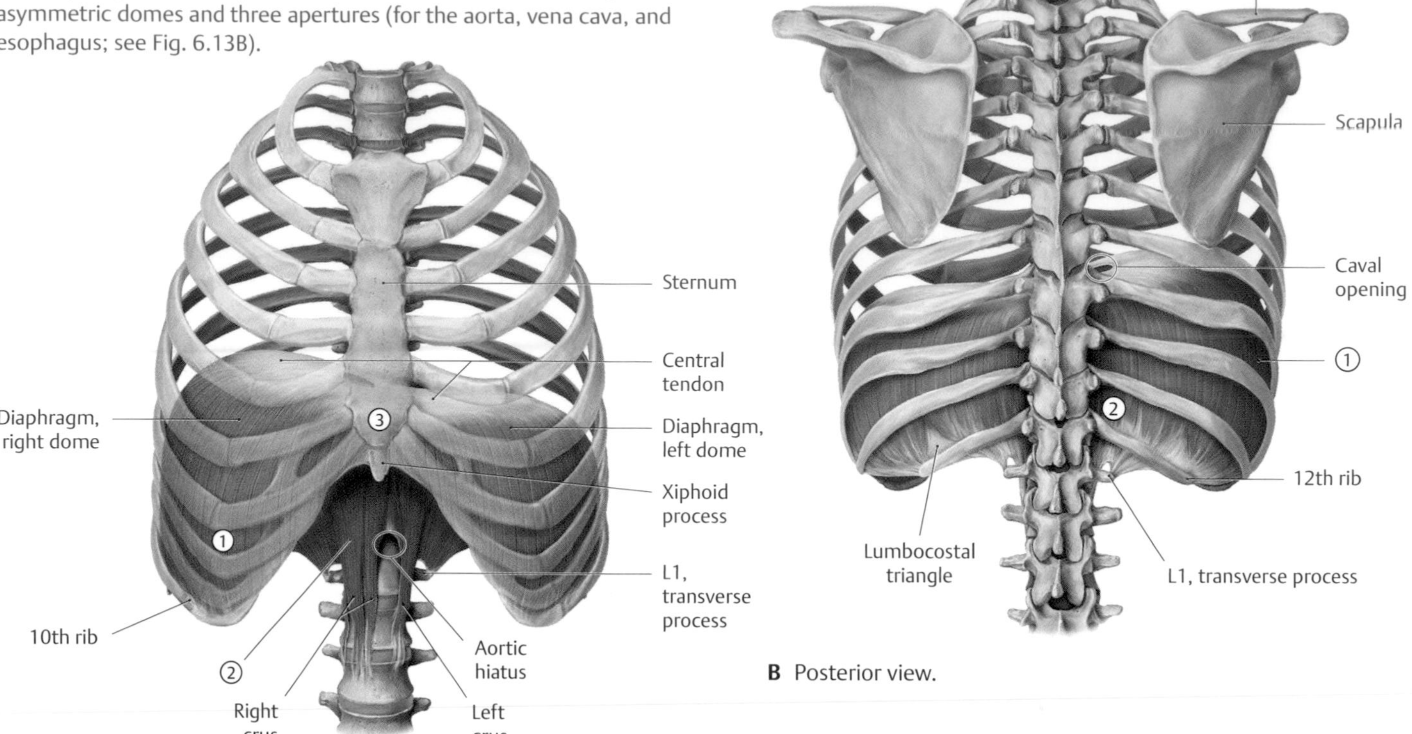
Sternum
Central tendon
Diaphragm, right dome
③
Diaphragm, left dome
Xiphoid process
①
L1, transverse process
10th rib
Aortic hiatus
②
Right crus
Left crus
Clavicle
Scapula
Caval opening
①
②
12th rib
Lumbocostal triangle
L1, transverse process

B Posterior view.

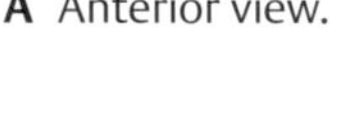

A Anterior view.

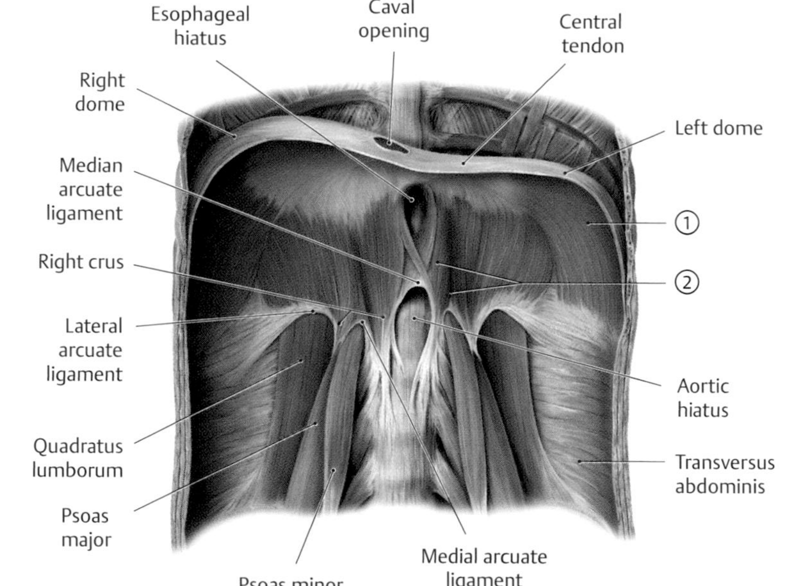
Esophageal hiatus
Caval opening
Central tendon
Right dome
Left dome
Median arcuate ligament
①
Right crus
②
Lateral arcuate ligament
Aortic hiatus
Quadratus lumborum
Transversus abdominis
Psoas major
Psoas minor
Medial arcuate ligament

C Coronal section with diaphragm in intermediate position.

Table 6.3 **Diaphragm**

Muscle		Origin	Insertion	Innervation	Action
Diaphragm	① Costal part	7th to 12th ribs (inner surface; lower margin of costal arch)	Central tendon	Phrenic n. (C3–C5, cervical plexus)	Principal muscle of respiration (diaphragmatic and thoracic breathing); aids in compressing abdominal viscera (abdominal press)
	② Lumbar part	Medial part: L1–L3 vertebral bodies, intervertebral disks, and anterior longitudinal ligament as right and left crura			
		Lateral parts: lateral and medial arcuate ligaments			
	③ Sternal part	Xiphoid process (posterior surface)			

Fig. 6.13 Diaphragm in situ

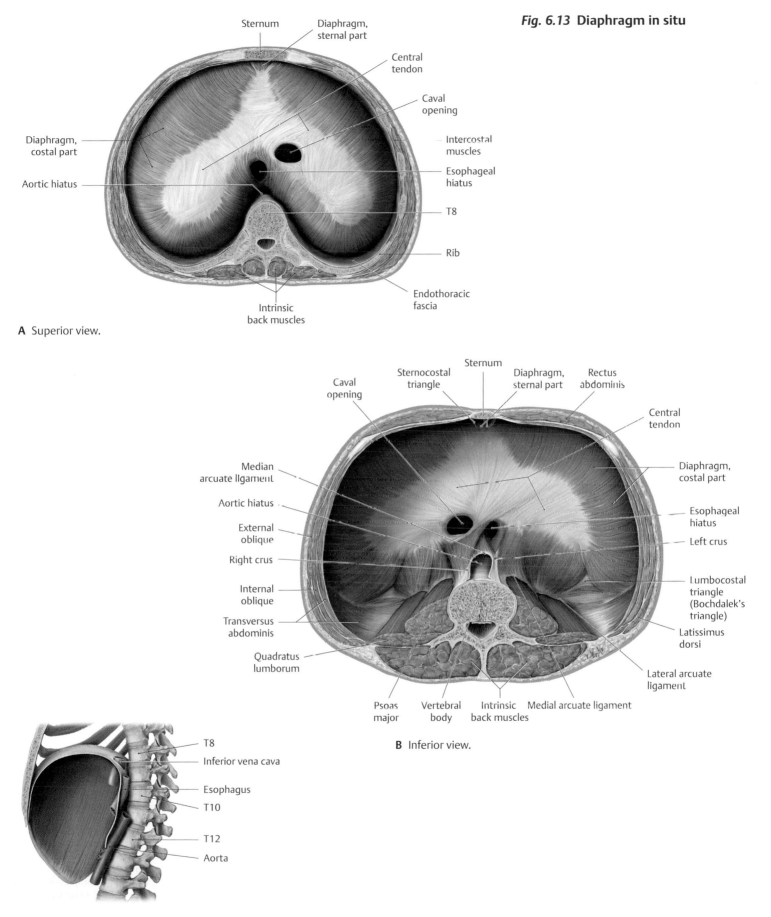

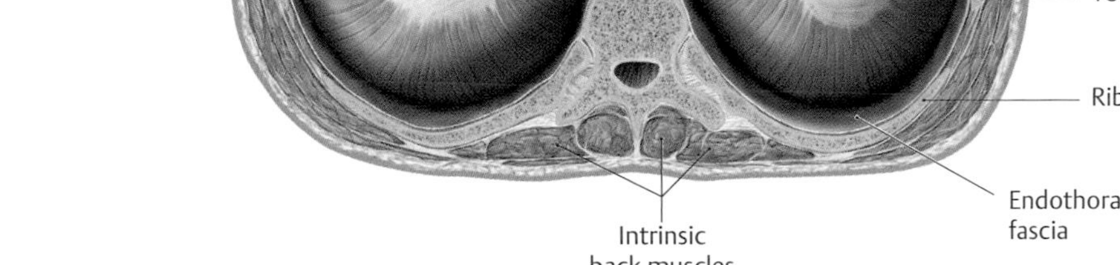
Sternum
Diaphragm, sternal part
Central tendon
Caval opening
Diaphragm, costal part
Intercostal muscles
Esophageal hiatus
Aortic hiatus
T8
Rib
Endothoracic fascia
Intrinsic back muscles

A Superior view.

Sternum
Sternocostal triangle
Caval opening
Diaphragm, sternal part
Rectus abdominis
Central tendon
Median arcuate ligament
Diaphragm, costal part
Aortic hiatus
Esophageal hiatus
External oblique
Left crus
Right crus
Internal oblique
Lumbocostal triangle (Bochdalek's triangle)
Transversus abdominis
Latissimus dorsi
Quadratus lumborum
Lateral arcuate ligament
Psoas major
Vertebral body
Intrinsic back muscles
Medial arcuate ligament

B Inferior view.

T8
Inferior vena cava
Esophagus
T10
T12
Aorta

C Diaphragmatic apertures, left lateral view.

Neurovasculature of the Diaphragm

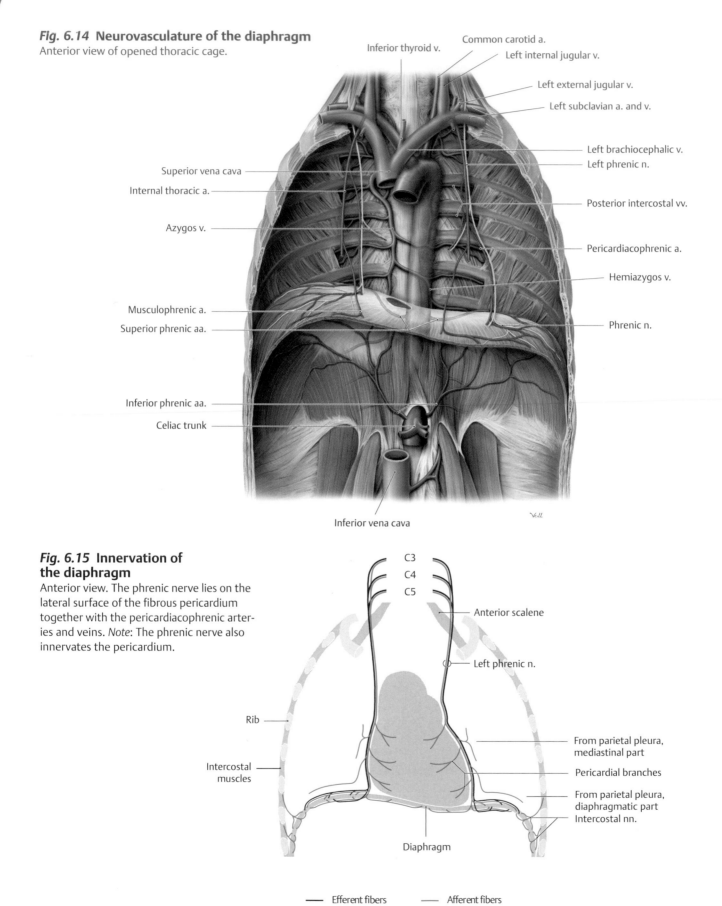

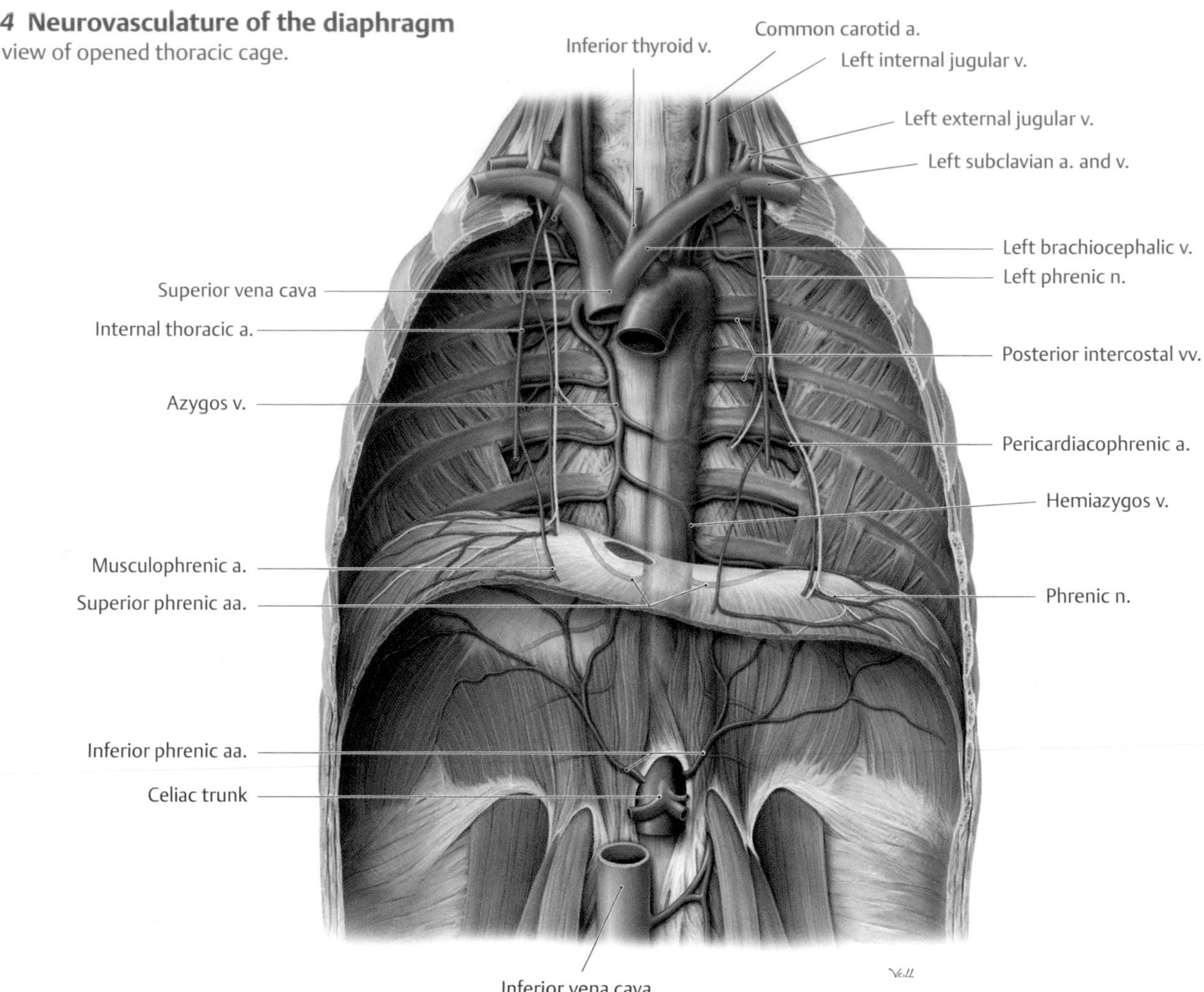
Inferior thyroid v.
Common carotid a.
Left internal jugular v.
Left external jugular v.
Left subclavian a. and v.
Left brachiocephalic v.
Left phrenic n.
Superior vena cava
Internal thoracic a.
Posterior intercostal vv.
Azygos v.
Pericardiacophrenic a.
Hemiazygos v.
Musculophrenic a.
Superior phrenic aa.
Phrenic n.
Inferior phrenic aa.
Celiac trunk
Inferior vena cava

Fig. 6.14 **Neurovasculature of the diaphragm**
Anterior view of opened thoracic cage.

Fig. 6.15 **Innervation of the diaphragm**
Anterior view. The phrenic nerve lies on the lateral surface of the fibrous pericardium together with the pericardiacophrenic arteries and veins. *Note*: The phrenic nerve also innervates the pericardium.

C3
C4
C5
Anterior scalene
Left phrenic n.
Rib
Intercostal muscles
From parietal pleura, mediastinal part
Pericardial branches
From parietal pleura, diaphragmatic part
Intercostal nn.
Diaphragm

Efferent fibers
Afferent fibers

Table 6.4 Blood vessels of the diaphragm

Artery	Origin	Vein	Drainage
Inferior phrenic aa. (chief blood supply)	Abdominal aorta; occasionally from celiac trunk	Inferior phrenic vv.	Inferior vena cava
Superior phrenic aa.	Thoracic aorta	Superior phrenic vv.	Azygos v. (right side), hemiazygos v. (left side)
Pericardiacophrenic aa.	Internal thoracic aa.	Pericardiacophrenic vv.	Internal thoracic vv. or brachiocephalic vv.
Musculophrenic aa.		Musculophrenic vv.	Internal thoracic vv.

Fig. 6.16 Arteries and nerves of the diaphragm

Note: The margins of the diaphragm receive sensory innervation from the lowest intercostal nerves.

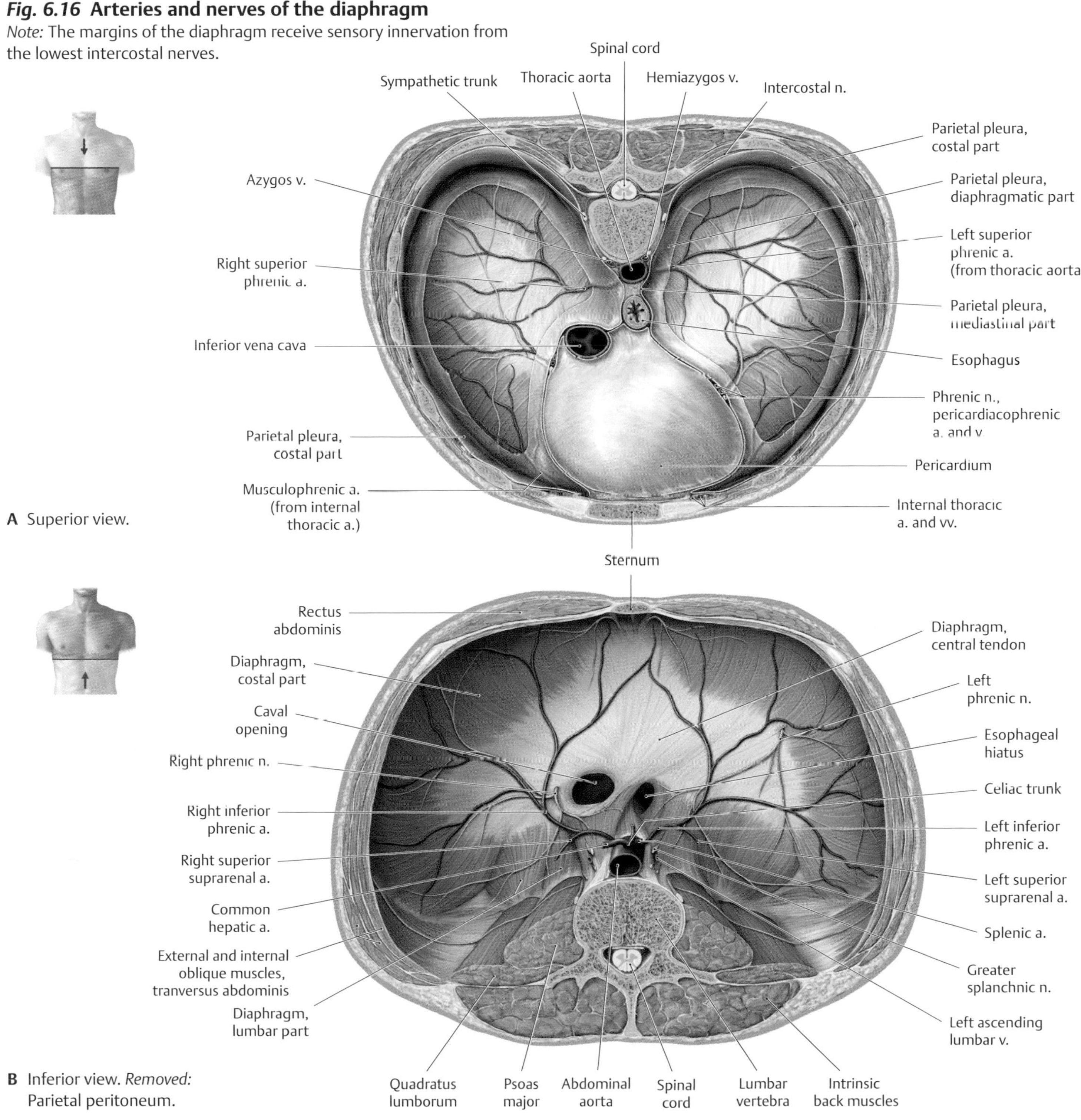

Spinal cord
Sympathetic trunk
Thoracic aorta
Hemiazygos v.
Intercostal n.
Parietal pleura, costal part
Azygos v.
Parietal pleura, diaphragmatic part
Left superior phrenic a. (from thoracic aorta)
Right superior phrenic a.
Parietal pleura, mediastinal part
Inferior vena cava
Esophagus
Phrenic n., pericardiacophrenic a. and v.
Parietal pleura, costal part
Pericardium
Musculophrenic a. (from internal thoracic a.)
Internal thoracic a. and vv.
Sternum
Rectus abdominis
Diaphragm, central tendon
Diaphragm, costal part
Left phrenic n.
Caval opening
Esophageal hiatus
Right phrenic n.
Celiac trunk
Right inferior phrenic a.
Left inferior phrenic a.
Right superior suprarenal a.
Left superior suprarenal a.
Common hepatic a.
Splenic a.
External and internal oblique muscles, tranversus abdominis
Greater splanchnic n.
Diaphragm, lumbar part
Left ascending lumbar v.
Quadratus lumborum
Psoas major
Abdominal aorta
Spinal cord
Lumbar vertebra
Intrinsic back muscles

A Superior view.

B Inferior view. *Removed:* Parietal peritoneum.

Arteries & Veins of the Thoracic Wall

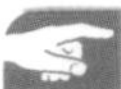

The posterior intercostal arteries anastomose with the anterior intercostal arteries to supply the structures of the thoracic wall. The posterior intercostal arteries branch from the thoracic aorta, with the exception of the 1st and 2nd, which arise from the superior intercostal artery (a branch of the costocervical trunk).

Table 6.5 Arteries of the thoracic wall

Origin	Branch
Axillary a.	Lateral thoracic a.
	Thoracoacromial a.
Subclavian a.	Posterior intercostal aa. (1st and 2nd; see p. 34)
	Superior thoracic a.
Thoracic aorta	Posterior intercostal aa. (3rd through 12th)
Internal thoracic a.	Anterior intercostal aa.
	Musculophrenic a.
	Superior epigastric a.

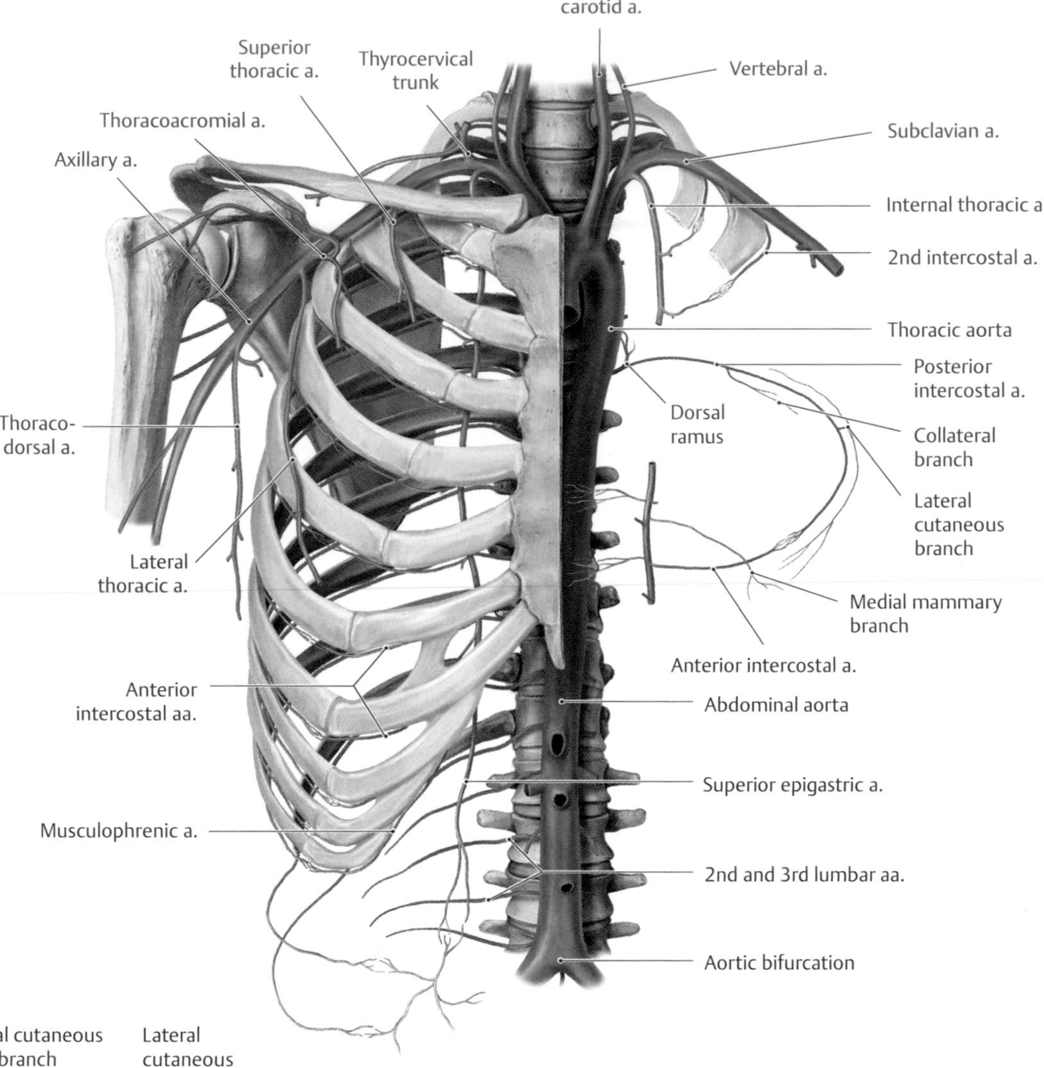

Common carotid a.
Superior thoracic a.
Thyrocervical trunk
Vertebral a.
Thoracoacromial a.
Subclavian a.
Axillary a.
Internal thoracic a.
2nd intercostal a.
Thoracic aorta
Posterior intercostal a.
Dorsal ramus
Collateral branch
Thoraco-dorsal a.
Lateral cutaneous branch
Lateral thoracic a.
Medial mammary branch
Anterior intercostal a.
Anterior intercostal aa.
Abdominal aorta
Superior epigastric a.
Musculophrenic a.
2nd and 3rd lumbar aa.
Aortic bifurcation

Fig. 6.17 **Arteries of the thoracic wall**
Anterior view.

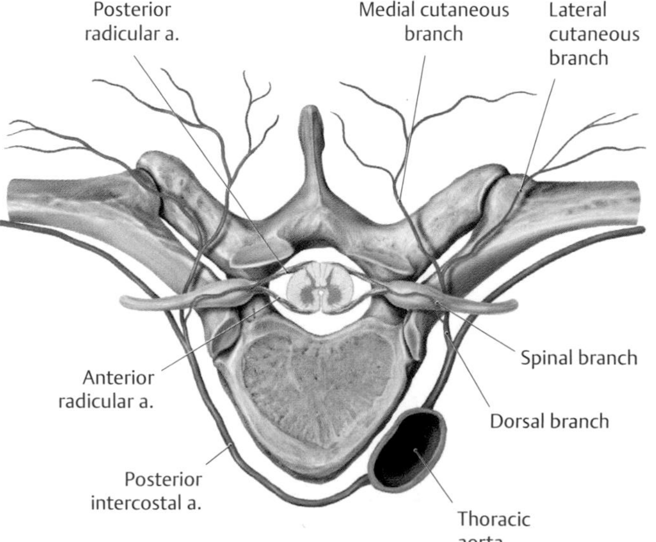

Posterior radicular a.
Medial cutaneous branch
Lateral cutaneous branch
Spinal branch
Anterior radicular a.
Dorsal branch
Posterior intercostal a.
Thoracic aorta

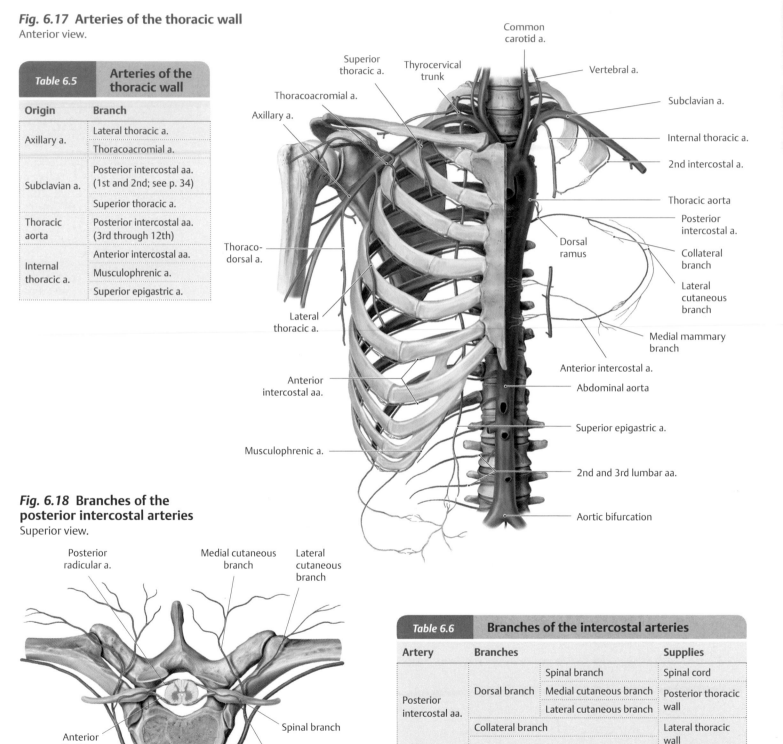

Fig. 6.18 **Branches of the posterior intercostal arteries**
Superior view.

Table 6.6 Branches of the intercostal arteries

Artery	Branches		Supplies
Posterior intercostal aa.	Dorsal branch	Spinal branch	Spinal cord
		Medial cutaneous branch	Posterior thoracic wall
		Lateral cutaneous branch	
	Collateral branch		Lateral thoracic wall
Anterior intercostal aa.	Lateral cutaneous branch*		Anterior thoracic wall

*The lateral mammary branch from the lateral cutaneous branch supplies the breast along with the medial mammary branch from the internal thoracic artery.

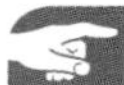

The intercostal veins drain primarily into the azygos system, but also into the internal thoracic vein. This blood ultimately returns to the heart via the superior vena cava. The intercostal veins follow a similar course to their arterial counterparts. However, the veins of the vertebral column form an external vertebral venous plexus that traverses the entire length of the spine (see p. 37).

Fig. 6.19 Veins of the thoracic wall

Internal jugular v.
Right brachiocephalic v.
Subclavian v.
Internal thoracic v.
Superior vena cava
Accessory hemiazygos v.
Azygos v.
Hemiazygos v.
Inferior vena cava
Anterior intercostal vv.
Internal thoracic vv.
Posterior intercostal vv.
Subcostal v. (12th intercostal v.)
1st lumbar v.

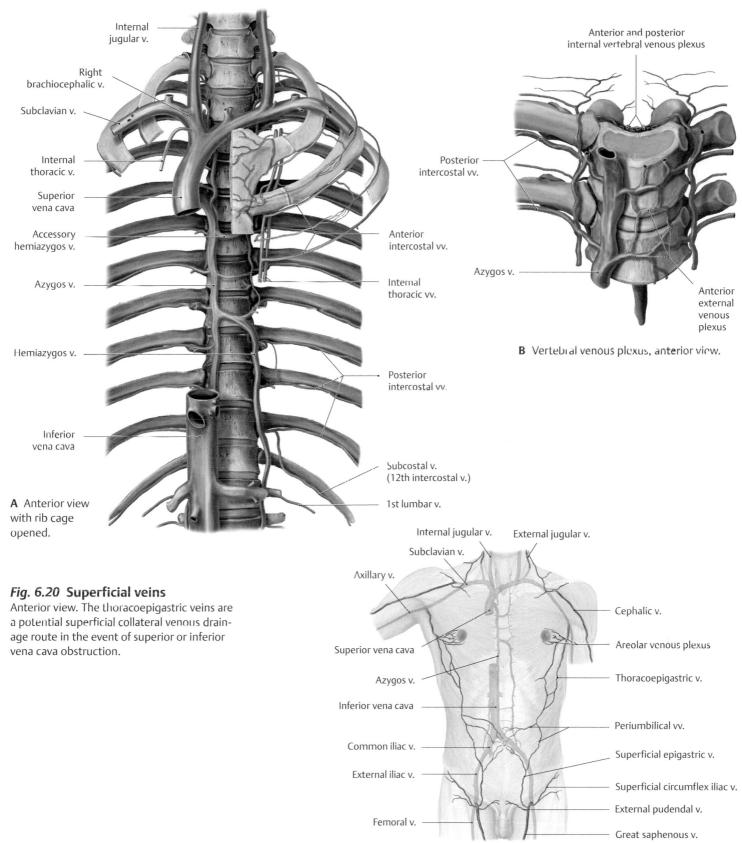

A Anterior view with rib cage opened.

Anterior and posterior internal vertebral venous plexus
Posterior intercostal vv.
Azygos v.
Anterior external venous plexus

B Vertebral venous plexus, anterior view.

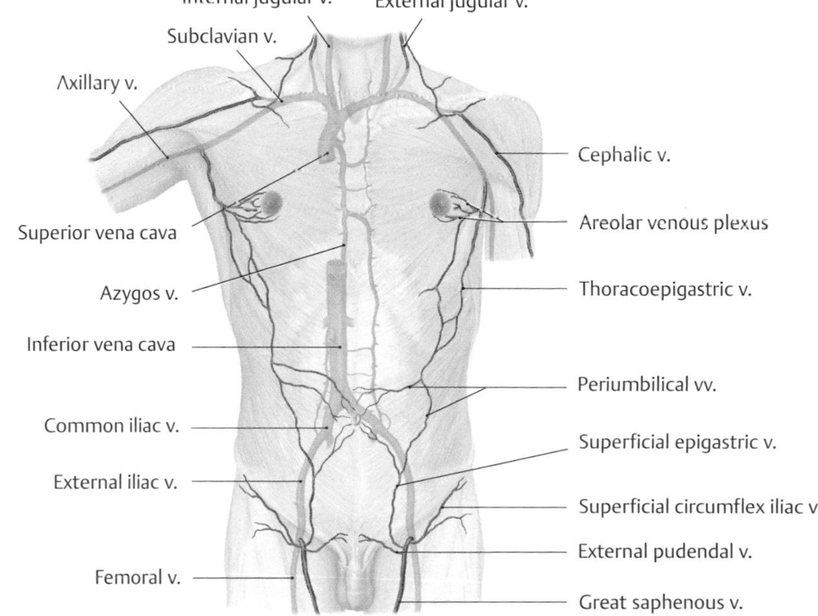

Internal jugular v.
External jugular v.
Subclavian v.
Axillary v.
Cephalic v.
Superior vena cava
Areolar venous plexus
Azygos v.
Thoracoepigastric v.
Inferior vena cava
Periumbilical vv.
Common iliac v.
Superficial epigastric v.
External iliac v.
Superficial circumflex iliac v.
External pudendal v.
Femoral v.
Great saphenous v.

Fig. 6.20 Superficial veins

Anterior view. The thoracoepigastric veins are a potential superficial collateral venous drainage route in the event of superior or inferior vena cava obstruction.

Nerves of the Thoracic Wall

Fig. 6.21 **Intercostal nerves**
Anterior view. The 1st rib has been removed to reveal the 1st and 2nd intercostal nerves.

Posterior (dorsal) ramus
1st and 2nd intercostal nn.
Lateral cutaneous branch
T1
Intercostobrachial nn.
Anterior cutaneous branch
3rd and 4th intercostal nn.
Anastomosis with medial brachial cutaneous n.
Sternal branches
Subcostal n. (12th intercostal n.)

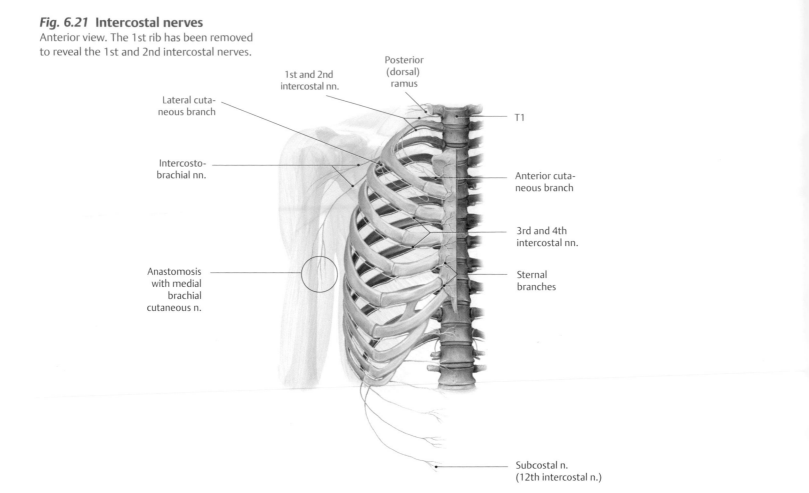

Fig. 6.22 **Cutaneous innervation of the thoracic wall**

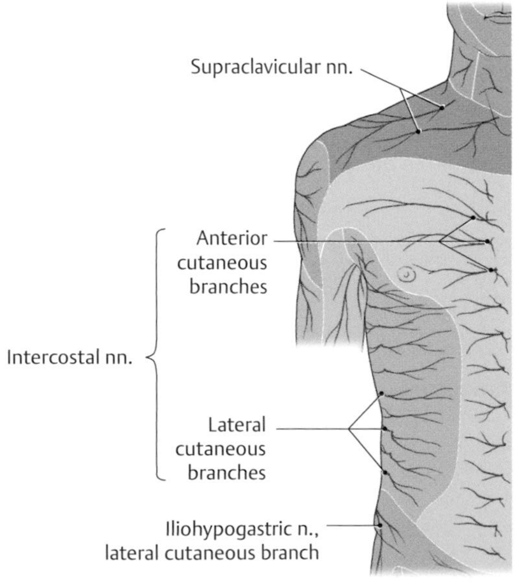

Supraclavicular nn.
Anterior cutaneous branches
Intercostal nn.
Lateral cutaneous branches
Iliohypogastric n., lateral cutaneous branch

A Anterior view.

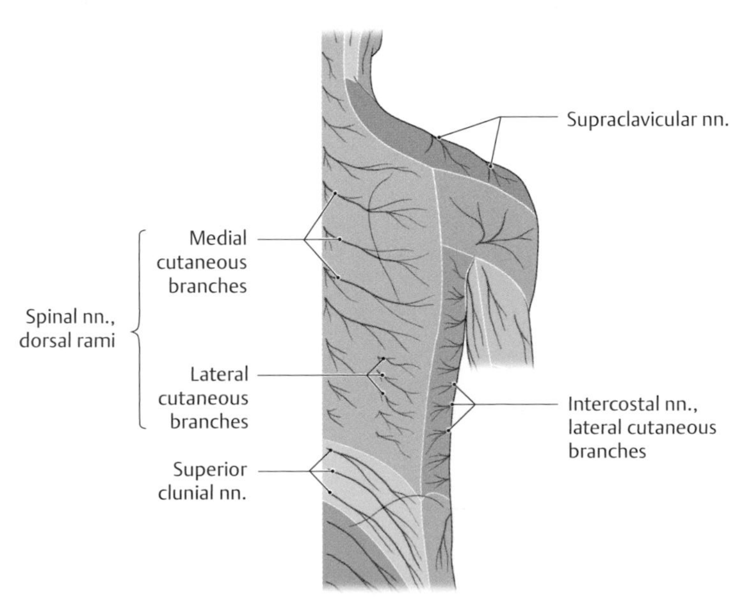

Supraclavicular nn.
Medial cutaneous branches
Spinal nn., dorsal rami
Lateral cutaneous branches
Intercostal nn., lateral cutaneous branches
Superior clunial nn.

B Posterior view.

Fig. 6.23 Spinal nerve branches

Superior view. The spinal nerve is formed by the union of posterior (dorsal) and anterior (ventral) roots. The posterior root contains sensory fibers and the anterior root contains motor fibers. The spinal nerve and all its subsequent branches are mixed nerves, containing both motor and sensory fibers. The spinal nerve exits the vertebral canal via the intervertebral foramen. Its posterior ramus innervates the skin and intrinsic muscles of the back; its anterior ramus forms the cervical, brachial, lumbar, and sacral plexuses, and the intercostal nerves. See p. 38 for more details.

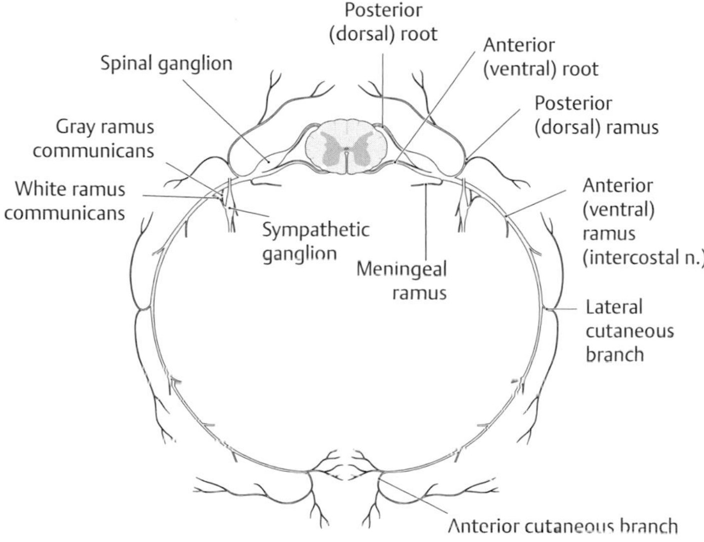
Posterior (dorsal) root
Anterior (ventral) root
Spinal ganglion
Posterior (dorsal) ramus
Gray ramus communicans
White ramus communicans
Anterior (ventral) ramus (intercostal n.)
Sympathetic ganglion
Meningeal ramus
Lateral cutaneous branch
Anterior cutaneous branch

Fig. 6.24 Course of the intercostal nerves

Coronal section, anterior view.

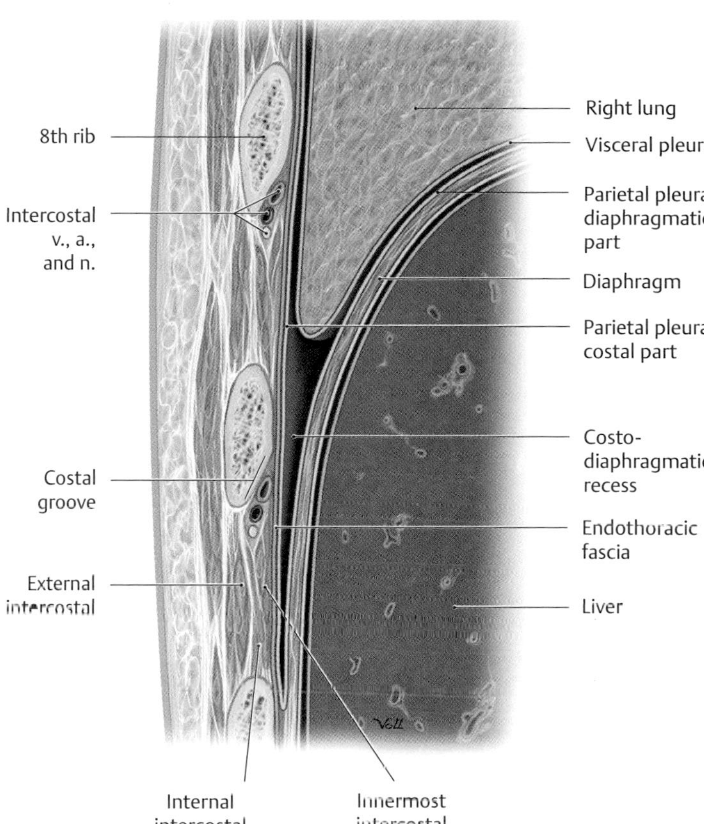
8th rib
Intercostal v., a., and n.
Costal groove
External intercostal
Internal intercostal
Innermost intercostal
Right lung
Visceral pleura
Parietal pleura, diaphragmatic part
Diaphragm
Parietal pleura, costal part
Costo-diaphragmatic recess
Endothoracic fascia
Liver

Fig. 6.25 Dermatomes of the thoracic wall

Landmarks: T4 generally includes the nipple; T6 innervates the skin over the xiphoid.

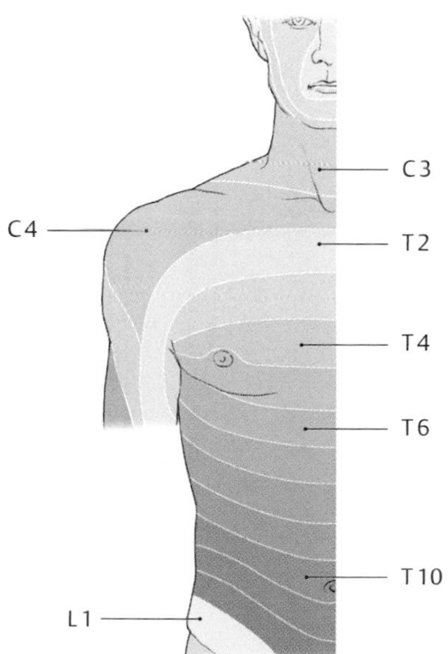
C3
C4
T2
T4
T6
T10
L1

A Anterior view.

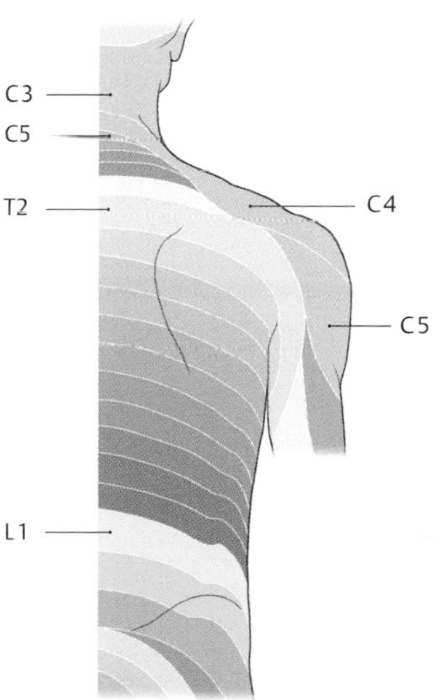
C3
C5
T2
C4
C5
L1

B Posterior view.

Neurovascular Topography of the Thoracic Wall

Fig. 6.26 **Anterior structures**
Anterior view (see Chapter 4 for neurovasculature of the back).

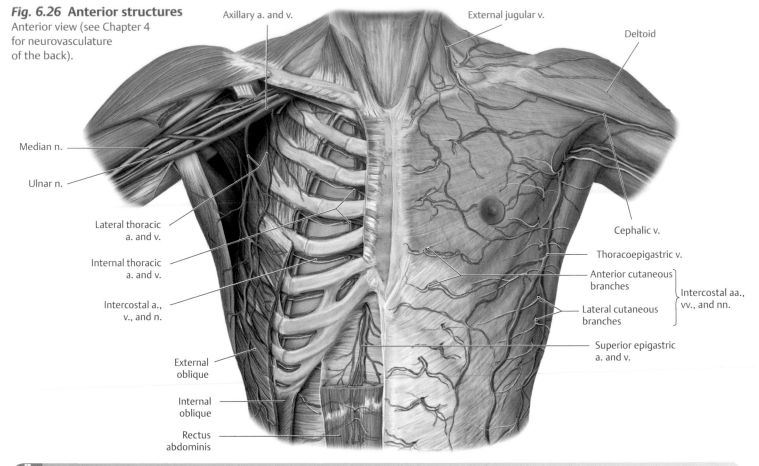

Axillary a. and v.
External jugular v.
Deltoid
Median n.
Ulnar n.
Lateral thoracic a. and v.
Internal thoracic a. and v.
Intercostal a., v., and n.
External oblique
Internal oblique
Rectus abdominis
Cephalic v.
Thoracoepigastric v.
Anterior cutaneous branches
Lateral cutaneous branches
Intercostal aa., vv., and nn.
Superior epigastric a. and v.

Clinical

Insertion of a chest tube

Abnormal fluid collection in the pleural space (e.g., pleural effusion due to bronchial carcinoma) may necessitate the insertion of a chest tube. Generally, the optimal puncture site in a sitting patient is at the level of the 7th or 8th intercostal space on the posterior axillary line. The drain should always be introduced at the upper margin of a rib to avoid injuring the intercostal vein, artery, and nerve. See p. 123 for details on collapsed lungs.

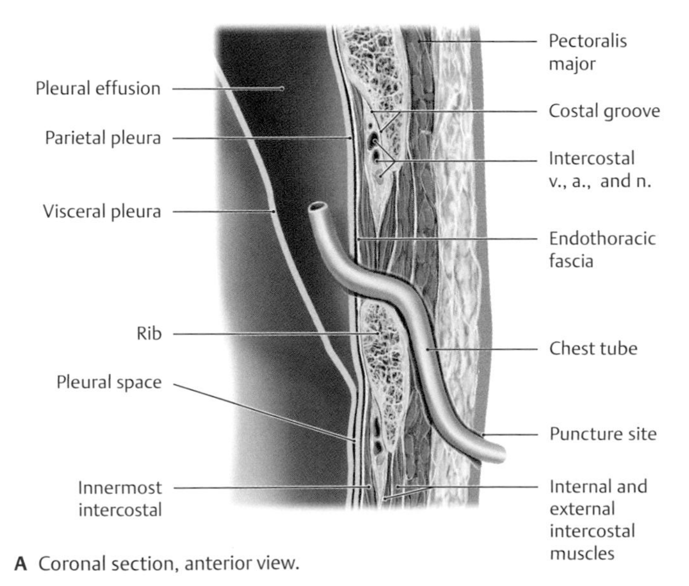
Pleural effusion
Parietal pleura
Visceral pleura
Rib
Pleural space
Innermost intercostal
Pectoralis major
Costal groove
Intercostal v., a., and n.
Endothoracic fascia
Chest tube
Puncture site
Internal and external intercostal muscles

A Coronal section, anterior view.

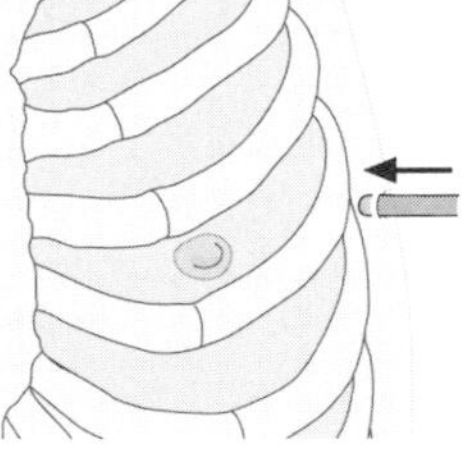

B Drainage tube is inserted perpendicular to chest wall.

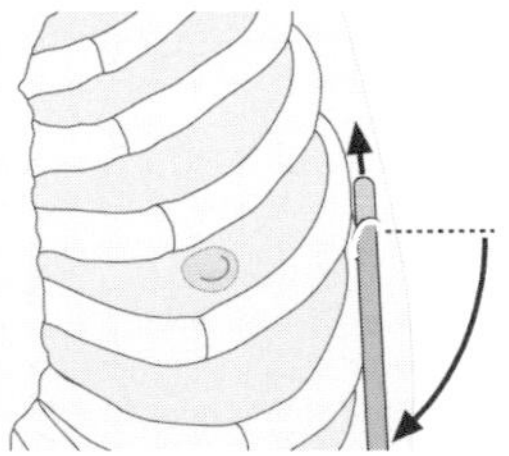

C At ribs, the tube is angled and advanced parallel to the chest wall in the subcutaneous plane.

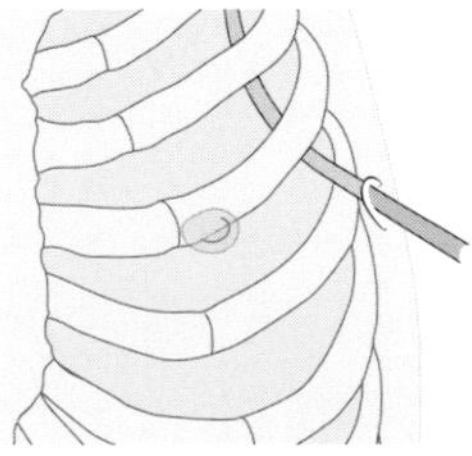

D At the superior margin of the rib, the tube is passed through the intercostal muscles and advanced into the pleural cavity.

Fig. 6.27 Intercostal structures in cross section
Transverse section, anterosuperior view. The relationship of the intercostal vessels in the costal groove, from superior to inferior, is vein, artery, and nerve (see clinical box, p. 68).

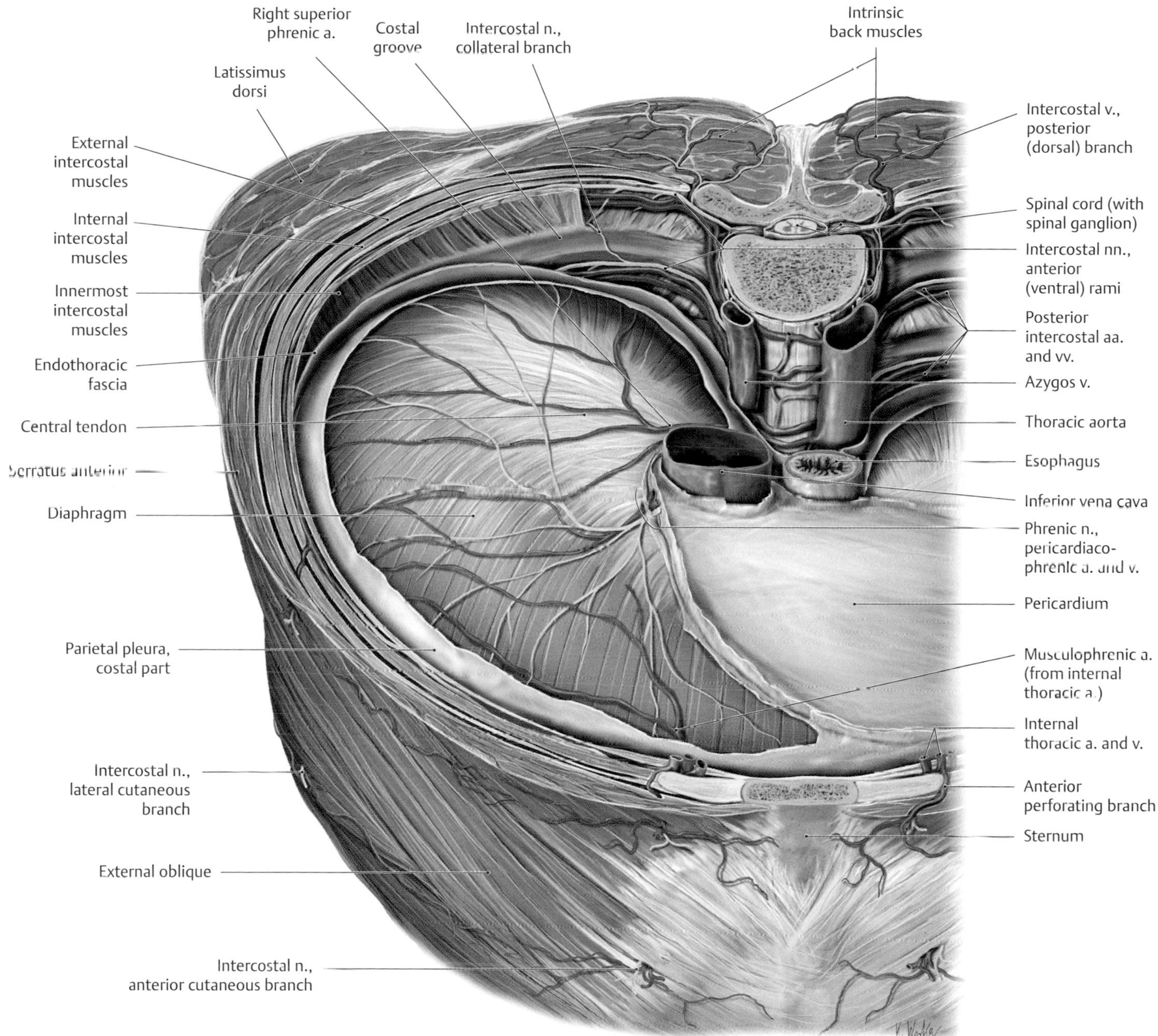
Right superior phrenic a.
Costal groove
Intercostal n., collateral branch
Intrinsic back muscles
Latissimus dorsi
External intercostal muscles
Internal intercostal muscles
Innermost intercostal muscles
Endothoracic fascia
Central tendon
Serratus anterior
Diaphragm
Parietal pleura, costal part
Intercostal n., lateral cutaneous branch
External oblique
Intercostal n., anterior cutaneous branch
Intercostal v., posterior (dorsal) branch
Spinal cord (with spinal ganglion)
Intercostal nn., anterior (ventral) rami
Posterior intercostal aa. and vv.
Azygos v.
Thoracic aorta
Esophagus
Inferior vena cava
Phrenic n., pericardiaco-phrenic a. and v.
Pericardium
Musculophrenic a. (from internal thoracic a.)
Internal thoracic a. and v.
Anterior perforating branch
Sternum

Female Breast

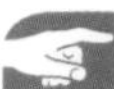

The female breast, a modified sweat gland in the subcutaneous tissue layer, consists of glandular tissue, fibrous stroma, and fat. The breast extends from the 2nd to the 6th rib and is loosely attached to the pectoral, axillary, and superficial abdominal fascia by connective tissue. The breast is additionally supported by suspensory ligaments. An extension of the breast tissue into the axilla, the axillary tail, is often present.

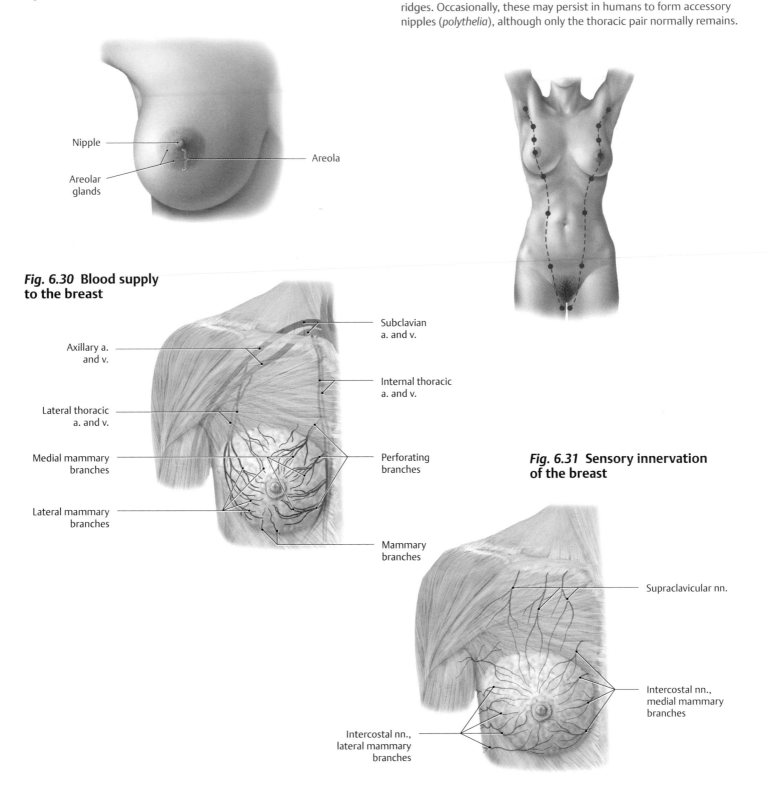

Fig. 6.28 **Female breast**
Right breast, anterior view.

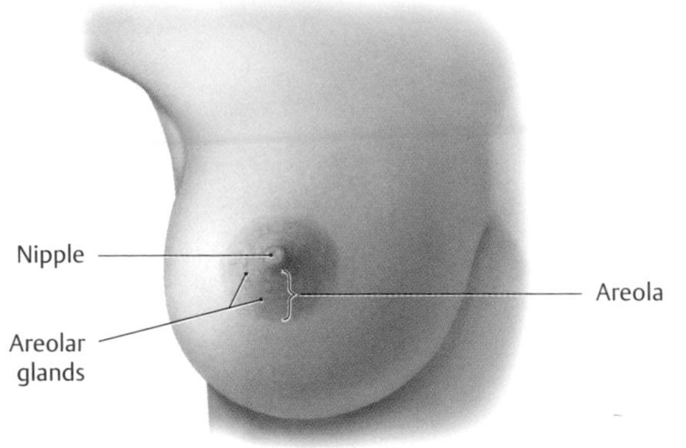
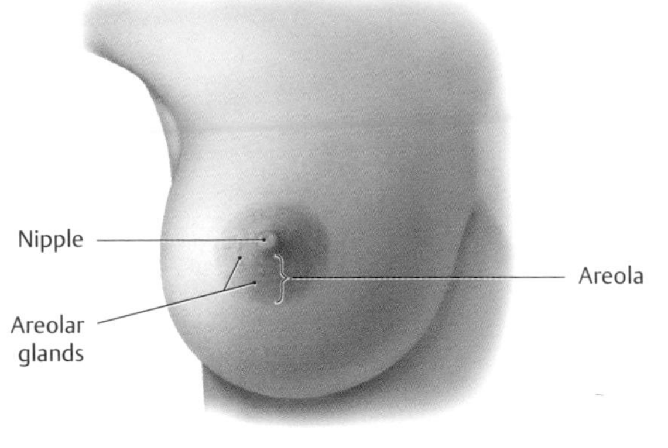
Nipple
Areola
Areolar glands

Fig. 6.29 **Mammary ridges**
Rudimentary mammary glands form in both sexes along the mammary ridges. Occasionally, these may persist in humans to form accessory nipples (*polythelia*), although only the thoracic pair normally remains.

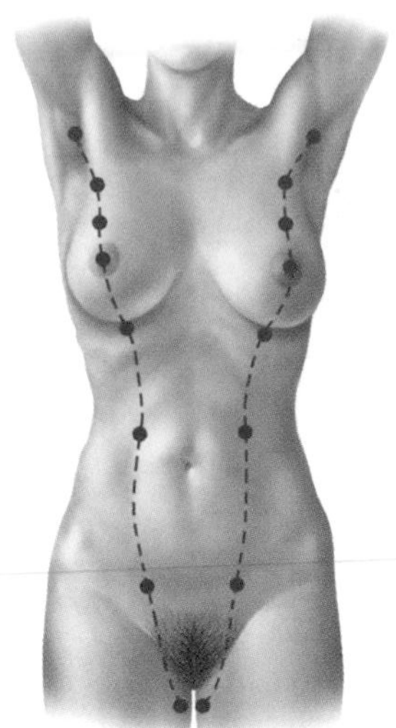

Fig. 6.30 **Blood supply to the breast**

Subclavian a. and v.
Axillary a. and v.
Internal thoracic a. and v.
Lateral thoracic a. and v.
Medial mammary branches
Perforating branches
Lateral mammary branches
Mammary branches

Fig. 6.31 **Sensory innervation of the breast**

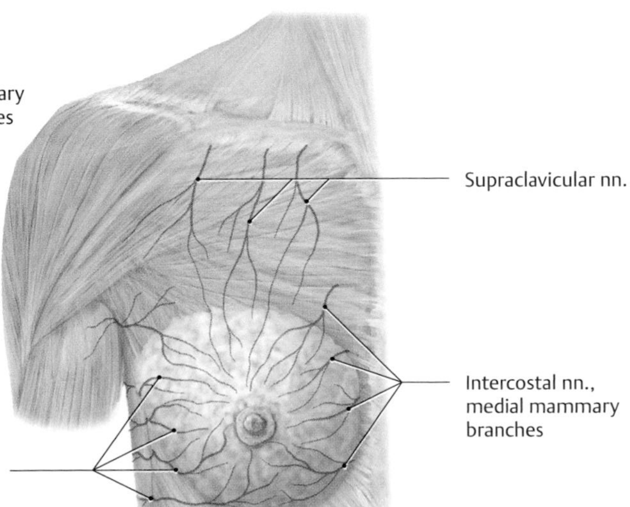
Supraclavicular nn.
Intercostal nn., medial mammary branches
Intercostal nn., lateral mammary branches

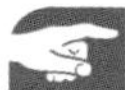

The glandular tissue is composed of 10 to 20 individual lobes, each with its own lactiferous duct. The gland ducts open on the elevated nipple at the center of the pigmented areola. Just proximal to the duct opening is a dilated portion called the lactiferous sinus. Areolar elevations are the openings of the areolar glands (sebaceous). The glands and lactiferous ducts are surrounded by firm, fibrofatty tissue with a rich blood supply.

Fig. 6.32 **Structures of the breast**

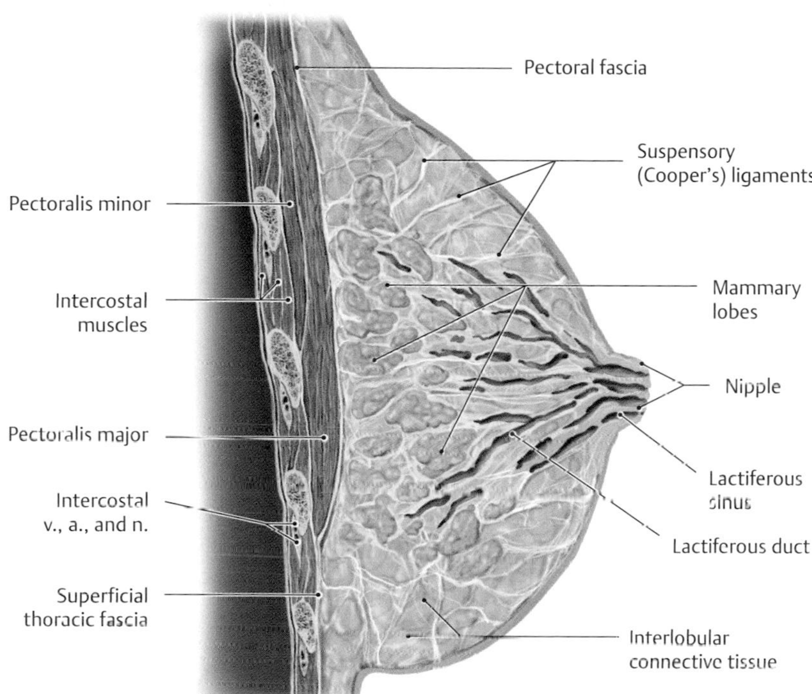
Pectoral fascia
Suspensory (Cooper's) ligaments
Pectoralis minor
Intercostal muscles
Mammary lobes
Nipple
Pectoralis major
Lactiferous sinus
Intercostal v., a., and n.
Lactiferous duct
Superficial thoracic fascia
Interlobular connective tissue

A Sagittal section along midclavicular line.

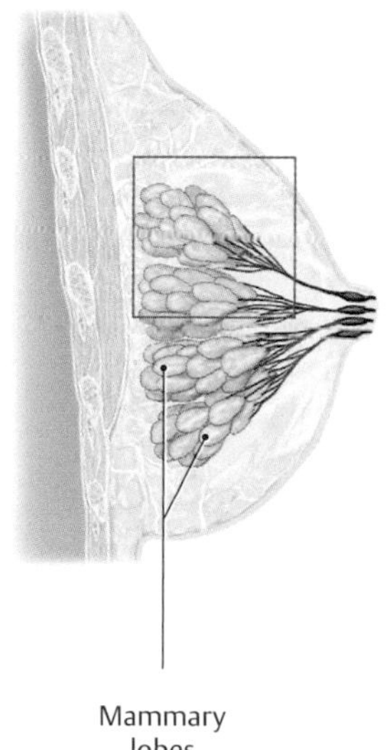
Mammary lobes

B Duct system and portions of a lobe, sagittal section. In the nonlactating breast (shown here), the lobules contain clusters of rudimentary acini.

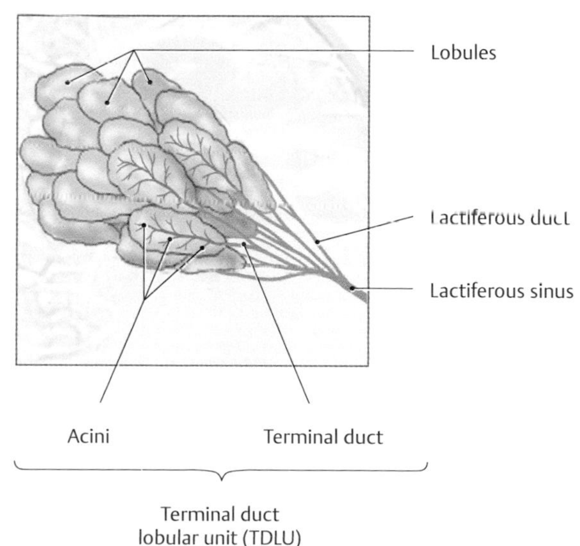
Lobules
Lactiferous duct
Lactiferous sinus
Acini
Terminal duct
Terminal duct lobular unit (TDLU)

C Terminal duct lobular unit (TDLU). The clustered acini composing the lobule empty into a terminal ductule; these structures are collectively known as the TDLU.

Lymphatics of the Female Breast

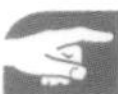

The lymphatic vessels of the breast (not shown) are divided into three systems: superficial, subcutaneous, and deep. These drain primarily into the axillary lymph nodes, which are classified based on their relationship to the pectoralis minor (Table 6.7). The medial portion of the breast is drained by the parasternal lymph nodes, which are associated with the internal thoracic vessels.

Fig. 6.33 Axillary lymph nodes

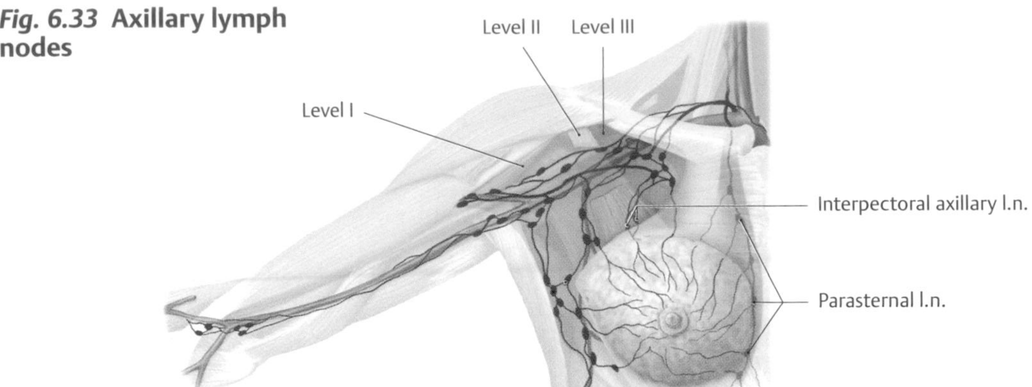
Level II
Level III
Level I
Interpectoral axillary l.n.
Parasternal l.n.

A Lymphatic drainage of the breast.

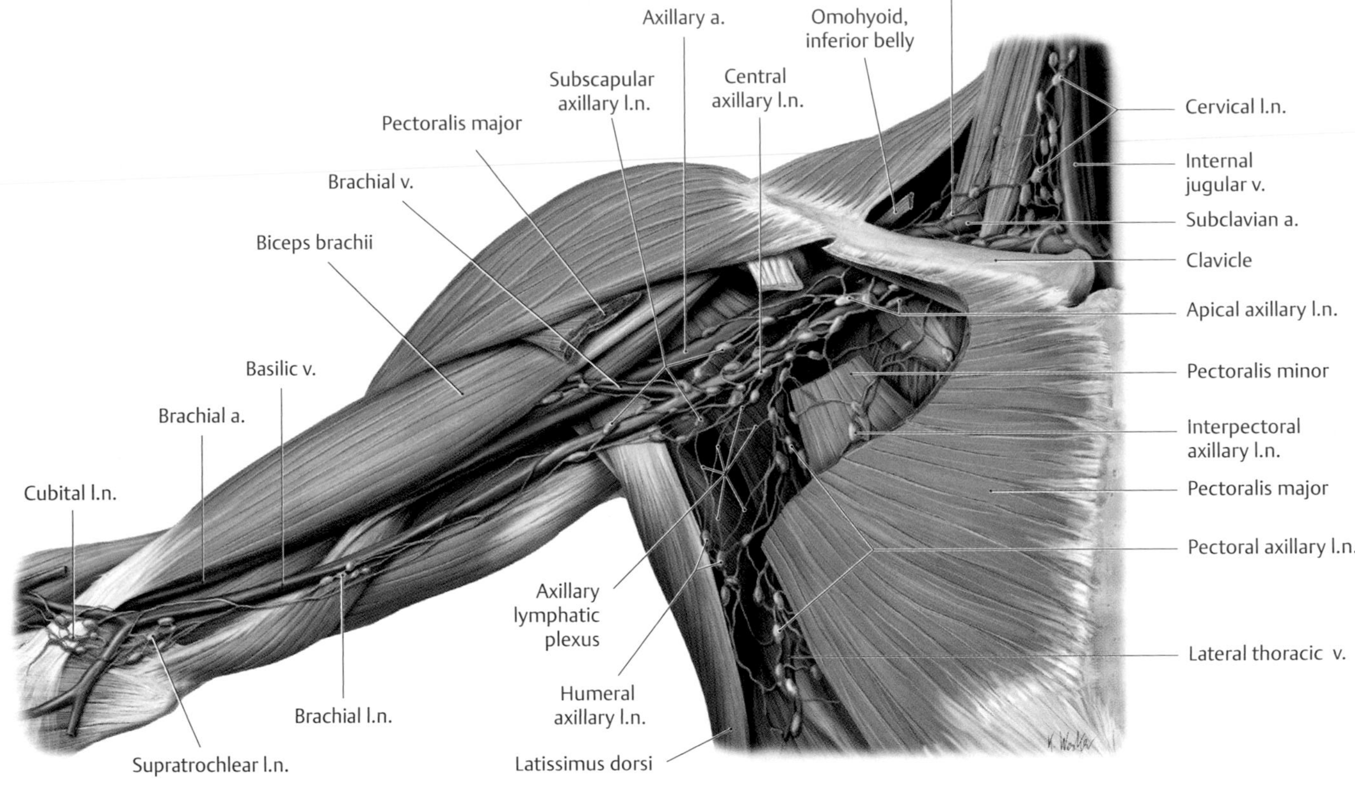
Supraclavicular l.n.
Axillary a.
Omohyoid, inferior belly
Subscapular axillary l.n.
Central axillary l.n.
Pectoralis major
Brachial v.
Biceps brachii
Basilic v.
Brachial a.
Cubital l.n.
Cervical l.n.
Internal jugular v.
Subclavian a.
Clavicle
Apical axillary l.n.
Pectoralis minor
Interpectoral axillary l.n.
Pectoralis major
Pectoral axillary l.n.
Lateral thoracic v.
Axillary lymphatic plexus
Humeral axillary l.n.
Brachial l.n.
Supratrochlear l.n.
Latissimus dorsi

B Anterior view.

Table 6.7 Levels of axillary lymph nodes

Level		Position	Lymph nodes (l.n.)
I	Lower axillary group	Lateral to pectoralis minor	Pectoral axillary l.n.
			Subscapular axillary l.n.
			Humeral axillary l.n.
II	Middle axillary group	Along pectoralis minor	Central l.n.
			Interpectoral axillary l.n.
III	Upper infraclavicular group	Medial to pectoralis minor	Apical axillary l.n.

Clinical

Breast cancer

Stem cells in the intralobular connective tissue give rise to tremendous cell growth, necessary for duct system proliferation and acini differentiation. This makes the terminal duct lobular unit (TDLU) the most common site of origin of malignant breast tumors.

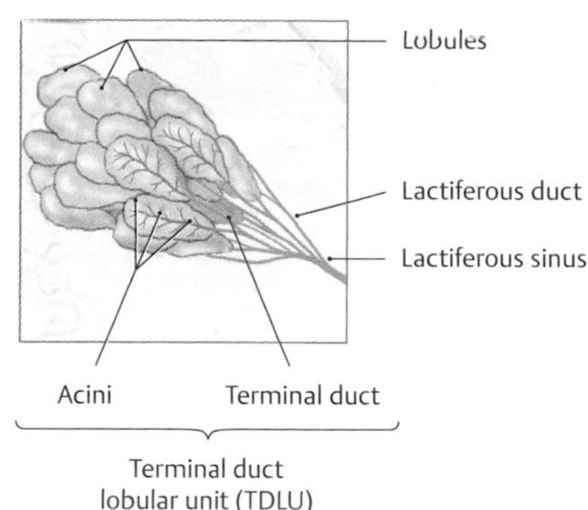
Lobules
Lactiferous duct
Lactiferous sinus
Acini
Terminal duct
Terminal duct
lobular unit (TDLU)

A Terminal duct lobular unit.

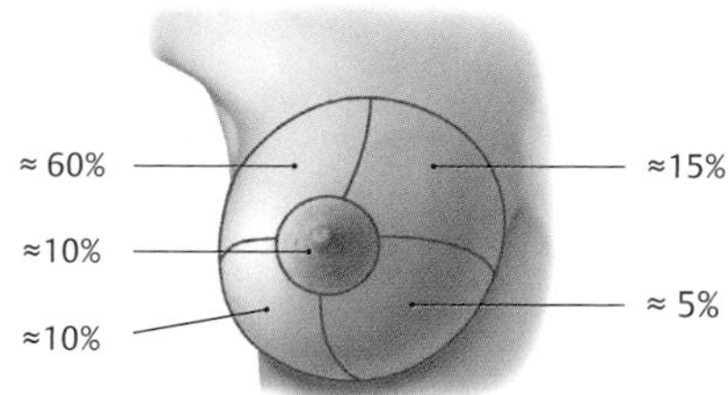
≈ 60%
≈10%
≈10%
≈15%
≈ 5%

B Origin of malignant tumors by quadrant.

Tumors originating in the breast spread via the lymphatic vessels. The deep system of lymphatic drainage (level III) is of particular importance, although the parasternal lymph nodes provide a route by which tumor cells may spread across the midline. The survival rate in breast cancer correlates most strongly with the number of lymph nodes involved at the axillary nodal level. Metastatic involvement is gauged through scintigraphic mapping with radiolabeled colloids (technetium [Tc] 99m sulfur microcolloid). The downstream sentinel node is the first to receive lymphatic drainage from the tumor and is therefore the first to be visualized with radiolabeling. Once identified, it can then be removed (via *sentinel lymphadenectomy*) and histologically examined for tumor cells. This method is 98% accurate in predicting the level of axillary nodal involvement.

Metastatic involvement	5-year survival rate
Level I	65%
Level II	31%
Level III	~0%

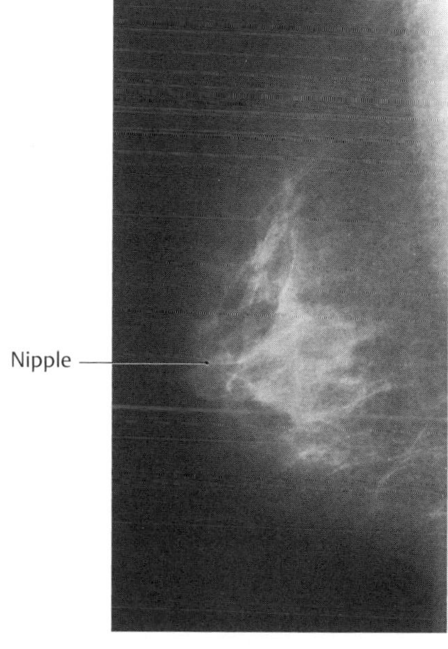
Nipple

C Normal mammogram.

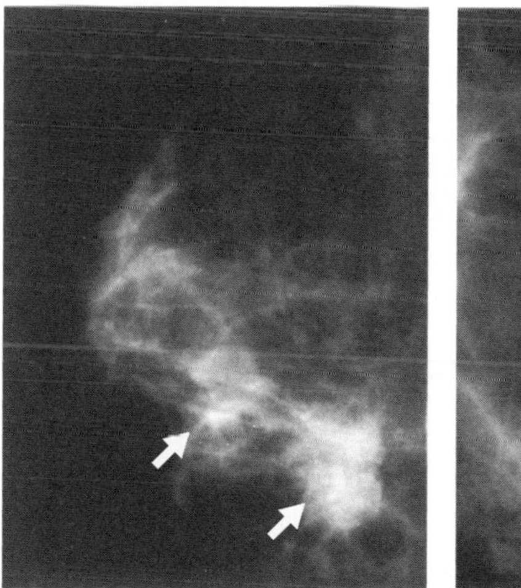

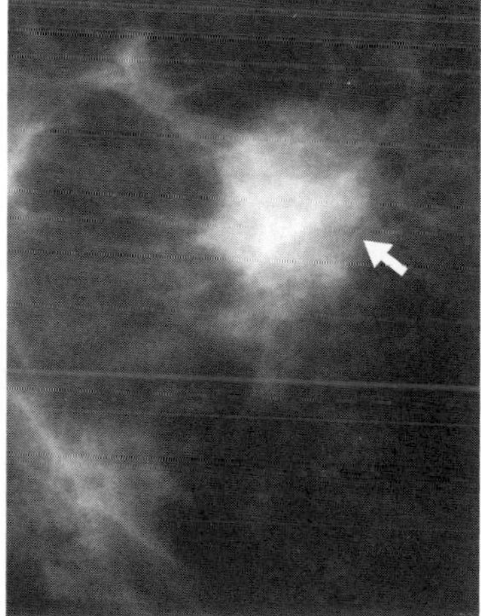

D Mammogram of invasive ductal carcinoma (irregular white areas, *arrows*). The large lesion has changed the architecture of the neighboring breast tissue.

Divisions of the Thoracic Cavity

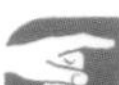

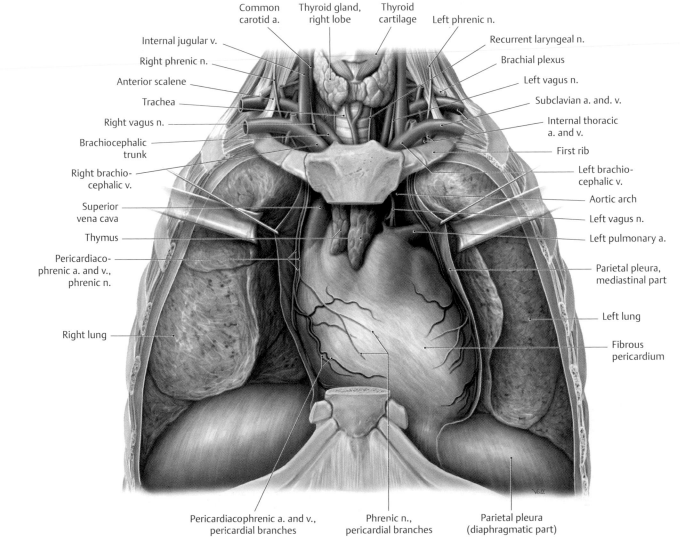

The thoracic cavity is divided into three large spaces: the mediastinum (p. 84) and the two pleural cavities (p. 110).

Fig. 7.1 Thoracic cavity
Coronal section, anterior view.

Superior mediastinum
Right pleural cavity (right lung)
Left pleural cavity (left lung)
Inferior mediastinum
Diaphragm

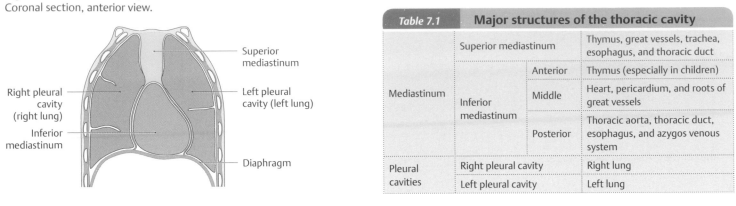

A Divisions of the thoracic cavity.

Table 7.1	Major structures of the thoracic cavity		
Mediastinum	Superior mediastinum		Thymus, great vessels, trachea, esophagus, and thoracic duct
	Inferior mediastinum	Anterior	Thymus (especially in children)
		Middle	Heart, pericardium, and roots of great vessels
		Posterior	Thoracic aorta, thoracic duct, esophagus, and azygos venous system
Pleural cavities	Right pleural cavity		Right lung
	Left pleural cavity		Left lung

Common carotid a.
Thyroid gland, right lobe
Thyroid cartilage
Left phrenic n.
Internal jugular v.
Recurrent laryngeal n.
Right phrenic n.
Brachial plexus
Anterior scalene
Left vagus n.
Trachea
Subclavian a. and v.
Right vagus n.
Internal thoracic a. and v.
Brachiocephalic trunk
First rib
Right brachio-cephalic v.
Left brachio-cephalic v.
Aortic arch
Superior vena cava
Left vagus n.
Thymus
Left pulmonary a.
Pericardiaco-phrenic a. and v., phrenic n.
Parietal pleura, mediastinal part
Left lung
Right lung
Fibrous pericardium
Pericardiacophrenic a. and v., pericardial branches
Phrenic n., pericardial branches
Parietal pleura (diaphragmatic part)

B Opened thoracic cavity. *Removed:* Thoracic wall; connective tissue of anterior mediastinum.

Fig. 7.2 Divisions of the mediastinum

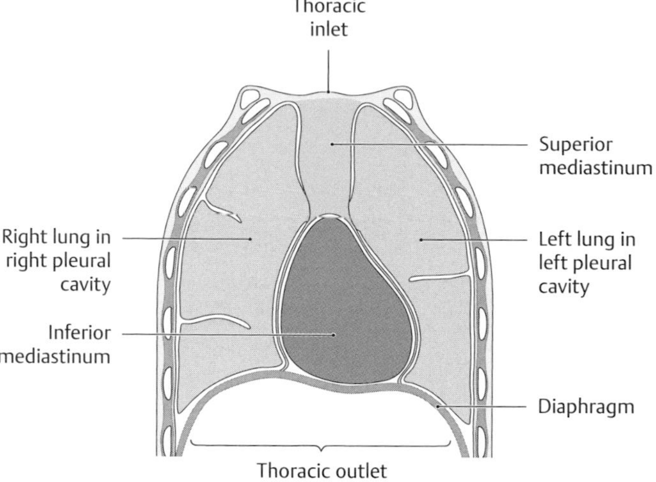
Thoracic inlet
Superior mediastinum
Right lung in right pleural cavity
Left lung in left pleural cavity
Inferior mediastinum
Diaphragm
Thoracic outlet

A Anterior view (coronal section).

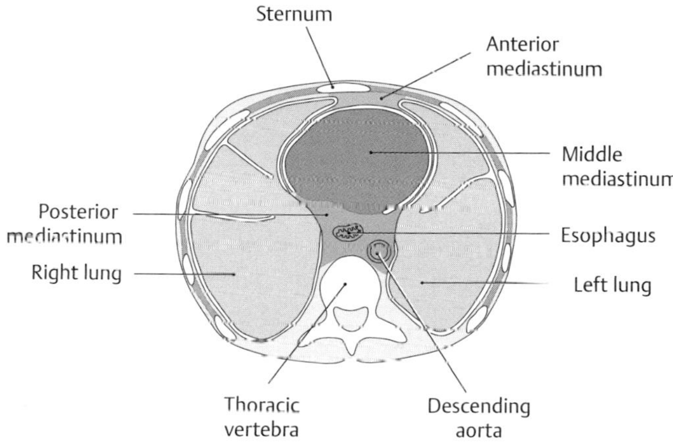
Sternum
Anterior mediastinum
Middle mediastinum
Posterior mediastinum
Esophagus
Right lung
Left lung
Thoracic vertebra
Descending aorta

C Inferior view (transverse section).

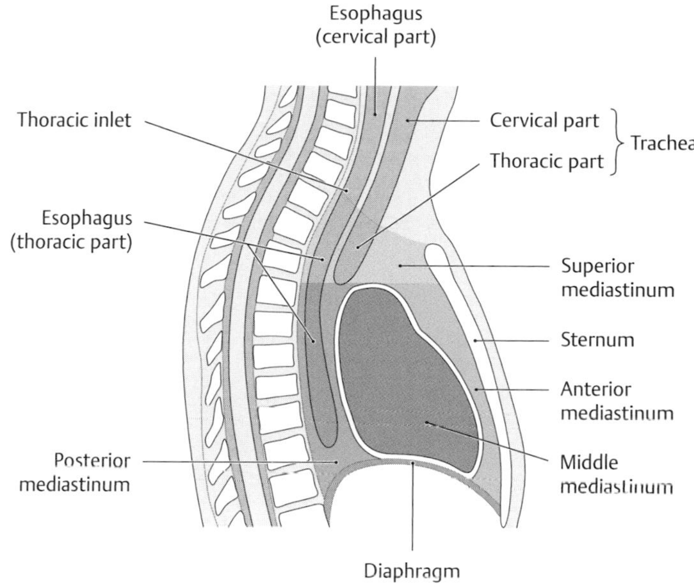
Esophagus (cervical part)
Thoracic inlet
Cervical part
Thoracic part
Trachea
Esophagus (thoracic part)
Superior mediastinum
Sternum
Anterior mediastinum
Posterior mediastinum
Middle mediastinum
Diaphragm

B Lateral view (midsagittal section).

Fig. 7.3 Transverse sections of the thorax

Computed tomography (CT) scan of thorax, inferior view.

Superior vena cava
Ascending aorta
Right and left main bronchii
Esophagus
Descending aorta

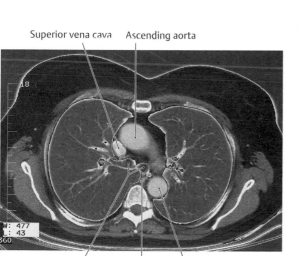

A Superior mediastinum.

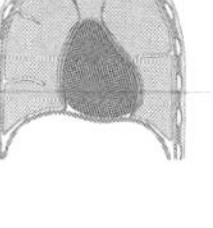

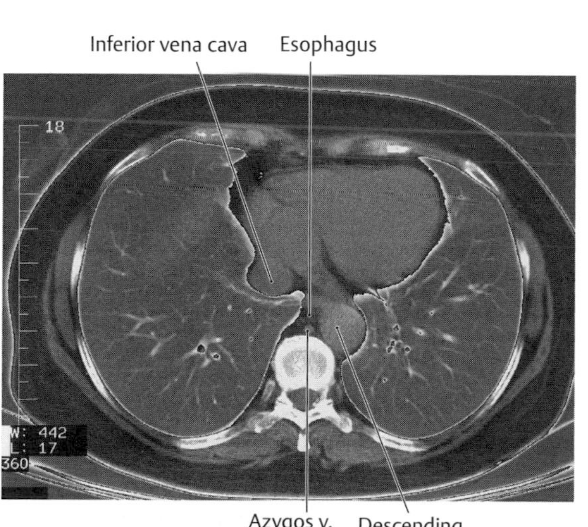
Inferior vena cava
Esophagus
Azygos v.
Descending aorta

B Inferior mediastinum.

Arteries of the Thoracic Cavity

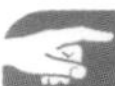

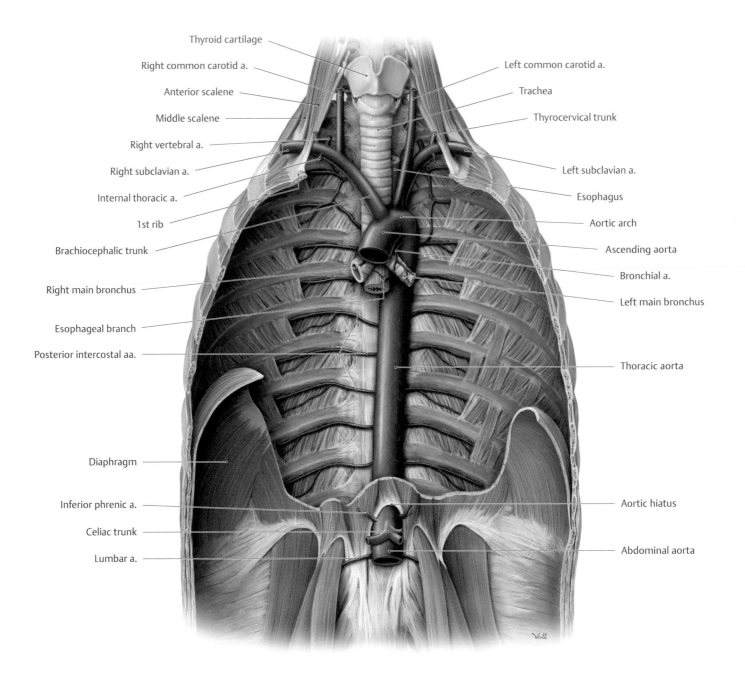

The arch of the aorta has three major branches: the brachiocephalic trunk, left common carotid artery, and left subclavian artery. After the aortic arch, the aorta begins its descent, becoming the thoracic aorta at the level of the sternal angle and the abdominal aorta once it passes through the aortic hiatus in the diaphragm.

Fig. 7.4 Thoracic aorta

Thyroid cartilage
Right common carotid a.
Anterior scalene
Middle scalene
Right vertebral a.
Right subclavian a.
Internal thoracic a.
1st rib
Brachiocephalic trunk
Right main bronchus
Esophageal branch
Posterior intercostal aa.
Diaphragm
Inferior phrenic a.
Celiac trunk
Lumbar a.
Left common carotid a.
Trachea
Thyrocervical trunk
Left subclavian a.
Esophagus
Aortic arch
Ascending aorta
Bronchial a.
Left main bronchus
Thoracic aorta
Aortic hiatus
Abdominal aorta

A Thoracic aorta in situ, anterior view. *Removed:* Heart, lungs, portions of diaphragm.

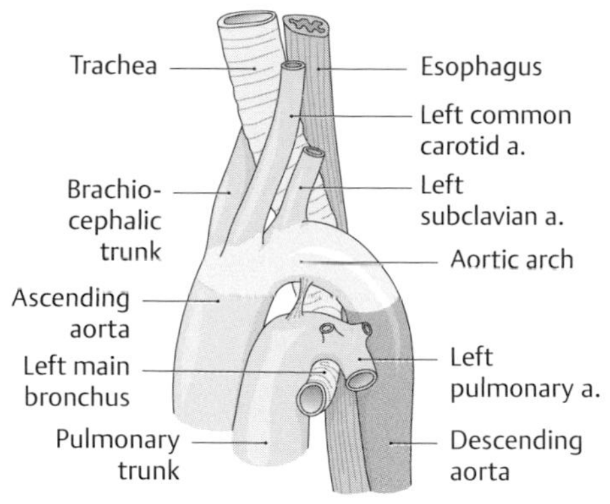
Trachea
Esophagus
Left common carotid a.
Brachio-cephalic trunk
Left subclavian a.
Aortic arch
Ascending aorta
Left main bronchus
Left pulmonary a.
Pulmonary trunk
Descending aorta

B Parts of the aorta, left lateral view. *Note:* The aortic arch begins and ends at the level of the sternal angle (see p. 54).

Table 7.2 Branches of the thoracic aorta

The thoracic organs are supplied by direct branches from the thoracic aorta, as well as indirect branches from the subclavian arteries.

Branches			Region supplied
Brachiocephalic trunk	Right subclavian a.		See left subclavian a.
	Right common carotid a.		Head and neck
Left common carotid a.			
Left subclavian a.	Vertebral a.		
	Internal thoracic a.	Anterior intercostal aa.	Anterior chest wall
		Thymic branches	Thymus
		Mediastinal branches	Posterior mediastinum
		Pericardiacophrenic a.	Pericardium, diaphragm
	Thyrocervical trunk	Inferior thyroid a.	Esophagus, trachea, thyroid gland
	Costocervical trunk	Superior intercostal a.	Chest wall
Descending thoracic aorta	Visceral branches		Bronchi, trachea, esophagus
	Parietal branches	Posterior intercostal aa.	Posterior chest wall
		Superior phrenic aa.	Diaphragm
Ascending aorta	Right and left coronary aa.		Heart

Clinical

Aortic dissection

A tear in the inner wall (intima) of the aorta allows blood to separate the layers of the aortic wall, creating a "false lumen" and potentially resulting in life-threatening aortic rupture. Symptoms are dyspnea (shortness of breath) and sudden onset of excruciating pain. Acute aortic dissections occur most often in the ascending aorta and generally require surgery. More distal aortic dissections may be treated conservatively, provided there are no complications (e.g., obstruction of blood supply to the organs, in which case a stent may be inserted to restore perfusion). Aortic dissections occurring at the base of a coronary artery may cause myocardial infarction.

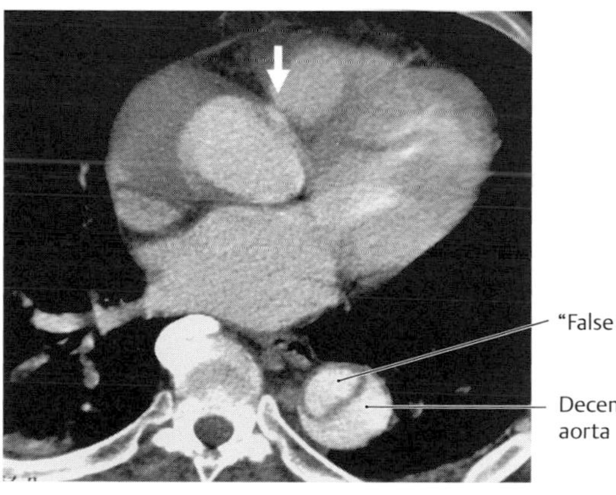
"False lumen"
Decending aorta

A Aortic dissection. Parts of the intima are still attached to the connective tissue in the wall of the aorta (*arrow*).

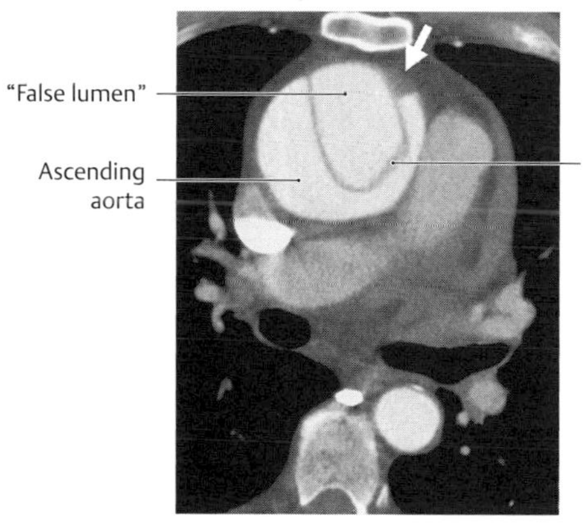
"False lumen"
Ascending aorta
Intima

B The flow in the coronary arteries is intact (*arrow*).

Veins of the Thoracic Cavity

The superior vena cava is formed by the union of the two brachiocephalic veins at the level of the T2–T3 junction. It receives blood drained by the azygos system (the inferior vena cava has no tributaries in the thorax).

Fig. 7.5 Superior vena cava and azygos system

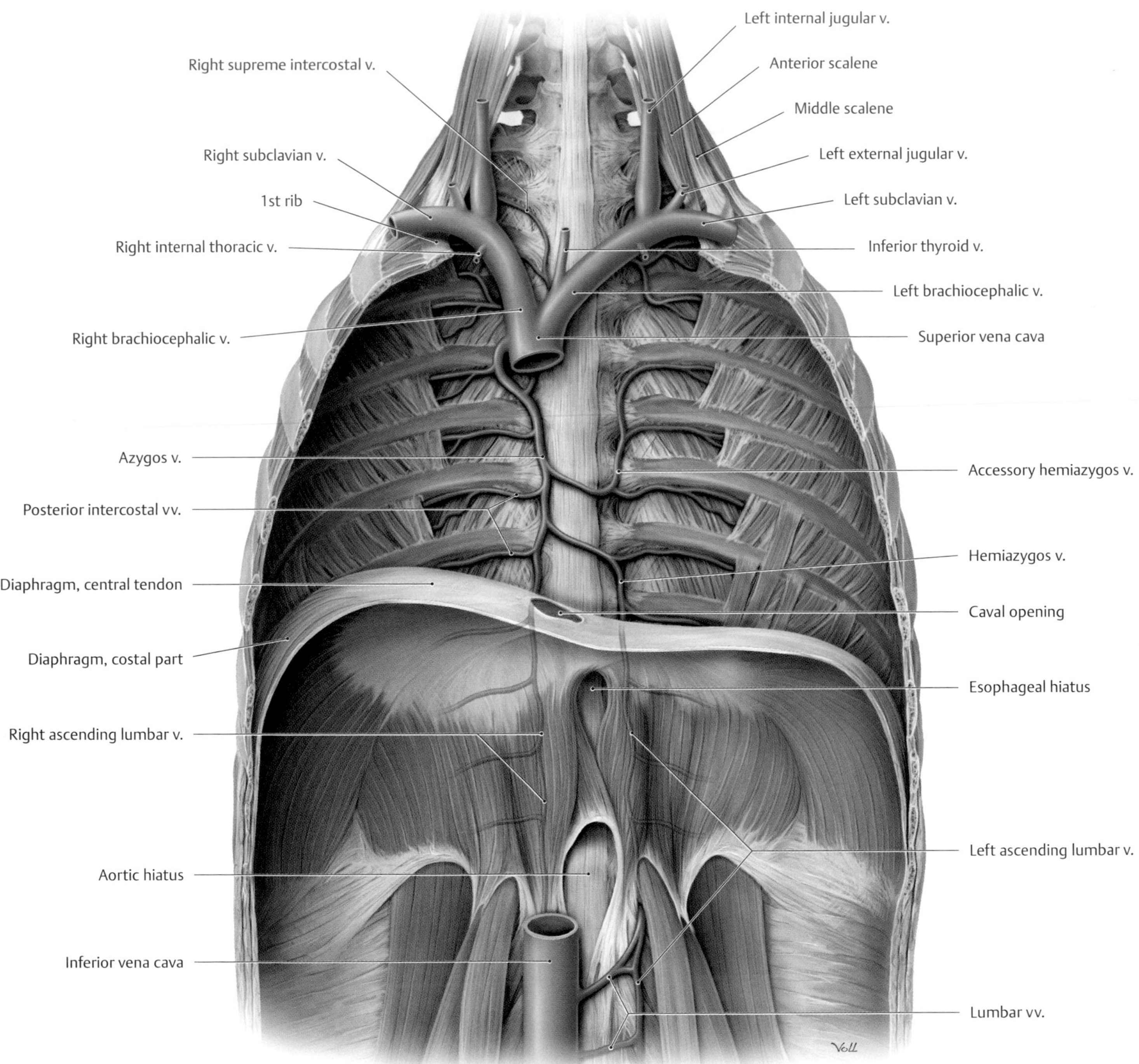

Left internal jugular v.
Anterior scalene
Middle scalene
Left external jugular v.
Left subclavian v.
Inferior thyroid v.
Left brachiocephalic v.
Superior vena cava
Accessory hemiazygos v.
Hemiazygos v.
Caval opening
Esophageal hiatus
Left ascending lumbar v.
Lumbar vv.
Right supreme intercostal v.
Right subclavian v.
1st rib
Right internal thoracic v.
Right brachiocephalic v.
Azygos v.
Posterior intercostal vv.
Diaphragm, central tendon
Diaphragm, costal part
Right ascending lumbar v.
Aortic hiatus
Inferior vena cava
Voll

A Veins of the thoracic cavity, anterior view of opened thorax.

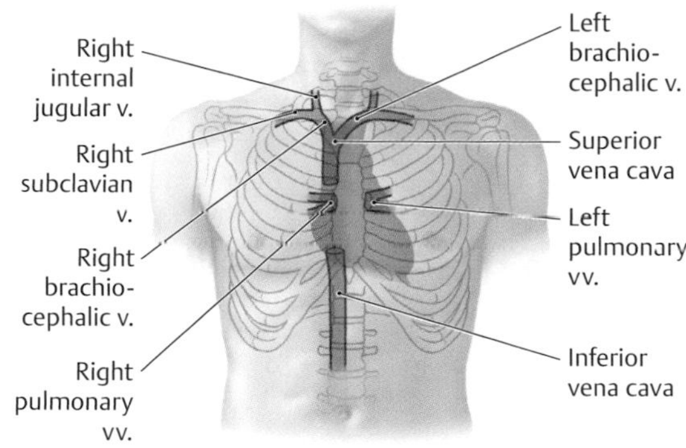

Right internal jugular v.
Right subclavian v.
Right brachio-cephalic v.
Right pulmonary vv.
Left brachio-cephalic v.
Superior vena cava
Left pulmonary vv.
Inferior vena cava

B Projection of venae cavae onto chest, anterior view.

Table 7.3 Thoracic tributaries of the superior vena cava

Major vein	Tributaries		Region drained
Brachiocephalic vv.	Inferior thyroid v.		Esophagus, trachea, thyroid gland
	Internal jugular vv.		Head, neck, upper limb
	External jugular vv.		
	Subclavian vv.		
	Supreme intercostal vv.		
	Pericardial vv.		
	Left superior intercostal v.		
Azygos system (left side: accessory hemiazygos v.; right side: azygos v.)	Visceral branches		Trachea, bronchi, esophagus
	Parietal branches	Posterior intercostal vv.	Inner chest wall and diaphragm
		Superior phrenic vv.	
		Right superior intercostal v.	
Internal thoracic v.	Thymic vv.		Thymus
	Mediastinal tributaries		Posterior mediastinum
	Anterior intercostal vv.		Anterior chest wall
	Pericardiacophrenic v.		Pericardium
	Musculophrenic v.		Diaphragm

Note: Structures of the superior mediastinum may also drain directly to the brachiocephalic veins via the tracheal, esophageal, and mediastinal veins.

Fig. 7.6 **Azygos system**
Anterior view.

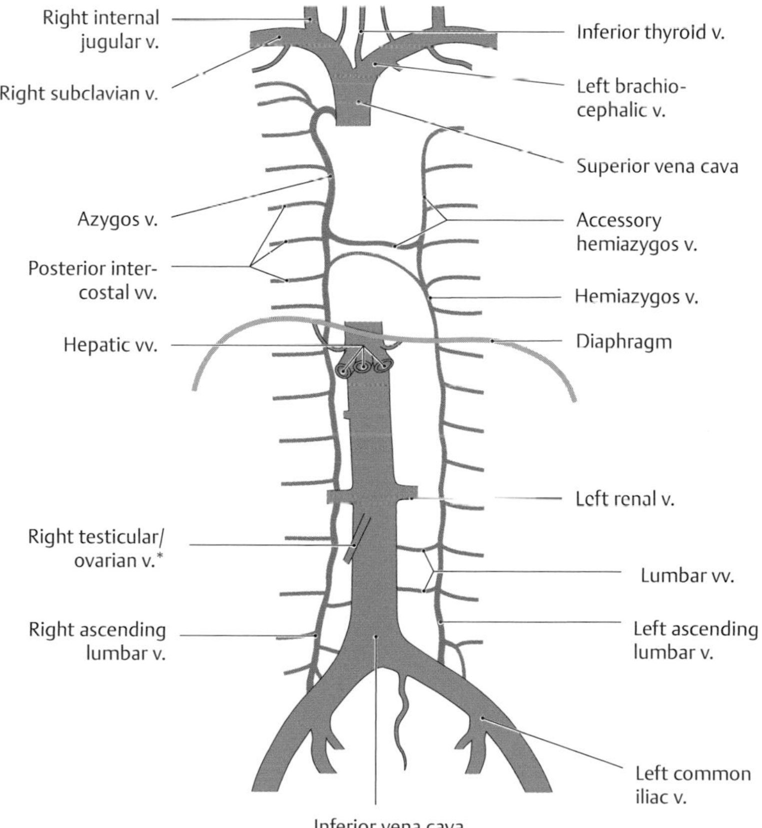

Right internal jugular v.
Right subclavian v.
Azygos v.
Posterior inter-costal vv.
Hepatic vv.
Right testicular/ ovarian v.*
Right ascending lumbar v.
Inferior vena cava
Inferior thyroid v.
Left brachio-cephalic v.
Superior vena cava
Accessory hemiazygos v.
Hemiazygos v.
Diaphragm
Left renal v.
Lumbar vv.
Left ascending lumbar v.
Left common iliac v.

*The left testicular/ovarian vein arises from the left renal vein.

Lymphatics of the Thoracic Cavity

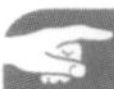

The body's chief lymph vessel is the thoracic duct. Beginning in the abdomen at the level of L1 as the *cisterna chyli*, the thoracic duct empties into the junction of the left internal jugular and subclavian veins. The right lymphatic duct drains to the right junction of the internal jugular and subclavian veins.

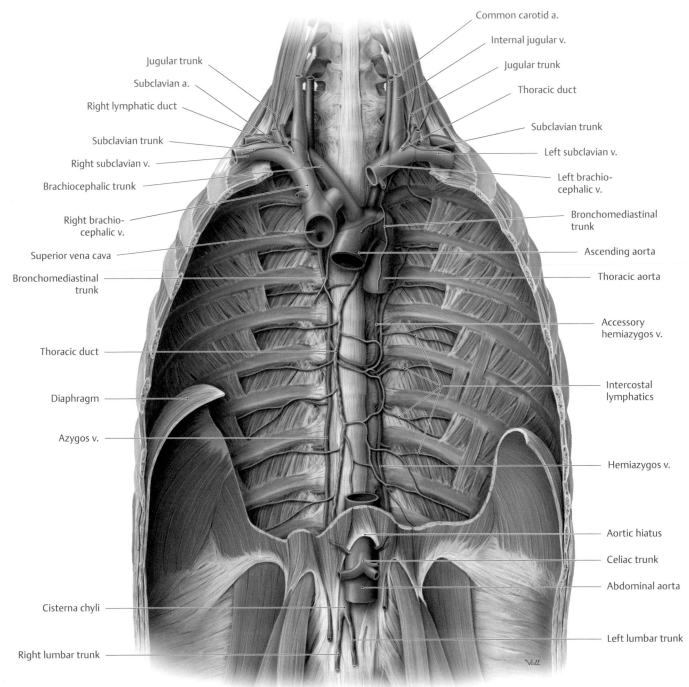

Common carotid a.
Internal jugular v.
Jugular trunk
Thoracic duct
Subclavian trunk
Left subclavian v.
Left brachio-cephalic v.
Bronchomediastinal trunk
Ascending aorta
Thoracic aorta
Accessory hemiazygos v.
Intercostal lymphatics
Hemiazygos v.
Aortic hiatus
Celiac trunk
Abdominal aorta
Left lumbar trunk
Jugular trunk
Subclavian a.
Right lymphatic duct
Subclavian trunk
Right subclavian v.
Brachiocephalic trunk
Right brachio-cephalic v.
Superior vena cava
Bronchomediastinal trunk
Thoracic duct
Diaphragm
Azygos v.
Cisterna chyli
Right lumbar trunk

Fig. 7.7 **Lymphatic trunks in the thorax**
Anterior view of opened thorax.

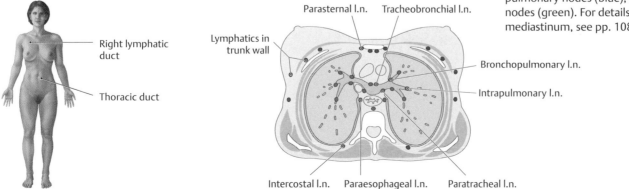

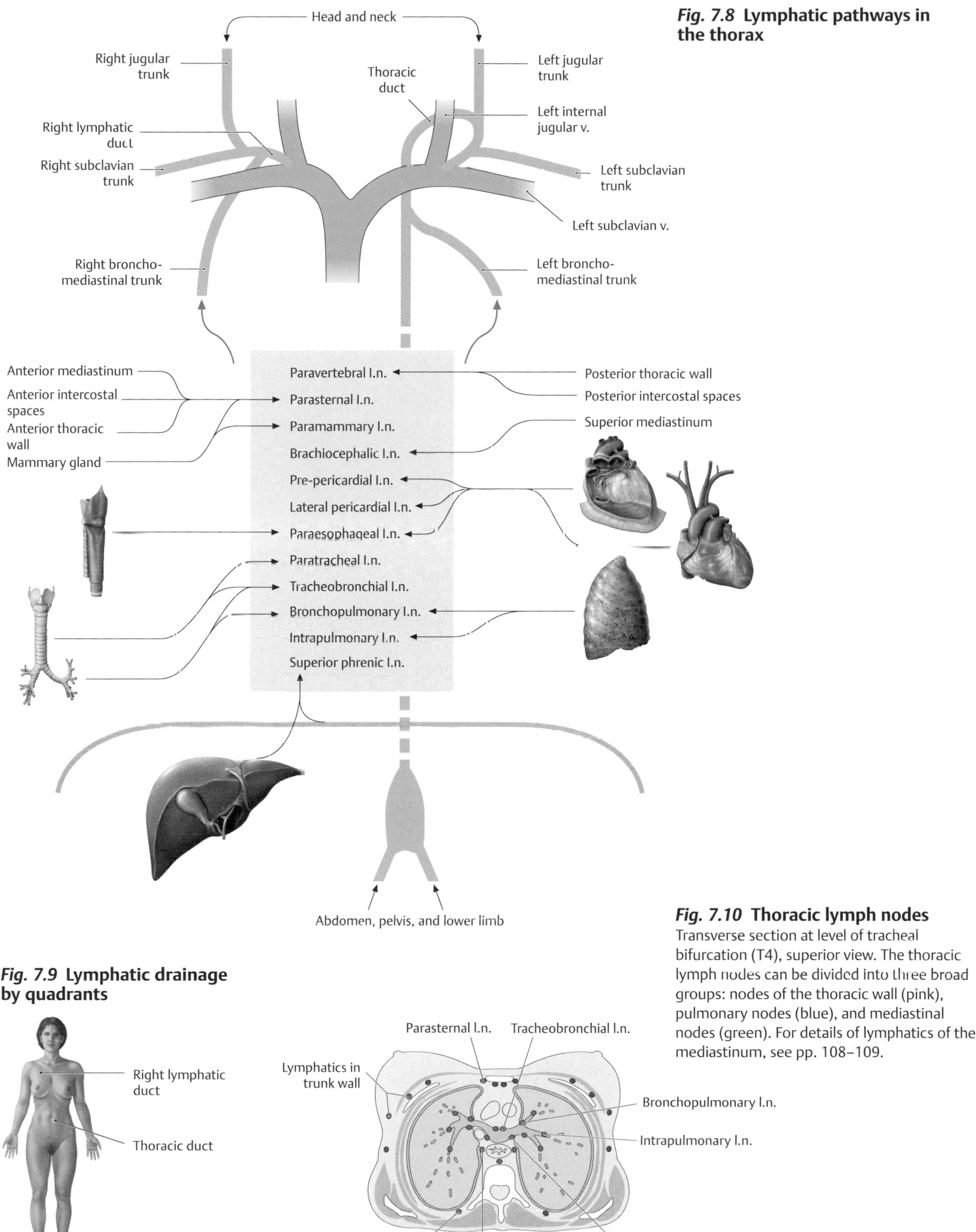
Head and neck
Right jugular trunk
Thoracic duct
Left jugular trunk
Left internal jugular v.
Right lymphatic duct
Right subclavian trunk
Left subclavian trunk
Left subclavian v.
Right broncho-mediastinal trunk
Left broncho-mediastinal trunk
Anterior mediastinum
Anterior intercostal spaces
Anterior thoracic wall
Mammary gland
Paravertebral l.n.
Parasternal l.n.
Paramammary l.n.
Brachiocephalic l.n.
Pre-pericardial l.n.
Lateral pericardial l.n.
Paraesophageal l.n.
Paratracheal l.n.
Tracheobronchial l.n.
Bronchopulmonary l.n.
Intrapulmonary l.n.
Superior phrenic l.n.
Posterior thoracic wall
Posterior intercostal spaces
Superior mediastinum
Abdomen, pelvis, and lower limb
Right lymphatic duct
Thoracic duct
Parasternal l.n.
Tracheobronchial l.n.
Lymphatics in trunk wall
Bronchopulmonary l.n.
Intrapulmonary l.n.
Intercostal l.n.
Paraesophageal l.n.
Paratracheal l.n.

Fig. 7.8 **Lymphatic pathways in the thorax**

Fig. 7.9 **Lymphatic drainage by quadrants**

Fig. 7.10 **Thoracic lymph nodes**
Transverse section at level of tracheal bifurcation (T4), superior view. The thoracic lymph nodes can be divided into three broad groups: nodes of the thoracic wall (pink), pulmonary nodes (blue), and mediastinal nodes (green). For details of lymphatics of the mediastinum, see pp. 108–109.

Nerves of the Thoracic Cavity

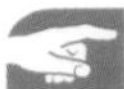

Thoracic innervation is mostly autonomic, arising from the paravertebral sympathetic trunks and parasympathetic vagus nerves. There are two exceptions: the phrenic nerves innervate the pericardium and diaphragm (p. 62) and the intercostal nerves innervate the thoracic wall (p. 66).

Fig. 7.11 Nerves in the thorax
Anterior view of opened thorax.

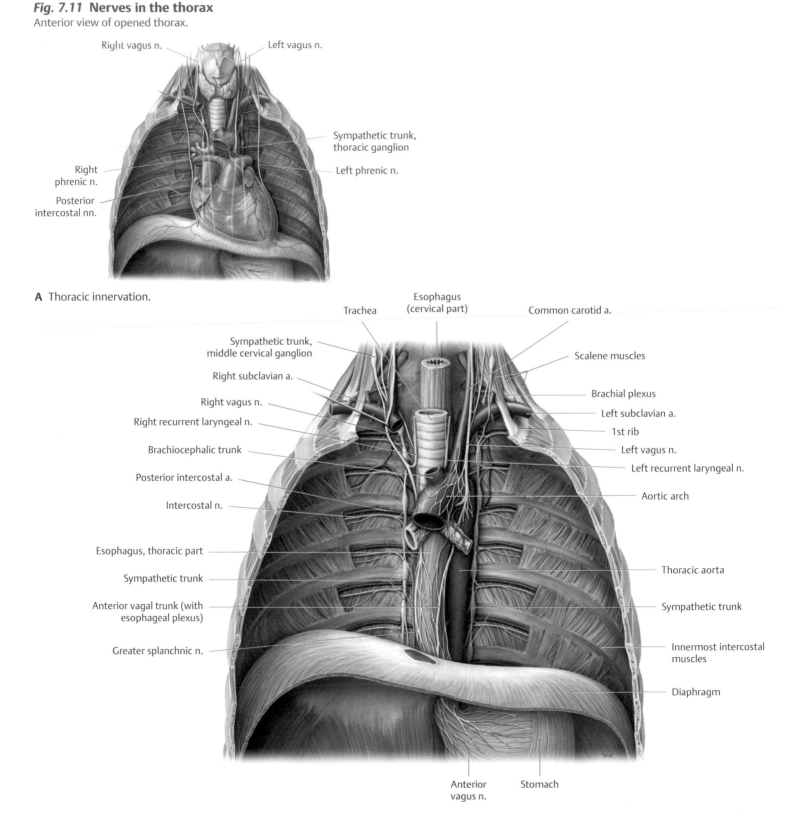

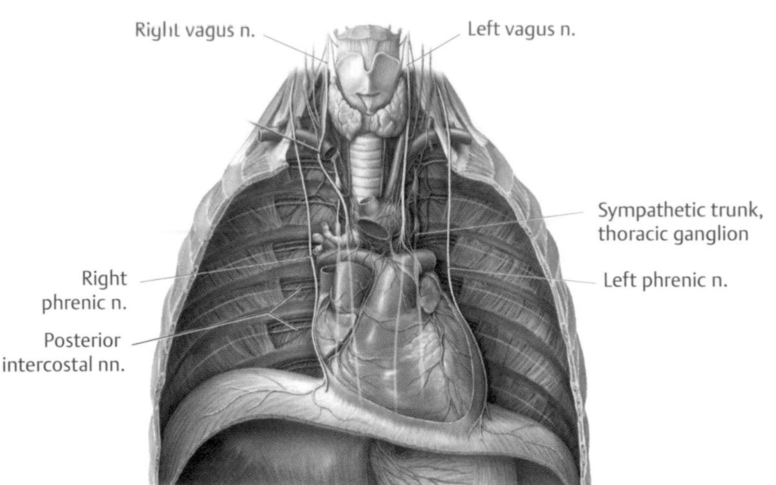
Right vagus n.
Left vagus n.
Sympathetic trunk, thoracic ganglion
Left phrenic n.
Right phrenic n.
Posterior intercostal nn.

A Thoracic innervation.

Trachea
Esophagus (cervical part)
Common carotid a.
Sympathetic trunk, middle cervical ganglion
Scalene muscles
Right subclavian a.
Brachial plexus
Right vagus n.
Left subclavian a.
Right recurrent laryngeal n.
1st rib
Brachiocephalic trunk
Left vagus n.
Left recurrent laryngeal n.
Posterior intercostal a.
Aortic arch
Intercostal n.
Esophagus, thoracic part
Thoracic aorta
Sympathetic trunk
Anterior vagal trunk (with esophageal plexus)
Sympathetic trunk
Innermost intercostal muscles
Greater splanchnic n.
Diaphragm
Anterior vagus n.
Stomach

B Nerves of the thorax in situ. *Note:* The recurrent laryngeal nerves have been slightly anteriorly retracted; normally, they occupy the groove between the trachea and the esophagus, making them vulnerable during thyroid gland surgery.

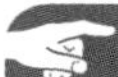

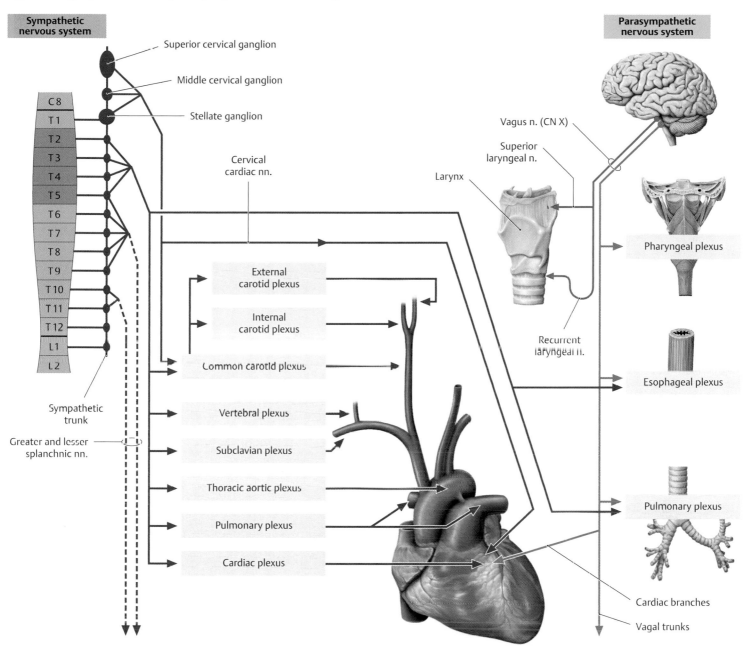

The autonomic nervous system innervates smooth muscle, cardiac muscle, and glands. It is subdivided into the sympathetic (red) and parasympathetic (blue) nervous systems, which together regulate blood flow, secretions, and organ function.

Fig. 7.12 Sympathetic and parasympathetic nervous systems in the thorax

Sympathetic nervous system
Superior cervical ganglion
Middle cervical ganglion
Stellate ganglion
C8
T1
T2
T3
T4
T5
T6
T7
T8
T9
T10
T11
T12
L1
L2
Cervical cardiac nn.
External carotid plexus
Internal carotid plexus
Common carotid plexus
Vertebral plexus
Subclavian plexus
Thoracic aortic plexus
Pulmonary plexus
Cardiac plexus
Sympathetic trunk
Greater and lesser splanchnic nn.
Parasympathetic nervous system
Vagus n. (CN X)
Superior laryngeal n.
Larynx
Pharyngeal plexus
Recurrent laryngeal n.
Esophageal plexus
Pulmonary plexus
Cardiac branches
Vagal trunks

Table 7.4 Peripheral sympathetic nervous system

Origin of preganglionic fibers*	Ganglion cells	Course of postganglionic fibers	Target
Spinal cord	Sympathetic trunk	Follow intercostal nn.	Blood vessels and glands in chest wall
		Accompany intrathoracic aa.	Visceral targets
		Gather in greater and lesser splanchnic nn.	Abdomen

*The axons of preganglionic neurons exit the spinal cord via the anterior roots and synapse with *post*ganglionic neurons in the sympathetic ganglia.

Table 7.5 Peripheral parasympathetic nervous system

Origin of preganglionic fibers	Course of preganglionic motor axons*		Target
Brainstem	Vagus n. (CN X)	Cardiac branches	Cardiac plexus
		Esophageal branches	Esophageal plexus
		Tracheal branches	Trachea
		Bronchial branches	Pulmonary plexus (bronchi, pulmonary vessels)

*The ganglion cells of the parasympathetic nervous system are scattered in microscopic groups in their target organs. The vagus nerve thus carries the *pre*ganglionic motor axons to these targets.
CN, cranial nerve.

Mediastinum: Overview

The mediastinum is the space in the thorax between the pleural sacs of the lungs. It is divided into two parts: superior and inferior. The inferior mediastinum is further divided into anterior, middle, and posterior portions.

Fig. 8.1 Divisions of the mediastinum

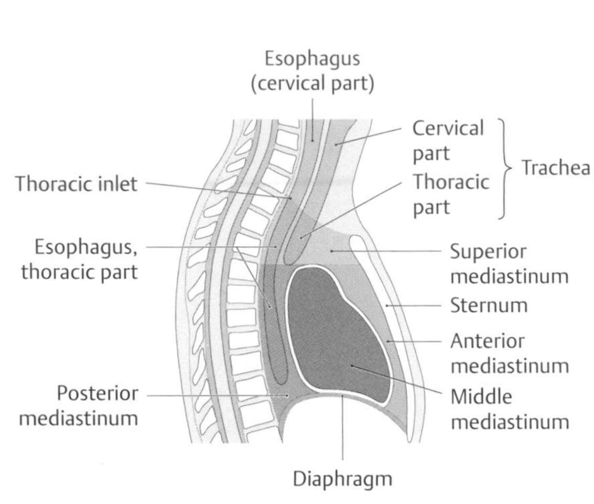

Esophagus (cervical part)
Cervical part
Thoracic part
Trachea
Thoracic inlet
Esophagus, thoracic part
Superior mediastinum
Sternum
Anterior mediastinum
Posterior mediastinum
Middle mediastinum
Diaphragm

A Schematic.

Table 8.1 Contents of the mediastinum

	Superior mediastinum	Inferior mediastinum		
		Anterior	*Middle*	*Posterior*
Organs	• Thymus • Trachea • Esophagus • Thoracic duct	• Thymus (in children, see Fig. 8.4B)	• Heart • Pericardium	• Esophagus
Arteries	• Aortic arch • Brachiocephalic trunk • Left common carotid a. • Left subclavian a.	• Smaller vessels	• Ascending aorta • Pulmonary trunk and branches • Pericardiacophrenic aa. and vv.	• Thoracic aorta and branches • Thoracic duct
Veins and lymph vessels	• Superior vena cava • Brachiocephalic vv. • Thoracic duct	• Smaller vessels, lymphatics, and lymph nodes	• Superior vena cava • Azygos v. • Pulmonary vv. • Pericardiacophrenic aa. and vv.	• Azygos v. • Hemiazygos v. • Thoracic duct
Nerves	• Vagus nn. • Left recurrent laryngeal n. • Cardiac nn. • Phrenic nn.	• None	• Phrenic nn.	• Vagus nn.

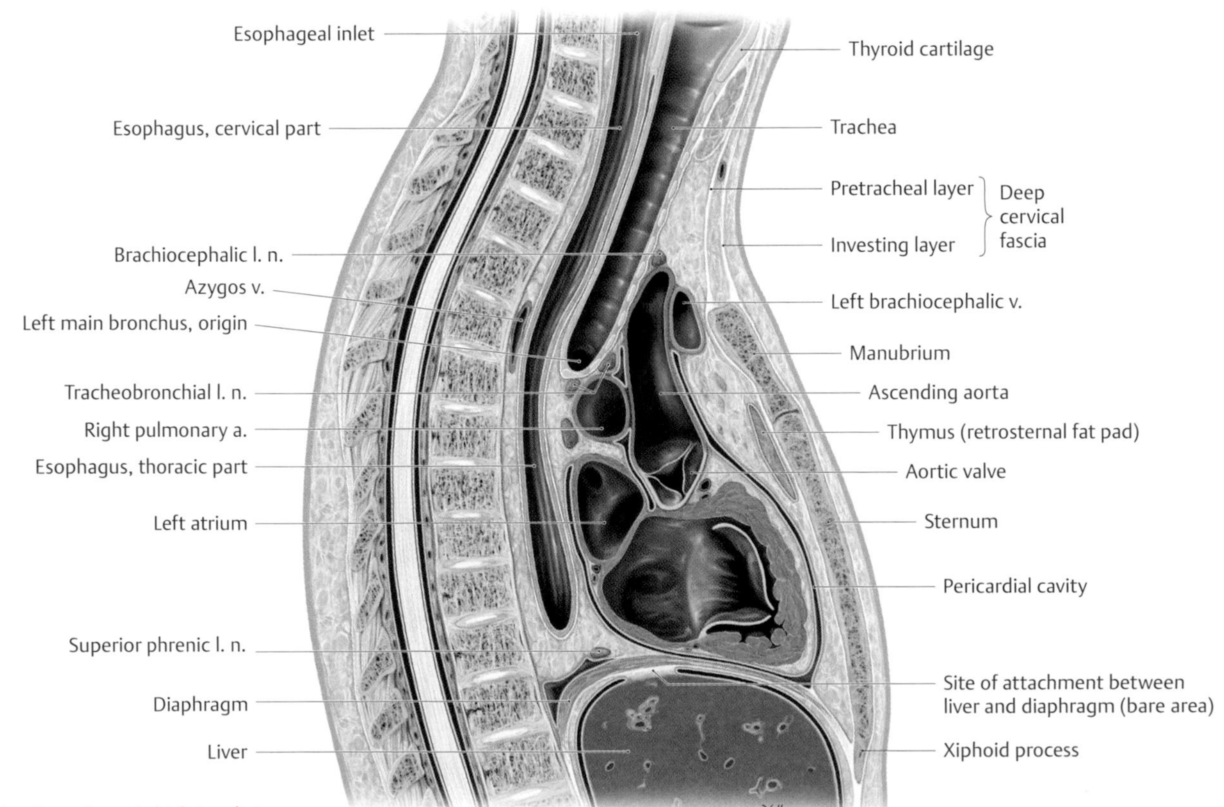

Esophageal inlet
Esophagus, cervical part
Brachiocephalic l. n.
Azygos v.
Left main bronchus, origin
Tracheobronchial l. n.
Right pulmonary a.
Esophagus, thoracic part
Left atrium
Superior phrenic l. n.
Diaphragm
Liver
Thyroid cartilage
Trachea
Pretracheal layer
Investing layer
Deep cervical fascia
Left brachiocephalic v.
Manubrium
Ascending aorta
Thymus (retrosternal fat pad)
Aortic valve
Sternum
Pericardial cavity
Site of attachment between liver and diaphragm (bare area)
Xiphoid process

B Midsagittal section, right lateral view.

Fig. 8.2 Contents of the mediastinum

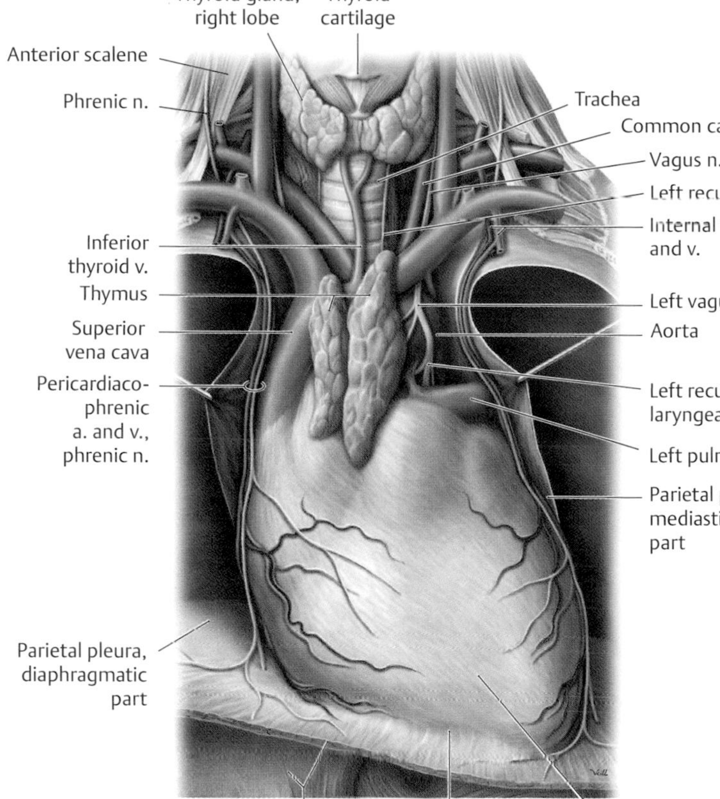
Thyroid gland, right lobe
Thyroid cartilage
Anterior scalene
Phrenic n.
Trachea
Common carotid a.
Vagus n. (CN X)
Left recurrent laryngeal n.
Internal thoracic a. and v.
Inferior thyroid v.
Thymus
Superior vena cava
Pericardiaco-phrenic a. and v., phrenic n.
Left vagus n.
Aorta
Left recurrent laryngeal n.
Left pulmonary a.
Parietal pleura, mediastinal part
Parietal pleura, diaphragmatic part
Diaphragm
Attachment between fibrous pericardium and diaphragmatic fascia
Fibrous pericardium

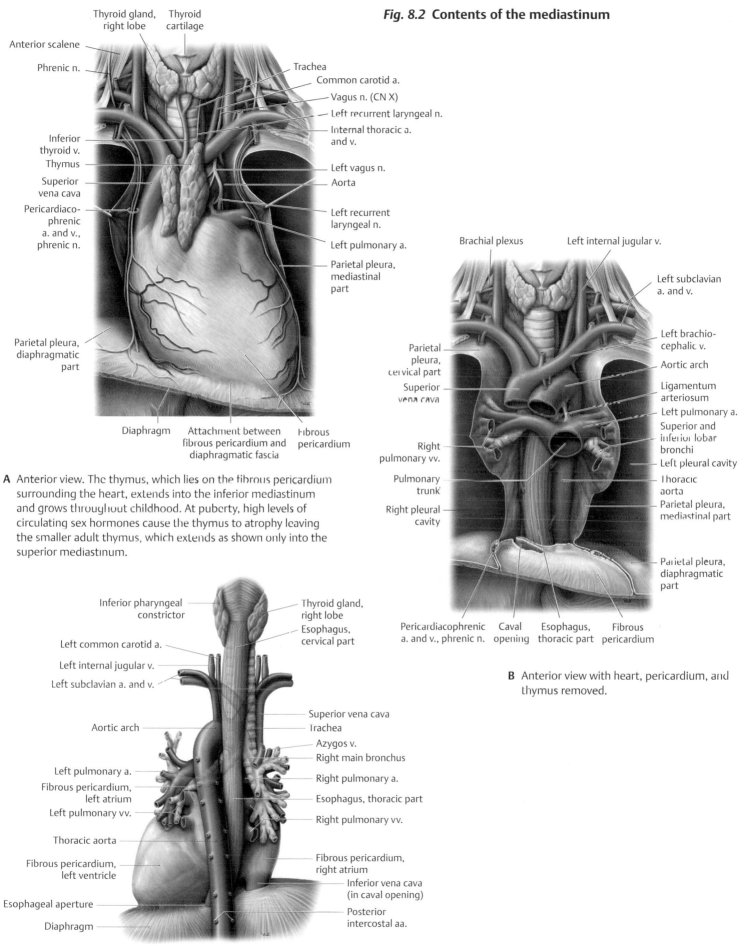

A Anterior view. The thymus, which lies on the fibrous pericardium surrounding the heart, extends into the inferior mediastinum and grows throughout childhood. At puberty, high levels of circulating sex hormones cause the thymus to atrophy leaving the smaller adult thymus, which extends as shown only into the superior mediastinum.

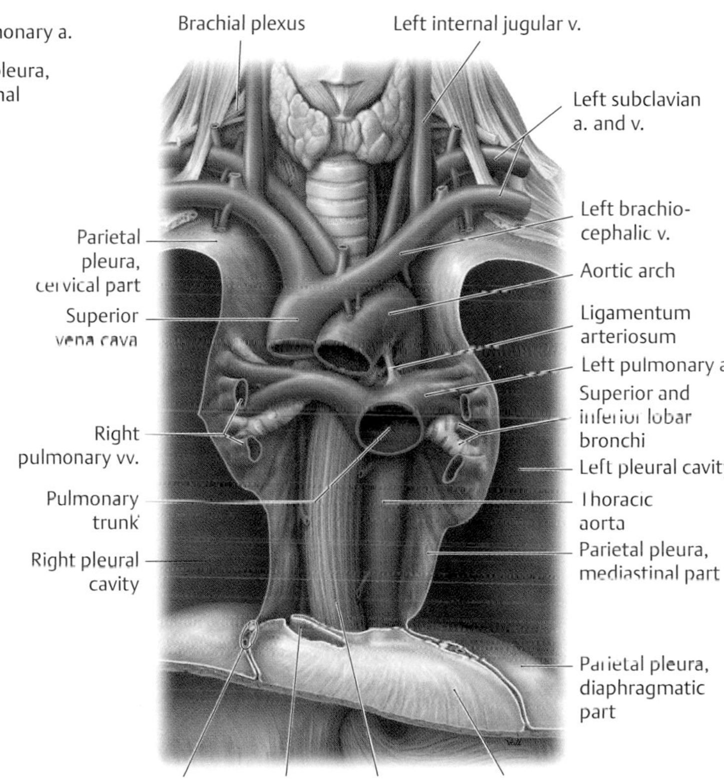
Brachial plexus
Left internal jugular v.
Left subclavian a. and v.
Left brachio-cephalic v.
Aortic arch
Ligamentum arteriosum
Left pulmonary a.
Superior and inferior lobar bronchi
Left pleural cavity
Thoracic aorta
Parietal pleura, mediastinal part
Parietal pleura, diaphragmatic part
Parietal pleura, cervical part
Superior vena cava
Right pulmonary vv.
Pulmonary trunk
Right pleural cavity
Pericardiacophrenic a. and v., phrenic n.
Caval opening
Esophagus, thoracic part
Fibrous pericardium

B Anterior view with heart, pericardium, and thymus removed.

Inferior pharyngeal constrictor
Thyroid gland, right lobe
Esophagus, cervical part
Left common carotid a.
Left internal jugular v.
Left subclavian a. and v.
Superior vena cava
Trachea
Aortic arch
Azygos v.
Right main bronchus
Left pulmonary a.
Right pulmonary a.
Fibrous pericardium, left atrium
Esophagus, thoracic part
Left pulmonary vv.
Right pulmonary vv.
Thoracic aorta
Fibrous pericardium, right atrium
Fibrous pericardium, left ventricle
Inferior vena cava (in caval opening)
Esophageal aperture
Posterior intercostal aa.
Diaphragm

C Posterior view.

Mediastinum: Structures

Fig. 8.3 Mediastinum

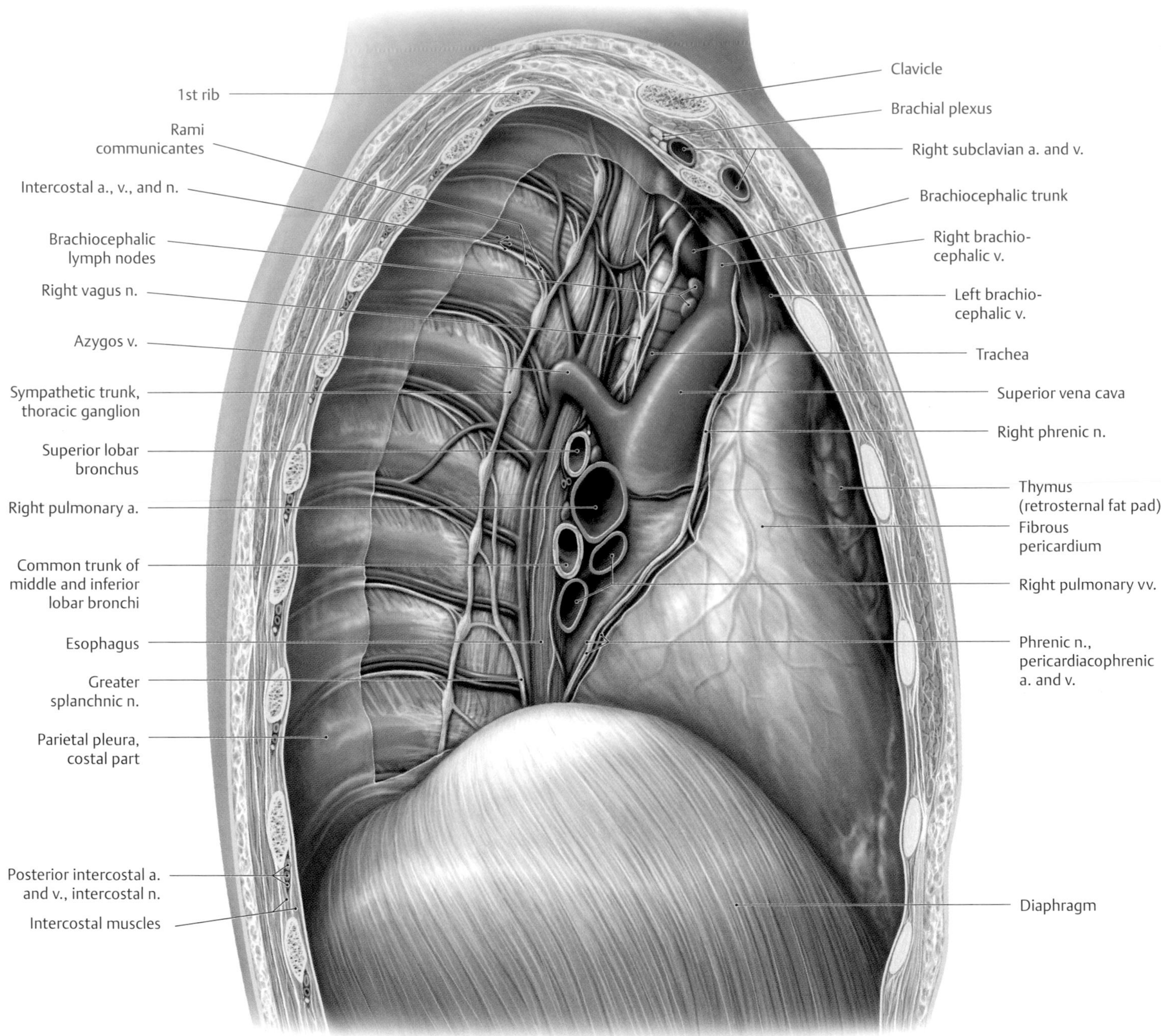
1st rib
Rami communicantes
Intercostal a., v., and n.
Brachiocephalic lymph nodes
Right vagus n.
Azygos v.
Sympathetic trunk, thoracic ganglion
Superior lobar bronchus
Right pulmonary a.
Common trunk of middle and inferior lobar bronchi
Esophagus
Greater splanchnic n.
Parietal pleura, costal part
Posterior intercostal a. and v., intercostal n.
Intercostal muscles
Clavicle
Brachial plexus
Right subclavian a. and v.
Brachiocephalic trunk
Right brachio-cephalic v.
Left brachio-cephalic v.
Trachea
Superior vena cava
Right phrenic n.
Thymus (retrosternal fat pad)
Fibrous pericardium
Right pulmonary vv.
Phrenic n., pericardiacophrenic a. and v.
Diaphragm

A Right lateral view, parasagittal section. Note the many structures passing between the superior and inferior (middle and posterior) mediastinum.

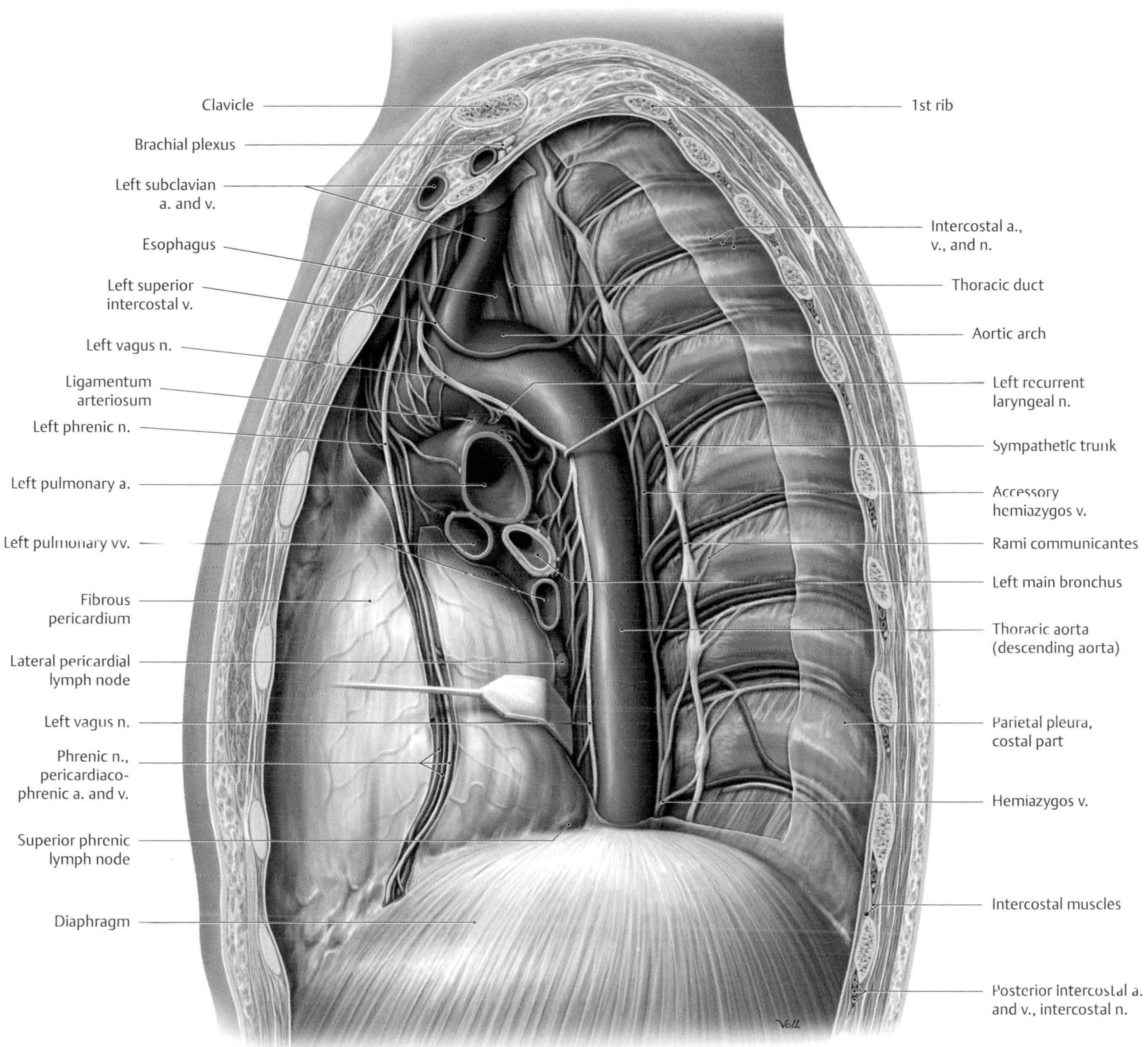
Clavicle
Brachial plexus
Left subclavian a. and v.
Esophagus
Left superior intercostal v.
Left vagus n.
Ligamentum arteriosum
Left phrenic n.
Left pulmonary a.
Left pulmonary vv.
Fibrous pericardium
Lateral pericardial lymph node
Left vagus n.
Phrenic n., pericardiaco-phrenic a. and v.
Superior phrenic lymph node
Diaphragm
1st rib
Intercostal a., v., and n.
Thoracic duct
Aortic arch
Left recurrent laryngeal n.
Sympathetic trunk
Accessory hemiazygos v.
Rami communicantes
Left main bronchus
Thoracic aorta (descending aorta)
Parietal pleura, costal part
Hemiazygos v.
Intercostal muscles
Posterior intercostal a. and v., intercostal n.

B Left lateral view, parasagittal section. *Removed:* Left lung and parietal pleura. *Revealed:* Posterior mediastinal structures.

Heart: Functions and Relations

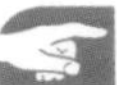

The heart pumps the blood: unoxygenated blood to the lungs and oxygenated blood throughout the body. It is located posterior to the sternum in the middle portion of the mediastinum in the pericardial cavity, located between the right and left pleural cavities containing the lungs. The cone-shaped heart points anteriorly and to the left in the thoracic cavity.

Fig. 8.4 Circulation

Oxygenated blood is shown in red; deoxygenated blood in blue. See p. 102 for prenatal circulation.

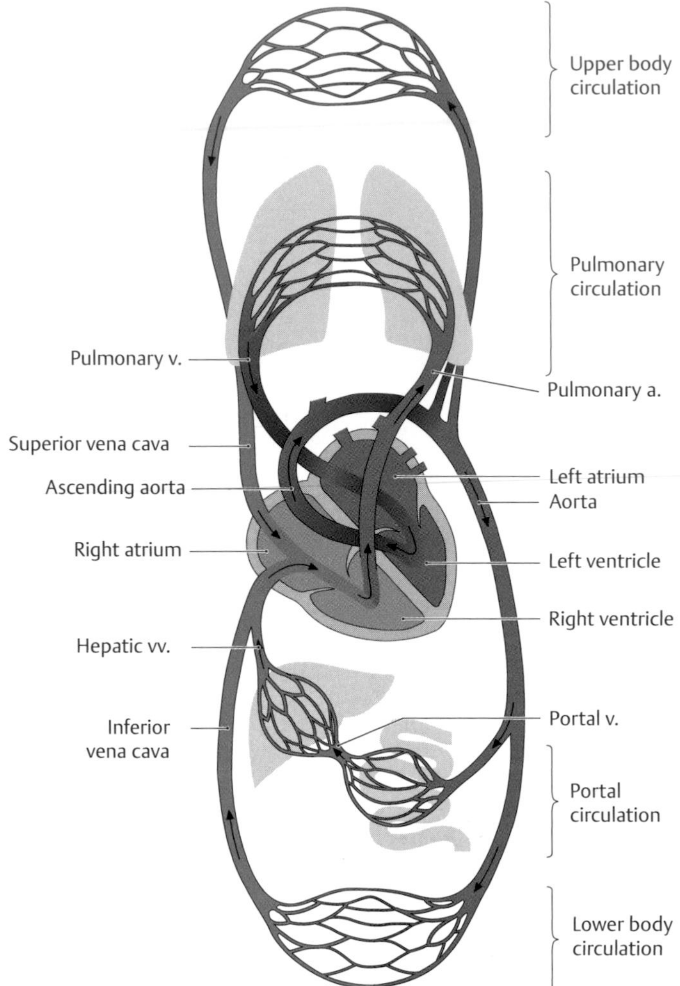

Upper body circulation
Pulmonary circulation
Pulmonary v.
Pulmonary a.
Superior vena cava
Ascending aorta
Left atrium
Aorta
Right atrium
Left ventricle
Right ventricle
Hepatic vv.
Inferior vena cava
Portal v.
Portal circulation
Lower body circulation

Fig. 8.5 Topographical relations of the heart

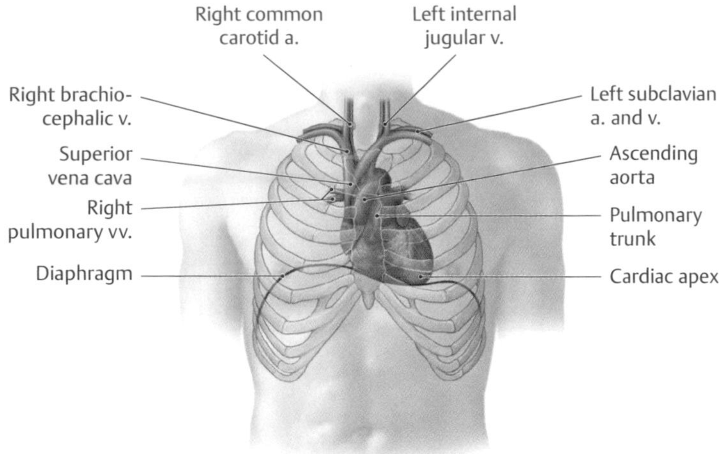

Right common carotid a.
Left internal jugular v.
Right brachio-cephalic v.
Left subclavian a. and v.
Superior vena cava
Ascending aorta
Right pulmonary vv.
Pulmonary trunk
Diaphragm
Cardiac apex

A Projection of the heart and great vessels onto chest, anterior view.

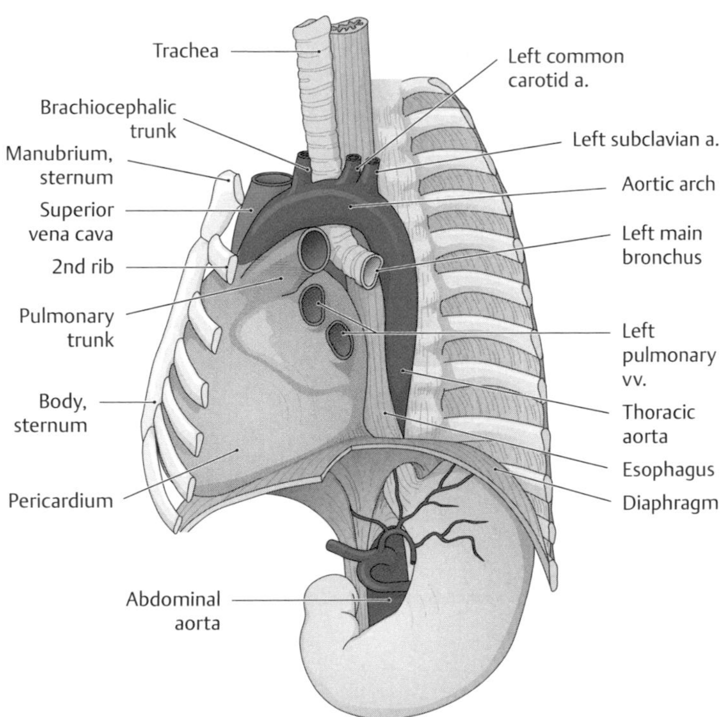

Trachea
Left common carotid a.
Brachiocephalic trunk
Left subclavian a.
Manubrium, sternum
Aortic arch
Superior vena cava
Left main bronchus
2nd rib
Pulmonary trunk
Left pulmonary vv.
Body, sternum
Thoracic aorta
Esophagus
Pericardium
Diaphragm
Abdominal aorta

B Left lateral view. *Removed:* Left thoracic wall and left lung.

Fig. 8.6 Heart in situ

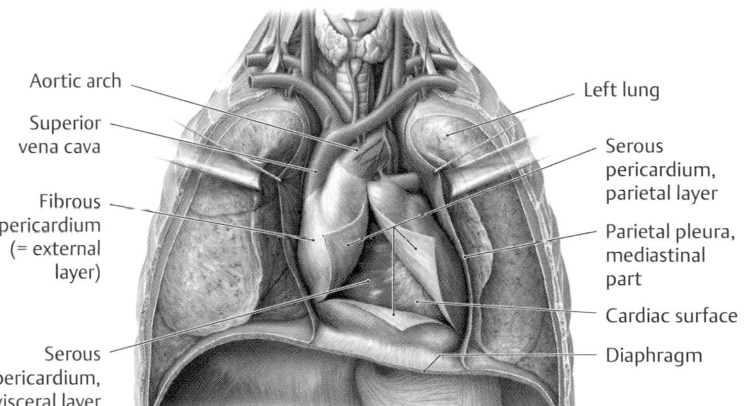

Aortic arch
Superior vena cava
Fibrous pericardium (= external layer)
Serous pericardium, visceral layer
Left lung
Serous pericardium, parietal layer
Parietal pleura, mediastinal part
Cardiac surface
Diaphragm

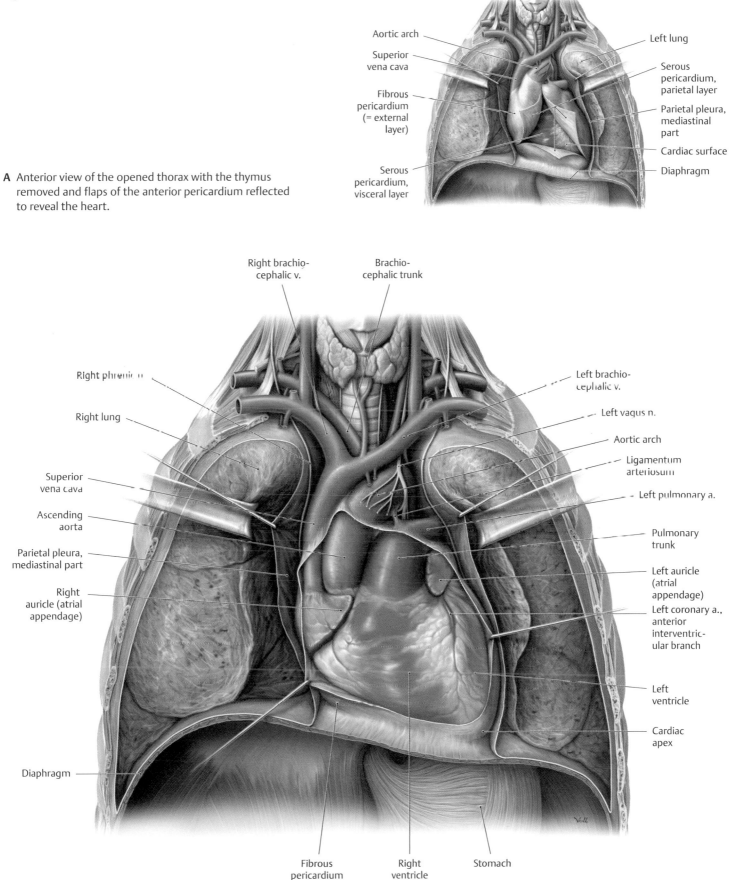

A Anterior view of the opened thorax with the thymus removed and flaps of the anterior pericardium reflected to reveal the heart.

Right brachio-cephalic v.
Brachio-cephalic trunk
Right phrenic n.
Right lung
Superior vena cava
Ascending aorta
Parietal pleura, mediastinal part
Right auricle (atrial appendage)
Diaphragm
Left brachio-cephalic v.
Left vagus n.
Aortic arch
Ligamentum arteriosum
Left pulmonary a.
Pulmonary trunk
Left auricle (atrial appendage)
Left coronary a., anterior interventric-ular branch
Left ventricle
Cardiac apex
Fibrous pericardium
Right ventricle
Stomach

B Anterior view of the opened thorax with thymus and anterior pericardium removed to reveal the heart.

Pericardium

Fig. 8.7 Posterior pericardial cavity

Anterior view of opened thorax with the anterior pericardium removed. The heart has been partially elevated to reveal the posterior pericardial cavity and the oblique pericardial sinus.

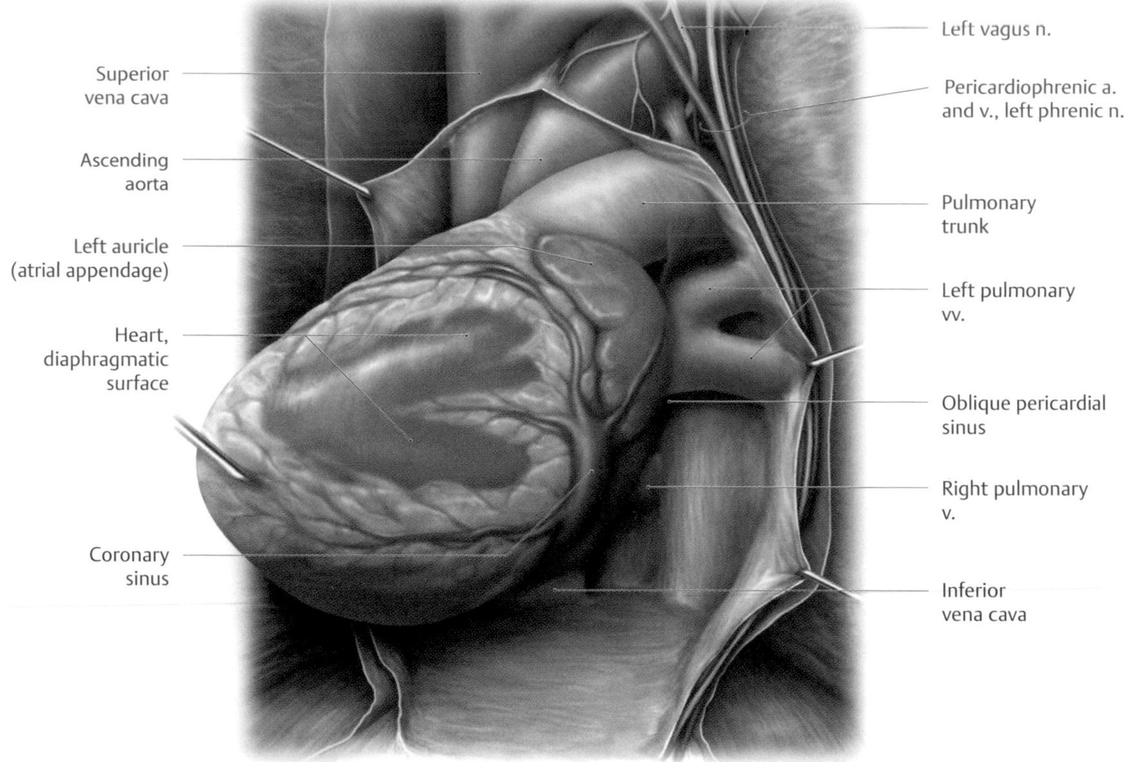
Superior vena cava
Ascending aorta
Left auricle (atrial appendage)
Heart, diaphragmatic surface
Coronary sinus
Left vagus n.
Pericardiophrenic a. and v., left phrenic n.
Pulmonary trunk
Left pulmonary vv.
Oblique pericardial sinus
Right pulmonary v.
Inferior vena cava

Fig. 8.8 Posterior pericardium

Anterior view of the opened thorax with the anterior pericardium and heart removed to reveal the posterior pericardium and the oblique pericardial sinus. The double-headed arrow illustrates the course of the tranverse pericardial sinus, the passage between the reflections of the serous layer of the pericardium around the arterial and venous great vessels of the heart.

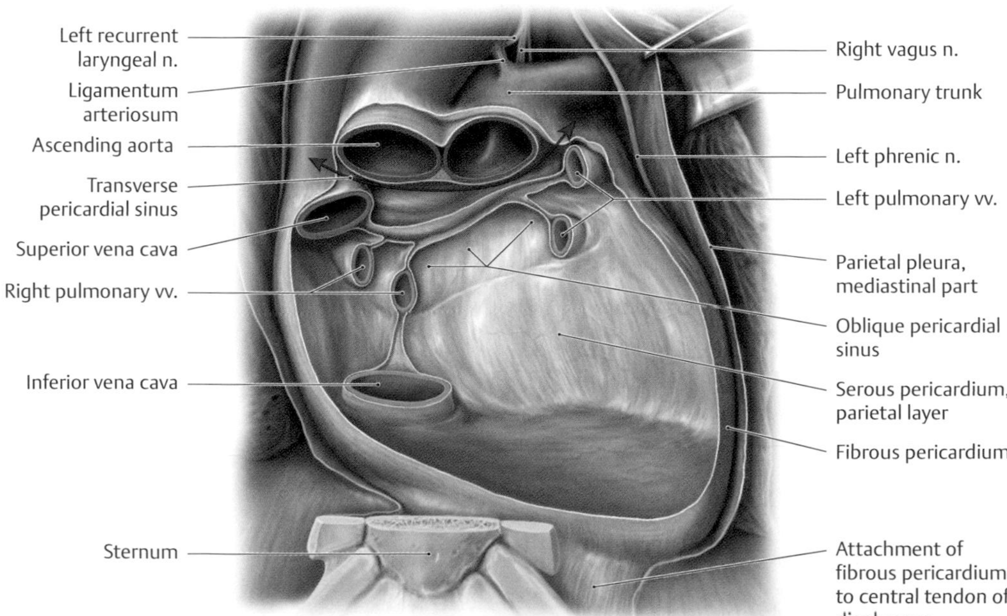
Left recurrent laryngeal n.
Ligamentum arteriosum
Ascending aorta
Transverse pericardial sinus
Superior vena cava
Right pulmonary vv.
Inferior vena cava
Sternum
Right vagus n.
Pulmonary trunk
Left phrenic n.
Left pulmonary vv.
Parietal pleura, mediastinal part
Oblique pericardial sinus
Serous pericardium, parietal layer
Fibrous pericardium
Attachment of fibrous pericardium to central tendon of diaphragm

Fig. 8.9 Posterior relations of the heart
Anterior view of the opened thorax with the anterior pericardium and heart removed and a window cut in the posterior pericardium to reveal the structures immediately posterior to the heart. This shows the close relationship of the esophagus to the heart, which is used in the transesophageal sonogram to assess the left atrium of the heart.

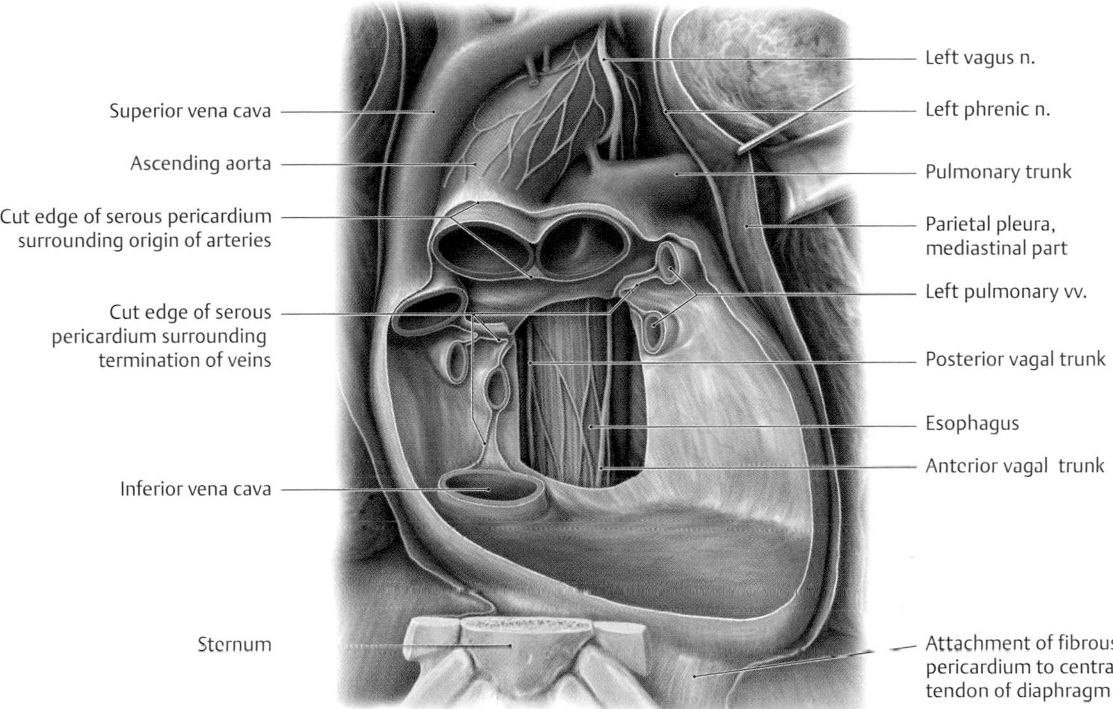
Superior vena cava
Ascending aorta
Cut edge of serous pericardium surrounding origin of arteries
Cut edge of serous pericardium surrounding termination of veins
Inferior vena cava
Sternum
Left vagus n.
Left phrenic n.
Pulmonary trunk
Parietal pleura, mediastinal part
Left pulmonary vv.
Posterior vagal trunk
Esophagus
Anterior vagal trunk
Attachment of fibrous pericardium to central tendon of diaphragm

Fig. 8.10 Pericardium, pericardial cavity, and transverse pericardial sinus
Sagittal section through the mediastinum. The fibrous pericardium is attached to the diaphragm and is continuous with the outer layer of the great vessels. The parietal layer of the serous pericardium lines the inner surface of the fibrous pericardium and the visceral layer adheres to the heart. The pericardial cavity, the space between the parietal and visceral layers of the serous pericardium around the heart, is filled with a thin layer of serous fluid that allows for frictionless movement. Where the parietal and visceral layers of the serous pericardium reach and reflect around the great vessels, they are continuous with one another. The passage between the arterial and venous reflections of the serous pericardium is the transverse pericardial sinus.

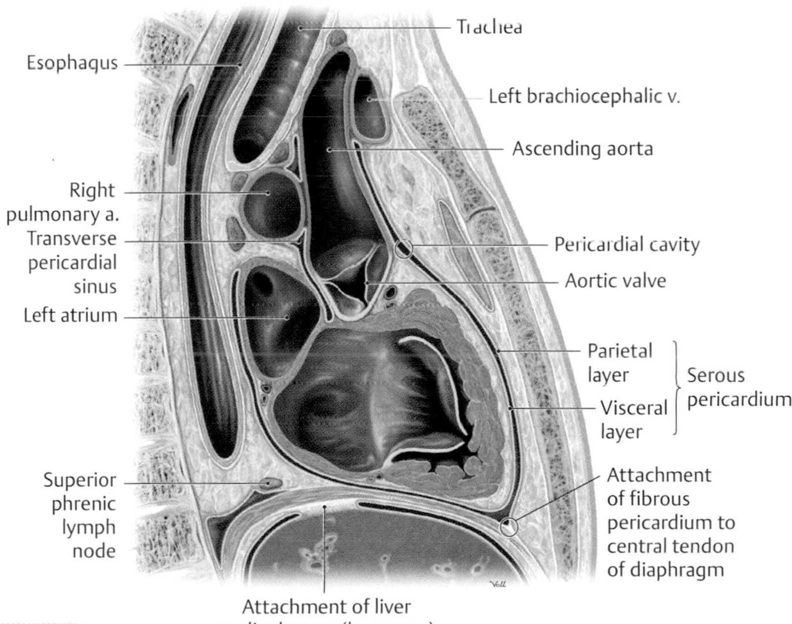
Esophagus
Right pulmonary a.
Transverse pericardial sinus
Left atrium
Superior phrenic lymph node
Trachea
Left brachiocephalic v.
Ascending aorta
Pericardial cavity
Aortic valve
Parietal layer
Visceral layer
Serous pericardium
Attachment of fibrous pericardium to central tendon of diaphragm
Attachment of liver to diaphragm (bare area)

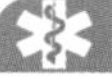 **Clinical**

Cardiac Tamponade
Rapid increases of fluid or blood within the pericardial sac inhibits full expansion of the heart, reducing cardiac blood return, thus decreasing cardiac output. This condition, cardiac tamponade (compression), is potentially fatal, unless relieved. The fluid or blood must first be removed to restore cardiac function and then the cause of the fluid or blood accumulation corrected.

Heart: Surfaces & Chambers

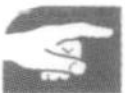

Note the reflection of visceral serous pericardium to become parietal serous pericardium.

***Fig. 8.11* Surfaces of the heart**
The heart has three surfaces: anterior (sternocostal), posterior (base), and inferior (diaphragmatic).

Left subclavian a.
Left common carotid a.
Aortic arch
Ligamentum arteriosum
Brachio-cephalic trunk
Left pulmonary a.
Right pulmonary a.
Left pulmonary vv.
Superior vena cava
Pulmonary trunk
Ascending aorta
Left auricle
Right auricle
Right atrium
Pericardium (reflected edge)
Coronary sulcus
Anterior inter-ventricular sulcus
Right ventricle
Left ventricle
Inferior vena cava
Cardiac apex

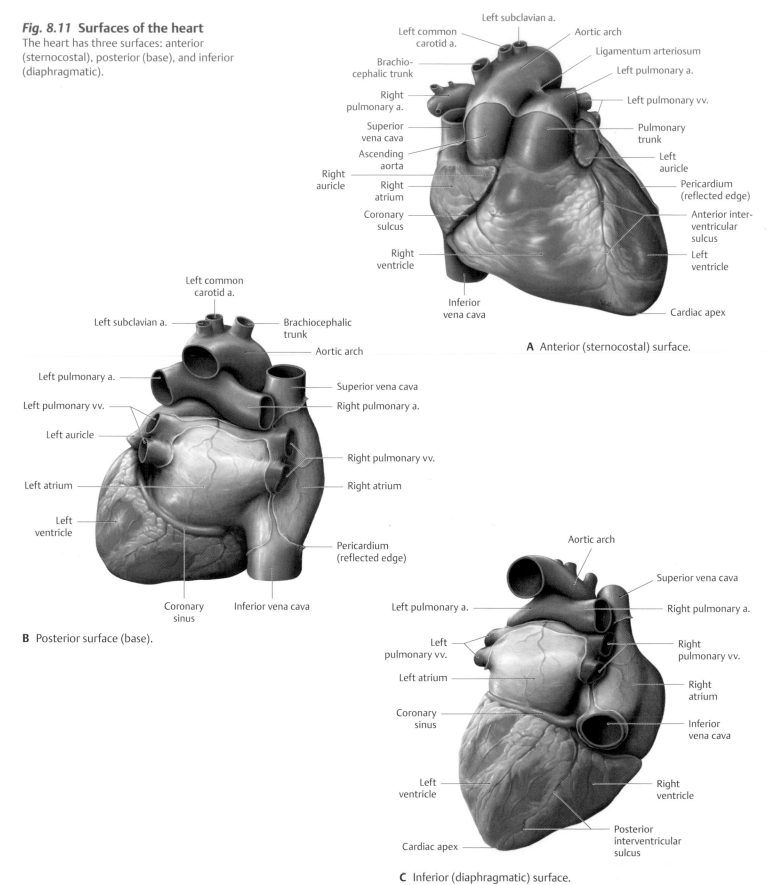

A Anterior (sternocostal) surface.

Left common carotid a.
Left subclavian a.
Brachiocephalic trunk
Aortic arch
Left pulmonary a.
Superior vena cava
Right pulmonary a.
Left pulmonary vv.
Left auricle
Right pulmonary vv.
Left atrium
Right atrium
Left ventricle
Pericardium (reflected edge)
Coronary sinus
Inferior vena cava

B Posterior surface (base).

Aortic arch
Superior vena cava
Left pulmonary a.
Right pulmonary a.
Left pulmonary vv.
Right pulmonary vv.
Left atrium
Right atrium
Coronary sinus
Inferior vena cava
Left ventricle
Right ventricle
Posterior interventricular sulcus
Cardiac apex

C Inferior (diaphragmatic) surface.

Fig. 8.12 Chambers of the heart

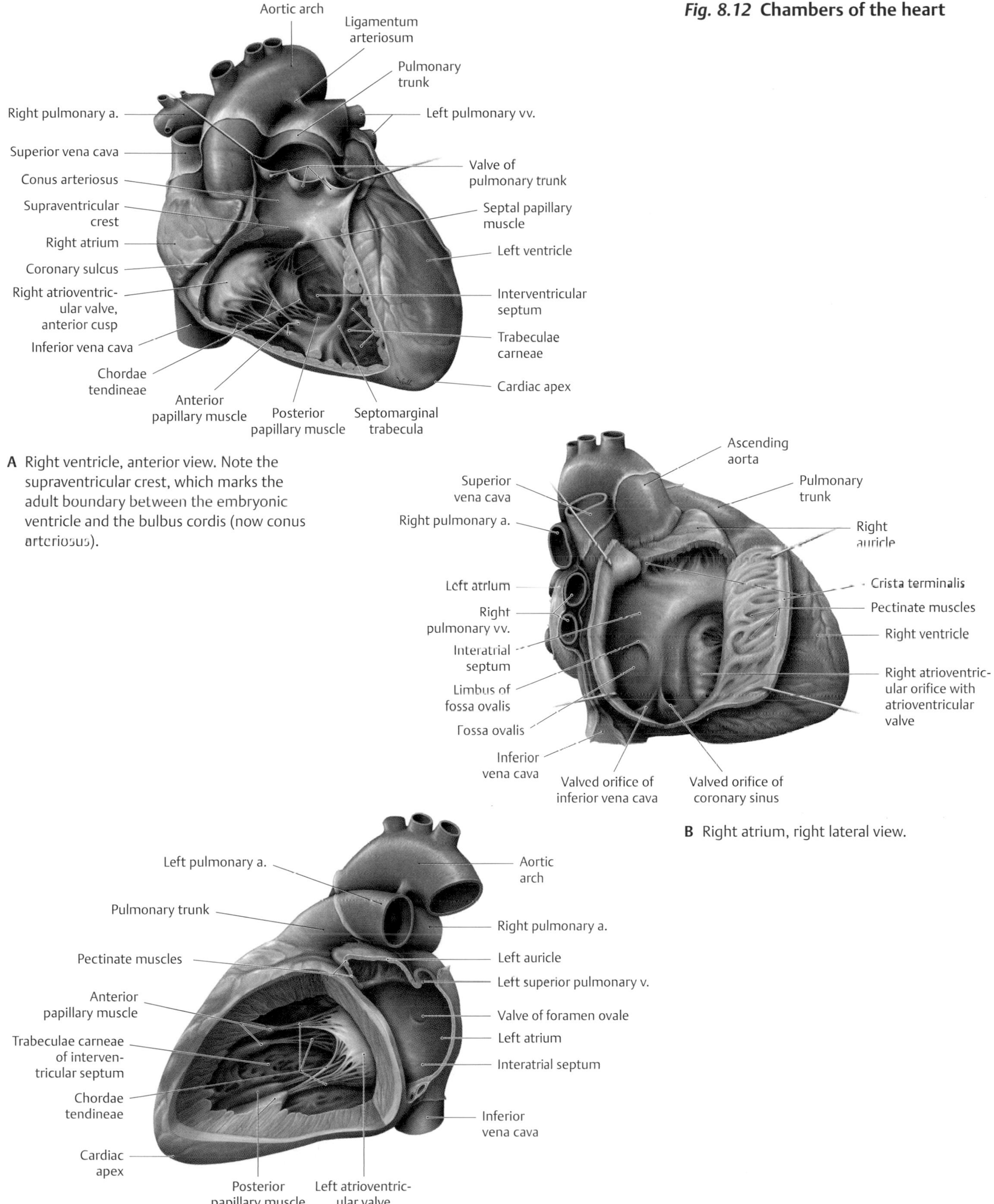

Aortic arch
Ligamentum arteriosum
Pulmonary trunk
Left pulmonary vv.
Right pulmonary a.
Superior vena cava
Conus arteriosus
Valve of pulmonary trunk
Supraventricular crest
Septal papillary muscle
Right atrium
Left ventricle
Coronary sulcus
Right atrioventricular valve, anterior cusp
Interventricular septum
Inferior vena cava
Trabeculae carneae
Chordae tendineae
Cardiac apex
Anterior papillary muscle
Posterior papillary muscle
Septomarginal trabecula
Ascending aorta
Superior vena cava
Pulmonary trunk
Right pulmonary a.
Right auricle
Left atrium
Crista terminalis
Pectinate muscles
Right pulmonary vv.
Right ventricle
Interatrial septum
Right atrioventricular orifice with atrioventricular valve
Limbus of fossa ovalis
Fossa ovalis
Inferior vena cava
Valved orifice of inferior vena cava
Valved orifice of coronary sinus
Left pulmonary a.
Aortic arch
Pulmonary trunk
Right pulmonary a.
Pectinate muscles
Left auricle
Left superior pulmonary v.
Anterior papillary muscle
Valve of foramen ovale
Left atrium
Trabeculae carneae of interventricular septum
Interatrial septum
Chordae tendineae
Inferior vena cava
Cardiac apex
Posterior papillary muscle
Left atrioventricular valve

A Right ventricle, anterior view. Note the supraventricular crest, which marks the adult boundary between the embryonic ventricle and the bulbus cordis (now conus arteriosus).

B Right atrium, right lateral view.

C Left atrium and ventricle, left lateral view. Note the irregular trabeculae carneae characteristic of the ventricular wall.

Heart: Valves

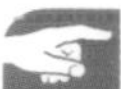

The cardiac valves are divided into two groups: semilunar and atrioventricular. The two semilunar valves (aortic and pulmonary) located at the base of the two great arteries of the heart regulate passage of blood from the ventricles to the aorta and pulmonary trunk. The two atrioventricular valves (left and right) lie at the interface between the atria and ventricles.

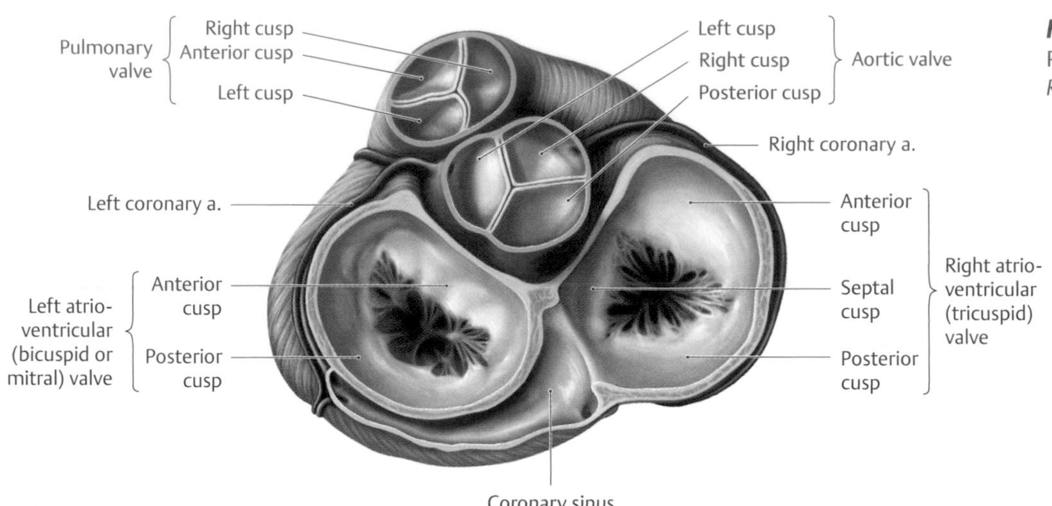
Pulmonary valve
Right cusp
Anterior cusp
Left cusp
Left cusp
Right cusp
Posterior cusp
Aortic valve
Right coronary a.
Left coronary a.
Anterior cusp
Septal cusp
Posterior cusp
Right atrioventricular (tricuspid) valve
Left atrioventricular (bicuspid or mitral) valve
Anterior cusp
Posterior cusp
Coronary sinus

A Ventricular diastole (relaxation of the ventricles). *Closed:* Semilunar valves. *Open:* Atrioventricular valves.

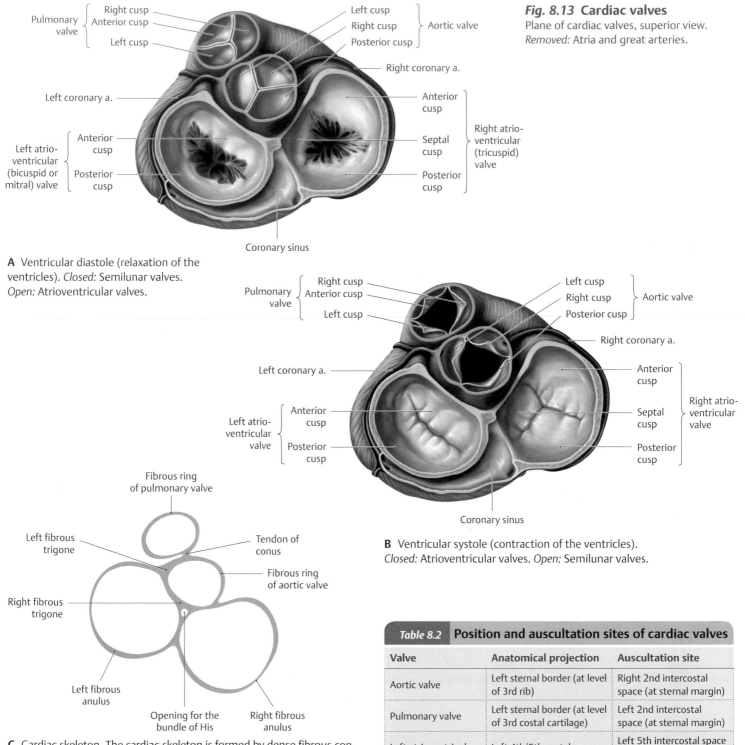

Fig. 8.13 **Cardiac valves**
Plane of cardiac valves, superior view. *Removed:* Atria and great arteries.

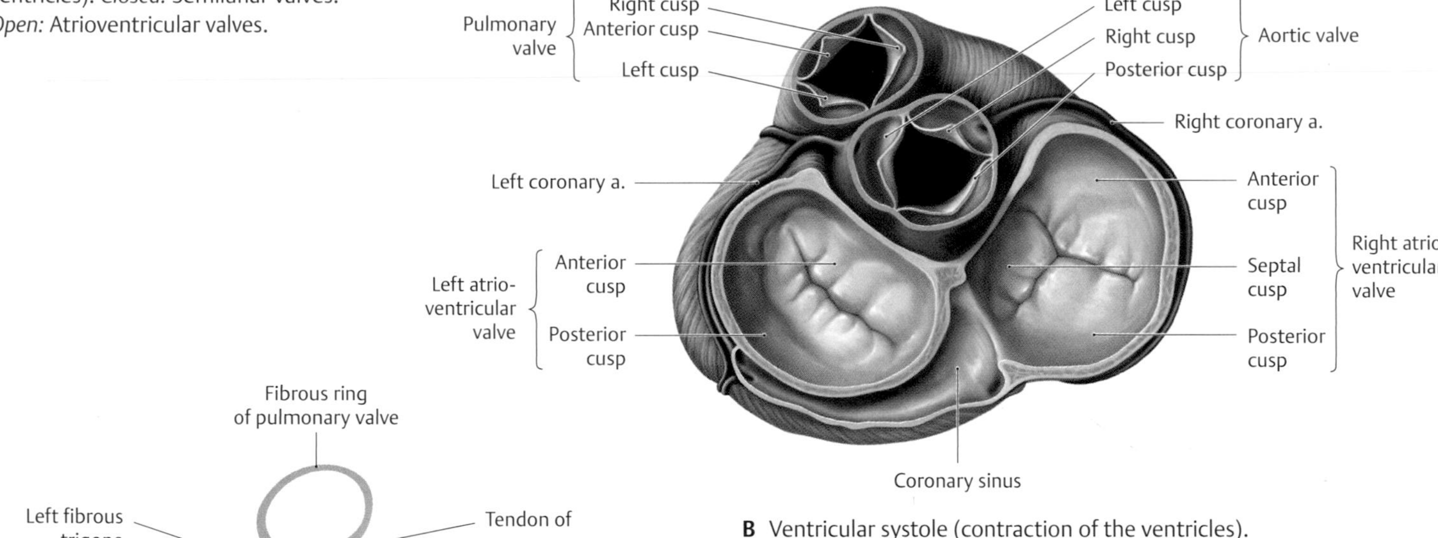
Pulmonary valve
Right cusp
Anterior cusp
Left cusp
Left cusp
Right cusp
Posterior cusp
Aortic valve
Right coronary a.
Left coronary a.
Anterior cusp
Septal cusp
Posterior cusp
Right atrioventricular valve
Left atrioventricular valve
Anterior cusp
Posterior cusp
Coronary sinus
Fibrous ring of pulmonary valve
Left fibrous trigone
Tendon of conus
Fibrous ring of aortic valve
Right fibrous trigone
Left fibrous anulus
Opening for the bundle of His
Right fibrous anulus

B Ventricular systole (contraction of the ventricles). *Closed:* Atrioventricular valves. *Open:* Semilunar valves.

C Cardiac skeleton. The cardiac skeleton is formed by dense fibrous connective tissue. The fibrous anuli (rings) and intervening trigones separate the atria from the ventricles. This provides mechanical stability, electrical insulation (see p. 98 for cardiac conduction system), and an attachment point for the cardiac muscles and valve cusps.

Table 8.2 Position and auscultation sites of cardiac valves

Valve	Anatomical projection	Auscultation site
Aortic valve	Left sternal border (at level of 3rd rib)	Right 2nd intercostal space (at sternal margin)
Pulmonary valve	Left sternal border (at level of 3rd costal cartilage)	Left 2nd intercostal space (at sternal margin)
Left atrioventricular valve	Left 4th/5th costal cartilage	Left 5th intercostal space (at midclavicular line) or cardiac apex
Right atrioventricular valve	Sternum (at level of 5th costal cartilage)	Left 5th intercostal space (at sternal margin)

Fig. 8.14 Semilunar valves

Valves have been longitudinally sectioned and opened.

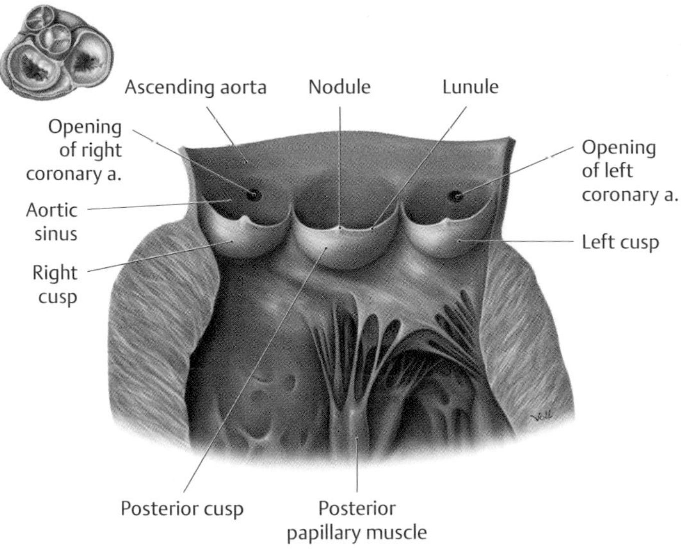

Ascending aorta
Nodule
Lunule
Opening of right coronary a.
Opening of left coronary a.
Aortic sinus
Left cusp
Right cusp
Posterior cusp
Posterior papillary muscle

A Aortic valve.

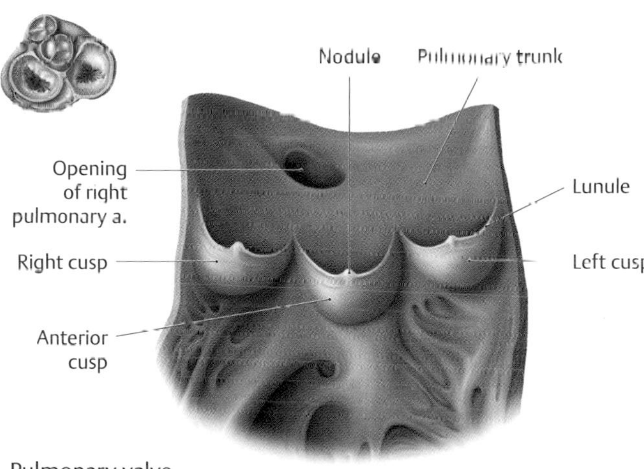

Nodule
Pulmonary trunk
Opening of right pulmonary a.
Lunule
Right cusp
Left cusp
Anterior cusp

B Pulmonary valve.

Fig. 8.15 Atrioventricular valves

Anterior view during ventricular systole.

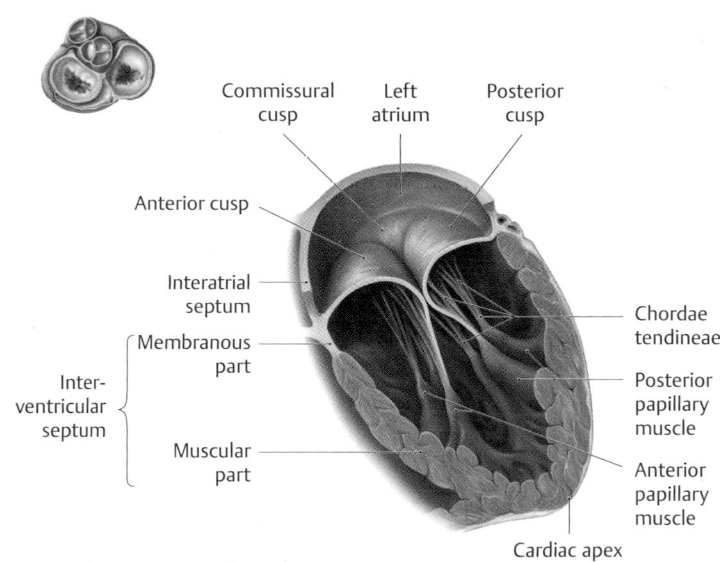

Commissural cusp
Left atrium
Posterior cusp
Anterior cusp
Interatrial septum
Membranous part
Inter-ventricular septum
Muscular part
Chordae tendineae
Posterior papillary muscle
Anterior papillary muscle
Cardiac apex

A Left atrioventricular valve.

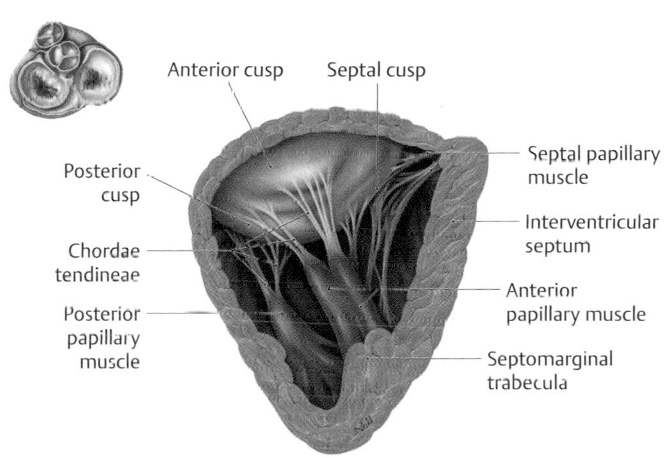

Anterior cusp
Septal cusp
Posterior cusp
Septal papillary muscle
Interventricular septum
Chordae tendineae
Anterior papillary muscle
Posterior papillary muscle
Septomarginal trabecula

B Right atrioventricular valve.

Clinical

Auscultation of the cardiac valves

Heart sounds, produced by closure of the semilunar and atrioventricular valves, are carried by the blood flowing through the valve. The resulting sounds are therefore best heard "downstream," at defined auscultation sites (dark circles). Valvular heart disease causes turbulent blood flow through the valve; this produces a murmur that may be detected in the colored regions.

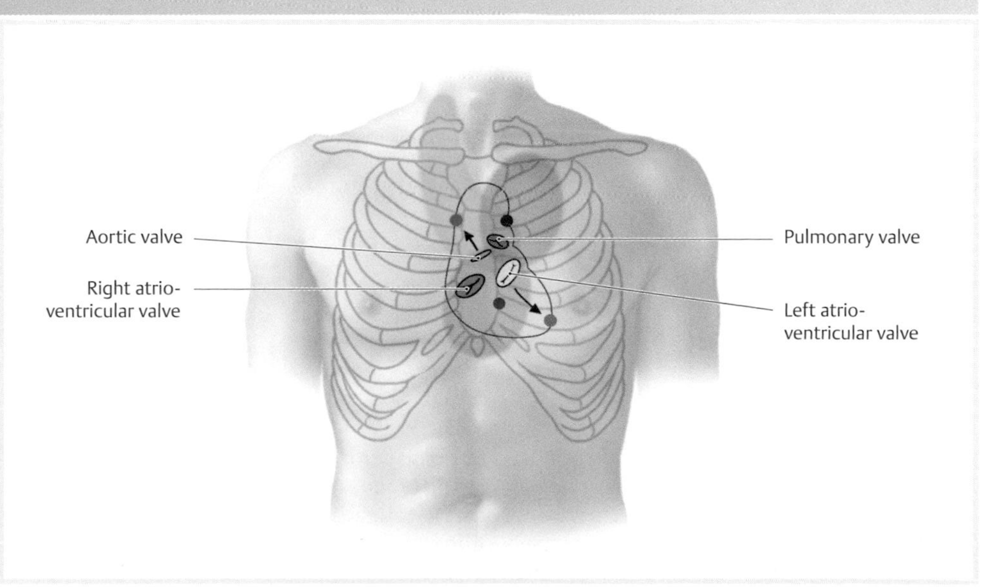

Aortic valve
Right atrio-ventricular valve
Pulmonary valve
Left atrio-ventricular valve

Arteries & Veins of the Heart

Fig. 8.16 Coronary arteries and cardiac veins

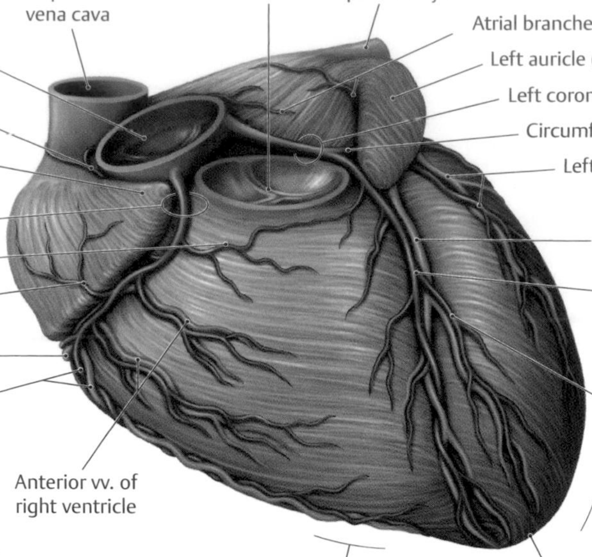

Superior vena cava
Pulmonary valve
Superior left pulmonary v.
Atrial branches
Ascending aorta with aortic sinus
Left auricle (atrial appendage)
Left coronary a.
Branch to sinoatrial node
Circumflex branch
Right auricle (atrial appendage)
Left marginal a. and v.
Right coronary a.
Great cardiac v.
Conus branch
Atrial branch
Anterior interventricular branch (left anterior descending)
Small cardiac v.
Right marginal a. and v.
Lateral branch
Anterior vv. of right ventricle
Left ventricle
Right ventricle
Cardiac apex

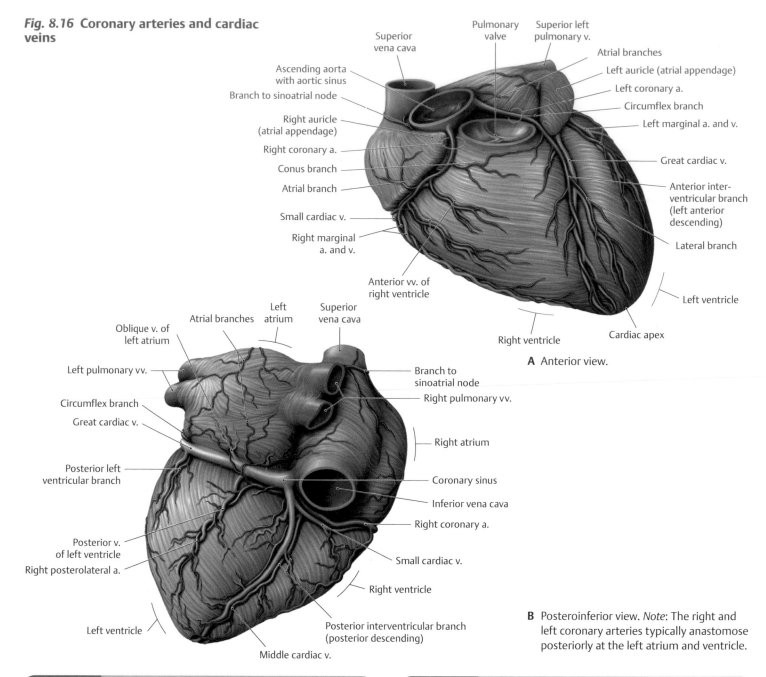

A Anterior view.

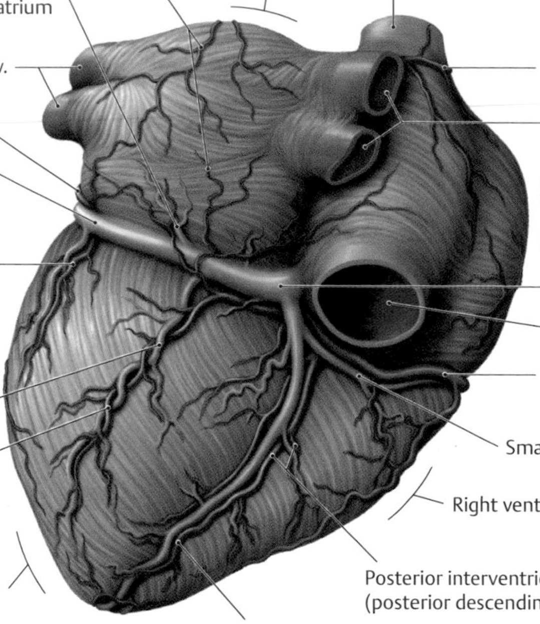

Oblique v. of left atrium
Atrial branches
Left atrium
Superior vena cava
Left pulmonary vv.
Branch to sinoatrial node
Right pulmonary vv.
Circumflex branch
Great cardiac v.
Right atrium
Posterior left ventricular branch
Coronary sinus
Inferior vena cava
Right coronary a.
Posterior v. of left ventricle
Small cardiac v.
Right posterolateral a.
Right ventricle
Left ventricle
Posterior interventricular branch (posterior descending)
Middle cardiac v.

B Posteroinferior view. *Note*: The right and left coronary arteries typically anastomose posteriorly at the left atrium and ventricle.

Table 8.3 Branches of the coronary arteries

Left coronary artery	Right coronary artery
Circumflex branch • Atrial branch • Left marginal a. • Posterior left ventricular branch	Branch to SA node Conus branch Atrial branch Right marginal a.
Anterior interventricular branch (left anterior descending) • Conus branch • Lateral branch • Interventricular septal branches	Posterior interventricular branch (posterior descending) • Interventricular septal branches Branch to AV node Right posterolateral a.
AV, atrioventricular; SA, sinoatrial.	

Table 8.4 Divisions of the cardiac veins

Vein	Tributaries	Drainage to
Anterior cardiac vv. (not shown)		Right atrium
Great cardiac v.	Anterior interventricular v.	Coronary sinus
	Left marginal v.	
	Oblique v. of left atrium	
Left posterior ventricular v.		
Middle cardiac v. (posterior interventricular v.)		
Small cardiac v.	Anterior vv. of right ventricle	
	Right marginal v.	

Fig. 8.17 Distribution of the coronary arteries

Anterior and posterior views of the heart, with superior views of transverse sections through the ventricles. The "distribution" of the coronary arteries refers to the area of the myocardium supplied by each artery, as seen in the transverse views, but the term "dominance" refers to the artery that gives rise to the posterior interventricular artery, as seen in the anterior and posterior views. Right coronary artery and branches (green); left coronary artery and branches (red).

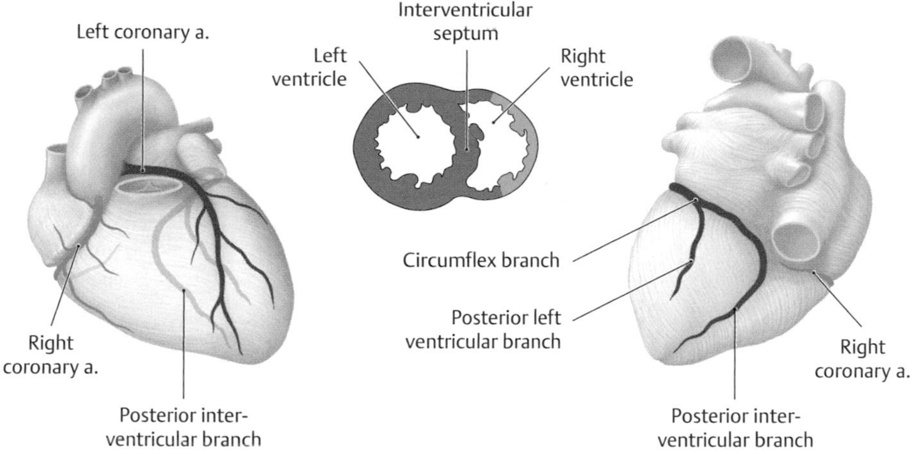
Left coronary a.
Left ventricle
Interventricular septum
Right ventricle
Circumflex branch
Posterior left ventricular branch
Right coronary a.
Posterior inter-ventricular branch
Right coronary a.
Posterior inter-ventricular branch

A Left coronary dominance (15–17%).

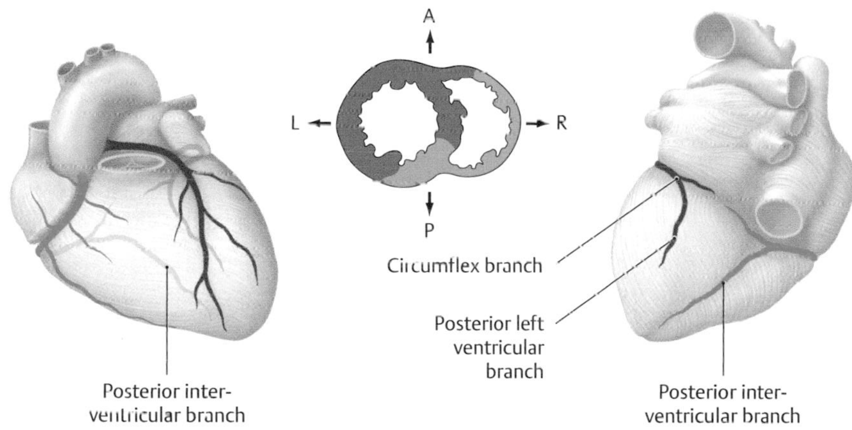
A
L
R
P
Circumflex branch
Posterior left ventricular branch
Posterior inter-ventricular branch
Posterior inter-ventricular branch

B Balanced distribution, right coronary artery dominance (67–70%).

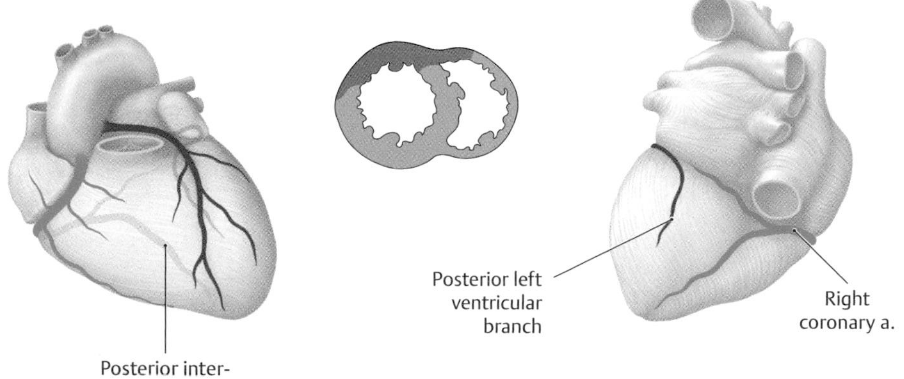
Posterior left ventricular branch
Right coronary a.
Posterior inter-ventricular branch

C Right coronary dominance (~15%).

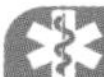

Clinical

Disturbed coronary blood flow

Although the coronary arteries are connected by structural anastomoses, they are end arteries from a functional standpoint. The most frequent cause of deficient blood flow is *atherosclerosis*, a narrowing of the coronary lumen due to plaque-like deposits on the vessel wall. When the decrease in luminal size (stenosis) reaches a critical point, coronary blood flow is restricted, causing chest pain (*angina pectoris*). Initially, this pain is induced by physical effort, but eventually it persists at rest, often radiating to characteristic sites (e.g., medial side of left upper limb, left side of head and neck). A myocardial infarction occurs when deficient blood supply causes myocardial tissue to die (necrosis). The location and extent of the infarction depends on the stenosed vessel (see **A–E**, after Heinecker).

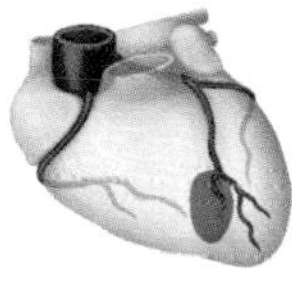

A Supra-apical anterior infarction.

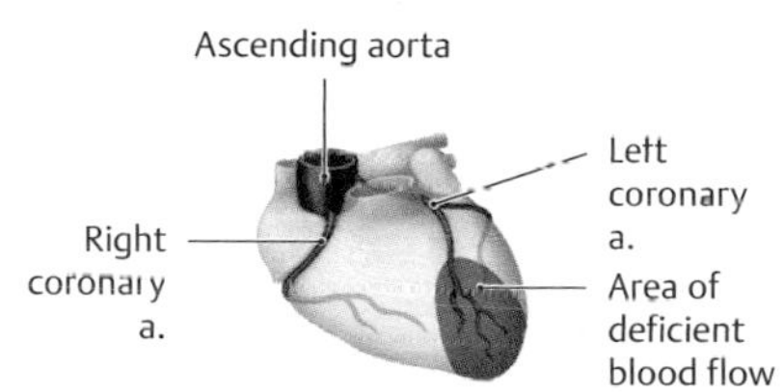
Ascending aorta
Right coronary a.
Left coronary a.
Area of deficient blood flow

B Apical anterior infarction.

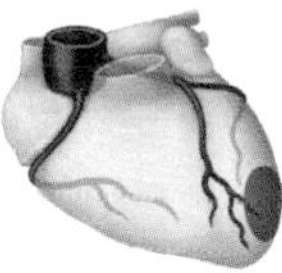

C Anterior lateral infarction.

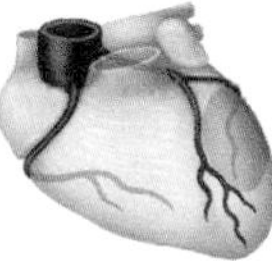

D Posterior lateral infarction.

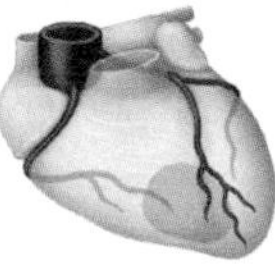

E Posterior infarction.

Conduction & Innervation of the Heart

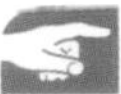

Contraction of cardiac muscle is modulated by the cardiac conduction system. This system of specialized myocardial cells (Purkinje fibers) generates and conducts excitatory impulses in the heart. The conduction system contains two nodes, both located in the atria: the sinoatrial (SA) node, known as the pacemaker, and the atrioventricular (AV) node.

Fig. 8.18 Cardiac conduction system

Superior vena cava
Sinoatrial (SA) node
Anterior, middle, and posterior internodal bundles
Atrioventricular (AV) node
Interatrial bundle
Atrioventricular bundle (of His)
Left bundle branch
Right bundle branch
Interventricular septum

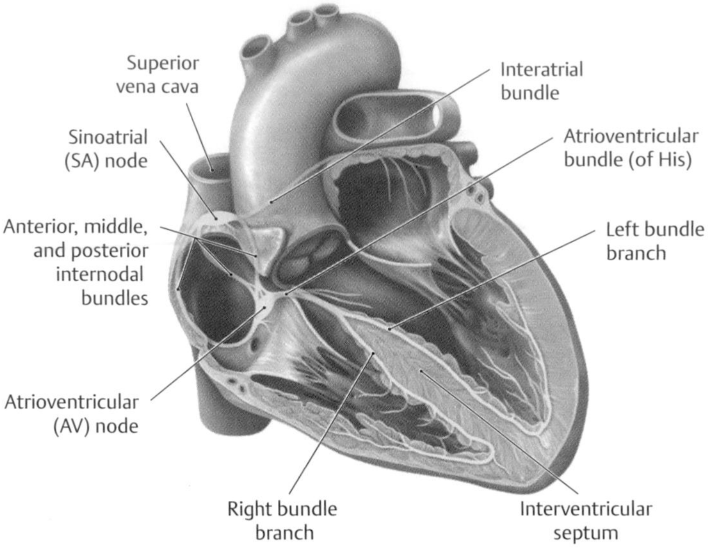

A Anterior view. *Opened:* All four chambers.

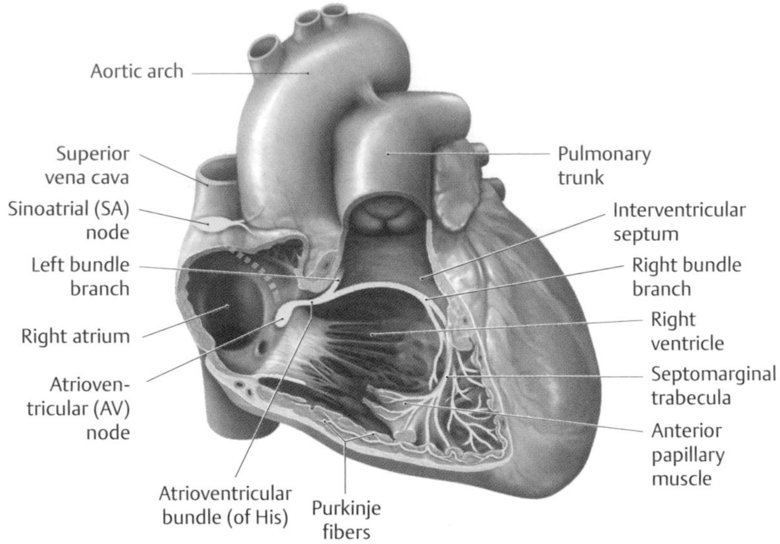

Aortic arch
Superior vena cava
Sinoatrial (SA) node
Left bundle branch
Right atrium
Atrioventricular (AV) node
Atrioventricular bundle (of His)
Purkinje fibers
Pulmonary trunk
Interventricular septum
Right bundle branch
Right ventricle
Septomarginal trabecula
Anterior papillary muscle

B Right lateral view. *Opened:* Right atrium and ventricle.

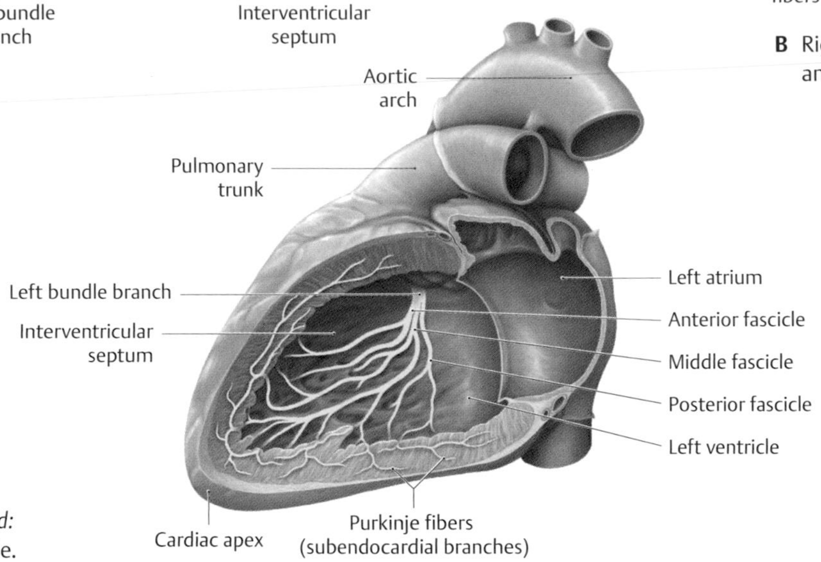

Aortic arch
Pulmonary trunk
Left bundle branch
Interventricular septum
Cardiac apex
Purkinje fibers (subendocardial branches)
Left atrium
Anterior fascicle
Middle fascicle
Posterior fascicle
Left ventricle

C Left lateral view. *Opened:* Left atrium and ventricle.

Clinical

Electrocardiogram (ECG)
The cardiac impulse (a physical dipole) travels across the heart and may be detected with electrodes. The use of three electrodes that separately record electrical activity of the heart along three axes or vectors (Einthoven limb leads) generates an electrocardiogram (ECG). The ECG graphs the cardiac cycle ("heartbeat"), reducing it to a series of waves, segments, and intervals. These ECG components can be used to determine whether cardiac impulses are normal or abnormal (e.g., myocardial infarction, chamber enlargement). *Note:* Although only three leads are required, a standard ECG examination includes at least two others (Goldberger, Wilson leads).

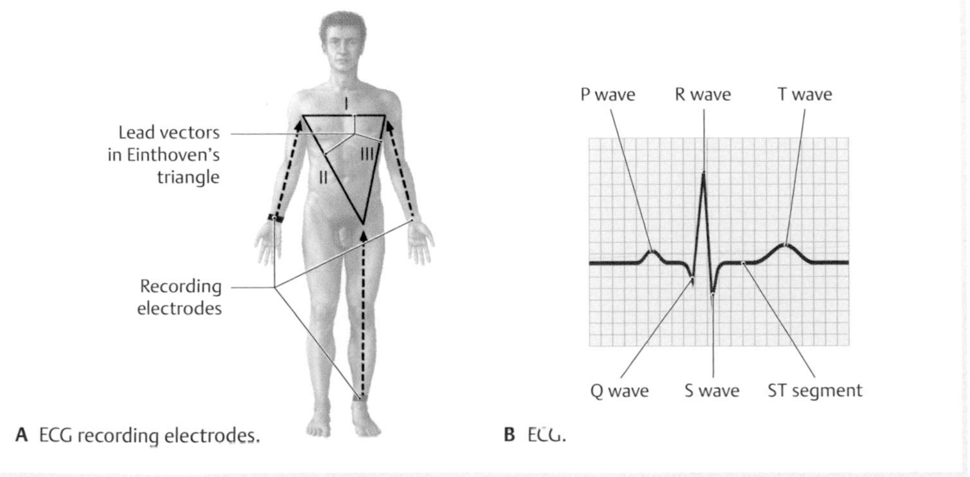
Lead vectors in Einthoven's triangle
I
II
III
Recording electrodes
P wave
R wave
T wave
Q wave
S wave
ST segment

A ECG recording electrodes.

B ECG.

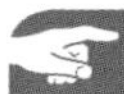

Sympathetic innervation: Preganglionic neurons from T1 to T6 spinal cord segments send fibers to synapse on postganglionic neurons in the cervical and upper thoracic sympathetic ganglia. The three cervical cardiac nerves and thoracic cardiac branches contribute to the cardiac plexus. Parasympathetic innervation: Preganglionic neurons and fibers reach the heart via cardiac branches, some of which also arise in the cervical region. They synapse on postganglionic neurons near the SA node and along the coronary arteries.

Fig. 8.19 Autonomic innervation of the heart

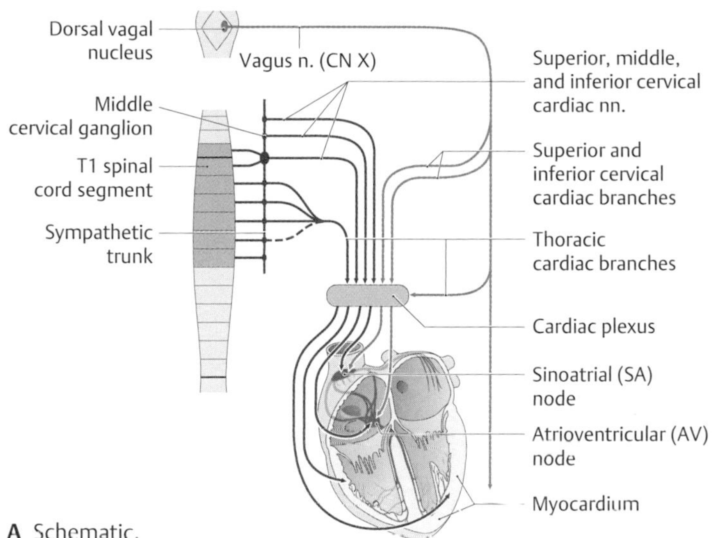

Dorsal vagal nucleus
Vagus n. (CN X)
Middle cervical ganglion
T1 spinal cord segment
Sympathetic trunk
Superior, middle, and inferior cervical cardiac nn.
Superior and inferior cervical cardiac branches
Thoracic cardiac branches
Cardiac plexus
Sinoatrial (SA) node
Atrioventricular (AV) node
Myocardium

A Schematic.

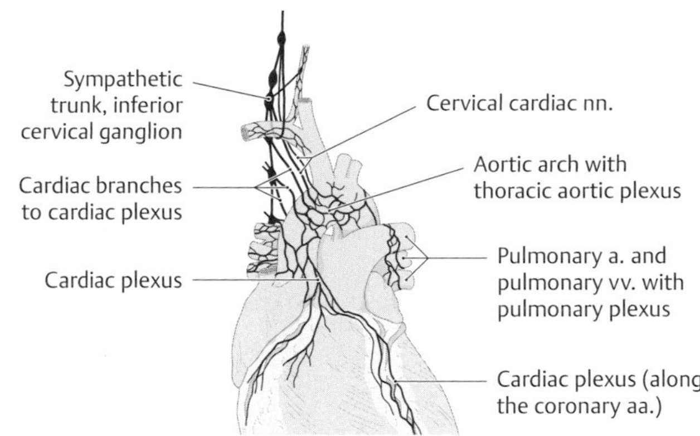

Sympathetic trunk, inferior cervical ganglion
Cardiac branches to cardiac plexus
Cardiac plexus
Cervical cardiac nn.
Aortic arch with thoracic aortic plexus
Pulmonary a. and pulmonary vv. with pulmonary plexus
Cardiac plexus (along the coronary aa.)

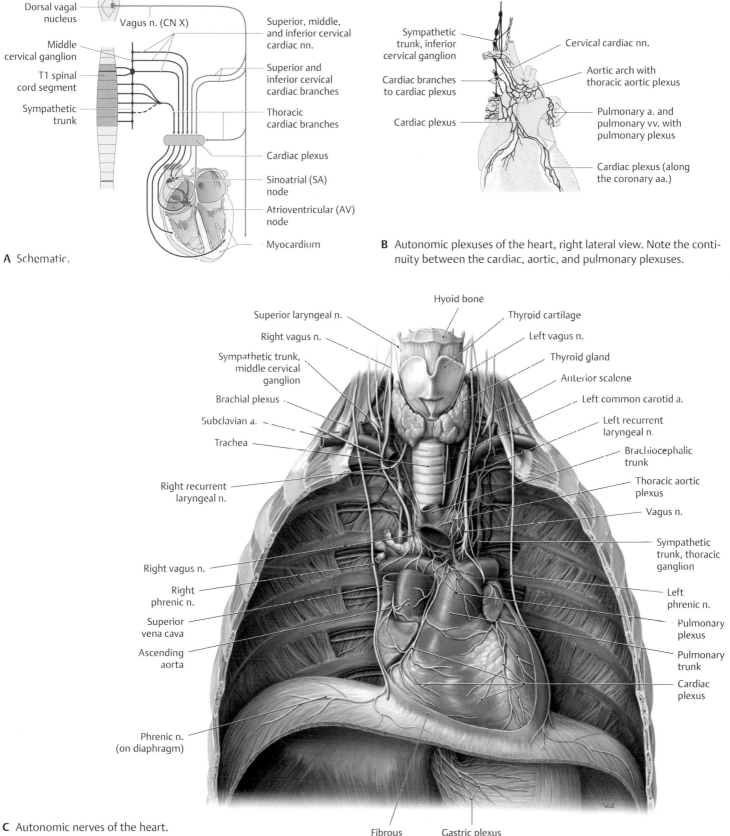

B Autonomic plexuses of the heart, right lateral view. Note the continuity between the cardiac, aortic, and pulmonary plexuses.

Hyoid bone
Superior laryngeal n.
Thyroid cartilage
Right vagus n.
Left vagus n.
Sympathetic trunk, middle cervical ganglion
Thyroid gland
Anterior scalene
Brachial plexus
Left common carotid a.
Subclavian a.
Left recurrent laryngeal n.
Trachea
Brachiocephalic trunk
Right recurrent laryngeal n.
Thoracic aortic plexus
Vagus n.
Sympathetic trunk, thoracic ganglion
Right vagus n.
Right phrenic n.
Left phrenic n.
Superior vena cava
Pulmonary plexus
Ascending aorta
Pulmonary trunk
Cardiac plexus
Phrenic n. (on diaphragm)
Fibrous pericardium (opened)
Gastric plexus

C Autonomic nerves of the heart. Anterior view of opened thorax.

Heart: Radiology

Table 8.5 Borders of the heart	
Border	**Defining structures**
Right cardiac border	Right atrium
	Superior vena cava
Apex	Left ventricle
Left cardiac border	Aortic arch ("aortic knob")
	Pulmonary trunk
	Left atrium
	Left ventricle
Inferior cardiac border	Left ventricle
	Right ventricle

Fig. 8.20 Cardiac borders and configurations

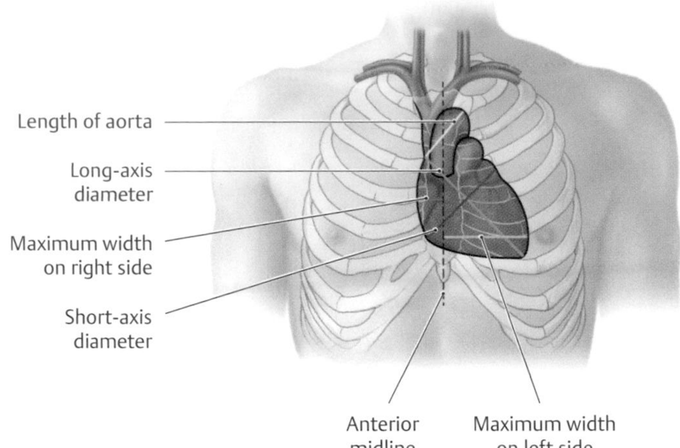
Length of aorta
Long-axis diameter
Maximum width on right side
Short-axis diameter
Anterior midline
Maximum width on left side

Fig. 8.21 Radiographic appearance of the heart

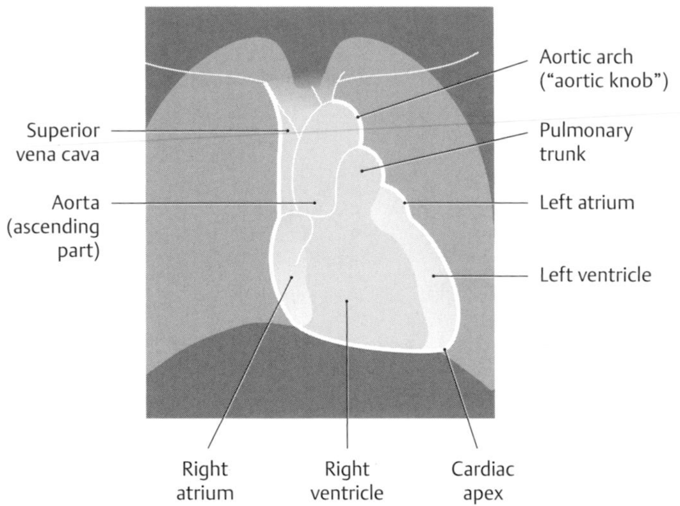
Superior vena cava
Aorta (ascending part)
Aortic arch ("aortic knob")
Pulmonary trunk
Left atrium
Left ventricle
Right atrium
Right ventricle
Cardiac apex

A Anterior view.

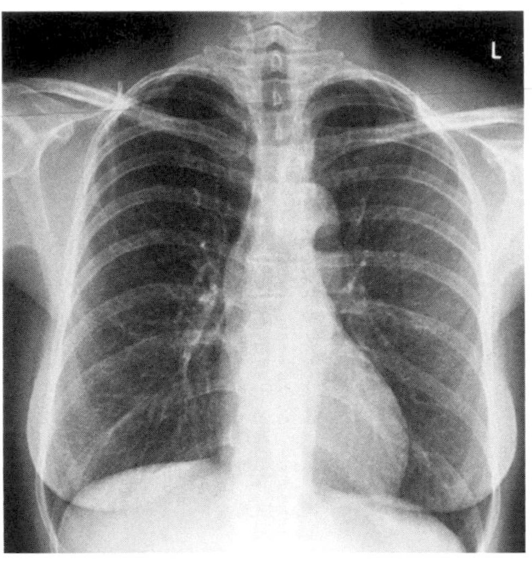
L

B Posteroanterior chest radiograph.

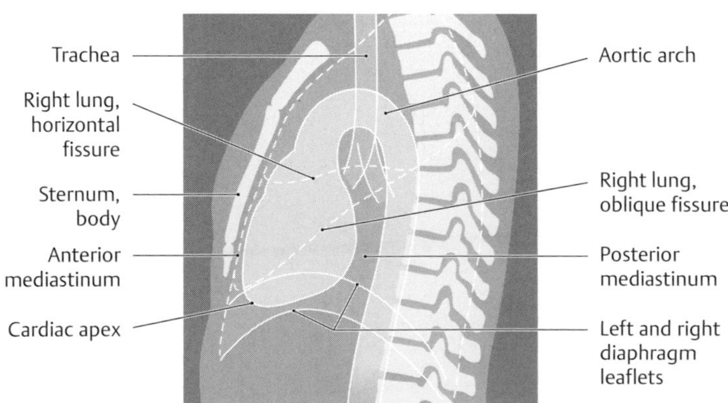
Trachea
Right lung, horizontal fissure
Sternum, body
Anterior mediastinum
Cardiac apex
Aortic arch
Right lung, oblique fissure
Posterior mediastinum
Left and right diaphragm leaflets

C Lateral view. *Visible:* Diaphragm leaflets and lungs. The aortic arch forms a sling over the left main bronchus. Note the narrowness of the anterior mediastinum relative to the posterior mediastinum.

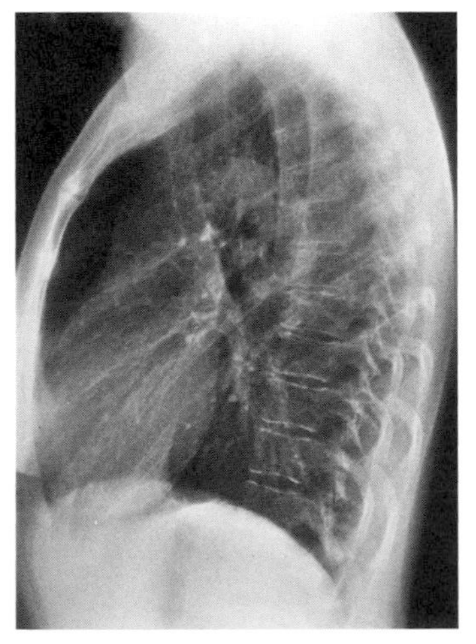

D Left lateral chest radiograph.

Fig. 8.22 Heart in transverse section

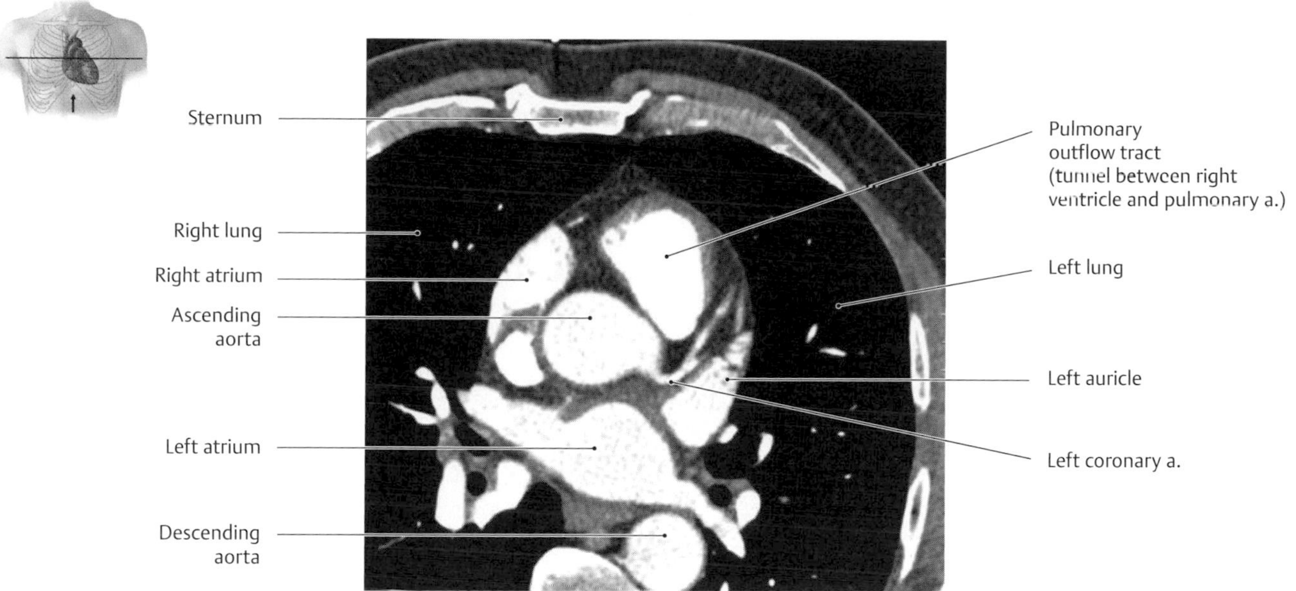
Sternum
Right lung
Right atrium
Ascending aorta
Left atrium
Descending aorta
Pulmonary outflow tract (tunnel between right ventricle and pulmonary a.)
Left lung
Left auricle
Left coronary a.

A Heart in normal chest magnetic resonance imaging (MRI). The cardiac chambers are clearly displayed owing to the high signal intensity, and the lungs are not visualized.

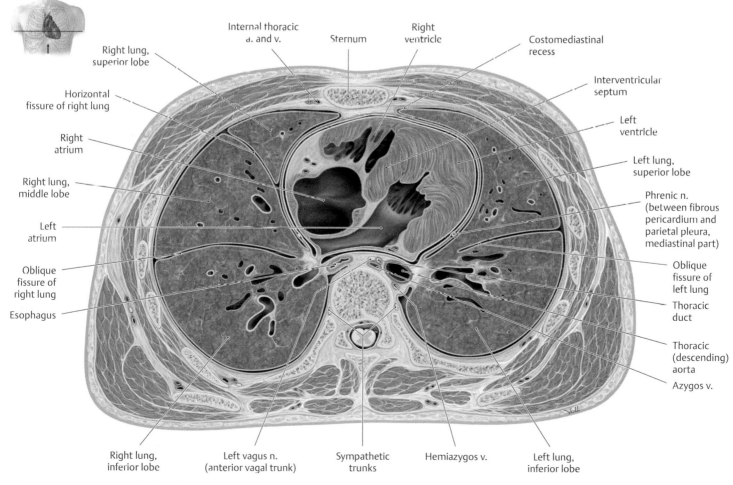

Internal thoracic a. and v.
Sternum
Right ventricle
Costomediastinal recess
Right lung, superior lobe
Horizontal fissure of right lung
Interventricular septum
Left ventricle
Right atrium
Left lung, superior lobe
Right lung, middle lobe
Phrenic n. (between fibrous pericardium and parietal pleura, mediastinal part)
Left atrium
Oblique fissure of left lung
Oblique fissure of right lung
Thoracic duct
Esophagus
Thoracic (descending) aorta
Azygos v.
Right lung, inferior lobe
Left vagus n. (anterior vagal trunk)
Sympathetic trunks
Hemiazygos v.
Left lung, inferior lobe

B Transverse section through T8, inferior view.

Pre- & Postnatal Circulation

Fig. 8.23 Prenatal circulation

After Fritsch and Kühnel.

① Oxygenated and nutrient-rich fetal blood from the placenta passes to the fetus via the umbilical *vein*.

② Approximately half of this blood bypasses the liver (via the ductus venosus) and enters the inferior vena cava. The remainder enters the portal vein to supply the liver with nutrients and oxygen.

③ Blood entering the right atrium from the inferior vena cava bypasses the right ventricle (as the lungs are not yet functioning) to enter the left atrium via the foramen ovale, a right-to-left shunt.

④ Blood from the superior vena cava enters the right atrium, passes to the right ventricle, and moves into the pulmonary trunk. Most of this blood enters the aorta via the ductus arteriosus, a right-to-left shunt.

⑤ The partially oxygenated blood in the aorta returns to the placenta via the paired umbilical arteries that arise from the internal iliac arteries.

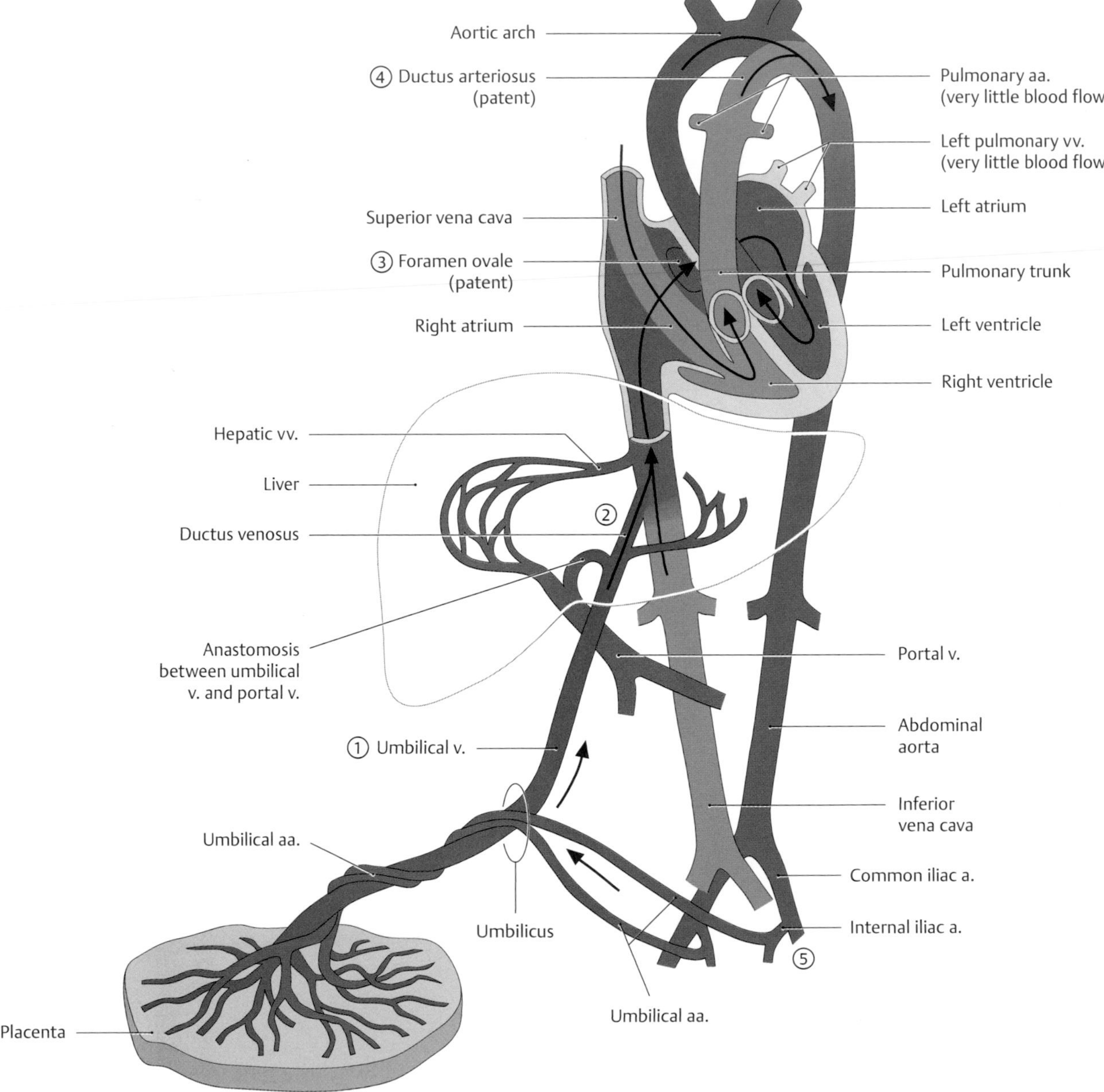

Aortic arch
④ Ductus arteriosus (patent)
Pulmonary aa. (very little blood flow)
Left pulmonary vv. (very little blood flow)
Left atrium
Superior vena cava
③ Foramen ovale (patent)
Pulmonary trunk
Right atrium
Left ventricle
Right ventricle
Hepatic vv.
Liver
②
Ductus venosus
Anastomosis between umbilical v. and portal v.
Portal v.
Abdominal aorta
① Umbilical v.
Inferior vena cava
Umbilical aa.
Common iliac a.
Umbilicus
Internal iliac a.
⑤
Umbilical aa.
Placenta

① As pulmonary respiration begins at birth, pulmonary blood pressure falls, causing blood from the right pulmonary trunk to enter the pulmonary arteries.

② The foramen ovale and ductus arteriosus close, eliminating the fetal right-to-left shunts. The pulmonary and systemic circulations in the heart are now separate.

③ As the infant is separated from the placenta, the umbilical arteries occlude (except for the proximal portions), along with the umbilical vein and ductus venosus.

④ Blood to be metabolized now passes through the liver.

Fig. 8.24 **Postnatal circulation**
After Fritsch and Kühnel.

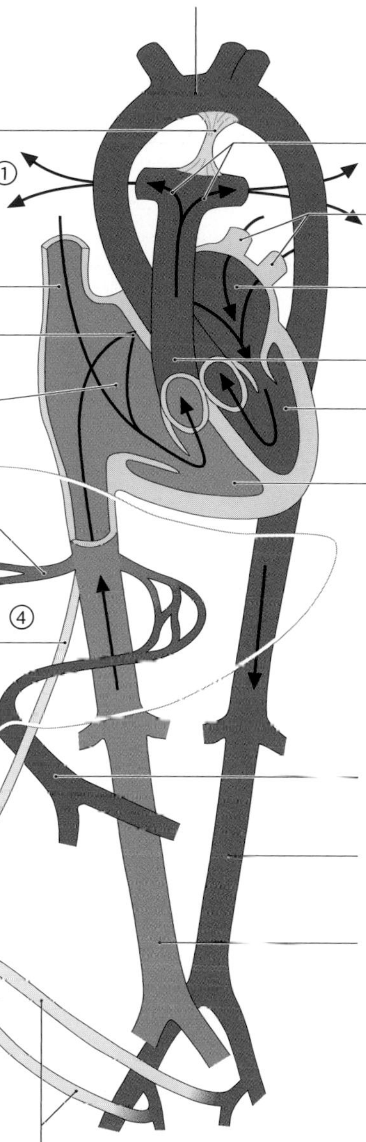

Aortic arch
② Ligamentum arteriosum (obliterated ductus arteriosus)
①
Pulmonary aa. (perfused)
Left pulmonary vv. (perfused)
Superior vena cava
Left atrium
② Foramen ovale (closed)
Pulmonary trunk
Right atrium
Left ventricle
Right ventricle
Hepatic vv.
Liver
④
Ligamentum venosum (obliterated ductus venosus)
Portal v.
Round ligament of liver (obliterated umbilical v.)
Abdominal aorta
③
Umbilical cord
Inferior vena cava
Umbilicus
Obliterated umbilical aa. (medial umbilical ligaments)

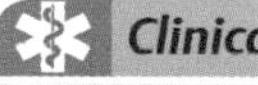
Clinical

Septal defects
Septal defects, the most common type of congenital heart defect, allow blood from the left chambers of the heart to improperly pass into the right chambers during systole. Ventrical septal defect (VSD, shown below) is the most common form. Patent foramen ovale, the most prevalent form of *atrial* septal defect (ASD), results from improper closure of the fetal shunt. LV, left ventricle; RV, right ventricle.

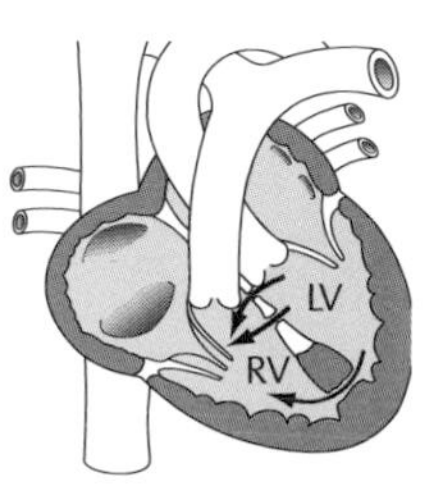
LV
RV

Table 8.6 Derivatives of fetal circulatory structures

Fetal structure	Adult remnant
Ductus arteriosus	Ligamentum arteriosum
Foramen ovale	Fossa ovalis
Ductus venosus	Ligamentum venosum
Umbilical v.	Round ligament of the liver (ligamentum teres)
Umbilical a.	Medial umbilical ligament

Esophagus

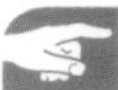

The esophagus is divided into three parts: cervical (C6–T1), thoracic (T1 to the esophageal hiatus of the diaphragm), and abdominal (the diaphragm to the cardiac orifice of the stomach). It descends slightly to the right of the thoracic aorta and pierces the diaphragm slightly to the left, just below the xiphoid process of the sternum.

Fig. 8.25 **Esophagus: Location and constrictions**

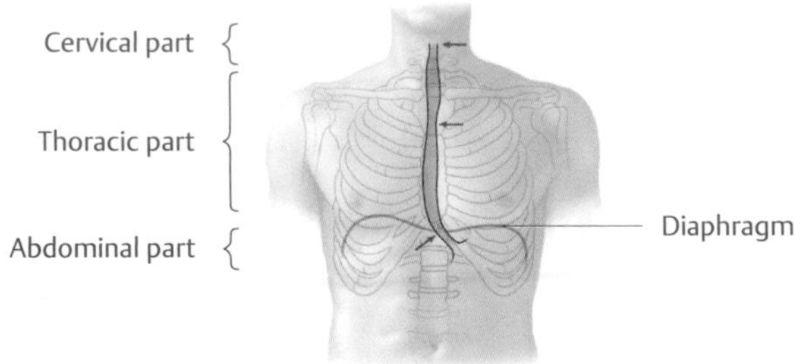
Cervical part
Thoracic part
Abdominal part
Diaphragm

A Projection of esophagus onto chest wall. Esophageal constrictions are indicated with arrows.

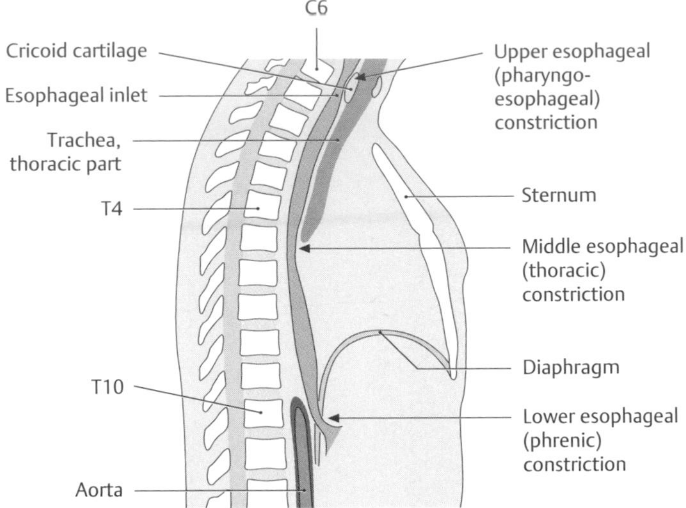
C6
Cricoid cartilage
Esophageal inlet
Trachea, thoracic part
T4
T10
Aorta
Upper esophageal (pharyngo-esophageal) constriction
Sternum
Middle esophageal (thoracic) constriction
Diaphragm
Lower esophageal (phrenic) constriction

B Esophageal constrictions, right lateral view.

Fig. 8.26 **Esophagus in situ**
Anterior view.

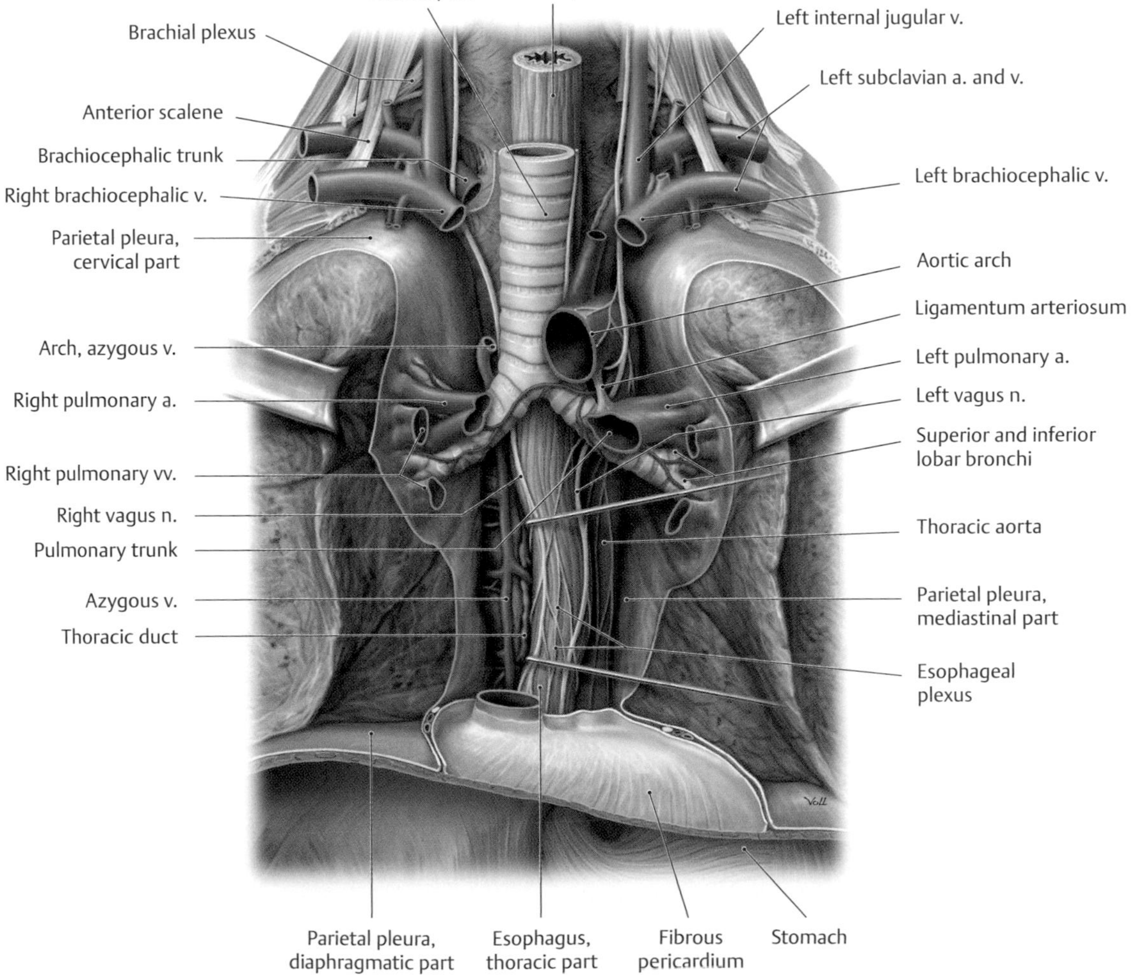

Trachea, cervical part
Esophagus, cervical part
Brachial plexus
Left internal jugular v.
Left subclavian a. and v.
Anterior scalene
Brachiocephalic trunk
Right brachiocephalic v.
Left brachiocephalic v.
Parietal pleura, cervical part
Aortic arch
Ligamentum arteriosum
Arch, azygous v.
Left pulmonary a.
Right pulmonary a.
Left vagus n.
Superior and inferior lobar bronchi
Right pulmonary vv.
Right vagus n.
Thoracic aorta
Pulmonary trunk
Azygous v.
Parietal pleura, mediastinal part
Thoracic duct
Esophageal plexus
Parietal pleura, diaphragmatic part
Esophagus, thoracic part
Fibrous pericardium
Stomach

Fig. 8.27 Structure of the esophagus

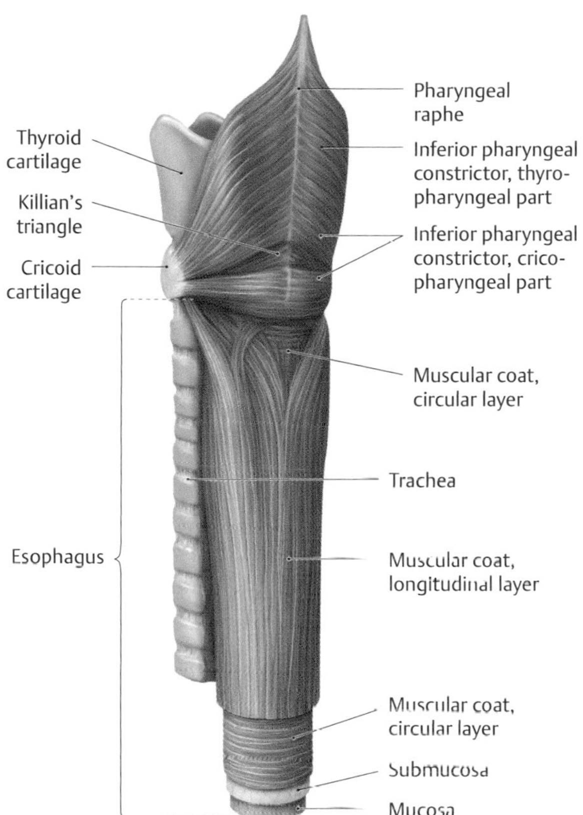
Pharyngeal raphe
Thyroid cartilage
Inferior pharyngeal constrictor, thyro-pharyngeal part
Killian's triangle
Cricoid cartilage
Inferior pharyngeal constrictor, crico-pharyngeal part
Muscular coat, circular layer
Trachea
Esophagus
Muscular coat, longitudinal layer
Muscular coat, circular layer
Submucosa
Mucosa

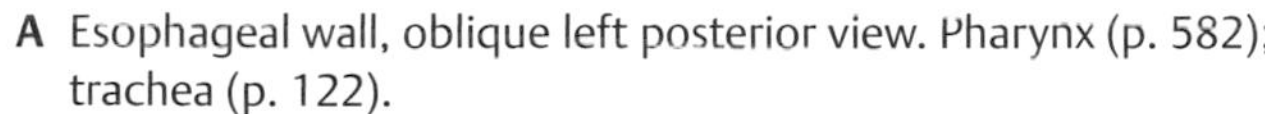

A Esophageal wall, oblique left posterior view. Pharynx (p. 582); trachea (p. 122).

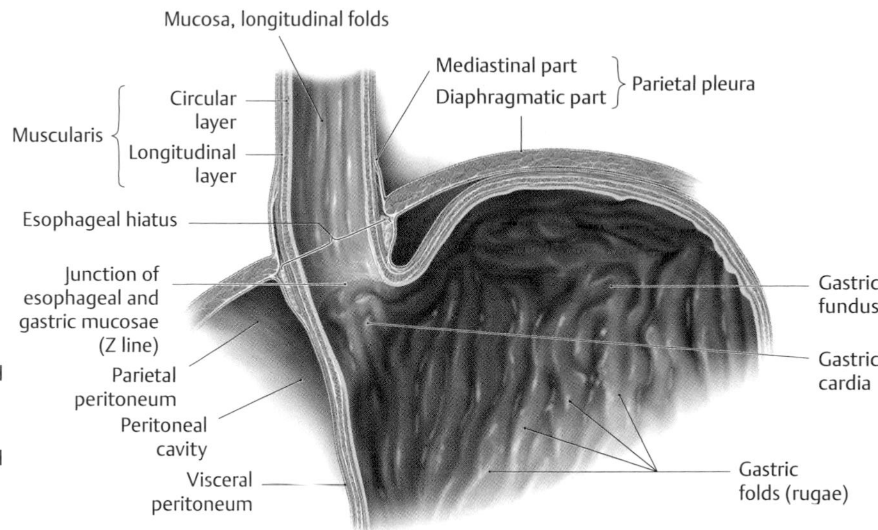
Mucosa, longitudinal folds
Mediastinal part
Diaphragmatic part
Parietal pleura
Muscularis
Circular layer
Longitudinal layer
Esophageal hiatus
Junction of esophageal and gastric mucosae (Z line)
Gastric fundus
Gastric cardia
Parietal peritoneum
Peritoneal cavity
Visceral peritoneum
Gastric folds (rugae)

B Esophagogastric junction, anterior view. A true sphincter is not identifiable at this junction; instead, the diaphragmatic muscle of the esophageal hiatus functions as a sphincter. It is often referred to as the "Z line" because of its zigzag form.

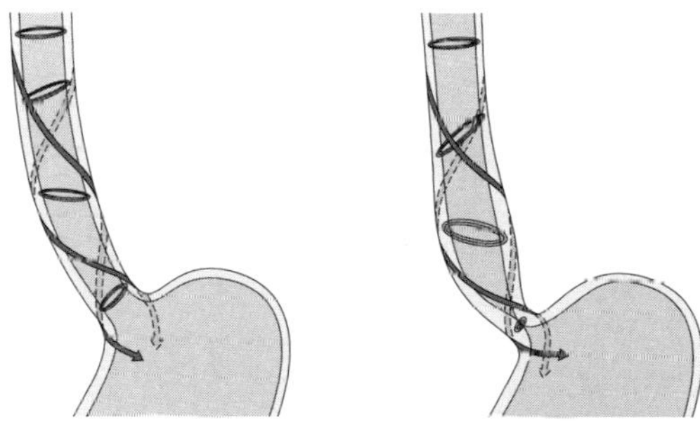

C Functional architecture of esophageal muscle.

Clinical

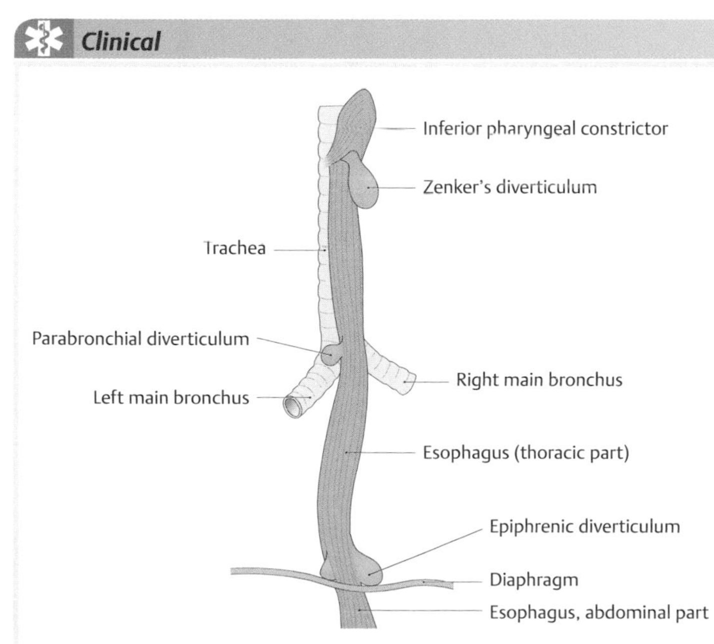
Inferior pharyngeal constrictor
Zenker's diverticulum
Trachea
Parabronchial diverticulum
Right main bronchus
Left main bronchus
Esophagus (thoracic part)
Epiphrenic diverticulum
Diaphragm
Esophagus, abdominal part

Esophageal diverticula

Diverticula (abnormal outpouchings or sacs) generally develop at weak spots in the esophageal wall. There are three main types of esophageal diverticula:

- Hypopharyngeal (pharyngo-esophageal) diverticula: Outpouchings occurring at the junction of the pharynx and the esophagus. These include Zenker's diverticula (70% of cases).
- "True" traction diverticula: Protrusion of all wall layers, not typically occurring at characteristic weak spots. However, they generally result from an inflammatory process (e.g., lymphangitis) and are thus common at sites where the esophagus closely approaches the bronchi and bronchial lymph nodes (thoracic or parabronchial diverticula).
- "False" pulsion diverticula: Herniations of the mucosa and submucosa through weak spots in the muscular coat due to a rise in esophageal pressure (e.g., during normal swallowing). These include parahiatal and epiphrenic diverticula occurring above the esophageal aperture of the diaphragm (10% of cases).

Neurovasculature of the Esophagus

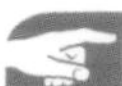

Sympathetic innervation: Preganglionic fibers arise from the T2–T6 spinal cord segments. Postganglionic fibers arise from the sympathetic chain to join the esophageal plexus. Parasympathetic innervation: Preganglionic fibers arise from the dorsal vagal nucleus and travel in the vagus nerves to form the extensive esophageal plexus. *Note:* The postganglionic neurons are in the wall of the esophagus. Fibers to the cervical portion of the esophagus travel in the recurrent laryngeal nerves.

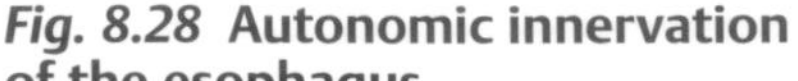

Fig. 8.28 **Autonomic innervation of the esophagus**

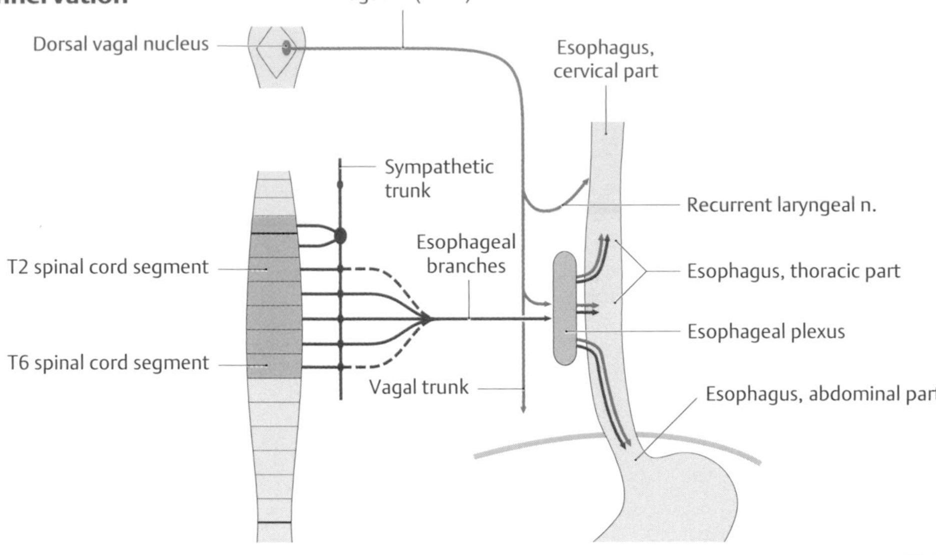
Vagus n. (CN X)
Dorsal vagal nucleus
Esophagus, cervical part
Sympathetic trunk
Recurrent laryngeal n.
Esophageal branches
T2 spinal cord segment
Esophagus, thoracic part
Esophageal plexus
T6 spinal cord segment
Vagal trunk
Esophagus, abdominal part

Fig. 8.29 **Esophageal plexus**

The left and right vagus nerves initially descend on the left and right sides of the esophagus. As they begin to contribute to the esophageal plexus, they shift to anterior and posterior positions, respectively. As the vagus nerves continue into the abdomen, they are named the anterior and posterior vagal trunks.

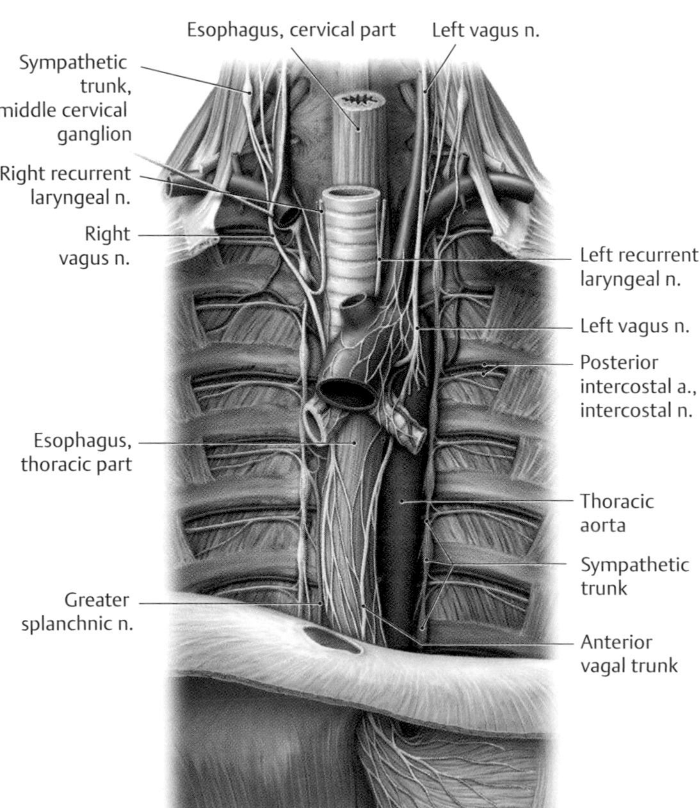
Esophagus, cervical part
Left vagus n.
Sympathetic trunk, middle cervical ganglion
Right recurrent laryngeal n.
Right vagus n.
Left recurrent laryngeal n.
Left vagus n.
Posterior intercostal a., intercostal n.
Esophagus, thoracic part
Thoracic aorta
Sympathetic trunk
Greater splanchnic n.
Anterior vagal trunk

A Esophageal plexus in situ. Anterior view.

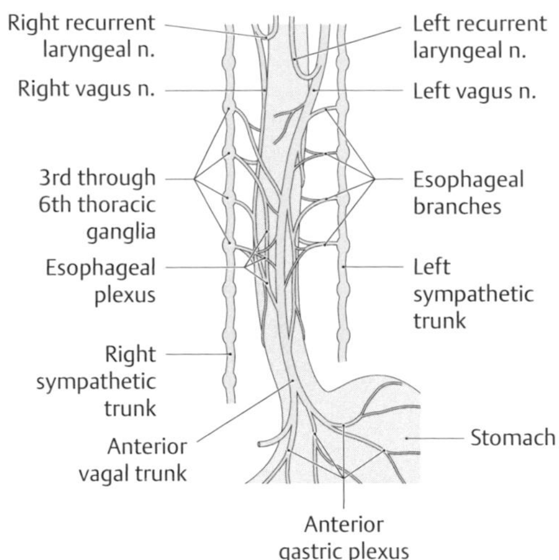
Right recurrent laryngeal n.
Left recurrent laryngeal n.
Right vagus n.
Left vagus n.
3rd through 6th thoracic ganglia
Esophageal branches
Esophageal plexus
Left sympathetic trunk
Right sympathetic trunk
Anterior vagal trunk
Stomach
Anterior gastric plexus

B Anterior view. Note the postganglionic sympathetic contribution to the esophageal plexus.

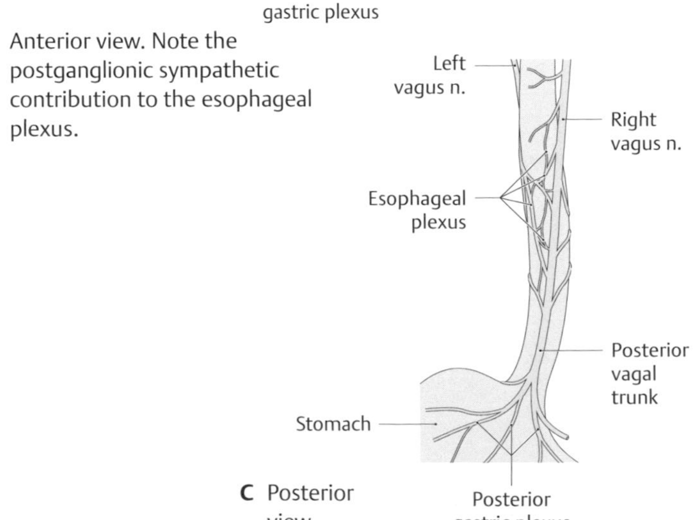
Left vagus n.
Right vagus n.
Esophageal plexus
Posterior vagal trunk
Stomach
Posterior gastric plexus

C Posterior view.

Fig. 8.30 Esophageal arteries
Anterior view.

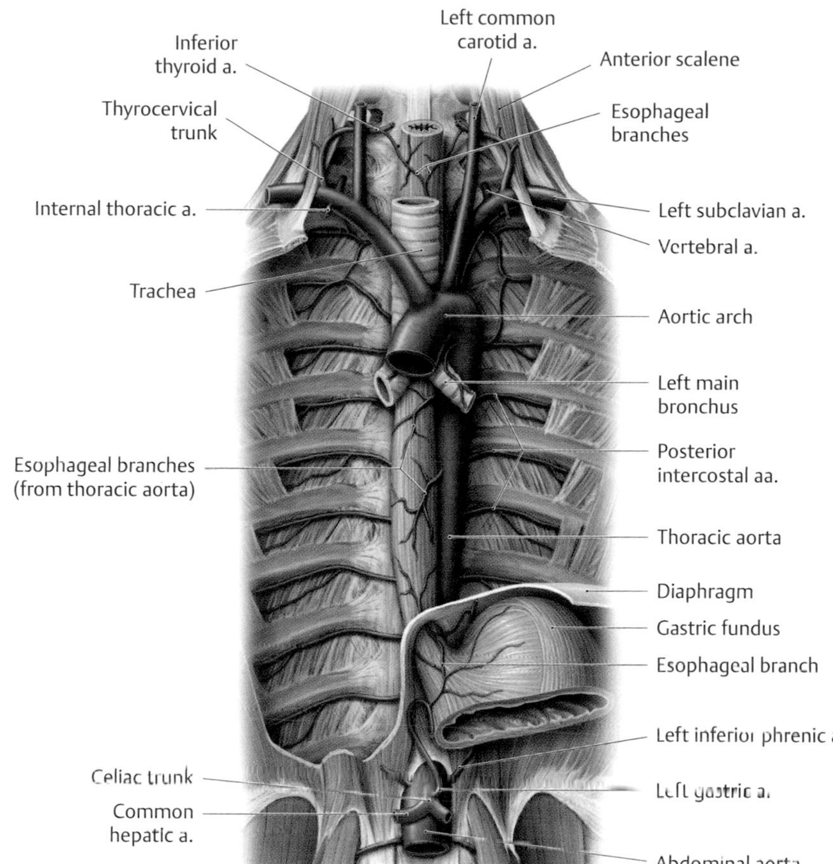
Left common carotid a.
Inferior thyroid a.
Anterior scalene
Esophageal branches
Thyrocervical trunk
Internal thoracic a.
Left subclavian a.
Vertebral a.
Trachea
Aortic arch
Left main bronchus
Posterior intercostal aa.
Esophageal branches (from thoracic aorta)
Thoracic aorta
Diaphragm
Gastric fundus
Esophageal branch
Left inferior phrenic a.
Celiac trunk
Left gastric a.
Common hepatic a.
Abdominal aorta

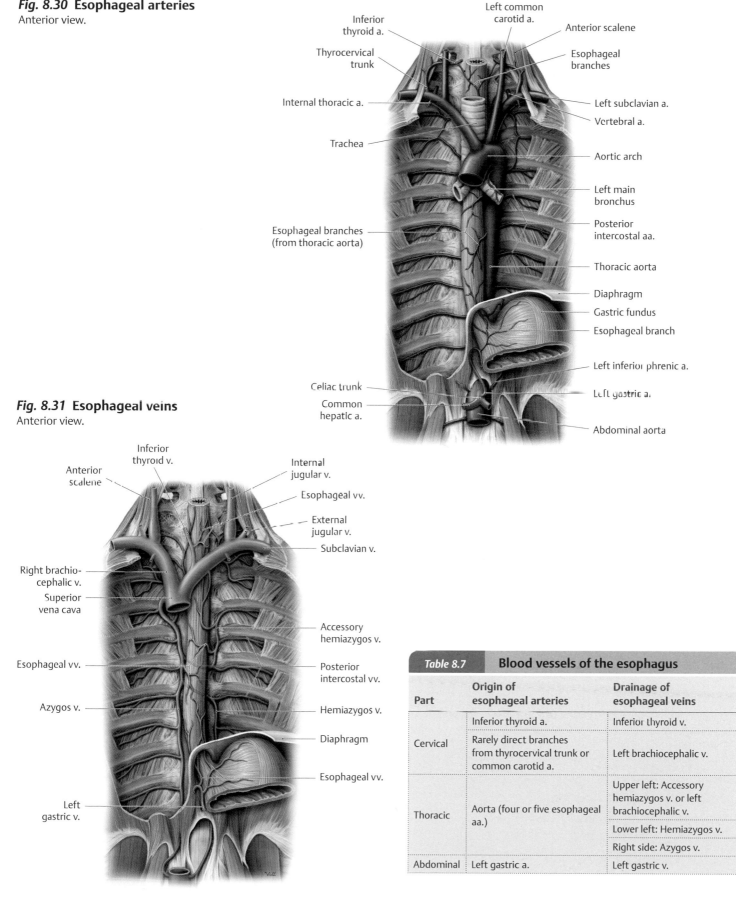

Fig. 8.31 Esophageal veins
Anterior view.

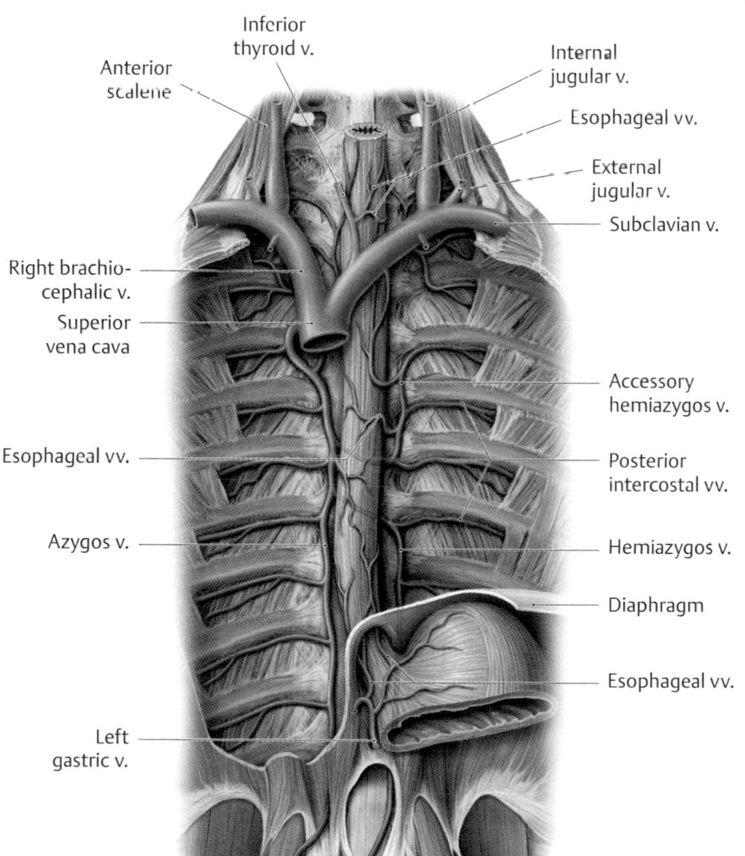
Inferior thyroid v.
Anterior scalene
Internal jugular v.
Esophageal vv.
External jugular v.
Subclavian v.
Right brachio-cephalic v.
Superior vena cava
Accessory hemiazygos v.
Esophageal vv.
Posterior intercostal vv.
Azygos v.
Hemiazygos v.
Diaphragm
Esophageal vv.
Left gastric v.

Table 8.7 Blood vessels of the esophagus

Part	Origin of esophageal arteries	Drainage of esophageal veins
Cervical	Inferior thyroid a.	Inferior thyroid v.
	Rarely direct branches from thyrocervical trunk or common carotid a.	Left brachiocephalic v.
Thoracic	Aorta (four or five esophageal aa.)	Upper left: Accessory hemiazygos v. or left brachiocephalic v.
		Lower left: Hemiazygos v.
		Right side: Azygos v.
Abdominal	Left gastric a.	Left gastric v.

Lymphatics of the Mediastinum

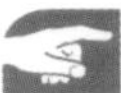

The superior phrenic lymph nodes drain lymph from the diaphragm, pericardium, lower esophagus, lung, and liver into the bronchomediastinal trunk. The inferior phrenic lymph nodes, found in the abdomen, collect lymph from the diaphragm and lower lobes of the lung and convey it to the lumbar trunk. *Note*: The pericardium may also drain superiorly to the brachiocephalic lymph nodes.

Fig. 8.32 **Lymph nodes of the mediastinum and thoracic cavity**
Left anterior oblique view.

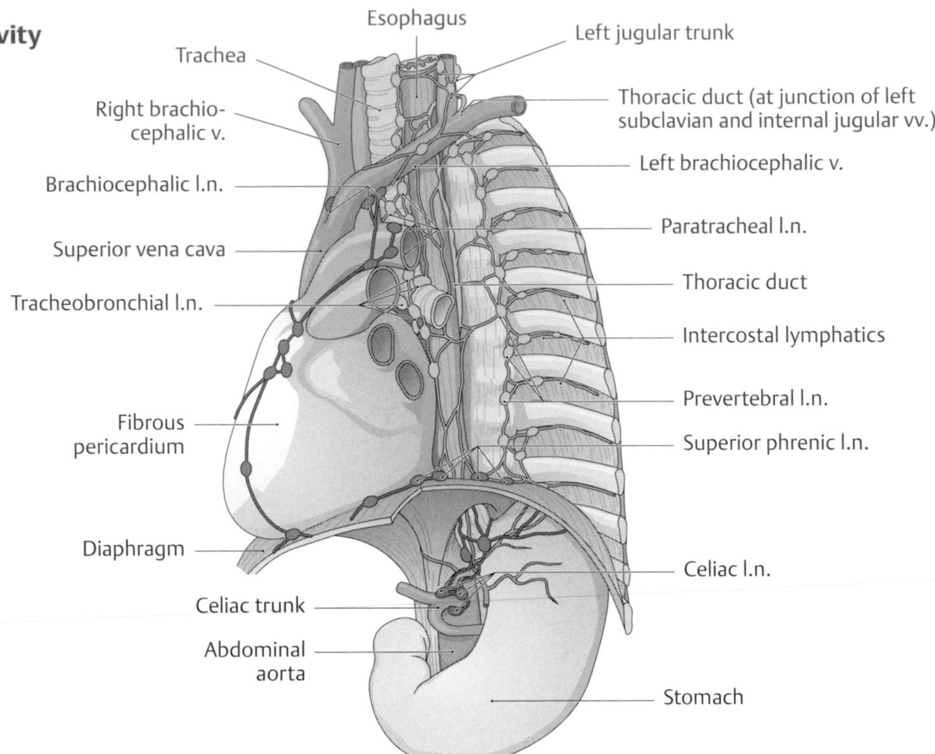
Esophagus
Left jugular trunk
Trachea
Thoracic duct (at junction of left subclavian and internal jugular vv.)
Right brachio-cephalic v.
Left brachiocephalic v.
Brachiocephalic l.n.
Paratracheal l.n.
Superior vena cava
Thoracic duct
Tracheobronchial l.n.
Intercostal lymphatics
Prevertebral l.n.
Fibrous pericardium
Superior phrenic l.n.
Diaphragm
Celiac l.n.
Celiac trunk
Abdominal aorta
Stomach

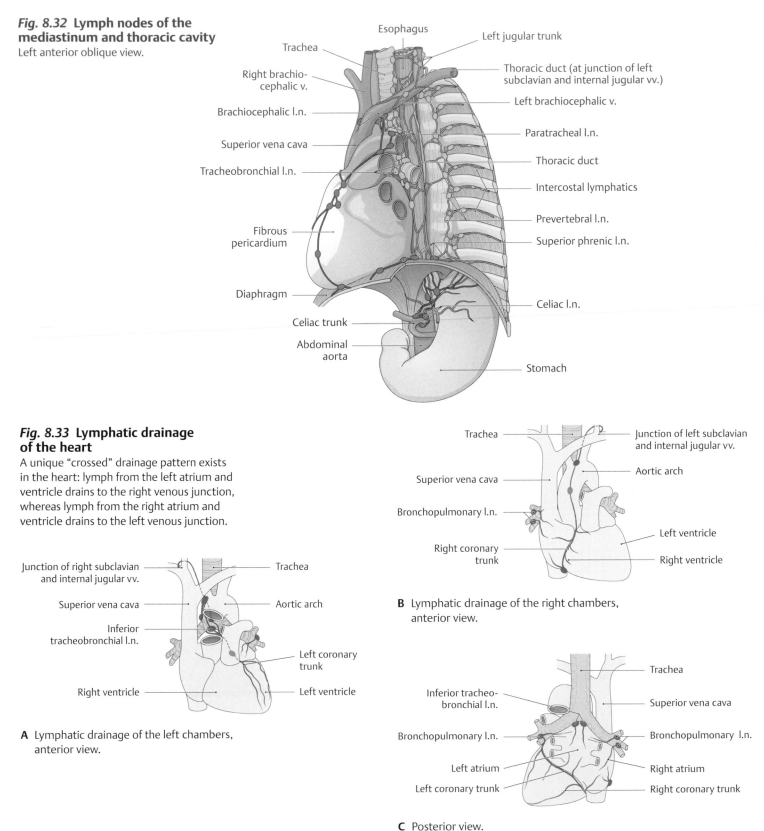

Fig. 8.33 **Lymphatic drainage of the heart**
A unique "crossed" drainage pattern exists in the heart: lymph from the left atrium and ventricle drains to the right venous junction, whereas lymph from the right atrium and ventricle drains to the left venous junction.

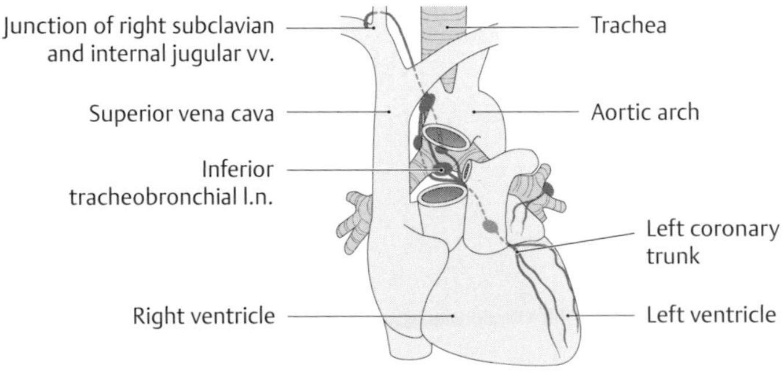
Junction of right subclavian and internal jugular vv.
Trachea
Superior vena cava
Aortic arch
Inferior tracheobronchial l.n.
Left coronary trunk
Right ventricle
Left ventricle

A Lymphatic drainage of the left chambers, anterior view.

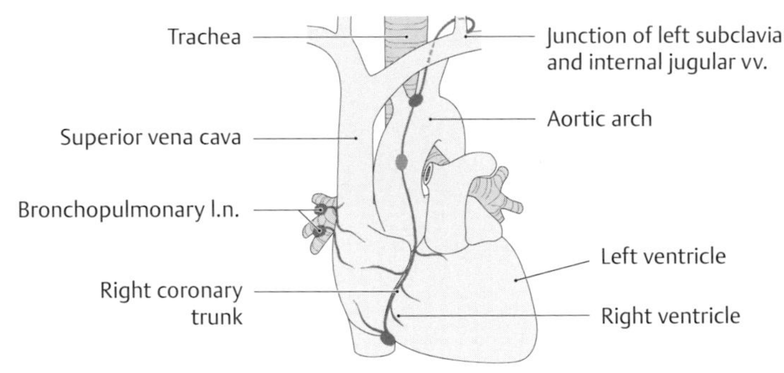
Trachea
Junction of left subclavian and internal jugular vv.
Aortic arch
Superior vena cava
Bronchopulmonary l.n.
Left ventricle
Right coronary trunk
Right ventricle

B Lymphatic drainage of the right chambers, anterior view.

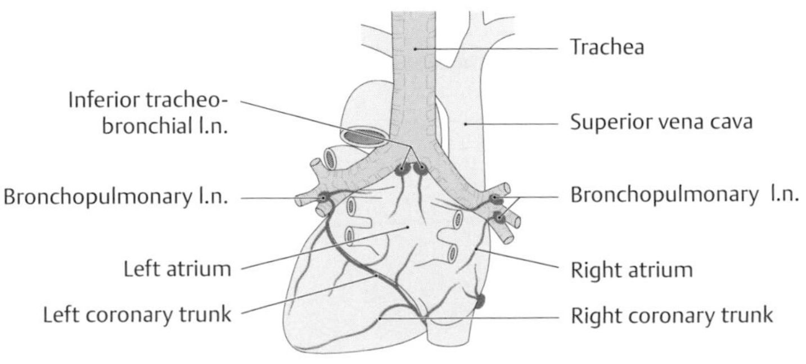
Trachea
Inferior tracheo-bronchial l.n.
Superior vena cava
Bronchopulmonary l.n.
Bronchopulmonary l.n.
Left atrium
Right atrium
Left coronary trunk
Right coronary trunk

C Posterior view.

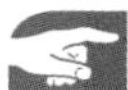

The paraesophageal nodes drain the esophagus. Lymphatic drainage of the cervical part of the esophagus is primarily cranial, to the deep cervical lymph nodes and then to the jugular trunk. The thoracic part of the esophagus drains to the bronchomediastinal trunks in two parts: the upper half drains cranially, and the lower half drains inferiorly via the superior phrenic lymph nodes. The bronchopulmonary and paratracheal nodes drain lymph from the lungs, bronchi, and trachea into the bronchomediastinal trunk (see p. 128).

Fig. 8.34 Mediastinal lymph nodes

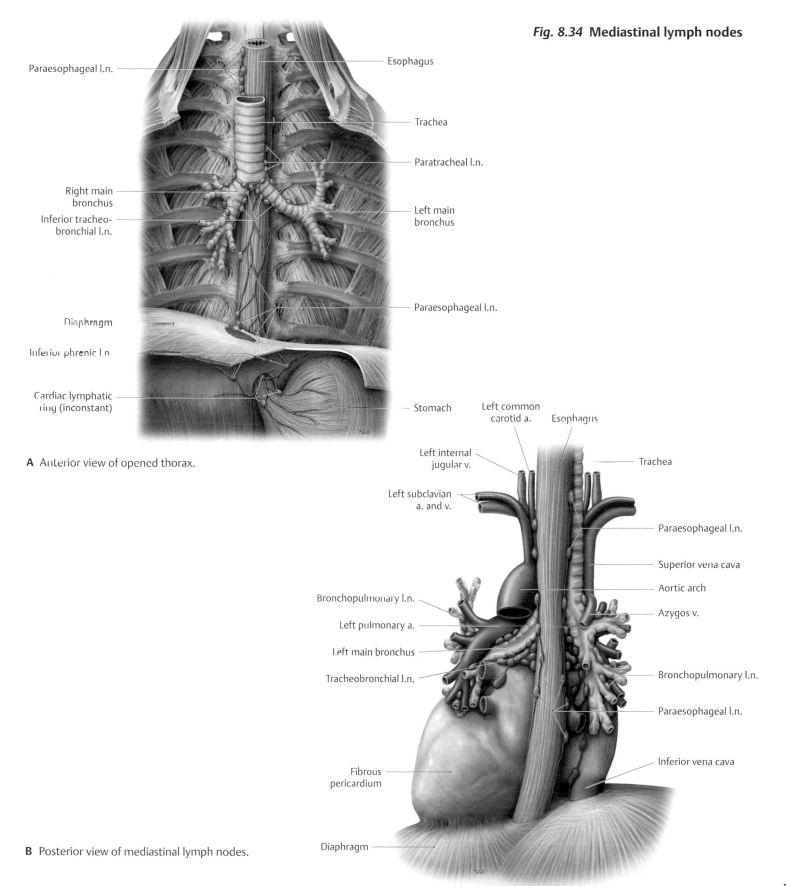

Paraesophageal l.n.
Esophagus
Trachea
Paratracheal l.n.
Right main bronchus
Inferior tracheo-bronchial l.n.
Left main bronchus
Paraesophageal l.n.
Diaphragm
Inferior phrenic l.n.
Cardiac lymphatic ring (inconstant)
Stomach

A Anterior view of opened thorax.

Left common carotid a.
Esophagus
Left internal jugular v.
Trachea
Left subclavian a. and v.
Paraesophageal l.n.
Superior vena cava
Aortic arch
Bronchopulmonary l.n.
Azygos v.
Left pulmonary a.
Left main bronchus
Tracheobronchial l.n.
Bronchopulmonary l.n.
Paraesophageal l.n.
Inferior vena cava
Fibrous pericardium
Diaphragm

B Posterior view of mediastinal lymph nodes.

Pleural Cavities

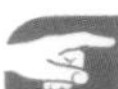

The paired pleural cavities contain the left and right lungs. They are completely separated from each other by the mediastinum and are under negative atmospheric pressure (see respiratory mechanics, pp. 122–123). The left pleural cavity is slightly smaller than the right, especially anteriorly, due to the asymmetrical position of the heart in the mediastinum, with the greater mass on the left . This causes a shift of some of the boundaries of the parietal pleura and lung on the left side at the level of the heart, as reflected in the difference in thoracic landmarks found at the intersection of the posterior border of the pleural cavities with certain reference lines on the left and right.

Fig. 9.1 **Boundaries of the lungs and pleural cavities**
The upper blue dot on each reference line is the inferior boundary of the lung and the lower red dot is the inferior boundary of the pleural cavity.

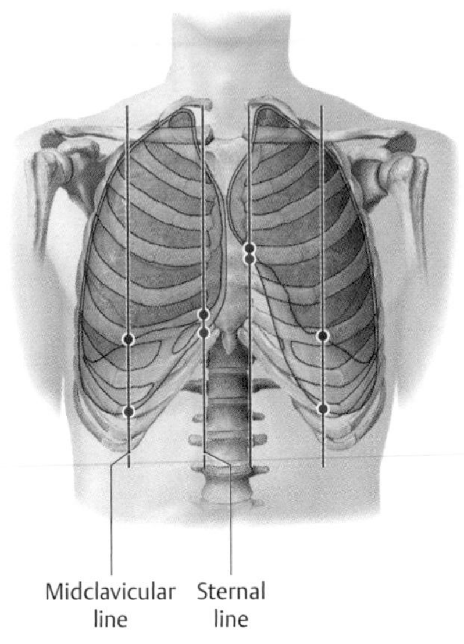
Midclavicular line
Sternal line

A Anterior view.

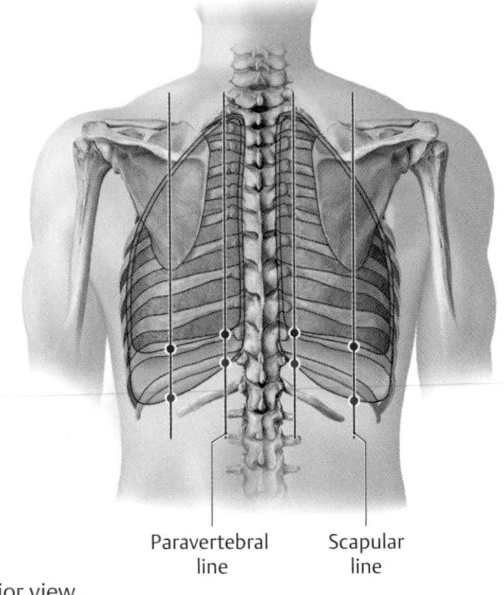
Paravertebral line
Scapular line

B Posterior view.

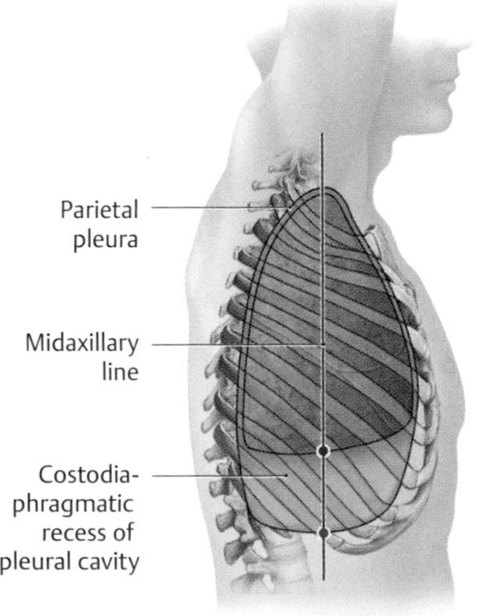
Parietal pleura
Midaxillary line
Costodia-phragmatic recess of pleural cavity

C Right lateral view.

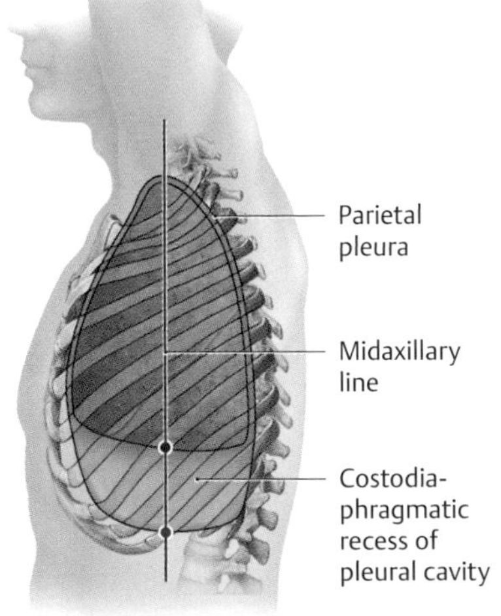
Parietal pleura
Midaxillary line
Costodia-phragmatic recess of pleural cavity

D Left lateral view.

Table 9.1 Pleural cavity boundaries and reference points

Reference line	Right lung	Right parietal pleura	Left lung	Left parietal pleura
Sternal line (STL)	6th rib	7th rib	4th rib	4th rib
Midclavicular line (MCL)	6th rib	8th costal cartilage	6th rib	8th rib
Midaxillary line (MAL)	8th rib	10th rib	8th rib	10th rib
Scapular line (SL)	10th rib	11th rib	10th rib	11th rib
Paravertebral line (PV)	10th rib	T12 vertebra	10th rib	T12 vertebra

Fig. 9.2 Parietal pleura

The pleural cavity is bounded by two serous layers. The visceral (pulmonary) pleura covers the lungs, and the parietal pleura lines the inner surface of the thoracic cavity. The four parts of the parietal pleura (costal, diaphragmatic, mediastinal, and cervical) are continuous.

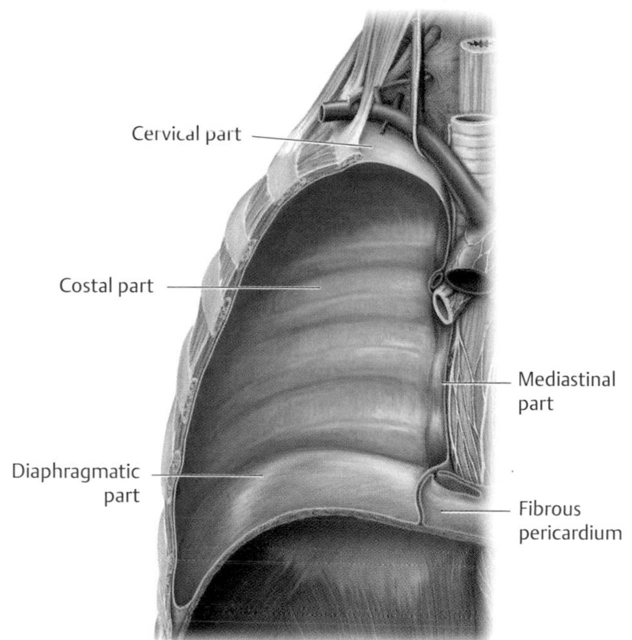

Cervical part
Costal part
Mediastinal part
Diaphragmatic part
Fibrous pericardium

A Parts of the parietal pleura. *Opened:* Right pleural cavity, anterior view.

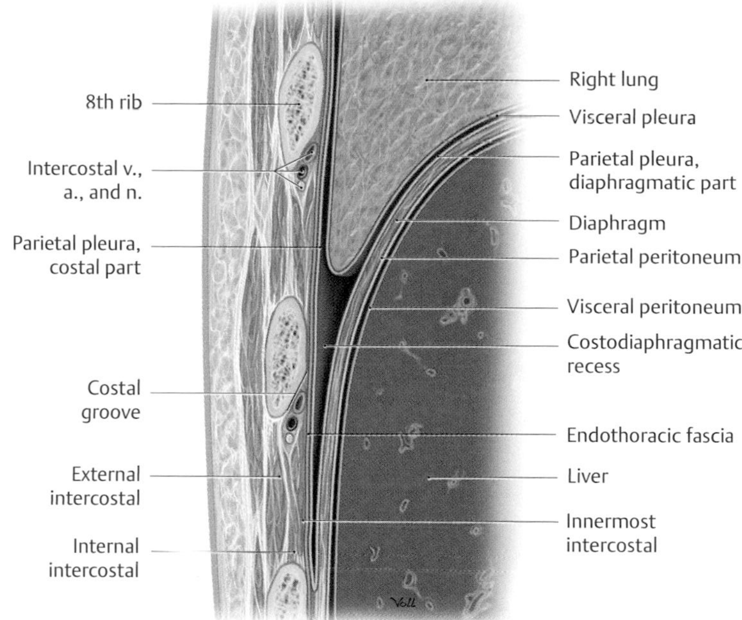

8th rib
Intercostal v., a., and n.
Parietal pleura, costal part
Costal groove
External intercostal
Internal intercostal
Right lung
Visceral pleura
Parietal pleura, diaphragmatic part
Diaphragm
Parietal peritoneum
Visceral peritoneum
Costodiaphragmatic recess
Endothoracic fascia
Liver
Innermost intercostal

B Costodiaphragmatic recess, coronal section, anterior view. Reflection of the diaphragmatic pleura onto the inner thoracic wall (becoming the costal pleura) forms the costodiaphragmatic recess.

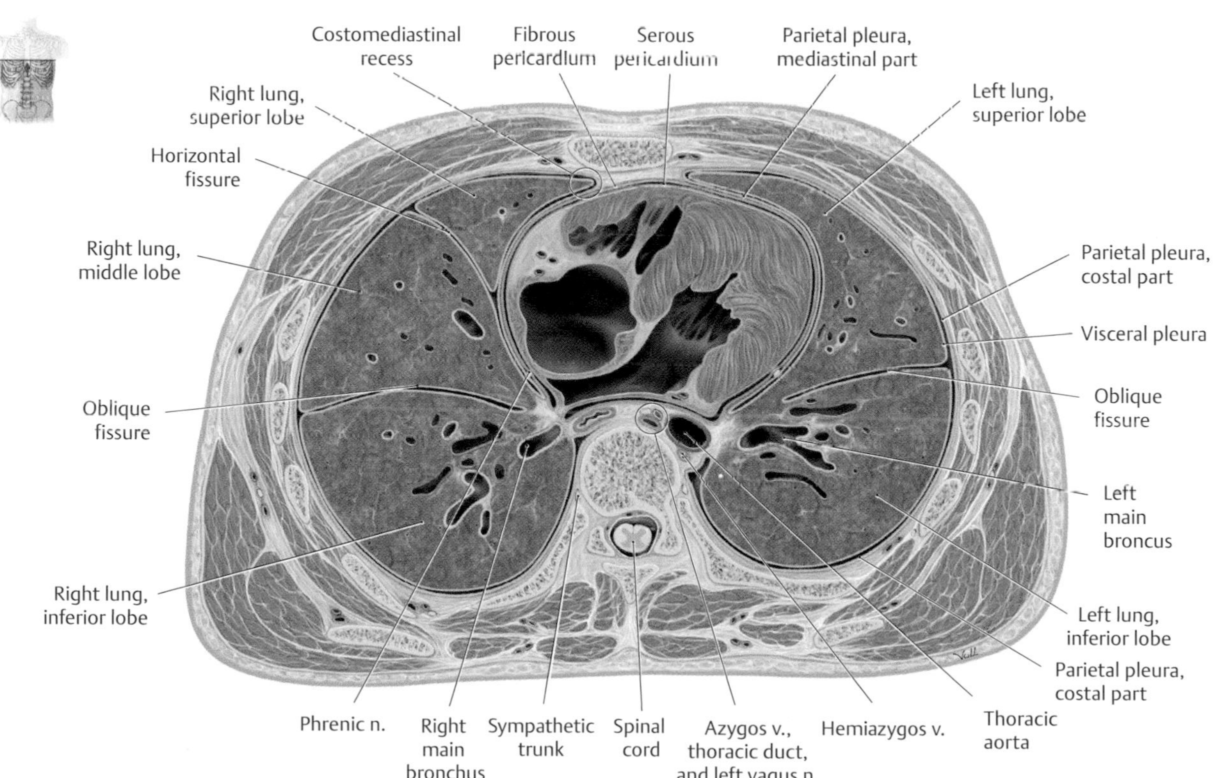

Costomediastinal recess
Fibrous pericardium
Serous pericardium
Parietal pleura, mediastinal part
Right lung, superior lobe
Left lung, superior lobe
Horizontal fissure
Right lung, middle lobe
Parietal pleura, costal part
Visceral pleura
Oblique fissure
Oblique fissure
Left main broncus
Right lung, inferior lobe
Left lung, inferior lobe
Parietal pleura, costal part
Phrenic n.
Right main bronchus
Sympathetic trunk
Spinal cord
Azygos v., thoracic duct, and left vagus n.
Hemiazygos v.
Thoracic aorta

C Transverse section, inferior view. Reflection of the costal pleura onto the pericardium forms the costomediastinal recess.

Pleura: Subdivisions, Recesses & Innervation

Fig. 9.3 **Pleura and its divisions**
The anterior thoracic wall and costal portion of the parietal pleura have been removed to show the lungs in situ.

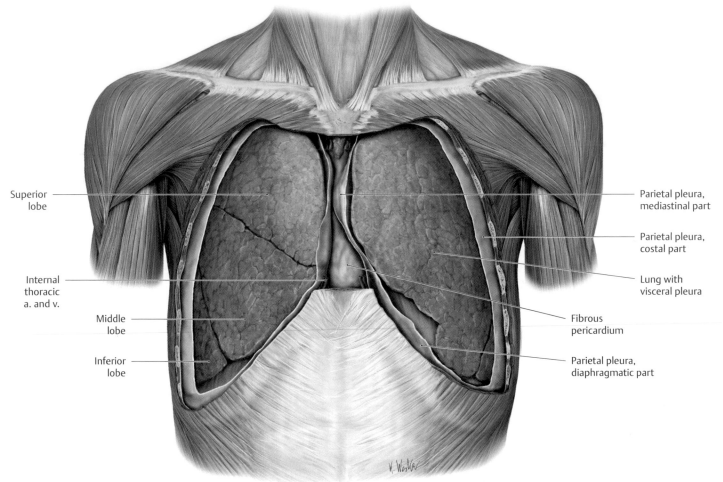

Superior lobe
Internal thoracic a. and v.
Middle lobe
Inferior lobe
Parietal pleura, mediastinal part
Parietal pleura, costal part
Lung with visceral pleura
Fibrous pericardium
Parietal pleura, diaphragmatic part

Clinical

Percutaneous liver biopsy
Percutaneous liver biopsy is usually performed 2–3 cm superior to the inferior border of the liver at the right midaxillary line. The biopsy needle traverses the skin, thoracic wall, costal parietal pleura, costodiaphragmatic recess, diaphragmatic parietal pleura, diaphragm, then enters the liver in the abdominal cavity. The lower margin of the right lung rarely descends into the costodiaphragmatic recess during quiet inspiration
and the costal and diaphragmatic parietal pleura are opposed by surface tension forces. Before inserting the biopsy needle, the physician will ask the patient to exhale and hold his or her breath. This increases the opposition of the costal and diaphragmatic pleura, more tightly closing the costodiaphragmatic recess, and further decreasing the risk of pneumothorax, the introduction of air in the interpleural space, when the biopsy needle is inserted. Pnemothorax, if severe, can produce lung collapse.

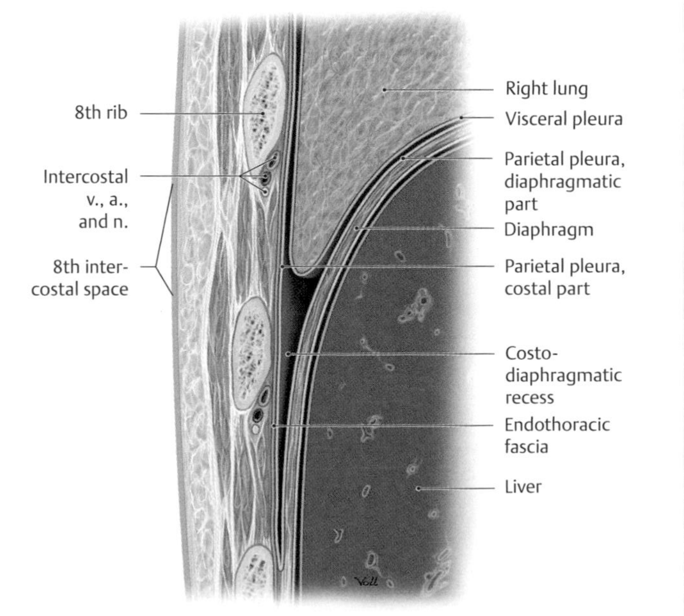
8th rib
Intercostal v., a., and n.
8th inter-costal space
Right lung
Visceral pleura
Parietal pleura, diaphragmatic part
Diaphragm
Parietal pleura, costal part
Costo-diaphragmatic recess
Endothoracic fascia
Liver

Fig. 9.4 Costomediastinal and costodiaphragmatic recesses
On the left side of the thorax, an examiner's fingertips are placed in the costomediastinal and costodiaphragmatic recesses. These recesses are formed by the acute reflection of the costal part of the parietal pleura onto the fibrous pericardium (costomediastinal) or diaphragm (costodiaphragmatic).

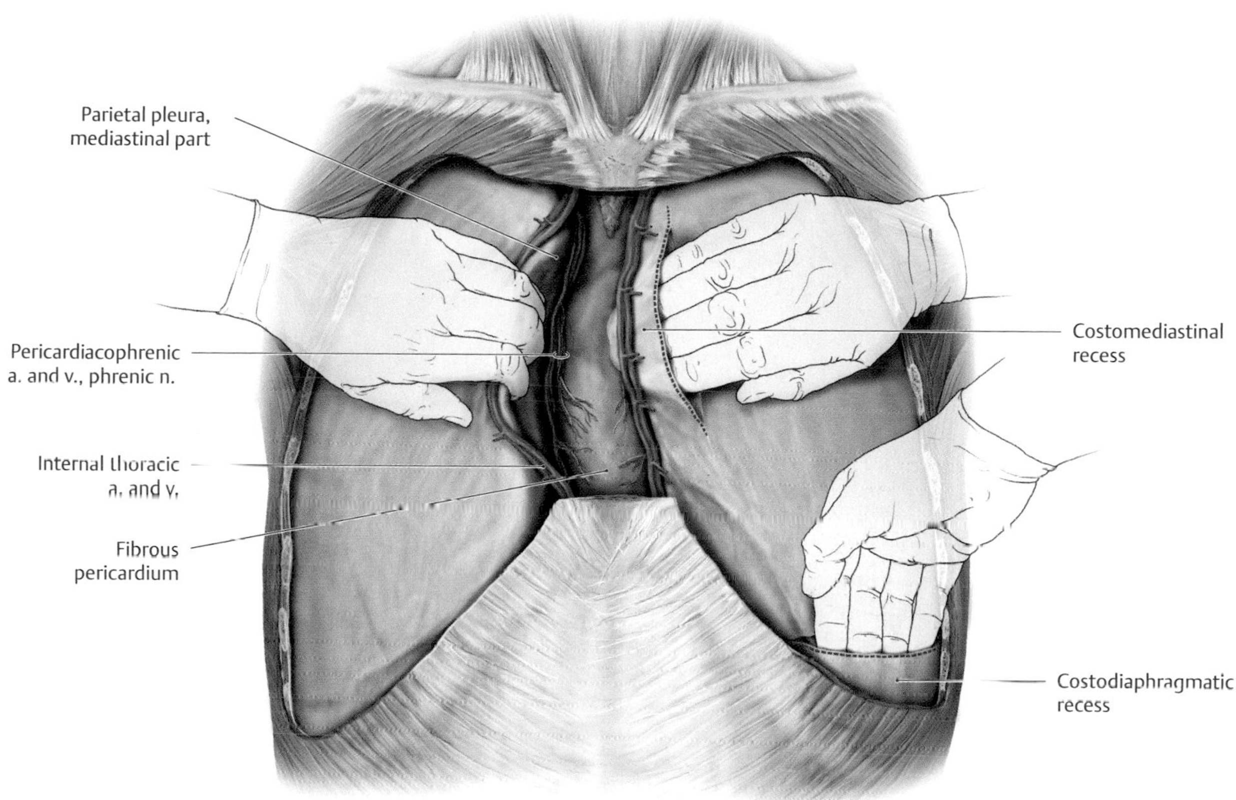

Parietal pleura, mediastinal part
Pericardiacophrenic a. and v., phrenic n.
Internal thoracic a. and v.
Fibrous pericardium
Costomediastinal recess
Costodiaphragmatic recess

Fig. 9.5 Innervation of the pleura
The costal and cervical portions and the periphery of the diaphragmatic portion of the parietal pleura are innervated by the intercostal nerves. The mediastinal and central portions of the diaphragmatic pleura are innervated by the phrenic nerves. The visceral pleura covering the lung itself receives its innervation from the autonomic nervous system.

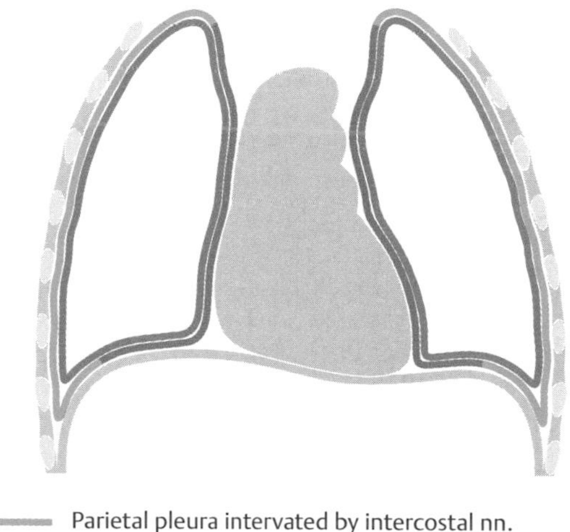

Parietal pleura intervated by intercostal nn.
Parietal pleura intervated by phrenic n.
Visceral pleura innervated by autonomic nn.

Lungs

Fig. 9.6 Lungs in situ
The left and right lungs occupy the full volume of the pleural cavity. Note that the left lung is slightly smaller than the right due to the asymmetrical position of the heart.

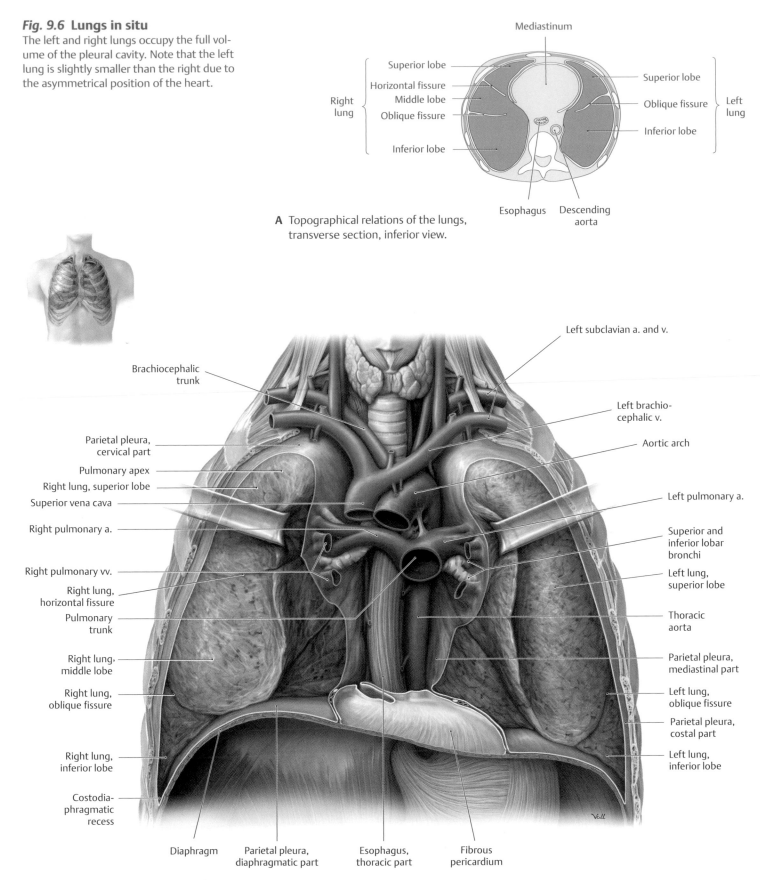

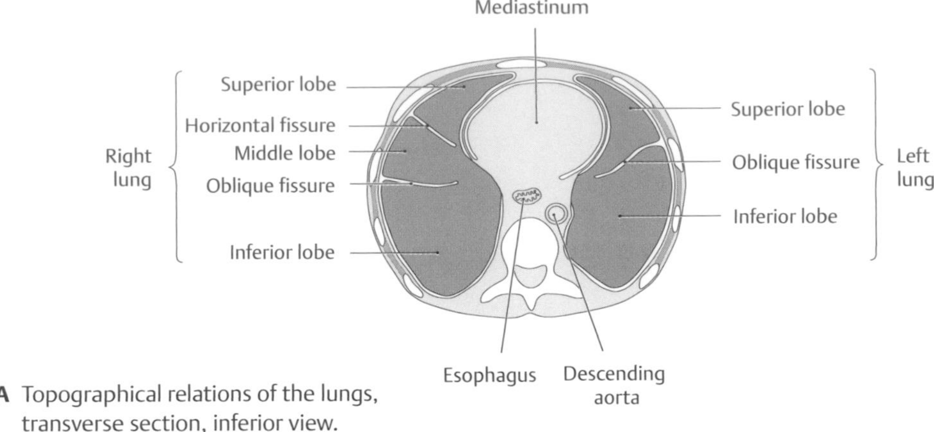
Mediastinum
Right lung
Superior lobe
Horizontal fissure
Middle lobe
Oblique fissure
Inferior lobe
Superior lobe
Oblique fissure
Inferior lobe
Left lung
Esophagus
Descending aorta

A Topographical relations of the lungs, transverse section, inferior view.

Left subclavian a. and v.
Brachiocephalic trunk
Left brachio-cephalic v.
Parietal pleura, cervical part
Aortic arch
Pulmonary apex
Right lung, superior lobe
Superior vena cava
Left pulmonary a.
Right pulmonary a.
Superior and inferior lobar bronchi
Right pulmonary vv.
Left lung, superior lobe
Right lung, horizontal fissure
Pulmonary trunk
Thoracic aorta
Right lung, middle lobe
Parietal pleura, mediastinal part
Right lung, oblique fissure
Left lung, oblique fissure
Parietal pleura, costal part
Right lung, inferior lobe
Left lung, inferior lobe
Costodia-phragmatic recess
Diaphragm
Parietal pleura, diaphragmatic part
Esophagus, thoracic part
Fibrous pericardium

B Anterior view with lungs retracted.

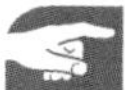

The oblique and horizontal fissures divide the right lung into three lobes: superior, middle, and inferior. The oblique fissure divides the left lung into two lobes: superior and inferior.

The apex of each lung extends into the root of the neck. The hilum is the location at which the bronchi and neurovascular structures connect to the lung.

Fig. 9.7 Gross anatomy of the lungs

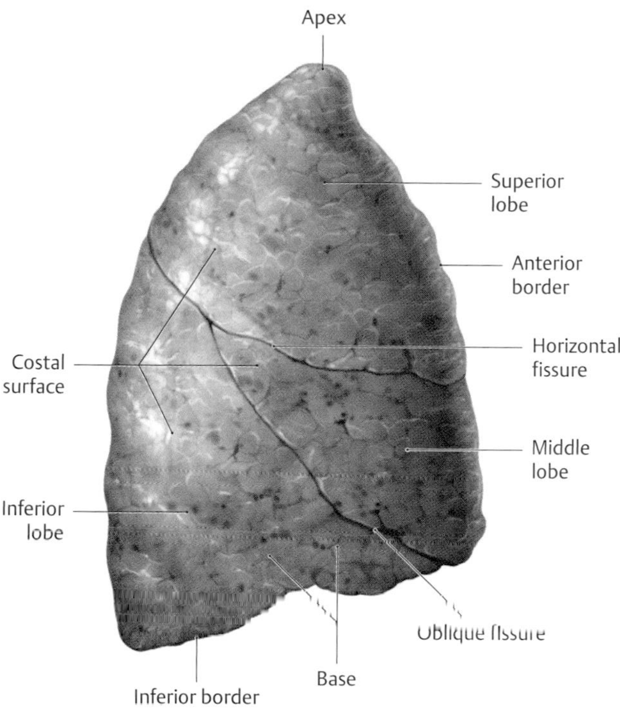
Apex
Superior lobe
Anterior border
Horizontal fissure
Costal surface
Middle lobe
Inferior lobe
Oblique fissure
Base
Inferior border

A Right lung, lateral view.

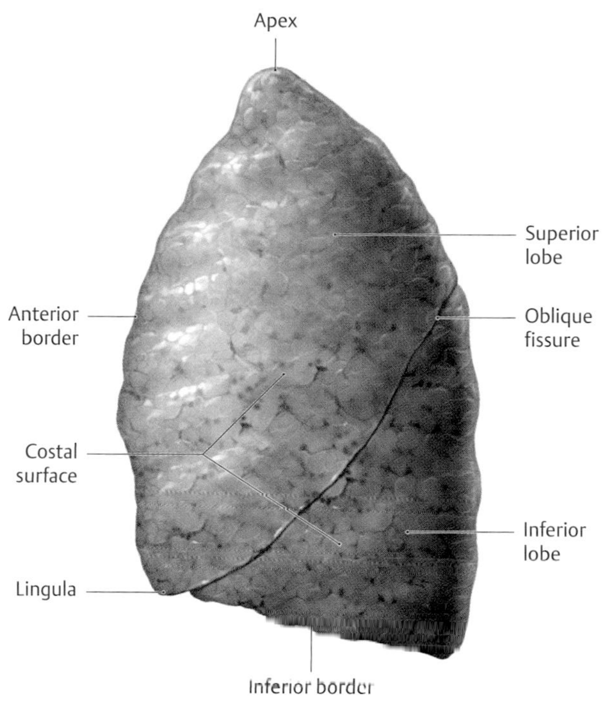
Apex
Superior lobe
Anterior border
Oblique fissure
Costal surface
Inferior lobe
Lingula
Inferior border

B Left lung, lateral view.

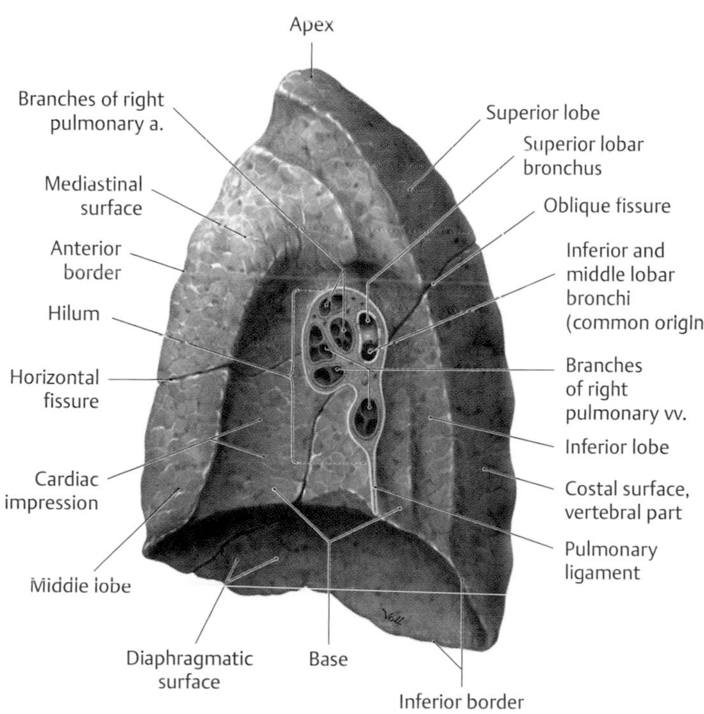
Apex
Branches of right pulmonary a.
Superior lobe
Superior lobar bronchus
Mediastinal surface
Oblique fissure
Anterior border
Inferior and middle lobar bronchi (common origin)
Hilum
Horizontal fissure
Branches of right pulmonary vv.
Inferior lobe
Cardiac impression
Costal surface, vertebral part
Pulmonary ligament
Middle lobe
Diaphragmatic surface
Base
Inferior border

C Right lung, medial view.

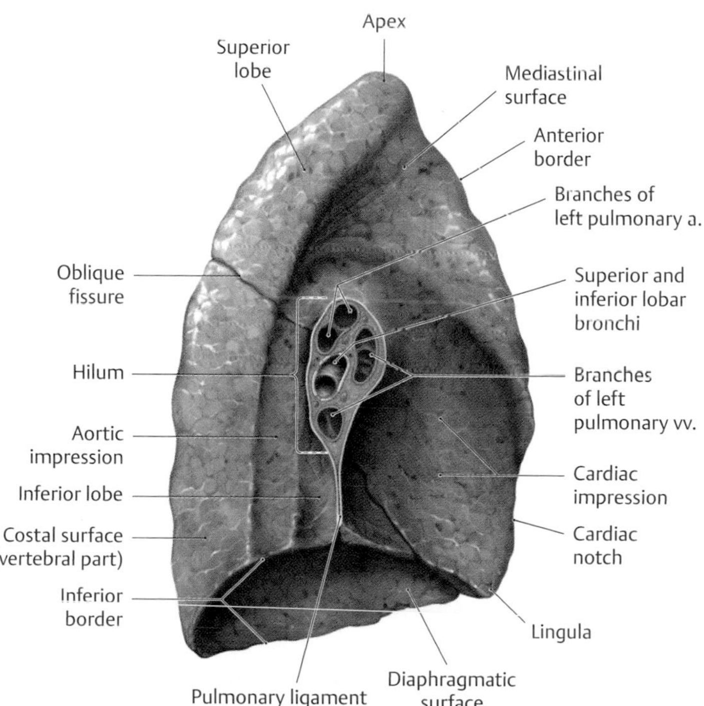
Apex
Superior lobe
Mediastinal surface
Anterior border
Branches of left pulmonary a.
Oblique fissure
Superior and inferior lobar bronchi
Hilum
Branches of left pulmonary vv.
Aortic impression
Cardiac impression
Inferior lobe
Cardiac notch
Costal surface (vertebral part)
Inferior border
Lingula
Pulmonary ligament
Diaphragmatic surface

D Left lung, medial view.

Lung: Radiology

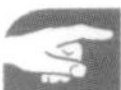

The regions of the lungs show varying degrees of lucency in chest radiographs. The perihilar region where the main bronchi and vessels enter and exit the lung is less radiolucent than the peripheral region, which contains small-caliber vascular branches and segmental bronchi. The perihilar lung region is also covered by the heart. These "shadows" appear as white or bright areas on the radiograph (radiographs are negatives: areas that are impermeable to light will appear bright).

Fig. 9.8 Radiographic appearance of the lungs

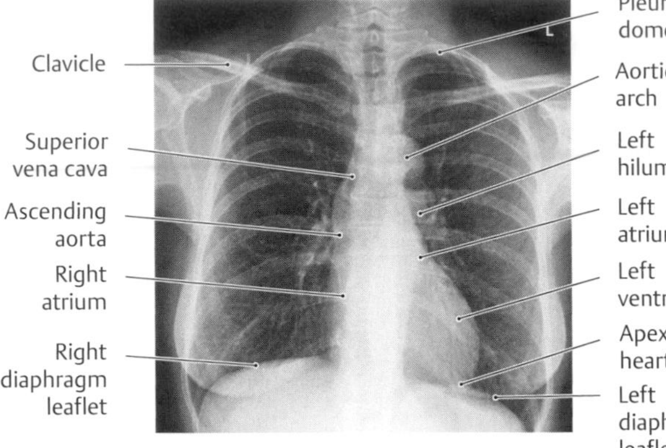
Clavicle
Superior vena cava
Ascending aorta
Right atrium
Right diaphragm leaflet
Pleural dome
Aortic arch
Left hilum
Left atrium
Left ventricle
Apex of heart
Left diaphragm leaflet

A Normal posteroanterior chest radiograph.

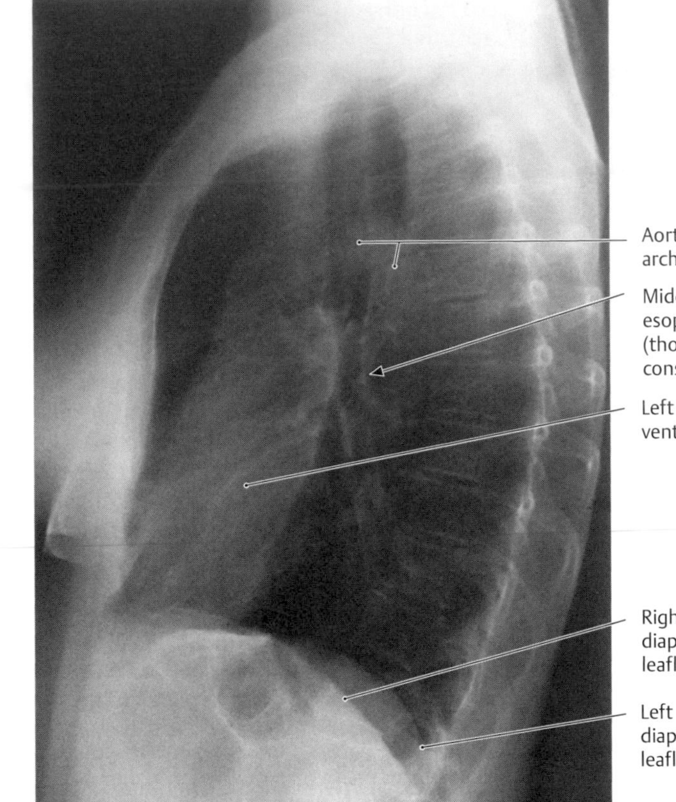
Aortic arch
Middle esophageal (thoracic) constriction
Left ventricle
Right diaphragm leaflet
Left diaphragm leaflet

B Normal lateral chest radiograph.

Fig. 9.9 Opacity in lung diseases

Lateral and anterior views of the right and left lungs. Opacity (decreased radiolucency) may be observed in diseased lung areas. Increased opacity may be due to fluid infiltration (inflammation) or tissue proliferation (neoplasia). These opacities are easier to detect in the peripheral part of the lung, which is inherently more radiolucent. *Note*: Opacities that conform to segmental lung boundaries are almost invariably due to pulmonary inflammation.

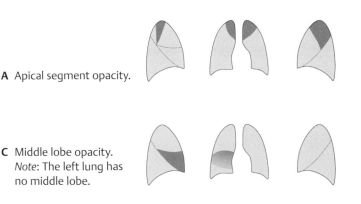

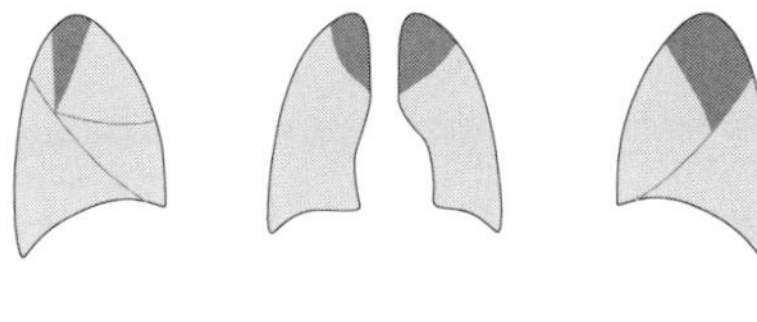

A Apical segment opacity.

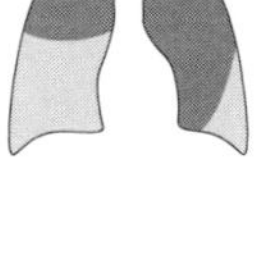
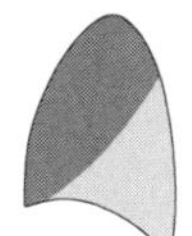

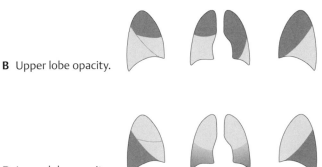

B Upper lobe opacity.

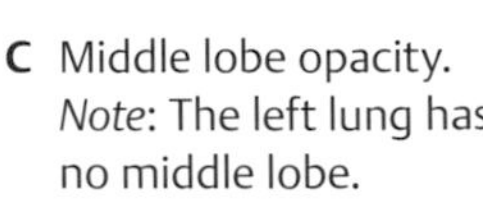

C Middle lobe opacity. *Note*: The left lung has no middle lobe.

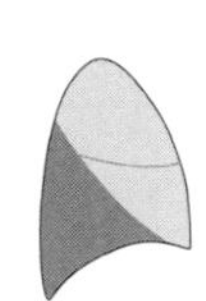
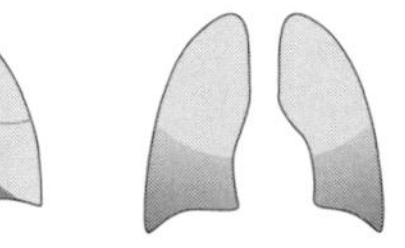

D Lower lobe opacity.

Clinical

Diseases of the lung

Increased opacity in the lungs does not necessarly correspond to segmental boundaries. Fluid accumulation in the lungs also creates characteristic "shadows" in pulmonary radiographs.

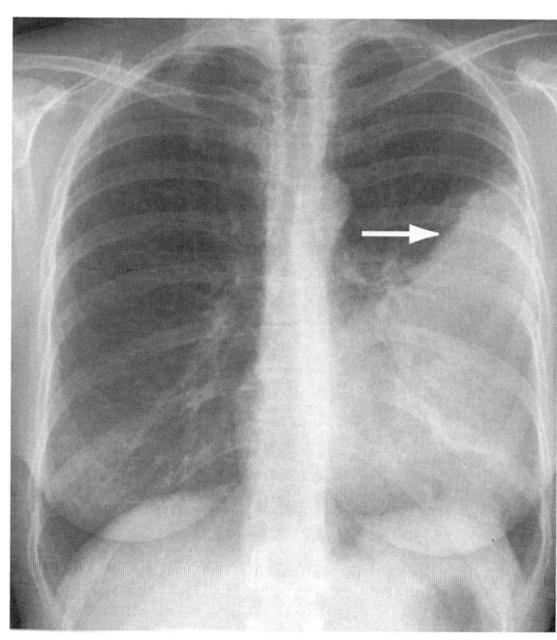

A Lingular pneumonia. The boundary between bronchopulmonary segments III and IV can be seen (*arrow*). *Note*: The heart is much more difficult to visualize here due to increased opacity of segments IV and V.

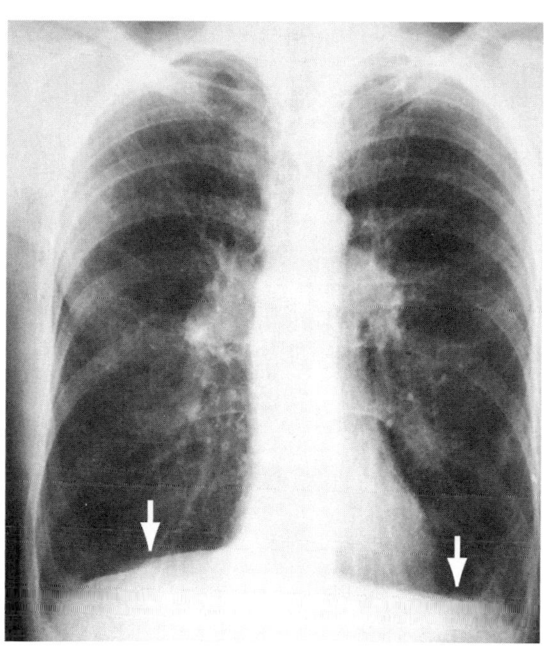

B Pulmonary emphysema. The chest radiograph reveals diaphragmatic depression (flattening of the domes of the diaphragm, *arrows*) with corresponding changes in the orientation of the cardiac shadow. The heart assumes a vertical orientation due to the low diaphragm (a lateral radiograph would reveal an increased retrosternal space). The central pulmonary arteries are dilated but taper dramatically at the segmental level.

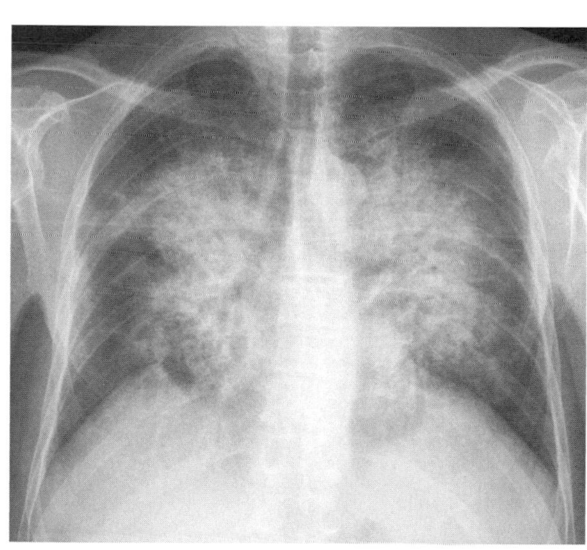

C Pulmonary edema complicating acute myocardial infarction. Dilation of vessels increases the number of visible vascular structures. This image shows a butterfly pattern of edema and bilateral pleural effusion.

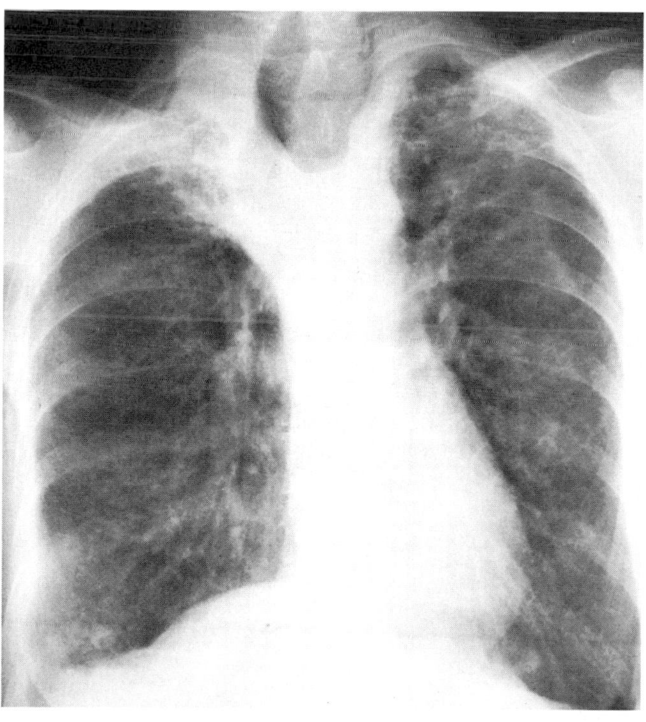

D Tuberculosis. Note the thickening of the pleura and the radiating fibrous bands. This image does not contain the small pulmonary nodules (tuberculomas) often found in the upper zones of the lung.

Bronchopulmonary Segments of the Lungs

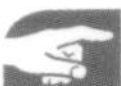

The lung lobes are subdivided into bronchopulmonary segments, each supplied by a tertiary (segmental) bronchus. *Note*: These subdivisions are not defined by surface boundaries but by origin.

Fig. 9.10 Segmentation of the lung
Anterior view. See pp. 120–121 for details of the trachea and bronchial tree.

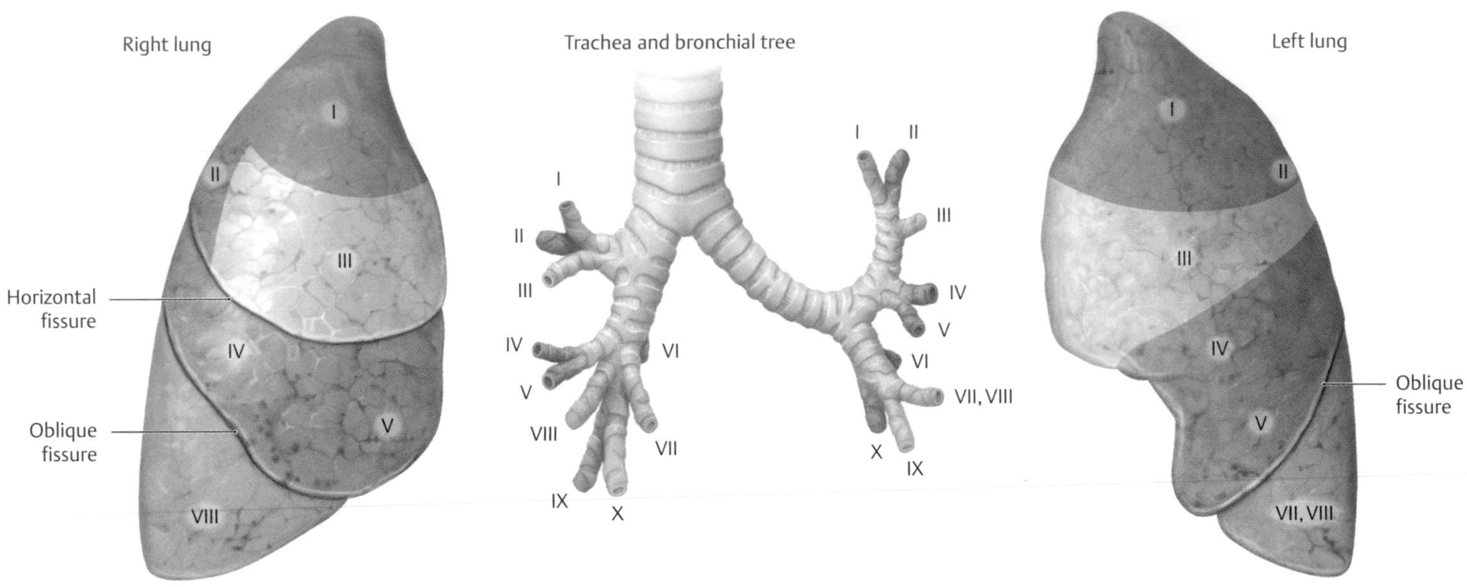

Right lung
I
II
III
Horizontal fissure
IV
V
Oblique fissure
VIII
Trachea and bronchial tree
I
II
III
IV
V
VI
VIII
VII
IX
X
I
II
III
IV
V
VI
VII, VIII
X
IX
Left lung
I
II
III
IV
V
Oblique fissure
VII, VIII

Fig. 9.11 Posteroanterior bronchogram
Anterior view of right lung.

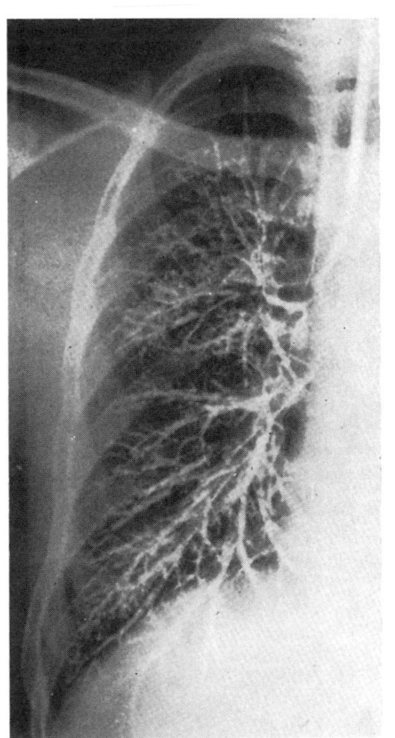

Table 9.2 Segmental architecture of the lungs

Each segment is supplied by a segmental bronchus of the same name (e.g., the apical segmental bronchus supplies the apical segment). See pp. 120–121 for details of the trachea and bronchial tree.

	Right lung	Left lung	
	Superior lobe		
I	Apical segment	Apicoposterior segment	I
II	Posterior segment		II
III	Anterior segment		III
	Middle lobe	**Lingula**	
IV	Lateral segment	Superior lingular segment	IV
V	Medial segment	Inferior lingular segment	V
	Inferior lobe		
VI	Superior segment		VI
VII	Medial basal segment		VII
VIII	Anterior basal segment		VIII
IX	Lateral basal segment		IX
X	Posterior basal segment		X

Fig. 9.12 Right lung: Bronchopulmonary segments

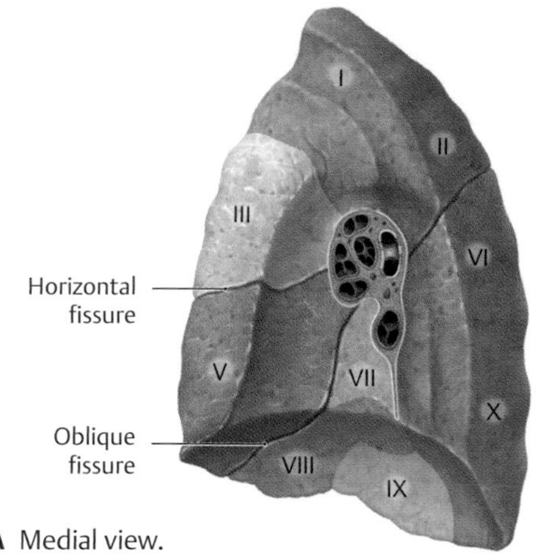
I
II
III
Horizontal fissure
VI
V
VII
X
Oblique fissure
VIII
IX

A Medial view.

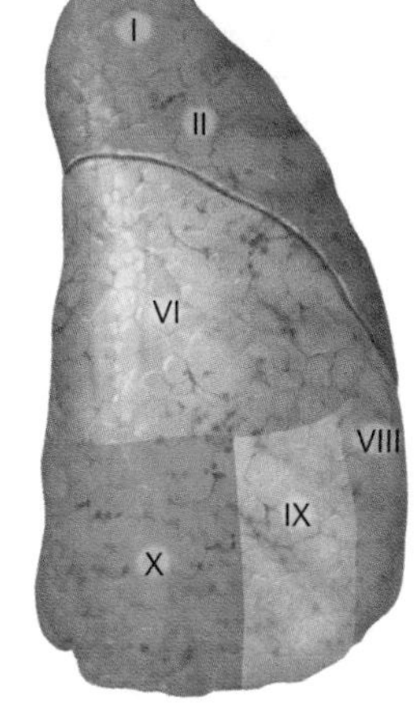
I
II
VI
VIII
IX
X

B Posterior view.

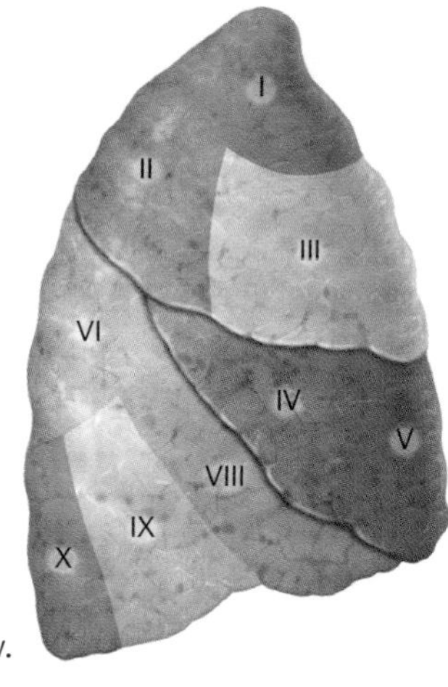
I
II
III
VI
IV
V
VIII
IX
X

C Lateral view.

Fig. 9.13 Left lung: Bronchopulmonary segments

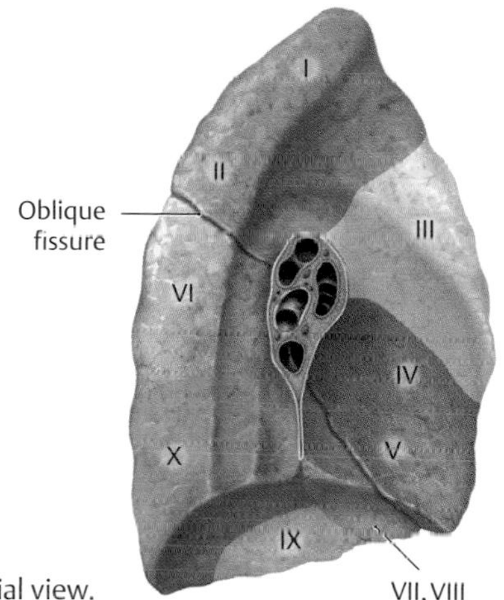
I
II
Oblique fissure
III
VI
IV
X
V
IX

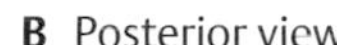
VII, VIII

A Medial view.

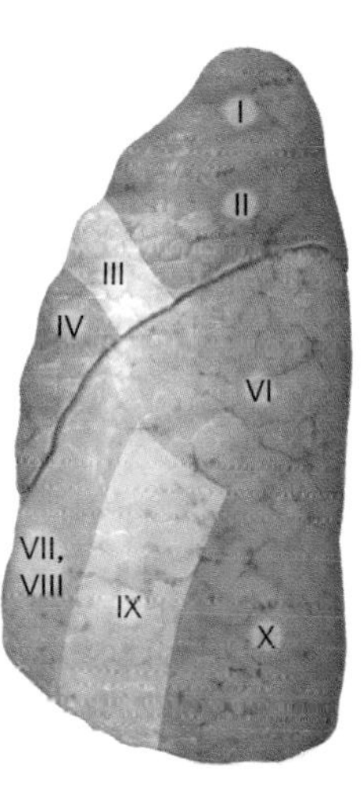
I
II
III
IV
VI
VII, VIII
IX
X

B Posterior view.

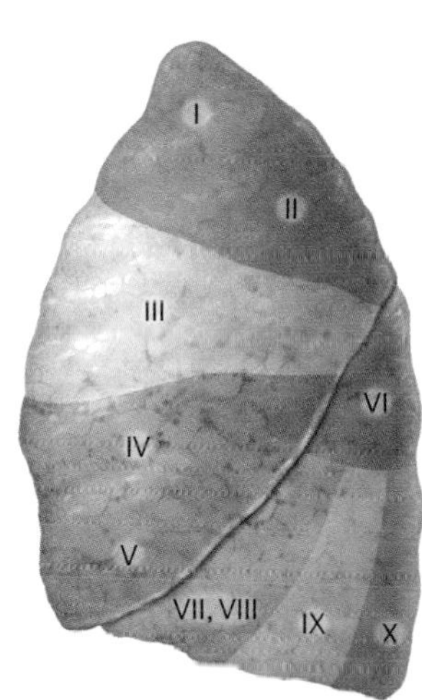
I
II
III
VI
IV
V
VII, VIII
IX
X

C Lateral view.

Clinical

Lung resections

Lung cancer, emphysema, or tuberculosis may necessitate the surgical removal of damaged portions of the lung. Surgeons exploit the anatomical subdivision of the lungs into lobes and segments when excising damaged tissue.

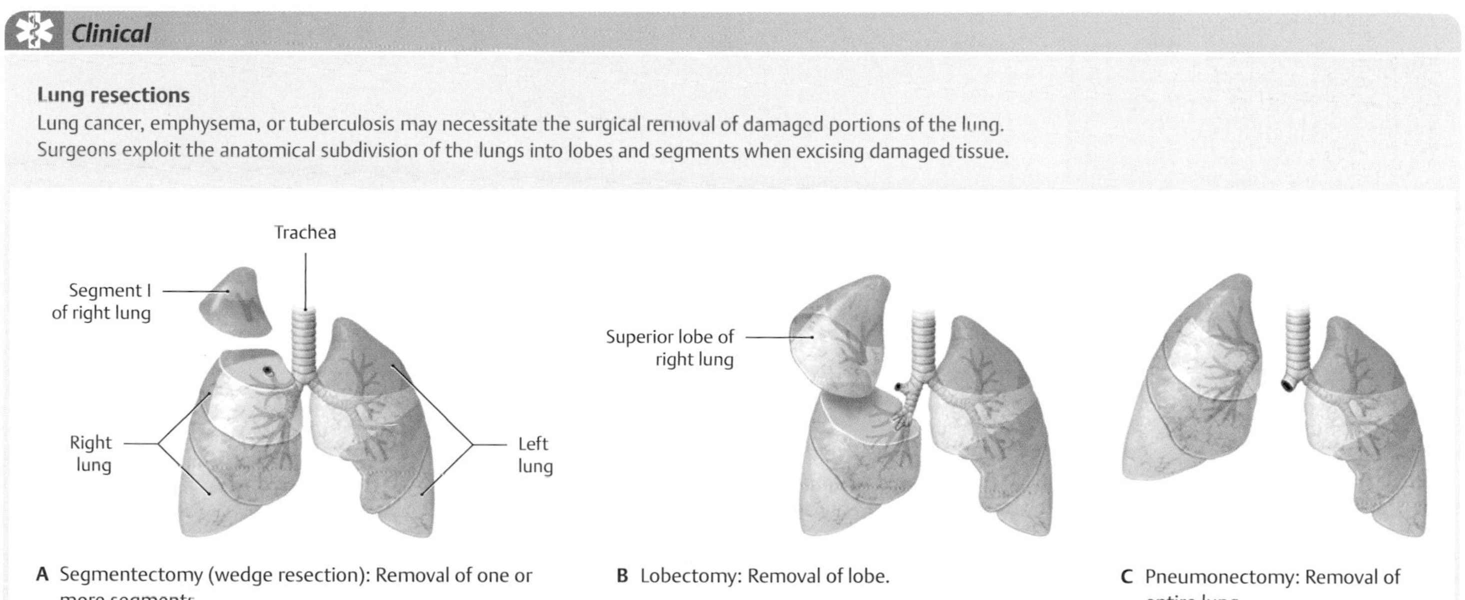
Trachea
Segment I of right lung
Right lung
Left lung
Superior lobe of right lung

A Segmentectomy (wedge resection): Removal of one or more segments.

B Lobectomy: Removal of lobe.

C Pneumonectomy: Removal of entire lung.

Trachea & Bronchial Tree

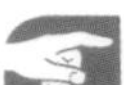

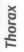

At or near the level of the sternal angle, the lowest tracheal cartilage extends anteroposteriorly, forming the carina. The trachea bifurcates at the carina into the right and left main bronchi. Each bronchus gives off lobar branches to the corresponding lung.

Fig. 9.14 Trachea

See p. 600 for the structures of the thyroid.

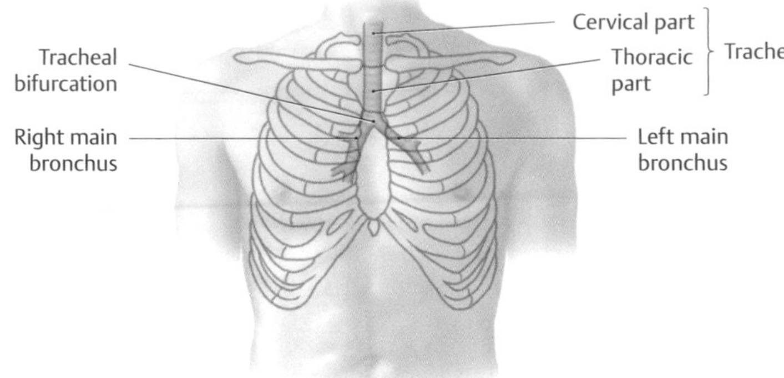

Cervical part
Thoracic part
Trachea
Tracheal bifurcation
Right main bronchus
Left main bronchus

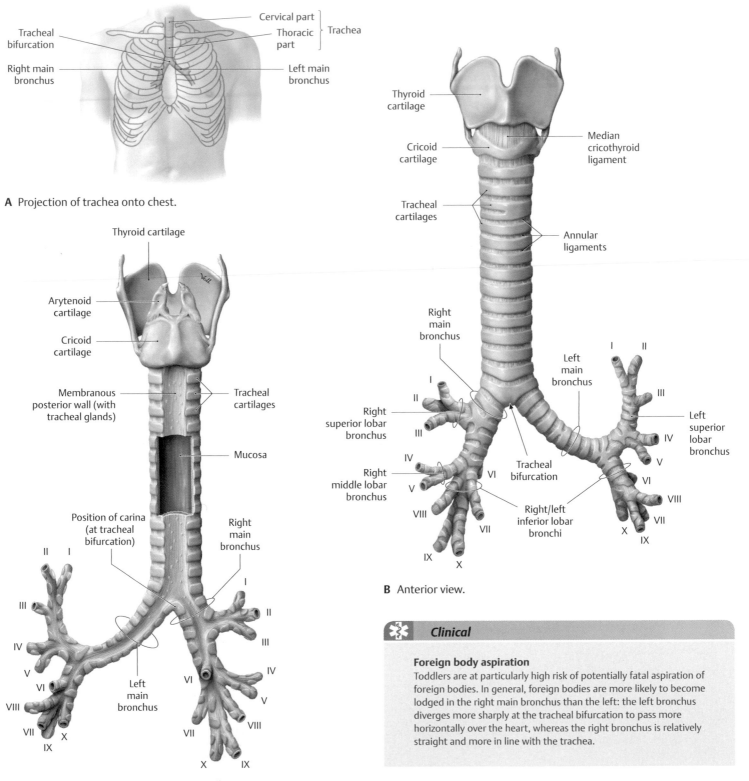

A Projection of trachea onto chest.

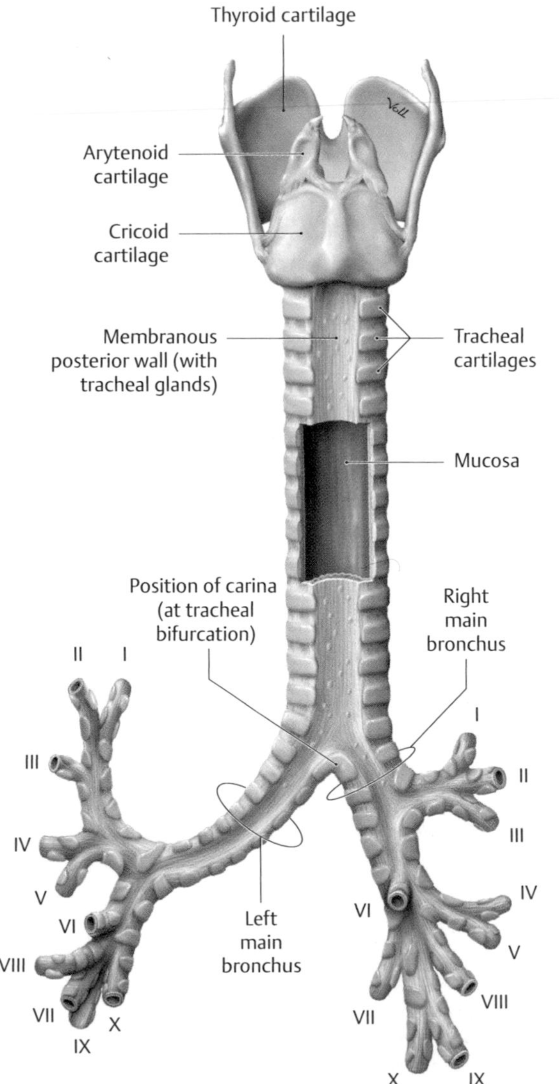

Thyroid cartilage
Arytenoid cartilage
Cricoid cartilage
Membranous posterior wall (with tracheal glands)
Tracheal cartilages
Mucosa
Position of carina (at tracheal bifurcation)
Right main bronchus
Left main bronchus
I
II
III
IV
V
VI
VII
VIII
IX
X

C Posterior view with opened posterior wall.

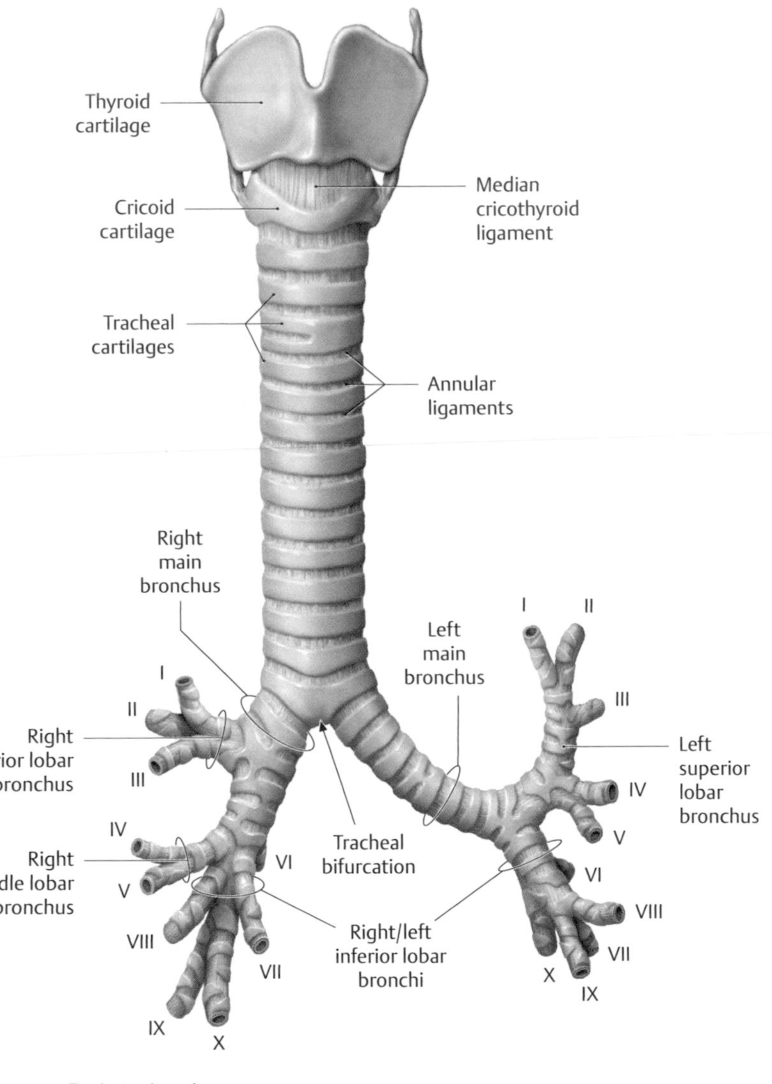

Thyroid cartilage
Cricoid cartilage
Median cricothyroid ligament
Tracheal cartilages
Annular ligaments
Right main bronchus
Left main bronchus
Right superior lobar bronchus
Right middle lobar bronchus
Tracheal bifurcation
Right/left inferior lobar bronchi
Left superior lobar bronchus
I
II
III
IV
V
VI
VII
VIII
IX
X

B Anterior view.

Clinical

Foreign body aspiration

Toddlers are at particularly high risk of potentially fatal aspiration of foreign bodies. In general, foreign bodies are more likely to become lodged in the right main bronchus than the left: the left bronchus diverges more sharply at the tracheal bifurcation to pass more horizontally over the heart, whereas the right bronchus is relatively straight and more in line with the trachea.

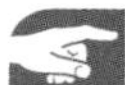

The conducting portion of the bronchial tree extends from the tracheal bifurcation to the terminal bronchiole, inclusive. The respiratory portion consists of the respiratory bronchiole, alveolar ducts, alveolar sacs, and alveoli.

Fig. 9.15 Bronchial tree

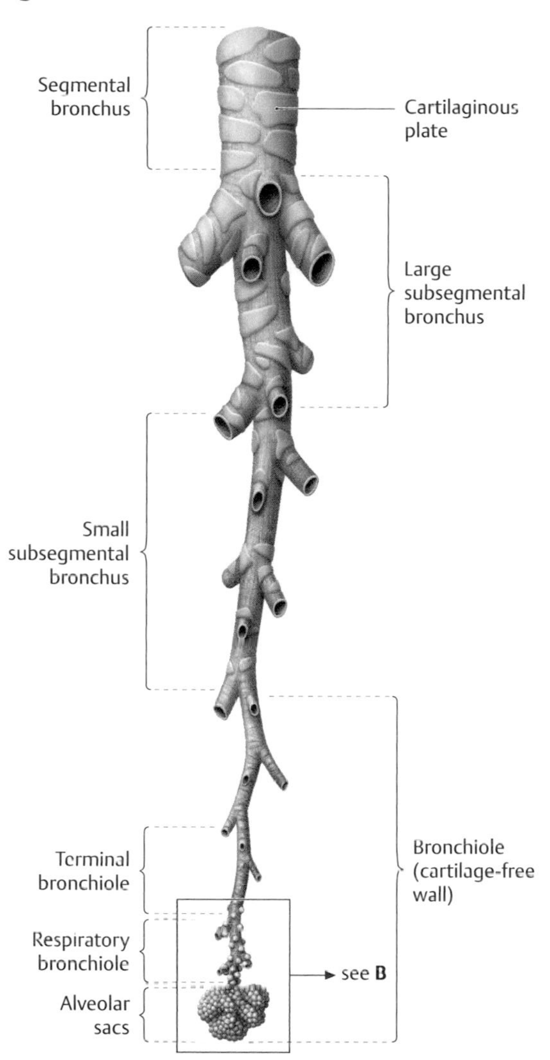

Segmental bronchus
Cartilaginous plate
Large subsegmental bronchus
Small subsegmental bronchus
Terminal bronchiole
Respiratory bronchiole
Alveolar sacs
Bronchiole (cartilage-free wall)
see B

A Divisions of the bronchial tree.

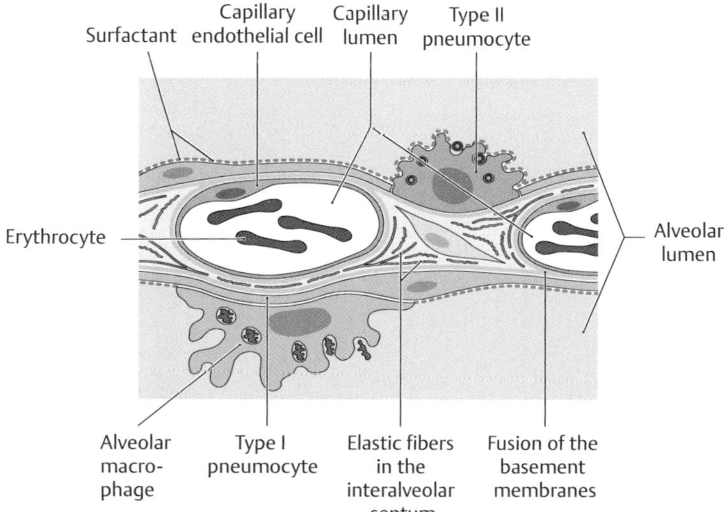

Surfactant
Capillary endothelial cell
Capillary lumen
Type II pneumocyte
Erythrocyte
Alveolar lumen
Alveolar macro-phage
Type I pneumocyte
Elastic fibers in the interalveolar septum
Fusion of the basement membranes

C Epithelial lining of the alveoli.

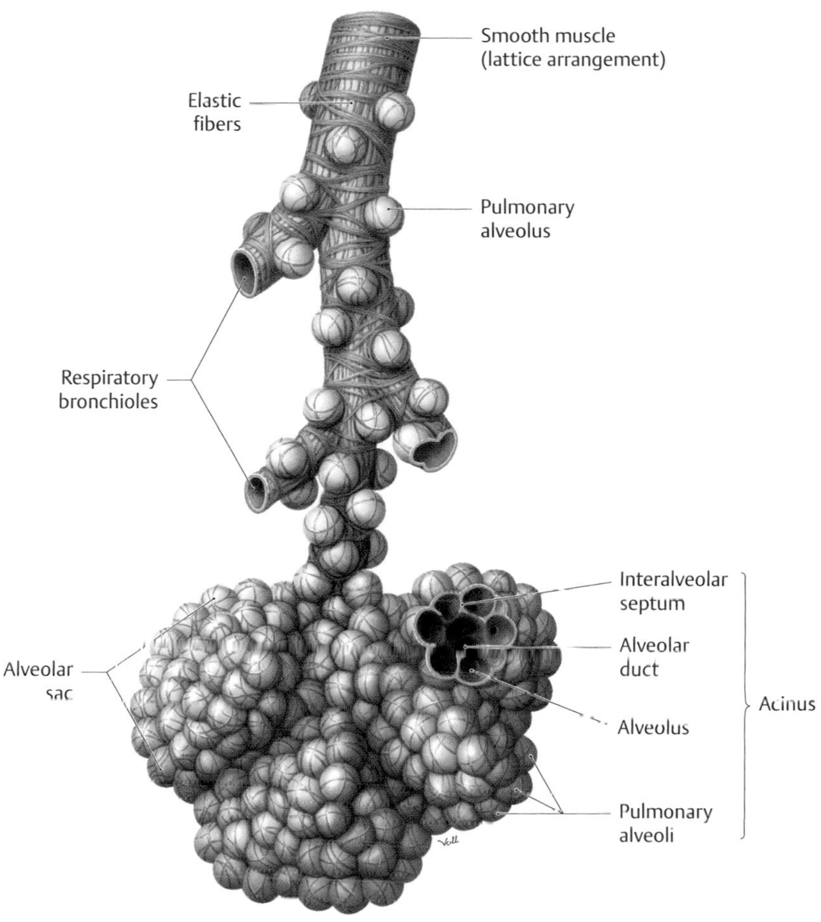

Smooth muscle (lattice arrangement)
Elastic fibers
Pulmonary alveolus
Respiratory bronchioles
Interalveolar septum
Alveolar duct
Alveolus
Alveolar sac
Acinus
Pulmonary alveoli

B Respiratory portion of the bronchial tree.

Clinical

Respiratory compromise

The most common cause of respiratory compromise at the bronchial level is asthma. Compromise at the alveolar level may result from increased diffusion distance, decreased aeration (emphysema), or fluid infiltration (e.g., pneumonia).

Diffusion distance: Gaseous exchange takes place between the alveolar and capillary lumens in the alveoli (see Fig. 9.15C). At these sites, the basement membranes of capillary endothelial cells are fused with those of type I alveolar epithelial cells, lowering the exchange distance to 0.5 µm. Diseases that increase this diffusion distance (e.g., edematous fluid collection or inflammation) result in compromised respiration.

Condition of alveoli: In diseases like emphysema, which occurs in chronic obstructive pulmonary disease (COPD), alveoli are destroyed or damaged. This reduces the surface area available for gaseous exchange.

Production of surfactant: Surfactant is a protein-phospholipid film that lowers the surface tension of the alveoli, making it easier for the lung to expand. The immature lungs of a preterm infant often fail to produce sufficient surfactant, leading to respiratory problems. Surfactant is produced and absorbed by alveolar epithelial cells (pneumocytes). Type I alveolar epithelial cells absorb surfactant; type II produce and distribute it.

Respiratory Mechanics

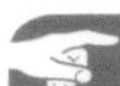

The mechanics of respiration are based on a rhythmic increase and decrease in thoracic volume, with an associated expansion and contraction of the lungs. *Inspiration* (red): Contraction of the diaphragm leaflets lowers the diaphragm into the inspiratory position, increasing the volume of the pleural cavity along the vertical axis. Contraction of the thoracic muscles (external intercostals with the scalene, intercartilaginous, and posterior serratus muscles) elevates the ribs, expanding the pleural cavity along the sagittal and transverse axes (Fig. 9.17A,B). Surface tension in the pleural space causes the visceral and parietal pleura to adhere; thus, changes in thoracic volume alter the volume of the lungs. This is particularly evident in the pleural recesses: at functional residual capacity (resting position between inspiration and expiration), the lung does not fully occupy the pleural cavity. As the pleural cavity expands, a negative intrapleural pressure is generated. The air pressure differential results in an influx of air (inspiration). *Expiration* (blue): During passive expiration, the muscles of the thoracic cage relax and the diaphragm returns to its expiratory position. Contraction of the lungs increases the pulmonary pressure and expels air from the lungs. For forcible expiration, the internal intercostal muscles (with the transverse thoracic and subcostal mucosa) can actively lower the rib cage more rapidly and to a greater extent than through passive elastic recoil.

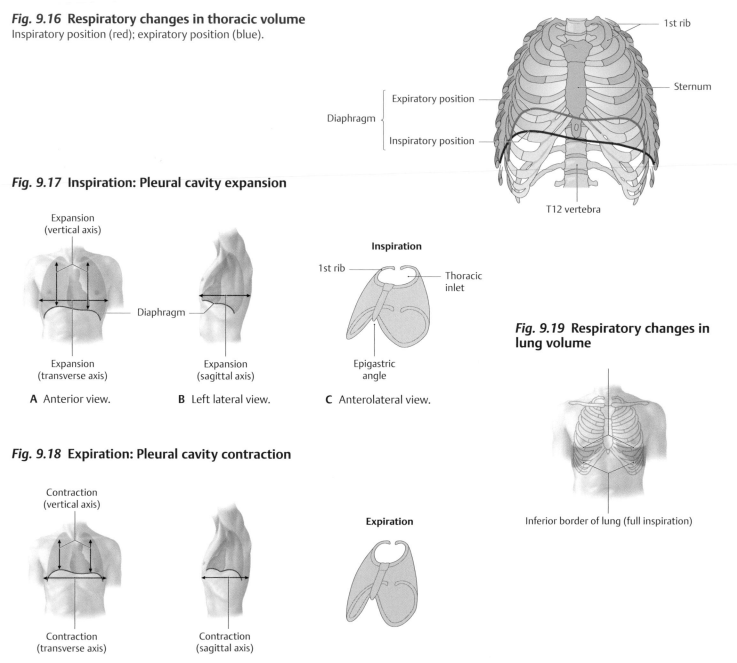

Fig. 9.16 Respiratory changes in thoracic volume
Inspiratory position (red); expiratory position (blue).

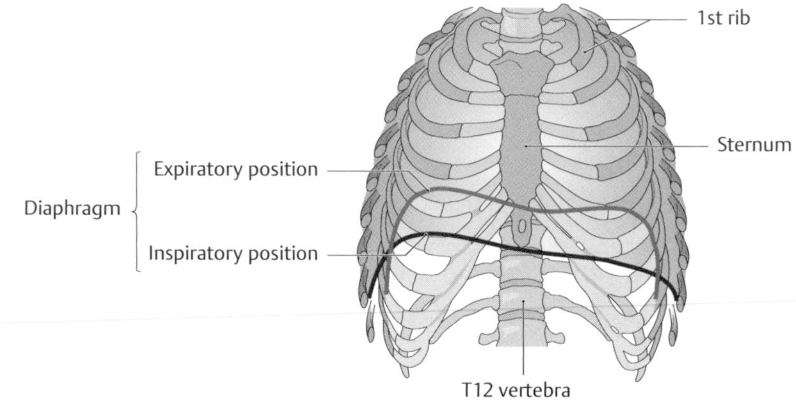
1st rib
Sternum
Diaphragm
Expiratory position
Inspiratory position
T12 vertebra

Fig. 9.17 Inspiration: Pleural cavity expansion

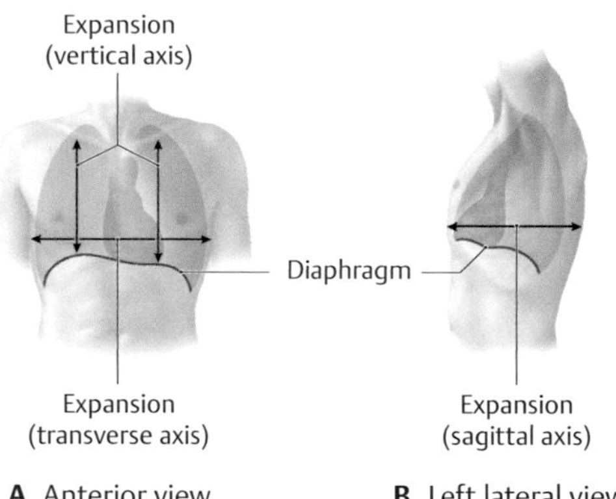
Expansion
(vertical axis)
Diaphragm
Expansion
(transverse axis)
Expansion
(sagittal axis)

A Anterior view.

B Left lateral view.

Inspiration

1st rib
Thoracic inlet
Epigastric angle

C Anterolateral view.

Fig. 9.18 Expiration: Pleural cavity contraction

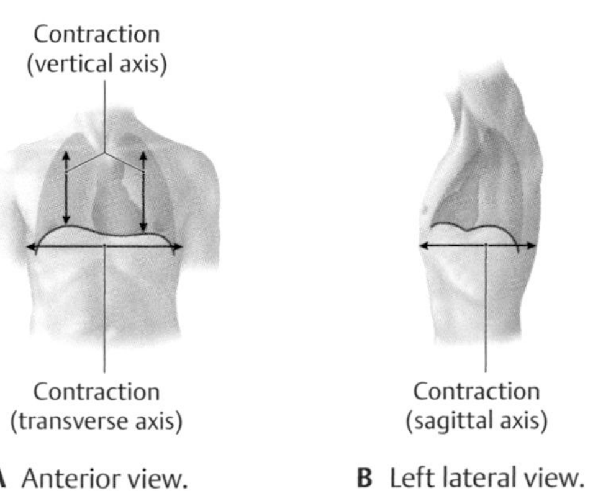
Contraction
(vertical axis)
Contraction
(transverse axis)
Contraction
(sagittal axis)

A Anterior view.

B Left lateral view.

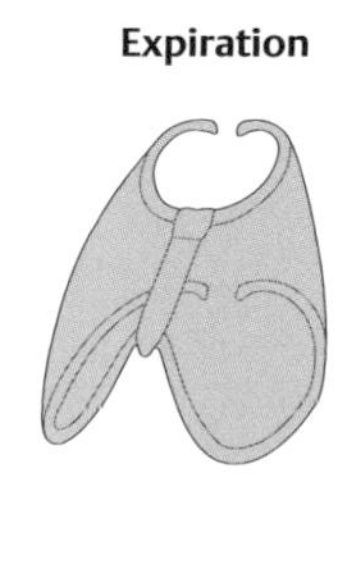
Expiration

C Anterolateral view.

Fig. 9.19 Respiratory changes in lung volume

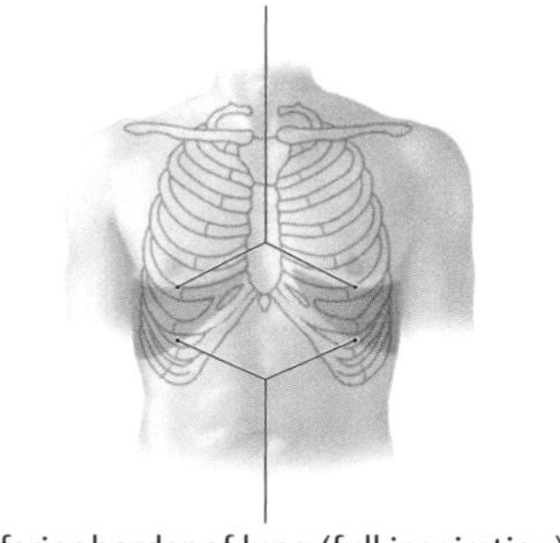
Inferior border of lung (full inspiration)

Fig. 9.20 Inspiration: Lung expansion

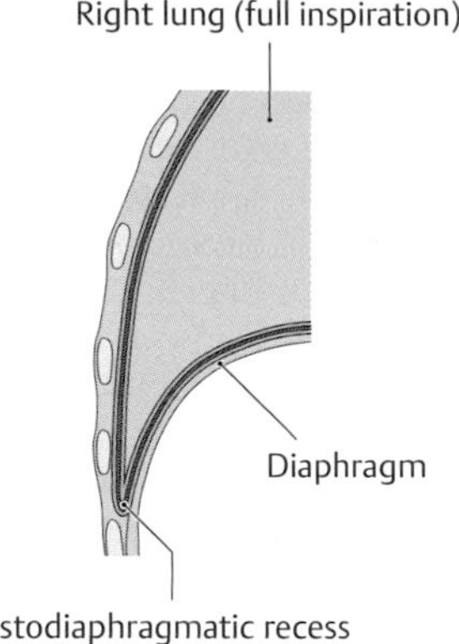
Right lung (full inspiration)
Diaphragm
Costodiaphragmatic recess

Fig. 9.21 Expiration: Lung contraction

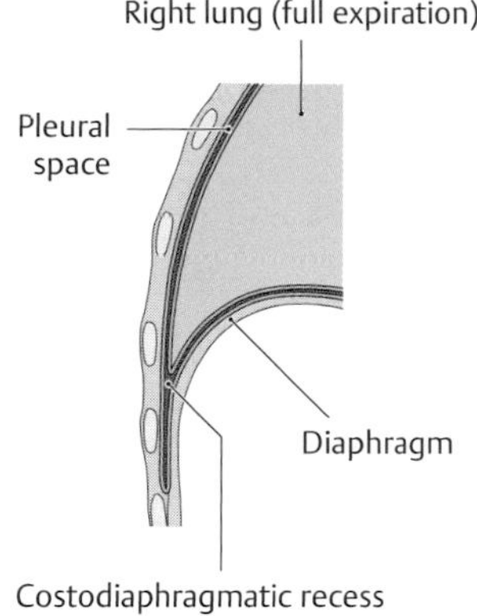
Right lung (full expiration)
Pleural space
Diaphragm
Costodiaphragmatic recess

Fig. 9.22 Movements of the lung and bronchial tree

As the volume of the lung changes with the thoracic cavity, the entire bronchial tree moves within the lung. These structural movements are more pronounced in portions of the bronchial tree distant from the pulmonary hilum.

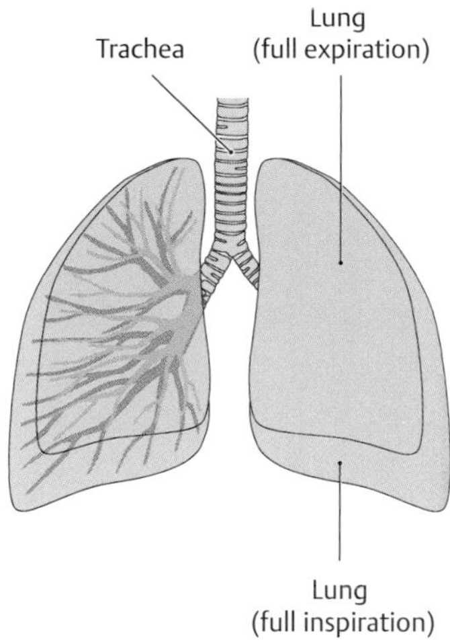
Trachea
Lung (full expiration)
Lung (full inspiration)

Clinical

Pneumothorax

The pleural space is normally sealed from the outside environment. Injury to the parietal pleura, visceral pleura, or lung allows air to enter the pleural cavity (pneumothorax). The lung collapses due to its inherent elasticity, and the patient's ability to breathe is compromised. The uninjured lung continues to function under normal pressure variations, resulting in "mediastinal flutter": the mediastinum shifts toward the normal side during inspiration and returns to the midline during expiration. Tension (valve) pneumothorax occurs when traumatically detached and displaced tissure covers the defect in the thoracic wall from the inside. This mobile flap allows air to enter, but not escape, the pleural cavity, causing a pressure buildup. The mediastinum shifts to the normal side, which may cause kinking of the great vessels and prevent the return of venous blood to the heart. Without treatment, tension pneumothorax is invariably fatal.

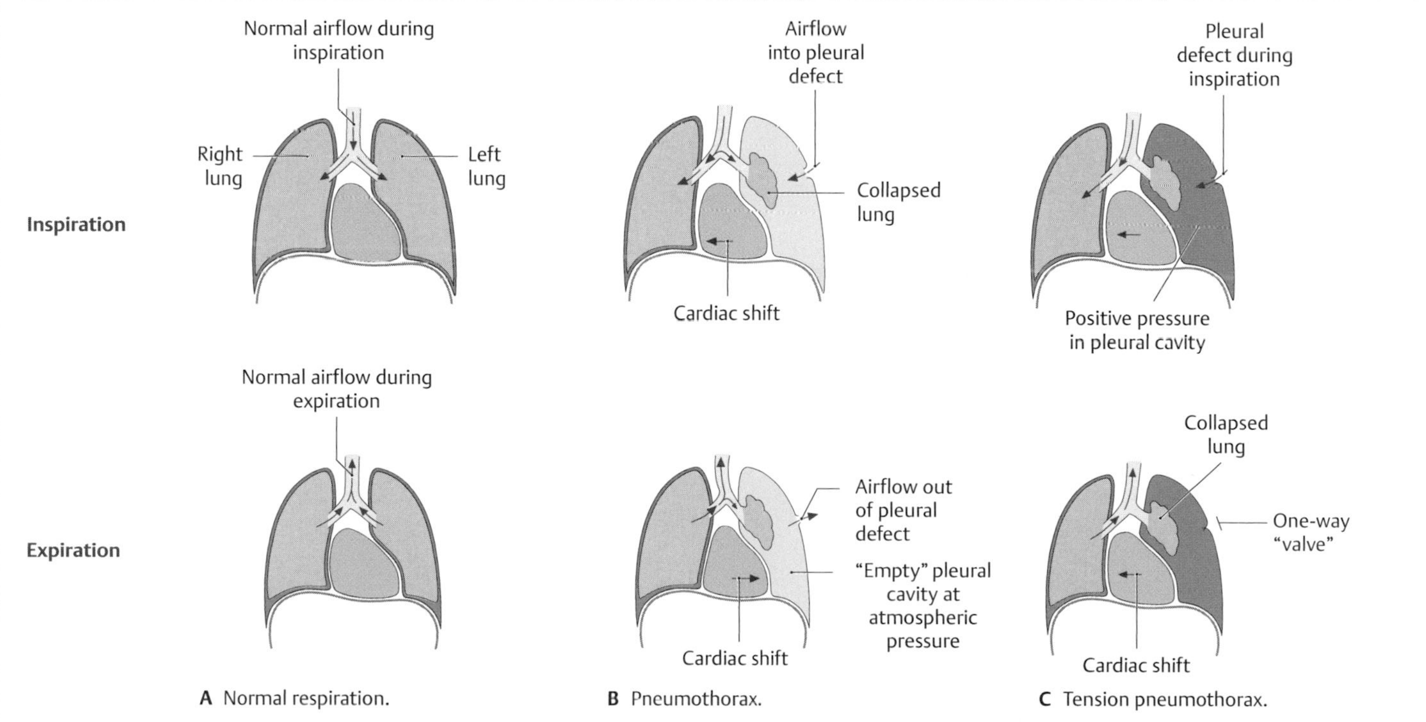
Normal airflow during inspiration
Right lung
Left lung
Inspiration
Airflow into pleural defect
Collapsed lung
Cardiac shift
Pleural defect during inspiration
Positive pressure in pleural cavity
Normal airflow during expiration
Expiration
Airflow out of pleural defect
"Empty" pleural cavity at atmospheric pressure
Cardiac shift
Collapsed lung
One-way "valve"
Cardiac shift

A Normal respiration.

B Pneumothorax.

C Tension pneumothorax.

Pulmonary Arteries & Veins

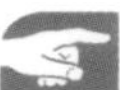

The pulmonary trunk arises from the right ventricle and divides into a left and right pulmonary artery for each lung. The paired pulmonary veins open into the left atrium on each side. The pulmonary arteries accompany and follow the branching of the bronchial tree, whereas the pulmonary veins do not, being located at the margins of the pulmonary lobules.

Fig. 9.23 **Pulmonary arteries and veins**
Anterior view.

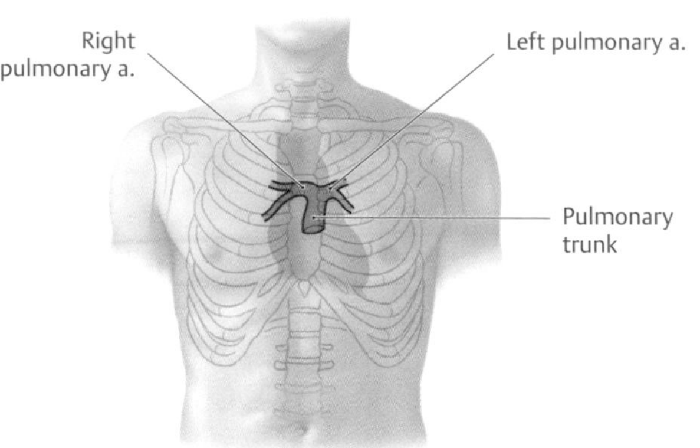
Right pulmonary a.
Left pulmonary a.
Pulmonary trunk

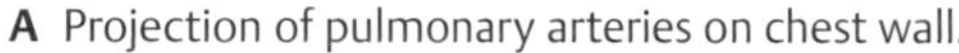
A Projection of pulmonary arteries on chest wall.

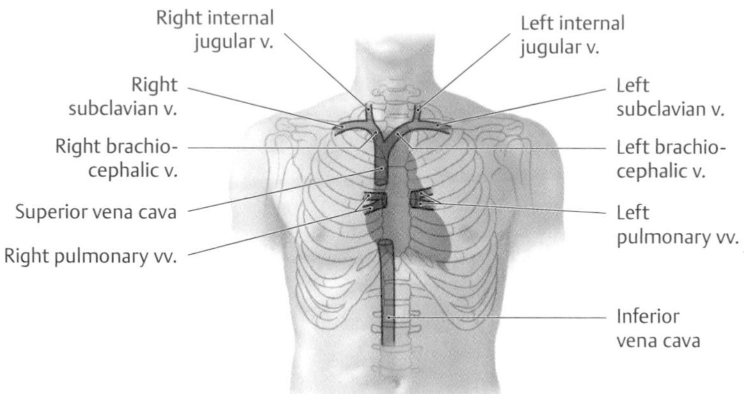
Right internal jugular v.
Left internal jugular v.
Right subclavian v.
Left subclavian v.
Right brachio-cephalic v.
Left brachio-cephalic v.
Superior vena cava
Left pulmonary vv.
Right pulmonary vv.
Inferior vena cava

B Projection of pulmonary veins on chest wall.

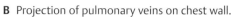

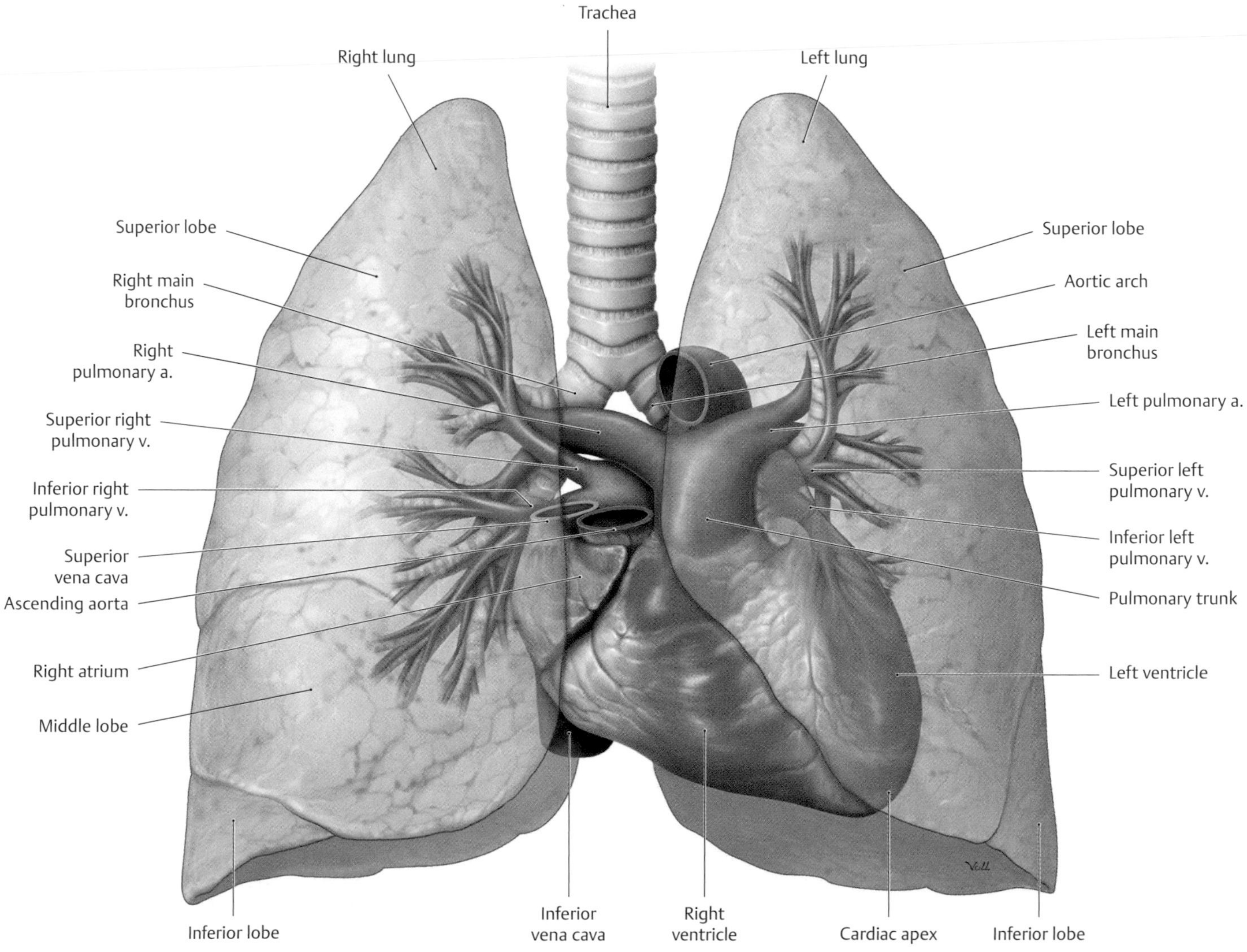

Trachea
Right lung
Left lung
Superior lobe
Superior lobe
Right main bronchus
Aortic arch
Right pulmonary a.
Left main bronchus
Left pulmonary a.
Superior right pulmonary v.
Superior left pulmonary v.
Inferior right pulmonary v.
Inferior left pulmonary v.
Superior vena cava
Pulmonary trunk
Ascending aorta
Right atrium
Left ventricle
Middle lobe
Inferior lobe
Inferior vena cava
Right ventricle
Cardiac apex
Inferior lobe

C Distribution of the pulmonary arteries and veins, anterior view.

Fig. 9.24 Pulmonary arteries

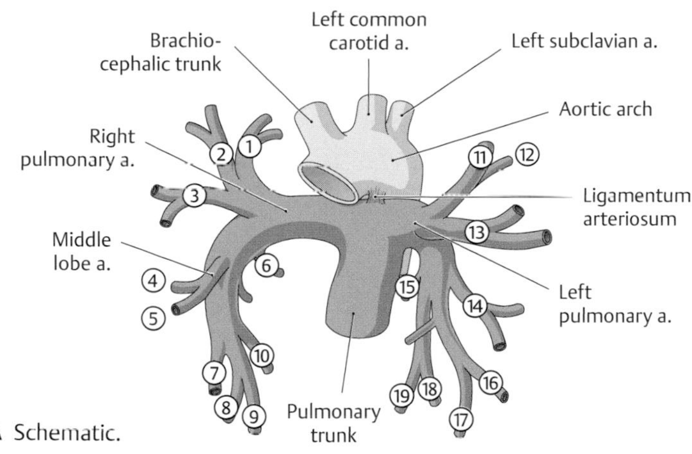
Left common carotid a.
Brachio-cephalic trunk
Left subclavian a.
Aortic arch
Right pulmonary a.
Ligamentum arteriosum
Middle lobe a.
Left pulmonary a.
Pulmonary trunk
1
2
3
4
5
6
7
8
9
10
11
12
13
14
15
16
17
18
19

A Schematic.

Fig. 9.25 Pulmonary veins

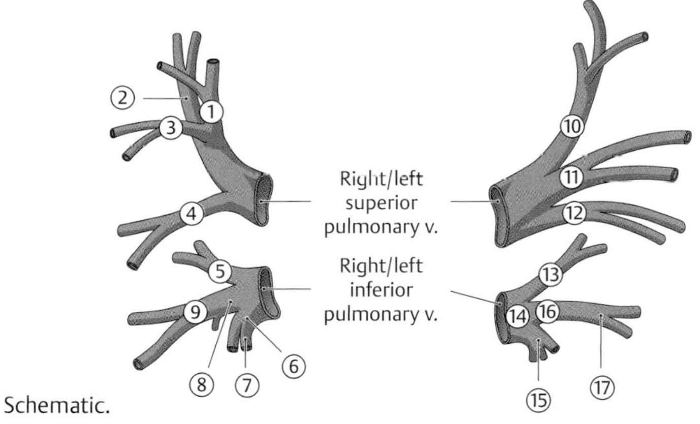
Right/left superior pulmonary v.
Right/left inferior pulmonary v.
1
2
3
4
5
6
7
8
9
10
11
12
13
14
15
16
17

A Schematic.

Table 9.3 Pulmonary arteries and their branches

Right pulmonary artery		Left pulmonary artery	
Superior lobe arteries			
①	Apical segmental a.		⑪
②	Posterior segmental a.		⑫
③	Anterior segmental a.		⑬
Middle lobe arteries			
④	Lateral segmental a.	Lingular a.	⑭
⑤	Medial segmental a.		
Inferior lobe arteries			
⑥	Superior segmental a.		⑮
⑦	Anterior basal segmental a.		⑯
⑧	Lateral basal segmental a.		⑰
⑨	Posterior basal segmental a.		⑱
⑩	Medial basal segmental a.		⑲

Table 9.4 Pulmonary veins and their tributaries

Right pulmonary vein		Left pulmonary vein	
Superior pulmonary veins			
①	Apical v.	Apicoposterior v.	⑩
②	Posterior v.		
③	Anterior v.	Anterior v.	⑪
④	Middle lobe v.	Lingular v.	⑫
Inferior pulmonary veins			
⑤	Superior v.		⑬
⑥	Common basal v.		⑭
⑦	Inferior basal v.		⑮
⑧	Superior basal v.		⑯
⑨	Anterior basal v.		⑰

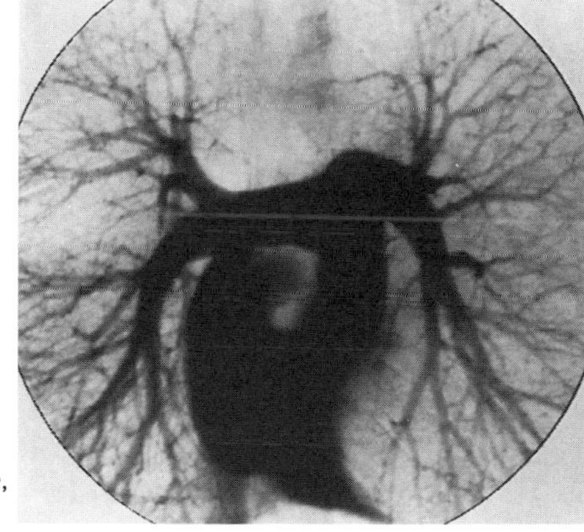

B Pulmonary arteriogram, arterial phase, anterior view.

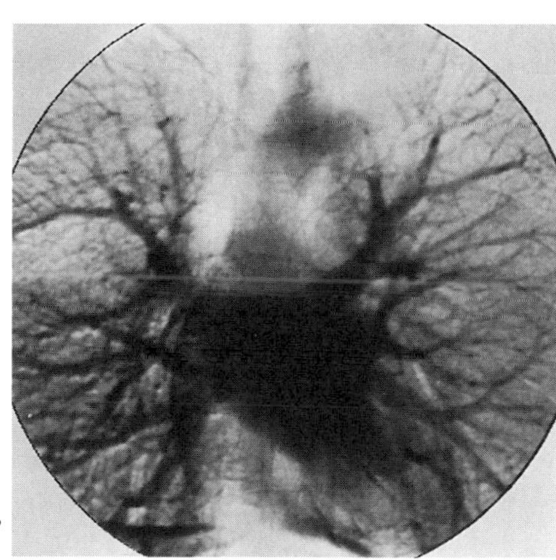

B Pulmonary arteriogram, venous phase, anterior view.

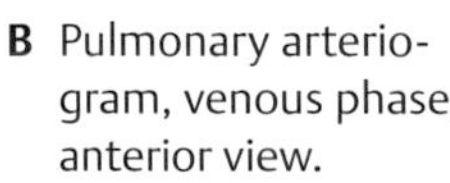

Clinical

Pulmonary embolism

Potentially life-threatening pulmonary embolism occurs when blood clots migrate through the venous system and become lodged in one of the arteries supplying the lungs. Symptoms include dyspnea (difficulty breathing) and tachycardia (increased heart rate). Most pulmonary emboli originate from stagnant blood in the veins of the lower limb and pelvis (venous thromboemboli). Causes include immobilization, disordered blood coagulation, and trauma. *Note*: A thromboembolus is a thrombus (blood clot) that has migrated (embolized).

Neurovasculature of the Tracheobronchial Tree

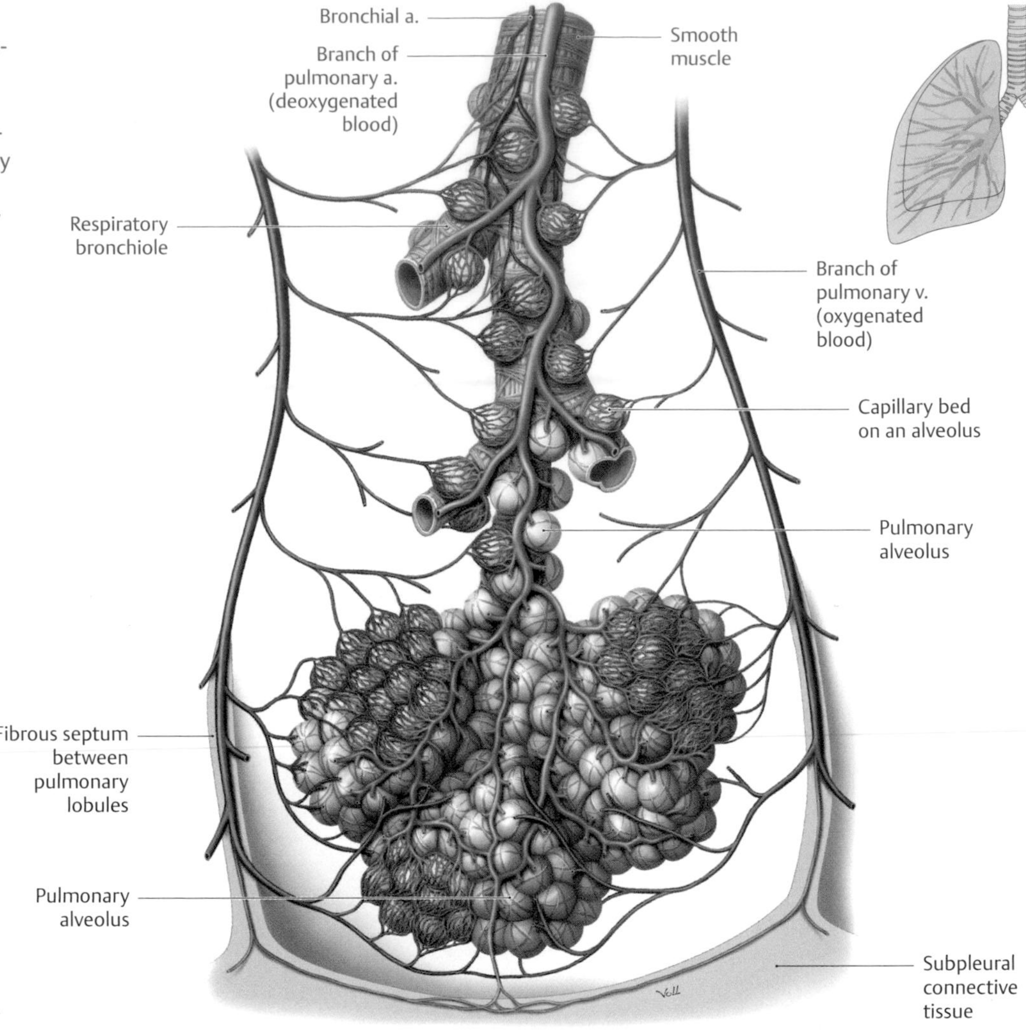

Bronchial a.
Branch of pulmonary a. (deoxygenated blood)
Smooth muscle
Respiratory bronchiole
Branch of pulmonary v. (oxygenated blood)
Capillary bed on an alveolus
Pulmonary alveolus
Fibrous septum between pulmonary lobules
Pulmonary alveolus
Subpleural connective tissue

Fig. 9.26 **Pulmonary vasculature**

The pulmonary system is responsible for gaseous exchange within the lung. Pulmonary arteries (shown in blue) carry *deoxygenated* blood and follow the bronchial tree. The pulmonary vein (red) is the only vein in the body carrying *oxygenated* blood, which it receives from the alveolar capillaries at the periphery of the lobule.

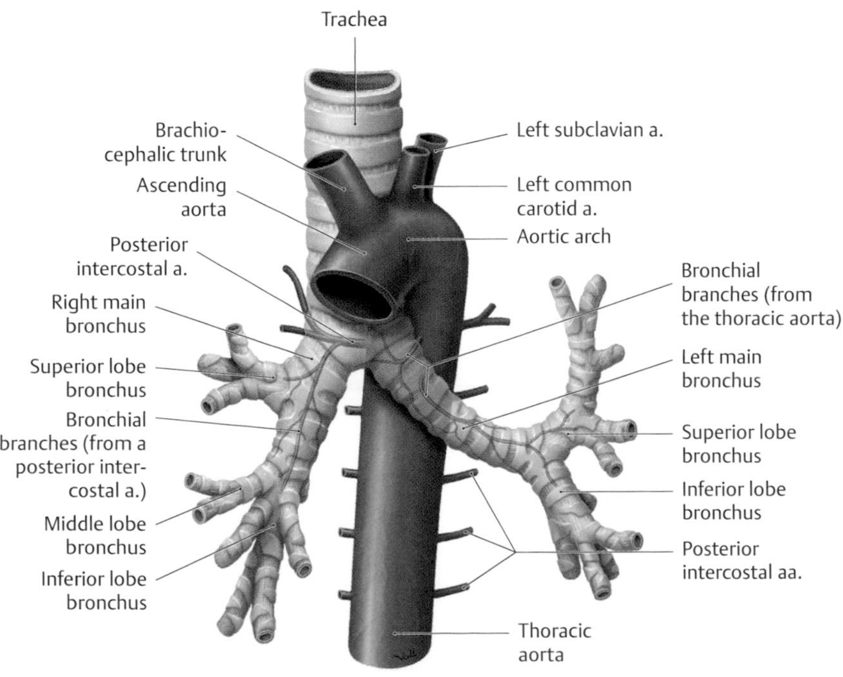

Trachea
Brachio-cephalic trunk
Left subclavian a.
Ascending aorta
Left common carotid a.
Aortic arch
Posterior intercostal a.
Bronchial branches (from the thoracic aorta)
Right main bronchus
Left main bronchus
Superior lobe bronchus
Bronchial branches (from a posterior inter-costal a.)
Superior lobe bronchus
Inferior lobe bronchus
Middle lobe bronchus
Posterior intercostal aa.
Inferior lobe bronchus
Thoracic aorta

Fig. 9.27 **Arteries of the tracheobronchial tree**

The bronchial tree receives its nutrients via the bronchial arteries, found in the adventitia of the airways. Typically, there are one to three bronchial arteries arising directly from the aorta. Origin from a posterior intercostal artery may also occur.

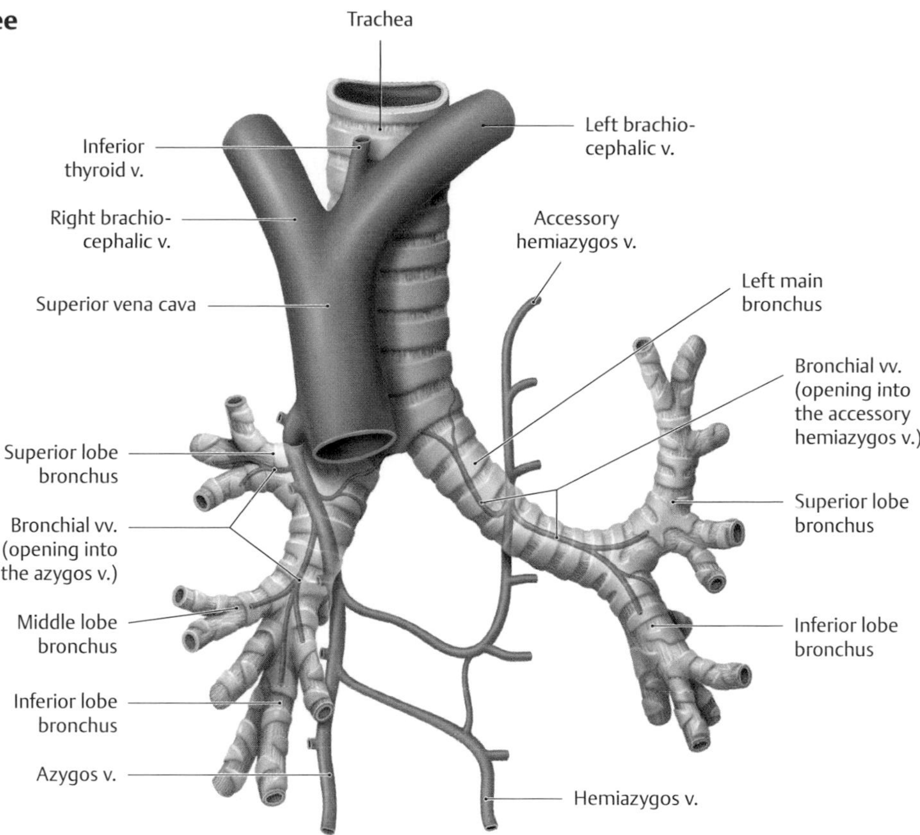
Trachea
Inferior thyroid v.
Left brachio-cephalic v.
Right brachio-cephalic v.
Accessory hemiazygos v.
Superior vena cava
Left main bronchus
Bronchial vv. (opening into the accessory hemiazygos v.)
Superior lobe bronchus
Bronchial vv. (opening into the azygos v.)
Superior lobe bronchus
Middle lobe bronchus
Inferior lobe bronchus
Inferior lobe bronchus
Azygos v.
Hemiazygos v.

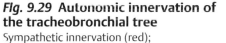

Fig. 9.28 **Veins of the tracheobronchial tree**

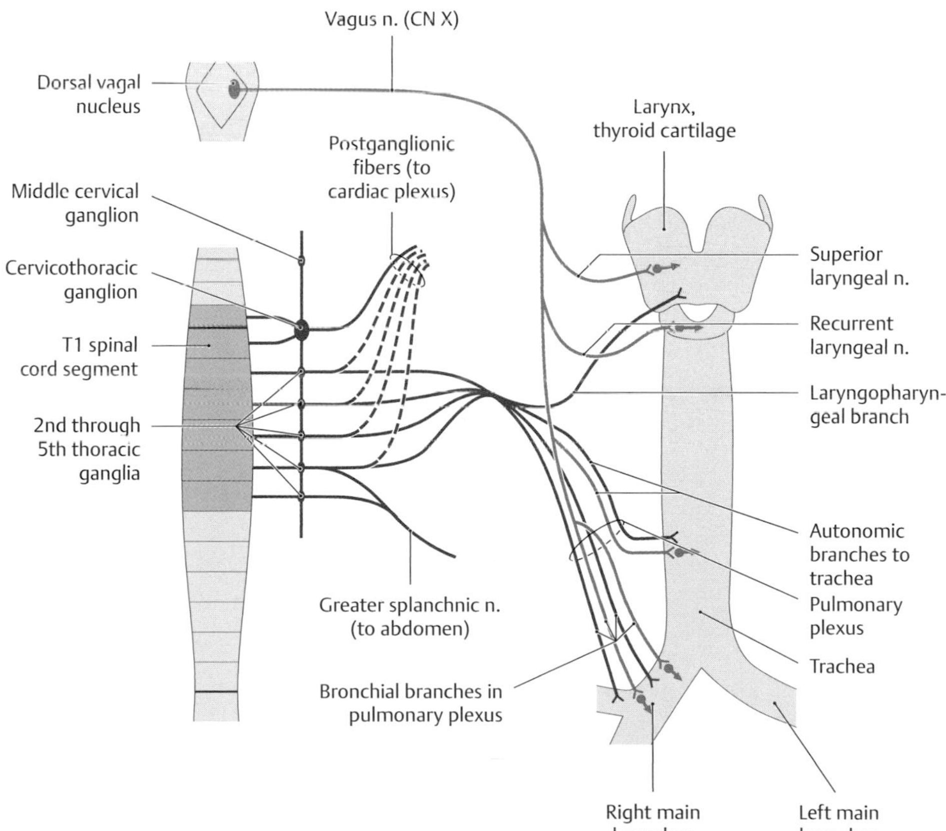
Vagus n. (CN X)
Dorsal vagal nucleus
Larynx, thyroid cartilage
Postganglionic fibers (to cardiac plexus)
Middle cervical ganglion
Superior laryngeal n.
Cervicothoracic ganglion
Recurrent laryngeal n.
T1 spinal cord segment
Laryngopharyngeal branch
2nd through 5th thoracic ganglia
Autonomic branches to trachea
Pulmonary plexus
Greater splanchnic n. (to abdomen)
Trachea
Bronchial branches in pulmonary plexus
Right main bronchus
Left main bronchus

Fig. 9.29 **Autonomic innervation of the tracheobronchial tree**
Sympathetic innervation (red); parasympathetic innervation (blue).

Lymphatics of the Pleural Cavity

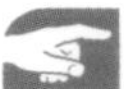

The lungs and bronchi are drained by two lymphatic drainage systems. The peribronchial network follows the bronchial tree, draining lymph from the bronchi and most of the lungs. The subpleural network collects lymph from the peripheral lung and visceral pleura.

Fig. 9.30 Lymphatic drainage of the pleural cavity

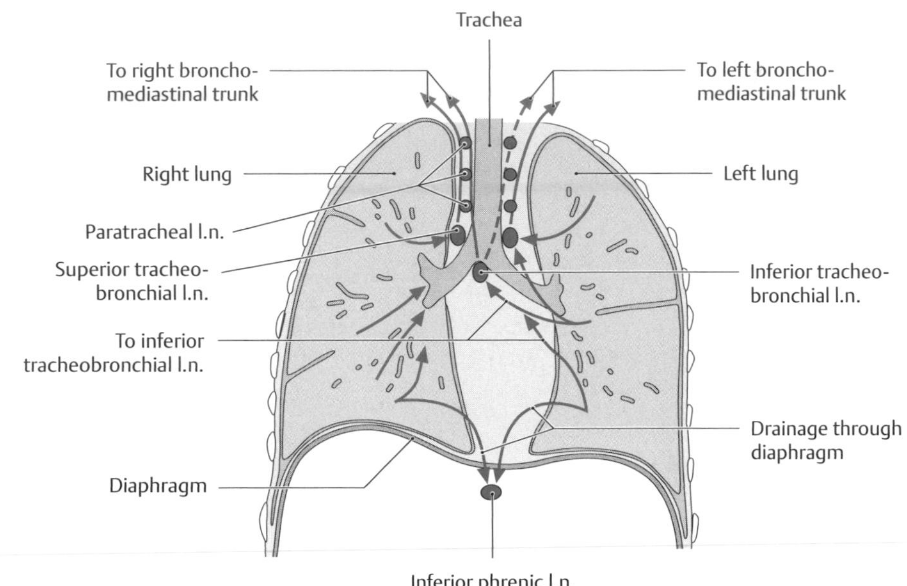
Trachea
To right broncho-mediastinal trunk
To left broncho-mediastinal trunk
Right lung
Left lung
Paratracheal l.n.
Superior tracheo-bronchial l.n.
Inferior tracheo-bronchial l.n.
To inferior tracheobronchial l.n.
Drainage through diaphragm
Diaphragm
Inferior phrenic l.n.

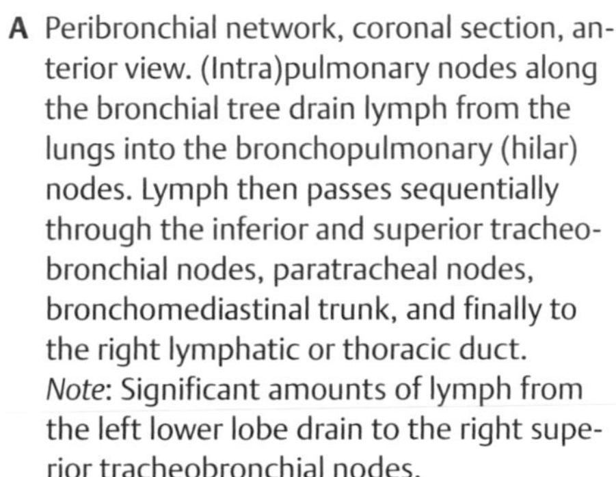

A Peribronchial network, coronal section, anterior view. (Intra)pulmonary nodes along the bronchial tree drain lymph from the lungs into the bronchopulmonary (hilar) nodes. Lymph then passes sequentially through the inferior and superior tracheobronchial nodes, paratracheal nodes, bronchomediastinal trunk, and finally to the right lymphatic or thoracic duct. *Note*: Significant amounts of lymph from the left lower lobe drain to the right superior tracheobronchial nodes.

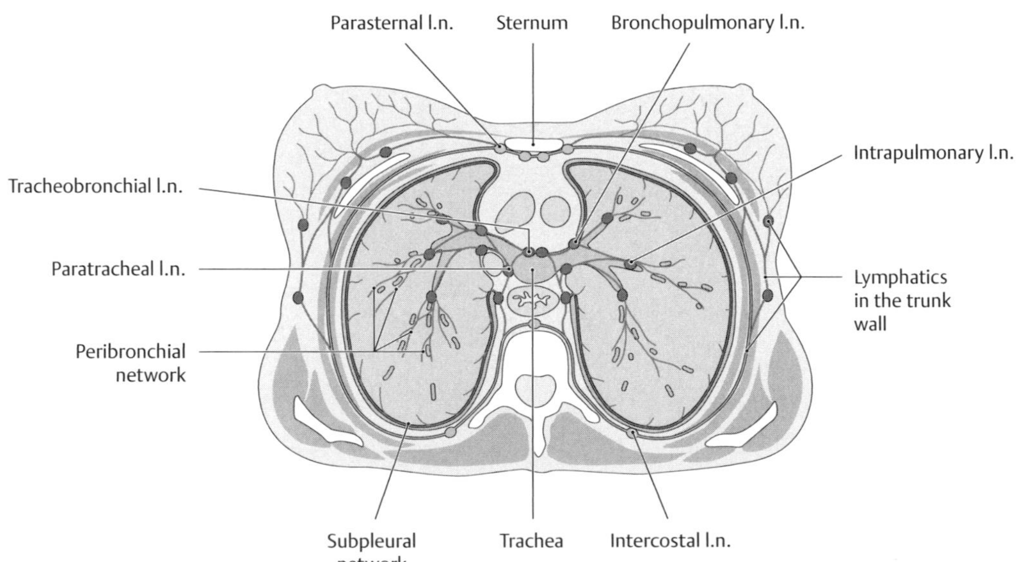
Parasternal l.n.
Sternum
Bronchopulmonary l.n.
Intrapulmonary l.n.
Tracheobronchial l.n.
Paratracheal l.n.
Lymphatics in the trunk wall
Peribronchial network
Subpleural network
Trachea
Intercostal l.n.

B Subpleural network, transverse section, superior view.

Fig. 9.31 **Lymph nodes of the pleural cavity**
Anterior view of pulmonary nodes.

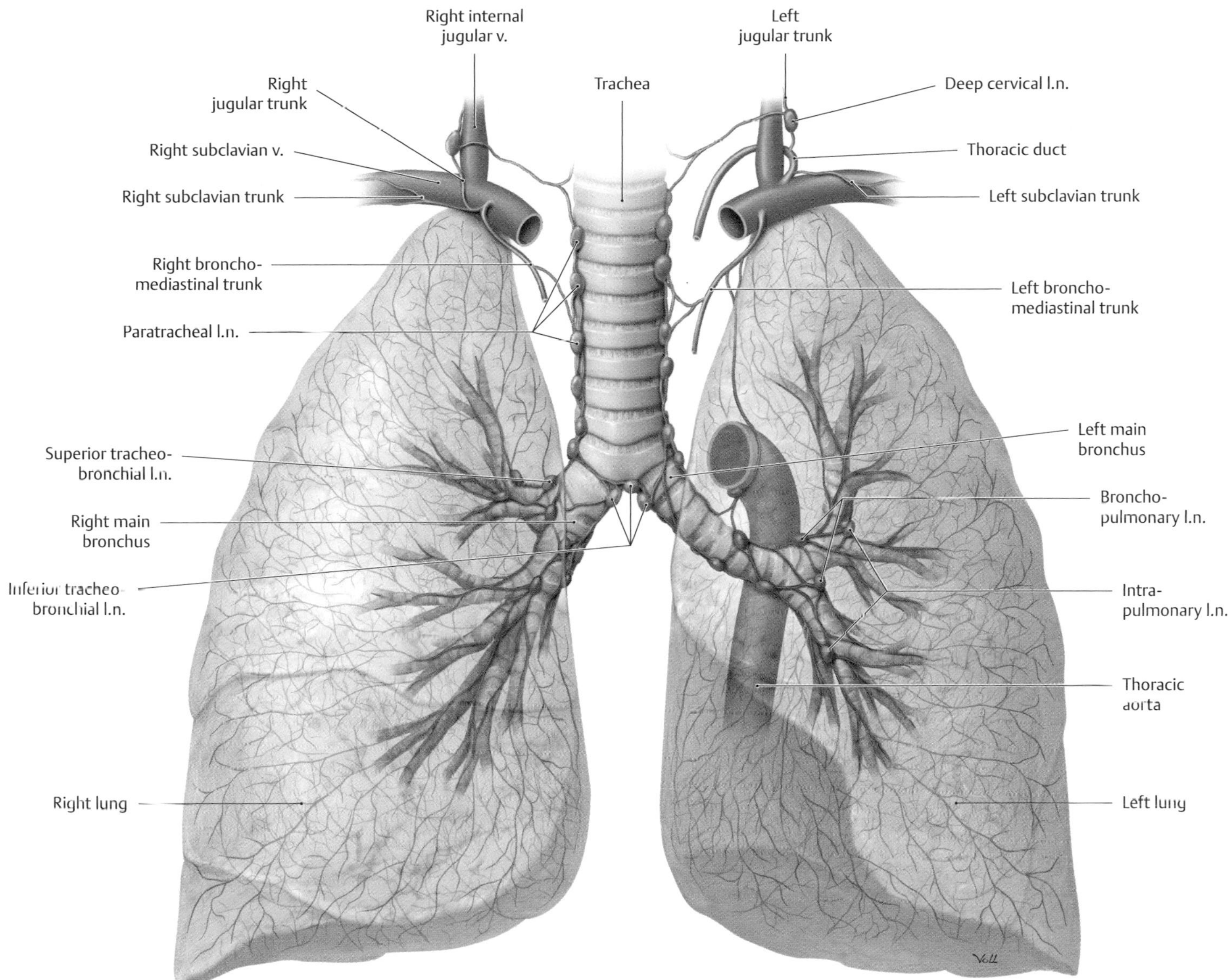

Right internal jugular v.
Left jugular trunk
Right jugular trunk
Trachea
Deep cervical l.n.
Right subclavian v.
Thoracic duct
Right subclavian trunk
Left subclavian trunk
Right broncho-mediastinal trunk
Left broncho-mediastinal trunk
Paratracheal l.n.
Left main bronchus
Superior tracheo-bronchial l.n.
Broncho-pulmonary l.n.
Right main bronchus
Inferior tracheo-bronchial l.n.
Intra-pulmonary l.n.
Thoracic aorta
Right lung
Left lung

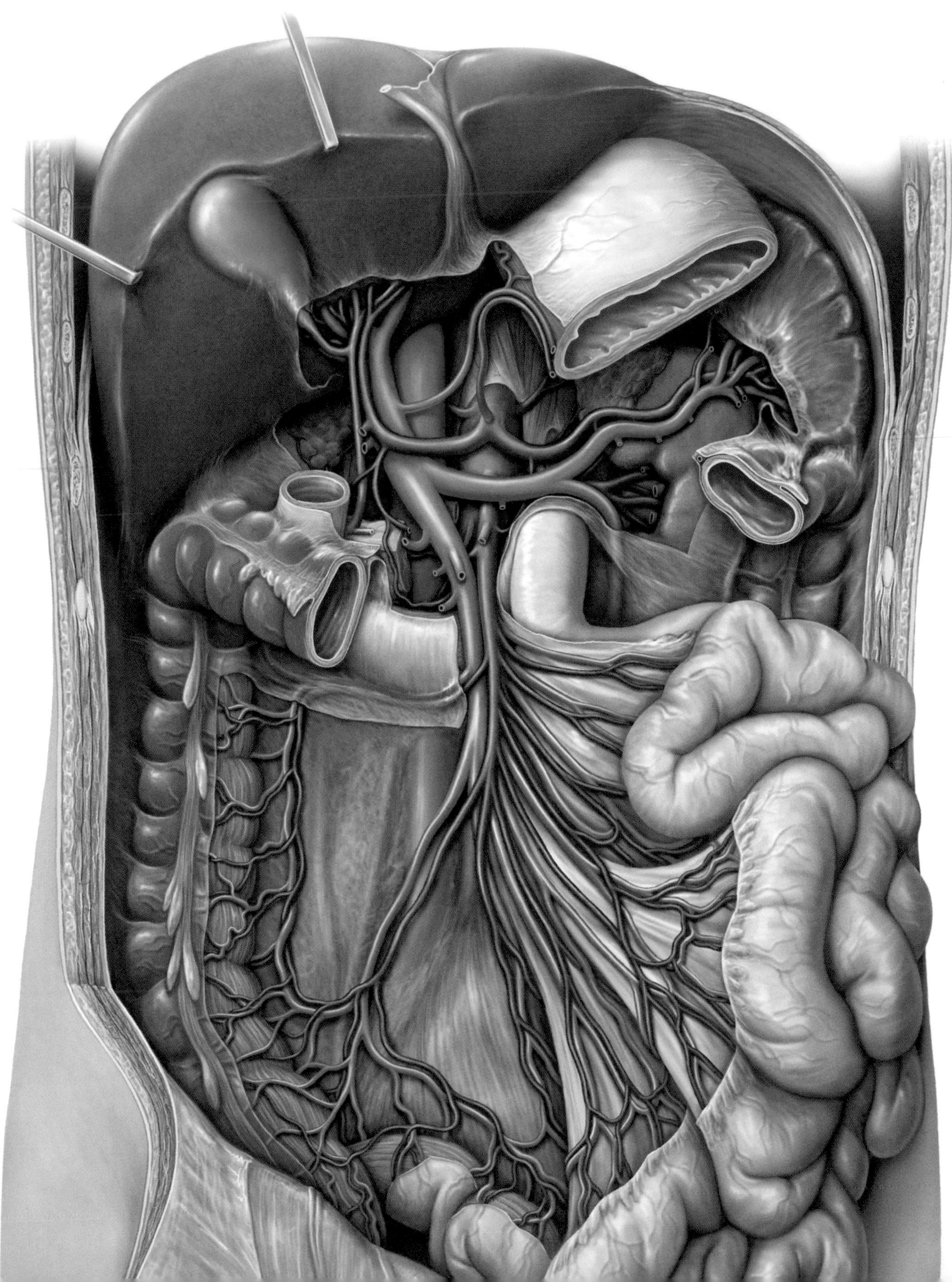

Abdomen

10 Surface Anatomy

Surface Anatomy 132

11 Abdominal Wall

Bony Framework for the Abdominal Wall 134
Muscles of the Anterolateral Abdominal Wall 136
Muscles of the Poeterior Abdominal Wall & Diaphragm . . . 138
Abdominal Wall Muscle Facts 140
Inguinal Region & Canal 142
Spermatic Cord, Scrotum & Testis 144
Anterior Abdominal Wall & Inguinal Hernias 146

12 Abdominal Cavity & Spaces

Divisions of the Abdominopelvic Cavity 148
Peritoneal Cavity & Greater Sac 150
Omental Bursa, or Lesser Sac 152
Mesenteries & Posterior Wall 154

13 Internal Organs

Stomach 156
Duodenum 158
Jejunum & Ileum 160
Cecum, Appendix & Colon 162
Liver: Overview 164
Liver: Segments & Lobes 166
Gallbladder & Bile Ducts 168
Pancreas & Spleen 170
Kidneys & Suprarenal Glands (I) 172
Kidneys & Suprarenal Glands (II) 174

14 Neurovasculature

Arteries of the Abdomen 176
Abdominal Aorta & Renal Arteries 178
Celiac Trunk 180
Superior & Inferior Mesenteric Arteries 182
Veins of the Abdomen 184
Inferior Vena Cava & Renal Veins 186
Portal Vein 188
Superior & Inferior Mesenteric Veins 190
Lymphatics of the Abdominal Organs 192
Lymph Nodes of the Posterior Abdominal Wall 194
Lymph Nodes of the Supracolic Organs 196
Lymph Nodes of the Infracolic Organs 198
Nerves of the Abdominal Wall 200
Autonomic Innervation: Overview 202
Autonomic Plexuses 204
Innervation of the Abdominal Organs 206
Innervation of the Intestines 208
Sectional Anatomy of the Abdomen 210

Surface Anatomy

Fig. 10.1 Palpable structures of the abdomen and pelvis

Anterior view. See pp. 2–3 for structures of the back.

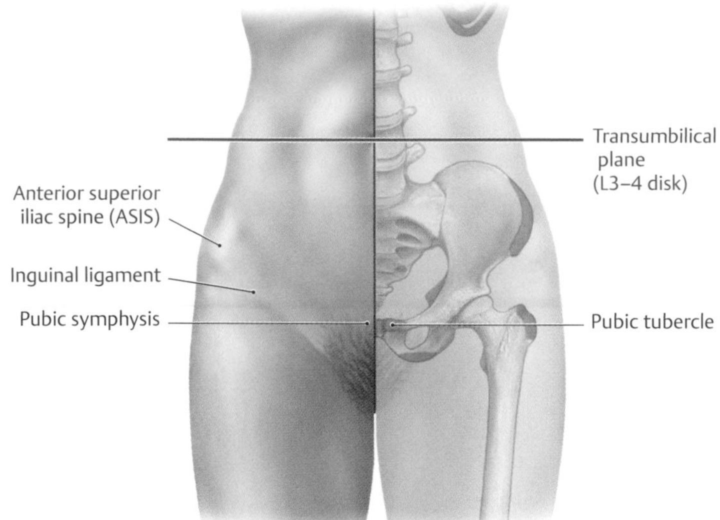
Transumbilical plane (L3–4 disk)
Anterior superior iliac spine (ASIS)
Inguinal ligament
Pubic symphysis
Pubic tubercle

A Bony prominences.

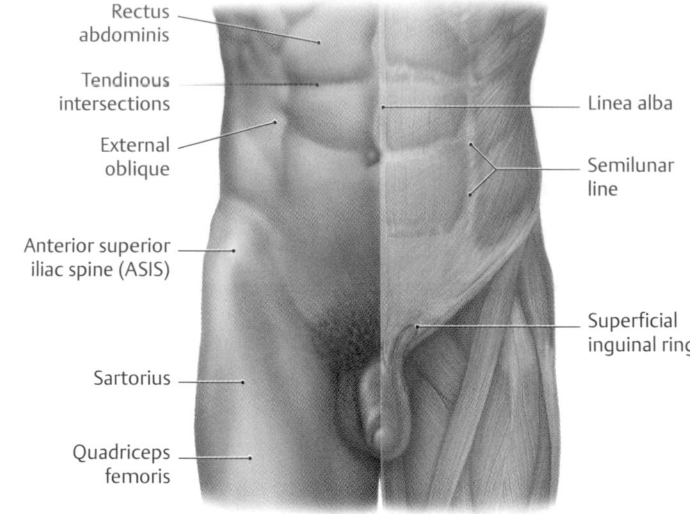
Rectus abdominis
Tendinous intersections
External oblique
Anterior superior iliac spine (ASIS)
Sartorius
Quadriceps femoris
Linea alba
Semilunar line
Superficial inguinal ring

B Musculature.

Fig. 10.2 Quadrants and layers of the abdominopelvic cavity

Anterior view. The location of the organs of the abdomen and pelvis can be described by quadrant and layer.

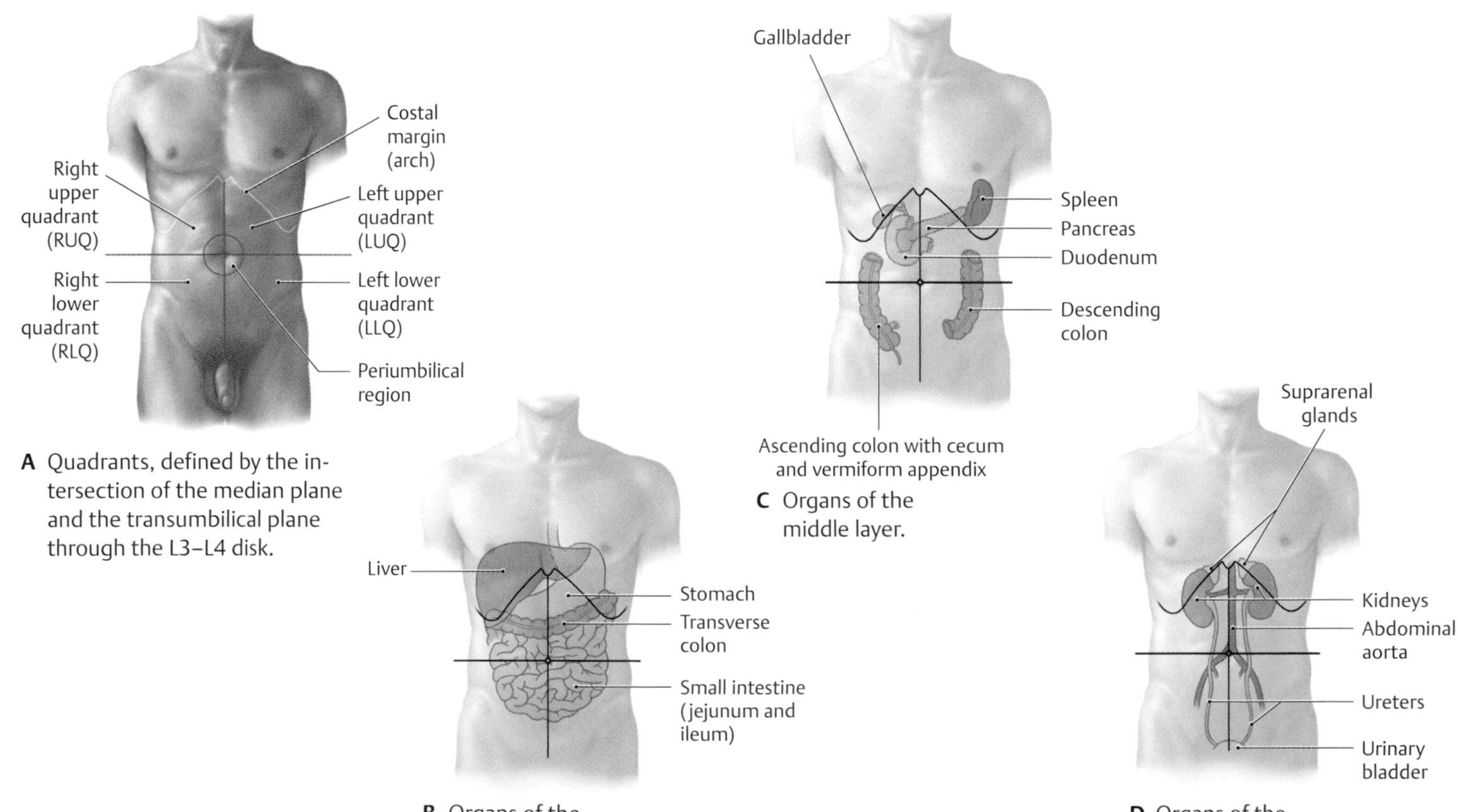
Right upper quadrant (RUQ)
Right lower quadrant (RLQ)
Costal margin (arch)
Left upper quadrant (LUQ)
Left lower quadrant (LLQ)
Periumbilical region
Liver
Stomach
Transverse colon
Small intestine (jejunum and ileum)
Gallbladder
Spleen
Pancreas
Duodenum
Descending colon
Ascending colon with cecum and vermiform appendix
Suprarenal glands
Kidneys
Abdominal aorta
Ureters
Urinary bladder

A Quadrants, defined by the intersection of the median plane and the transumbilical plane through the L3–L4 disk.

B Organs of the anterior layer.

C Organs of the middle layer.

D Organs of the posterior layer.

Table 10.1	Transverse planes through the abdomen
① Transpyloric plane	Transverse plane midway between the superior borders of the pubic symphysis and the manubrium
② Subcostal plane	Plane at the lowest level of the costal margin (the inferior margin of the tenth costal cartilage)
③ Supracrestal plane	Plane passing through the summits of the iliac crests
④ Transtubercular plane	Plane at the level of the iliac tubercles (the iliac tubercle lies ~5 cm posterolateral to the anterior superior iliac spine)
⑤ Interspinous plane	Plane at the level of the anterior superior iliac spine

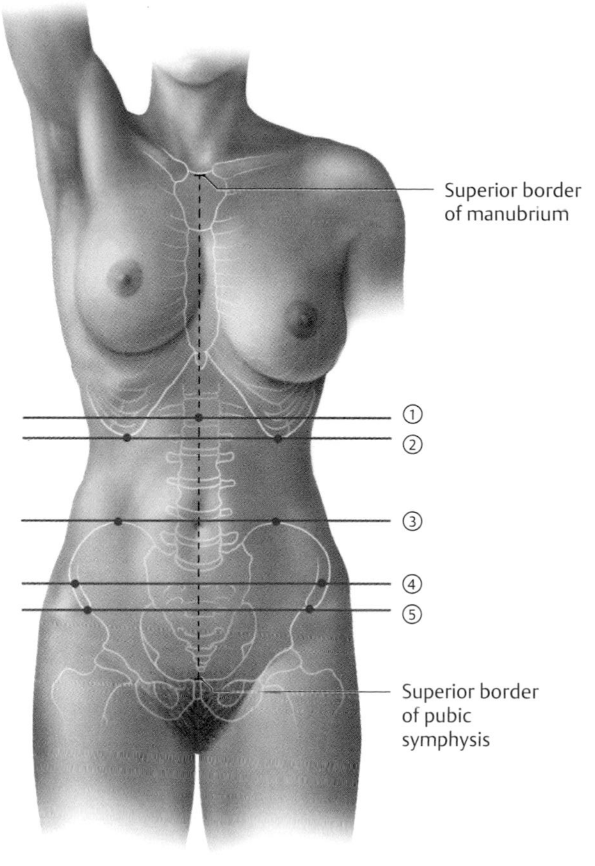
Superior border of manubrium
①
②
③
④
⑤
Superior border of pubic symphysis

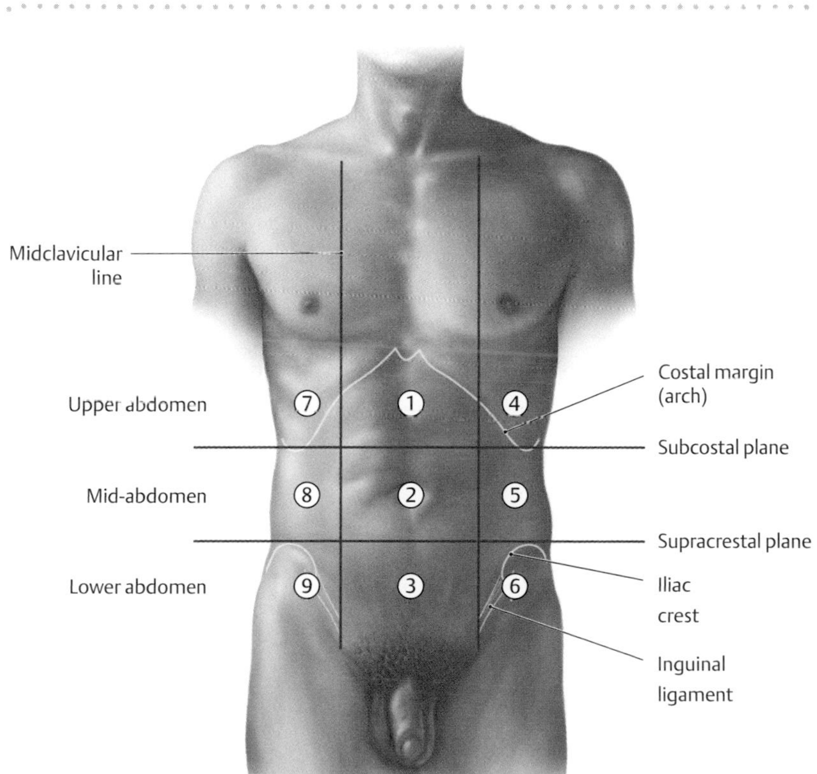
Midclavicular line
Upper abdomen
Mid-abdomen
Lower abdomen
⑦
①
④
⑧
②
⑤
⑨
③
⑥
Costal margin (arch)
Subcostal plane
Supracrestal plane
Iliac crest
Inguinal ligament

Table 10.2	Regions of the abdomen
① Epigastric region	
② Umbilical region	
③ Pubic region	
④ Left hypochondriac region	
⑤ Left lateral (lumbar) region	
⑥ Left inguinal region	
⑦ Right hypochondriac region	
⑧ Right lateral (lumbar) region	
⑨ Right inguinal region	

Bony Framework for the Abdominal Wall

Fig. 11.1 **Bony framework of the abdomen**
Anterior view. These bones are the site of attachment for the muscles and ligaments of the anterolateral abdominal wall and form a bony cage that protects certain abdominal organs.

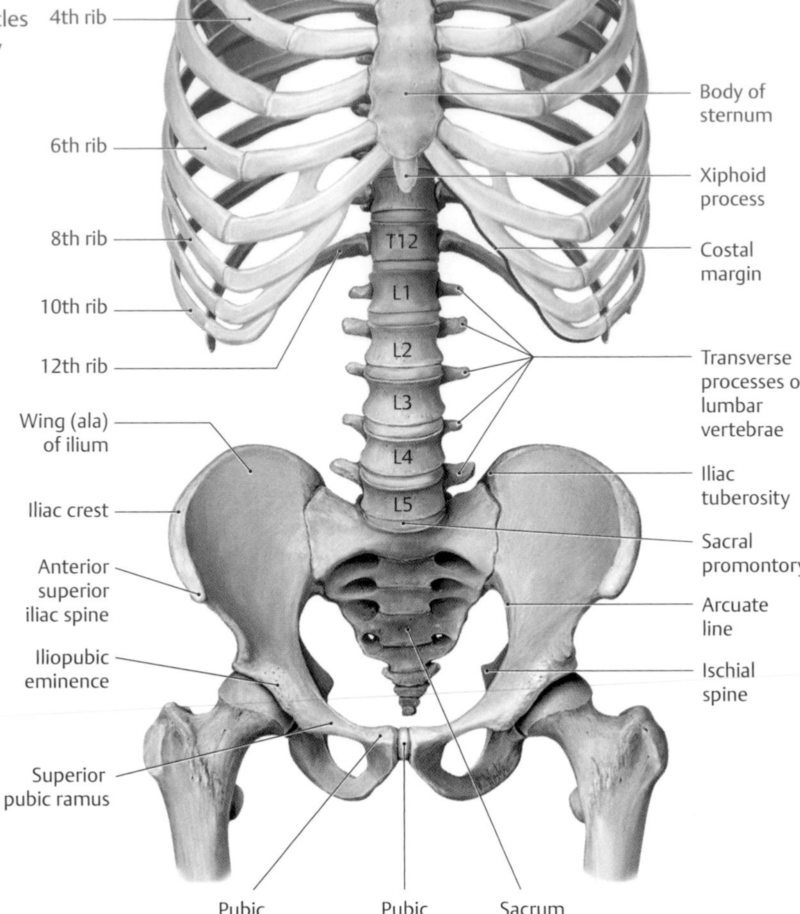
4th rib
6th rib
8th rib
10th rib
12th rib
Wing (ala) of ilium
Iliac crest
Anterior superior iliac spine
Iliopubic eminence
Superior pubic ramus
Pubic tubercle
Pubic symphysis
Sacrum
Body of sternum
Xiphoid process
Costal margin
Transverse processes of lumbar vertebrae
Iliac tuberosity
Sacral promontory
Arcuate line
Ischial spine
T12
L1
L2
L3
L4
L5

Fig. 11.2 **Ligaments of the pelvis**

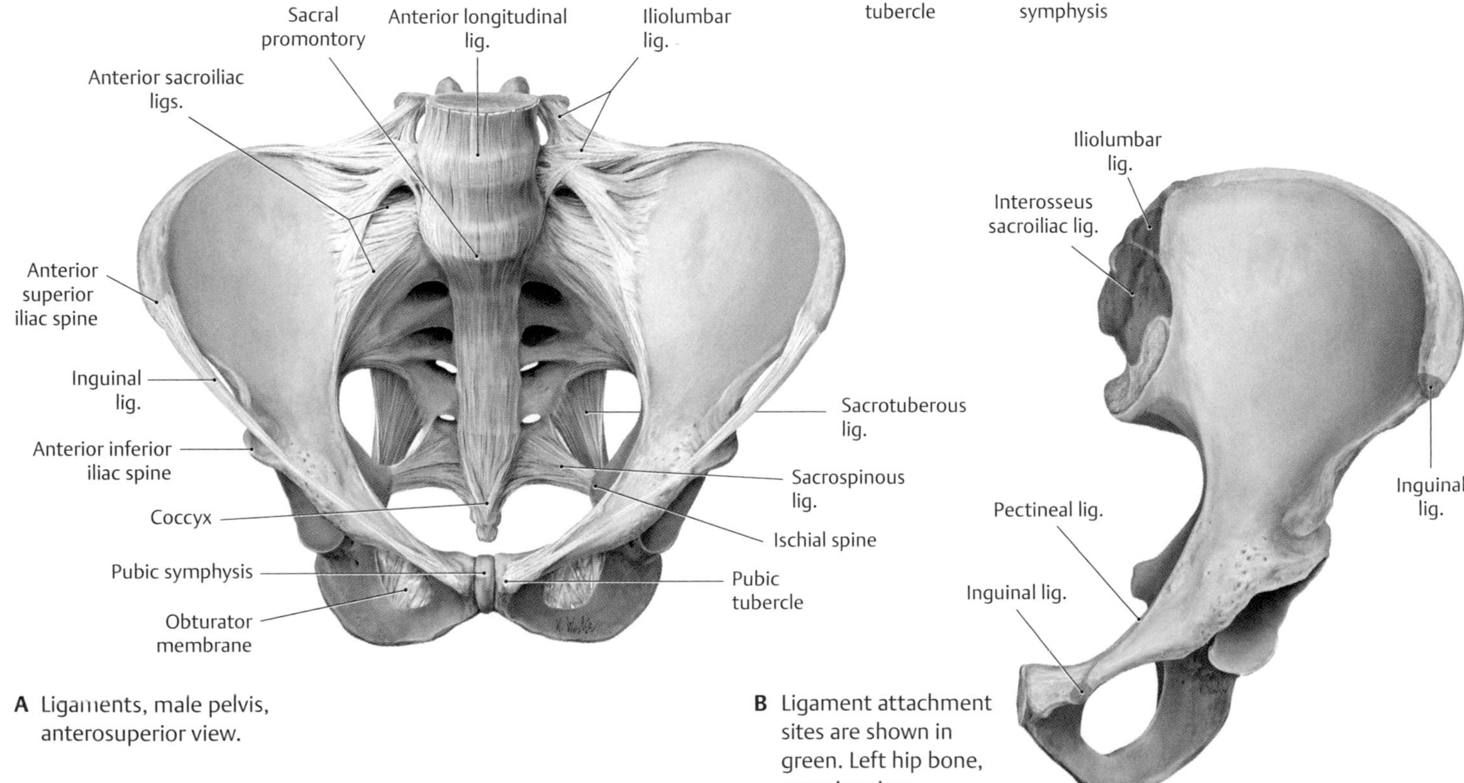
Sacral promontory
Anterior longitudinal lig.
Iliolumbar lig.
Anterior sacroiliac ligs.
Anterior superior iliac spine
Inguinal lig.
Anterior inferior iliac spine
Coccyx
Pubic symphysis
Obturator membrane
Sacrotuberous lig.
Sacrospinous lig.
Ischial spine
Pubic tubercle
Iliolumbar lig.
Interosseus sacroiliac lig.
Pectineal lig.
Inguinal lig.
Inguinal lig.

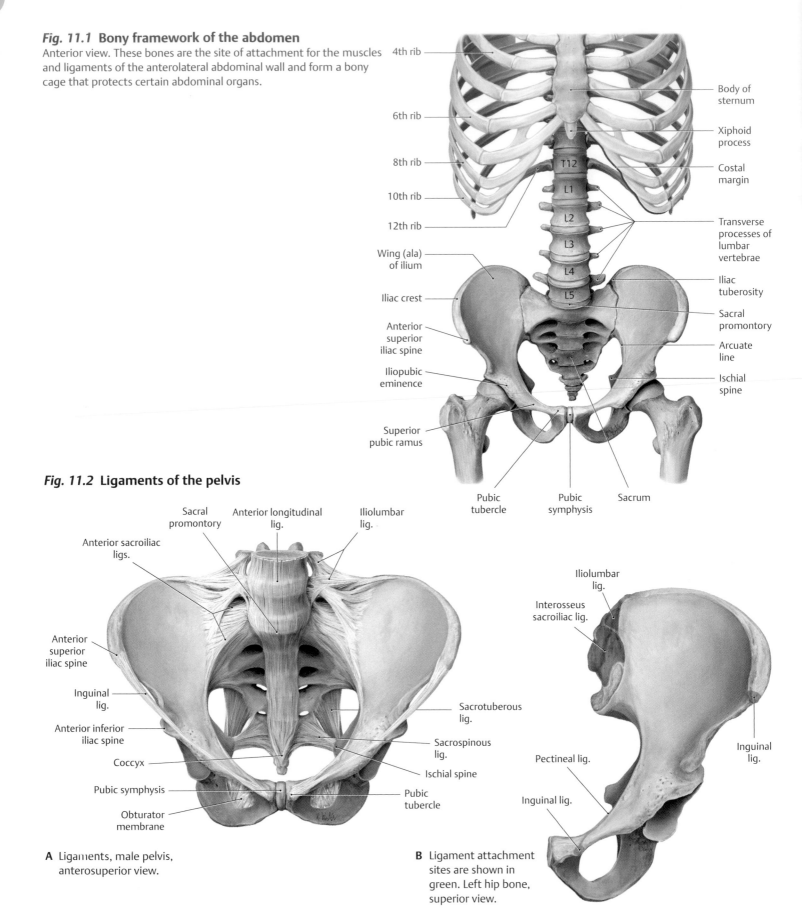

A Ligaments, male pelvis, anterosuperior view.

B Ligament attachment sites are shown in green. Left hip bone, superior view.

Fig. 11.3 Abdominal-wall muscle attachment sites

Left hip bone. Muscle origins are in red, insertions in blue.

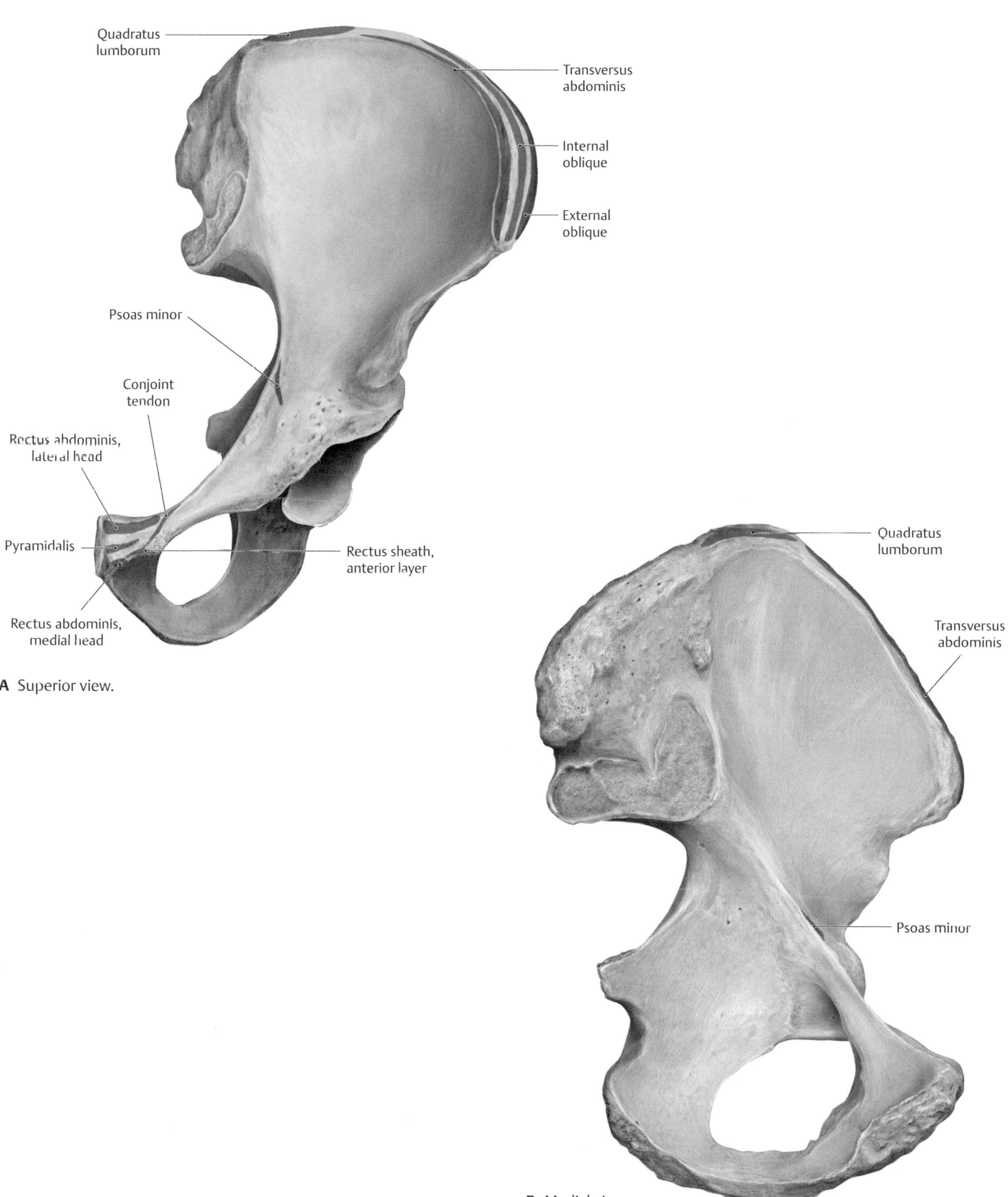
Quadratus lumborum
Transversus abdominis
Internal oblique
External oblique
Psoas minor
Conjoint tendon
Rectus abdominis, lateral head
Pyramidalis
Rectus sheath, anterior layer
Rectus abdominis, medial head
Quadratus lumborum
Transversus abdominis
Psoas minor

A Superior view.

B Medial view.

Muscles of the Anterolateral Abdominal Wall

The oblique muscles of the anterolateral abdominal wall consist of the external and internal obliques and the transversus abdominis. The posterior or deep abdominal wall muscles (notably the psoas major) are functionally hip muscles (see p. 140).

Fig. 11.4 **Muscles of the abdominal wall**
Right side, anterior view.

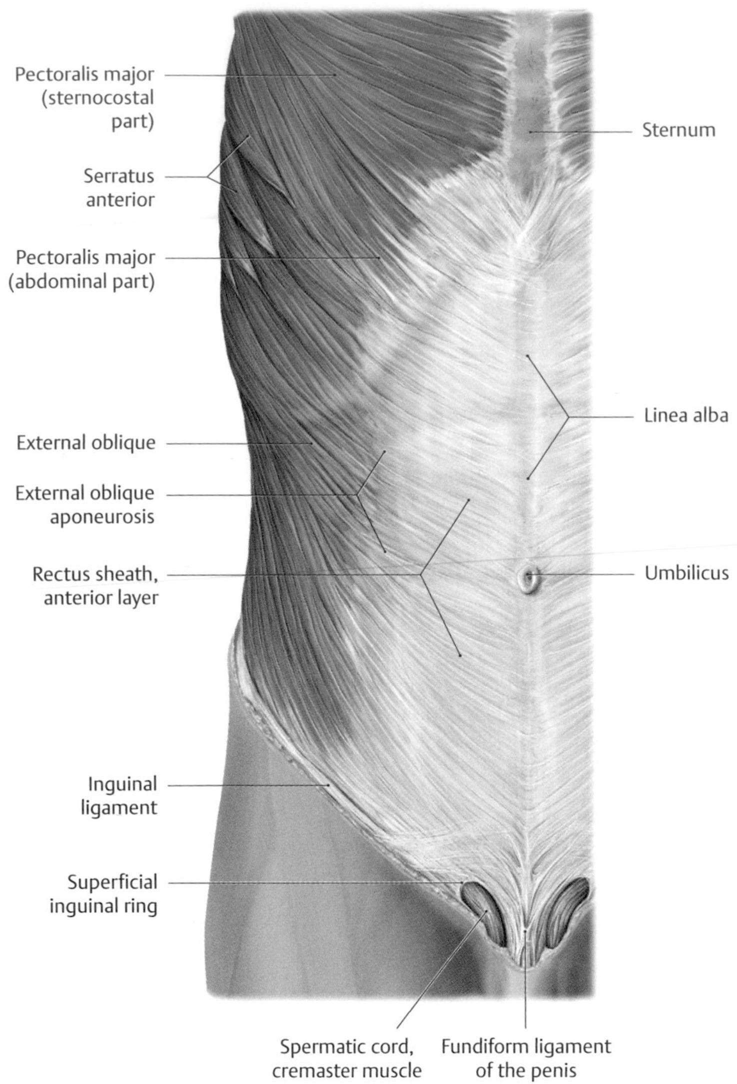
Pectoralis major (sternocostal part)
Serratus anterior
Pectoralis major (abdominal part)
External oblique
External oblique aponeurosis
Rectus sheath, anterior layer
Inguinal ligament
Superficial inguinal ring
Sternum
Linea alba
Umbilicus
Spermatic cord, cremaster muscle
Fundiform ligament of the penis

A Superficial abdominal wall muscles.

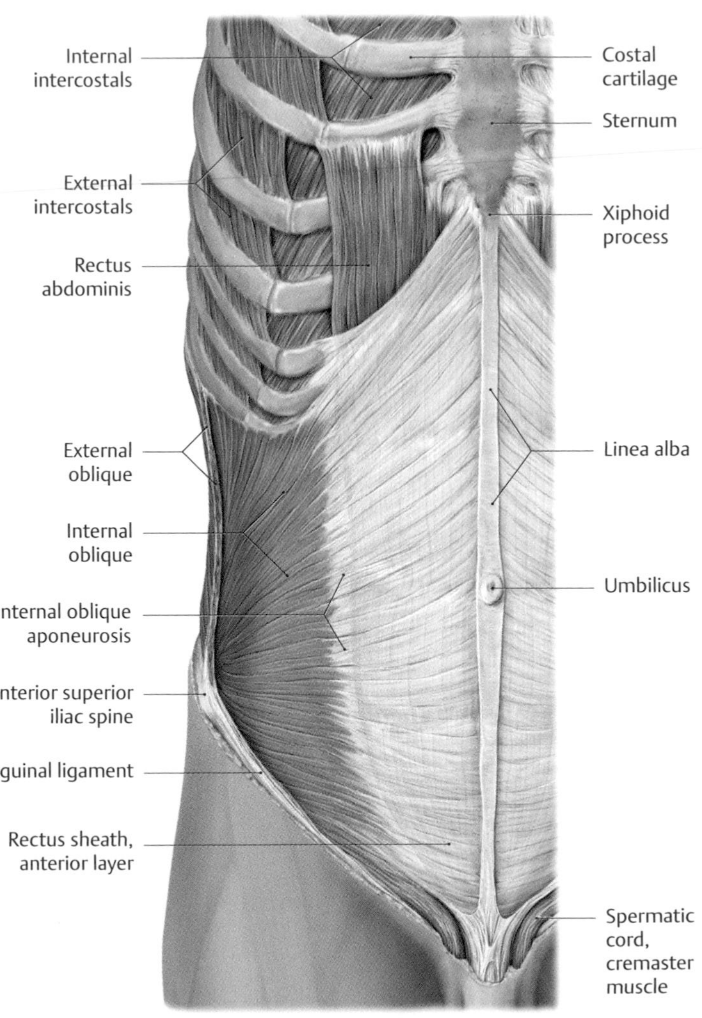
Internal intercostals
External intercostals
Rectus abdominis
External oblique
Internal oblique
Internal oblique aponeurosis
Anterior superior iliac spine
Inguinal ligament
Rectus sheath, anterior layer
Costal cartilage
Sternum
Xiphoid process
Linea alba
Umbilicus
Spermatic cord, cremaster muscle

B *Removed:* External oblique, pectoralis major, and serratus anterior.

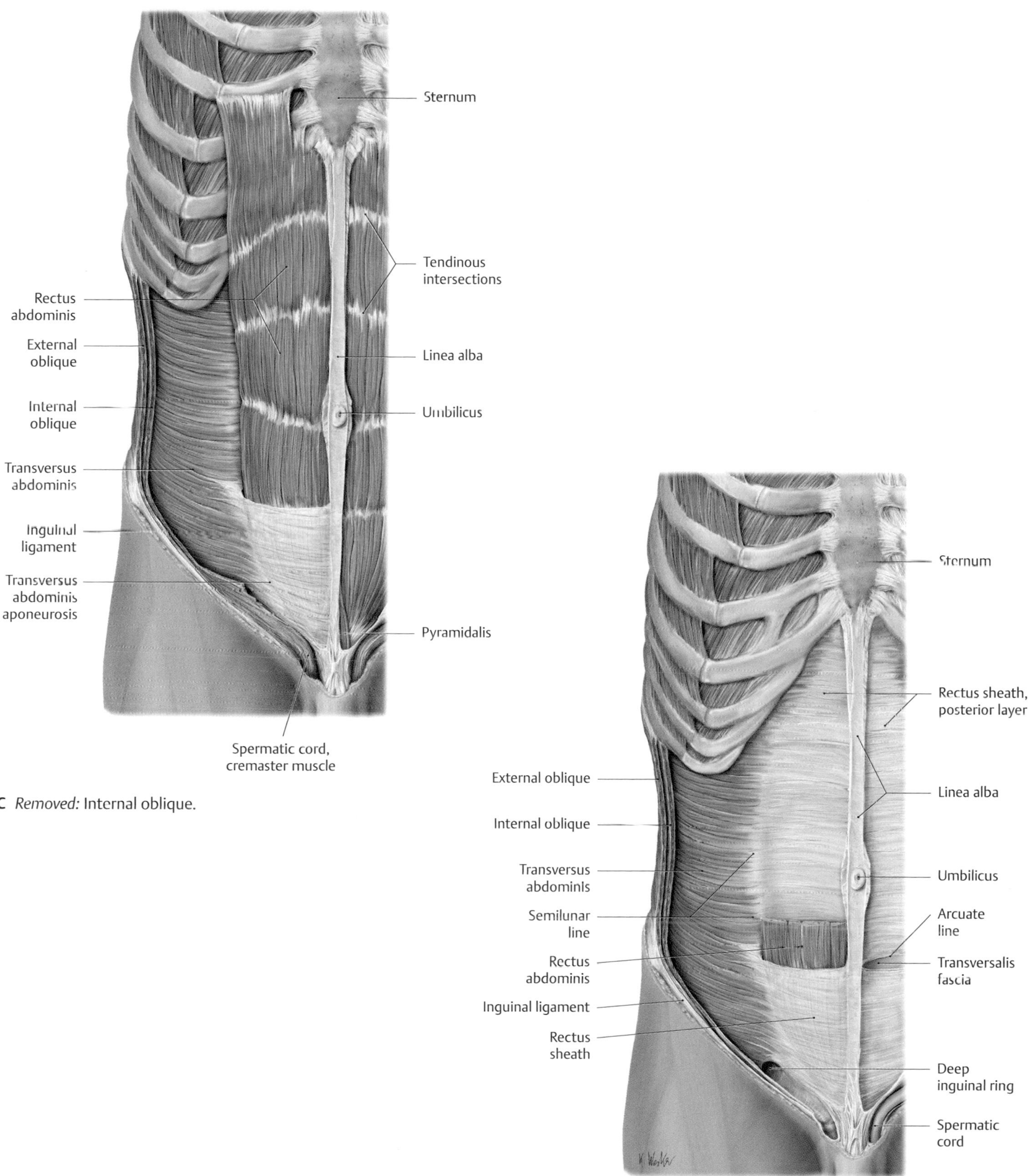
Sternum
Tendinous intersections
Rectus abdominis
External oblique
Linea alba
Internal oblique
Umbilicus
Transversus abdominis
Inguinal ligament
Transversus abdominis aponeurosis
Pyramidalis
Spermatic cord, cremaster muscle
Sternum
Rectus sheath, posterior layer
External oblique
Linea alba
Internal oblique
Transversus abdominis
Umbilicus
Semilunar line
Arcuate line
Rectus abdominis
Transversalis fascia
Inguinal ligament
Rectus sheath
Deep inguinal ring
Spermatic cord

C *Removed:* Internal oblique.

D *Removed:* Rectus abdominis.

Muscles of the Posterior Abdominal Wall & Diaphragm

Fig. 11.5 **Muscles of the posterior abdominal wall.**

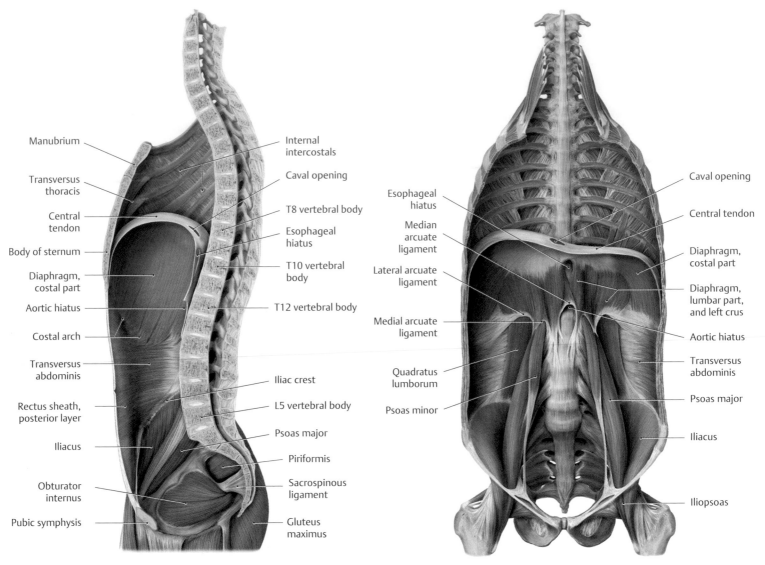

Manubrium
Transversus thoracis
Central tendon
Body of sternum
Diaphragm, costal part
Aortic hiatus
Costal arch
Transversus abdominis
Rectus sheath, posterior layer
Iliacus
Obturator internus
Pubic symphysis
Internal intercostals
Caval opening
T8 vertebral body
Esophageal hiatus
T10 vertebral body
T12 vertebral body
Iliac crest
L5 vertebral body
Psoas major
Piriformis
Sacrospinous ligament
Gluteus maximus

A Midsagittal section with diagraphm in intermediate position.

Esophageal hiatus
Median arcuate ligament
Lateral arcuate ligament
Medial arcuate ligament
Quadratus lumborum
Psoas minor
Caval opening
Central tendon
Diaphragm, costal part
Diaphragm, lumbar part, and left crus
Aortic hiatus
Transversus abdominis
Psoas major
Iliacus
Iliopsoas

B Coronal section with diaphragm in intermediate position.

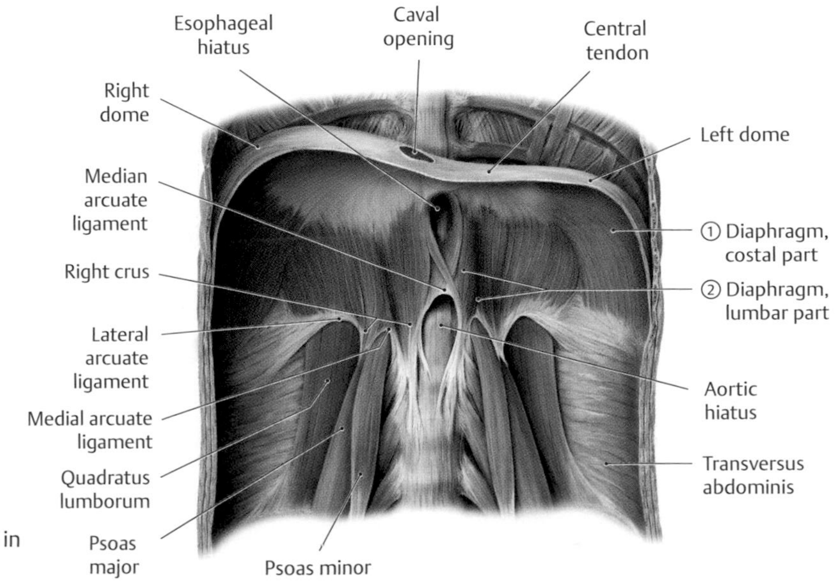
Esophageal hiatus
Caval opening
Central tendon
Right dome
Left dome
Median arcuate ligament
① Diaphragm, costal part
Right crus
② Diaphragm, lumbar part
Lateral arcuate ligament
Aortic hiatus
Medial arcuate ligament
Transversus abdominis
Quadratus lumborum
Psoas major
Psoas minor

C Coronal section with diaphragm in intermediate position.

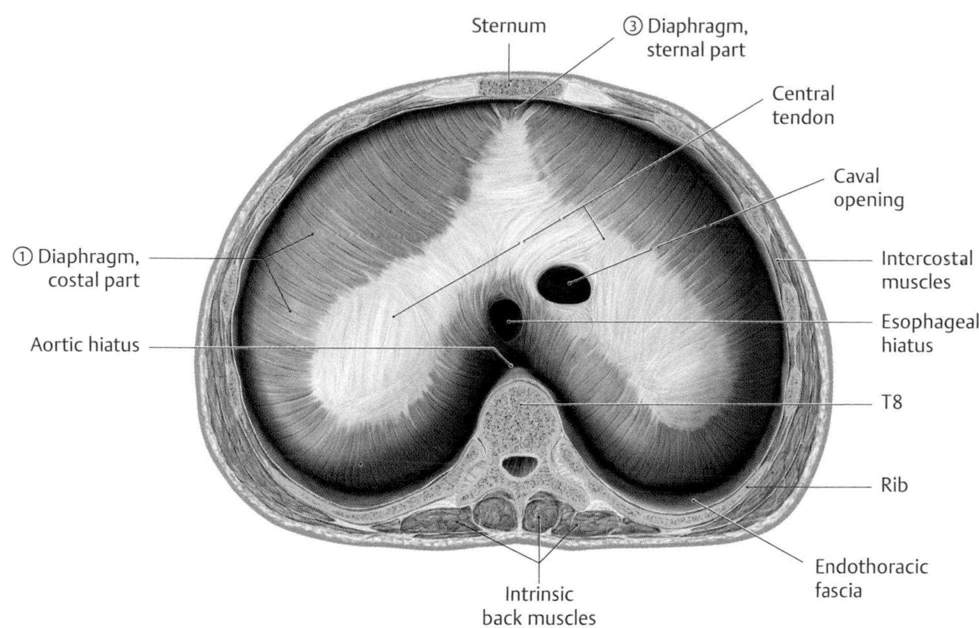
Sternum
③ Diaphragm, sternal part
Central tendon
Caval opening
① Diaphragm, costal part
Intercostal muscles
Esophageal hiatus
Aortic hiatus
T8
Rib
Endothoracic fascia
Intrinsic back muscles

A Superior view.

Fig. 11.6 **Diaphragm in situ**
The diaphragm, which separates the thorax from the abdomen, has two asymmetric domes and three apertures (for the aorta, vena cava, and esophagus).

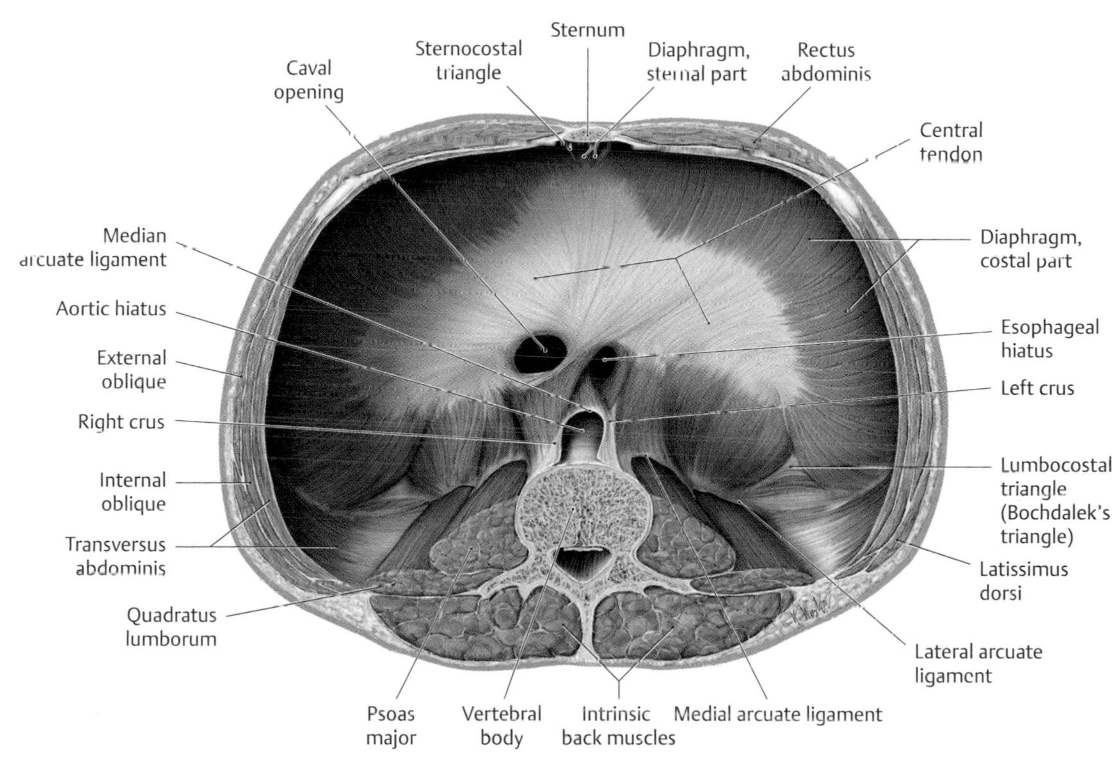
Sternum
Caval opening
Sternocostal triangle
Diaphragm, sternal part
Rectus abdominis
Central tendon
Median arcuate ligament
Diaphragm, costal part
Aortic hiatus
Esophageal hiatus
External oblique
Left crus
Right crus
Lumbocostal triangle (Bochdalek's triangle)
Internal oblique
Transversus abdominis
Latissimus dorsi
Quadratus lumborum
Lateral arcuate ligament
Psoas major
Vertebral body
Intrinsic back muscles
Medial arcuate ligament

B Inferior view.

Table 11.1 **Diaphragm**

Muscle		Origin	Insertion	Innervation	Action
Diaphragm	① Costal part	7th to 12th ribs (inner surface; lower margin of costal arch)	Central tendon	Phrenic n. (C3–C5, cervical plexus)	Principal muscle of respiration (diaphragmatic and thoracic breathing); aids in compressing abdominal viscera (abdominal press)
	② Lumbar part	Medial part: L1–L3 vertebral bodies, intervertebral disks, and anterior longitudinal ligament as right and left crura			
		Lateral parts: lateral and medial arcuate ligaments			
	③ Sternal part	Xiphoid process (posterior surface)			

Abdominal Wall Muscle Facts

Fig. 11.7 Anterior abdominal wall muscles
Anterior view.

Linea alba
②
①

Fig. 11.8 Anterolateral abdominal wall muscles
Anterior view.

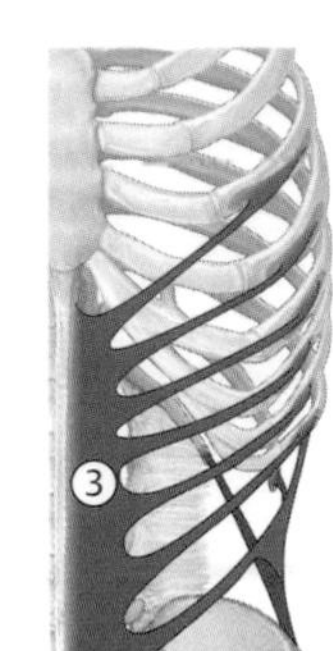
③
A External oblique.

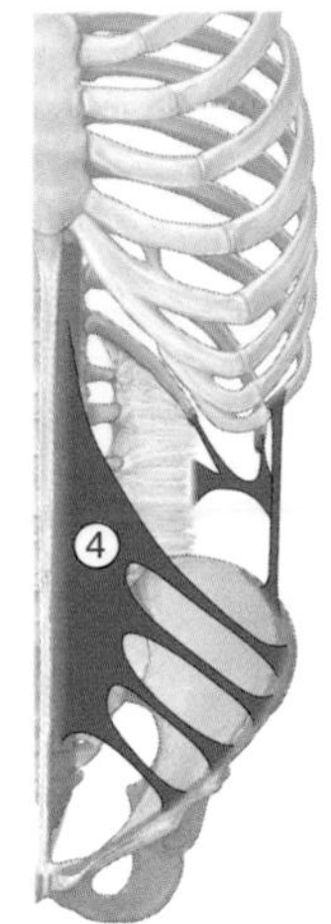
④
B Internal oblique.

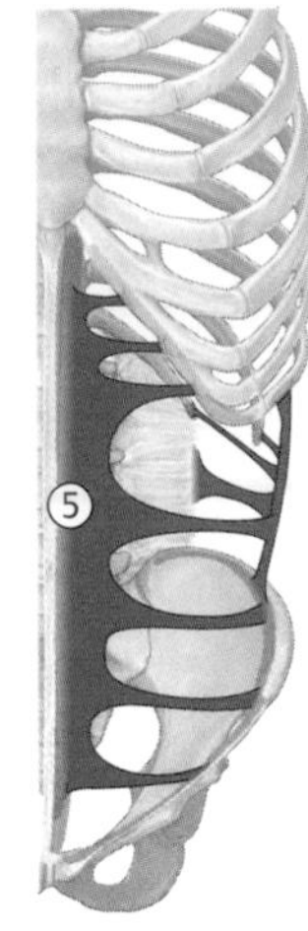
⑤
C Transversus abdominis.

Fig. 11.9 Posterior abdominal wall muscles
Anterior view. The psoas major and iliacus are together known as the iliopsoas.

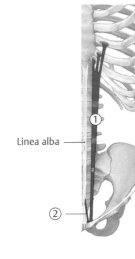

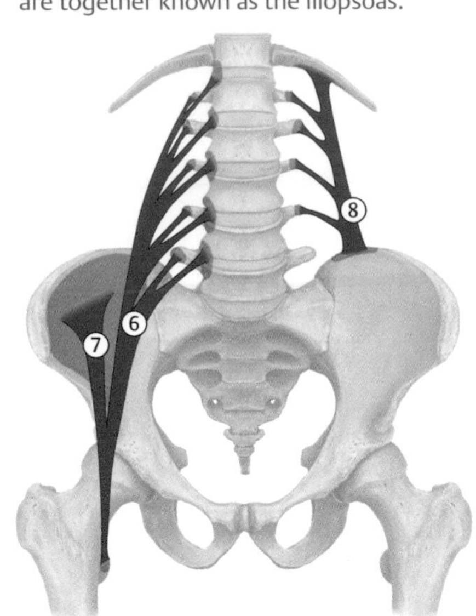
⑥
⑦
⑧

Table 11.2 Abdominal wall muscles

Muscle	Origin	Insertion	Innervation	Action
Anterior abdominal wall muscles				
① Rectus abdominis	*Lateral head:* Crest of pubis to pubic tubercle *Medial head:* Anterior region of pubic symphysis	Cartilages of 5th to 7th ribs, xiphoid process of sternum	Intercostal nn. (T5–T12)	Flexes trunk, compresses abdomen, stabilizes pelvis
② Pyramidalis	Pubis (anterior to rectus abdominis)	Linea alba (runs within the rectus sheath)	Subcostal n. (12th intercostal n.)	Tenses linea alba
Anterolateral abdominal wall muscles				
③ External oblique	5th to 12th ribs (outer surface)	Linea alba, pubic tubercle, anterior iliac crest	Intercostal nn. (T7–T12)	*Unilateral:* Bends trunk to same side, rotates trunk to opposite side *Bilateral:* Flexes trunk, compresses abdomen, stabilizes pelvis
④ Internal oblique	Thoracolumbar fascia (deep layer), iliac crest (intermediate line), anterior superior iliac spine, iliopsoas fascia	10th to 12th ribs (lower borders), linea alba (anterior and posterior layers)	Intercostal nn. (T7–T12), iliohypogastric n., ilioinguinal n.	
⑤ Transversus abdominis	7th to 12th costal cartilages (inner surfaces), thoracolumbar fascia (deep layer), iliac crest, anterior superior iliac spine (inner lip), iliopsoas fascia	Linea alba, pubic crest		*Unilateral:* Rotates trunk to same side *Bilateral:* Compresses abdomen
Posterior abdominal wall muscles				
⑥ Psoas major – Superficial layer	T12–L4 vertebral bodies and associated intervertebral disks (lateral surfaces)	Femur (lesser trochanter), joint insertion as iliopsoas muscle	Direct branches from lumbar plexus (L2–L4)	Hip joint: Flexion and external rotation Lumbar spine (with femur fixed): *Unilateral:* Contraction bends trunk laterally *Bilateral:* Contraction raises trunk from supine position
⑥ Psoas major – Deep layer	L1–L5 (costal processes)			
Psoas minor* (see Fig. 26.17)	T12, L1 vertebrae and intervertebral disk (lateral surfaces)	Pecten pubis, iliopubic ramus, iliac fascia; lowermost fibers may reach inguinal ligament	Direct branches from lumbar plexus (L2–L4)	Weak flexor of the trunk
⑦ Iliacus	Iliac fossa		Femoral n. (L2–L4)	
⑧ Quadratus lumborum	Iliac crest and iliolumbar ligament (not shown)	12th rib, L1–L4 vertebrae (transverse processes)	T12, L1–L4 spinal nn.	*Unilateral:* Bends trunk to same side *Bilateral:* Bearing down and expiration, stabilizes 12th rib

* Approximately 50% of the population has this muscle. For the diaphragm see p. 60–61.

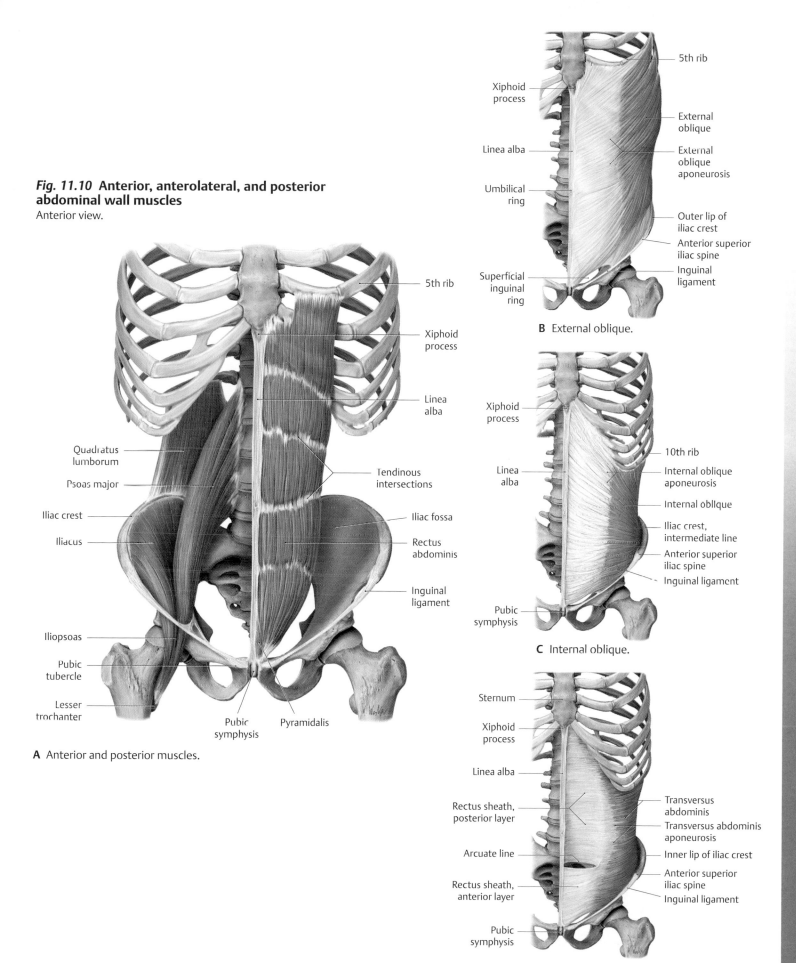

Fig. 11.10 Anterior, anterolateral, and posterior abdominal wall muscles
Anterior view.

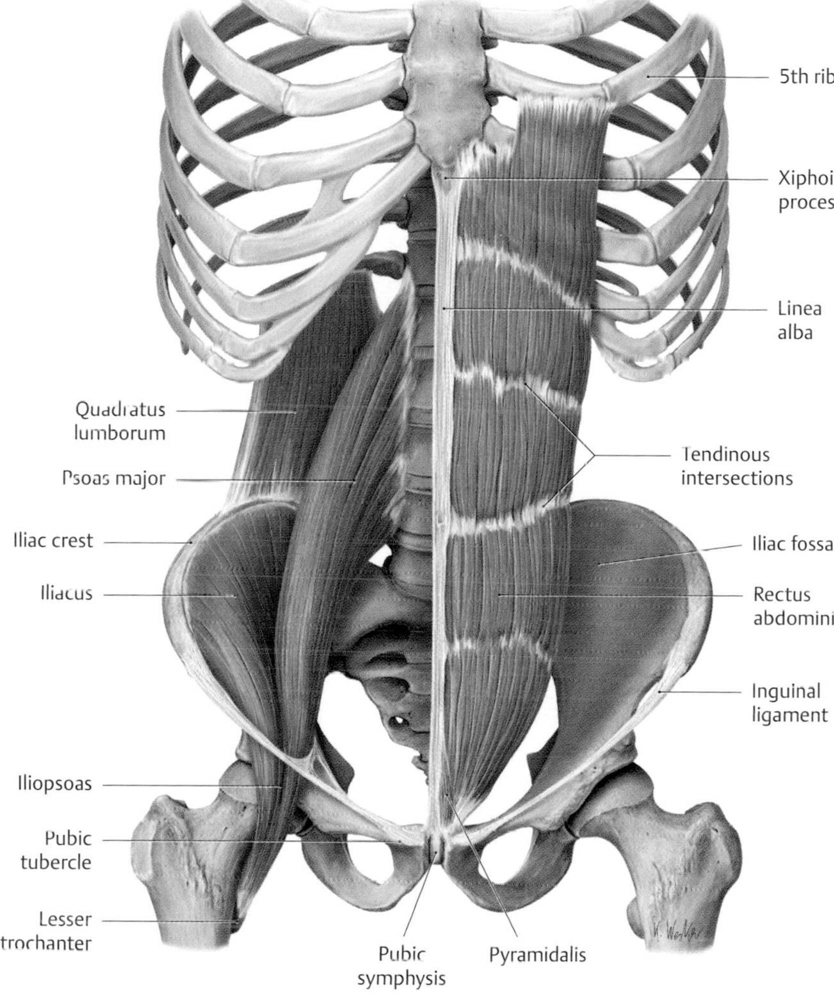
5th rib
Xiphoid process
Linea alba
Quadratus lumborum
Tendinous intersections
Psoas major
Iliac crest
Iliac fossa
Iliacus
Rectus abdominis
Inguinal ligament
Iliopsoas
Pubic tubercle
Lesser trochanter
Pubic symphysis
Pyramidalis

A Anterior and posterior muscles.

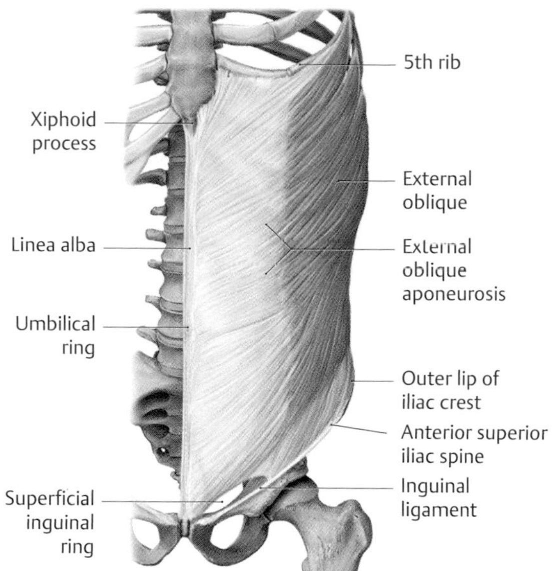
5th rib
Xiphoid process
External oblique
Linea alba
External oblique aponeurosis
Umbilical ring
Outer lip of iliac crest
Anterior superior iliac spine
Superficial inguinal ring
Inguinal ligament

B External oblique.

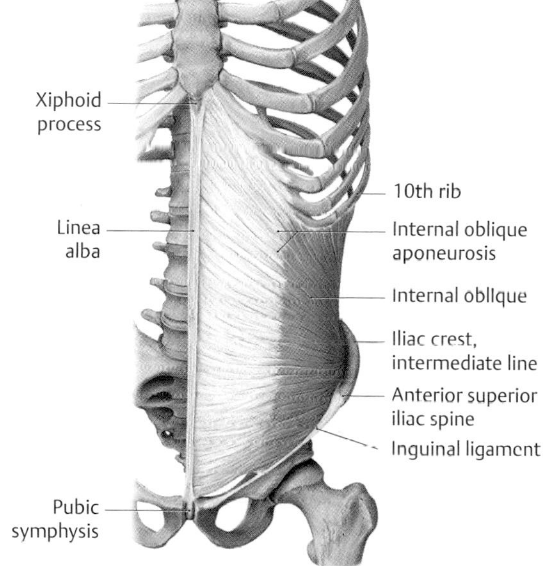
Xiphoid process
10th rib
Linea alba
Internal oblique aponeurosis
Internal oblique
Iliac crest, intermediate line
Anterior superior iliac spine
Inguinal ligament
Pubic symphysis

C Internal oblique.

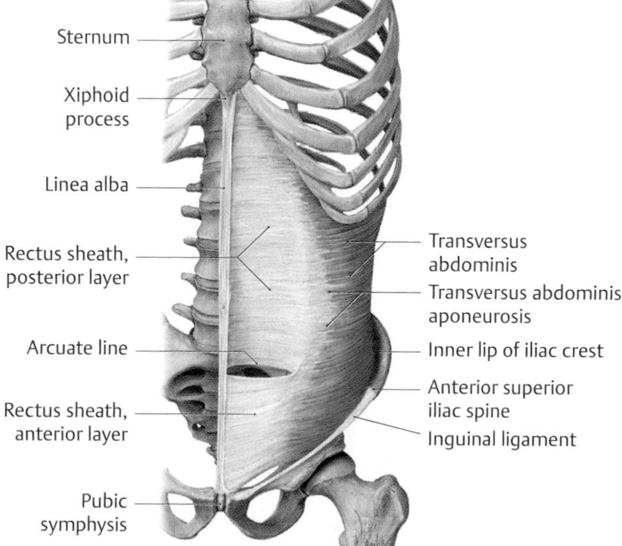
Sternum
Xiphoid process
Linea alba
Rectus sheath, posterior layer
Transversus abdominis
Transversus abdominis aponeurosis
Arcuate line
Inner lip of iliac crest
Anterior superior iliac spine
Rectus sheath, anterior layer
Inguinal ligament
Pubic symphysis

D Transversus abdominis.

Inguinal Region & Canal

The inguinal region is the junction of the anterior abdominal wall and the anterior thigh. The inguinal canal is an important site for the passage of structures into and out of the abdominal cavity (e.g., components of the spermatic cord).

Fig. 11.11 ***Inguinal region***
Right side, anterior view.

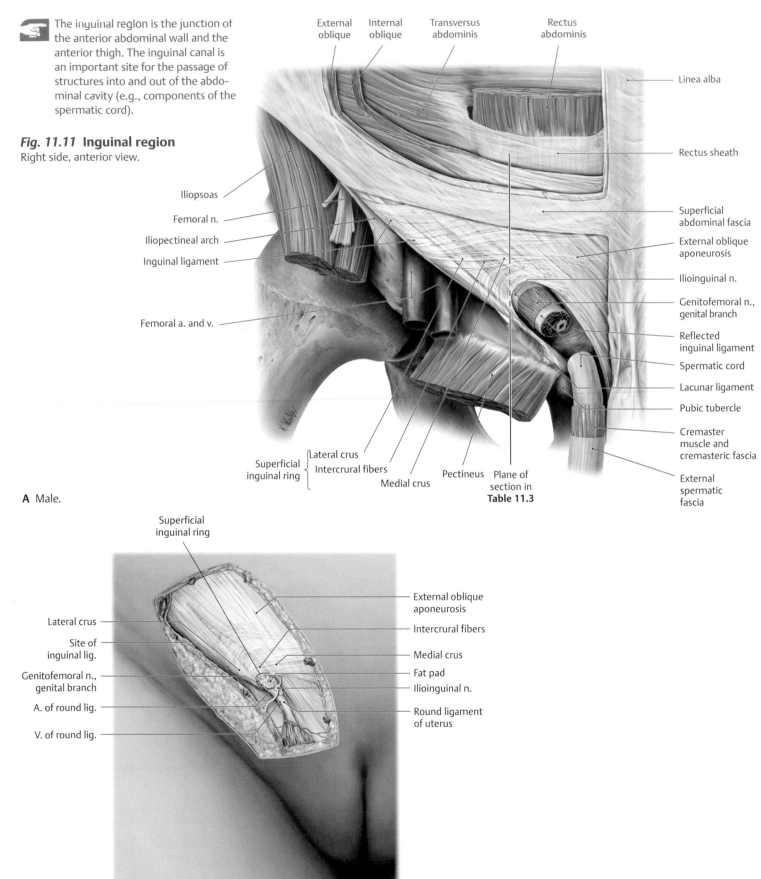

External oblique
Internal oblique
Transversus abdominis
Rectus abdominis
Linea alba
Rectus sheath
Iliopsoas
Femoral n.
Iliopectineal arch
Inguinal ligament
Femoral a. and v.
Superficial abdominal fascia
External oblique aponeurosis
Ilioinguinal n.
Genitofemoral n., genital branch
Reflected inguinal ligament
Spermatic cord
Lacunar ligament
Pubic tubercle
Cremaster muscle and cremasteric fascia
External spermatic fascia
Superficial inguinal ring
Lateral crus
Intercrural fibers
Medial crus
Pectineus
Plane of section in **Table 11.3**

A Male.

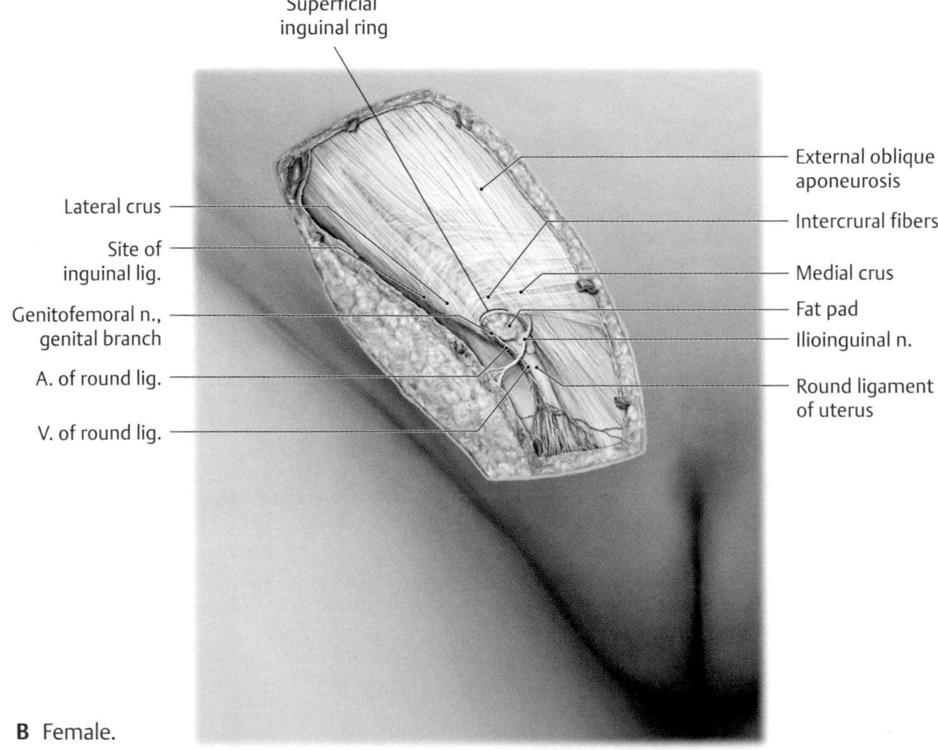

Superficial inguinal ring
Lateral crus
Site of inguinal lig.
Genitofemoral n., genital branch
A. of round lig.
V. of round lig.
External oblique aponeurosis
Intercrural fibers
Medial crus
Fat pad
Ilioinguinal n.
Round ligament of uterus

B Female.

Table 11.3 Structures of the inguinal canal

Structures			Formed by
Wall	Anterior wall	①	External oblique aponeurosis
	Roof	②	Internal oblique muscle
		③	Transversus abdominis
	Posterior wall	④	Transversalis fascia
		⑤	Parietal peritoneum
	Floor	⑥	Inguinal ligament (densely interwoven fibers of the lower external oblique aponeurosis and adjacent fascia lata of thigh)
Openings	Superficial inguinal ring		Opening in external oblique aponeurosis; bounded by medial and lateral crus, intercrural fibers, and reflected inguinal ligament
	Deep inguinal ring		Outpouching of the transversalis fascia lateral to the lateral umbilical fold (inferior epigastric vessels)

Sagittal section through plane in Fig. 11.11A.

②
③
Superficial abdominal fascia
④
⑤
①
Ilioinguinal n.
Spermatic cord
⑥
Pectineal ligament
Lacunar ligament
Superior pubic ramus
Pectineus
Fascia lata

Fig. 11.12 Dissection of the inguinal region
Right side, anterior view.

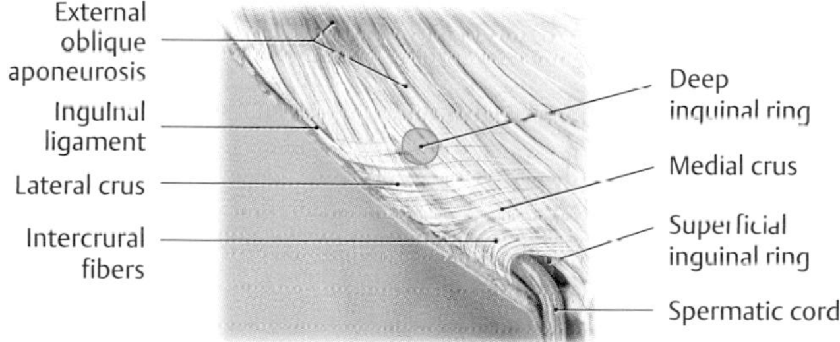
External oblique aponeurosis
Inguinal ligament
Lateral crus
Intercrural fibers
Deep inguinal ring
Medial crus
Superficial inguinal ring
Spermatic cord

A Superficial layer.

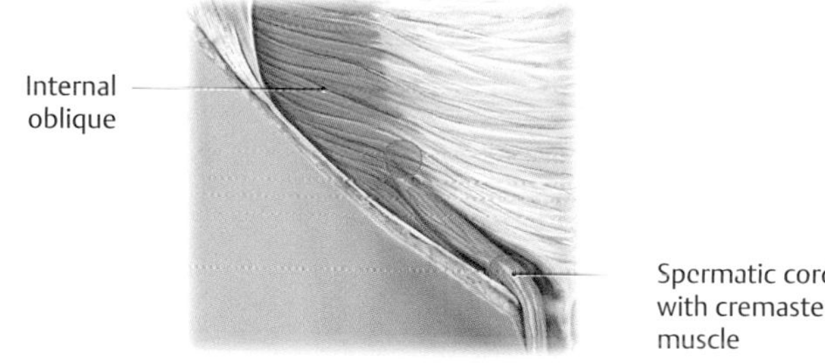
Internal oblique
Spermatic cord with cremaster muscle

B *Removed:* External oblique aponeurosis.

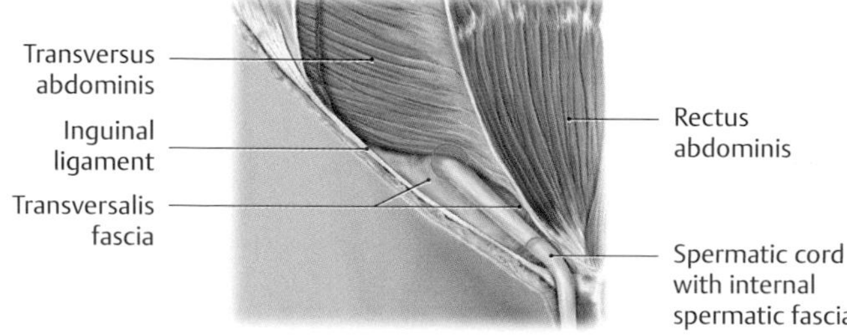
Transversus abdominis
Inguinal ligament
Transversalis fascia
Rectus abdominis
Spermatic cord with internal spermatic fascia

C *Removed:* Internal oblique.

Fig. 11.13 Opening of the inguinal canal
Right side, anterior view.

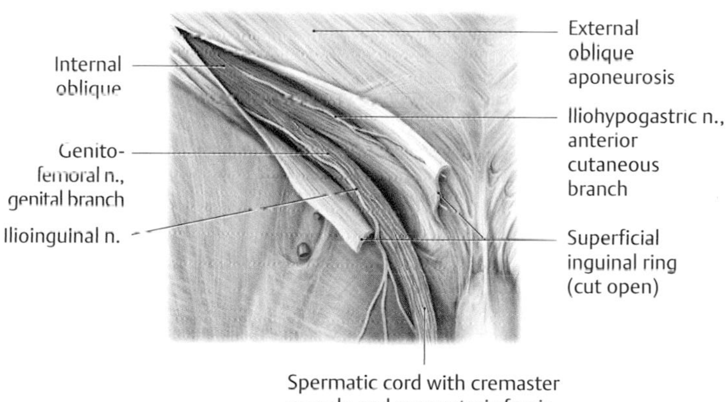
Internal oblique
Genito-femoral n., genital branch
Ilioinguinal n.
External oblique aponeurosis
Iliohypogastric n., anterior cutaneous branch
Superficial inguinal ring (cut open)
Spermatic cord with cremaster muscle and cremasteric fascia

A *Divided:* External oblique aponeurosis.

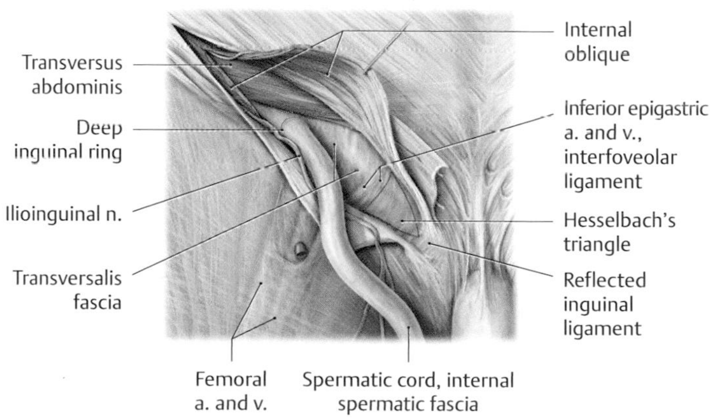
Transversus abdominis
Deep inguinal ring
Ilioinguinal n.
Transversalis fascia
Internal oblique
Inferior epigastric a. and v., interfoveolar ligament
Hesselbach's triangle
Reflected inguinal ligament
Femoral a. and v.
Spermatic cord, internal spermatic fascia

B *Divided:* Internal oblique and cremaster.

Spermatic Cord, Scrotum & Testis

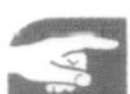

The coverings of the scrotum, testis, and spermatic cord are continuations of muscular and fascial layers of the anterior abdominal wall, as are those of the inguinal canal.

Fig. 11.14 Scrotum and spermatic cord
Anterior view. *Removed:* Skin over the scrotum and spermatic cord.

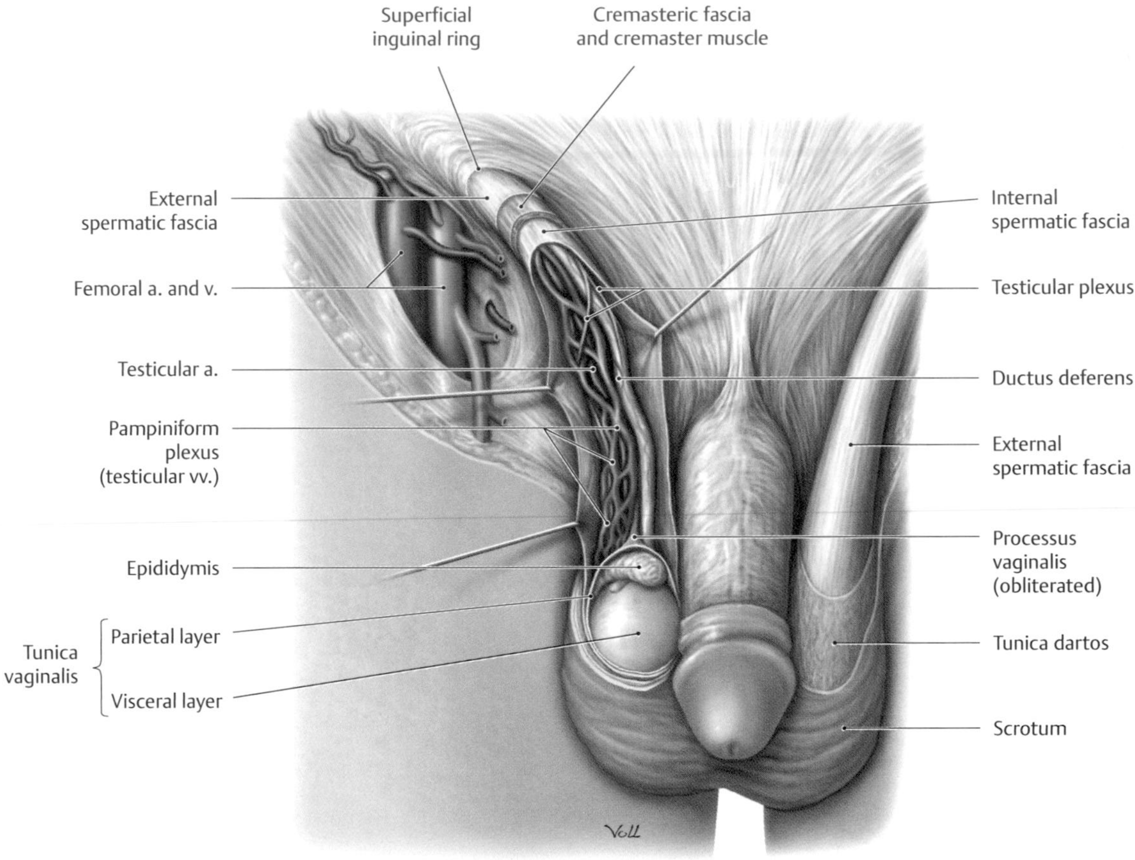

Superficial inguinal ring
Cremasteric fascia and cremaster muscle
External spermatic fascia
Femoral a. and v.
Testicular a.
Pampiniform plexus (testicular vv.)
Epididymis
Tunica vaginalis
Parietal layer
Visceral layer
Internal spermatic fascia
Testicular plexus
Ductus deferens
External spermatic fascia
Processus vaginalis (obliterated)
Tunica dartos
Scrotum

Fig. 11.15 Spermatic cord: Contents
Cross section.

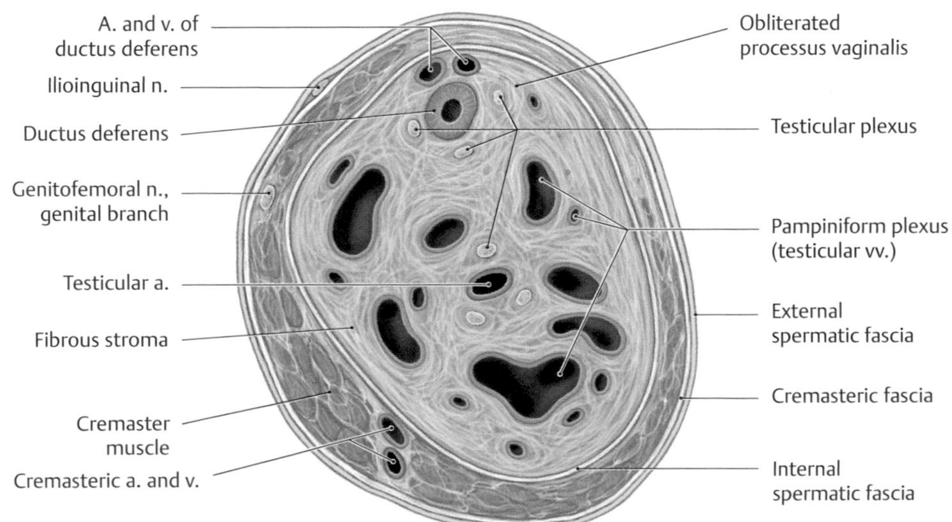

A. and v. of ductus deferens
Ilioinguinal n.
Ductus deferens
Genitofemoral n., genital branch
Testicular a.
Fibrous stroma
Cremaster muscle
Cremasteric a. and v.
Obliterated processus vaginalis
Testicular plexus
Pampiniform plexus (testicular vv.)
External spermatic fascia
Cremasteric fascia
Internal spermatic fascia

***Fig. 11.16* Testis and epididymis**
Left lateral view.

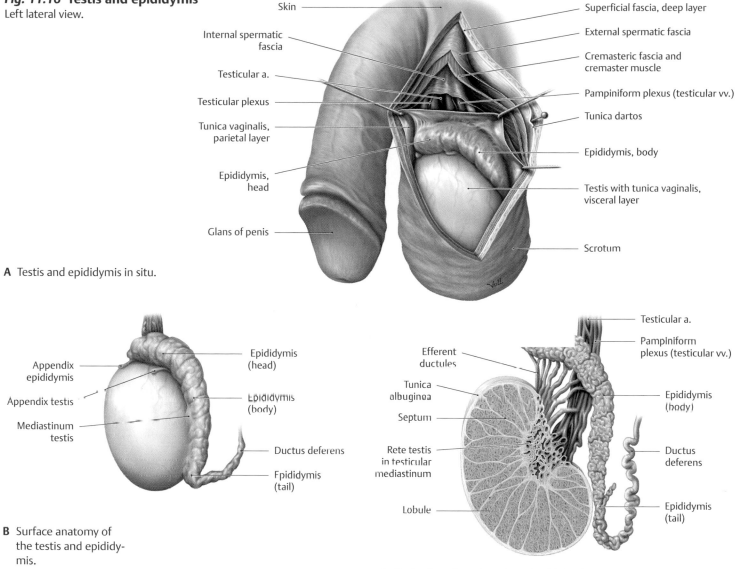

Skin
Internal spermatic fascia
Testicular a.
Testicular plexus
Tunica vaginalis, parietal layer
Epididymis, head
Glans of penis
Superficial fascia, deep layer
External spermatic fascia
Cremasteric fascia and cremaster muscle
Pampiniform plexus (testicular vv.)
Tunica dartos
Epididymis, body
Testis with tunica vaginalis, visceral layer
Scrotum

A Testis and epididymis in situ.

Appendix epididymis
Appendix testis
Mediastinum testis
Epididymis (head)
Epididymis (body)
Ductus deferens
Epididymis (tail)

B Surface anatomy of the testis and epididymis.

Efferent ductules
Tunica albuginea
Septum
Rete testis in testicular mediastinum
Lobule
Testicular a.
Pampiniform plexus (testicular vv.)
Epididymis (body)
Ductus deferens
Epididymis (tail)

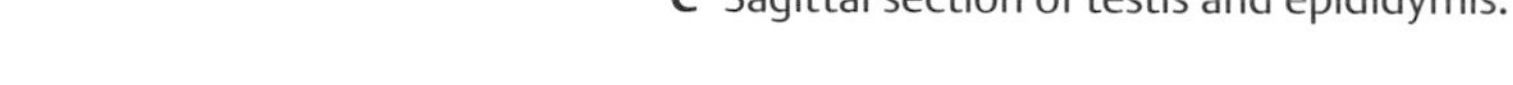

C Sagittal section of testis and epididymis.

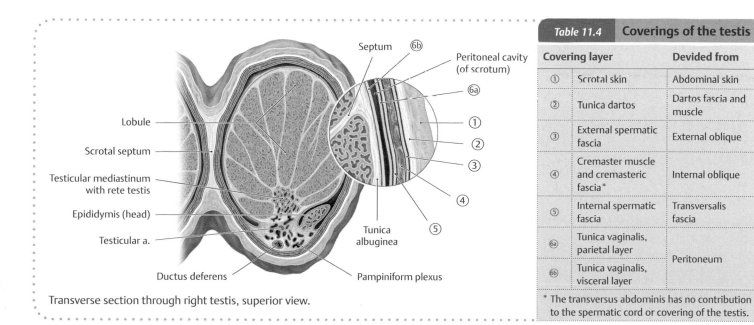

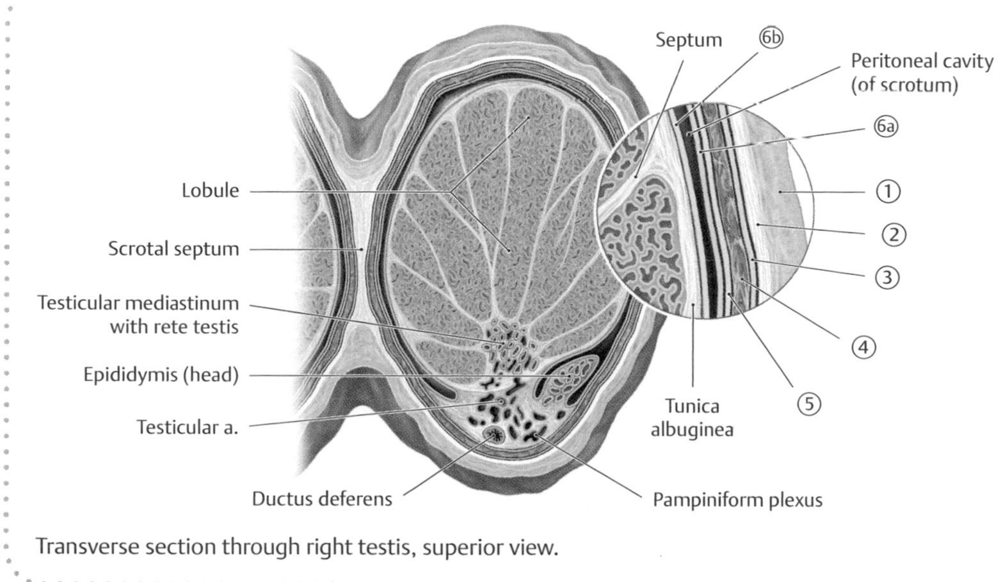
Septum
6b
Peritoneal cavity (of scrotum)
6a
1
2
3
4
5
Lobule
Scrotal septum
Testicular mediastinum with rete testis
Epididymis (head)
Testicular a.
Tunica albuginea
Ductus deferens
Pampiniform plexus

Transverse section through right testis, superior view.

Table 11.4 Coverings of the testis

	Covering layer	Devided from
①	Scrotal skin	Abdominal skin
②	Tunica dartos	Dartos fascia and muscle
③	External spermatic fascia	External oblique
④	Cremaster muscle and cremasteric fascia*	Internal oblique
⑤	Internal spermatic fascia	Transversalis fascia
6a	Tunica vaginalis, parietal layer	Peritoneum
6b	Tunica vaginalis, visceral layer	

* The transversus abdominis has no contribution to the spermatic cord or covering of the testis.

Anterior Abdominal Wall & Inguinal Hernias

The rectus sheath is created by fusion of the aponeuroses of the transversus abdominis and abdominal oblique muscles. The inferior edge of the posterior layer of the rectus sheath is called the arcuate line.

***Fig. 11.17* Anterior abdominal wall and rectus sheath**

Diaphragm
Parietal peritoneum
Falciform ligament of the liver
Round ligament of liver, paraumbilical veins
Transversalis fascia
Plane of section in **B**
Umbilicus
Rectus sheath, posterior layer
Median umbilical fold
Arcuate line
Medial umbilical fold
Rectus abdominis
Lateral umbilical fold
Inferior epigastric a. and v.
Lateral inguinal fossa (deep inguinal ring)
Deep circumflex iliac a. and v.
Iliacus
Testicular a. and v.
Plane of section in **C**
A. and v. of ductus deferens
Psoas major
Femoral a. and v.
Medial inguinal fossa (Hesselbach's triangle)
Ductus deferens
Supravesical fossa
Obturator branch, inferior epigastric a.
Bladder
Prostate
Obturator n., a., and v.

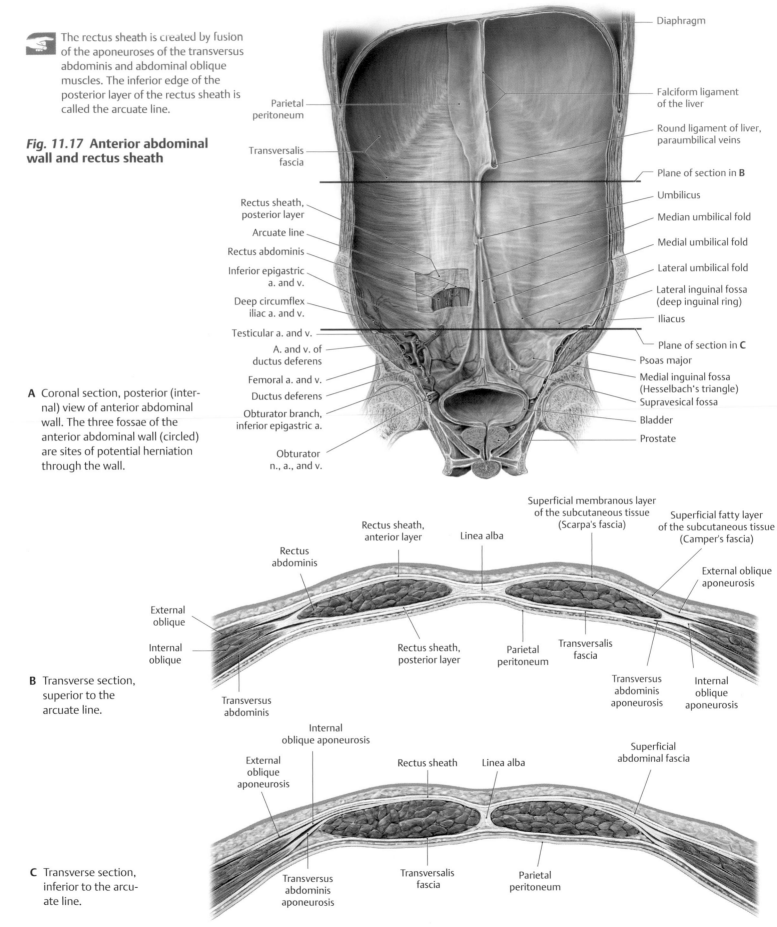

A Coronal section, posterior (internal) view of anterior abdominal wall. The three fossae of the anterior abdominal wall (circled) are sites of potential herniation through the wall.

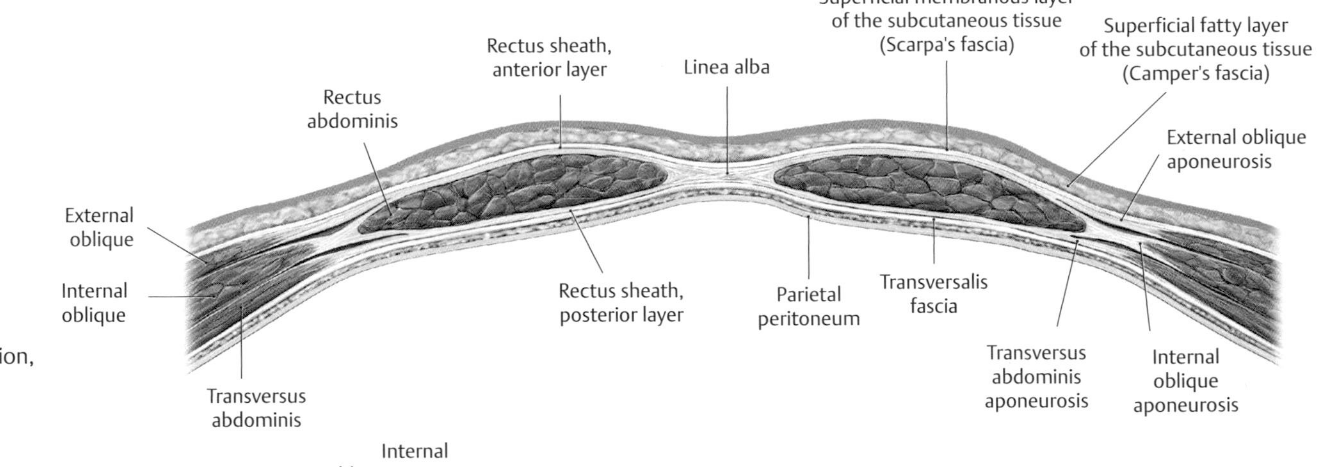
Superficial membranous layer of the subcutaneous tissue (Scarpa's fascia)
Superficial fatty layer of the subcutaneous tissue (Camper's fascia)
Rectus sheath, anterior layer
Linea alba
Rectus abdominis
External oblique aponeurosis
External oblique
Internal oblique
Rectus sheath, posterior layer
Parietal peritoneum
Transversalis fascia
Transversus abdominis aponeurosis
Internal oblique aponeurosis
Transversus abdominis

B Transverse section, superior to the arcuate line.

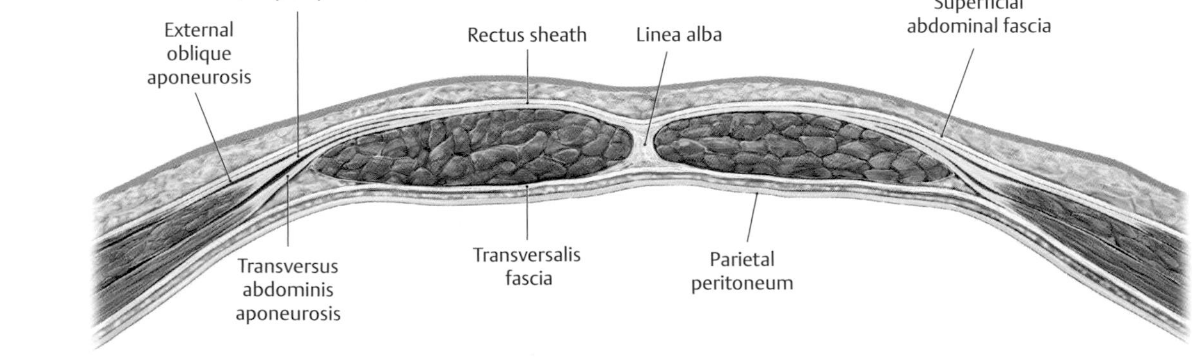
Internal oblique aponeurosis
External oblique aponeurosis
Rectus sheath
Linea alba
Superficial abdominal fascia
Transversus abdominis aponeurosis
Transversalis fascia
Parietal peritoneum

C Transverse section, inferior to the arcuate line.

Fig. 11.18 Inferior anterior abdominal wall: Structure and fossae

Coronal section, posterior (internal) view of left inferior portion of the anterior abdominal wall.

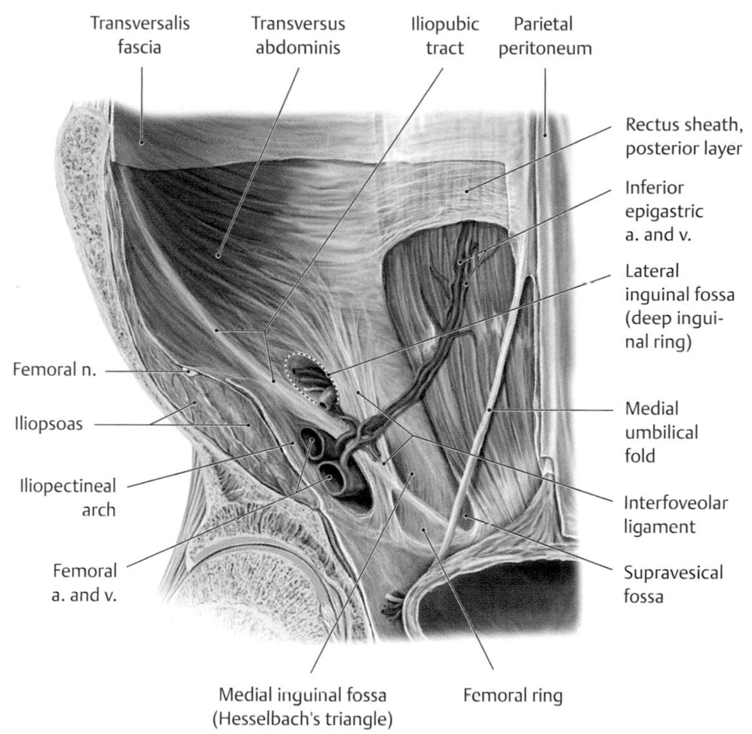
Transversalis fascia
Transversus abdominis
Iliopubic tract
Parietal peritoneum
Rectus sheath, posterior layer
Inferior epigastric a. and v.
Lateral inguinal fossa (deep inguinal ring)
Femoral n.
Iliopsoas
Iliopectineal arch
Femoral a. and v.
Medial umbilical fold
Interfoveolar ligament
Supravesical fossa
Medial inguinal fossa (Hesselbach's triangle)
Femoral ring

Clinical

Inguinal and femoral hernias

Indirect inguinal hernias occur in younger males and may be congenital or acquired; direct inguinal hernias generally occur in older males and are always acquired. Femoral hernias are acquired and more common in females.

Deep inguinal ring
Inguinal lig.
Inguinal canal
Femoral a. and vv.
Superficial inguinal ring
Peritoneum of hernial sac
Transversalis fascia (= internal spermatic fascia)
Cremaster muscle and spermatic cord

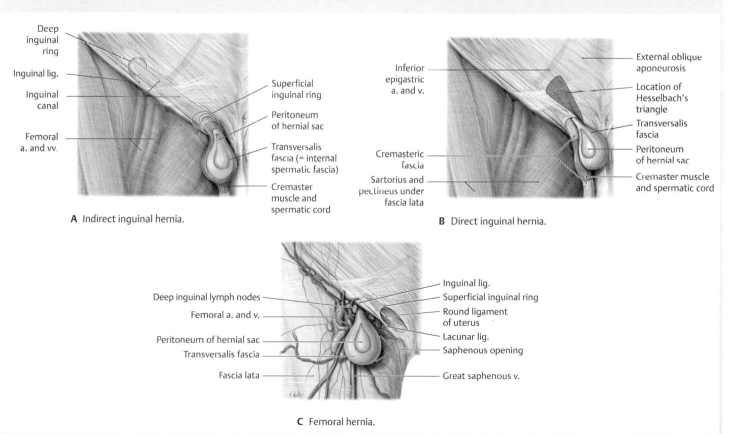

A Indirect inguinal hernia.

Inferior epigastric a. and v.
Cremasteric fascia
Sartorius and pectineus under fascia lata
External oblique aponeurosis
Location of Hesselbach's triangle
Transversalis fascia
Peritoneum of hernial sac
Cremaster muscle and spermatic cord

B Direct inguinal hernia.

Deep inguinal lymph nodes
Femoral a. and v.
Peritoneum of hernial sac
Transversalis fascia
Fascia lata
Inguinal lig.
Superficial inguinal ring
Round ligament of uterus
Lacunar lig.
Saphenous opening
Great saphenous v.

C Femoral hernia.

Divisions of the Abdominopelvic Cavity

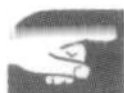

Organs in the abdominopelvic cavity are classified by the presence of surrounding peritoneum (the serous membrane lining the cavity) and a mesentery (a double layer of peritoneum that connects the organ to the abdominal wall) (see Table 12.1).

Fig. 12.1 Peritoneal cavity

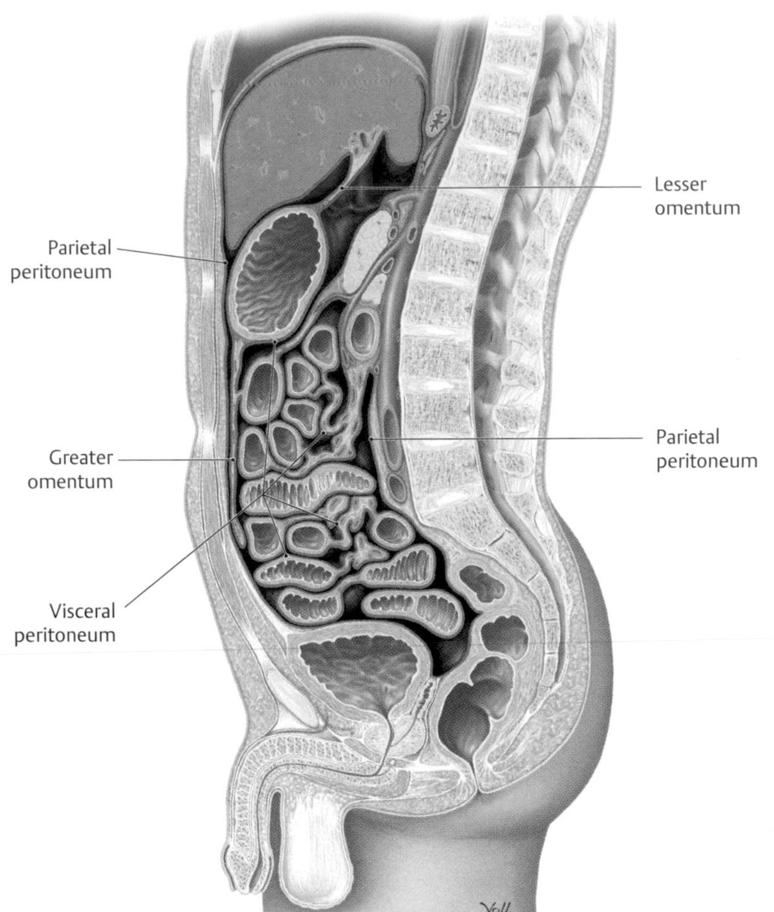

Lesser omentum
Parietal peritoneum
Greater omentum
Parietal peritoneum
Visceral peritoneum

A Midsagittal section through the male abdominopelvic cavity, viewed from the left. The peritoneum is shown in red.

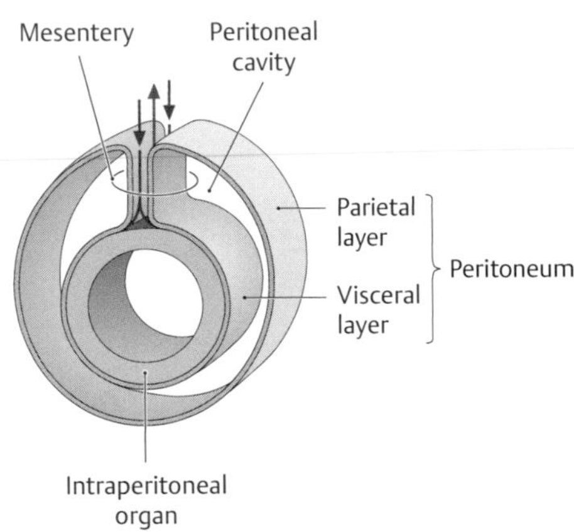

Mesentery
Peritoneal cavity
Parietal layer
Visceral layer
Peritoneum
Intraperitoneal organ

B An intraperitoneal organ, showing the mesentery and surrounding peritoneum. Arrows indicate location of blood vessels in the mesentery.

Table 12.1 Organs of the abdominopelvic cavity classified by their relationship to the peritoneum

Location		Organs		
Intraperitoneal organs: These organs have a mesentery and are completely covered by the peritoneum.				
Abdominal peritoneal		• Stomach • Small intestine (jejunum, ileum, some of the superior part of the duodenum) • Spleen • Liver		• Gallbladder • Cecum with vermiform appendix (portions of variable size may be retroperitoneal) • Large intestine (transverse and sigmoid colons)
Pelvic peritoneal		• Uterus (fundus and body)	• Ovaries	• Uterine tubes
Extraperitoneal organs: These organs either have no mesentery or lost it during development.				
Retroperitoneal	Primarily	• Kidneys and ureters	• Suprarenal glands	• Uterine cervix
	Secondarily	• Duodenum (descending, horizontal, and ascending) • Pancreas		• Ascending and descending colon and cecum • Rectum (upper 2/3)
Infraperitoneal/subperitoneal		• Urinary bladder • Distal ureters • Prostate	• Seminal vesicle • Uterine cervix	• Vagina • Rectum (lower 1/3)

Fig. 12.2 **Peritoneal relationships of the abdominopelvic organs**
Midsagittal section through the male abdominopelvic cavity, viewed from the left.

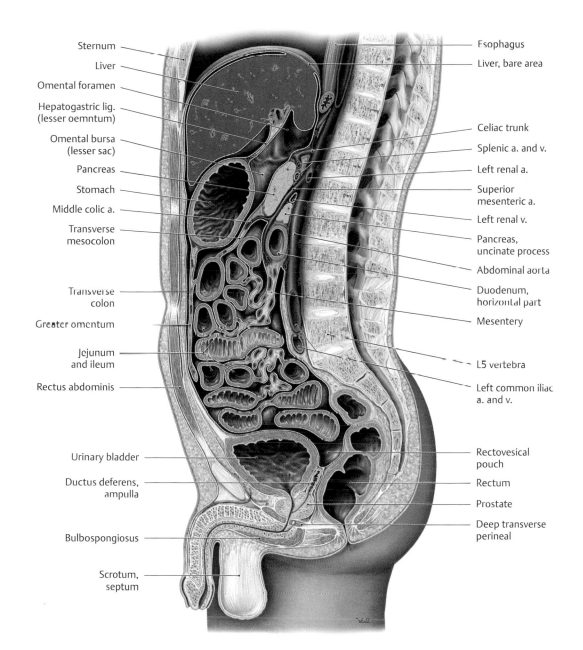

Sternum
Liver
Omental foramen
Hepatogastric lig. (lesser oemntum)
Omental bursa (lesser sac)
Pancreas
Stomach
Middle colic a.
Transverse mesocolon
Transverse colon
Greater omentum
Jejunum and ileum
Rectus abdominis
Urinary bladder
Ductus deferens, ampulla
Bulbospongiosus
Scrotum, septum
Esophagus
Liver, bare area
Celiac trunk
Splenic a. and v.
Left renal a.
Superior mesenteric a.
Left renal v.
Pancreas, uncinate process
Abdominal aorta
Duodenum, horizontal part
Mesentery
L5 vertebra
Left common iliac a. and v.
Rectovesical pouch
Rectum
Prostate
Deep transverse perineal

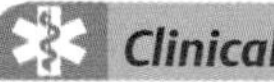 *Clinical*

Acute abdominal pain

Acute abdominal pain ("acute abdomen") may be so severe that the abdominal wall becomes extremely sensitive to touch ("guarding") and the intestines stop functioning. Causes include organ inflammation such as appendicitis, perforation due to a gastric ulcer (see p. 157), or organ blockage by a stone, tumor, etc. In women, gynecological processes or ectopic pregnancies may produce severe abdominal pain.

Peritoneal Cavity & Greater Sac

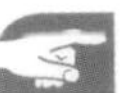

The peritoneal cavity is divided into the large greater sac and small omental bursa (lesser sac). The greater omentum is an apron-like fold of peritoneum suspended from the greater curvature of the stomach and covering the anterior surface of the transverse colon. The attachment of the transverse mesocolon on the anterior surface of the descending part of the duodenum and the pancreas divides the peritoneal cavity into a supracolic compartment (liver, gallbladder, and stomach) and an infracolic compartment (intestines).

Fig. 12.3 **Dissection of the peritoneal cavity**
Anterior view.

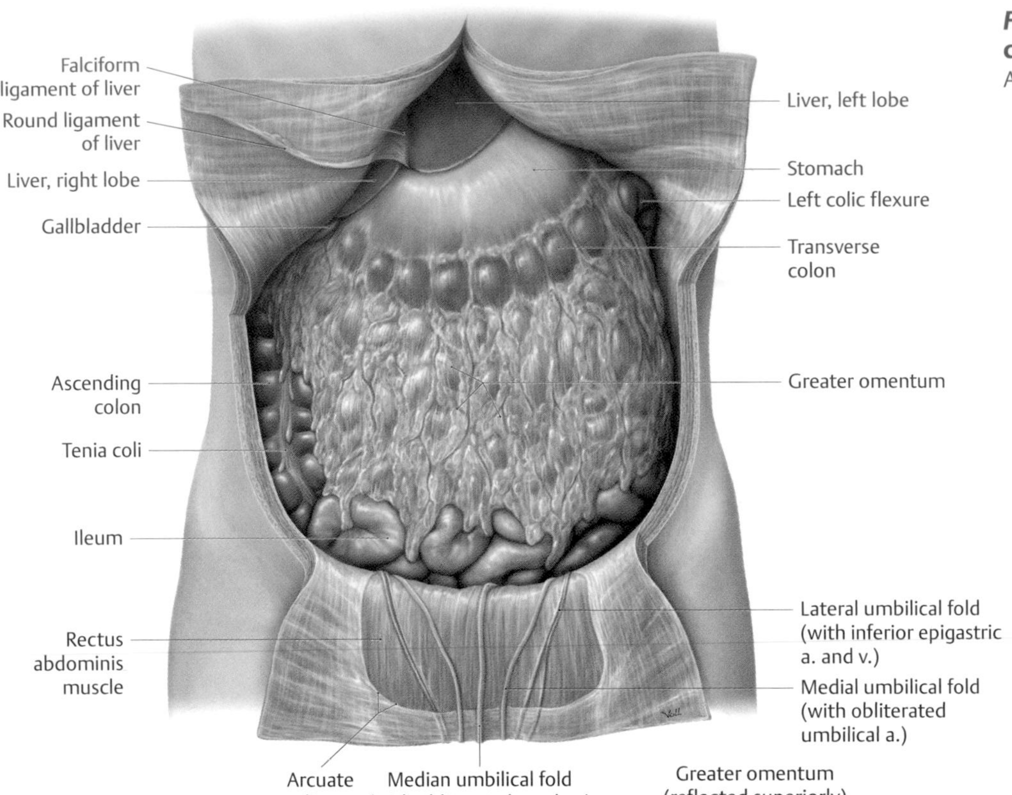
Falciform ligament of liver
Round ligament of liver
Liver, right lobe
Gallbladder
Ascending colon
Tenia coli
Ileum
Rectus abdominis muscle
Arcuate line
Median umbilical fold (with obliterated urachus)
Liver, left lobe
Stomach
Left colic flexure
Transverse colon
Greater omentum
Lateral umbilical fold (with inferior epigastric a. and v.)
Medial umbilical fold (with obliterated umbilical a.)

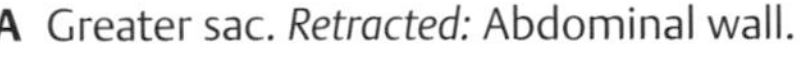

A Greater sac. *Retracted:* Abdominal wall.

Greater omentum (reflected superiorly)
Transverse colon
Transverse mesocolon with middle colic a. and v.
Parietal peritoneum
Jejunum (covered by visceral peritoneum)
Ascending colon
Tenia coli
Ileum
Rectus abdominis muscle
Lateral umbilical fold (with inferior epigastric a. and v.)
Medial umbilical fold (with obliterated umbilical a.)
Arcuate line
Median umbilical fold (with obliterated urachus)

B Infracolic compartment, the portion of the peritoneal cavity below the attachement of the transverse mesocolon. *Reflected:* Greater omentum and transverse colon.

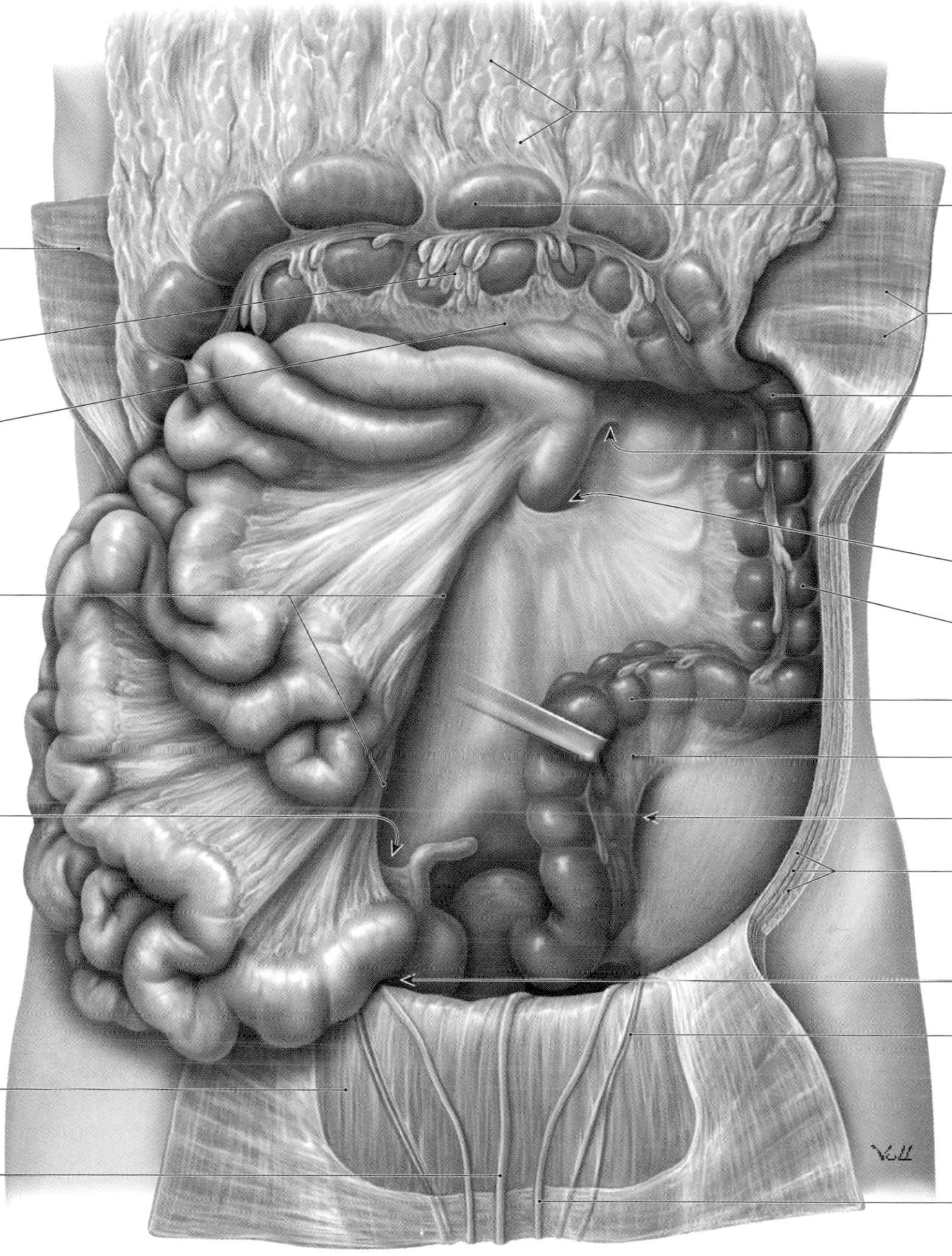

Greater omentum (reflected superiorly)
Transverse colon
Round ligament of liver
Parietal peritoneum
Epiploic appendices
Transverse mesocolon
Left colic flexure
Superior duodenal recess
Inferior duodenal recess
Mesentery, root
Descending colon
Sigmoid colon
Sigmoid mesocolon
Inferior iliocecal recess
Intersigmoidal recess
Transversus abdominis, internal and external obliques
Retrocecal recess
Lateral umbilical fold (with inferior epigastric a. and v.)
Rectus abdominis
Median umbilical fold (with obliterated urachus)
Medial umbilical fold (with obliterated umbilical a.)

C Mesenteries and mesenteric recesses in the infracolic compartment. *Reflected:* Greater omentum, transverse colon, small intestines, and sigmoid colon.

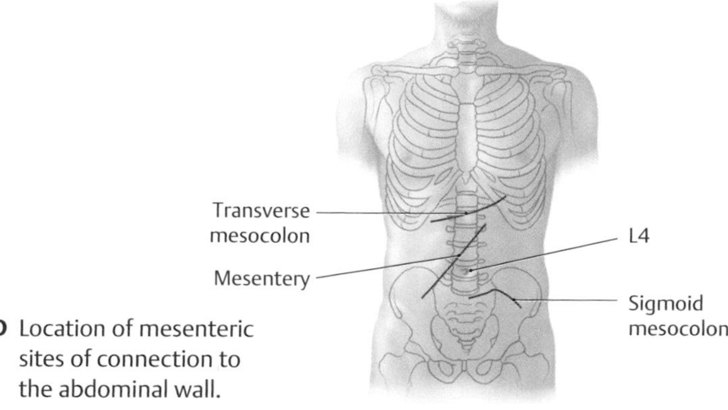
Transverse mesocolon
L4
Mesentery
Sigmoid mesocolon

D Location of mesenteric sites of connection to the abdominal wall.

Omental Bursa, or Lesser Sac

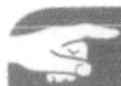

The omental bursa, or lesser sac, is the portion of the peritoneal cavity behind the stomach and the lesser omentum (a double-layerd peritoneal structure connecting the lesser curvature of the stomach and the proximal part of the duodenum to the liver). The omental bursa communicates with the greater sac via the omental (epiploic) foramen, located posterior to the free edge of the lesser omentum.

Fig. 12.4 Omental bursa (lesser sac)

Anterior view. The omental bursa (lesser sac) is the portion of the peritoneal cavity located behind the lesser omentum and stomach.

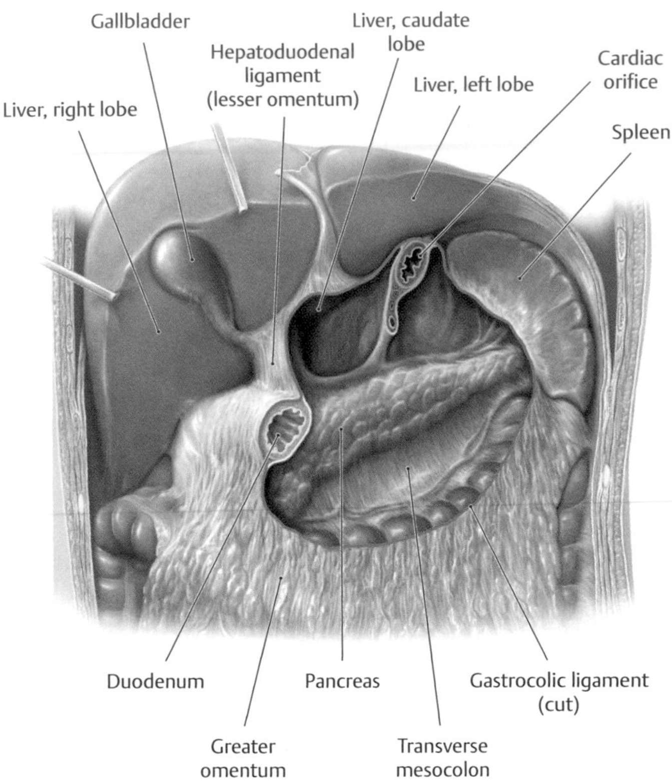
Gallbladder
Liver, caudate lobe
Hepatoduodenal ligament (lesser omentum)
Cardiac orifice
Liver, left lobe
Liver, right lobe
Spleen
Duodenum
Pancreas
Gastrocolic ligament (cut)
Greater omentum
Transverse mesocolon

A Boundaries of the omental bursa (lesser sac).

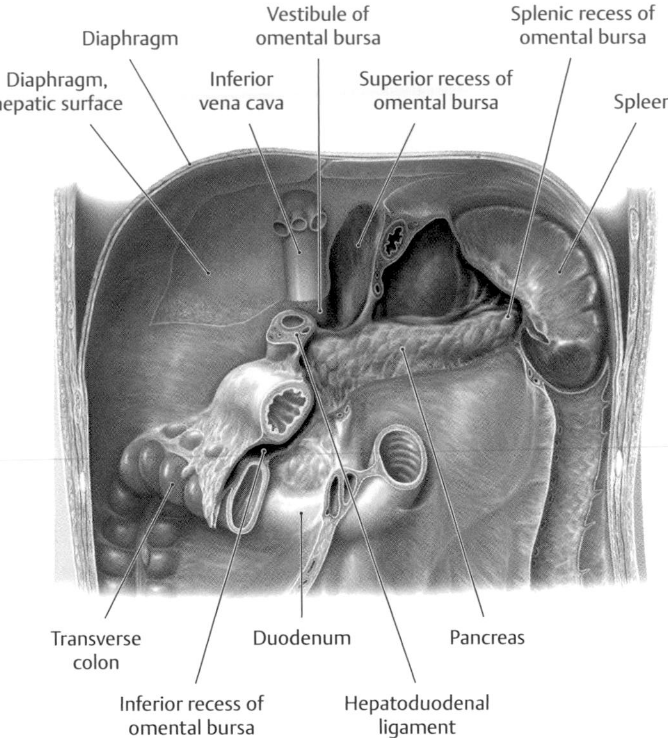
Vestibule of omental bursa
Splenic recess of omental bursa
Diaphragm
Diaphragm, hepatic surface
Inferior vena cava
Superior recess of omental bursa
Spleen
Transverse colon
Duodenum
Pancreas
Inferior recess of omental bursa
Hepatoduodenal ligament

B Posterior wall of the omental bursa (lesser sac).

Fig. 12.5 Location of the omental bursa

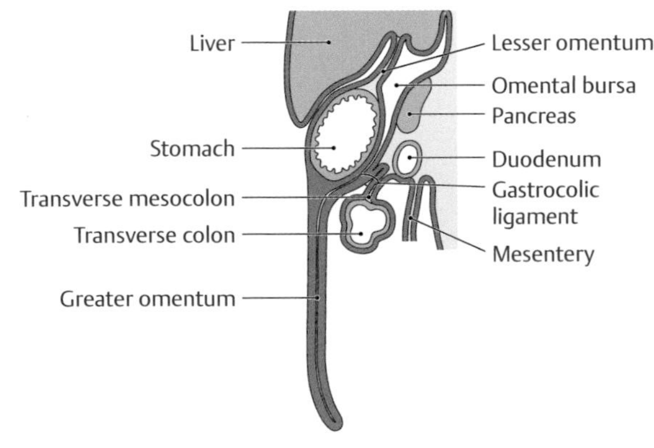
Liver
Lesser omentum
Omental bursa
Pancreas
Stomach
Duodenum
Gastrocolic ligament
Transverse mesocolon
Transverse colon
Mesentery
Greater omentum

A Sagittal section.

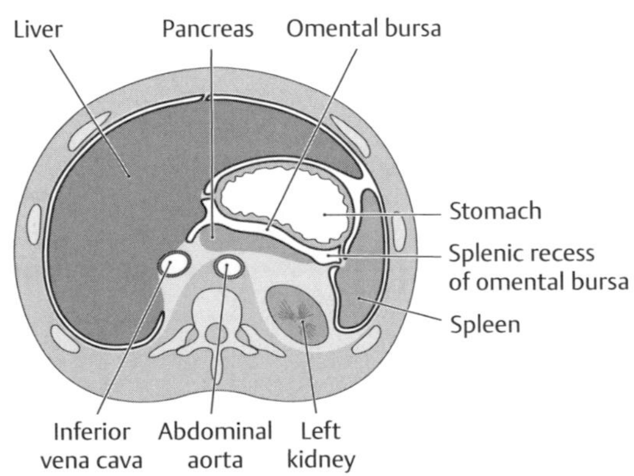
Liver
Pancreas
Omental bursa
Stomach
Splenic recess of omental bursa
Spleen
Inferior vena cava
Abdominal aorta
Left kidney

B Transverse section, inferior view.

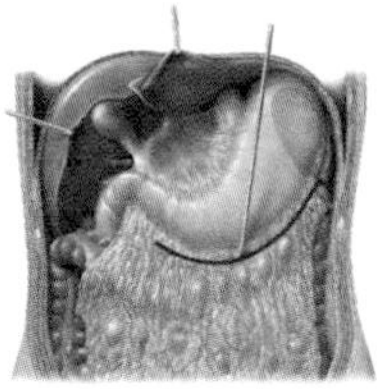

Fig. 12.6 Omental bursa in situ
Anterior view. *Divided:* Gastrocolic ligament. *Retracted:* Liver. *Reflected:* Stomach.

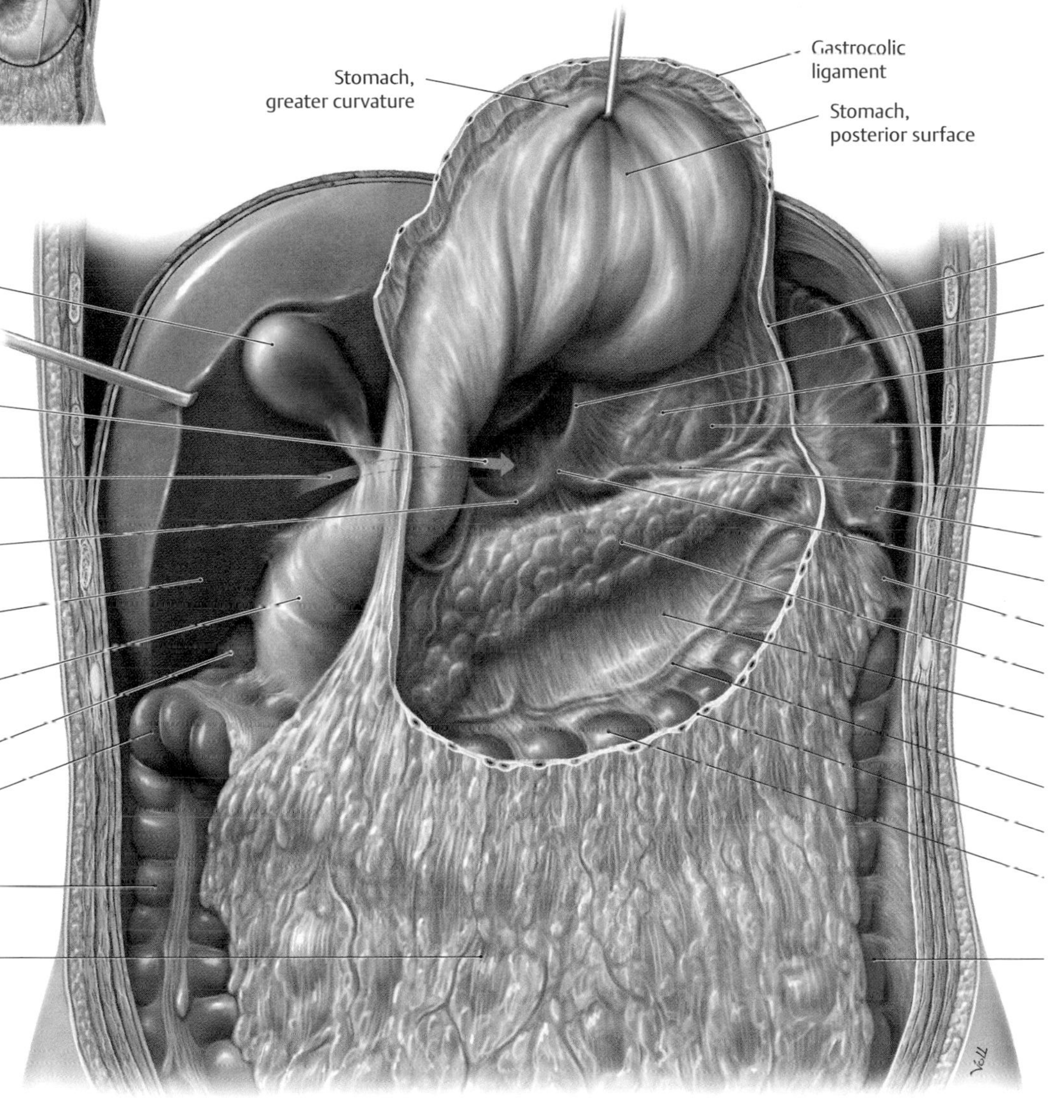

Stomach, greater curvature
Gastrocolic ligament
Stomach, posterior surface
Gallbladder
Vestibule of omental bursa
Omental foramen
Common hepatic a.
Liver, right lobe
Duodenum, descending part
Right kidney
Right colic flexure
Ascending colon
Greater omentum
Gastrosplenic ligament
Left gastric a.
Left suprarenal gland
Left kidney, superior pole
Splenic a.
Spleen
Celiac trunk
Phrenicocolic ligament
Pancreas
Transverse mesocolon
Middle colic a. and v.
Gastrocolic ligament
Transverse colon
Descending colon

Table 12.2 Boundaries of the omental bursa

Direction	Boundary	Recess
Anterior	Lesser omentum, gastrocolic ligament	–
Inferior	Transverse mesocolon	Inferior recess
Superior	Liver (with caudate lobe)	Superior recess
Posterior	Pancreas, aorta (abdominal part), celiac trunk, splenic a. and v., gastrosplenic fold, left suprarenal gland, left kidney (superior pole)	–
Right	Liver, duodenal bulb	–
Left	Spleen, gastrosplenic ligament	Splenic recess

Table 12.3 Boundaries of the omental foramen

The communication between the greater sac and lesser sac (omental bursa) is the omental (epiploic) foramen (see arrow in Fig. 12.6).

Direction	Boundary
Anterior	Hepatoduodenal ligament with the portal v., proper hepatic a., and bile duct
Inferior	Duodenum (superior part)
Posterior	Inferior vena cava, diaphragm (right crus)
Superior	Liver (caudate lobe)

Mesenteries & Posterior Wall

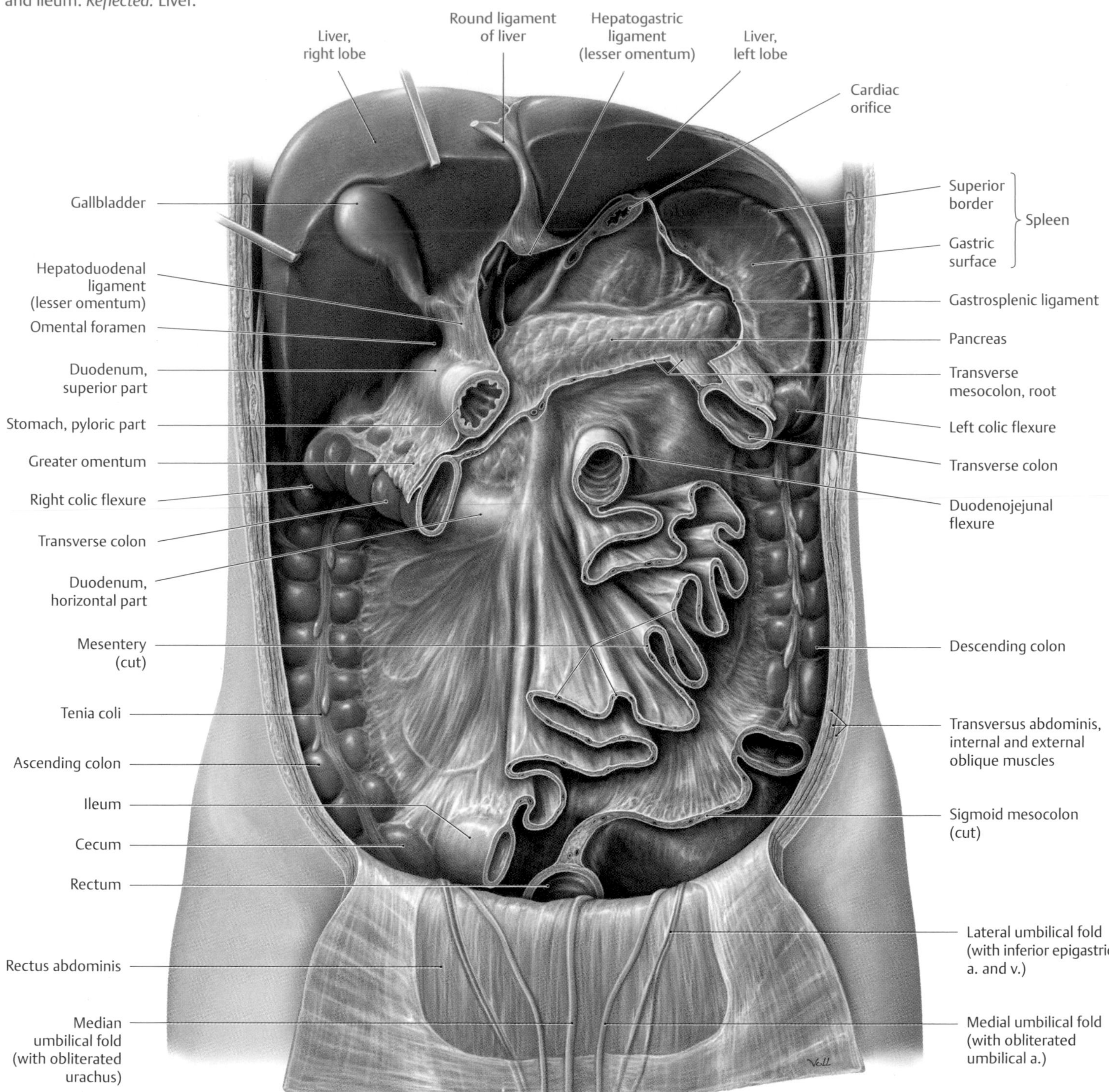

Liver, right lobe
Round ligament of liver
Hepatogastric ligament (lesser omentum)
Liver, left lobe
Cardiac orifice
Gallbladder
Superior border
Gastric surface
Spleen
Hepatoduodenal ligament (lesser omentum)
Gastrosplenic ligament
Omental foramen
Pancreas
Duodenum, superior part
Transverse mesocolon, root
Stomach, pyloric part
Left colic flexure
Greater omentum
Transverse colon
Right colic flexure
Duodenojejunal flexure
Transverse colon
Duodenum, horizontal part
Mesentery (cut)
Descending colon
Tenia coli
Transversus abdominis, internal and external oblique muscles
Ascending colon
Ileum
Sigmoid mesocolon (cut)
Cecum
Rectum
Lateral umbilical fold (with inferior epigastric a. and v.)
Rectus abdominis
Median umbilical fold (with obliterated urachus)
Medial umbilical fold (with obliterated umbilical a.)

Fig. 12.7 **Mesenteries and organs of the peritoneal cavity**
Anterior view. *Removed:* Stomach, jejunum, and ileum. *Reflected:* Liver.

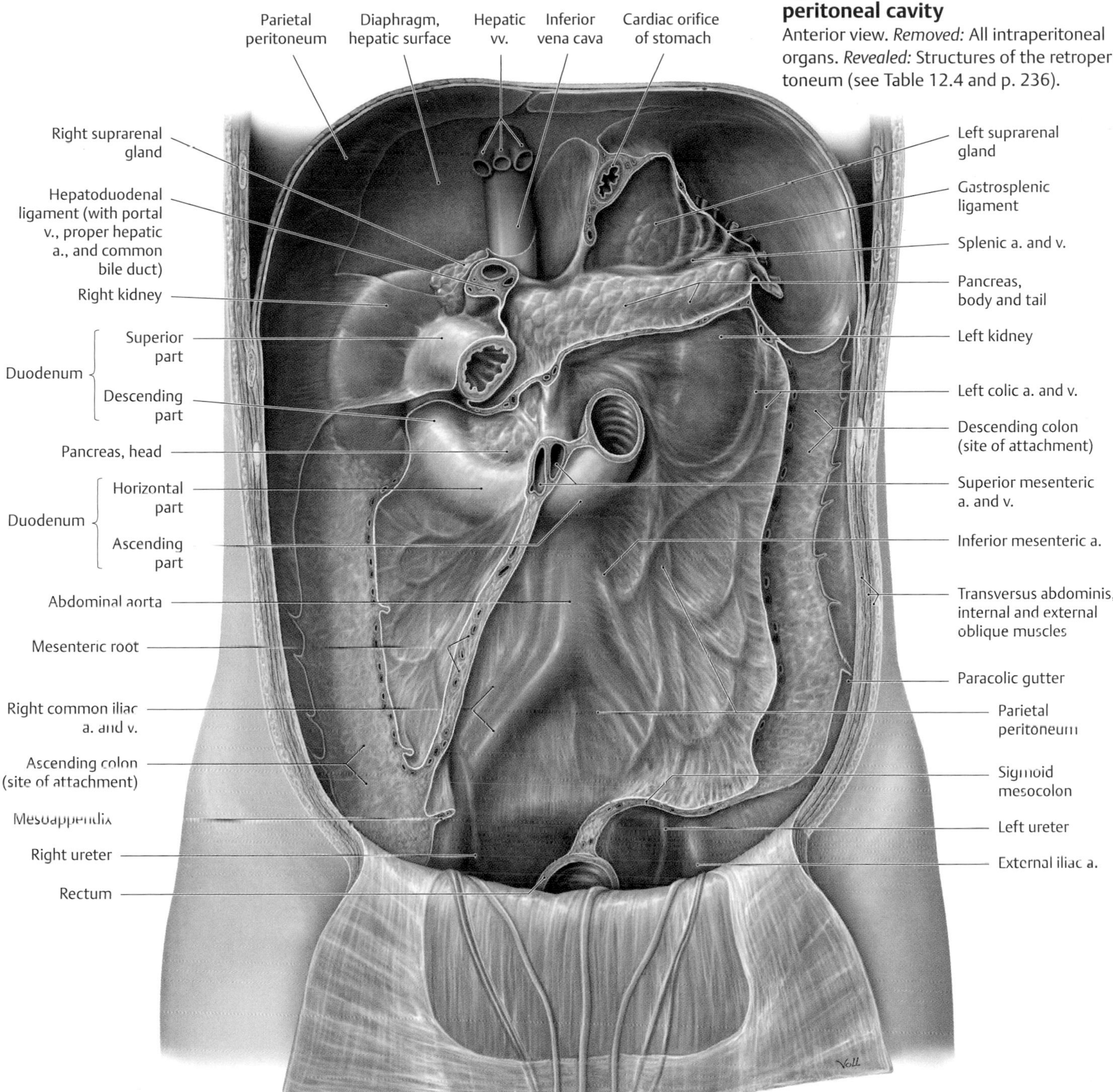

Parietal peritoneum
Diaphragm, hepatic surface
Hepatic vv.
Inferior vena cava
Cardiac orifice of stomach
Right suprarenal gland
Hepatoduodenal ligament (with portal v., proper hepatic a., and common bile duct)
Right kidney
Duodenum
Superior part
Descending part
Pancreas, head
Duodenum
Horizontal part
Ascending part
Abdominal aorta
Mesenteric root
Right common iliac a. and v.
Ascending colon (site of attachment)
Mesoappendix
Right ureter
Rectum
Left suprarenal gland
Gastrosplenic ligament
Splenic a. and v.
Pancreas, body and tail
Left kidney
Left colic a. and v.
Descending colon (site of attachment)
Superior mesenteric a. and v.
Inferior mesenteric a.
Transversus abdominis, internal and external oblique muscles
Paracolic gutter
Parietal peritoneum
Sigmoid mesocolon
Left ureter
External iliac a.

***Fig. 12.8* Posterior wall of the peritoneal cavity**
Anterior view. *Removed:* All intraperitoneal organs. *Revealed:* Structures of the retroperitoneum (see Table 12.4 and p. 236).

Table 12.4 Structures of the retroperitoneum

See pp. 186, 194, 207 for neurovascular structures of the retroperitoneum.

Classification	Organs	Vessels	Nerves
Primarily retroperitoneal (no mesentery; retroperitoneal when formed)	• Kidneys • Suprarenal glands • Ureters	• Aorta (abdominal part) • Inferior vena cava and tributaries • Ascending lumbar vv. • Portal v. and tributaries • Lumbar, sacral, and iliac lymph nodes • Lumbar trunks and cisterna chyli	• Lumbar plexus branches ∘ Iliohypogastric n. ∘ Ilioinguinal n. ∘ Genitofemoral n. ∘ Lateral femoral cutaneous n. ∘ Femoral n. ∘ Obturator n. • Sympathetic trunk • Autonomic ganglia and plexuses
Secondarily retroperitoneal (mesentery lost during development)	• Pancreas • Duodenum (descending and horizontal parts; some of ascending part) • Ascending and descending colon • Cecum (portions; variable) • Rectum (upper 2/3)		

Stomach

Fig. 13.1 Stomach: Location

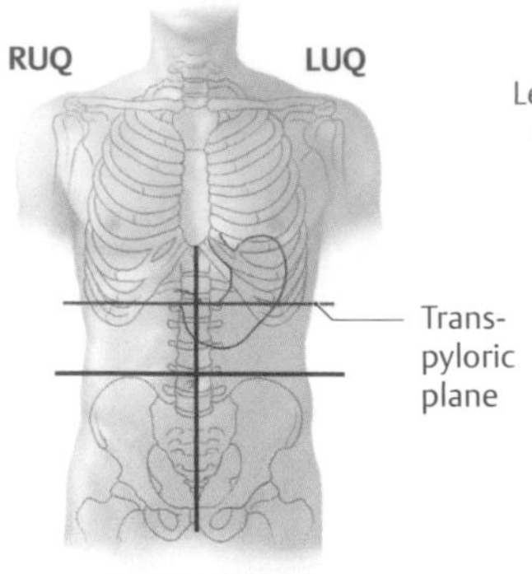

RUQ
LUQ
Trans-pyloric plane

A Anterior view.

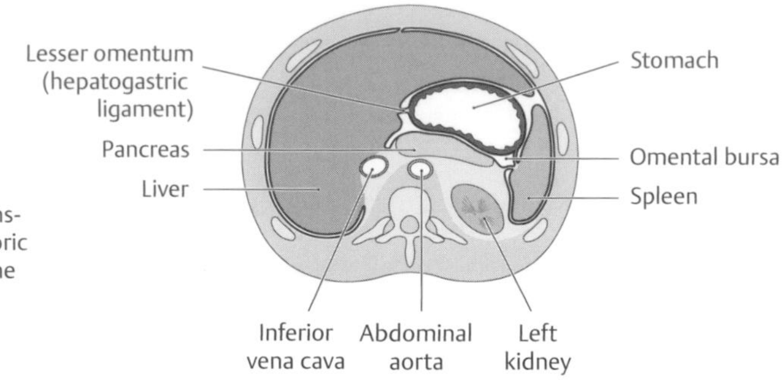

Lesser omentum (hepatogastric ligament)
Pancreas
Liver
Stomach
Omental bursa
Spleen
Inferior vena cava
Abdominal aorta
Left kidney

B Transverse section, inferior view.

Fig. 13.2 Relations of the stomach

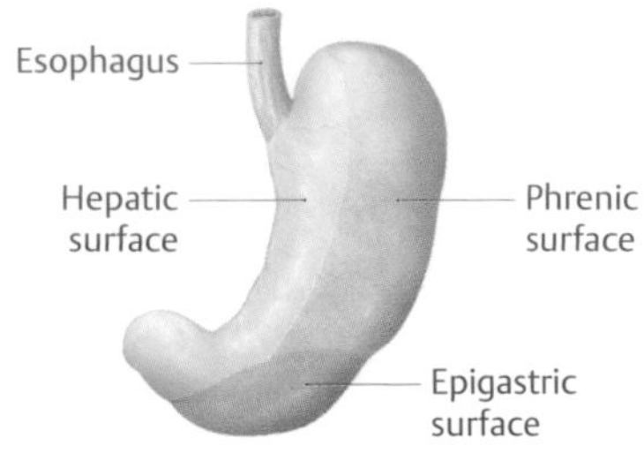

Esophagus
Hepatic surface
Phrenic surface
Epigastric surface

A Anterior view.

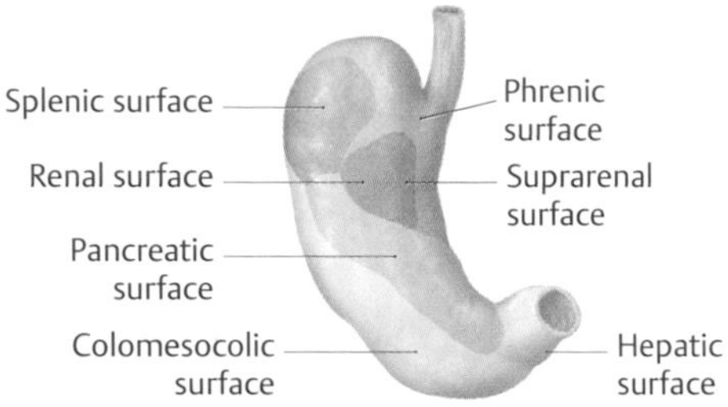

Splenic surface
Renal surface
Pancreatic surface
Colomesocolic surface
Phrenic surface
Suprarenal surface
Hepatic surface

B Posterior view.

Fig. 13.3 Stomach

Anterior view.

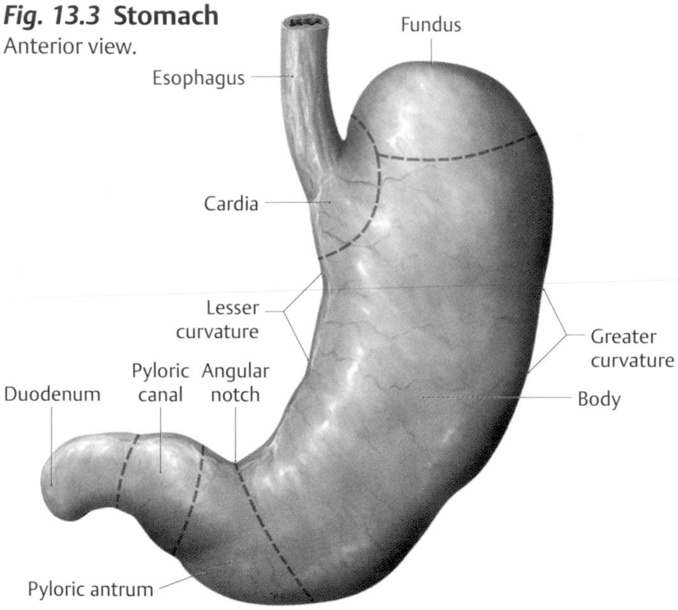

Fundus
Esophagus
Cardia
Lesser curvature
Greater curvature
Duodenum
Pyloric canal
Angular notch
Body
Pyloric antrum

A Anterior wall.

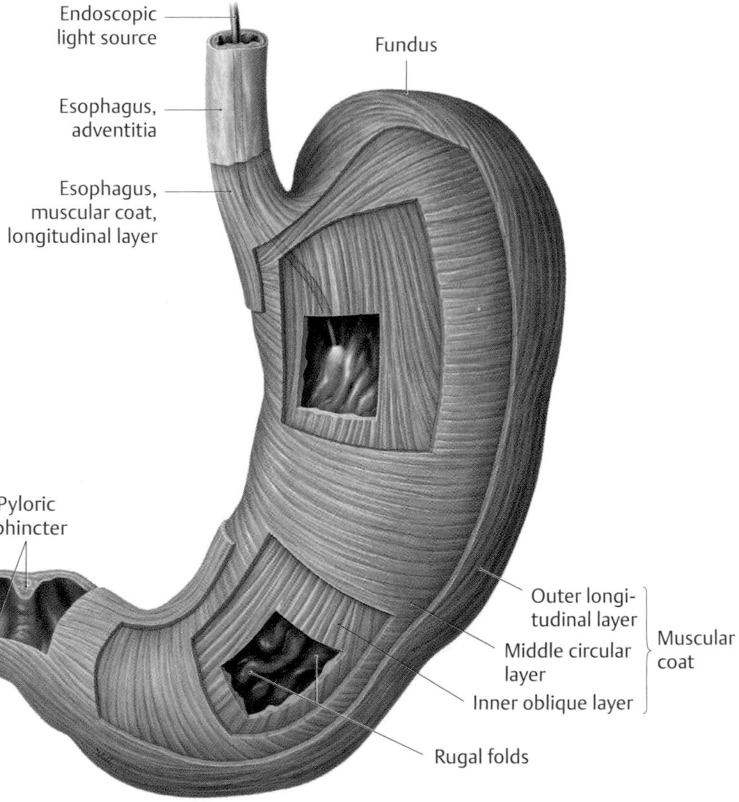

Endoscopic light source
Esophagus, adventitia
Esophagus, muscular coat, longitudinal layer
Fundus
Duodenum, superior part
Pyloric sphincter
Outer longitudinal layer
Middle circular layer
Inner oblique layer
Muscular coat
Rugal folds

B Muscular layers. *Removed:* Serosa and subserosa. *Windowed:* Muscular coat.

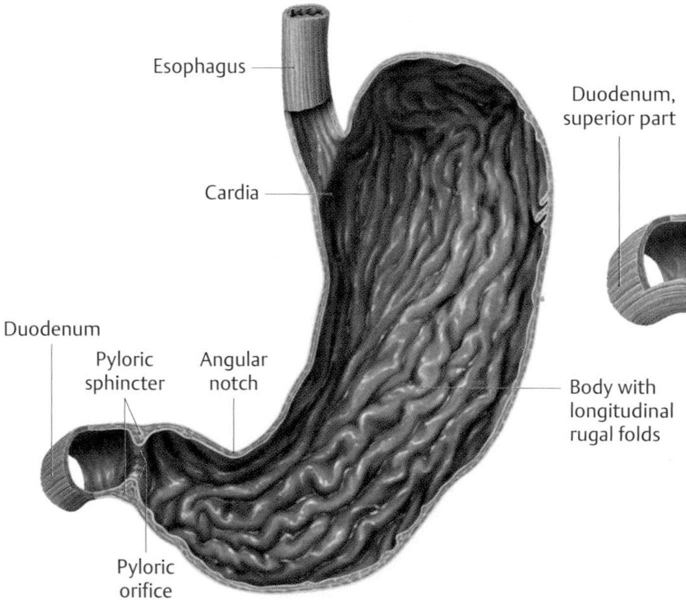

Esophagus
Cardia
Duodenum
Pyloric sphincter
Angular notch
Body with longitudinal rugal folds
Pyloric orifice

C Interior. *Removed:* Anterior wall.

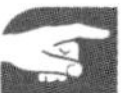

The stomach resides primarily in the left upper quadrant. It is intraperitoneal, its mesenteries being the lesser and greater omenta.

Fig. 13.4 Stomach in situ
Anterior view of the opened upper abdomen. Arrow indicates the omental foramen.

Falciform ligament of liver
Round ligament of liver
Liver, right lobe
Liver, left lobe
Esophagus
Parietal peritoneum
Diaphragm
Gallbladder
Lesser omentum
Hepato-duodenal ligament
Hepato-gastric ligament
Right kidney
Right colic flexure
Ascending colon
Stomach, fundus
Stomach, cardia
Hepato-esophageal ligament
Stomach, body
Spleen
Lesser curvature
Greater curvature
Descending colon
Transversus abdominis, internal and external obliques
Duodenum
Pyloric canal
Pyloric antrum
Greater omentum

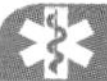

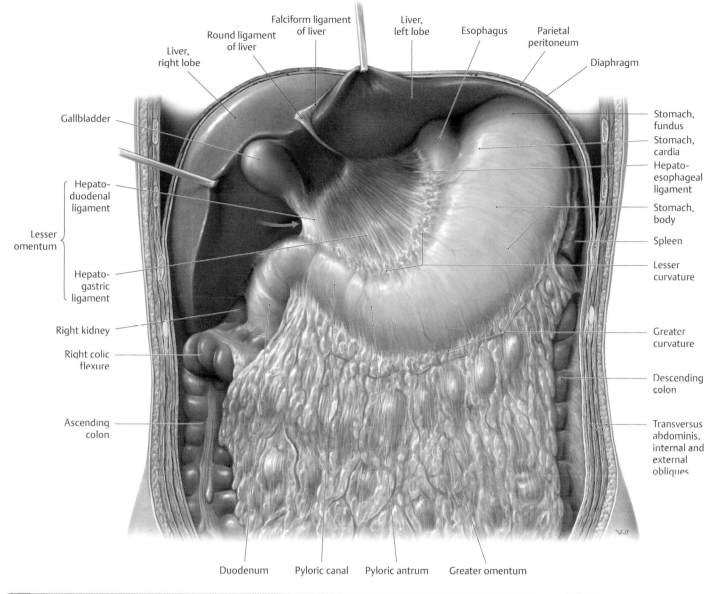

Clinical

Gastritis and gastric ulcers

Gastritis and gastric ulcers, the two most common diseases of the stomach, are associated with increased acid production and are caused by alcohol, drugs such as aspirin, and the bacterium *Helicobacter pylori*. Symptoms include lessened appetite, pain, and even bleeding, which manifests as black stool or dark brown material in vomit. Gastritis is limited to the inner surface of the stomach, while gastric ulcers extend into the stomach wall. The gastric ulcer in **C** is covered with fibrin and shows hematin spots.

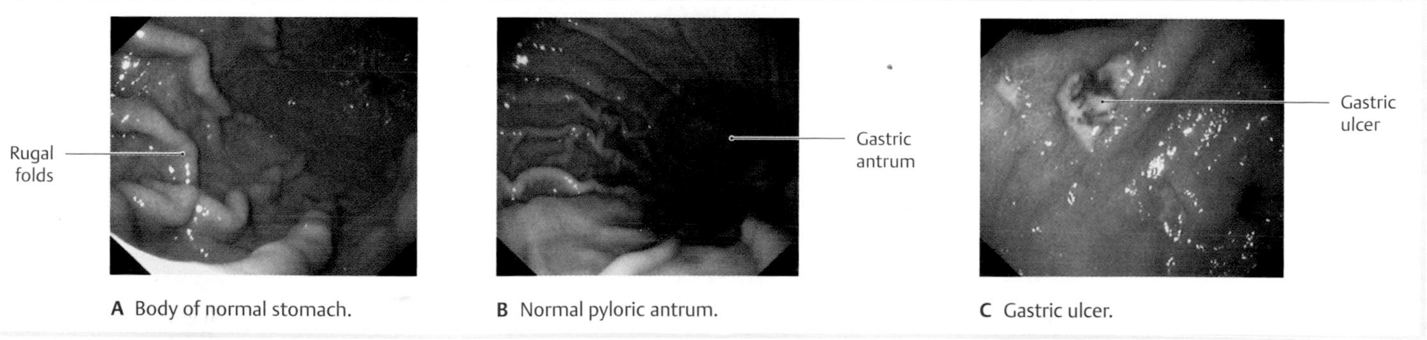

Rugal folds
Gastric antrum
Gastric ulcer

A Body of normal stomach.

B Normal pyloric antrum.

C Gastric ulcer.

Duodenum

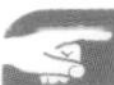

The small intestine consists of the duodenum, jejunum, and ileum (see p. 160). The duodenum is primarily retroperitoneal and is divided into four parts: superior, descending, horizontal, and ascending.

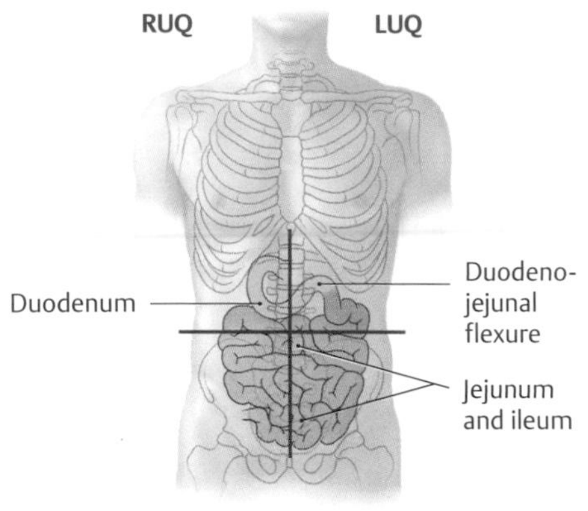
RUQ
LUQ
Duodenum
Duodeno-jejunal flexure
Jejunum and ileum

Fig. 13.5 **Duodenum: Location**
Anterior view.

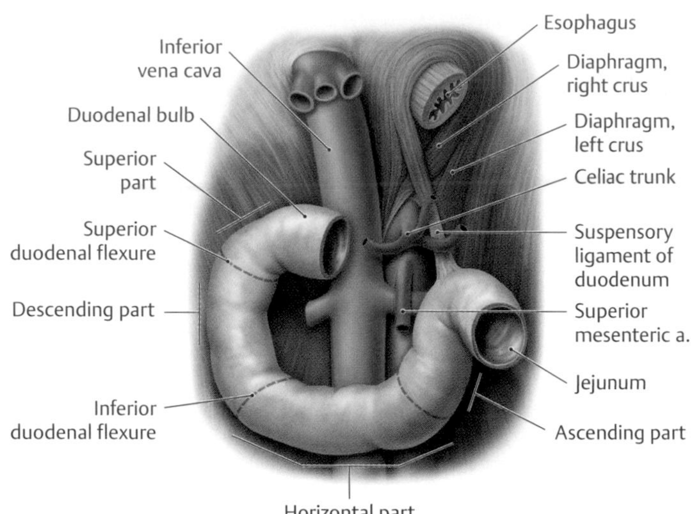
Esophagus
Inferior vena cava
Diaphragm, right crus
Duodenal bulb
Diaphragm, left crus
Superior part
Celiac trunk
Superior duodenal flexure
Suspensory ligament of duodenum
Descending part
Superior mesenteric a.
Jejunum
Inferior duodenal flexure
Ascending part
Horizontal part

Fig. 13.6 **Parts of the duodenum**
Anterior view

Fig. 13.7 **Duodenum**
Anterior view with the anterior wall opened.

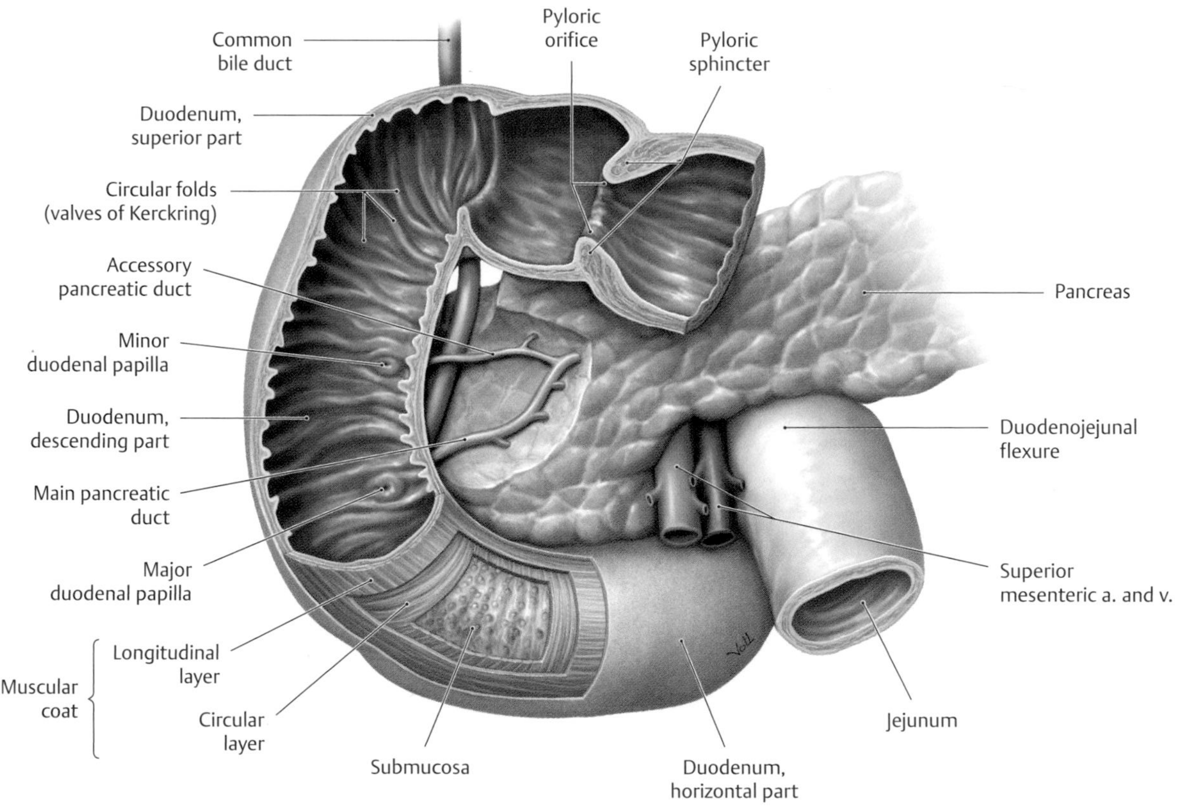
Common bile duct
Pyloric orifice
Pyloric sphincter
Duodenum, superior part
Circular folds (valves of Kerckring)
Accessory pancreatic duct
Pancreas
Minor duodenal papilla
Duodenum, descending part
Duodenojejunal flexure
Main pancreatic duct
Major duodenal papilla
Superior mesenteric a. and v.
Muscular coat
Longitudinal layer
Circular layer
Submucosa
Duodenum, horizontal part
Jejunum

Fig. 13.8 Duodenum in situ

Anterior view. *Removed:* Stomach, liver, small intestine, and large portions of the transverse colon. *Thinned:* Retroperitoneal fat and connective tissue.

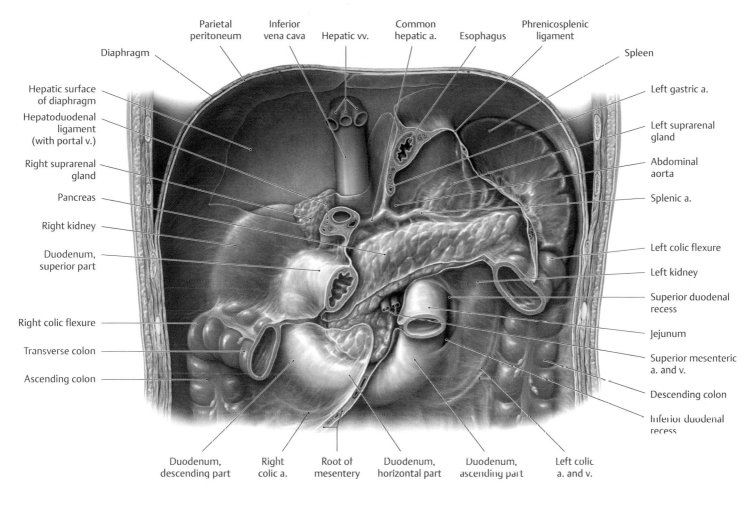

Parietal peritoneum
Inferior vena cava
Hepatic vv.
Common hepatic a.
Esophagus
Phrenicosplenic ligament
Diaphragm
Spleen
Hepatic surface of diaphragm
Left gastric a.
Hepatoduodenal ligament (with portal v.)
Left suprarenal gland
Right suprarenal gland
Abdominal aorta
Pancreas
Splenic a.
Right kidney
Duodenum, superior part
Left colic flexure
Left kidney
Superior duodenal recess
Right colic flexure
Jejunum
Transverse colon
Superior mesenteric a. and v.
Ascending colon
Descending colon
Inferior duodenal recess
Duodenum, descending part
Right colic a.
Root of mesentery
Duodenum, horizontal part
Duodenum, ascending part
Left colic a. and v.

Clinical

Endoscopy of the papillary region

Two important ducts end in the papillary region of the duodenum: the common bile duct and the pancreatic duct (see Fig. 13.7). These ducts may be examined by X-ray through endoscopic retrograde cholangiopancreatography (ERCP), in which dye is injected endoscopically into the duodenal papilla. Duodenal diverticula (generally harmless outpouchings) may complicate the procedure.

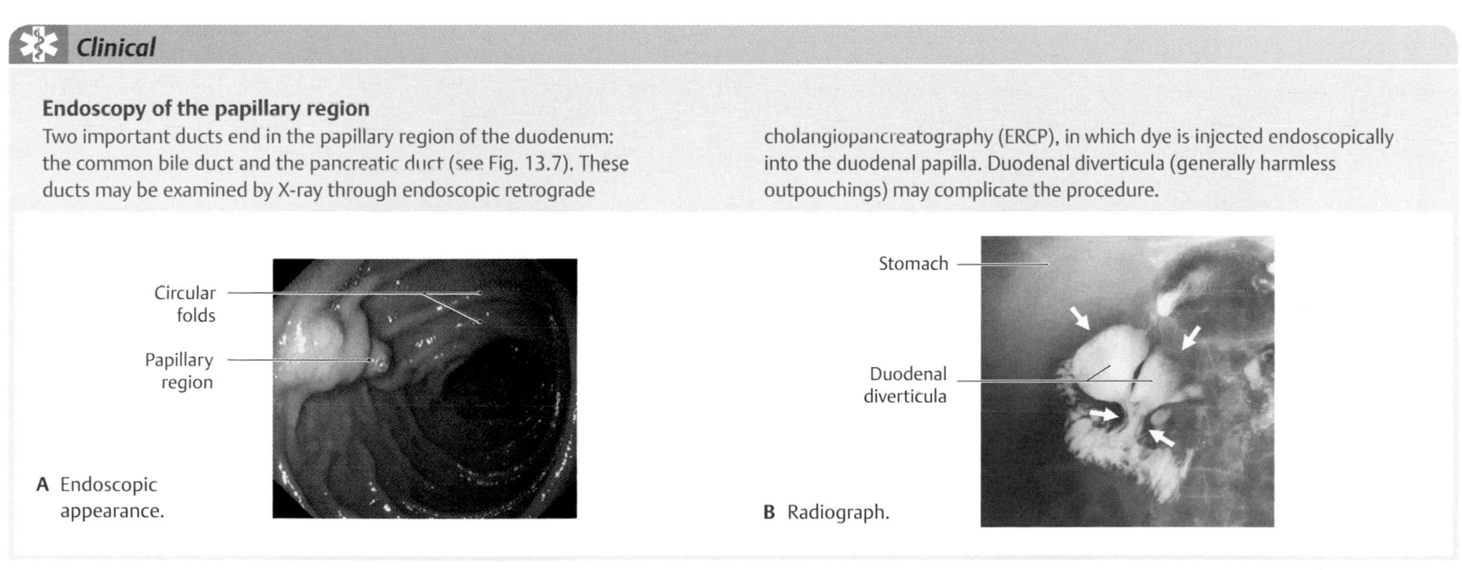
Circular folds
Papillary region
Stomach
Duodenal diverticula

A Endoscopic appearance.

B Radiograph.

Jejunum & Ileum

Fig. 13.9 Jejunum and ileum: Location
Anterior view. The intraperitoneal jejunum and ileum are enclosed by the mesentery proper.

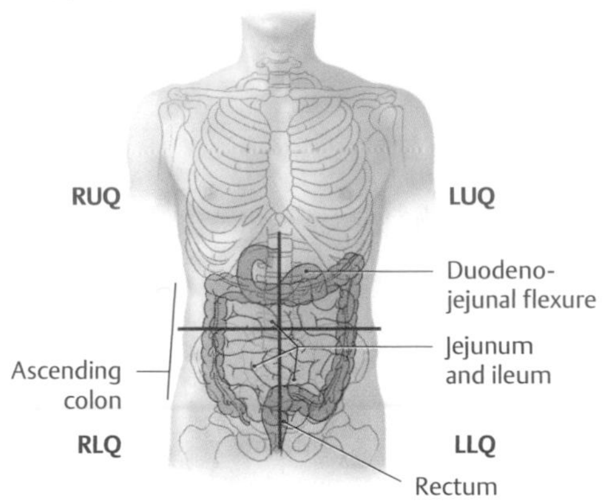
RUQ
LUQ
Duodeno-jejunal flexure
Jejunum and ileum
Ascending colon
RLQ
LLQ
Rectum

Fig. 13.10 Wall structure of the jejunum and ileum
Macroscopic views of the longitudinally opened small intestine.

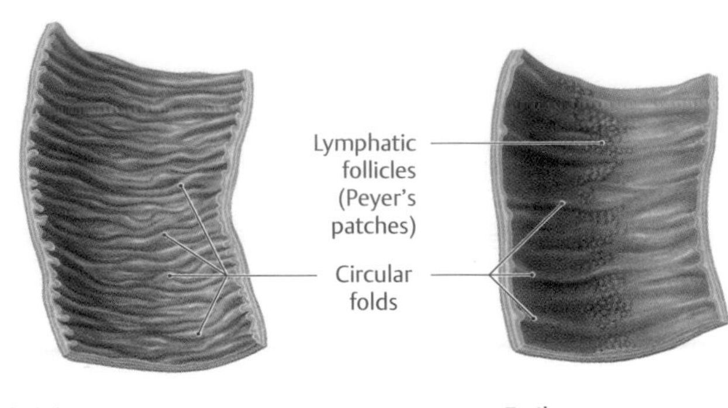
Lymphatic follicles (Peyer's patches)
Circular folds

A Jejunum.

B Ileum.

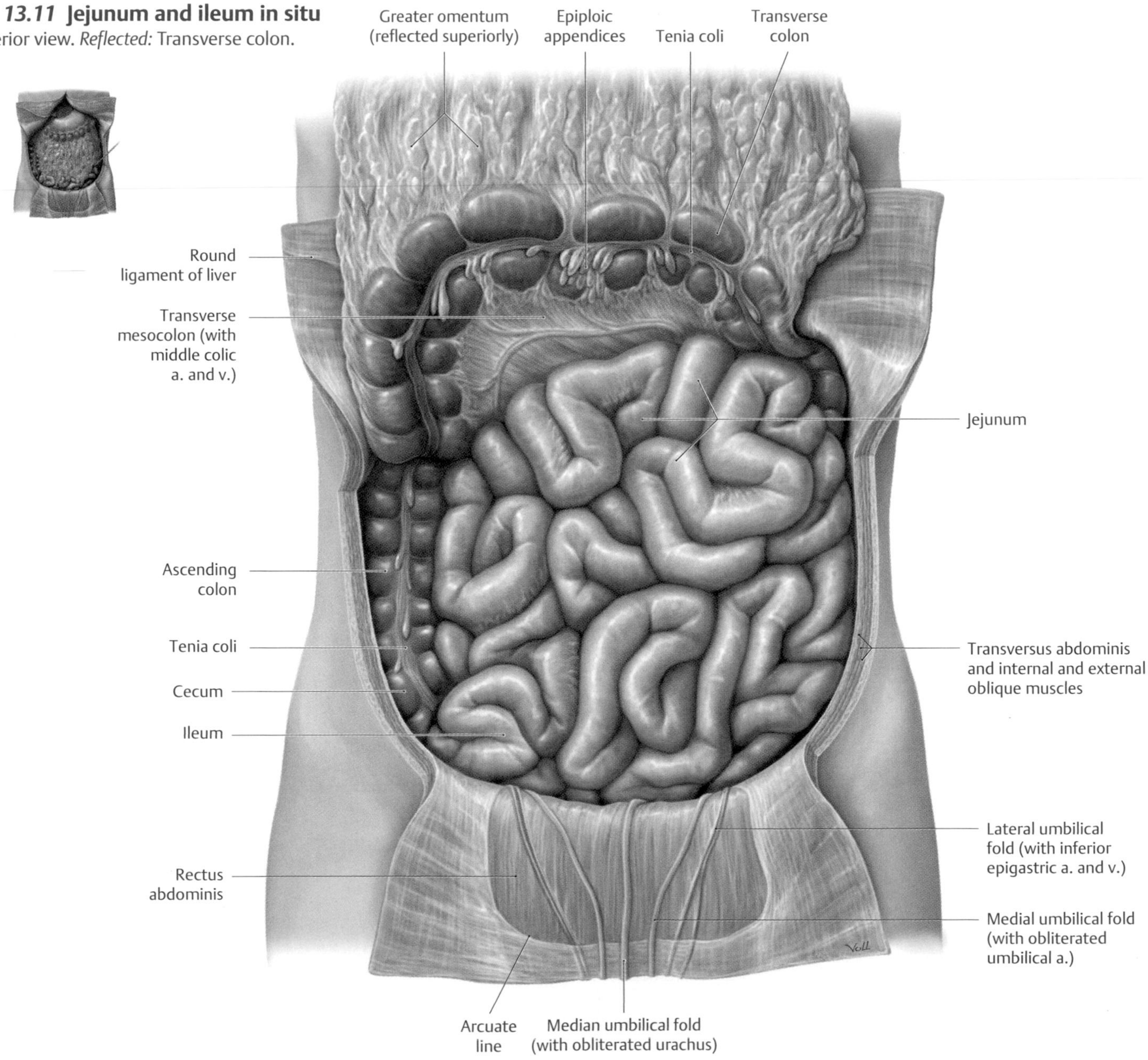

Fig. 13.11 Jejunum and ileum in situ
Anterior view. *Reflected:* Transverse colon.

Greater omentum (reflected superiorly)
Epiploic appendices
Tenia coli
Transverse colon
Round ligament of liver
Transverse mesocolon (with middle colic a. and v.)
Jejunum
Ascending colon
Tenia coli
Cecum
Ileum
Transversus abdominis and internal and external oblique muscles
Lateral umbilical fold (with inferior epigastric a. and v.)
Rectus abdominis
Medial umbilical fold (with obliterated umbilical a.)
Arcuate line
Median umbilical fold (with obliterated urachus)

Clinical

Crohn's disease

Crohn's disease, a chronic inflammation of the digestive tract, occurs most often in the terminal ileum (30% of cases). Patients are generally young and suffer from abdominal pain, nausea, elevated body temperature, and diarrhea. Initially, these symptoms can be confused with appendicitis.

Complications of the chronic inflammation in Crohn's disease often lead to fistula formation (in this case, an abnormal passage between two gastrointestinal regions) (**B**).

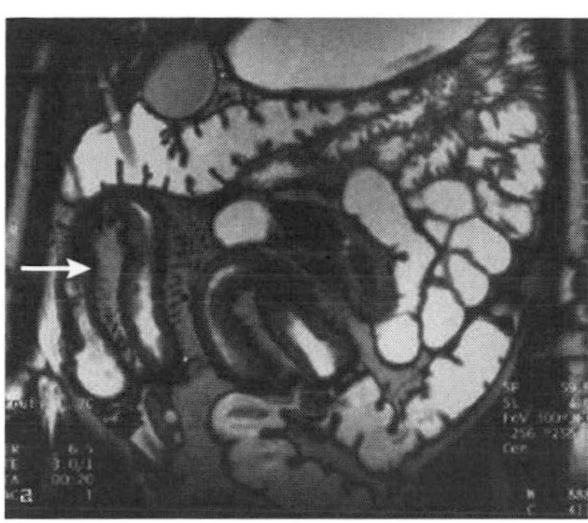

A MRI showing thickened wall of terminal ileum.

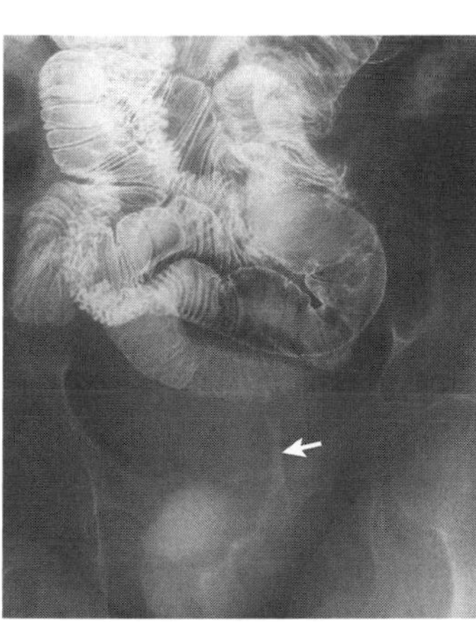

B Double-contrast radiograph. Arrow indicates ileorectal fistula.

Fig. 13.12 **Mesentery of the small intestine**

Anterior view. *Removed:* Stomach, jejunum, and ileum. *Reflected:* Liver.

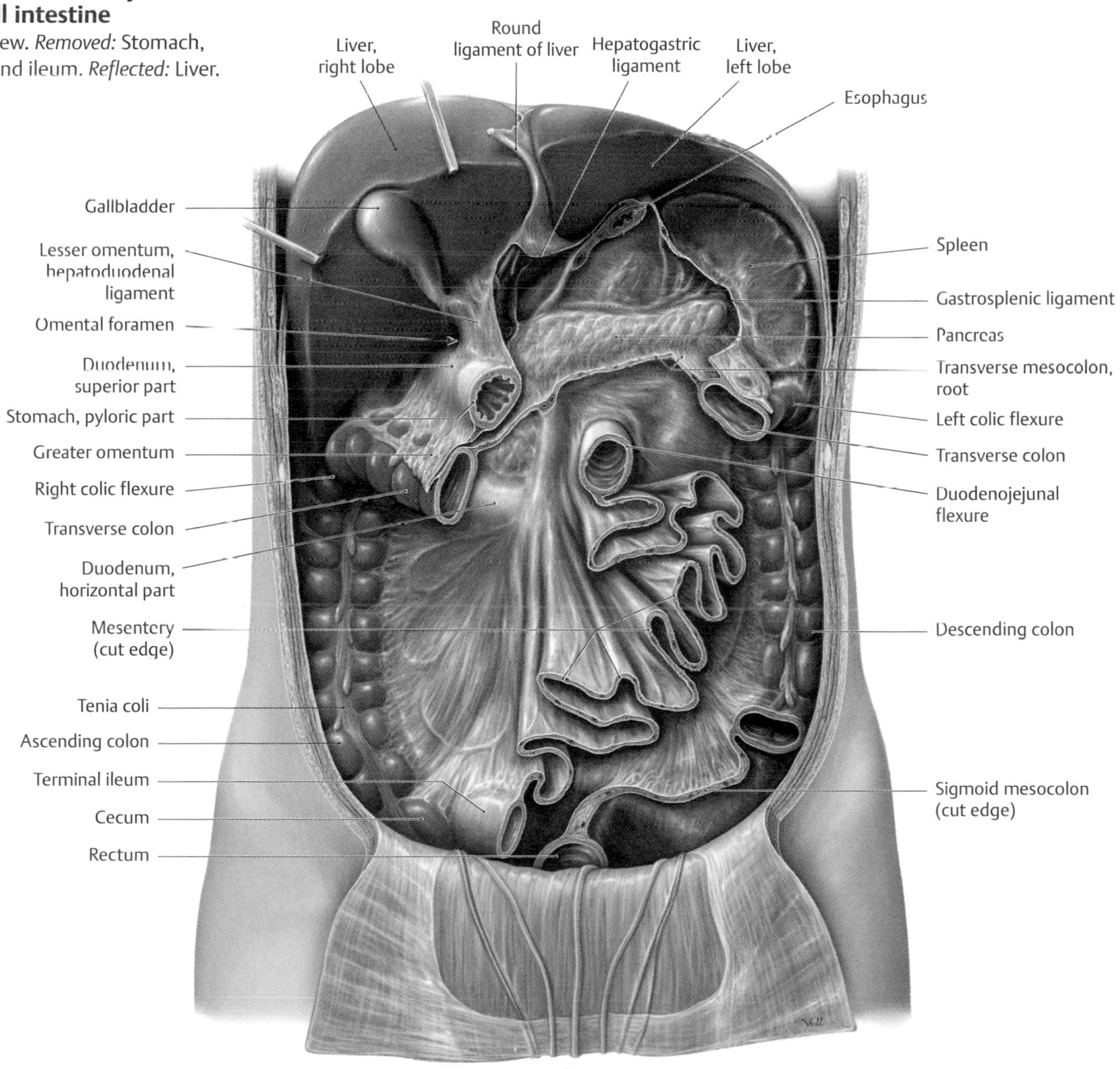

Liver, right lobe
Round ligament of liver
Hepatogastric ligament
Liver, left lobe
Esophagus
Gallbladder
Lesser omentum, hepatoduodenal ligament
Omental foramen
Duodenum, superior part
Stomach, pyloric part
Greater omentum
Right colic flexure
Transverse colon
Duodenum, horizontal part
Mesentery (cut edge)
Tenia coli
Ascending colon
Terminal ileum
Cecum
Rectum
Spleen
Gastrosplenic ligament
Pancreas
Transverse mesocolon, root
Left colic flexure
Transverse colon
Duodenojejunal flexure
Descending colon
Sigmoid mesocolon (cut edge)

Cecum, Appendix & Colon

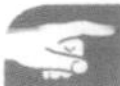

The ascending and descending colon are normally secondarily retroperitoneal, but sometimes they are suspended by a short mesentery from the posterior abdominal wall. *Note*: In the clinical setting, the left colic flexure is often referred to as the splenic flexure and the right colic flexure, as the hepatic flexure.

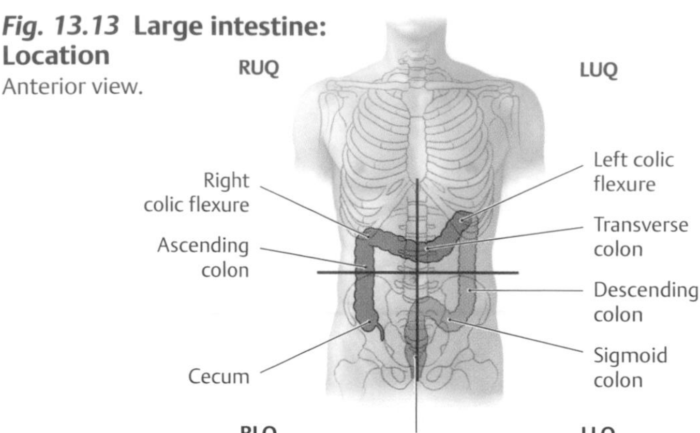
RUQ
LUQ
Right colic flexure
Ascending colon
Cecum
Left colic flexure
Transverse colon
Descending colon
Sigmoid colon
RLQ
Rectum
LLQ

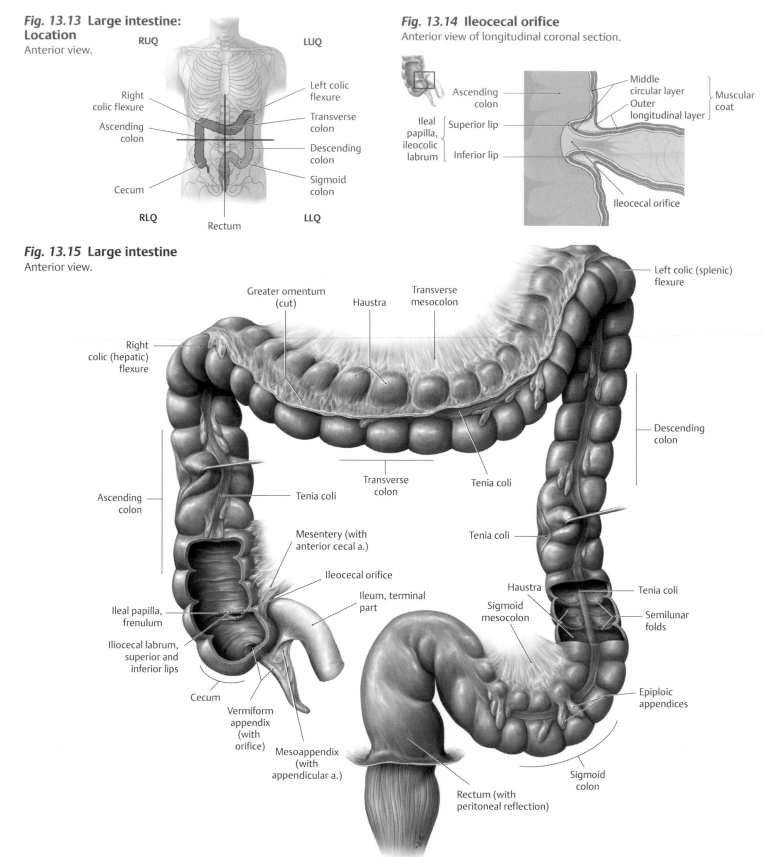

Fig. 13.13 **Large intestine: Location**
Anterior view.

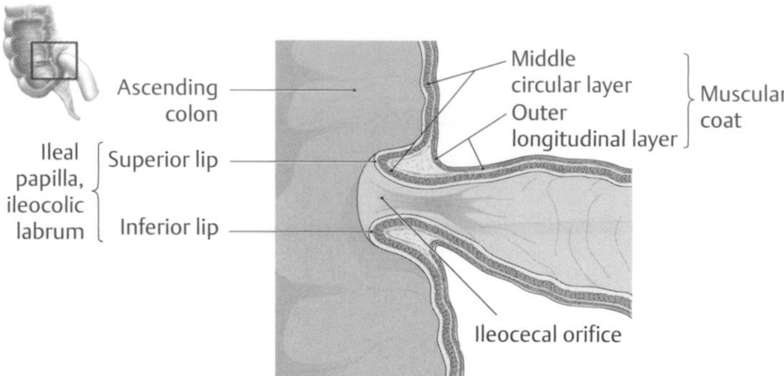
Ascending colon
Ileal papilla, ileocolic labrum
Superior lip
Inferior lip
Middle circular layer
Outer longitudinal layer
Muscular coat
Ileocecal orifice

Fig. 13.14 **Ileocecal orifice**
Anterior view of longitudinal coronal section.

Fig. 13.15 **Large intestine**
Anterior view.

Greater omentum (cut)
Haustra
Transverse mesocolon
Left colic (splenic) flexure
Right colic (hepatic) flexure
Descending colon
Transverse colon
Tenia coli
Ascending colon
Tenia coli
Tenia coli
Mesentery (with anterior cecal a.)
Ileocecal orifice
Ileum, terminal part
Haustra
Sigmoid mesocolon
Tenia coli
Semilunar folds
Ileal papilla, frenulum
Iliocecal labrum, superior and inferior lips
Cecum
Vermiform appendix (with orifice)
Mesoappendix (with appendicular a.)
Epiploic appendices
Rectum (with peritoneal reflection)
Sigmoid colon

Fig. 13.16 Large intestine in situ

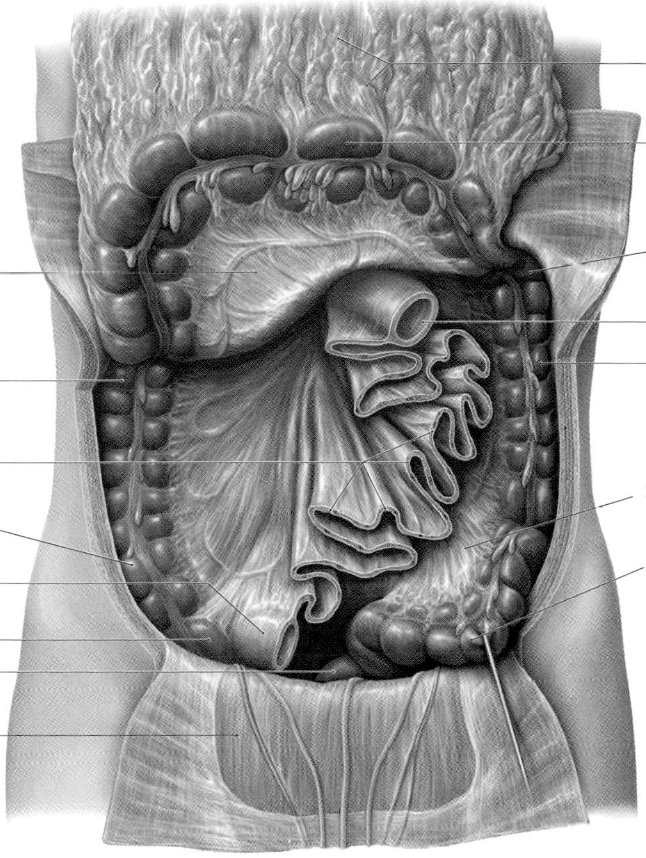

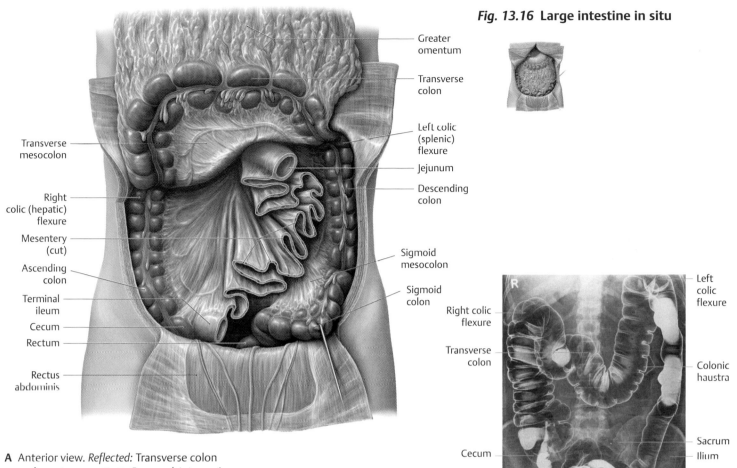

Greater omentum
Transverse colon
Transverse mesocolon
Left colic (splenic) flexure
Jejunum
Right colic (hepatic) flexure
Descending colon
Mesentery (cut)
Sigmoid mesocolon
Ascending colon
Sigmoid colon
Terminal ileum
Cecum
Rectum
Rectus abdominis

A Anterior view. *Reflected:* Transverse colon and greater omentum. *Removed:* Intraperitoneal small intestine.

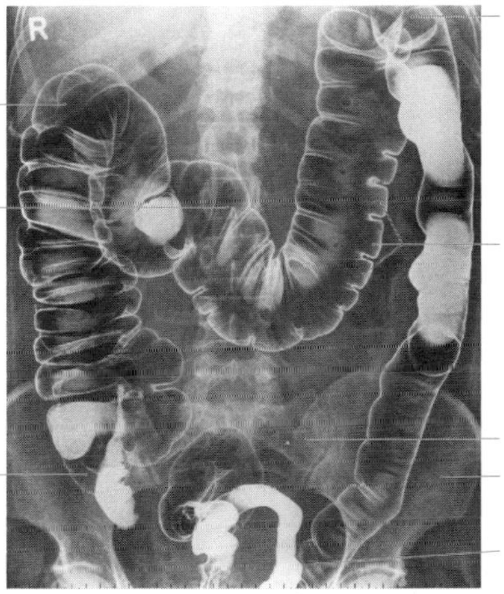

Right colic flexure
Transverse colon
Cecum
Left colic flexure
Colonic haustra
Sacrum
Ilium
Sigmoid colon

B Normal radiographic appearance. Double-contrast radiograph, anterior view.

Clinical

Colitis

Ulcerative colitis is a chronic inflammation of the large intestine, often starting in the rectum. Typical symptoms include diarrhea (sometimes with blood), pain, weight loss, and inflammation of other organs. Patients are also at higher risk for colorectal carcinomas.

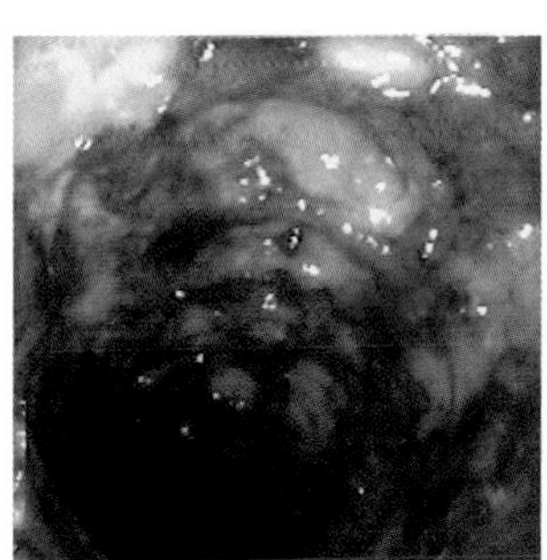

A Colonoscopy of ulcerative colitis.

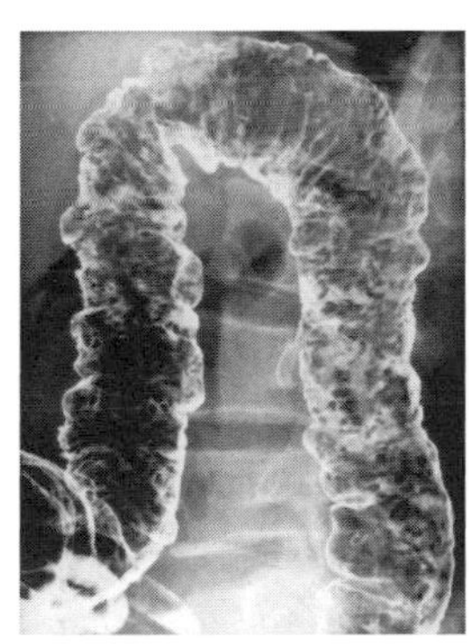

B Early-phase colitis. Residual normal mucosa appears as pseudopolyps.

Clinical

Colon carcinoma

Malignant tumors of the colon and rectum are among the most frequent solid tumors. More than 90% occur in patients over the age of 50. In early stages, the tumor may be asymptomatic; later symptoms include loss of appetite, changes in bowel movements, and weight loss. Blood in the stools is particularly incriminating, necessitating a thorough examination. Hemorrhoids are not a sufficient explanation for blood in stools unless all other tests (including a colonoscopy) are negative.

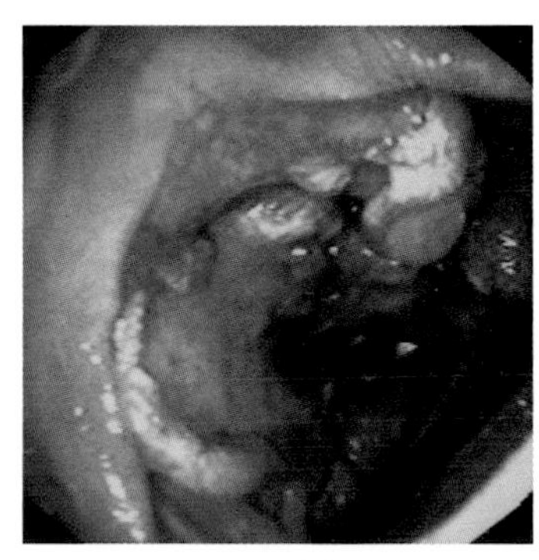

Colonoscopy of colon carcinoma. The tumor partially blocks the lumen of the colon.

Liver: Overview

Fig. 13.17 **Liver: Location**

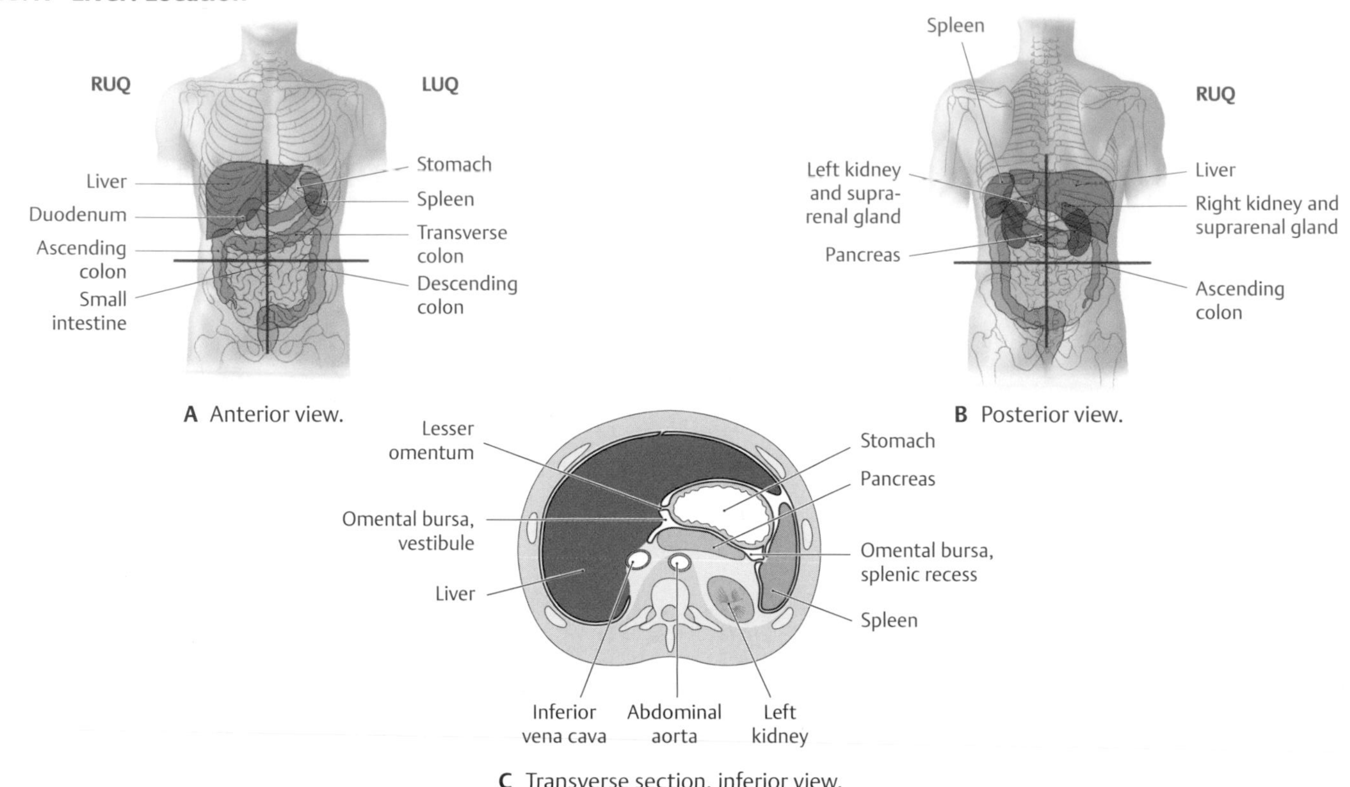
RUQ
LUQ
Liver
Duodenum
Ascending colon
Small intestine
Stomach
Spleen
Transverse colon
Descending colon
A Anterior view.
Spleen
RUQ
Left kidney and supra-renal gland
Pancreas
Liver
Right kidney and suprarenal gland
Ascending colon
B Posterior view.
Lesser omentum
Omental bursa, vestibule
Liver
Stomach
Pancreas
Omental bursa, splenic recess
Spleen
Inferior vena cava
Abdominal aorta
Left kidney
C Transverse section, inferior view.

Fig. 13.18 **Liver in situ**

Anterior view. The liver is intraperitoneal except for its "bare area" (see Fig. 13.22A); its mesenteries include the falciform, coronary, and triangular ligaments (see Fig. 13.23). *Inset:* Liver retracted to show inferior surface and gallbladder.

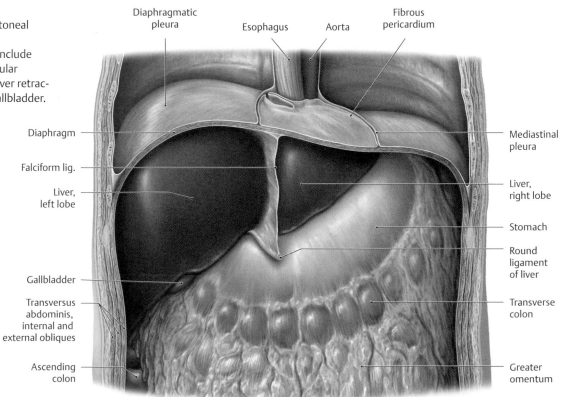

Diaphragmatic pleura
Esophagus
Aorta
Fibrous pericardium
Diaphragm
Falciform lig.
Liver, left lobe
Gallbladder
Transversus abdominis, internal and external obliques
Ascending colon
Mediastinal pleura
Liver, right lobe
Stomach
Round ligament of liver
Transverse colon
Greater omentum

Fig. 13.19 **Abdominal MRI**
Inferior view.

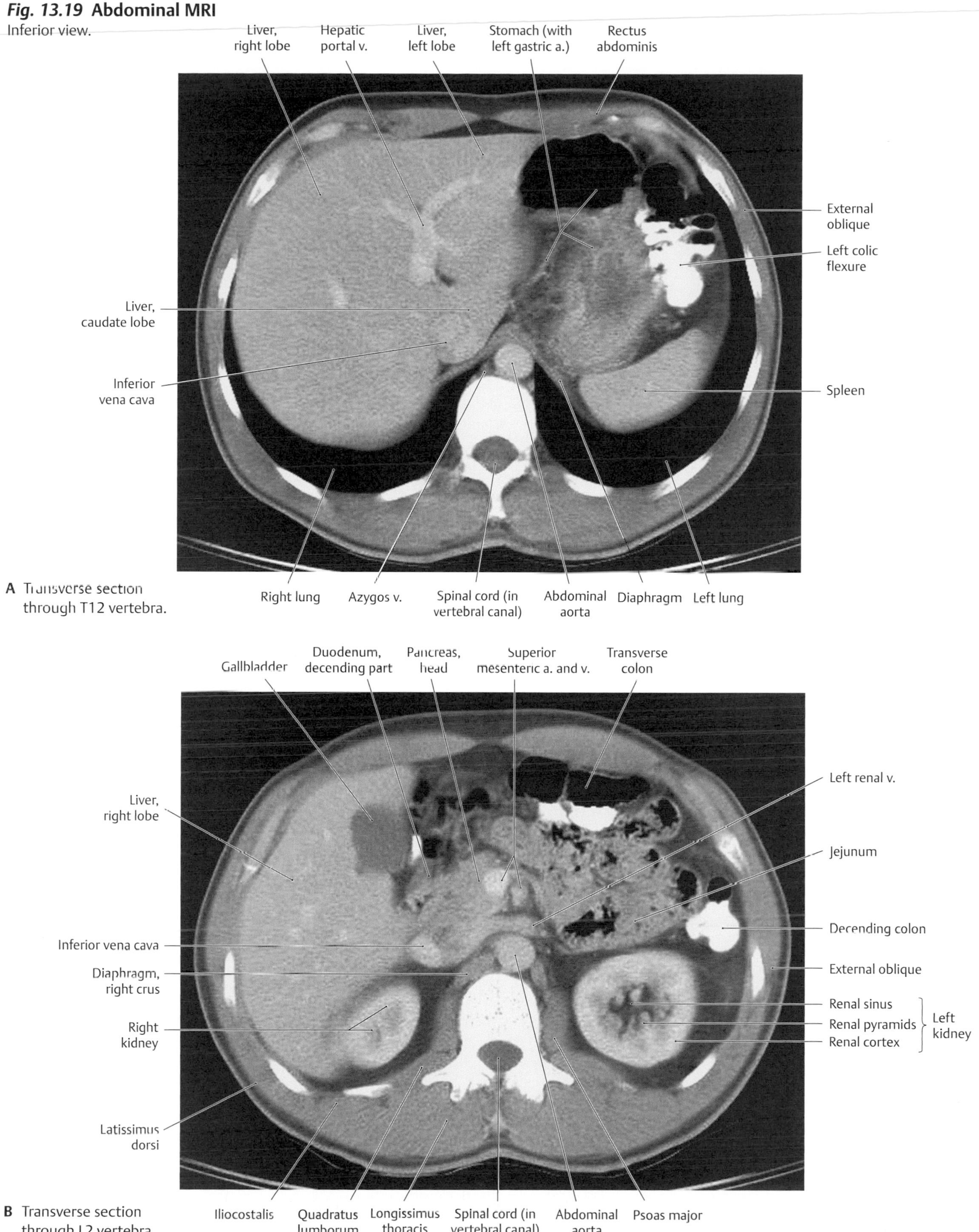
Liver, right lobe
Hepatic portal v.
Liver, left lobe
Stomach (with left gastric a.)
Rectus abdominis
External oblique
Left colic flexure
Liver, caudate lobe
Inferior vena cava
Spleen
Right lung
Azygos v.
Spinal cord (in vertebral canal)
Abdominal aorta
Diaphragm
Left lung
Gallbladder
Duodenum, decending part
Pancreas, head
Superior mesenteric a. and v.
Transverse colon
Left renal v.
Liver, right lobe
Jejunum
Decending colon
Inferior vena cava
External oblique
Diaphragm, right crus
Renal sinus
Renal pyramids
Renal cortex
Left kidney
Right kidney
Latissimus dorsi
Iliocostalis
Quadratus lumborum
Longissimus thoracis
Spinal cord (in vertebral canal)
Abdominal aorta
Psoas major

A Transverse section through T12 vertebra.

B Transverse section through L2 vertebra.

Liver: Segments & Lobes

***Fig. 13.20* Segmentation of the liver**
The liver is divided into functional divisions, which are further divided into segments (see Table 13.1). Each segment is served by tertiary branches of the hepatic artery, the portal vein, and the common hepatic duct, which together make up the portal triad.

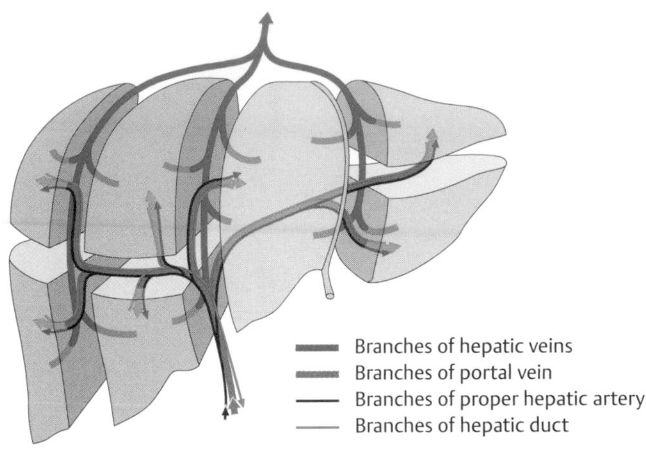

Branches of hepatic veins
Branches of portal vein
Branches of proper hepatic artery
Branches of hepatic duct

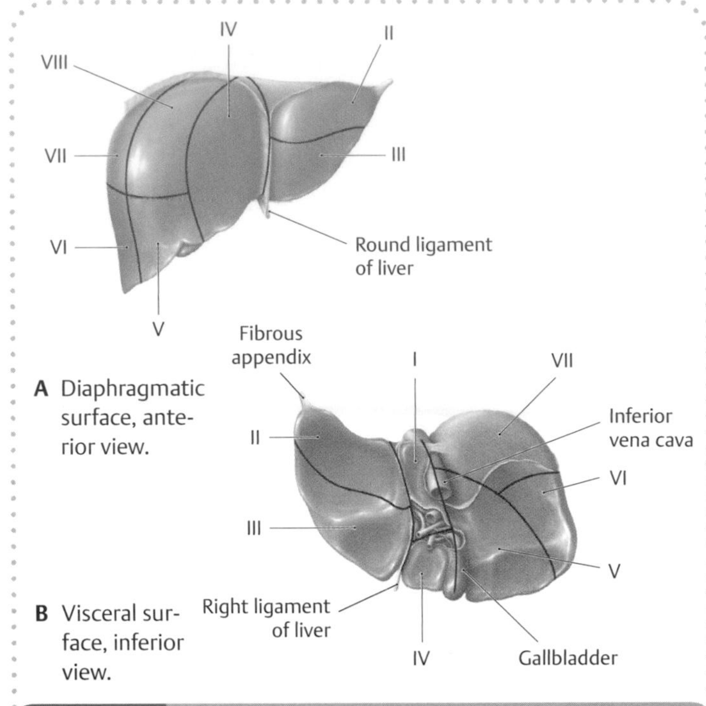

IV
II
VIII
VII
III
VI
Round ligament of liver
V
Fibrous appendix
I
VII
Inferior vena cava
II
VI
III
V
Right ligament of liver
IV
Gallbladder

A Diaphragmatic surface, anterior view.

B Visceral surface, inferior view.

***Fig. 13.21* Relations of the liver**
Visceral surface, inferior view.

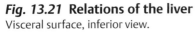

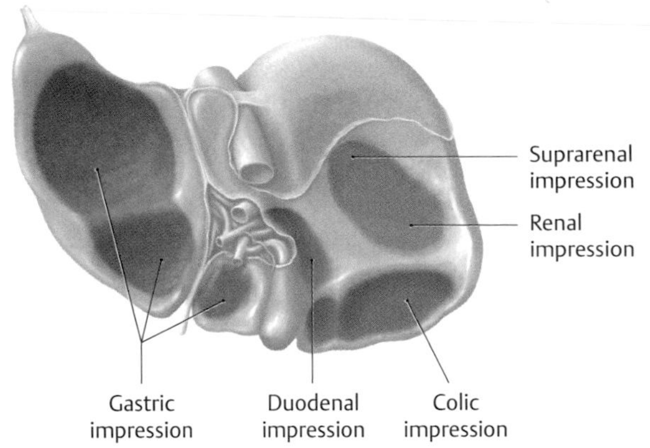

Suprarenal impression
Renal impression
Gastric impression
Duodenal impression
Colic impression

***Table 13.1* Hepatic segments**

Part	Division	Segment	
Left part	Posterior part	I	Caudate lobe
	Left lateral division	II	Left posterolateral
		III	Left anterolateral
	Left medial division	IV	Left medial
Right part	Right medial division	V	Right anteromedial
		VI	Right anterolateral
	Right lateral division	VII	Right posterolateral
		VIII	Right posteromedial

***Fig. 13.22* Attachment of liver to diaphragm**

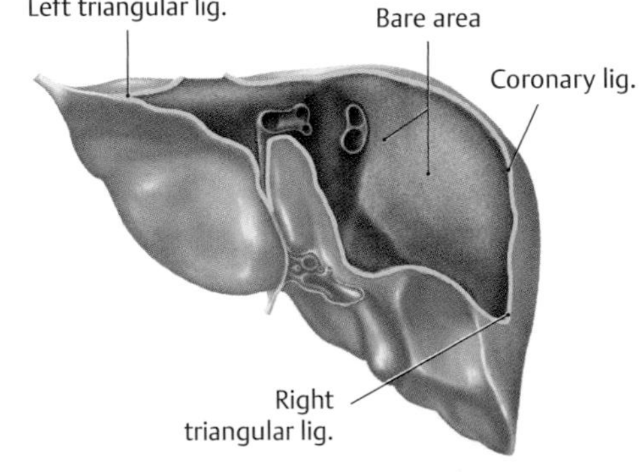

Left triangular lig.
Bare area
Coronary lig.
Right triangular lig.

A Diaphragmatic surface of the liver, posterior view.

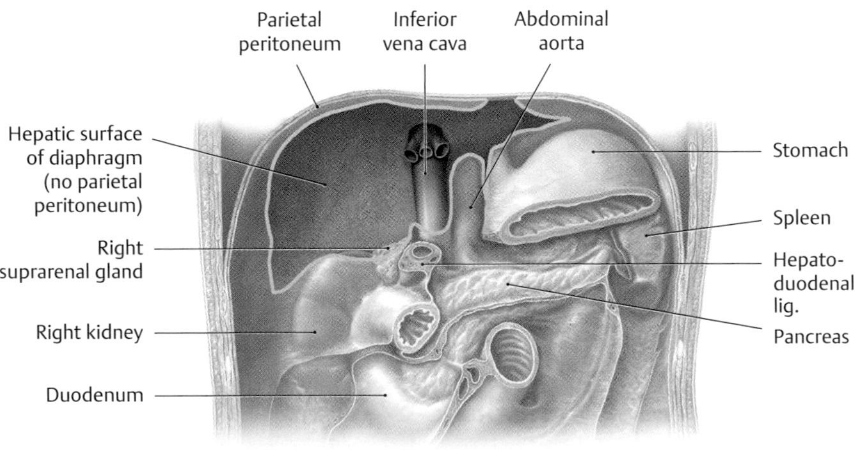

Parietal peritoneum
Inferior vena cava
Abdominal aorta
Hepatic surface of diaphragm (no parietal peritoneum)
Right suprarenal gland
Right kidney
Duodenum
Stomach
Spleen
Hepato-duodenal lig.
Pancreas

B Hepatic surface of the diaphragm, anterior view.

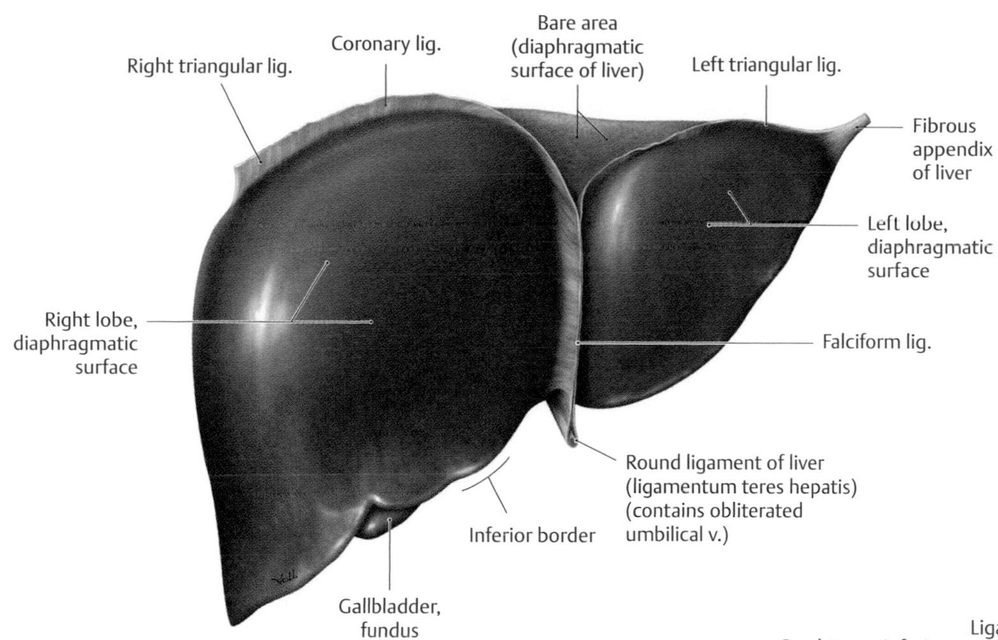

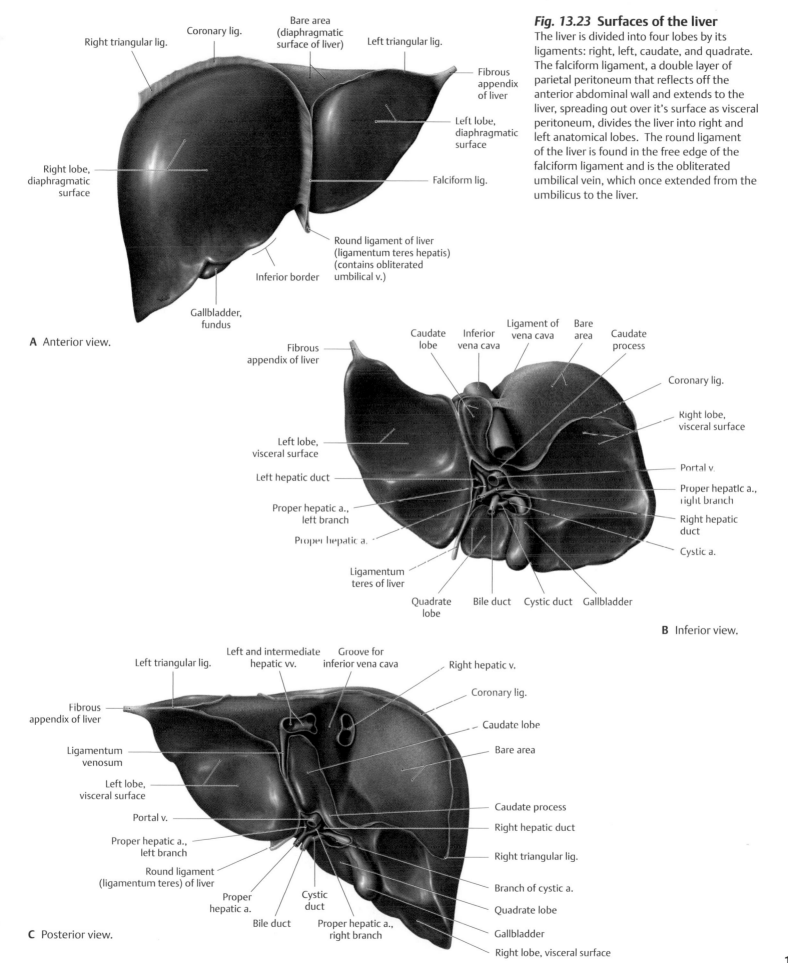

Right triangular lig.
Coronary lig.
Bare area (diaphragmatic surface of liver)
Left triangular lig.
Fibrous appendix of liver
Left lobe, diaphragmatic surface
Right lobe, diaphragmatic surface
Falciform lig.
Round ligament of liver (ligamentum teres hepatis) (contains obliterated umbilical v.)
Inferior border
Gallbladder, fundus

A Anterior view.

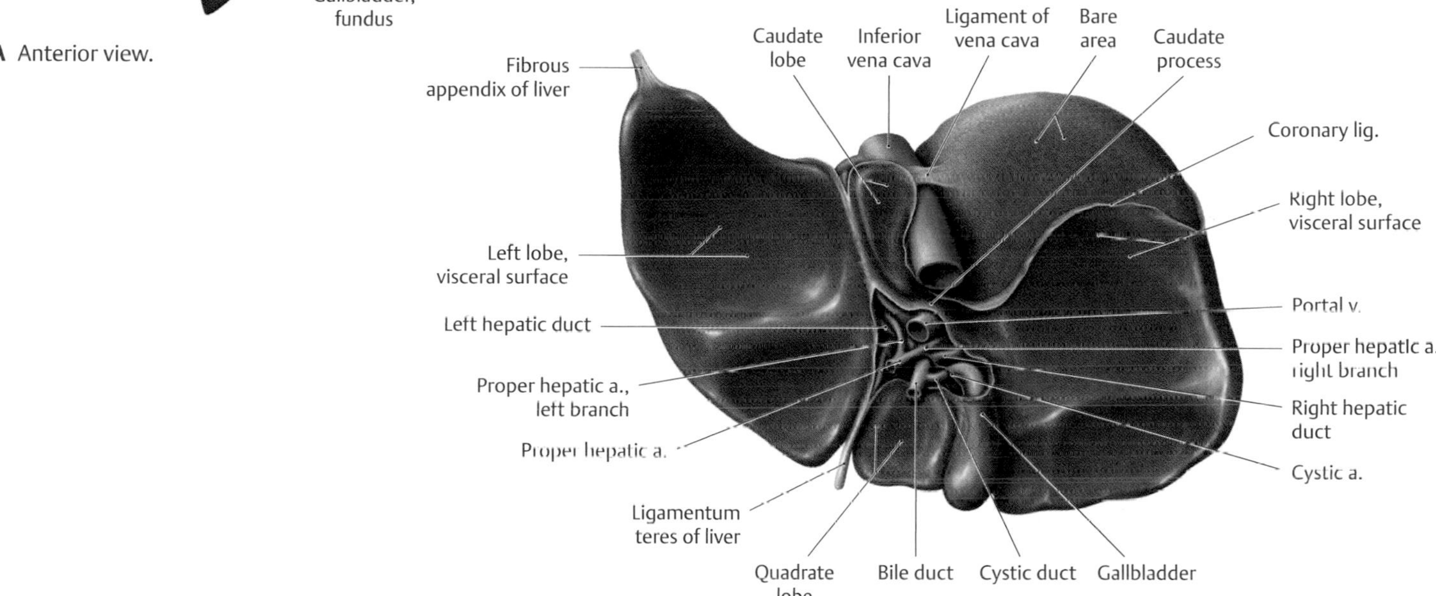

Fibrous appendix of liver
Caudate lobe
Inferior vena cava
Ligament of vena cava
Bare area
Caudate process
Coronary lig.
Right lobe, visceral surface
Left lobe, visceral surface
Left hepatic duct
Portal v.
Proper hepatic a., right branch
Proper hepatic a., left branch
Right hepatic duct
Proper hepatic a.
Cystic a.
Ligamentum teres of liver
Quadrate lobe
Bile duct
Cystic duct
Gallbladder

B Inferior view.

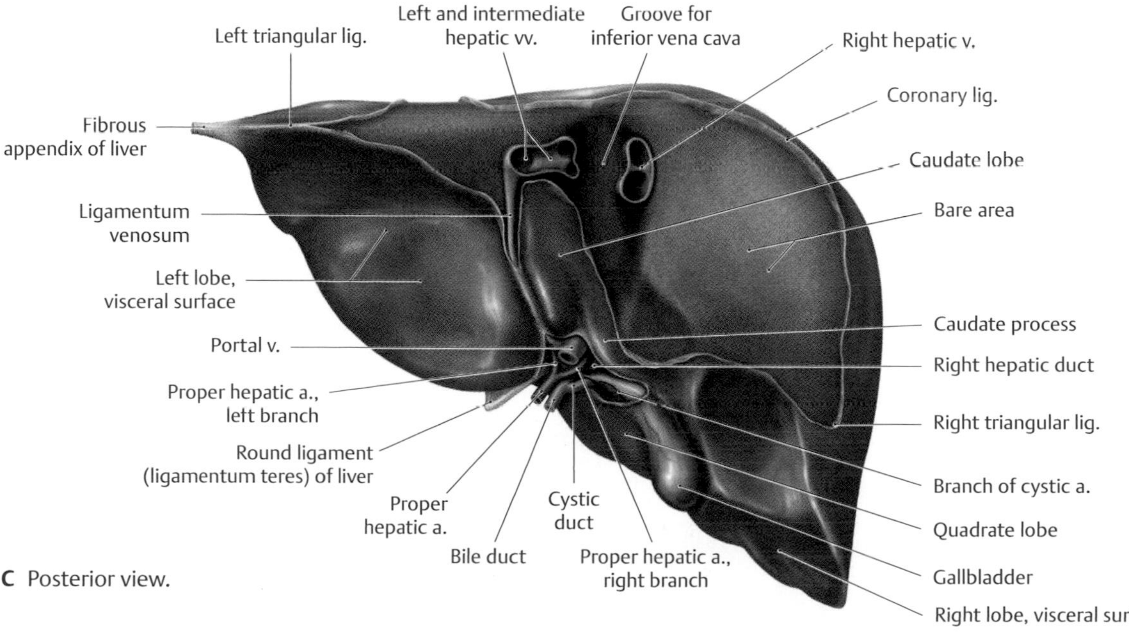

Left triangular lig.
Left and intermediate hepatic vv.
Groove for inferior vena cava
Right hepatic v.
Coronary lig.
Fibrous appendix of liver
Caudate lobe
Ligamentum venosum
Bare area
Left lobe, visceral surface
Caudate process
Portal v.
Right hepatic duct
Proper hepatic a., left branch
Right triangular lig.
Round ligament (ligamentum teres) of liver
Branch of cystic a.
Proper hepatic a.
Cystic duct
Quadrate lobe
Bile duct
Proper hepatic a., right branch
Gallbladder
Right lobe, visceral surface

C Posterior view.

Fig. 13.23 **Surfaces of the liver**
The liver is divided into four lobes by its ligaments: right, left, caudate, and quadrate. The falciform ligament, a double layer of parietal peritoneum that reflects off the anterior abdominal wall and extends to the liver, spreading out over it's surface as visceral peritoneum, divides the liver into right and left anatomical lobes. The round ligament of the liver is found in the free edge of the falciform ligament and is the obliterated umbilical vein, which once extended from the umbilicus to the liver.

Gallbladder & Bile Ducts

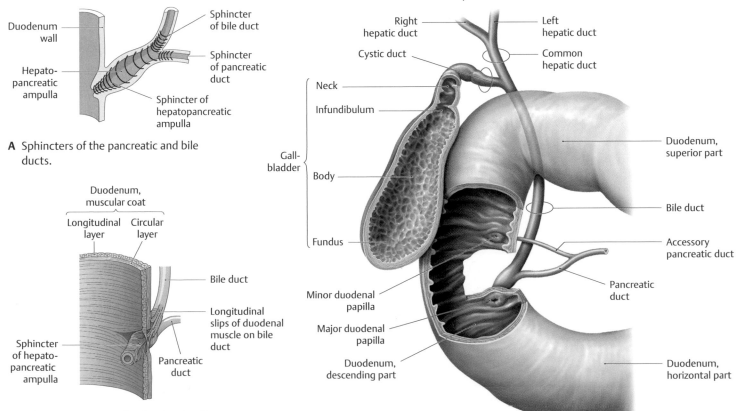

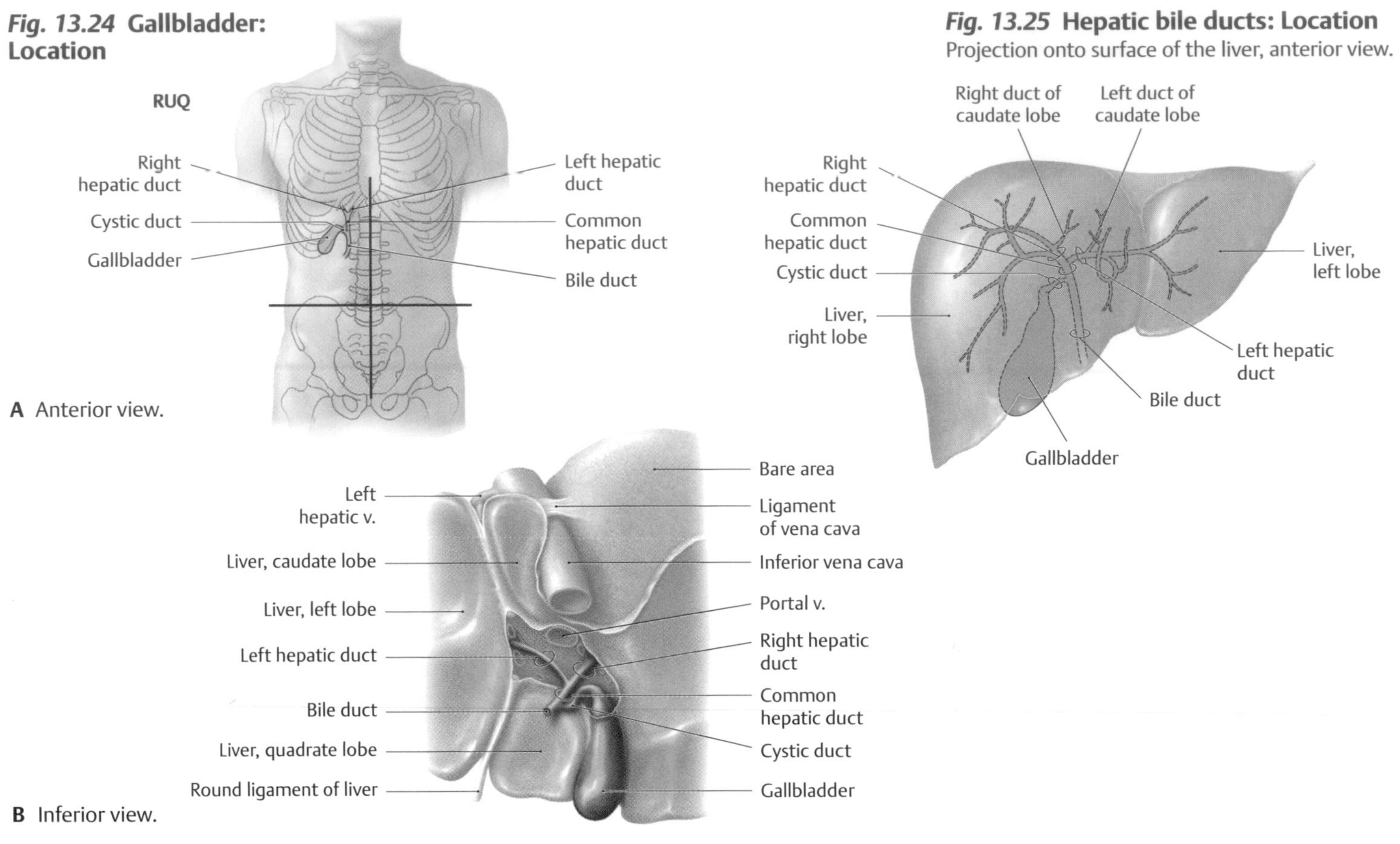
RUQ
Right hepatic duct
Cystic duct
Gallbladder
Left hepatic duct
Common hepatic duct
Bile duct
Left hepatic v.
Liver, caudate lobe
Liver, left lobe
Left hepatic duct
Bile duct
Liver, quadrate lobe
Round ligament of liver
Bare area
Ligament of vena cava
Inferior vena cava
Portal v.
Right hepatic duct
Common hepatic duct
Cystic duct
Gallbladder
Right duct of caudate lobe
Left duct of caudate lobe
Right hepatic duct
Common hepatic duct
Cystic duct
Liver, right lobe
Liver, left lobe
Left hepatic duct
Bile duct
Gallbladder

Fig. 13.24 **Gallbladder: Location**

A Anterior view.

B Inferior view.

Fig. 13.25 **Hepatic bile ducts: Location**

Projection onto surface of the liver, anterior view.

Fig. 13.26 **Biliary sphincter system**

Duodenum wall

Hepato-pancreatic ampulla

Sphincter of bile duct

Sphincter of pancreatic duct

Sphincter of hepatopancreatic ampulla

A Sphincters of the pancreatic and bile ducts.

Duodenum, muscular coat

Longitudinal layer

Circular layer

Bile duct

Longitudinal slips of duodenal muscle on bile duct

Sphincter of hepato-pancreatic ampulla

Pancreatic duct

B Sphincter system in the duodenal wall.

Fig. 13.27 **Extrahepatic bile ducts**

Anterior view. *Opened:* Gallbladder and duodenum.

Right hepatic duct

Cystic duct

Left hepatic duct

Common hepatic duct

Gall-bladder

Neck

Infundibulum

Body

Fundus

Minor duodenal papilla

Major duodenal papilla

Duodenum, descending part

Duodenum, superior part

Bile duct

Accessory pancreatic duct

Pancreatic duct

Duodenum, horizontal part

Fig. 13.28 Biliary tract in situ
Anterior view. *Removed:* Stomach, small intestine, transverse colon, and large portions of the liver. The gallbladder is intraperitoneal, covered by visceral peritoneum where it is not attached to the liver.

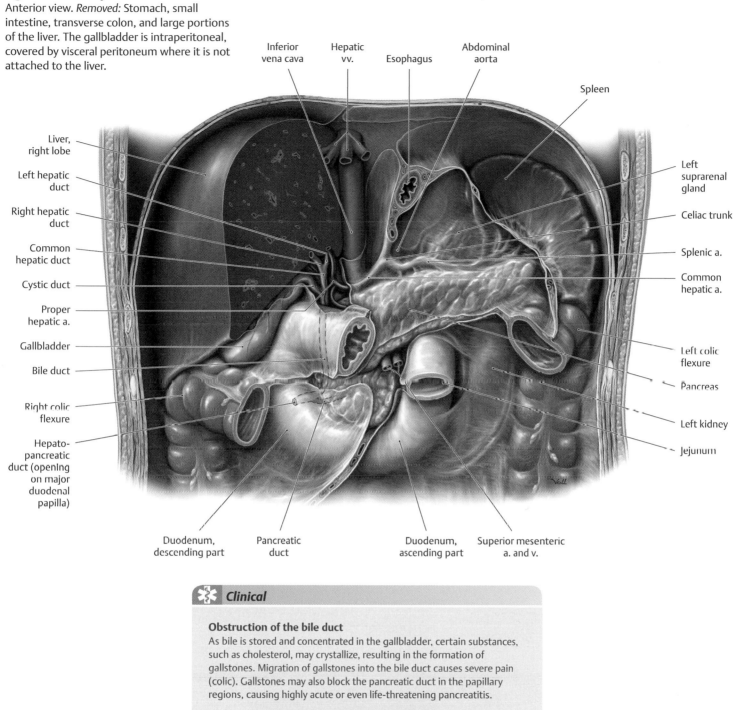

Inferior vena cava
Hepatic vv.
Esophagus
Abdominal aorta
Spleen
Liver, right lobe
Left hepatic duct
Right hepatic duct
Common hepatic duct
Cystic duct
Proper hepatic a.
Gallbladder
Bile duct
Right colic flexure
Hepato-pancreatic duct (opening on major duodenal papilla)
Left suprarenal gland
Celiac trunk
Splenic a.
Common hepatic a.
Left colic flexure
Pancreas
Left kidney
Jejunum
Duodenum, descending part
Pancreatic duct
Duodenum, ascending part
Superior mesenteric a. and v.

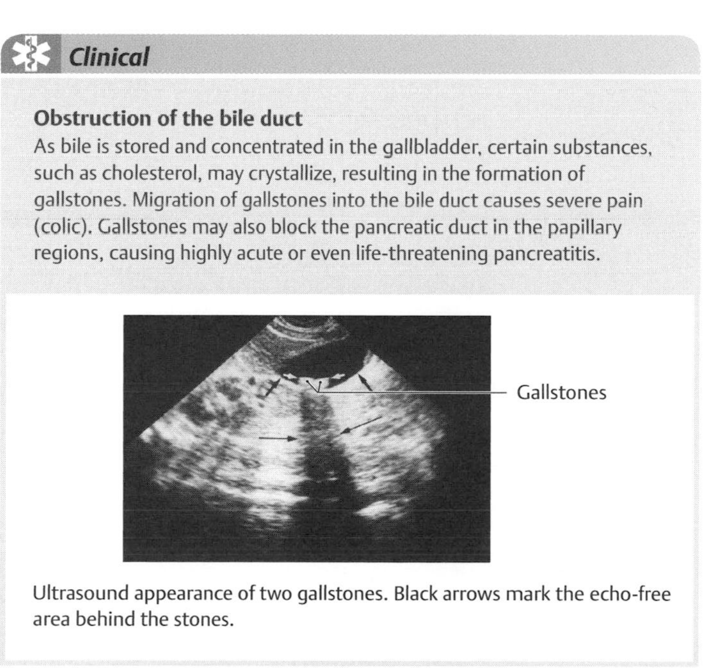
Gallstones

Clinical

Obstruction of the bile duct

As bile is stored and concentrated in the gallbladder, certain substances, such as cholesterol, may crystallize, resulting in the formation of gallstones. Migration of gallstones into the bile duct causes severe pain (colic). Gallstones may also block the pancreatic duct in the papillary regions, causing highly acute or even life-threatening pancreatitis.

Ultrasound appearance of two gallstones. Black arrows mark the echo-free area behind the stones.

Pancreas & Spleen

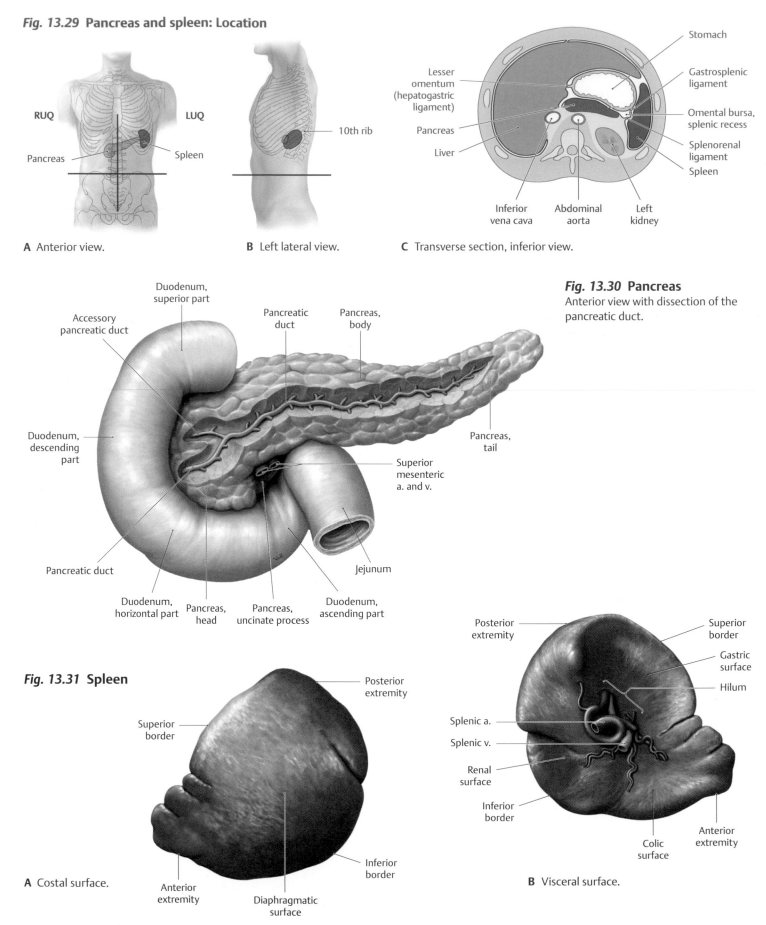

Fig. 13.29 **Pancreas and spleen: Location**

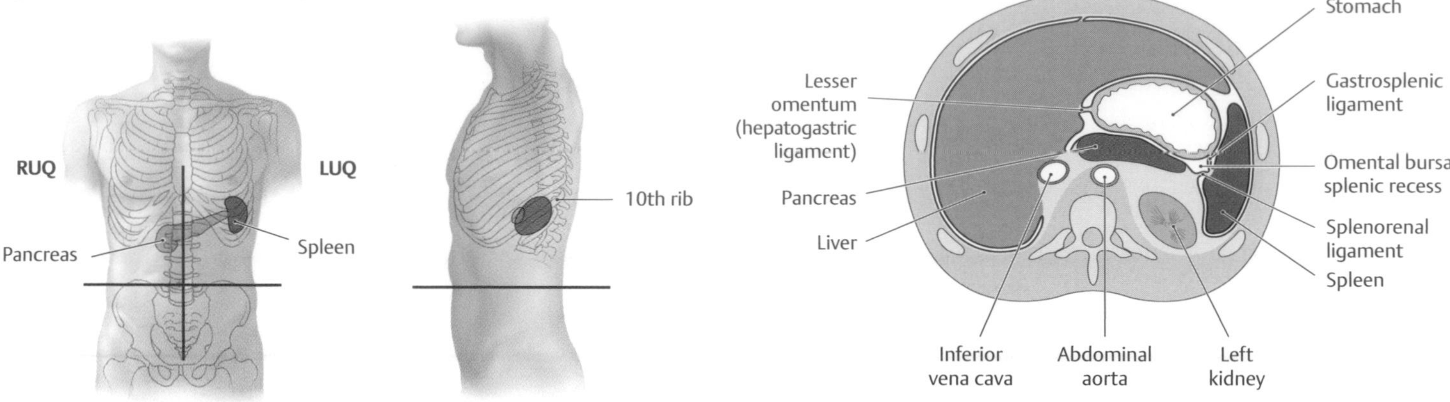
RUQ
LUQ
Pancreas
Spleen
10th rib
Lesser omentum (hepatogastric ligament)
Pancreas
Liver
Stomach
Gastrosplenic ligament
Omental bursa, splenic recess
Splenorenal ligament
Spleen
Inferior vena cava
Abdominal aorta
Left kidney

A Anterior view. **B** Left lateral view. **C** Transverse section, inferior view.

Fig. 13.30 **Pancreas**
Anterior view with dissection of the pancreatic duct.

Duodenum, superior part
Accessory pancreatic duct
Pancreatic duct
Pancreas, body
Duodenum, descending part
Pancreas, tail
Superior mesenteric a. and v.
Jejunum
Pancreatic duct
Duodenum, horizontal part
Pancreas, head
Pancreas, uncinate process
Duodenum, ascending part

Fig. 13.31 **Spleen**

Posterior extremity
Superior border
Anterior extremity
Diaphragmatic surface
Inferior border

A Costal surface.

Posterior extremity
Superior border
Gastric surface
Hilum
Splenic a.
Splenic v.
Renal surface
Inferior border
Colic surface
Anterior extremity

B Visceral surface.

Fig. 13.32 Pancreas and spleen in situ

Anterior view. *Removed:* Liver, stomach, small intestine, and large intestine. The pancreas is retroperitoneal, while the spleen is intraperitoneal.

Fig. 13.33 Pancreas and spleen: Transverse section

Inferior view. Section through L1 vertebra.

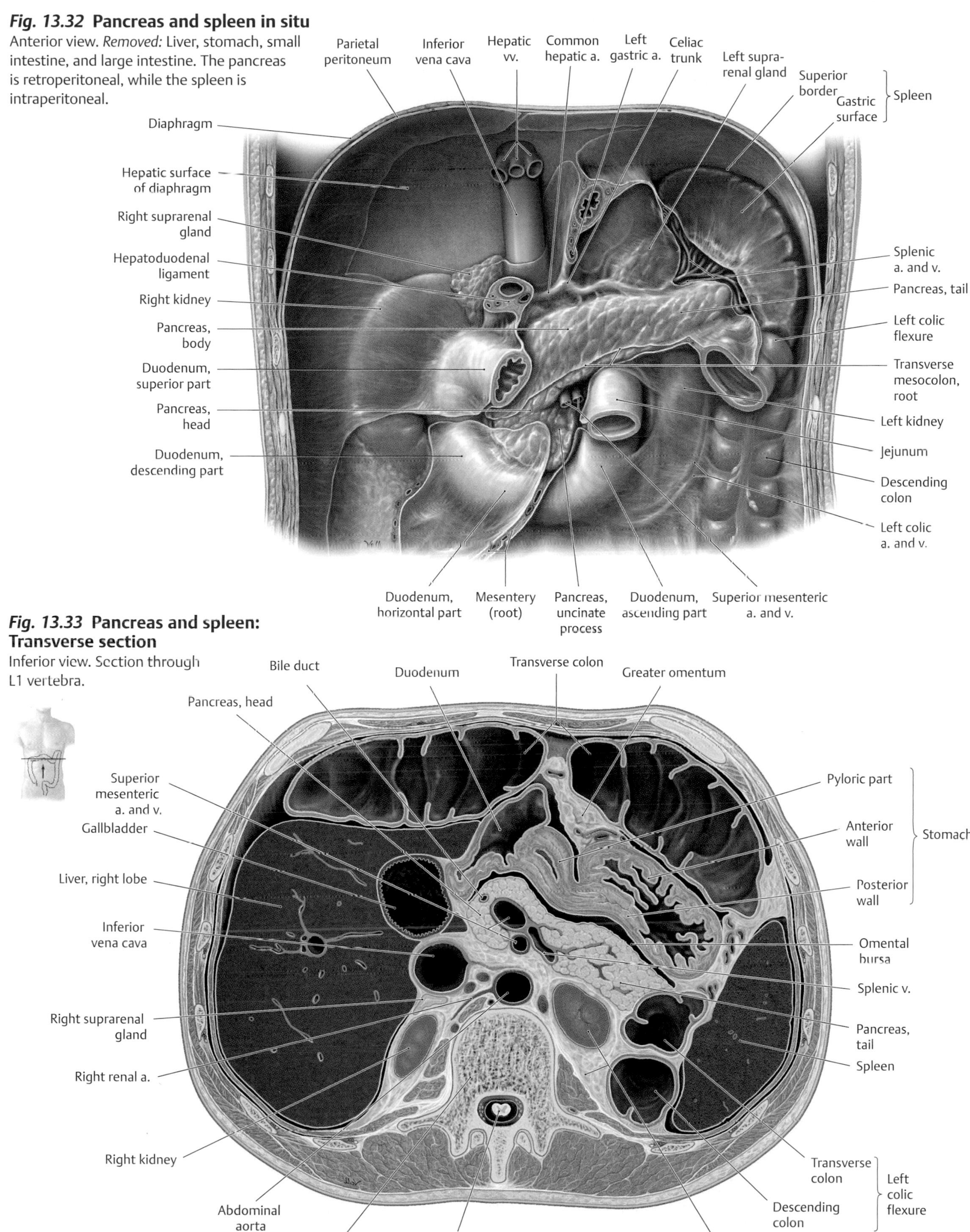

Parietal peritoneum
Inferior vena cava
Hepatic vv.
Common hepatic a.
Left gastric a.
Celiac trunk
Left suprarenal gland
Superior border
Gastric surface
Spleen
Diaphragm
Hepatic surface of diaphragm
Right suprarenal gland
Hepatoduodenal ligament
Right kidney
Pancreas, body
Duodenum, superior part
Pancreas, head
Duodenum, descending part
Splenic a. and v.
Pancreas, tail
Left colic flexure
Transverse mesocolon, root
Left kidney
Jejunum
Descending colon
Left colic a. and v.
Duodenum, horizontal part
Mesentery (root)
Pancreas, uncinate process
Duodenum, ascending part
Superior mesenteric a. and v.
Bile duct
Duodenum
Transverse colon
Greater omentum
Pancreas, head
Superior mesenteric a. and v.
Gallbladder
Liver, right lobe
Inferior vena cava
Right suprarenal gland
Right renal a.
Right kidney
Abdominal aorta
L1 vertebra
Spinal cord (in vertebral canal)
Left kidney and perirenal fat capsule
Pyloric part
Anterior wall
Posterior wall
Stomach
Omental bursa
Splenic v.
Pancreas, tail
Spleen
Transverse colon
Descending colon
Left colic flexure

Kidneys & Suprarenal Glands (I)

Fig. 13.34 Kidneys and suprarenal glands: Location

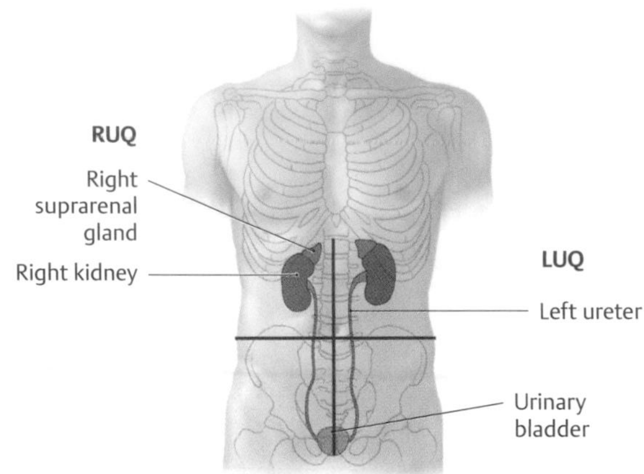
RUQ
Right suprarenal gland
Right kidney
LUQ
Left ureter
Urinary bladder

A Anterior view.

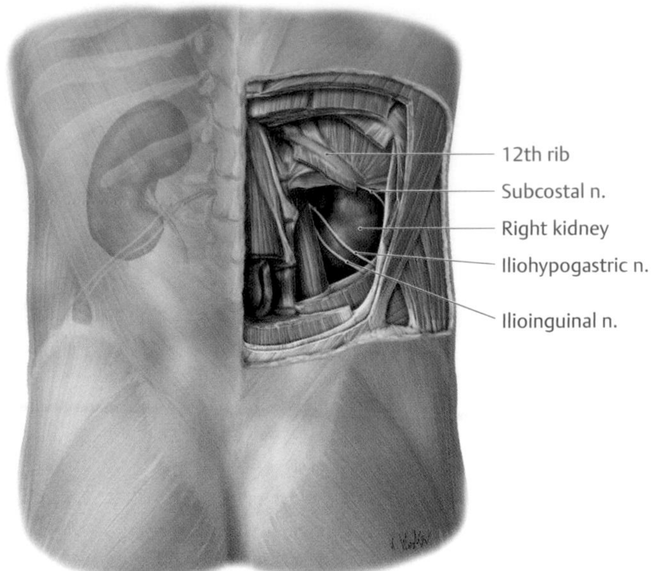
12th rib
Subcostal n.
Right kidney
Iliohypogastric n.
Ilioinguinal n.

B Posterior view. Right side windowed.

Fig. 13.35 Relations of the kidneys
Anterior view.

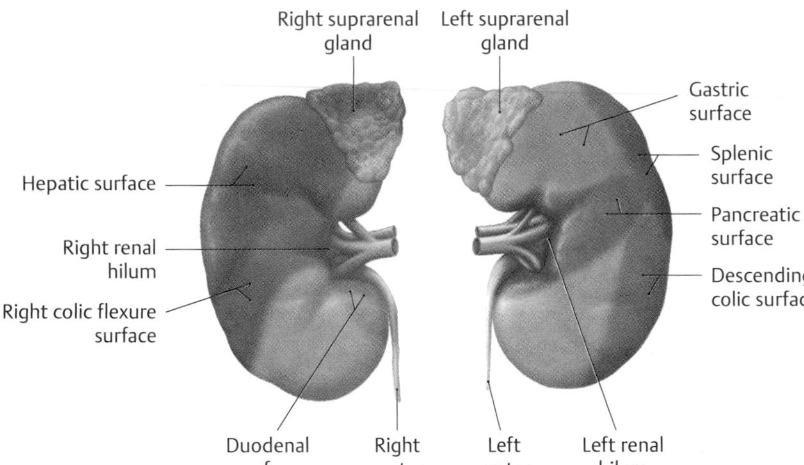
Right suprarenal gland
Left suprarenal gland
Gastric surface
Splenic surface
Hepatic surface
Pancreatic surface
Right renal hilum
Descending colic surface
Right colic flexure surface
Duodenal surface
Right ureter
Left ureter
Left renal hilum

Fig. 13.36 Right kidney in the renal bed
Sagittal section through the right renal bed.

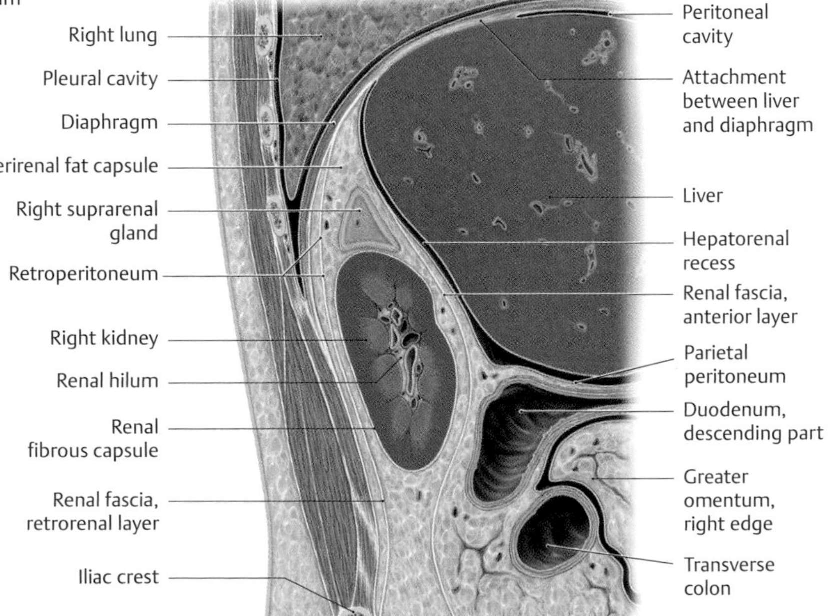
Right lung
Pleural cavity
Diaphragm
Perirenal fat capsule
Right suprarenal gland
Retroperitoneum
Right kidney
Renal hilum
Renal fibrous capsule
Renal fascia, retrorenal layer
Iliac crest
Peritoneal cavity
Attachment between liver and diaphragm
Liver
Hepatorenal recess
Renal fascia, anterior layer
Parietal peritoneum
Duodenum, descending part
Greater omentum, right edge
Transverse colon

***Fig. 13.37* Kidneys and suprarenal glands in the retroperitoneum**

Anterior view. Both the kidneys and suprarenal glands are retroperitoneal.

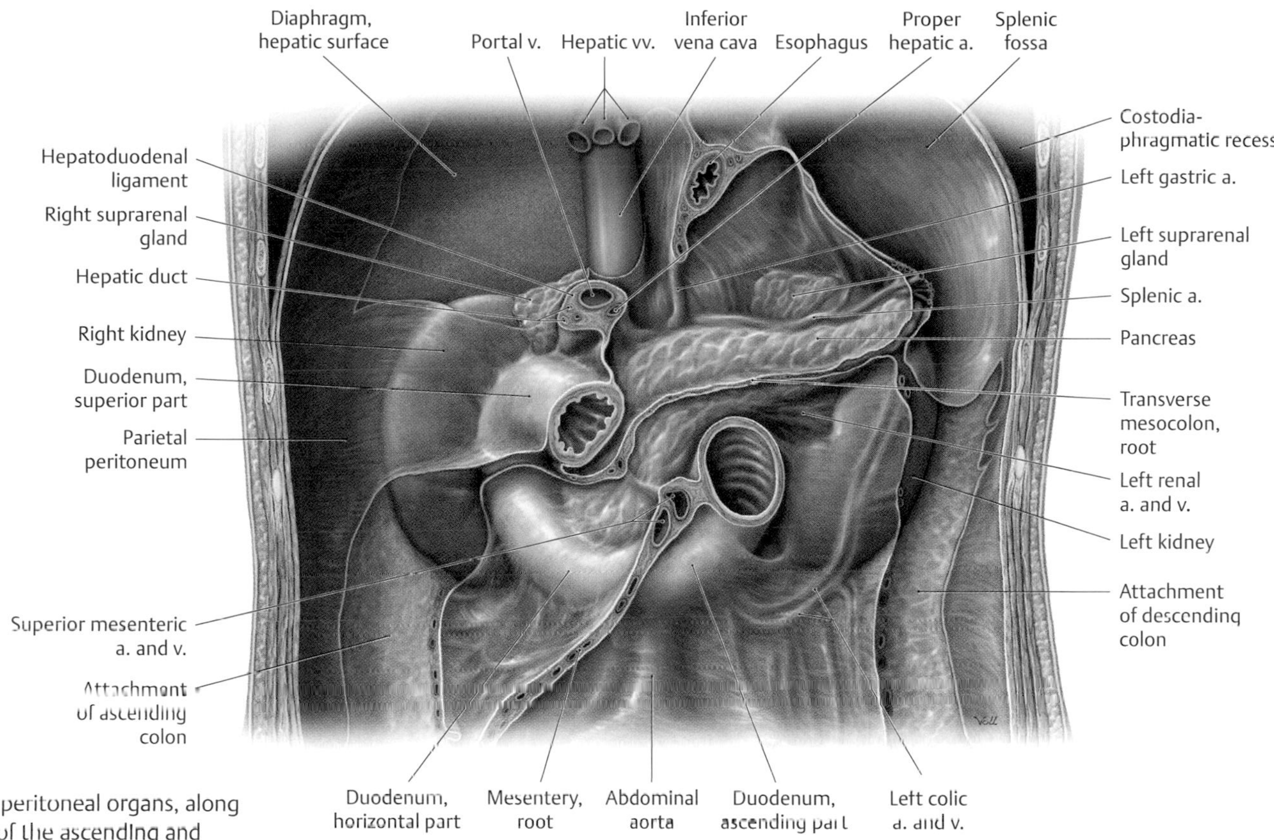

Diaphragm, hepatic surface
Portal v.
Hepatic vv.
Inferior vena cava
Esophagus
Proper hepatic a.
Splenic fossa
Costodiaphragmatic recess
Left gastric a.
Left suprarenal gland
Splenic a.
Pancreas
Transverse mesocolon, root
Left renal a. and v.
Left kidney
Attachment of descending colon
Left colic a. and v.
Duodenum, ascending part
Abdominal aorta
Mesentery, root
Duodenum, horizontal part
Hepatoduodenal ligament
Right suprarenal gland
Hepatic duct
Right kidney
Duodenum, superior part
Parietal peritoneum
Superior mesenteric a. and v.
Attachment of ascending colon

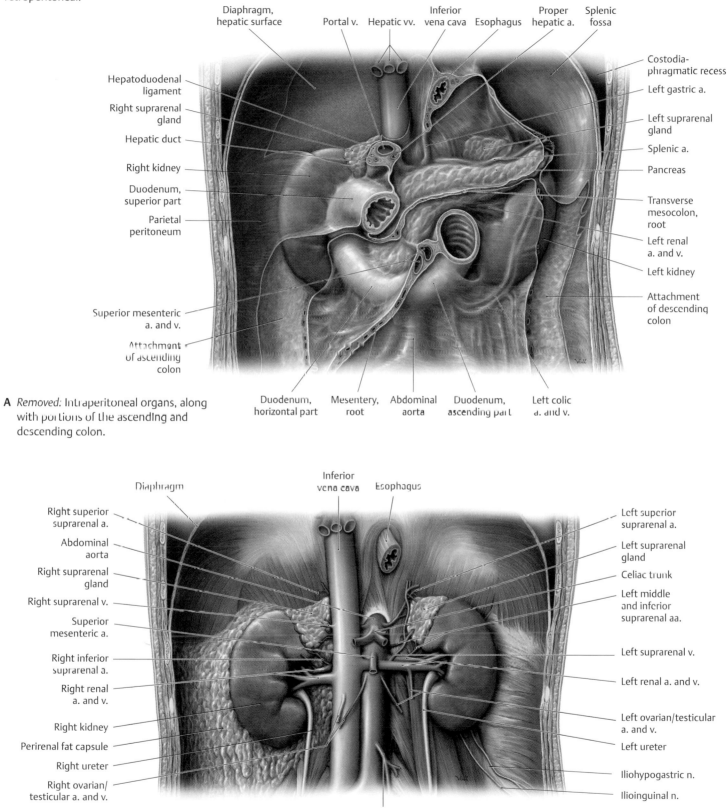

A *Removed:* Intraperitoneal organs, along with portions of the ascending and descending colon.

Diaphragm
Inferior vena cava
Esophagus
Right superior suprarenal a.
Abdominal aorta
Right suprarenal gland
Right suprarenal v.
Superior mesenteric a.
Right inferior suprarenal a.
Right renal a. and v.
Right kidney
Perirenal fat capsule
Right ureter
Right ovarian/testicular a. and v.
Inferior mesenteric a.
Left superior suprarenal a.
Left suprarenal gland
Celiac trunk
Left middle and inferior suprarenal aa.
Left suprarenal v.
Left renal a. and v.
Left ovarian/testicular a. and v.
Left ureter
Iliohypogastric n.
Ilioinguinal n.

B *Removed:* Peitoneum, spleen and gastrointestinal organs, along with fat capsule (left side) *Retracted:* Esophagus

Kidneys & Suprarenal Glands (II)

Fig. 13.38 **Kidney: Structure**
Right kidney with suprarenal gland.

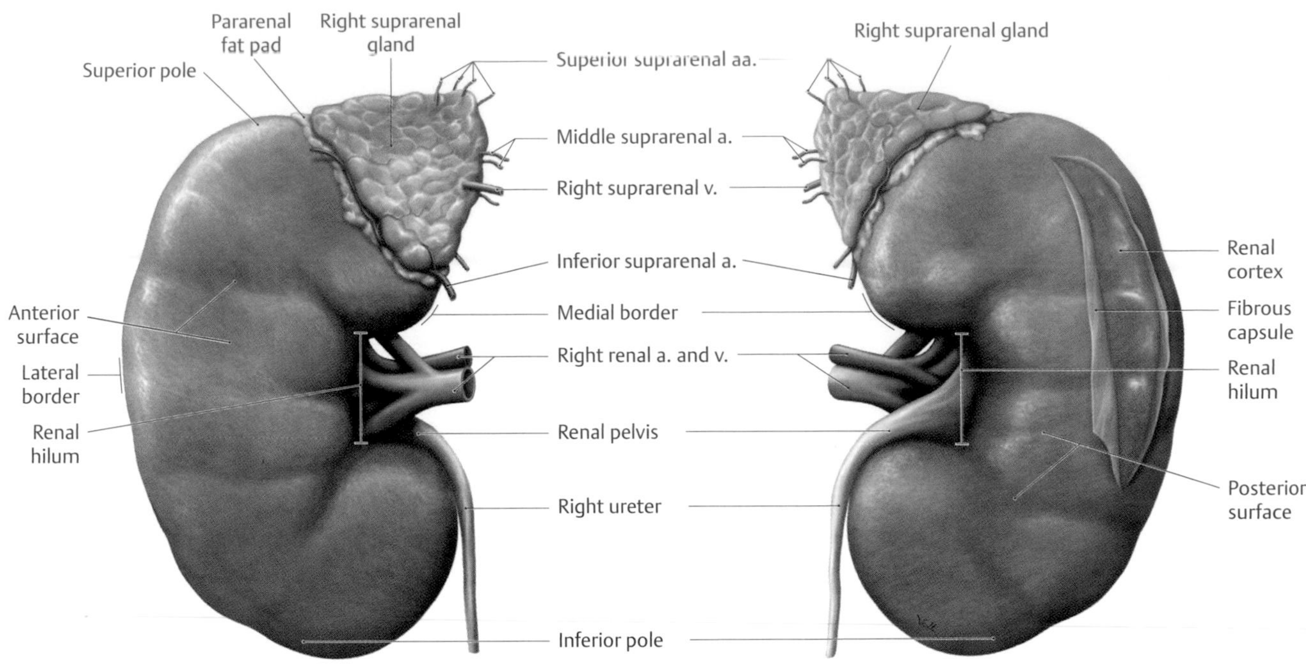
Pararenal fat pad
Right suprarenal gland
Superior pole
Superior suprarenal aa.
Middle suprarenal a.
Right suprarenal v.
Inferior suprarenal a.
Anterior surface
Medial border
Lateral border
Right renal a. and v.
Renal hilum
Renal pelvis
Right ureter
Inferior pole
Right suprarenal gland
Renal cortex
Fibrous capsule
Renal hilum
Posterior surface

A Anterior view.

B Posterior view.

Renal cortex
Renal pyramid
Renal papilla
Renal medulla
Minor calyx
Major calyx
Medullary rays
Arcuate a. and v.
Interlobar a. and v.
Renal a. and v.
Renal column
Renal pelvis
Fibrous capsule
Ureter

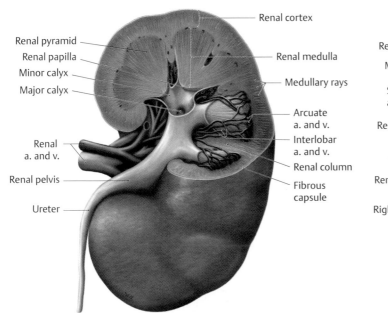

C Posterior view with upper half partially removed.

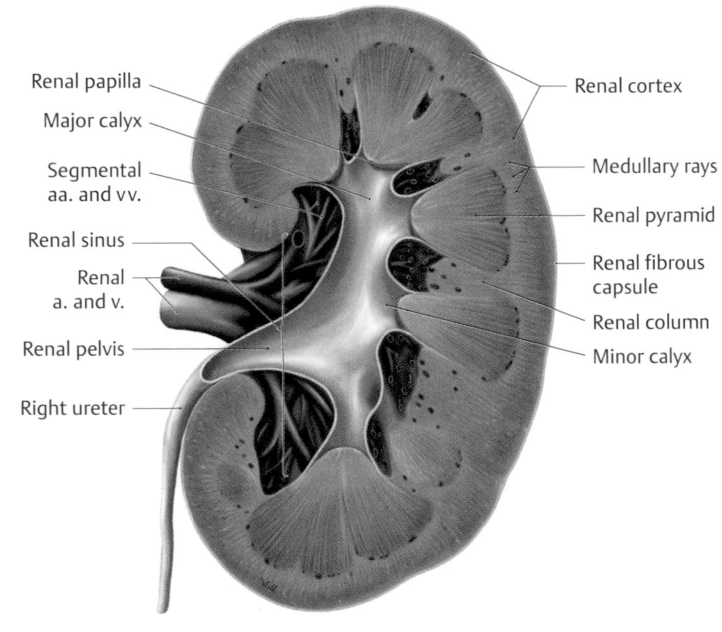
Renal papilla
Renal cortex
Major calyx
Segmental aa. and vv.
Medullary rays
Renal pyramid
Renal sinus
Renal fibrous capsule
Renal a. and v.
Renal column
Renal pelvis
Minor calyx
Right ureter

D Posterior view, midlongitudinal section.

Fig. 13.39 Right kidney and suprarenal gland.
Anterior view. *Removed:* Perirenal fat capsule.
Retracted: Inferior vena cava.

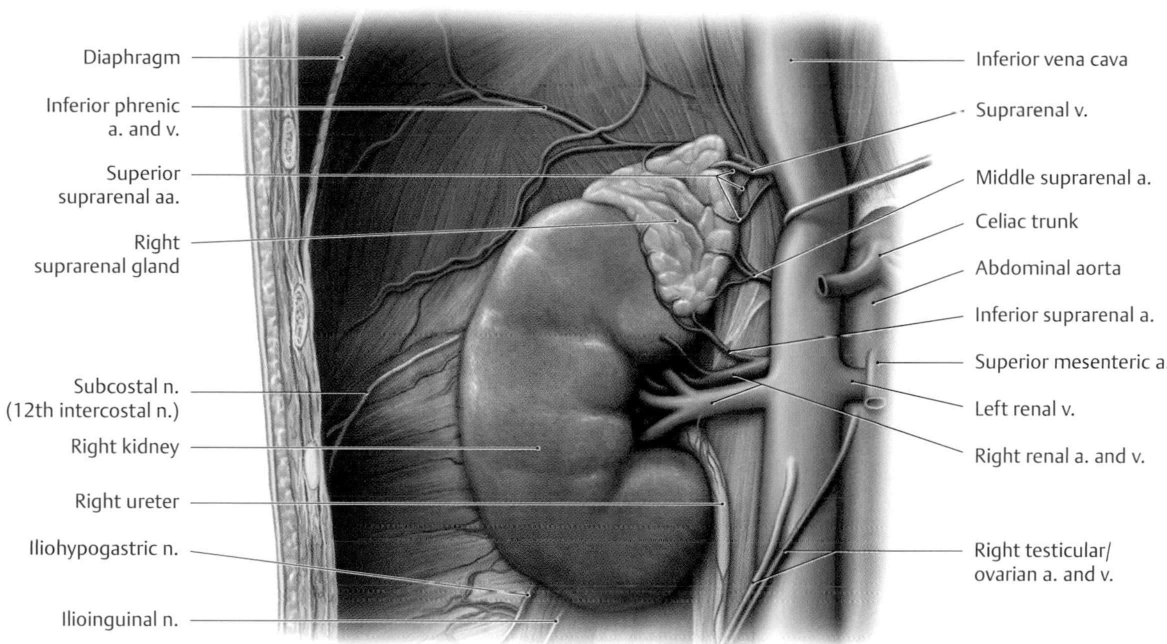

Diaphragm
Inferior phrenic a. and v.
Superior suprarenal aa.
Right suprarenal gland
Subcostal n. (12th intercostal n.)
Right kidney
Right ureter
Iliohypogastric n.
Ilioinguinal n.
Inferior vena cava
Suprarenal v.
Middle suprarenal a.
Celiac trunk
Abdominal aorta
Inferior suprarenal a.
Superior mesenteric a.
Left renal v.
Right renal a. and v.
Right testicular/ ovarian a. and v.

Fig. 13.40 Left kidney and suprarenal gland.
Anterior view. *Removed:* Perirenal fat capsule.
Retracted: Pancreas.

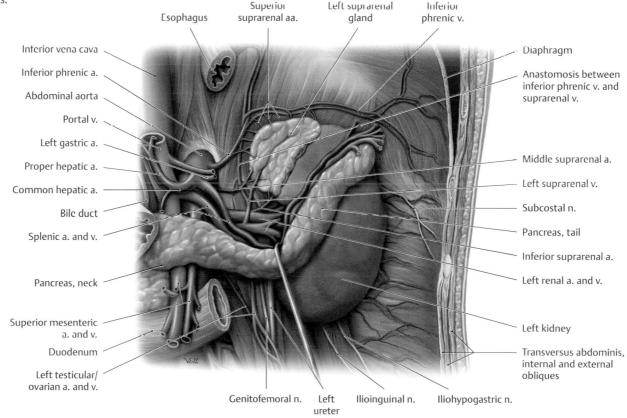

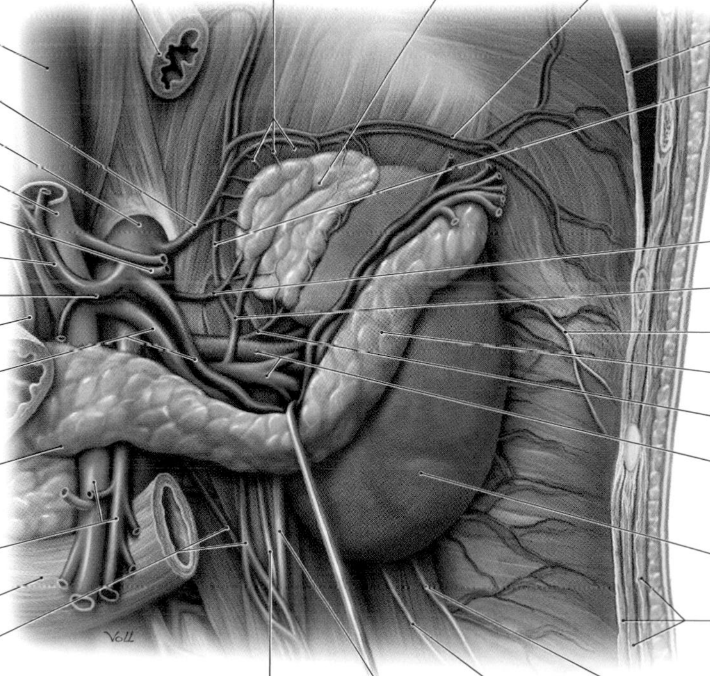

Esophagus
Superior suprarenal aa.
Left suprarenal gland
Inferior phrenic v.
Inferior vena cava
Inferior phrenic a.
Abdominal aorta
Portal v.
Left gastric a.
Proper hepatic a.
Common hepatic a.
Bile duct
Splenic a. and v.
Pancreas, neck
Superior mesenteric a. and v.
Duodenum
Left testicular/ ovarian a. and v.
Diaphragm
Anastomosis between inferior phrenic v. and suprarenal v.
Middle suprarenal a.
Left suprarenal v.
Subcostal n.
Pancreas, tail
Inferior suprarenal a.
Left renal a. and v.
Left kidney
Transversus abdominis, internal and external obliques
Genitofemoral n.
Left ureter
Ilioinguinal n.
Iliohypogastric n.

Arteries of the Abdomen

Fig. 14.1 Abdominal aorta and major branches

Anterior view. The abdominal aorta enters the abdomen at the T12 level through the aortic hiatus of the diaphragm (see p. 62). Before bifurcating at L4 into its terminal branches, the common iliac arteries, the abdominal aorta gives off the renal arteries (see p. 175) and three major trunks that supply the organs of the alimentary canal:

Celiac trunk: Supplies the structures of the foregut, the anterior portion of the alimentary canal. The foregut consists of the esophagus (abdominal 1.25 cm), stomach, duodenum (proximal half), liver, gallbladder, and pancreas (superior portion).

Superior mesenteric artery: Supplies the structures of the midgut: the duodenum (distal half), jejunum and ileum, cecum and appendix, ascending colon, right colic flexure, and the proximal one half of the transverse colon.

Inferior mesenteric artery: Supplies the structures of the hindgut: the transverse colon (distal half), left colic flexure, descending and sigmoid colons, rectum, and anal canal (upper part).

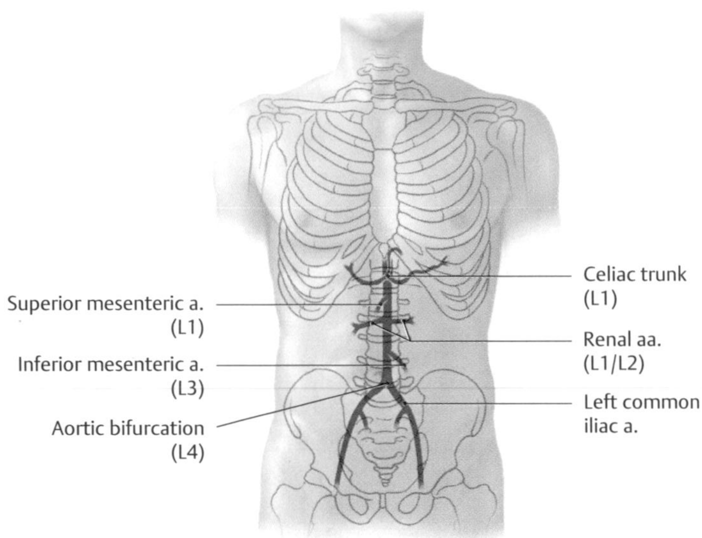

Superior mesenteric a. (L1)
Inferior mesenteric a. (L3)
Aortic bifurcation (L4)
Celiac trunk (L1)
Renal aa. (L1/L2)
Left common iliac a.

Fig. 14.2 Arteries of the abdominal wall

The superior and inferior epigastric arteries form a potential anastomosis, or bypass for blood, from the subclavian and femoral arteries. This effectively allows blood to bypass the abdominal aorta.

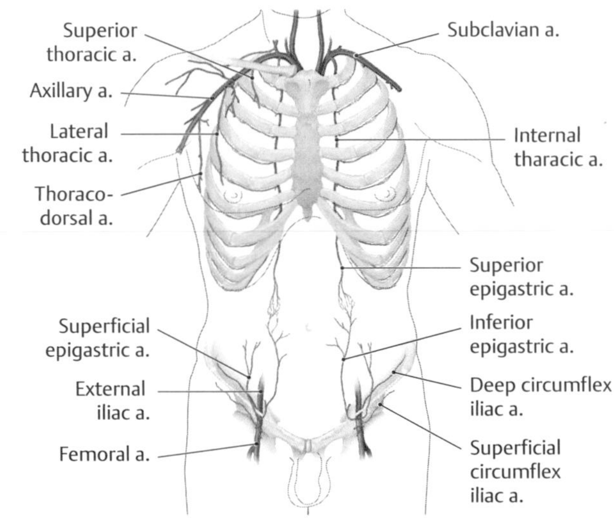

Superior thoracic a.
Axillary a.
Lateral thoracic a.
Thoraco-dorsal a.
Subclavian a.
Internal tharacic a.
Superior epigastric a.
Inferior epigastric a.
Superficial epigastric a.
External iliac a.
Femoral a.
Deep circumflex iliac a.
Superficial circumflex iliac a.

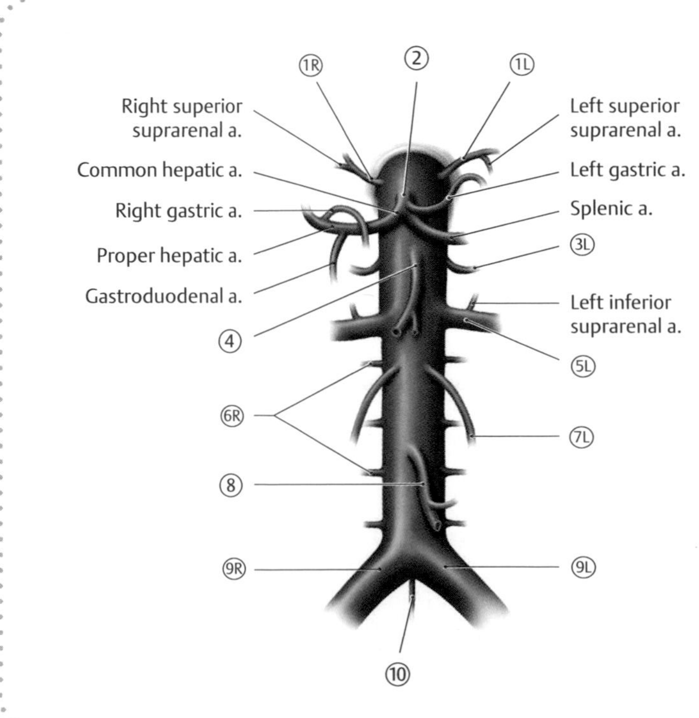

①R
②
①L
Right superior suprarenal a.
Common hepatic a.
Right gastric a.
Proper hepatic a.
Gastroduodenal a.
④
⑥R
⑧
⑨R
⑩
Left superior suprarenal a.
Left gastric a.
Splenic a.
③L
Left inferior suprarenal a.
⑤L
⑦L
⑨L

Table 14.1 Branches of the abdominal aorta

The abdominal aorta gives rise to three major unpaired trunks (bold) and the unpaired median sacral artery, as well as six paired branches.

Branch from abdominal aorta			Branches	
①R	①L	Inferior phrenic aa. (paired)	Superior suprarenal aa.	
②		**Celiac trunk**	Left gastric a.	
			Splenic a.	
			Common hepatic a.	Proper hepatic a.
				Right gastric a.
				Gastroduodenal a.
③R	③L	Middle suprarenal aa. (paired)		
④		**Superior mesenteric a.**		
⑤R	⑤L	Renal aa. (paired)	Inferior suprarenal aa.	
⑥R	⑥L	Lumbar aa. (1st through 4th, paired)		
⑦R	⑦L	Testicular/ovarian aa. (paired)		
⑧		**Inferior mesenteric a.**		
⑨R	⑨L	Common iliac aa. (paired)	External iliac a.	
			Internal iliac a.	
⑩		Median sacral a.		

Fig. 14.3 Celiac trunk

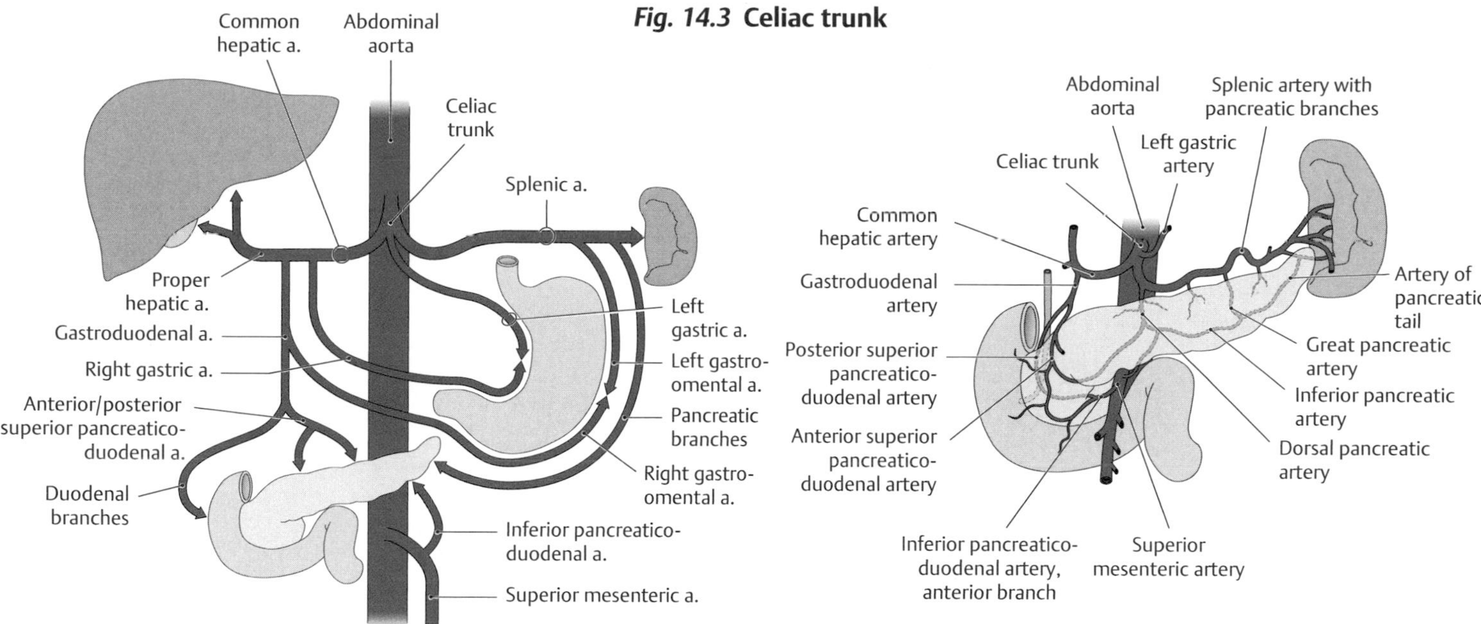
Common
hepatic a.
Abdominal
aorta
Celiac
trunk
Splenic a.
Proper
hepatic a.
Gastroduodenal a.
Right gastric a.
Anterior/posterior
superior pancreatico-
duodenal a.
Duodenal
branches
Left
gastric a.
Left gastro-
omental a.
Pancreatic
branches
Right gastro-
omental a.
Inferior pancreatico-
duodenal a.
Superior mesenteric a.
Abdominal
aorta
Splenic artery with
pancreatic branches
Left gastric
artery
Celiac trunk
Common
hepatic artery
Gastroduodenal
artery
Posterior superior
pancreatico-
duodenal artery
Anterior superior
pancreatico-
duodenal artery
Artery of
pancreatic
tail
Great pancreatic
artery
Inferior pancreatic
artery
Dorsal pancreatic
artery
Inferior pancreatico-
duodenal artery,
anterior branch
Superior
mesenteric artery

A Celiac trunk distribution.

B Arterial supply to the pancreas

Fig. 14.4 Superior mesenteric artery

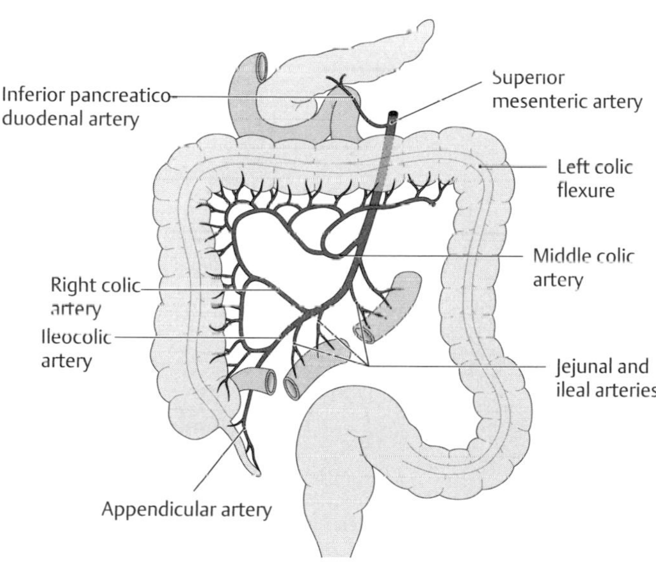
Inferior pancreatico-
duodenal artery
Superior
mesenteric artery
Left colic
flexure
Middle colic
artery
Right colic
artery
Ileocolic
artery
Jejunal and
ileal arteries
Appendicular artery

Fig. 14.5 Inferior mesenteric artery

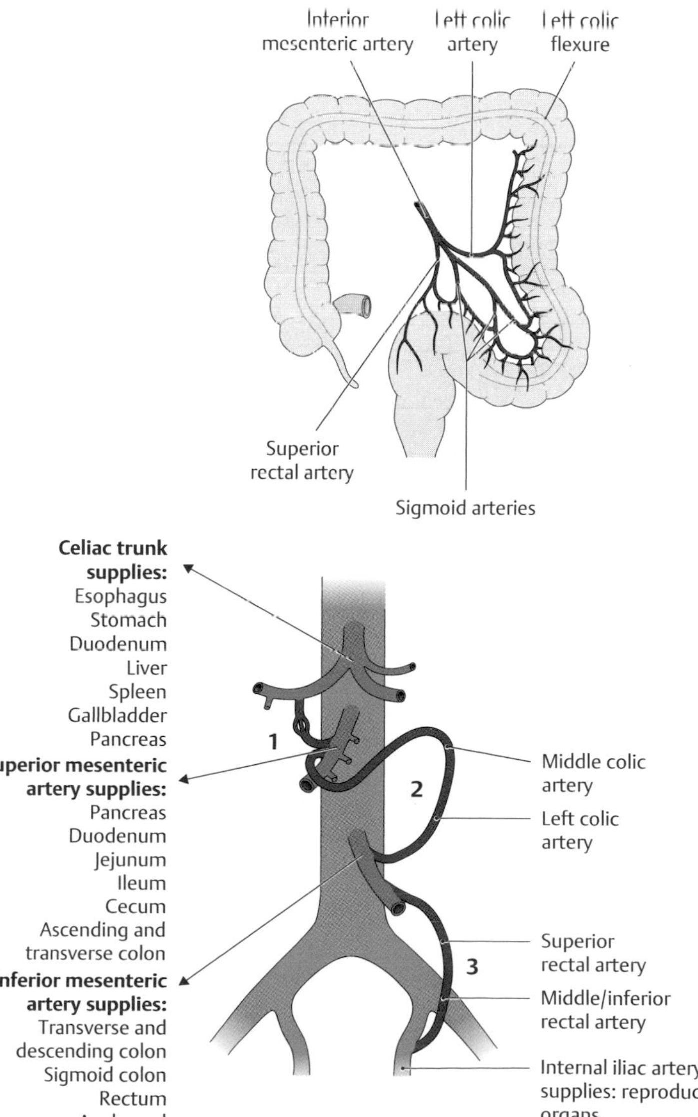
Inferior
mesenteric artery
Left colic
artery
Left colic
flexure
Superior
rectal artery
Sigmoid arteries
Celiac trunk supplies:
Esophagus
Stomach
Duodenum
Liver
Spleen
Gallbladder
Pancreas
Superior mesenteric artery supplies:
Pancreas
Duodenum
Jejunum
Ileum
Cecum
Ascending and
transverse colon
Inferior mesenteric artery supplies:
Transverse and
descending colon
Sigmoid colon
Rectum
Anal canal
1
2
3
Middle colic
artery
Left colic
artery
Superior
rectal artery
Middle/inferior
rectal artery
Internal iliac artery
supplies: reproductive
organs

Fig. 14.6 Abdominal arterial anastomoses

The three major arterial anastomoses of the abdomen – (1) between the celiac trunk and the superior mesenteric artery via the pancreaticoduodenal arteries, (2) between the superior and inferior mesenteric arteries via the middle and left colic arteries, and (3) between the inferior mesenteric and the internal iliac arteries via the superior and middle or inferior rectal arteries– provide overlap in the arterial supply to abdominal areas to ensure adequate blood flow.

Abdominal Aorta & Renal Arteries

Fig. 14.7 **Abdominal aorta**
Anterior view of the female abdomen. *Removed:* All organs except the left kidney and suprarenal gland. The abdominal aorta is the distal continuation of the thoracic aorta (see p. 76). It enters the abdomen at the T12 level and bifurcates into the common iliac arteries at L4.

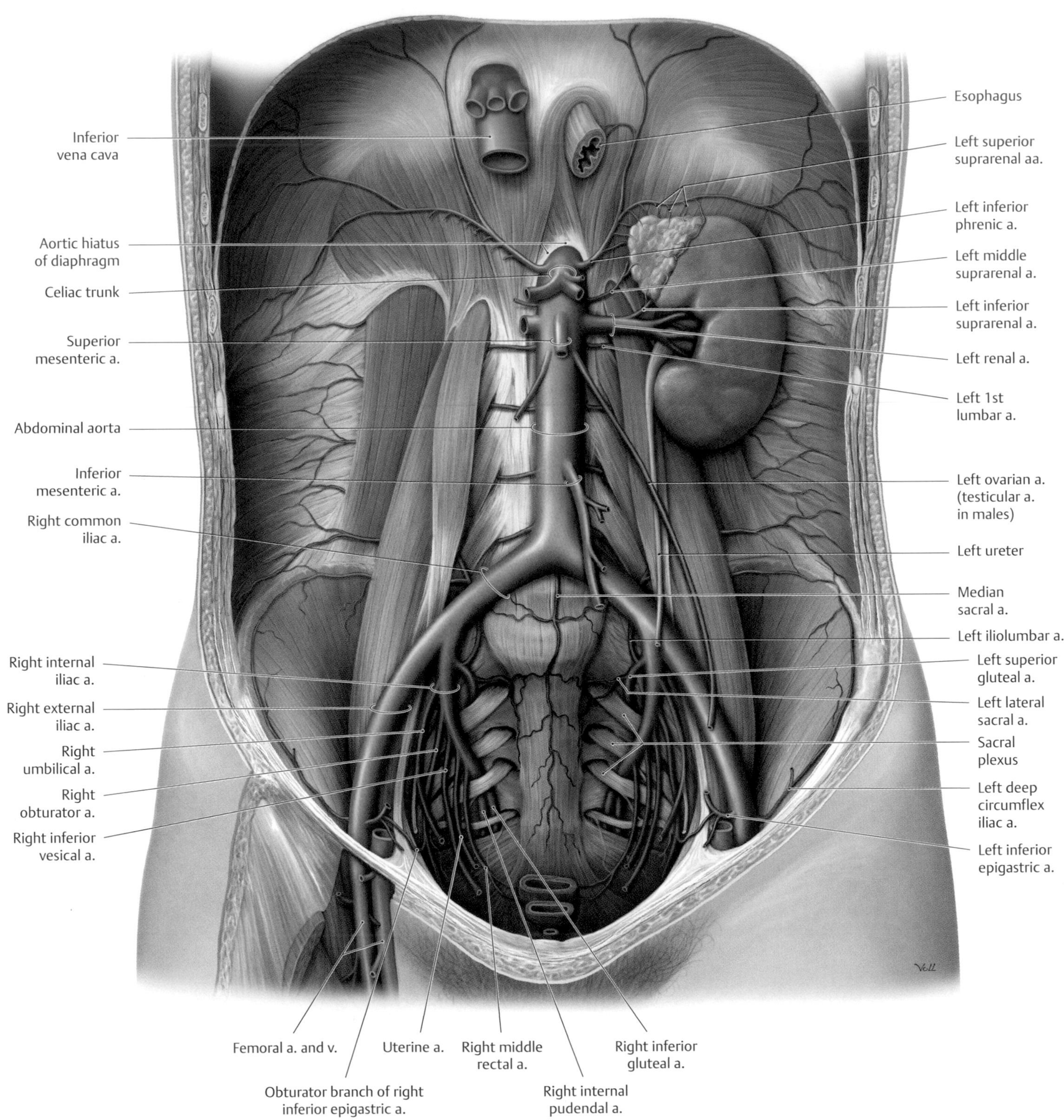
Inferior vena cava
Aortic hiatus of diaphragm
Celiac trunk
Superior mesenteric a.
Abdominal aorta
Inferior mesenteric a.
Right common iliac a.
Right internal iliac a.
Right external iliac a.
Right umbilical a.
Right obturator a.
Right inferior vesical a.
Esophagus
Left superior suprarenal aa.
Left inferior phrenic a.
Left middle suprarenal a.
Left inferior suprarenal a.
Left renal a.
Left 1st lumbar a.
Left ovarian a. (testicular a. in males)
Left ureter
Median sacral a.
Left iliolumbar a.
Left superior gluteal a.
Left lateral sacral a.
Sacral plexus
Left deep circumflex iliac a.
Left inferior epigastric a.
Femoral a. and v.
Uterine a.
Right middle rectal a.
Right inferior gluteal a.
Obturator branch of right inferior epigastric a.
Right internal pudendal a.

Fig. 14.8 Renal arteries

Left kidney, anterior view. The renal arteries arise at approximately the level of L2. Each renal artery divides into an anterior and a posterior branch. The anterior branch further divides into four segmental arteries (circled).

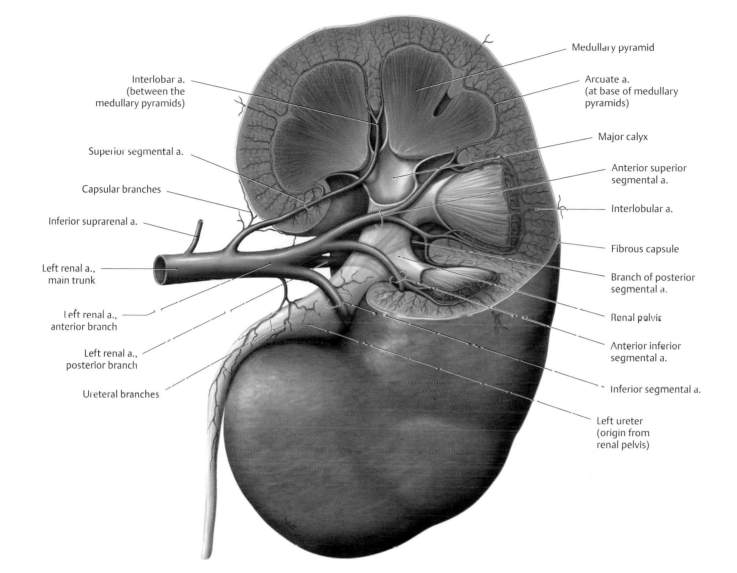

Interlobar a. (between the medullary pyramids)
Superior segmental a.
Capsular branches
Inferior suprarenal a.
Left renal a., main trunk
Left renal a., anterior branch
Left renal a., posterior branch
Ureteral branches
Medullary pyramid
Arcuate a. (at base of medullary pyramids)
Major calyx
Anterior superior segmental a.
Interlobular a.
Fibrous capsule
Branch of posterior segmental a.
Renal pelvis
Anterior inferior segmental a.
Inferior segmental a.
Left ureter (origin from renal pelvis)

Clinical

Renal hypertension

The kidney is an important blood pressure sensor and regulator. Stenosis (narrowing) of the renal artery reduces blood flow through the kidney and stimulates increased production of renin, an enzyme that cleaves angiotensinogen to form angiotensin I. Subsequent cleavage yields angiotensin II, which induces vasoconstriction and an increase in blood pressure. Renal hypertension must be excluded (or confirmed) when diagnosing high blood pressure.

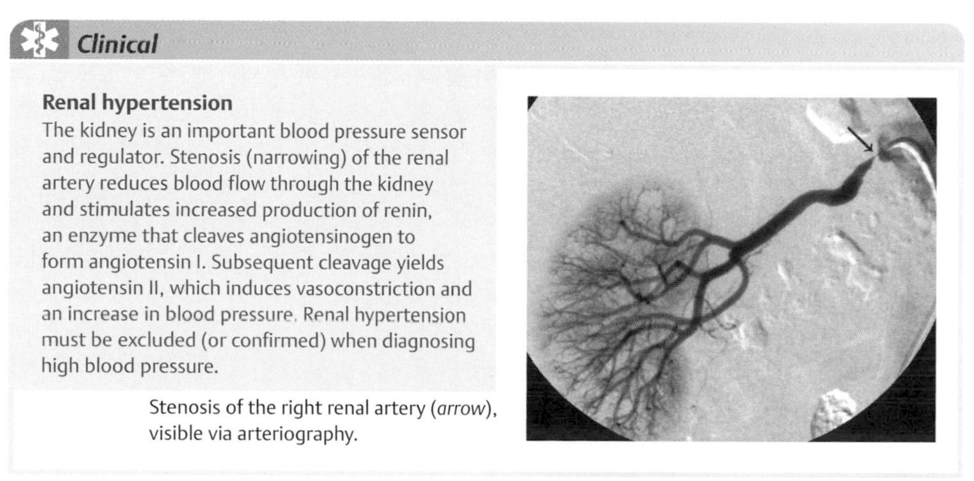

Stenosis of the right renal artery (*arrow*), visible via arteriography.

Celiac Trunk

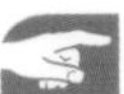
The distribution of the celiac trunk is shown on p. 177.

Fig. 14.9 **Celiac trunk: Stomach, liver, and gallbladder**
Anterior view. *Opened:* Lesser omentum. *Incised:* Greater omentum. The celiac trunk arises from the abdominal aorta at about the level of L1.

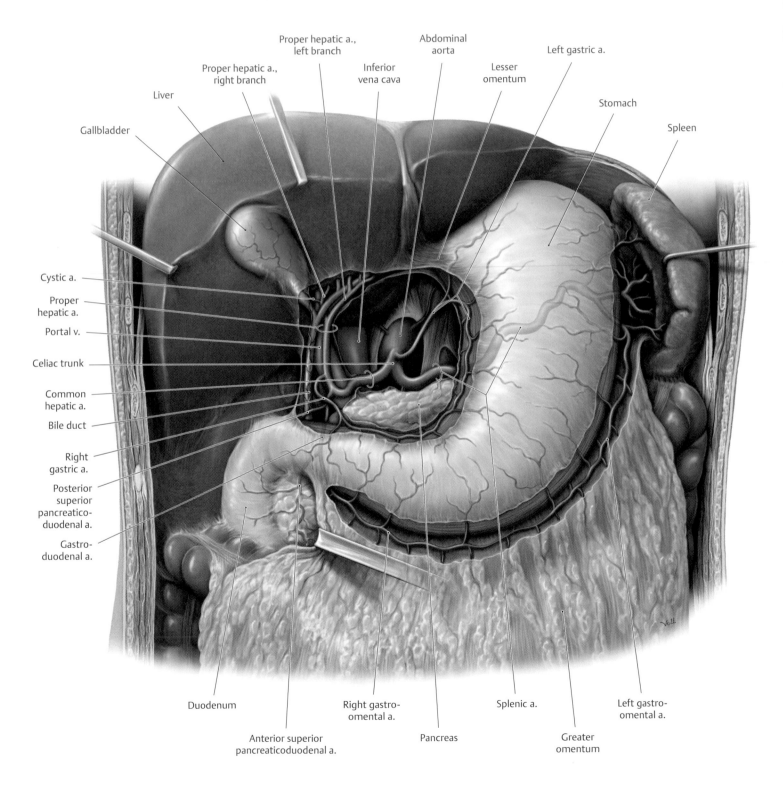

Proper hepatic a., left branch
Abdominal aorta
Left gastric a.
Proper hepatic a., right branch
Inferior vena cava
Lesser omentum
Liver
Stomach
Gallbladder
Spleen
Cystic a.
Proper hepatic a.
Portal v.
Celiac trunk
Common hepatic a.
Bile duct
Right gastric a.
Posterior superior pancreaticoduodenal a.
Gastroduodenal a.
Duodenum
Right gastro-omental a.
Splenic a.
Left gastro-omental a.
Anterior superior pancreaticoduodenal a.
Pancreas
Greater omentum

Fig. 14.10 **Celiac trunk: Pancreas, duodenum, and spleen**
Anterior view. *Removed:* Stomach (body) and lesser omentum.

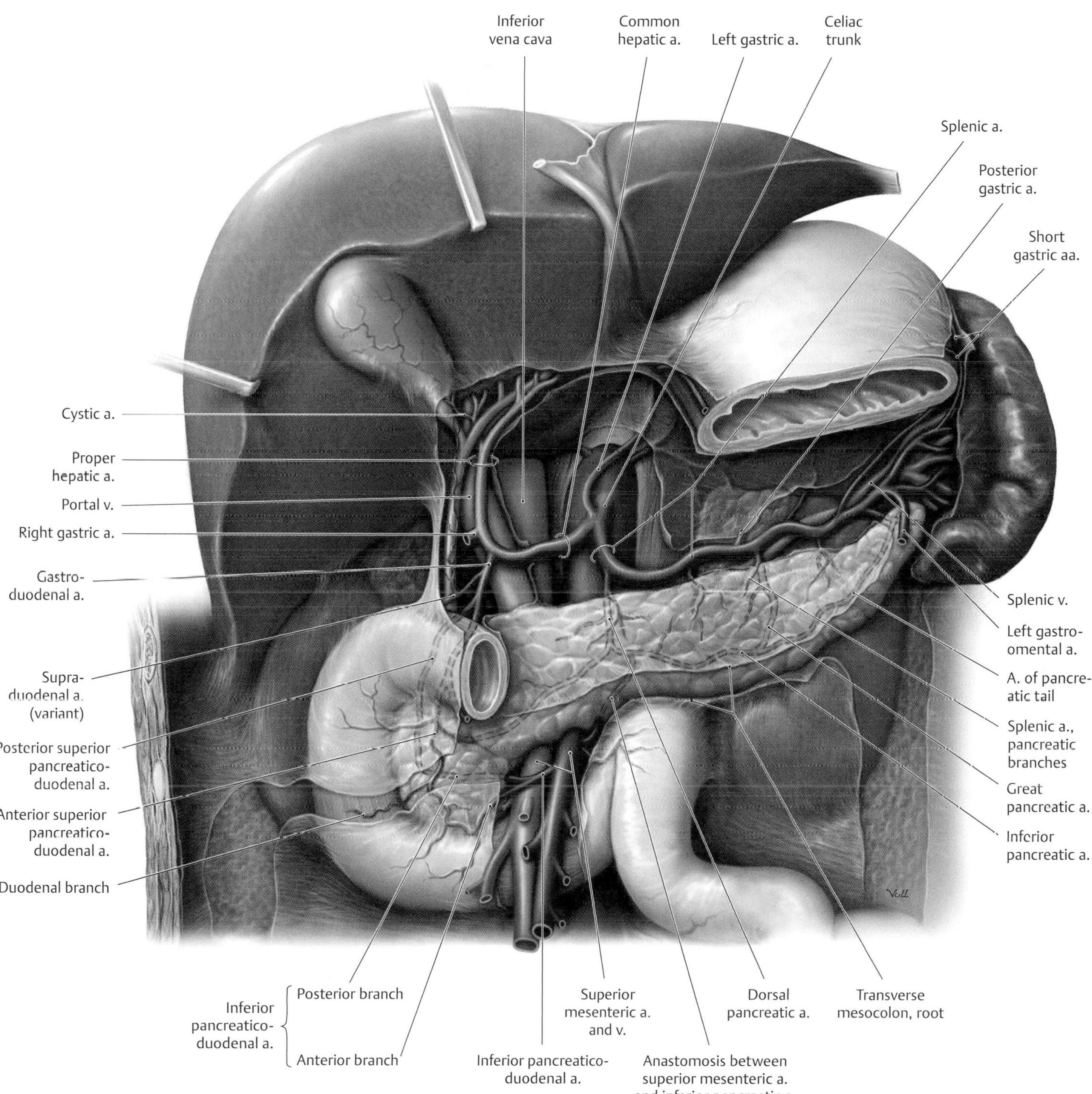
Inferior vena cava
Common hepatic a.
Left gastric a.
Celiac trunk
Splenic a.
Posterior gastric a.
Short gastric aa.
Cystic a.
Proper hepatic a.
Portal v.
Right gastric a.
Gastro-duodenal a.
Supra-duodenal a. (variant)
Posterior superior pancreatico-duodenal a.
Anterior superior pancreatico-duodenal a.
Duodenal branch
Splenic v.
Left gastro-omental a.
A. of pancre-atic tail
Splenic a., pancreatic branches
Great pancreatic a.
Inferior pancreatic a.
Inferior pancreatico-duodenal a.
Posterior branch
Anterior branch
Superior mesenteric a. and v.
Inferior pancreatico-duodenal a.
Dorsal pancreatic a.
Anastomosis between superior mesenteric a. and inferior pancreatic a.
Transverse mesocolon, root

Superior & Inferior Mesenteric Arteries

***Fig. 14.11* Superior mesenteric artery**
Anterior view. *Partially removed:* Stomach, duodenum, and peritoneum. *Reflected:* Liver and gallbladder. *Note:* The middle colic artery has been truncated (see Fig. 14.12). The superior and inferior mesenteric arteries arise from the aorta opposite L2 and L3, respectively.

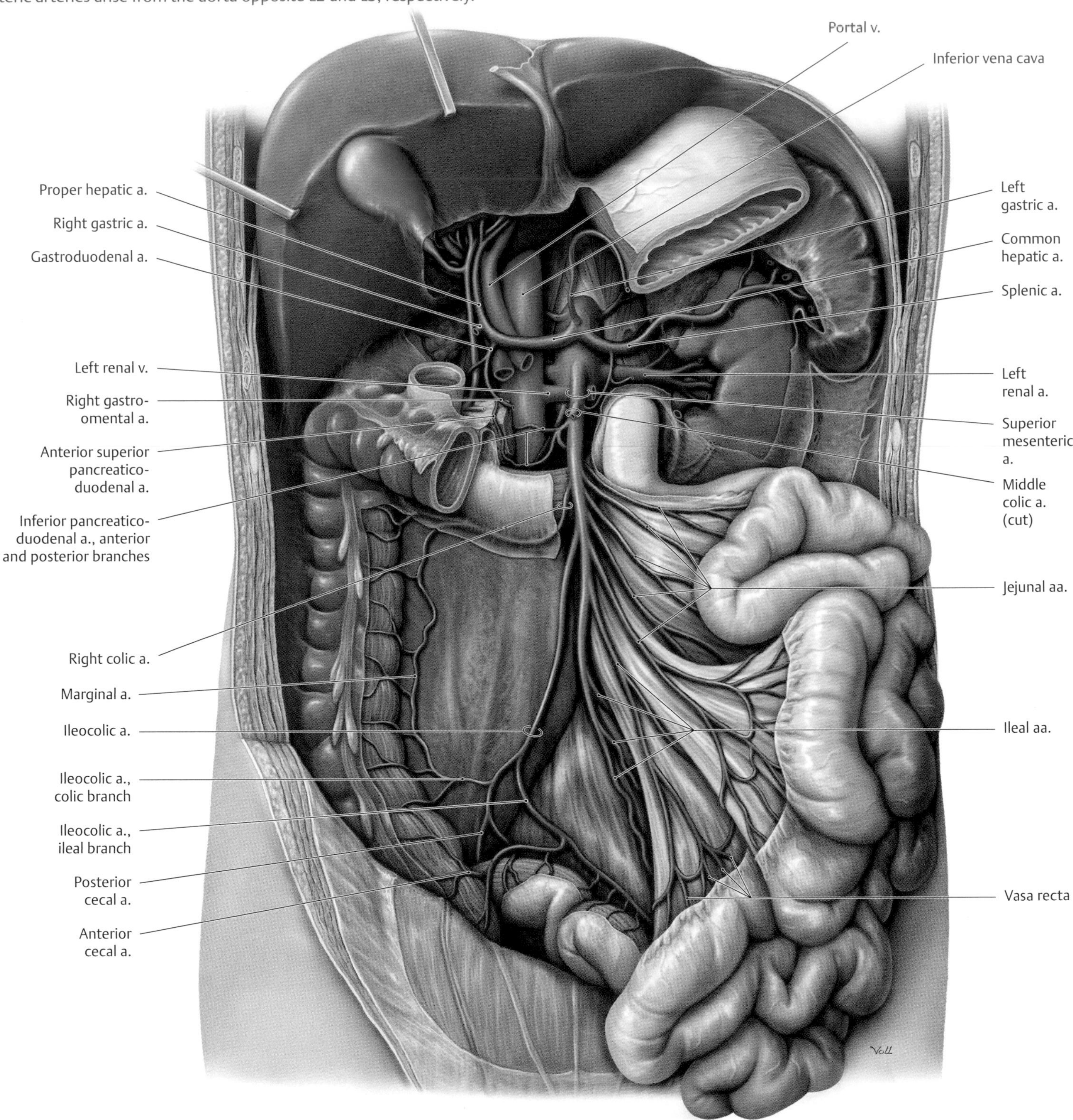
Portal v.
Inferior vena cava
Proper hepatic a.
Right gastric a.
Gastroduodenal a.
Left gastric a.
Common hepatic a.
Splenic a.
Left renal v.
Right gastro-omental a.
Anterior superior pancreatico-duodenal a.
Inferior pancreatico-duodenal a., anterior and posterior branches
Left renal a.
Superior mesenteric a.
Middle colic a. (cut)
Jejunal aa.
Right colic a.
Marginal a.
Ileocolic a.
Ileocolic a., colic branch
Ileocolic a., ileal branch
Posterior cecal a.
Anterior cecal a.
Ileal aa.
Vasa recta
Voll

Fig. 14.12 Inferior mesenteric artery
Anterior view. *Removed:* Jejunum and ileum. *Reflected:* Transverse colon.

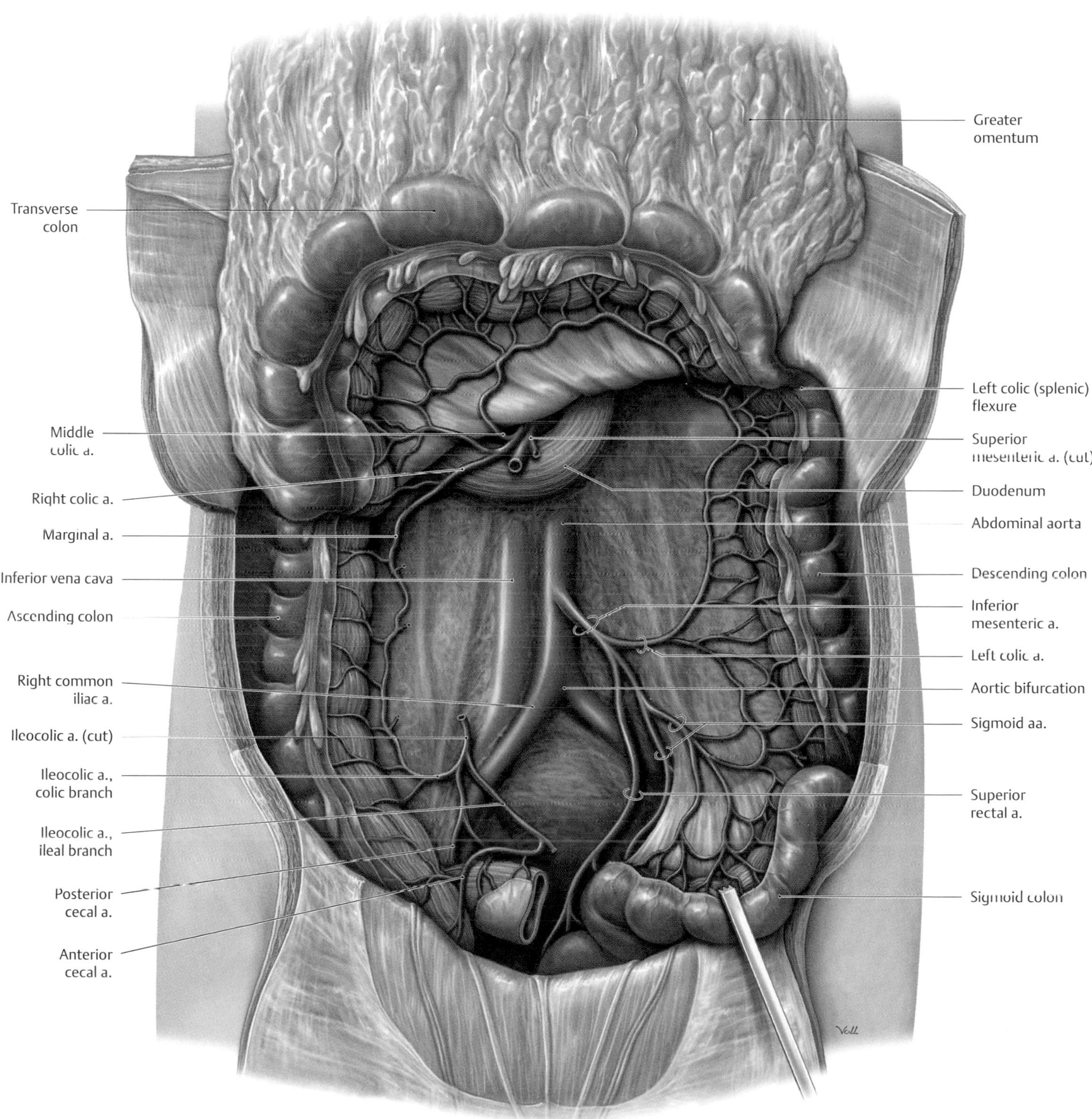
Greater omentum
Transverse colon
Left colic (splenic) flexure
Middle colic a.
Superior mesenteric a. (cut)
Right colic a.
Duodenum
Marginal a.
Abdominal aorta
Inferior vena cava
Descending colon
Ascending colon
Inferior mesenteric a.
Left colic a.
Right common iliac a.
Aortic bifurcation
Ileocolic a. (cut)
Sigmoid aa.
Ileocolic a., colic branch
Superior rectal a.
Ileocolic a., ileal branch
Posterior cecal a.
Sigmoid colon
Anterior cecal a.

Veins of the Abdomen

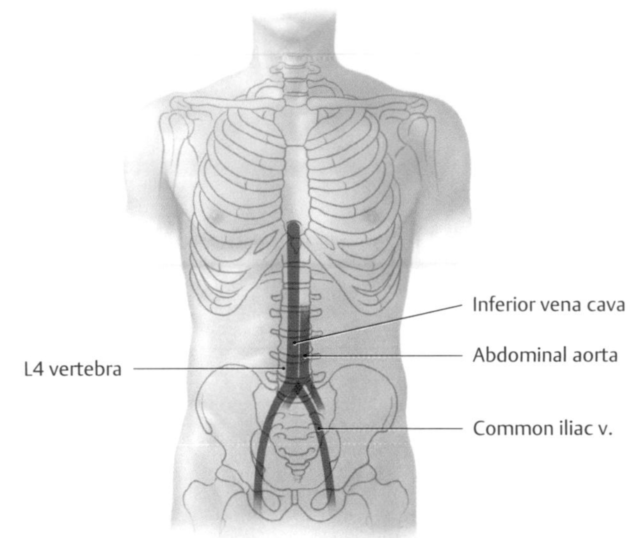
Inferior vena cava
Abdominal aorta
L4 vertebra
Common iliac v.

Fig. 14.13 **Inferior vena cava: Location**
Anterior view.

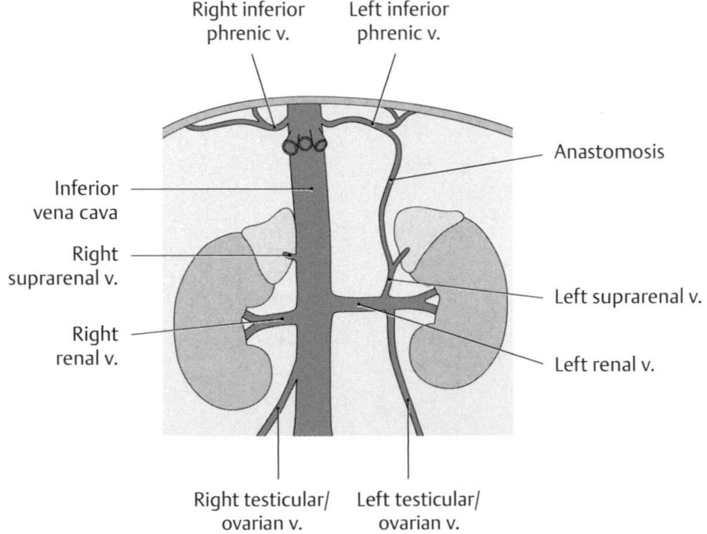
Right inferior phrenic v.
Left inferior phrenic v.
Anastomosis
Inferior vena cava
Right suprarenal v.
Left suprarenal v.
Right renal v.
Left renal v.
Right testicular/ ovarian v.
Left testicular/ ovarian v.

Fig. 14.14 **Tributaries of the renal veins**
Anterior view.

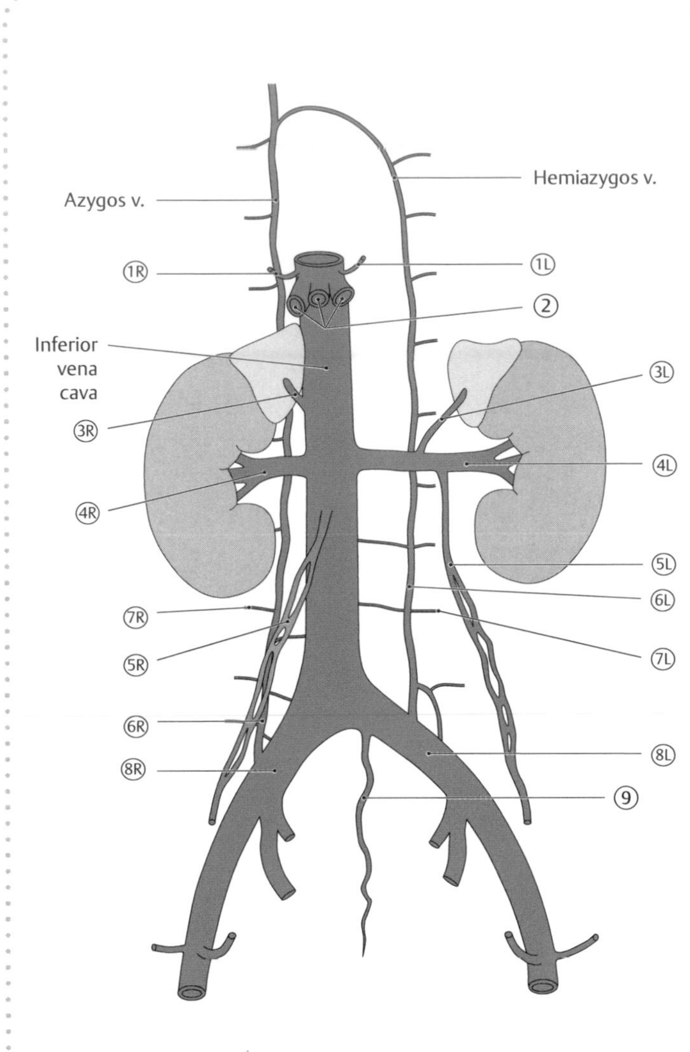
Azygos v.
Hemiazygos v.
1R
1L
2
Inferior vena cava
3R
3L
4R
4L
5L
6L
7R
7L
5R
6R
8R
8L
9

Table 14.2		Tributaries of the inferior vena cava
1R	1L	Inferior phrenic vv. (paired)
2		Hepatic vv. (3)
3R	3L	Suprarenal vv. (the right vein is a direct tributary)
4R	4L	Renal vv. (paired)
5R	5L	Testicular/ovarian vv. (the right vein is a direct tributary)
6R	6L	Ascending lumbar vv. (paired), not direct tributaries
7R	7L	Lumbar vv.
8R	8L	Common iliac vv. (paired)
9		Median sacral v.

Fig. 14.15 Portal vein

The portal vein (see p. 188) drains venous blood from the abdominopelvic organs supplied by the celiac trunk and superior and inferior mesenteric arteries.

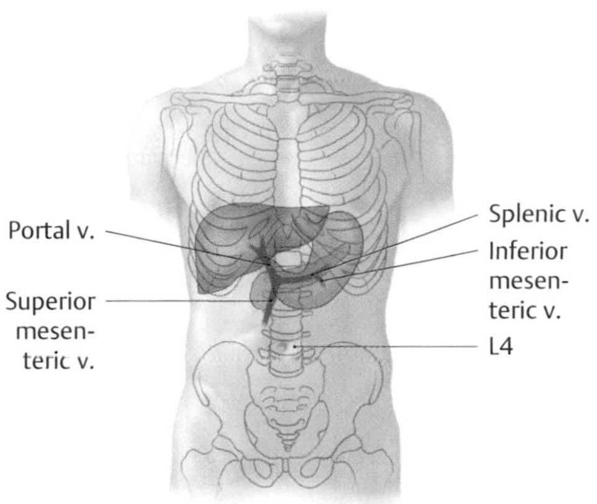
Portal v.
Superior mesenteric v.
Splenic v.
Inferior mesenteric v.
L4

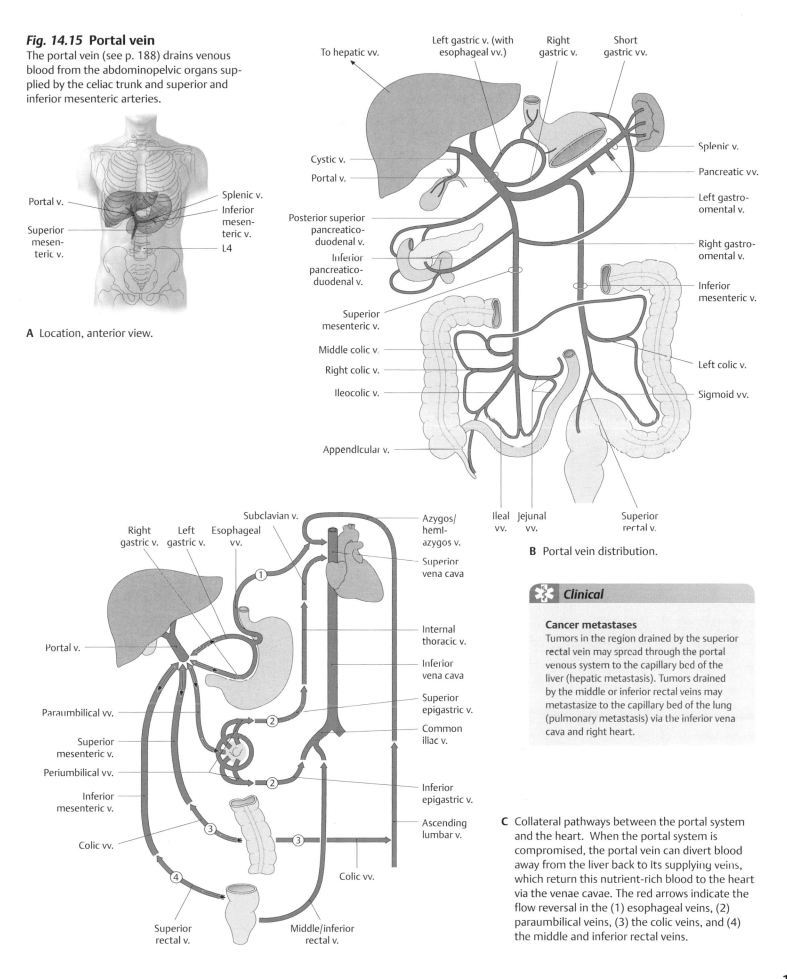

A Location, anterior view.

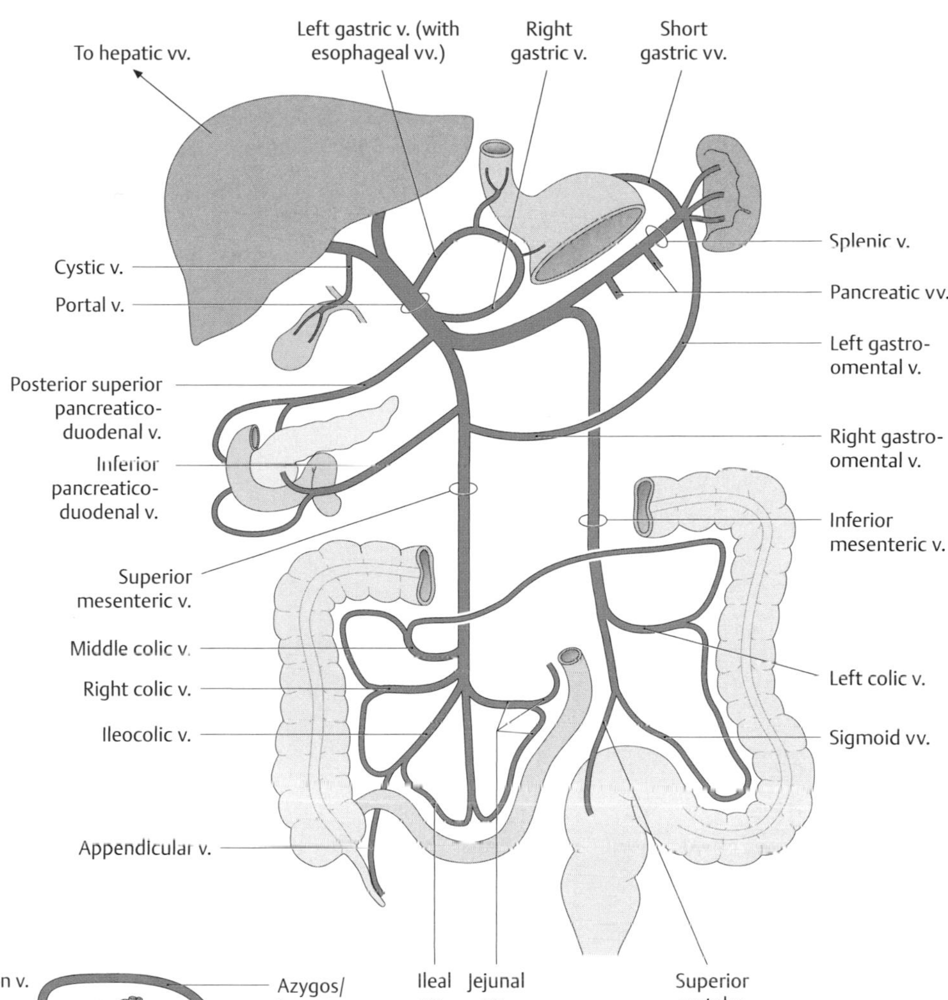
To hepatic vv.
Left gastric v. (with esophageal vv.)
Right gastric v.
Short gastric vv.
Cystic v.
Portal v.
Splenic v.
Pancreatic vv.
Left gastro-omental v.
Posterior superior pancreaticoduodenal v.
Inferior pancreaticoduodenal v.
Right gastro-omental v.
Inferior mesenteric v.
Superior mesenteric v.
Middle colic v.
Right colic v.
Ileocolic v.
Left colic v.
Sigmoid vv.
Appendicular v.
Ileal vv.
Jejunal vv.
Superior rectal v.

B Portal vein distribution.

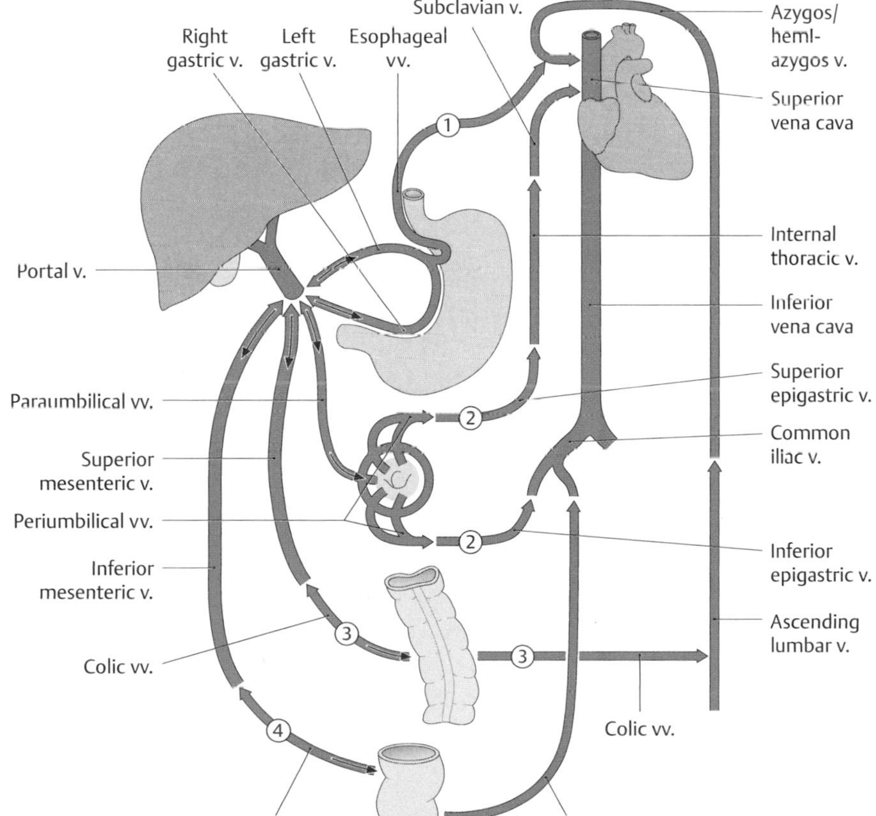
Subclavian v.
Right gastric v.
Left gastric v.
Esophageal vv.
Azygos/hemiazygos v.
Superior vena cava
Portal v.
Internal thoracic v.
Inferior vena cava
Paraumbilical vv.
Superior epigastric v.
Common iliac v.
Superior mesenteric v.
Periumbilical vv.
Inferior mesenteric v.
Inferior epigastric v.
Colic vv.
Ascending lumbar v.
Colic vv.
Superior rectal v.
Middle/inferior rectal v.
1
2
2
3
3
4

C Collateral pathways between the portal system and the heart. When the portal system is compromised, the portal vein can divert blood away from the liver back to its supplying veins, which return this nutrient-rich blood to the heart via the venae cavae. The red arrows indicate the flow reversal in the (1) esophageal veins, (2) paraumbilical veins, (3) the colic veins, and (4) the middle and inferior rectal veins.

> ***Clinical***
>
> **Cancer metastases**
>
> Tumors in the region drained by the superior rectal vein may spread through the portal venous system to the capillary bed of the liver (hepatic metastasis). Tumors drained by the middle or inferior rectal veins may metastasize to the capillary bed of the lung (pulmonary metastasis) via the inferior vena cava and right heart.

Inferior Vena Cava & Renal Veins

Fig. 14.16 **Inferior vena cava**
Anterior view of the female abdomen. *Removed:* All organs except the left kidney and suprarenal gland.

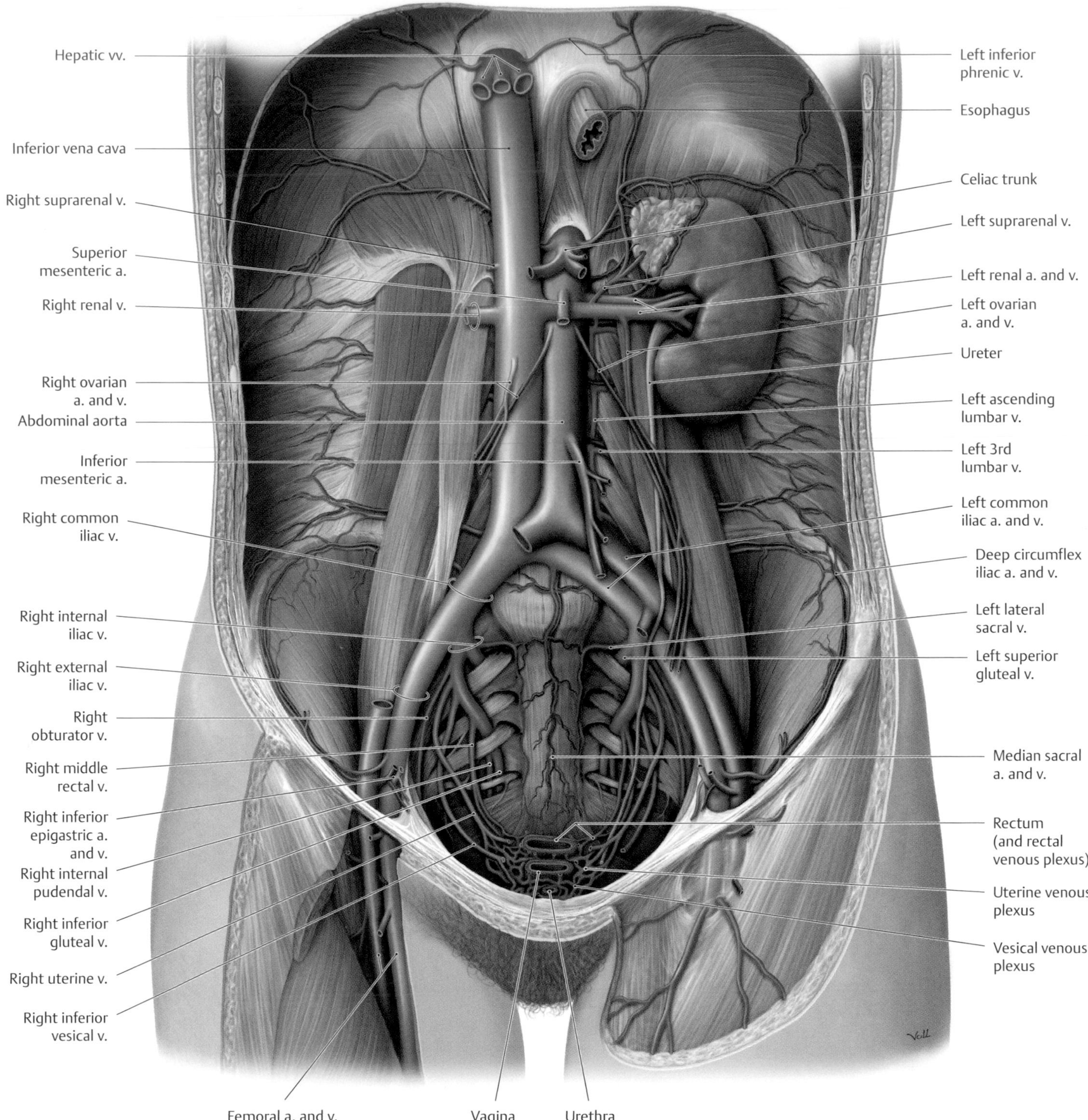
Hepatic vv.
Inferior vena cava
Right suprarenal v.
Superior mesenteric a.
Right renal v.
Right ovarian a. and v.
Abdominal aorta
Inferior mesenteric a.
Right common iliac v.
Right internal iliac v.
Right external iliac v.
Right obturator v.
Right middle rectal v.
Right inferior epigastric a. and v.
Right internal pudendal v.
Right inferior gluteal v.
Right uterine v.
Right inferior vesical v.
Femoral a. and v.
Vagina
Urethra
Left inferior phrenic v.
Esophagus
Celiac trunk
Left suprarenal v.
Left renal a. and v.
Left ovarian a. and v.
Ureter
Left ascending lumbar v.
Left 3rd lumbar v.
Left common iliac a. and v.
Deep circumflex iliac a. and v.
Left lateral sacral v.
Left superior gluteal v.
Median sacral a. and v.
Rectum (and rectal venous plexus)
Uterine venous plexus
Vesical venous plexus

Fig. 14.17 **Renal veins**
Anterior view. See p. 179 for the renal arteries in isolation.
Removed: All organs except kidneys and suprarenal glands.

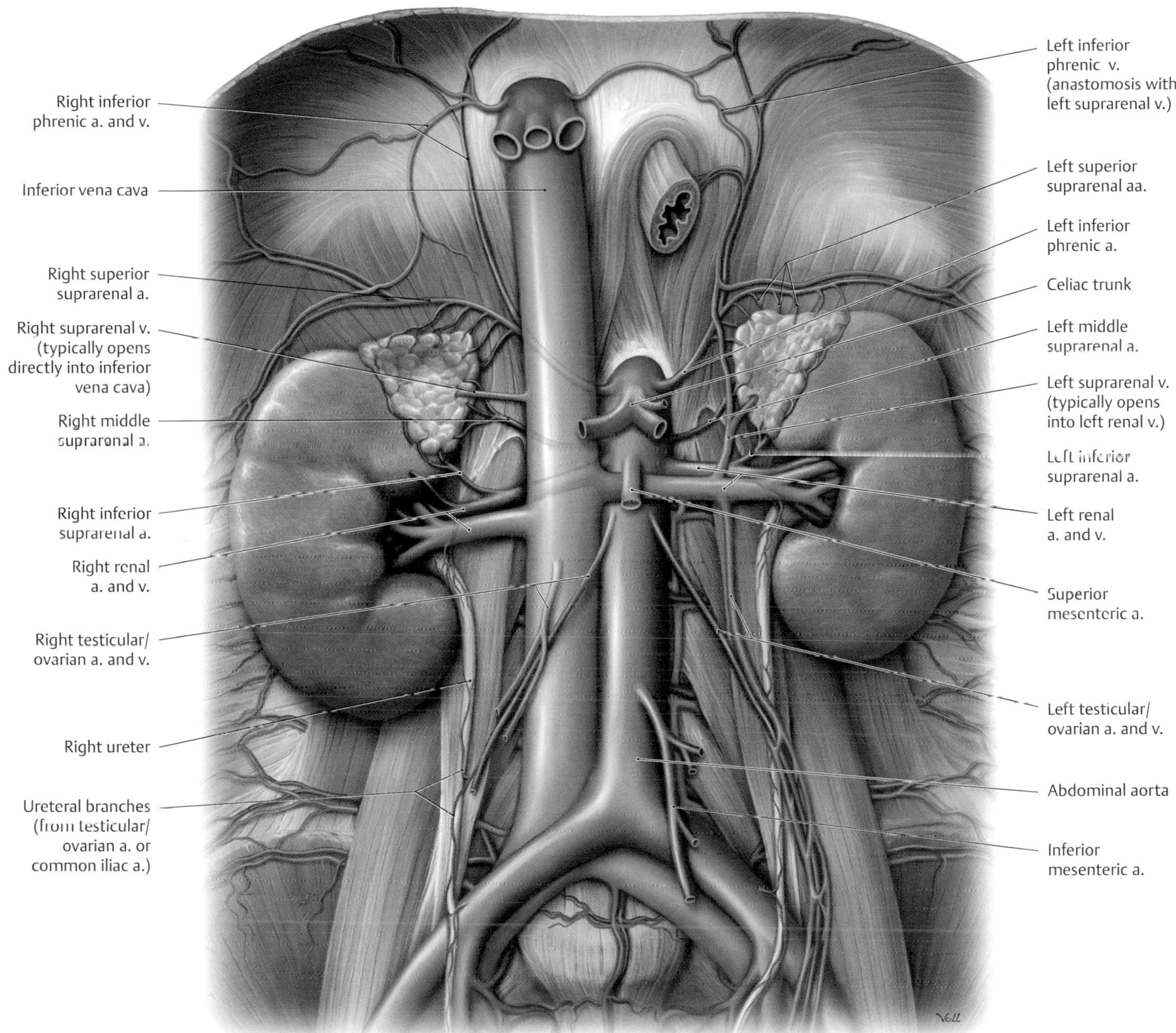

Right inferior phrenic a. and v.
Inferior vena cava
Right superior suprarenal a.
Right suprarenal v. (typically opens directly into inferior vena cava)
Right middle suprarenal a.
Right inferior suprarenal a.
Right renal a. and v.
Right testicular/ ovarian a. and v.
Right ureter
Ureteral branches (from testicular/ ovarian a. or common iliac a.)
Left inferior phrenic v. (anastomosis with left suprarenal v.)
Left superior suprarenal aa.
Left inferior phrenic a.
Celiac trunk
Left middle suprarenal a.
Left suprarenal v. (typically opens into left renal v.)
Left inferior suprarenal a.
Left renal a. and v.
Superior mesenteric a.
Left testicular/ ovarian a. and v.
Abdominal aorta
Inferior mesenteric a.

Portal Vein

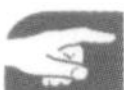

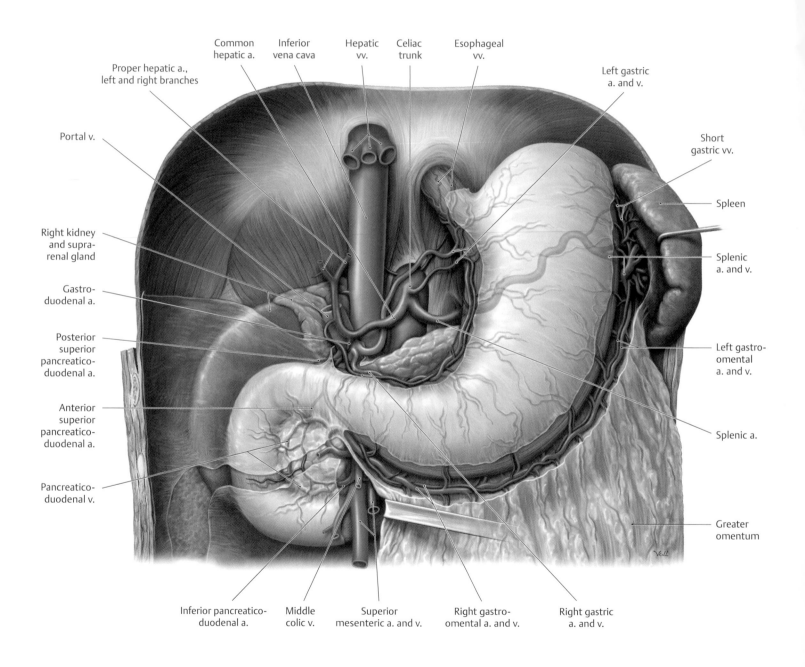

The portal vein is typically formed by the union of the superior mesenteric and the splenic veins posterior to the neck of the pancreas. The distribution of the portal vein is shown on p. 185.

Fig. 14.18 Portal vein: Stomach and duodenum
Anterior view. *Removed:* Liver, lesser omentum, and peritoneum. *Opened:* Greater omentum.

Common hepatic a.
Inferior vena cava
Hepatic vv.
Celiac trunk
Esophageal vv.
Proper hepatic a., left and right branches
Left gastric a. and v.
Portal v.
Short gastric vv.
Spleen
Right kidney and supra-renal gland
Splenic a. and v.
Gastro-duodenal a.
Posterior superior pancreatico-duodenal a.
Left gastro-omental a. and v.
Anterior superior pancreatico-duodenal a.
Splenic a.
Pancreatico-duodenal v.
Greater omentum
Inferior pancreatico-duodenal a.
Middle colic v.
Superior mesenteric a. and v.
Right gastro-omental a. and v.
Right gastric a. and v.

Fig. 14.19 Portal vein: Pancreas and spleen
Anterior view. *Partially removed:* Liver, stomach, pancreas, and peritoneum.

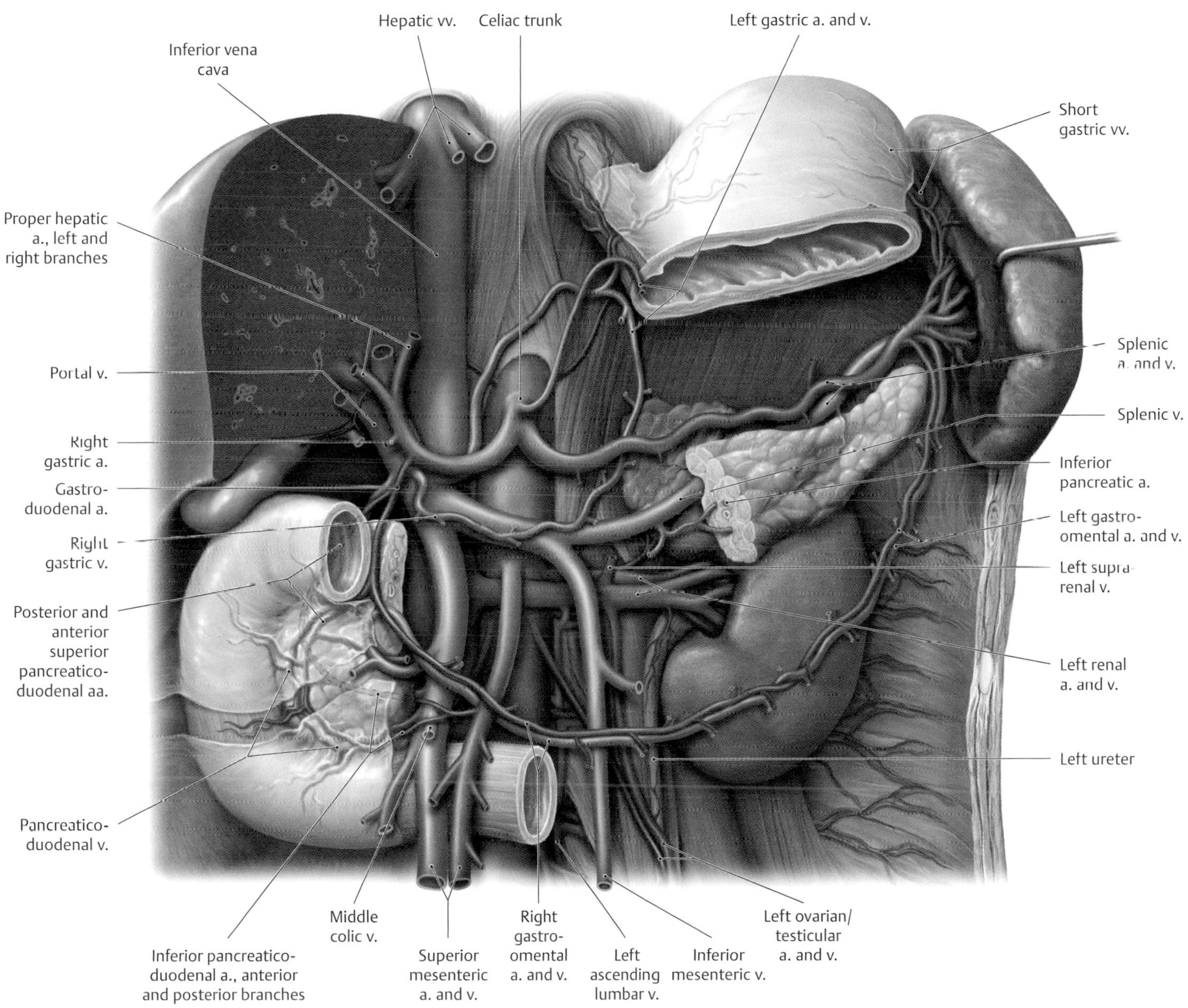

Hepatic vv.
Celiac trunk
Left gastric a. and v.
Inferior vena cava
Short gastric vv.
Proper hepatic a., left and right branches
Splenic a. and v.
Portal v.
Splenic v.
Right gastric a.
Inferior pancreatic a.
Gastro-duodenal a.
Left gastro-omental a. and v.
Right gastric v.
Left supra-renal v.
Posterior and anterior superior pancreatico-duodenal aa.
Left renal a. and v.
Left ureter
Pancreatico-duodenal v.
Middle colic v.
Right gastro-omental a. and v.
Left ovarian/testicular a. and v.
Inferior pancreatico-duodenal a., anterior and posterior branches
Superior mesenteric a. and v.
Left ascending lumbar v.
Inferior mesenteric v.

Superior & Inferior Mesenteric Veins

Fig. 14.20 Superior mesenteric vein
Anterior view. *Partially removed*: Stomach, duodenum, and peritoneum. *Removed*: Pancreas, greater omentum, and transverse colon. *Reflected*: Liver and gallbladder. *Displaced*: Small intestine.

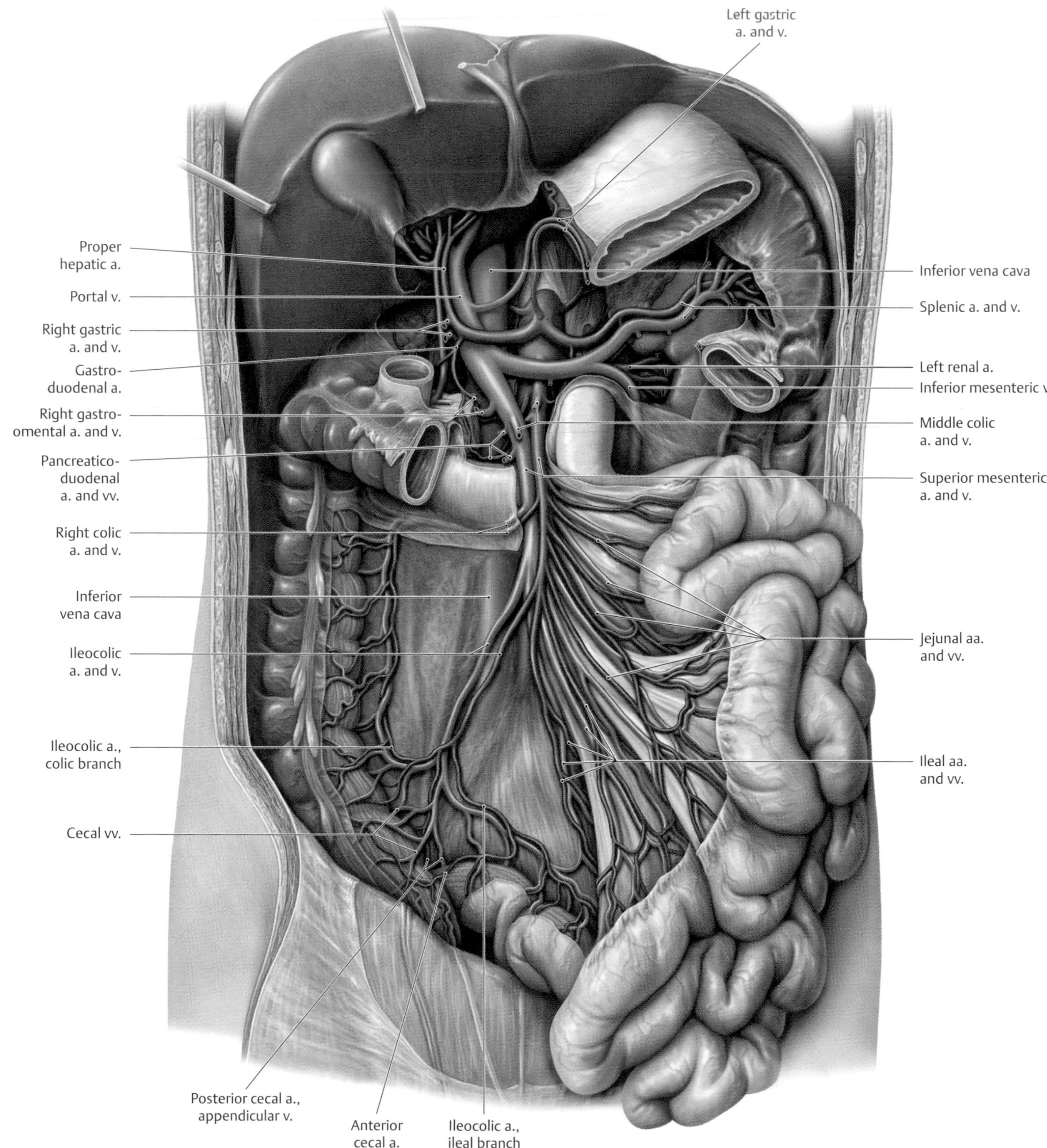

Left gastric a. and v.
Proper hepatic a.
Portal v.
Right gastric a. and v.
Gastro-duodenal a.
Right gastro-omental a. and v.
Pancreatico-duodenal a. and vv.
Right colic a. and v.
Inferior vena cava
Ileocolic a. and v.
Ileocolic a., colic branch
Cecal vv.
Posterior cecal a., appendicular v.
Anterior cecal a.
Ileocolic a., ileal branch
Inferior vena cava
Splenic a. and v.
Left renal a.
Inferior mesenteric v.
Middle colic a. and v.
Superior mesenteric a. and v.
Jejunal aa. and vv.
Ileal aa. and vv.

Fig. 14.21 **Inferior mesenteric vein**
Anterior view. *Partially removed*: Stomach, duodenum, and peritoneum. *Removed*: Pancreas, greater omentum, transverse colon, and small intestine. *Reflected*: Liver and gallbladder.

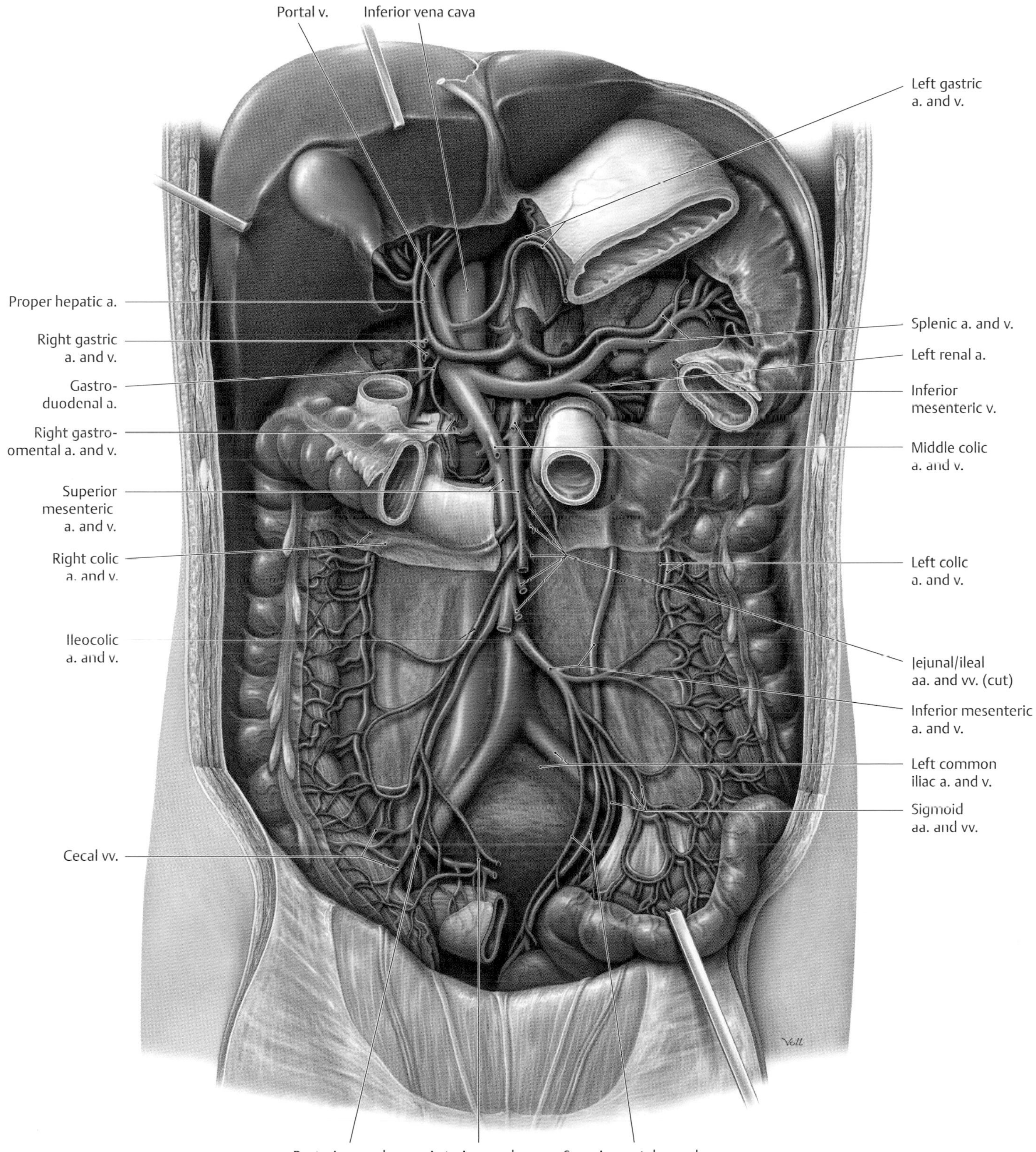
Portal v.
Inferior vena cava
Left gastric a. and v.
Proper hepatic a.
Splenic a. and v.
Right gastric a. and v.
Left renal a.
Gastro-duodenal a.
Inferior mesenteric v.
Right gastro-omental a. and v.
Middle colic a. and v.
Superior mesenteric a. and v.
Right colic a. and v.
Left colic a. and v.
Ileocolic a. and v.
Jejunal/ileal aa. and vv. (cut)
Inferior mesenteric a. and v.
Left common iliac a. and v.
Sigmoid aa. and vv.
Cecal vv.
Posterior cecal a.
Anterior cecal a.
Superior rectal a. and v.

Lymphatics of the Abdominal Organs

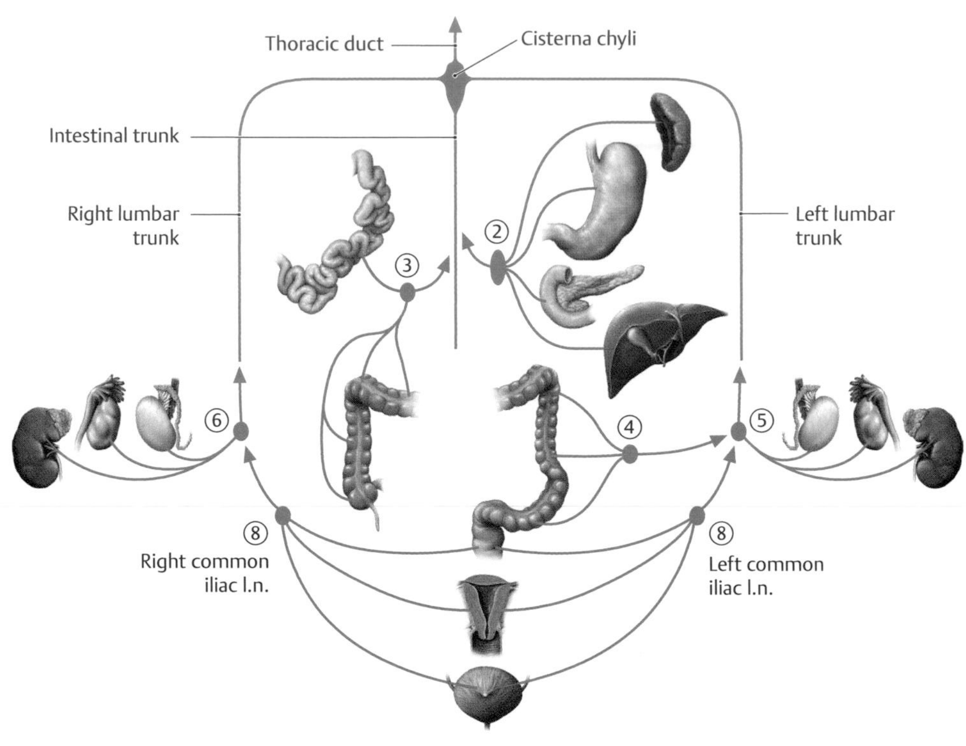

Thoracic duct
Cisterna chyli
Intestinal trunk
Right lumbar trunk
Left lumbar trunk
②
③
④
⑤
⑥
⑧
Right common iliac l.n.
⑧
Left common iliac l.n.

Fig. 14.22 Lymphatic drainage of the internal organs
See Table 14.3 for numbering. Lymph drainage from the abdomen, pelvis, and lower limb ultimately passes through the lumbar lymph nodes (clinically, the aortic nodes). The lumbar lymph nodes consist of the right lateral aortic (caval) and left lateral aortic nodes, the preaortic nodes, and the retroaortic nodes.

Efferent lymph vessels from the lateral aortic lymph nodes and the retroaortic nodes form the lumbar trunks and those from the preaortic nodes form the intestinal trunks, respectively. The lumbar and intestinal trunks terminate into the cisterna chyli.

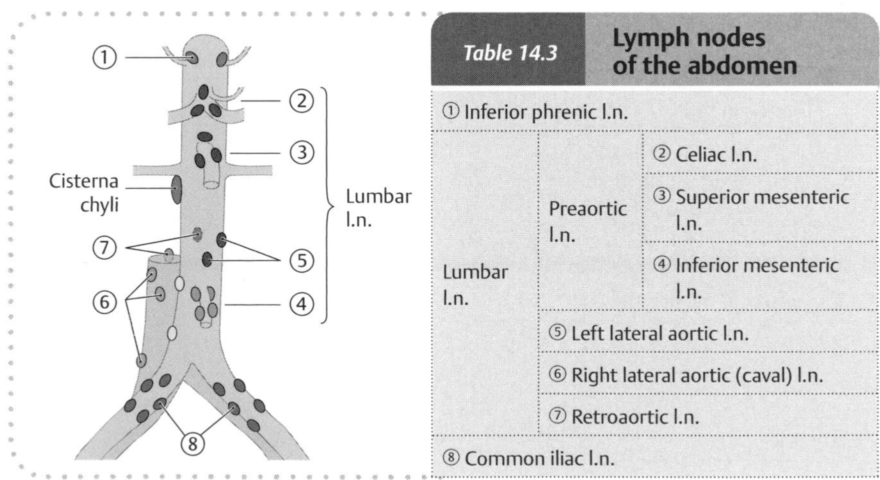

①
②
③
Cisterna chyli
Lumbar l.n.
⑦
⑤
⑥
④
⑧

Table 14.3	Lymph nodes of the abdomen	
① Inferior phrenic l.n.		
Lumbar l.n.	Preaortic l.n.	② Celiac l.n.
		③ Superior mesenteric l.n.
		④ Inferior mesenteric l.n.
	⑤ Left lateral aortic l.n.	
	⑥ Right lateral aortic (caval) l.n.	
	⑦ Retroaortic l.n.	
⑧ Common iliac l.n.		

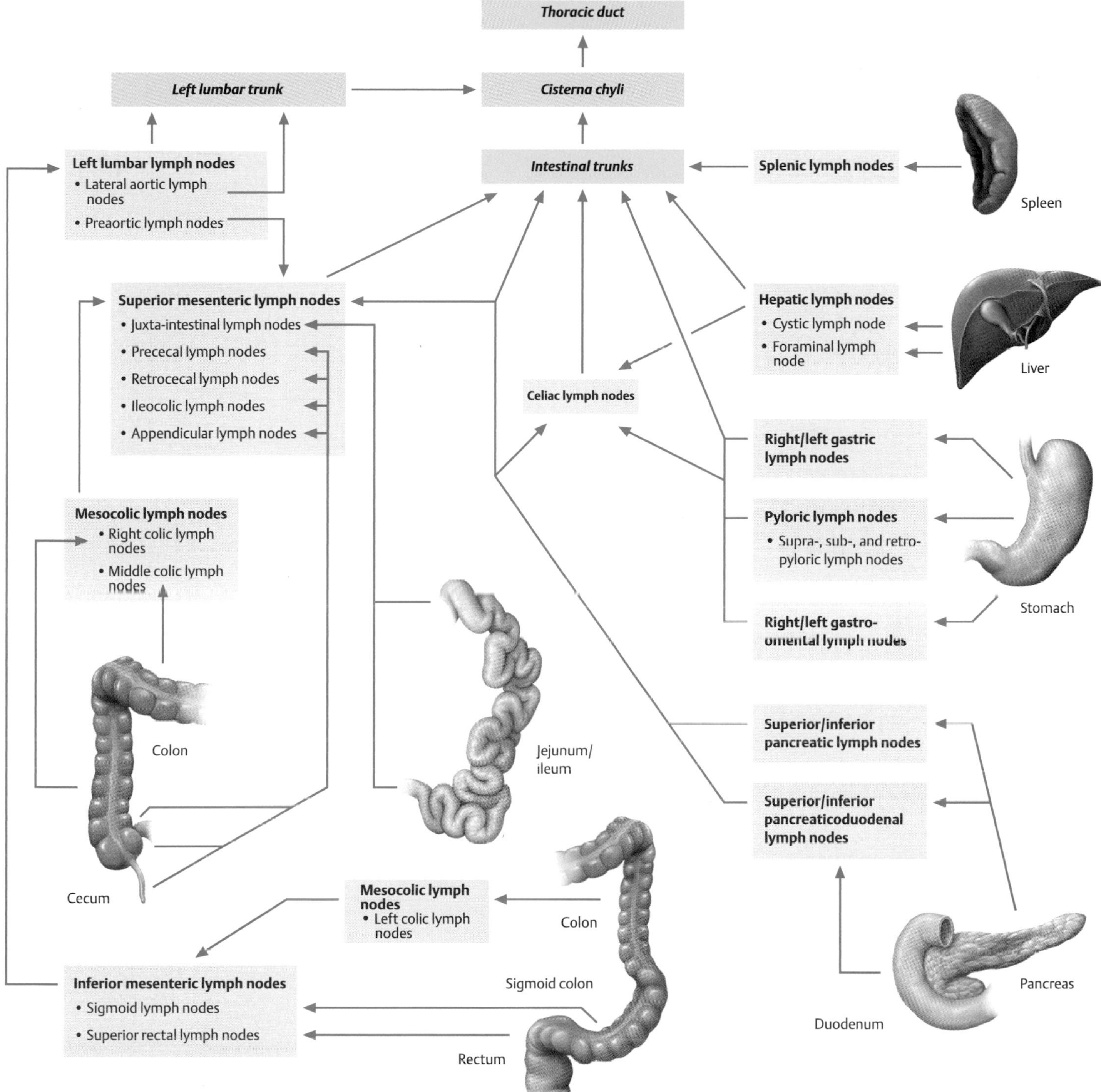
Thoracic duct
Left lumbar trunk
Cisterna chyli
Left lumbar lymph nodes
• Lateral aortic lymph nodes
• Preaortic lymph nodes
Intestinal trunks
Splenic lymph nodes
Spleen
Superior mesenteric lymph nodes
• Juxta-intestinal lymph nodes
• Prececal lymph nodes
• Retrocecal lymph nodes
• Ileocolic lymph nodes
• Appendicular lymph nodes
Hepatic lymph nodes
• Cystic lymph node
• Foraminal lymph node
Liver
Celiac lymph nodes
Right/left gastric lymph nodes
Pyloric lymph nodes
• Supra-, sub-, and retro-pyloric lymph nodes
Stomach
Right/left gastro-omental lymph nodes
Mesocolic lymph nodes
• Right colic lymph nodes
• Middle colic lymph nodes
Colon
Jejunum/ileum
Superior/inferior pancreatic lymph nodes
Superior/inferior pancreaticoduodenal lymph nodes
Cecum
Mesocolic lymph nodes
• Left colic lymph nodes
Colon
Pancreas
Duodenum
Inferior mesenteric lymph nodes
• Sigmoid lymph nodes
• Superior rectal lymph nodes
Sigmoid colon
Rectum

Fig. 14.23 **Principal lymphatic pathways draining the digestive organs and spleen**

Lymph from the spleen and most digestive organs drains directly from regional lymph nodes or through intervening collecting nodes to the intestinal trunks, except for the descending and sigmoid colon and the upper part of the rectum, which are drained by the left lumbar trunk.

The three large collecting nodes are:

- *Celiac lymph nodes* collect lymph from the stomach, duodenum, pancreas, spleen, and liver. Topographically and at dissection they are often indistinguishable from the regional lymph nodes of the nearby upper abdominal organs.
- *Superior mesenteric lymph nodes* collect lymph from the jejunum, ileum, ascending and transverse colon.
- *Inferior mesenteric lymph nodes* collect lymph from the descending and sigmoid colon and rectum.

These nodes drain principally through the intestinal trunks to the cisterna chyli, but there is an accessory drainage route by way of the left lumbar lymph nodes. Lymph from the pelvis also drains up into the inferior mesenteric and lateral aortic lymph nodes. A complete drainage pathway for lymph from the pelvis can be found on p. 259.

Lymph Nodes of the Posterior Abdominal Wall

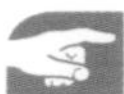

Lymph nodes in the abdomen and pelvis may be classified as either parietal or visceral. The majority of the parietal lymph nodes are located on the posterior abdominal wall.

Fig. 14.24 Parietal lymph nodes in the abdomen and pelvis
Anterior view. *Removed:* All visceral structures except vessels.

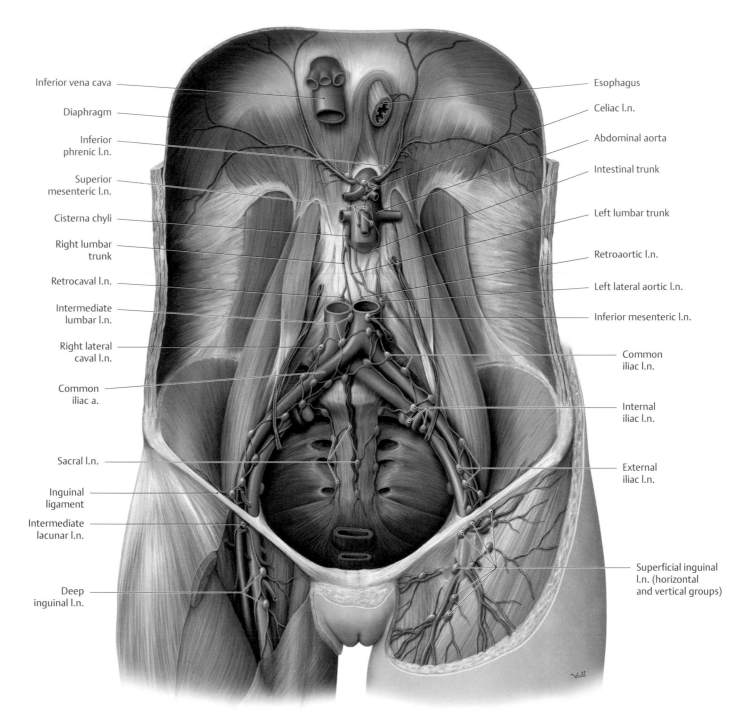

Inferior vena cava
Diaphragm
Inferior phrenic l.n.
Superior mesenteric l.n.
Cisterna chyli
Right lumbar trunk
Retrocaval l.n.
Intermediate lumbar l.n.
Right lateral caval l.n.
Common iliac a.
Sacral l.n.
Inguinal ligament
Intermediate lacunar l.n.
Deep inguinal l.n.
Esophagus
Celiac l.n.
Abdominal aorta
Intestinal trunk
Left lumbar trunk
Retroaortic l.n.
Left lateral aortic l.n.
Inferior mesenteric l.n.
Common iliac l.n.
Internal iliac l.n.
External iliac l.n.
Superficial inguinal l.n. (horizontal and vertical groups)
Voll

***Fig. 14.25* Lymph nodes of the urinary organs**
Anterior view.

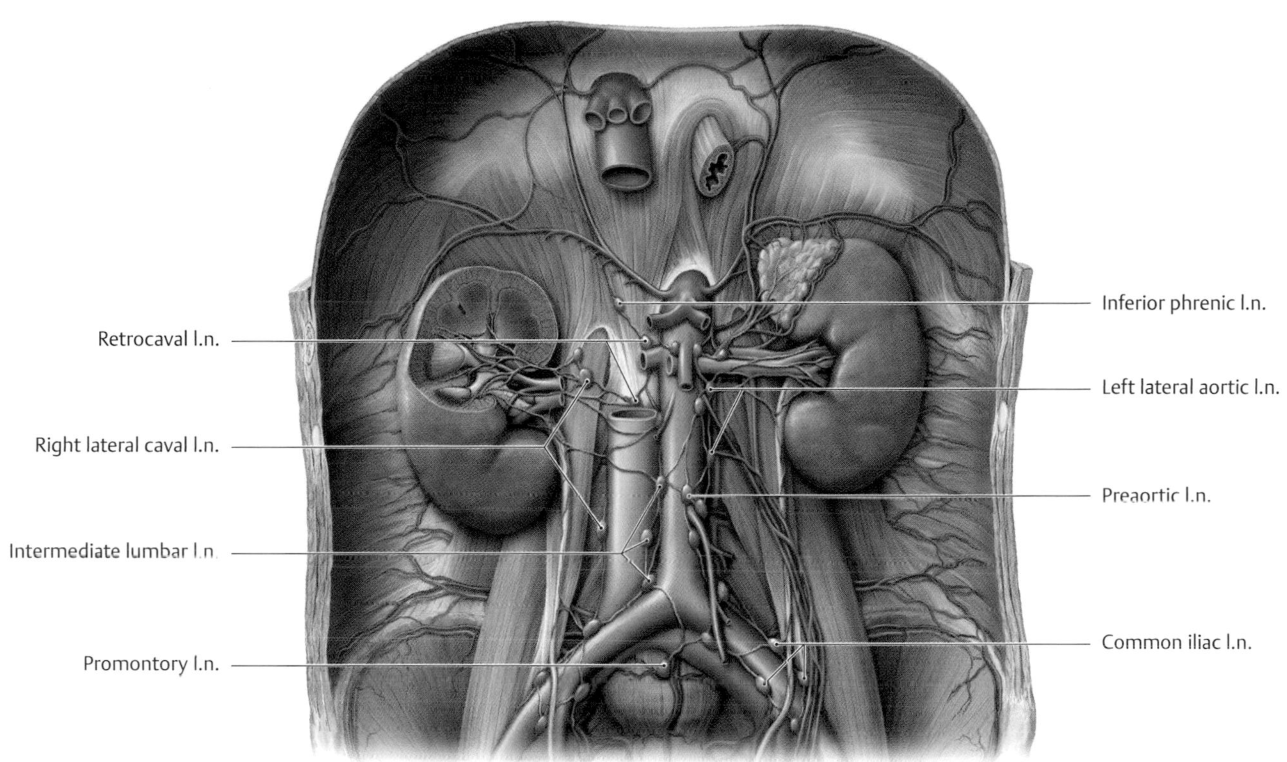
Inferior phrenic l.n.
Retrocaval l.n.
Left lateral aortic l.n.
Right lateral caval l.n.
Preaortic l.n.
Intermediate lumbar l.n.
Common iliac l.n.
Promontory l.n.

***Fig. 14.26* Lymphatic drainage of the kidneys (with pelvic organs)**

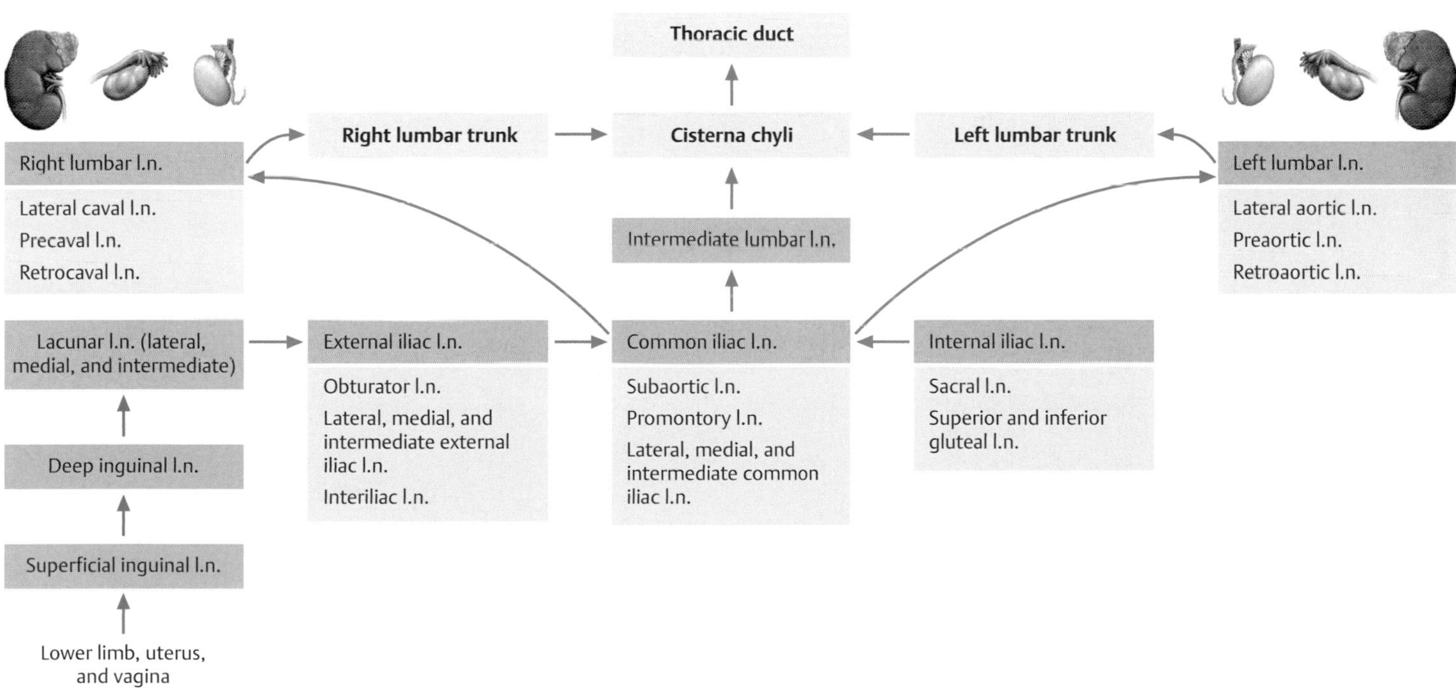
Thoracic duct
Right lumbar trunk
Cisterna chyli
Left lumbar trunk
Right lumbar l.n.
Lateral caval l.n.
Precaval l.n.
Retrocaval l.n.
Intermediate lumbar l.n.
Left lumbar l.n.
Lateral aortic l.n.
Preaortic l.n.
Retroaortic l.n.
Lacunar l.n. (lateral, medial, and intermediate)
External iliac l.n.
Obturator l.n.
Lateral, medial, and intermediate external iliac l.n.
Interiliac l.n.
Common iliac l.n.
Subaortic l.n.
Promontory l.n.
Lateral, medial, and intermediate common iliac l.n.
Internal iliac l.n.
Sacral l.n.
Superior and inferior gluteal l.n.
Deep inguinal l.n.
Superficial inguinal l.n.
Lower limb, uterus, and vagina

Lymph Nodes of the Supracolic Organs

Fig. 14.27 **Lymph nodes of the stomach and liver**
Anterior view. *Removed:* Lesser omentum. *Opened:* Greater omentum. Arrows show direction of lymphatic drainage.

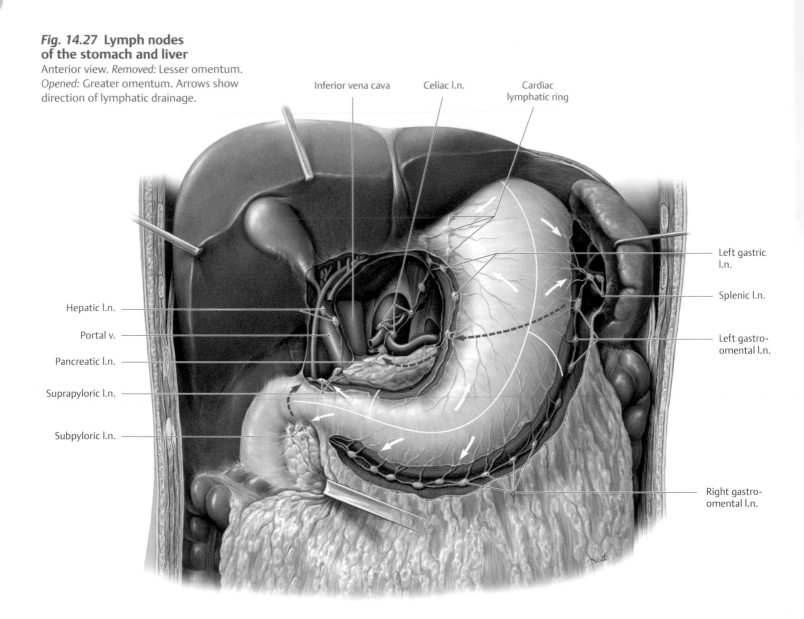

Inferior vena cava
Celiac l.n.
Cardiac lymphatic ring
Left gastric l.n.
Splenic l.n.
Left gastro-omental l.n.
Right gastro-omental l.n.
Hepatic l.n.
Portal v.
Pancreatic l.n.
Suprapyloric l.n.
Subpyloric l.n.

Fig. 14.28 **Lymphatic pathways for the liver and biliary tract**
Anterior view. In the region of the liver, the major lymph-producing organ, the important pathways are:

- *Liver and intrahepatic bile ducts:* Most lymph drains inferiorly through the hepatic nodes to the celiac nodes and then to the intestinal trunk and cisterna chyli, but it may take a more direct route bypassing the celiac nodes. A small amount drains cranially through the inferior phrenic nodes to the lumbar trunk. It also can drain through the diaphragm to the superior phrenic nodes and on to the bronchomediastinal trunk.
- *Gallbladder:* Lymph drains initially to the cystic node, then follows one of the pathways described above.
- *Common bile duct:* Lymph drains through the pyloric nodes (supra-, sub-, and retropyloric) and the foraminal node to the celiac nodes, then to the intestinal trunk.

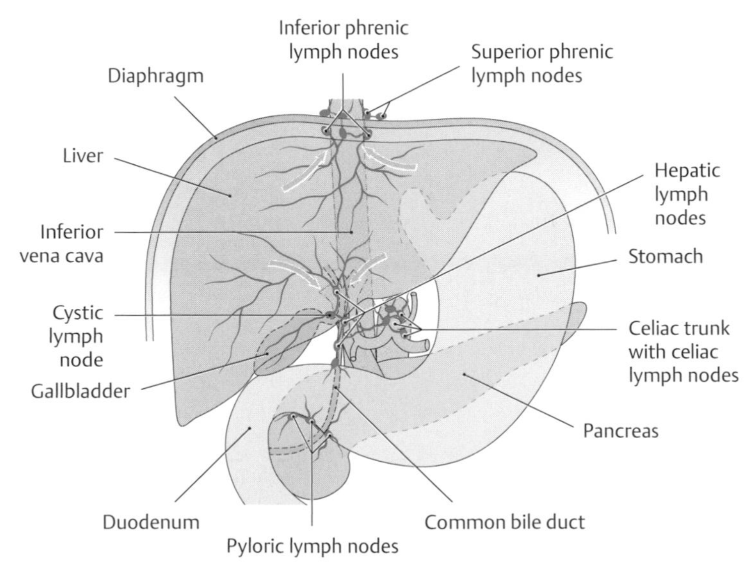

Inferior phrenic lymph nodes
Superior phrenic lymph nodes
Diaphragm
Liver
Inferior vena cava
Cystic lymph node
Gallbladder
Hepatic lymph nodes
Stomach
Celiac trunk with celiac lymph nodes
Pancreas
Duodenum
Pyloric lymph nodes
Common bile duct

Fig. 14.29 **Lymph nodes of the spleen, pancreas, and duodenum**

Anterior view. *Removed:* Stomach and colon.

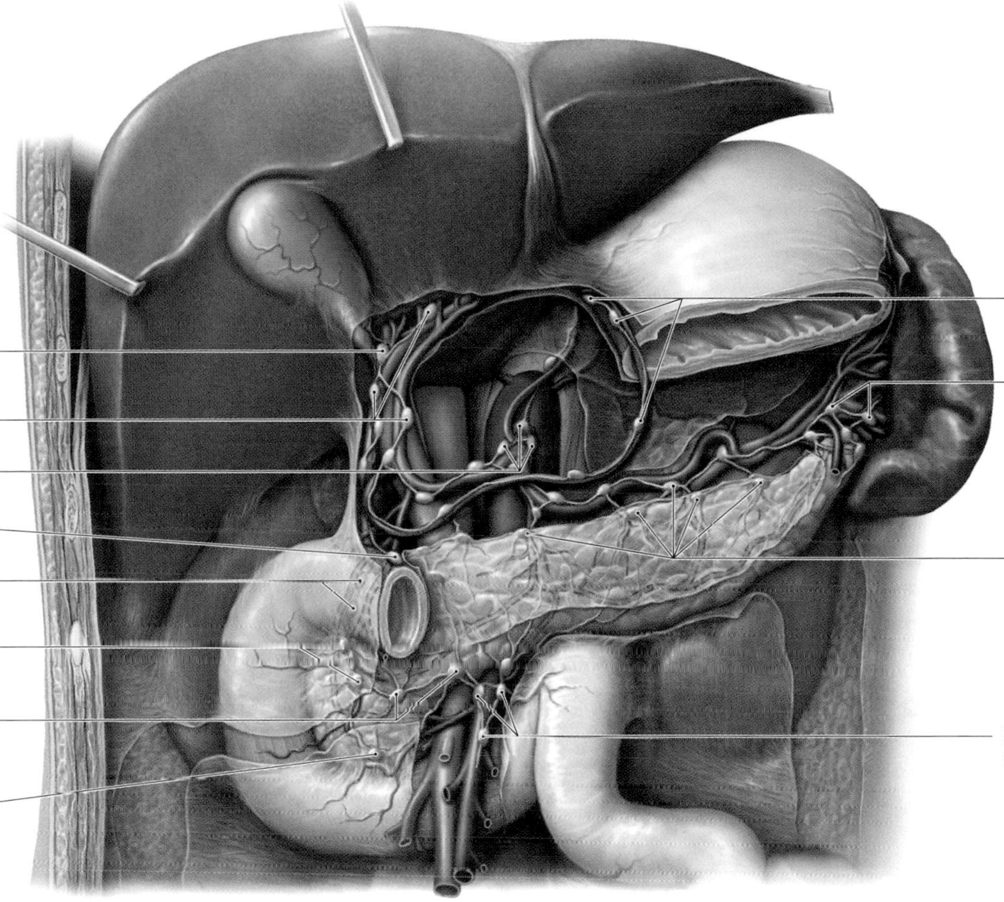

Cystic l.n.
Hepatic l.n.
Celiac l.n.
Suprapyloric l.n.
Retropyloric l.n.
Subpyloric l.n.
Pancreatic l.n. (inferior)
Pancreaticoduodenal l.n.
Left gastric l.n.
Splenic l.n.
Pancreatic l.n. (superior)
Superior mesenteric l.n.

Fig. 14.30 **Lymphatic drainage of the stomach, liver, spleen, pancreas, and duodenum**

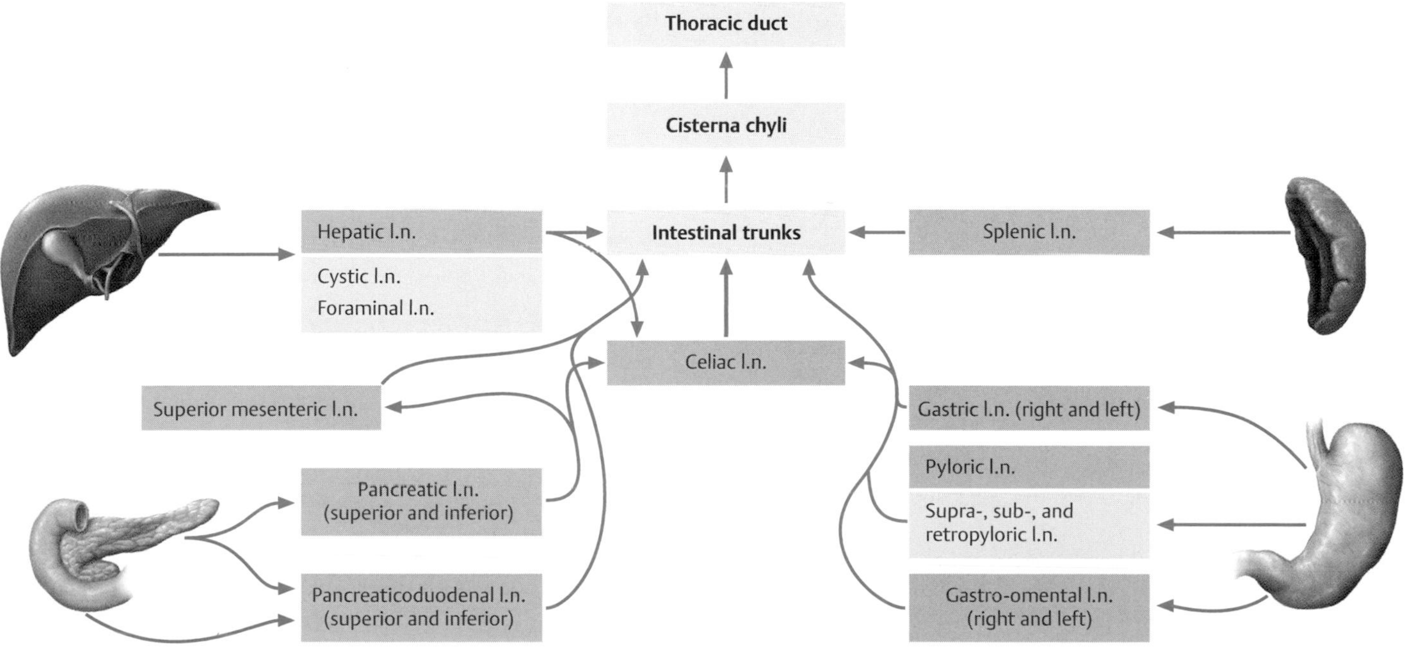
Thoracic duct
Cisterna chyli
Hepatic l.n.
Cystic l.n.
Foraminal l.n.
Intestinal trunks
Splenic l.n.
Celiac l.n.
Superior mesenteric l.n.
Gastric l.n. (right and left)
Pyloric l.n.
Supra-, sub-, and retropyloric l.n.
Pancreatic l.n. (superior and inferior)
Pancreaticoduodenal l.n. (superior and inferior)
Gastro-omental l.n. (right and left)

Lymph Nodes of the Infracolic Organs

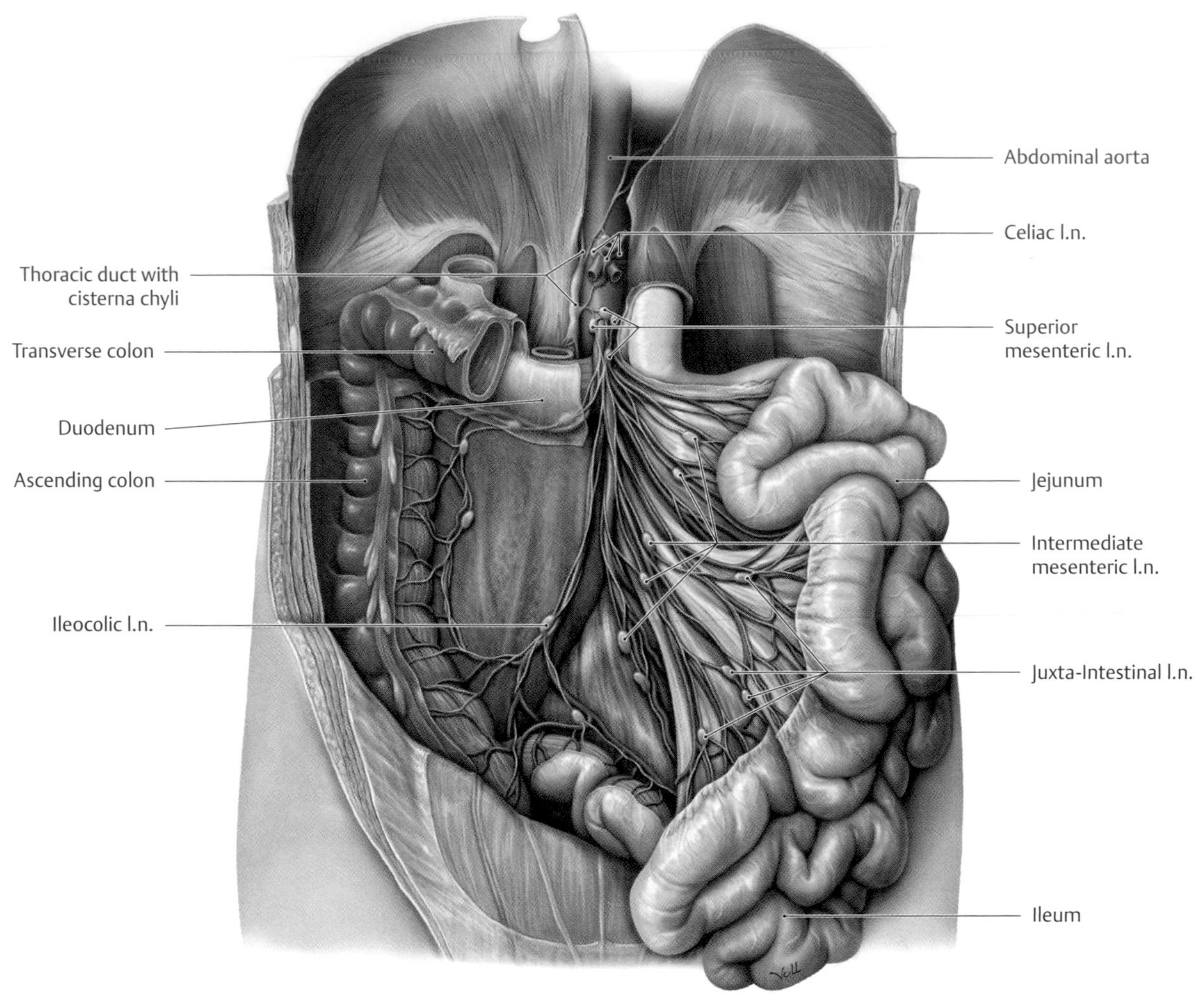
Abdominal aorta
Celiac l.n.
Thoracic duct with cisterna chyli
Transverse colon
Superior mesenteric l.n.
Duodenum
Ascending colon
Jejunum
Intermediate mesenteric l.n.
Ileocolic l.n.
Juxta-Intestinal l.n.
Ileum

Fig. 14.31 **Lymph nodes of the jejunum and ileum**
Anterior view. *Removed:* Stomach, liver, pancreas, and colon.

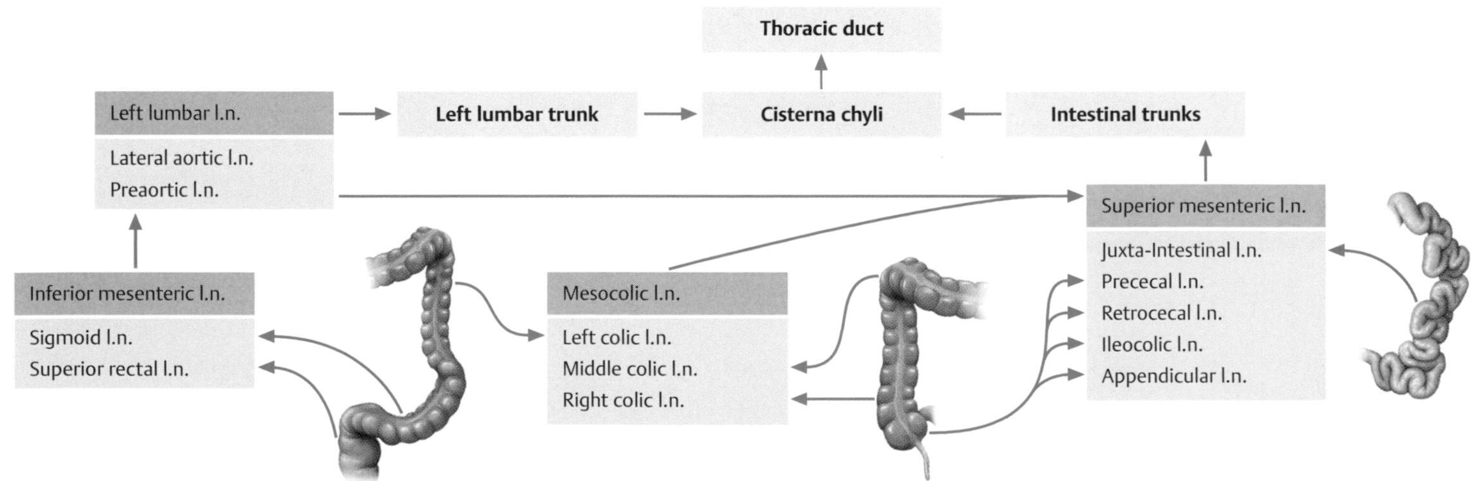
Thoracic duct
Left lumbar l.n.
Left lumbar trunk
Cisterna chyli
Intestinal trunks
Lateral aortic l.n.
Preaortic l.n.
Superior mesenteric l.n.
Juxta-Intestinal l.n.
Prececal l.n.
Retrocecal l.n.
Ileocolic l.n.
Appendicular l.n.
Inferior mesenteric l.n.
Sigmoid l.n.
Superior rectal l.n.
Mesocolic l.n.
Left colic l.n.
Middle colic l.n.
Right colic l.n.

Fig. 14.32 **Lymphatic drainage of the intestines**

Fig. 14.33 **Lymph nodes of the large intestine**
Anterior view. *Reflected:* Transverse colon and greater omentum.

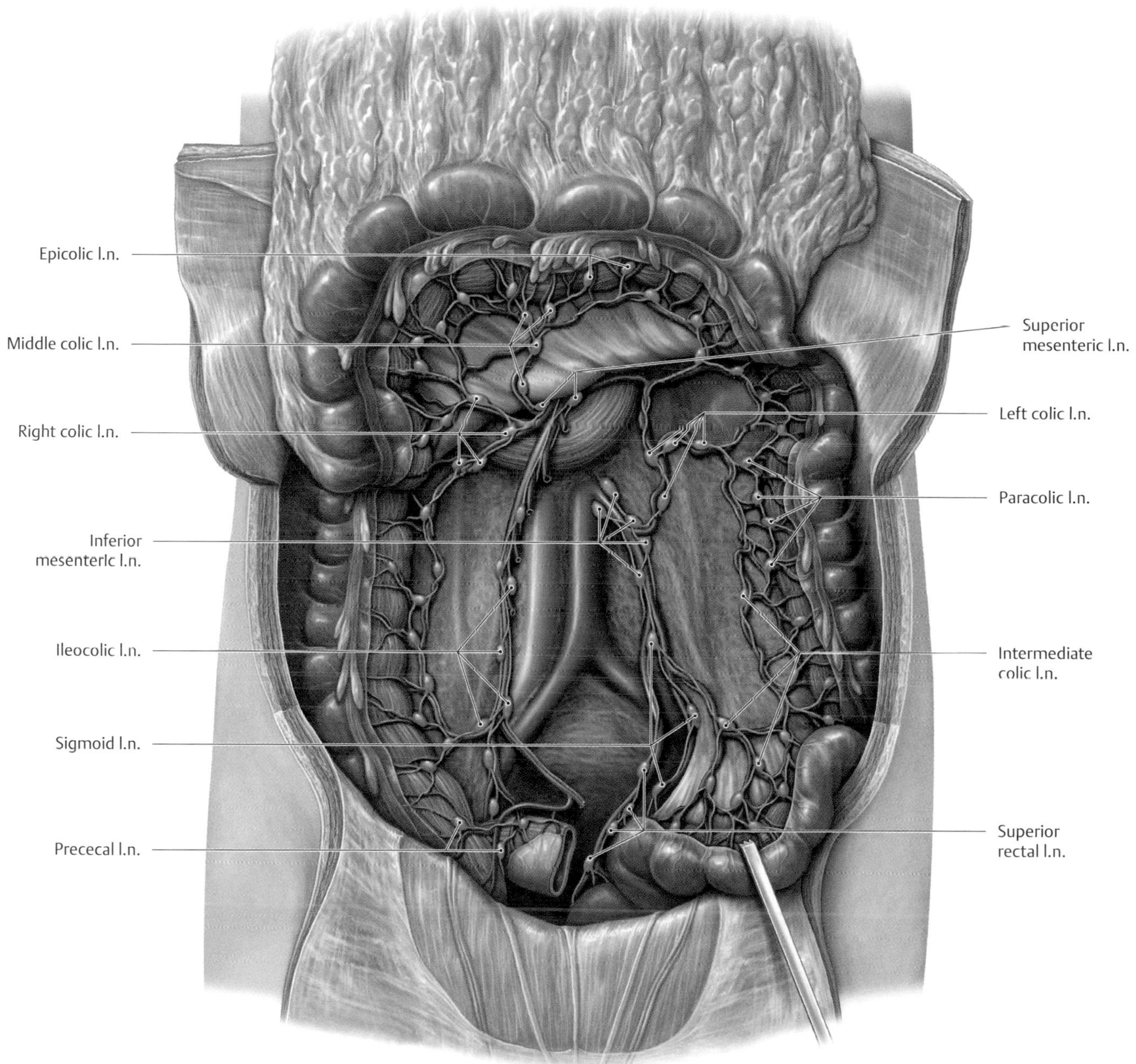
Epicolic l.n.
Middle colic l.n.
Right colic l.n.
Inferior mesenteric l.n.
Ileocolic l.n.
Sigmoid l.n.
Prececal l.n.
Superior mesenteric l.n.
Left colic l.n.
Paracolic l.n.
Intermediate colic l.n.
Superior rectal l.n.

Nerves of the Abdominal Wall

Fig. 14.34 **Somatic nerves of the abdomen and pelvis**
Anterior view.

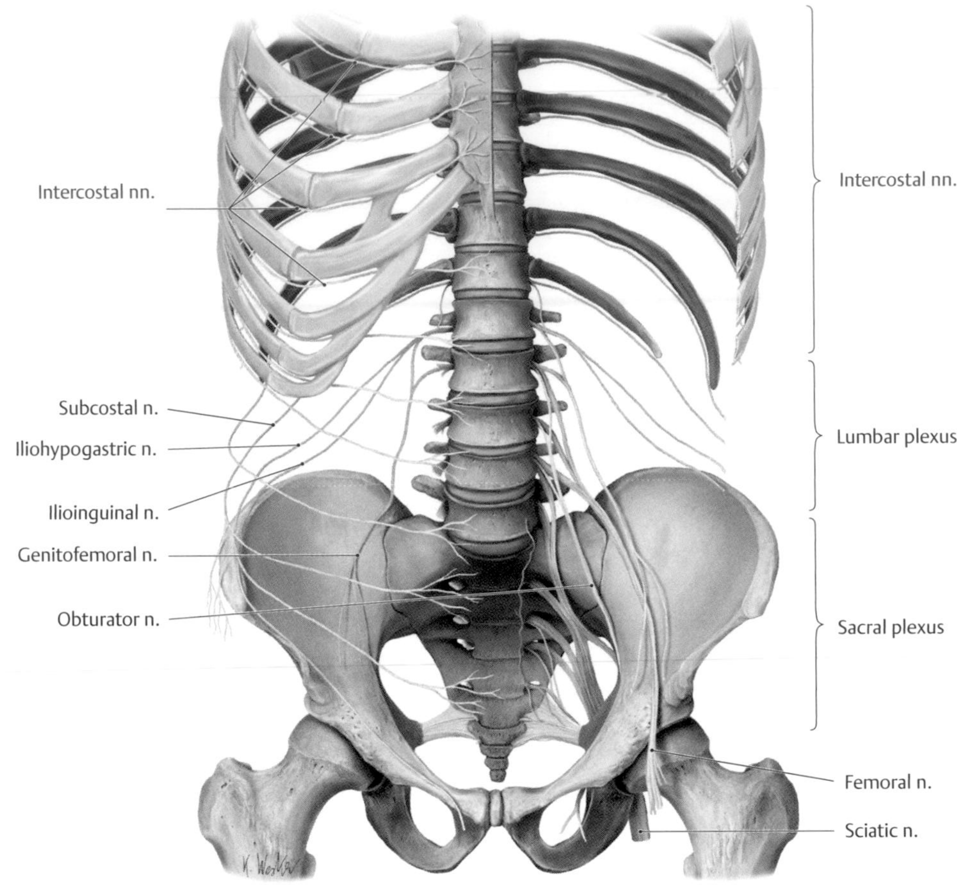
Intercostal nn.
Subcostal n.
Iliohypogastric n.
Ilioinguinal n.
Genitofemoral n.
Obturator n.
Intercostal nn.
Lumbar plexus
Sacral plexus
Femoral n.
Sciatic n.

Fig. 14.35 **Cutaneous innervation of the anterior trunk**
Anterior view.

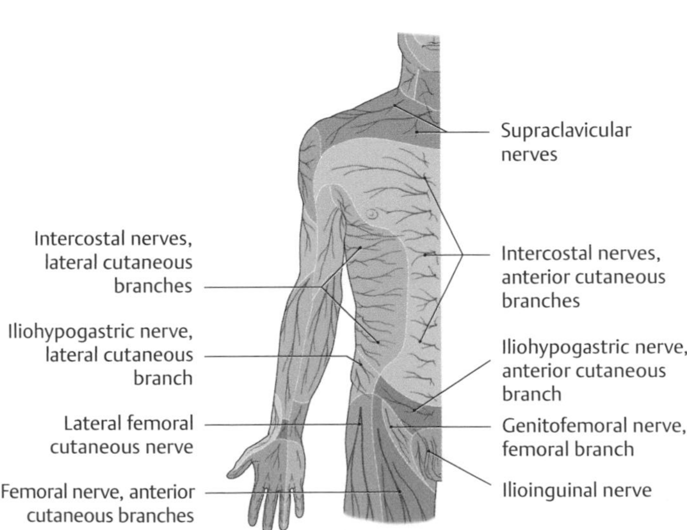
Supraclavicular nerves
Intercostal nerves, lateral cutaneous branches
Iliohypogastric nerve, lateral cutaneous branch
Lateral femoral cutaneous nerve
Femoral nerve, anterior cutaneous branches
Intercostal nerves, anterior cutaneous branches
Iliohypogastric nerve, anterior cutaneous branch
Genitofemoral nerve, femoral branch
Ilioinguinal nerve

Fig. 14.36 **Dermatomes of the anterior trunk**
Anterior view.

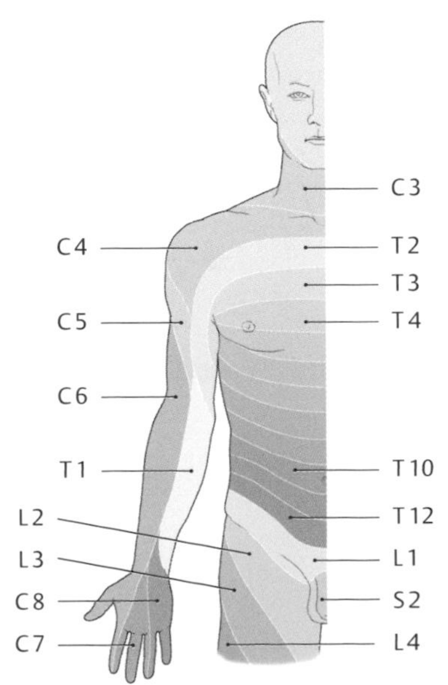
C3
C4
T2
T3
C5
T4
C6
T1
T10
L2
T12
L3
L1
C8
S2
C7
L4

Fig. 14.37 Nerves of the lumbar plexus.

Anterior view.

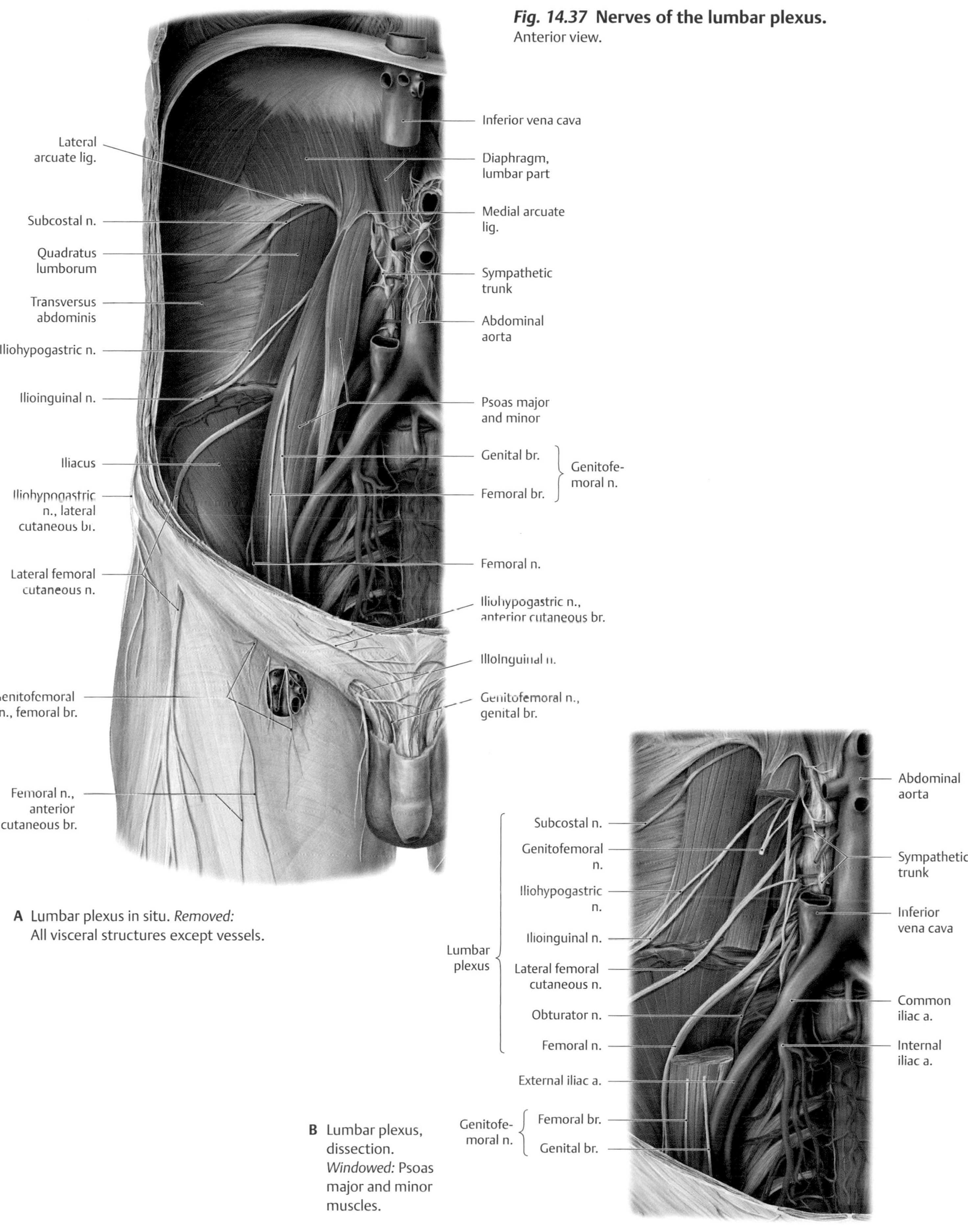

Inferior vena cava
Lateral arcuate lig.
Diaphragm, lumbar part
Subcostal n.
Medial arcuate lig.
Quadratus lumborum
Sympathetic trunk
Transversus abdominis
Abdominal aorta
Iliohypogastric n.
Ilioinguinal n.
Psoas major and minor
Iliacus
Genital br.
Genitofemoral n.
Femoral br.
Iliohypogastric n., lateral cutaneous br.
Femoral n.
Lateral femoral cutaneous n.
Iliohypogastric n., anterior cutaneous br.
Ilioinguinal n.
Genitofemoral n., femoral br.
Genitofemoral n., genital br.
Femoral n., anterior cutaneous br.
Abdominal aorta
Subcostal n.
Genitofemoral n.
Sympathetic trunk
Iliohypogastric n.
Inferior vena cava
Ilioinguinal n.
Lumbar plexus
Lateral femoral cutaneous n.
Common iliac a.
Obturator n.
Femoral n.
Internal iliac a.
External iliac a.
Genitofemoral n.
Femoral br.
Genital br.

A Lumbar plexus in situ. *Removed:* All visceral structures except vessels.

B Lumbar plexus, dissection. *Windowed:* Psoas major and minor muscles.

Autonomic Innervation: Overview

Fig. 14.38 Sympathetic and parasympathetic nervous systems in the abdomen and pelvis

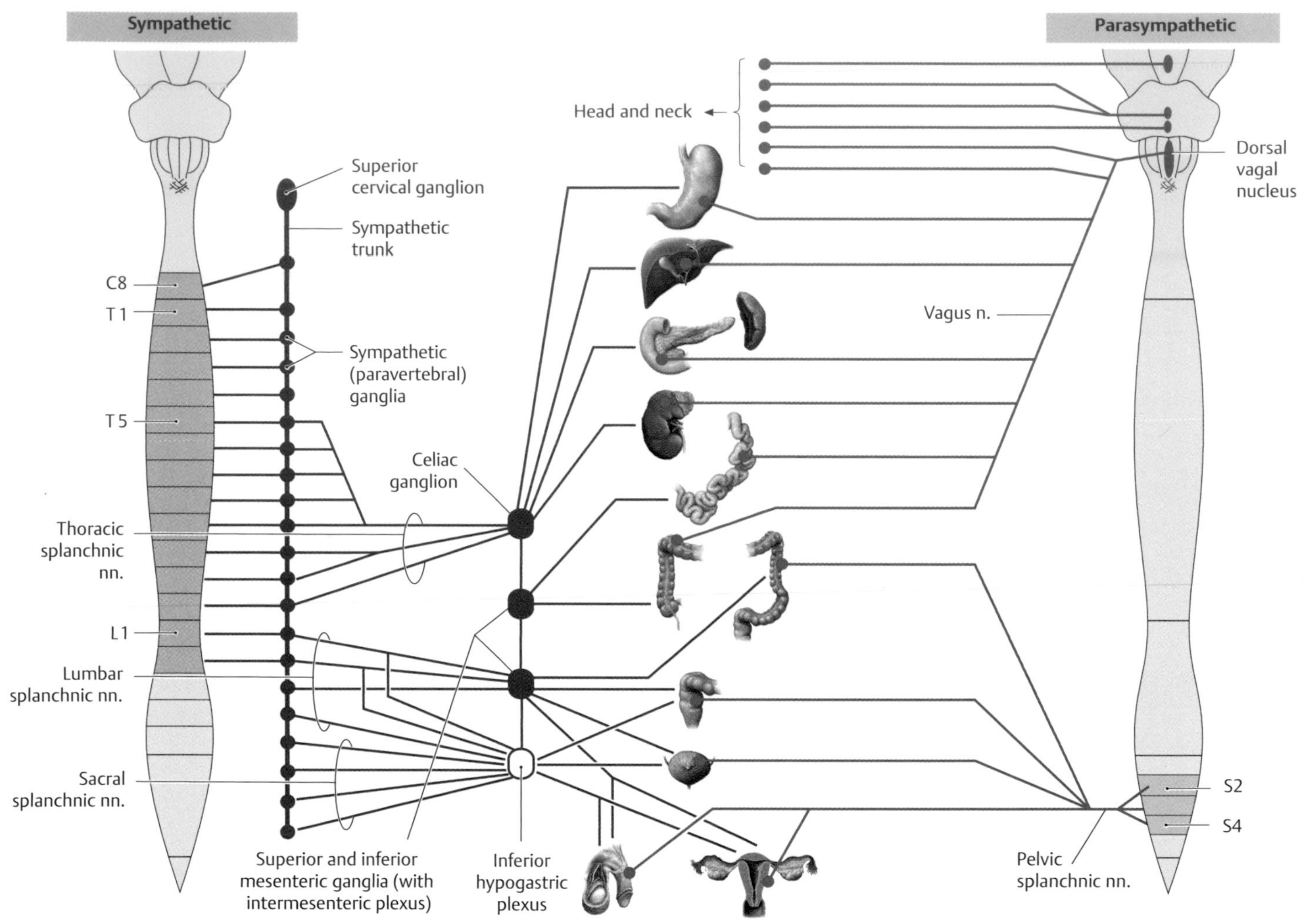
Sympathetic
Parasympathetic
Superior cervical ganglion
Sympathetic trunk
C8
T1
Sympathetic (paravertebral) ganglia
T5
Celiac ganglion
Thoracic splanchnic nn.
L1
Lumbar splanchnic nn.
Sacral splanchnic nn.
Superior and inferior mesenteric ganglia (with intermesenteric plexus)
Inferior hypogastric plexus
Head and neck
Dorsal vagal nucleus
Vagus n.
S2
S4
Pelvic splanchnic nn.

A Sympathetic nervous system.

B Parasympathetic nervous system.

Table 14.4 Effects of the autonomic nervous system in the abdomen and pelvis

Organ (organ system)		Sympathetic effect	Parasympathetic effect
Gastrointestinal tract	Longitudinal and circular muscle fibers	↓ motility	↑ motility
	Sphincter muscles	Contraction	Relaxation
	Glands	↓ secretions	↑ secretions
Splenic capsule		Contraction	No effect
Liver		↑ glycogenolysis/gluconeogenesis	
Pancreas	Endocrine pancreas	↓ insulin secretion	
	Exocrine pancreas	↓ secretion	↑ secretion
Urinary bladder	Detrusor vesicae	Relaxation	Contraction
	Functional bladder sphincter	Contraction	Inhibits contraction
Seminal vesicle and ductus deferens		Contraction (ejaculation)	No effect
Uterus		Contraction or relaxation, depending on hormonal status	
Arteries		Vasoconstriction	Vasodilation of the arteries of the penis and clitoris (erection)
Suprarenal glands (medulla)		Release of adrenalin	No effect
Urinary tract	Kidney	Vasoconstriction (↓ urine formation)	Vasodilation

***Fig. 14.39* Autonomic innervation of the intraperitoneal organs**

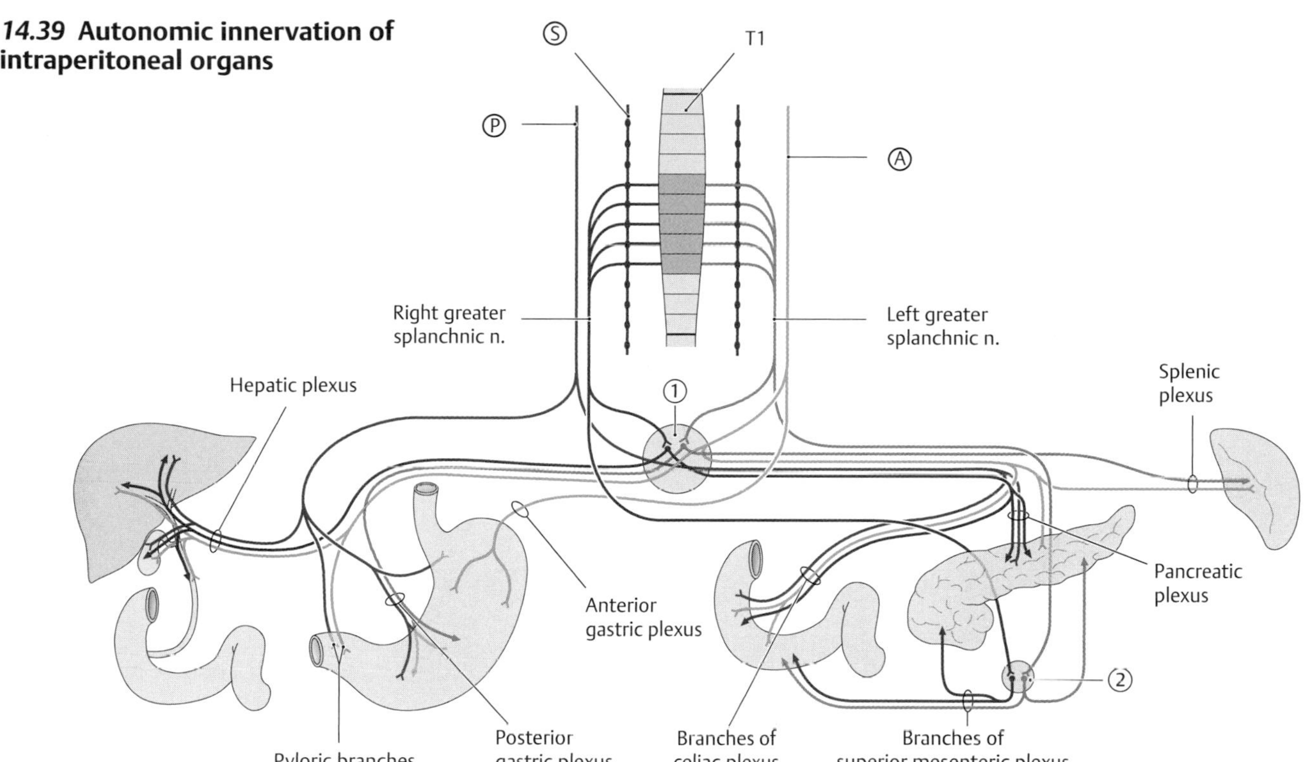
Ⓢ
T1
Ⓟ
Ⓐ
Right greater splanchnic n.
Left greater splanchnic n.
Hepatic plexus
①
Splenic plexus
Pancreatic plexus
Anterior gastric plexus
②
Pyloric branches
Posterior gastric plexus
Branches of celiac plexus
Branches of superior mesenteric plexus

A Innervation of the foregut. As the left and right vagus nerves descend along the esophagus, they become the anterior and posterior vagal trunks, respectively. Each trunk produces a celiac, pyloric, and hepatic branch, and a gastric plexus.

Ⓢ	Sympathetic trunk
Ⓟ	Posterior vagal trunk (from right vagus n.)
Ⓐ	Anterior vagal trunk (from left vagus n.)
①	Celiac ganglia
②	Superior mesenteric ganglion
③	Inferior mesenteric ganglion
④	Greater splanchnic n. (T5–T9)
⑤	Lesser splanchnic n. (T10–T11)
⑥	Least splanchnic n. (T12)
⑦	Lumbar splanchnic nn. (L1–L2)
⑧	Lumbar splanchnic nn. (from 3rd to 5th lumbar ganglia)
⑨	Sacral splanchnic nn. (from 1st to 3rd sacral ganglia)
⑩	Pelvic splanchnic nn. (S2–S4)

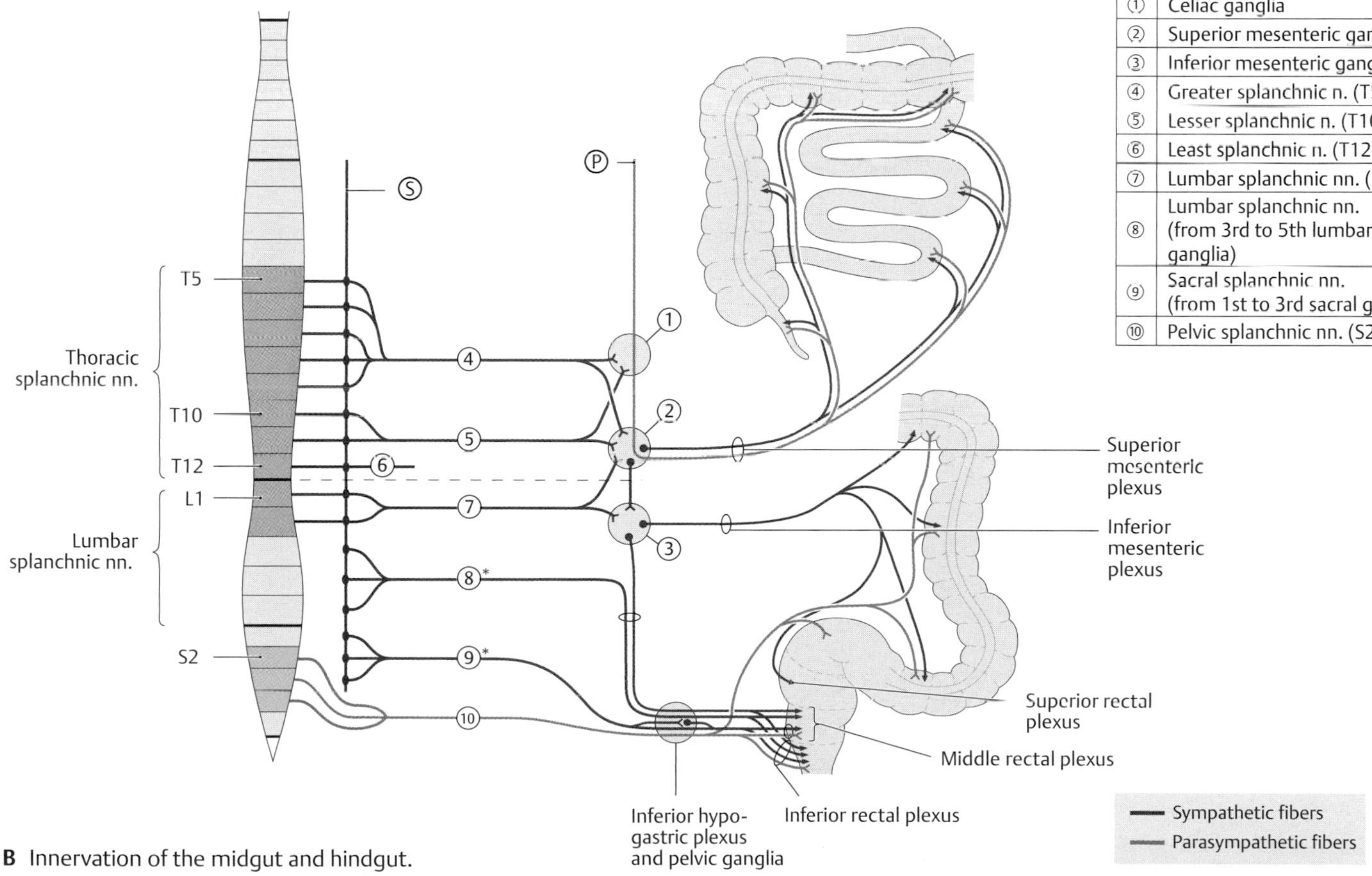

Ⓢ
Ⓟ
T5
Thoracic splanchnic nn.
T10
T12
L1
Lumbar splanchnic nn.
S2
①
②
③
④
⑤
⑥
⑦
⑧*
⑨*
⑩
Superior mesenteric plexus
Inferior mesenteric plexus
Superior rectal plexus
Middle rectal plexus
Inferior hypogastric plexus and pelvic ganglia
Inferior rectal plexus
Sympathetic fibers
Parasympathetic fibers

B Innervation of the midgut and hindgut.

*Synapse in the lumbar sympathetic ganglia.

Autonomic Plexuses

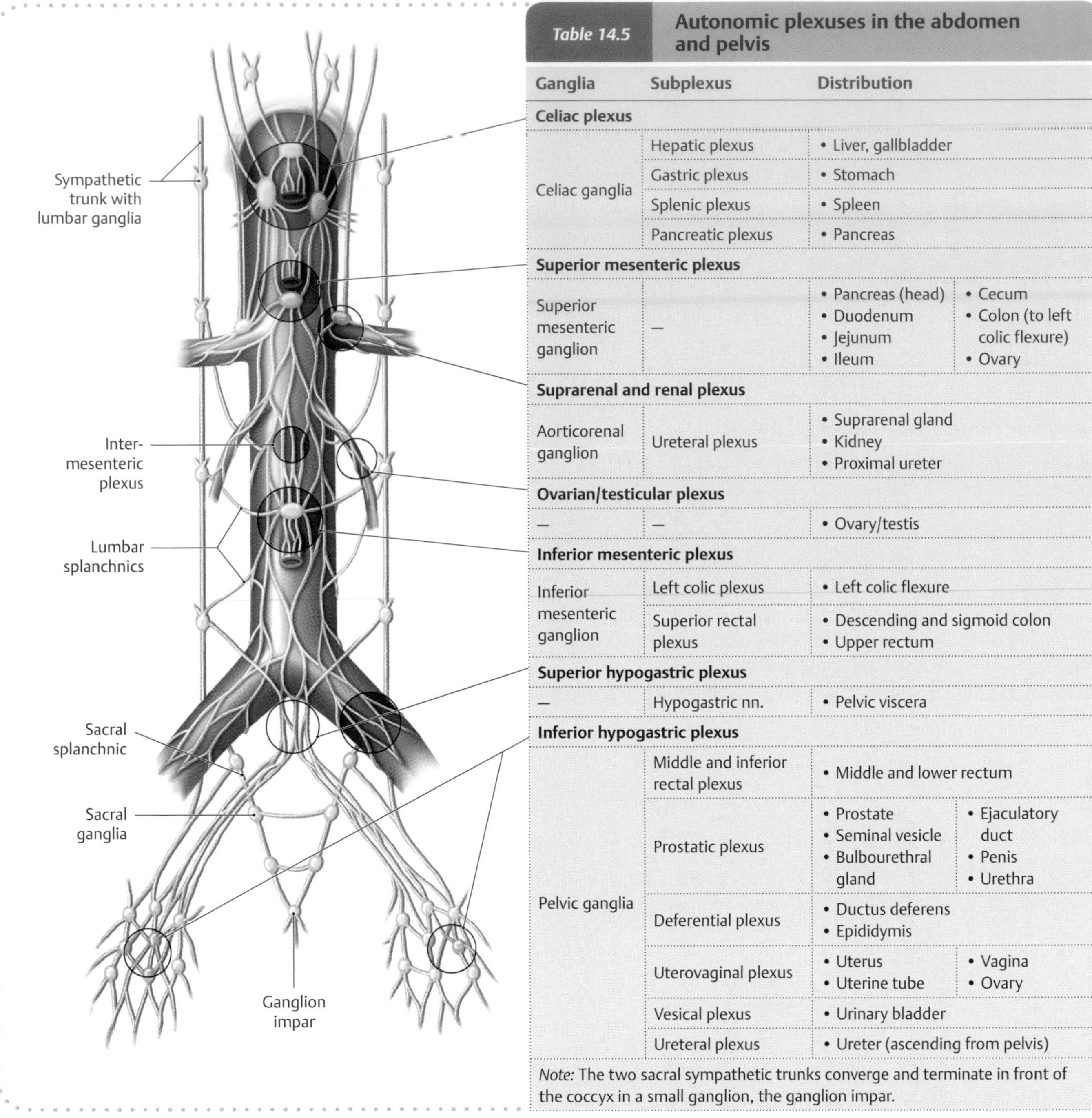
Sympathetic trunk with lumbar ganglia
Inter-mesenteric plexus
Lumbar splanchnics
Sacral splanchnic
Sacral ganglia
Ganglion impar

Table 14.5 Autonomic plexuses in the abdomen and pelvis

Ganglia	Subplexus	Distribution	
Celiac plexus			
Celiac ganglia	Hepatic plexus	• Liver, gallbladder	
	Gastric plexus	• Stomach	
	Splenic plexus	• Spleen	
	Pancreatic plexus	• Pancreas	
Superior mesenteric plexus			
Superior mesenteric ganglion	—	• Pancreas (head) • Duodenum • Jejunum • Ileum	• Cecum • Colon (to left colic flexure) • Ovary
Suprarenal and renal plexus			
Aorticorenal ganglion	Ureteral plexus	• Suprarenal gland • Kidney • Proximal ureter	
Ovarian/testicular plexus			
—	—	• Ovary/testis	
Inferior mesenteric plexus			
Inferior mesenteric ganglion	Left colic plexus	• Left colic flexure	
	Superior rectal plexus	• Descending and sigmoid colon • Upper rectum	
Superior hypogastric plexus			
—	Hypogastric nn.	• Pelvic viscera	
Inferior hypogastric plexus			
Pelvic ganglia	Middle and inferior rectal plexus	• Middle and lower rectum	
	Prostatic plexus	• Prostate • Seminal vesicle • Bulbourethral gland	• Ejaculatory duct • Penis • Urethra
	Deferential plexus	• Ductus deferens • Epididymis	
	Uterovaginal plexus	• Uterus • Uterine tube	• Vagina • Ovary
	Vesical plexus	• Urinary bladder	
	Ureteral plexus	• Ureter (ascending from pelvis)	

Note: The two sacral sympathetic trunks converge and terminate in front of the coccyx in a small ganglion, the ganglion impar.

Fig. 14.40 **Autonomic plexuses in the abdomen and pelvis**
Anterior view of the male abdomen and pelvis. *Removed:* Peritoneum, majority of the stomach, and all other abdominal organs except kidneys and suprarenal glands.

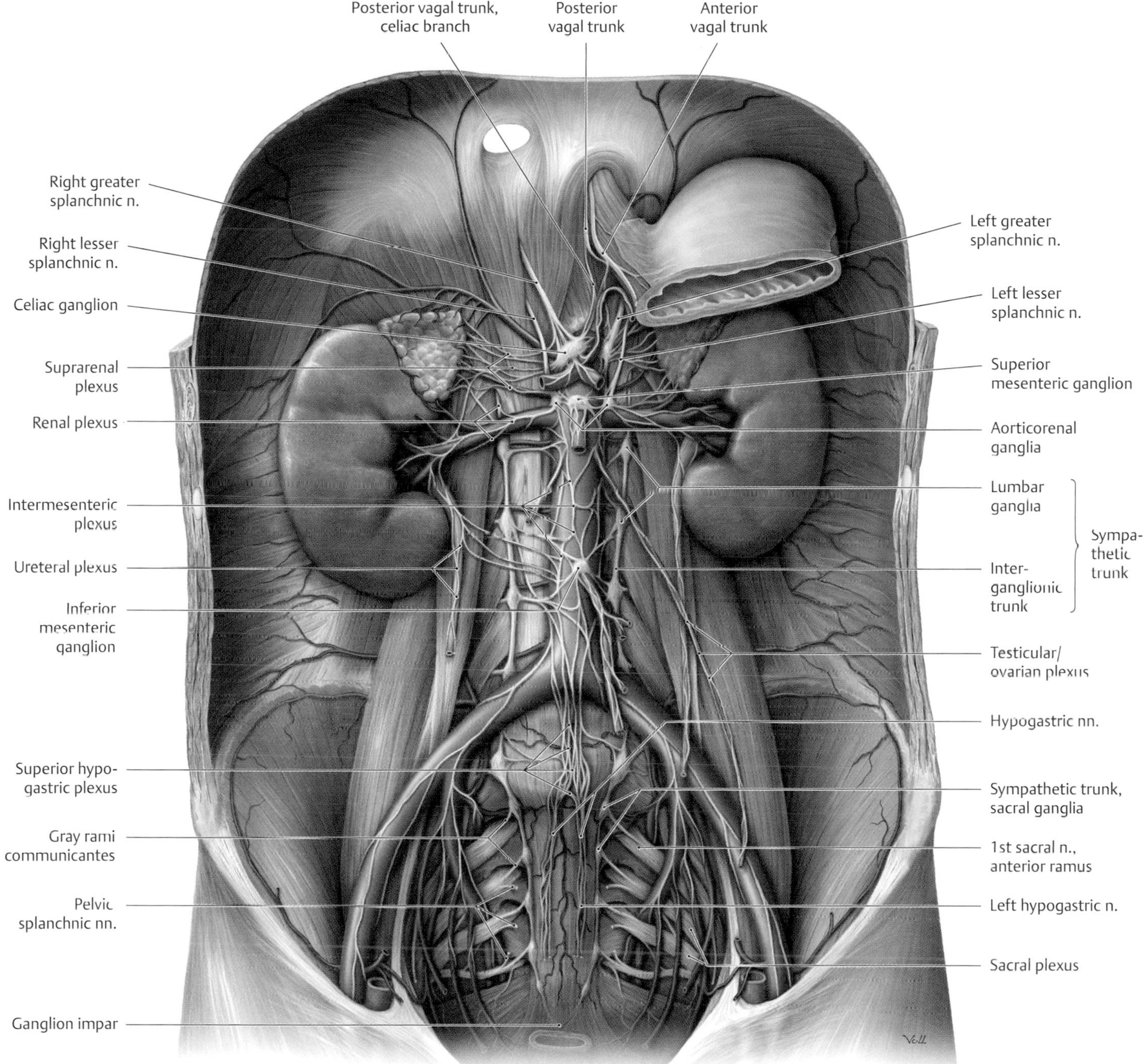
Posterior vagal trunk, celiac branch
Posterior vagal trunk
Anterior vagal trunk
Right greater splanchnic n.
Right lesser splanchnic n.
Celiac ganglion
Suprarenal plexus
Renal plexus
Intermesenteric plexus
Ureteral plexus
Inferior mesenteric ganglion
Superior hypogastric plexus
Gray rami communicantes
Pelvic splanchnic nn.
Ganglion impar
Left greater splanchnic n.
Left lesser splanchnic n.
Superior mesenteric ganglion
Aorticorenal ganglia
Lumbar ganglia
Inter-ganglionic trunk
Sympathetic trunk
Testicular/ ovarian plexus
Hypogastric nn.
Sympathetic trunk, sacral ganglia
1st sacral n., anterior ramus
Left hypogastric n.
Sacral plexus

Innervation of the Abdominal Organs

Fig. 14.41 **Innervation of the anterior abdominal organs**
Anterior view. *Removed:* Lesser omentum, ascending colon, and parts of the transverse colon. *Opened:* Omental bursa. The anterior and posterior vagal trunks each produce a celiac, hepatic, and pyloric branch, and a gastric plexus. See p. 203 for schematic.

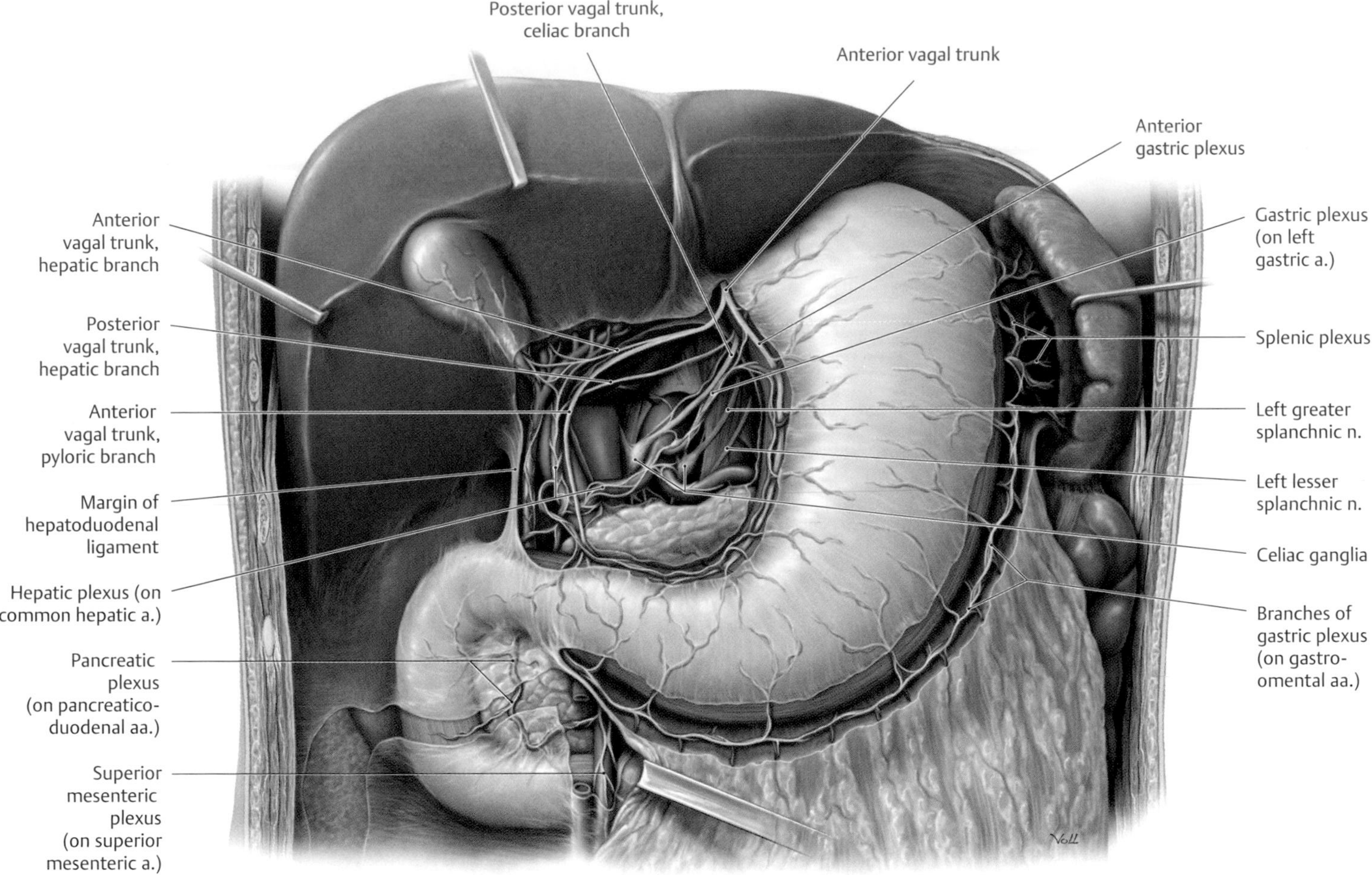
Posterior vagal trunk, celiac branch
Anterior vagal trunk
Anterior gastric plexus
Anterior vagal trunk, hepatic branch
Gastric plexus (on left gastric a.)
Posterior vagal trunk, hepatic branch
Splenic plexus
Anterior vagal trunk, pyloric branch
Left greater splanchnic n.
Margin of hepatoduodenal ligament
Left lesser splanchnic n.
Celiac ganglia
Hepatic plexus (on common hepatic a.)
Branches of gastric plexus (on gastro-omental aa.)
Pancreatic plexus (on pancreatico-duodenal aa.)
Superior mesenteric plexus (on superior mesenteric a.)
Voll

Fig. 14.42 **Innervation of the urinary organs**
Anterior view of the male abdomen and pelvis. *Removed:* Peritoneum, majority of stomach, and abdominal organs except kidneys, suprarenal glands, and bladder. See p. 264 for schematic.

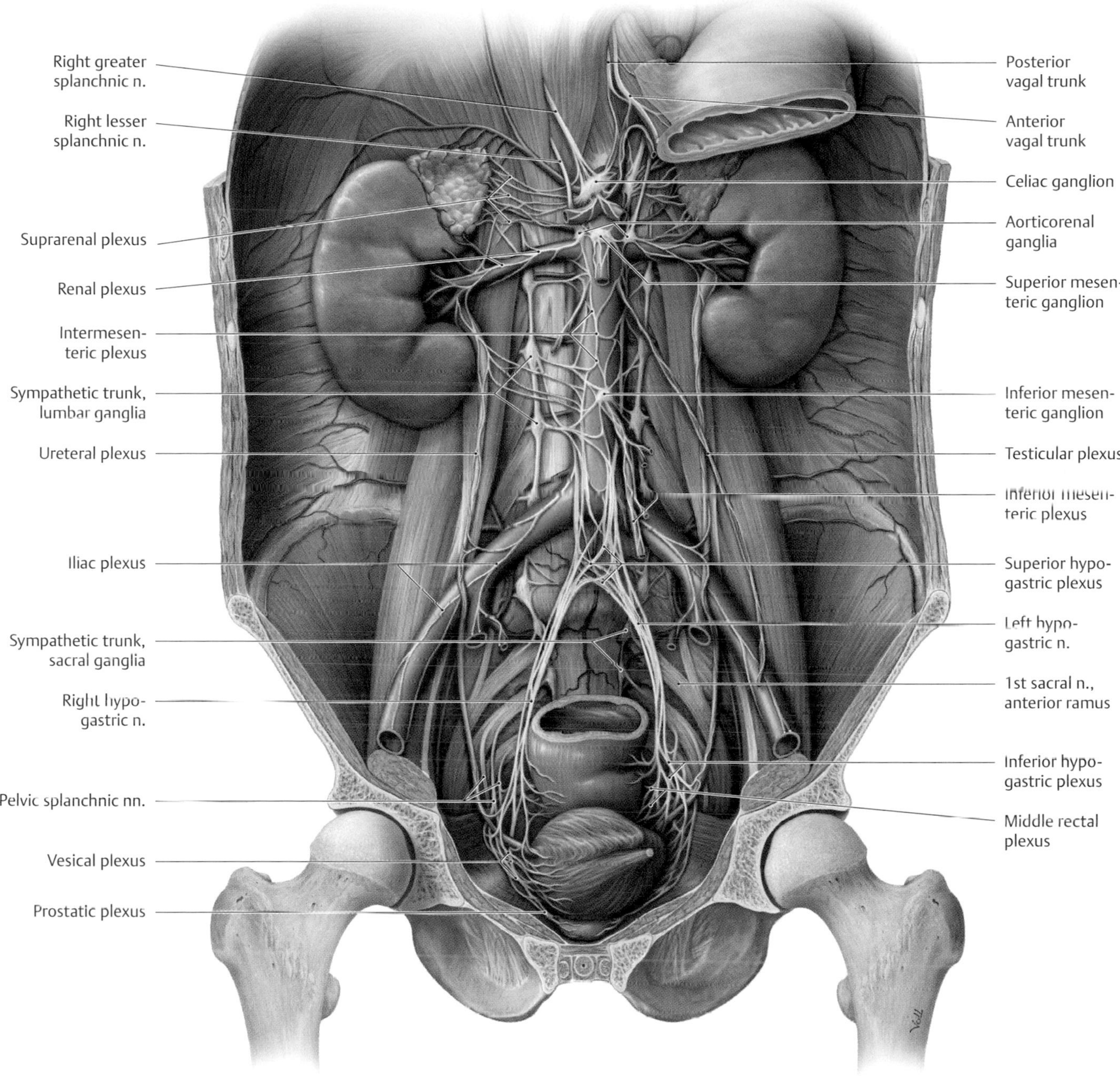
Right greater splanchnic n.
Right lesser splanchnic n.
Suprarenal plexus
Renal plexus
Intermesenteric plexus
Sympathetic trunk, lumbar ganglia
Ureteral plexus
Iliac plexus
Sympathetic trunk, sacral ganglia
Right hypogastric n.
Pelvic splanchnic nn.
Vesical plexus
Prostatic plexus
Posterior vagal trunk
Anterior vagal trunk
Celiac ganglion
Aorticorenal ganglia
Superior mesenteric ganglion
Inferior mesenteric ganglion
Testicular plexus
Inferior mesenteric plexus
Superior hypogastric plexus
Left hypogastric n.
1st sacral n., anterior ramus
Inferior hypogastric plexus
Middle rectal plexus

Innervation of the Intestines

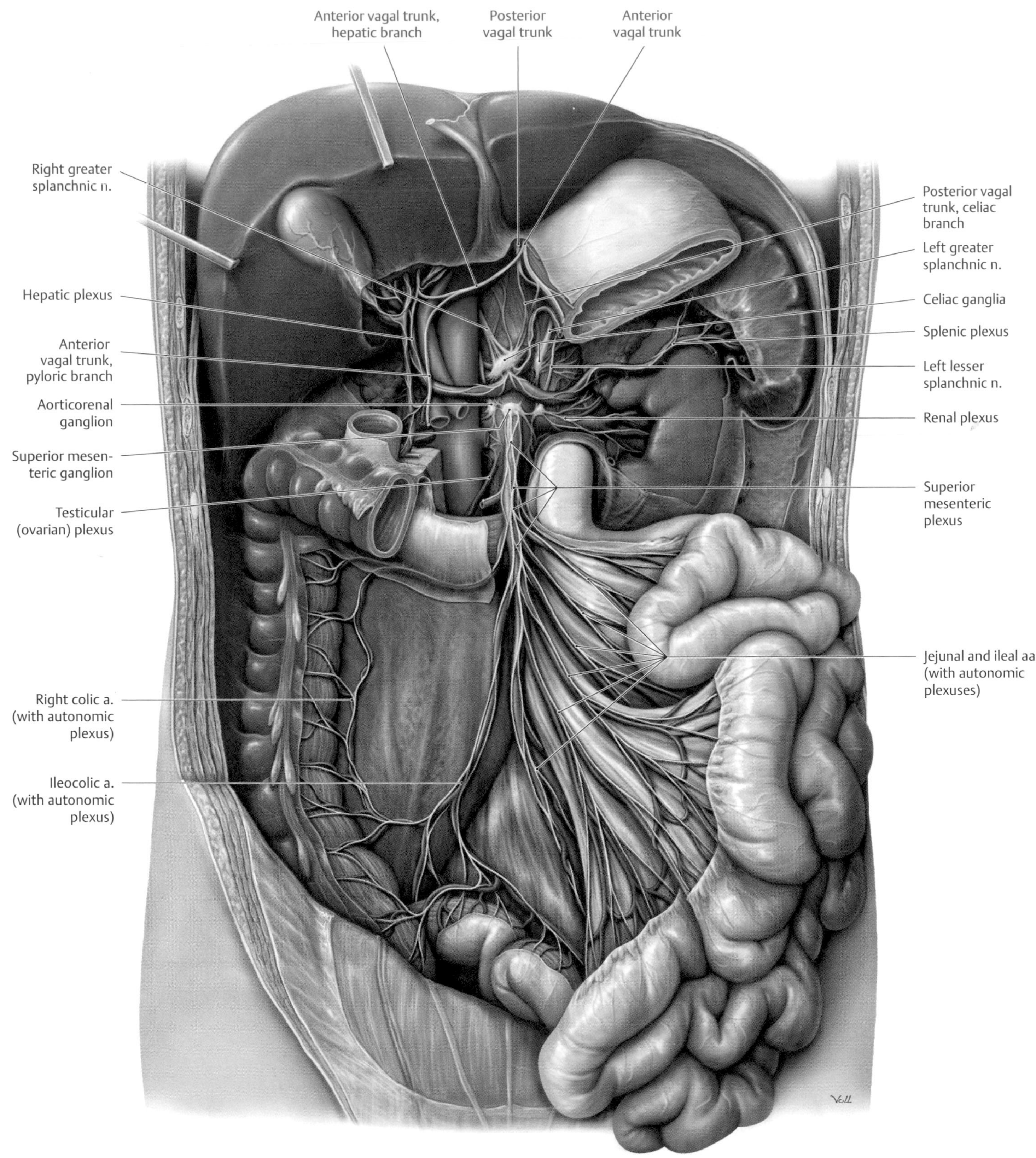
Anterior vagal trunk, hepatic branch
Posterior vagal trunk
Anterior vagal trunk
Right greater splanchnic n.
Hepatic plexus
Anterior vagal trunk, pyloric branch
Aorticorenal ganglion
Superior mesenteric ganglion
Testicular (ovarian) plexus
Right colic a. (with autonomic plexus)
Ileocolic a. (with autonomic plexus)
Posterior vagal trunk, celiac branch
Left greater splanchnic n.
Celiac ganglia
Splenic plexus
Left lesser splanchnic n.
Renal plexus
Superior mesenteric plexus
Jejunal and ileal aa. (with autonomic plexuses)

Fig. 14.43 **Innervation of the small intestine**
Anterior view. *Partially removed:* Stomach, pancreas, and transverse colon (distal part). See p. 203 for schematic.

Fig. 14.44 Innervation of the large intestine
Anterior view. *Removed:* Jejunum, ileum, and small intestine. *Reflected*: Transverse and sigmoid colons. See p. 203 for schematic.

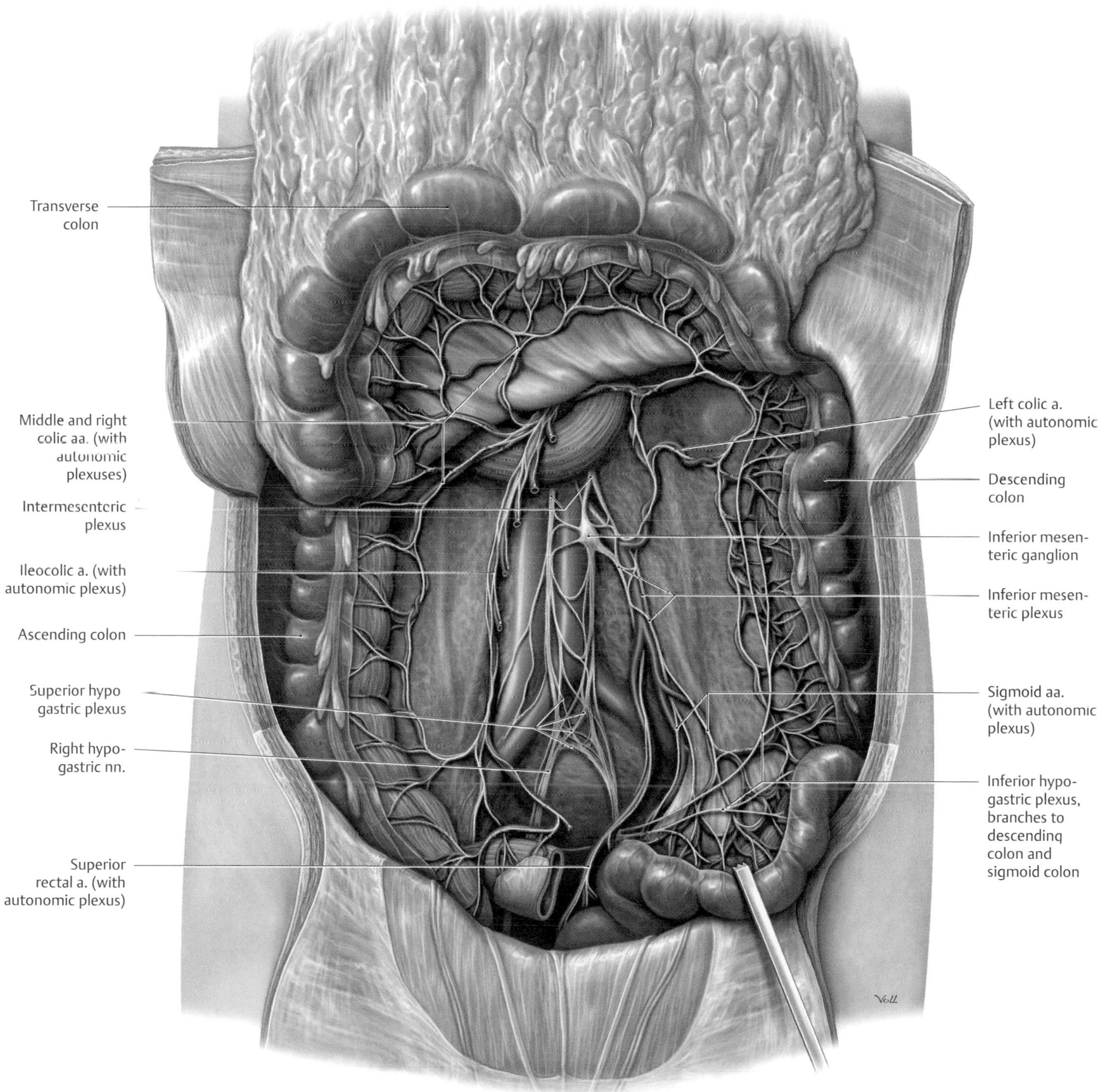
Transverse colon
Middle and right colic aa. (with autonomic plexuses)
Intermesenteric plexus
Ileocolic a. (with autonomic plexus)
Ascending colon
Superior hypo gastric plexus
Right hypo-gastric nn.
Superior rectal a. (with autonomic plexus)
Left colic a. (with autonomic plexus)
Descending colon
Inferior mesen-teric ganglion
Inferior mesen-teric plexus
Sigmoid aa. (with autonomic plexus)
Inferior hypo-gastric plexus, branches to descending colon and sigmoid colon

Sectional Anatomy of the Abdomen

Fig. 14.45 **Transverse sections of the abdomen**

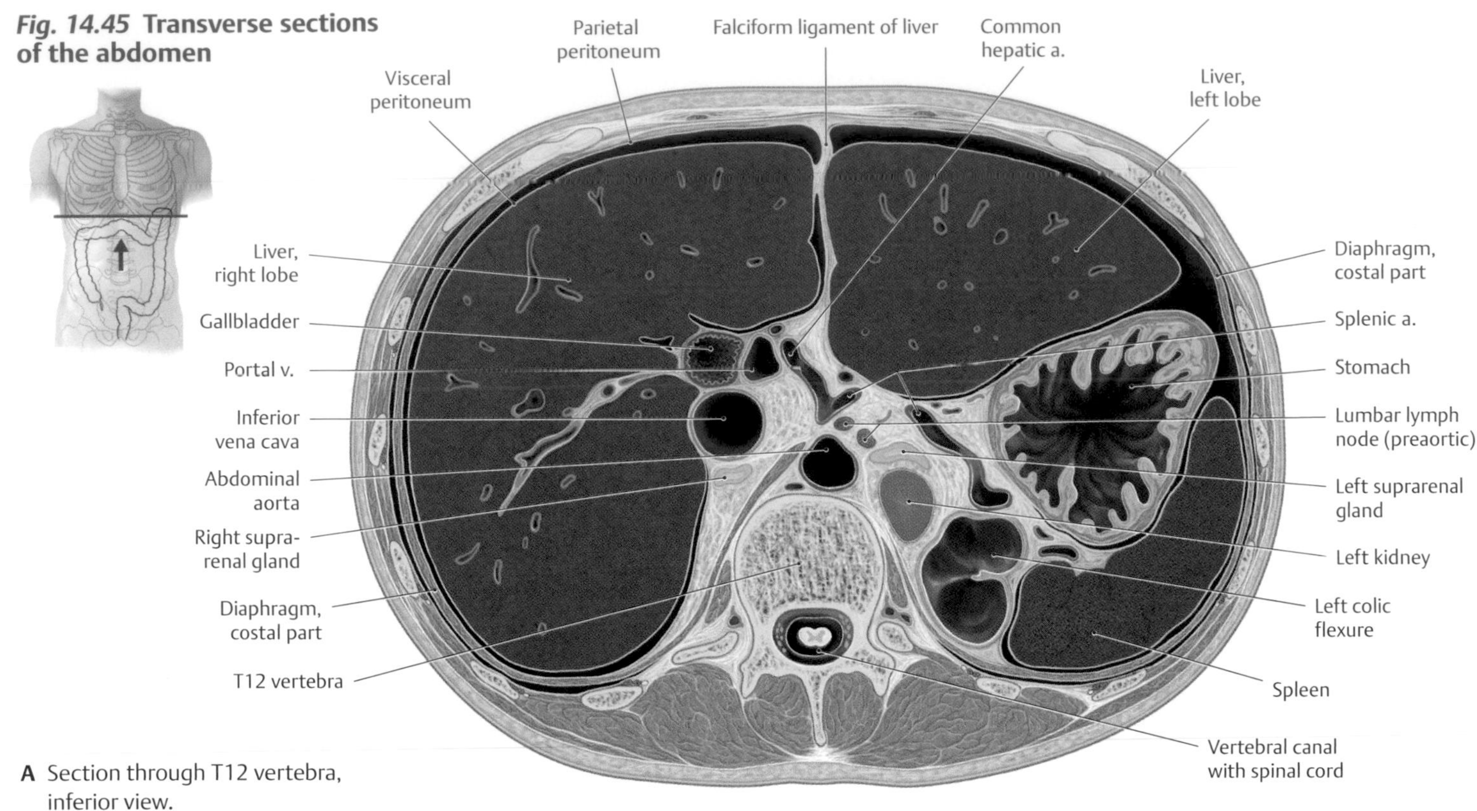
Visceral peritoneum
Parietal peritoneum
Falciform ligament of liver
Common hepatic a.
Liver, left lobe
Liver, right lobe
Gallbladder
Portal v.
Inferior vena cava
Abdominal aorta
Right supra-renal gland
Diaphragm, costal part
T12 vertebra
Diaphragm, costal part
Splenic a.
Stomach
Lumbar lymph node (preaortic)
Left suprarenal gland
Left kidney
Left colic flexure
Spleen
Vertebral canal with spinal cord

A Section through T12 vertebra, inferior view.

Internal thoracic a. and v.
Common bile duct
Duodenum
Transverse colon
Greater omentum
Superior mesenteric a. and v.
Gallbladder
Liver, right lobe
Inferior vena cava
Intercostal a., v., and n.
Intermediate lumbar lymph nodes
Right suprarenal gland
Kidney (with right renal a.)
Pyloric part
Anterior wall
Posterior wall
Stomach
Omental bursa
Splenic v.
Pancreas
Spleen
Transverse colon
Descending colon
Left colic flexure
Abdominal aorta
L1 vertebra
Spinal cord (in vertebral canal)
Lateral lumbar lymph node
Perirenal fat capsule
Left kidney
Vertebral venous plexus

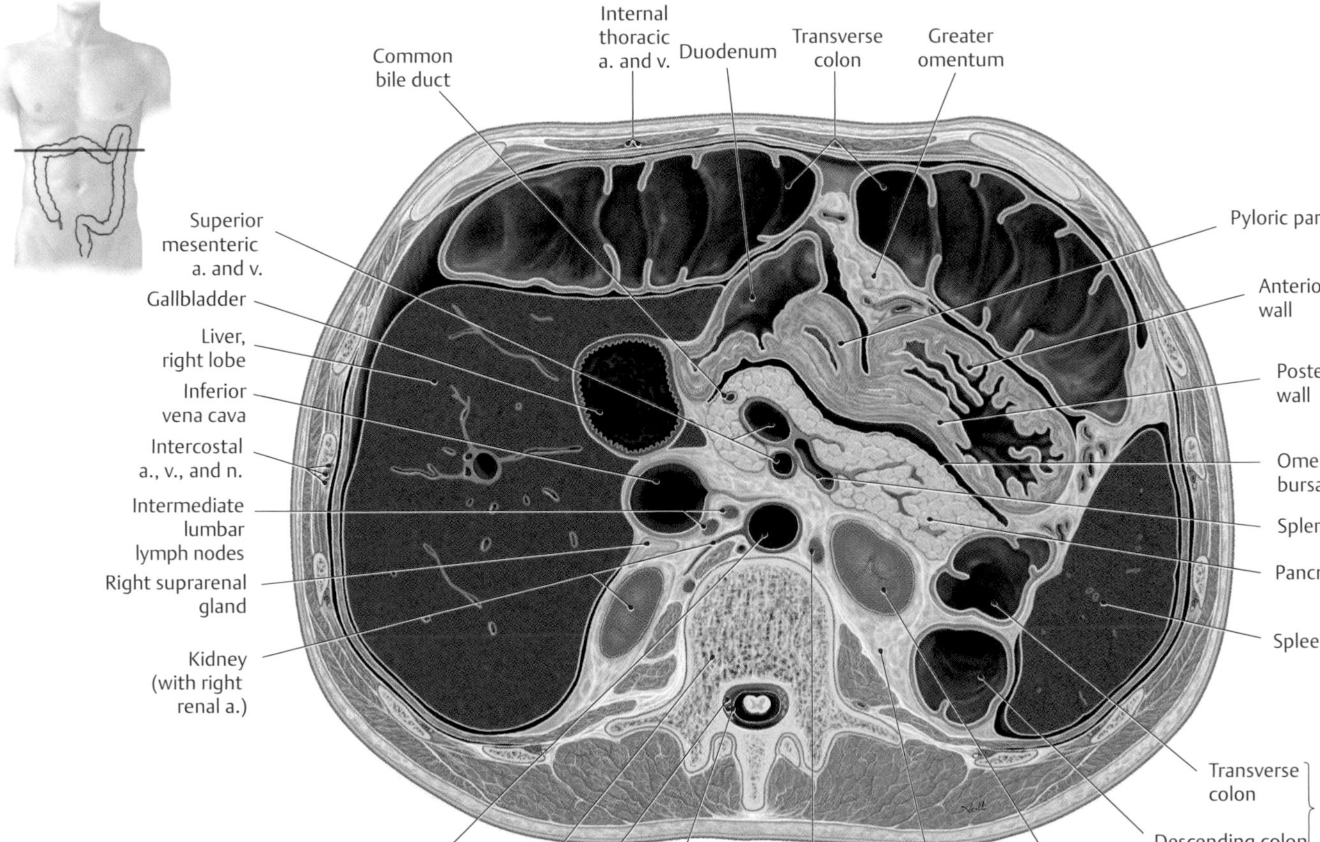

B Section through L1 vertebra, inferior view.

Transverse colon
Pancreas, head
Superior mesenteric a. and v.
Stomach, body
Jejunal a.
Celiac lymph nodes
Transverse mesocolon
Jejunum
Duodenum, descending part
Gallbladder
Liver
Right kidney
Psoas major
Inferior vena cava
Spinal cord
Abdominal aorta
Ureter
Duodenojejunal flexure

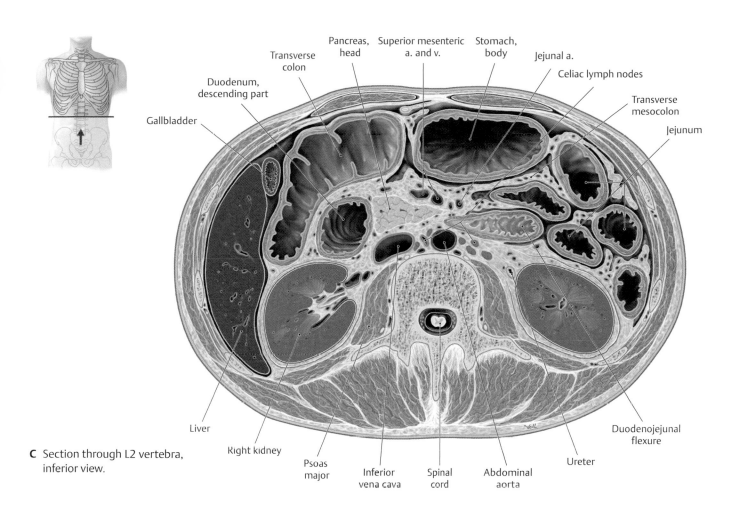

C Section through L2 vertebra, inferior view.

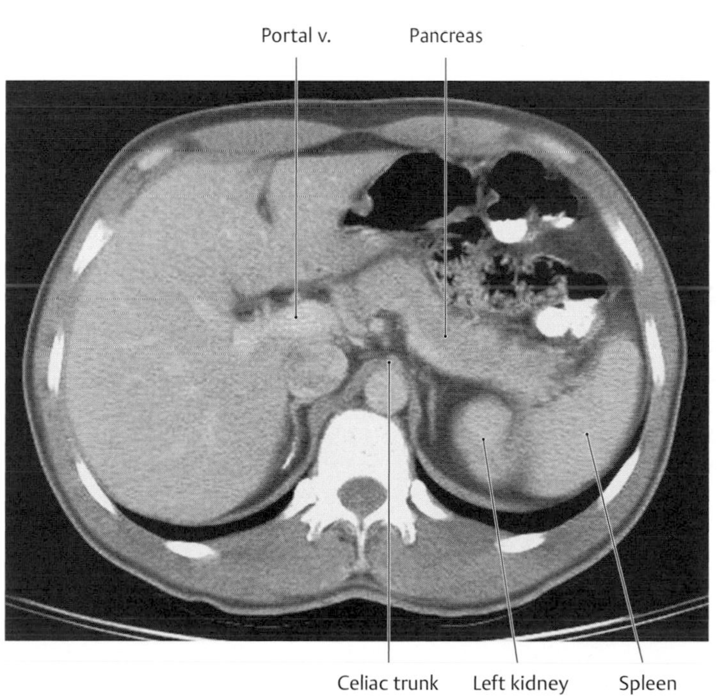
Portal v.
Pancreas
Celiac trunk
Left kidney
Spleen

D Axial CT scan through L1 vertebra.

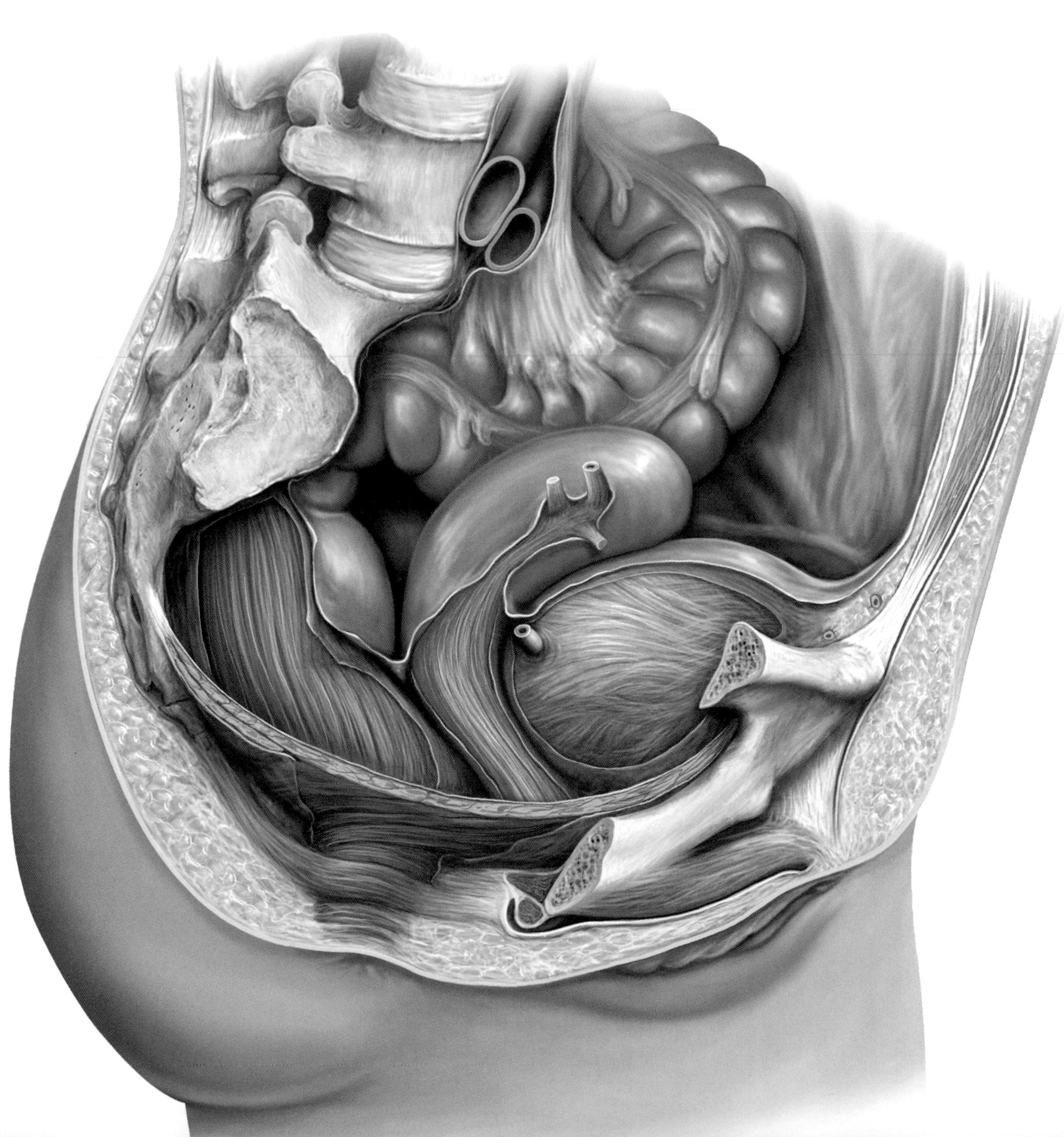

Pelvis and Perineum

15 Surface Anatomy

Surface Anatomy 214

16 Bones, Ligaments & Muscles

Pelvic Girdle 216
Female & Male Pelvis 218
Female & Male Pelvic Measurements 220
Pelvic Ligaments 222
Muscles of the Pelvic Floor & Perineum 224
Pelvic Floor & Perineal Muscle Facts 226

17 Spaces

Contents of the Pelvis 228
Peritoneal Relationships 230
Pelvis & Perineum 232

18 Internal Organs

Rectum & Anal Canal 234
Ureters 236
Urinary Bladder & Urethra 238
Overview of the Genital Organs 240
Uterus & Ovaries 242
Ligaments & Fascia of the Deep Pelvis 244
Vagina 246
Female External Genitalia 248
Penis, Testis & Epididymis 250
Male Accessory Sex Glands 252

19 Neurovasculature

Arteries & Veins of the Pelvis. 254
Arteries & Veins of the Rectum & Genitalia 256
Lymph Nodes of the Abdomen & Pelvis 258
Lymph Nodes of the Genitalia. 260
Autonomic Plexuses of the Pelvis 262
Autonomic Innervation: Urinary & Genital Organs 264
Neurovasculature of the Female Perineum & Genitalia 266
Neurovasculature of the Male Perineum & Genitalia 268
Sectional Anatomy of the Pelvis & Perineum 270

Surface Anatomy

Fig. 15.1 Palpable structures of the pelvis
Anterior view. The structures are common to both male and female. See pp. 2–3 for structures of the back.

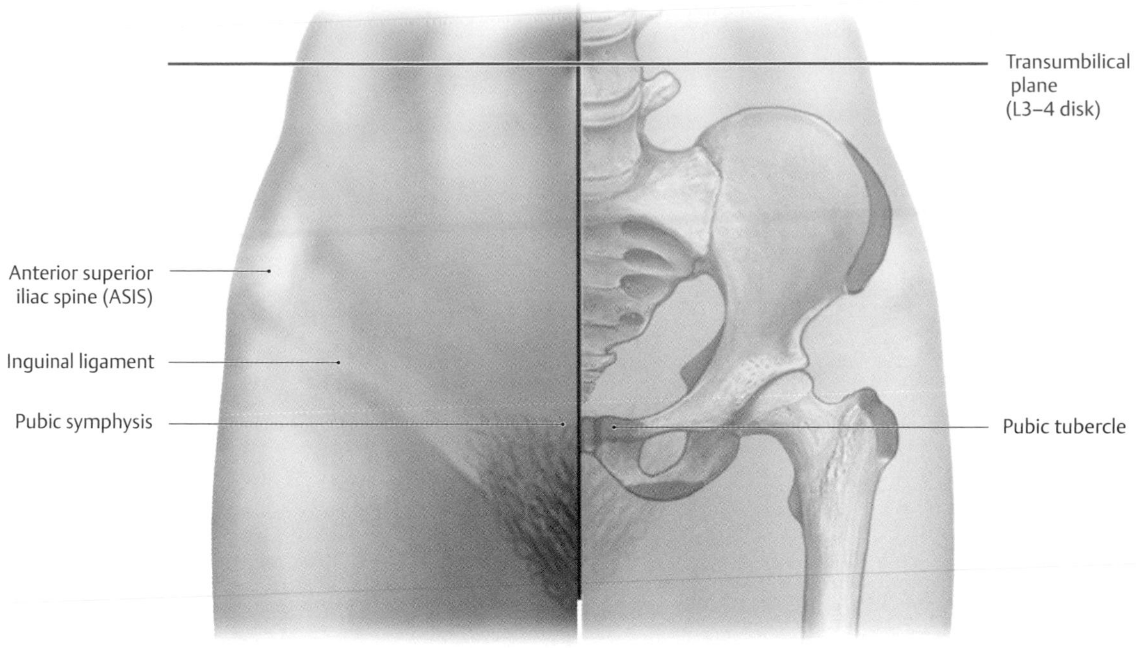

Transumbilical plane (L3–4 disk)
Anterior superior iliac spine (ASIS)
Inguinal ligament
Pubic symphysis
Pubic tubercle

A Bony prominences, female pelvis.

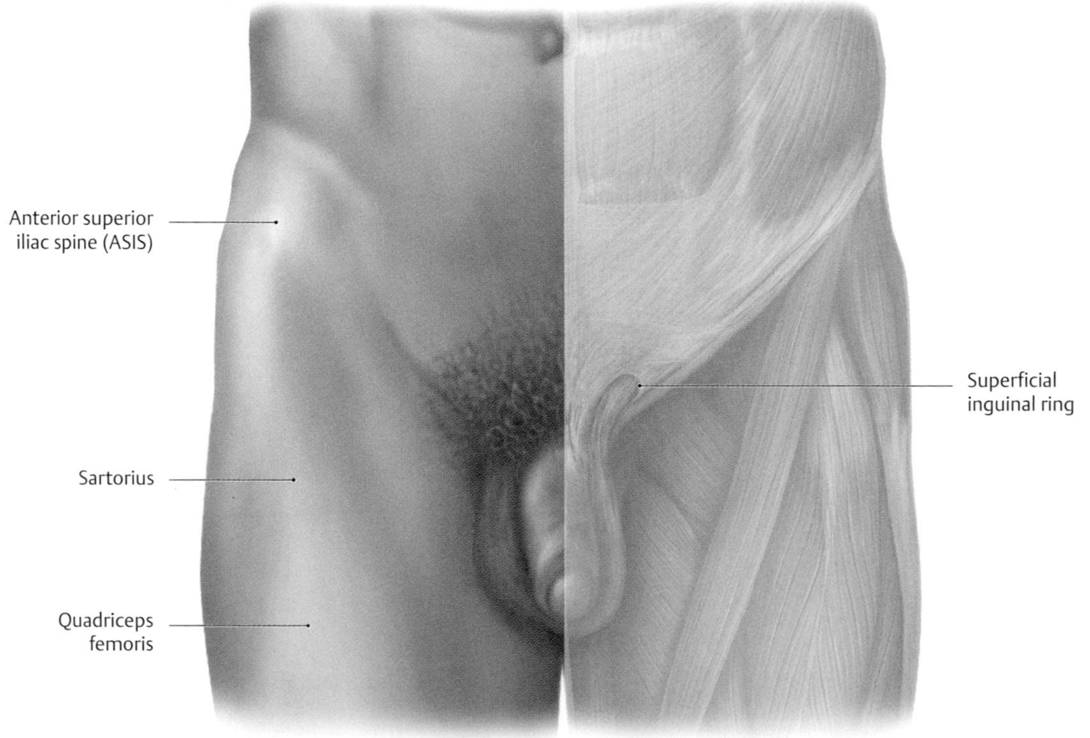

Anterior superior iliac spine (ASIS)
Superficial inguinal ring
Sartorius
Quadriceps femoris

B Musculature, male pelvis.

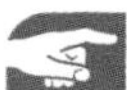

The *perineum* is the inferiormost portion of the trunk, between the thighs and buttocks, extending from the pubis to the coccyx and superiorly to the inferior fascia of the pelvic diaphragm, including all of the structures of the anal and urogenital triangles (Fig. 15.2A). The bilateral boundaries of the perineum are the pubic symphysis, ischiopubic ramus, ischial tuberosity, sacrotuberous ligament, and coccyx.

Fig. 15.2 **Regions of the female perineum**
Lithotomy position.

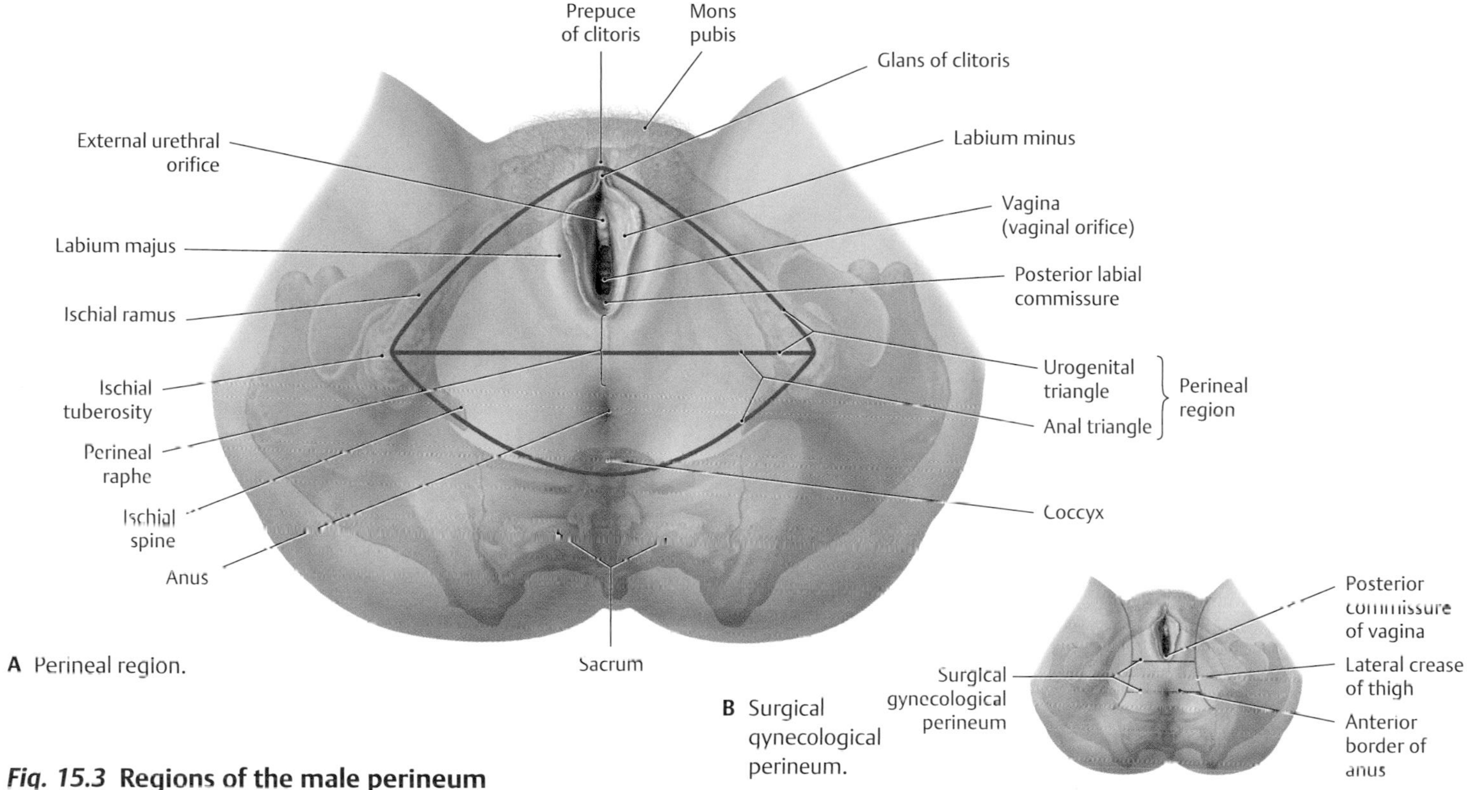

Prepuce of clitoris
Mons pubis
Glans of clitoris
External urethral orifice
Labium minus
Vagina (vaginal orifice)
Labium majus
Posterior labial commissure
Ischial ramus
Ischial tuberosity
Urogenital triangle
Anal triangle
Perineal region
Perineal raphe
Coccyx
Ischial spine
Anus
Sacrum
Posterior commissure of vagina
Lateral crease of thigh
Surgical gynecological perineum
Anterior border of anus

A Perineal region.

B Surgical gynecological perineum.

Fig. 15.3 **Regions of the male perineum**
Lithotomy position.

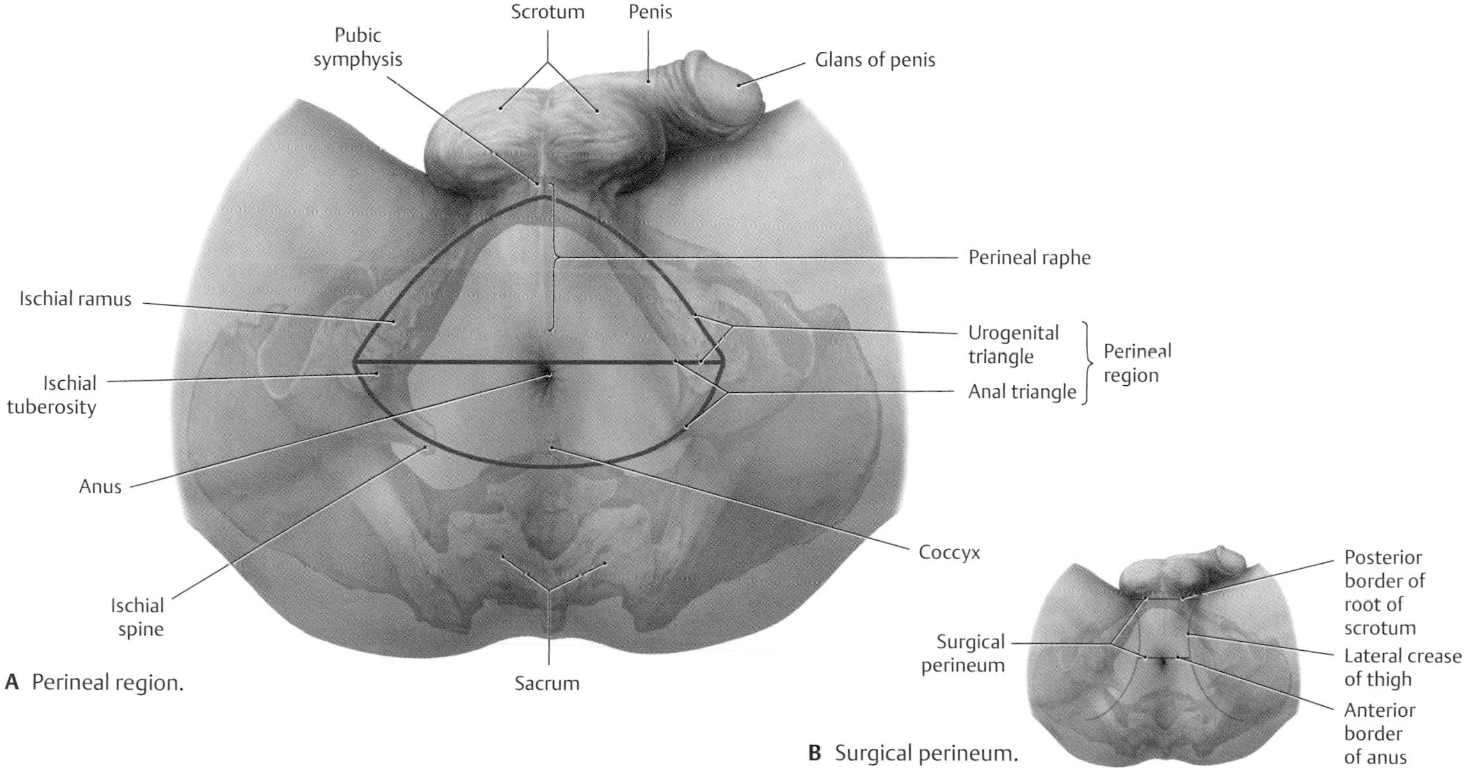

Scrotum
Penis
Pubic symphysis
Glans of penis
Perineal raphe
Ischial ramus
Urogenital triangle
Perineal region
Ischial tuberosity
Anal triangle
Anus
Coccyx
Ischial spine
Sacrum
Posterior border of root of scrotum
Surgical perineum
Lateral crease of thigh
Anterior border of anus

A Perineal region.

B Surgical perineum.

Pelvic Girdle

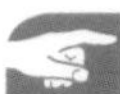

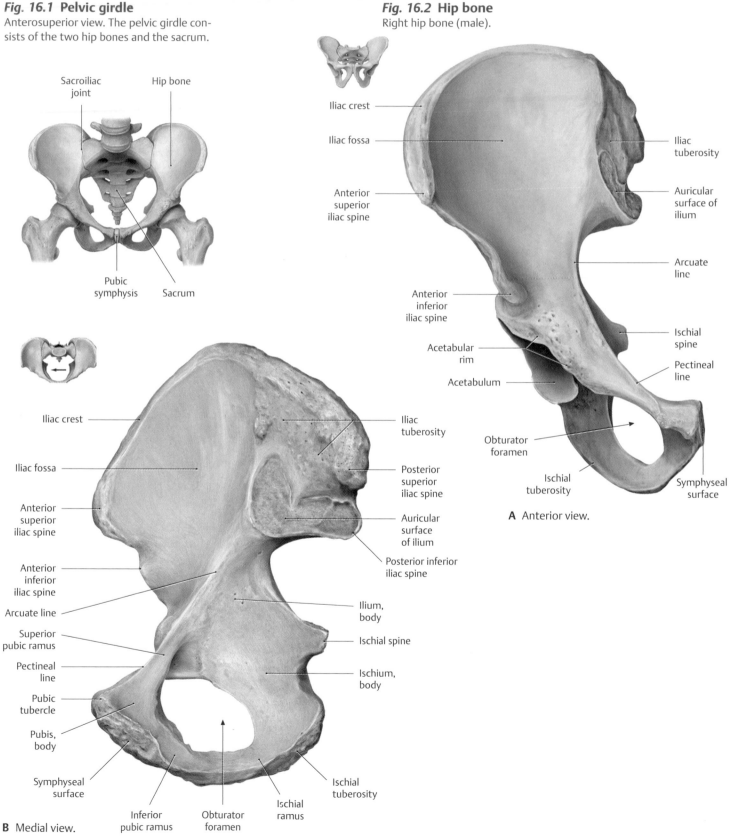

The pelvis is the region of the body inferior to the abdomen and surrounded by the pelvic girdle, which is the two hip bones and the sacrum that connect the vertebral column to the femur. The two hip bones are connected to each other at the cartilaginous pubic symphysis and to the sacrum via the sacroiliac joints, creating the pelvic brim (red, Fig. 16.1). The stability of the pelvic girdle is necessary for the transfer of trunk loads to the lower limb, which occurs in normal gait.

Fig. 16.1 **Pelvic girdle**
Anterosuperior view. The pelvic girdle consists of the two hip bones and the sacrum.

Sacroiliac joint
Hip bone
Pubic symphysis
Sacrum

Fig. 16.2 **Hip bone**
Right hip bone (male).

Iliac crest
Iliac fossa
Anterior superior iliac spine
Iliac tuberosity
Auricular surface of ilium
Arcuate line
Anterior inferior iliac spine
Ischial spine
Acetabular rim
Pectineal line
Acetabulum
Obturator foramen
Ischial tuberosity
Symphyseal surface

A Anterior view.

Iliac crest
Iliac fossa
Anterior superior iliac spine
Anterior inferior iliac spine
Arcuate line
Superior pubic ramus
Pectineal line
Pubic tubercle
Pubis, body
Symphyseal surface
Inferior pubic ramus
Obturator foramen
Ischial ramus
Ischial tuberosity
Ischium, body
Ischial spine
Ilium, body
Posterior inferior iliac spine
Auricular surface of ilium
Posterior superior iliac spine
Iliac tuberosity

B Medial view.

Fig. 16.3 Triradiate cartilage of the hip bone

Right hip bone, lateral view. The hip bone consists of the ilium, ischium, and pubis.

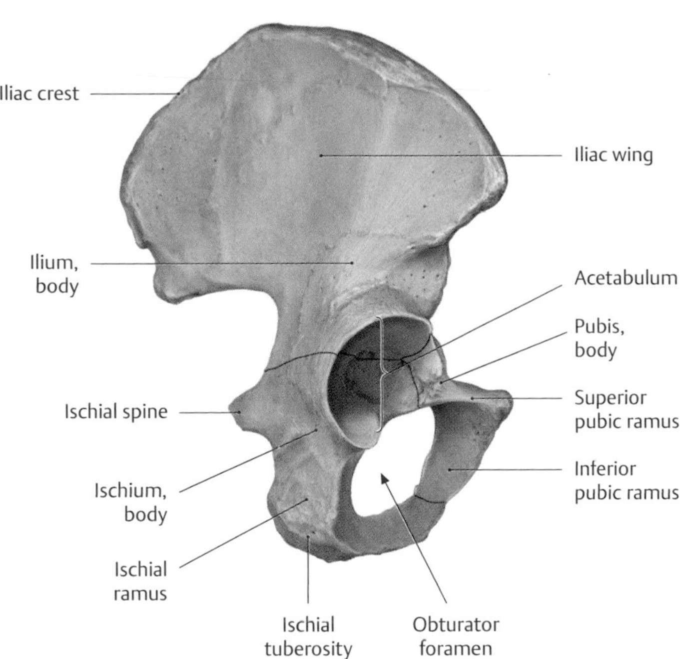
Iliac crest
Iliac wing
Ilium, body
Acetabulum
Pubis, body
Ischial spine
Superior pubic ramus
Ischium, body
Inferior pubic ramus
Ischial ramus
Ischial tuberosity
Obturator foramen

A Junction of the triradiate cartilage.

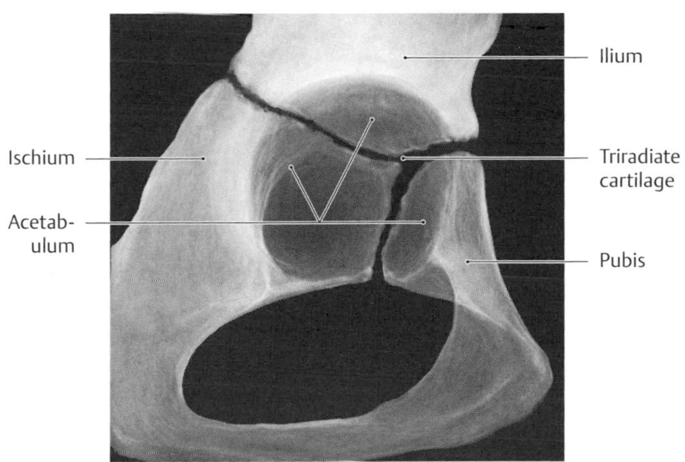
Ilium
Ischium
Triradiate cartilage
Acetab-ulum
Pubis

B Radiograph of a child's acetabulum. Right hip bone, lateral view.

Fig. 16.4 Hip bone: Lateral view

Right hip bone (male).

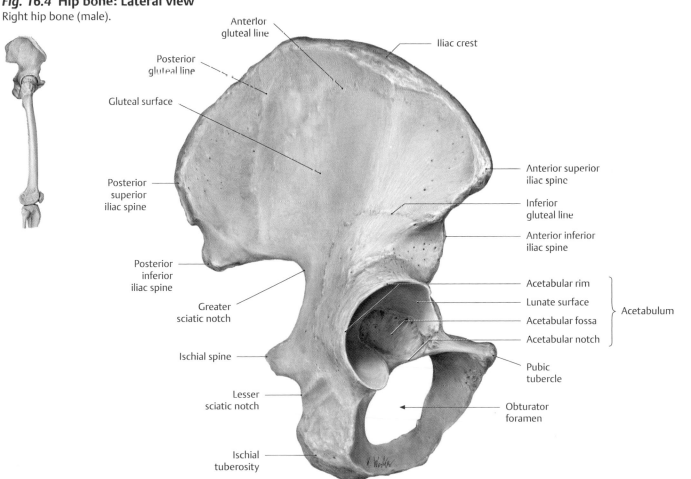

Anterior gluteal line
Iliac crest
Posterior gluteal line
Gluteal surface
Anterior superior iliac spine
Posterior superior iliac spine
Inferior gluteal line
Anterior inferior iliac spine
Posterior inferior iliac spine
Acetabular rim
Lunate surface
Acetabular fossa
Acetabular notch
Acetabulum
Greater sciatic notch
Ischial spine
Pubic tubercle
Lesser sciatic notch
Obturator foramen
Ischial tuberosity

Female & Male Pelvis

Fig. 16.5 Female pelvis

Iliac crest
Sacroiliac joint
Pubic tubercle
Iliac fossa
Sacrum
Anterior superior iliac spine
Anterior inferior iliac spine
Superior and inferior pubic rami
Acetabular margin
Ischial spine
Pubic symphysis
Obturator foramen
Coccyx
Pubic arch
Ischial ramus

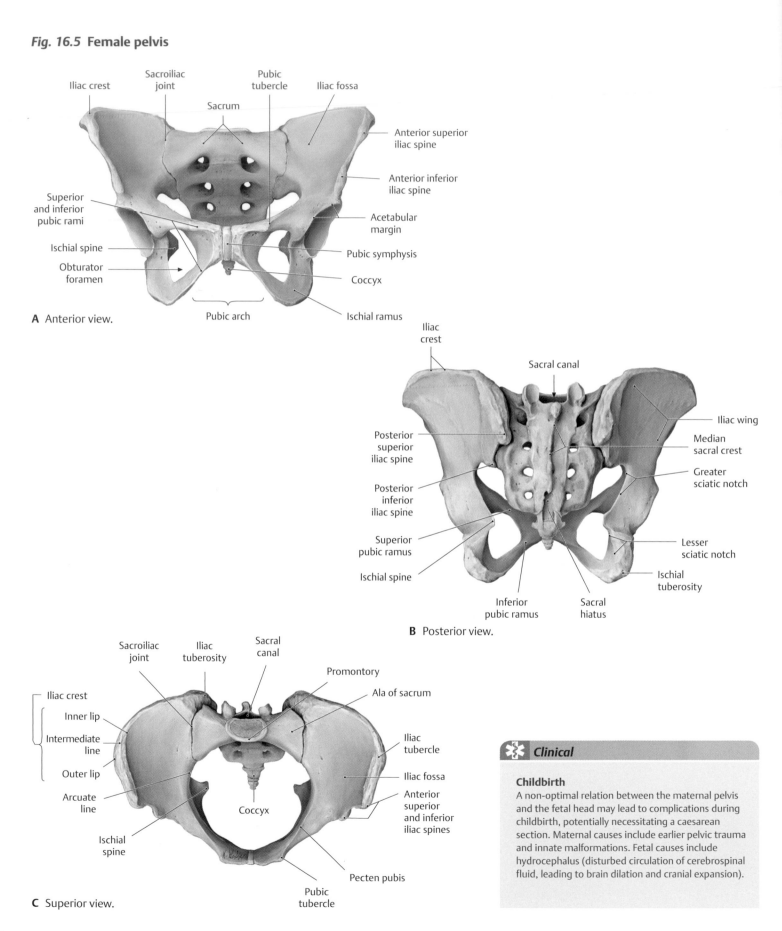

A Anterior view.

Iliac crest
Sacral canal
Iliac wing
Median sacral crest
Posterior superior iliac spine
Greater sciatic notch
Posterior inferior iliac spine
Superior pubic ramus
Lesser sciatic notch
Ischial spine
Ischial tuberosity
Inferior pubic ramus
Sacral hiatus

B Posterior view.

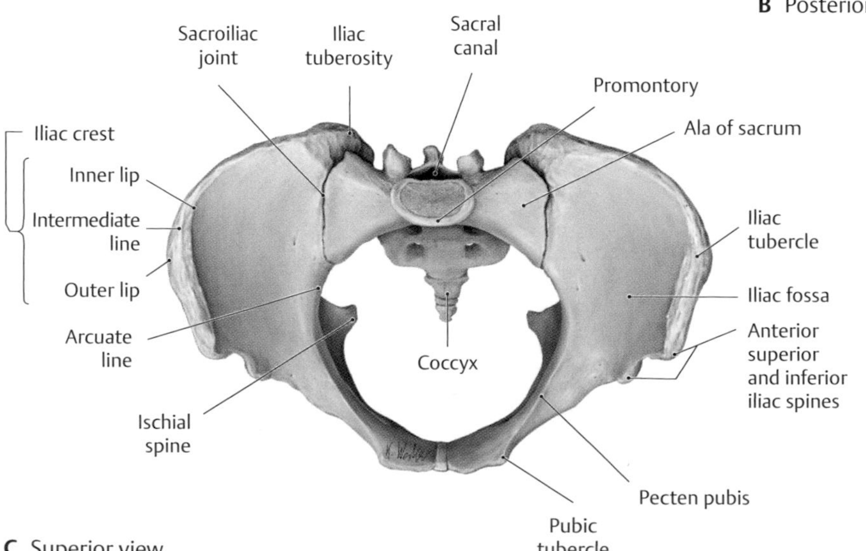
Sacroiliac joint
Iliac tuberosity
Sacral canal
Promontory
Iliac crest
Ala of sacrum
Inner lip
Intermediate line
Iliac tubercle
Outer lip
Iliac fossa
Arcuate line
Anterior superior and inferior iliac spines
Coccyx
Ischial spine
Pecten pubis
Pubic tubercle

C Superior view.

Clinical

Childbirth

A non-optimal relation between the maternal pelvis and the fetal head may lead to complications during childbirth, potentially necessitating a caesarean section. Maternal causes include earlier pelvic trauma and innate malformations. Fetal causes include hydrocephalus (disturbed circulation of cerebrospinal fluid, leading to brain dilation and cranial expansion).

Fig. 16.6 Male pelvis

Sacrum
Superior articular process
Pelvic surface
Ala
Iliac crest
Promontory
Anterior superior and inferior iliac spines
Posterior inferior iliac spine
Anterior sacral foramina
Pecten pubis
Pubic tubercle
Acetabulum
Ischial spine
Pubic symphysis
Obturator foramen
Pubic arch

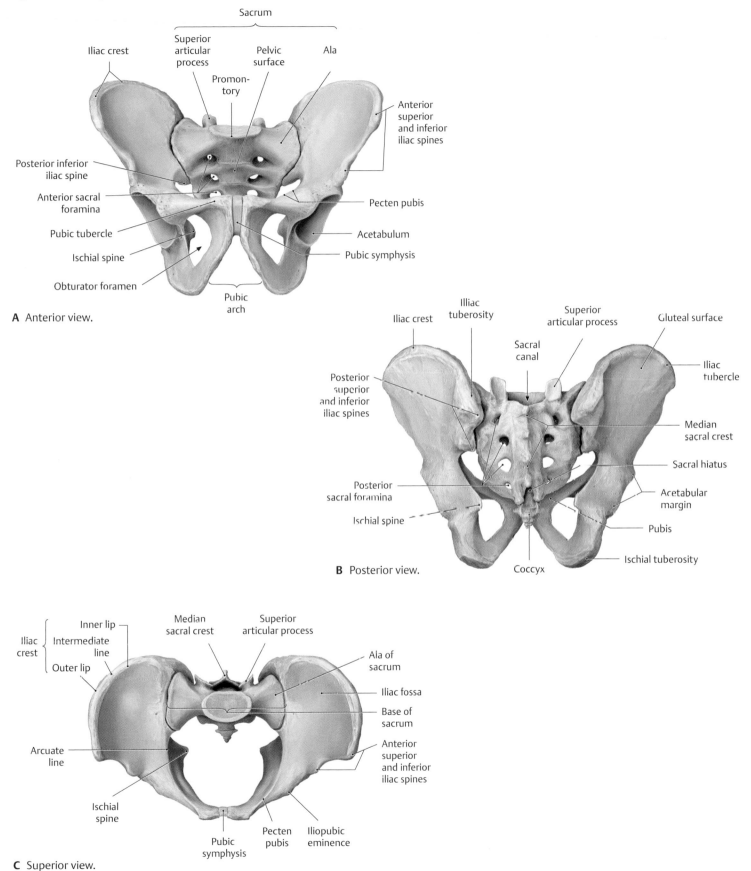

A Anterior view.

Iliac crest
Illiac tuberosity
Superior articular process
Gluteal surface
Sacral canal
Iliac tubercle
Posterior superior and inferior iliac spines
Median sacral crest
Sacral hiatus
Posterior sacral foramina
Acetabular margin
Ischial spine
Pubis
Ischial tuberosity
Coccyx

B Posterior view.

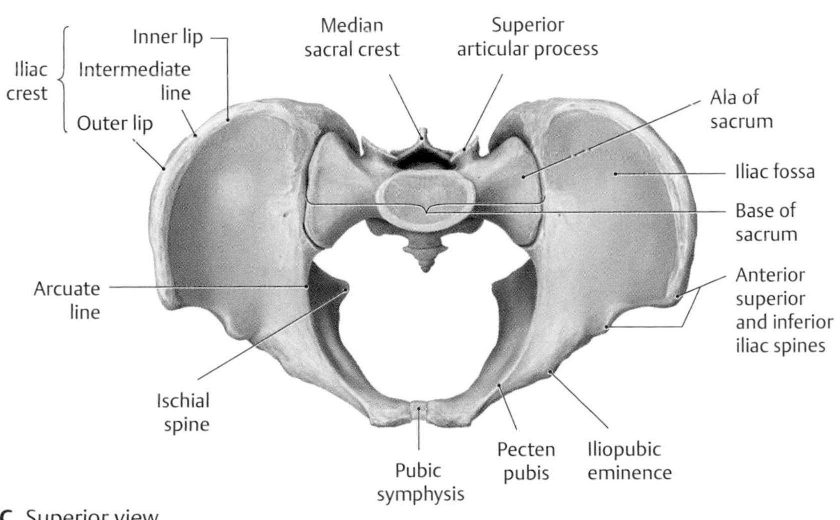
Iliac crest
Inner lip
Intermediate line
Outer lip
Median sacral crest
Superior articular process
Ala of sacrum
Iliac fossa
Base of sacrum
Arcuate line
Anterior superior and inferior iliac spines
Ischial spine
Pubic symphysis
Pecten pubis
Iliopubic eminence

C Superior view.

Female & Male Pelvic Measurements

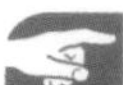

The *pelvic inlet*, the superior aperture of the pelvis, is the boundary between the abdominal and pelvic cavities. It is defined by the plane that passes through its edge, the *pelvic brim*, which is the prominence of the sacrum, the arcuate and pectineal lines, and the upper margin of the pubic symphysis. Occasionally, the terms *pelvic inlet* and *pelvic brim* are used interchangeably. The *pelvic outlet* is the plane of the inferior aperture, passing through the pubic arch, the ischial tuberosities, the inferior margin of the sacrotuberous ligament, and the tip of the coccyx.

Table 16.1 Gender-specific features of the pelvis

Structure	♀	♂
False pelvis	Wide and shallow	Narrow and deep
Pelvic inlet	Transversely oval	Heart-shaped
Pelvic outlet	Roomy and round	Narrow and oblong
Ischial tuberosities	Everted	Inverted
Pelvic cavity	Roomy and shallow	Narrow and deep
Sacrum	Short, wide, and flat	Long, narrow, and convex
Subpubic angle	90–100 degrees	70 degrees

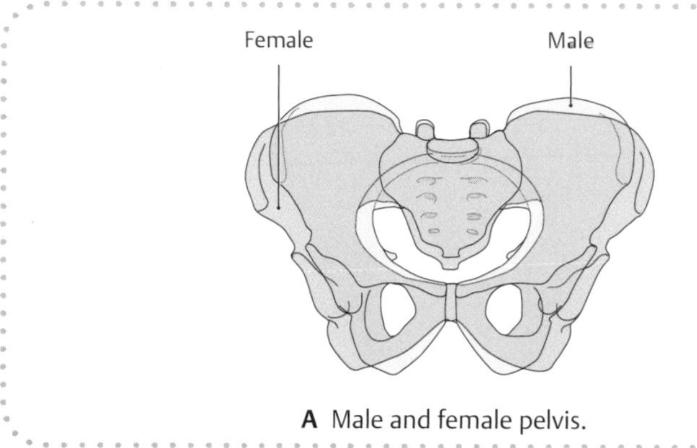
Female
Male

A Male and female pelvis.

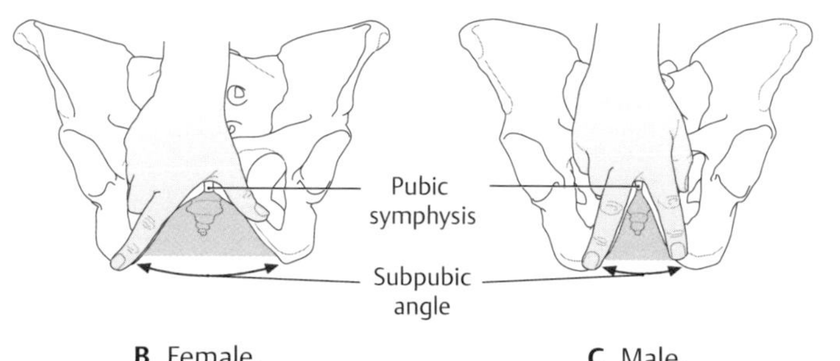
Pubic symphysis
Subpubic angle

B Female.

C Male.

Fig. 16.7 Pelvic inlet and outlet

The measurements shown are applicable to both male and female. The transverse and oblique diameters of the female pelvic inlet are obstetrically important, as they are the measure of the diameter of the pelvic (birth) canal. The interspinous distance is the narrowest diameter of the pelvic outlet.

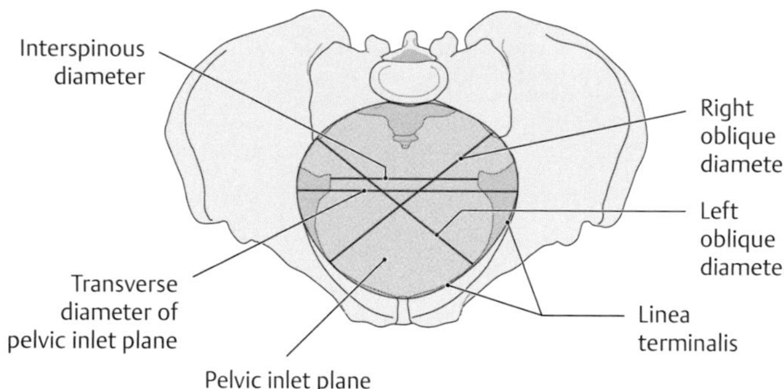
Interspinous diameter
Right oblique diameter
Left oblique diameter
Transverse diameter of pelvic inlet plane
Linea terminalis
Pelvic inlet plane

A Female pelvis, superior view. Pelvic inlet outlined in red.

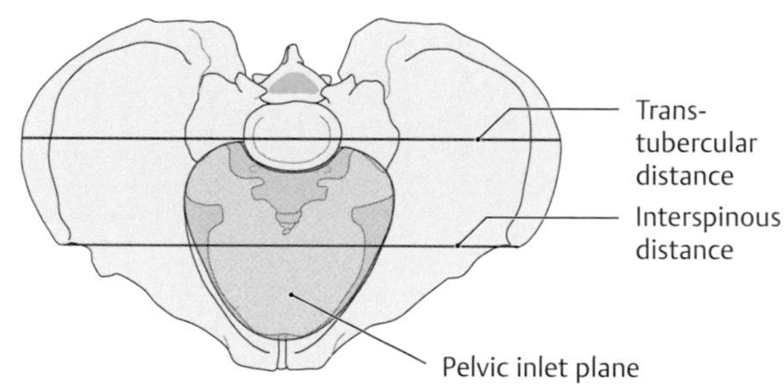
Trans-tubercular distance
Interspinous distance
Pelvic inlet plane

B Male pelvis, superior view. Pelvic inlet outlined in red.

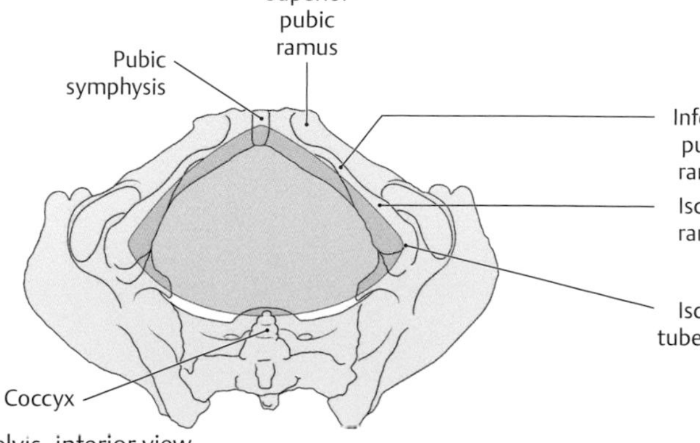
Superior pubic ramus
Pubic symphysis
Inferior pubic ramus
Ischial ramus
Ischial tuberosity
Coccyx

C Female pelvis, inferior view. Pelvic outlet outlined in red.

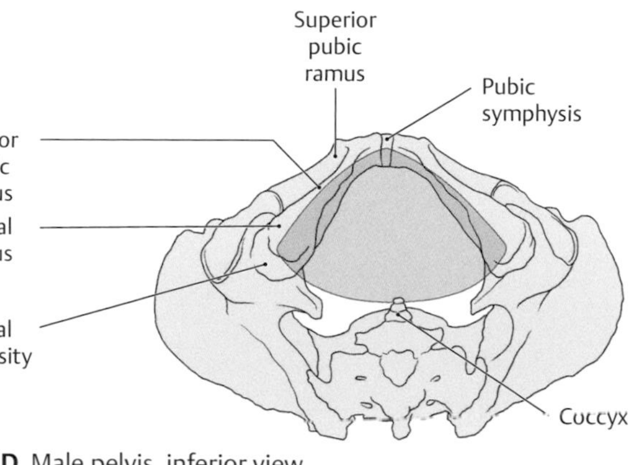
Superior pubic ramus
Pubic symphysis
Coccyx

D Male pelvis, inferior view. Pelvic outlet outlined in red.

Fig. 16.8 Narrowest diameter of female pelvic canal

The true conjugate, the distance between the promontory and the most posterosuperior point of the pubic symphysis, is the narrowest AP (anteroposterior) diameter of the pelvic (birth) canal. This diameter is difficult to measure due to the viscera, so the diagonal conjugate, the distance between the promontory and the inferior border of the pubic symphysis, is used to estimate it. The linea terminalis is part of the border defining the pelvic inlet.

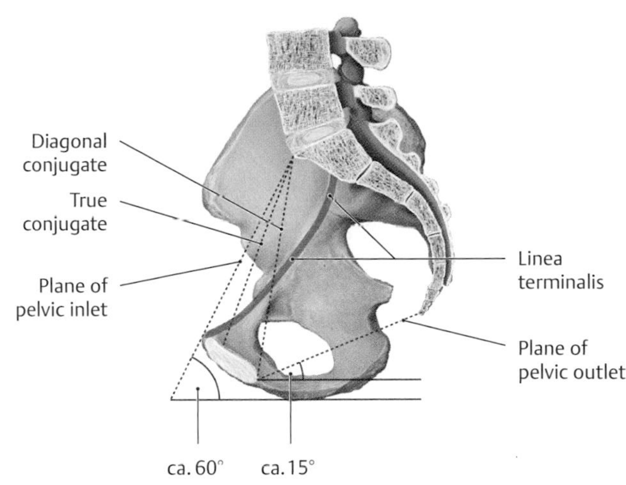

Diagonal conjugate
True conjugate
Plane of pelvic inlet
Linea terminalis
Plane of pelvic outlet
ca. 60°
ca. 15°

Fig. 16.9 True and false pelvis

The pelvis is the region of the body inferior to the abdomen, surrounded by the pelvic girdle. The *false*, or greater, *pelvis* is immediately inferior to the abdominal cavity, between the iliac alae, and superior to the pelvic inlet. The *true*, or lesser, *pelvis* is the bony-walled space between the pelvic inlet and the pelvic outlet. It is bounded inferiorly by the pelvic diaphragm, also called the pelvic floor.

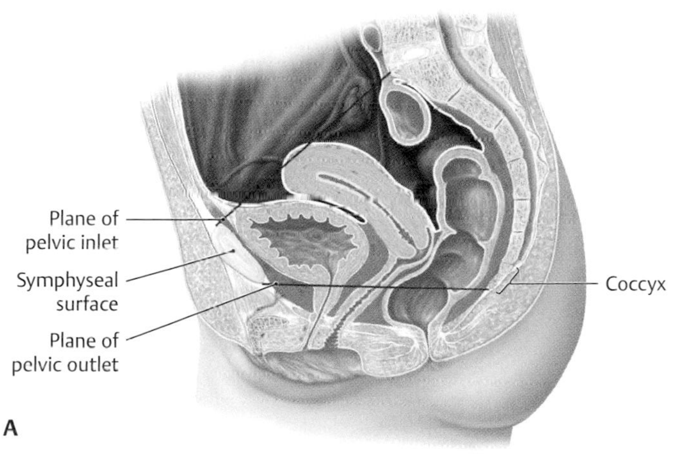

Plane of pelvic inlet
Symphyseal surface
Plane of pelvic outlet
Coccyx
A

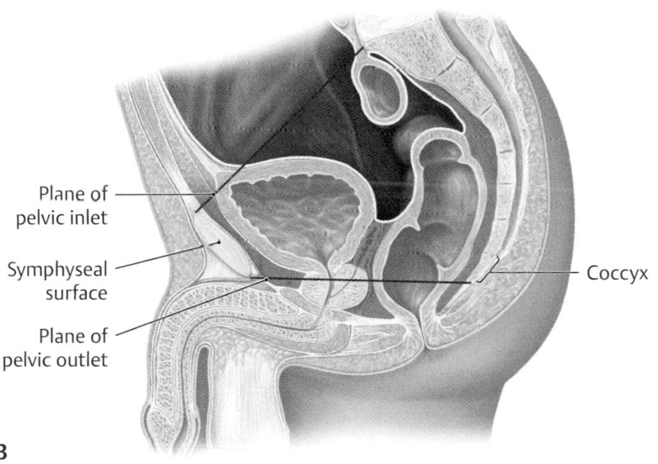

Plane of pelvic inlet
Symphyseal surface
Plane of pelvic outlet
Coccyx
B

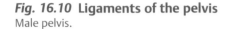

Pelvic Ligaments

Fig. 16.10 **Ligaments of the pelvis**
Male pelvis.

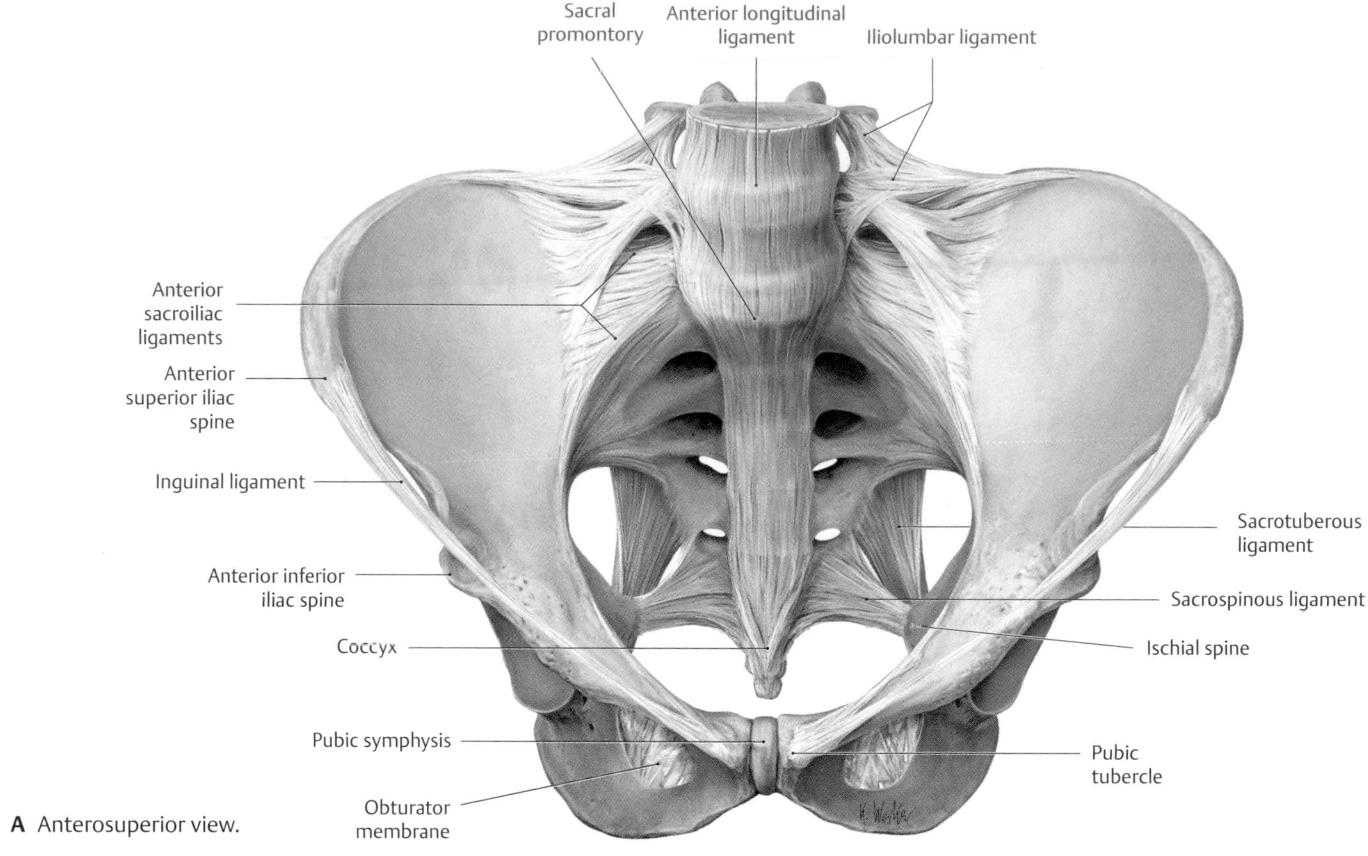

Sacral promontory
Anterior longitudinal ligament
Iliolumbar ligament
Anterior sacroiliac ligaments
Anterior superior iliac spine
Inguinal ligament
Anterior inferior iliac spine
Coccyx
Pubic symphysis
Obturator membrane
Sacrotuberous ligament
Sacrospinous ligament
Ischial spine
Pubic tubercle

A Anterosuperior view.

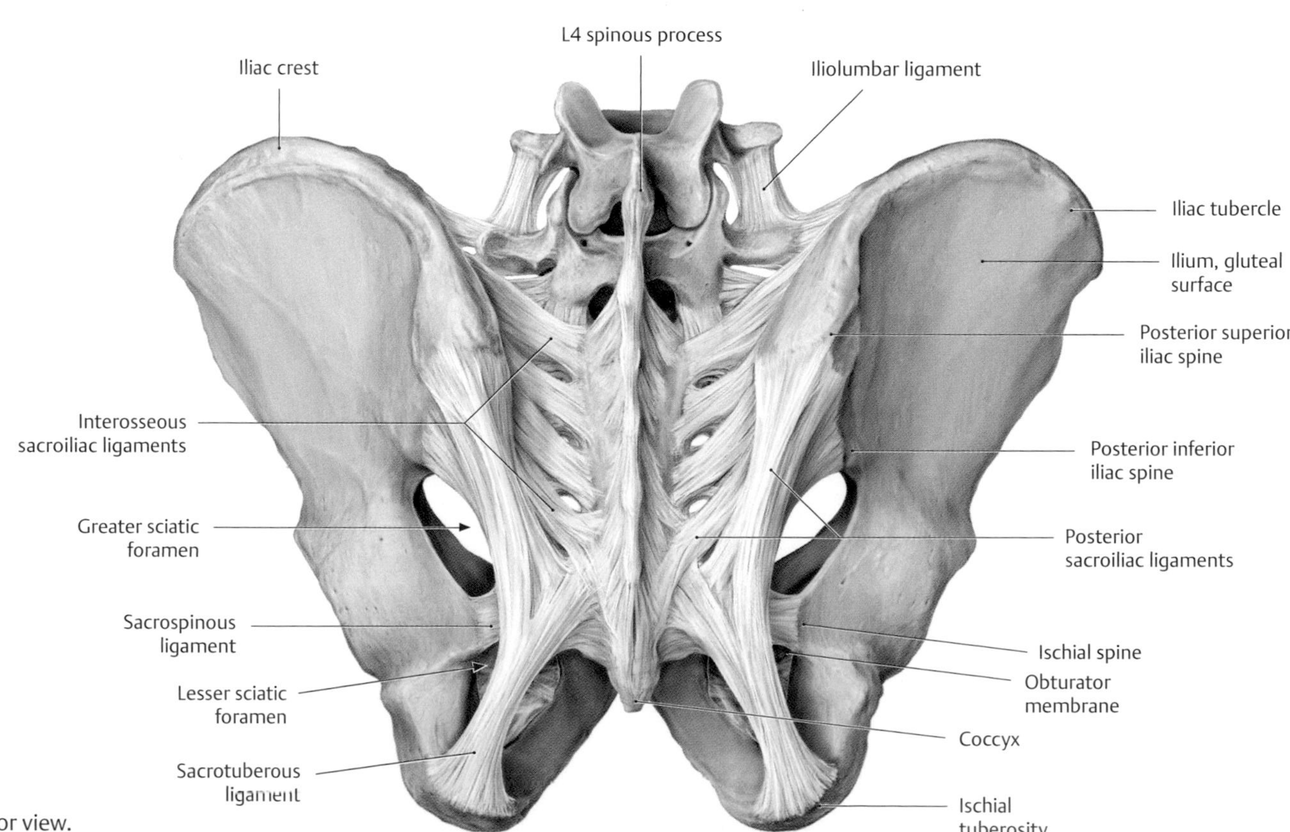

L4 spinous process
Iliac crest
Iliolumbar ligament
Iliac tubercle
Ilium, gluteal surface
Posterior superior iliac spine
Interosseous sacroiliac ligaments
Posterior inferior iliac spine
Greater sciatic foramen
Posterior sacroiliac ligaments
Sacrospinous ligament
Ischial spine
Obturator membrane
Lesser sciatic foramen
Coccyx
Sacrotuberous ligament
Ischial tuberosity

B Posterior view.

Fig. 16.11 **Ligaments of the sacroiliac joint**
Male pelvis.

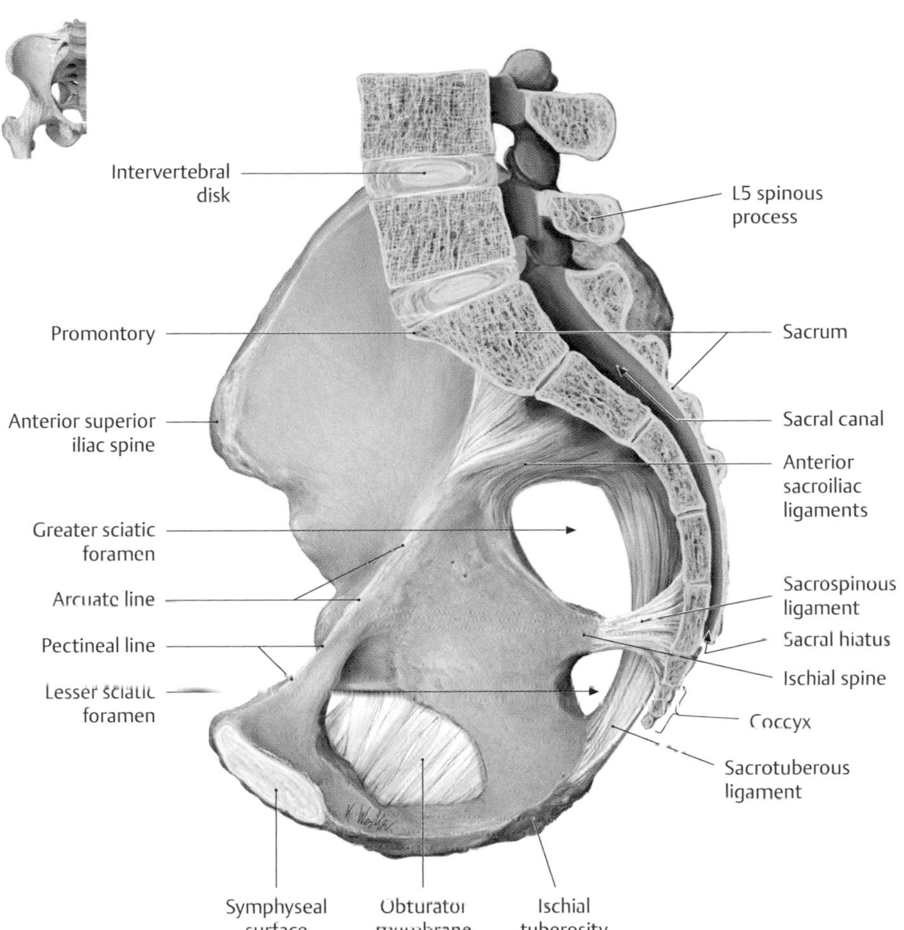

Intervertebral disk
L5 spinous process
Promontory
Sacrum
Anterior superior iliac spine
Sacral canal
Anterior sacroiliac ligaments
Greater sciatic foramen
Arcuate line
Sacrospinous ligament
Pectineal line
Sacral hiatus
Ischial spine
Lesser sciatic foramen
Coccyx
Sacrotuberous ligament
Symphyseal surface
Obturator membrane
Ischial tuberosity

A Right half of pelvis, medial view.

Fig. 16.12 **Pelvic ligament attachment sites on hip bone**
Left hip bone, medial view. Ligament attachments are shown in green.

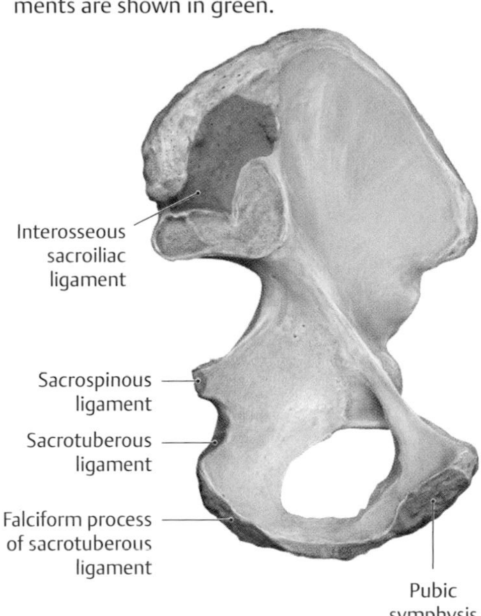

Interosseous sacroiliac ligament
Sacrospinous ligament
Sacrotuberous ligament
Falciform process of sacrotuberous ligament
Pubic symphysis

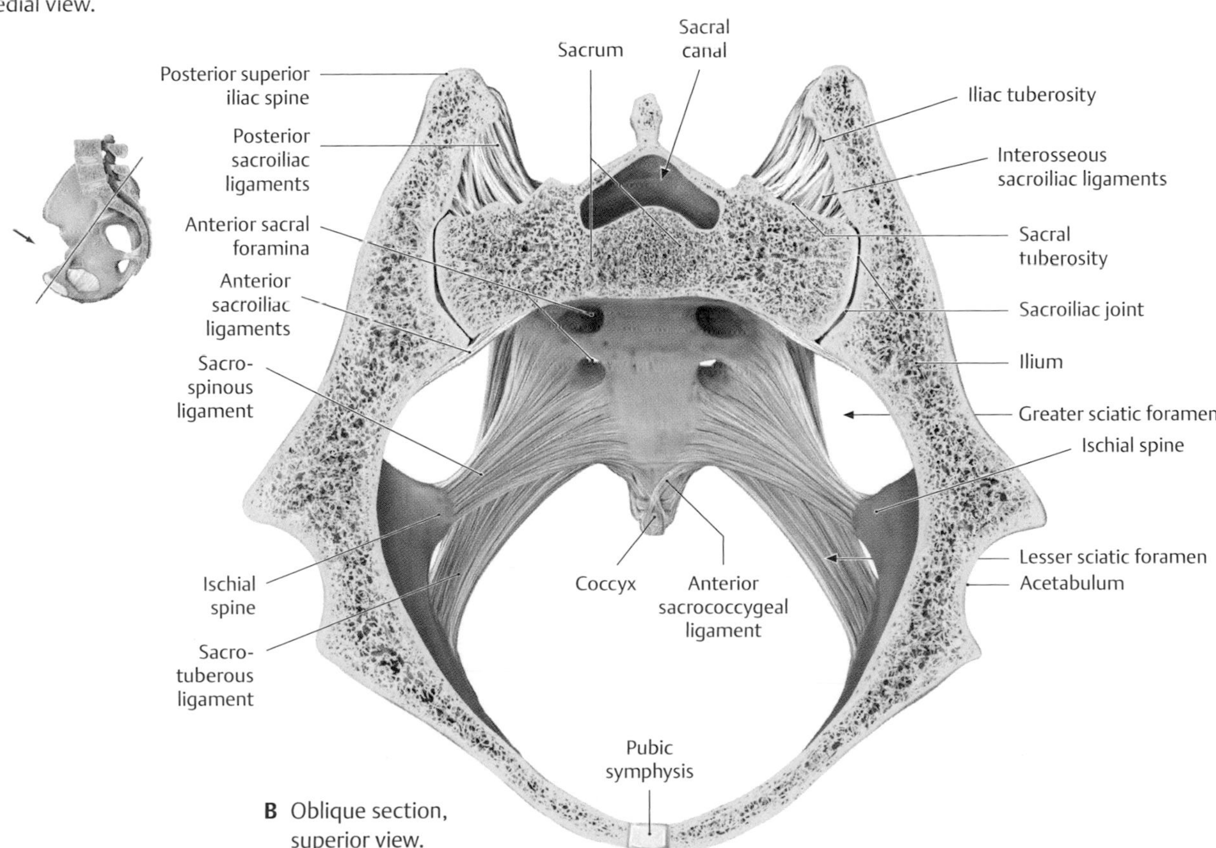

Sacrum
Sacral canal
Posterior superior iliac spine
Iliac tuberosity
Posterior sacroiliac ligaments
Interosseous sacroiliac ligaments
Anterior sacral foramina
Sacral tuberosity
Anterior sacroiliac ligaments
Sacroiliac joint
Sacro-spinous ligament
Ilium
Greater sciatic foramen
Ischial spine
Lesser sciatic foramen
Acetabulum
Ischial spine
Coccyx
Anterior sacrococcygeal ligament
Sacro-tuberous ligament
Pubic symphysis

B Oblique section, superior view.

Muscles of the Pelvic Floor & Perineum

Fig. 16.13 Muscles of the pelvic floor

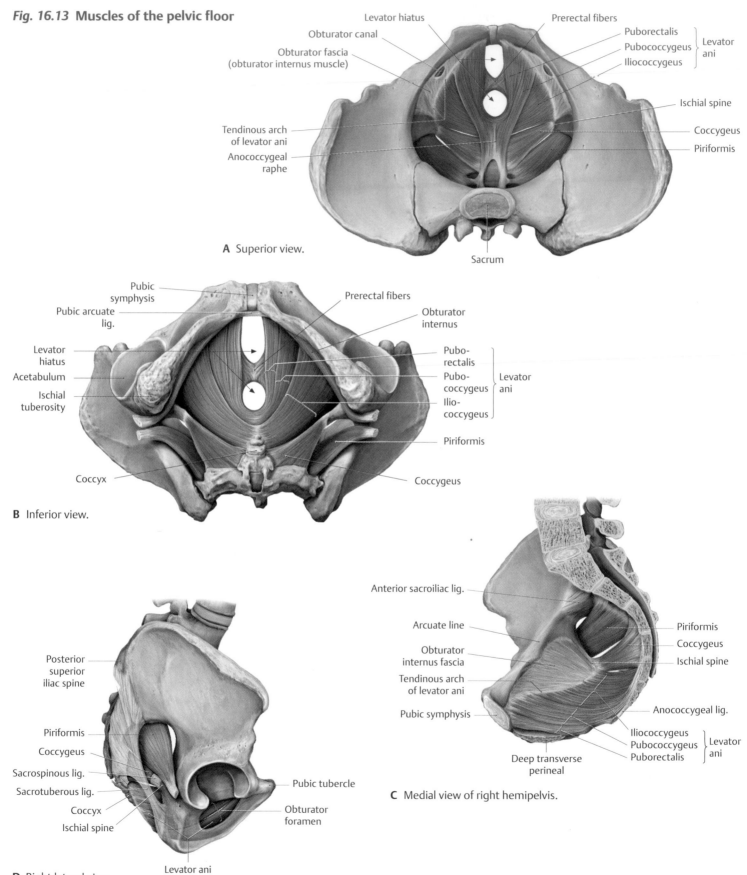

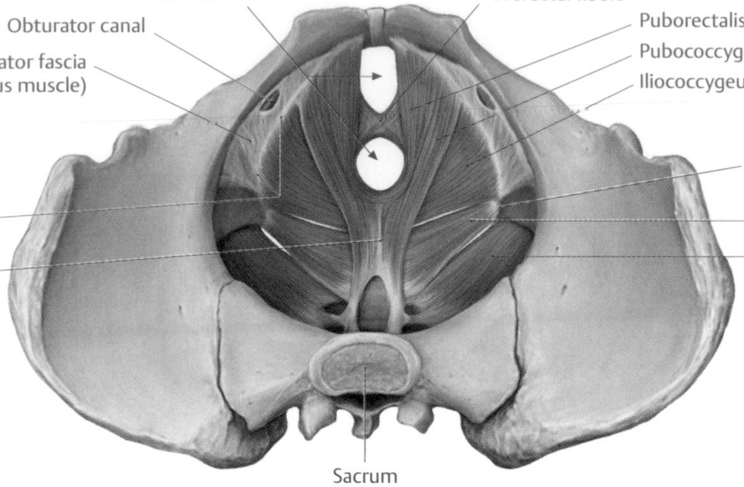

A Superior view.

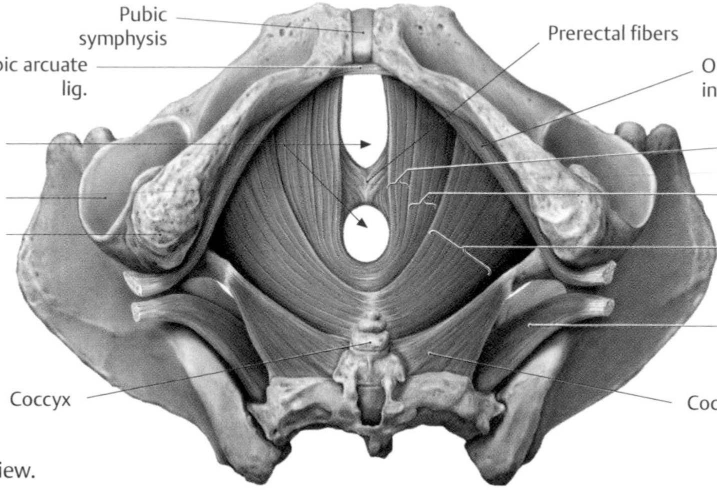

Levator hiatus
Obturator canal
Obturator fascia (obturator internus muscle)
Tendinous arch of levator ani
Anococcygeal raphe
Prerectal fibers
Puborectalis
Pubococcygeus
Iliococcygeus
Levator ani
Ischial spine
Coccygeus
Piriformis
Sacrum

B Inferior view.

Pubic symphysis
Pubic arcuate lig.
Levator hiatus
Acetabulum
Ischial tuberosity
Coccyx
Prerectal fibers
Obturator internus
Pubo-rectalis
Pubo-coccygeus
Ilio-coccygeus
Levator ani
Piriformis
Coccygeus

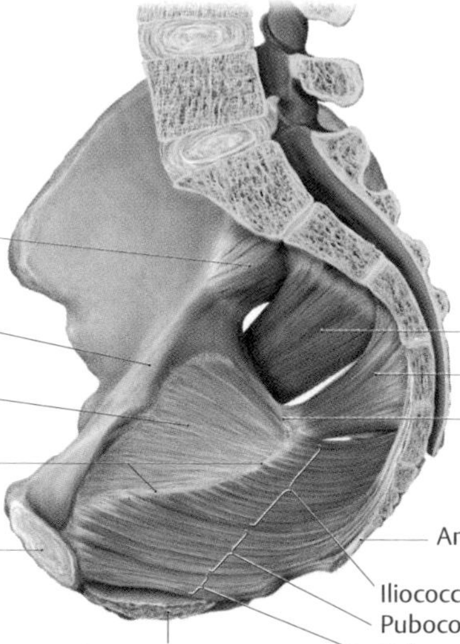

C Medial view of right hemipelvis.

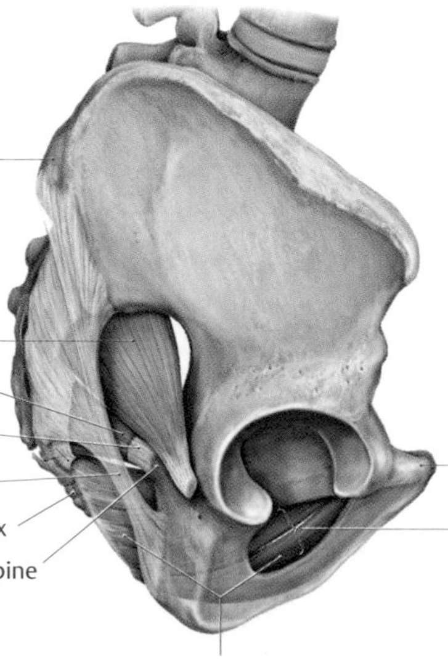

Anterior sacroiliac lig.
Arcuate line
Obturator internus fascia
Tendinous arch of levator ani
Pubic symphysis
Deep transverse perineal
Piriformis
Coccygeus
Ischial spine
Anococcygeal lig.
Iliococcygeus
Pubococcygeus
Puborectalis
Levator ani

D Right lateral view.

Posterior superior iliac spine
Piriformis
Coccygeus
Sacrospinous lig.
Sacrotuberous lig.
Coccyx
Ischial spine
Levator ani
Pubic tubercle
Obturator foramen

Fig. 16.14 Muscles and fascia of the pelvic floor and perineum, in situ
Lithotomy position. Removed on left side: Superficial perineal (Colle's) fascia, inferior fascia of the pelvic diaphragm, and obturator fascia.
Note: The green arrows are pointing forward to the anterior recess of the ischioanal fossa.

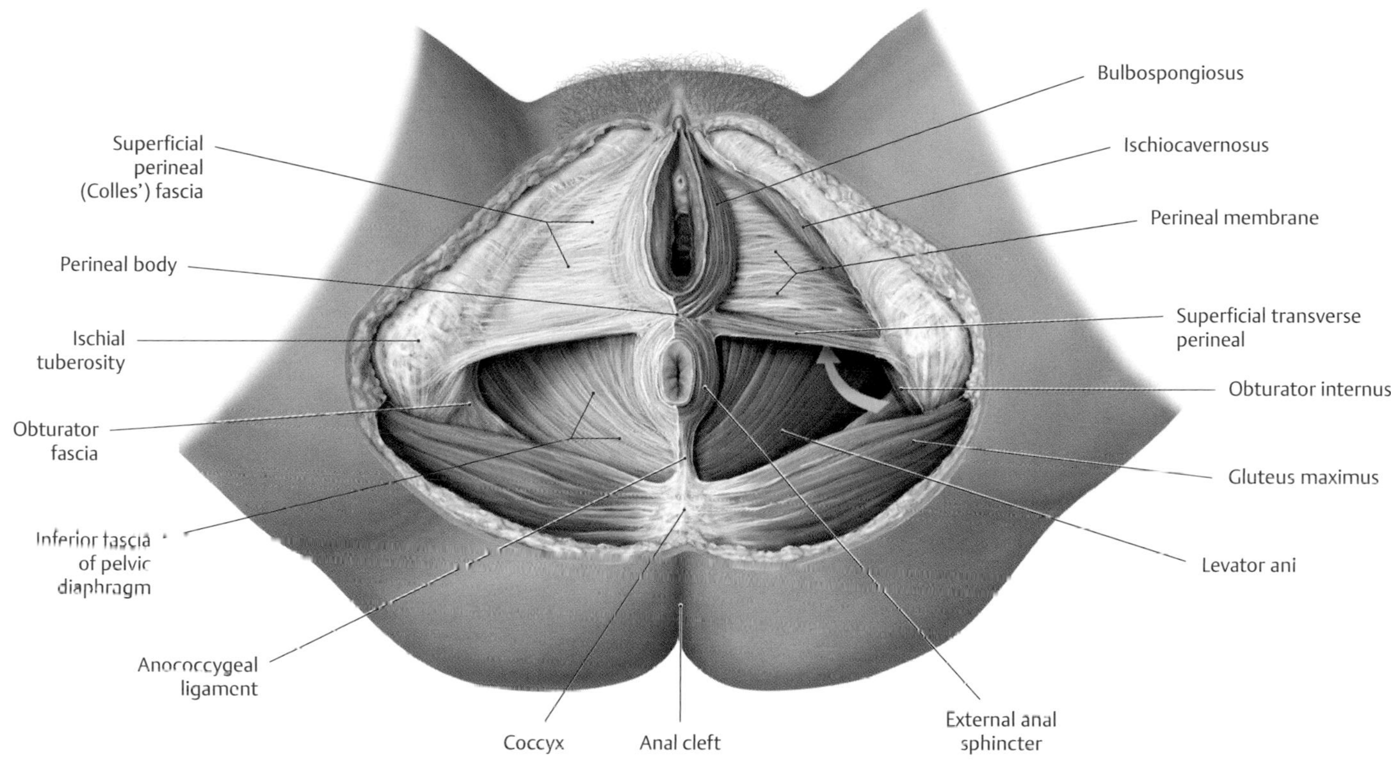
Superficial perineal (Colles') fascia
Perineal body
Ischial tuberosity
Obturator fascia
Inferior fascia of pelvic diaphragm
Anococcygeal ligament
Coccyx
Anal cleft
External anal sphincter
Bulbospongiosus
Ischiocavernosus
Perineal membrane
Superficial transverse perineal
Obturator internus
Gluteus maximus
Levator ani

A Female.

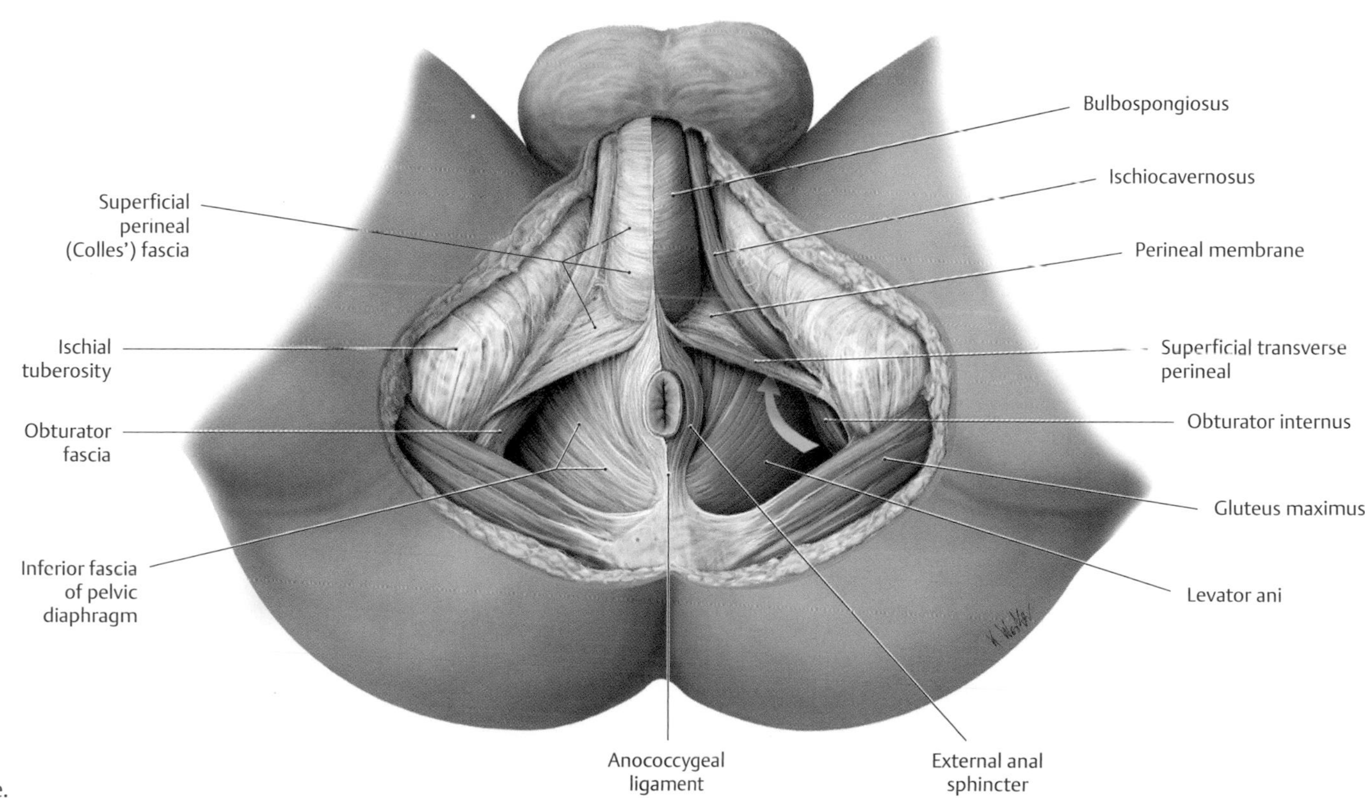
Superficial perineal (Colles') fascia
Ischial tuberosity
Obturator fascia
Inferior fascia of pelvic diaphragm
Anococcygeal ligament
External anal sphincter
Bulbospongiosus
Ischiocavernosus
Perineal membrane
Superficial transverse perineal
Obturator internus
Gluteus maximus
Levator ani

B Male.

Pelvic Floor & Perineal Muscle Facts

Fig. 16.15 Muscles of the pelvic floor
Superior view.

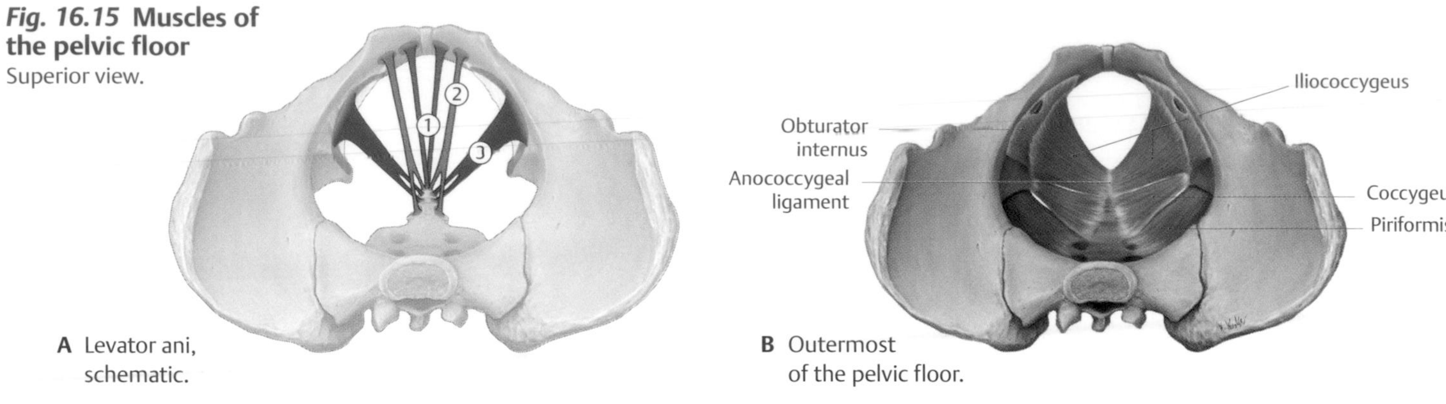
1
2
3
Obturator internus
Anococcygeal ligament
Iliococcygeus
Coccygeus
Piriformis

A Levator ani, schematic.

B Outermost of the pelvic floor.

Table 16.2 Muscles of the pelvic floor

Muscle		Origin	Insertion	Innervation	Action
Muscles of the pelvic diaphragm					
Levator ani	① Puborectalis	Superior pubic ramus (both sides of pubic symphysis)	Anococcygeal ligament	Direct branches of sacral plexus (S4), inferior anal n.	Pelvic diaphragm: Supports pelvic viscera
	② Pubococcygeus	Pubis (lateral to origin of puborectalis)	Anococcygeal ligament, coccyx		
	③ Iliococcygeus	Internal obturator fascia of levator ani (tendinous arch)			
Coccygeus		Sacrum (inferior end)	Ischial spine	Direct branches from sacral plexus (S4–S5)	Supports pelvic viscera, flexes coccyx
Muscles of the pelvic wall (parietal muscles)					
Piriformis*		Sacrum (pelvic surface)	Femur (apex of greater trochanter)	Direct branches from sacral plexus (S1–S2)	Hip joint: External rotation, stabilization, and abduction of flexed hip
Obturator internus*		Obturator membrane and bony boundaries (inner surface)	Femur (greater trochanter, medial surface)	Direct branches from sacral plexus (L5–S1)	Hip joint: External rotation and abduction of flexed hip

*The piriformis and obturator internus are considered muscles of the hip (see p. 398).
The female and male external genitalia are shown on pp. 266, 268.

Fig. 16.16 Muscles of the perineum
Inferior view.

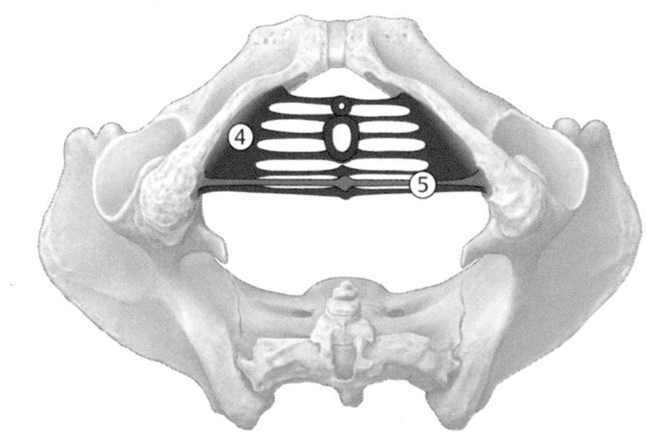
4
5

A Superficial and deep transverse perineal muscles, schematic.

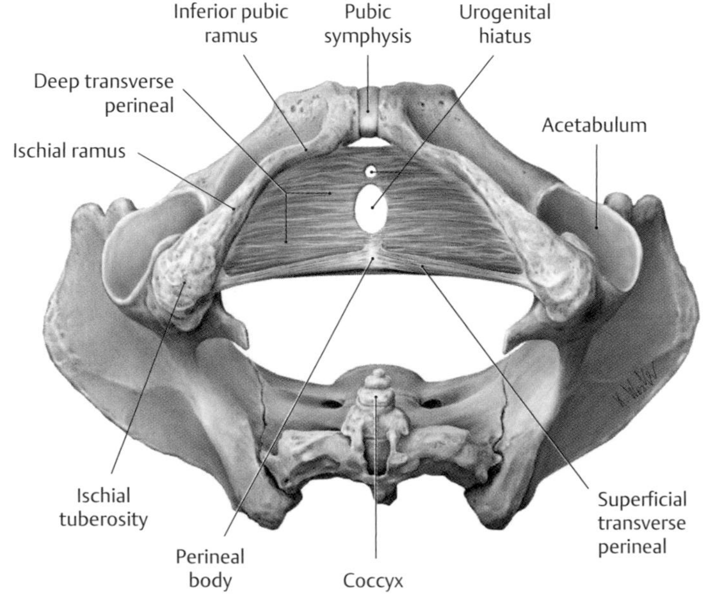
Inferior pubic ramus
Pubic symphysis
Urogenital hiatus
Deep transverse perineal
Ischial ramus
Acetabulum
Ischial tuberosity
Perineal body
Coccyx
Superficial transverse perineal

B Superficial and deep transverse perineal muscles.

Table 16.3	**Muscles of the perineum**			
Muscle	**Origin**	**Insertion**	**Innervation**	**Action**
④ Deep transverse perineal	Inferior pubic ramus, ischial ramus	Wall of vagina or prostate, perineal body		
⑤ Superficial transverse perineal	Ischial ramus	Perineal body		Holds the pelvic organs in place, closes the urethra
⑥ External anal sphincter	Encircles anus (runs posteriorly from perineal body to anococcygeal ligament)			Closes anus
⑦ External urethral sphincter	Encircles urethra (division of deep transverse perineal muscle)		Pudendal n. (S2–S4)	Closes urethra
⑧ Bulbospongiosus	Runs anteriorly from perineal body to clitoris (females) or penile raphe (males)			Females: Compresses greater vestibular gland Males: Assists in erection
⑨ Ischiocavernosus	Ischial ramus	Crus of clitoris or penis		Maintains erection by squeezing blood into corpus cavernosum of clitoris or penis

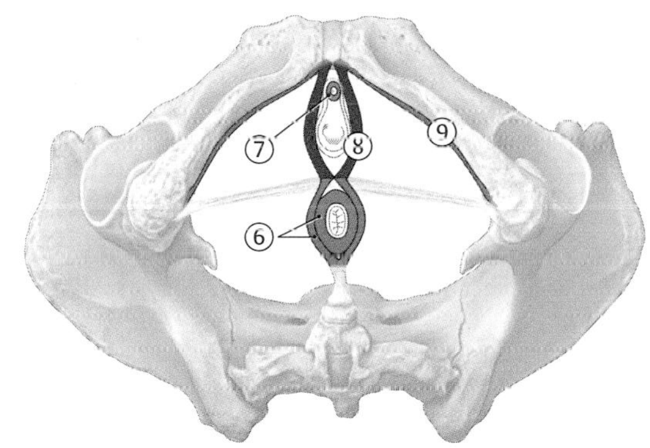

⑦
⑧
⑨
⑥

C Sphincter and erector muscles, schematic.

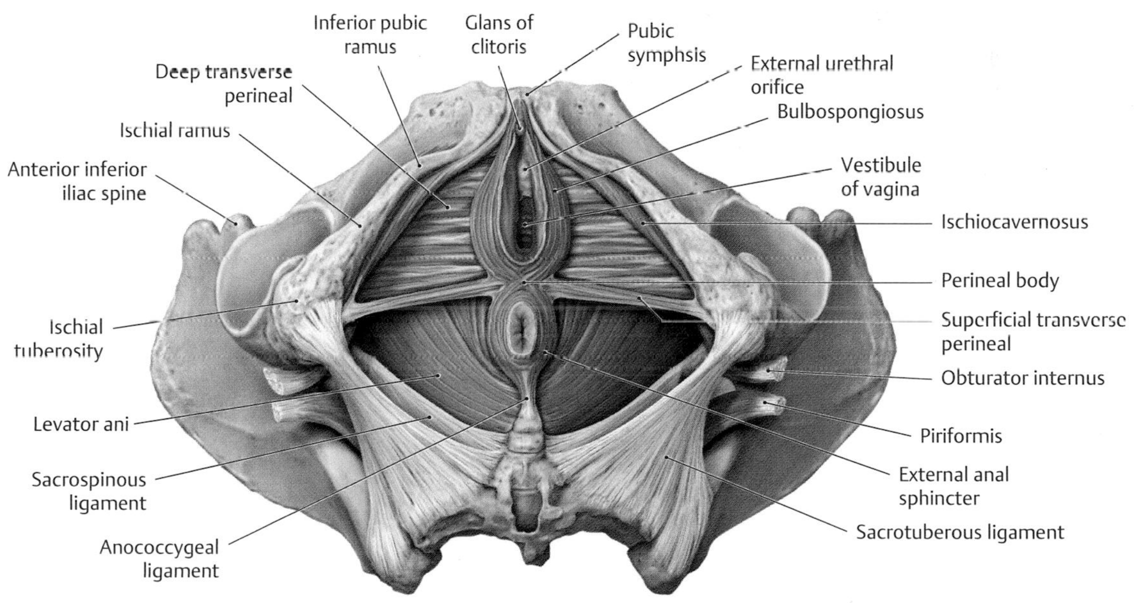

Inferior pubic ramus
Glans of clitoris
Pubic symphysis
Deep transverse perineal
External urethral orifice
Bulbospongiosus
Ischial ramus
Anterior inferior iliac spine
Vestibule of vagina
Ischiocavernosus
Perineal body
Ischial tuberosity
Superficial transverse perineal
Obturator internus
Levator ani
Piriformis
Sacrospinous ligament
External anal sphincter
Sacrotuberous ligament
Anococcygeal ligament

D Sphincter and erector muscles.

Contents of the Pelvis

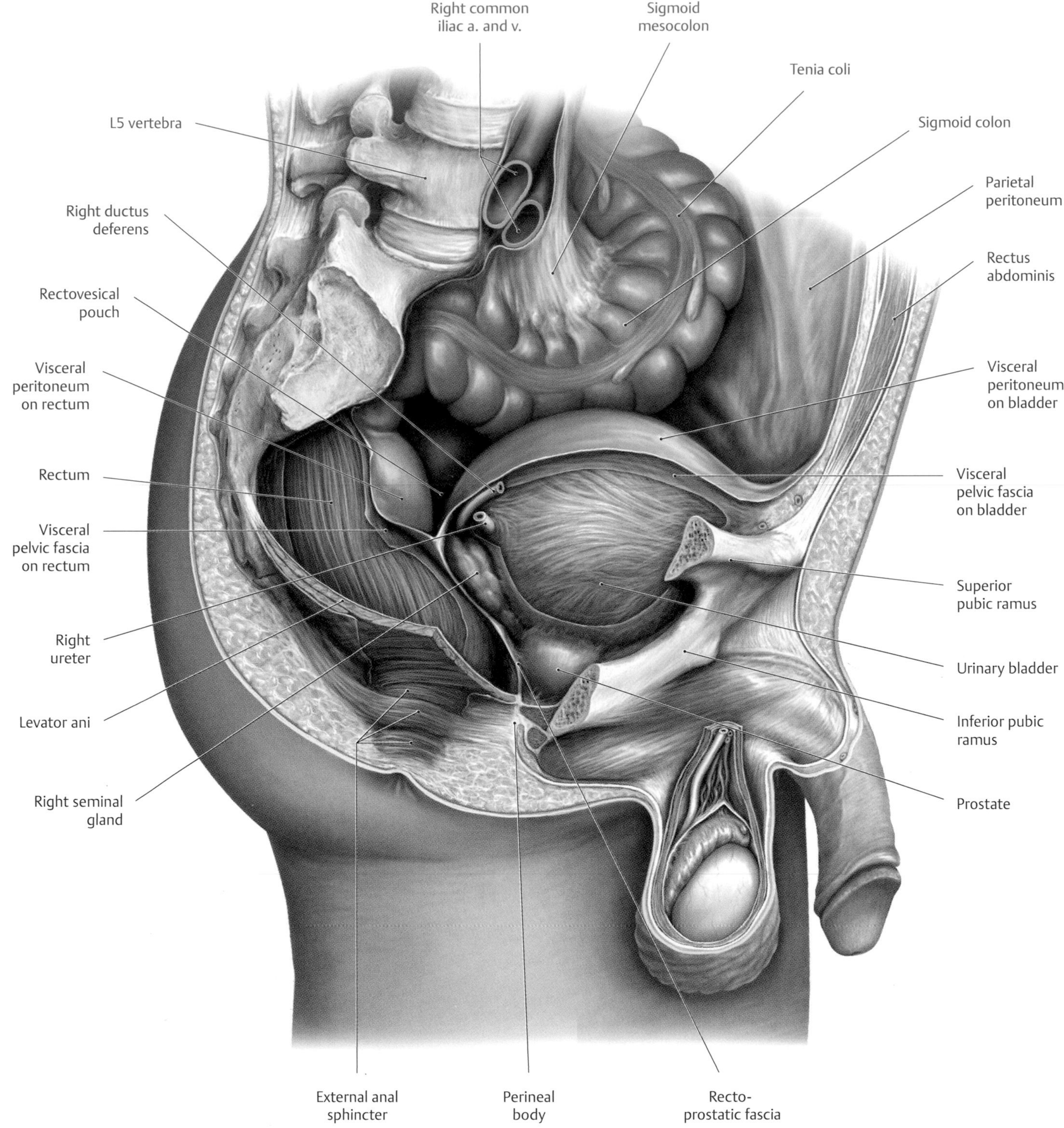
Right common iliac a. and v.
Sigmoid mesocolon
Tenia coli
Sigmoid colon
L5 vertebra
Parietal peritoneum
Right ductus deferens
Rectus abdominis
Rectovesical pouch
Visceral peritoneum on rectum
Visceral peritoneum on bladder
Rectum
Visceral pelvic fascia on bladder
Visceral pelvic fascia on rectum
Superior pubic ramus
Right ureter
Urinary bladder
Levator ani
Inferior pubic ramus
Right seminal gland
Prostate
External anal sphincter
Perineal body
Recto-prostatic fascia

Fig. 17.1 **Male pelvis**
Parasagittal section, viewed from the right side.

Fig. 17.2 **Female pelvis**
Parasagittal section, viewed from the right side.

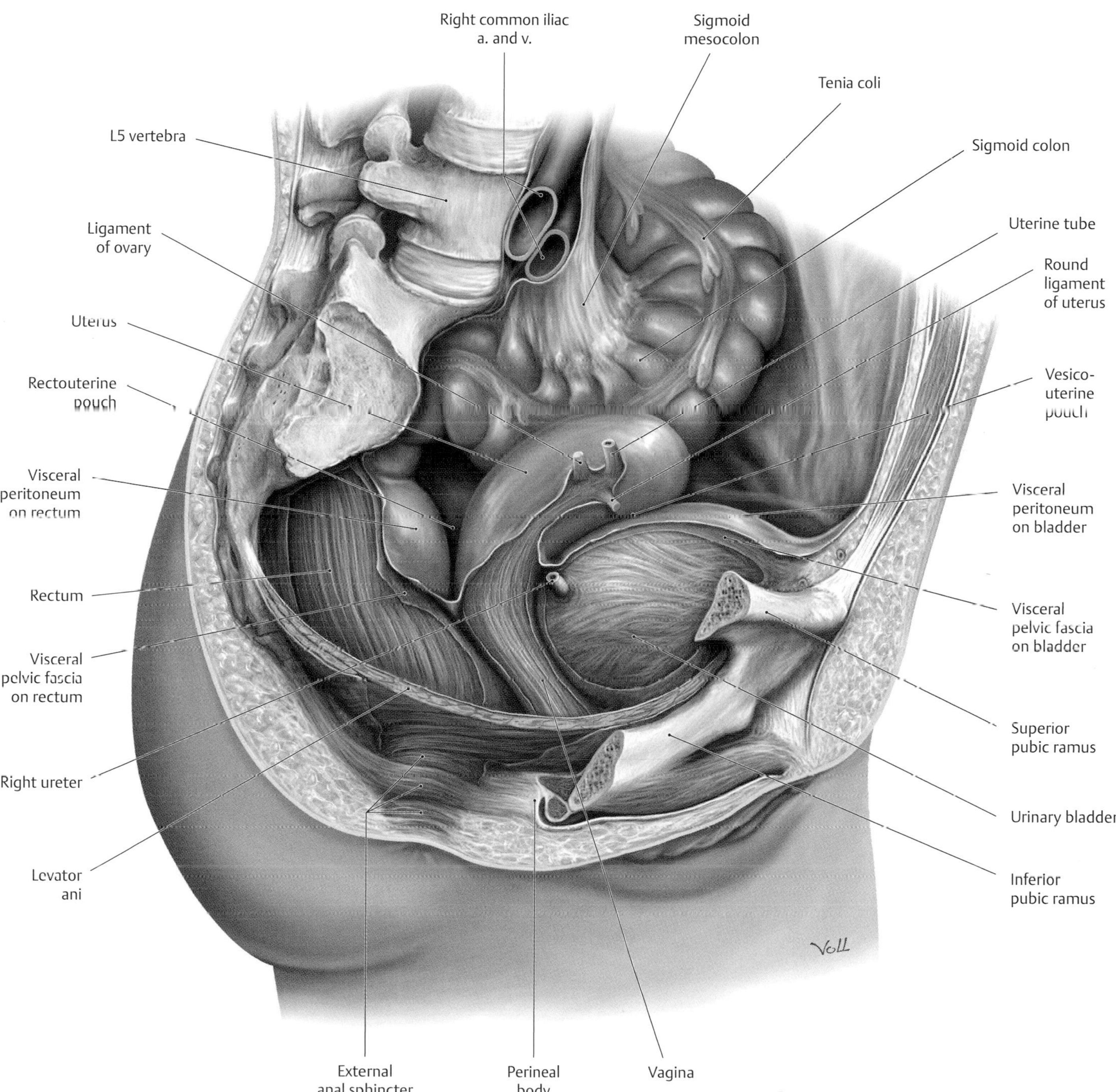
Right common iliac a. and v.
Sigmoid mesocolon
Tenia coli
Sigmoid colon
L5 vertebra
Ligament of ovary
Uterine tube
Round ligament of uterus
Uterus
Rectouterine pouch
Vesico-uterine pouch
Visceral peritoneum on rectum
Visceral peritoneum on bladder
Rectum
Visceral pelvic fascia on bladder
Visceral pelvic fascia on rectum
Superior pubic ramus
Right ureter
Urinary bladder
Levator ani
Inferior pubic ramus
External anal sphincter
Perineal body
Vagina

Peritoneal Relationships

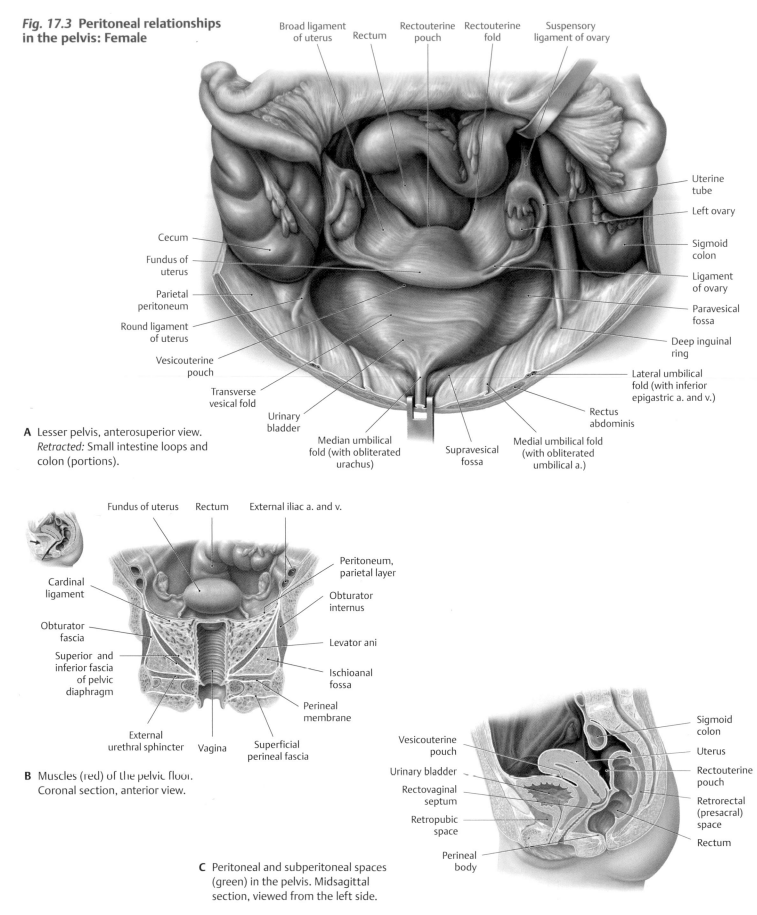

Fig. 17.3 **Peritoneal relationships in the pelvis: Female**

Broad ligament of uterus
Rectum
Rectouterine pouch
Rectouterine fold
Suspensory ligament of ovary
Uterine tube
Left ovary
Sigmoid colon
Ligament of ovary
Paravesical fossa
Deep inguinal ring
Lateral umbilical fold (with inferior epigastric a. and v.)
Rectus abdominis
Medial umbilical fold (with obliterated umbilical a.)
Supravesical fossa
Median umbilical fold (with obliterated urachus)
Urinary bladder
Transverse vesical fold
Vesicouterine pouch
Round ligament of uterus
Parietal peritoneum
Fundus of uterus
Cecum

A Lesser pelvis, anterosuperior view. *Retracted:* Small intestine loops and colon (portions).

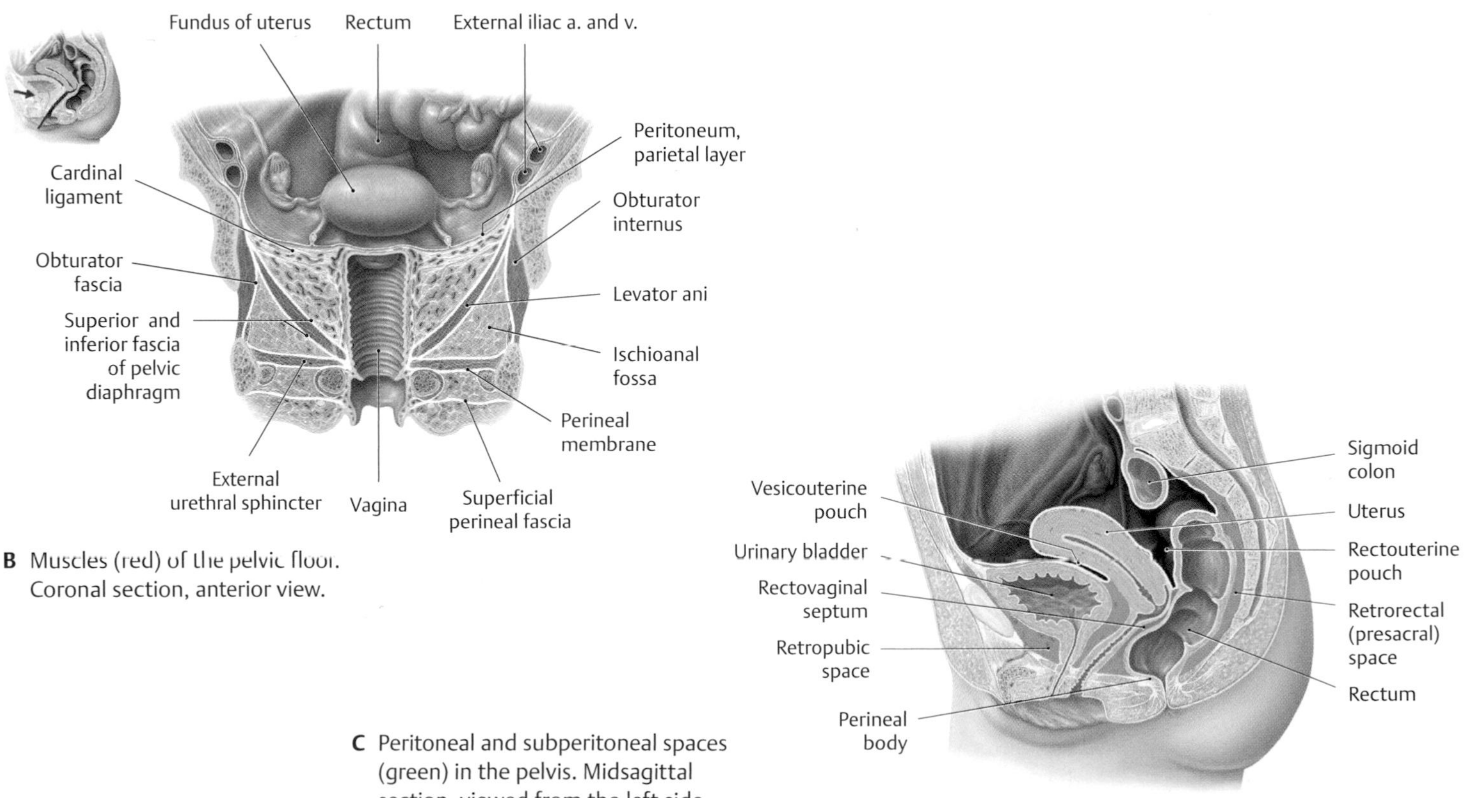
Fundus of uterus
Rectum
External iliac a. and v.
Peritoneum, parietal layer
Obturator internus
Levator ani
Ischioanal fossa
Perineal membrane
Superficial perineal fascia
Vagina
External urethral sphincter
Superior and inferior fascia of pelvic diaphragm
Obturator fascia
Cardinal ligament
Sigmoid colon
Uterus
Rectouterine pouch
Retrorectal (presacral) space
Rectum
Vesicouterine pouch
Urinary bladder
Rectovaginal septum
Retropubic space
Perineal body

B Muscles (red) of the pelvic floor. Coronal section, anterior view.

C Peritoneal and subperitoneal spaces (green) in the pelvis. Midsagittal section, viewed from the left side.

Fig. 17.4 Peritoneal relationships in the pelvis: Male

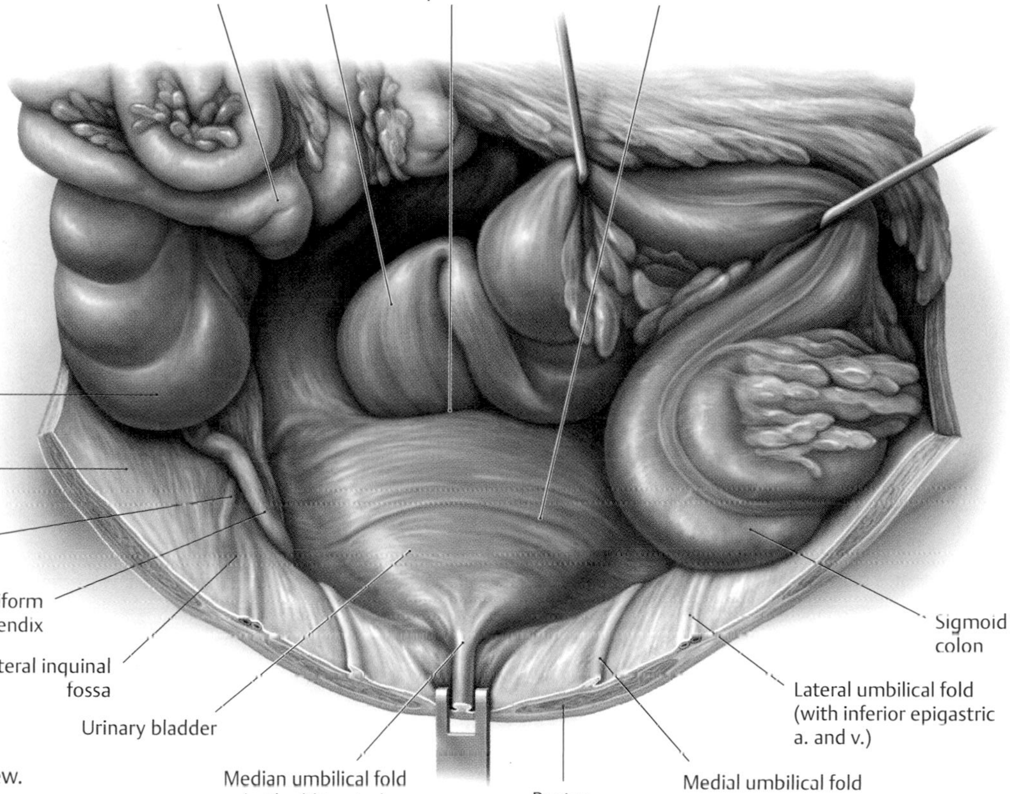

Ileum
Rectum
Rectovesical pouch
Transverse vesical fold
Cecum
Parietal peritoneum
Ductus deferens
Vermiform appendix
Lateral inquinal fossa
Urinary bladder
Median umbilical fold (with obliterated urachus)
Rectus abdominis
Medial umbilical fold (with obliterated umbilical a.)
Lateral umbilical fold (with inferior epigastric a. and v.)
Sigmoid colon

A Lesser pelvis, anterosuperior view. *Retracted:* Small intestine and colon (portions).

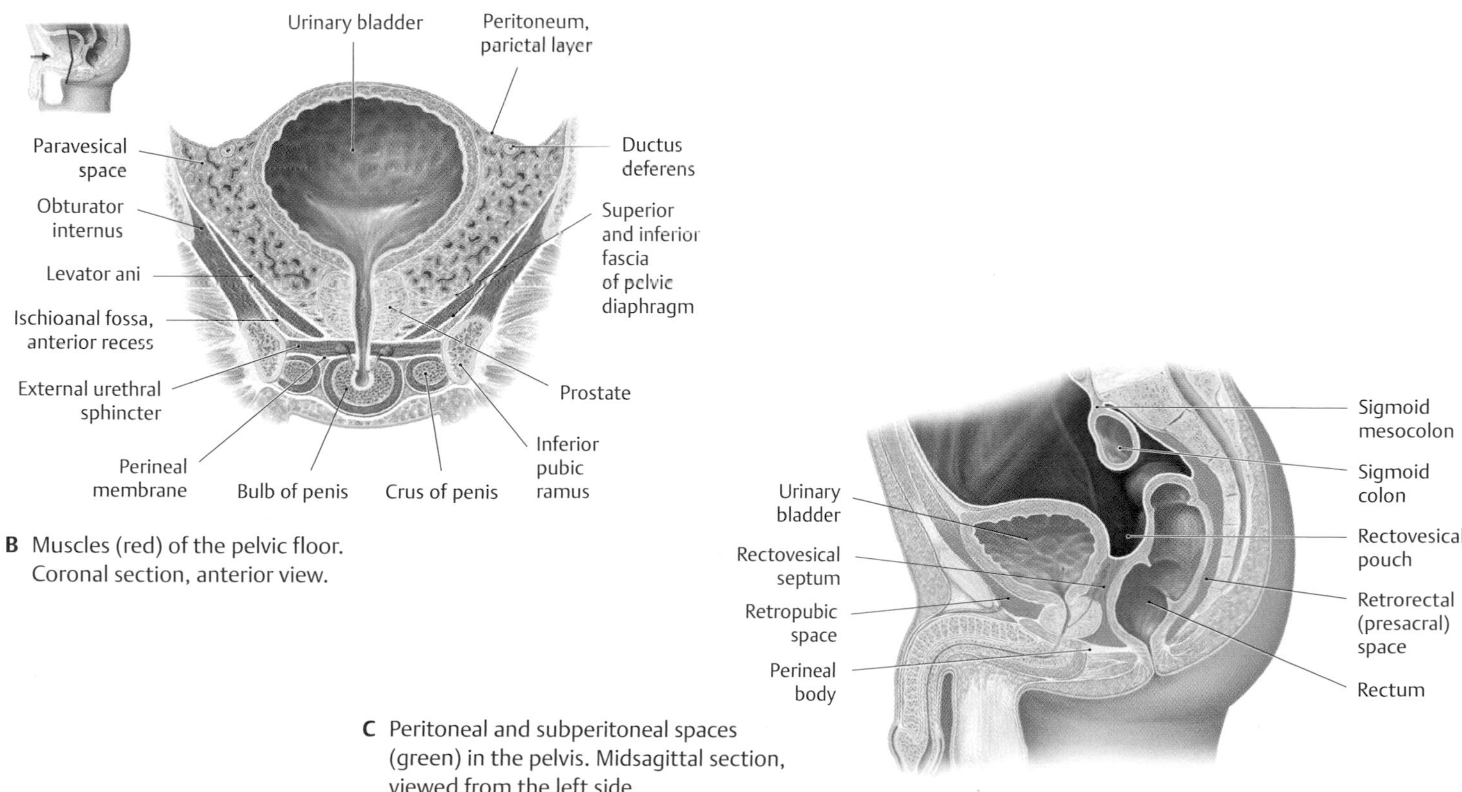
Urinary bladder
Peritoneum, parietal layer
Paravesical space
Obturator internus
Levator ani
Ischioanal fossa, anterior recess
External urethral sphincter
Perineal membrane
Bulb of penis
Crus of penis
Inferior pubic ramus
Prostate
Superior and inferior fascia of pelvic diaphragm
Ductus deferens
Urinary bladder
Rectovesical septum
Retropubic space
Perineal body
Sigmoid mesocolon
Sigmoid colon
Rectovesical pouch
Retrorectal (presacral) space
Rectum

B Muscles (red) of the pelvic floor. Coronal section, anterior view.

C Peritoneal and subperitoneal spaces (green) in the pelvis. Midsagittal section, viewed from the left side.

Pelvis & Perineum

The *pelvis* is the region of the body inferior to the abdomen, surrounded by the pelvic girdle. The *false*, or greater, *pelvis* is immediately inferior to the abdominal cavity, between the iliac alae, and superior to the pelvic inlet. The *true*, or lesser, *pelvis* is found between the pelvic inlet and the pelvic outlet and extends inferiorly to the pelvic diaphragm, a muscular sling attached to the boundaries of the pelvic outlet. The *perineum* is the inferior most portion of the trunk, between the thighs and buttocks, extending from the pubis to the coccyx and superiorly to the pelvic diaphragm. The *superficial perineal* pouch lies between the membranous layer of the subcutaneous tissue (Colle's fascia) and the perineal membrane. The *deep perineal* pouch lies between the perineal membrane and the inferior fascia of the pelvic diaphragm

Table 17.1 Divisions of the pelvis and perineum

The levels of the pelvis are determined by bony landmarks (iliac alae and pelvic inlet/brim). The contents of the perineum are separated from the true pelvis by the pelvic diaphragm and two fascial layers.

Iliac crest		
Pelvis	**False pelvis**	• Ileum (coils)
		• Cecum and appendix
		• Sigmoid colon
		• Common and external iliac aa. and vv.
		• Lumbar plexus (branches)
	Pelvic inlet	
	True pelvis	• Distal ureters
		• Urinary bladder
		• Rectum
		♀: Vagina, uterus, uterine tubes, and ovaries
		♂: Ductus deferens, seminal gland, and prostate
		• Internal iliac a. and v. and branches
		• Sacral plexus
		• Inferior hypogastric plexus
Pelvic diaphragm (levator ani with superior and inferior fascia of pelvic diaphragm)		
Perineum	**Deep pouch**	• Sphincter urethrae and deep transverse perineal mm.
		• Urethra (membranous)
		• Vagina
		• Rectum
		• Bulbourethral gland
		• Ischioanal fossa
		• Internal pudendal a. and v., pudendal n. and branches
	Perineal membrane	
	Superficial pouch	• Ischiocavernosus, bulbocavernosus, and superficial transverse perineal mm.
		• Urethra (penile)
		• Clitoris and penis
		• Internal pudendal a. and v., pudendal n. and branches
	Superficial perineal (Colles') fascia	
	Subcutaneous perineal space	• Fat
Skin		

Fig. 17.5 **Pelvis and urogenital triangle**
Coronal section, anterior view.

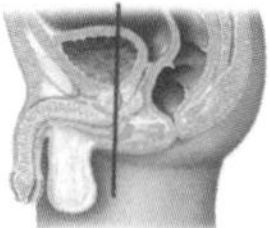

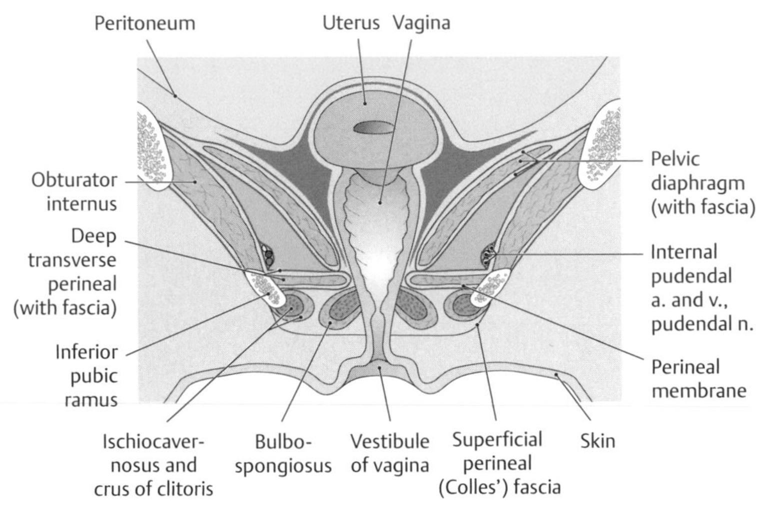

Peritoneum
Uterus
Vagina
Obturator internus
Deep transverse perineal (with fascia)
Inferior pubic ramus
Ischiocavernosus and crus of clitoris
Bulbospongiosus
Vestibule of vagina
Superficial perineal (Colles') fascia
Skin
Pelvic diaphragm (with fascia)
Internal pudendal a. and v., pudendal n.
Perineal membrane

A Female.

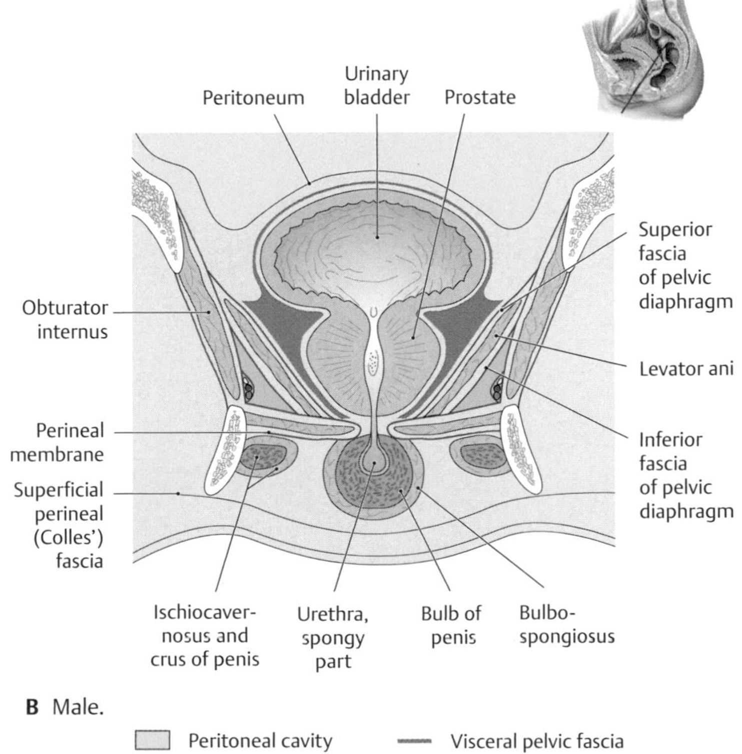

Peritoneum
Urinary bladder
Prostate
Obturator internus
Perineal membrane
Superficial perineal (Colles') fascia
Ischiocavernosus and crus of penis
Urethra, spongy part
Bulb of penis
Bulbospongiosus
Superior fascia of pelvic diaphragm
Levator ani
Inferior fascia of pelvic diaphragm

B Male.

Peritoneal cavity
Subperitoneal space
Ischioanal fossa
Visceral pelvic fascia
Parietal pelvic fascia

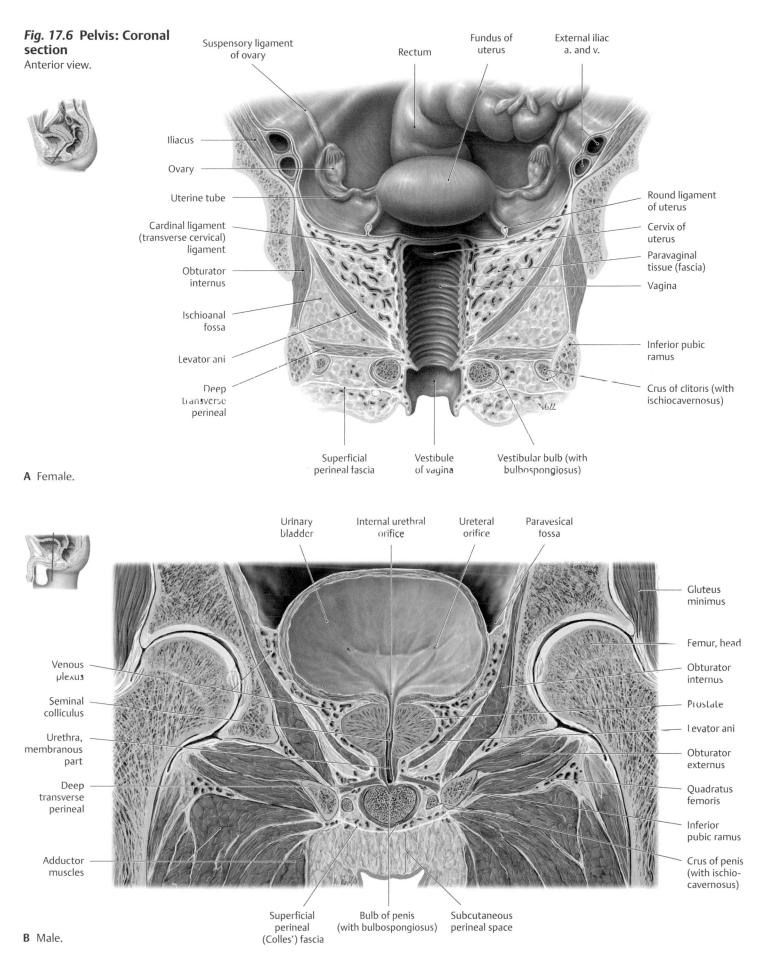

Fig. 17.6 **Pelvis: Coronal section**
Anterior view.

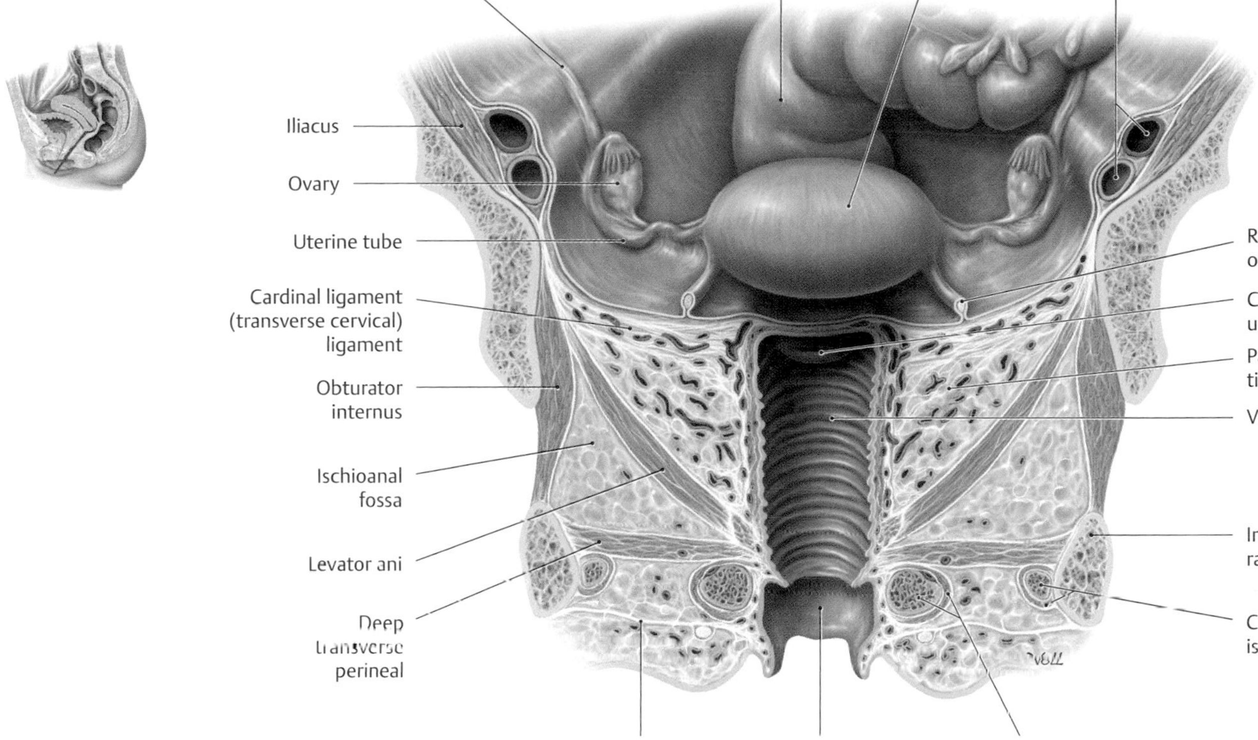

Suspensory ligament of ovary
Rectum
Fundus of uterus
External iliac a. and v.
Iliacus
Ovary
Uterine tube
Cardinal ligament (transverse cervical) ligament
Obturator internus
Ischioanal fossa
Levator ani
Deep transverse perineal
Round ligament of uterus
Cervix of uterus
Paravaginal tissue (fascia)
Vagina
Inferior pubic ramus
Crus of clitoris (with ischiocavernosus)
Superficial perineal fascia
Vestibule of vagina
Vestibular bulb (with bulbospongiosus)

A Female.

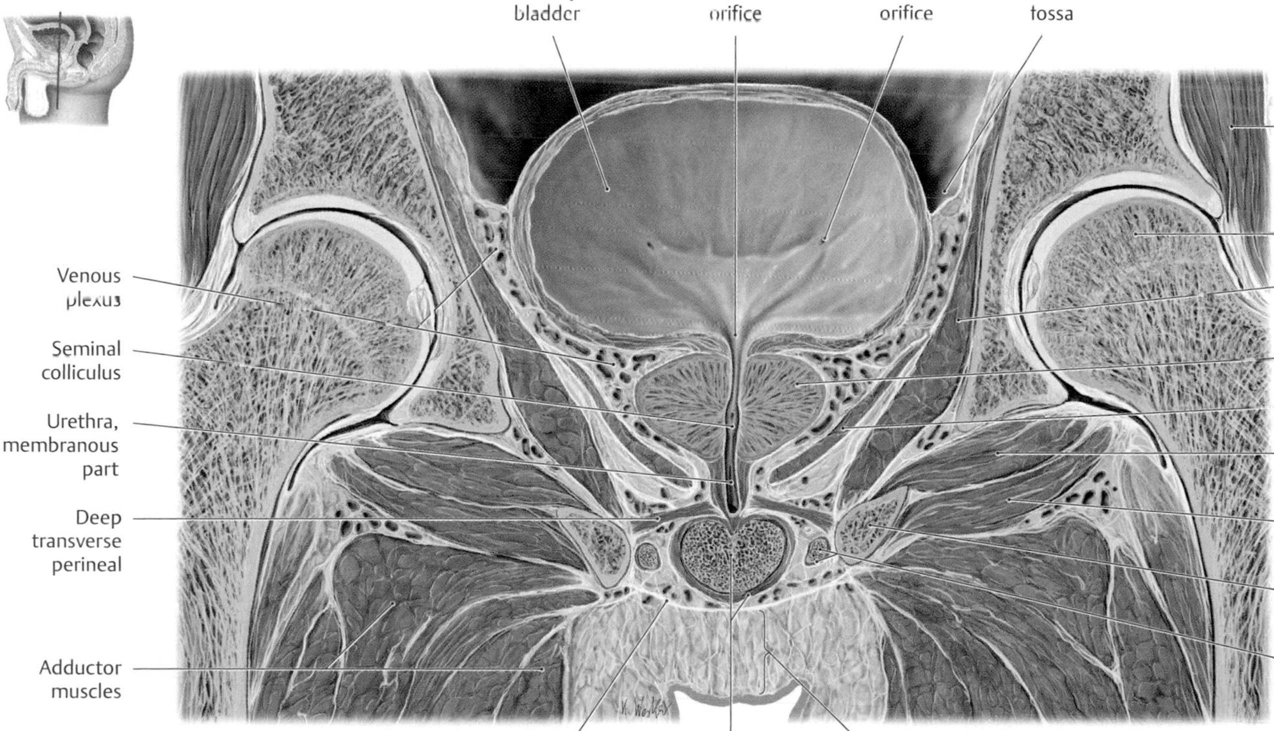

Urinary bladder
Internal urethral orifice
Ureteral orifice
Paravesical fossa
Gluteus minimus
Femur, head
Obturator internus
Prostate
Levator ani
Obturator externus
Quadratus femoris
Inferior pubic ramus
Crus of penis (with ischiocavernosus)
Venous plexus
Seminal colliculus
Urethra, membranous part
Deep transverse perineal
Adductor muscles
Superficial perineal (Colles') fascia
Bulb of penis (with bulbospongiosus)
Subcutaneous perineal space

B Male.

Rectum & Anal Canal

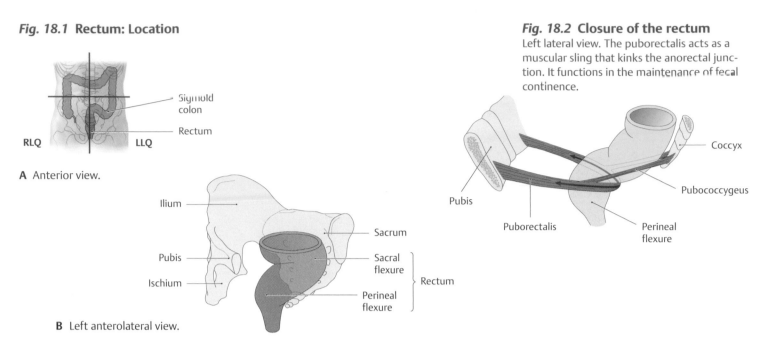

Fig. 18.1 Rectum: Location

Sigmoid colon
Rectum
RLQ
LLQ

A Anterior view.

Ilium
Pubis
Ischium
Sacrum
Sacral flexure
Perineal flexure
Rectum

B Left anterolateral view.

Fig. 18.2 Closure of the rectum

Left lateral view. The puborectalis acts as a muscular sling that kinks the anorectal junction. It functions in the maintenance of fecal continence.

Coccyx
Pubococcygeus
Pubis
Puborectalis
Perineal flexure

Fig. 18.3 Rectum in situ

Coronal section, anterior view of the female pelvis. The upper third of the rectum is covered with visceral peritoneum on its anterior and lateral sides. The middle third is covered only anteriorly and the lower third is inferior to the parietal peritoneum.

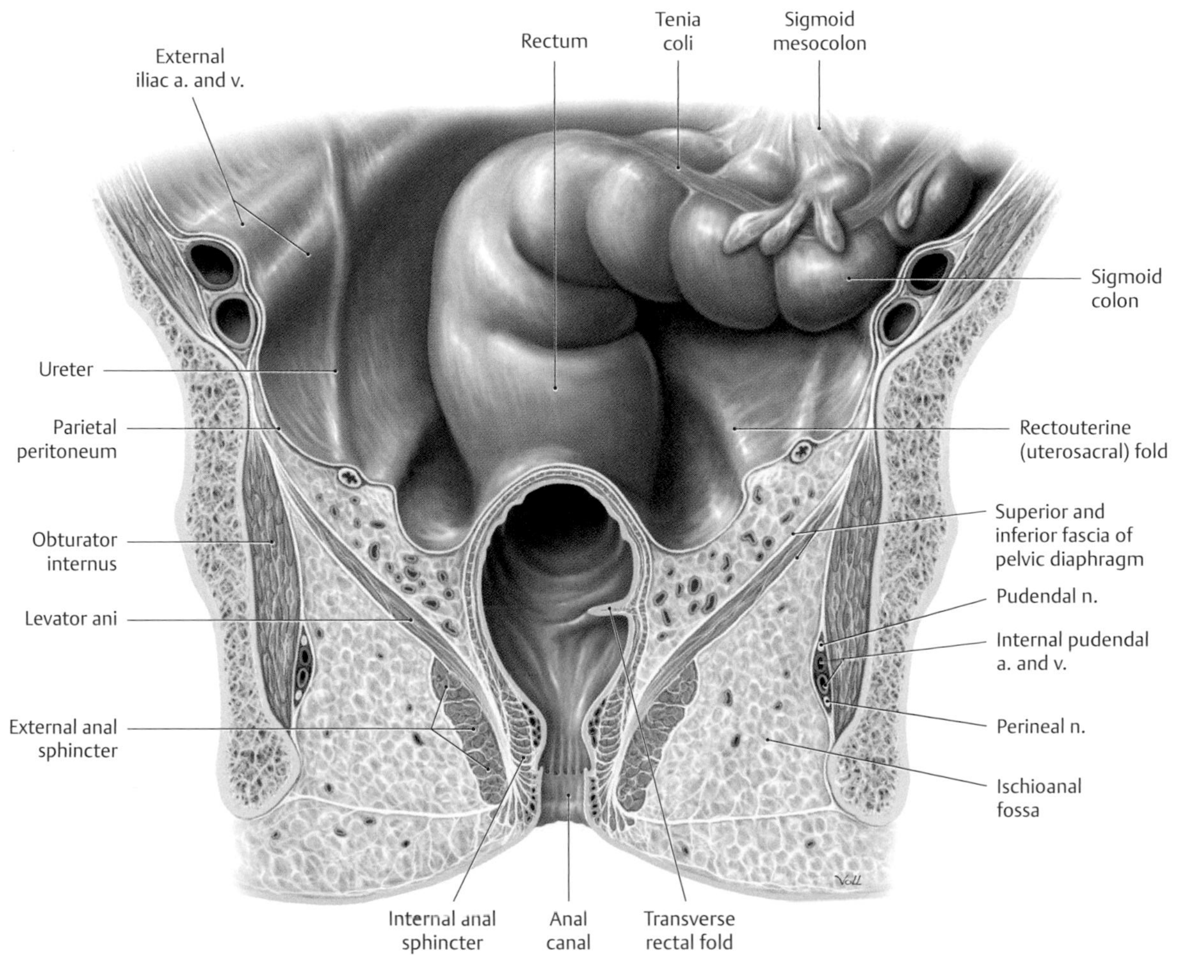
External iliac a. and v.
Rectum
Tenia coli
Sigmoid mesocolon
Sigmoid colon
Ureter
Parietal peritoneum
Rectouterine (uterosacral) fold
Obturator internus
Superior and inferior fascia of pelvic diaphragm
Levator ani
Pudendal n.
Internal pudendal a. and v.
External anal sphincter
Perineal n.
Ischioanal fossa
Internal anal sphincter
Anal canal
Transverse rectal fold

Fig. 18.4 Rectum and anal canal
Coronal section, anterior view with the anterior wall removed.

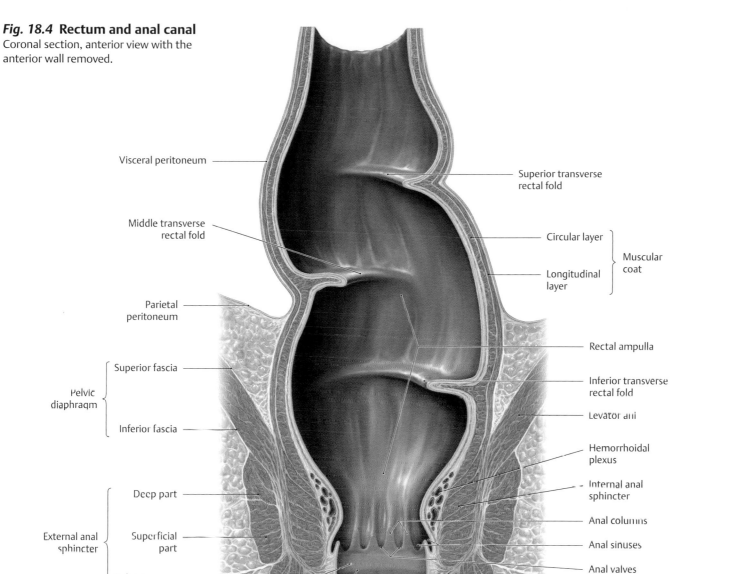

Visceral peritoneum
Superior transverse rectal fold
Middle transverse rectal fold
Circular layer
Longitudinal layer
Muscular coat
Parietal peritoneum
Rectal ampulla
Superior fascia
Pelvic diaphragm
Inferior fascia
Inferior transverse rectal fold
Levator ani
Hemorrhoidal plexus
Internal anal sphincter
Deep part
External anal sphincter
Superficial part
Subcutaneous part
Anal columns
Anal sinuses
Anal valves
Corrugator cutis ani
Subcutaneous venous plexus
Anal pecten (white zone)
Anocutaneous line
Anus
Perianal skin

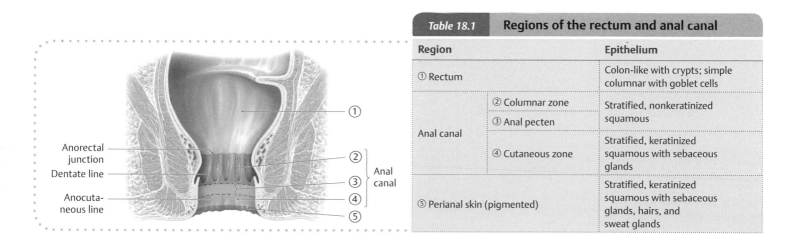

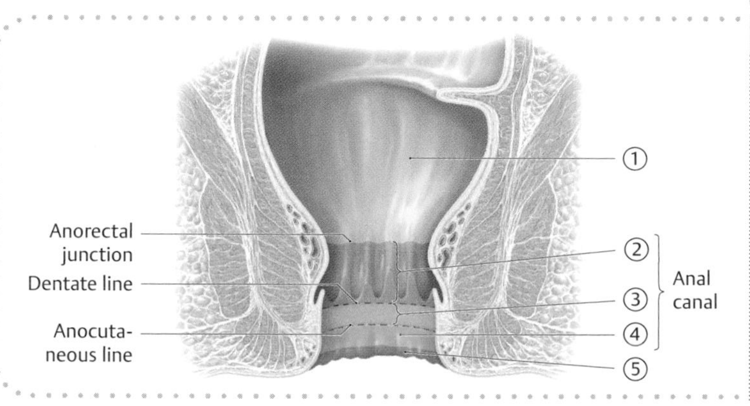

Anorectal junction
Dentate line
Anocuta-neous line
①
②
③
④
⑤
Anal canal

Table 18.1 Regions of the rectum and anal canal

Region		Epithelium
① Rectum		Colon-like with crypts; simple columnar with goblet cells
Anal canal	② Columnar zone	Stratified, nonkeratinized squamous
	③ Anal pecten	
	④ Cutaneous zone	Stratified, keratinized squamous with sebaceous glands
⑤ Perianal skin (pigmented)		Stratified, keratinized squamous with sebaceous glands, hairs, and sweat glands

Ureters

The ureters cross the common iliac artery at its bifurcation into the external and internal iliac arteries.

Fig. 18.5 Ureters in situ
Anterior view, male abdomen. *Removed:* Non-urinary organs and rectal stump. The ureters are retroperitoneal.

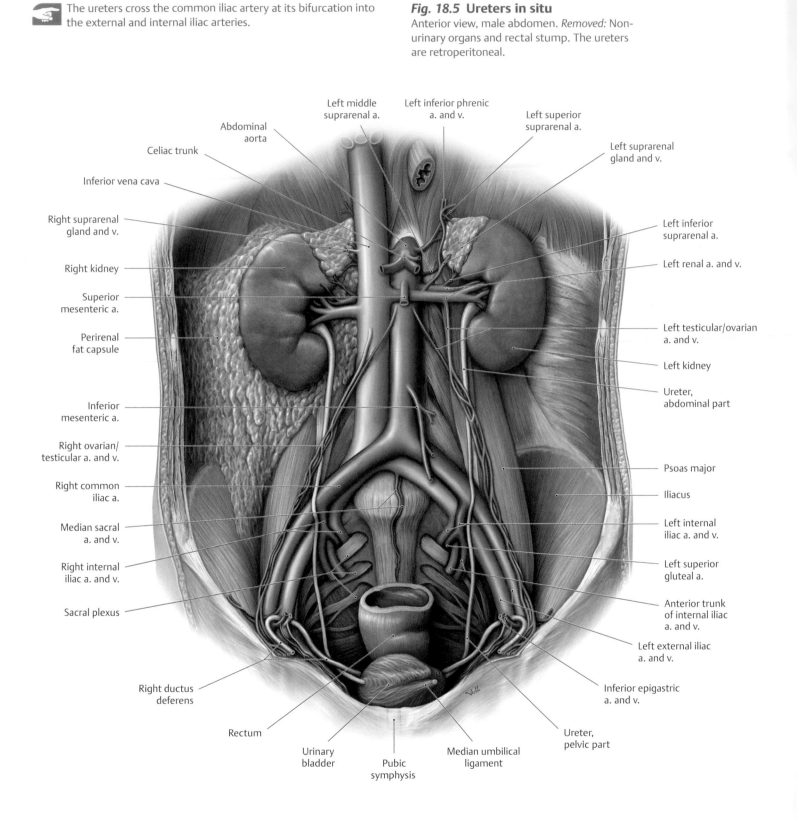

Left middle suprarenal a.
Left inferior phrenic a. and v.
Left superior suprarenal a.
Abdominal aorta
Left suprarenal gland and v.
Celiac trunk
Inferior vena cava
Right suprarenal gland and v.
Left inferior suprarenal a.
Right kidney
Left renal a. and v.
Superior mesenteric a.
Left testicular/ovarian a. and v.
Perirenal fat capsule
Left kidney
Ureter, abdominal part
Inferior mesenteric a.
Right ovarian/testicular a. and v.
Psoas major
Right common iliac a.
Iliacus
Median sacral a. and v.
Left internal iliac a. and v.
Right internal iliac a. and v.
Left superior gluteal a.
Sacral plexus
Anterior trunk of internal iliac a. and v.
Left external iliac a. and v.
Right ductus deferens
Inferior epigastric a. and v.
Rectum
Ureter, pelvic part
Urinary bladder
Pubic symphysis
Median umbilical ligament

Fig. 18.6 **Ureter in the male pelvis**
Superior view.

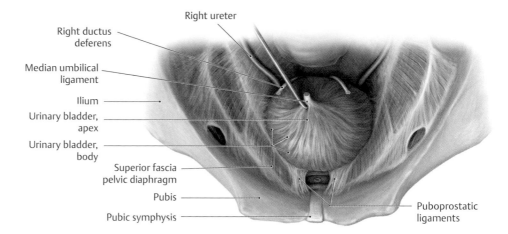

Right ureter
Right ductus deferens
Median umbilical ligament
Ilium
Urinary bladder, apex
Urinary bladder, body
Superior fascia pelvic diaphragm
Pubis
Pubic symphysis
Puboprostatic ligaments

Fig. 18.7 **Ureter in the female pelvis**
Pelvis viewed from above. *Removed from right side:* Peritoneum and broad ligament of uterus. The pelvic ureters pass under the uterine artery approximately 2 cm lateral to the cervix.

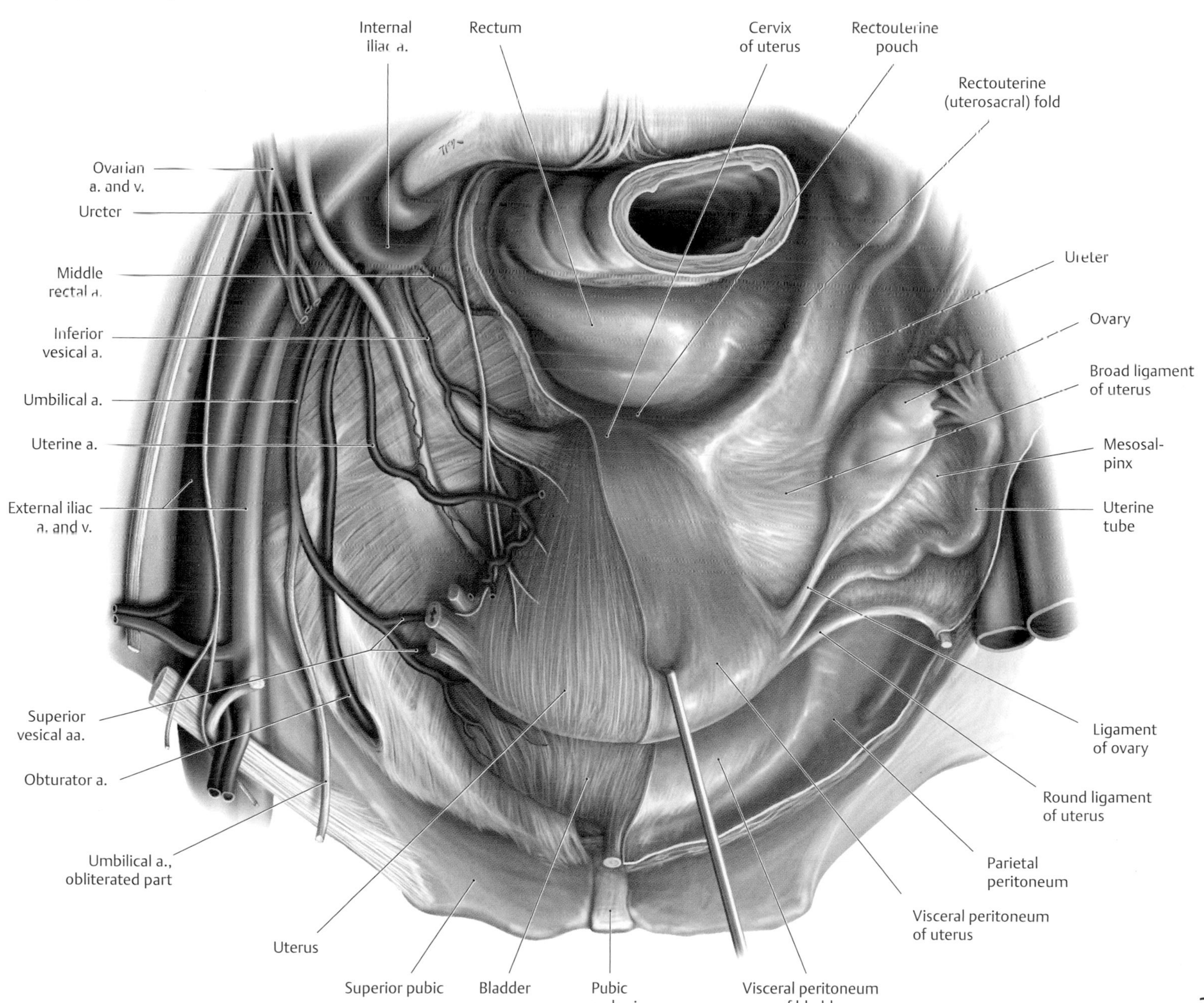
Internal iliac a.
Rectum
Cervix of uterus
Rectouterine pouch
Rectouterine (uterosacral) fold
Ovarian a. and v.
Ureter
Middle rectal a.
Inferior vesical a.
Umbilical a.
Uterine a.
External iliac a. and v.
Ureter
Ovary
Broad ligament of uterus
Mesosal-pinx
Uterine tube
Superior vesical aa.
Obturator a.
Umbilical a., obliterated part
Uterus
Superior pubic ramus
Bladder
Pubic symphysis
Visceral peritoneum of bladder
Visceral peritoneum of uterus
Parietal peritoneum
Round ligament of uterus
Ligament of ovary

Urinary Bladder & Urethra

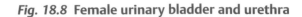

Fig. 18.8 Female urinary bladder and urethra

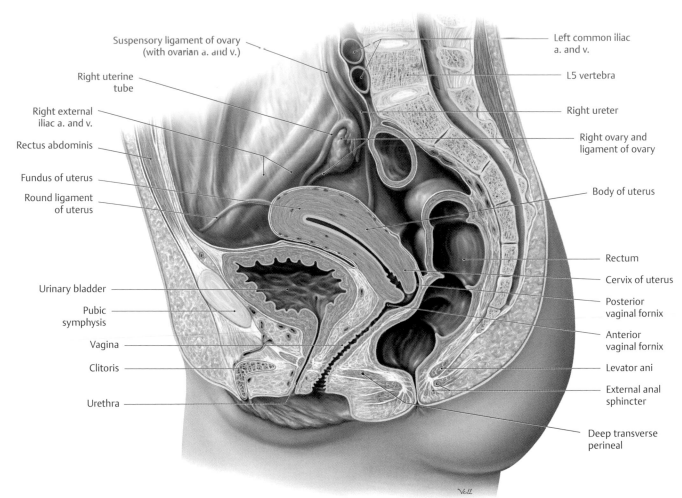

Suspensory ligament of ovary (with ovarian a. and v.)
Right uterine tube
Right external iliac a. and v.
Rectus abdominis
Fundus of uterus
Round ligament of uterus
Urinary bladder
Pubic symphysis
Vagina
Clitoris
Urethra
Left common iliac a. and v.
L5 vertebra
Right ureter
Right ovary and ligament of ovary
Body of uterus
Rectum
Cervix of uterus
Posterior vaginal fornix
Anterior vaginal fornix
Levator ani
External anal sphincter
Deep transverse perineal

A Midsagittal section of pelvis, viewed from the left side. Right hemipelvis.

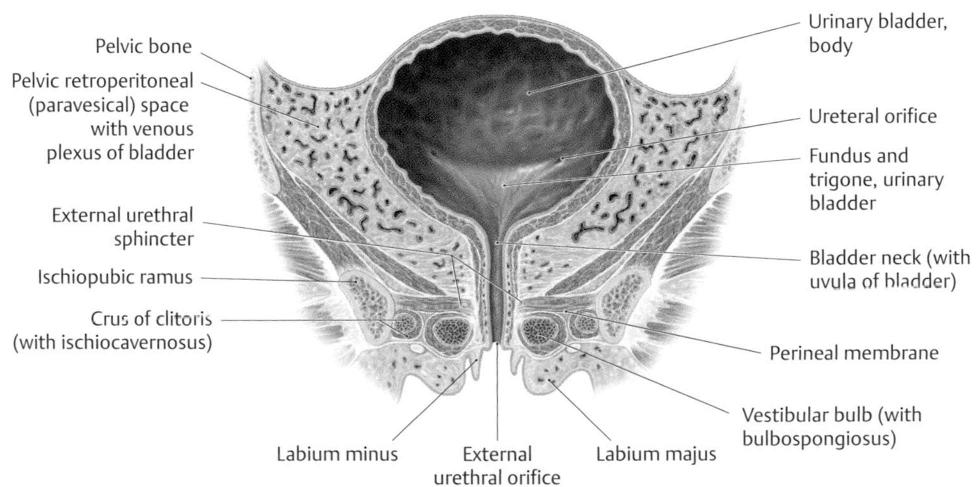
Pelvic bone
Pelvic retroperitoneal (paravesical) space with venous plexus of bladder
External urethral sphincter
Ischiopubic ramus
Crus of clitoris (with ischiocavernosus)
Labium minus
External urethral orifice
Labium majus
Urinary bladder, body
Ureteral orifice
Fundus and trigone, urinary bladder
Bladder neck (with uvula of bladder)
Perineal membrane
Vestibular bulb (with bulbospongiosus)

B Coronal section of pelvis, anterior view.

Fig. 18.9 Male urinary bladder and urethra

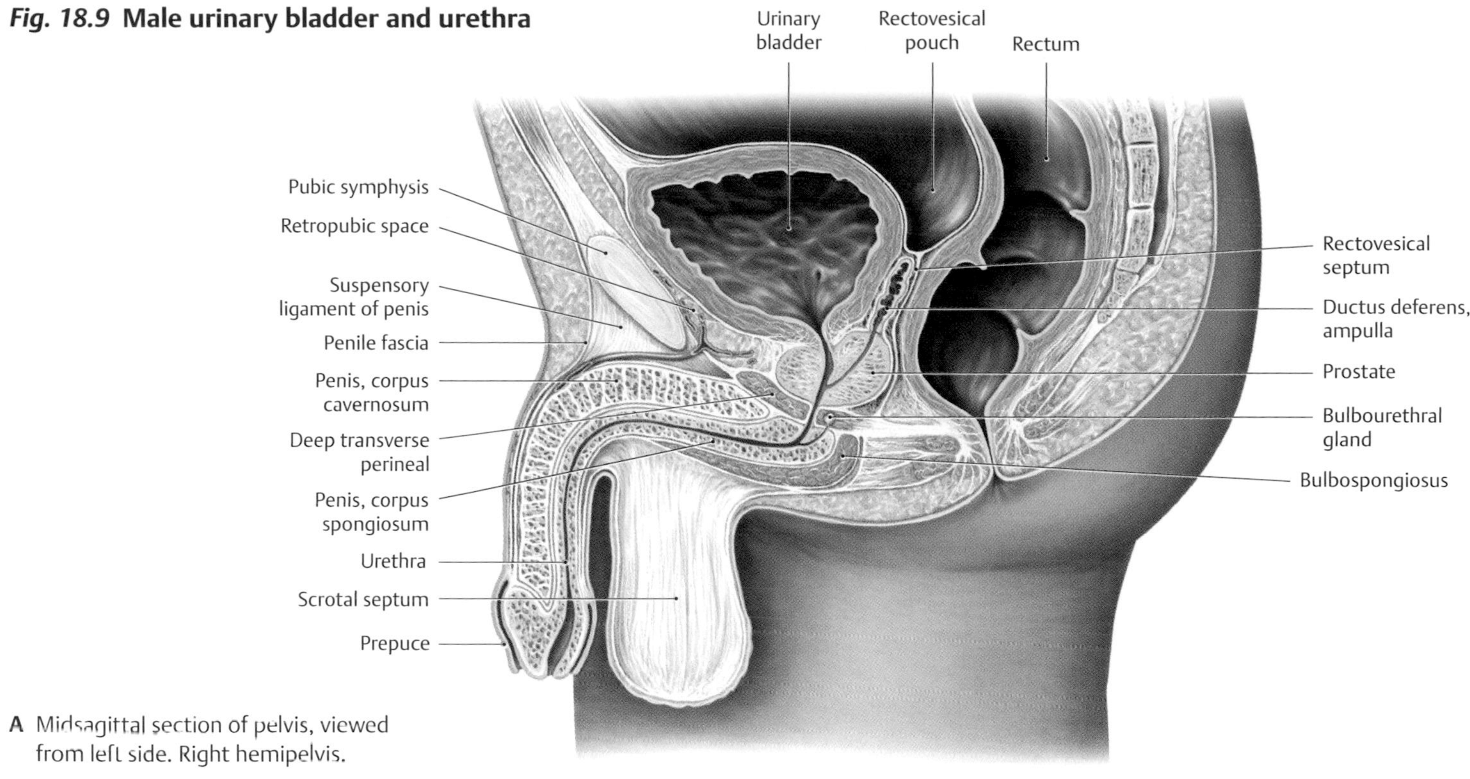

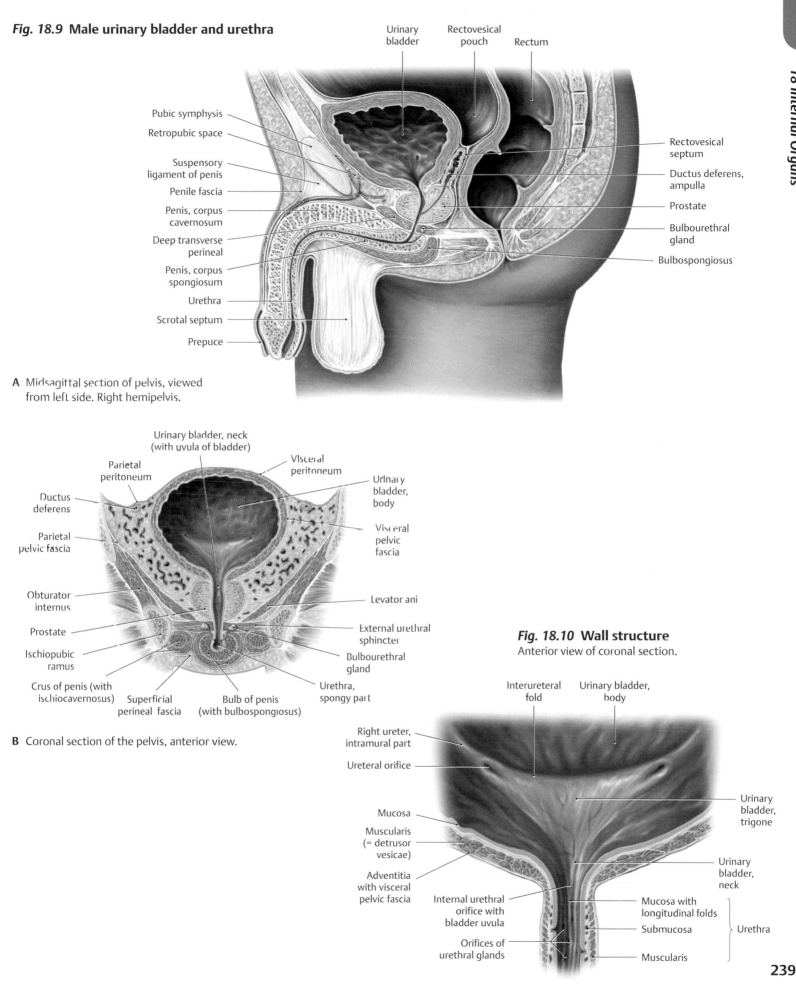

Urinary bladder
Rectovesical pouch
Rectum
Pubic symphysis
Retropubic space
Suspensory ligament of penis
Penile fascia
Penis, corpus cavernosum
Deep transverse perineal
Penis, corpus spongiosum
Urethra
Scrotal septum
Prepuce
Rectovesical septum
Ductus deferens, ampulla
Prostate
Bulbourethral gland
Bulbospongiosus

A Midsagittal section of pelvis, viewed from left side. Right hemipelvis.

Urinary bladder, neck (with uvula of bladder)
Parietal peritoneum
Visceral peritoneum
Ductus deferens
Urinary bladder, body
Parietal pelvic fascia
Visceral pelvic fascia
Obturator internus
Levator ani
Prostate
External urethral sphincter
Ischiopubic ramus
Bulbourethral gland
Crus of penis (with ischiocavernosus)
Superficial perineal fascia
Bulb of penis (with bulbospongiosus)
Urethra, spongy part

B Coronal section of the pelvis, anterior view.

Fig. 18.10 Wall structure

Anterior view of coronal section.

Interureteral fold
Urinary bladder, body
Right ureter, intramural part
Ureteral orifice
Urinary bladder, trigone
Mucosa
Muscularis (= detrusor vesicae)
Adventitia with visceral pelvic fascia
Urinary bladder, neck
Internal urethral orifice with bladder uvula
Mucosa with longitudinal folds
Submucosa
Muscularis
Urethra
Orifices of urethral glands

Overview of the Genital Organs

The genital organs can be classified topographically (external versus internal) and functionally (Tables 18.2 and 18.3).

Table 18.2 Female genital organs

	Organ		Function
Internal genitalia	Ovary		Germ cell and hormone production
	Uterine tube		Site of conception and transport organ for zygote
	Uterus		Organ of incubation and parturition
	Vagina (upper portion)		Organ of copulation and parturition
External genitalia	Vulva	Vagina (vestibule)	
		Labia majora and minora	Accessory copulatory organ
		Clitoris	
		Greater and lesser vestibular glands	Production of mucoid secretions
		Mons pubis	Protection of the pubic bone

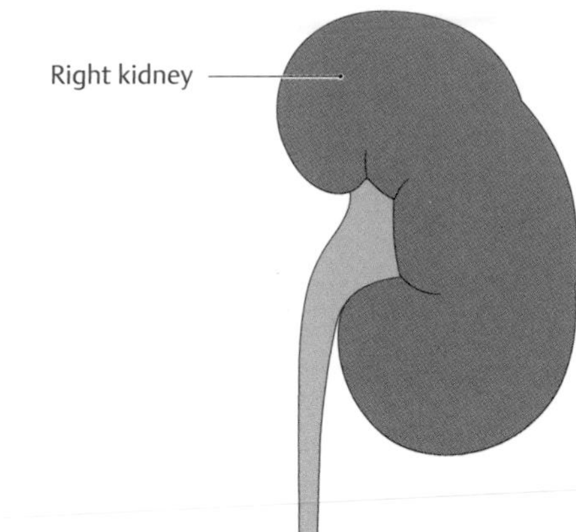
Right kidney
Right ureter

Fig. 18.11 **Female genital organs**

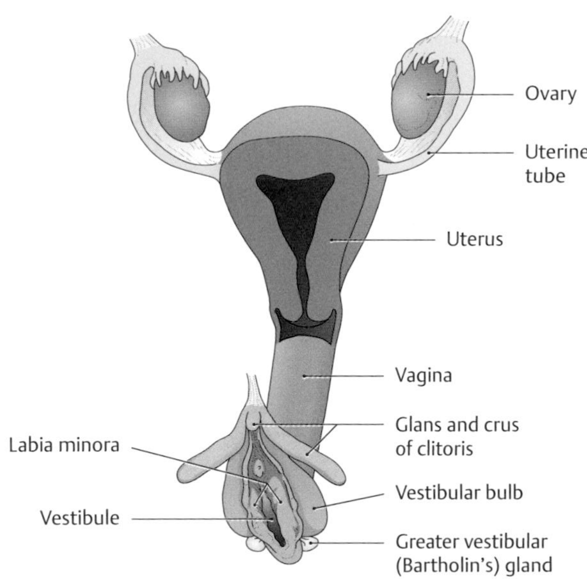
Ovary
Uterine tube
Uterus
Vagina
Glans and crus of clitoris
Labia minora
Vestibular bulb
Vestibule
Greater vestibular (Bartholin's) gland

A Internal and external genitalia.

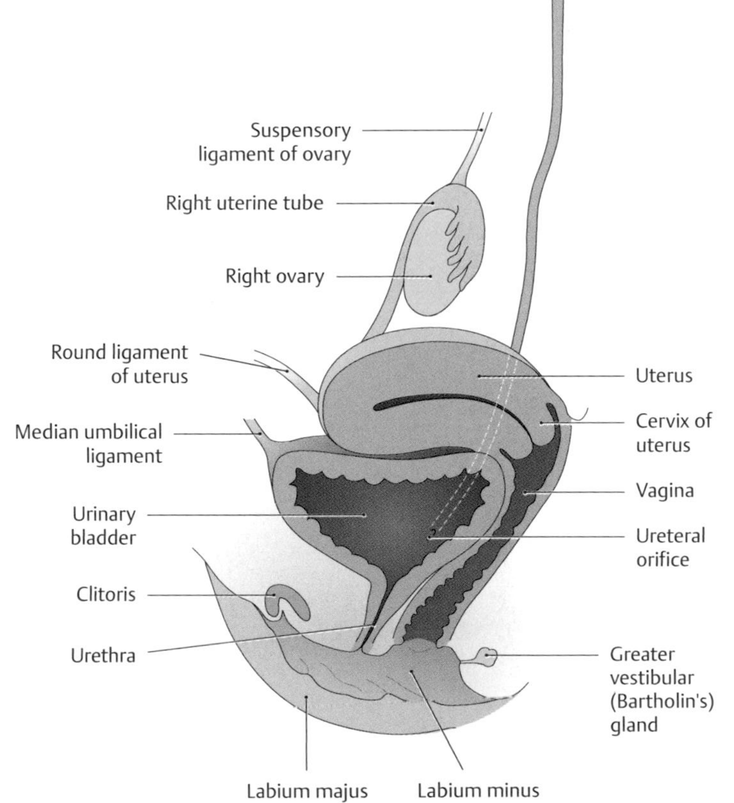
Suspensory ligament of ovary
Right uterine tube
Right ovary
Round ligament of uterus
Uterus
Cervix of uterus
Median umbilical ligament
Vagina
Urinary bladder
Ureteral orifice
Clitoris
Urethra
Greater vestibular (Bartholin's) gland
Labium majus
Labium minus

B Urogenital system. *Note:* The female urinary and genital tracts are functionally separate, though topographically close.

	Table 18.3 Male genital organs		
	Organ		**Function**
Internal genitalia	Testis		Germ cell and hormone production
	Epididymis		Reservoir for sperm
	Ductus deferens		Transport organ for sperm
	Accessory sex glands	Prostate	Production of secretions (semen)
		Seminal glands	
		Bulbourethral gland	
External genitalia	Penis		Copulatory and urinary organ
	Urethra		Conduit for urine and semen
	Scrotum		Protection of testis
	Coverings of the testis		

Fig. 18.12 Male genital organs

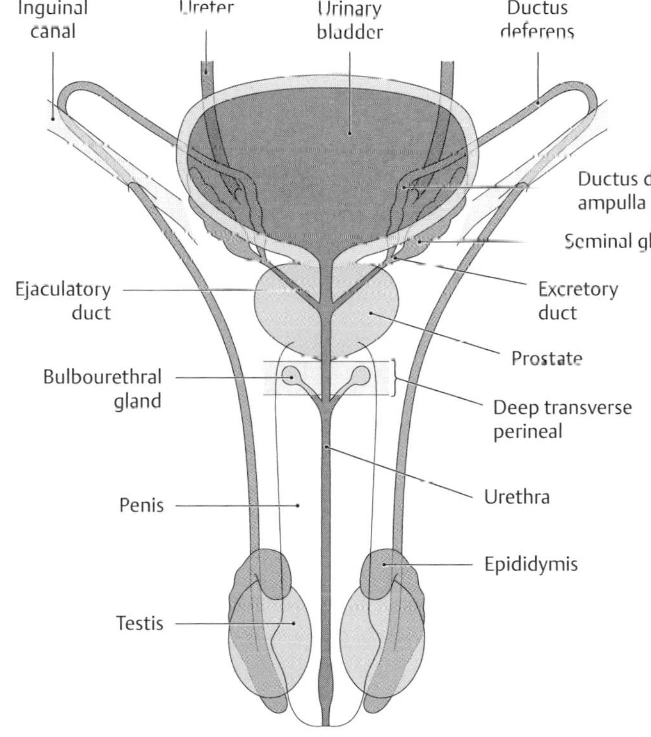
Inguinal canal
Ureter
Urinary bladder
Ductus deferens
Ductus deferens, ampulla
Seminal gland
Ejaculatory duct
Excretory duct
Prostate
Bulbourethral gland
Deep transverse perineal
Penis
Urethra
Epididymis
Testis

A Seminiferous structures.

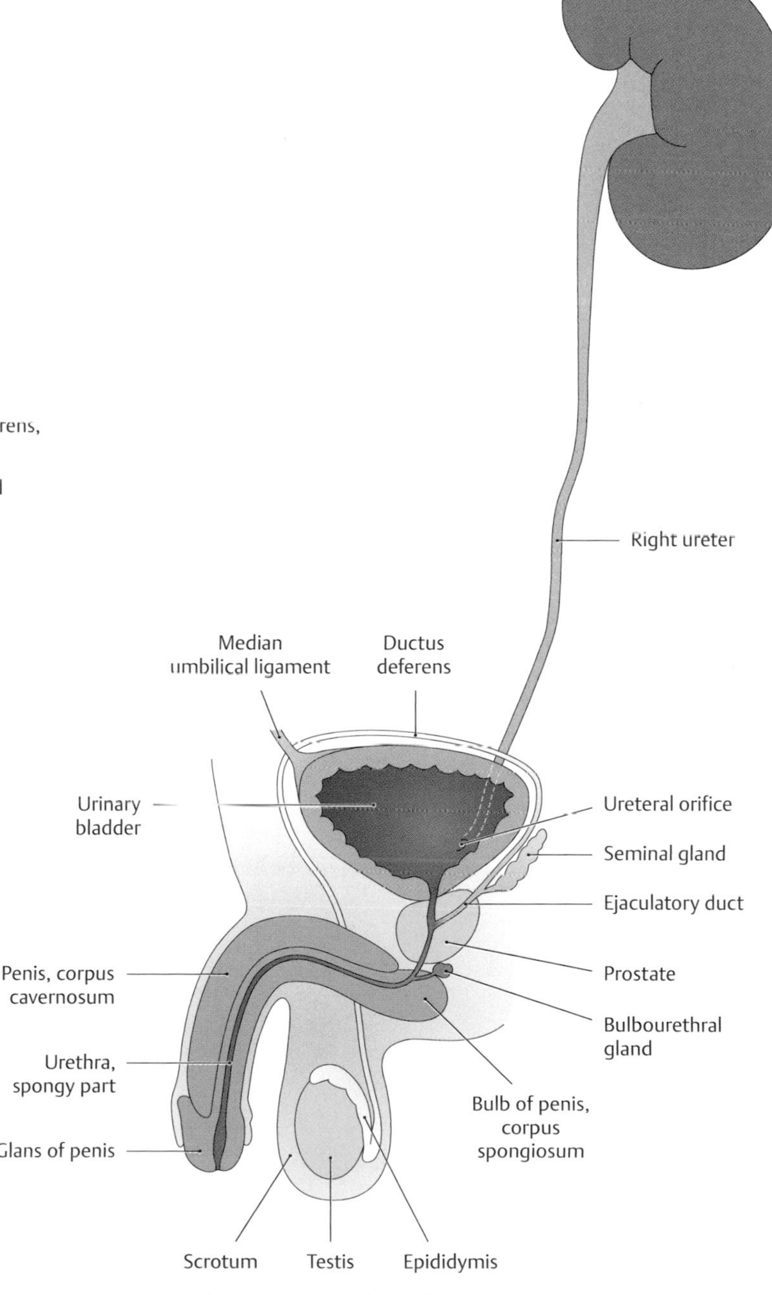
Right kidney
Right ureter
Median umbilical ligament
Ductus deferens
Urinary bladder
Ureteral orifice
Seminal gland
Ejaculatory duct
Prostate
Penis, corpus cavernosum
Bulbourethral gland
Urethra, spongy part
Bulb of penis, corpus spongiosum
Glans of penis
Scrotum
Testis
Epididymis

B Urogenital system. *Note:* The male urethra serves as a common urinary and genital passage.

Uterus & Ovaries

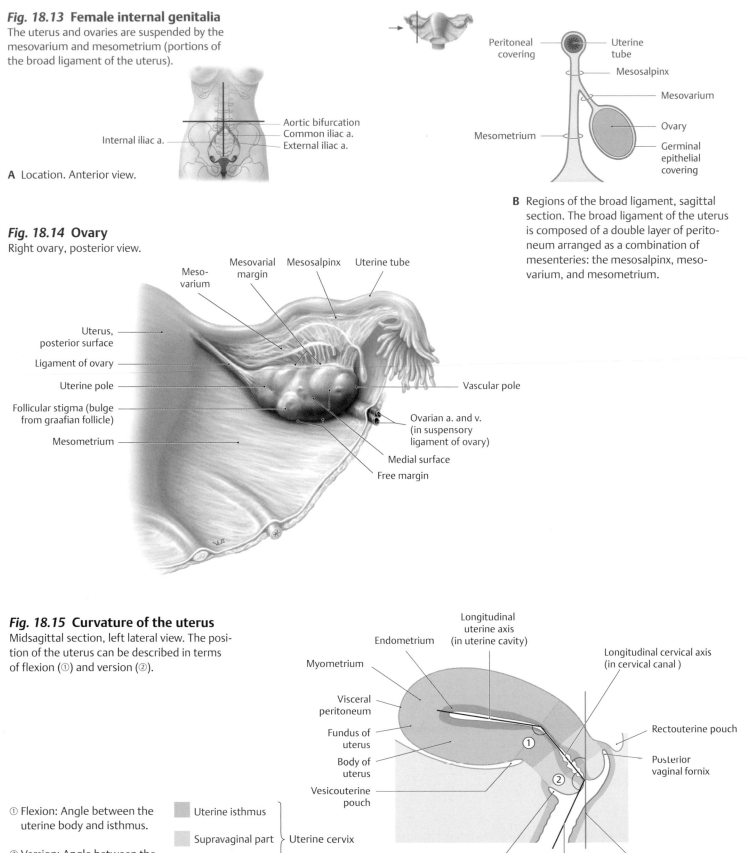

Fig. 18.13 **Female internal genitalia**
The uterus and ovaries are suspended by the mesovarium and mesometrium (portions of the broad ligament of the uterus).

A Location. Anterior view.

B Regions of the broad ligament, sagittal section. The broad ligament of the uterus is composed of a double layer of peritoneum arranged as a combination of mesenteries: the mesosalpinx, mesovarium, and mesometrium.

Fig. 18.14 **Ovary**
Right ovary, posterior view.

Fig. 18.15 **Curvature of the uterus**
Midsagittal section, left lateral view. The position of the uterus can be described in terms of flexion (①) and version (②).

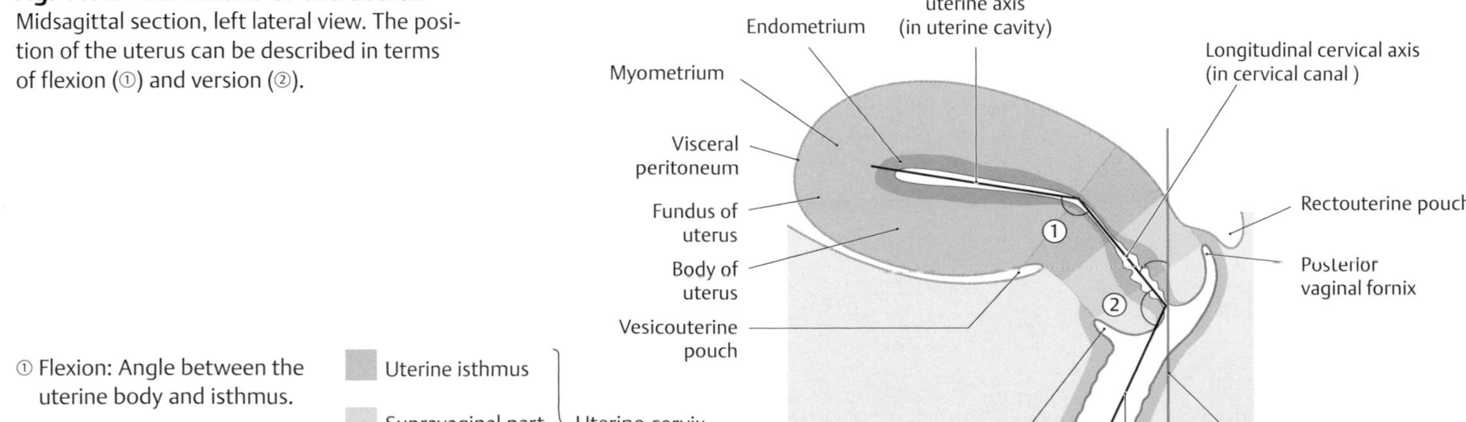

① Flexion: Angle between the uterine body and isthmus.
② Version: Angle between the cervical canal and the vagina.
Uterine isthmus
Supravaginal part
Vaginal part
Uterine cervix
Endometrium
Longitudinal uterine axis (in uterine cavity)
Longitudinal cervical axis (in cervical canal)
Myometrium
Visceral peritoneum
Fundus of uterus
Body of uterus
Vesicouterine pouch
Rectouterine pouch
Posterior vaginal fornix
Anterior vaginal fornix
Longitudinal vaginal axis
Longitudinal body axis
1
2

Fig. 18.16 **Uterus and uterine tube**

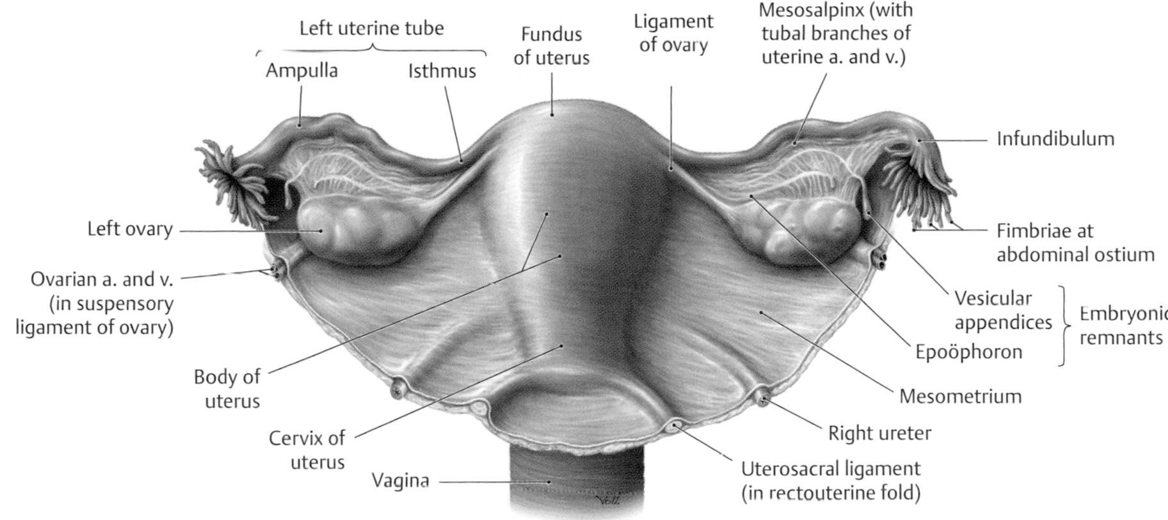
Left uterine tube
Ampulla
Isthmus
Fundus of uterus
Ligament of ovary
Mesosalpinx (with tubal branches of uterine a. and v.)
Infundibulum
Left ovary
Fimbriae at abdominal ostium
Ovarian a. and v. (in suspensory ligament of ovary)
Vesicular appendices
Epoöphoron
Embryonic remnants
Body of uterus
Mesometrium
Right ureter
Cervix of uterus
Vagina
Uterosacral ligament (in rectouterine fold)

A Posterosuperior view.

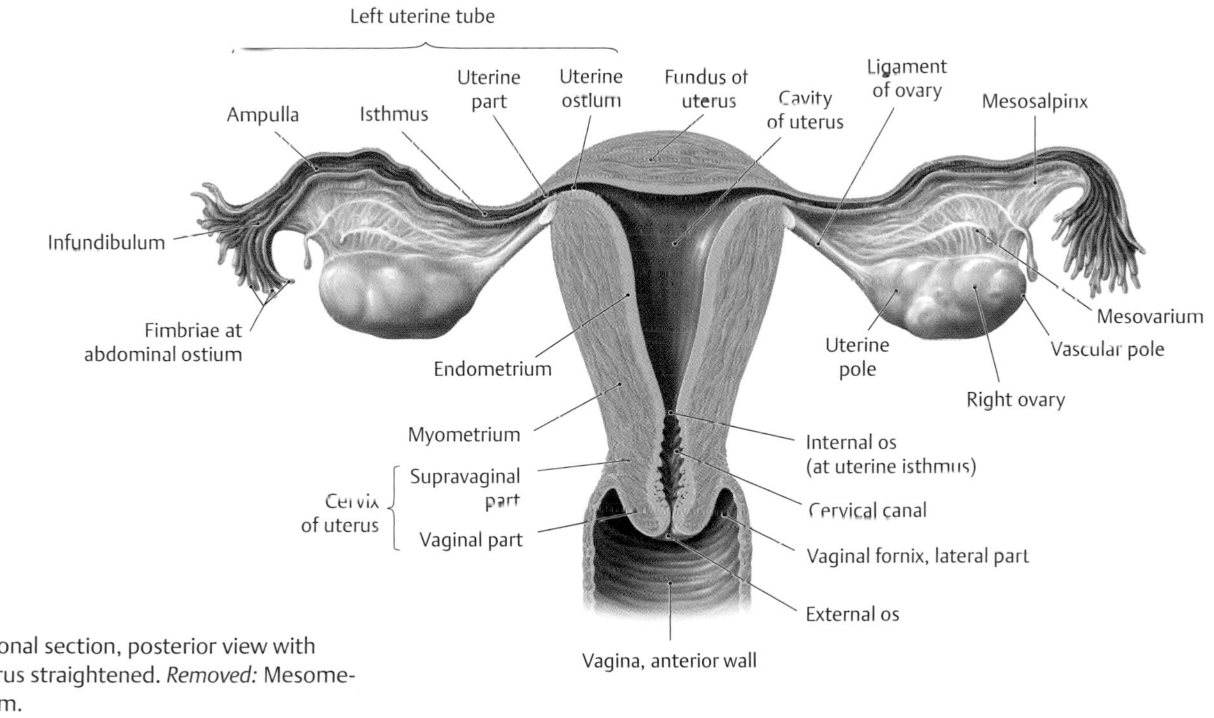
Left uterine tube
Ampulla
Isthmus
Uterine part
Uterine ostium
Fundus of uterus
Cavity of uterus
Ligament of ovary
Mesosalpinx
Infundibulum
Mesovarium
Fimbriae at abdominal ostium
Uterine pole
Vascular pole
Endometrium
Right ovary
Myometrium
Internal os (at uterine isthmus)
Cervix of uterus
Supravaginal part
Vaginal part
Cervical canal
Vaginal fornix, lateral part
External os
Vagina, anterior wall

B Coronal section, posterior view with uterus straightened. *Removed:* Mesometrium.

Clinical

Ectopic pregnancy

After fertilization in the ampulla of the uterine tube, the ovum usually implants in the wall of the uterine cavity. However, it may become implanted at other sites (e.g., the uterine tube or even the peritoneal cavity). Tubal pregnancies, the most common type of ectopic pregnancy, pose the risk of tubal wall rupture and potentially life-threatening bleeding into the peritoneal cavity. Tubal pregnancies are promoted by adhesion of the tubal mucosa, mostly due to inflammation.

Ligaments & Fascia of the Deep Pelvis

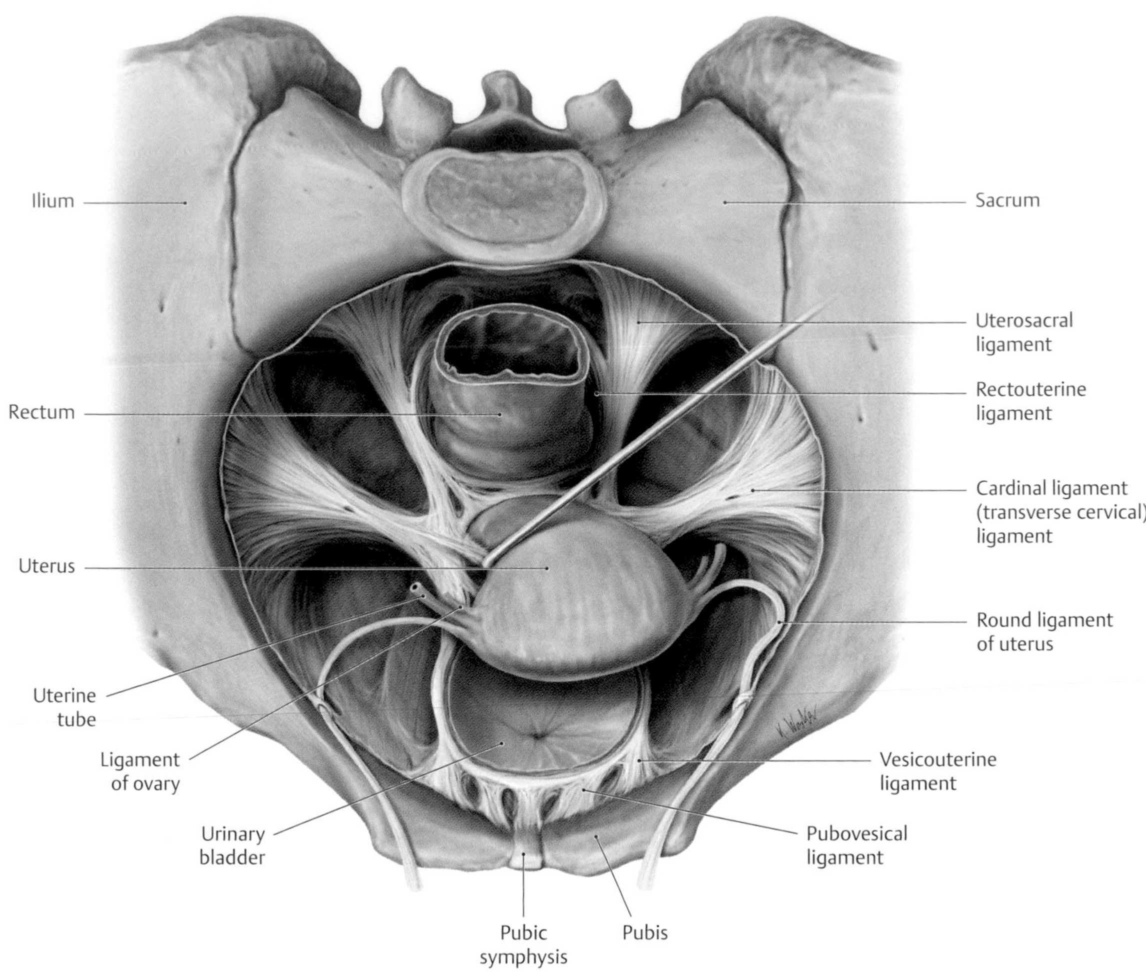
Ilium
Sacrum
Uterosacral ligament
Rectouterine ligament
Rectum
Cardinal ligament (transverse cervical) ligament
Uterus
Round ligament of uterus
Uterine tube
Ligament of ovary
Vesicouterine ligament
Urinary bladder
Pubovesical ligament
Pubic symphysis
Pubis

***Fig. 18.17* Ligaments of the female pelvis**
Superior view. *Removed:* Peritoneum, neurovasculature, and superior portion of the bladder to demonstrate only the fascial condensations (ligaments). Deep pelvic ligaments support the uterus within the pelvic cavity and prevent uterine prolapse, the downward displacement of the uterus into the vagina.

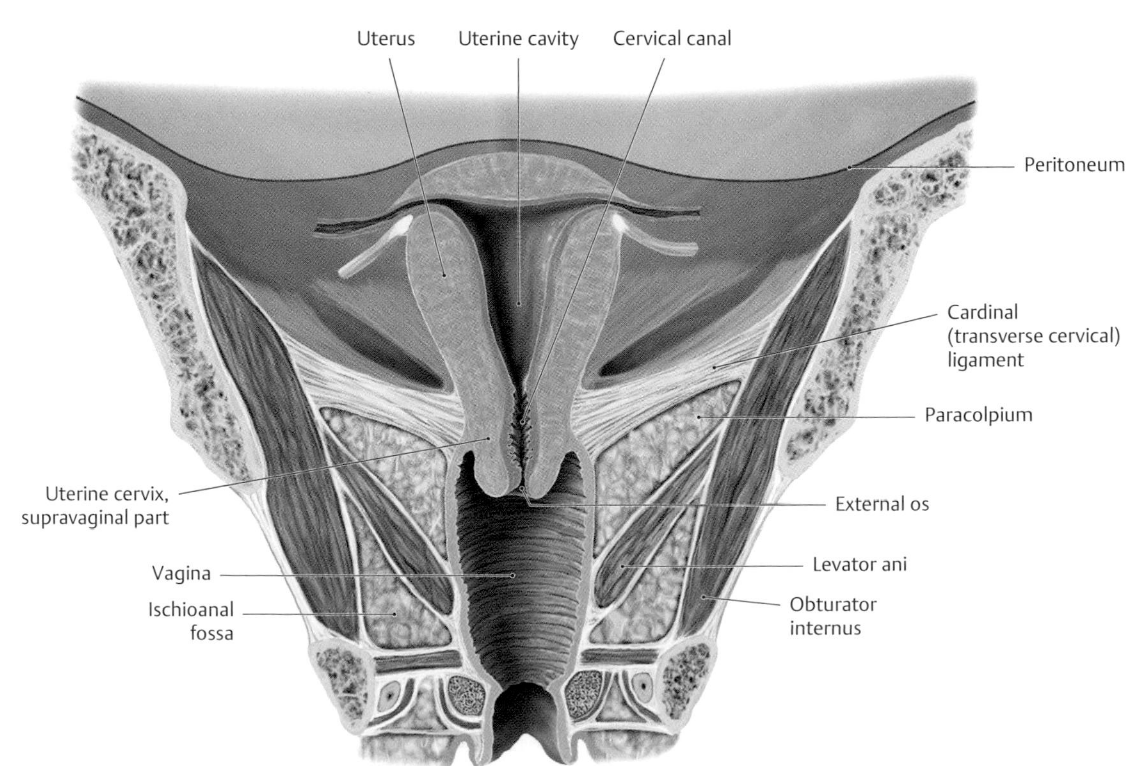
Uterus
Uterine cavity
Cervical canal
Peritoneum
Cardinal (transverse cervical) ligament
Paracolpium
Uterine cervix, supravaginal part
External os
Levator ani
Vagina
Ischioanal fossa
Obturator internus

***Fig. 18.18* Cardinal (transverse cervical) ligaments of the uterus.**
Coronal section, through uterus and vagina. Each of the cardinal ligaments, major ligaments of the uterus, is located at the base of the broad ligament and contains a uterine artery and vein. These paired ligaments attach the cervix of the uterus to the lateral pelvic wall, providing major uterine support. Clinically, ligation of the ligament during hysterectomy may damage the ureters, which lie in close proximity (see Fig. 18.7).

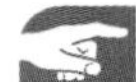

Fascia of the pelvis plays an important role in the support of pelvic viscera. On either side of the pelvic floor, where the visceral fascia of the pelvic organs is continuous with the parietal fascia of the muscular walls, thickenings called tendinous arches of the pelvic fascia are formed. In females, the paracolpium – lateral connections between the visceral fascia and the tendinous arches – suspends and supports the vagina. Pubovesical ligaments (and puboprostatic ligaments in the male) are extensions of the tendinous arches that support the bladder and prostate. Endopelvic fascia, a loose areolar (fatty) tissue that fills the spaces between pelvic viscera, condenses to form "ligaments" (cardinal ligaments, lateral ligaments of the bladder, lateral rectal ligaments ;see Fig 18.17) that provide passage for the ureters and neurovascular elements within the pelvis.

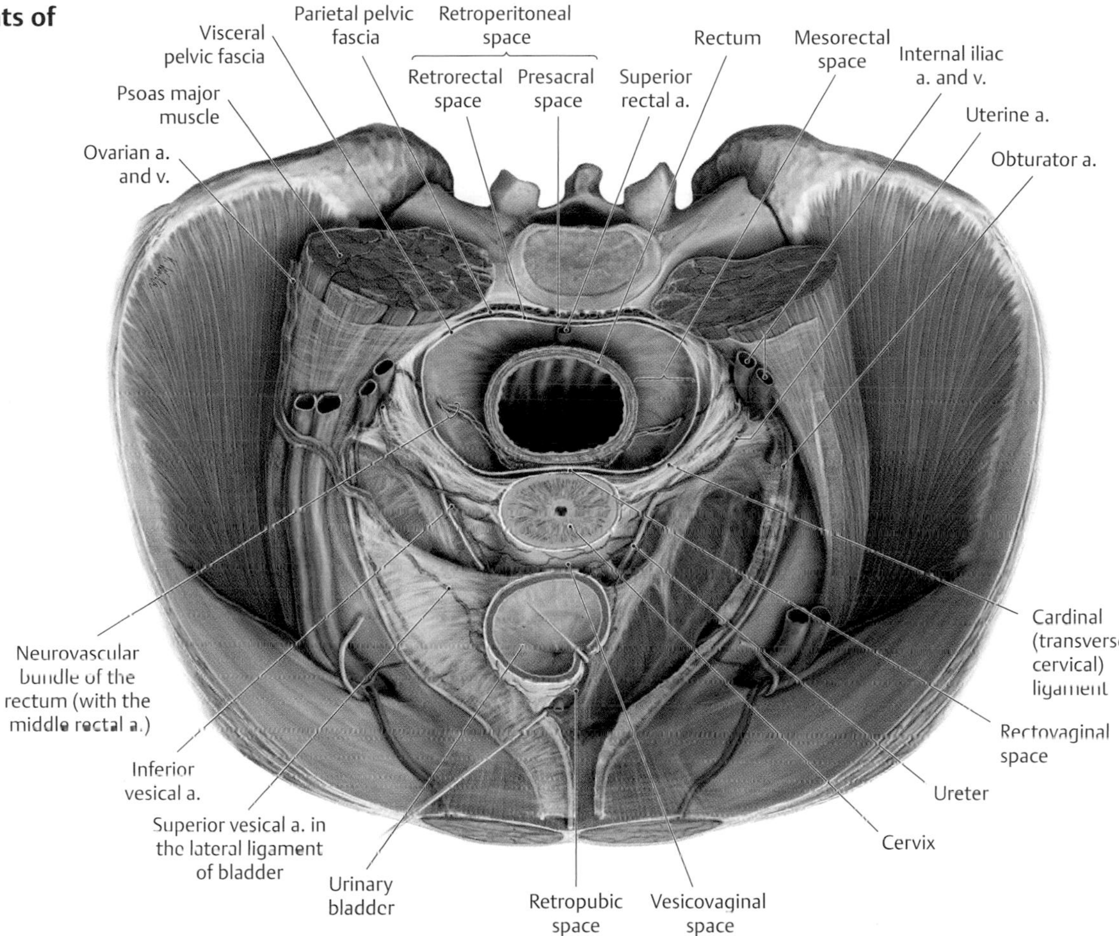
Visceral pelvic fascia
Parietal pelvic fascia
Retroperitoneal space
Retrorectal space
Presacral space
Superior rectal a.
Rectum
Mesorectal space
Internal iliac a. and v.
Uterine a.
Obturator a.
Psoas major muscle
Ovarian a. and v.
Neurovascular bundle of the rectum (with the middle rectal a.)
Inferior vesical a.
Superior vesical a. in the lateral ligament of bladder
Urinary bladder
Retropubic space
Vesicovaginal space
Cervix
Ureter
Rectovaginal space
Cardinal (transverse cervical) ligament

Fig. 18.19 **Fascia and ligaments of the female pelvis**
Transverse section, through cervix, superior view.

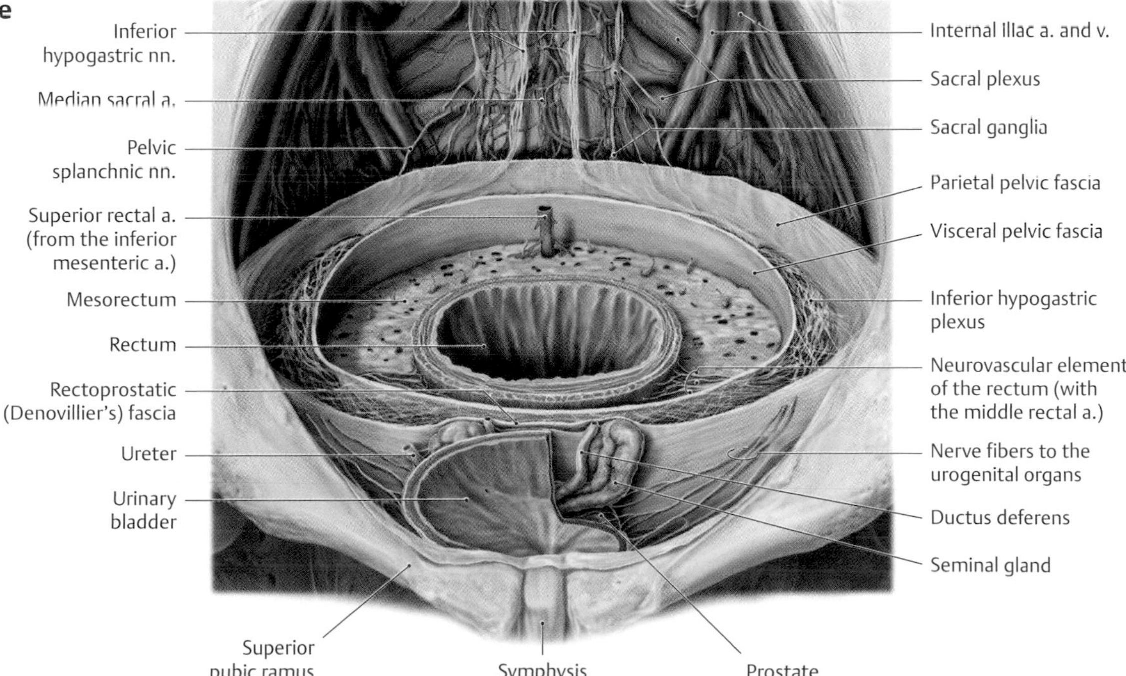
Inferior hypogastric nn.
Median sacral a.
Pelvic splanchnic nn.
Superior rectal a. (from the inferior mesenteric a.)
Mesorectum
Rectum
Rectoprostatic (Denovillier's) fascia
Ureter
Urinary bladder
Superior pubic ramus
Symphysis
Prostate
Internal Iliac a. and v.
Sacral plexus
Sacral ganglia
Parietal pelvic fascia
Visceral pelvic fascia
Inferior hypogastric plexus
Neurovascular elements of the rectum (with the middle rectal a.)
Nerve fibers to the urogenital organs
Ductus deferens
Seminal gland

Fig. 18.20 **Fascia and course of neurovascular elements in the male pelvis**
Anterosuperior view. *Removed:* Upper two thirds of the rectum and bladder.

Vagina

Fig. 18.21 Location of vagina
Midsagittal section, left lateral view.

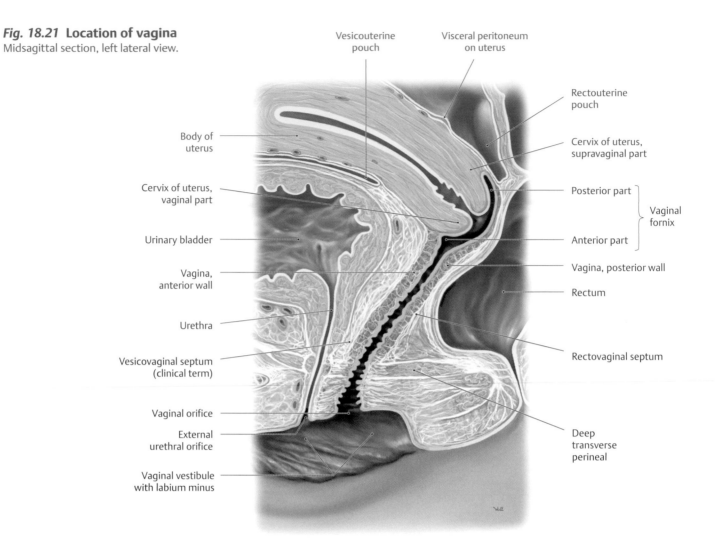

Vesicouterine pouch
Visceral peritoneum on uterus
Rectouterine pouch
Body of uterus
Cervix of uterus, supravaginal part
Cervix of uterus, vaginal part
Posterior part
Vaginal fornix
Anterior part
Urinary bladder
Vagina, anterior wall
Vagina, posterior wall
Rectum
Urethra
Rectovaginal septum
Vesicovaginal septum (clinical term)
Vaginal orifice
External urethral orifice
Deep transverse perineal
Vaginal vestibule with labium minus

Fig. 18.22 Structure of vagina
Posteriorly angled coronal section, posterior view.

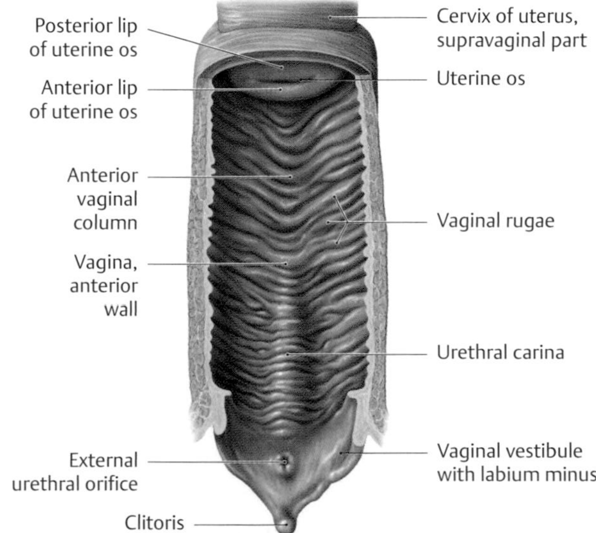
Posterior lip of uterine os
Cervix of uterus, supravaginal part
Uterine os
Anterior lip of uterine os
Anterior vaginal column
Vaginal rugae
Vagina, anterior wall
Urethral carina
External urethral orifice
Vaginal vestibule with labium minus
Clitoris

Fig. 18.23 Female genital organs: Coronal section

Anterior view. The vagina is both pelvic and perineal in location. It is also retroperitoneal.

Suspensory ligament of ovary
Fundus of the uterus
Rectum
Sigmoid colon
Parietal peritoneum
Ilium
Right external iliac a. and v.
Iliacus
Left ovary
Cardinal (transverse cervical) ligament (with sections of the uterine a. and uterine venous plexus)
Left uterine tube
Round ligament of uterus
Cervix with uterine os
Pelvic retro-peritoneal space
Vaginal arterial branches and venous plexus
Obturator internus (with obturator fascia)
Levator ani (with superior and inferior fascia of pelvic diaphragm)
Vagina, posterior wall with vaginal rugae
Deep transverse perineal
Ischiopubic ramus
Superficial perineal (Colles') fascia
Crus of clitoris with ischiocavernosus
Perineal a.
Round ligament of uterus
Labium minus
A. of vestibular bulb
Labium majus
Vestibule of vagina (with vaginal orifice)
Vestibular bulb with bulbospongiosus

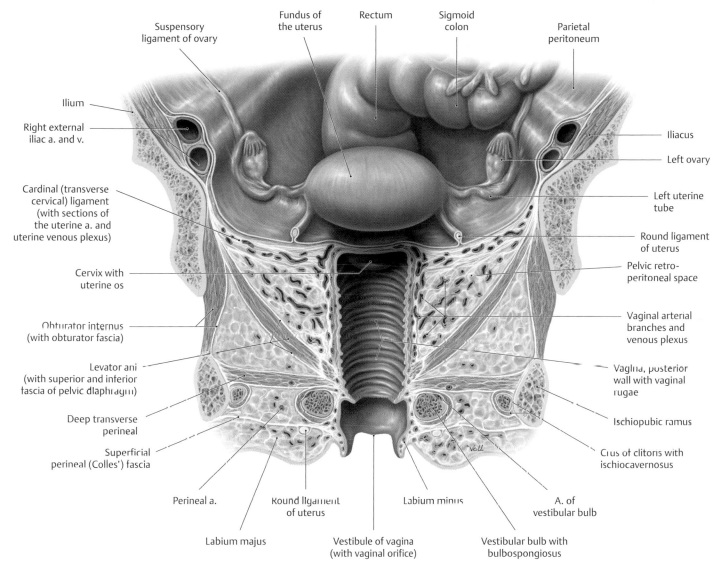

Fig. 18.24 Vagina: Location in the perineum

Inferior view.

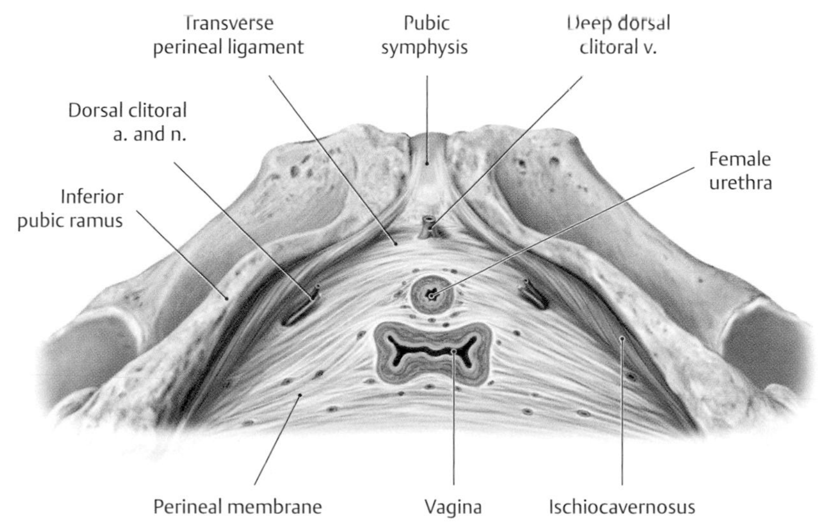
Transverse perineal ligament
Pubic symphysis
Deep dorsal clitoral v.
Dorsal clitoral a. and n.
Female urethra
Inferior pubic ramus
Perineal membrane
Vagina
Ischiocavernosus

Female External Genitalia

Fig. 18.25 **Female external genitalia**
Lithotomy position with labia minora separated.

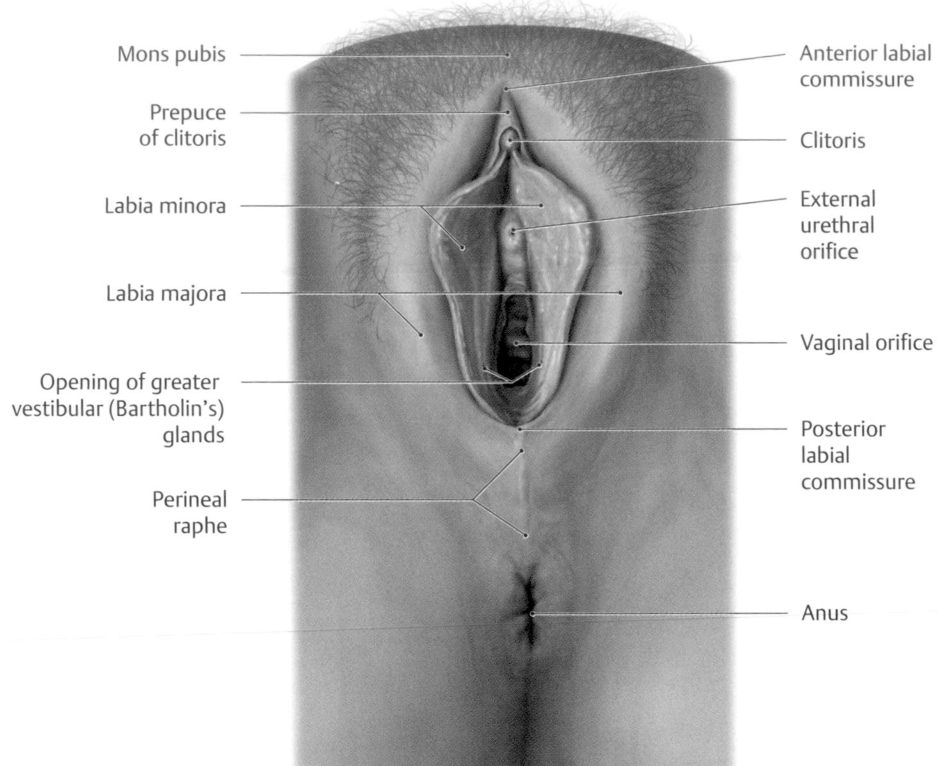
Mons pubis
Prepuce of clitoris
Labia minora
Labia majora
Opening of greater vestibular (Bartholin's) glands
Perineal raphe
Anterior labial commissure
Clitoris
External urethral orifice
Vaginal orifice
Posterior labial commissure
Anus

Fig. 18.26 **Vestibule and vestibular glands**
Lithotomy position with labia minora separated.

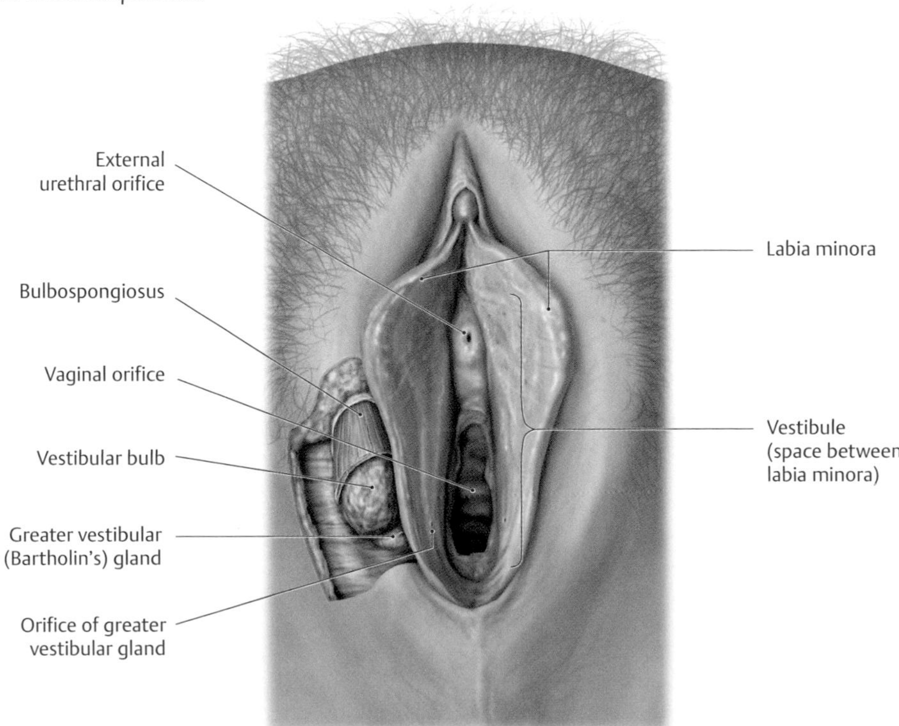
External urethral orifice
Bulbospongiosus
Vaginal orifice
Vestibular bulb
Greater vestibular (Bartholin's) gland
Orifice of greater vestibular gland
Labia minora
Vestibule (space between labia minora)

Fig. 18.27 **Erectile tissue and muscles of the female**
Lithotomy position. *Removed:* Labia, skin, and perineal membrane. *Removed from left side:* Ischiocavernosus and bulbospongiosus muscle and greater vestibular (Bartholin's) gland.

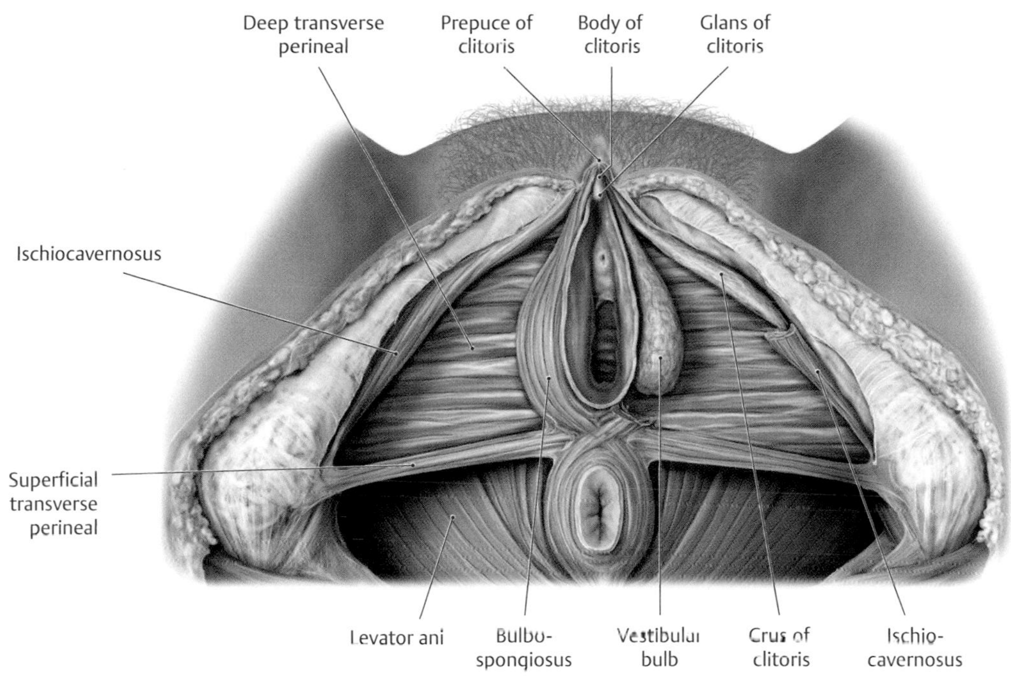
Deep transverse perineal
Prepuce of clitoris
Body of clitoris
Glans of clitoris
Ischiocavernosus
Superficial transverse perineal
Levator ani
Bulbo-spongiosus
Vestibular bulb
Crus of clitoris
Ischio-cavernosus

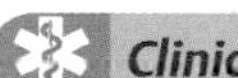

Clinical

Episiotomy

Episiotomy is a common obstetric procedure used to enlarge the birth canal during the expulsive stage of labor. The procedure is generally used to expedite the delivery of a baby at risk for hypoxia during the expulsive stage. Alternately, if the perineal skin turns white (indicating diminished blood flow), there is imminent danger of perineal laceration, and an episiotomy is often performed. More lateral incisions gain more room, but they are more difficult to repair.

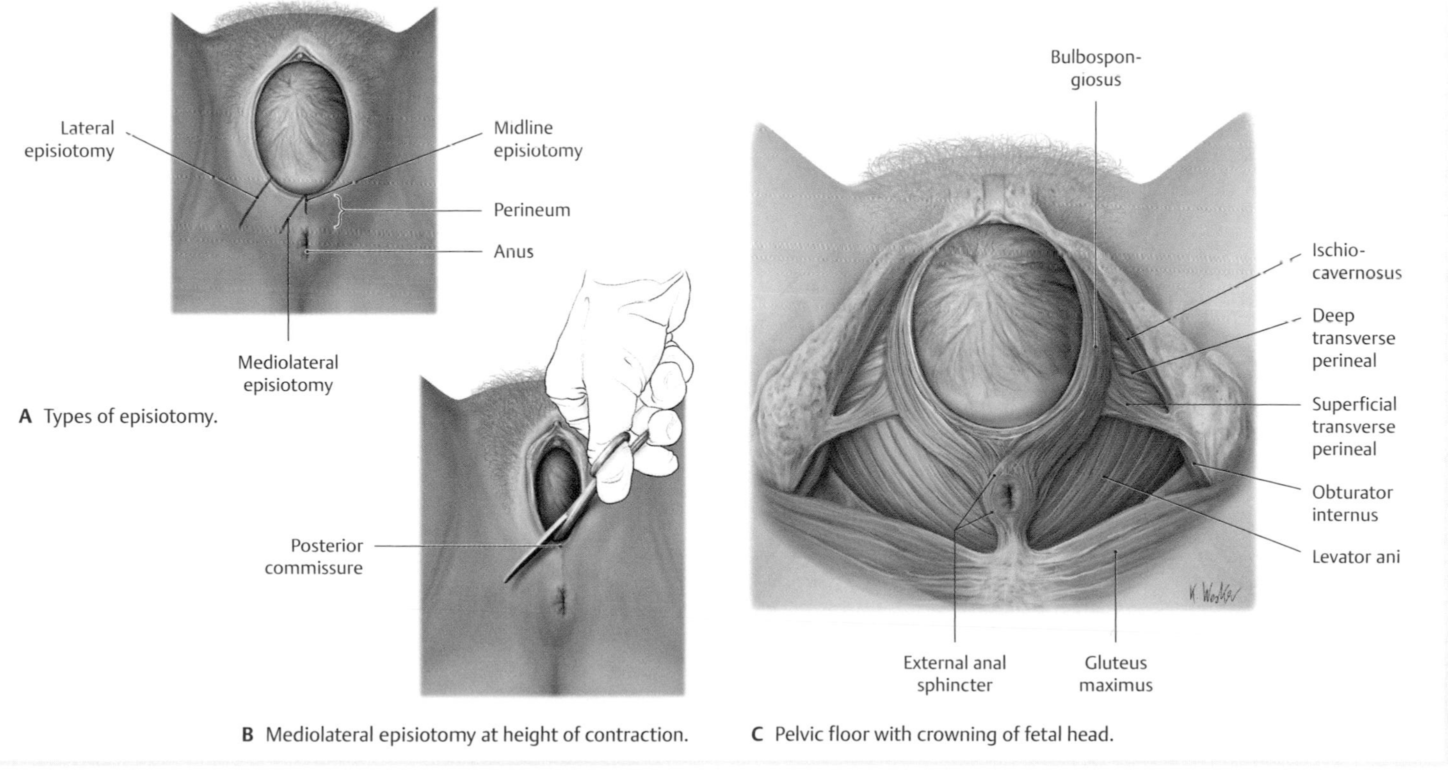
Lateral episiotomy
Midline episiotomy
Perineum
Anus
Mediolateral episiotomy
Posterior commissure
Bulbospon-giosus
Ischio-cavernosus
Deep transverse perineal
Superficial transverse perineal
Obturator internus
Levator ani
External anal sphincter
Gluteus maximus

A Types of episiotomy.

B Mediolateral episiotomy at height of contraction.

C Pelvic floor with crowning of fetal head.

Penis, Testis & Epididymis

Fig. 18.28 **Penis**

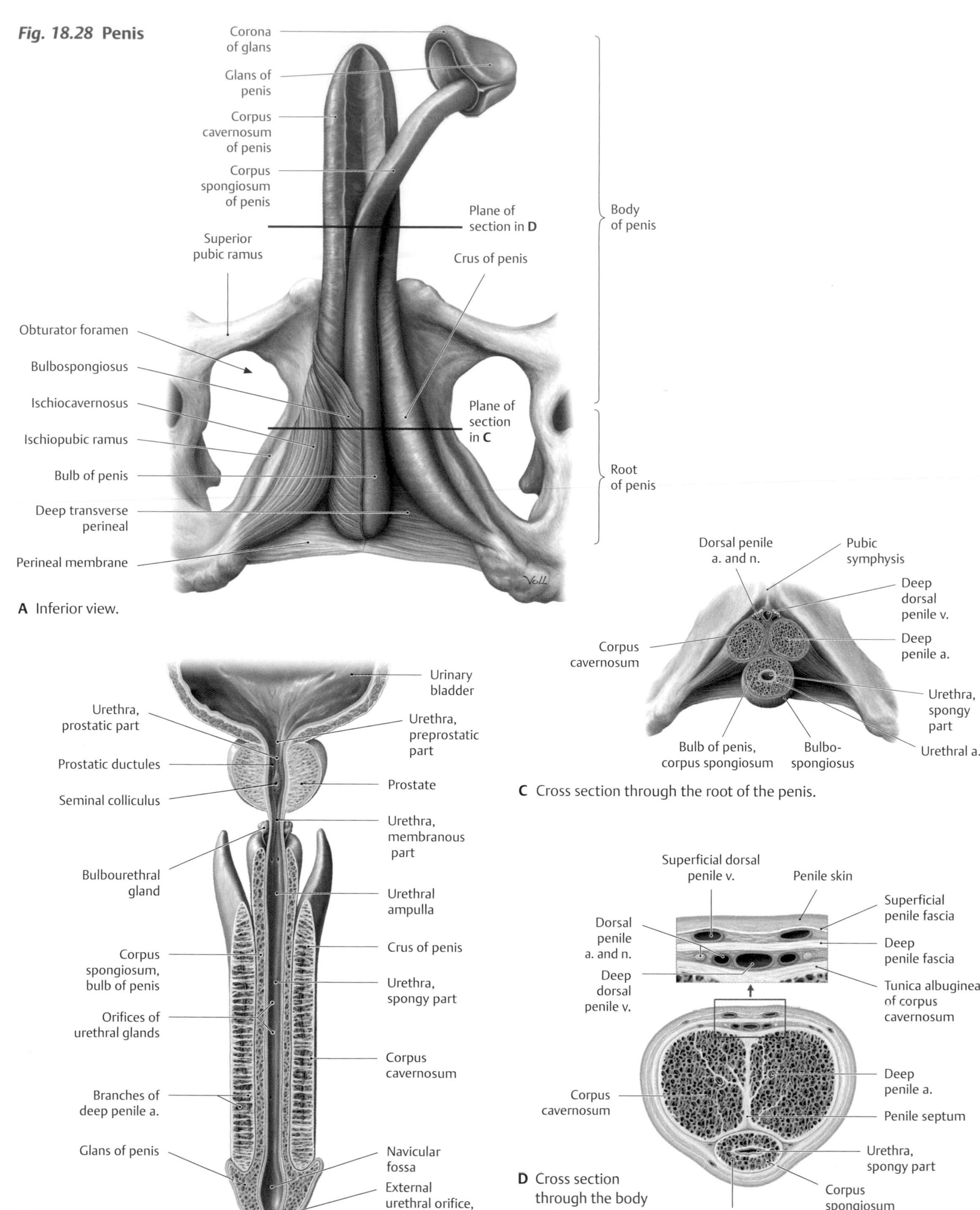
Corona of glans
Glans of penis
Corpus cavernosum of penis
Corpus spongiosum of penis
Superior pubic ramus
Plane of section in **D**
Crus of penis
Body of penis
Obturator foramen
Bulbospongiosus
Ischiocavernosus
Ischiopubic ramus
Bulb of penis
Deep transverse perineal
Perineal membrane
Plane of section in **C**
Root of penis
Voll
Dorsal penile a. and n.
Pubic symphysis
Deep dorsal penile v.
Deep penile a.
Corpus cavernosum
Urethra, spongy part
Urethral a.
Bulb of penis, corpus spongiosum
Bulbo-spongiosus
Urinary bladder
Urethra, prostatic part
Urethra, preprostatic part
Prostatic ductules
Prostate
Seminal colliculus
Urethra, membranous part
Bulbourethral gland
Urethral ampulla
Crus of penis
Corpus spongiosum, bulb of penis
Urethra, spongy part
Orifices of urethral glands
Corpus cavernosum
Branches of deep penile a.
Glans of penis
Navicular fossa
External urethral orifice, urethral crest
Superficial dorsal penile v.
Penile skin
Superficial penile fascia
Dorsal penile a. and n.
Deep penile fascia
Deep dorsal penile v.
Tunica albuginea of corpus cavernosum
Corpus cavernosum
Deep penile a.
Penile septum
Urethra, spongy part
Corpus spongiosum of penis
Urethral a.

A Inferior view.

B Longitudinal section.

C Cross section through the root of the penis.

D Cross section through the body of the penis.

Fig. 18.29 Testis and epididymis

Left lateral view.

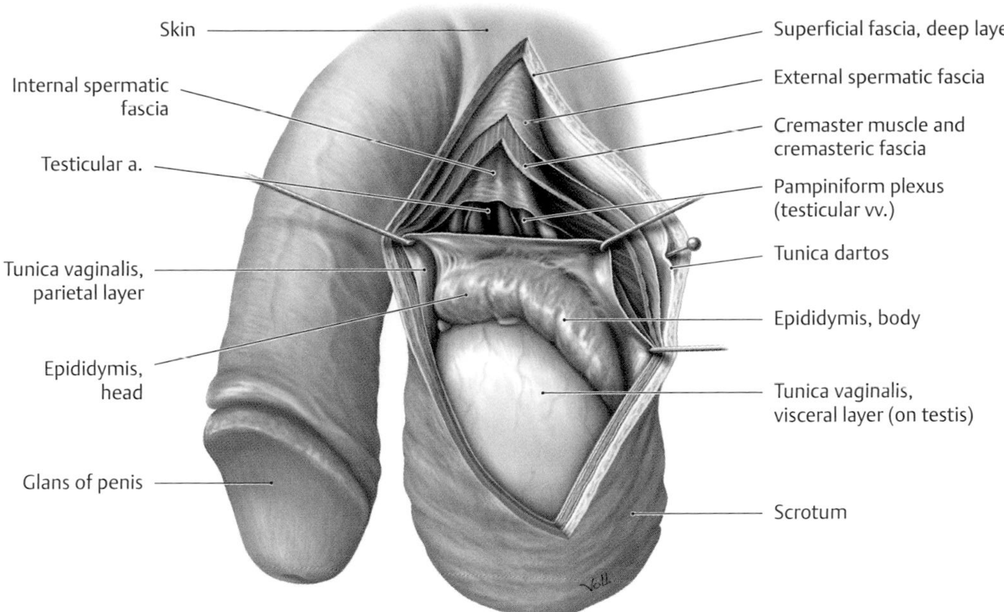
Skin
Internal spermatic fascia
Testicular a.
Tunica vaginalis, parietal layer
Epididymis, head
Glans of penis
Superficial fascia, deep layer
External spermatic fascia
Cremaster muscle and cremasteric fascia
Pampiniform plexus (testicular vv.)
Tunica dartos
Epididymis, body
Tunica vaginalis, visceral layer (on testis)
Scrotum

A Testis and epididymis in situ.

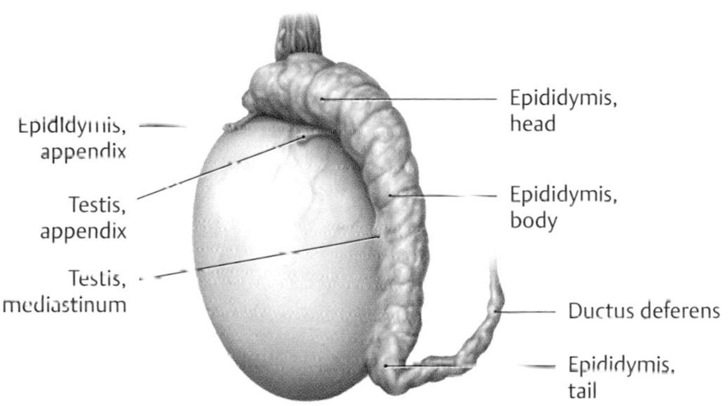
Epididymis, appendix
Testis, appendix
Testis, mediastinum
Epididymis, head
Epididymis, body
Ductus deferens
Epididymis, tail

B Surface anatomy of the testis and epididymis.

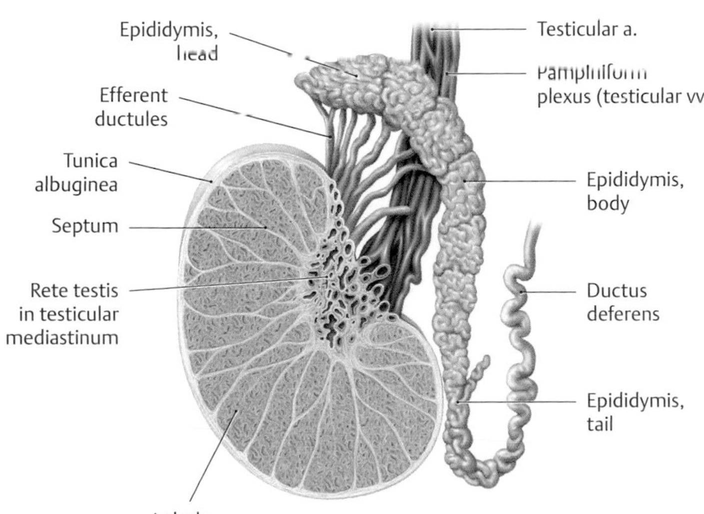
Epididymis, head
Efferent ductules
Tunica albuginea
Septum
Rete testis in testicular mediastinum
Lobule
Testicular a.
Pampiniform plexus (testicular vv.)
Epididymis, body
Ductus deferens
Epididymis, tail

C Sagittal section of the testis and epididymis.

Fig. 18.30 Blood vessels of the testis

Left lateral view.

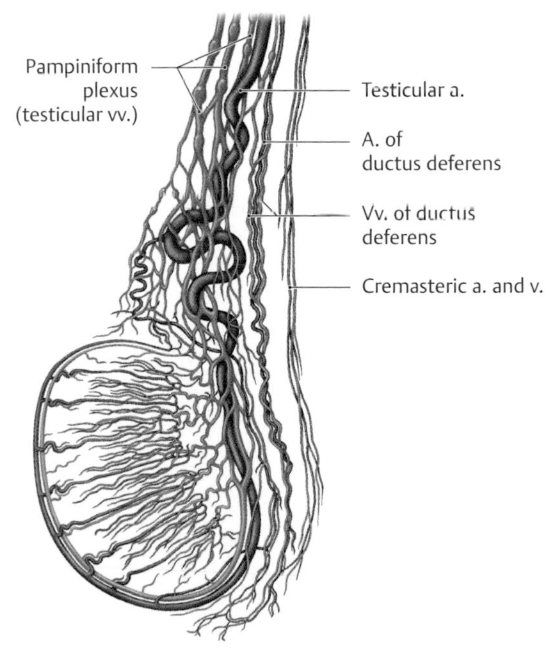
Pampiniform plexus (testicular vv.)
Testicular a.
A. of ductus deferens
Vv. of ductus deferens
Cremasteric a. and v.

Male Accessory Sex Glands

The accessory male sex glands consist of the seminal, prostate, and bulbourethral glands, which contribute fluid to the ejaculate that provides nourishment for the spermatozoa as well as neutralizes the pH of the male urethra and the vaginal environment.

Fig. 18.31 Accessory sex glands
The ducts of the seminal gland and ductus deferens combine to form the ejaculatory duct.

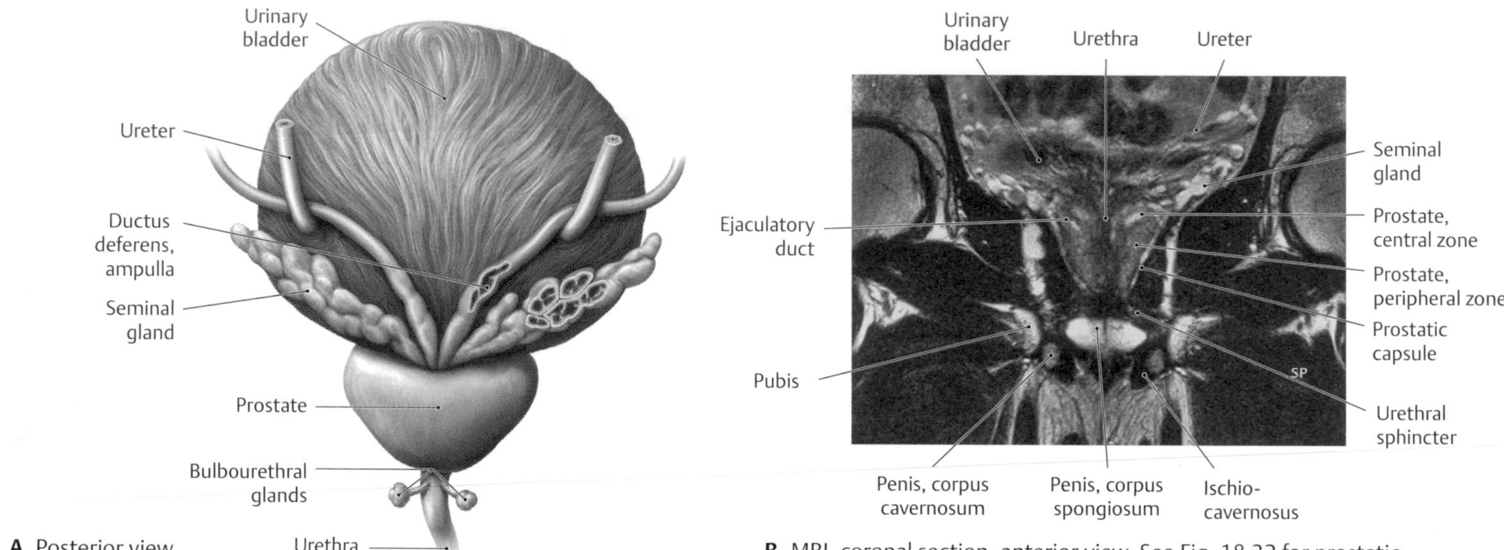
Urinary bladder
Ureter
Ductus deferens, ampulla
Seminal gland
Prostate
Bulbourethral glands
Urethra
Urinary bladder
Urethra
Ureter
Seminal gland
Prostate, central zone
Prostate, peripheral zone
Prostatic capsule
Urethral sphincter
SP
Ejaculatory duct
Pubis
Penis, corpus cavernosum
Penis, corpus spongiosum
Ischio-cavernosus

A Posterior view.

B MRI, coronal section, anterior view. See Fig. 18.32 for prostatic capsule and zones of prostate.

Fig. 18.32 Structure of prostate
The prostate may be divided anatomically (top row) or clinically (bottom row).

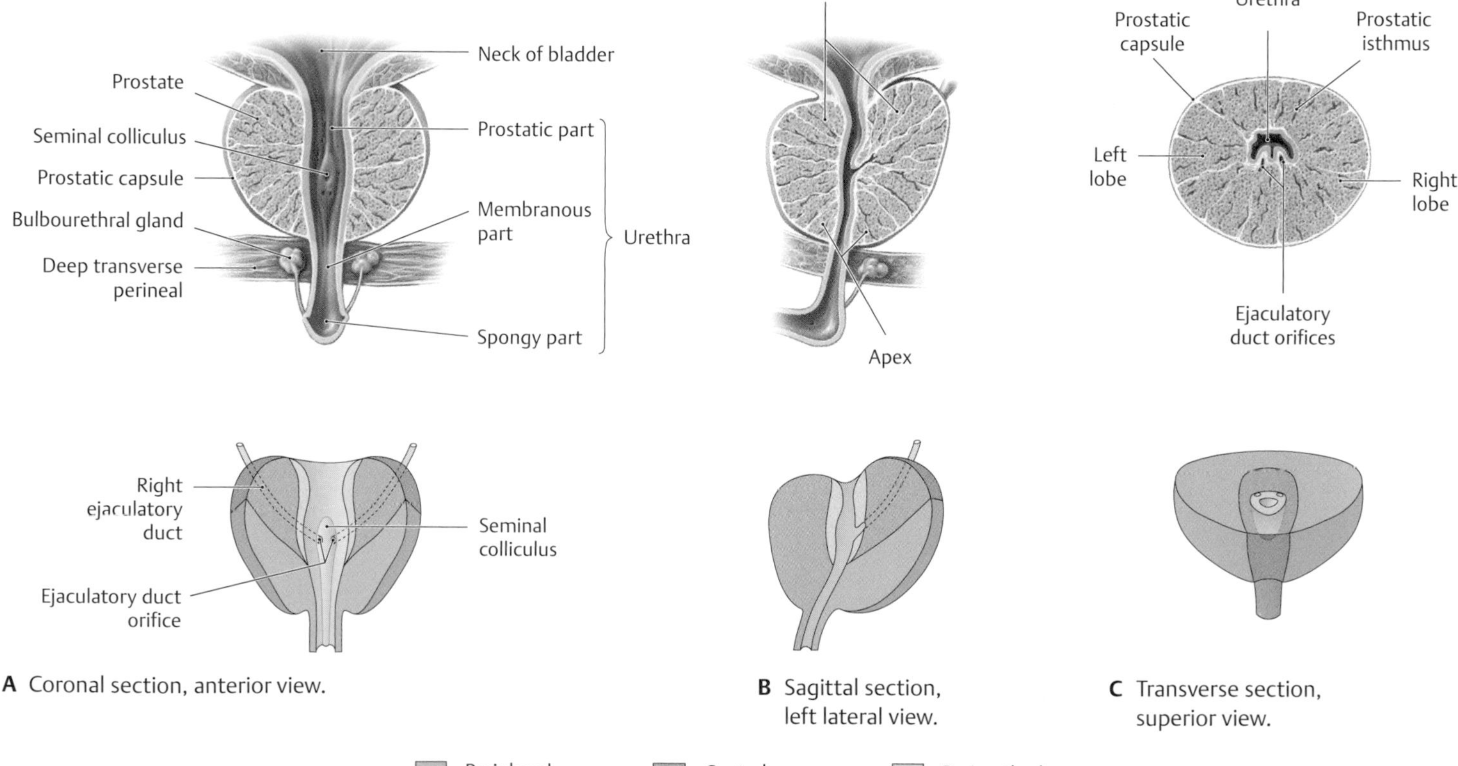
Prostate
Seminal colliculus
Prostatic capsule
Bulbourethral gland
Deep transverse perineal
Neck of bladder
Prostatic part
Membranous part
Spongy part
Urethra
Base
Apex
Urethra
Prostatic capsule
Prostatic isthmus
Left lobe
Right lobe
Ejaculatory duct orifices
Right ejaculatory duct
Ejaculatory duct orifice
Seminal colliculus
Peripheral zone (outer zone)
Central zone (inner zone)
Periurethral zone

A Coronal section, anterior view.

B Sagittal section, left lateral view.

C Transverse section, superior view.

Fig. 18.33 **Prostate in situ**
Sagittal section through the male pelvis, left lateral view.

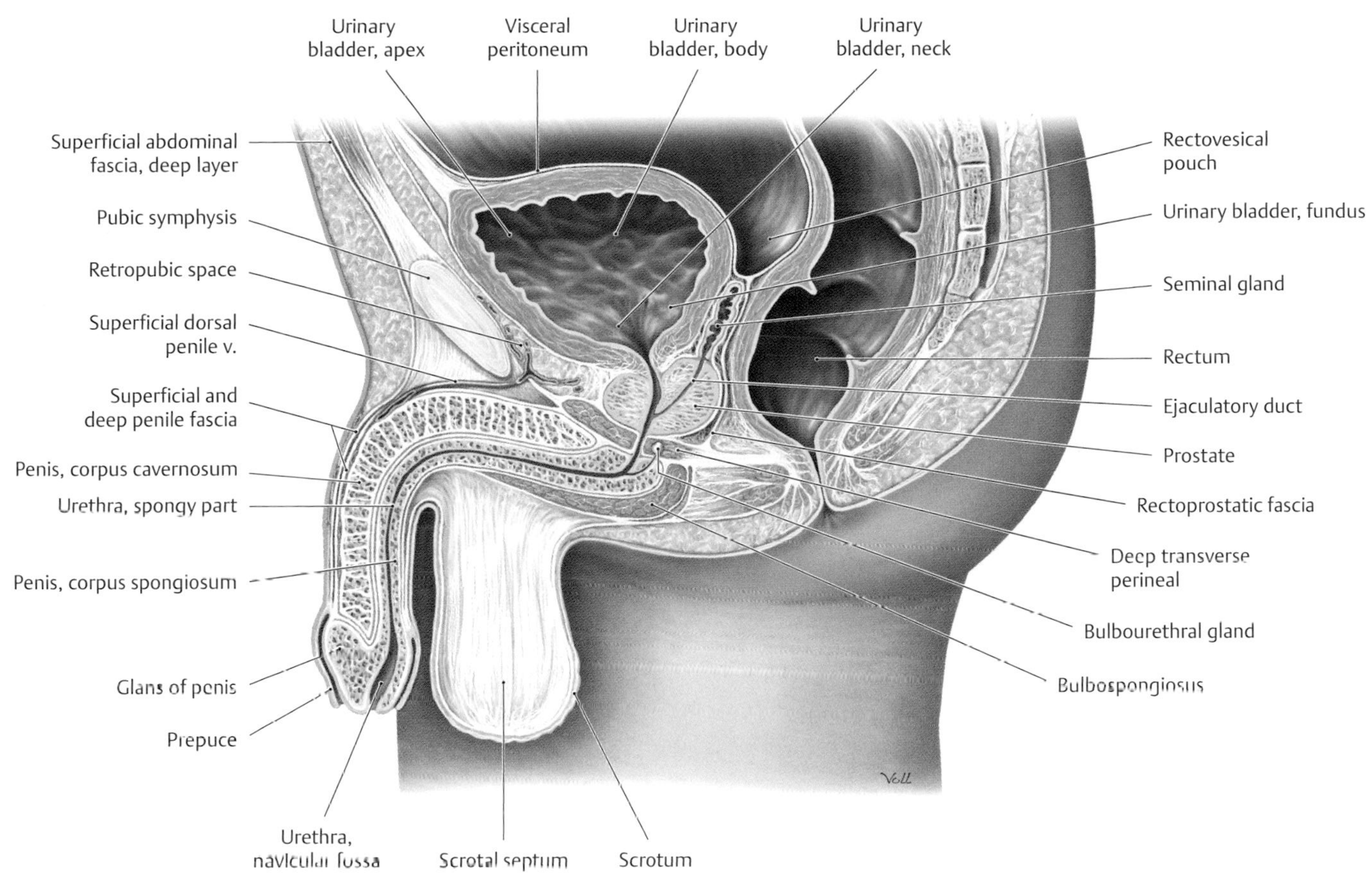
Urinary bladder, apex
Visceral peritoneum
Urinary bladder, body
Urinary bladder, neck
Superficial abdominal fascia, deep layer
Pubic symphysis
Retropubic space
Superficial dorsal penile v.
Superficial and deep penile fascia
Penis, corpus cavernosum
Urethra, spongy part
Penis, corpus spongiosum
Glans of penis
Prepuce
Urethra, navicular fossa
Scrotal septum
Scrotum
Rectovesical pouch
Urinary bladder, fundus
Seminal gland
Rectum
Ejaculatory duct
Prostate
Rectoprostatic fascia
Deep transverse perineal
Bulbourethral gland
Bulbospongiosus

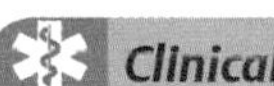
Clinical

Prostatic carcinoma and hypertrophy

Prostatic carcinoma is one of the most common malignant tumors in older men, often growing at a subcapsular location (deep to the prostatic capsule) in the peripheral zone of the prostate. Unlike benign prostatic hyperplasia, which begins in the central part of the gland, prostatic carcinoma does not cause urinary outflow obstruction in its early stages. Being in the peripheral zone, the tumor is palpable as a firm mass through the anterior wall of the rectum during rectal examination.

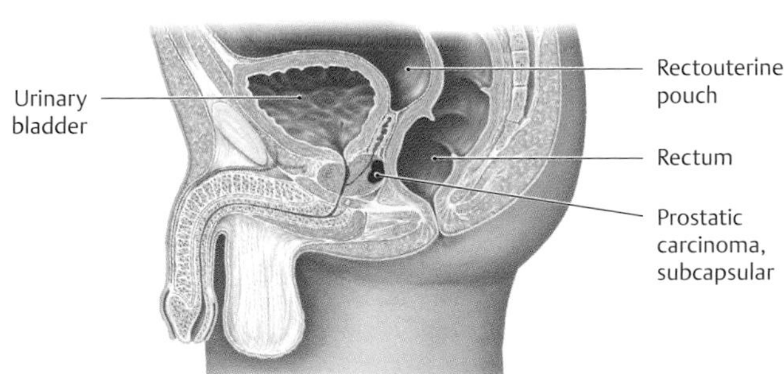
Urinary bladder
Rectouterine pouch
Rectum
Prostatic carcinoma, subcapsular

A Common site of prostatic carcinoma.

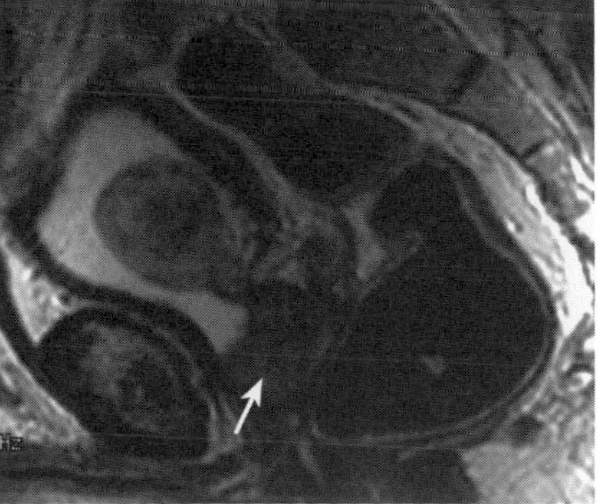

B Prostatic carcinoma (*arrow*) with bladder infiltration.

In certain prostate diseases, especially cancer, increased amounts of a protein, prostate-specific antigen or PSA, appear in the blood. This protein can be measured by a simple blood test.

Arteries & Veins of the Pelvis

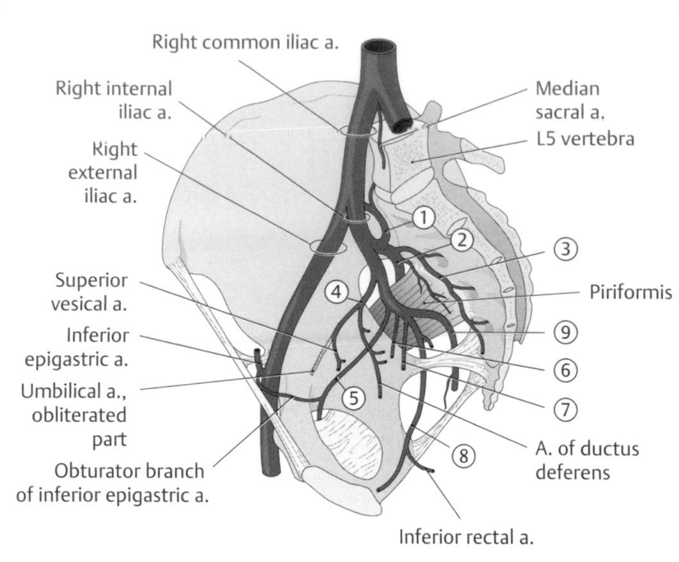

Right common iliac a.
Right internal iliac a.
Right external iliac a.
Superior vesical a.
Inferior epigastric a.
Umbilical a., obliterated part
Obturator branch of inferior epigastric a.
Median sacral a.
L5 vertebra
Piriformis
A. of ductus deferens
Inferior rectal a.
1
2
3
4
5
6
7
8
9

A Male pelvis.

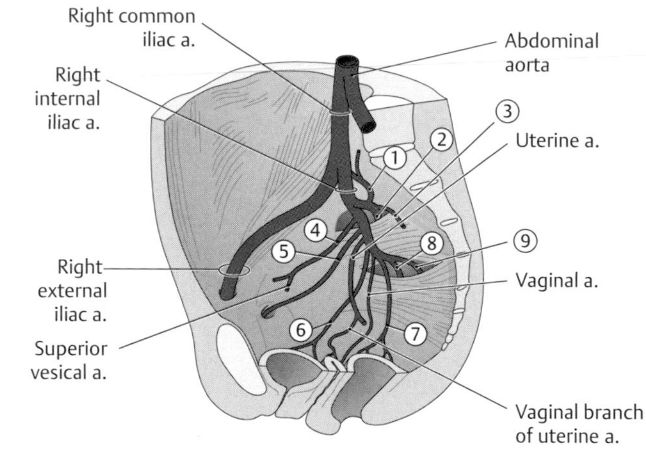

Right common iliac a.
Right internal iliac a.
Right external iliac a.
Superior vesical a.
Abdominal aorta
Uterine a.
Vaginal a.
Vaginal branch of uterine a.
1
2
3
4
5
6
7
8
9

B Female pelvis.

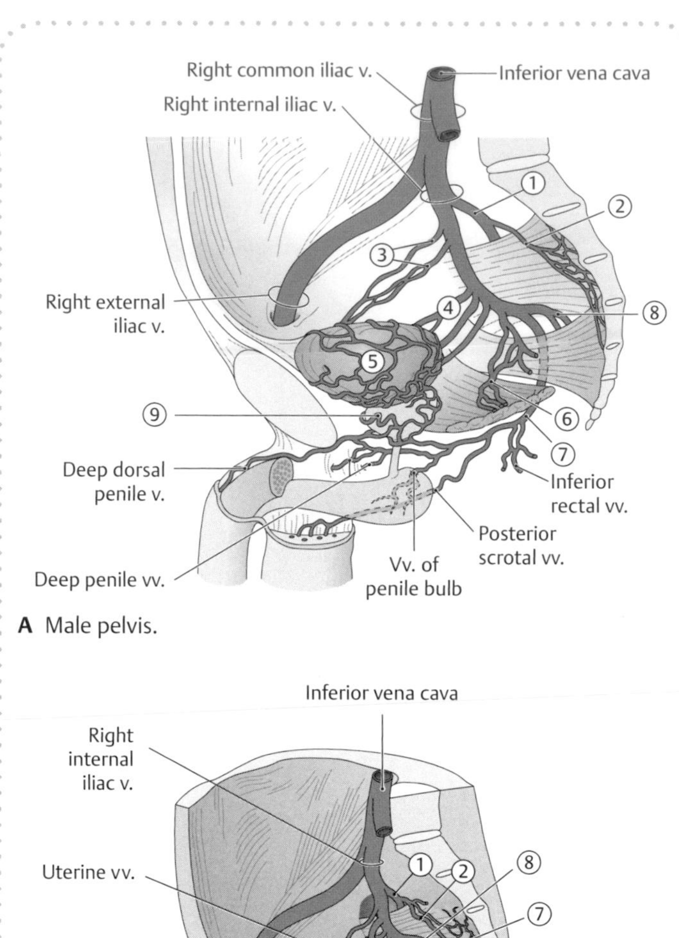

Right common iliac v.
Right internal iliac v.
Inferior vena cava
Right external iliac v.
Deep dorsal penile v.
Deep penile vv.
Vv. of penile bulb
Posterior scrotal vv.
Inferior rectal vv.
1
2
3
4
5
6
7
8
9
Inferior vena cava
Right internal iliac v.
Uterine vv.
Right external iliac v.
10

A Male pelvis.

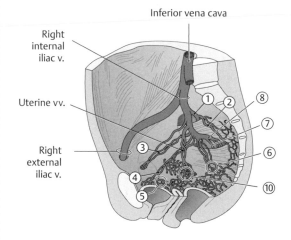

B Female pelvis.

Table 19.1 Branches of the internal iliac artery

The internal iliac artery gives off five parietal (pelvic wall) and four visceral (pelvic organs) branches.* Parietal branches are shown in italics.

Branches		
①	*Iiolumbar a.*	
②	*Superior gluteal a.*	
③	*Lateral sacral a.*	
④	Umbilical a.	A. of ductus deferens
		Superior vesical a.
⑤	*Obturator a.*	
⑥	Inferior vesical a.	
⑦	Middle rectal a.	
⑧	Internal pudendal a.	Inferior rectal a.
⑨	*Inferior gluteal a.*	

* In the female pelvis, the uterine and vaginal arteries arise directly from the anterior division of the internal iliac artery.

Table 19.2 Venous drainage of the pelvis

Tributaries	
①	Superior gluteal v.
②	Lateral sacral v.
③	Obturator vv.
④	Vesical vv.
⑤	Vesical venous plexus
⑥	Middle rectal vv. (rectal venous plexus) (also superior and inferior rectal vv., not shown)
⑦	Internal pudendal v.
⑧	Inferior gluteal vv.
⑨	Prostatic venous plexus
⑩	Uterine and vaginal venous plexus

The male pelvis also contains veins draining the penis and scrotum.

Fig. 19.1 Blood vessels of the pelvis
Idealized right hemipelvis, left lateral view.

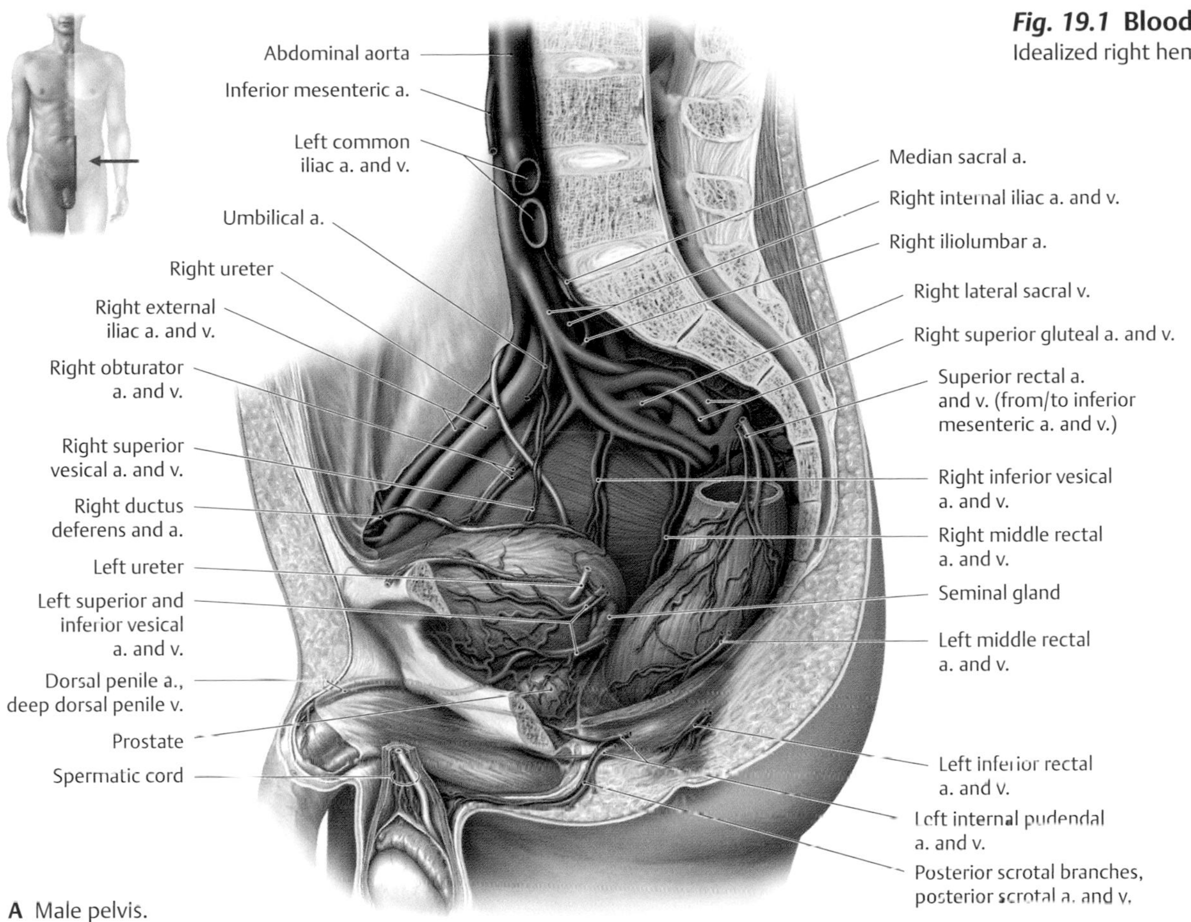
Abdominal aorta
Inferior mesenteric a.
Left common iliac a. and v.
Umbilical a.
Right ureter
Right external iliac a. and v.
Right obturator a. and v.
Right superior vesical a. and v.
Right ductus deferens and a.
Left ureter
Left superior and inferior vesical a. and v.
Dorsal penile a., deep dorsal penile v.
Prostate
Spermatic cord
Median sacral a.
Right internal iliac a. and v.
Right iliolumbar a.
Right lateral sacral v.
Right superior gluteal a. and v.
Superior rectal a. and v. (from/to inferior mesenteric a. and v.)
Right inferior vesical a. and v.
Right middle rectal a. and v.
Seminal gland
Left middle rectal a. and v.
Left inferior rectal a. and v.
Left internal pudendal a. and v.
Posterior scrotal branches, posterior scrotal a. and v.

A Male pelvis.

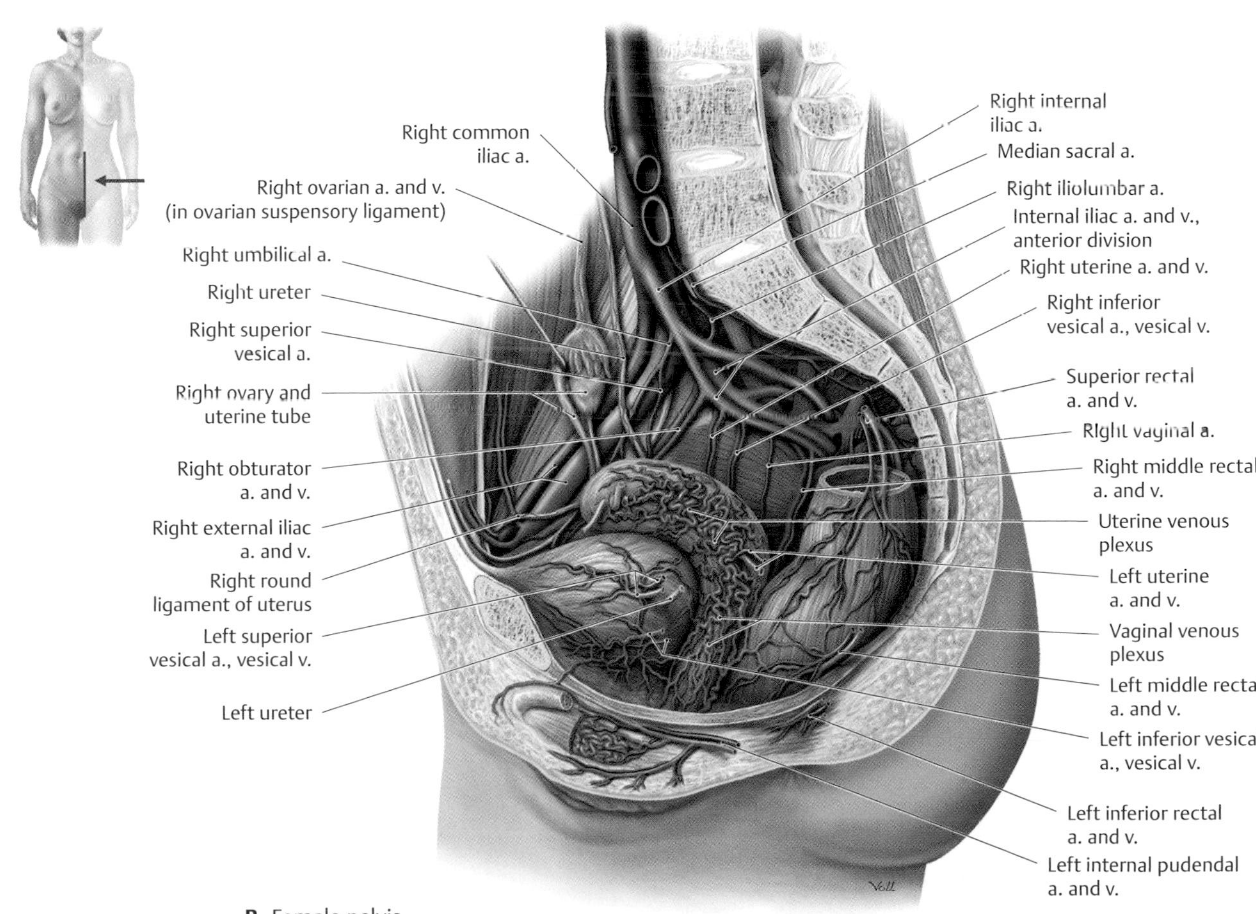
Right common iliac a.
Right ovarian a. and v. (in ovarian suspensory ligament)
Right umbilical a.
Right ureter
Right superior vesical a.
Right ovary and uterine tube
Right obturator a. and v.
Right external iliac a. and v.
Right round ligament of uterus
Left superior vesical a., vesical v.
Left ureter
Right internal iliac a.
Median sacral a.
Right iliolumbar a.
Internal iliac a. and v., anterior division
Right uterine a. and v.
Right inferior vesical a., vesical v.
Superior rectal a. and v.
Right vaginal a.
Right middle rectal a. and v.
Uterine venous plexus
Left uterine a. and v.
Vaginal venous plexus
Left middle rectal a. and v.
Left inferior vesical a., vesical v.
Left inferior rectal a. and v.
Left internal pudendal a. and v.

B Female pelvis.

Arteries & Veins of the Rectum & Genitalia

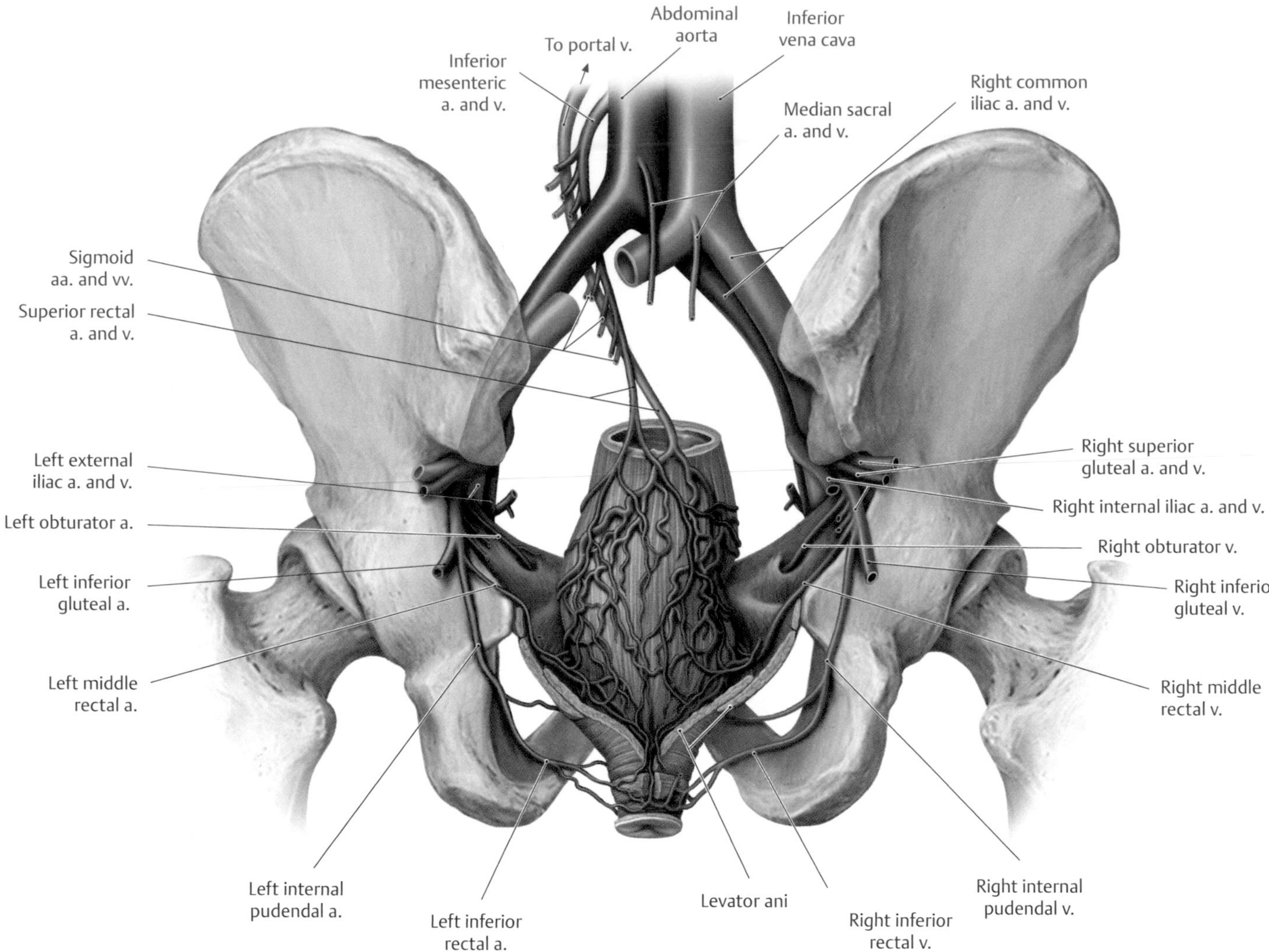

To portal v.
Abdominal aorta
Inferior vena cava
Inferior mesenteric a. and v.
Median sacral a. and v.
Right common iliac a. and v.
Sigmoid aa. and vv.
Superior rectal a. and v.
Left external iliac a. and v.
Left obturator a.
Left inferior gluteal a.
Left middle rectal a.
Right superior gluteal a. and v.
Right internal iliac a. and v.
Right obturator v.
Right inferior gluteal v.
Right middle rectal v.
Left internal pudendal a.
Left inferior rectal a.
Levator ani
Right inferior rectal v.
Right internal pudendal v.

Fig. 19.2 **Blood vessels of the rectum**
Posterior view. The main blood supply to the rectum is from the superior rectal arteries; the middle rectal arteries serve as an anastomosis between the superior and inferior rectal arteries.

Fig. 19.3 **Blood vessels of the genitalia**

Anterior view. *Retracted and partially removed:* Uterus.

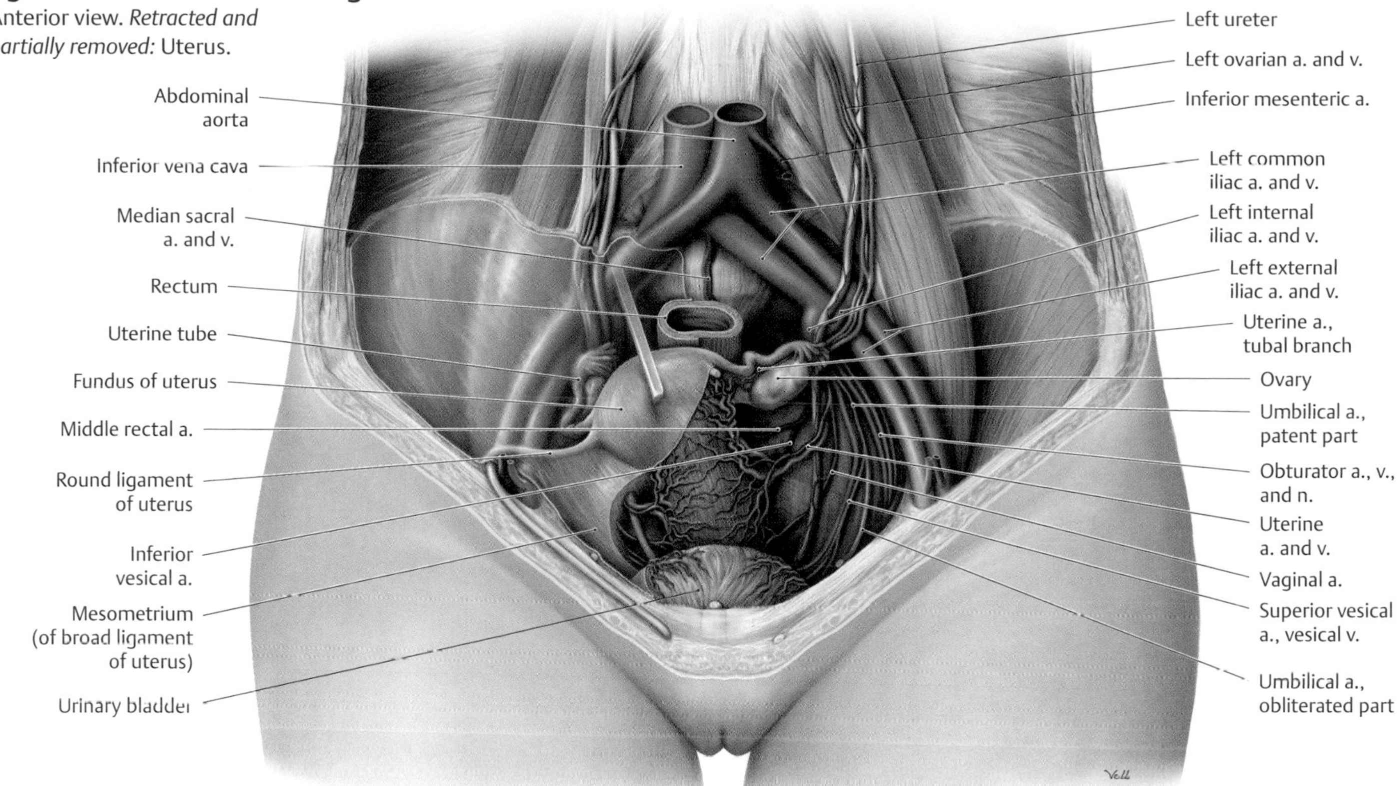
Abdominal aorta
Inferior vena cava
Median sacral a. and v.
Rectum
Uterine tube
Fundus of uterus
Middle rectal a.
Round ligament of uterus
Inferior vesical a.
Mesometrium (of broad ligament of uterus)
Urinary bladder
Left ureter
Left ovarian a. and v.
Inferior mesenteric a.
Left common iliac a. and v.
Left internal iliac a. and v.
Left external iliac a. and v.
Uterine a., tubal branch
Ovary
Umbilical a., patent part
Obturator a., v., and n.
Uterine a. and v.
Vaginal a.
Superior vesical a., vesical v.
Umbilical a., obliterated part

A Female pelvis. *Removed:* Peritoneum (left side). *Displaced:* Uterus.

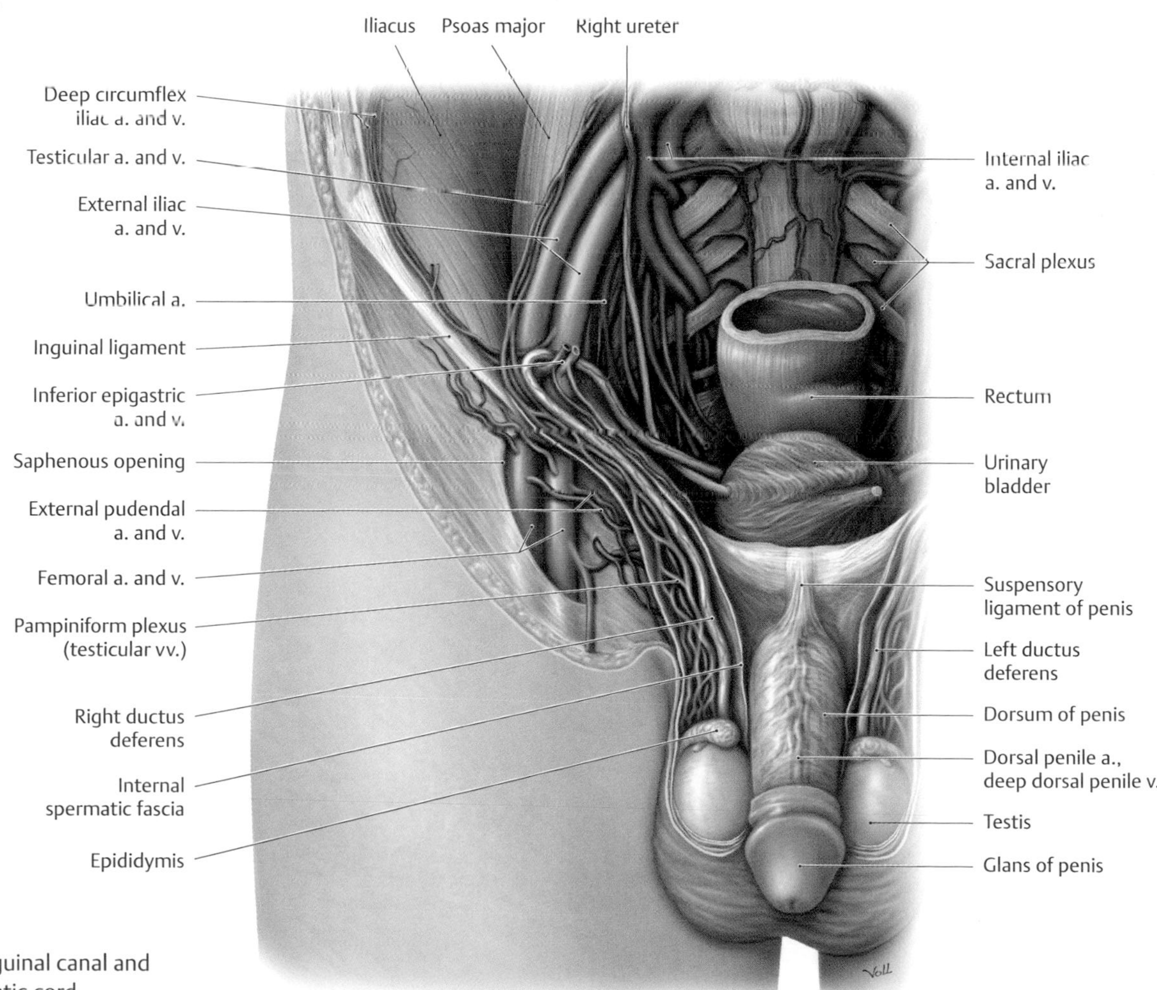
Iliacus
Psoas major
Right ureter
Deep circumflex iliac a. and v.
Testicular a. and v.
External iliac a. and v.
Umbilical a.
Inguinal ligament
Inferior epigastric a. and v.
Saphenous opening
External pudendal a. and v.
Femoral a. and v.
Pampiniform plexus (testicular vv.)
Right ductus deferens
Internal spermatic fascia
Epididymis
Internal iliac a. and v.
Sacral plexus
Rectum
Urinary bladder
Suspensory ligament of penis
Left ductus deferens
Dorsum of penis
Dorsal penile a., deep dorsal penile v.
Testis
Glans of penis

B Male pelvis. *Opened:* Inguinal canal and coverings of the spermatic cord.

Lymph Nodes of the Abdomen & Pelvis

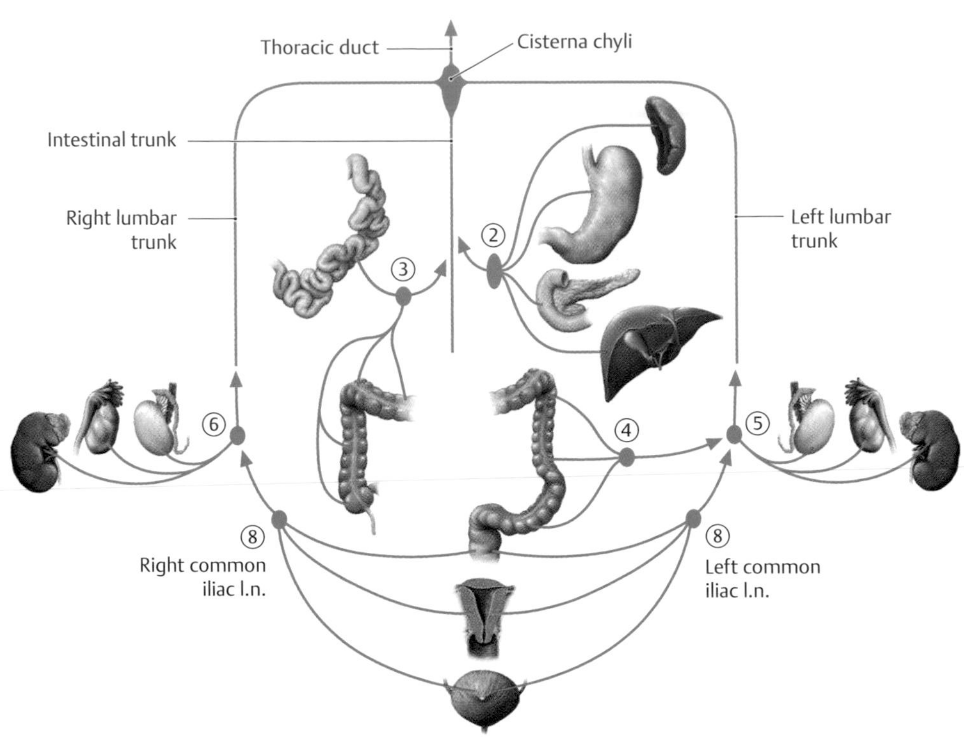

Thoracic duct
Cisterna chyli
Intestinal trunk
Right lumbar trunk
Left lumbar trunk
②
③
④
⑤
⑥
⑧
Right common iliac l.n.
⑧
Left common iliac l.n.

Fig. 19.4 **Lymphatic drainage of the internal organs**
Lymph draining from the abdomen, pelvis, and lower limb, ultimately passes through the lumbar lymph nodes (clinically, the aortic lymph nodes). (See Table 19.1 for numbering.) The lumbar lymph nodes consist of the right lateral aortic (caval) and left lateral aortic nodes, the preaortic nodes, and the retroaortic nodes. Efferent lymph vessels from the lateral aortic lymph nodes and the retroaortic nodes form the lumbar trunks and those from the preaortic nodes form the intestinal trunks. The lumbar and intestinal trunks terminate in the cistern chyli.

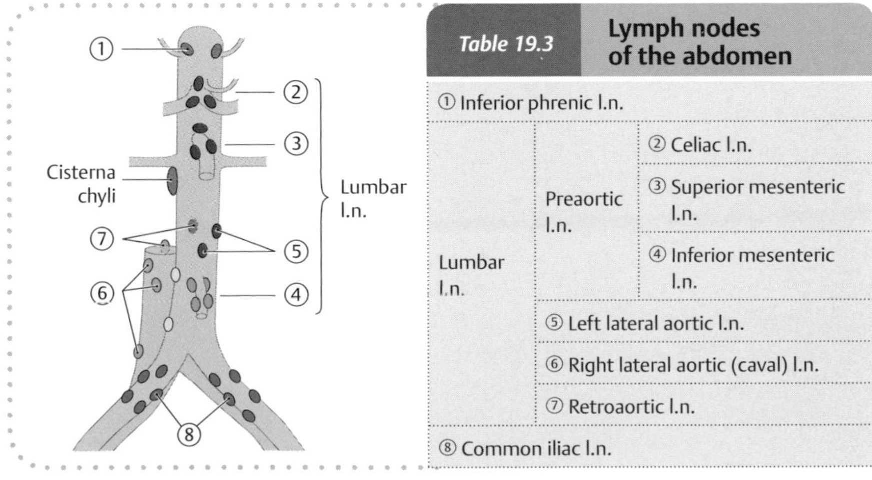

①
②
③
Cisterna chyli
Lumbar l.n.
⑦
⑤
⑥
④
⑧

Table 19.3	**Lymph nodes of the abdomen**	
① Inferior phrenic l.n.		
Lumbar l.n.	Preaortic l.n.	② Celiac l.n.
		③ Superior mesenteric l.n.
		④ Inferior mesenteric l.n.
	⑤ Left lateral aortic l.n.	
	⑥ Right lateral aortic (caval) l.n.	
	⑦ Retroaortic l.n.	
⑧ Common iliac l.n.		

Fig. 19.5 **Lymphatic drainage of the rectum**
Anterior view.

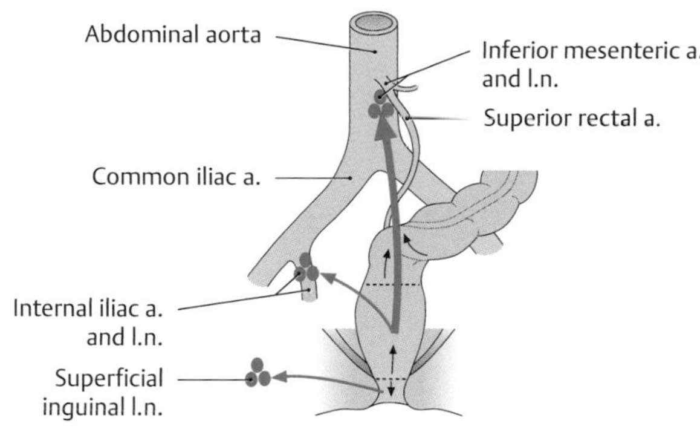
Abdominal aorta
Inferior mesenteric a. and l.n.
Superior rectal a.
Common iliac a.
Internal iliac a. and l.n.
Superficial inguinal l.n.

Fig. 19.6 **Lymphatic drainage of the bladder and urethra**
Anterior view.

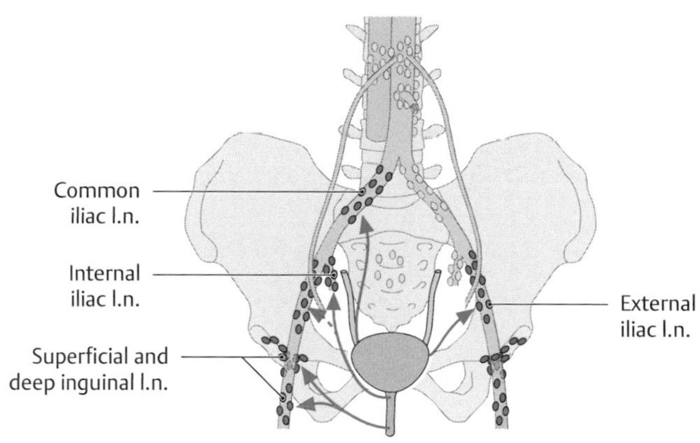
Common iliac l.n.
Internal iliac l.n.
Superficial and deep inguinal l.n.
External iliac l.n.

Fig. 19.7 **Lymphatic drainage of the male genitalia**
Anterior view.

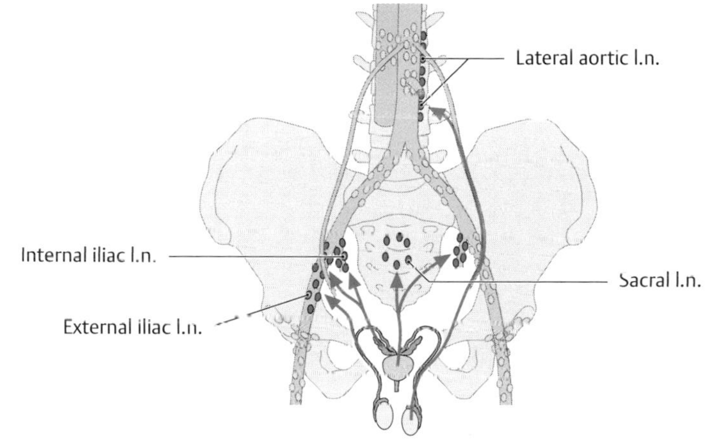
Lateral aortic l.n.
Internal iliac l.n.
Sacral l.n.
External iliac l.n.

Fig. 19.8 **Lymphatic drainage of the female genitalia**
Anterior view.

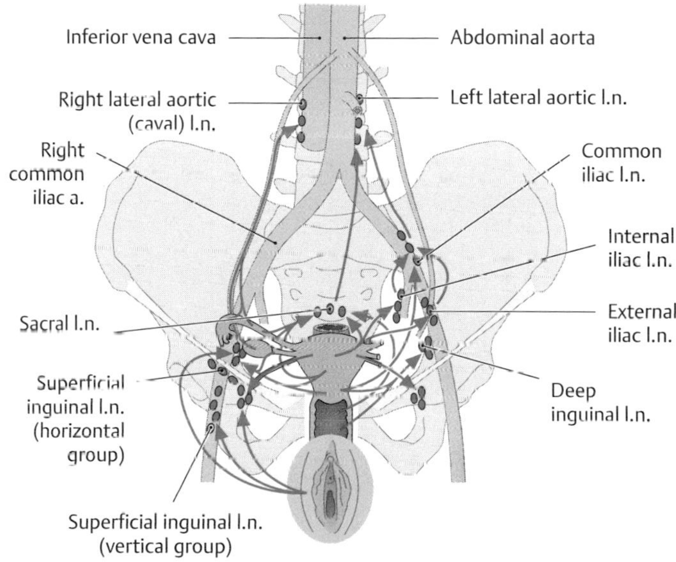
Inferior vena cava
Abdominal aorta
Right lateral aortic (caval) l.n.
Left lateral aortic l.n.
Right common iliac a.
Common iliac l.n.
Internal iliac l.n.
External iliac l.n.
Sacral l.n.
Superficial inguinal l.n. (horizontal group)
Deep inguinal l.n.
Superficial inguinal l.n. (vertical group)

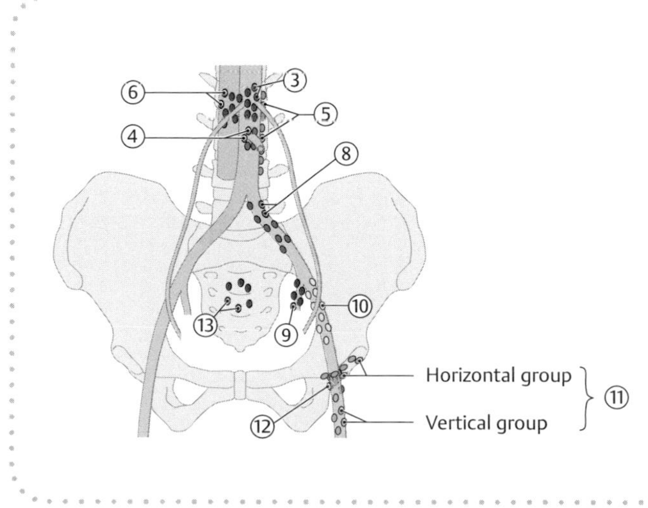
⑥
③
⑤
④
⑧
⑩
⑬
⑨
Horizontal group
⑪
⑫
Vertical group

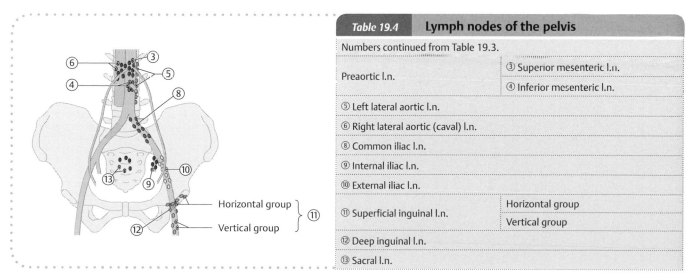

Table 19.4 Lymph nodes of the pelvis

Numbers continued from Table 19.3.	
Preaortic l.n.	③ Superior mesenteric l.n.
	④ Inferior mesenteric l.n.
⑤ Left lateral aortic l.n.	
⑥ Right lateral aortic (caval) l.n.	
⑧ Common iliac l.n.	
⑨ Internal iliac l.n.	
⑩ External iliac l.n.	
⑪ Superficial inguinal l.n.	Horizontal group
	Vertical group
⑫ Deep inguinal l.n.	
⑬ Sacral l.n.	

Lymph Nodes of the Genitalia

Fig. 19.9 **Lymph nodes of the male genitalia**
Anterior view. *Removed:* Gastrointestinal tract (except rectal stump) and peritoneum.

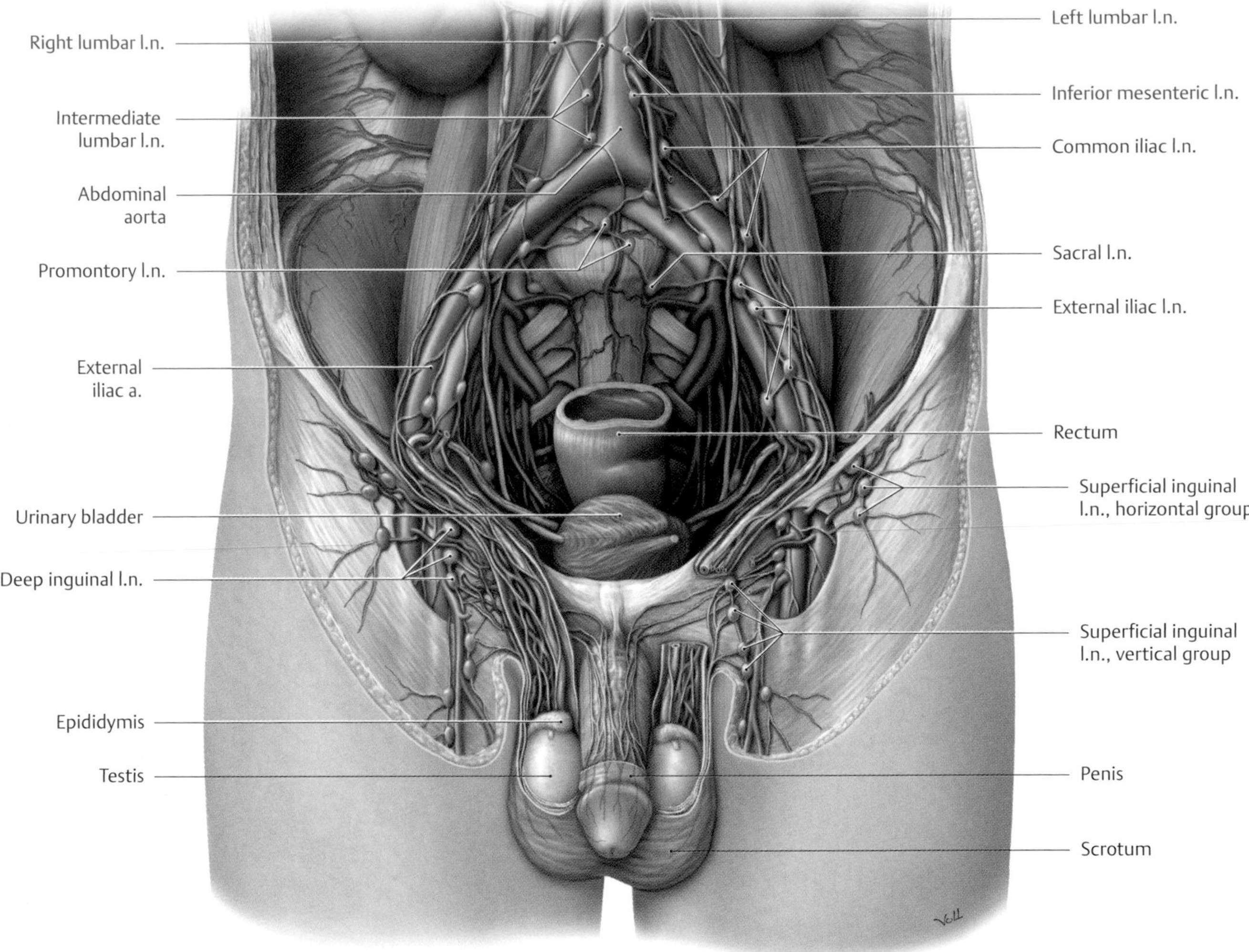
Right lumbar l.n.
Intermediate lumbar l.n.
Abdominal aorta
Promontory l.n.
External iliac a.
Urinary bladder
Deep inguinal l.n.
Epididymis
Testis
Left lumbar l.n.
Inferior mesenteric l.n.
Common iliac l.n.
Sacral l.n.
External iliac l.n.
Rectum
Superficial inguinal l.n., horizontal group
Superficial inguinal l.n., vertical group
Penis
Scrotum

Fig. 19.10 Lymph nodes of the female genitalia
Anterior view. *Removed:* Gastrointestinal tract (except rectal stump) and peritoneum. *Retracted:* Uterus.

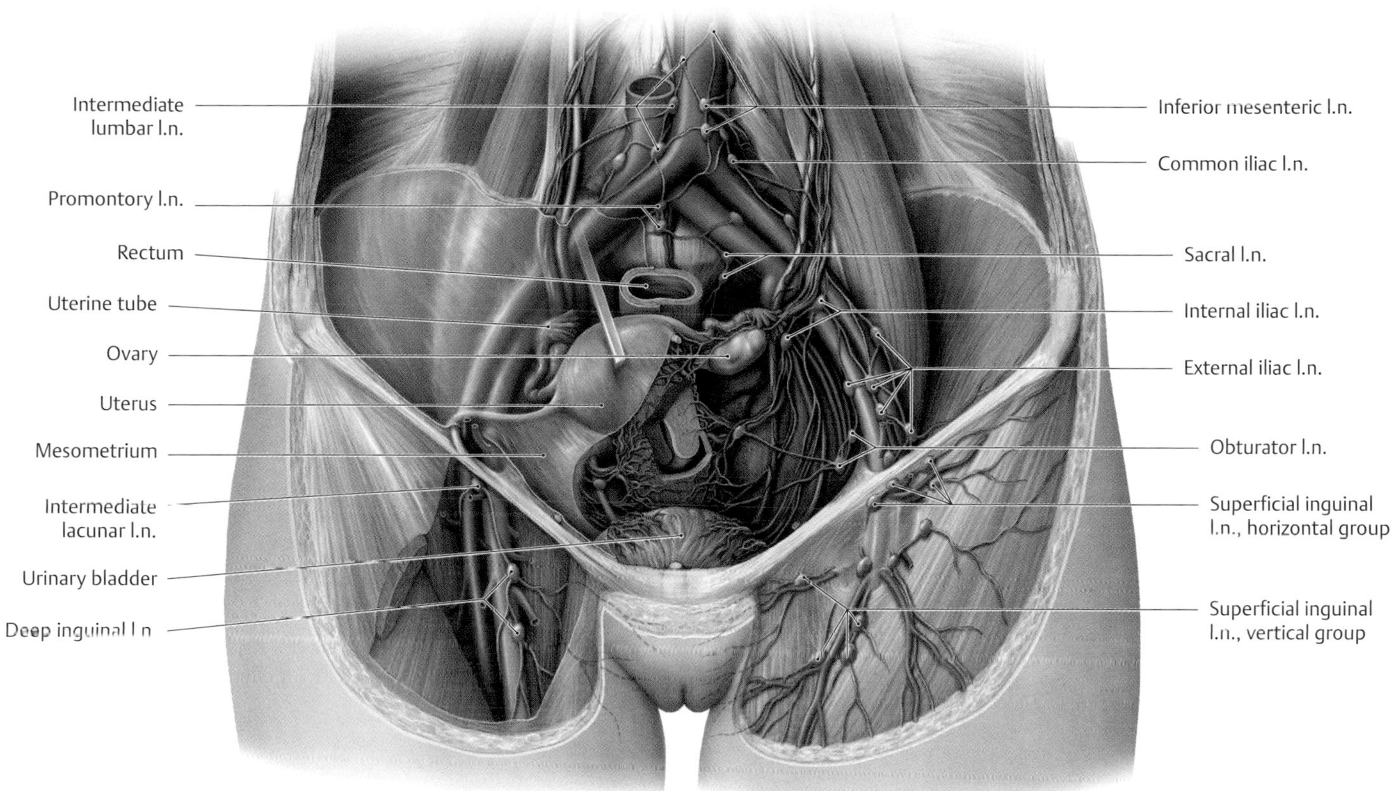
Intermediate lumbar l.n.
Promontory l.n.
Rectum
Uterine tube
Ovary
Uterus
Mesometrium
Intermediate lacunar l.n.
Urinary bladder
Deep inguinal l.n.
Inferior mesenteric l.n.
Common iliac l.n.
Sacral l.n.
Internal iliac l.n.
External iliac l.n.
Obturator l.n.
Superficial inguinal l.n., horizontal group
Superficial inguinal l.n., vertical group

Fig. 19.11 Lymphatic drainage of the pelvic organs

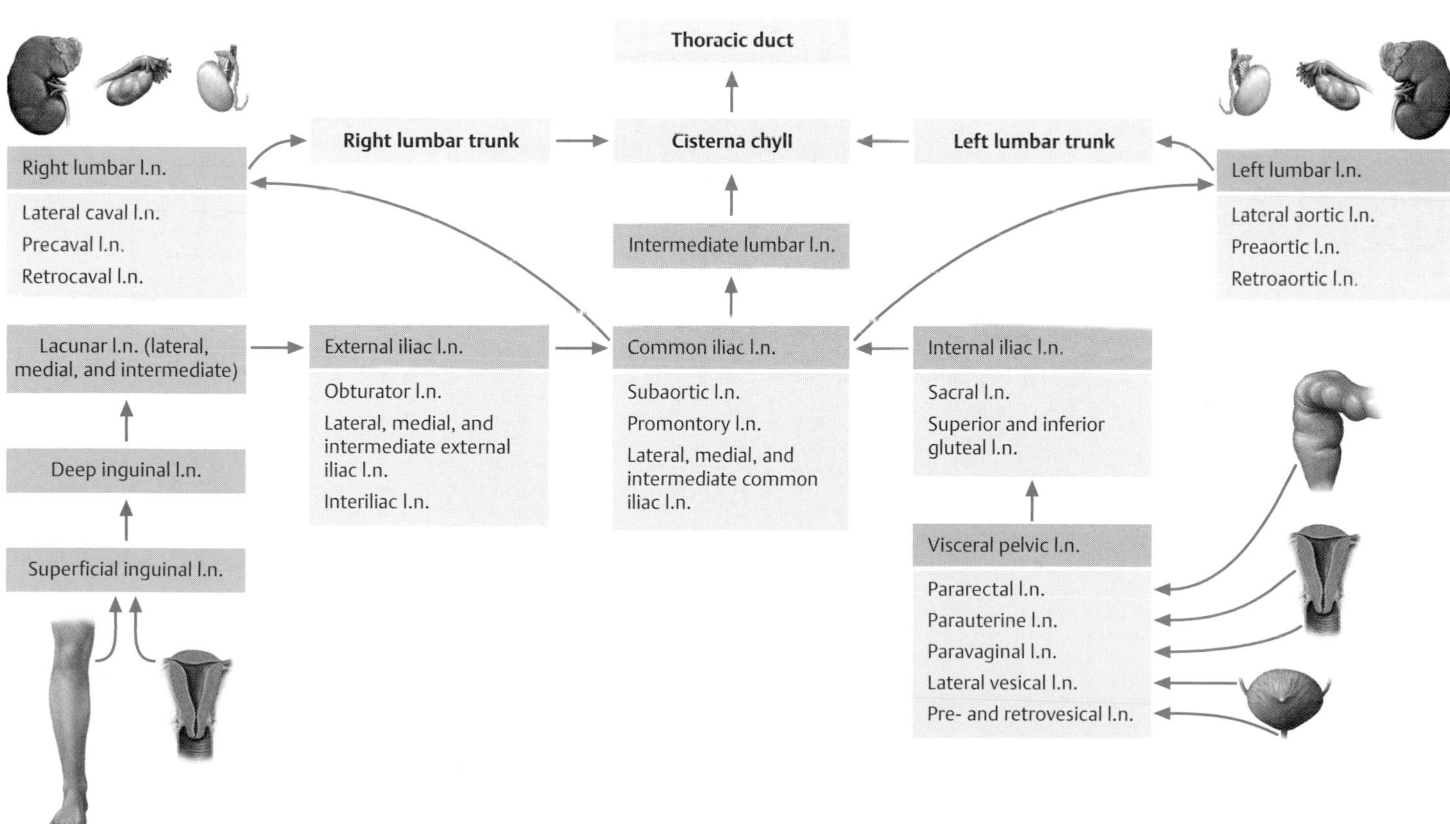
Thoracic duct
Right lumbar trunk
Cisterna chyli
Left lumbar trunk
Right lumbar l.n.
Lateral caval l.n.
Precaval l.n.
Retrocaval l.n.
Intermediate lumbar l.n.
Left lumbar l.n.
Lateral aortic l.n.
Preaortic l.n.
Retroaortic l.n.
Lacunar l.n. (lateral, medial, and intermediate)
External iliac l.n.
Obturator l.n.
Lateral, medial, and intermediate external iliac l.n.
Interiliac l.n.
Common iliac l.n.
Subaortic l.n.
Promontory l.n.
Lateral, medial, and intermediate common iliac l.n.
Internal iliac l.n.
Sacral l.n.
Superior and inferior gluteal l.n.
Deep inguinal l.n.
Superficial inguinal l.n.
Visceral pelvic l.n.
Pararectal l.n.
Parauterine l.n.
Paravaginal l.n.
Lateral vesical l.n.
Pre- and retrovesical l.n.

Autonomic Plexuses of the Pelvis

Fig. 19.12 Autonomic plexuses in the pelvis
Anterior view of the male lower abdomen. *Removed:* Peritoneum and abdominopelvic organs except kidneys, suprarenal glands, and part of stomach.

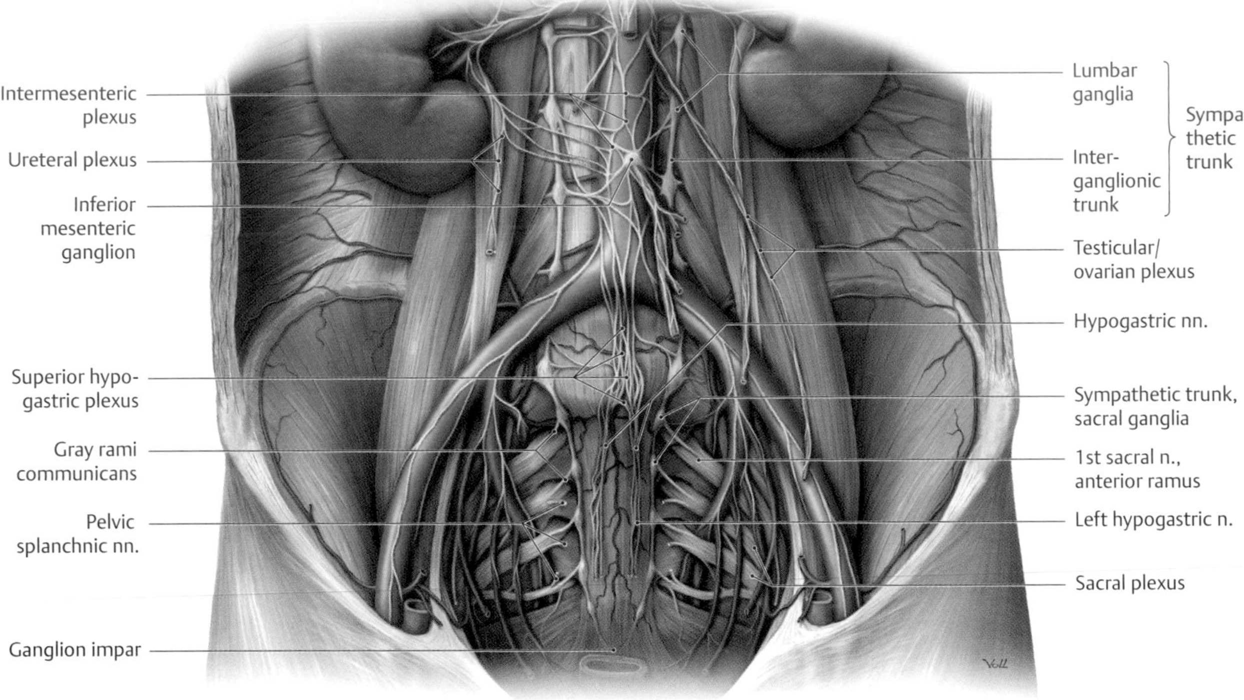

Intermesenteric plexus
Ureteral plexus
Inferior mesenteric ganglion
Superior hypogastric plexus
Gray rami communicans
Pelvic splanchnic nn.
Ganglion impar
Lumbar ganglia
Inter-ganglionic trunk
Sympathetic trunk
Testicular/ ovarian plexus
Hypogastric nn.
Sympathetic trunk, sacral ganglia
1st sacral n., anterior ramus
Left hypogastric n.
Sacral plexus

Fig. 19.13 Innervation of the urinary organs
Anterior view of the male lower abdomen and pelvis. *Removed:* Peritoneum and abdominopelvic organs except kidneys, suprarenal glands, rectal stump, and bladder. See p. 264 for schematic of innervation of urinary organs.

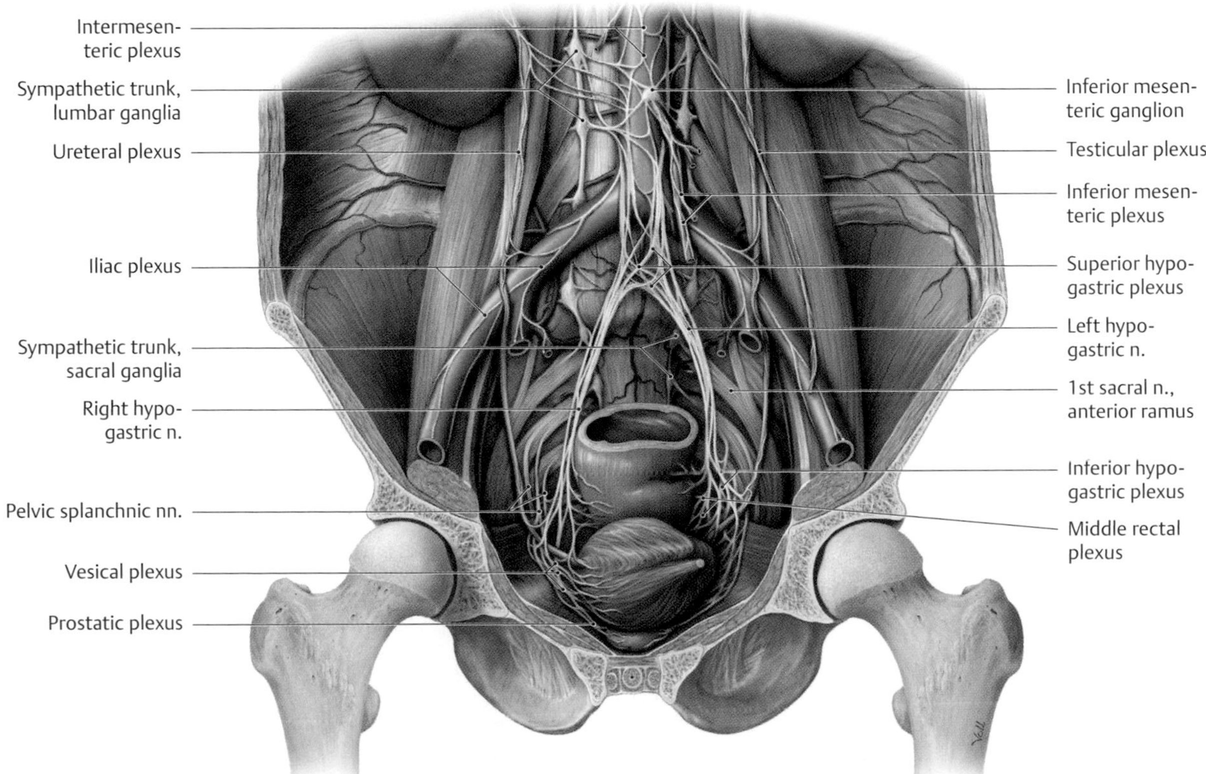

Intermesenteric plexus
Sympathetic trunk, lumbar ganglia
Ureteral plexus
Iliac plexus
Sympathetic trunk, sacral ganglia
Right hypogastric n.
Pelvic splanchnic nn.
Vesical plexus
Prostatic plexus
Inferior mesenteric ganglion
Testicular plexus
Inferior mesenteric plexus
Superior hypogastric plexus
Left hypogastric n.
1st sacral n., anterior ramus
Inferior hypogastric plexus
Middle rectal plexus

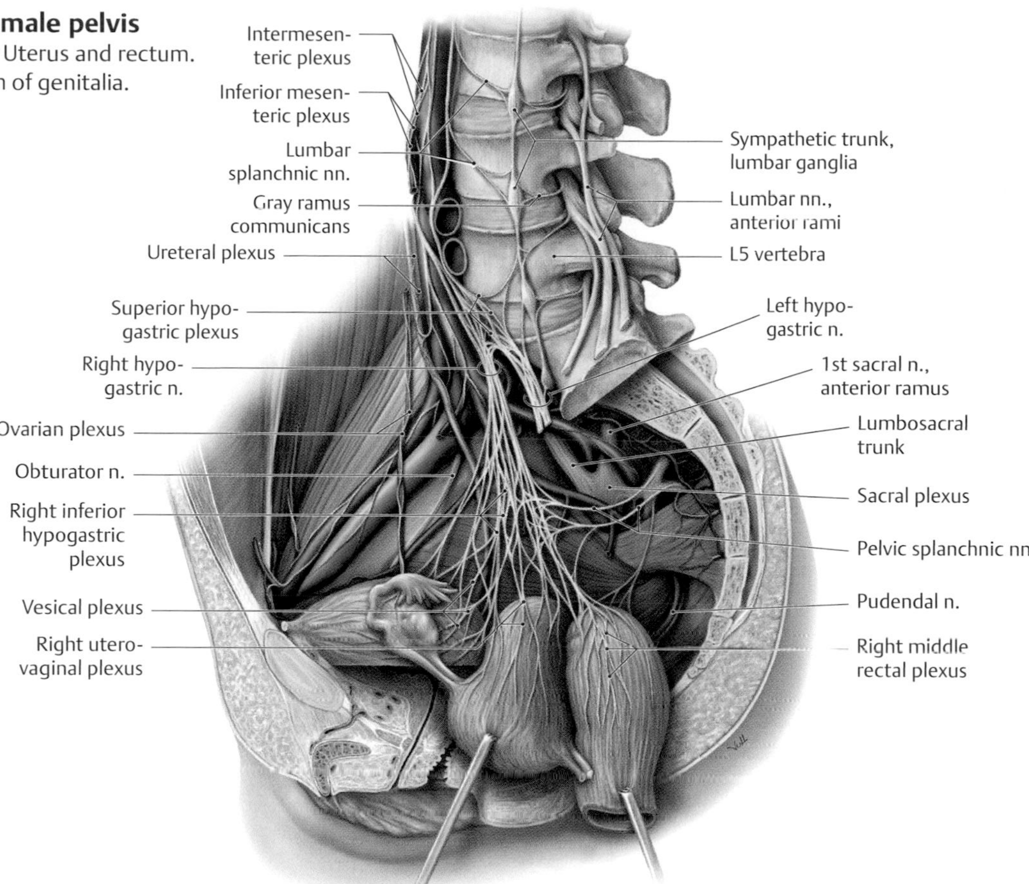
Intermesen-
teric plexus
Inferior mesen-
teric plexus
Lumbar
splanchnic nn.
Gray ramus
communicans
Ureteral plexus
Superior hypo-
gastric plexus
Right hypo-
gastric n.
Ovarian plexus
Obturator n.
Right inferior
hypogastric
plexus
Vesical plexus
Right utero-
vaginal plexus
Sympathetic trunk,
lumbar ganglia
Lumbar nn.,
anterior rami
L5 vertebra
Left hypo-
gastric n.
1st sacral n.,
anterior ramus
Lumbosacral
trunk
Sacral plexus
Pelvic splanchnic nn.
Pudendal n.
Right middle
rectal plexus

Fig. 19.14 **Innervation of the female pelvis**
Right pelvis, left lateral view. *Reflected:* Uterus and rectum. See p. 265 for schematic of innervation of genitalia.

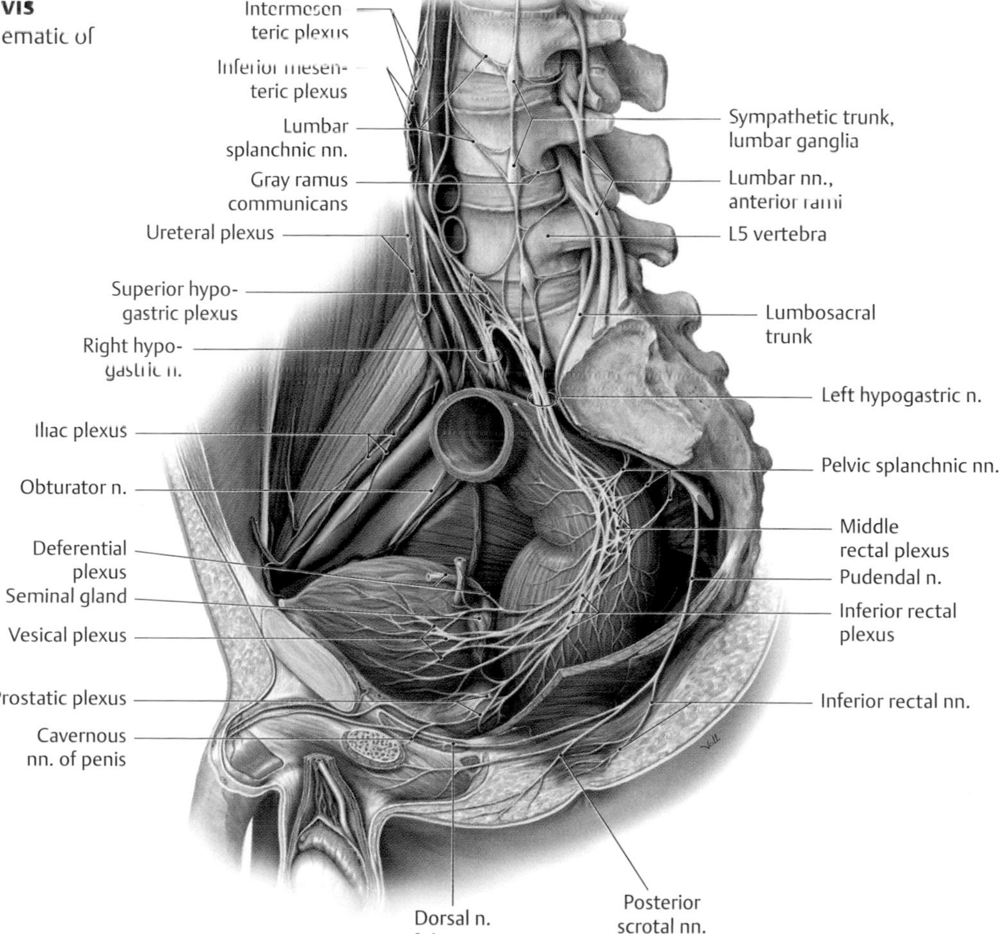
Intermesen-
teric plexus
Inferior mesen-
teric plexus
Lumbar
splanchnic nn.
Gray ramus
communicans
Ureteral plexus
Superior hypo-
gastric plexus
Right hypo-
gastric n.
Iliac plexus
Obturator n.
Deferential
plexus
Seminal gland
Vesical plexus
Prostatic plexus
Cavernous
nn. of penis
Dorsal n.
of the penis
Posterior
scrotal nn.
Sympathetic trunk,
lumbar ganglia
Lumbar nn.,
anterior rami
L5 vertebra
Lumbosacral
trunk
Left hypogastric n.
Pelvic splanchnic nn.
Middle
rectal plexus
Pudendal n.
Inferior rectal
plexus
Inferior rectal nn.

Fig. 19.15 **Innervation of the male pelvis**
Right pelvis, left lateral view. See p. 265 for schematic of innervation of genitalia.

Autonomic Innervation: Urinary & Genital Organs

Fig. 19.16 Autonomic innervation of the urinary organs

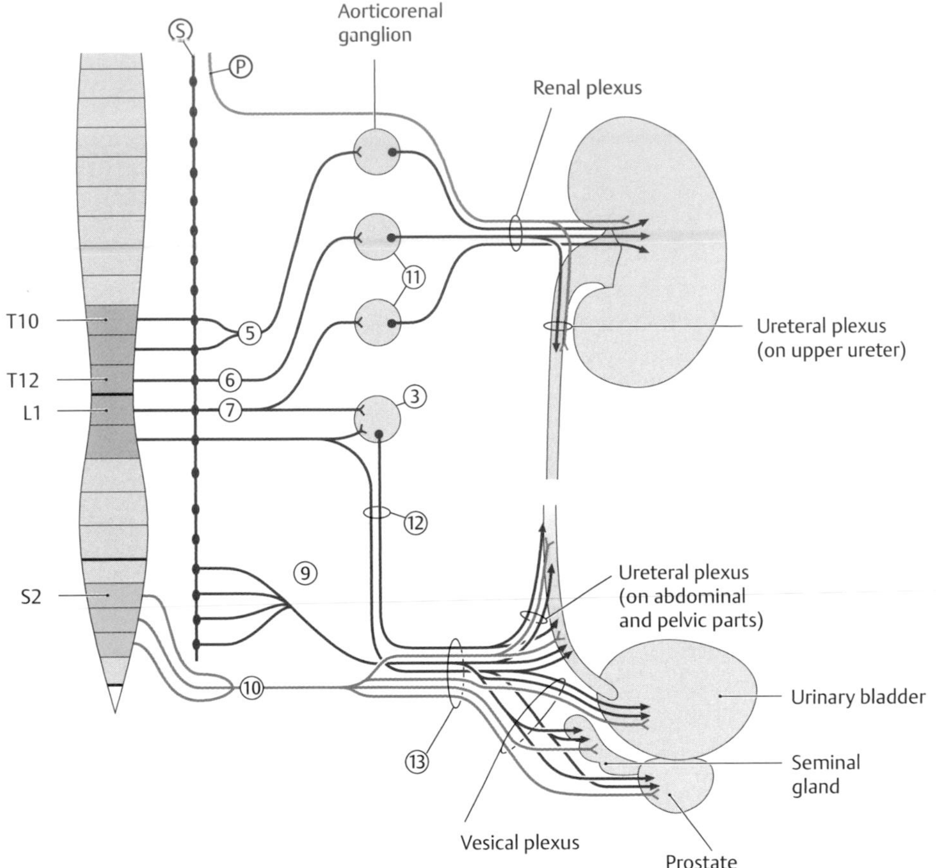

Sympathetic fibers
Parasympathetic fibers
Aorticorenal ganglion
Renal plexus
Ureteral plexus (on upper ureter)
Ureteral plexus (on abdominal and pelvic parts)
Urinary bladder
Seminal gland
Prostate
Vesical plexus
T10
T12
L1
S2

Numbering continued from p. 203.	
Ⓢ	Sympathetic trunk
Ⓟ	Posterior vagal trunk (from right vagus n.)
③	Inferior mesenteric ganglion
⑤	Lesser splanchnic n. (T10–T11)
⑥	Least splanchnic n. (T12)
⑦	Lumbar splanchnic nn. (L1–L2)
⑨	Sacral splanchnic nn. (from 1st to 3rd sacral ganglia)
⑩	Pelvic splanchnic nn. (S2–S4)
⑪	Renal ganglia
⑫	Superior hypogastric plexus
⑬	Inferior hypogastric plexus

Clinical

Referred pain from the internal organs

The convergence of somatic and visceral afferent fibers to a common level of the spinal cord confuses the relationship between the perceived and actual sites of pain, a phenomenon known as referred pain. Pain impulses from a particular organ are consistently projected to the same well-defined skin area.

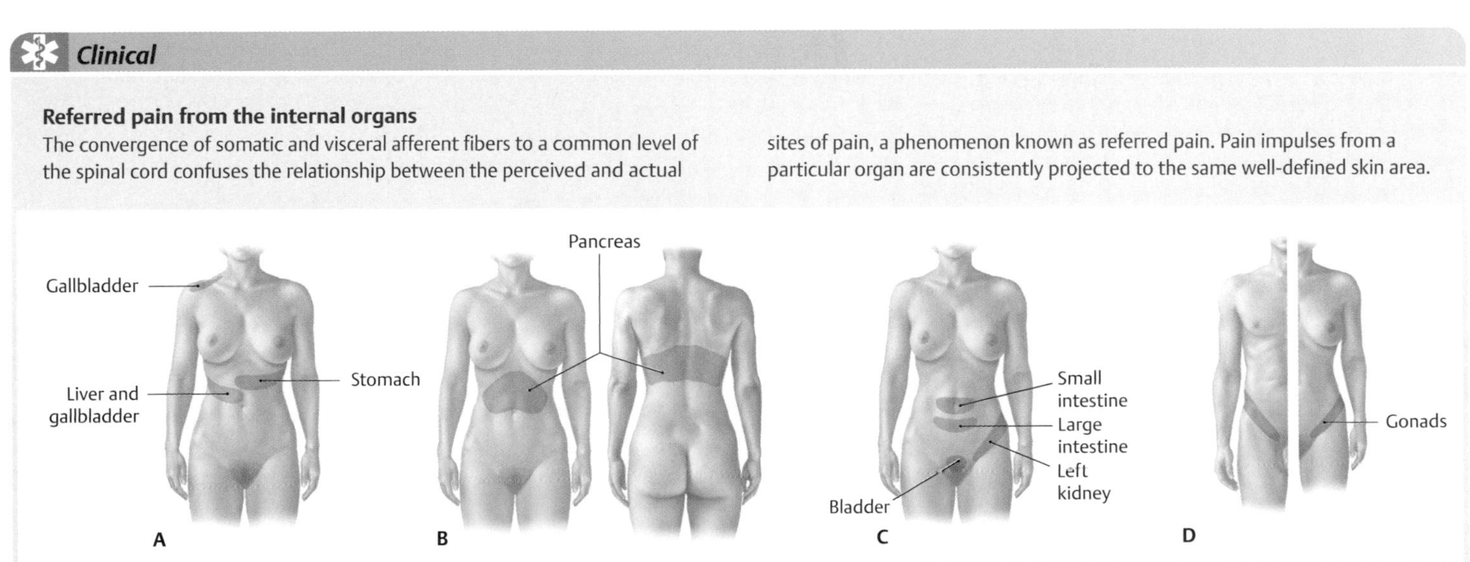

Gallbladder
Liver and gallbladder
Stomach
Pancreas
Small intestine
Large intestine
Left kidney
Bladder
Gonads
A
B
C
D

Fig. 19.17 **Autonomic innervation of the genitalia**

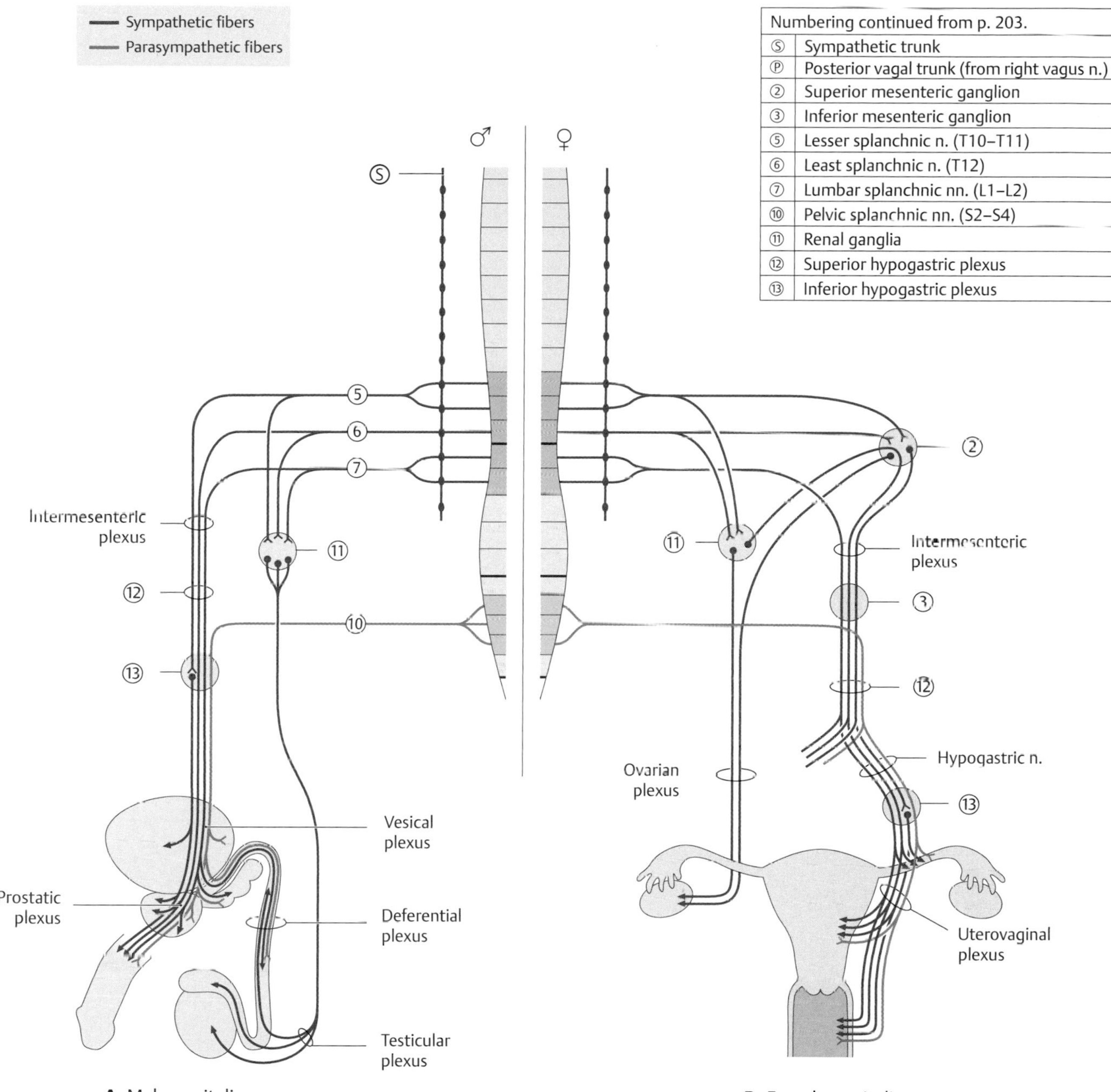
Sympathetic fibers
Parasympathetic fibers
♂
♀
Ⓢ
⑤
⑥
⑦
Intermesenteric plexus
⑫
⑪
⑩
⑬
Vesical plexus
Prostatic plexus
Deferential plexus
Testicular plexus
②
⑪
Intermesenteric plexus
③
⑫
Hypogastric n.
Ovarian plexus
⑬
Uterovaginal plexus

Numbering continued from p. 203.	
Ⓢ	Sympathetic trunk
Ⓟ	Posterior vagal trunk (from right vagus n.)
②	Superior mesenteric ganglion
③	Inferior mesenteric ganglion
⑤	Lesser splanchnic n. (T10–T11)
⑥	Least splanchnic n. (T12)
⑦	Lumbar splanchnic nn. (L1–L2)
⑩	Pelvic splanchnic nn. (S2–S4)
⑪	Renal ganglia
⑫	Superior hypogastric plexus
⑬	Inferior hypogastric plexus

A Male genitalia.

B Female genitalia.

Neurovasculature of the Female Perineum & Genitalia

Fig. 19.18 **Nerves of the female perineum and genitalia**

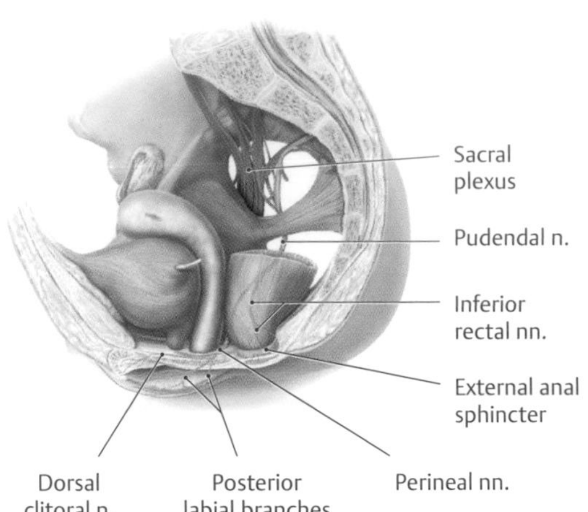
Sacral plexus
Pudendal n.
Inferior rectal nn.
External anal sphincter
Dorsal clitoral n.
Posterior labial branches
Perineal nn.

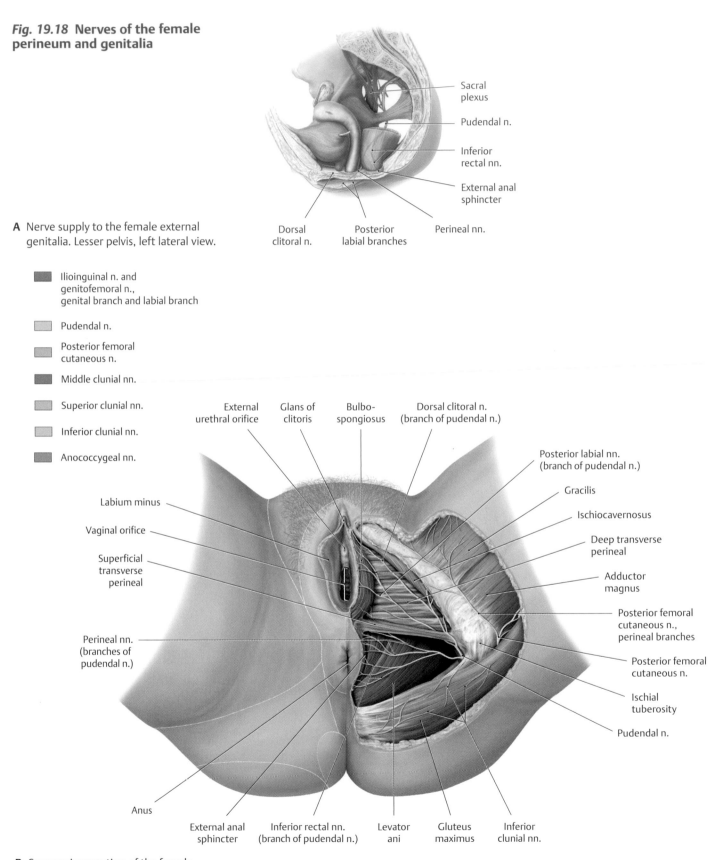

A Nerve supply to the female external genitalia. Lesser pelvis, left lateral view.

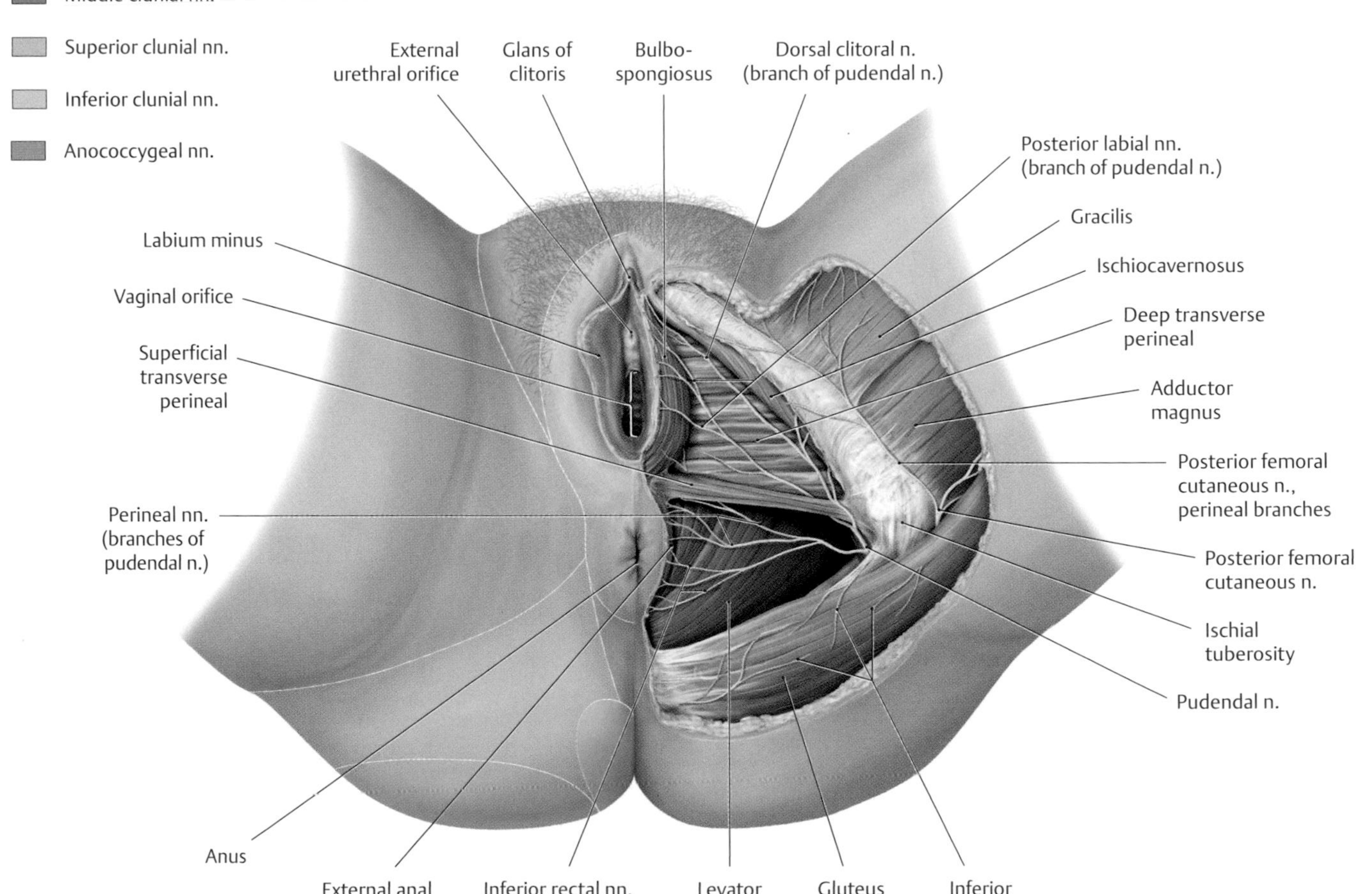
Ilioinguinal n. and genitofemoral n., genital branch and labial branch
Pudendal n.
Posterior femoral cutaneous n.
Middle clunial nn.
Superior clunial nn.
Inferior clunial nn.
Anococcygeal nn.
External urethral orifice
Glans of clitoris
Bulbo-spongiosus
Dorsal clitoral n. (branch of pudendal n.)
Posterior labial nn. (branch of pudendal n.)
Gracilis
Ischiocavernosus
Deep transverse perineal
Adductor magnus
Posterior femoral cutaneous n., perineal branches
Posterior femoral cutaneous n.
Ischial tuberosity
Pudendal n.
Labium minus
Vaginal orifice
Superficial transverse perineal
Perineal nn. (branches of pudendal n.)
Anus
External anal sphincter
Inferior rectal nn. (branch of pudendal n.)
Levator ani
Gluteus maximus
Inferior clunial nn.

B Sensory innervation of the female perineum. Lithotomy position.

Fig. 19.19 **Blood vessels of the female external genitalia**
Inferior view.

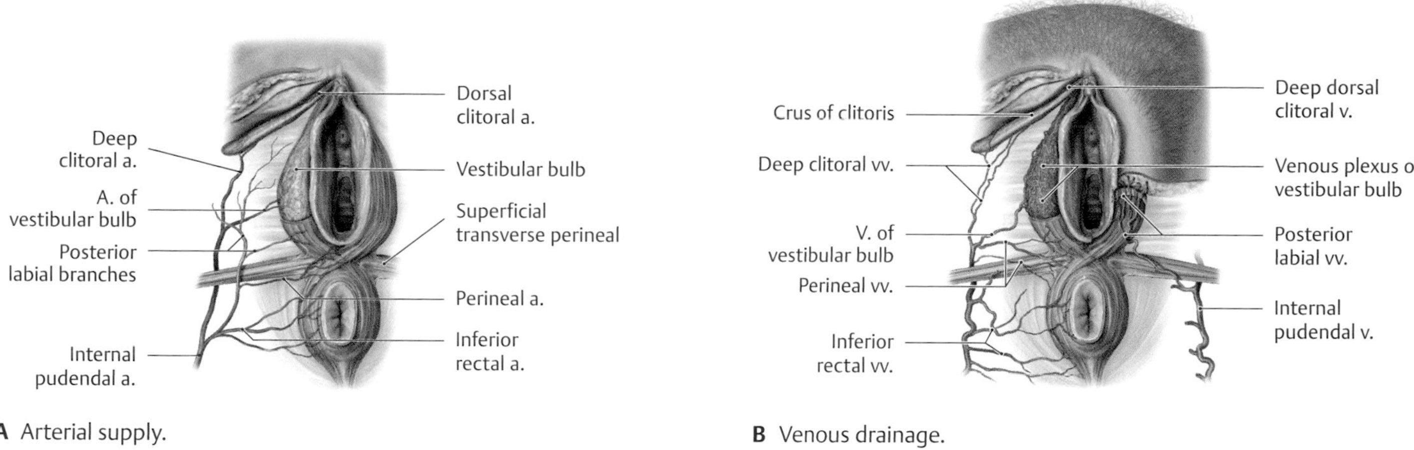

Dorsal clitoral a.
Deep clitoral a.
Vestibular bulb
A. of vestibular bulb
Superficial transverse perineal
Posterior labial branches
Perineal a.
Inferior rectal a.
Internal pudendal a.
Crus of clitoris
Deep dorsal clitoral v.
Deep clitoral vv.
Venous plexus of vestibular bulb
V. of vestibular bulb
Posterior labial vv.
Perineal vv.
Internal pudendal v.
Inferior rectal vv.

A Arterial supply.

B Venous drainage.

Fig. 19.20 **Neurovasculature of the female perineum**
Lithotomy position. *Removed from left side*: Bulbospongiosus, ischiocavernosus, and greater vestibular (Bartholin's) gland.

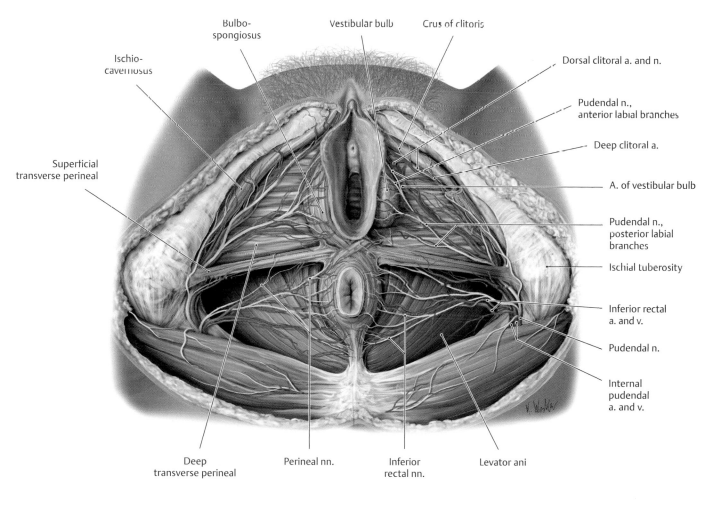

Bulbo-spongiosus
Vestibular bulb
Crus of clitoris
Ischio-cavernosus
Dorsal clitoral a. and n.
Pudendal n., anterior labial branches
Deep clitoral a.
Superficial transverse perineal
A. of vestibular bulb
Pudendal n., posterior labial branches
Ischial tuberosity
Inferior rectal a. and v.
Pudendal n.
Internal pudendal a. and v.
Deep transverse perineal
Perineal nn.
Inferior rectal nn.
Levator ani

Neurovasculature of the Male Perineum & Genitalia

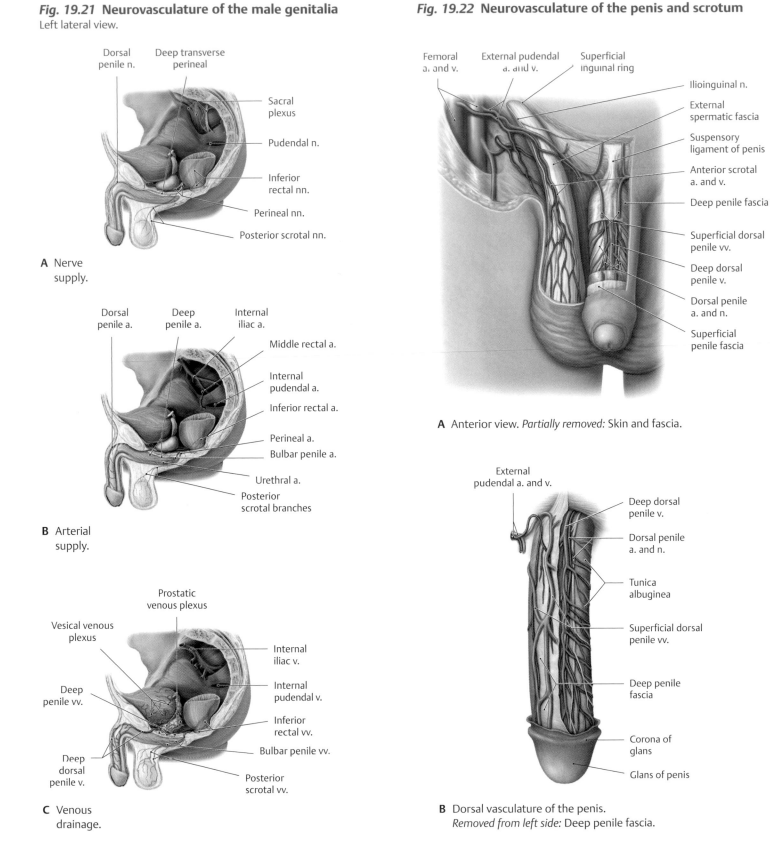

Fig. 19.21 Neurovasculature of the male genitalia

Left lateral view.

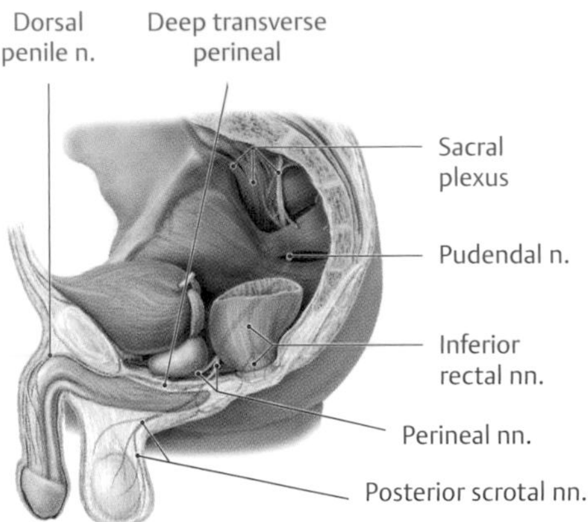
Dorsal penile n.
Deep transverse perineal
Sacral plexus
Pudendal n.
Inferior rectal nn.
Perineal nn.
Posterior scrotal nn.

A Nerve supply.

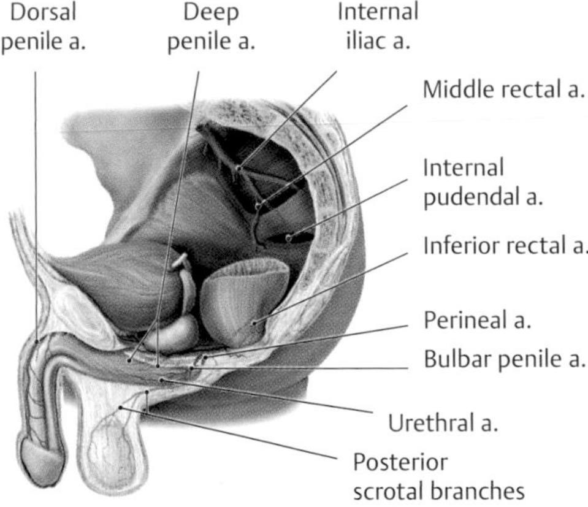
Dorsal penile a.
Deep penile a.
Internal iliac a.
Middle rectal a.
Internal pudendal a.
Inferior rectal a.
Perineal a.
Bulbar penile a.
Urethral a.
Posterior scrotal branches

B Arterial supply.

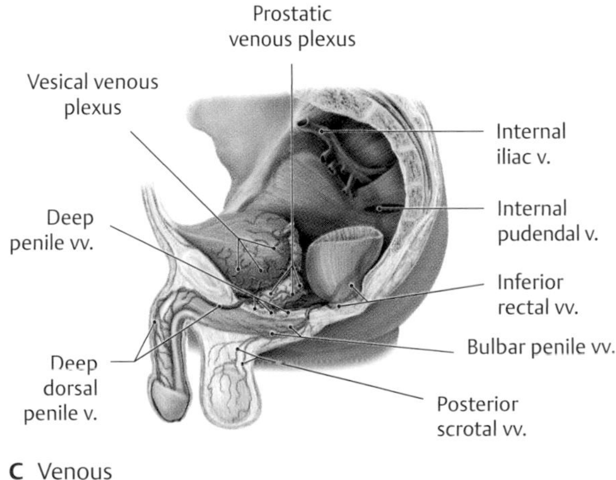
Prostatic venous plexus
Vesical venous plexus
Internal iliac v.
Internal pudendal v.
Deep penile vv.
Inferior rectal vv.
Bulbar penile vv.
Deep dorsal penile v.
Posterior scrotal vv.

C Venous drainage.

Fig. 19.22 Neurovasculature of the penis and scrotum

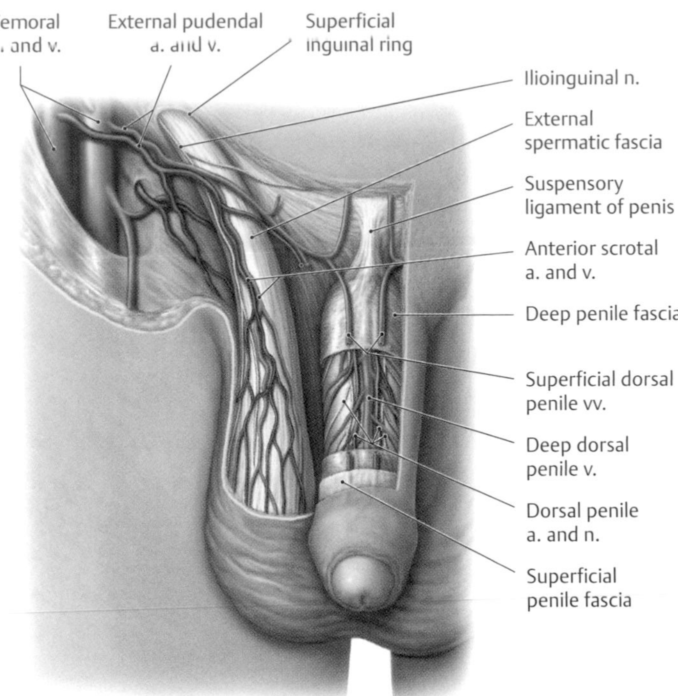
Femoral a. and v.
External pudendal a. and v.
Superficial inguinal ring
Ilioinguinal n.
External spermatic fascia
Suspensory ligament of penis
Anterior scrotal a. and v.
Deep penile fascia
Superficial dorsal penile vv.
Deep dorsal penile v.
Dorsal penile a. and n.
Superficial penile fascia

A Anterior view. *Partially removed:* Skin and fascia.

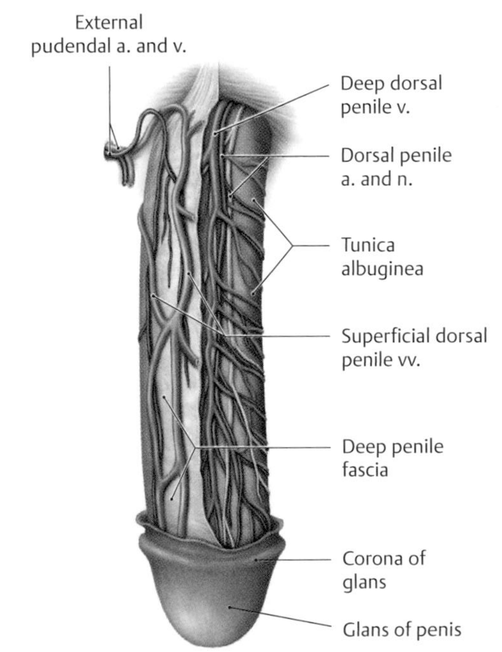
External pudendal a. and v.
Deep dorsal penile v.
Dorsal penile a. and n.
Tunica albuginea
Superficial dorsal penile vv.
Deep penile fascia
Corona of glans
Glans of penis

B Dorsal vasculature of the penis.
Removed from left side: Deep penile fascia.

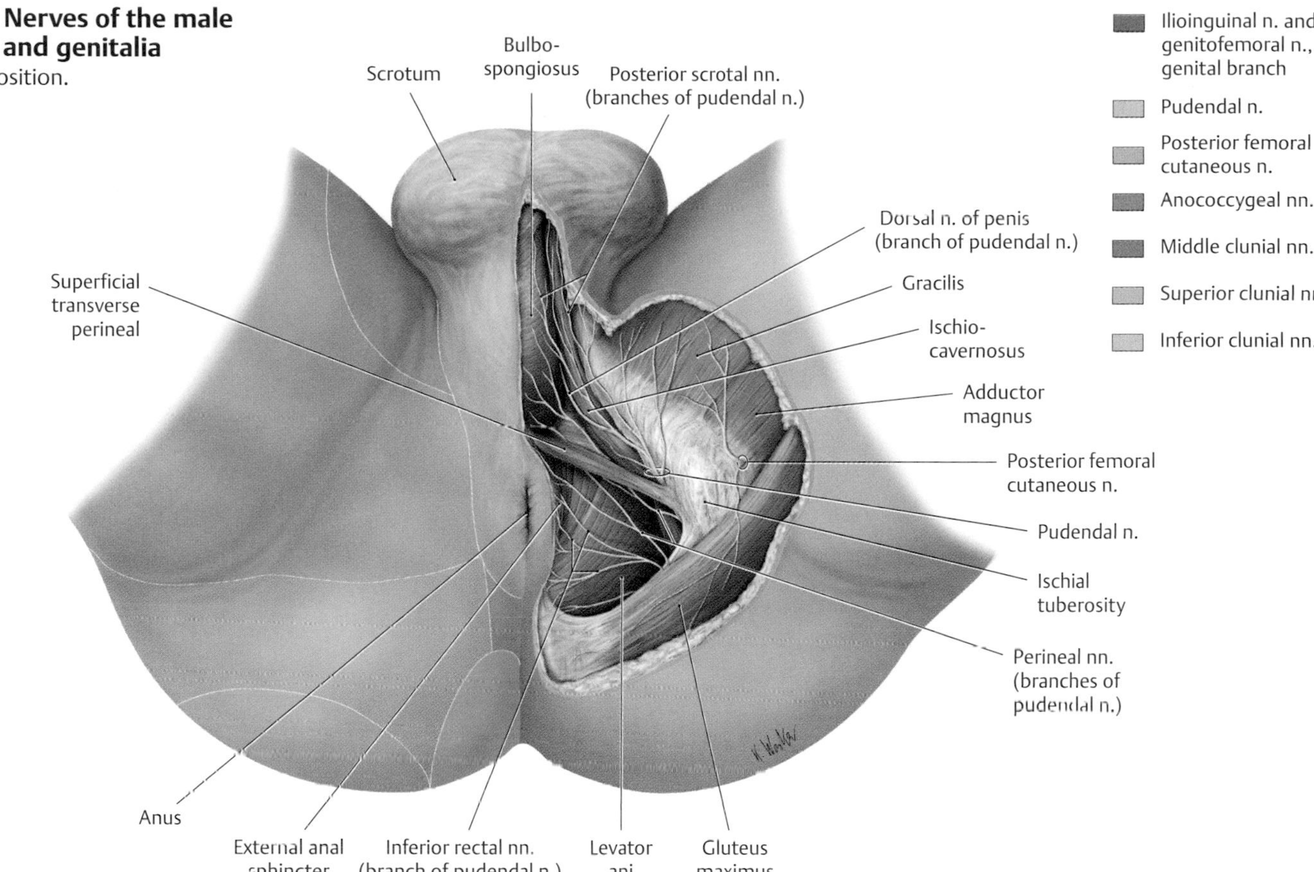
Scrotum
Bulbo-
spongiosus
Posterior scrotal nn.
(branches of pudendal n.)
Superficial
transverse
perineal
Dorsal n. of penis
(branch of pudendal n.)
Gracilis
Ischio-
cavernosus
Adductor
magnus
Posterior femoral
cutaneous n.
Pudendal n.
Ischial
tuberosity
Perineal nn.
(branches of
pudendal n.)
Anus
External anal
sphincter
Inferior rectal nn.
(branch of pudendal n.)
Levator
ani
Gluteus
maximus
Ilioinguinal n. and
genitofemoral n.,
genital branch
Pudendal n.
Posterior femoral
cutaneous n.
Anococcygeal nn.
Middle clunial nn.
Superior clunial nn.
Inferior clunial nn.

Fig. 19.23 **Nerves of the male perineum and genitalia**
Lithotomy position.

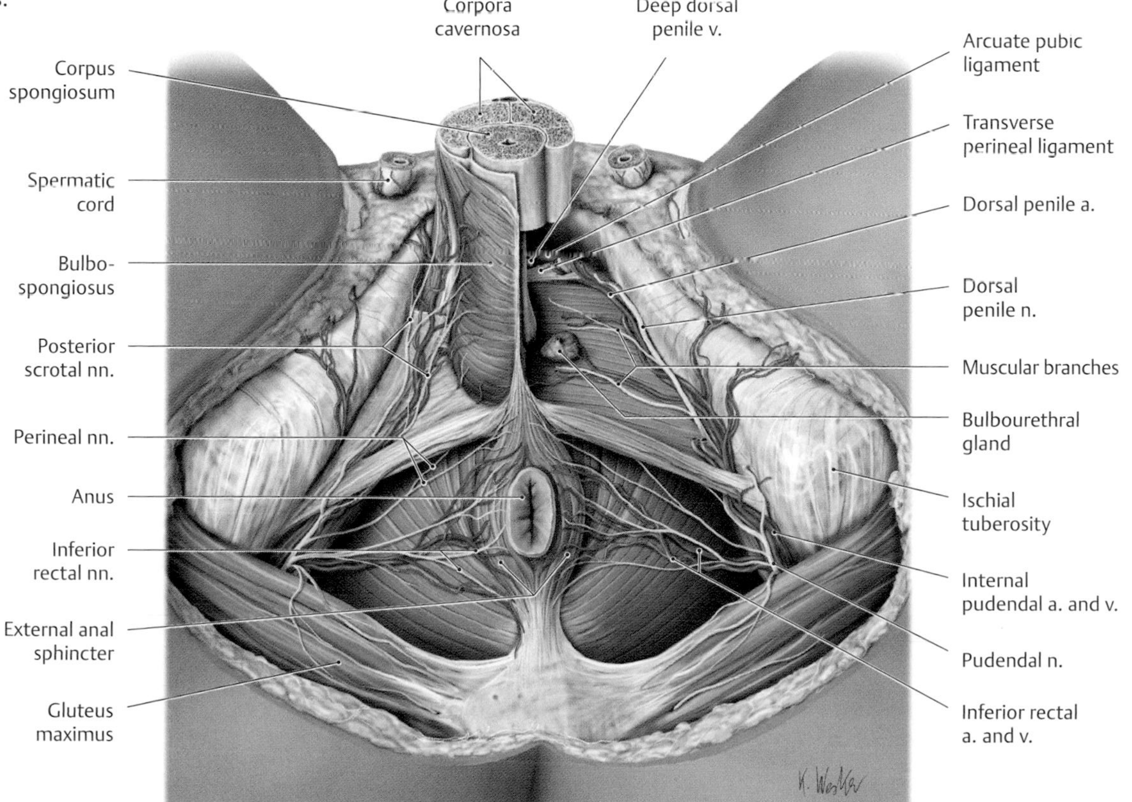
Corpora
cavernosa
Deep dorsal
penile v.
Corpus
spongiosum
Spermatic
cord
Bulbo-
spongiosus
Posterior
scrotal nn.
Perineal nn.
Anus
Inferior
rectal nn.
External anal
sphincter
Gluteus
maximus
Arcuate pubic
ligament
Transverse
perineal ligament
Dorsal penile a.
Dorsal
penile n.
Muscular branches
Bulbourethral
gland
Ischial
tuberosity
Internal
pudendal a. and v.
Pudendal n.
Inferior rectal
a. and v.

Fig. 19.24 **Neurovasculature of the male perineum**
Lithotomy position. *Removed from left side*: Perineal membrane, bulbospongiosus, and root of penis.

Sectional Anatomy of the Pelvis & Perineum

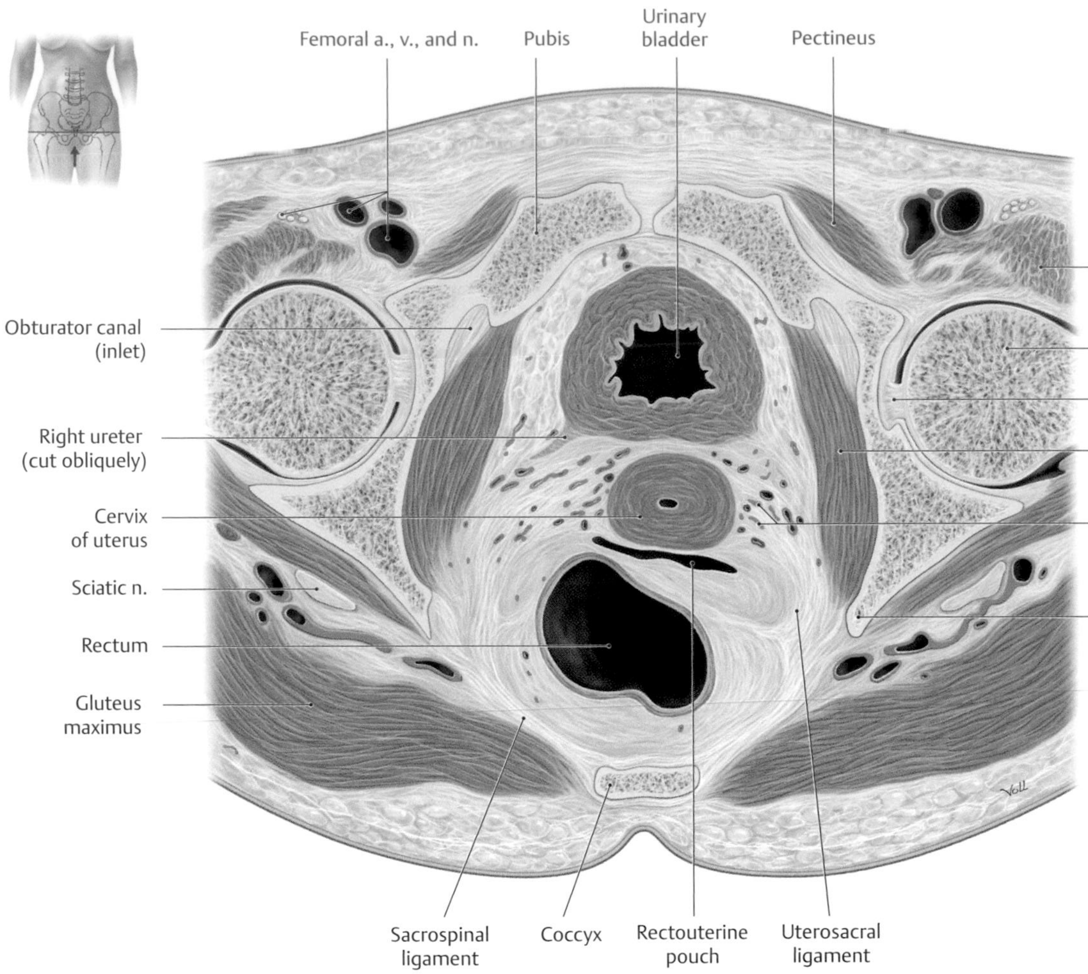

Fig. 19.25 **Female pelvis**
Transverse section through the bladder and cervix of the uterus. Inferior view..

Femoral a., v., and n.
Pubis
Urinary bladder
Pectineus
Iliopsoas
Obturator canal (inlet)
Head of femur
Ligament of head of femur
Right ureter (cut obliquely)
Obturator internus
Cervix of uterus
Uterovaginal venous plexus
Sciatic n.
Ischial spine
Rectum
Gluteus maximus
Sacrospinal ligament
Coccyx
Rectouterine pouch
Uterosacral ligament

Fig. 19.26 **Male pelvis**
Transverse section through the bladder and seminal glands. Inferior view.

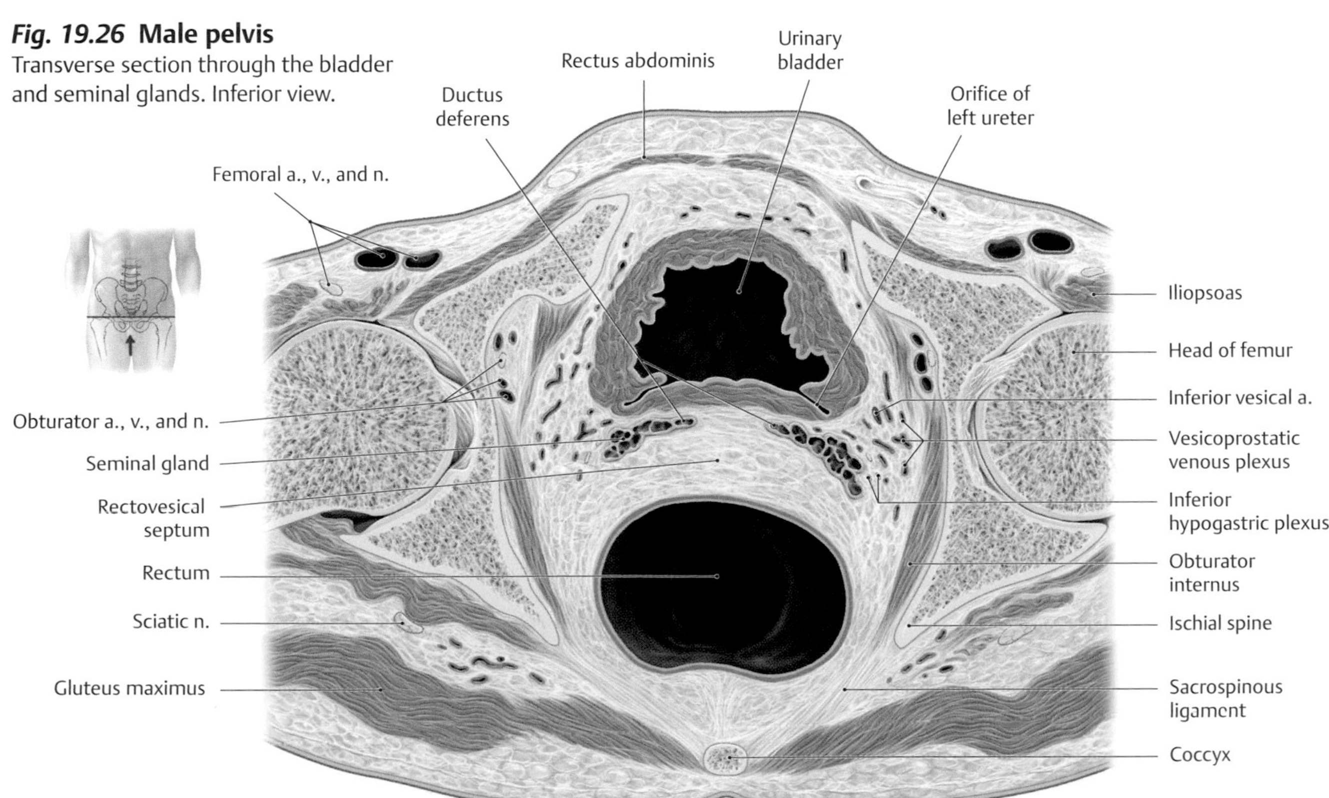
Rectus abdominis
Urinary bladder
Ductus deferens
Orifice of left ureter
Femoral a., v., and n.
Iliopsoas
Head of femur
Inferior vesical a.
Obturator a., v., and n.
Vesicoprostatic venous plexus
Seminal gland
Inferior hypogastric plexus
Rectovesical septum
Obturator internus
Rectum
Ischial spine
Sciatic n.
Sacrospinous ligament
Gluteus maximus
Coccyx

Fig. 19.27 Male pelvis
Transverse section through the prostate gland and anal canal. Inferior view.

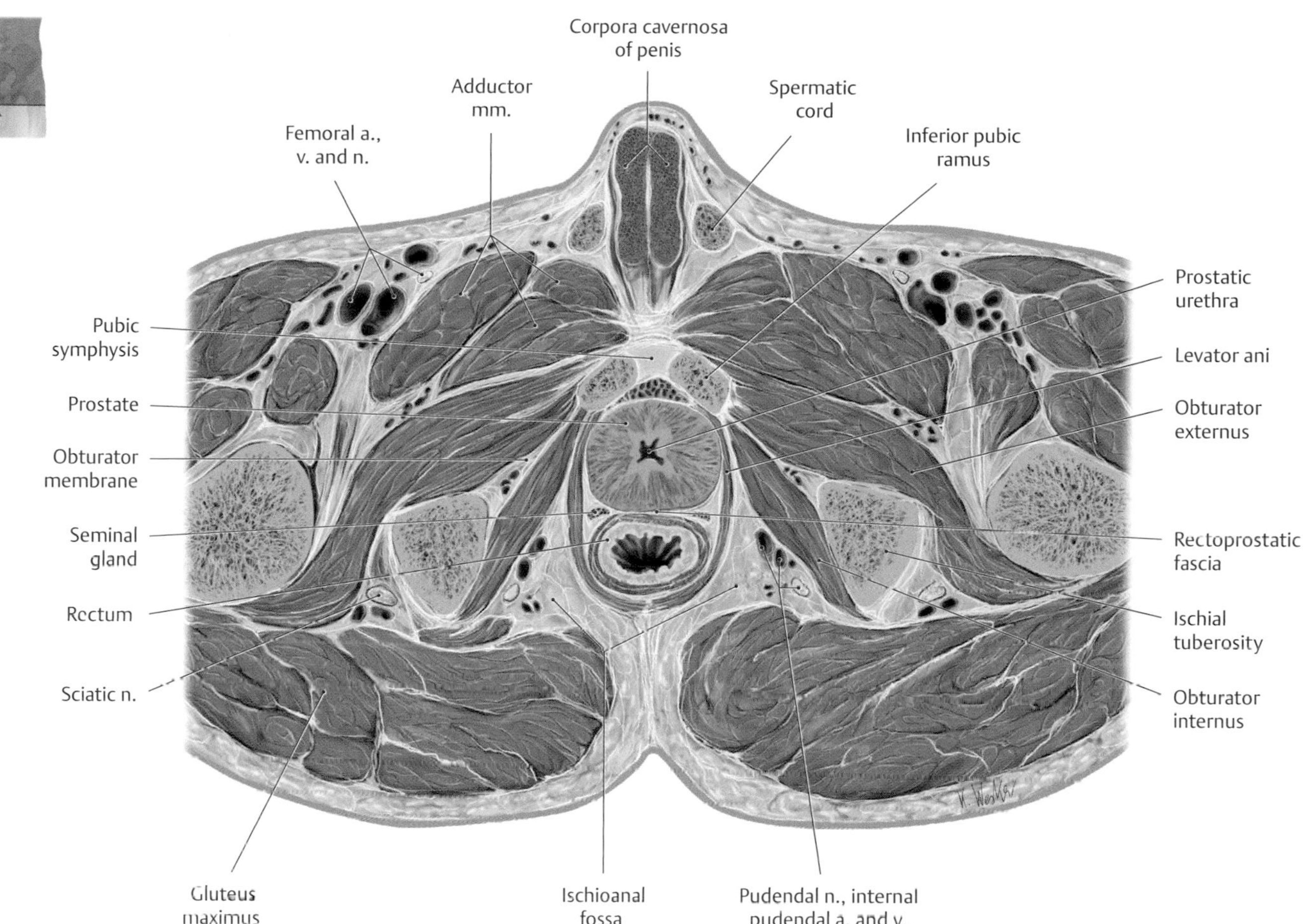

Corpora cavernosa of penis
Adductor mm.
Spermatic cord
Femoral a., v. and n.
Inferior pubic ramus
Pubic symphysis
Prostatic urethra
Levator ani
Prostate
Obturator externus
Obturator membrane
Seminal gland
Rectoprostatic fascia
Rectum
Ischial tuberosity
Sciatic n.
Obturator internus
Gluteus maximus
Ischioanal fossa
Pudendal n., internal pudendal a. and v.

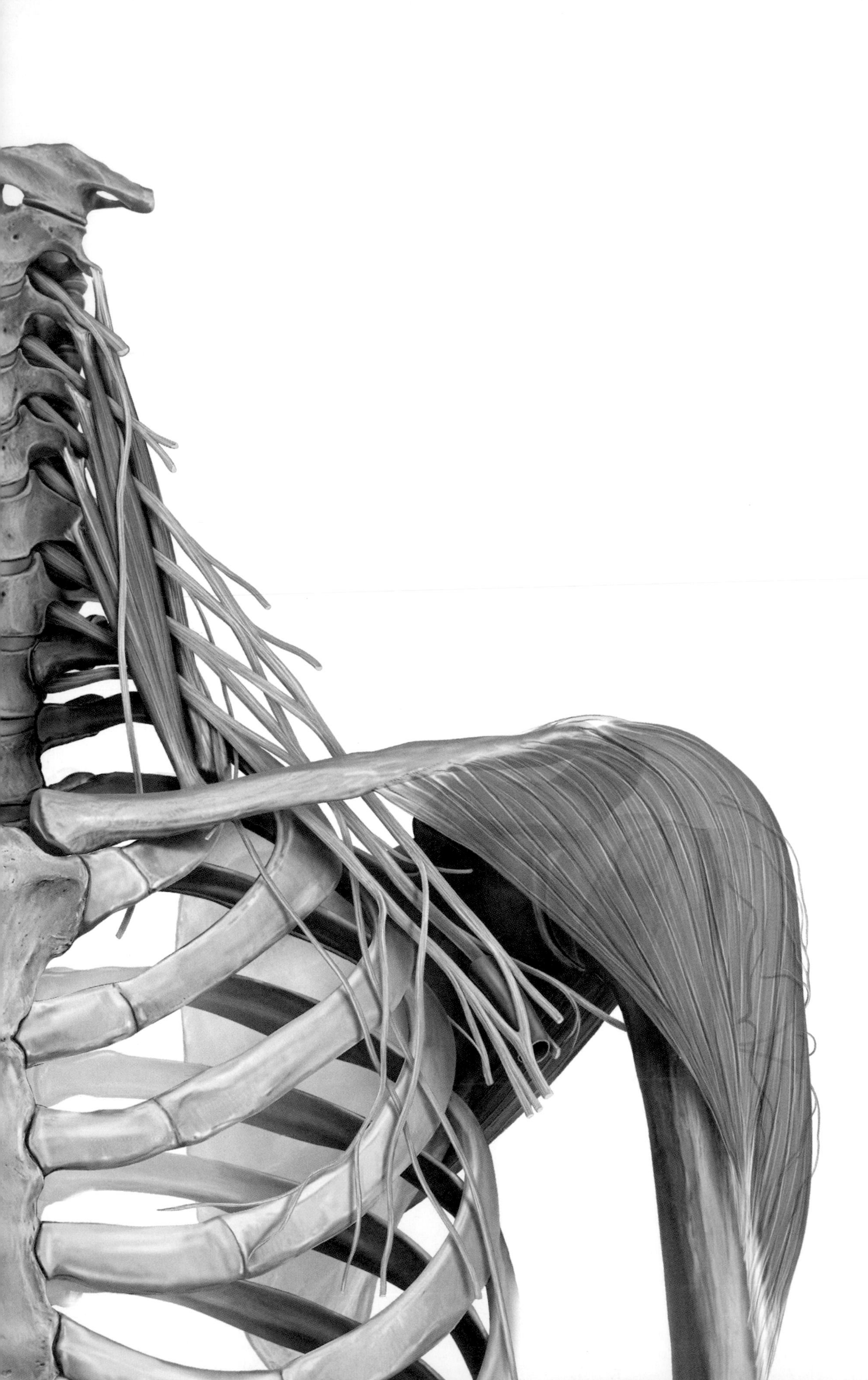

Upper Limb

20 Surface Anatomy

Surface Anatomy 274

21 Shoulder & Arm

Bones of the Upper Limb 276
Clavicle & Scapula 278
Humerus 280
Joints of the Shoulder 282
Joints of the Shoulder: Glenohumeral Joint 284
Subacromial Space & Bursae 286
Anterior Muscles of the Shoulder & Arm (I) 288
Anterior Muscles of the Shoulder & Arm (II) 290
Posterior Muscles of the Shoulder & Arm (I) 292
Posterior Muscles of the Shoulder & Arm (II) 294
Muscle Facts (I) 296
Muscle Facts (II) 298
Muscle Facts (III) 300
Muscle Facts (IV) 302

22 Elbow & Forearm

Radius & Ulna 304
Elbow Joint 306
Ligaments of the Elbow Joint 308
Radioulnar Joints 310
Muscles of the Forearm (I) 312
Muscles of the Forearm (II) 314
Muscle Facts (I) 316
Muscle Facts (II) 318
Muscle Facts (III) 320

23 Wrist & Hand

Bones of the Wrist & Hand 322
The Carpal Bones 324
Joints of the Wrist & Hand 326
Ligaments of the Hand 328
Ligaments of the Wrist 330
Ligaments of the Fingers 332
Muscles of the Hand: Superficial & Middle Layers 334
Muscles of the Hand: Middle & Deep Layers 336
Dorsum of the Hand 338
Muscle Facts (I) 340
Muscle Facts (II) 342

24 Neurovasculature

Arteries of the Upper Limb 344
Veins & Lymphatics of the Upper Limb 346
Nerves of the Brachial Plexus 348
Supraclavicular Branches & Posterior Cord 350
Posterior Cord: Axillary & Radial Nerves 352
Medial & Lateral Cords 354
Median & Ulnar Nerves 356
Superficial Veins & Nerves of the Upper Limb 358
Posterior Shoulder & Axilla 360
Anterior Shoulder 362
Topography of the Axilla 364
Topography of the Brachial & Cubital Regions 366
Topography of the Forearm 368
Topography of the Carpal Region 370
Topography of the Palm of the Hand 372
Topography of the Dorsum of the Hand 374
Sectional Anatomy of the Upper Limb 376

Surface Anatomy

Fig. 20.1 Regions of the upper limb

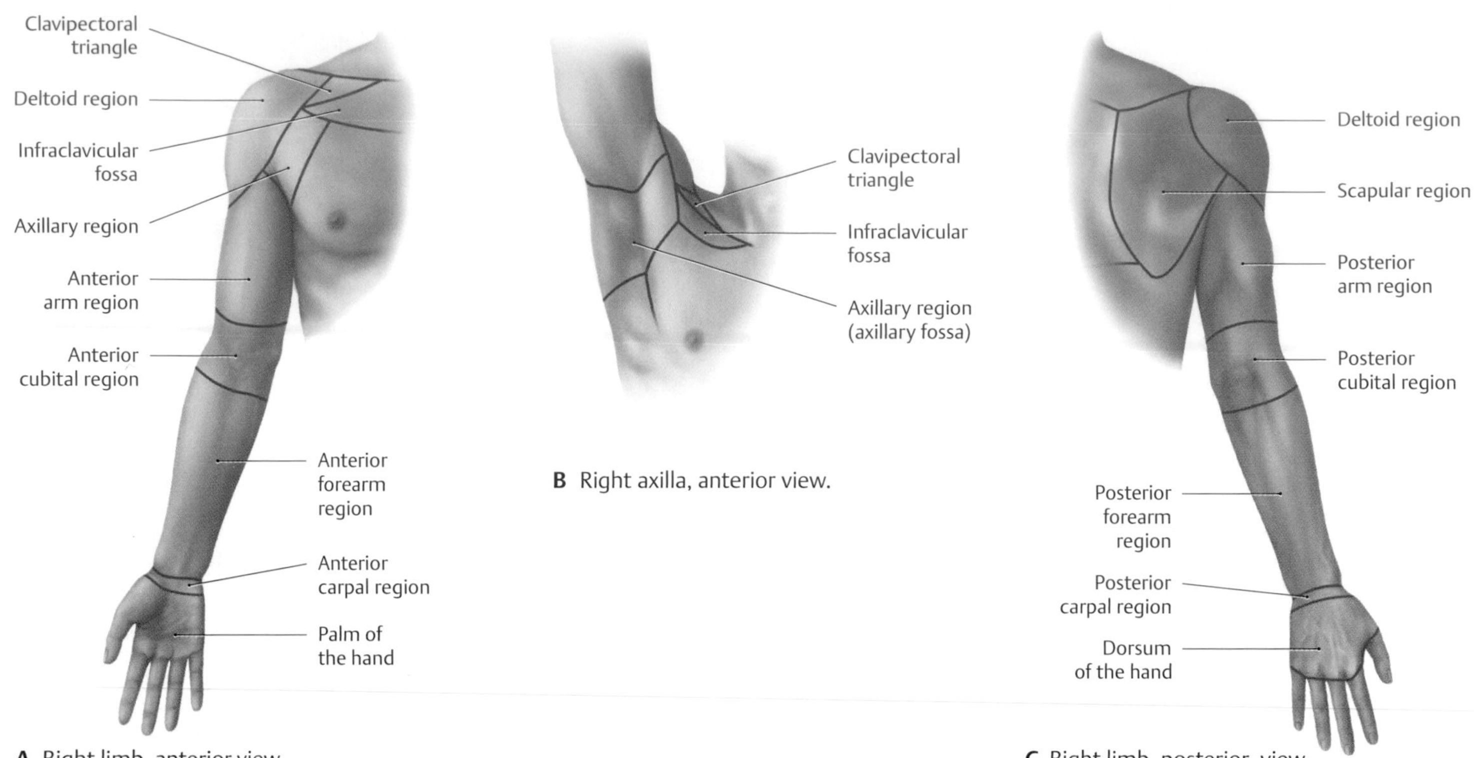

Clavipectoral triangle
Deltoid region
Infraclavicular fossa
Axillary region
Anterior arm region
Anterior cubital region
Anterior forearm region
Anterior carpal region
Palm of the hand
Clavipectoral triangle
Infraclavicular fossa
Axillary region (axillary fossa)
Deltoid region
Scapular region
Posterior arm region
Posterior cubital region
Posterior forearm region
Posterior carpal region
Dorsum of the hand

A Right limb, anterior view.

B Right axilla, anterior view.

C Right limb, posterior view.

Fig. 20.2 Palpable musculature of the upper limb

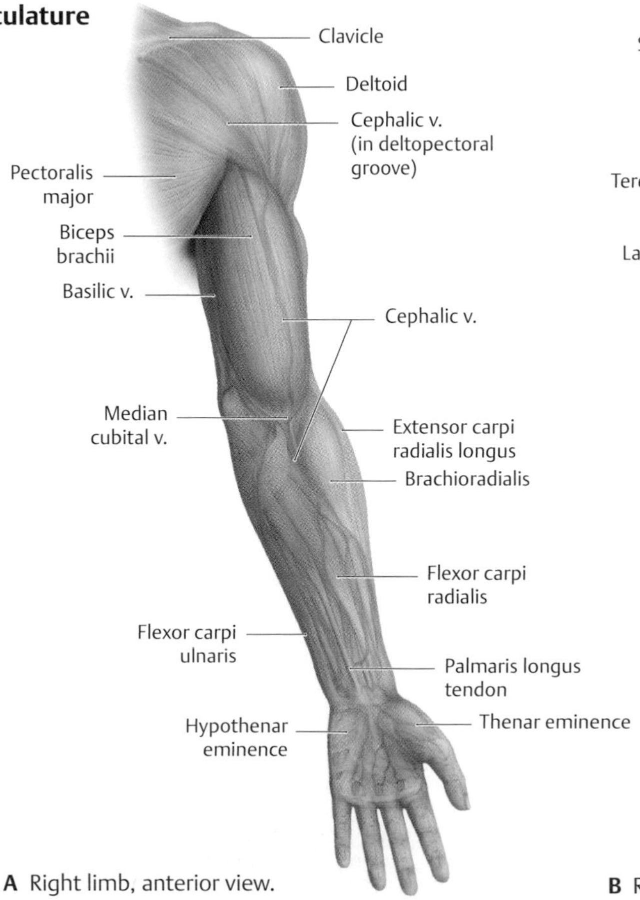

Clavicle
Deltoid
Cephalic v. (in deltopectoral groove)
Pectoralis major
Biceps brachii
Basilic v.
Cephalic v.
Median cubital v.
Extensor carpi radialis longus
Brachioradialis
Flexor carpi radialis
Flexor carpi ulnaris
Palmaris longus tendon
Hypothenar eminence
Thenar eminence

A Right limb, anterior view.

Scapular spine
Deltoid
Teres major
Long head, Lateral head — Triceps brachii
Latissimus dorsi
Olecranon
Extensor carpi radialis longus
Basilic v.
Cephalic v.
Extensor carpi ulnaris
Flexor carpi ulnaris
Extensor digitorum
Extensor digitorum tendons, dorsal venous network

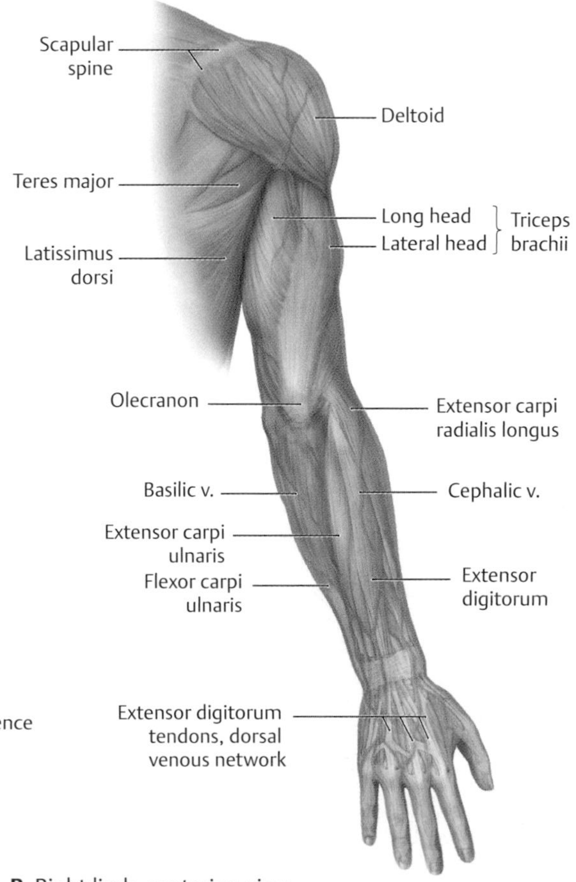

B Right limb, posterior view.

Fig. 20.3 Palpable bony prominences of the upper limb

Except for the lunate and trapezoid bones, all of the bones in the upper limb are palpable to some degree through the skin and soft tissues.

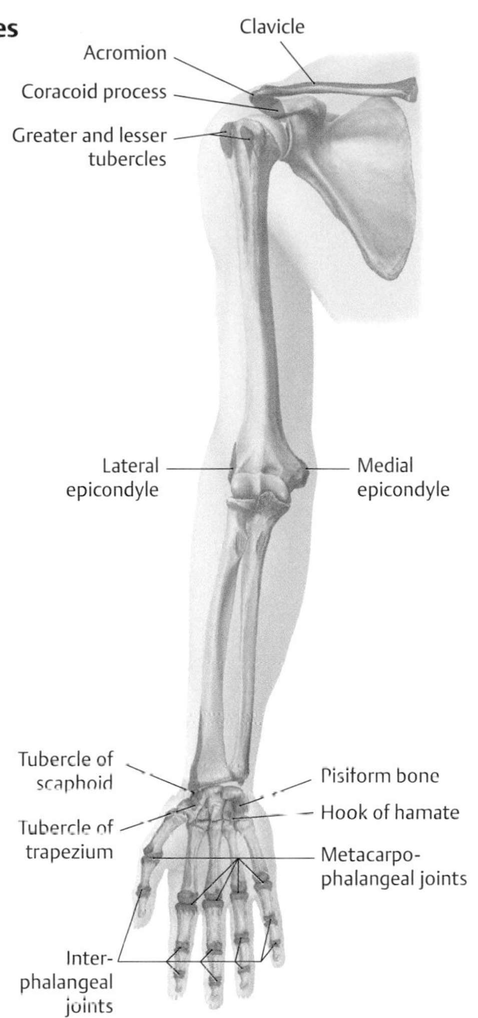

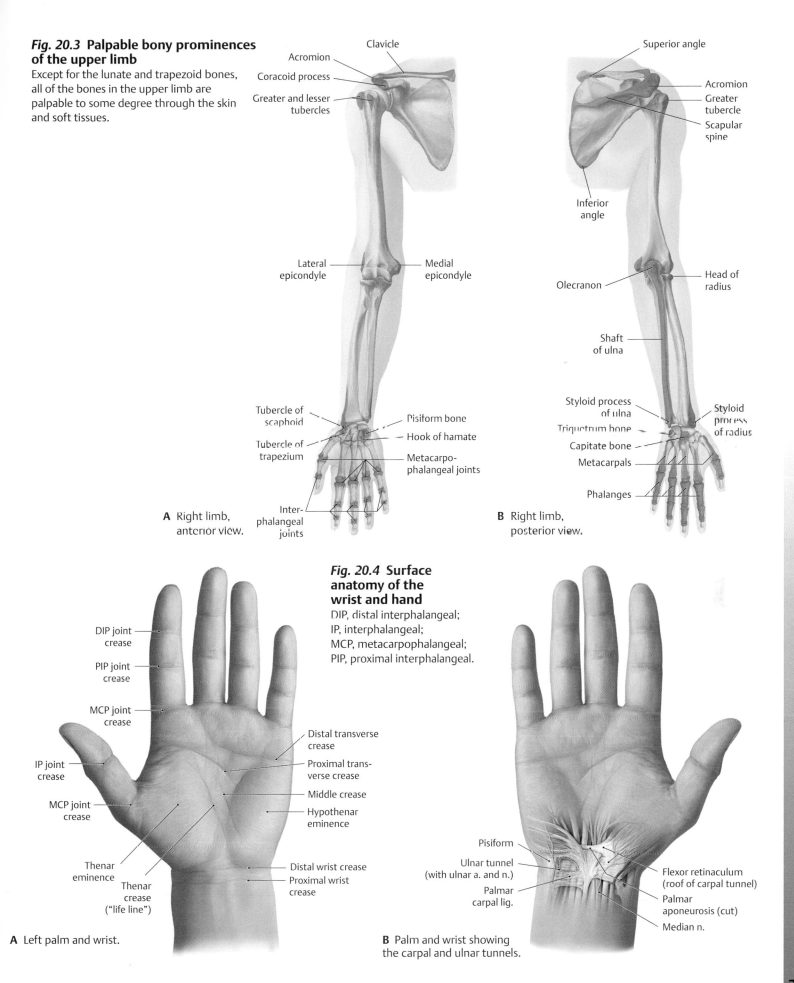

Clavicle
Acromion
Coracoid process
Greater and lesser tubercles
Lateral epicondyle
Medial epicondyle
Tubercle of scaphoid
Pisiform bone
Tubercle of trapezium
Hook of hamate
Metacarpo-phalangeal joints
Inter-phalangeal joints

A Right limb, anterior view.

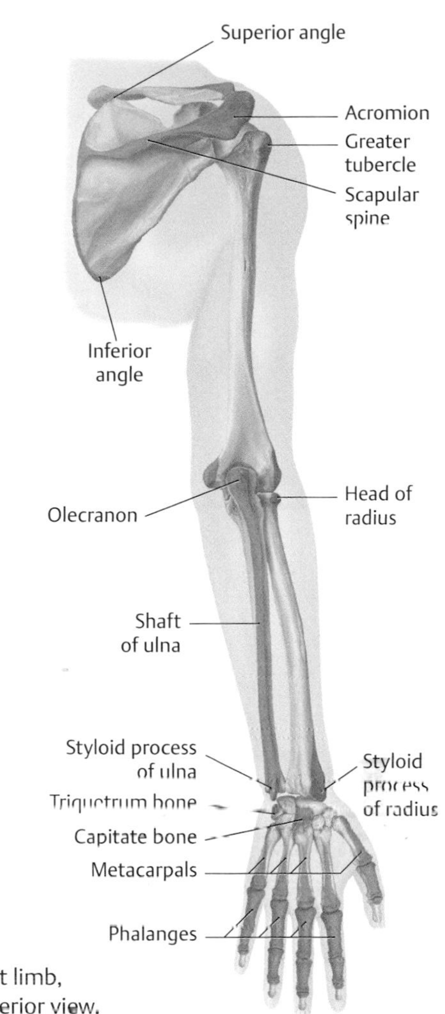

Superior angle
Acromion
Greater tubercle
Scapular spine
Inferior angle
Olecranon
Head of radius
Shaft of ulna
Styloid process of ulna
Styloid process of radius
Triquetrum bone
Capitate bone
Metacarpals
Phalanges

B Right limb, posterior view.

Fig. 20.4 Surface anatomy of the wrist and hand

DIP, distal interphalangeal; IP, interphalangeal; MCP, metacarpophalangeal; PIP, proximal interphalangeal.

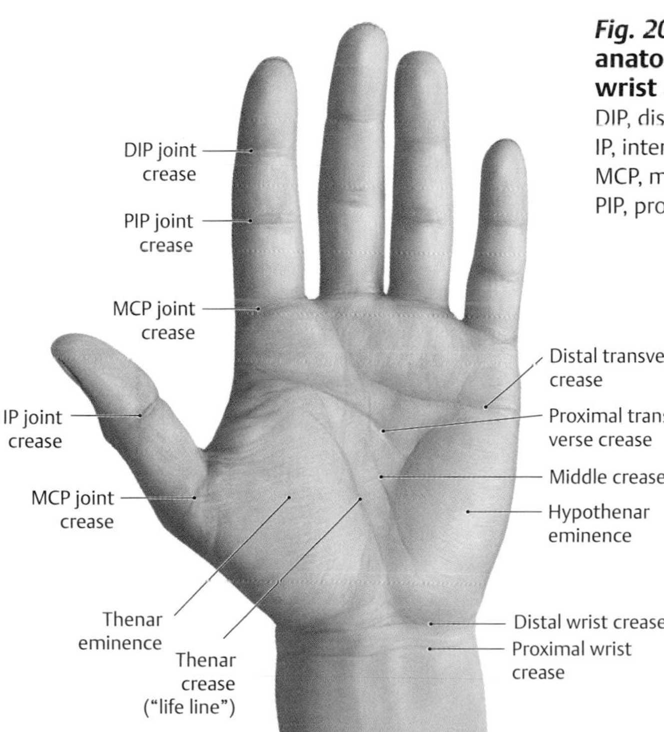

DIP joint crease
PIP joint crease
MCP joint crease
IP joint crease
MCP joint crease
Thenar eminence
Thenar crease ("life line")
Distal transverse crease
Proximal trans-verse crease
Middle crease
Hypothenar eminence
Distal wrist crease
Proximal wrist crease

A Left palm and wrist.

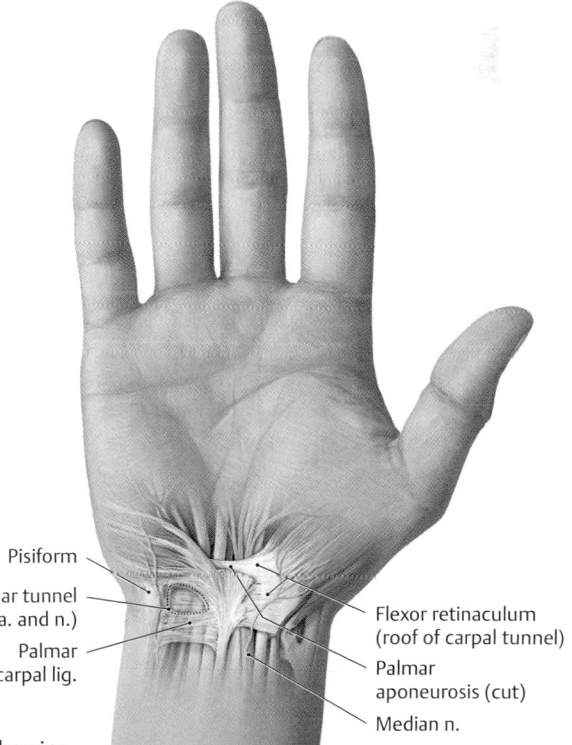

Pisiform
Ulnar tunnel (with ulnar a. and n.)
Palmar carpal lig.
Flexor retinaculum (roof of carpal tunnel)
Palmar aponeurosis (cut)
Median n.

B Palm and wrist showing the carpal and ulnar tunnels.

Bones of the Upper Limb

Fig. 21.1 Skeleton of the upper limb
Right limb. The upper limb is subdivided into three regions: arm, forearm, and hand. The shoulder girdle (clavicle and scapula) joins the upper limb to the thorax at the sternoclavicular joint.

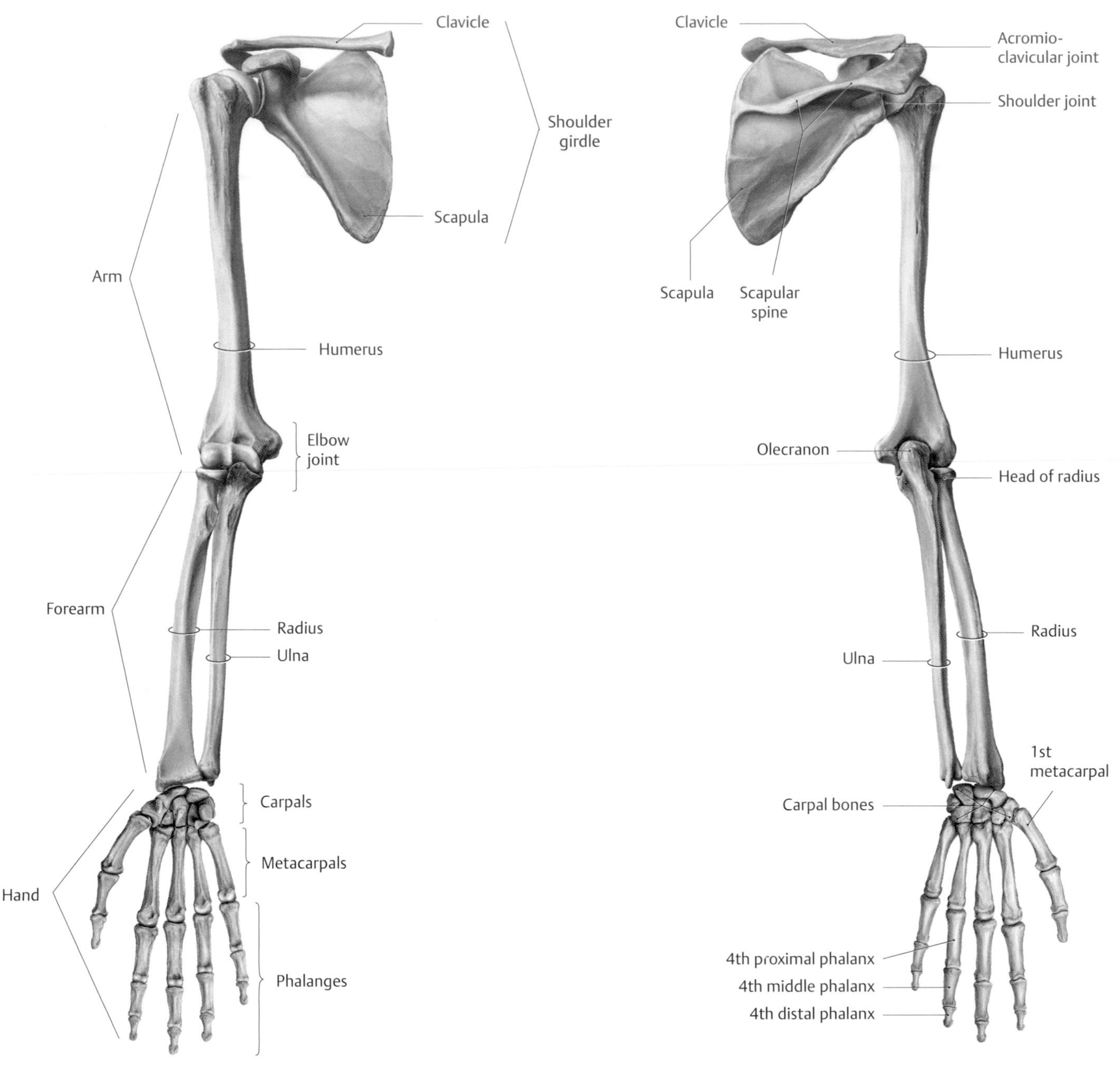
Clavicle
Shoulder girdle
Scapula
Arm
Humerus
Elbow joint
Forearm
Radius
Ulna
Carpals
Metacarpals
Hand
Phalanges
Clavicle
Acromio-clavicular joint
Shoulder joint
Scapula
Scapular spine
Humerus
Olecranon
Head of radius
Radius
Ulna
1st metacarpal
Carpal bones
4th proximal phalanx
4th middle phalanx
4th distal phalanx

A Anterior view.

B Posterior view.

Fig. 21.2 **Bones of the right shoulder girdle in their normal relation to the skeleton of the trunk**

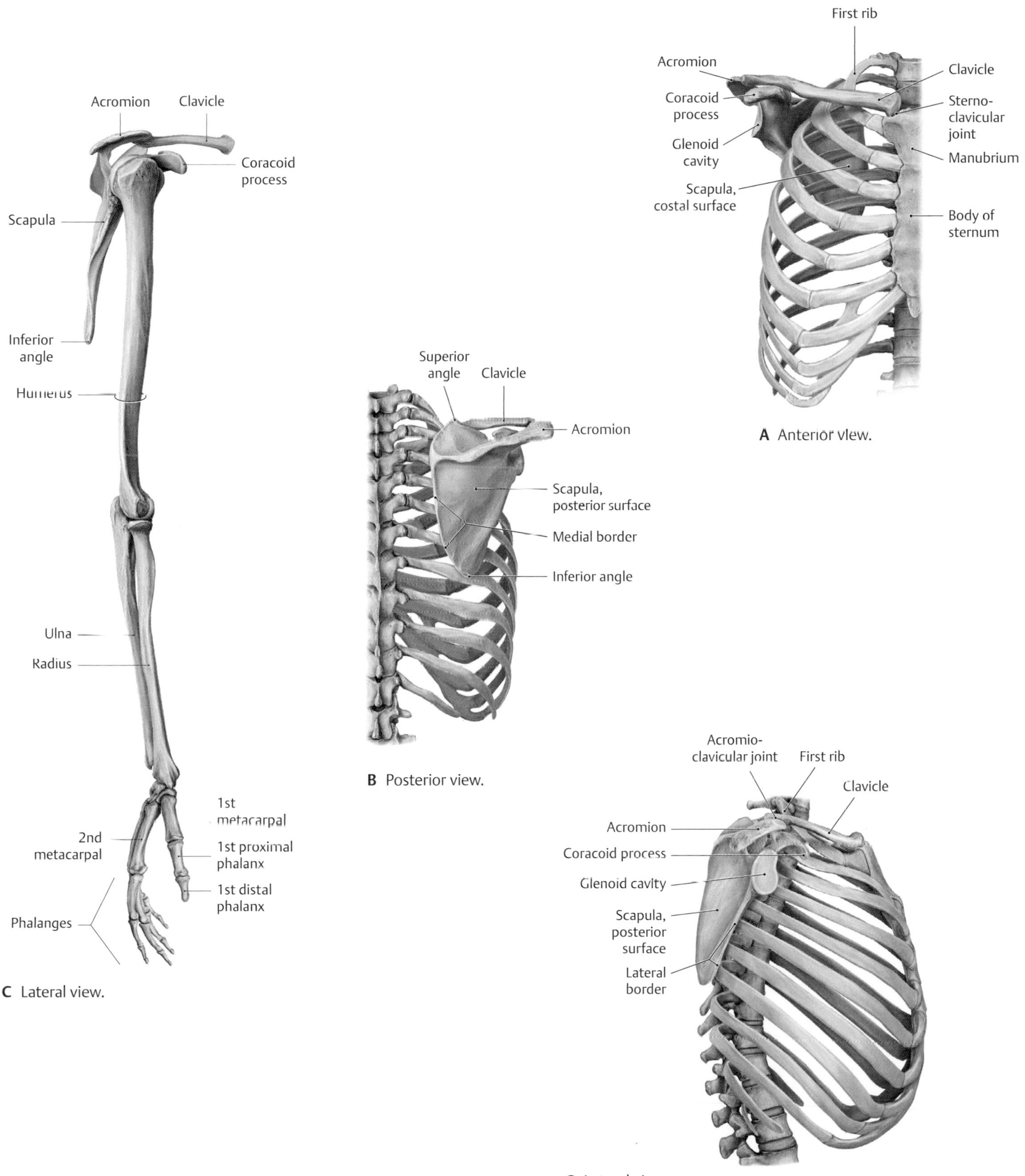
First rib
Acromion
Clavicle
Coracoid process
Sterno-clavicular joint
Glenoid cavity
Manubrium
Scapula, costal surface
Body of sternum
Superior angle
Clavicle
Acromion
Scapula, posterior surface
Medial border
Inferior angle
Acromion
Clavicle
Coracoid process
Scapula
Inferior angle
Humerus
Ulna
Radius
1st metacarpal
2nd metacarpal
1st proximal phalanx
1st distal phalanx
Phalanges
Acromio-clavicular joint
First rib
Clavicle
Acromion
Coracoid process
Glenoid cavity
Scapula, posterior surface
Lateral border

A Anterior view.

B Posterior view.

C Lateral view.

C Lateral view.

Clavicle & Scapula

The shoulder girdle (clavicle and scapula) connects the bones of the upper limb to the thoracic cage. Whereas the pelvic girdle (paired hip bones) is firmly integrated into the axial skeleton (see pp. 216–217), the shoulder girdle is extremely mobile.

Fig. 21.3 Clavicle

Right clavicle. The S-shaped clavicle is visible and palpable along its entire length (generally 12 to 15 cm). Its medial end articulates with the sternum at the sternoclavicular joint (see p. 283). Its lateral end articulates with the scapula at the acromioclavicular joint (see p. 283).

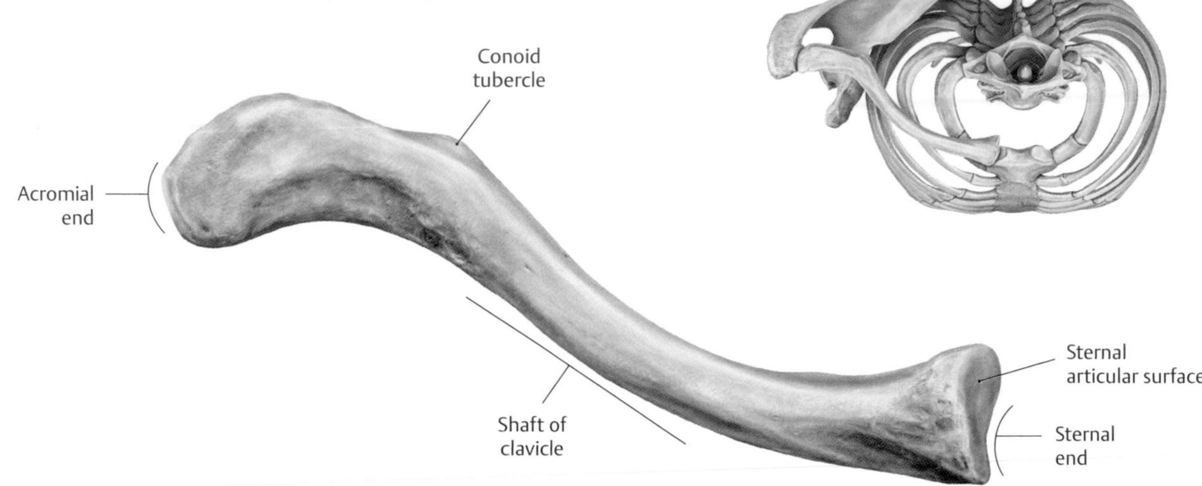
Conoid tubercle
Acromial end
Sternal articular surface
Sternal end
Shaft of clavicle

A Superior view.

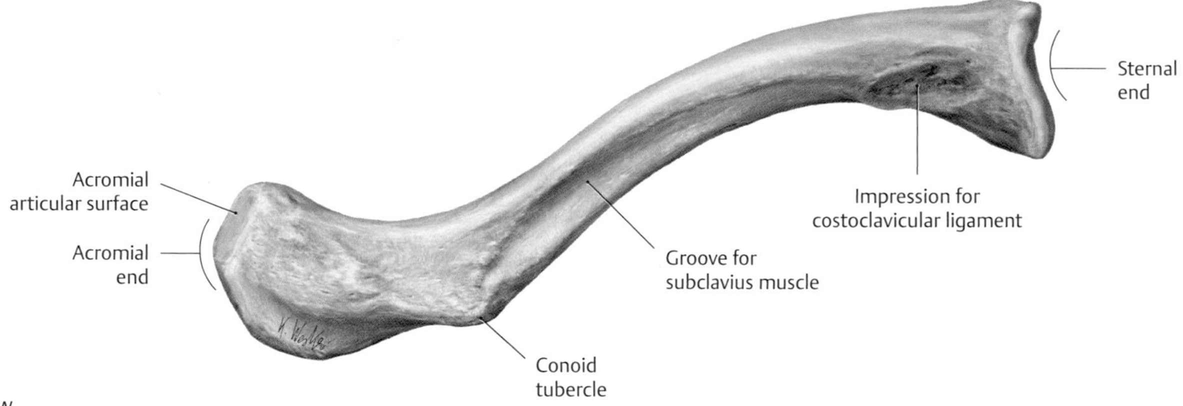
Sternal end
Acromial articular surface
Acromial end
Impression for costoclavicular ligament
Groove for subclavius muscle
Conoid tubercle

B Inferior view.

Clinical

Scapular foramen

The superior transverse ligament of the scapula (see Fig. 21.13, p. 285) may become ossified, transforming the scapular notch into an anomalous bony canal, the scapular foramen. This can lead to compression of the suprascapular nerve as it passes through the canal (see p. 361).

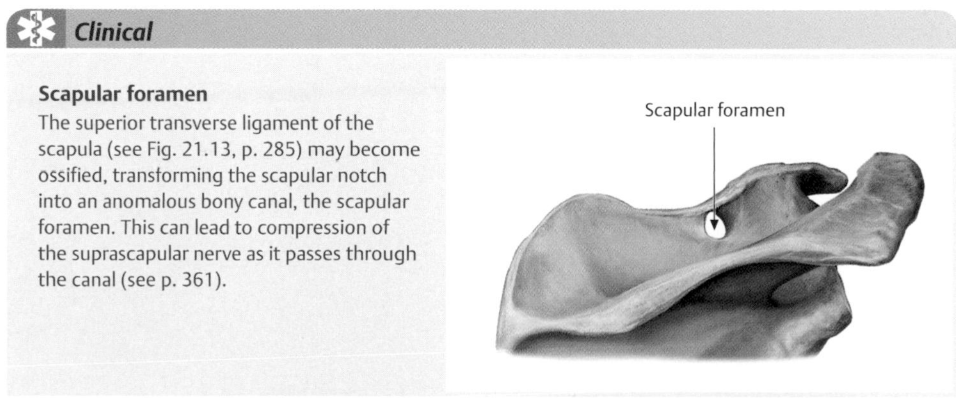
Scapular foramen

Fig. 21.4 Scapula
Right scapula. In its normal anatomical position, the scapula extends from the 2nd to the 7th rib.

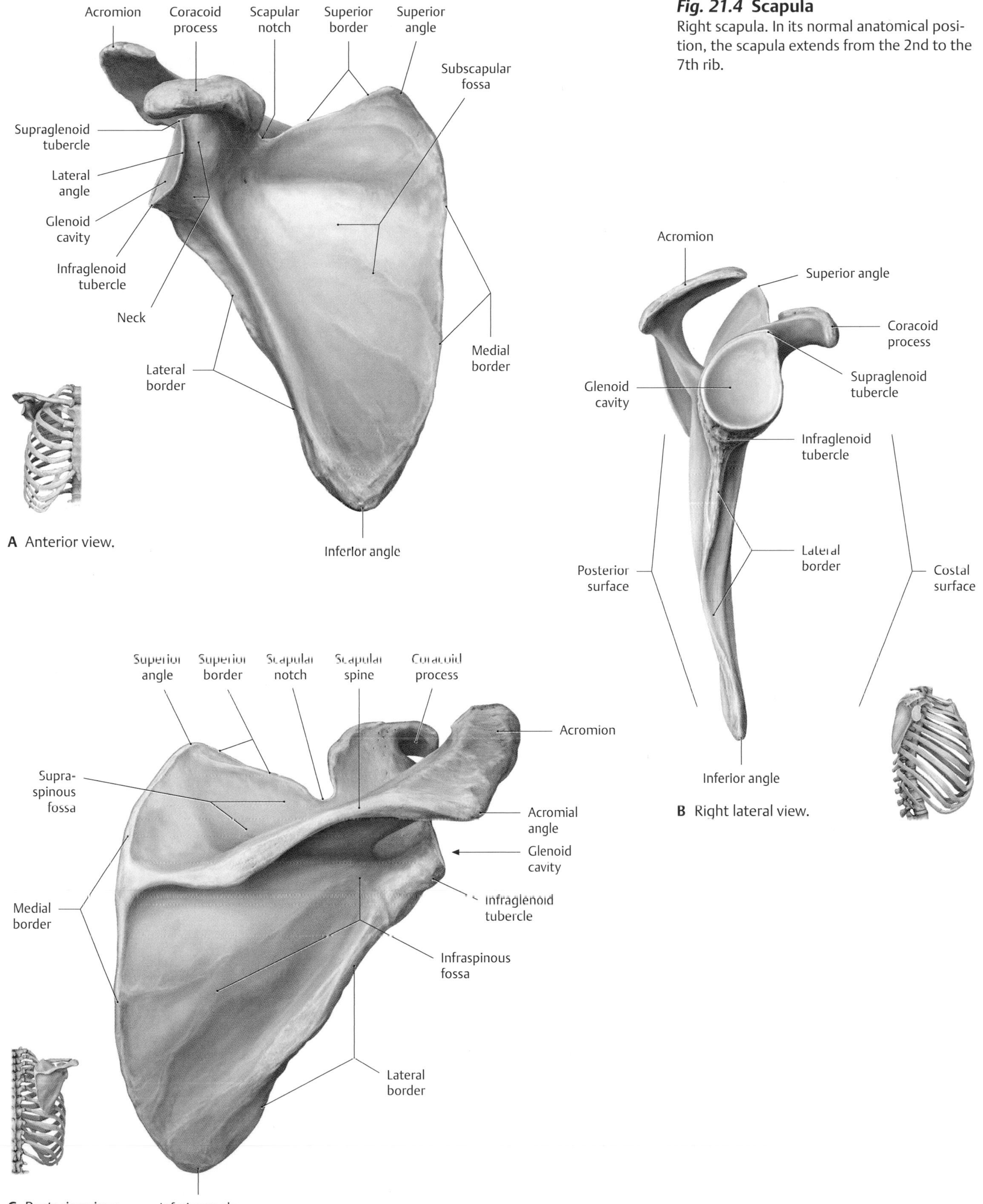
Acromion
Coracoid process
Scapular notch
Superior border
Superior angle
Subscapular fossa
Supraglenoid tubercle
Lateral angle
Glenoid cavity
Infraglenoid tubercle
Neck
Lateral border
Medial border
Inferior angle
Acromion
Superior angle
Coracoid process
Supraglenoid tubercle
Glenoid cavity
Infraglenoid tubercle
Lateral border
Posterior surface
Costal surface
Inferior angle
Superior angle
Superior border
Scapular notch
Scapular spine
Coracoid process
Acromion
Supra-spinous fossa
Acromial angle
Glenoid cavity
Infraglenoid tubercle
Medial border
Infraspinous fossa
Lateral border
Inferior angle

A Anterior view.

B Right lateral view.

C Posterior view.

Humerus

Fig. 21.5 Humerus

Right humerus. The head of the humerus articulates with the scapula at the glenohumeral joint (see p. 284). The capitellum and trochlea of the humerus articulate with the radius and ulna, respectively, at the elbow (cubital) joint (see p. 306).

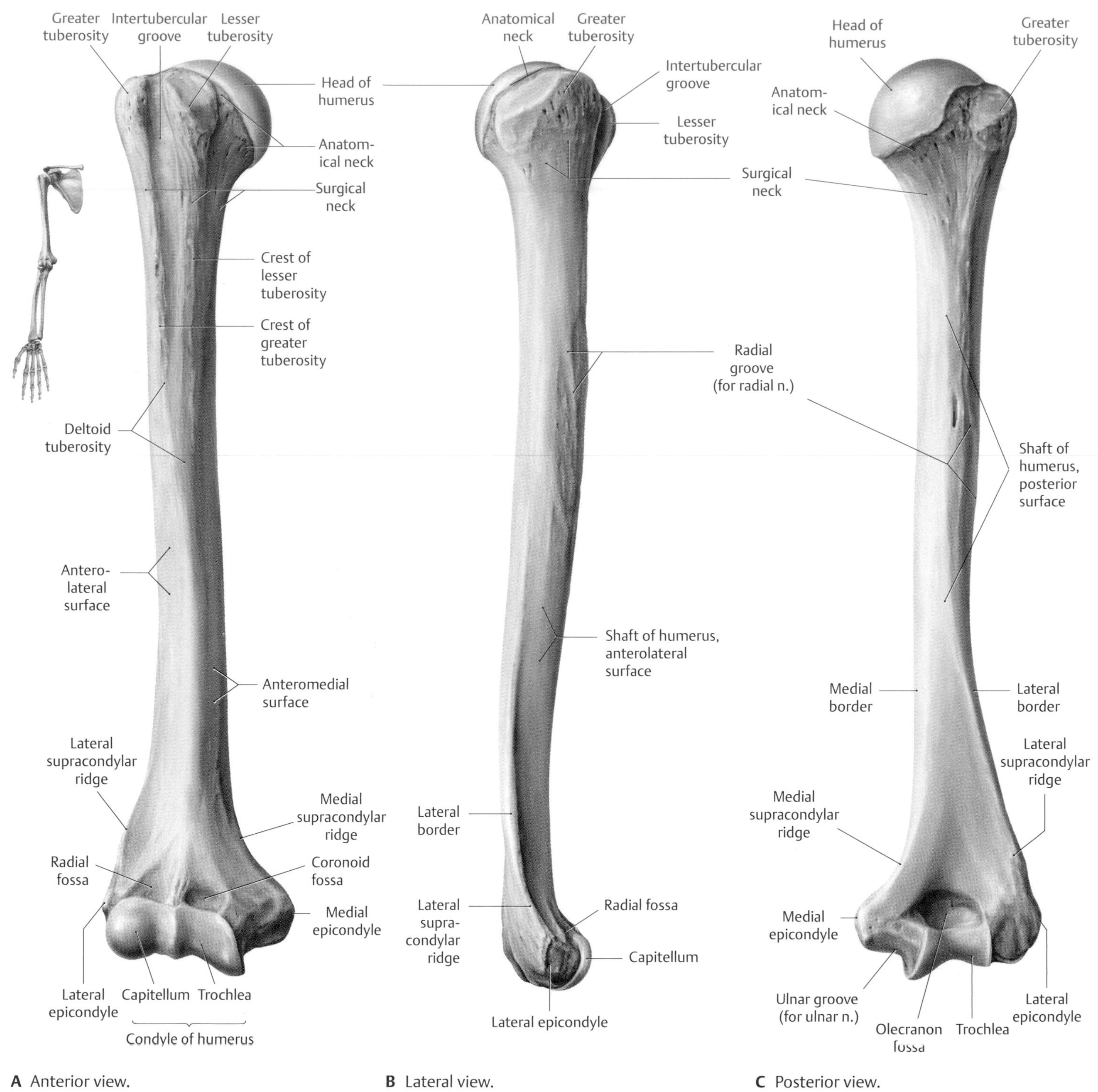

Greater tuberosity
Intertubercular groove
Lesser tuberosity
Head of humerus
Anatomical neck
Surgical neck
Crest of lesser tuberosity
Crest of greater tuberosity
Deltoid tuberosity
Anterolateral surface
Anteromedial surface
Lateral supracondylar ridge
Medial supracondylar ridge
Radial fossa
Coronoid fossa
Medial epicondyle
Lateral epicondyle
Capitellum
Trochlea
Condyle of humerus
Anatomical neck
Greater tuberosity
Intertubercular groove
Lesser tuberosity
Surgical neck
Radial groove (for radial n.)
Shaft of humerus, anterolateral surface
Lateral border
Lateral supracondylar ridge
Radial fossa
Capitellum
Lateral epicondyle
Head of humerus
Greater tuberosity
Anatomical neck
Surgical neck
Shaft of humerus, posterior surface
Medial border
Lateral border
Lateral supracondylar ridge
Medial supracondylar ridge
Medial epicondyle
Ulnar groove (for ulnar n.)
Olecranon fossa
Trochlea
Lateral epicondyle

A Anterior view.

B Lateral view.

C Posterior view.

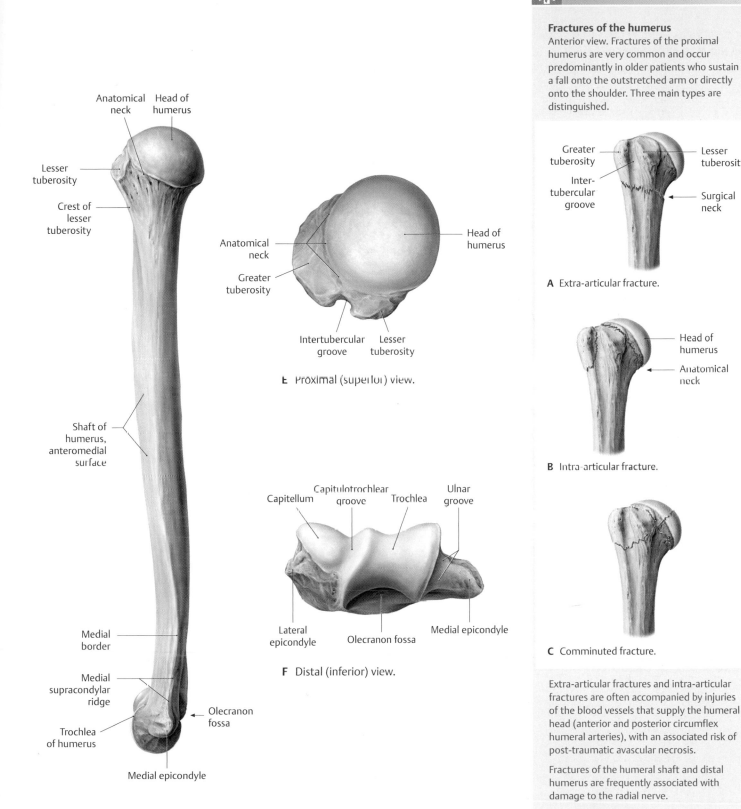

Anatomical neck
Head of humerus
Lesser tuberosity
Crest of lesser tuberosity
Shaft of humerus, anteromedial surface
Medial border
Medial supracondylar ridge
Olecranon fossa
Trochlea of humerus
Medial epicondyle

D Medial view.

Anatomical neck
Greater tuberosity
Head of humerus
Intertubercular groove
Lesser tuberosity

E Proximal (superior) view.

Capitellum
Capitulotrochlear groove
Trochlea
Ulnar groove
Lateral epicondyle
Olecranon fossa
Medial epicondyle

F Distal (inferior) view.

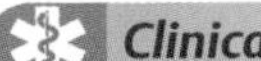

Clinical

Fractures of the humerus

Anterior view. Fractures of the proximal humerus are very common and occur predominantly in older patients who sustain a fall onto the outstretched arm or directly onto the shoulder. Three main types are distinguished.

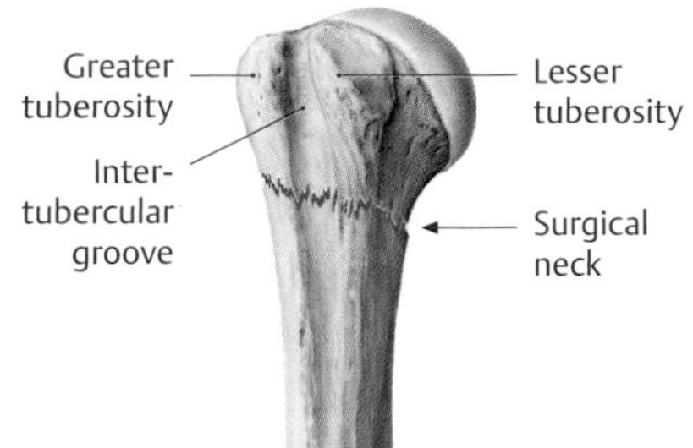

Greater tuberosity
Inter-tubercular groove
Lesser tuberosity
Surgical neck

A Extra-articular fracture.

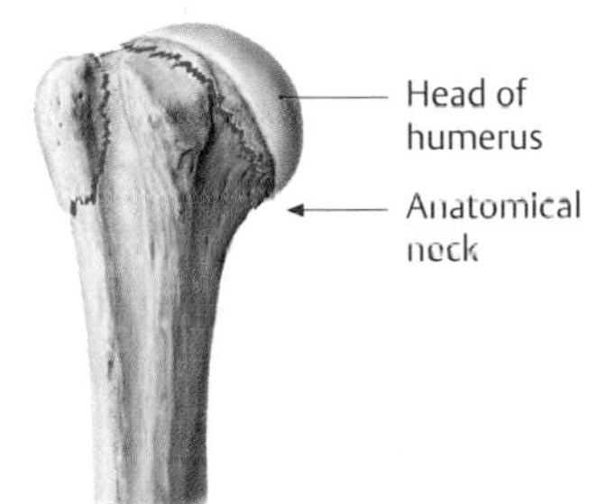

Head of humerus
Anatomical neck

B Intra-articular fracture.

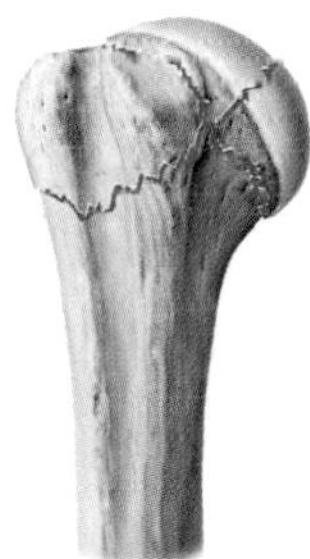

C Comminuted fracture.

Extra-articular fractures and intra-articular fractures are often accompanied by injuries of the blood vessels that supply the humeral head (anterior and posterior circumflex humeral arteries), with an associated risk of post-traumatic avascular necrosis.

Fractures of the humeral shaft and distal humerus are frequently associated with damage to the radial nerve.

Joints of the Shoulder

Fig. 21.6 Joints of the shoulder: Overview
Right shoulder, anterior view.

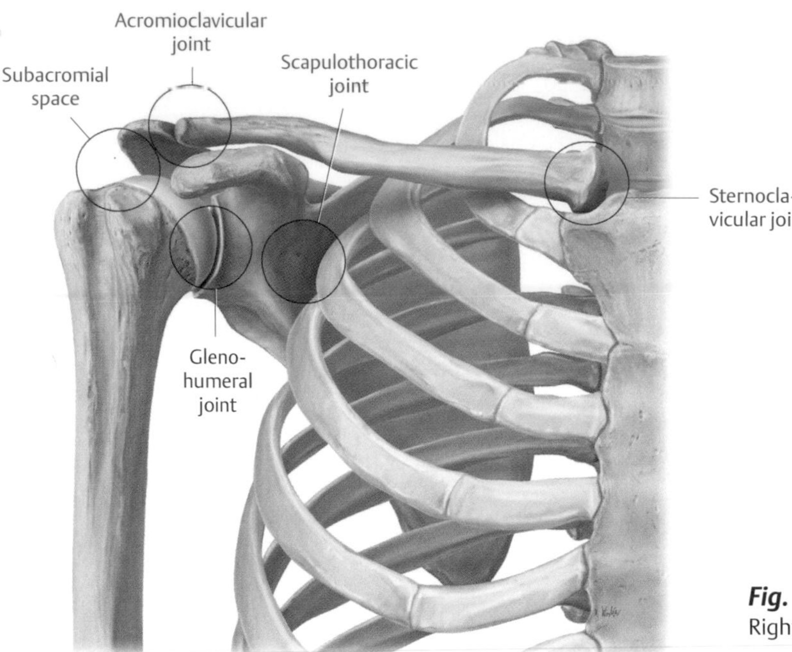
Acromioclavicular joint
Subacromial space
Scapulothoracic joint
Sternoclavicular joint
Glenohumeral joint

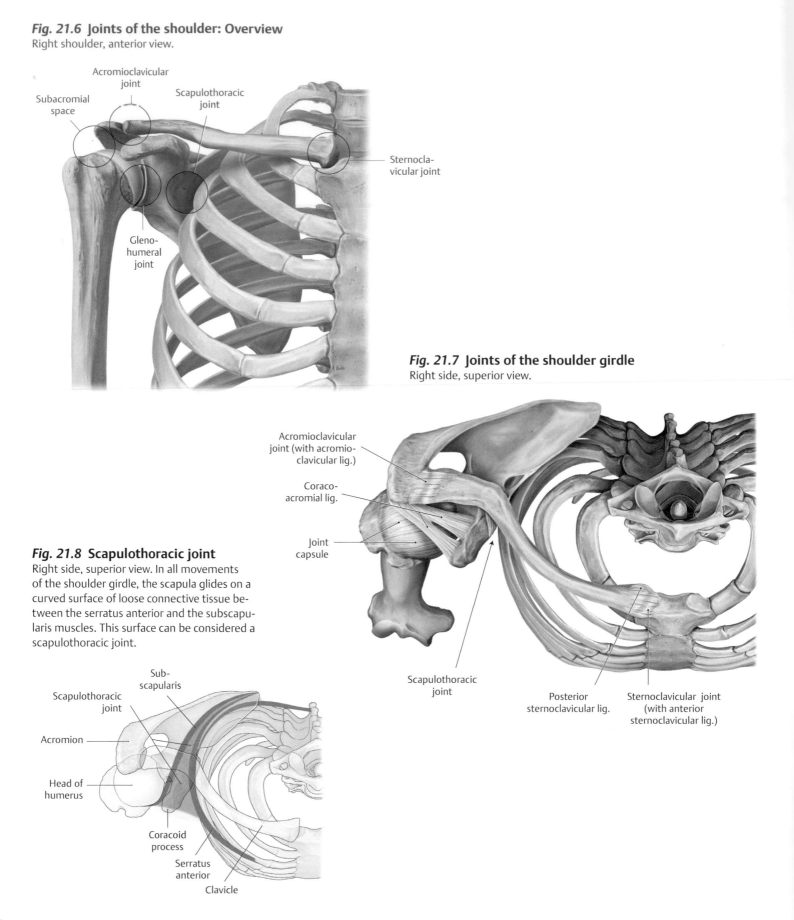

Fig. 21.7 Joints of the shoulder girdle
Right side, superior view.

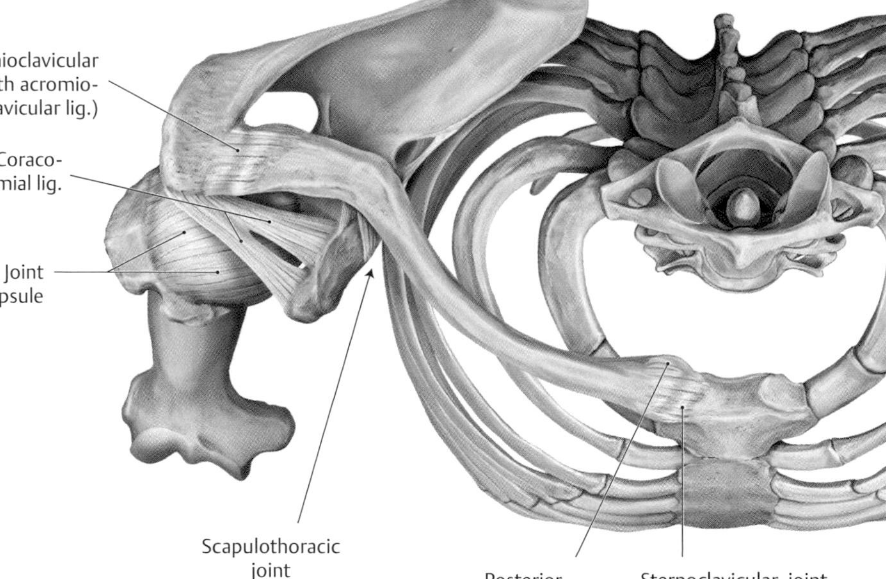
Acromioclavicular joint (with acromioclavicular lig.)
Coracoacromial lig.
Joint capsule
Scapulothoracic joint
Posterior sternoclavicular lig.
Sternoclavicular joint (with anterior sternoclavicular lig.)

Fig. 21.8 Scapulothoracic joint
Right side, superior view. In all movements of the shoulder girdle, the scapula glides on a curved surface of loose connective tissue between the serratus anterior and the subscapularis muscles. This surface can be considered a scapulothoracic joint.

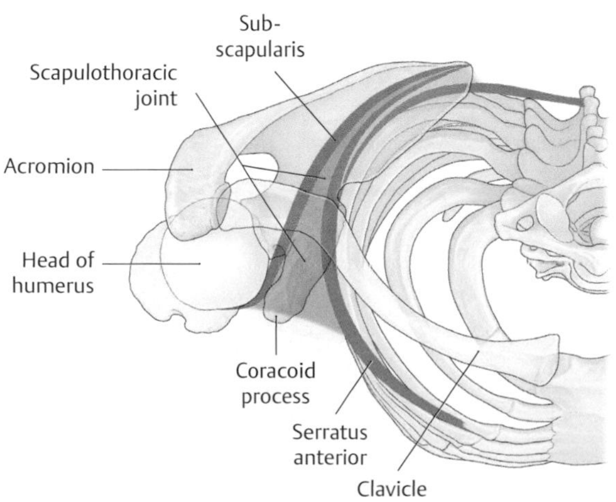
Subscapularis
Scapulothoracic joint
Acromion
Head of humerus
Coracoid process
Serratus anterior
Clavicle

Fig. 21.9 Sternoclavicular joint
Anterior view with sternum coronally sectioned (left). *Note:* A fibrocartilaginous articular disk compensates for the mismatch of surfaces between the two saddle-shaped articular facets of the clavicle and manubrium of the sternum.

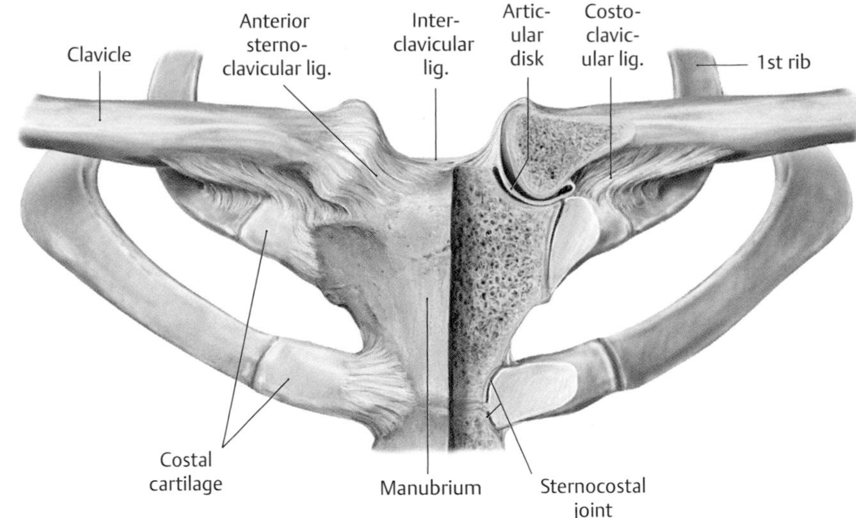
Clavicle
Anterior sterno-clavicular lig.
Inter-clavicular lig.
Artic-ular disk
Costo-clavic-ular lig.
1st rib
Costal cartilage
Manubrium
Sternocostal joint

Fig. 21.10 Acromioclavicular joint
Anterior view. The acromioclavicular joint is a plane joint. Because the articulating surfaces are flat, they must be held in place by strong ligaments, greatly limiting the mobility of the joint.

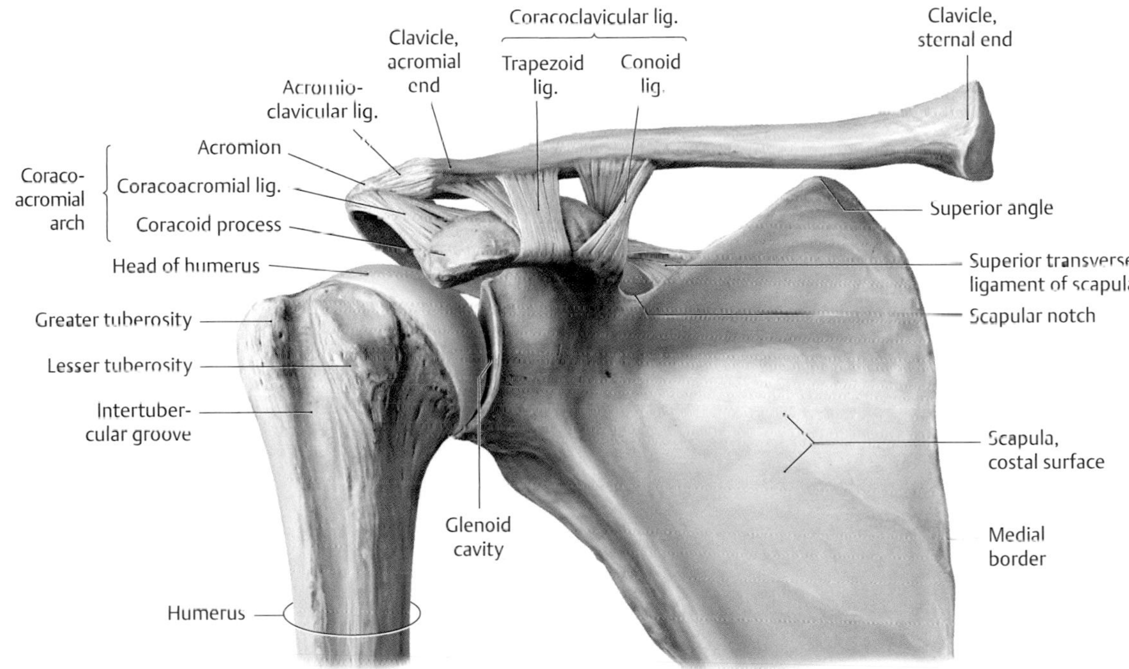
Coracoclavicular lig.
Clavicle, acromial end
Trapezoid lig.
Conoid lig.
Clavicle, sternal end
Acromio-clavicular lig.
Coraco-acromial arch
Acromion
Coracoacromial lig.
Coracoid process
Head of humerus
Greater tuberosity
Lesser tuberosity
Intertuber-cular groove
Humerus
Glenoid cavity
Superior angle
Superior transverse ligament of scapula
Scapular notch
Scapula, costal surface
Medial border

Clinical

Injuries of the acromioclavicular joint
A fall onto the outstretched arm or shoulder frequently causes dislocation of the acromioclavicular joint and damage to the coracoclavicular ligaments.

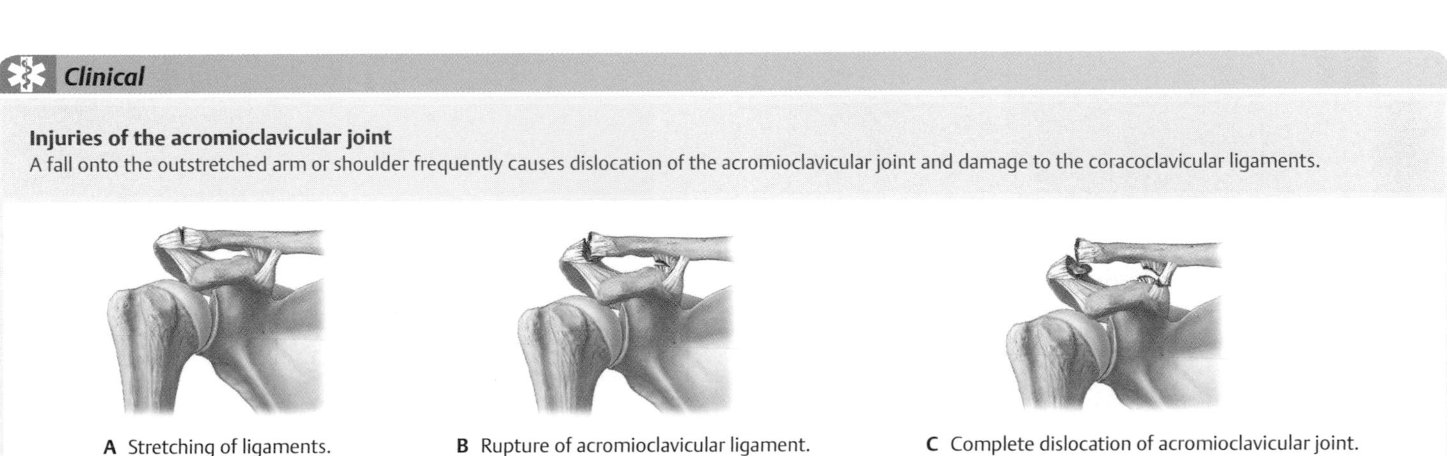

A Stretching of ligaments.
B Rupture of acromioclavicular ligament.
C Complete dislocation of acromioclavicular joint.

Joints of the Shoulder: Glenohumeral Joint

Fig. 21.11 **Glenohumeral joint: Bony elements**
Right shoulder.

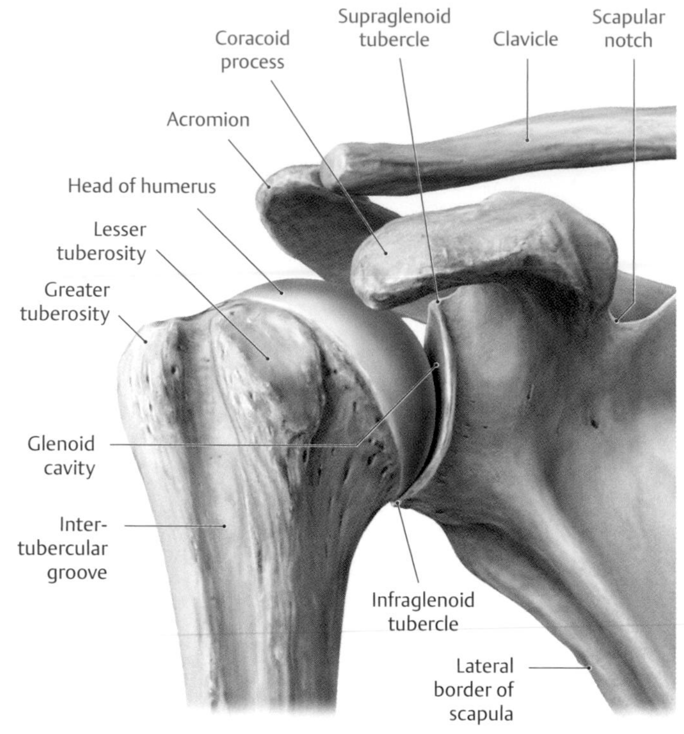
Coracoid process
Supraglenoid tubercle
Clavicle
Scapular notch
Acromion
Head of humerus
Lesser tuberosity
Greater tuberosity
Glenoid cavity
Inter-tubercular groove
Infraglenoid tubercle
Lateral border of scapula

A Anterior view.

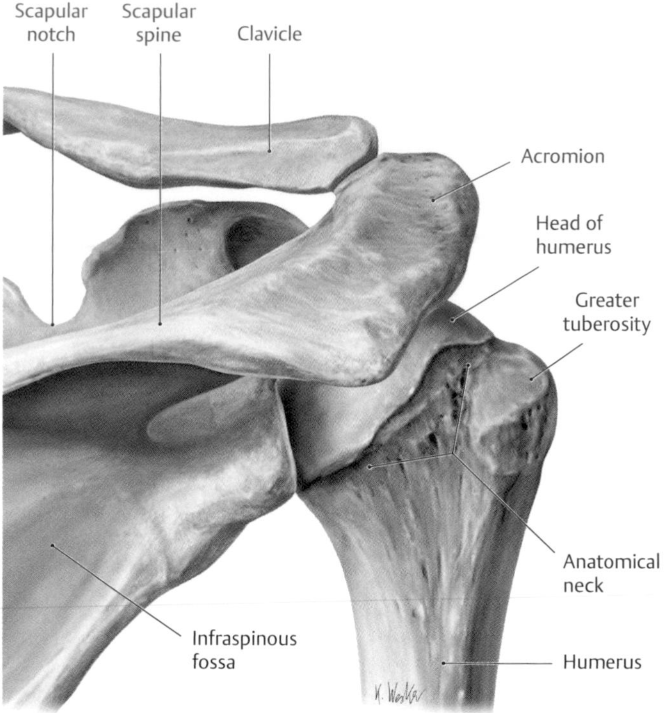
Scapular notch
Scapular spine
Clavicle
Acromion
Head of humerus
Greater tuberosity
Anatomical neck
Infraspinous fossa
Humerus

B Posterior view.

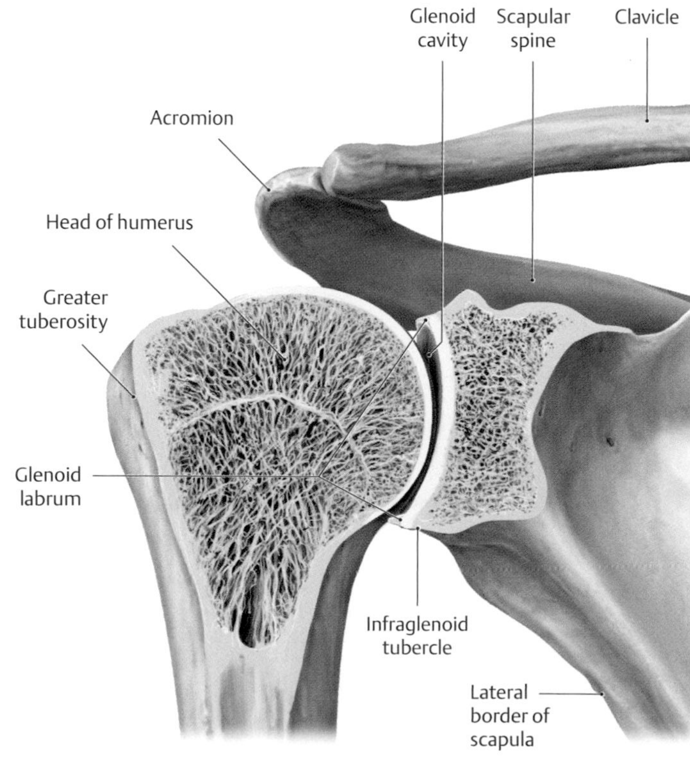
Glenoid cavity
Scapular spine
Clavicle
Acromion
Head of humerus
Greater tuberosity
Glenoid labrum
Infraglenoid tubercle
Lateral border of scapula

C Coronal section through the shoulder joint, anterior view.

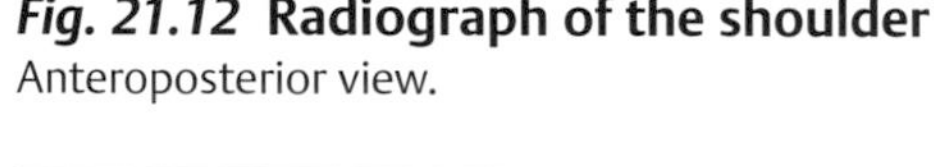

Fig. 21.12 **Radiograph of the shoulder**
Anteroposterior view.

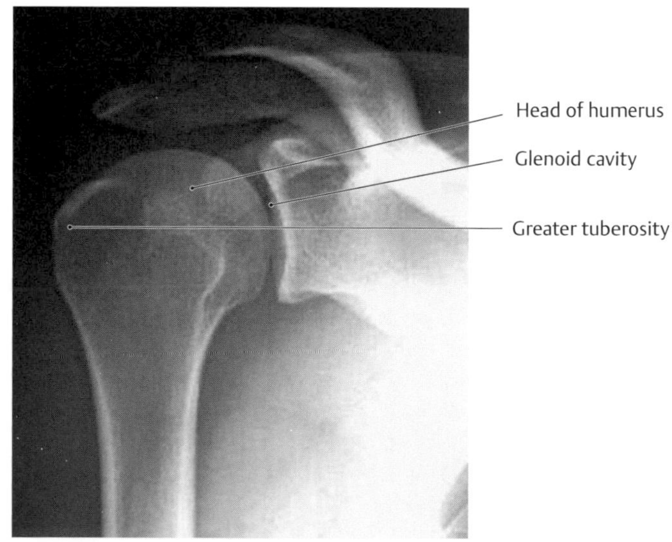
Head of humerus
Glenoid cavity
Greater tuberosity

Fig. 21.13 Glenohumeral joint: Capsule and ligaments
Right shoulder.

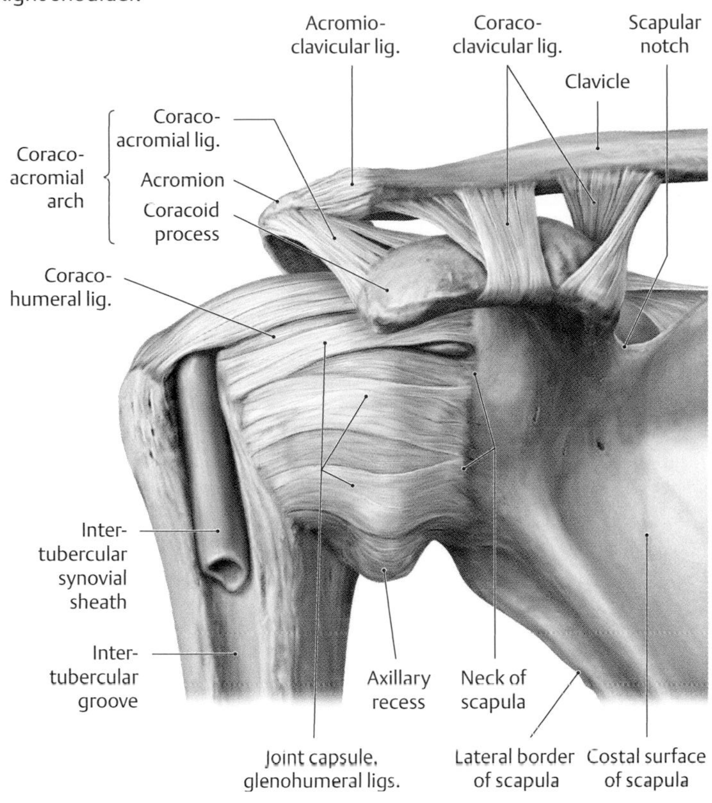

Acromio-clavicular lig.
Coraco-clavicular lig.
Scapular notch
Clavicle
Coraco-acromial lig.
Coraco-acromial arch
Acromion
Coracoid process
Coraco-humeral lig.
Inter-tubercular synovial sheath
Inter-tubercular groove
Axillary recess
Neck of scapula
Joint capsule, glenohumeral ligs.
Lateral border of scapula
Costal surface of scapula

A Anterior view.

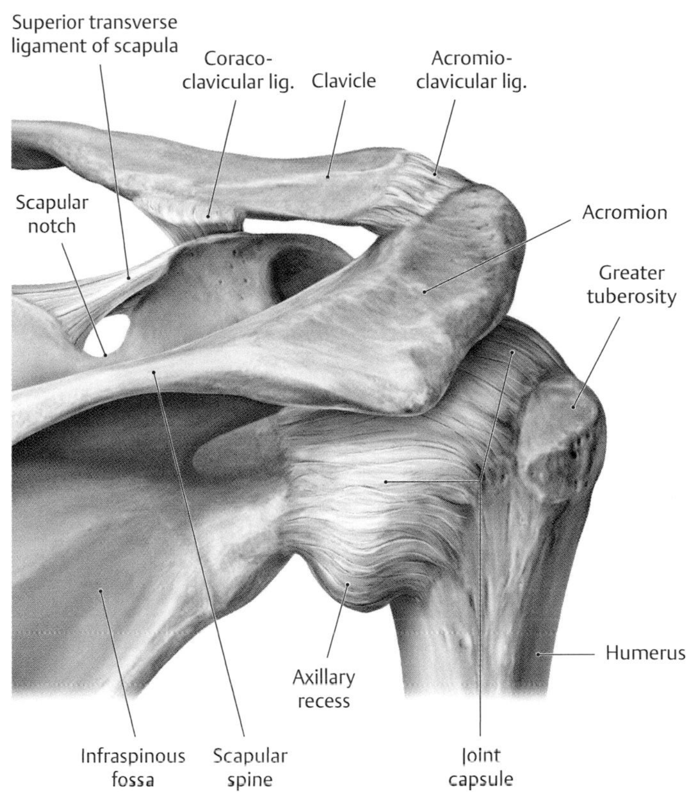

Superior transverse ligament of scapula
Coraco-clavicular lig.
Clavicle
Acromio-clavicular lig.
Scapular notch
Acromion
Greater tuberosity
Humerus
Axillary recess
Infraspinous fossa
Scapular spine
Joint capsule

B Posterior view.

Fig. 21.14 Glenohumeral joint cavity
Anterior view.

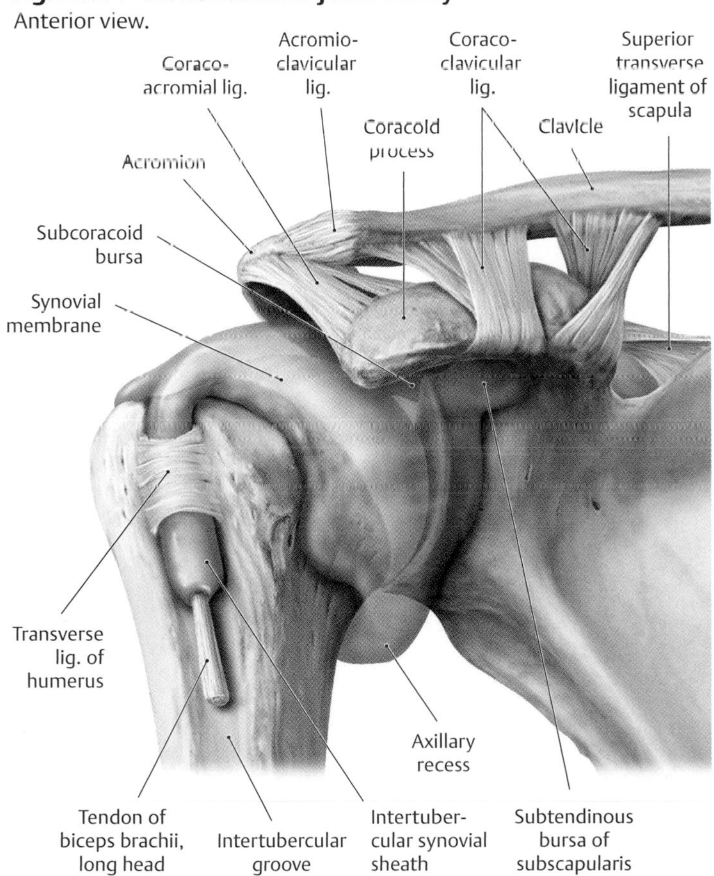

Coraco-acromial lig.
Acromio-clavicular lig.
Coraco-clavicular lig.
Superior transverse ligament of scapula
Coracoid process
Clavicle
Acromion
Subcoracoid bursa
Synovial membrane
Transverse lig. of humerus
Axillary recess
Tendon of biceps brachii, long head
Intertubercular groove
Intertuber-cular synovial sheath
Subtendinous bursa of subscapularis

Fig. 21.15 MRI of the shoulder
Coronal section, anterior view.

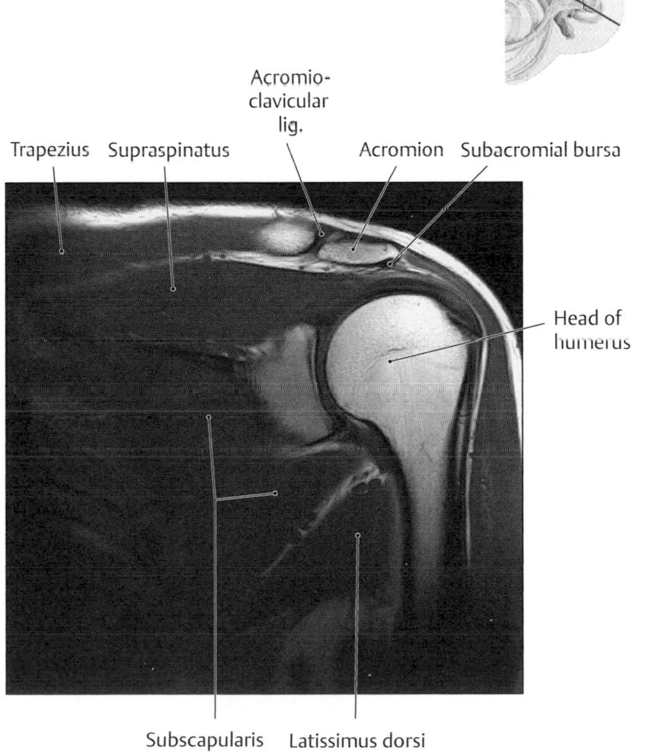

Acromio-clavicular lig.
Trapezius
Supraspinatus
Acromion
Subacromial bursa
Head of humerus
Subscapularis
Latissimus dorsi

Subacromial Space & Bursae

Fig. 21.16 Subacromial space

Right shoulder.

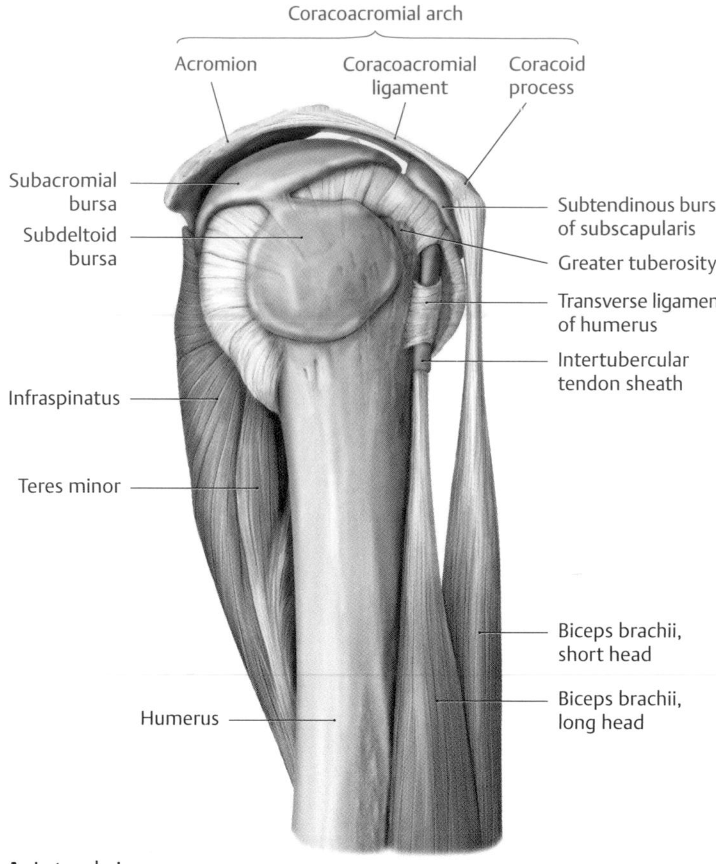

Coracoacromial arch
Acromion
Coracoacromial ligament
Coracoid process
Subacromial bursa
Subdeltoid bursa
Subtendinous bursa of subscapularis
Greater tuberosity
Transverse ligament of humerus
Intertubercular tendon sheath
Infraspinatus
Teres minor
Biceps brachii, short head
Biceps brachii, long head
Humerus

A Lateral view.

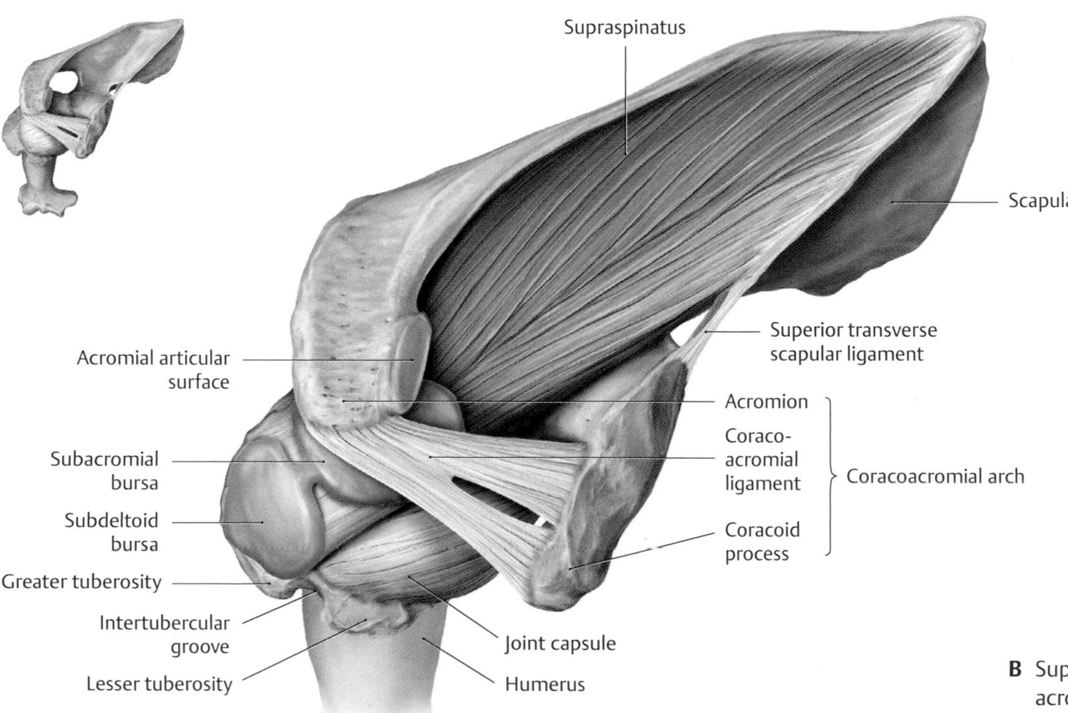

Supraspinatus
Scapula
Superior transverse scapular ligament
Acromial articular surface
Acromion
Coraco-acromial ligament
Coracoacromial arch
Coracoid process
Subacromial bursa
Subdeltoid bursa
Greater tuberosity
Intertubercular groove
Lesser tuberosity
Joint capsule
Humerus

B Superior view. Note the position of the subacromial bursa between the supraspinatus muscle and the coracoacromial arch.

Fig. 21.17 Subacromial bursa and glenoid cavity

Right shoulder, lateral view of sagittal section with humerus removed.

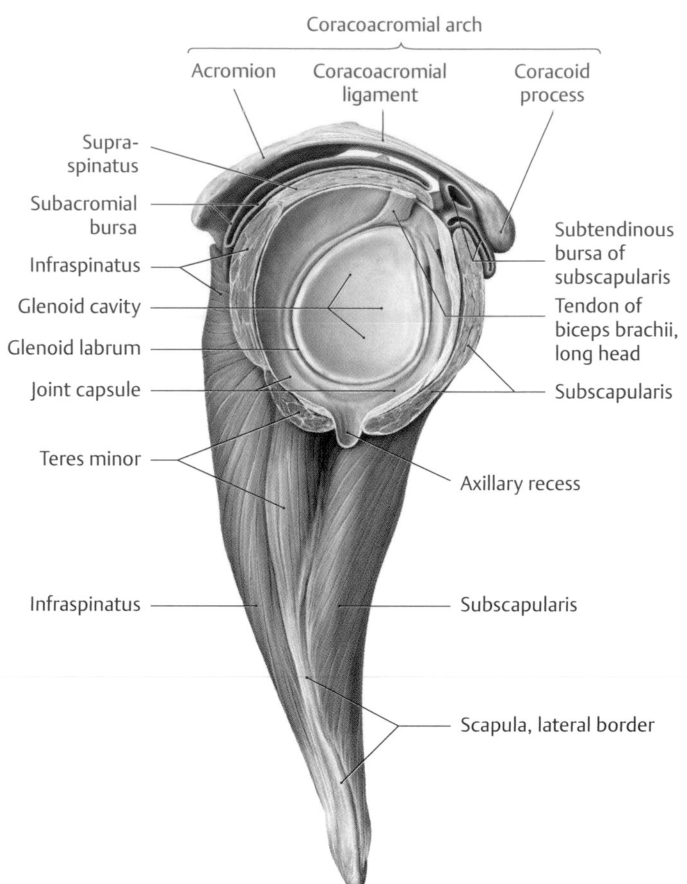

Coracoacromial arch
Acromion
Coracoacromial ligament
Coracoid process
Supra-spinatus
Subacromial bursa
Infraspinatus
Glenoid cavity
Glenoid labrum
Joint capsule
Teres minor
Infraspinatus
Subtendinous bursa of subscapularis
Tendon of biceps brachii, long head
Subscapularis
Axillary recess
Subscapularis
Scapula, lateral border

Fig. 21.18 **Subacromial and subdeltoid bursae**
Right shoulder, anterior view.

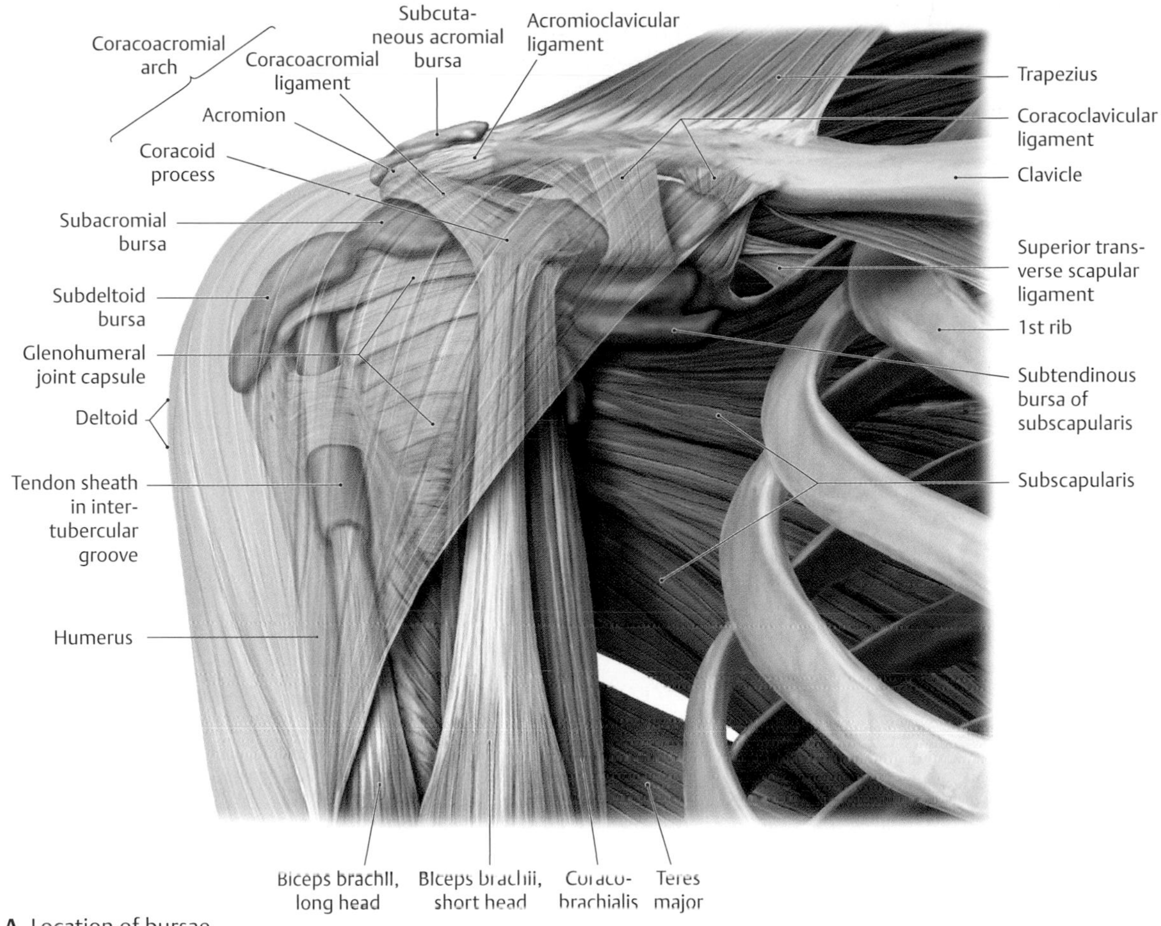
Coracoacromial arch
Coracoacromial ligament
Subcutaneous acromial bursa
Acromioclavicular ligament
Acromion
Coracoid process
Subacromial bursa
Subdeltoid bursa
Glenohumeral joint capsule
Deltoid
Tendon sheath in intertubercular groove
Humerus
Trapezius
Coracoclavicular ligament
Clavicle
Superior transverse scapular ligament
1st rib
Subtendinous bursa of subscapularis
Subscapularis
Biceps brachii, long head
Biceps brachii, short head
Coracobrachialis
Teres major

A Location of bursae.

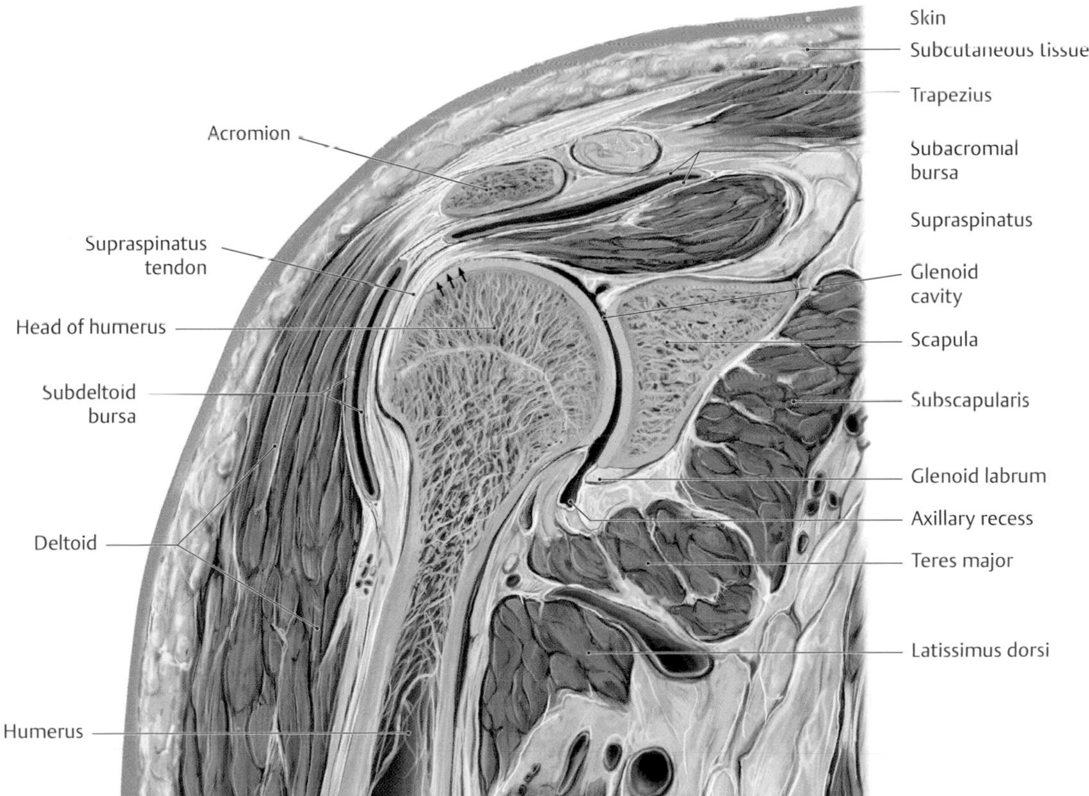
Skin
Subcutaneous tissue
Trapezius
Acromion
Subacromial bursa
Supraspinatus
Supraspinatus tendon
Glenoid cavity
Head of humerus
Scapula
Subdeltoid bursa
Subscapularis
Glenoid labrum
Axillary recess
Deltoid
Teres major
Latissimus dorsi
Humerus

B Coronal section. The arrows are pointing at the supraspinatus tendon, which is frequently injured in a "rotator cuff tear" (for rotator cuff, see p. 296).

Anterior Muscles of the Shoulder & Arm (I)

Fig. 21.19 **Anterior muscles of the shoulder and arm**
Right side, anterior view. Muscle origins are shown in red, insertions in blue.

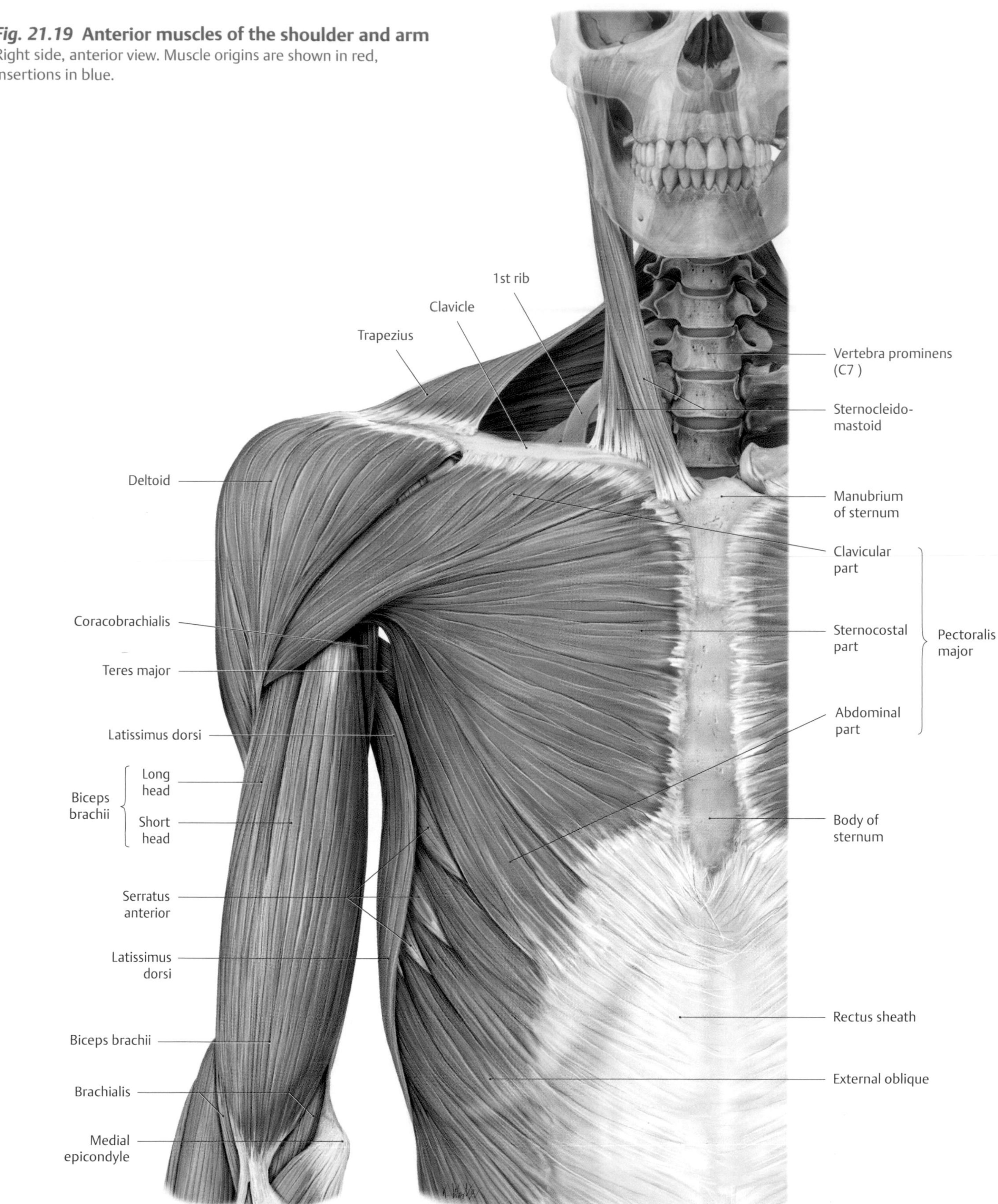
1st rib
Clavicle
Trapezius
Vertebra prominens (C7)
Sternocleido-mastoid
Deltoid
Manubrium of sternum
Clavicular part
Sternocostal part
Abdominal part
Pectoralis major
Coracobrachialis
Teres major
Latissimus dorsi
Biceps brachii
Long head
Short head
Body of sternum
Serratus anterior
Latissimus dorsi
Rectus sheath
Biceps brachii
External oblique
Brachialis
Medial epicondyle

A Superficial dissection.

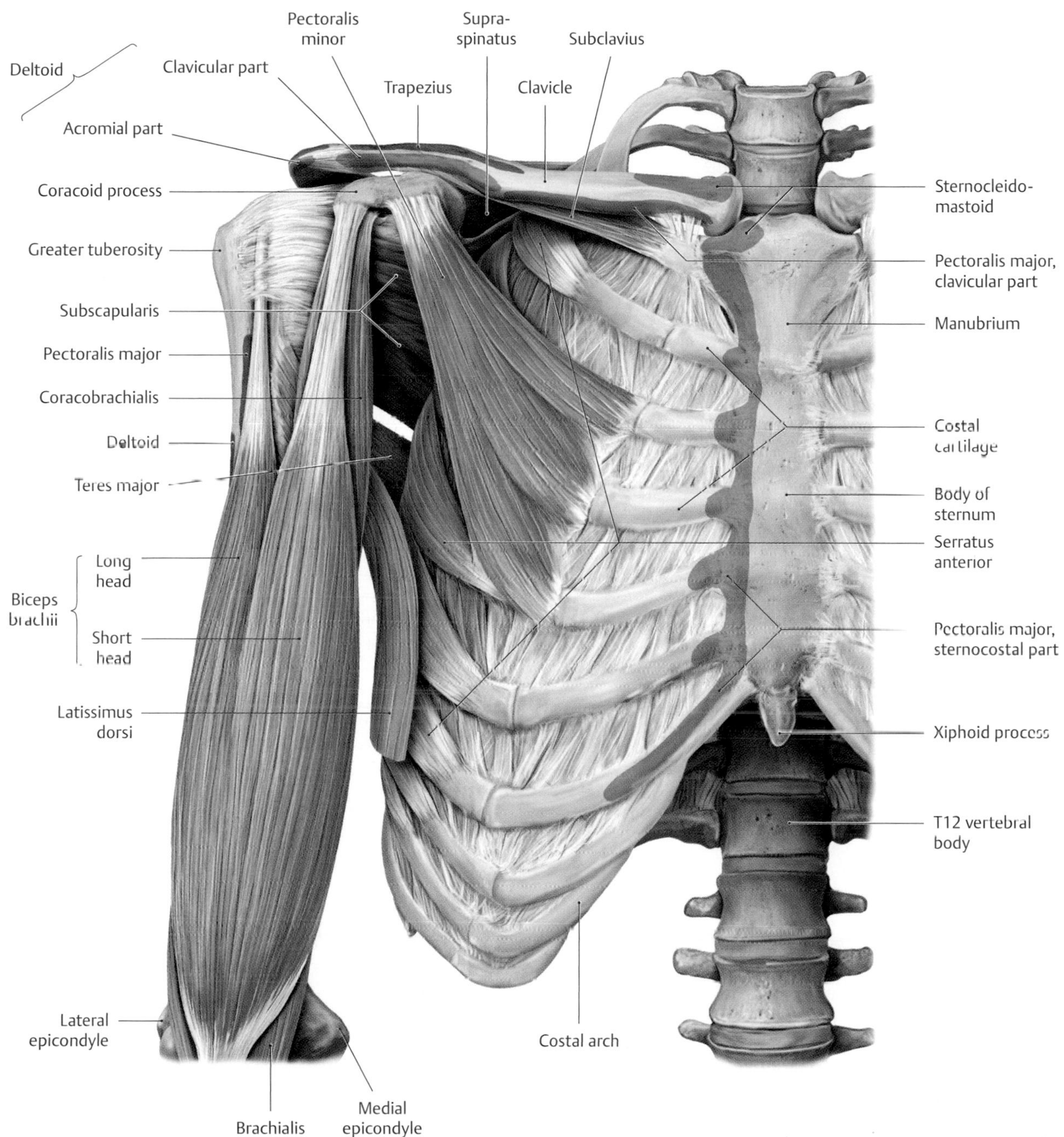

Pectoralis minor
Supra-spinatus
Subclavius
Deltoid
Clavicular part
Trapezius
Clavicle
Acromial part
Coracoid process
Sternocleido-mastoid
Greater tuberosity
Pectoralis major, clavicular part
Subscapularis
Manubrium
Pectoralis major
Coracobrachialis
Costal cartilage
Deltoid
Teres major
Body of sternum
Serratus anterior
Biceps brachii
Long head
Short head
Pectoralis major, sternocostal part
Latissimus dorsi
Xiphoid process
T12 vertebral body
Lateral epicondyle
Costal arch
Brachialis
Medial epicondyle

B Deep dissection. *Removed:* Sternocleidomastoid, trapezius, pectoralis major, deltoid, and external oblique muscles.

Anterior Muscles of the Shoulder & Arm (II)

Fig. 21.20 Anterior muscles of the shoulder and arm: Dissection
Right arm, anterior view. Muscle origins are shown in red, insertions in blue.

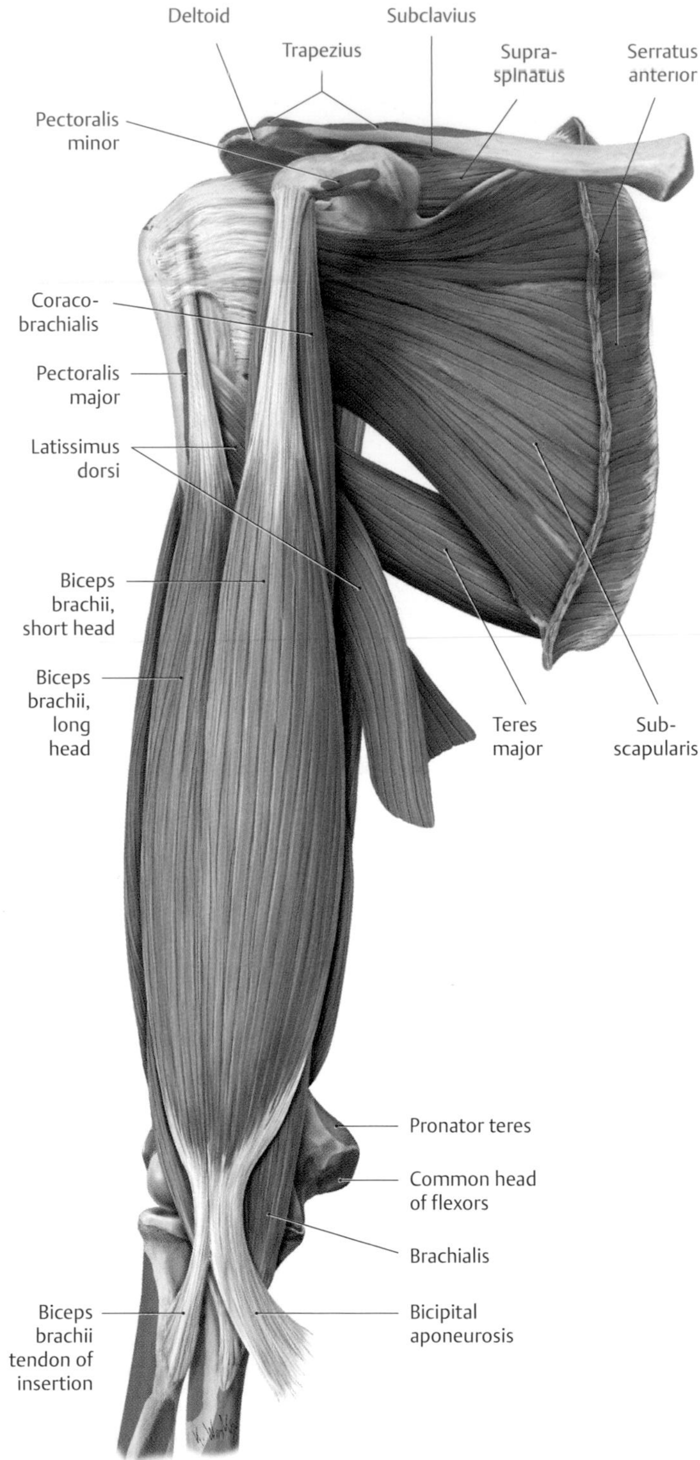
Deltoid
Subclavius
Trapezius
Supra-
spinatus
Serratus
anterior
Pectoralis
minor
Coraco-
brachialis
Pectoralis
major
Latissimus
dorsi
Biceps
brachii,
short head
Biceps
brachii,
long
head
Teres
major
Sub-
scapularis
Pronator teres
Common head
of flexors
Brachialis
Biceps
brachii
tendon of
insertion
Bicipital
aponeurosis

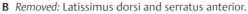

A *Removed:* Thoracic skeleton. *Partially removed:* Latissimus dorsi and serratus anterior.

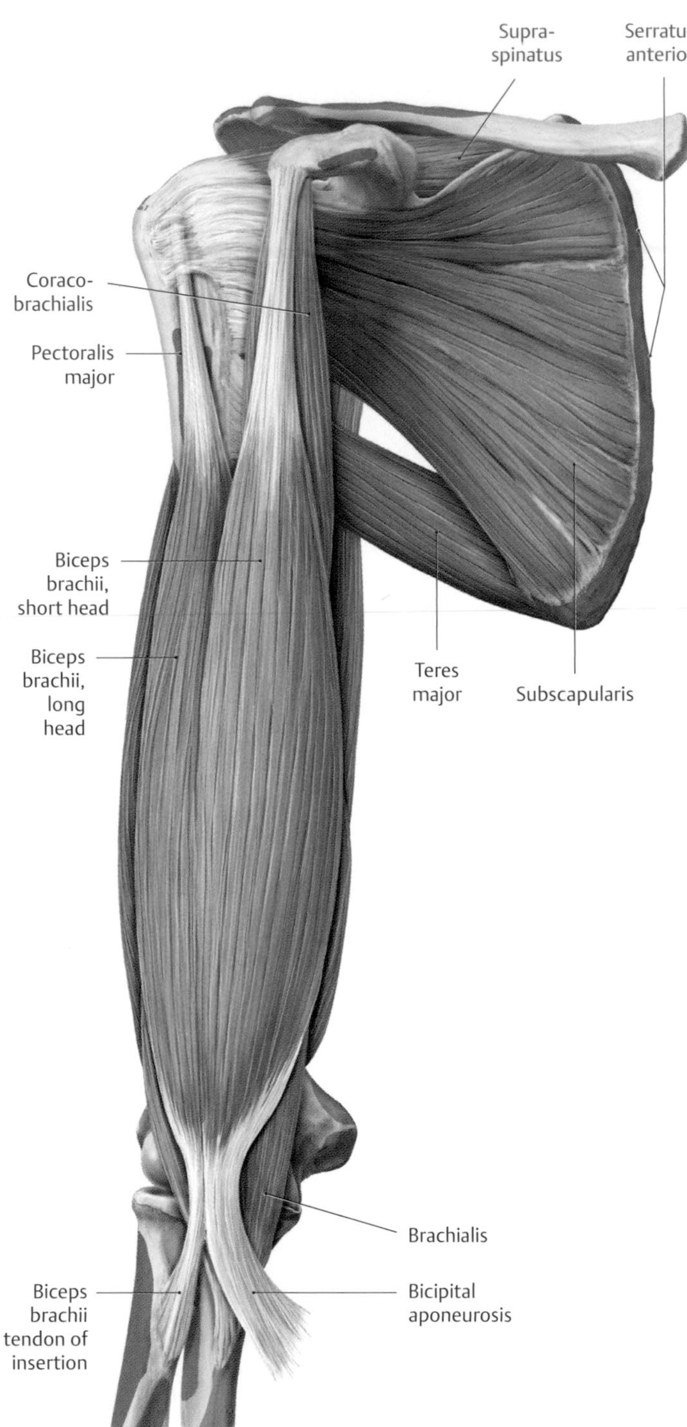
Supra-
spinatus
Serratus
anterior
Coraco-
brachialis
Pectoralis
major
Biceps
brachii,
short head
Biceps
brachii,
long
head
Teres
major
Subscapularis
Brachialis
Biceps
brachii
tendon of
insertion
Bicipital
aponeurosis

B *Removed:* Latissimus dorsi and serratus anterior.

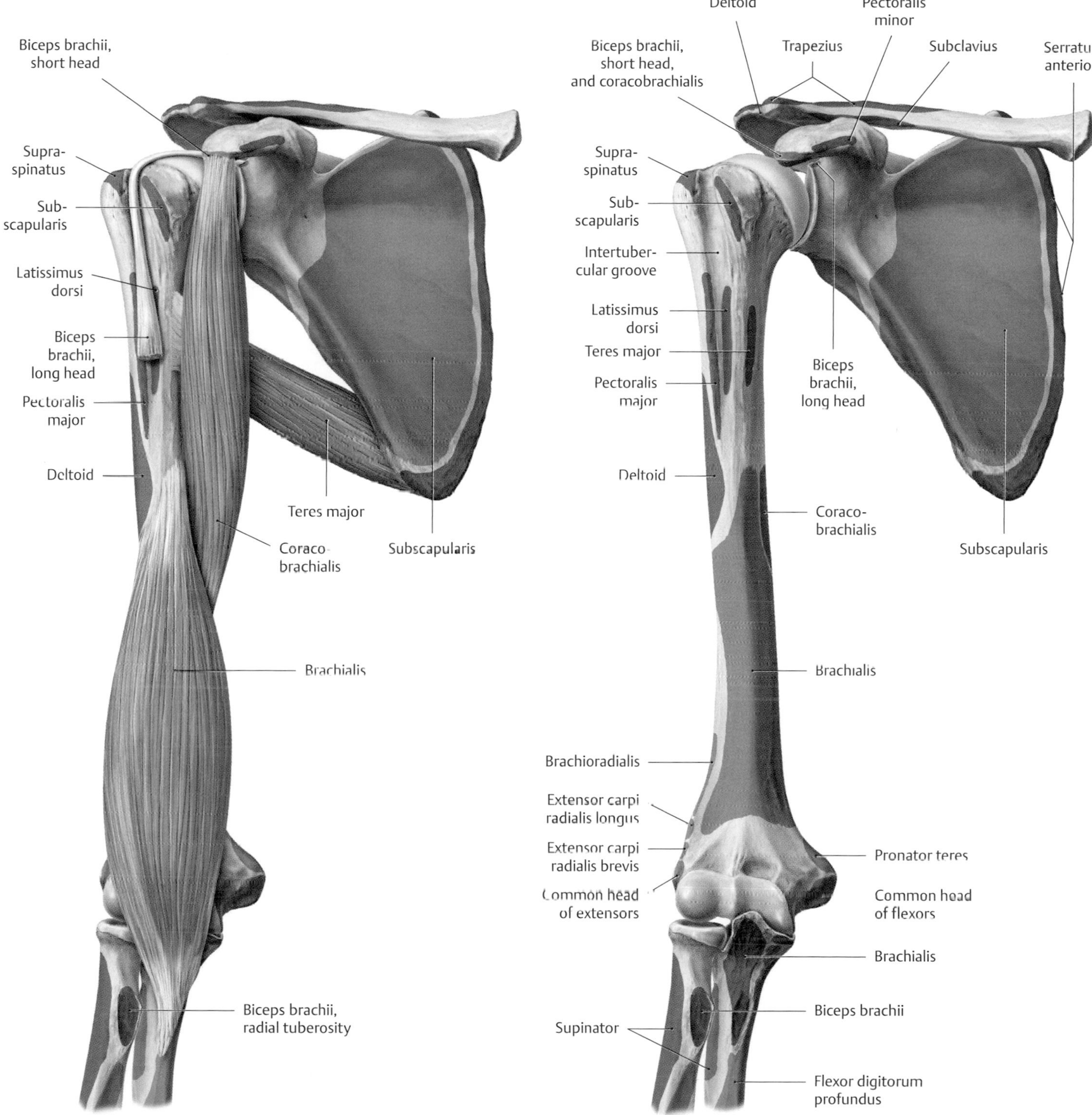

Biceps brachii, short head
Supra-spinatus
Sub-scapularis
Latissimus dorsi
Biceps brachii, long head
Pectoralis major
Deltoid
Teres major
Coraco-brachialis
Subscapularis
Brachialis
Biceps brachii, radial tuberosity
Deltoid
Pectoralis minor
Biceps brachii, short head, and coracobrachialis
Trapezius
Subclavius
Serratus anterior
Supra-spinatus
Sub-scapularis
Intertuber-cular groove
Latissimus dorsi
Teres major
Pectoralis major
Biceps brachii, long head
Deltoid
Coraco-brachialis
Subscapularis
Brachialis
Brachioradialis
Extensor carpi radialis longus
Extensor carpi radialis brevis
Common head of extensors
Pronator teres
Common head of flexors
Brachialis
Biceps brachii
Supinator
Flexor digitorum profundus

C *Removed:* Subscapularis and supraspinatus muscles. *Partially removed:* Biceps brachii.

D *Removed:* Biceps brachii, coracobrachialis, and teres major.

Posterior Muscles of the Shoulder & Arm (I)

Fig. 21.21 **Posterior muscles of the shoulder and arm**
Right side, posterior view.

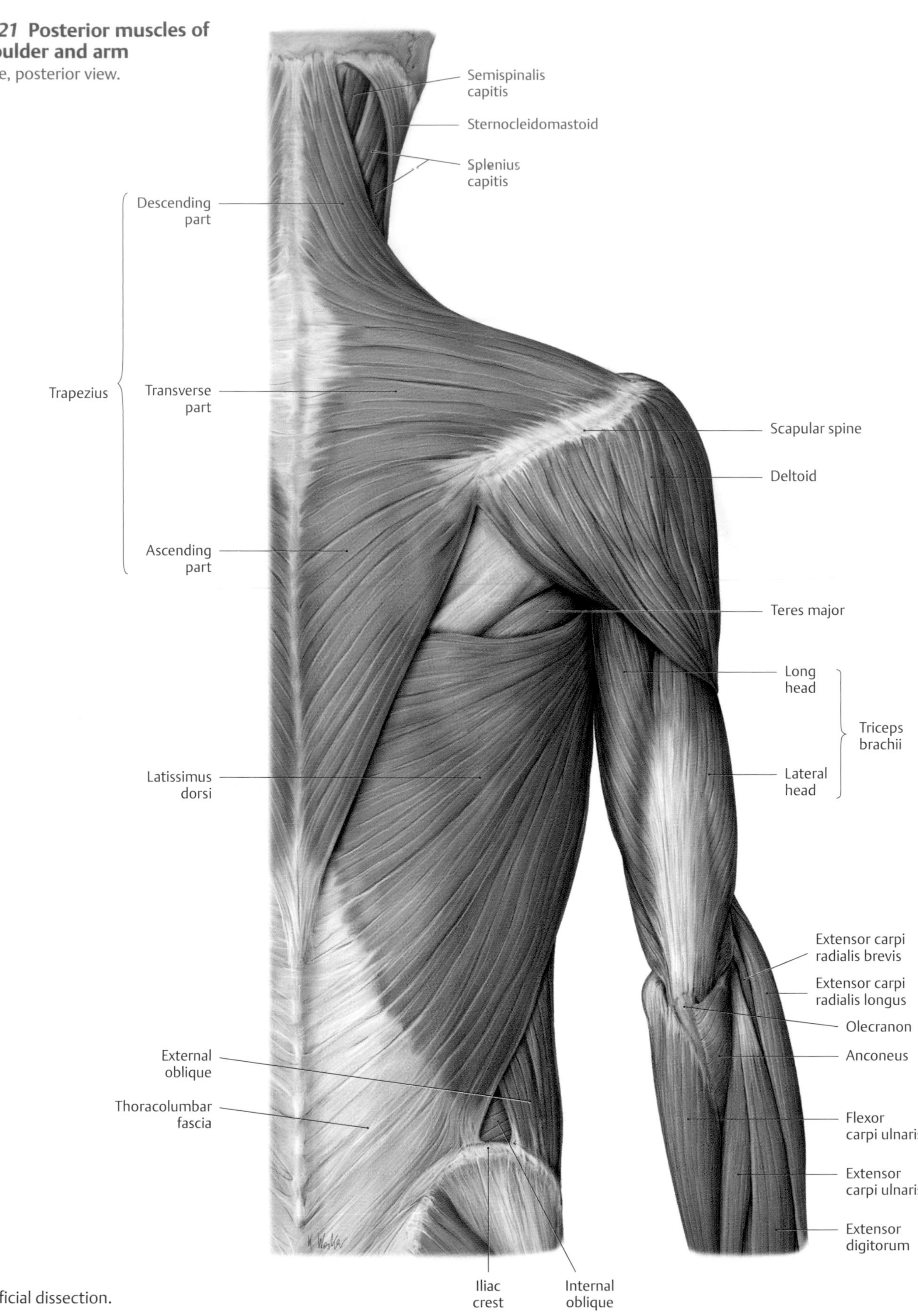
Semispinalis capitis
Sternocleidomastoid
Splenius capitis
Trapezius
Descending part
Transverse part
Ascending part
Scapular spine
Deltoid
Teres major
Long head
Lateral head
Triceps brachii
Latissimus dorsi
Extensor carpi radialis brevis
Extensor carpi radialis longus
Olecranon
Anconeus
External oblique
Thoracolumbar fascia
Flexor carpi ulnaris
Extensor carpi ulnaris
Extensor digitorum
Iliac crest
Internal oblique

A Superficial dissection.

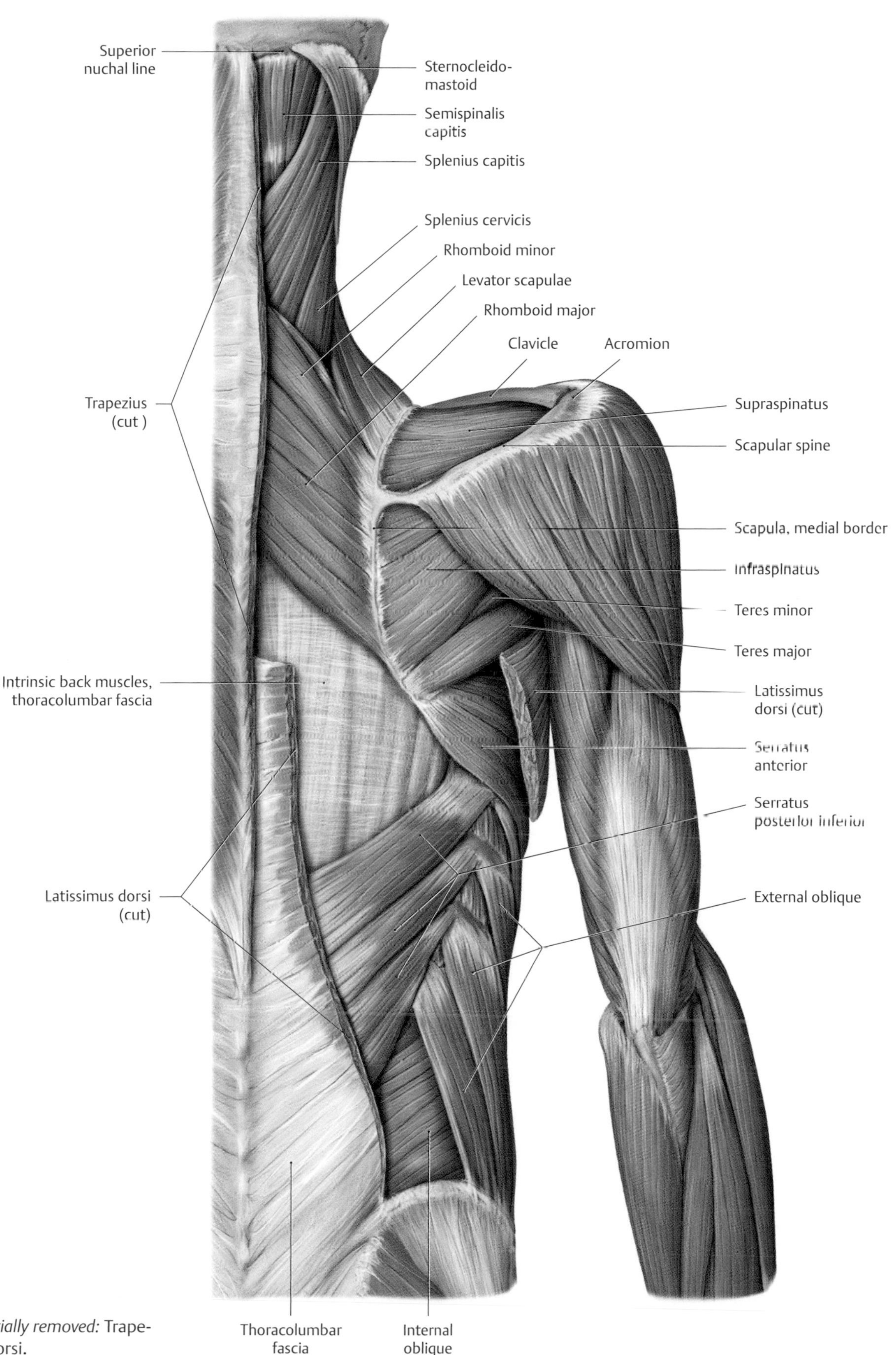
Superior nuchal line
Sternocleido-mastoid
Semispinalis capitis
Splenius capitis
Splenius cervicis
Rhomboid minor
Levator scapulae
Rhomboid major
Clavicle
Acromion
Trapezius (cut)
Supraspinatus
Scapular spine
Scapula, medial border
Infraspinatus
Teres minor
Teres major
Intrinsic back muscles, thoracolumbar fascia
Latissimus dorsi (cut)
Serratus anterior
Serratus posterior inferior
Latissimus dorsi (cut)
External oblique
Thoracolumbar fascia
Internal oblique

B Deep dissection. *Partially removed:* Trapezius and latissimus dorsi.

Posterior Muscles of the Shoulder & Arm (II)

***Fig. 21.22* Posterior muscles of the shoulder and arm: Dissection**
Right arm, posterior view. Muscle origins are shown in red, insertions in blue.

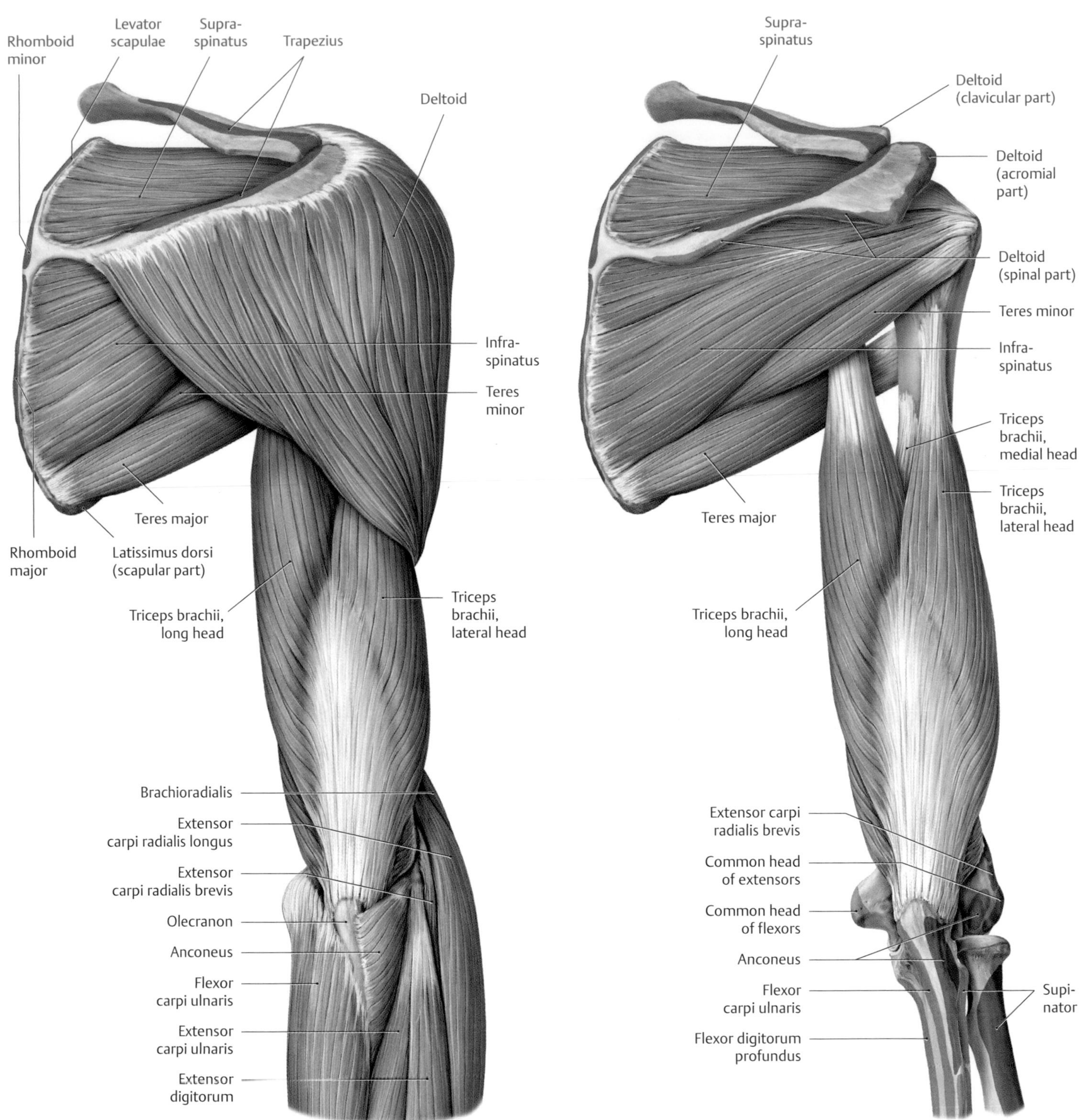

Rhomboid minor
Levator scapulae
Supra-spinatus
Trapezius
Deltoid
Infra-spinatus
Teres minor
Teres major
Rhomboid major
Latissimus dorsi (scapular part)
Triceps brachii, long head
Triceps brachii, lateral head
Brachioradialis
Extensor carpi radialis longus
Extensor carpi radialis brevis
Olecranon
Anconeus
Flexor carpi ulnaris
Extensor carpi ulnaris
Extensor digitorum
Supra-spinatus
Deltoid (clavicular part)
Deltoid (acromial part)
Deltoid (spinal part)
Teres minor
Infra-spinatus
Triceps brachii, medial head
Triceps brachii, lateral head
Teres major
Triceps brachii, long head
Extensor carpi radialis brevis
Common head of extensors
Common head of flexors
Anconeus
Flexor carpi ulnaris
Flexor digitorum profundus
Supi-nator

A *Removed:* Rhomboids major and minor, serratus anterior, and levator scapulae.

B *Removed:* Deltoid and forearm muscles.

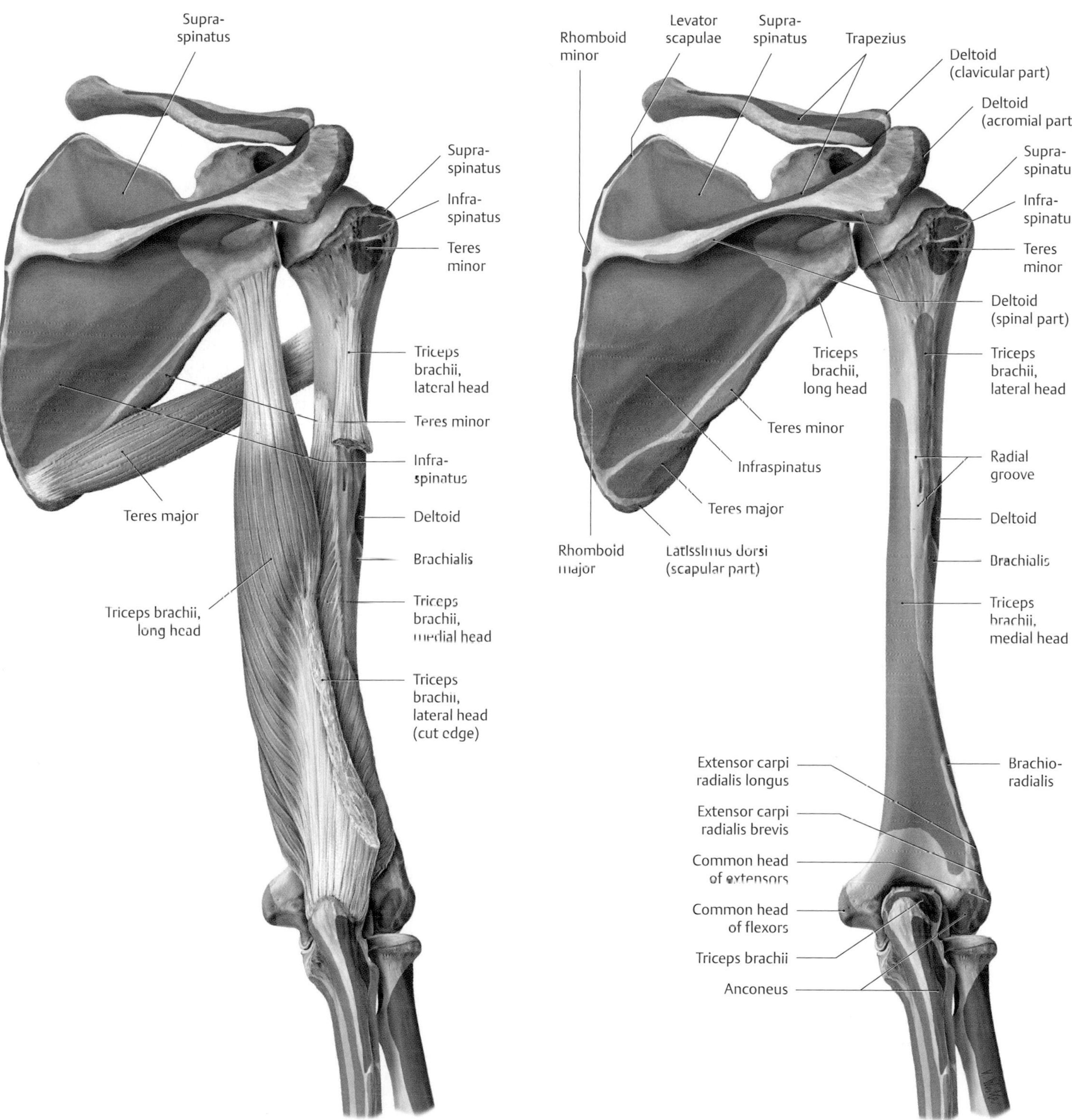
Supra-
spinatus
Supra-
spinatus
Infra-
spinatus
Teres
minor
Triceps
brachii,
lateral head
Teres minor
Infra-
spinatus
Teres major
Deltoid
Brachialis
Triceps brachii,
long head
Triceps
brachii,
medial head
Triceps
brachii,
lateral head
(cut edge)
Rhomboid
minor
Levator
scapulae
Supra-
spinatus
Trapezius
Deltoid
(clavicular part)
Deltoid
(acromial part)
Supra-
spinatus
Infra-
spinatus
Teres
minor
Deltoid
(spinal part)
Triceps
brachii,
long head
Triceps
brachii,
lateral head
Teres minor
Infraspinatus
Radial
groove
Teres major
Deltoid
Rhomboid
major
Latissimus dorsi
(scapular part)
Brachialis
Triceps
brachii,
medial head
Extensor carpi
radialis longus
Brachio-
radialis
Extensor carpi
radialis brevis
Common head
of extensors
Common head
of flexors
Triceps brachii
Anconeus

C *Removed:* Supraspinatus, infraspinatus, and teres minor. *Partially removed:* Triceps brachii.

D *Removed:* Triceps brachii and teres major.

Muscle Facts (I)

The actions of the three parts of the deltoid muscle depend on their relationship to the position of the humerus and its axis of motion. At less than 60 degrees, the muscles act as adductors, but at greater than 60 degrees, they act as abductors. As a result, the parts of the deltoid can act antagonistically as well as synergistically.

Fig. 21.23 **Deltoid**
Right shoulder.

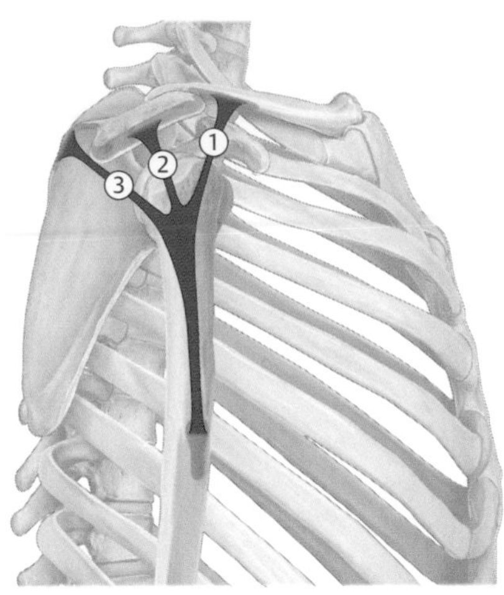

①
②
③

A Parts of the deltoid, right lateral view, schematic.

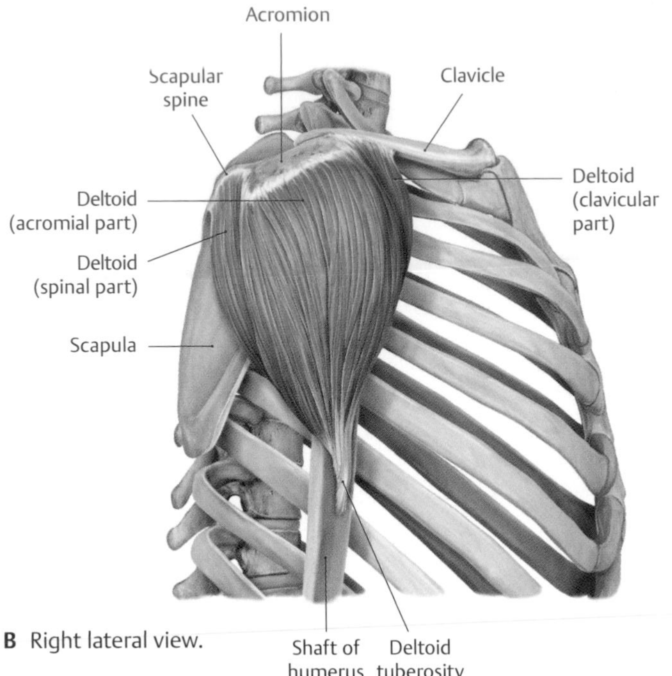

Acromion
Scapular spine
Clavicle
Deltoid (acromial part)
Deltoid (clavicular part)
Deltoid (spinal part)
Scapula
Shaft of humerus
Deltoid tuberosity

B Right lateral view.

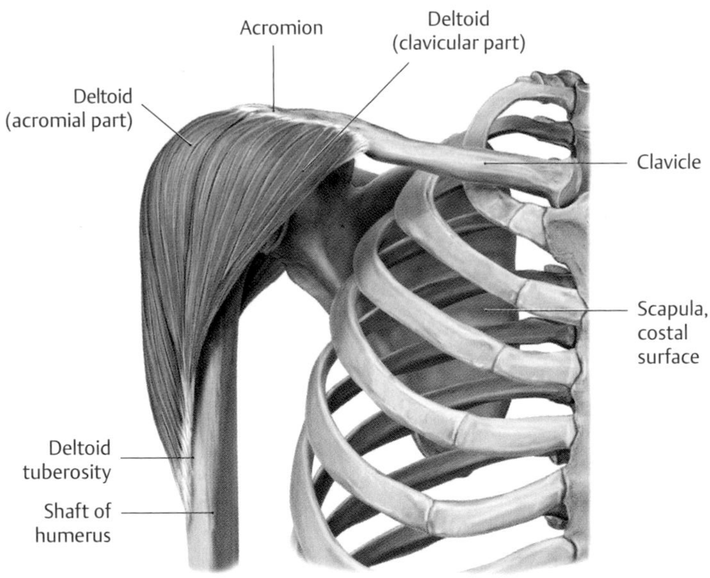

Acromion
Deltoid (clavicular part)
Deltoid (acromial part)
Clavicle
Scapula, costal surface
Deltoid tuberosity
Shaft of humerus

C Anterior view.

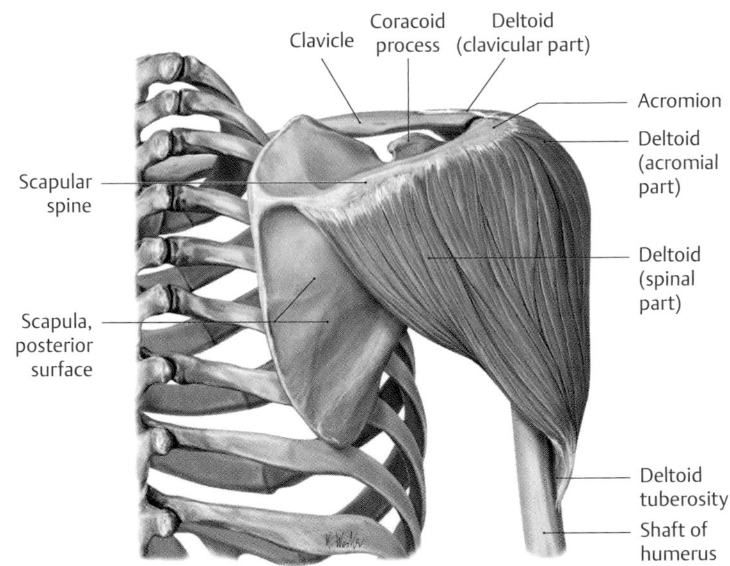

Clavicle
Coracoid process
Deltoid (clavicular part)
Acromion
Deltoid (acromial part)
Scapular spine
Deltoid (spinal part)
Scapula, posterior surface
Deltoid tuberosity
Shaft of humerus

D Posterior view.

Table 21.1 Parts of the deltoid

Muscle		Origin	Insertion	Innervation	Action*
Deltoid	① Clavicular part	Lateral one third of clavicle	Humerus (deltoid tuberosity)	Axillary n. (C5, C6)	Flexion, internal rotation, adduction
	② Acromial part	Acromion			Abduction
	③ Spinal part	Scapular spine			Extension, external rotation, adduction

* Between 60 and 90 degrees of abduction, the clavicular and spinal parts assist the acromial part with abduction.

Fig. 21.24 Rotator cuff

Right shoulder. The rotator cuff consists of four muscles: supraspinatus, infraspinatus, teres minor, and subscapularis.

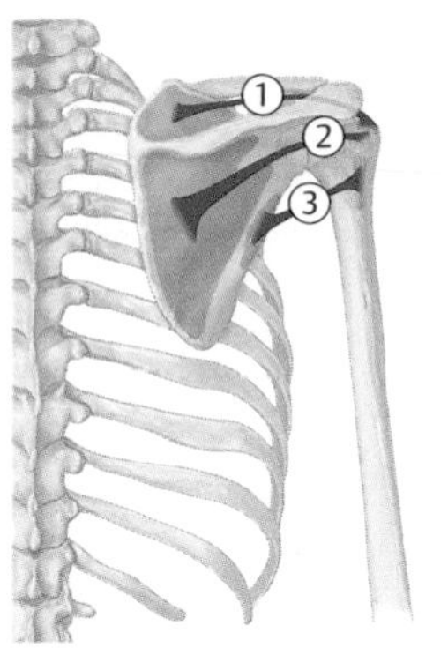

①
②
③

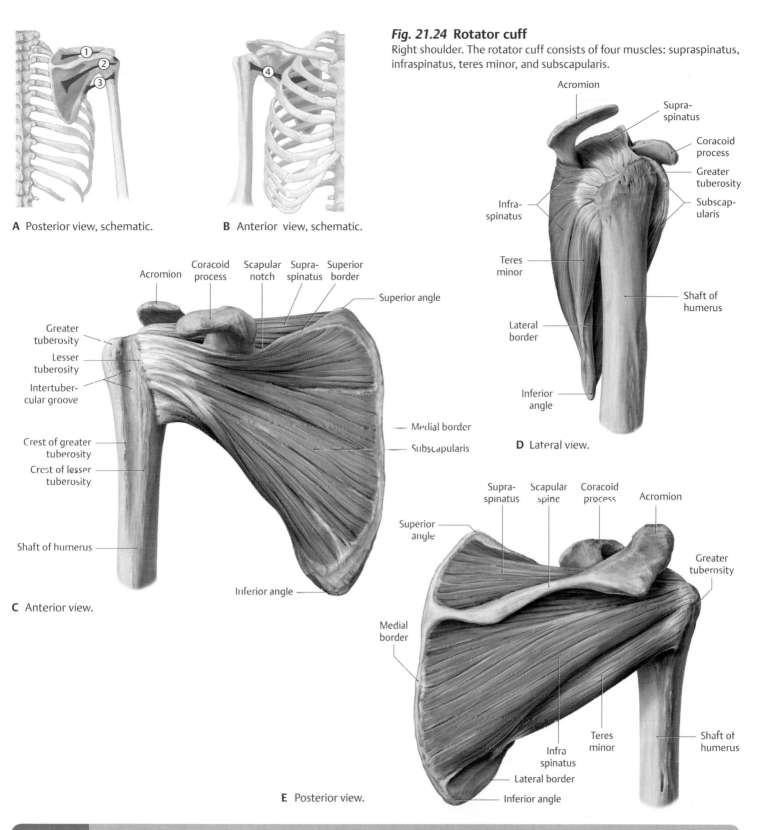

A Posterior view, schematic.

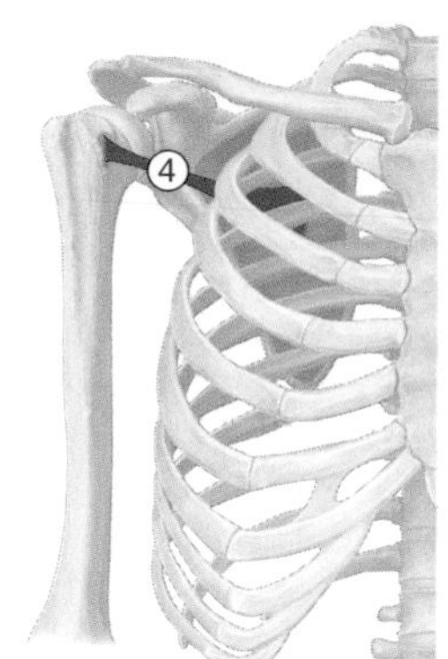

④

B Anterior view, schematic.

Acromion
Coracoid process
Scapular notch
Supra-spinatus
Superior border
Superior angle
Greater tuberosity
Lesser tuberosity
Intertuber-cular groove
Crest of greater tuberosity
Crest of lesser tuberosity
Shaft of humerus
Medial border
Subscapularis
Inferior angle

C Anterior view.

Acromion
Supra-spinatus
Coracoid process
Greater tuberosity
Subscap-ularis
Infra-spinatus
Teres minor
Shaft of humerus
Lateral border
Inferior angle

D Lateral view.

Supra-spinatus
Scapular spine
Coracoid process
Acromion
Superior angle
Greater tuberosity
Medial border
Teres minor
Infra spinatus
Shaft of humerus
Lateral border
Inferior angle

E Posterior view.

Table 21.2 **Muscles of the rotator cuff**

Muscle	Origin		Insertion		Innervation	Action
① Supraspinatus	Scapula	Supraspinous fossa	Humerus	Greater tuberosity	Suprascapular n. (C4–C6)	Abduction
② Infraspinatus		Infraspinous fossa				External rotation
③ Teres minor		Lateral border			Axillary n. (C5, C6)	External rotation, weak adduction
④ Subscapularis		Subscapular fossa		Lesser tuberosity	Subscapular n. (C5, C6)	Internal rotation

Muscle Facts (II)

Fig. 21.25 **Pectoralis major and coracobrachialis**
Anterior view.

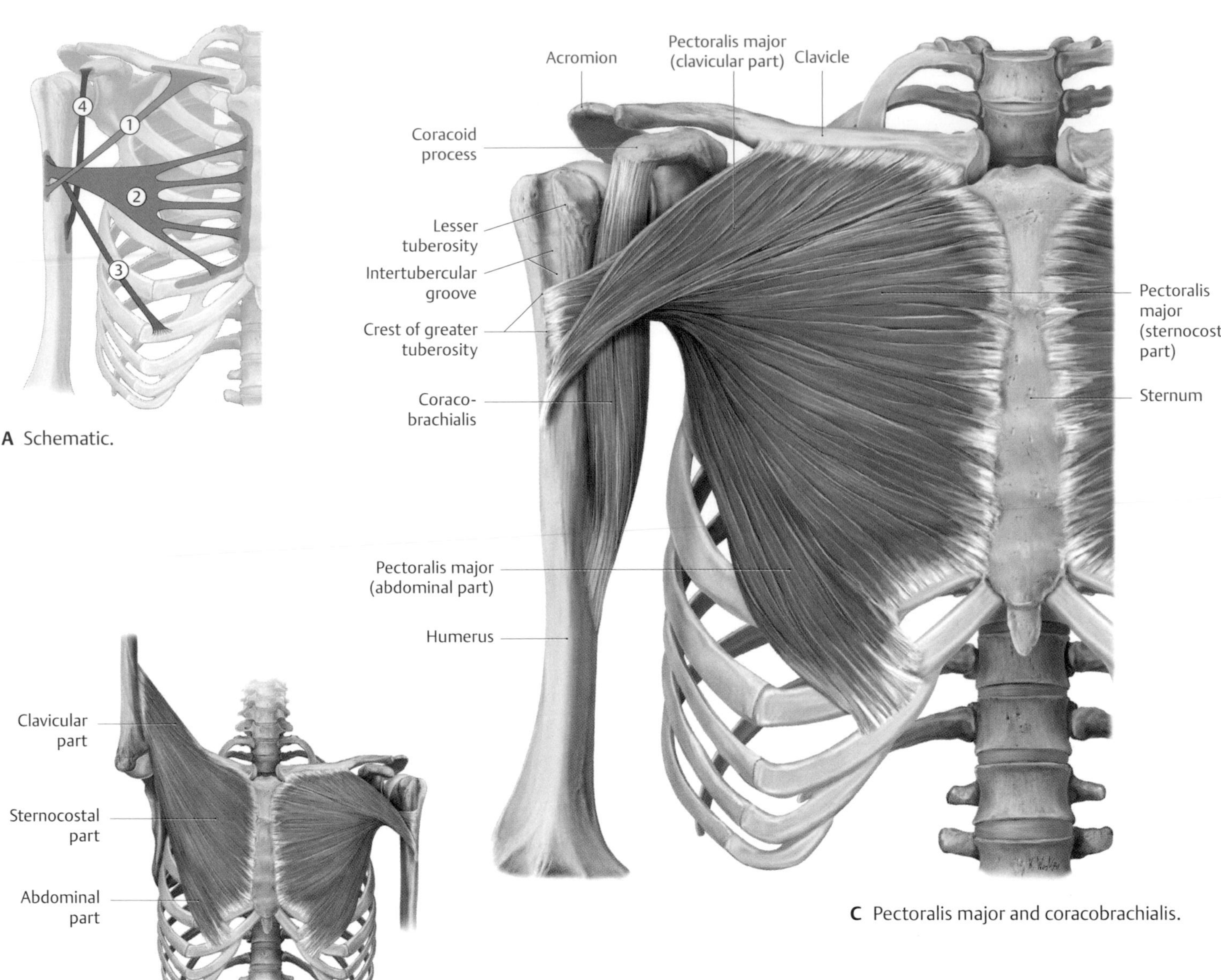

④
①
②
③
Acromion
Pectoralis major
(clavicular part)
Clavicle
Coracoid
process
Lesser
tuberosity
Intertubercular
groove
Crest of greater
tuberosity
Coraco-
brachialis
Pectoralis
major
(sternocostal
part)
Sternum
Pectoralis major
(abdominal part)
Humerus
Clavicular
part
Sternocostal
part
Abdominal
part

A Schematic.

B Pectoralis major in neutral position (left) and elevation (right).

C Pectoralis major and coracobrachialis.

Table 21.3	**Pectoralis major and coracobrachialis**				
Muscle		**Origin**	**Insertion**	**Innervation**	**Action**
Pectoralis major	① Clavicular part	Clavicle (medial half)	Humerus (crest of greater tuberosity)	Medial and lateral pectoral nn. (C5–T1)	Entire muscle: adduction, internal rotation Clavicular and sternocostal parts: flexion; assist in respiration when shoulder is fixed
	② Sternocostal part	Sternum and costal cartilages 1–6			
	③ Abdominal part	Rectus sheath (anterior layer)			
④ Coracobrachialis		Scapula (coracoid process)	Humerus (in line with crest of lesser tuberosity)	Musculocutaneous nn. (C5–C7)	Flexion, adduction, internal rotation

***Fig. 21.26* Subclavius and pectoralis minor**
Right side, anterior view.

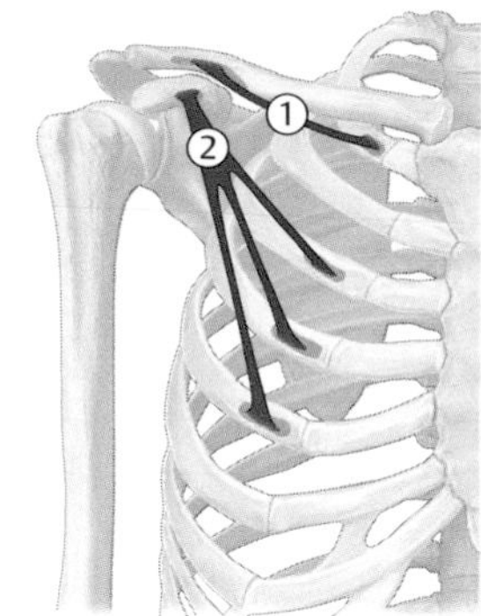

①
②

A Schematic.

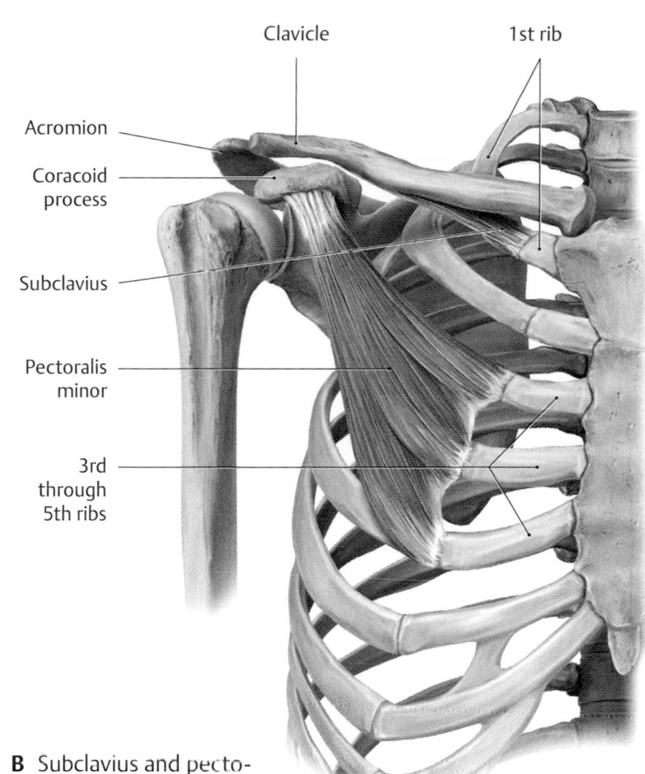

Clavicle
1st rib
Acromion
Coracoid process
Subclavius
Pectoralis minor
3rd through 5th ribs

B Subclavius and pectoralis minor.

***Fig. 21.27* Serratus anterior**
Right lateral view.

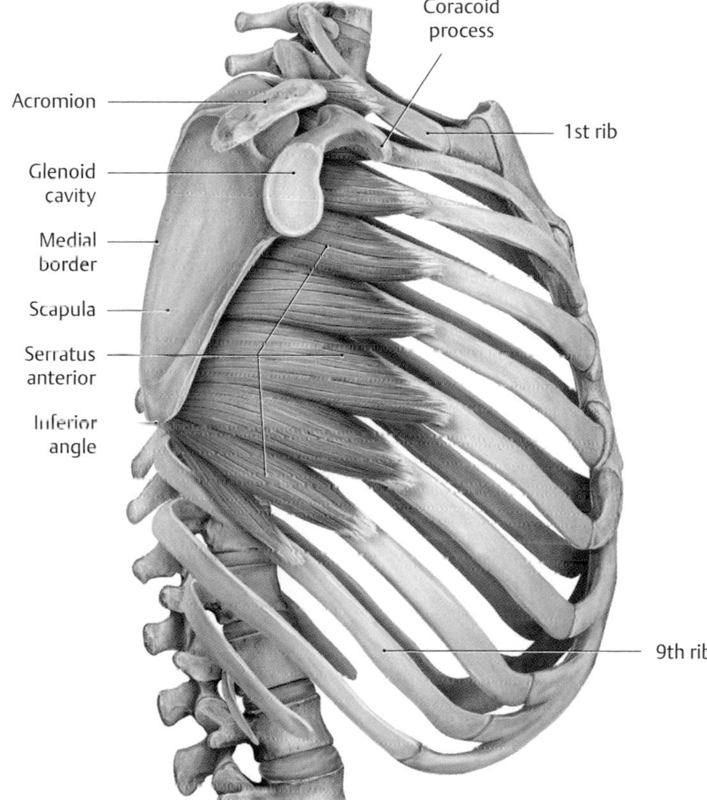

Coracoid process
Acromion
1st rib
Glenoid cavity
Medial border
Scapula
Serratus anterior
Inferior angle
9th rib

A Serratus anterior.

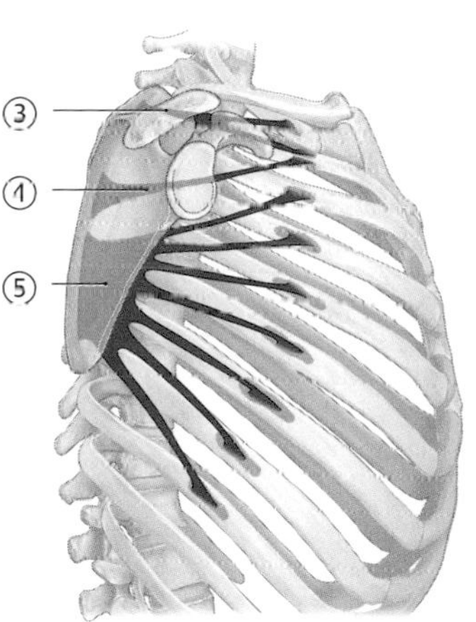

③
④
⑤

B Schematic.

Table 21.4 Subclavius, pectoralis minor, and serratus anterior

Muscle		Origin	Insertion	Innervation	Action
① Subclavius		1st rib	Clavicle (inferior surface)	N. to subclavius (C5, C6)	Steadies the clavicle in the sternoclavicular joint
② Pectoralis minor		3rd to 5th ribs	Coracoid process	Medial pectoral n. (C8, T1)	Draws scapula downward, causing inferior angle to move posteromedially; rotates glenoid inferiorly; assists in respiration
Serratus anterior	③ Superior part	1st to 9th ribs	Scapula (medial border)	Long thoracic n. (C5–C7)	Superior part: lowers the raised arm
	④ Intermediate part				Entire muscle: draws scapula laterally forward; elevates ribs when shoulder is fixed
	⑤ Inferior part				Inferior part: rotates scapula laterally

Muscle Facts (III)

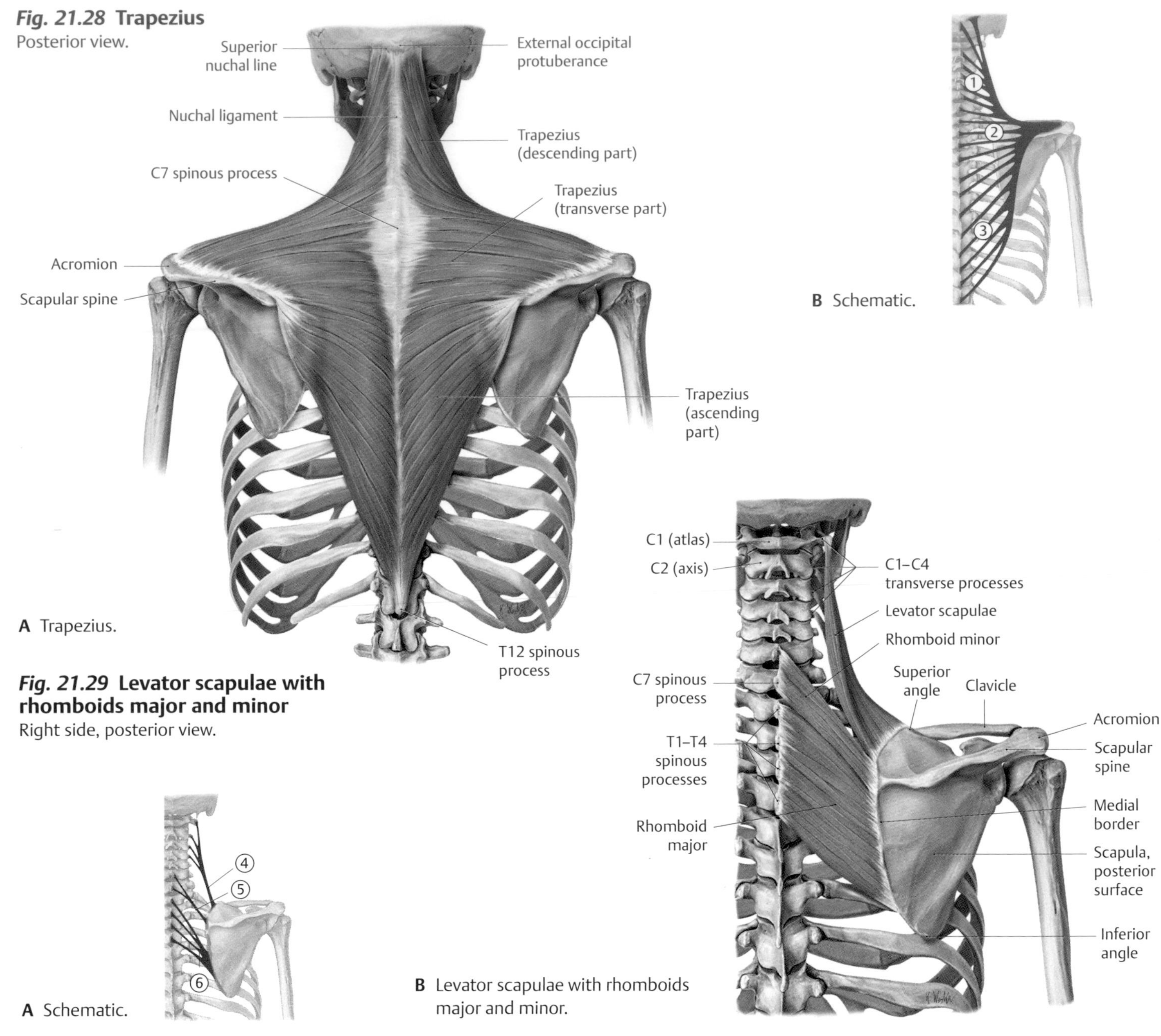

Superior nuchal line
External occipital protuberance
Nuchal ligament
Trapezius (descending part)
C7 spinous process
Trapezius (transverse part)
Acromion
Scapular spine
Trapezius (ascending part)
T12 spinous process
①
②
③
④
⑤
⑥
C1 (atlas)
C2 (axis)
C1–C4 transverse processes
Levator scapulae
Rhomboid minor
C7 spinous process
Superior angle
Clavicle
Acromion
Scapular spine
T1–T4 spinous processes
Medial border
Rhomboid major
Scapula, posterior surface
Inferior angle

Fig. 21.28 **Trapezius**
Posterior view.

A Trapezius.

B Schematic.

Fig. 21.29 **Levator scapulae with rhomboids major and minor**
Right side, posterior view.

A Schematic.

B Levator scapulae with rhomboids major and minor.

Table 21.5 Trapezius, levator scapulae, and rhomboids major and minor

Muscle		Origin	Insertion	Innervation	Action
Trapezius	① Descending part	Occipital bone; spinous process of C1–C7	Clavicle (lateral one third)	Accessory n. (CN XI); C3–C4 of cervical plexus	Draws scapula obliquely upward; rotates glenoid cavity superiorly; tilts head to same side and rotates it to opposite
	② Transverse part	Aponeurosis at T1–T4 spinous processes	Acromion		Draws scapula medially
	③ Ascending part	Spinous process of T5–T12	Scapular spine		Draws scapula medially downward
					Entire muscle: steadies scapula on thorax
④ Levator scapulae		Transverse process of C1–C4	Scapula (superior angle)	Dorsal scapular n. (C4–C5)	Draws scapula medially upward while moving inferior angle medially; inclines neck to same side
⑤ Rhomboid minor		Spinous process of C6, C7	Medial border of scapula above (minor) and below (major) scapular spine		Steadies scapula; draws scapula medially upward
⑥ Rhomboid major		Spinous process of T1–T4 vertebrae			

CN, cranial nerve.

Fig. 21.30 Latissimus dorsi and teres major
Posterior view.

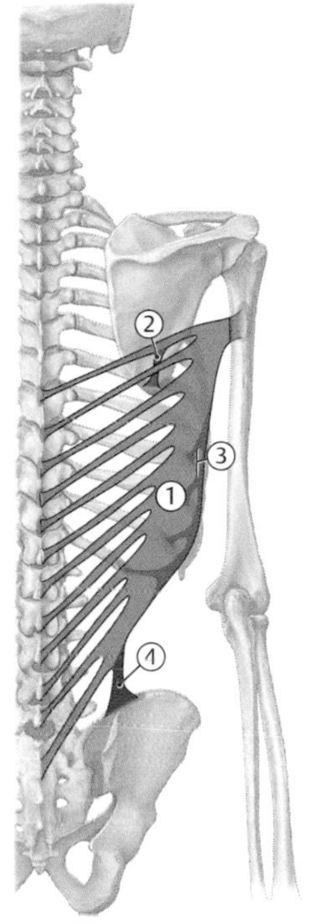
2
3
1
4

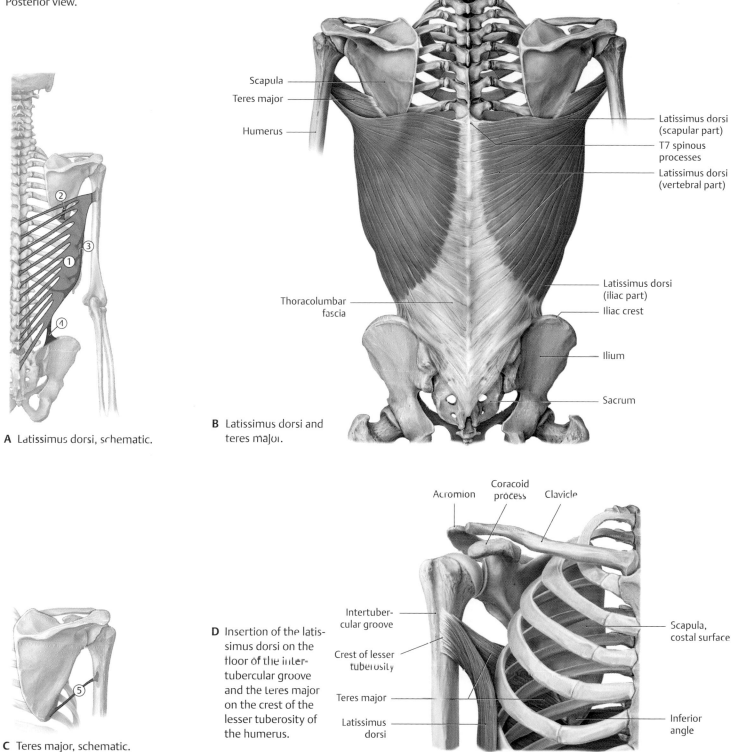

A Latissimus dorsi, schematic.

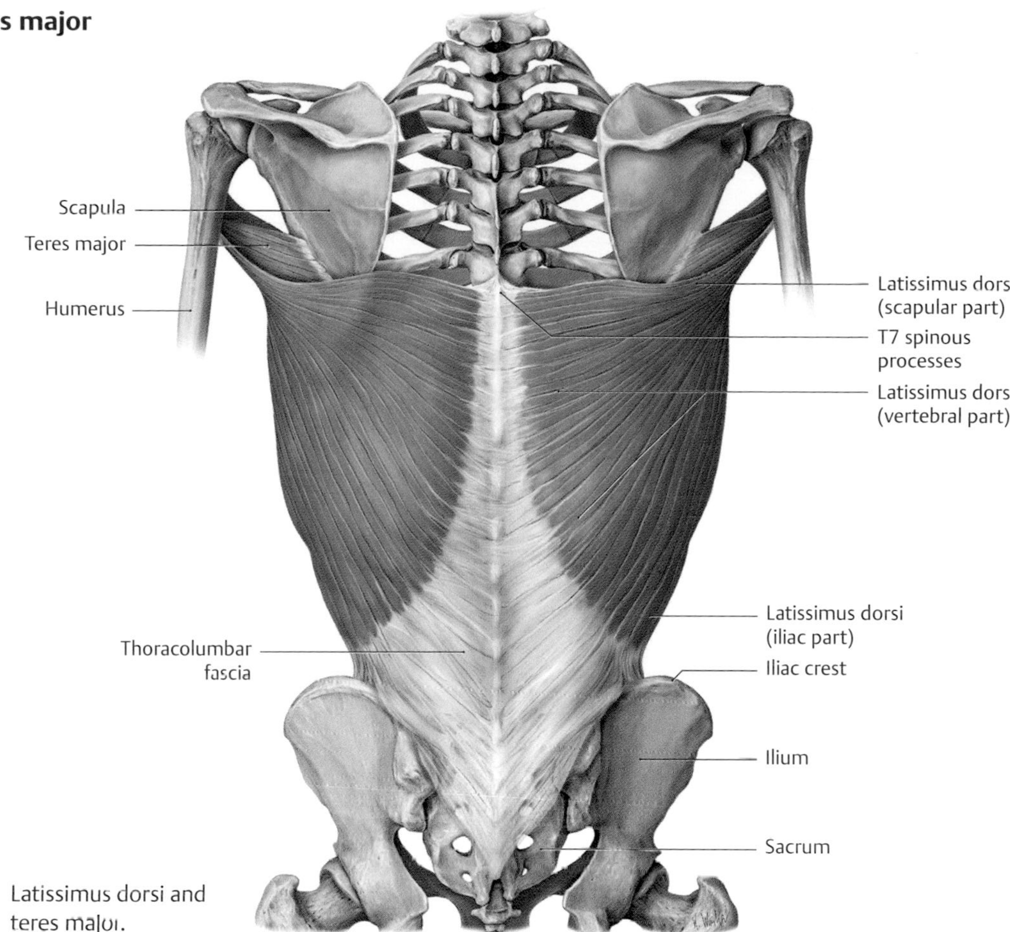
Scapula
Teres major
Humerus
Latissimus dorsi (scapular part)
T7 spinous processes
Latissimus dorsi (vertebral part)
Thoracolumbar fascia
Latissimus dorsi (iliac part)
Iliac crest
Ilium
Sacrum

B Latissimus dorsi and teres major.

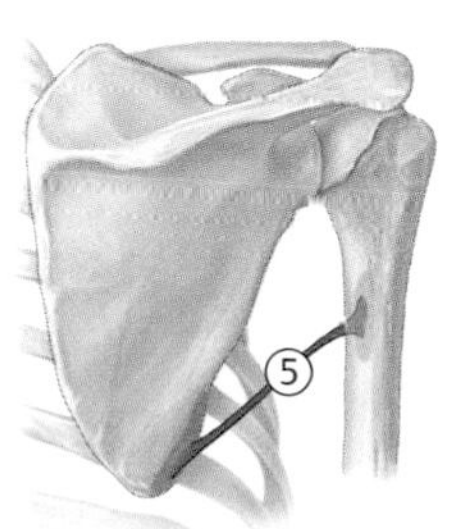
5

C Teres major, schematic.

D Insertion of the latissimus dorsi on the floor of the intertubercular groove and the teres major on the crest of the lesser tuberosity of the humerus.

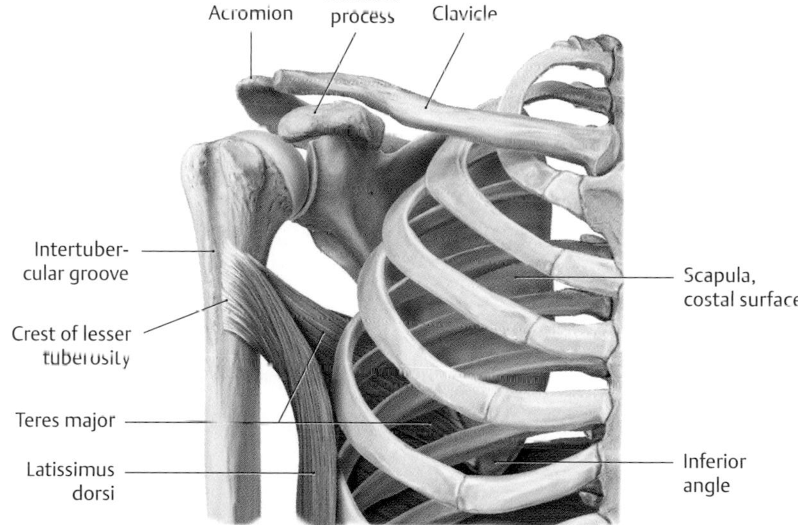
Acromion
Coracoid process
Clavicle
Intertuber-cular groove
Crest of lesser tuberosity
Teres major
Latissimus dorsi
Scapula, costal surface
Inferior angle

Table 21.6 Latissimus dorsi and teres major

Muscle		Origin	Insertion	Innervation	Action
Latissimus dorsi	① Vertebral part	Spinous process of T7–T12 vertebrae; thoracolumbar fascia	Floor of the intertubercular groove of the humerus	Thoracodorsal n. (C6–C8)	Internal rotation, adduction, extension, respiration ("cough muscle")
	② Scapular part	Scapula (inferior angle)			
	③ Costal part	9th to 12th ribs			
	④ Iliac part	Iliac crest (posterior one third)			
⑤ Teres major		Scapula (inferior angle)	Crest of lesser tuberosity of the humerus (anterior angle)	Lower subscapular n. (C5–C7)	Internal rotation, adduction, extension

Muscle Facts (IV)

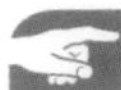

The anterior and posterior muscles of the arm may be classified respectively as flexors and extensors relative to the movement of the elbow joint. Although the coracobrachialis is topographically part of the anterior compartment, it is functionally grouped with the muscles of the shoulder (see p. 298).

***Fig. 21.31* Biceps brachii and brachialis**
Right arm, anterior view.

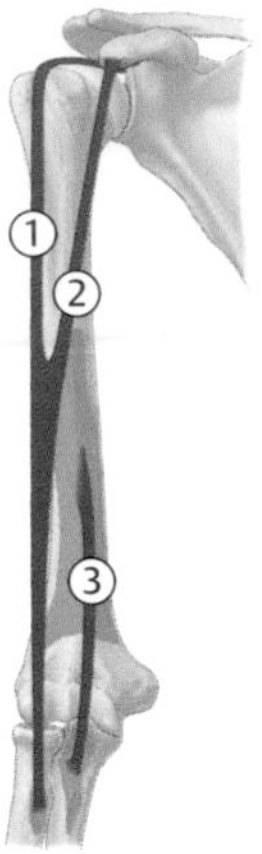

①
②
③

A Schematic.

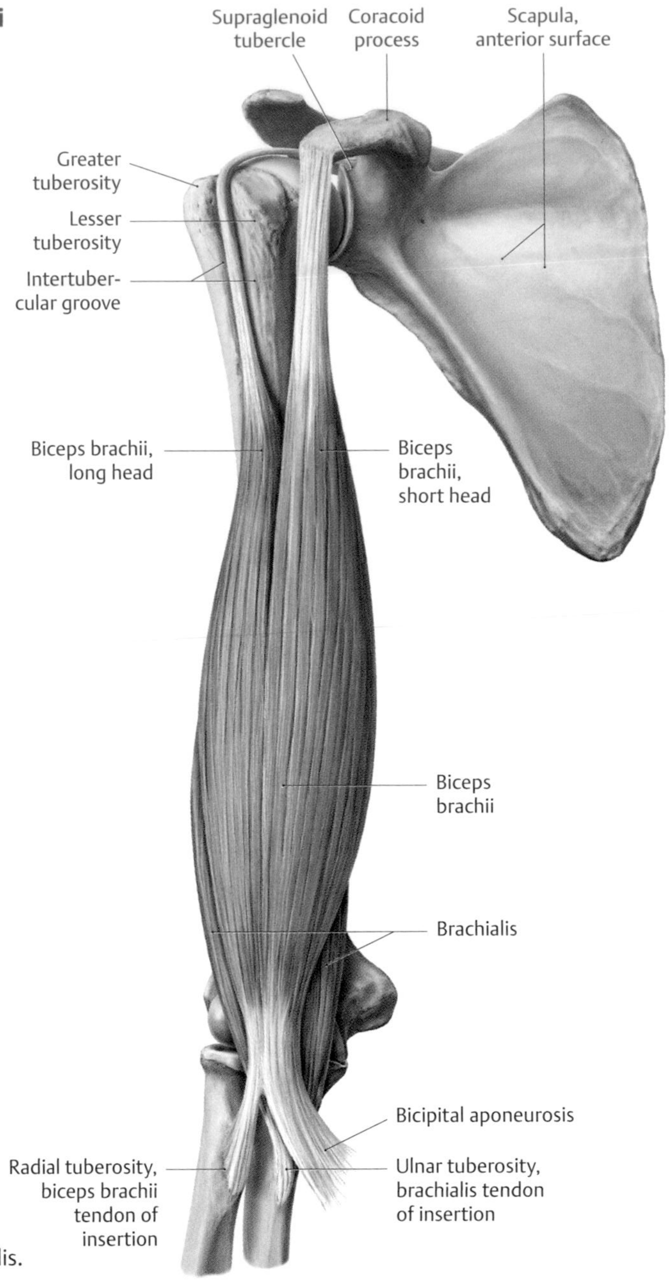

Supraglenoid tubercle
Coracoid process
Scapula, anterior surface
Greater tuberosity
Lesser tuberosity
Intertuber-cular groove
Biceps brachii, long head
Biceps brachii, short head
Biceps brachii
Brachialis
Bicipital aponeurosis
Radial tuberosity, biceps brachii tendon of insertion
Ulnar tuberosity, brachialis tendon of insertion

B Biceps brachii and brachialis.

Shaft of humerus
Brachialis
Medial epicondyle
Lateral epicondyle
Radial tuberosity
Ulnar tuberosity

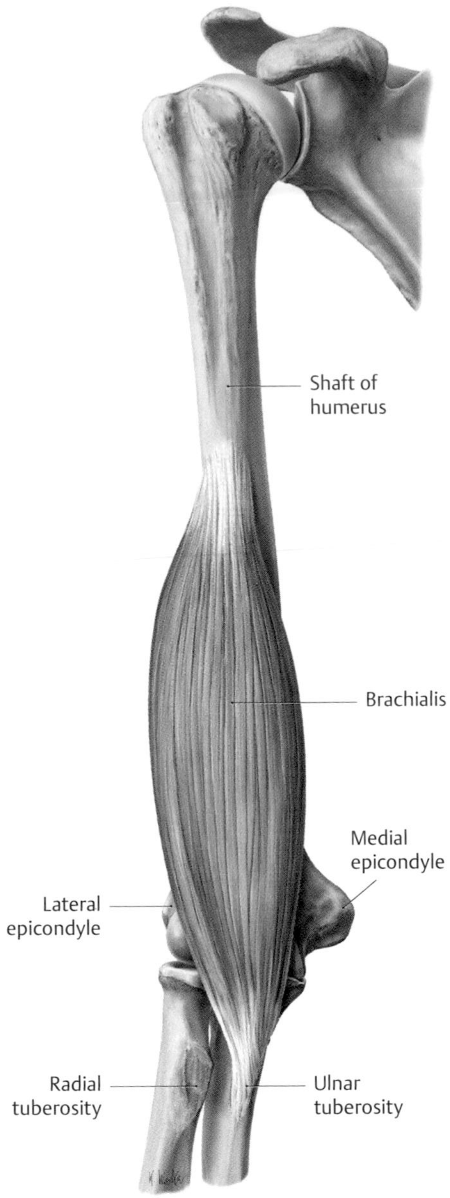

C Brachialis.

Table 21.7 **Anterior muscles: Biceps brachii and brachialis**

Muscle		Origin	Insertion	Innervation	Action
Biceps brachii	① Long head	Supraglenoid tubercle of scapula	Radial tuberosity	Musculocutaneous n. (C5–C6)	Elbow joint: flexion; supination* Shoulder joint: flexion; stabilization of humeral head during deltoid contraction; abduction and internal rotation of the humerus
	② Short head	Coracoid process of scapula			
③ Brachialis		Humerus (distal half of anterior surface)	Ulnar tuberosity	Musculocutaneous n. (C5–C6) and radial n. (C7, minor)	Flexion at the elbow joint

* *Note:* When the elbow is flexed, the biceps brachii acts as a powerful supinator because the lever arm is almost perpendicular to the axis of pronation/supination.

***Fig. 21.32* Triceps brachii and anconeus**
Right arm, posterior view.

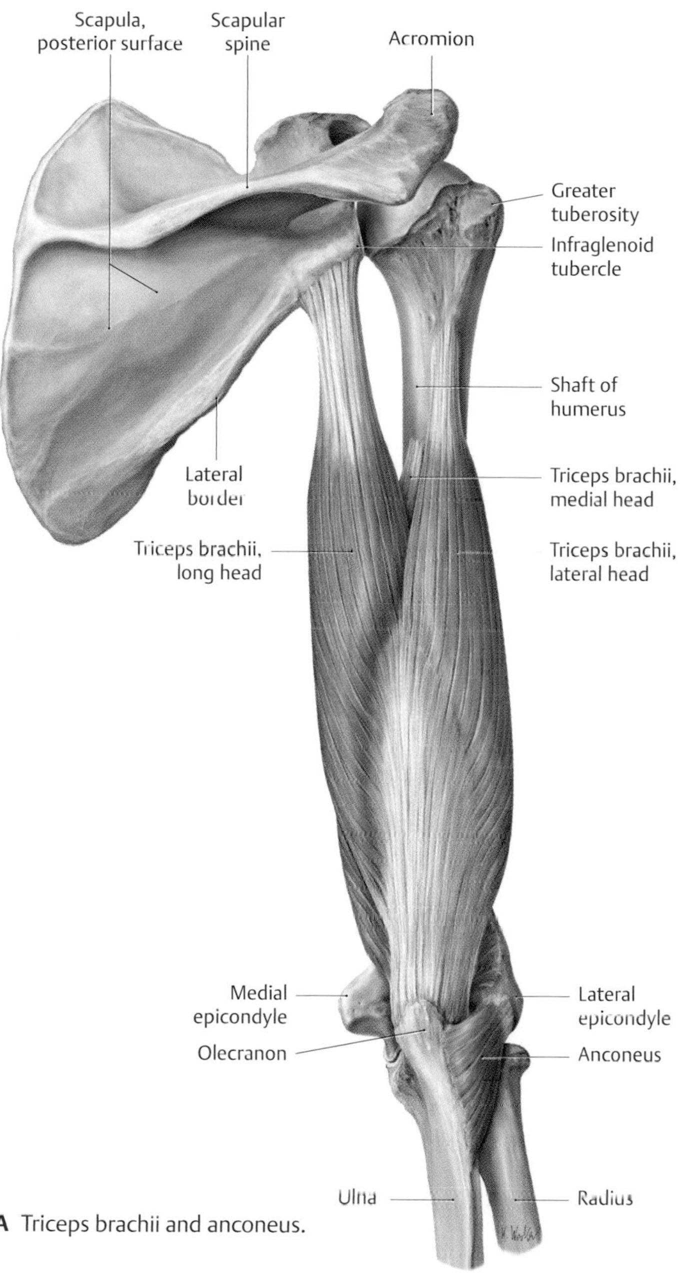
Scapula,
posterior surface
Scapular
spine
Acromion
Greater
tuberosity
Infraglenoid
tubercle
Shaft of
humerus
Lateral
border
Triceps brachii,
medial head
Triceps brachii,
long head
Triceps brachii,
lateral head
Medial
epicondyle
Lateral
epicondyle
Olecranon
Anconeus
Ulna
Radius

A Triceps brachii and anconeus.

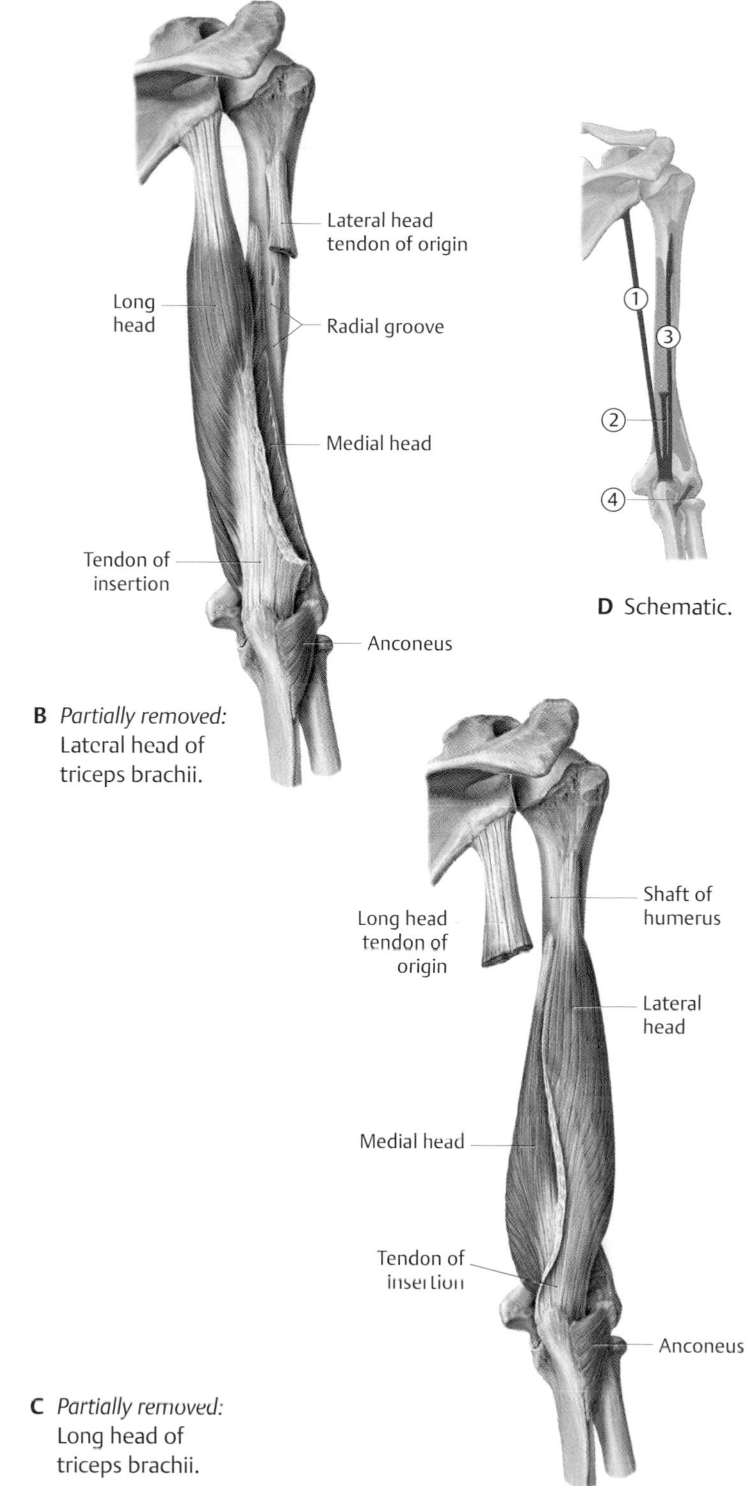
Lateral head
tendon of origin
Long
head
Radial groove
Medial head
Tendon of
insertion
Anconeus
1
2
3
4
Shaft of
humerus
Long head
tendon of
origin
Lateral
head
Medial head
Tendon of
insertion
Anconeus

B *Partially removed:* Lateral head of triceps brachii.

C *Partially removed:* Long head of triceps brachii.

D Schematic.

Table 21.8 Posterior muscles: Triceps brachii and anconeus

Muscle		Origin	Insertion	Innervation	Action
Triceps brachii	① Long head	Scapula (infraglenoid tubercle)	Olecranon of ulna	Radial n. (C6–C8)	Elbow joint: extension Shoulder joint, long head: extension and adduction
	② Medial head	Posterior humerus, inferior to radial groove; medial intermuscular septum			
	③ Lateral head	Posterior humerus, proximal to radial groove; lateral intermuscular septum			
④ Anconeus		Lateral epicondyle of humerus (variance: posterior joint capsule)	Olecranon of ulna (radial surface)		Extends the elbow and tightens its joint

Radius & Ulna

Fig. 22.1 Radius and ulna
Right forearm.

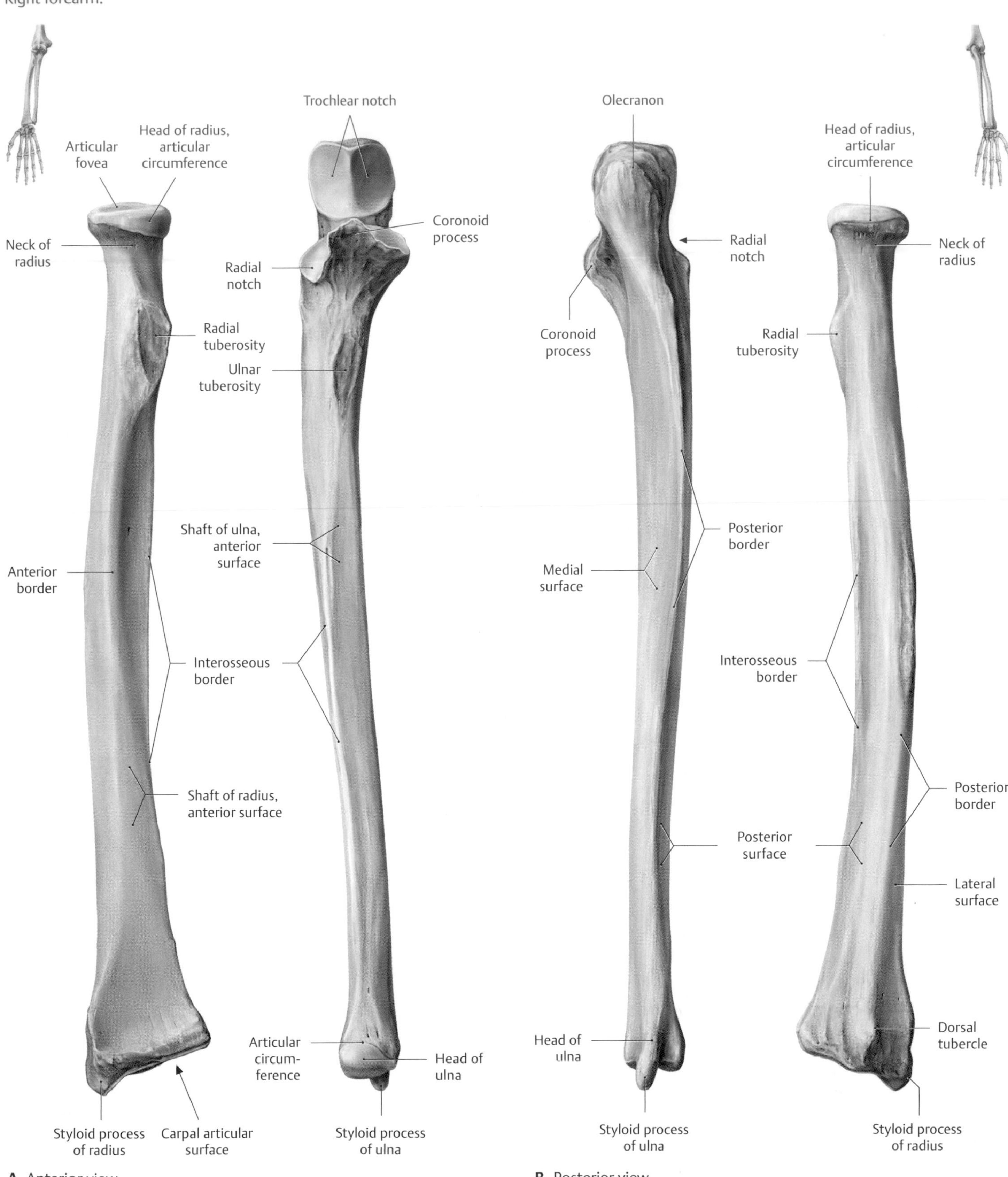

Articular fovea
Head of radius, articular circumference
Neck of radius
Radial tuberosity
Anterior border
Interosseous border
Shaft of radius, anterior surface
Styloid process of radius
Carpal articular surface
Trochlear notch
Coronoid process
Radial notch
Ulnar tuberosity
Shaft of ulna, anterior surface
Interosseous border
Articular circum-ference
Head of ulna
Styloid process of ulna
Olecranon
Radial notch
Coronoid process
Posterior border
Medial surface
Posterior surface
Head of ulna
Styloid process of ulna
Head of radius, articular circumference
Neck of radius
Radial tuberosity
Interosseous border
Posterior border
Posterior surface
Lateral surface
Dorsal tubercle
Styloid process of radius

A Anterior view.

B Posterior view.

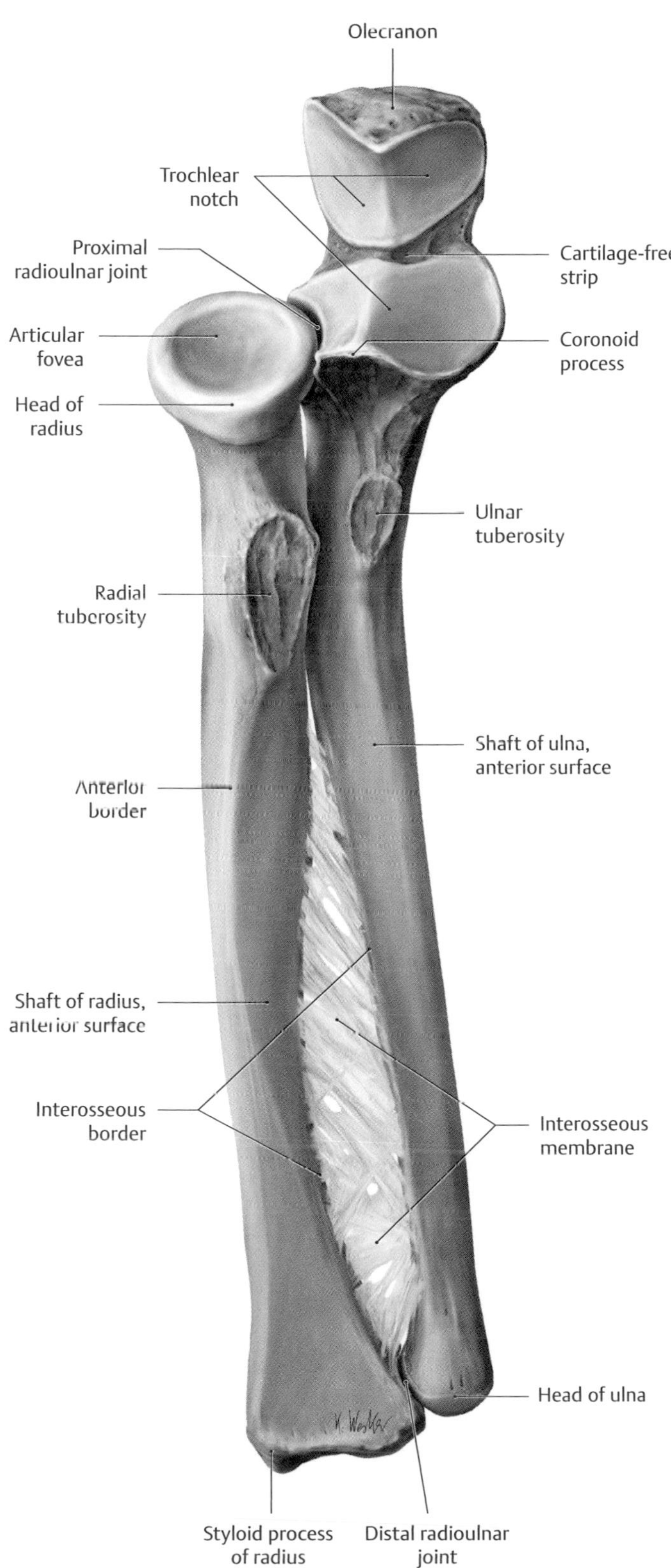
Olecranon
Trochlear notch
Proximal radioulnar joint
Cartilage-free strip
Articular fovea
Coronoid process
Head of radius
Ulnar tuberosity
Radial tuberosity
Shaft of ulna, anterior surface
Anterior border
Shaft of radius, anterior surface
Interosseous border
Interosseous membrane
Head of ulna
Styloid process of radius
Distal radioulnar joint

C Anterosuperior view.

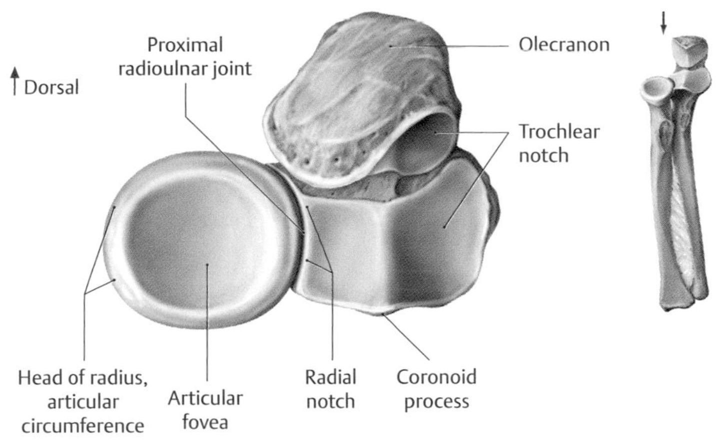
Dorsal
Proximal radioulnar joint
Olecranon
Trochlear notch
Head of radius, articular circumference
Articular fovea
Radial notch
Coronoid process

D Proximal view.

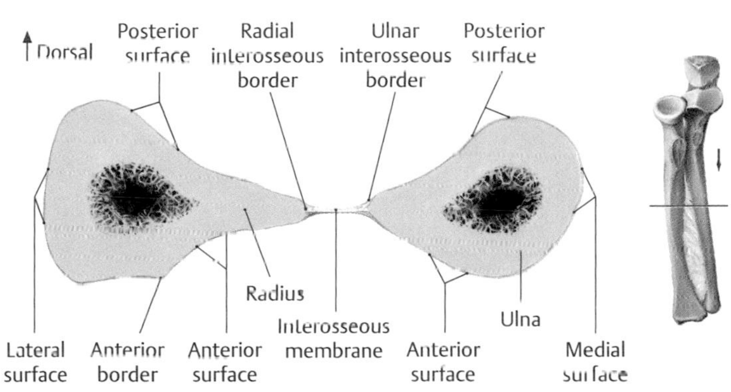
Dorsal
Posterior surface
Radial interosseous border
Ulnar interosseous border
Posterior surface
Radius
Interosseous membrane
Ulna
Lateral surface
Anterior border
Anterior surface
Anterior surface
Medial surface

E Transverse section, proximal view.

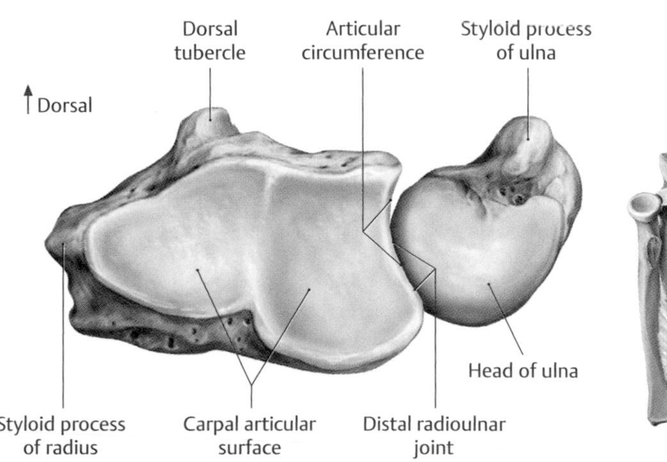
Dorsal
Dorsal tubercle
Articular circumference
Styloid process of ulna
Head of ulna
Styloid process of radius
Carpal articular surface
Distal radioulnar joint

F Distal view.

Elbow Joint

Fig. 22.2 **Elbow (cubital) joint**
Right limb. The elbow consists of three articulations between the humerus, ulna, and radius: the humeroulnar, humeroradial, and proximal radioulnar joints.

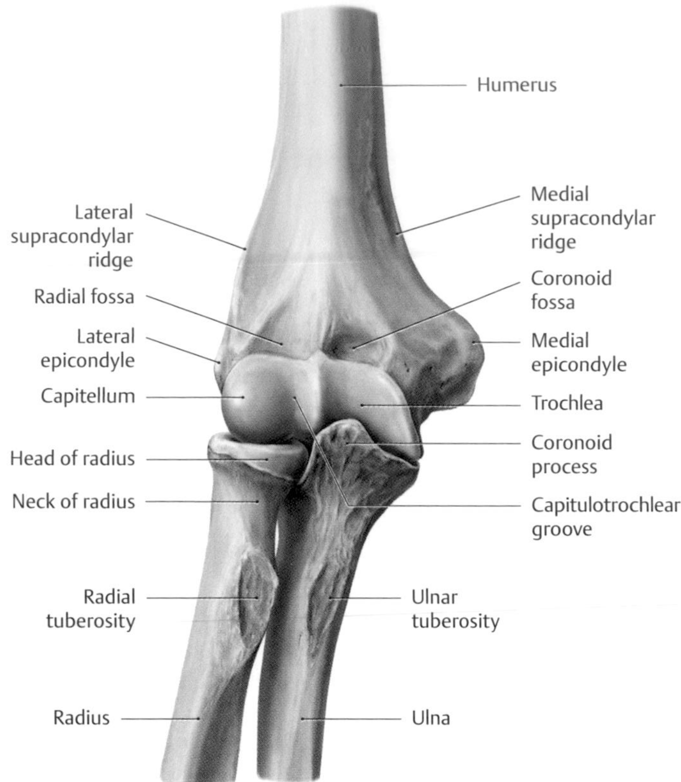
Humerus
Lateral supracondylar ridge
Medial supracondylar ridge
Radial fossa
Coronoid fossa
Lateral epicondyle
Medial epicondyle
Capitellum
Trochlea
Head of radius
Coronoid process
Neck of radius
Capitulotrochlear groove
Radial tuberosity
Ulnar tuberosity
Radius
Ulna

A Anterior view.

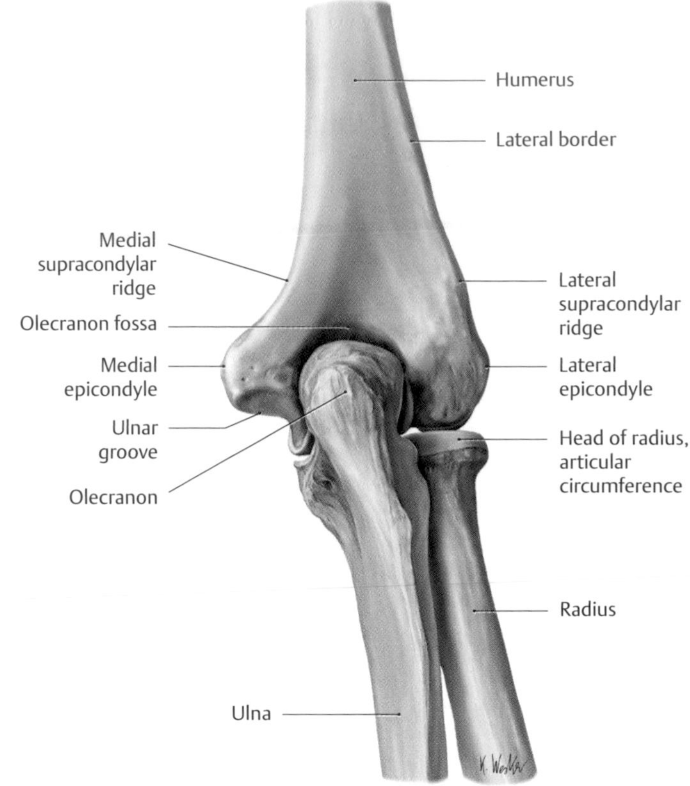
Humerus
Lateral border
Medial supracondylar ridge
Lateral supracondylar ridge
Olecranon fossa
Medial epicondyle
Lateral epicondyle
Ulnar groove
Head of radius, articular circumference
Olecranon
Radius
Ulna

B Posterior view.

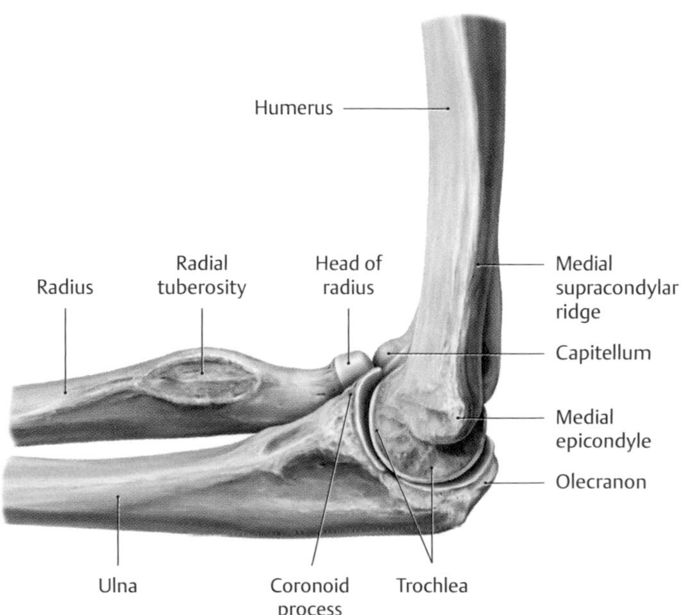
Humerus
Radius
Radial tuberosity
Head of radius
Medial supracondylar ridge
Capitellum
Medial epicondyle
Olecranon
Ulna
Coronoid process
Trochlea

C Medial view.

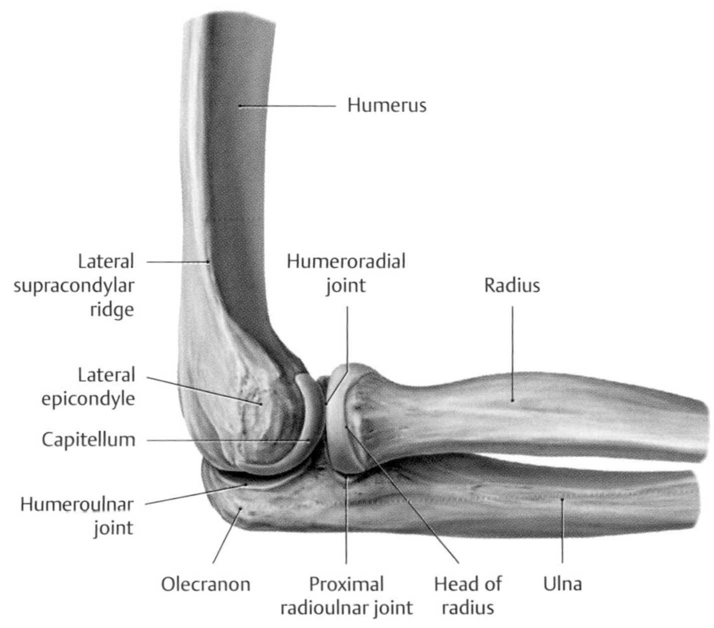
Humerus
Lateral supracondylar ridge
Humeroradial joint
Radius
Lateral epicondyle
Capitellum
Humeroulnar joint
Olecranon
Proximal radioulnar joint
Head of radius
Ulna

D Lateral view.

Fig. 22.3 MRI of the elbow joint

Sagittal section.

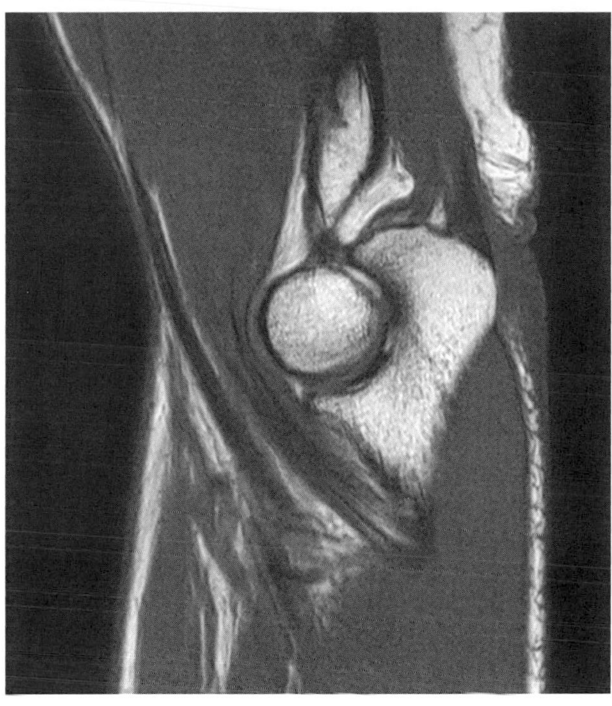

Fig. 22.4 Humeroulnar joint

Sagittal section through the humeroulnar joint, medial view.

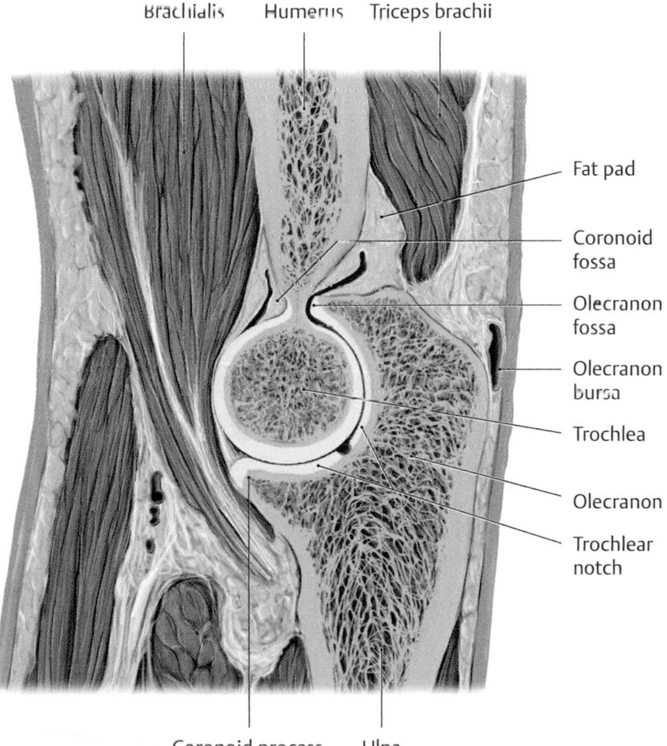

Brachialis
Humerus
Triceps brachii
Fat pad
Coronoid fossa
Olecranon fossa
Olecranon bursa
Trochlea
Olecranon
Trochlear notch
Coronoid process
Ulna

Clinical

Assessing elbow injuries

The fat pads between the fibrous capsule and synovial membrane are part of the normal anatomy of the elbow joint. The anterior pad is most readily seen on a sagittal MRI while the posterior pad is often hidden within the bony fossa (see Figs. 22.3 and 22.4). With an effusion of the joint space, the inferior edge of the anterior pad appears concave as it gets pushed superiorly by the intra-articular fluid. This causes the pad to resemble the shape of a ship's sail, thus creating a characteristic "sail sign." The alignment of the prominences in the elbow also aids in the identification of fractures and dislocations.

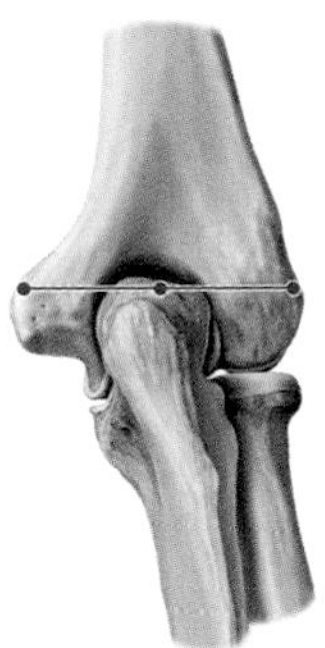

A Posterior view of extended elbow: The epicondyles and olecranon lie in a straight line.

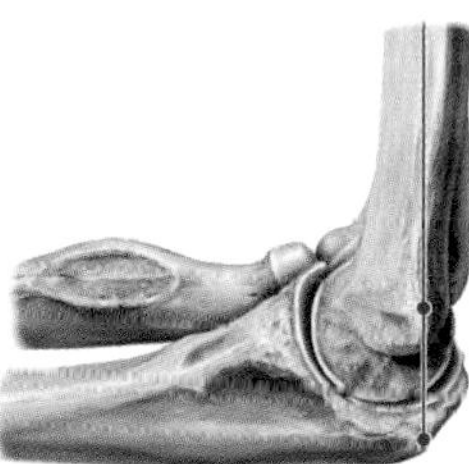

B Lateral view of flexed elbow: The epicondyles and olecranon lie in a straight line.

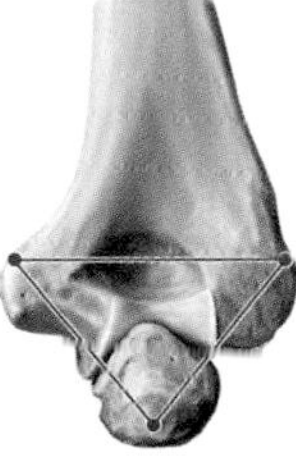

C Posterior view of flexed elbow: The two epicondyles and the tip of the olecranon form an equilateral triangle. Fractures and dislocations alter the shape of the triangle.

Ligaments of the Elbow Joint

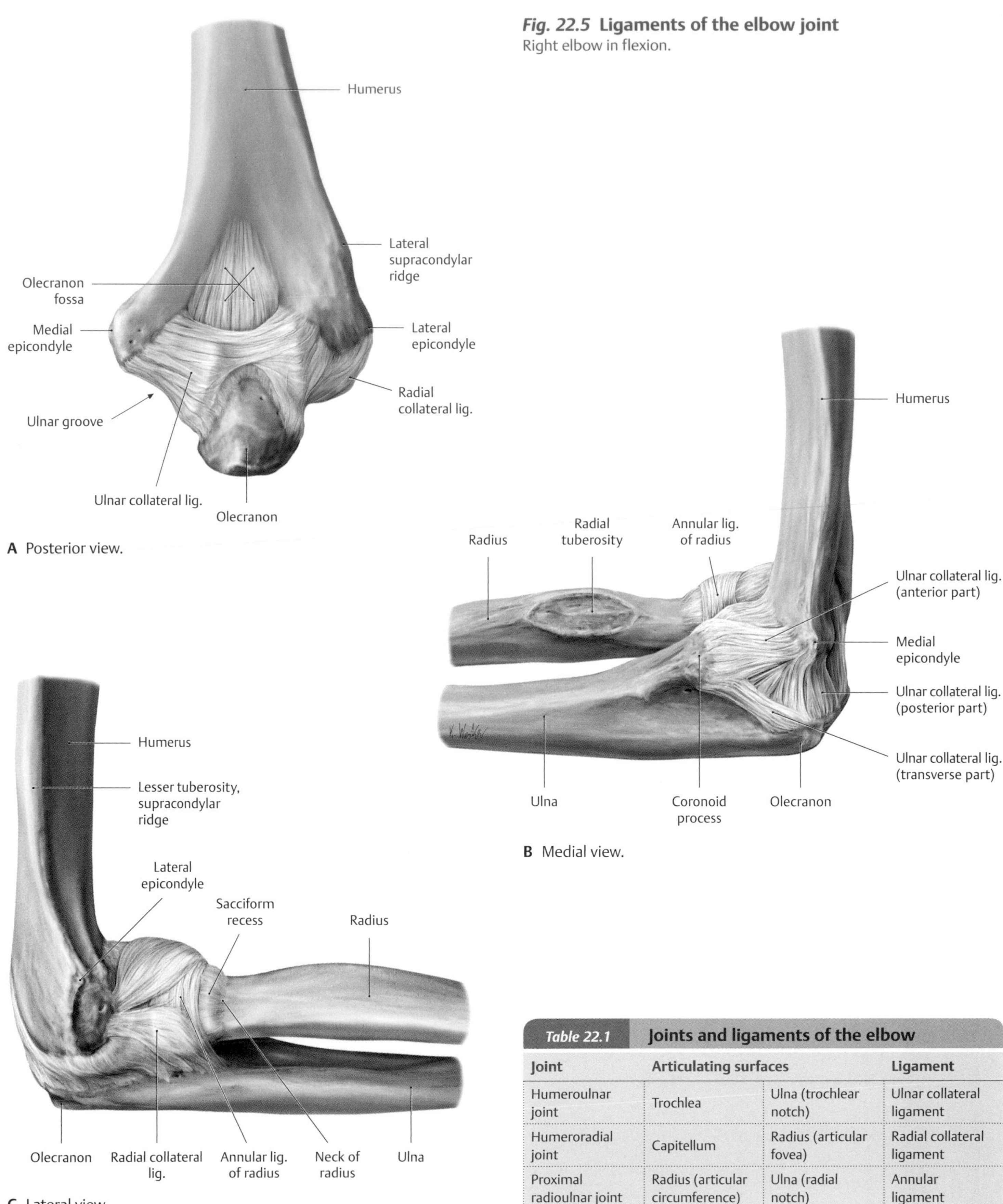
Humerus
Olecranon fossa
Lateral supracondylar ridge
Medial epicondyle
Lateral epicondyle
Radial collateral lig.
Ulnar groove
Ulnar collateral lig.
Olecranon
A Posterior view.
Humerus
Radius
Radial tuberosity
Annular lig. of radius
Ulnar collateral lig. (anterior part)
Medial epicondyle
Ulnar collateral lig. (posterior part)
Ulnar collateral lig. (transverse part)
Ulna
Coronoid process
Olecranon
B Medial view.
Humerus
Lesser tuberosity, supracondylar ridge
Lateral epicondyle
Sacciform recess
Radius
Olecranon
Radial collateral lig.
Annular lig. of radius
Neck of radius
Ulna
C Lateral view.

Fig. 22.5 **Ligaments of the elbow joint**
Right elbow in flexion.

Table 22.1 Joints and ligaments of the elbow

Joint	Articulating surfaces		Ligament
Humeroulnar joint	Trochlea	Ulna (trochlear notch)	Ulnar collateral ligament
Humeroradial joint	Capitellum	Radius (articular fovea)	Radial collateral ligament
Proximal radioulnar joint	Radius (articular circumference)	Ulna (radial notch)	Annular ligament

Fig. 22.6 Joint capsule of the elbow
Right elbow in extension, anterior view.

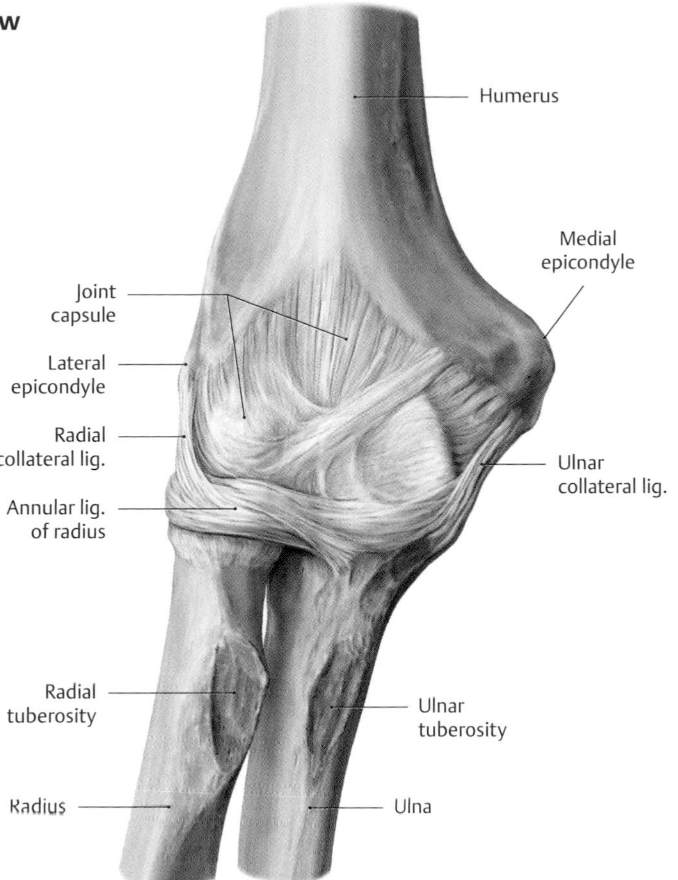
Humerus
Medial epicondyle
Joint capsule
Lateral epicondyle
Radial collateral lig.
Ulnar collateral lig.
Annular lig. of radius
Radial tuberosity
Ulnar tuberosity
Radius
Ulna

A Intact joint capsule.

Clinical

Subluxation of the radial head (Nursemaid's Elbow)
A common and painful injury of small children occurs when the arm is jerked upward with the forearm pronated, tearing the annular ligament from its loose attachment on the radial neck. As the immature radial head slips out of the socket, the ligament may become trapped between the radial head and the capitulum of the humerus. Supinating the forearm and flexing the elbow usually returns the radial head to the normal position.

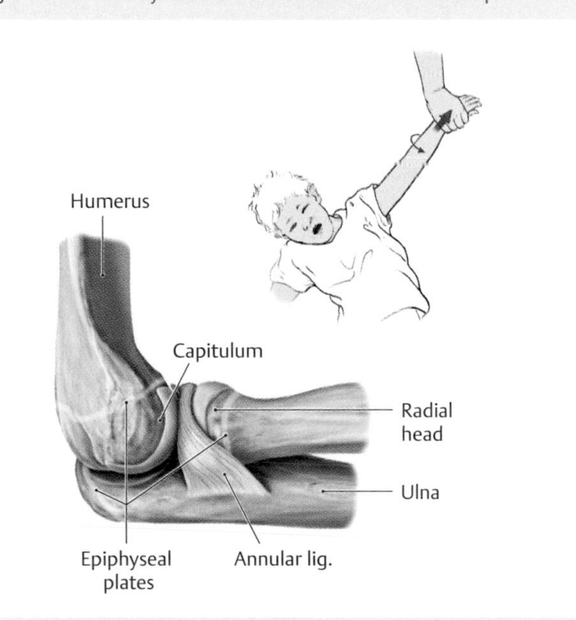
Humerus
Capitulum
Radial head
Ulna
Epiphyseal plates
Annular lig.

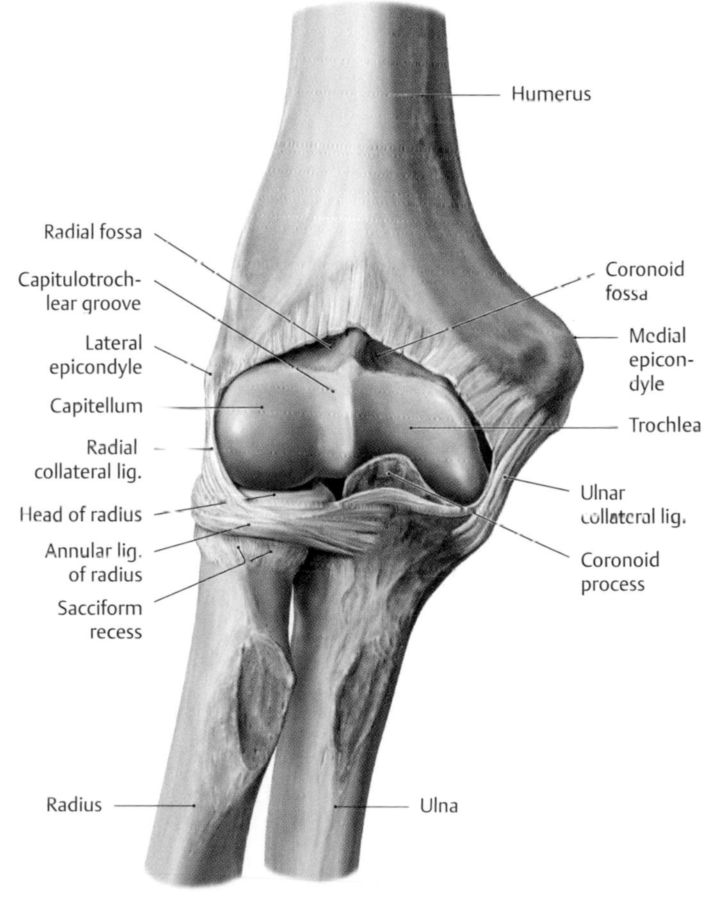
Humerus
Radial fossa
Coronoid fossa
Capitulotroch-lear groove
Lateral epicondyle
Medial epicon-dyle
Capitellum
Trochlea
Radial collateral lig.
Head of radius
Ulnar collateral lig.
Annular lig. of radius
Coronoid process
Sacciform recess
Radius
Ulna

B Windowed joint capsule.

Radioulnar Joints

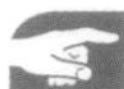

The proximal and distal radioulnar joints function together to enable pronation and supination movements of the hand. The joints are functionally linked by the interosseous membrane. The axis for pronation and supination runs obliquely from the center of the humeral capitellum through the center of the radial articular fovea down to the styloid process of the ulna.

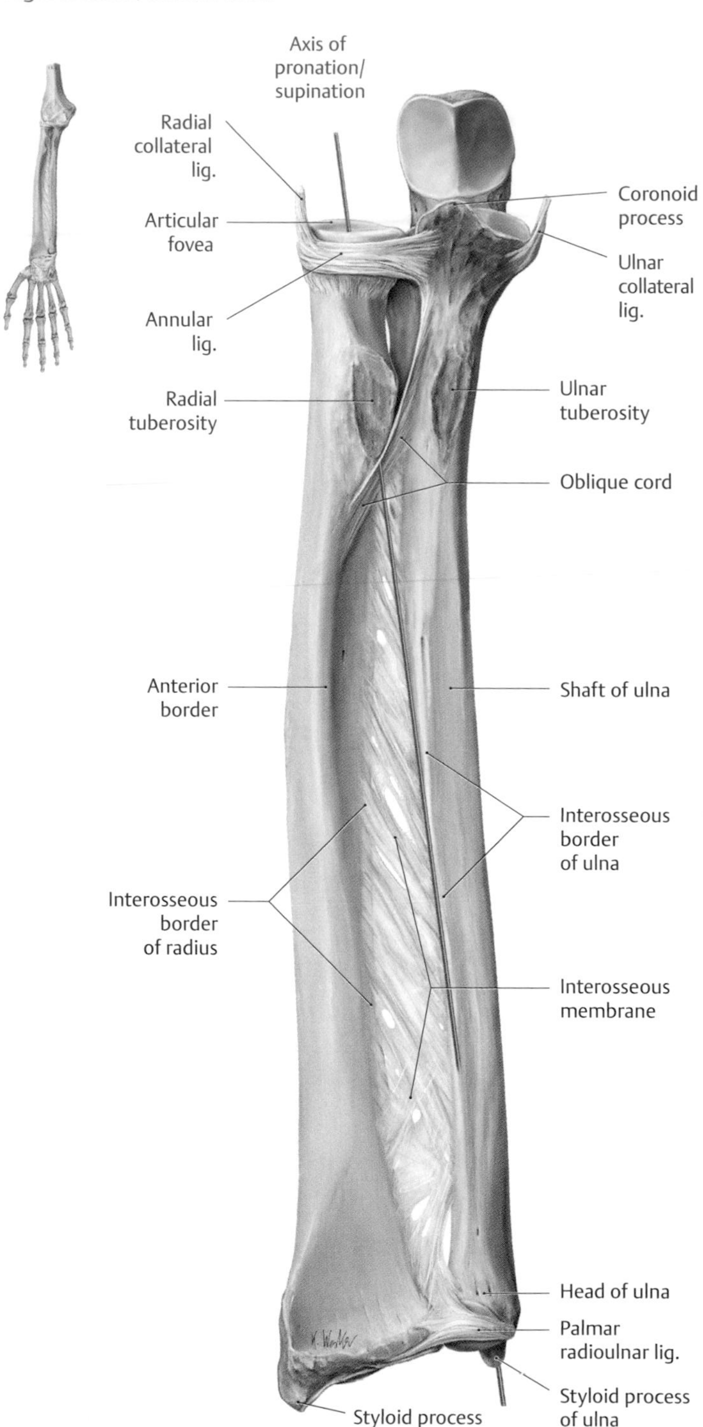

Axis of pronation/ supination
Radial collateral lig.
Articular fovea
Annular lig.
Radial tuberosity
Coronoid process
Ulnar collateral lig.
Ulnar tuberosity
Oblique cord
Anterior border
Shaft of ulna
Interosseous border of ulna
Interosseous border of radius
Interosseous membrane
Head of ulna
Palmar radioulnar lig.
Styloid process of ulna
Styloid process of radius

Fig. 22.7 **Supination**
Right forearm, anterior view.

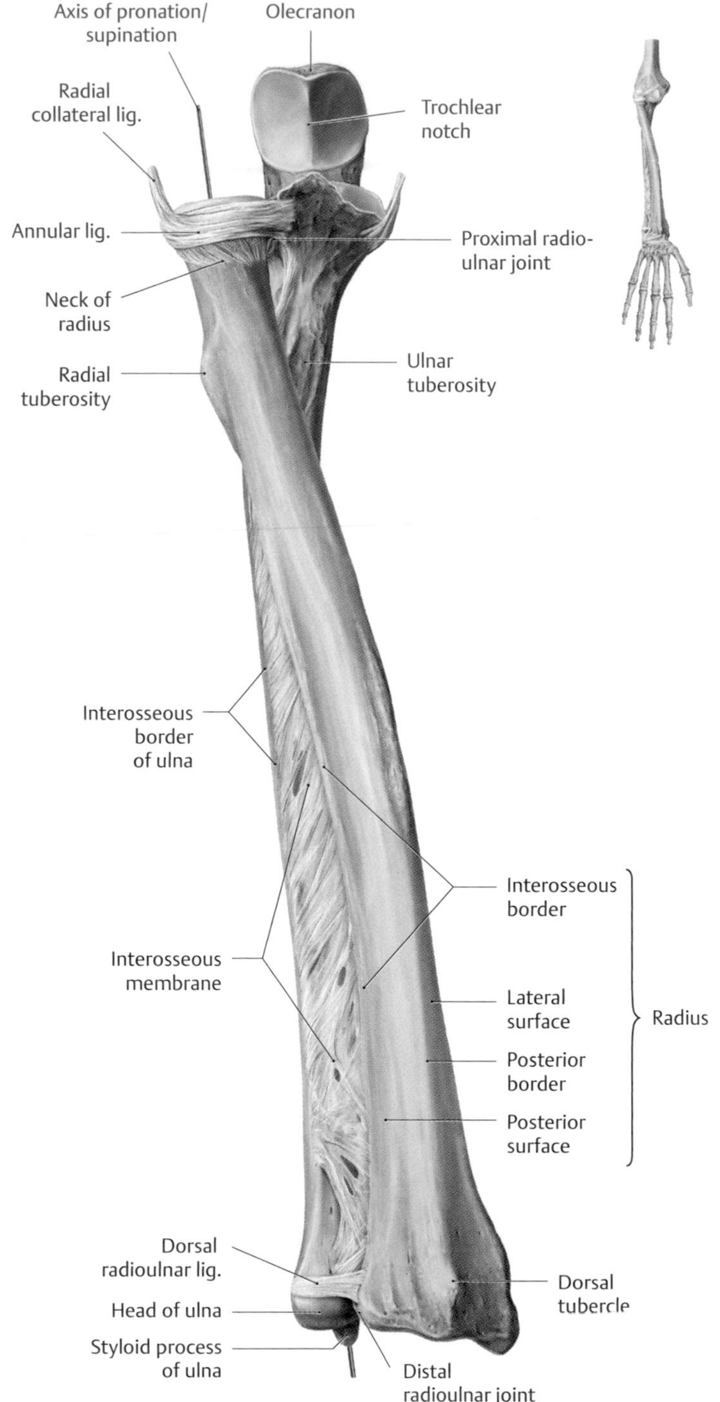

Axis of pronation/ supination
Olecranon
Radial collateral lig.
Trochlear notch
Annular lig.
Proximal radio-ulnar joint
Neck of radius
Radial tuberosity
Ulnar tuberosity
Interosseous border of ulna
Interosseous border
Interosseous membrane
Lateral surface
Radius
Posterior border
Posterior surface
Dorsal radioulnar lig.
Head of ulna
Styloid process of ulna
Dorsal tubercle
Distal radioulnar joint

Fig. 22.8 **Pronation**
Right forearm, anterior view.

Fig. 22.9 Proximal radioulnar joint

Right elbow, proximal (superior) view.

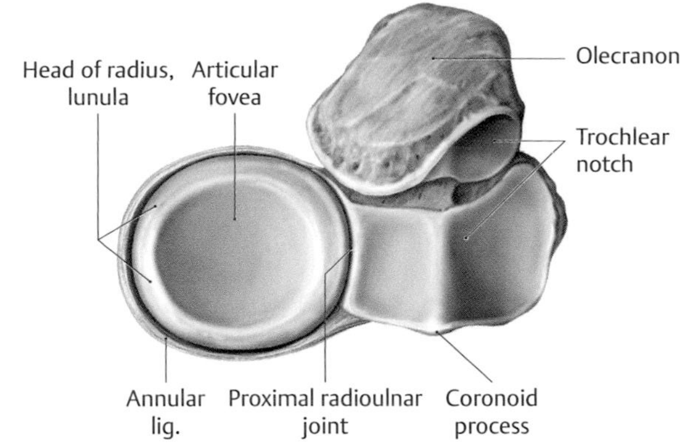

Head of radius, lunula
Articular fovea
Olecranon
Trochlear notch
Annular lig.
Proximal radioulnar joint
Coronoid process

A Proximal articular surfaces of radius and ulna.

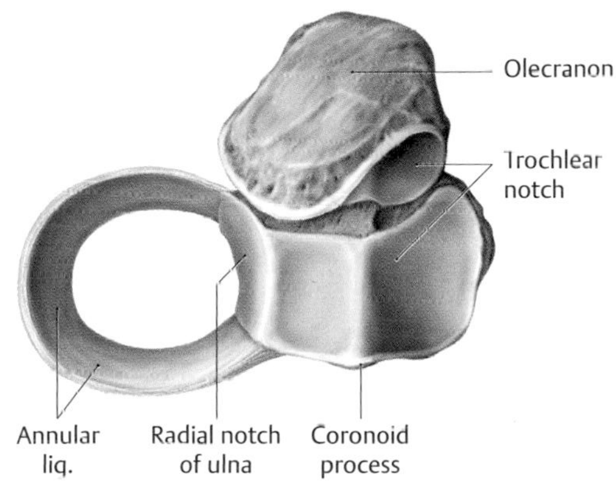

Olecranon
Trochlear notch
Annular lig.
Radial notch of ulna
Coronoid process

B Radius removed.

Clinical

Radius fracture

Falls onto the outstretched arm often result in fractures of the distal radius. In a "Colles' fracture," the distal fragment is tilted dorsally.

Dorsal ←

Styloid process of radius

A B

Fig. 22.10 Distal radioulnar joint rotation

Right forearm, distal view of articular surfaces of radius and ulna. The dorsal and palmar radioulnar ligaments stabilize the distal radioulnar joint.

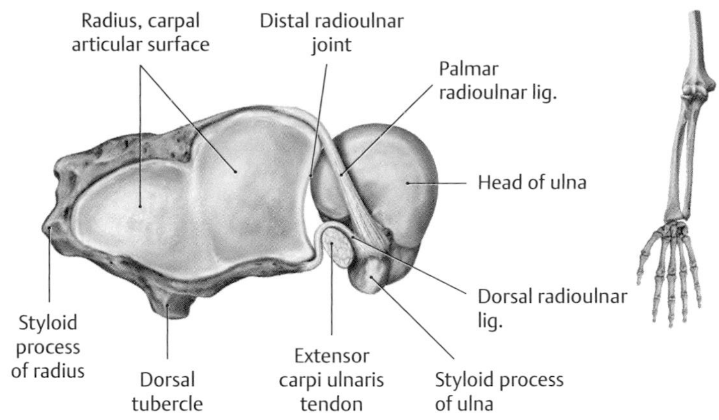

Radius, carpal articular surface
Distal radioulnar joint
Palmar radioulnar lig.
Head of ulna
Dorsal radioulnar lig.
Styloid process of radius
Dorsal tubercle
Extensor carpi ulnaris tendon
Styloid process of ulna

A Supination.

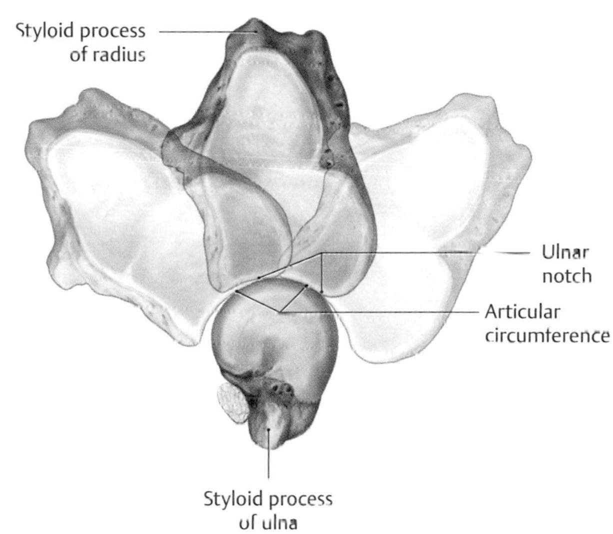

Styloid process of radius
Ulnar notch
Articular circumference
Styloid process of ulna

B Semipronation.

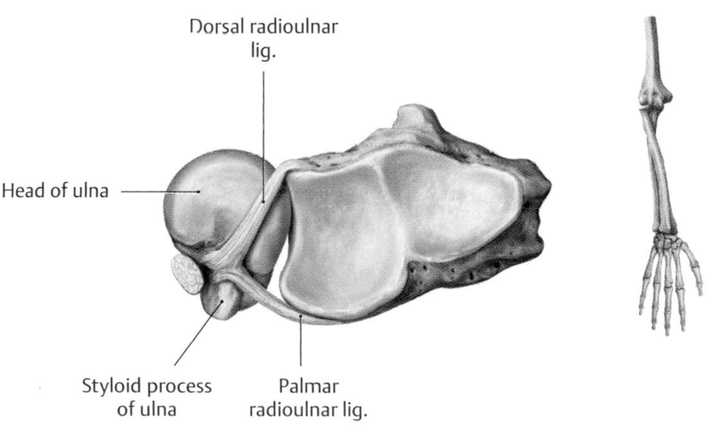

Dorsal radioulnar lig.
Head of ulna
Styloid process of ulna
Palmar radioulnar lig.

C Pronation.

Muscles of the Forearm (I)

Fig. 22.11 **Anterior muscles of the forearm: Dissection**
Right forearm, anterior view. Muscle origins are shown in red, insertions in blue.

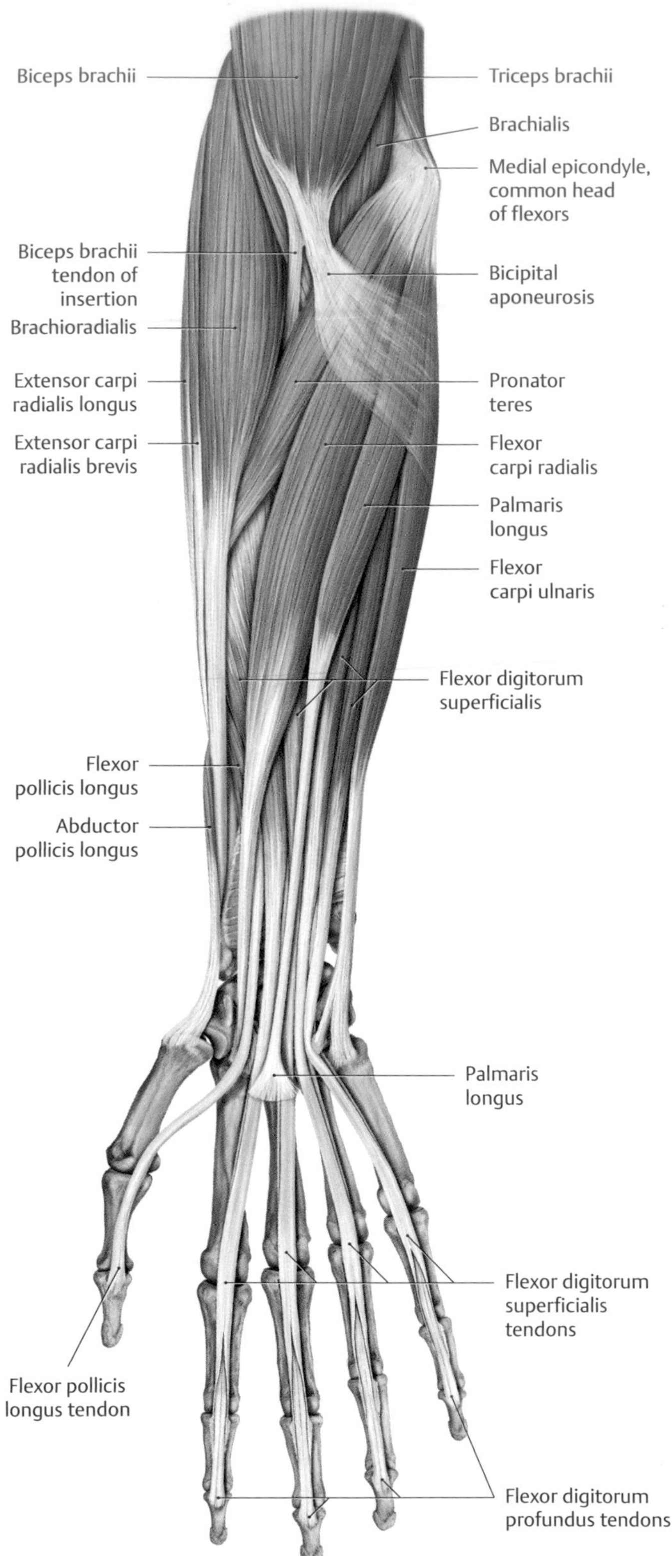

Biceps brachii
Triceps brachii
Brachialis
Medial epicondyle, common head of flexors
Biceps brachii tendon of insertion
Bicipital aponeurosis
Brachioradialis
Extensor carpi radialis longus
Pronator teres
Extensor carpi radialis brevis
Flexor carpi radialis
Palmaris longus
Flexor carpi ulnaris
Flexor digitorum superficialis
Flexor pollicis longus
Abductor pollicis longus
Palmaris longus
Flexor digitorum superficialis tendons
Flexor pollicis longus tendon
Flexor digitorum profundus tendons

A Superficial flexors and radialis group.

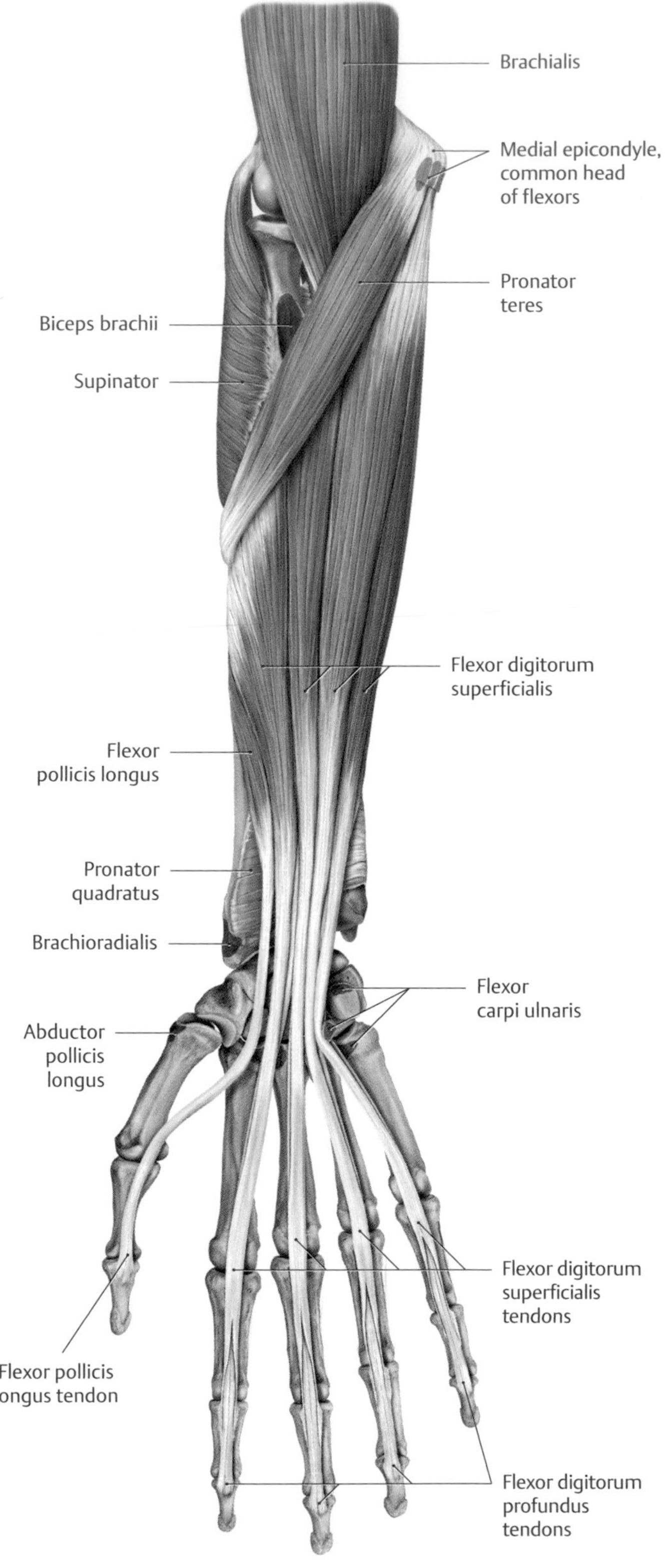

Brachialis
Medial epicondyle, common head of flexors
Pronator teres
Biceps brachii
Supinator
Flexor digitorum superficialis
Flexor pollicis longus
Pronator quadratus
Brachioradialis
Flexor carpi ulnaris
Abductor pollicis longus
Flexor digitorum superficialis tendons
Flexor pollicis longus tendon
Flexor digitorum profundus tendons

B *Removed:* Radialis group (brachioradialis, extensor carpi radialis longus, and extensor carpi radialis brevis), flexor carpi radialis, flexor carpi ulnaris, abductor pollicis longus, palmaris longus, and biceps brachii.

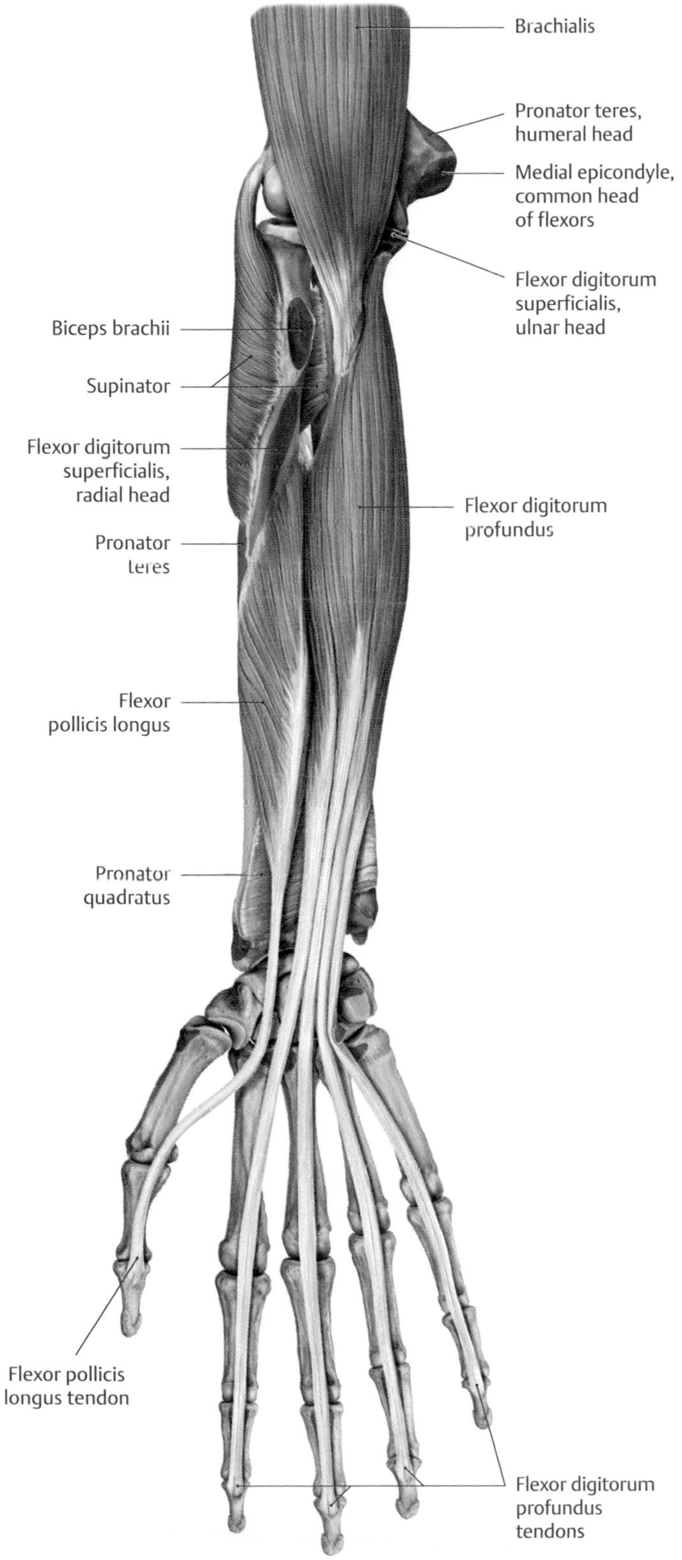

Brachialis
Pronator teres, humeral head
Medial epicondyle, common head of flexors
Flexor digitorum superficialis, ulnar head
Biceps brachii
Supinator
Flexor digitorum superficialis, radial head
Flexor digitorum profundus
Pronator teres
Flexor pollicis longus
Pronator quadratus
Flexor pollicis longus tendon
Flexor digitorum profundus tendons

C *Removed:* Pronator teres and flexor digitorum superficialis.

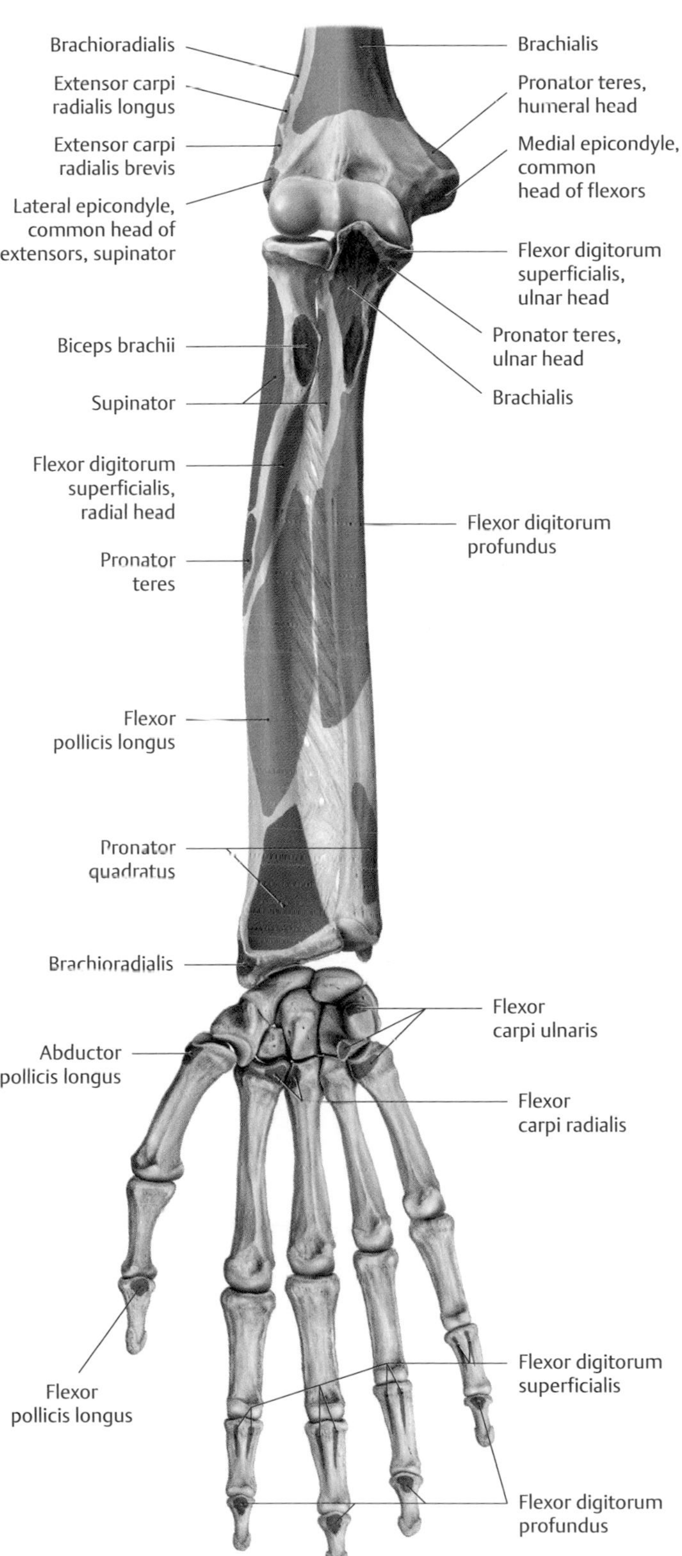
Brachioradialis
Extensor carpi radialis longus
Extensor carpi radialis brevis
Lateral epicondyle, common head of extensors, supinator
Biceps brachii
Supinator
Flexor digitorum superficialis, radial head
Pronator teres
Flexor pollicis longus
Pronator quadratus
Brachioradialis
Abductor pollicis longus
Flexor pollicis longus
Brachialis
Pronator teres, humeral head
Medial epicondyle, common head of flexors
Flexor digitorum superficialis, ulnar head
Pronator teres, ulnar head
Brachialis
Flexor digitorum profundus
Flexor carpi ulnaris
Flexor carpi radialis
Flexor digitorum superficialis
Flexor digitorum profundus

D *Removed:* Brachialis, supinator, pronator quadratus, and deep flexors.

Muscles of the Forearm (II)

Fig. 22.12 Posterior muscles of the forearm: Dissection
Right forearm, posterior view. Muscle origins are shown in red, insertions in blue.

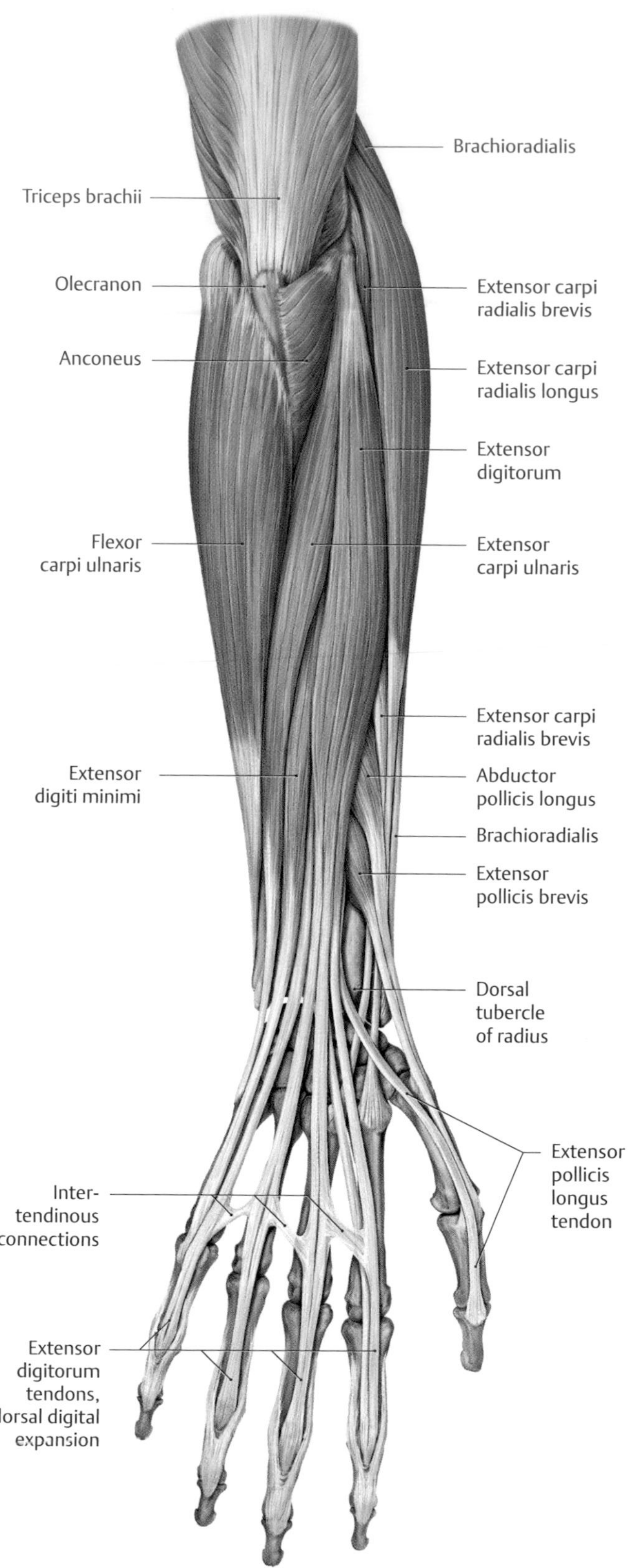

Brachioradialis
Triceps brachii
Olecranon
Extensor carpi radialis brevis
Anconeus
Extensor carpi radialis longus
Extensor digitorum
Flexor carpi ulnaris
Extensor carpi ulnaris
Extensor carpi radialis brevis
Extensor digiti minimi
Abductor pollicis longus
Brachioradialis
Extensor pollicis brevis
Dorsal tubercle of radius
Extensor pollicis longus tendon
Inter-tendinous connections
Extensor digitorum tendons, dorsal digital expansion

A Superficial extensors and radialis group.

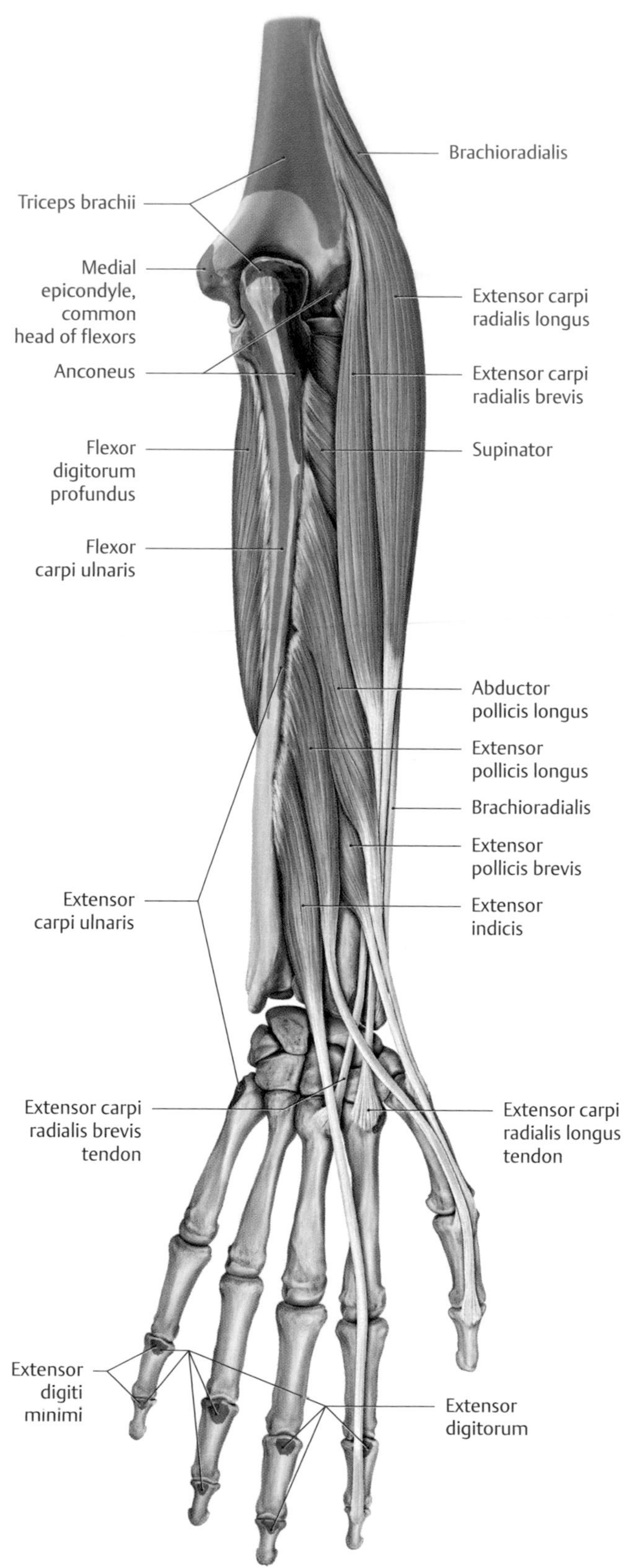

Brachioradialis
Triceps brachii
Medial epicondyle, common head of flexors
Extensor carpi radialis longus
Anconeus
Extensor carpi radialis brevis
Flexor digitorum profundus
Supinator
Flexor carpi ulnaris
Abductor pollicis longus
Extensor pollicis longus
Brachioradialis
Extensor pollicis brevis
Extensor carpi ulnaris
Extensor indicis
Extensor carpi radialis brevis tendon
Extensor carpi radialis longus tendon
Extensor digiti minimi
Extensor digitorum

B *Removed:* Triceps brachii, anconeus, flexor carpi ulnaris, extensor carpi ulnaris, and extensor digitorum.

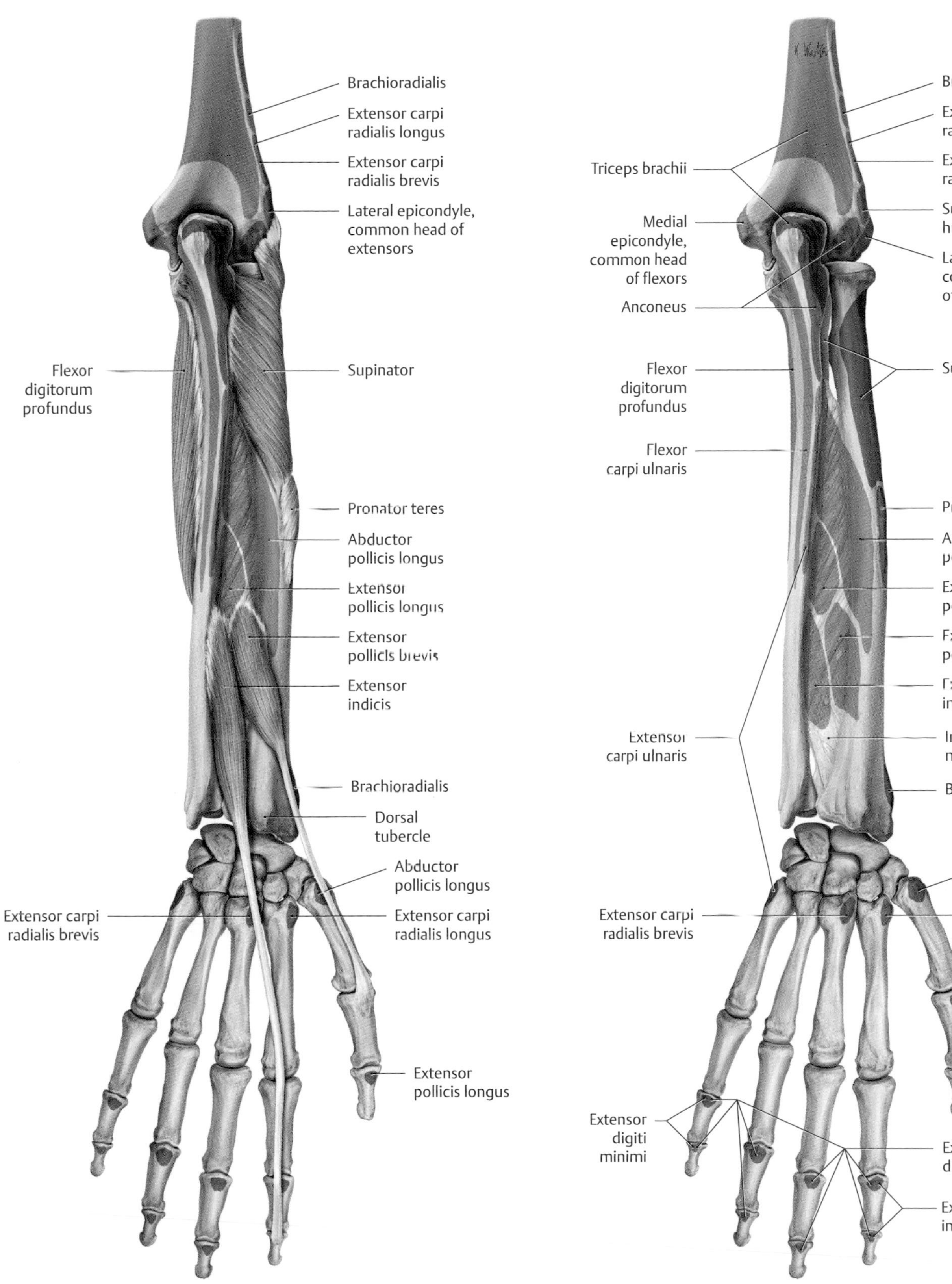
Brachioradialis
Extensor carpi radialis longus
Extensor carpi radialis brevis
Lateral epicondyle, common head of extensors
Flexor digitorum profundus
Supinator
Pronator teres
Abductor pollicis longus
Extensor pollicis longus
Extensor pollicis brevis
Extensor indicis
Brachioradialis
Dorsal tubercle
Abductor pollicis longus
Extensor carpi radialis brevis
Extensor carpi radialis longus
Extensor pollicis longus
Brachioradialis
Extensor carpi radialis longus
Triceps brachii
Extensor carpi radialis brevis
Medial epicondyle, common head of flexors
Supinator, humeral head
Lateral epicondyle, common head of extensors
Anconeus
Flexor digitorum profundus
Supinator
Flexor carpi ulnaris
Pronator teres
Abductor pollicis longus
Extensor pollicis longus
Extensor pollicis brevis
Extensor indicis
Extensor carpi ulnaris
Interosseous membrane
Brachioradialis
Abductor pollicis longus
Extensor carpi radialis brevis
Extensor carpi radialis longus
Extensor pollicis brevis
Extensor pollicis longus
Extensor digiti minimi
Extensor digitorum
Extensor indicis

C *Removed:* Abductor pollicis longus, extensor pollicis longus, and radialis group.

D *Removed:* Flexor digitorum profundus, supinator, extensor pollicis brevis, and extensor indicis.

Muscle Facts (I)

Fig. 22.13 **Muscles of the anterior compartment of the forearm**
Right forearm, anterior view.

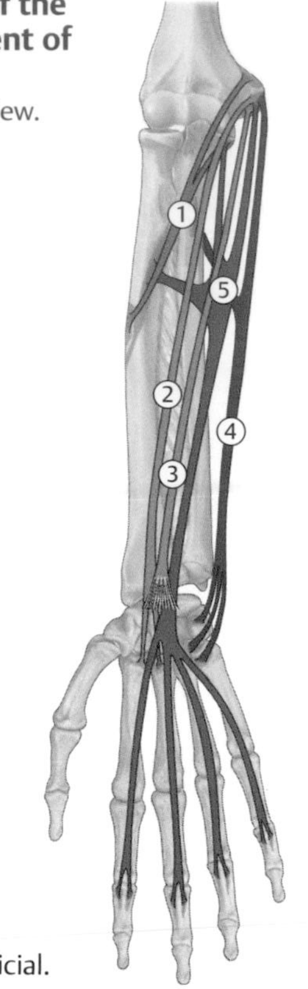

1
5
2
4
3

A Superficial.

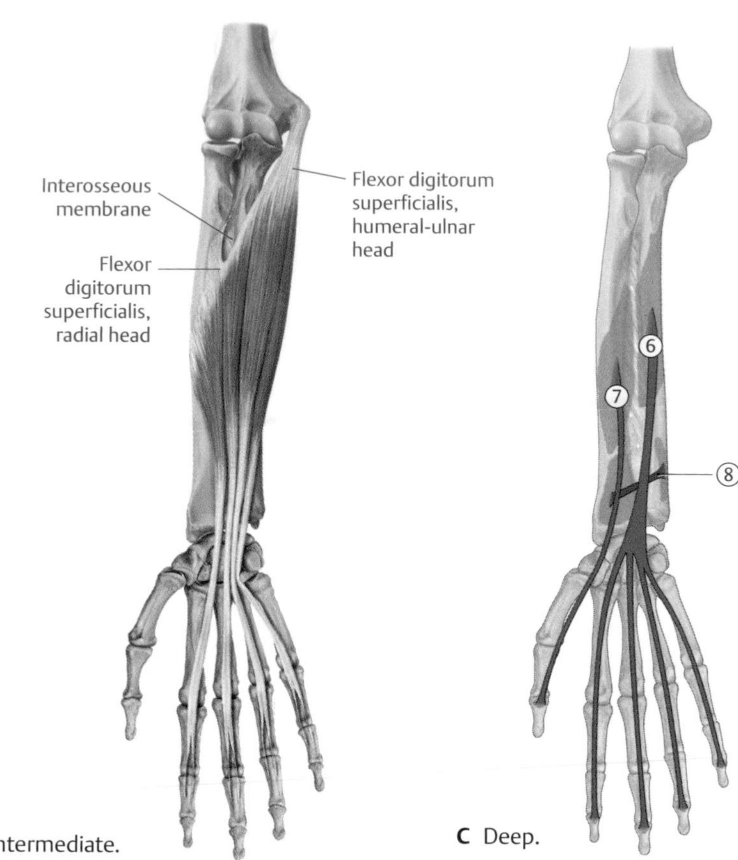

Interosseous membrane
Flexor digitorum superficialis, radial head
Flexor digitorum superficialis, humeral-ulnar head
6
7
8

B Intermediate.

C Deep.

Table 22.2 **Anterior compartment of the forearm**

Muscle	Origin	Insertion	Innervation	Action
Superficial muscles				
① Pronator teres	Humeral head: medial epicondyle of humerus Ulnar head: coronoid process	Lateral radius (distal to supinator insertion)	Median n. (C6, C7)	Elbow: weak flexor Forearm: pronation
② Flexor carpi radialis	Medial epicondyle of humerus	Base of 2nd metacarpal (variance: base of 3rd metacarpal)		Wrist: flexion and abduction (radial deviation) of hand
③ Palmaris longus		Palmar aponeurosis	Median n. (C7, C8)	Elbow: weak flexion Wrist: flexion tightens palmar aponeurosis
④ Flexor carpi ulnaris	Humeral head: medial epicondyle Ulnar head: olecranon	Pisiform; hook of hamate; base of 5th metacarpal	Ulnar n. (C7–T1)	Wrist: flexion and adduction (ulnar deviation) of hand
Intermediate muscles				
⑤ Flexor digitorum superficialis	Humeral-ulnar head: medial epicondyle of humerus Radial head: upper half of anterior border of radius	Sides of middle phalanges of 2nd to 5th digits	Median n. (C8, T1)	Elbow: weak flexor Wrist, MCP, and PIP joints of 2nd to 5th digits: flexion
Deep muscles				
⑥ Flexor digitorum profundus	Ulna (proximal two thirds of flexor surface) and interosseous membrane	Distal phalanges of 2nd to 5th digits (palmar surface)	Median n. (C8, T1) Ulnar n. (C8, T1)	Wrist, MCP, PIP, and DIP of 2nd to 5th digits: flexion
⑦ Flexor pollicis longus	Radius (midanterior surface) and adjacent interosseous membrane	Distal phalanx of thumb (palmar surface)	Median n. (C8, T1)	Wrist: flexion and abduction (radial deviation) of hand Carpometacarpal of thumb: flexion MCP and IP of thumb: flexion
⑧ Pronator quadratus	Distal quarter of ulna (anterior surface)	Distal quarter of radius (anterior surface)		Hand: pronation Distal radioulnar joint: stabilization

DIP, distal interphalangeal; IP, interphalangeal; MCP, metacarpophalangeal; PIP, proximal interphalangeal.

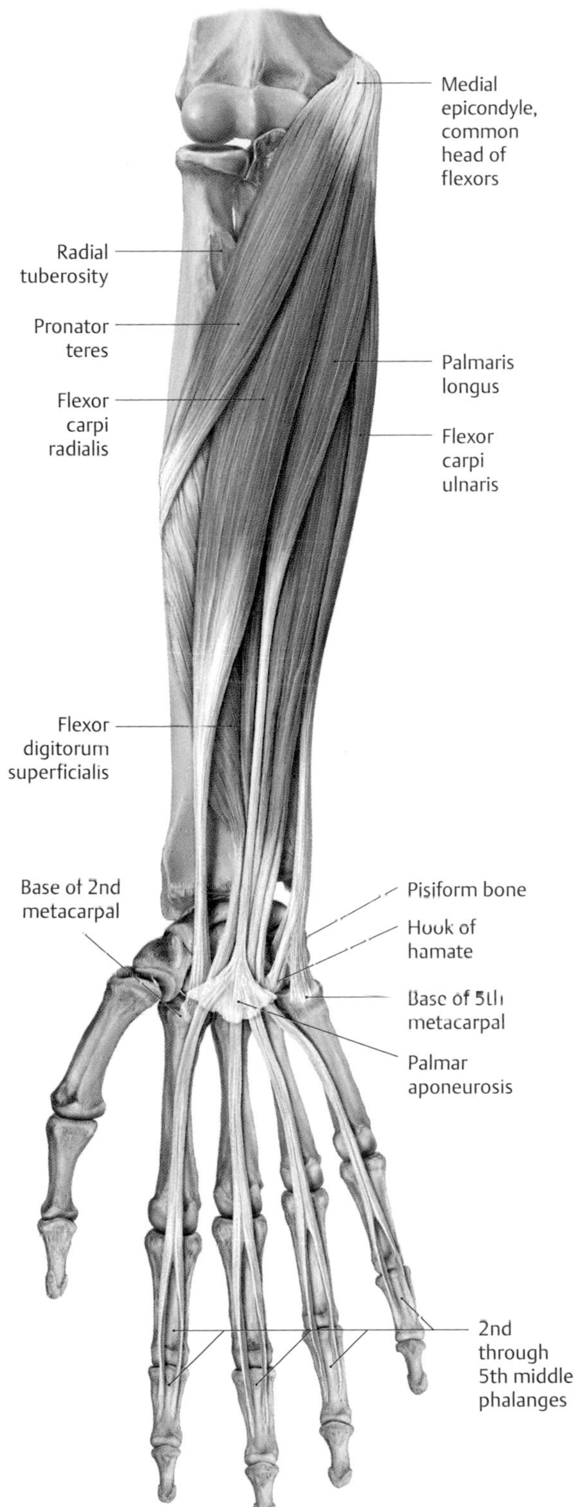
Medial
epicondyle,
common
head of
flexors
Radial
tuberosity
Pronator
teres
Palmaris
longus
Flexor
carpi
radialis
Flexor
carpi
ulnaris
Flexor
digitorum
superficialis
Base of 2nd
metacarpal
Pisiform bone
Hook of
hamate
Base of 5th
metacarpal
Palmar
aponeurosis
2nd
through
5th middle
phalanges

Fig. 22.14 **Anterior compartment of the forearm: Superficial and intermediate muscles**
Right forearm, anterior view.

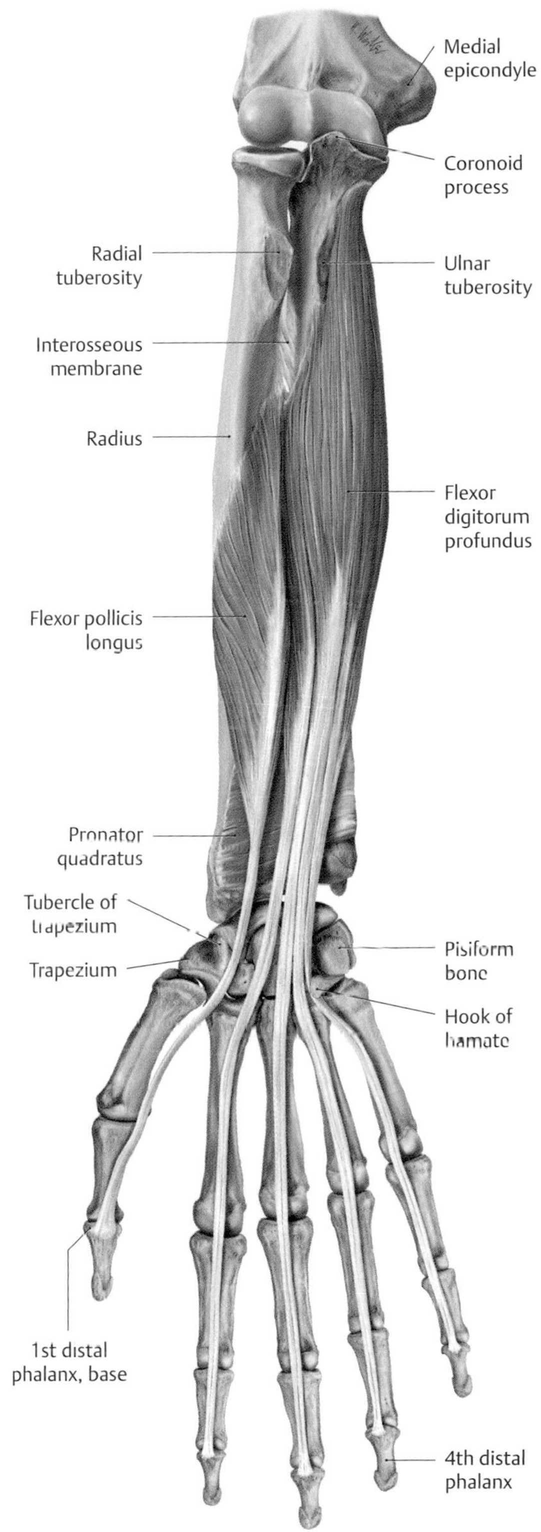
Medial
epicondyle
Coronoid
process
Radial
tuberosity
Ulnar
tuberosity
Interosseous
membrane
Radius
Flexor
digitorum
profundus
Flexor pollicis
longus
Pronator
quadratus
Tubercle of
trapezium
Pisiform
bone
Trapezium
Hook of
hamate
1st distal
phalanx, base
4th distal
phalanx

Fig. 22.15 **Anterior compartment of the forearm: Deep muscles**
Right forearm, anterior view.

Muscle Facts (II)

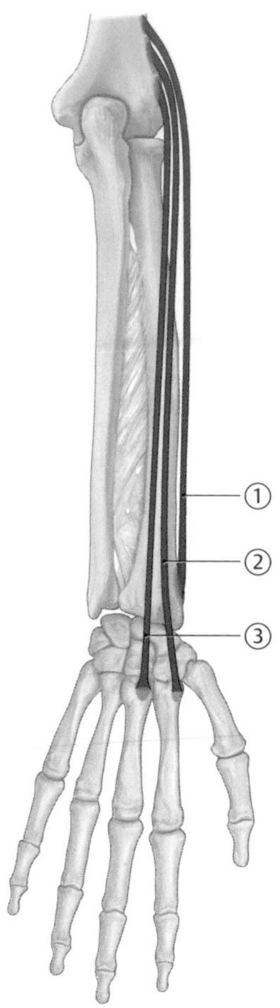
①
②
③

Fig. 22.16 Posterior compartment of the forearm: Radialis muscles
Right forearm, posterior view, schematic.

Clinical

Lateral epicondylitis

Lateral epicondylitis, or tennis elbow, involves the extensor muscles and tendons of the forearm that attach on the lateral epicondyle. The tendon most commonly involved is that of the extensor carpi radialis brevis, a muscle that helps stabilize the wrist when the elbow is extended. When the extensor carpi radialis brevis is weakened from overuse, microscopic tears form in the tendon where it attaches to the lateral epicondyle. This leads to inflammation and pain. There is some evidence that the inflammation can extend back along the tendon to the periosteum of the lateral epicondyle.

Athletes are not the only people who get tennis elbow and are actually in the minority — leading some to suggest the condition be referred to as "lateral elbow syndrome". Workers whose activities require repetitive and vigorous use of the forearm muscles, such as common to painters, plumbers, and carpenters, are particularly prone to developing this pathology. Studies show a high incidence also among auto workers, cooks, and butchers. Common signs and symptoms of tennis elbow include pain with wrist extension against resistance, point tenderness or burning on the lateral epicondyle, and weak grip strength. Symptoms are intensified with forearm activity.

Table 22.3 Posterior compartment of the forearm: Radialis muscles

Muscle	Origin	Insertion	Innervation	Action
① Brachioradialis	Distal humerus (distal surface), lateral intermuscular septum	Styloid process of the radius	Radial n. (C5, C6)	Elbow: flexion Forearm: semipronation
② Extensor carpi radialis longus	Lateral supracondylar ridge of distal humerus, lateral intermuscular septum	2nd metacarpal (base)	Radial n. (C6, C7)	Elbow: weak flexion Wrist: extension and abduction
③ Extensor carpi radialis brevis	Lateral epicondyle of humerus	3rd metacarpal (base)	Radial n. (C7, C8)	

Fig. 22.17 Posterior compartment of the forearm: Radialis muscles

Right forearm.

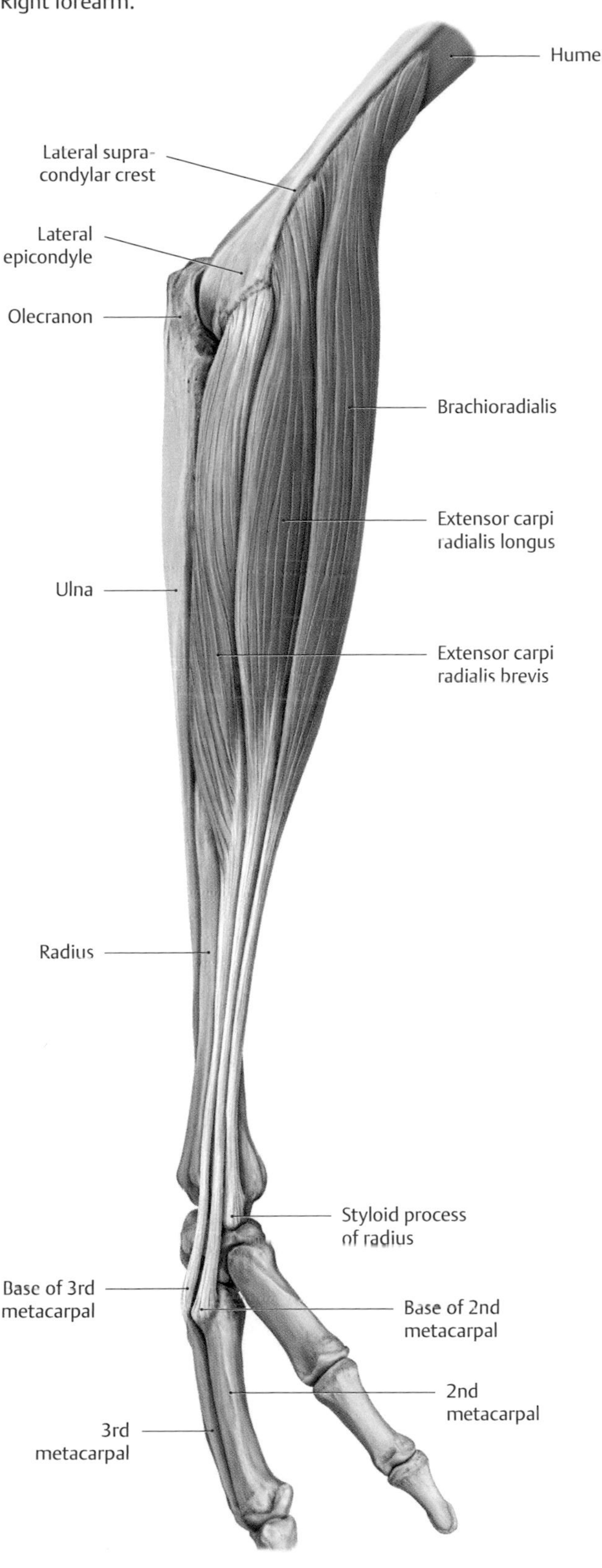
Humerus
Lateral supra-
condylar crest
Lateral
epicondyle
Olecranon
Brachioradialis
Extensor carpi
radialis longus
Ulna
Extensor carpi
radialis brevis
Radius
Styloid process
of radius
Base of 3rd
metacarpal
Base of 2nd
metacarpal
2nd
metacarpal
3rd
metacarpal

A Lateral (radial) view.

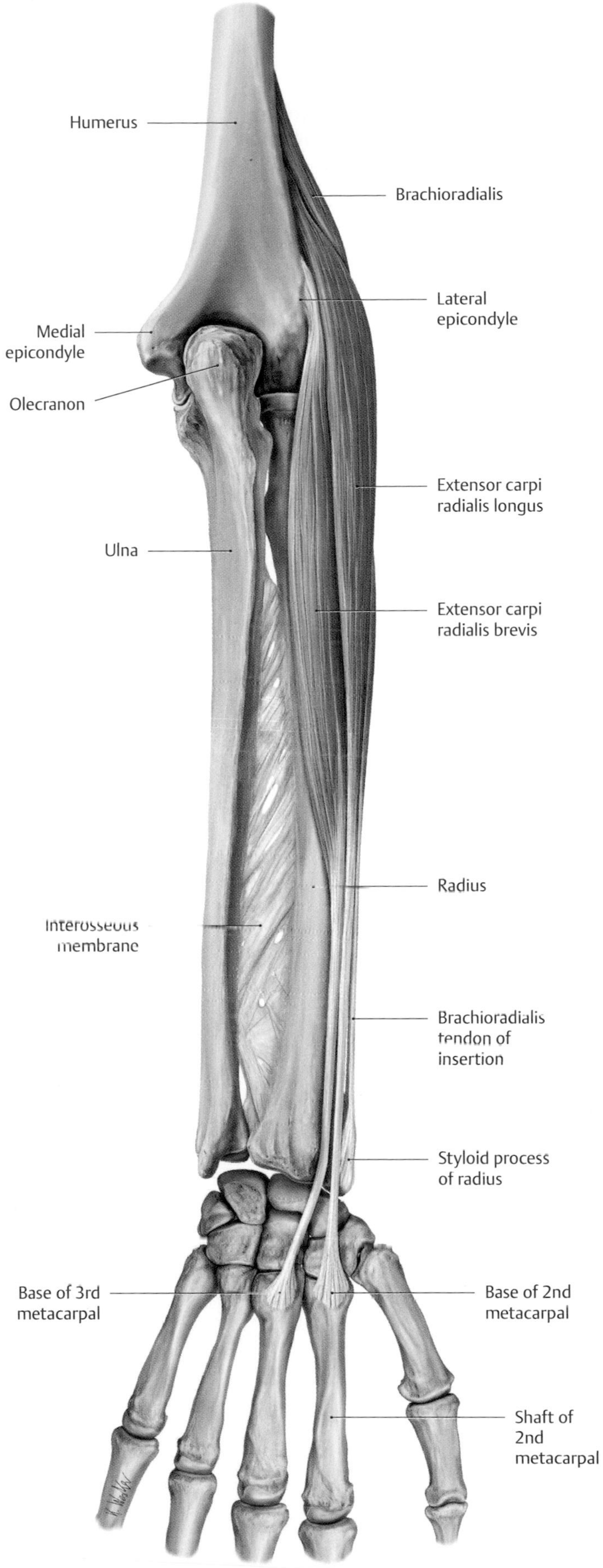

Humerus
Brachioradialis
Lateral
epicondyle
Medial
epicondyle
Olecranon
Extensor carpi
radialis longus
Ulna
Extensor carpi
radialis brevis
Radius
Interosseous
membrane
Brachioradialis
tendon of
insertion
Styloid process
of radius
Base of 3rd
metacarpal
Base of 2nd
metacarpal
Shaft of
2nd
metacarpal

B Posterior view.

Muscle Facts (III)

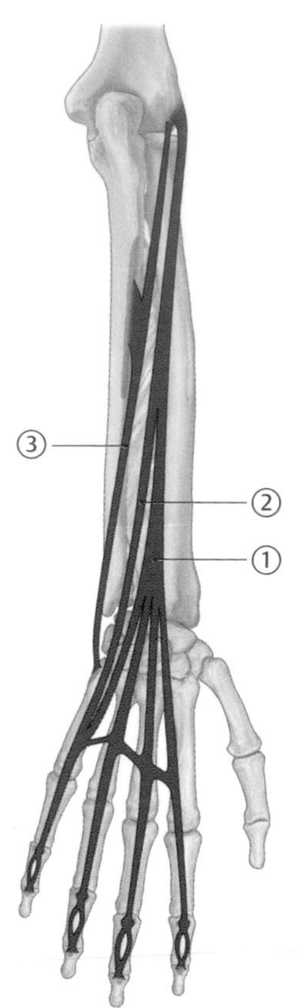
③
②
①

Fig. 22.18 **Posterior compartment of the forearm: Superficial muscles**
Right forearm, posterior view, schematic.

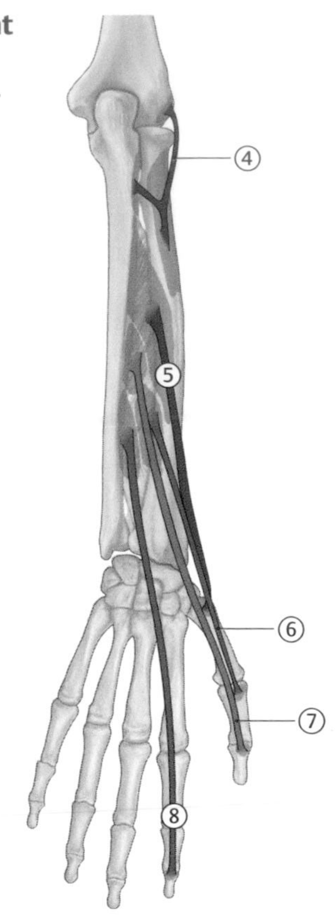
④
⑤
⑥
⑦
⑧

Fig. 22.19 **Posterior compartment of the forearm: Deep muscles**
Right forearm, posterior view, schematic.

Table 22.4 **Posterior compartment of the forearm**

Muscle	Origin	Insertion	Innervation	Action
Superficial muscles				
① Extensor digitorum	Common head (lateral epicondyle of humerus)	Dorsal digital expansion of 2nd to 5th digits	Radial n. (C7, C8)	Wrist: extension MCP, PIP, and DIP of 2nd to 5th digits: extension/abduction of fingers
② Extensor digiti minimi		Dorsal digital expansion of 5th digit		Wrist: extension, ulnar abduction of hand MCP, PIP, and DIP of 5th digit: extension and abduction of 5th digit
③ Extensor carpi ulnaris	Common head (lateral epicondyle of humerus) Ulnar head (dorsal surface)	Base of 5th metacarpal		Wrist: extension, adduction (ulnar deviation) of hand
Deep muscles				
④ Supinator	Olecranon, lateral epicondyle of humerus, radial collateral ligament, annular ligament of radius	Radius (between radial tuberosity and insertion of pronator teres)	Radial n. (C6, C7)	Radioulnar joints: supination
⑤ Abductor pollicis longus	Radius and ulna (dorsal surfaces, interosseous membrane)	Base of 1st metacarpal	Radial n. (C7, C8)	Radiocarpal joint: abduction of the hand Carpometacarpal joint of thumb: abduction
⑥ Extensor pollicis brevis	Radius (posterior surface) and interosseous membrane	Base of proximal phalanx of thumb		Radiocarpal joint: abduction (radial deviation) of hand Carpometacarpal and MCP of thumb: extension
⑦ Extensor pollicis longus	Ulna (posterior surface) and interosseous membrane	Base of distal phalanx of thumb		Wrist: extension and abduction (radial deviation) of hand Carpometacarpal of thumb: adduction MCP and IP of thumb: extension
⑧ Extensor indicis	Ulna (posterior surface) and interosseous membrane	Posterior digital extension of 2nd digit		Wrist: extension MCP, PIP, and DIP of 2nd digit: extension

DIP, distal interphalangeal; IP, interphalangeal; MCP, metacarpophalangeal; PIP, proximal interphalangeal.

Fig. 22.20 Muscles of the posterior compartment of the forearm

Right forearm, posterior view.

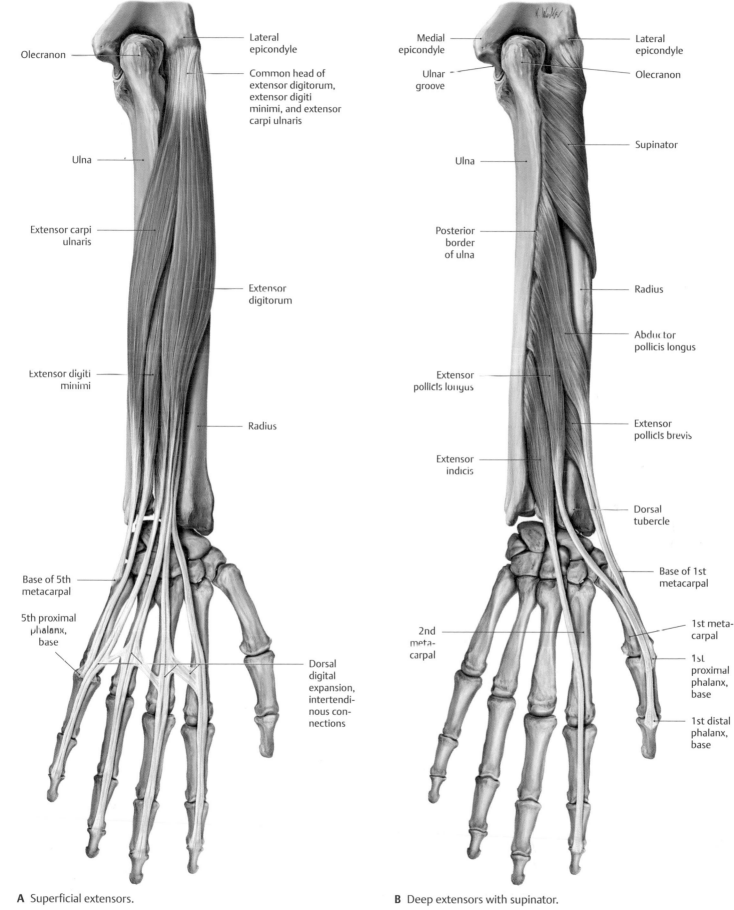

Olecranon
Lateral epicondyle
Common head of extensor digitorum, extensor digiti minimi, and extensor carpi ulnaris
Ulna
Extensor carpi ulnaris
Extensor digitorum
Extensor digiti minimi
Radius
Base of 5th metacarpal
5th proximal phalanx, base
Dorsal digital expansion, intertendinous connections

A Superficial extensors.

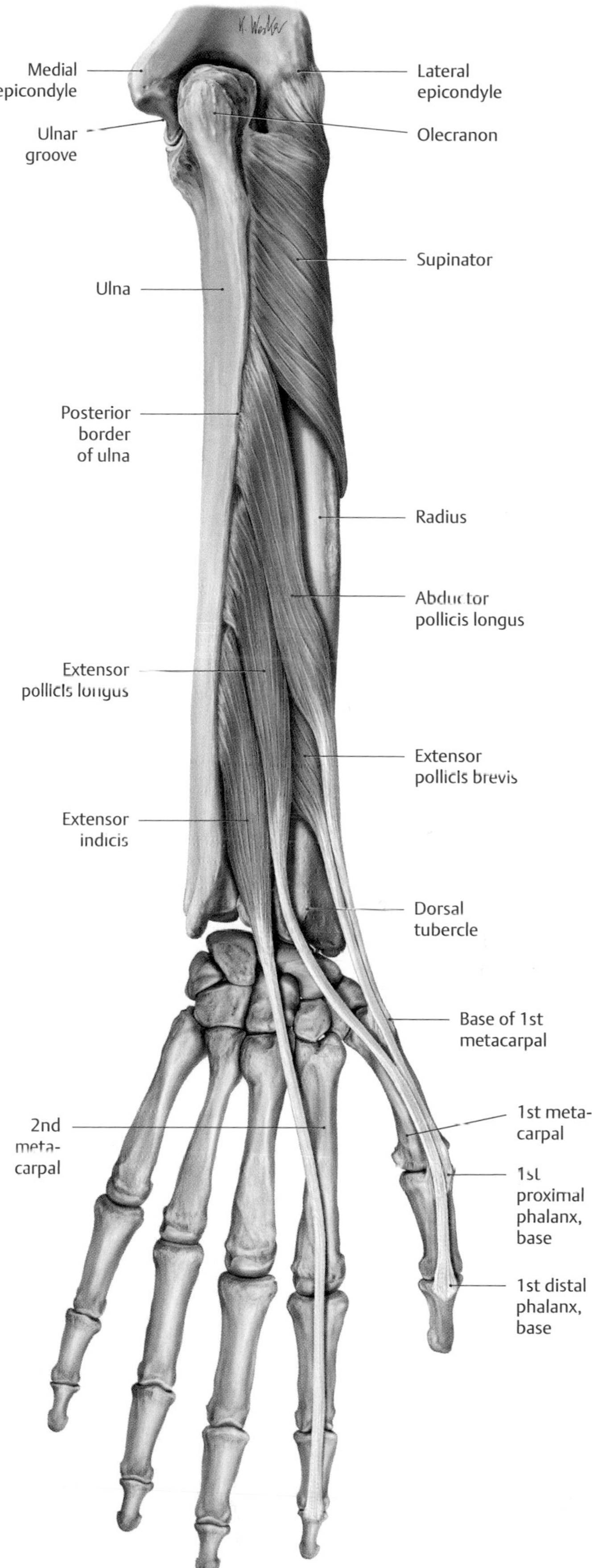
Medial epicondyle
Ulnar groove
Lateral epicondyle
Olecranon
Supinator
Ulna
Posterior border of ulna
Radius
Abductor pollicis longus
Extensor pollicis longus
Extensor pollicis brevis
Extensor indicis
Dorsal tubercle
Base of 1st metacarpal
2nd metacarpal
1st metacarpal
1st proximal phalanx, base
1st distal phalanx, base

B Deep extensors with supinator.

Bones of the Wrist & Hand

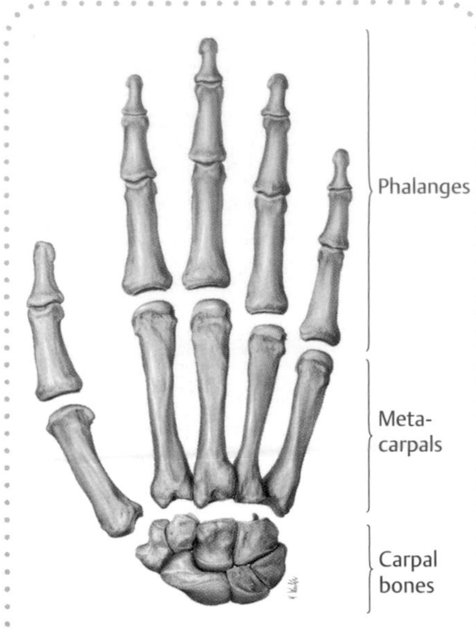
Phalanges
Meta-
carpals
Carpal
bones

Table 23.1 Bones of the wrist and hand

Phalanges	1st to 5th proximal phalanges	
	2nd to 5th middle phalanges*	
	1st to 5th distal phalanges	
Metacarpal bones	1st to 5th metacarpals	
Carpal bones	Trapezium	Scaphoid
	Trapezoid	Lunate
	Capitate	Triquetrum
	Hamate	Pisiform

*There are only four middle phalanges (the thumb has only a proximal and a distal phalanx).

Fig. 23.1 **Dorsal view**
Right hand.

2nd distal phalanx
2nd middle phalanx
2nd proximal phalanx
1st metacarpal
Trapezoid
Trapezium
Scaphoid
Styloid process of radius
Radius
Capitate
Hamate
Triquetrum
Lunate
Styloid process of ulna
Ulna

Fig. 23.2 **Palmar view**
Right hand.

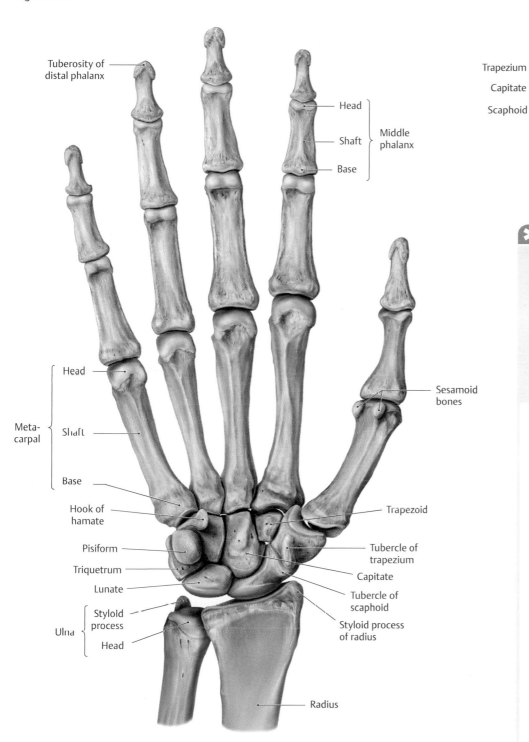

Tuberosity of distal phalanx
Head
Shaft
Base
Middle phalanx
Meta-carpal
Head
Shaft
Base
Sesamoid bones
Hook of hamate
Trapezoid
Pisiform
Tubercle of trapezium
Triquetrum
Capitate
Lunate
Tubercle of scaphoid
Ulna
Styloid process
Head
Styloid process of radius
Radius

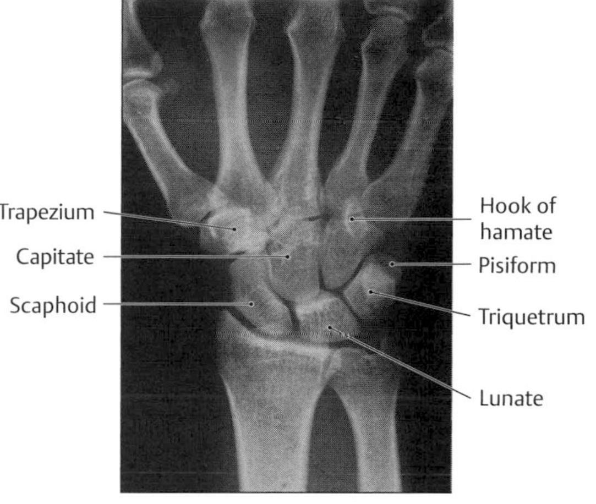
Trapezium
Capitate
Scaphoid
Hook of hamate
Pisiform
Triquetrum
Lunate

Fig. 23.3 **Radiograph of the wrist**
Anteroposterior view of left limb.

Clinical

Scaphoid Fractures
Scaphoid fractures are the most common carpal bone fractures, generally occurring at the narrowed waist between the proximal and distal poles (**A**, right scaphoid). Because blood supply to the scaphoid is transmitted via the distal segment, fractures at the waist can compromise the supply to the proximal segment, often resulting in nonunion and avascular necrosis.

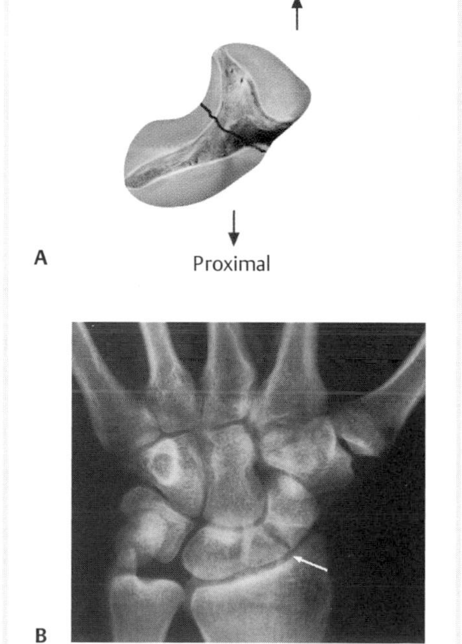
Distal
A
Proximal
B

The Carpal Bones

Fig. 23.4 **Carpal bones of the right wrist**

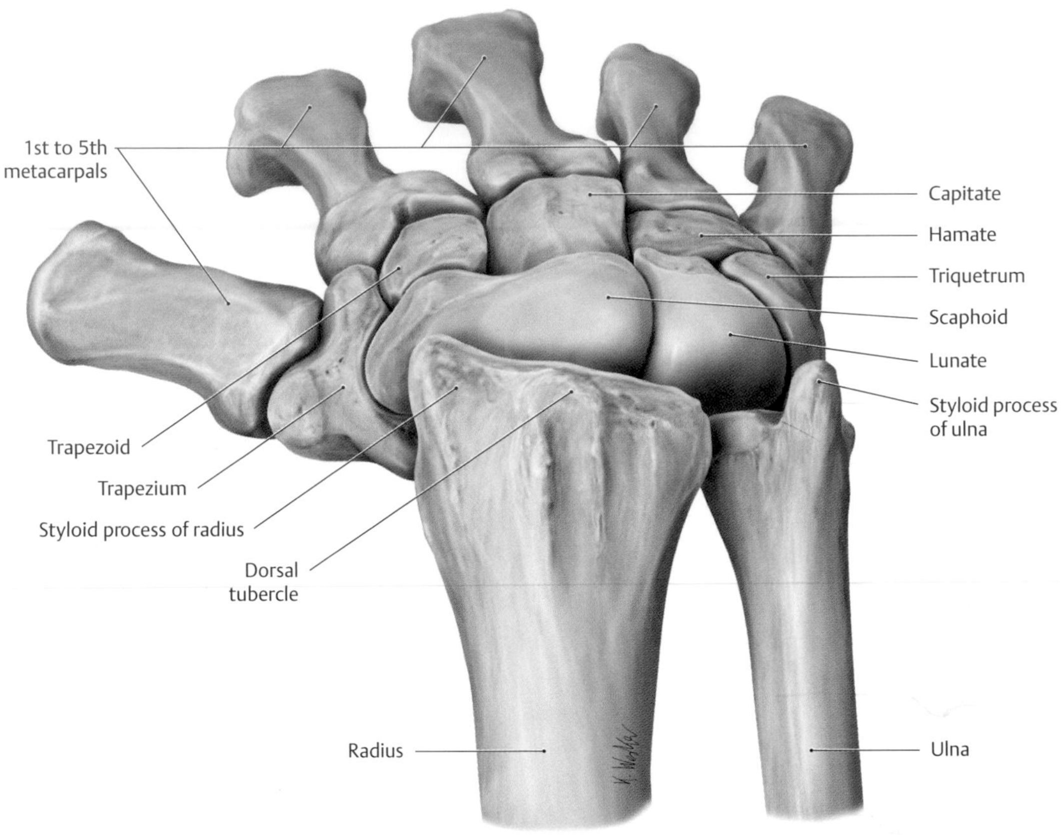
1st to 5th metacarpals
Capitate
Hamate
Triquetrum
Scaphoid
Lunate
Styloid process of ulna
Trapezoid
Trapezium
Styloid process of radius
Dorsal tubercle
Radius
Ulna

A Carpal bones of the right wrist with the wrist in flexion, proximal view.

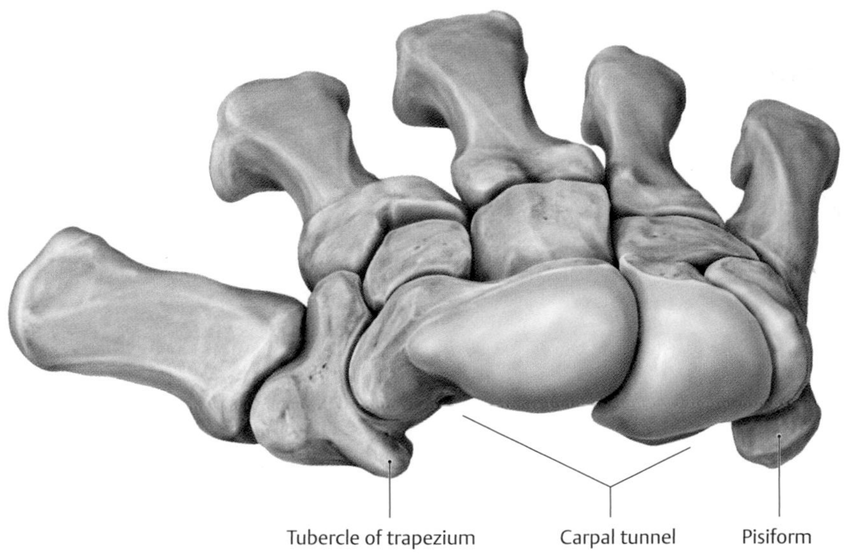
Tubercle of trapezium
Carpal tunnel
Pisiform

B Carpal and metacarpal bones of the right wrist with radius and ulna removed, proximal view.

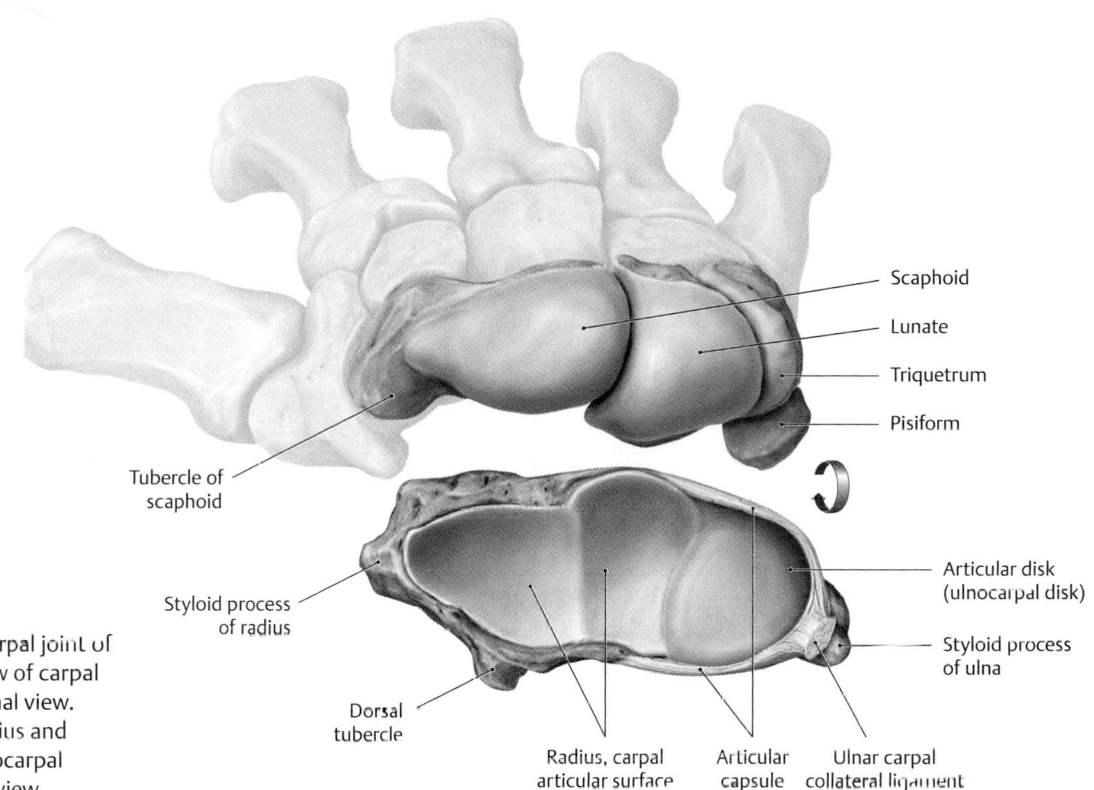
Scaphoid
Lunate
Triquetrum
Pisiform
Tubercle of scaphoid
Articular disk (ulnocarpal disk)
Styloid process of radius
Styloid process of ulna
Dorsal tubercle
Radius, carpal articular surface
Articular capsule
Ulnar carpal collateral ligament

C Articular surfaces of the radiocarpal joint of the right wrist. The proximal row of carpal bones is shown from the proximal view. The articular surfaces of the radius and ulna, and the articular disk (ulnocarpal disk) are shown from the distal view.

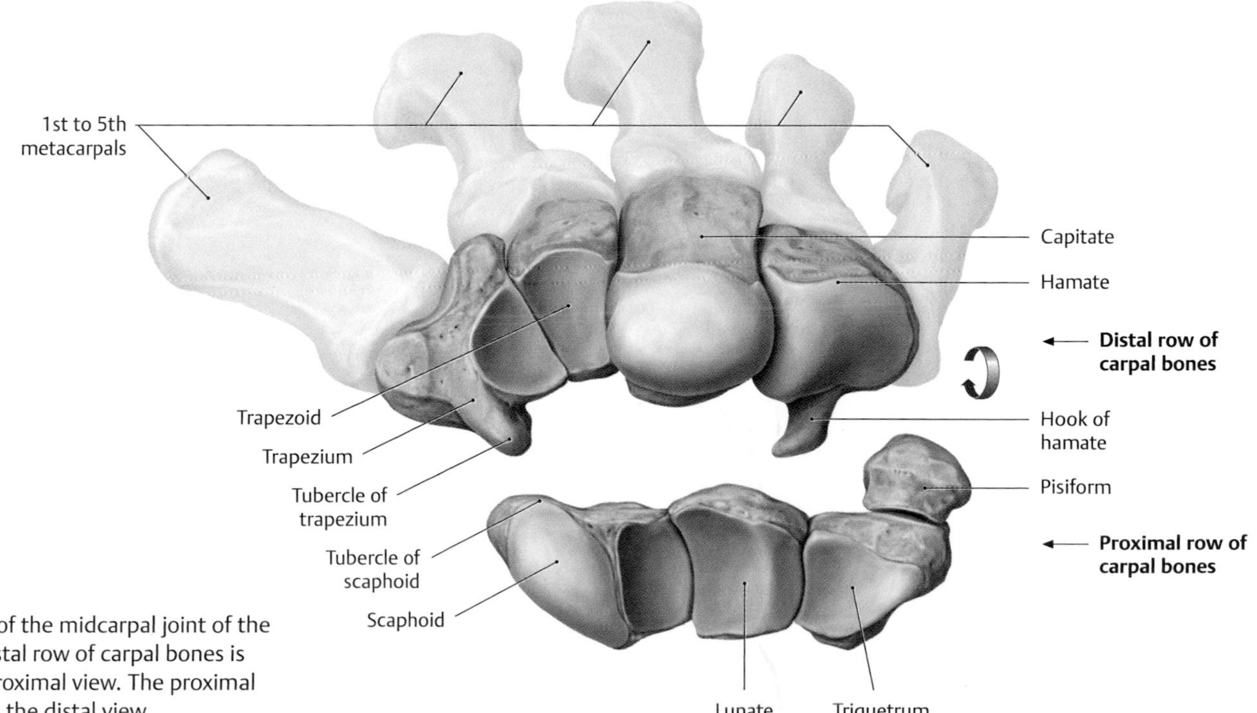
1st to 5th metacarpals
Capitate
Hamate
Distal row of carpal bones
Hook of hamate
Pisiform
Proximal row of carpal bones
Trapezoid
Trapezium
Tubercle of trapezium
Tubercle of scaphoid
Scaphoid
Lunate
Triquetrum

D Articular surfaces of the midcarpal joint of the right wrist. The distal row of carpal bones is shown from the proximal view. The proximal row is shown from the distal view.

Joints of the Wrist & Hand

Fig. 23.5 Joints of the wrist and hand

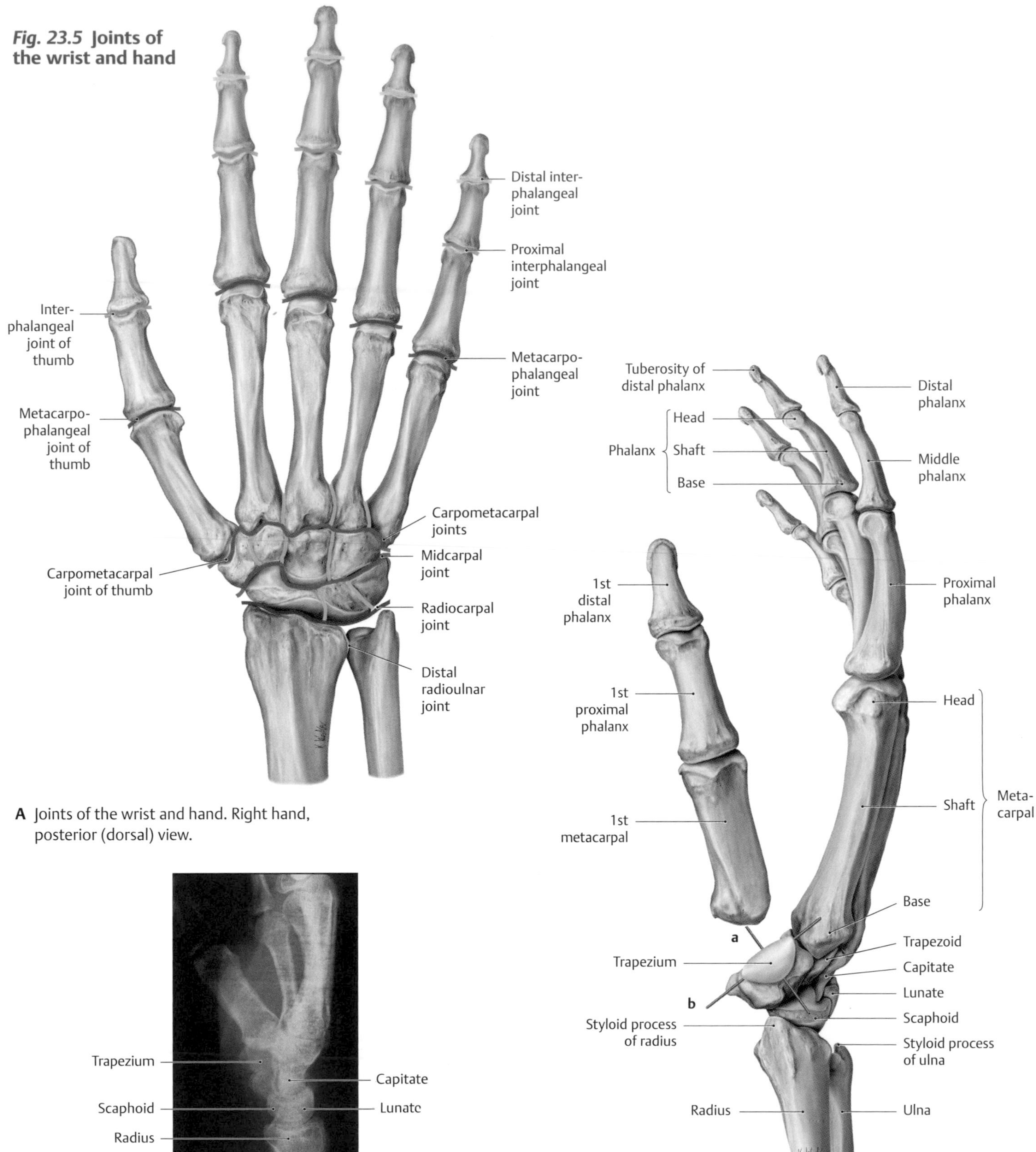
Distal interphalangeal joint
Proximal interphalangeal joint
Interphalangeal joint of thumb
Metacarpophalangeal joint
Metacarpophalangeal joint of thumb
Carpometacarpal joints
Midcarpal joint
Carpometacarpal joint of thumb
Radiocarpal joint
Distal radioulnar joint
Tuberosity of distal phalanx
Phalanx
Head
Shaft
Base
Distal phalanx
Middle phalanx
1st distal phalanx
Proximal phalanx
1st proximal phalanx
Head
Shaft
Meta-carpal
1st metacarpal
Base
a
Trapezoid
Trapezium
Capitate
Lunate
b
Scaphoid
Styloid process of radius
Styloid process of ulna
Radius
Ulna
Trapezium
Capitate
Scaphoid
Lunate
Radius

A Joints of the wrist and hand. Right hand, posterior (dorsal) view.

B Carpometacarpal joint of the thumb. Radial view. The 1st metacarpal bone has been moved slightly distally to expose the articular surface of the trapezium. Two cardinal axes of motion are shown here: (**a**) abduction/adduction and (**b**) flexion/extension.

C Radiograph of wrist. Radial view.

Fig. 23.6 Wrist and hand: Coronal section
Right hand, posterior (dorsal) view.

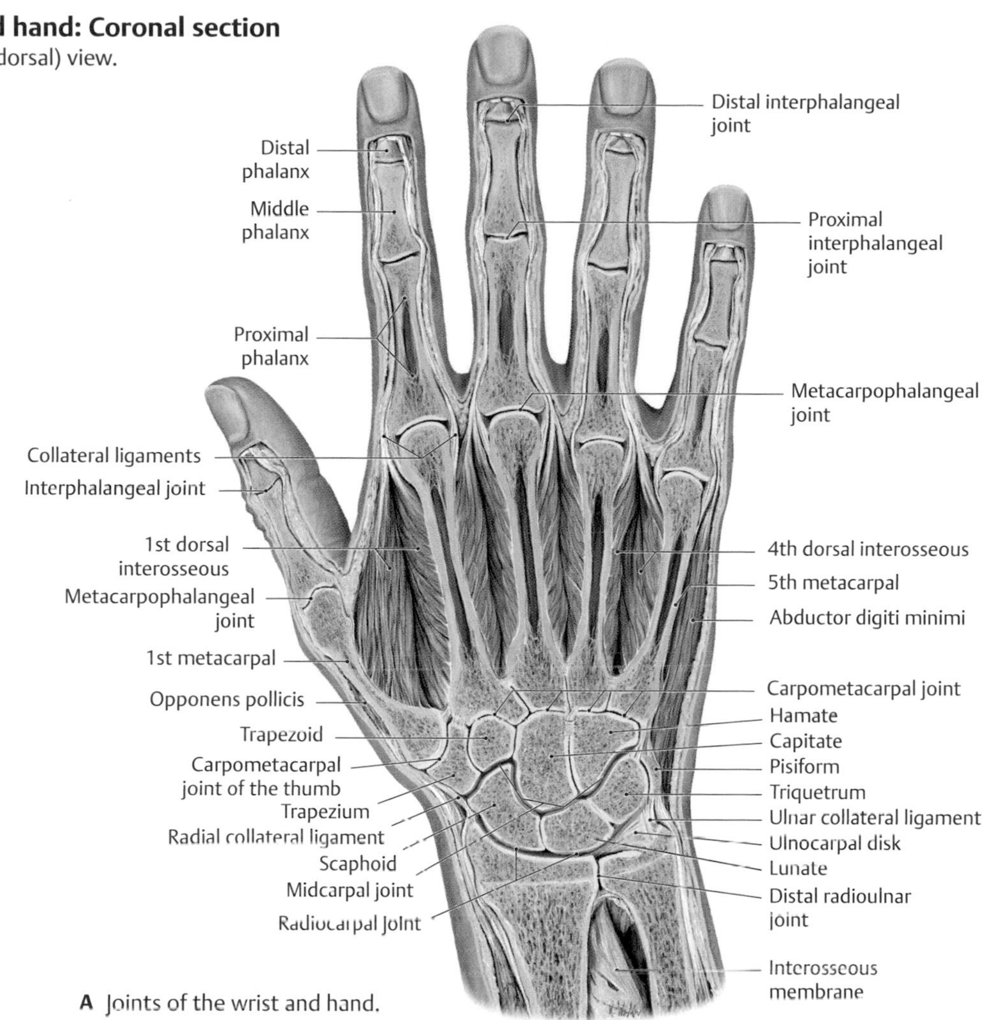
Distal phalanx
Middle phalanx
Proximal phalanx
Collateral ligaments
Interphalangeal joint
1st dorsal interosseous
Metacarpophalangeal joint
1st metacarpal
Opponens pollicis
Trapezoid
Carpometacarpal joint of the thumb
Trapezium
Radial collateral ligament
Scaphoid
Midcarpal joint
Radiocarpal joint
Distal interphalangeal joint
Proximal interphalangeal joint
Metacarpophalangeal joint
4th dorsal interosseous
5th metacarpal
Abductor digiti minimi
Carpometacarpal joint
Hamate
Capitate
Pisiform
Triquetrum
Ulnar collateral ligament
Ulnocarpal disk
Lunate
Distal radioulnar joint
Interosseous membrane

A Joints of the wrist and hand.

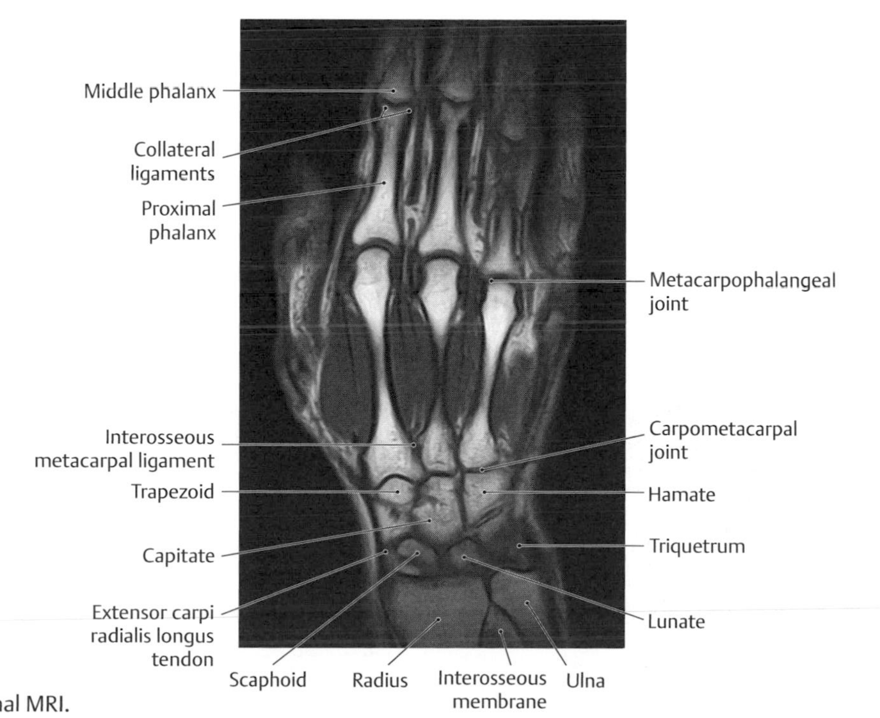
Middle phalanx
Collateral ligaments
Proximal phalanx
Interosseous metacarpal ligament
Trapezoid
Capitate
Extensor carpi radialis longus tendon
Scaphoid
Radius
Interosseous membrane
Ulna
Metacarpophalangeal joint
Carpometacarpal joint
Hamate
Triquetrum
Lunate

B Coronal MRI.

Ligaments of the Hand

Fig. 23.7 **Ligaments of the hand**
Right hand.

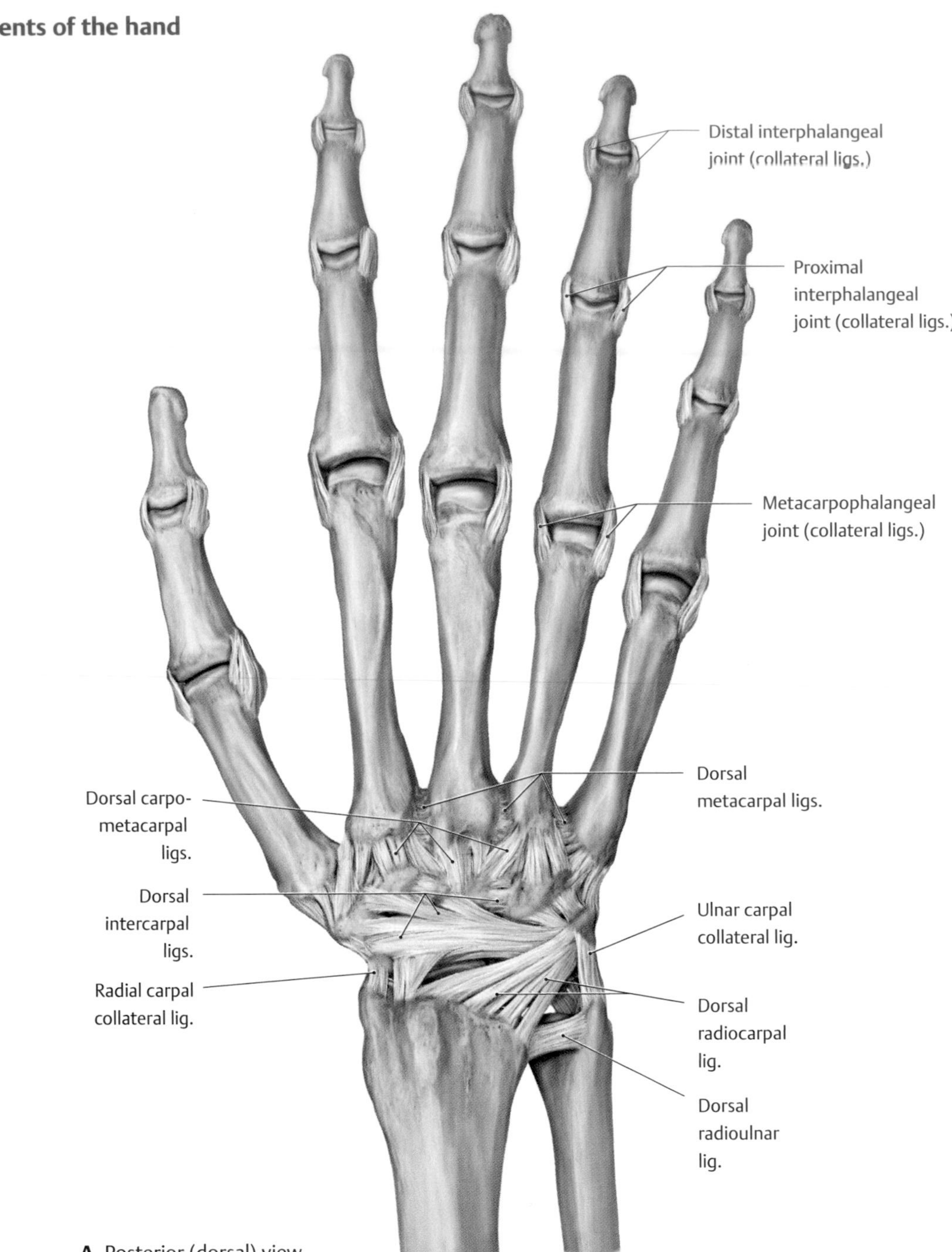
Distal interphalangeal joint (collateral ligs.)
Proximal interphalangeal joint (collateral ligs.)
Metacarpophalangeal joint (collateral ligs.)
Dorsal metacarpal ligs.
Dorsal carpo-metacarpal ligs.
Dorsal intercarpal ligs.
Radial carpal collateral lig.
Ulnar carpal collateral lig.
Dorsal radiocarpal lig.
Dorsal radioulnar lig.

A Posterior (dorsal) view.

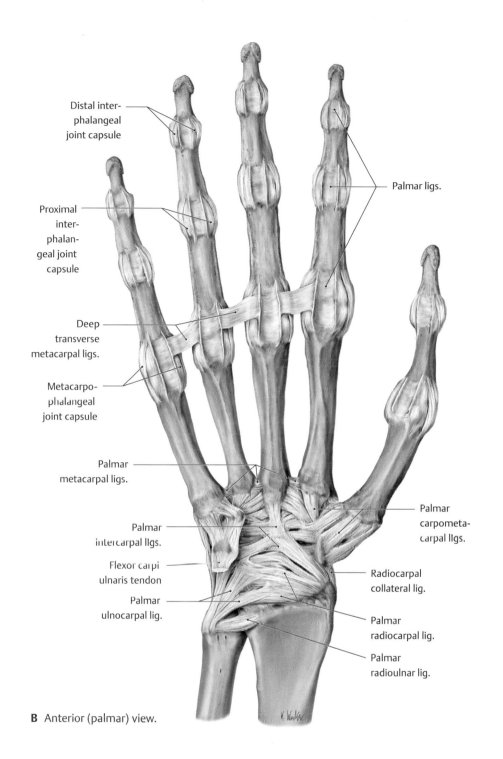

Distal interphalangeal joint capsule

Palmar ligs.

Proximal interphalangeal joint capsule

Deep transverse metacarpal ligs.

Metacarpophalangeal joint capsule

Palmar metacarpal ligs.

Palmar carpometacarpal ligs.

Palmar intercarpal ligs.

Flexor carpi ulnaris tendon

Radiocarpal collateral lig.

Palmar ulnocarpal lig.

Palmar radiocarpal lig.

Palmar radioulnar lig.

B Anterior (palmar) view.

Clinical

Functional position of the hand

The anatomic position of the hand, in which the palm is flat, the fingers are extended, and the forearm is supinated (palm facing forward), differs from the normal relaxed position of the hand. At rest, the forearm is in mid-supination/pronation (palm facing the body), the wrist is slightly extended, the fingers form an arcade of flexion, and the thumb is in the neutral position. Postoperative immobilization of the hand (by a cast or splint) fixes the wrist and fingers in the flexed position to prevent shortening of the ligaments and to maintain the ability of the hand to assume normal resting position.

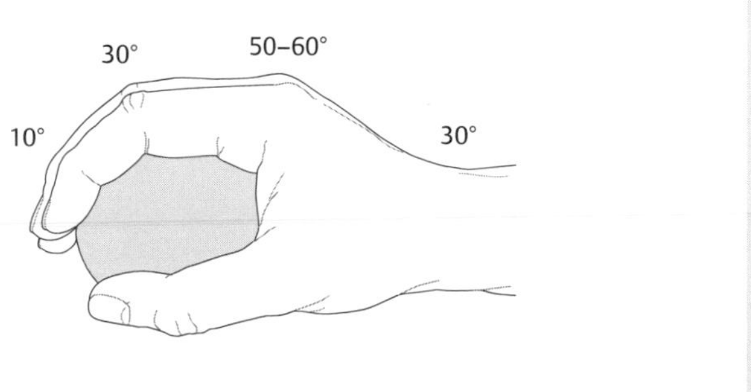

30°
50–60°
10°
30°

Ligaments of the Wrist

Fig. 23.8 **Ligaments of the carpal tunnel**
Right hand, anterior view.

Hook of hamate
Pisiform bone
Carpal tunnel entrance
Ulna
Flexor retinaculum (transverse carpal lig.)
Tubercle of trapezium
Radius

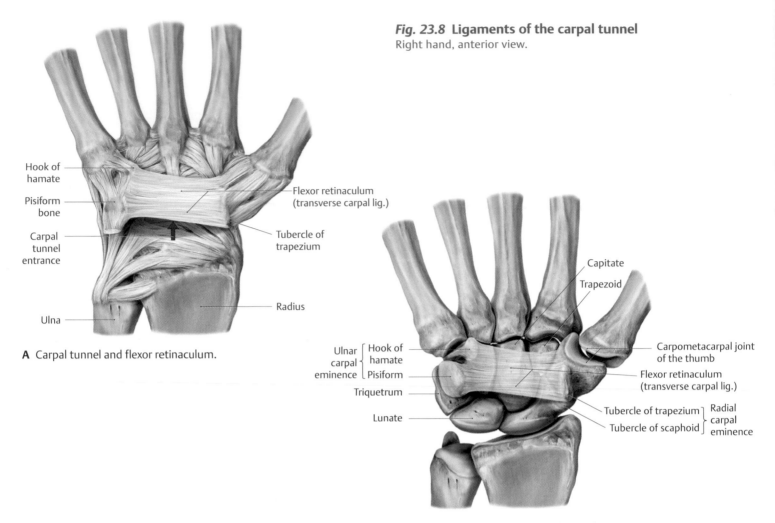

A Carpal tunnel and flexor retinaculum.

Capitate
Trapezoid
Ulnar carpal eminence
Hook of hamate
Pisiform
Triquetrum
Lunate
Carpometacarpal joint of the thumb
Flexor retinaculum (transverse carpal lig.)
Tubercle of trapezium
Tubercle of scaphoid
Radial carpal eminence

B Bony boundaries of the carpal tunnel.

Fig. 23.9 **Carpal tunnel**
Right hand, transverse section. The contents of the carpal tunnel are discussed on p. 370. See p. 371 for the ulnar tunnel and palmar carpal ligament.

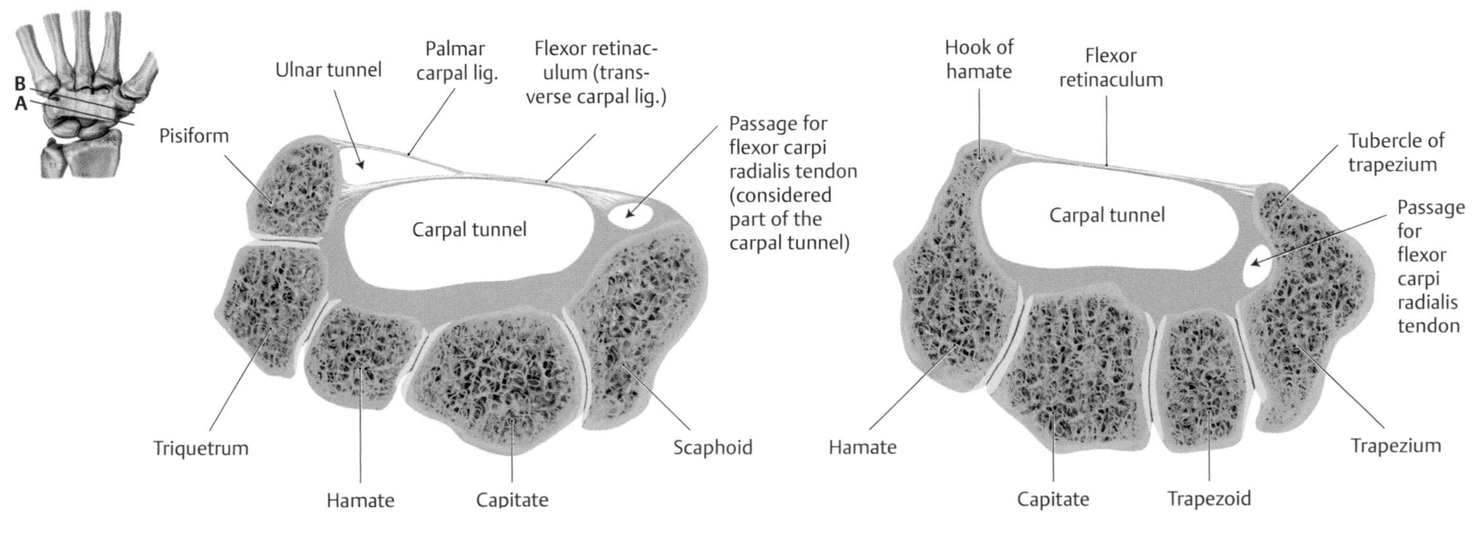
B
A
Pisiform
Ulnar tunnel
Palmar carpal lig.
Flexor retinaculum (transverse carpal lig.)
Passage for flexor carpi radialis tendon (considered part of the carpal tunnel)
Carpal tunnel
Triquetrum
Hamate
Capitate
Scaphoid
Hook of hamate
Flexor retinaculum
Carpal tunnel
Tubercle of trapezium
Passage for flexor carpi radialis tendon
Hamate
Capitate
Trapezoid
Trapezium

A Proximal part of the carpal tunnel.

B Distal part of the carpal tunnel.

Fig. 23.10 Ligaments of the ulnocarpal region
Right hand, anterior view.

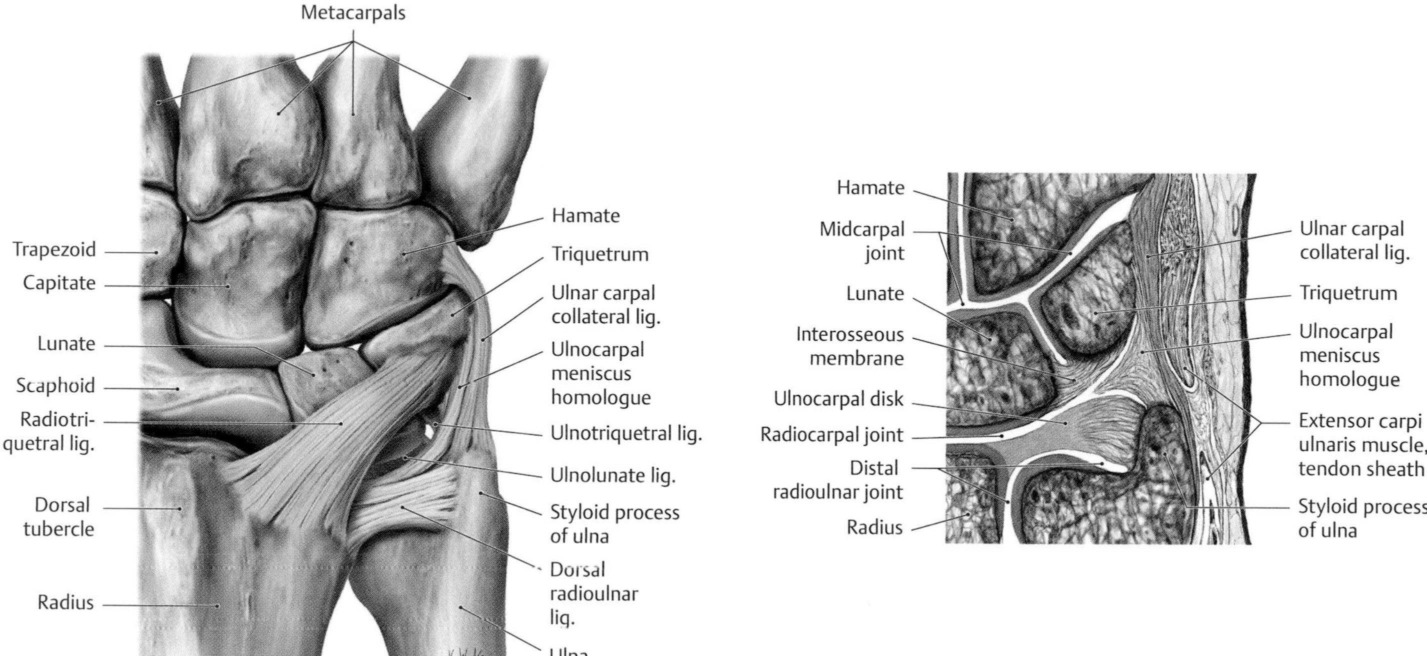
Metacarpals
Trapezoid
Capitate
Lunate
Scaphoid
Radiotri-quetral lig.
Dorsal tubercle
Radius
Hamate
Triquetrum
Ulnar carpal collateral lig.
Ulnocarpal meniscus homologue
Ulnotriquetral lig.
Ulnolunate lig.
Styloid process of ulna
Dorsal radioulnar lig.
Ulna
Hamate
Midcarpal joint
Lunate
Interosseous membrane
Ulnocarpal disk
Radiocarpal joint
Distal radioulnar joint
Radius
Ulnar carpal collateral lig.
Triquetrum
Ulnocarpal meniscus homologue
Extensor carpi ulnaris muscle, tendon sheath
Styloid process of ulna

A Right wrist, posterior view.

B Schematic of a histologic preparation of the triangular fibrocartilage (ulnocarpal) complex.

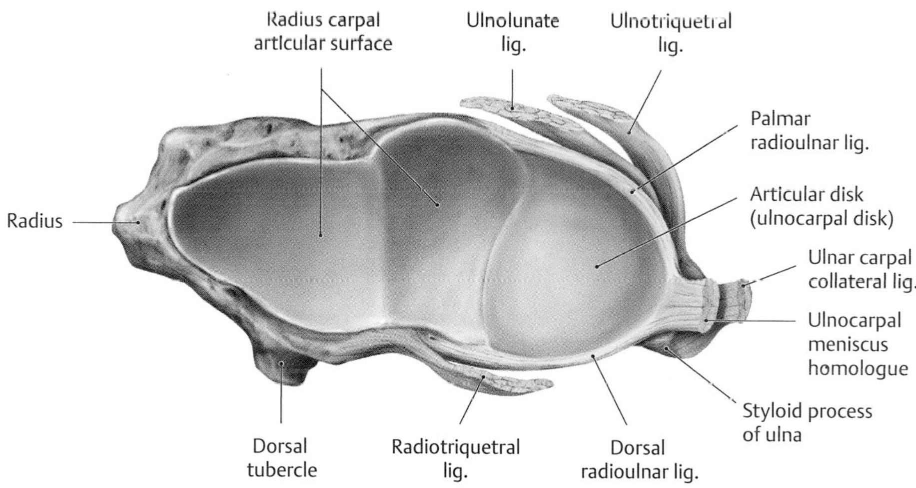
Radius carpal articular surface
Ulnolunate lig.
Ulnotriquetral lig.
Palmar radioulnar lig.
Articular disk (ulnocarpal disk)
Ulnar carpal collateral lig.
Ulnocarpal meniscus homologue
Styloid process of ulna
Radius
Dorsal tubercle
Radiotriquetral lig.
Dorsal radioulnar lig.

C Right wrist, distal view.

Ligaments of the Fingers

Fig. 23.11 **Ligaments of the fingers: Lateral view**
Right middle finger. The outer fibrous layer of the tendon sheaths (stratum fibrosum) is strengthened by the annular and cruciform ligaments, which also bind the sheaths to the palmar surface of the phalanx and prevent palmar deviation of the sheaths during flexion.

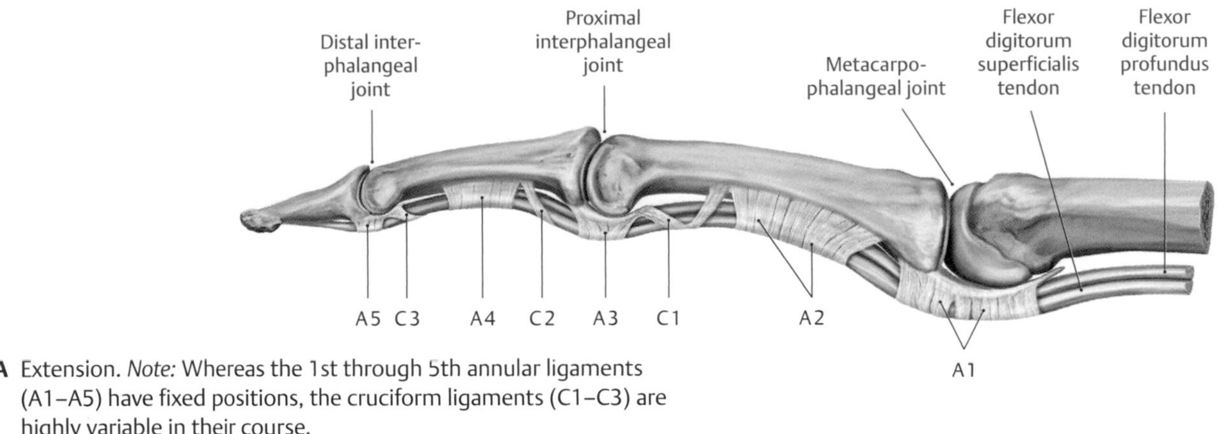
Distal inter-
phalangeal
joint
Proximal
interphalangeal
joint
Metacarpo-
phalangeal joint
Flexor
digitorum
superficialis
tendon
Flexor
digitorum
profundus
tendon
A5
C3
A4
C2
A3
C1
A2
A1

A Extension. *Note:* Whereas the 1st through 5th annular ligaments (A1–A5) have fixed positions, the cruciform ligaments (C1–C3) are highly variable in their course.

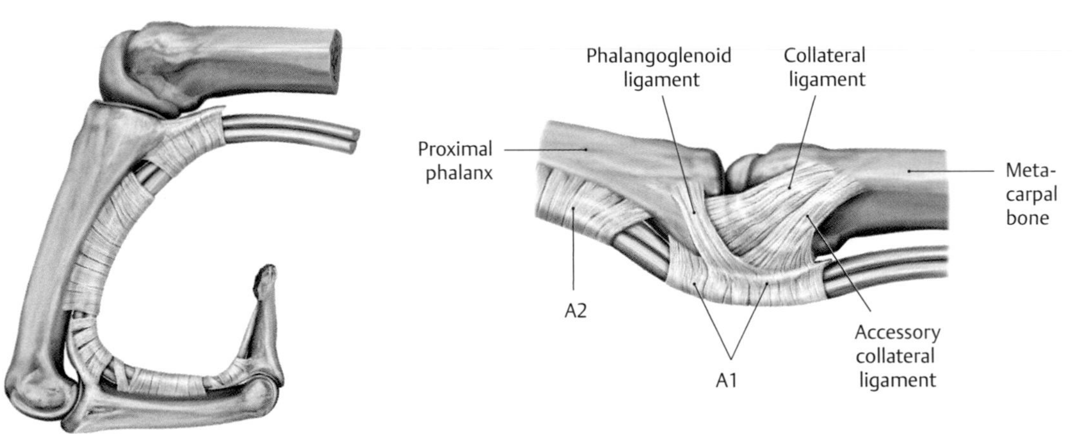
Phalangoglenoid
ligament
Collateral
ligament
Proximal
phalanx
Meta-
carpal
bone
A2
A1
Accessory
collateral
ligament

B Flexion.

C Extension of the metacarpophalangeal joint. *Note:* The collateral ligament is lax.

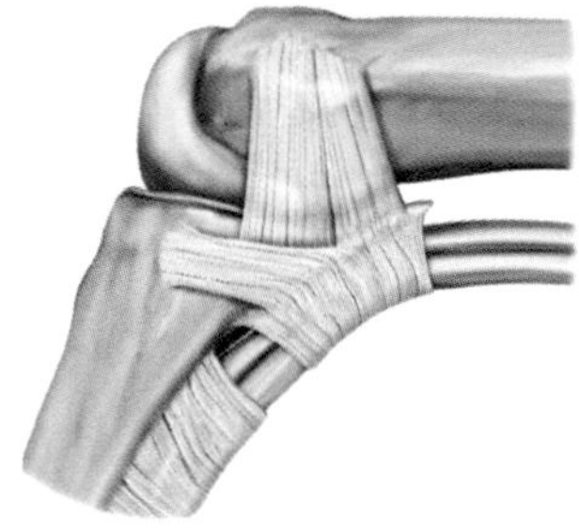

D Flexion of the metacarpophalangeal joint. *Note:* The collateral ligament is taut.

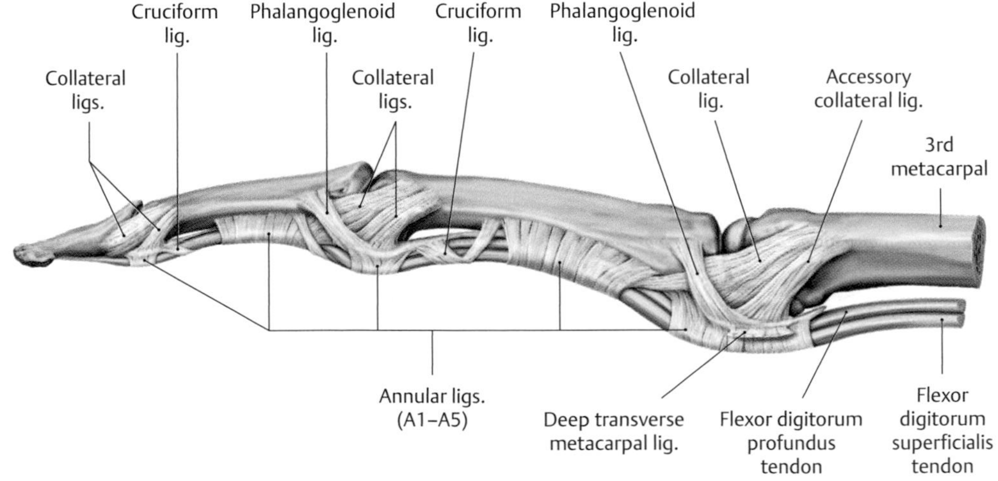
Cruciform
lig.
Phalangoglenoid
lig.
Cruciform
lig.
Phalangoglenoid
lig.
Collateral
ligs.
Collateral
ligs.
Collateral
lig.
Accessory
collateral lig.
3rd
metacarpal
Annular ligs.
(A1–A5)
Deep transverse
metacarpal lig.
Flexor digitorum
profundus
tendon
Flexor
digitorum
superficialis
tendon

E Joint capsules, ligaments, and digital tendon sheaths.

Fig. 23.12 Ligaments of the fingers: Anterior view

Right middle finger, palmar view.

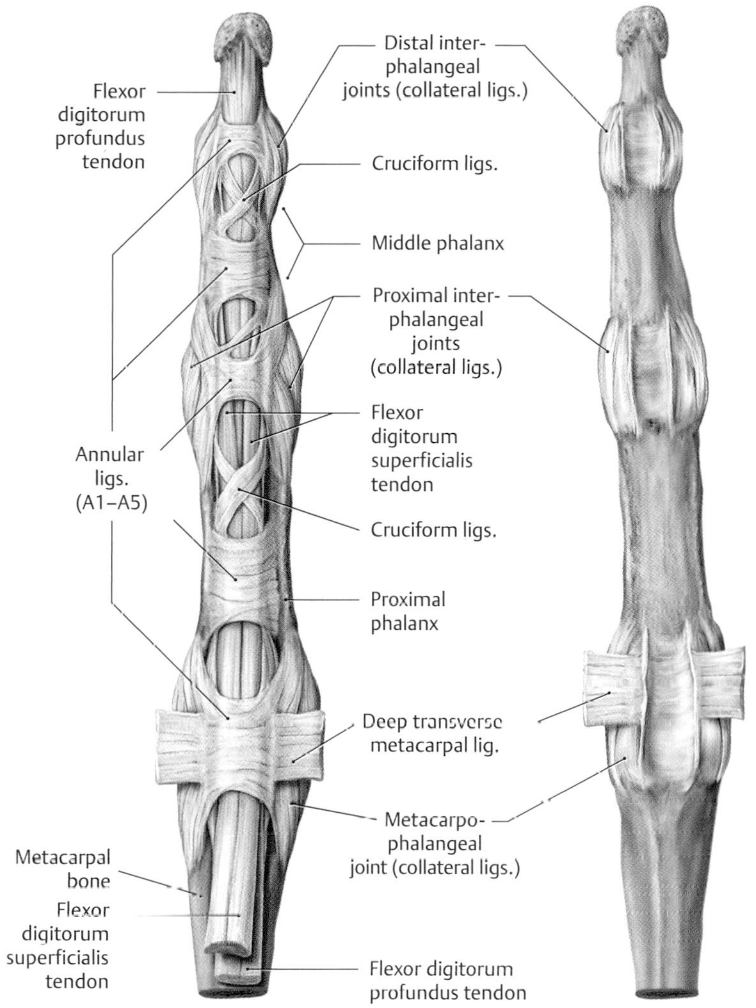

Flexor digitorum profundus tendon
Distal interphalangeal joints (collateral ligs.)
Cruciform ligs.
Middle phalanx
Proximal interphalangeal joints (collateral ligs.)
Flexor digitorum superficialis tendon
Annular ligs. (A1–A5)
Cruciform ligs.
Proximal phalanx
Deep transverse metacarpal lig.
Metacarpophalangeal joint (collateral ligs.)
Metacarpal bone
Flexor digitorum superficialis tendon
Flexor digitorum profundus tendon

A Superficial ligaments.

B Deep ligaments with digital tendon sheath removed.

Fig. 23.13 Third metacarpal: Transverse section

Proximal view.

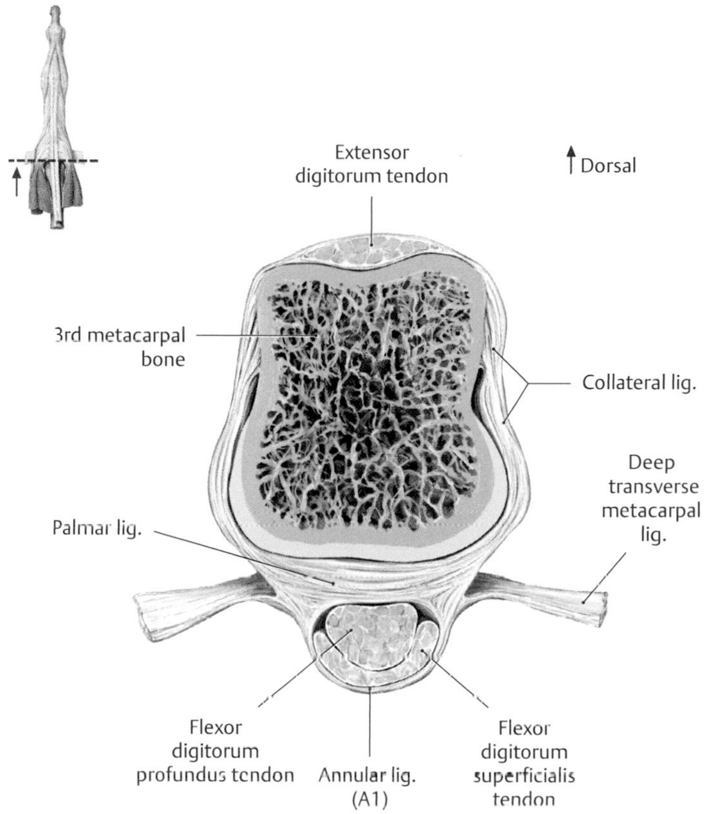

Extensor digitorum tendon
Dorsal
3rd metacarpal bone
Collateral lig.
Deep transverse metacarpal lig.
Palmar lig.
Flexor digitorum profundus tendon
Annular lig. (A1)
Flexor digitorum superficialis tendon

Fig. 23.14 Fingertip: Longitudinal section

The palmar articular surfaces of the phalanges are enlarged proximally at the joints by the palmar ligament. This fibrocartilaginous plate, also known as the volar plate, forms the floor of the digital tendon sheaths.

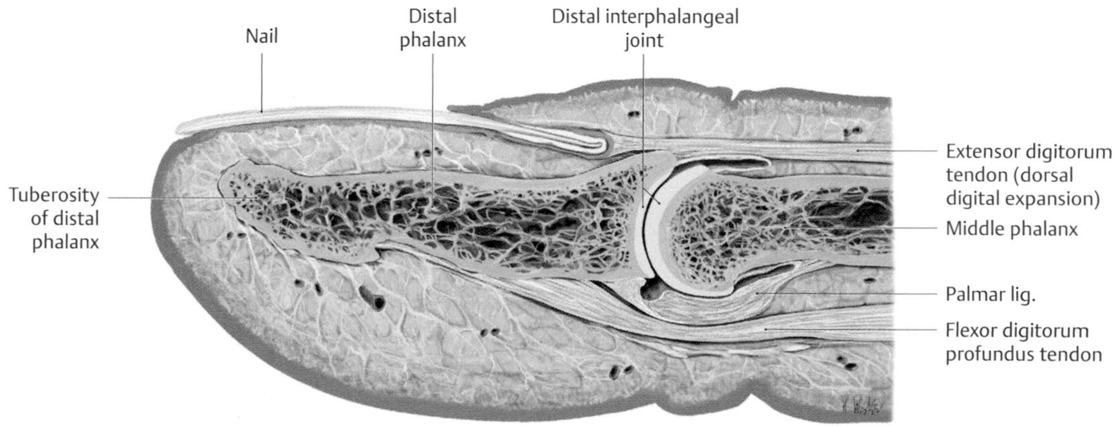
Nail
Distal phalanx
Distal interphalangeal joint
Tuberosity of distal phalanx
Extensor digitorum tendon (dorsal digital expansion)
Middle phalanx
Palmar lig.
Flexor digitorum profundus tendon

Muscles of the Hand: Superficial & Middle Layers

Fig. 23.15 Intrinsic muscles of the hand: Superficial and middle layers
Right hand, palmar surface.

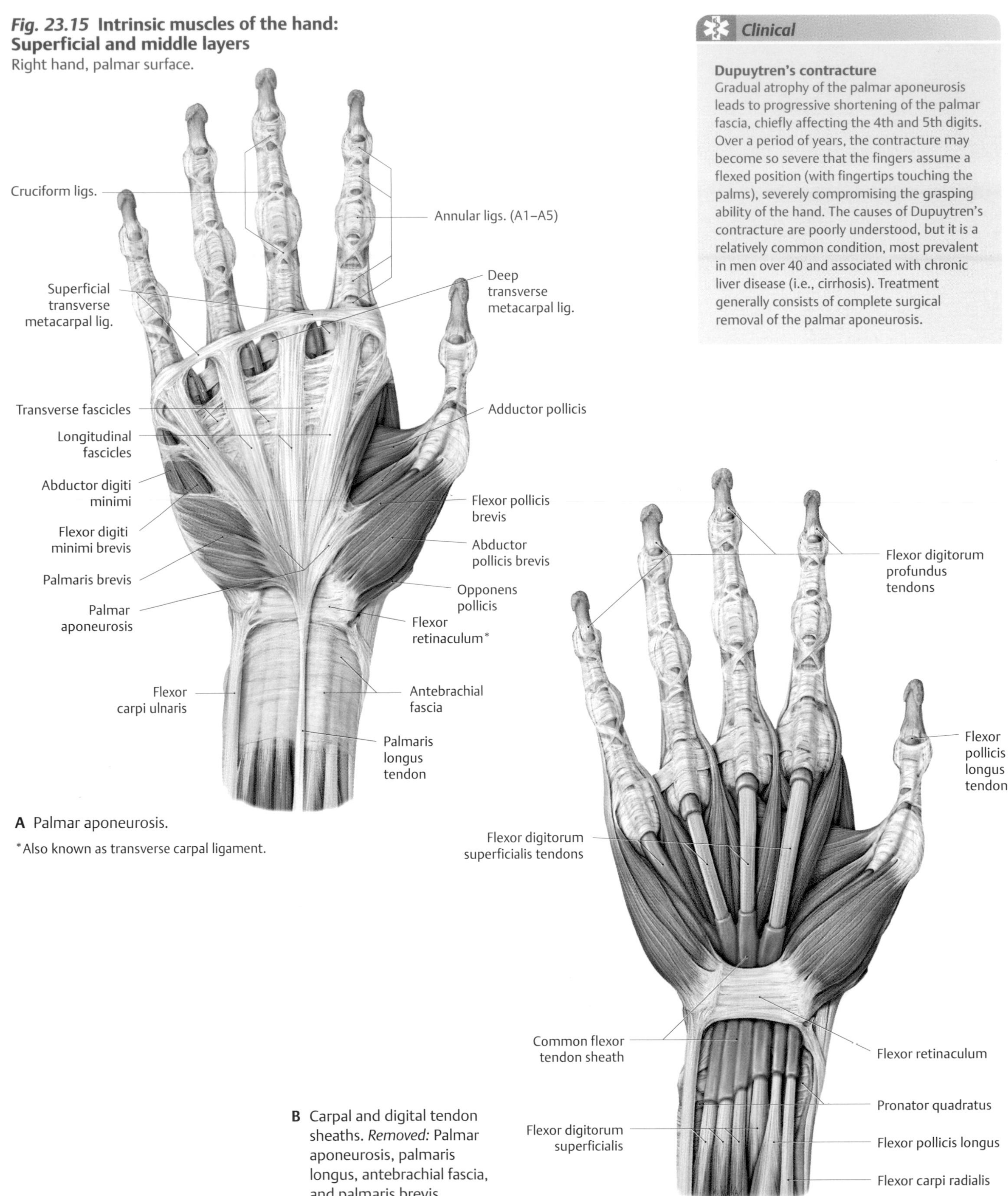
Cruciform ligs.
Annular ligs. (A1–A5)
Superficial transverse metacarpal lig.
Deep transverse metacarpal lig.
Transverse fascicles
Adductor pollicis
Longitudinal fascicles
Abductor digiti minimi
Flexor pollicis brevis
Flexor digiti minimi brevis
Abductor pollicis brevis
Palmaris brevis
Opponens pollicis
Palmar aponeurosis
Flexor retinaculum*
Flexor carpi ulnaris
Antebrachial fascia
Palmaris longus tendon
Flexor digitorum profundus tendons
Flexor pollicis longus tendon
Flexor digitorum superficialis tendons
Common flexor tendon sheath
Flexor retinaculum
Pronator quadratus
Flexor digitorum superficialis
Flexor pollicis longus
Flexor carpi radialis

A Palmar aponeurosis.

*Also known as transverse carpal ligament.

B Carpal and digital tendon sheaths. *Removed:* Palmar aponeurosis, palmaris longus, antebrachial fascia, and palmaris brevis.

Clinical

Dupuytren's contracture
Gradual atrophy of the palmar aponeurosis leads to progressive shortening of the palmar fascia, chiefly affecting the 4th and 5th digits. Over a period of years, the contracture may become so severe that the fingers assume a flexed position (with fingertips touching the palms), severely compromising the grasping ability of the hand. The causes of Dupuytren's contracture are poorly understood, but it is a relatively common condition, most prevalent in men over 40 and associated with chronic liver disease (i.e., cirrhosis). Treatment generally consists of complete surgical removal of the palmar aponeurosis.

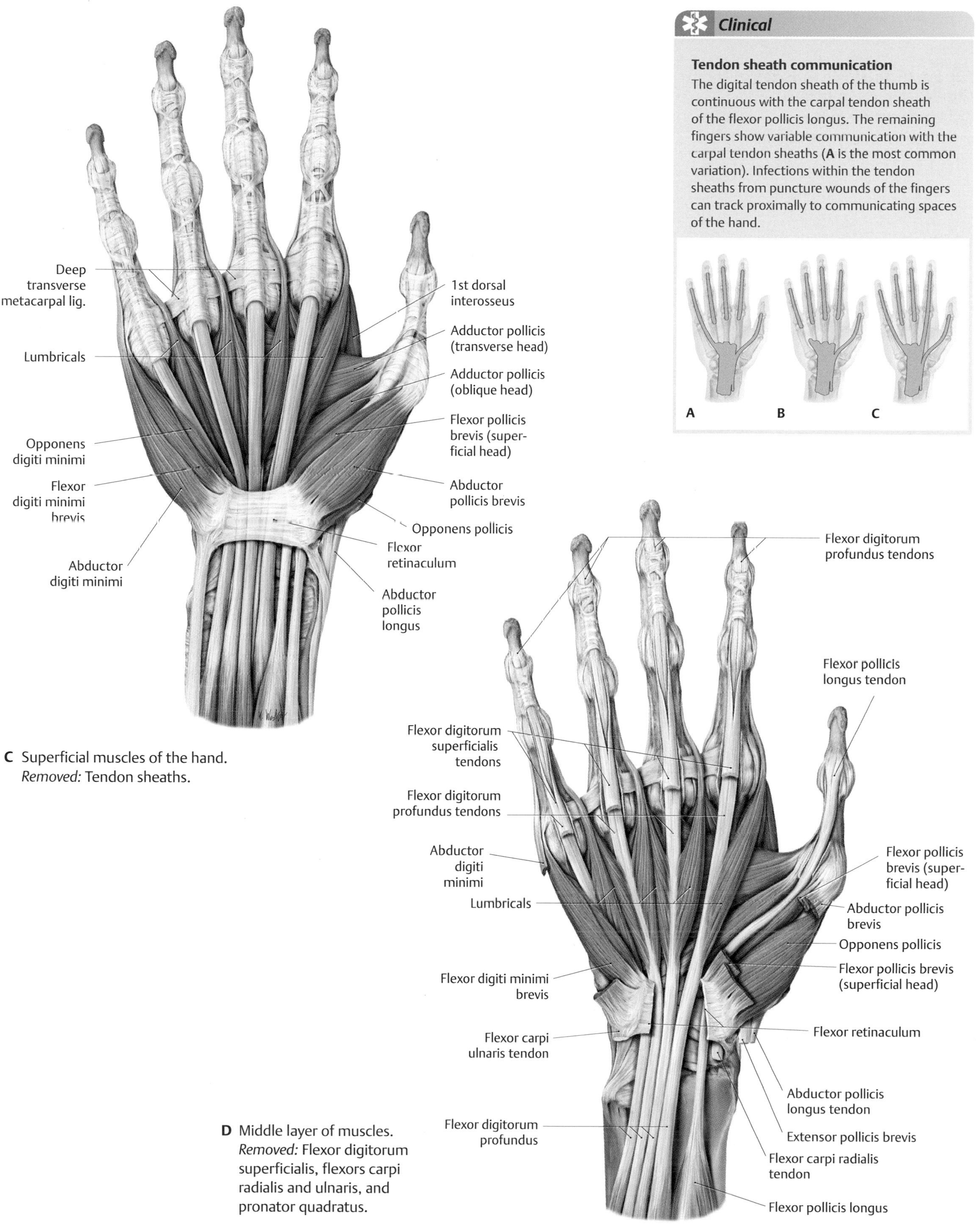
Deep
transverse
metacarpal lig.
Lumbricals
Opponens
digiti minimi
Flexor
digiti minimi
brevis
Abductor
digiti minimi
1st dorsal
interosseus
Adductor pollicis
(transverse head)
Adductor pollicis
(oblique head)
Flexor pollicis
brevis (super-
ficial head)
Abductor
pollicis brevis
Opponens pollicis
Flexor
retinaculum
Abductor
pollicis
longus
Flexor digitorum
profundus tendons
Flexor pollicis
longus tendon
Flexor digitorum
superficialis
tendons
Flexor digitorum
profundus tendons
Abductor
digiti
minimi
Lumbricals
Flexor digiti minimi
brevis
Flexor carpi
ulnaris tendon
Flexor digitorum
profundus
Flexor pollicis
brevis (super-
ficial head)
Abductor pollicis
brevis
Opponens pollicis
Flexor pollicis brevis
(superficial head)
Flexor retinaculum
Abductor pollicis
longus tendon
Extensor pollicis brevis
Flexor carpi radialis
tendon
Flexor pollicis longus

C Superficial muscles of the hand.
Removed: Tendon sheaths.

D Middle layer of muscles.
Removed: Flexor digitorum superficialis, flexors carpi radialis and ulnaris, and pronator quadratus.

Clinical

Tendon sheath communication

The digital tendon sheath of the thumb is continuous with the carpal tendon sheath of the flexor pollicis longus. The remaining fingers show variable communication with the carpal tendon sheaths (**A** is the most common variation). Infections within the tendon sheaths from puncture wounds of the fingers can track proximally to communicating spaces of the hand.

A **B** **C**

Muscles of the Hand: Middle & Deep Layers

Fig. 23.16 **Intrinsic muscles: Middle and deep layers**
Right hand, palmar surface.

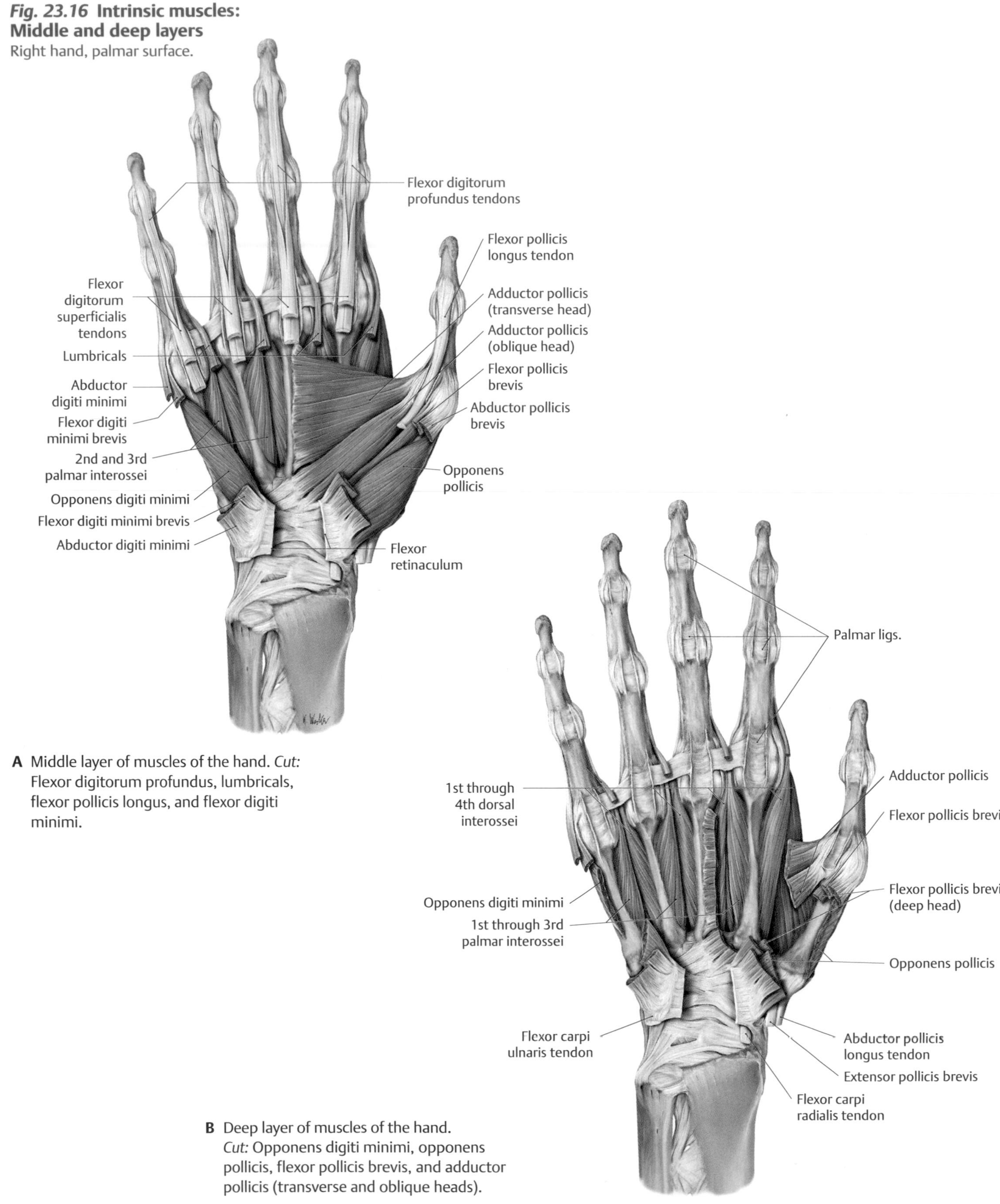

Flexor digitorum profundus tendons
Flexor pollicis longus tendon
Flexor digitorum superficialis tendons
Adductor pollicis (transverse head)
Adductor pollicis (oblique head)
Lumbricals
Flexor pollicis brevis
Abductor digiti minimi
Flexor digiti minimi brevis
Abductor pollicis brevis
2nd and 3rd palmar interossei
Opponens pollicis
Opponens digiti minimi
Flexor digiti minimi brevis
Abductor digiti minimi
Flexor retinaculum
Palmar ligs.
Adductor pollicis
1st through 4th dorsal interossei
Flexor pollicis brevis
Flexor pollicis brevis (deep head)
Opponens digiti minimi
1st through 3rd palmar interossei
Opponens pollicis
Flexor carpi ulnaris tendon
Abductor pollicis longus tendon
Extensor pollicis brevis
Flexor carpi radialis tendon

A Middle layer of muscles of the hand. *Cut:* Flexor digitorum profundus, lumbricals, flexor pollicis longus, and flexor digiti minimi.

B Deep layer of muscles of the hand. *Cut:* Opponens digiti minimi, opponens pollicis, flexor pollicis brevis, and adductor pollicis (transverse and oblique heads).

***Fig. 23.17* Origins and insertions of muscles of the hand**

Right hand. Muscle origins shown in red, insertions in blue.

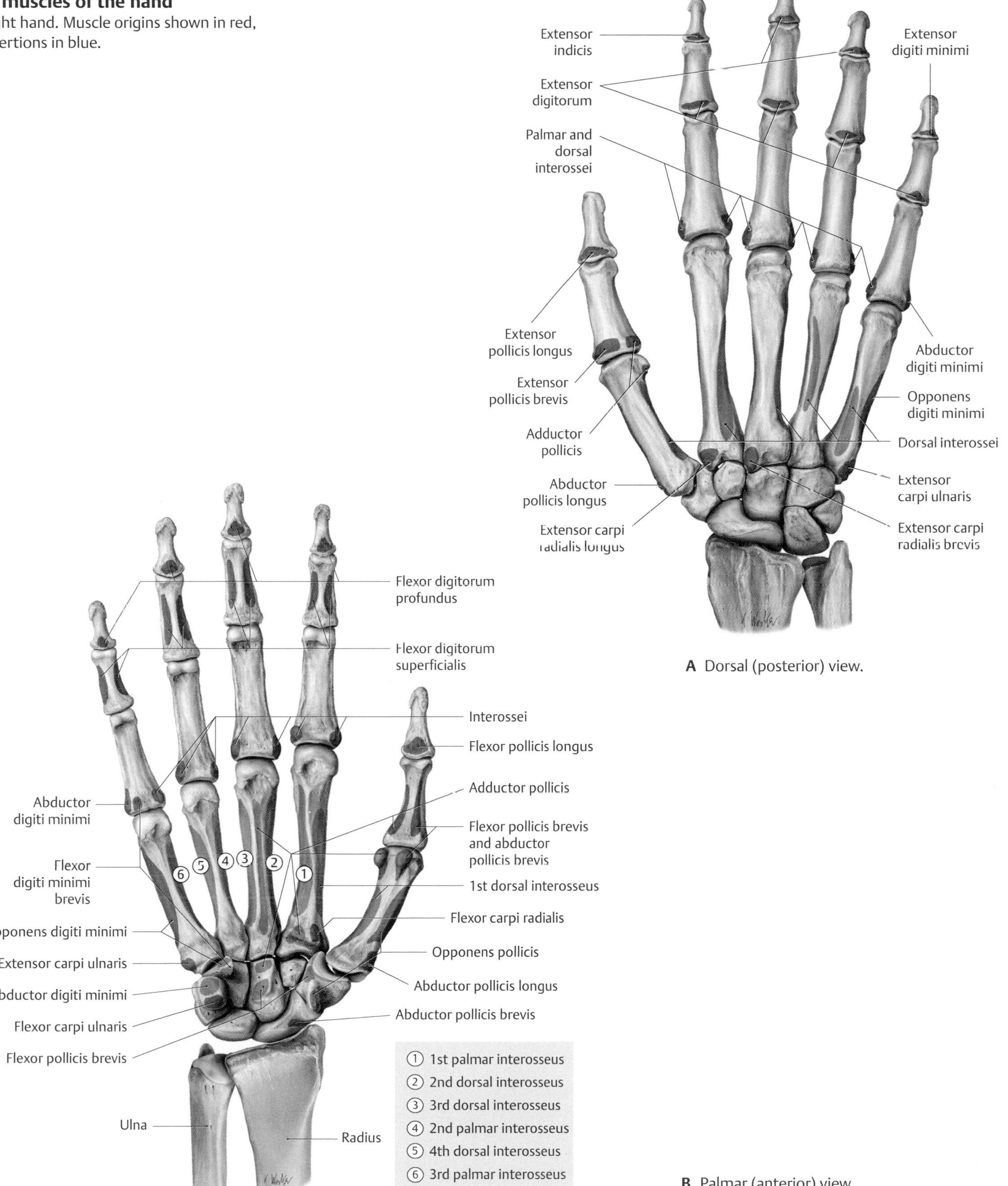
Extensor indicis
Extensor digitorum
Palmar and dorsal interossei
Extensor digiti minimi
Extensor pollicis longus
Extensor pollicis brevis
Adductor pollicis
Abductor pollicis longus
Extensor carpi radialis longus
Abductor digiti minimi
Opponens digiti minimi
Dorsal interossei
Extensor carpi ulnaris
Extensor carpi radialis brevis
Flexor digitorum profundus
Flexor digitorum superficialis
Interossei
Flexor pollicis longus
Adductor pollicis
Flexor pollicis brevis and abductor pollicis brevis
1st dorsal interosseus
Flexor carpi radialis
Opponens pollicis
Abductor pollicis longus
Abductor pollicis brevis
Abductor digiti minimi
Flexor digiti minimi brevis
Opponens digiti minimi
Extensor carpi ulnaris
Abductor digiti minimi
Flexor carpi ulnaris
Flexor pollicis brevis
Ulna
Radius
① 1st palmar interosseus
② 2nd dorsal interosseus
③ 3rd dorsal interosseus
④ 2nd palmar interosseus
⑤ 4th dorsal interosseus
⑥ 3rd palmar interosseus

A Dorsal (posterior) view.

B Palmar (anterior) view.

Dorsum of the Hand

Fig. 23.18 Extensor retinaculum and dorsal carpal tendon sheaths
Right hand, posterior (dorsal) view.

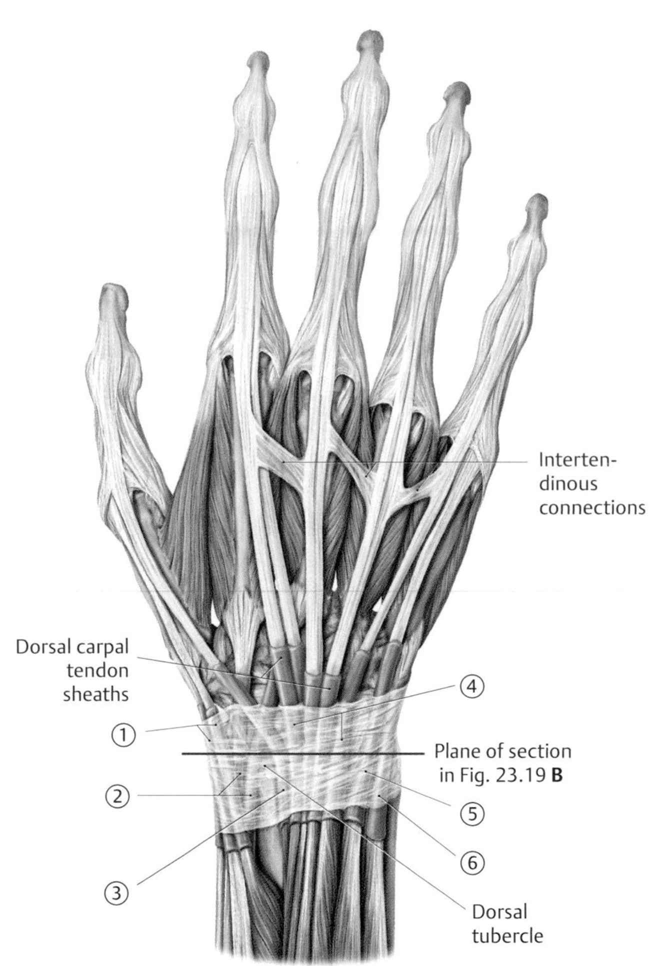
Interten-
dinous
connections
Dorsal carpal
tendon
sheaths
④
①
Plane of section
in Fig. 23.19 B
②
⑤
⑥
③
Dorsal
tubercle

Fig. 23.19 Muscles and tendons of the dorsum
Right hand.

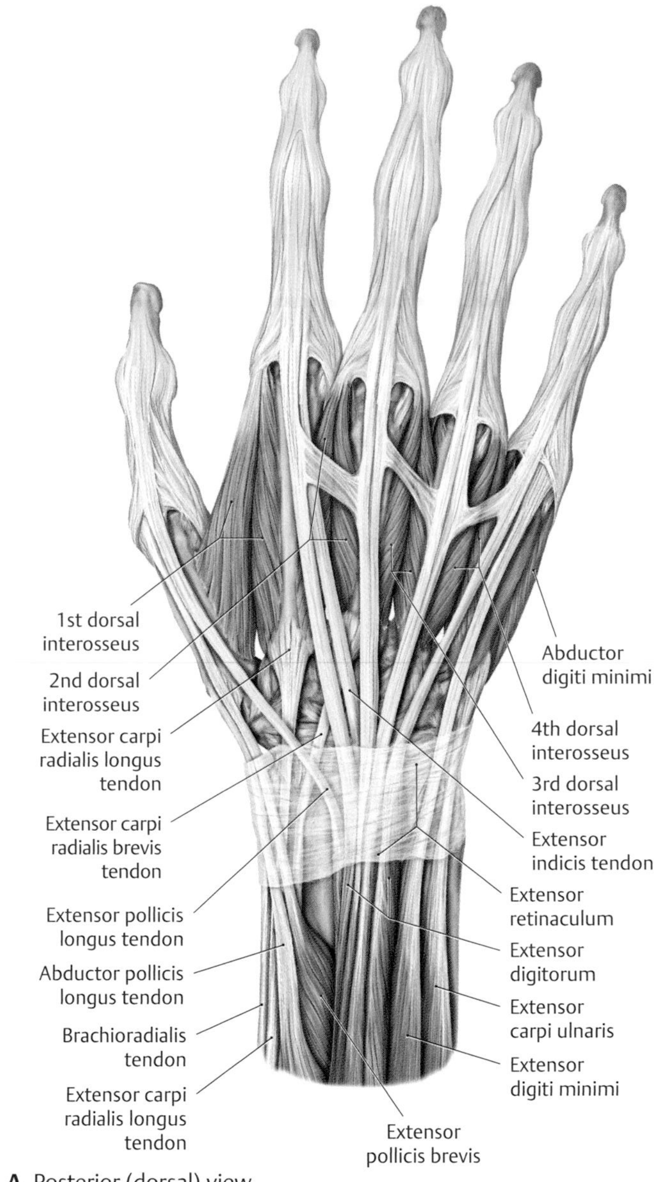
1st dorsal
interosseus
2nd dorsal
interosseus
Extensor carpi
radialis longus
tendon
Extensor carpi
radialis brevis
tendon
Extensor pollicis
longus tendon
Abductor pollicis
longus tendon
Brachioradialis
tendon
Extensor carpi
radialis longus
tendon
Abductor
digiti minimi
4th dorsal
interosseus
3rd dorsal
interosseus
Extensor
indicis tendon
Extensor
retinaculum
Extensor
digitorum
Extensor
carpi ulnaris
Extensor
digiti minimi
Extensor
pollicis brevis

A Posterior (dorsal) view.

Table 23.2	Dorsal compartments for extensor tendons
①	Abductor pollicis longus
	Extensor pollicis brevis
②	Extensor carpi radialis longus
	Extensor carpi radialis brevis
③	Extensor pollicis longus
④	Extensor digitorum
	Extensor indicis
⑤	Extensor digiti minimi
⑥	Extensor carpi ulnaris

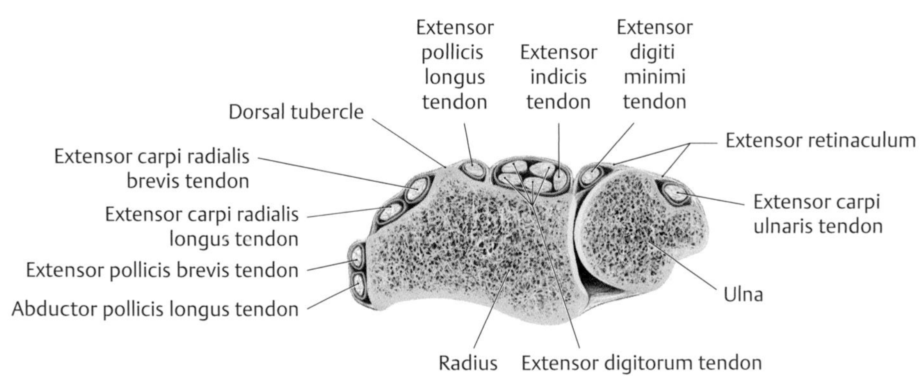
Extensor
pollicis
longus
tendon
Extensor
indicis
tendon
Extensor
digiti
minimi
tendon
Dorsal tubercle
Extensor retinaculum
Extensor carpi radialis
brevis tendon
Extensor carpi radialis
longus tendon
Extensor carpi
ulnaris tendon
Extensor pollicis brevis tendon
Abductor pollicis longus tendon
Ulna
Radius
Extensor digitorum tendon

B Dorsal compartments, proximal view of section in Fig. 23.18.

Fig. 23.20 **Dorsal digital expansion**

Right hand, middle finger. The dorsal digital expansion permits the long digital flexors and the short muscles of the hand to act on all three finger joints.

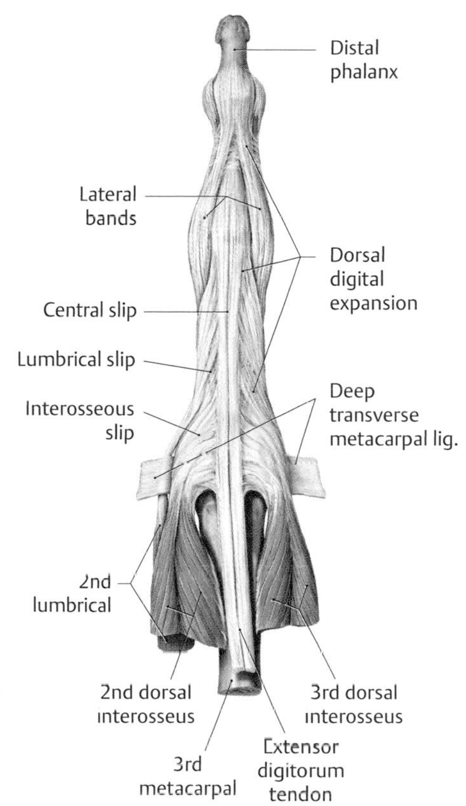
Distal phalanx
Lateral bands
Dorsal digital expansion
Central slip
Lumbrical slip
Interosseous slip
Deep transverse metacarpal lig.
2nd lumbrical
2nd dorsal interosseus
3rd dorsal interosseus
3rd metacarpal
Extensor digitorum tendon

A Posterior view.

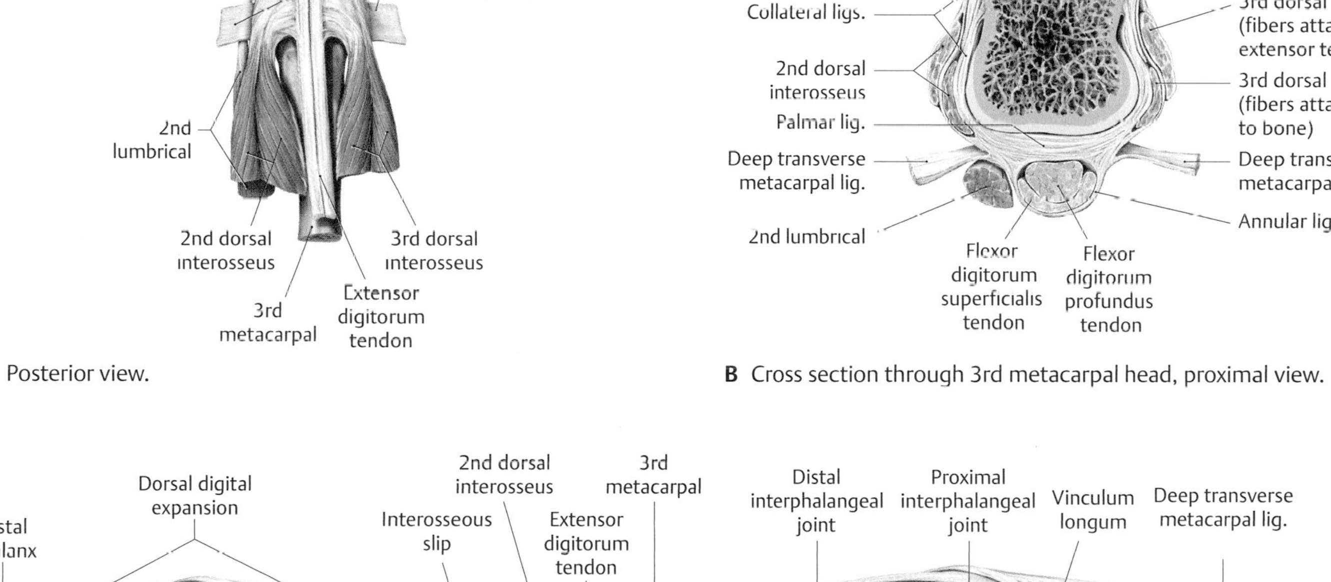
Extensor digitorum tendon
Dorsal
3rd metacarpal
3rd dorsal interosseus (fibers attached to extensor tendon)
Collateral ligs.
2nd dorsal interosseus
Palmar lig.
3rd dorsal interosseus (fibers attached to bone)
Deep transverse metacarpal lig.
Deep transverse metacarpal lig.
2nd lumbrical
Annular lig. (A1)
Flexor digitorum superficialis tendon
Flexor digitorum profundus tendon

B Cross section through 3rd metacarpal head, proximal view.

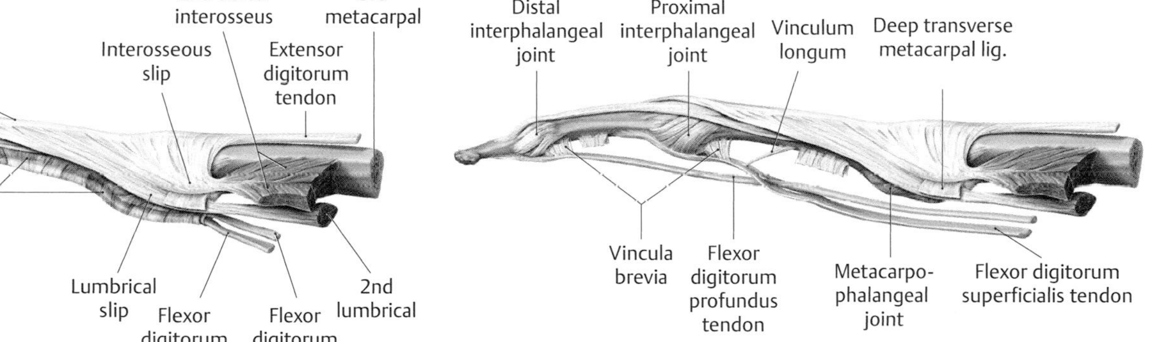
Dorsal digital expansion
Distal phalanx
2nd dorsal interosseus
3rd metacarpal
Interosseous slip
Extensor digitorum tendon
Annular ligs.
Lumbrical slip
Flexor digitorum superficialis tendon
Flexor digitorum profundus tendon
2nd lumbrical
Distal interphalangeal joint
Proximal interphalangeal joint
Vinculum longum
Deep transverse metacarpal lig.
Vincula brevia
Flexor digitorum profundus tendon
Metacarpo-phalangeal joint
Flexor digitorum superficialis tendon

C Radial view.

D Radial view with common tendon sheath of flexor digitorum superficialis and profundus opened.

Muscle Facts (I)

The intrinsic muscles of the hand are divided into three groups: the thenar, hypothenar, and metacarpal muscles (see p. 342). The thenar muscles are responsible for movement of the thumb, while the hypothenar muscles move the 5th digit.

Table 23.3 Thenar muscles

Muscle	Origin	Insertion		Innervation		Action
① Adductor pollicis	Transverse head: 3rd metacarpal (palmar surface)	Thumb (base of proximal phalanx)	Via the ulnar sesamoid	Ulnar n.	C8, T1	CMC joint of thumb: adduction MCP joint of thumb: flexion
	Oblique head: capitate bone, 2nd and 3rd metacarpals (bases)					
② Abductor pollicis brevis	Scaphoid bone and trapezium, flexor retinaculum		Via the radial sesamoid	Median n.		CMC joint of thumb: abduction
③ Flexor pollicis brevis	Superficial head: flexor retinaculum			Superficial head: median n.		CMC joint of thumb: flexion
	Deep head: capitate bone, trapezium			Deep head: ulnar n.		
④ Opponens pollicis	Trapezium	First metacarpal (radial border)		Median n.		CMC joint of thumb: opposition
CMC, carpometacarpal; MCP, metacarpophalangeal.						

Fig. 23.21 Thenar and hypothenar muscles
Right hand, palmar (anterior) view, schematic.

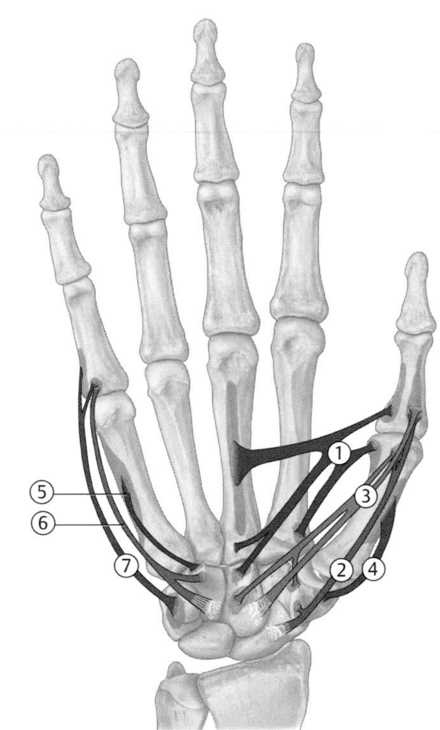

①
②
③
④
⑤
⑥
⑦

Table 23.4 Hypothenar muscles

Muscle	Origin	Insertion	Innervation	Action
⑤ Opponens digiti minimi	Hook of hamate, flexor retinaculum	5th metacarpal (ulnar border)	Ulnar n. (C8, T1)	Draws metacarpal in palmar direction (opposition)
⑥ Flexor digiti minimi brevis		5th proximal phalanx (base)		MCP joint of little finger: flexion
⑦ Abductor digiti minimi	Pisiform bone	5th proximal phalanx (ulnar base) and dorsal digital expansion of 5th digit		MCP joint of little finger: flexion and abduction of little finger PIP and DIP joints of little finger: extension
Palmaris brevis	Palmar aponeurosis (ulnar border)	Skin of hypothenar eminence		Tightens the palmar aponeurosis (protective function)
DIP, distal interphalangeal; MCP, metacarpophalangeal; PIP, proximal interphalangeal.				

Fig. 23.22 Thenar and hypothenar muscles
Right hand, palmar (anterior) view.

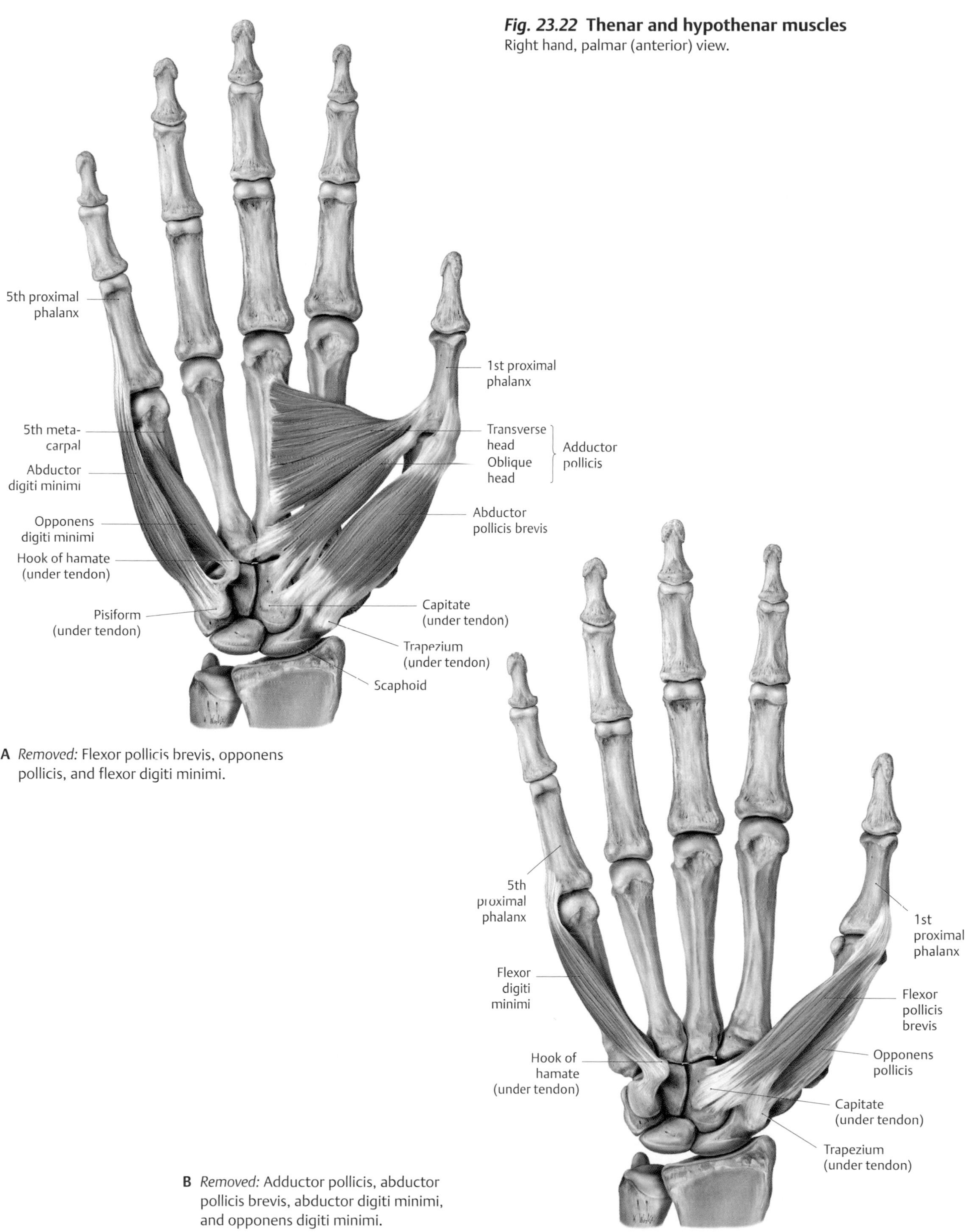
5th proximal phalanx
1st proximal phalanx
5th meta-carpal
Transverse head
Oblique head
Adductor pollicis
Abductor digiti minimi
Abductor pollicis brevis
Opponens digiti minimi
Hook of hamate (under tendon)
Capitate (under tendon)
Pisiform (under tendon)
Trapezium (under tendon)
Scaphoid
5th proximal phalanx
1st proximal phalanx
Flexor digiti minimi
Flexor pollicis brevis
Hook of hamate (under tendon)
Opponens pollicis
Capitate (under tendon)
Trapezium (under tendon)

A *Removed:* Flexor pollicis brevis, opponens pollicis, and flexor digiti minimi.

B *Removed:* Adductor pollicis, abductor pollicis brevis, abductor digiti minimi, and opponens digiti minimi.

Muscle Facts (II)

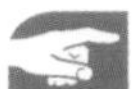

The metacarpal muscles of the hand consist of the lumbricals and interossei. They are responsible for the movement of the digits (with the hypothenars, which act on the 5th digit).

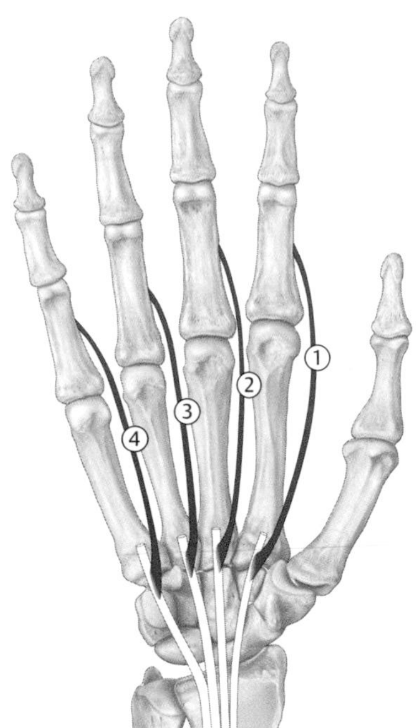
①
②
③
④

Fig. 23.23 **Lumbricals**
Right hand, palmar view, schematic.

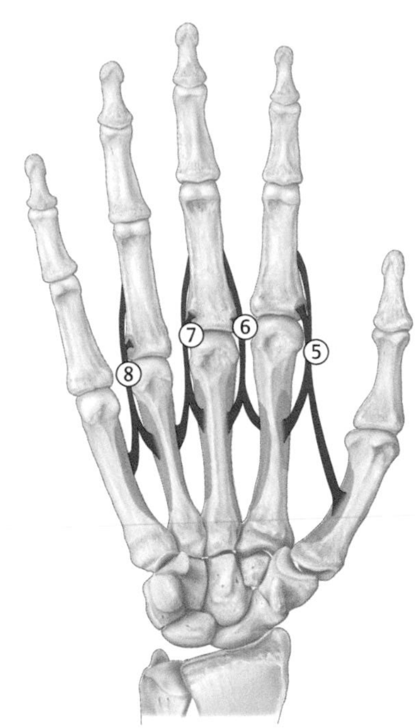
⑤
⑥
⑦
⑧

Fig. 23.24 **Dorsal interossei**
Right hand, palmar view, schematic.

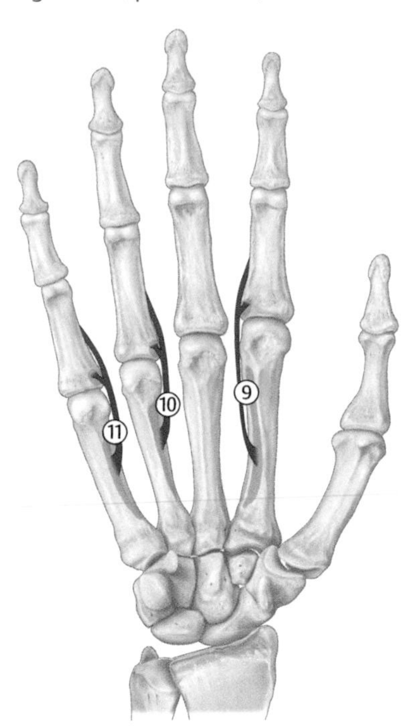
⑨
⑩
⑪

Fig. 23.25 **Palmar interossei**
Right hand, palmar view, schematic.

Table 23.5 **Metacarpal muscles**

Muscle group	Muscle	Origin	Insertion	Innervation	Action
Lumbricals	① 1st	Tendons of flexor digitorum profundus (radial sides)	2nd digit (dde)	Median n. (C8, T1)	2nd to 5th digits: • MCP joints: flexion • Proximal and distal IP joints: extension
	② 2nd		3rd digit (dde)		
	③ 3rd	Tendons of flexor digitorum profundus (bipennate from medial and lateral sides)	4th digit (dde)	Ulnar n. (C8, T1)	
	④ 4th		5th digit (dde)		
Dorsal interossei	⑤ 1st	1st and 2nd metacarpals (adjacent sides, two heads)	2nd digit (dde) 2nd proximal phalanx (radial side)		2nd to 4th digits: • MCP joints: flexion • Proximal and distal IP joints: extension and abduction from 3rd digit
	⑥ 2nd	2nd and 3rd metacarpals (adjacent sides, two heads)	3rd digit (dde) 3rd proximal phalanx (radial side)		
	⑦ 3rd	3rd and 4th metacarpals (adjacent sides, two heads)	3rd digit (dde) 3rd proximal phalanx (ulnar side)		
	⑧ 4th	4th and 5th metacarpals (adjacent sides, two heads)	4th digit (dde) 4th proximal phalanx (ulnar side)		
Palmar interossei	⑨ 1st	2nd metacarpal (ulnar side)	2nd digit (dde) 2nd proximal phalanx (base)		2nd, 4th, and 5th digits: • MCP joints: flexion • Proximal and distal IP joints: extension and adduction toward 3rd digit
	⑩ 2nd	4th metacarpal (radial side)	4th digit (dde) 4th proximal phalanx (base)		
	⑪ 3rd	5th metacarpal (radial side)	5th digit (dde) 5th proximal phalanx (base)		

dde, dorsal digital expansion; IP, interphalangeal; MCP, metacarpophalangeal.

***Fig. 23.26* Metacarpal muscles**
Right hand, palmar (anterior) view.

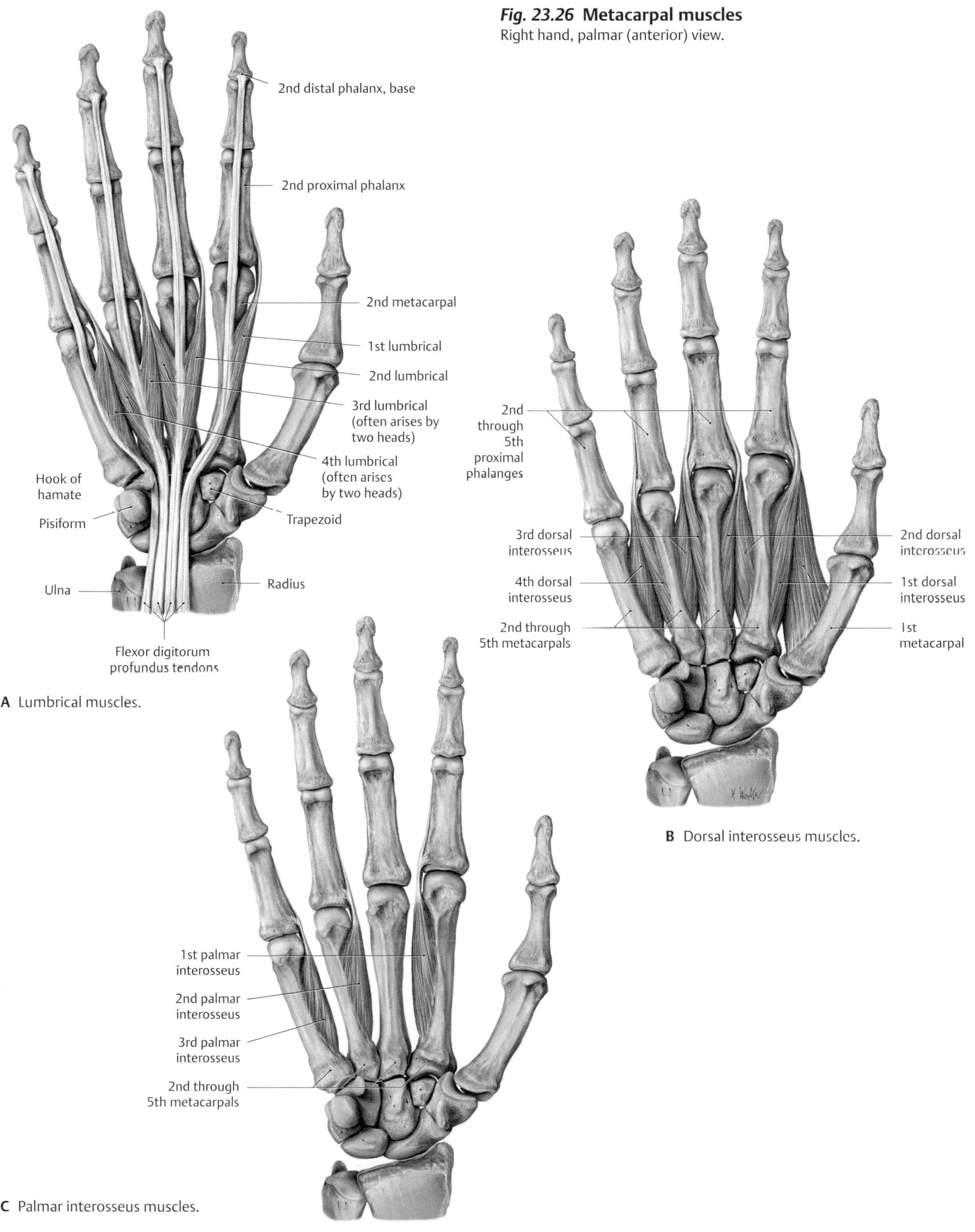
2nd distal phalanx, base
2nd proximal phalanx
2nd metacarpal
1st lumbrical
2nd lumbrical
3rd lumbrical (often arises by two heads)
4th lumbrical (often arises by two heads)
Hook of hamate
Pisiform
Trapezoid
Ulna
Radius
Flexor digitorum profundus tendons
2nd through 5th proximal phalanges
3rd dorsal interosseus
4th dorsal interosseus
2nd through 5th metacarpals
2nd dorsal interosseus
1st dorsal interosseus
1st metacarpal
1st palmar interosseus
2nd palmar interosseus
3rd palmar interosseus
2nd through 5th metacarpals

A Lumbrical muscles.

B Dorsal interosseus muscles.

C Palmar interosseus muscles.

Arteries of the Upper Limb

Fig. 24.1 Arteries of the upper limb
Right limb, anterior view.

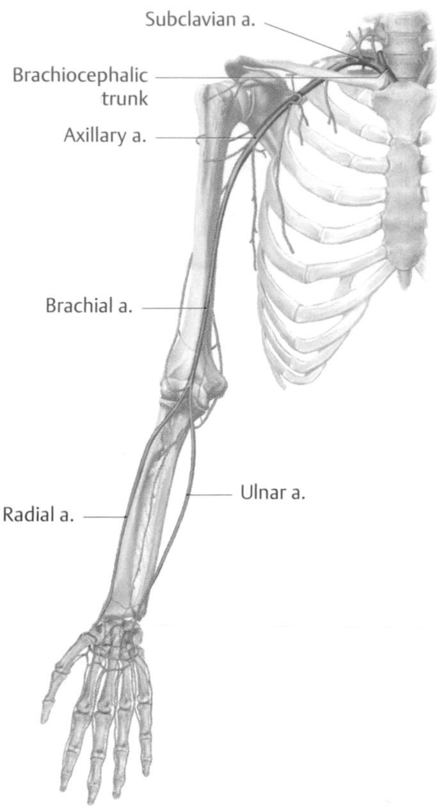

Subclavian a.
Brachiocephalic trunk
Axillary a.
Brachial a.
Ulnar a.
Radial a.

A Main arterial segments.

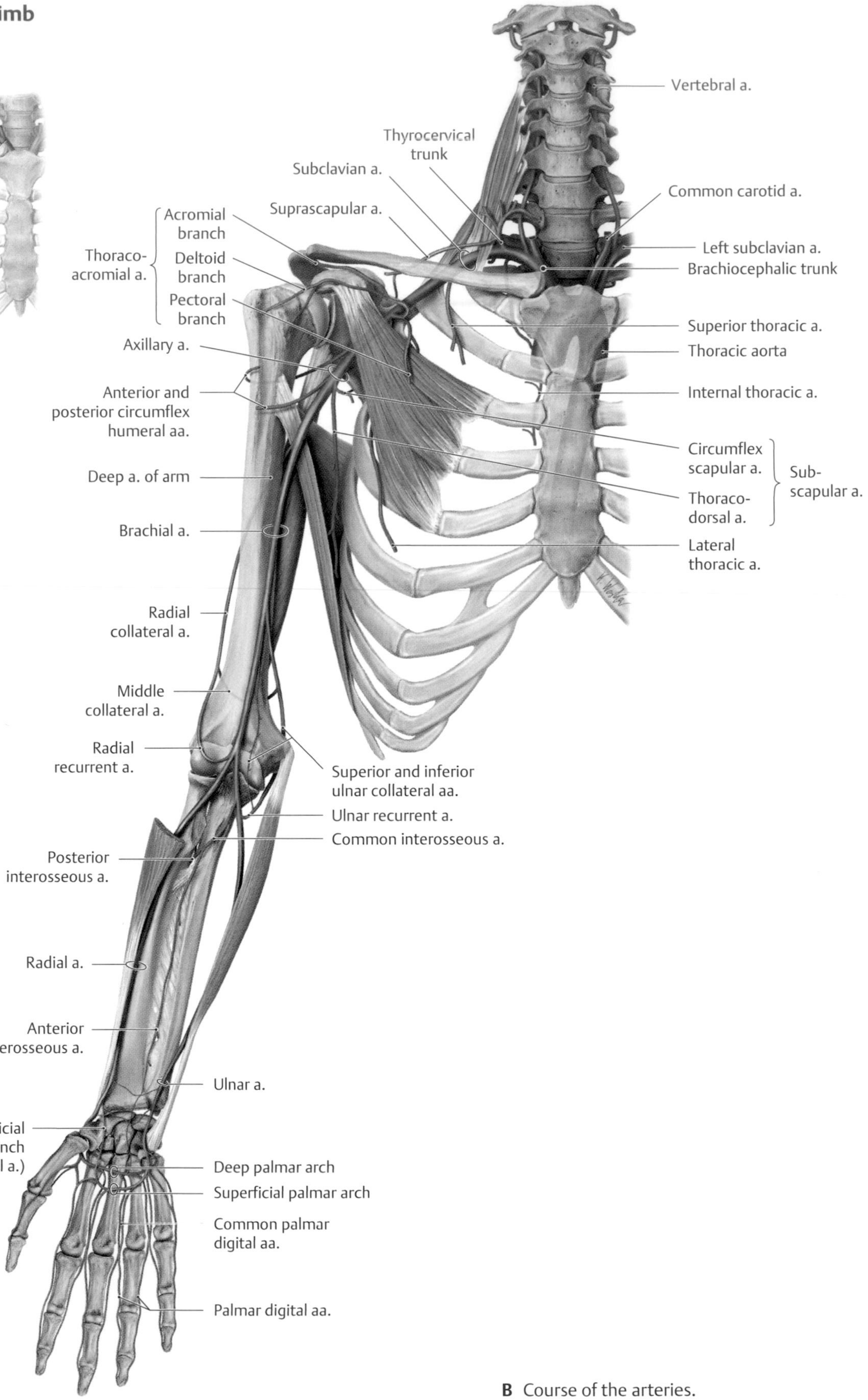

Vertebral a.
Thyrocervical trunk
Subclavian a.
Suprascapular a.
Common carotid a.
Thoraco-acromial a.: Acromial branch, Deltoid branch, Pectoral branch
Left subclavian a.
Brachiocephalic trunk
Superior thoracic a.
Thoracic aorta
Axillary a.
Anterior and posterior circumflex humeral aa.
Internal thoracic a.
Sub-scapular a.: Circumflex scapular a., Thoraco-dorsal a.
Deep a. of arm
Brachial a.
Lateral thoracic a.
Radial collateral a.
Middle collateral a.
Radial recurrent a.
Superior and inferior ulnar collateral aa.
Ulnar recurrent a.
Common interosseous a.
Posterior interosseous a.
Radial a.
Anterior interosseous a.
Ulnar a.
Superficial palmar branch (radial a.)
Deep palmar arch
Superficial palmar arch
Common palmar digital aa.
Palmar digital aa.

B Course of the arteries.

Fig. 24.2 Branches of the subclavian artery
Right side, anterior view.

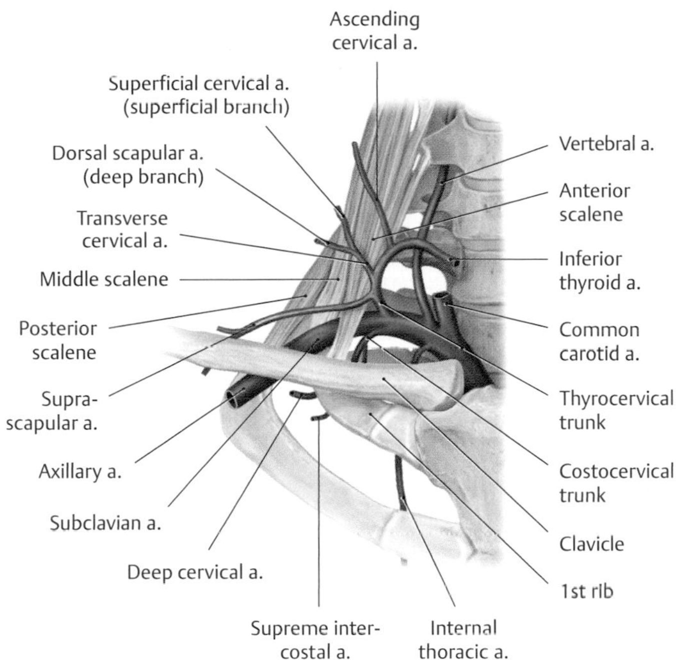
Ascending cervical a.
Superficial cervical a. (superficial branch)
Dorsal scapular a. (deep branch)
Transverse cervical a.
Middle scalene
Posterior scalene
Supra-scapular a.
Axillary a.
Subclavian a.
Deep cervical a.
Supreme inter-costal a.
Internal thoracic a.
Vertebral a.
Anterior scalene
Inferior thyroid a.
Common carotid a.
Thyrocervical trunk
Costocervical trunk
Clavicle
1st rib

Fig. 24.3 Scapular arcade
Right side, posterior view.

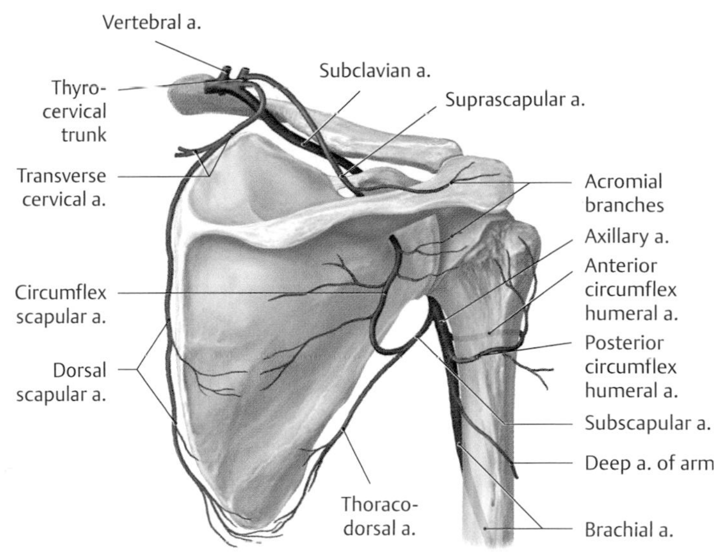
Vertebral a.
Thyro-cervical trunk
Subclavian a.
Suprascapular a.
Transverse cervical a.
Acromial branches
Axillary a.
Anterior circumflex humeral a.
Circumflex scapular a.
Posterior circumflex humeral a.
Dorsal scapular a.
Subscapular a.
Deep a. of arm
Thoraco-dorsal a.
Brachial a.

Fig. 24.4 Arteries of the forearm and hand
Right limb. The ulnar and radial arteries are interconnected by the superficial and deep palmar arches, the perforating branches, and the dorsal carpal network.

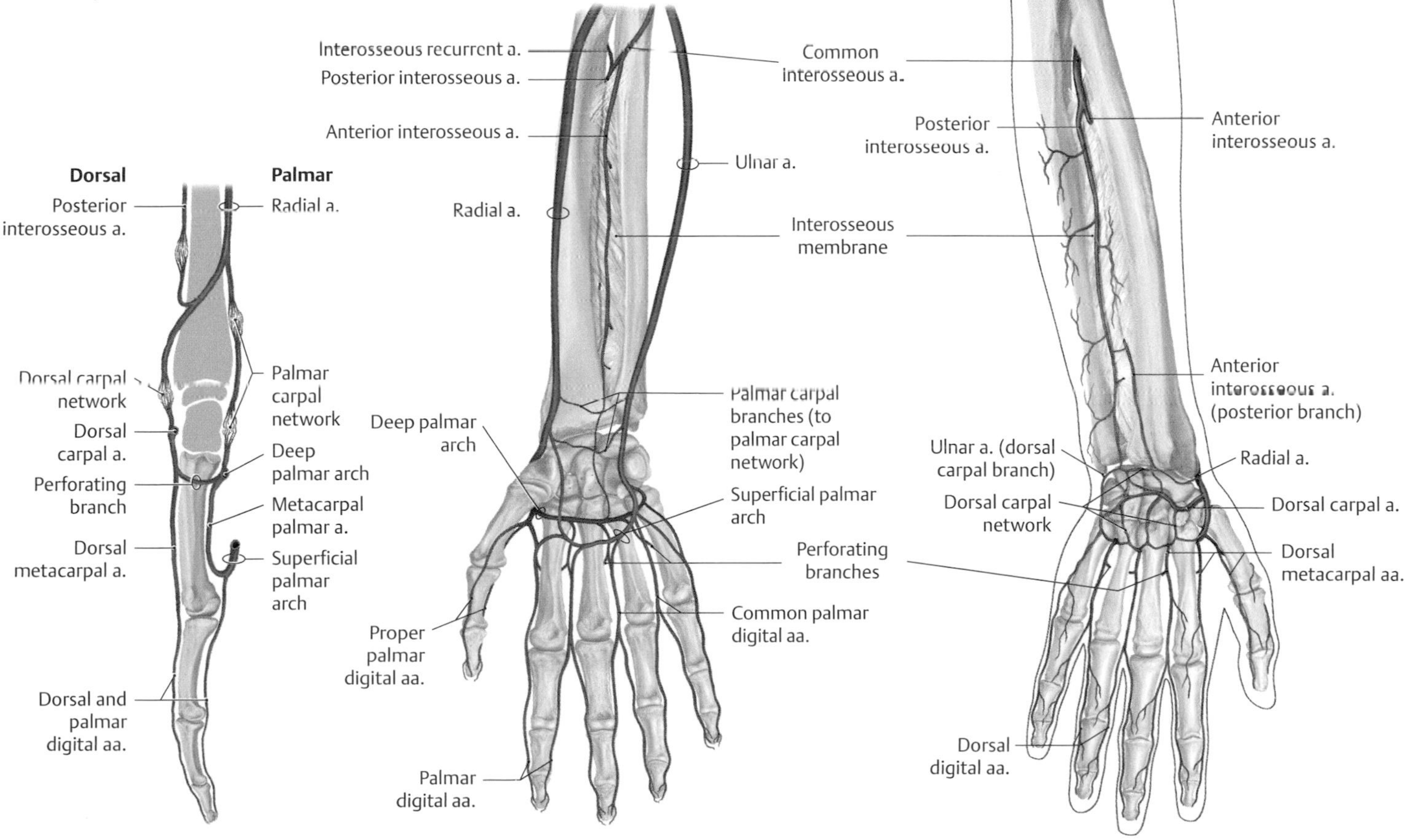

Dorsal
Palmar
Posterior interosseous a.
Radial a.
Dorsal carpal network
Palmar carpal network
Dorsal carpal a.
Deep palmar arch
Perforating branch
Metacarpal palmar a.
Dorsal metacarpal a.
Superficial palmar arch
Dorsal and palmar digital aa.

A Right middle finger, lateral view.

Interosseous recurrent a.
Posterior interosseous a.
Anterior interosseous a.
Common interosseous a.
Ulnar a.
Radial a.
Interosseous membrane
Deep palmar arch
Palmar carpal branches (to palmar carpal network)
Superficial palmar arch
Perforating branches
Common palmar digital aa.
Proper palmar digital aa.
Palmar digital aa.

B Anterior (palmar) view.

Posterior interosseous a.
Anterior interosseous a.
Anterior interosseous a. (posterior branch)
Ulnar a. (dorsal carpal branch)
Radial a.
Dorsal carpal network
Dorsal carpal a.
Dorsal metacarpal aa.
Dorsal digital aa.

C Posterior (dorsal) view.

Veins & Lymphatics of the Upper Limb

Fig. 24.5 **Veins of the upper limb**
Right limb, anterior view.

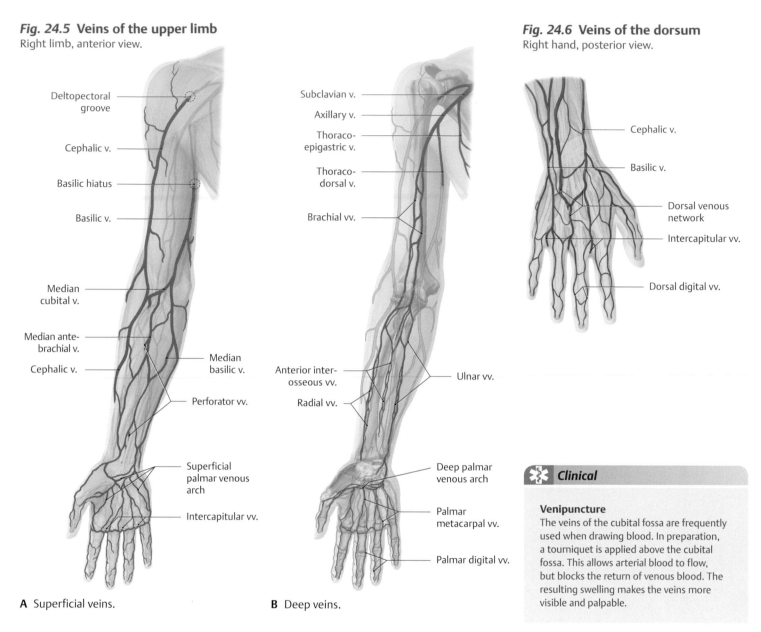

Deltopectoral groove
Cephalic v.
Basilic hiatus
Basilic v.
Median cubital v.
Median antebrachial v.
Cephalic v.
Median basilic v.
Perforator vv.
Superficial palmar venous arch
Intercapitular vv.

A Superficial veins.

Subclavian v.
Axillary v.
Thoraco-epigastric v.
Thoraco-dorsal v.
Brachial vv.
Anterior interosseous vv.
Radial vv.
Ulnar vv.
Deep palmar venous arch
Palmar metacarpal vv.
Palmar digital vv.

B Deep veins.

Fig. 24.6 **Veins of the dorsum**
Right hand, posterior view.

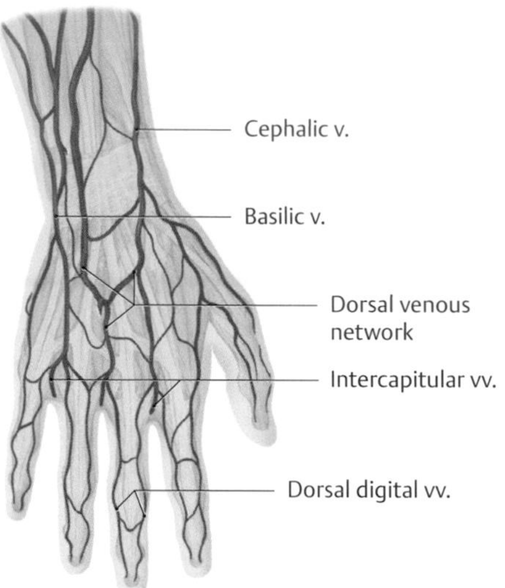
Cephalic v.
Basilic v.
Dorsal venous network
Intercapitular vv.
Dorsal digital vv.

Clinical

Venipuncture
The veins of the cubital fossa are frequently used when drawing blood. In preparation, a tourniquet is applied above the cubital fossa. This allows arterial blood to flow, but blocks the return of venous blood. The resulting swelling makes the veins more visible and palpable.

Fig. 24.7 **Cubital fossa**
Right limb, anterior view. The subcutaneous veins of the cubital fossa have a highly variable course.

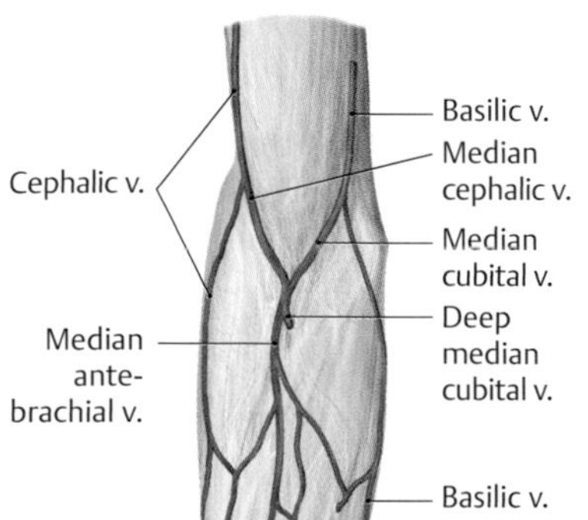
Cephalic v.
Basilic v.
Median cephalic v.
Median cubital v.
Deep median cubital v.
Median antebrachial v.
Basilic v.

A M-shaped.

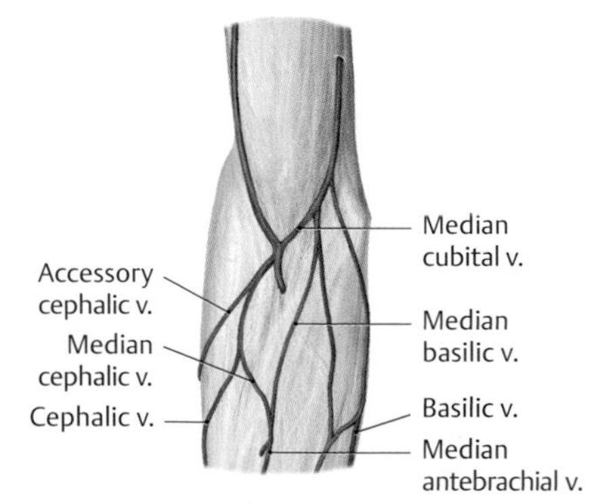
Median cubital v.
Accessory cephalic v.
Median cephalic v.
Median basilic v.
Cephalic v.
Basilic v.
Median antebrachial v.

B Accessory cephalic vein.

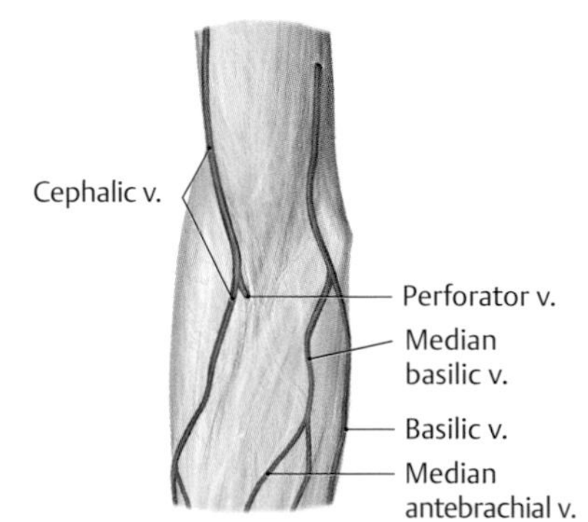
Cephalic v.
Perforator v.
Median basilic v.
Basilic v.
Median antebrachial v.

C Absent median cubital vein.

Lymph from the upper limb and breast drains to the axillary lymph nodes. The superficial lymphatics of the upper limb lie in the subcutaneous tissue, while the deep lymphatics accompany the arteries and deep veins. Numerous anastomoses exist between the two systems.

Fig. 24.8 **Lymph vessels of the upper limb**
Right limb.

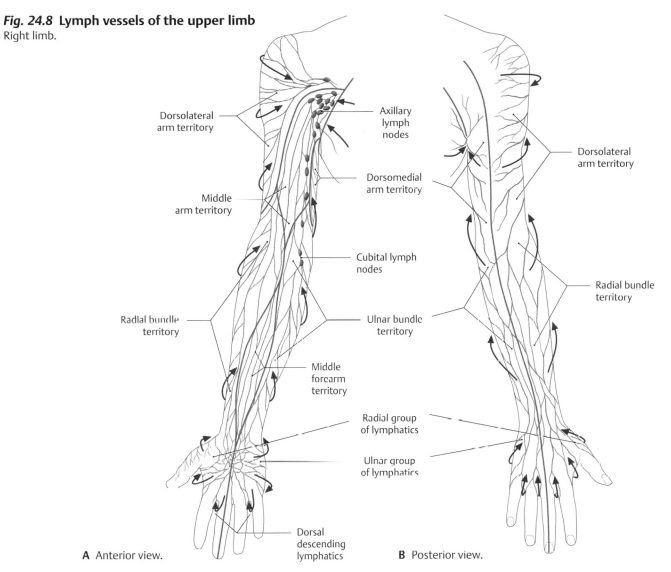

Dorsolateral arm territory
Axillary lymph nodes
Dorsomedial arm territory
Middle arm territory
Cubital lymph nodes
Radial bundle territory
Ulnar bundle territory
Middle forearm territory
Radial group of lymphatics
Ulnar group of lymphatics
Dorsal descending lymphatics
Dorsolateral arm territory
Radial bundle territory

A Anterior view.

B Posterior view.

Fig. 24.9 **Lymphatic drainage of the hand**
Right hand, radial view. Most of the hand drains to the axillary nodes via cubital nodes. However, the thumb, index finger, and dorsum of the hand drain directly.

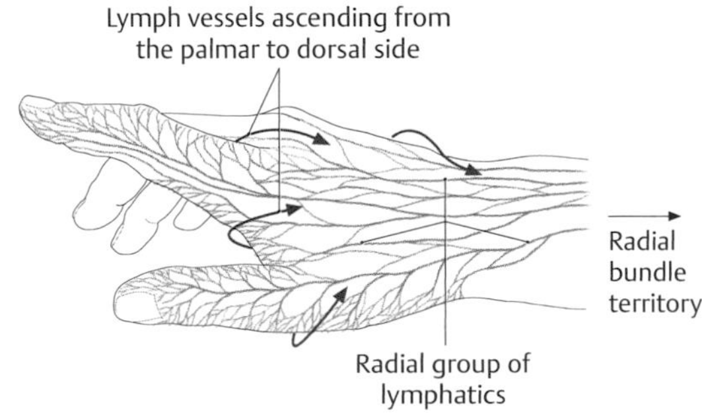
Lymph vessels ascending from the palmar to dorsal side
Radial bundle territory
Radial group of lymphatics

Fig. 24.10 **Axillary lymph nodes**
Right side, anterior view. For surgical purposes, the axillary lymph nodes are divided into three levels with respect to their relationship with the pectoralis minor: lateral (level I), posterior (level II), or medial (level III). They have major clinical importance in breast cancer (see p. 73).

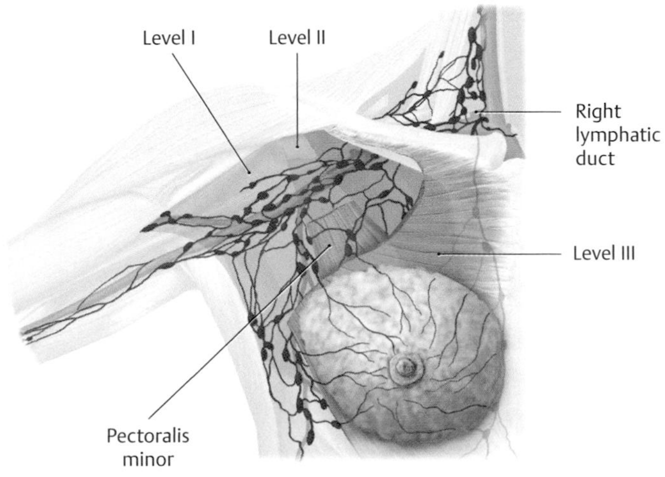
Level I
Level II
Right lymphatic duct
Level III
Pectoralis minor

Nerves of the Brachial Plexus

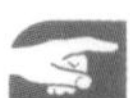

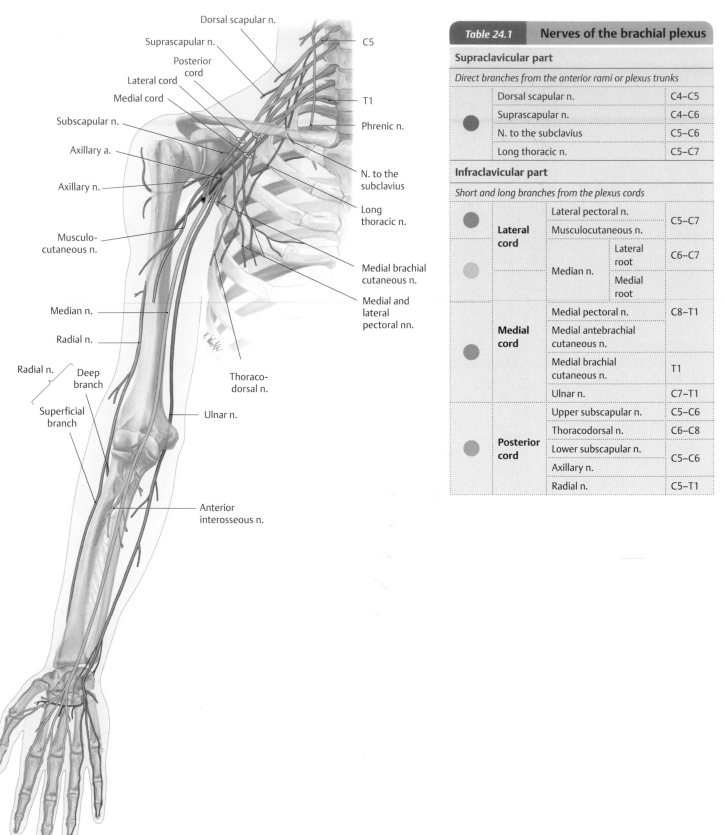

Almost all muscles in the upper limb are innervated by the brachial plexus, which arises from spinal cord segments C5 to T1. The anterior rami of the spinal nerves give off direct branches (supraclavicular part of the brachial plexus) and merge to form three trunks, six divisions (three anterior and three posterior), and three cords. The infraclavicular part of the brachial plexus consists of short branches that arise directly from the cords and long (terminal) branches that traverse the limb.

Dorsal scapular n.
Suprascapular n.
Posterior cord
Lateral cord
Medial cord
Subscapular n.
Axillary a.
Axillary n.
Musculo-cutaneous n.
Median n.
Radial n.
Radial n.
Deep branch
Superficial branch
C5
T1
Phrenic n.
N. to the subclavius
Long thoracic n.
Medial brachial cutaneous n.
Medial and lateral pectoral nn.
Thoraco-dorsal n.
Ulnar n.
Anterior interosseous n.

Table 24.1 Nerves of the brachial plexus

		Nerve		Segments
Supraclavicular part				
Direct branches from the anterior rami or plexus trunks				
●		Dorsal scapular n.		C4–C5
		Suprascapular n.		C4–C6
		N. to the subclavius		C5–C6
		Long thoracic n.		C5–C7
Infraclavicular part				
Short and long branches from the plexus cords				
●	**Lateral cord**	Lateral pectoral n.		C5–C7
		Musculocutaneous n.		
●		Median n.	Lateral root	C6–C7
			Medial root	
●	**Medial cord**	Medial pectoral n.		C8–T1
		Medial antebrachial cutaneous n.		
		Medial brachial cutaneous n.		T1
		Ulnar n.		C7–T1
●	**Posterior cord**	Upper subscapular n.		C5–C6
		Thoracodorsal n.		C6–C8
		Lower subscapular n.		C5–C6
		Axillary n.		
		Radial n.		C5–T1

Fig. 24.11 Brachial plexus
Right side, anterior view.

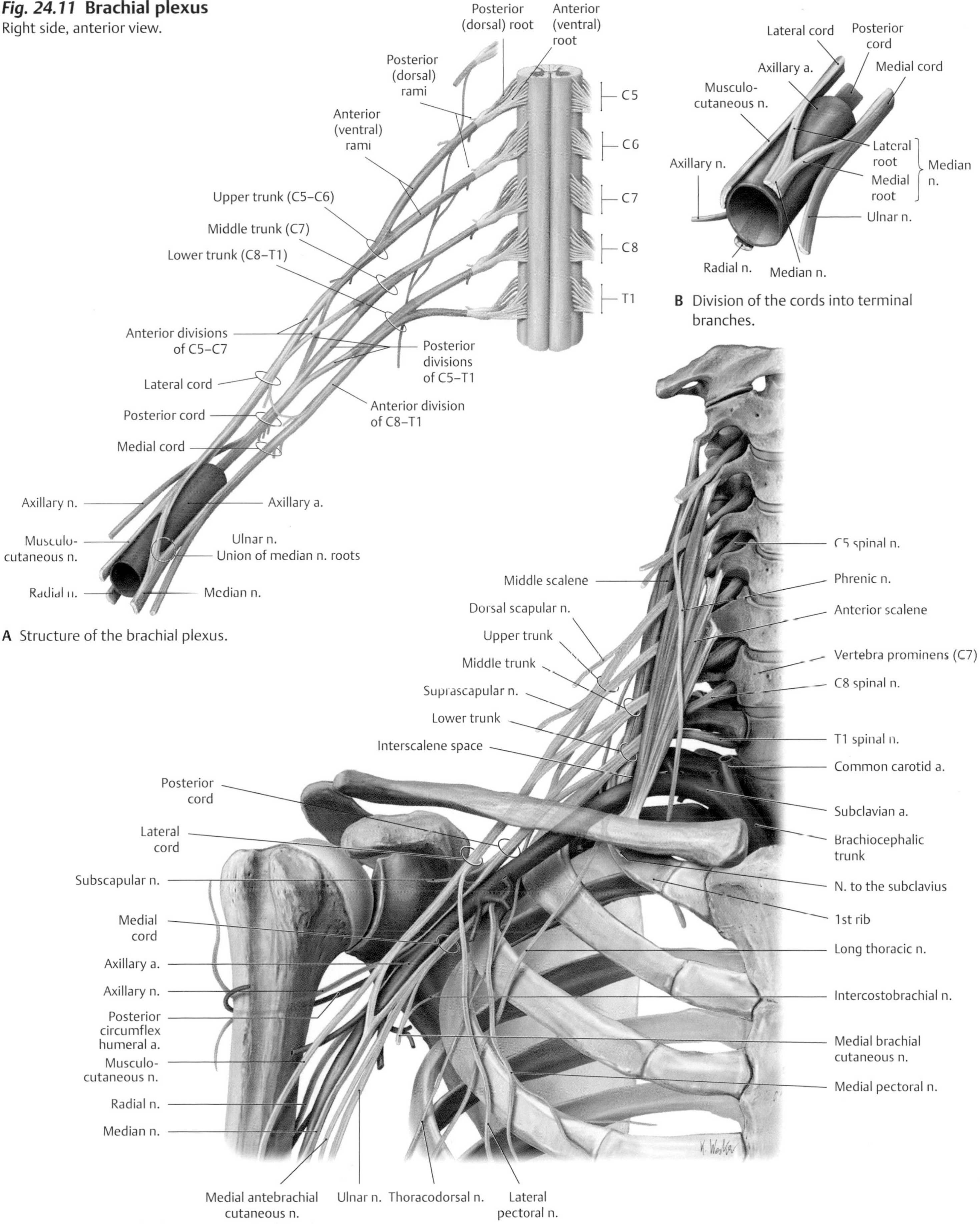
Posterior (dorsal) root
Anterior (ventral) root
Posterior (dorsal) rami
Anterior (ventral) rami
C5
C6
C7
C8
T1
Upper trunk (C5–C6)
Middle trunk (C7)
Lower trunk (C8–T1)
Anterior divisions of C5–C7
Posterior divisions of C5–T1
Lateral cord
Posterior cord
Medial cord
Anterior division of C8–T1
Axillary n.
Axillary a.
Musculo-cutaneous n.
Ulnar n.
Union of median n. roots
Radial n.
Median n.
Lateral cord
Posterior cord
Axillary a.
Medial cord
Musculo-cutaneous n.
Lateral root
Medial root
Median n.
Axillary n.
Ulnar n.
Radial n.
Median n.
Middle scalene
Dorsal scapular n.
Upper trunk
Middle trunk
Suprascapular n.
Lower trunk
Interscalene space
C5 spinal n.
Phrenic n.
Anterior scalene
Vertebra prominens (C7)
C8 spinal n.
T1 spinal n.
Common carotid a.
Subclavian a.
Brachiocephalic trunk
N. to the subclavius
1st rib
Long thoracic n.
Intercostobrachial n.
Medial brachial cutaneous n.
Medial pectoral n.
Posterior cord
Lateral cord
Subscapular n.
Medial cord
Axillary a.
Axillary n.
Posterior circumflex humeral a.
Musculo-cutaneous n.
Radial n.
Median n.
Medial antebrachial cutaneous n.
Ulnar n.
Thoracodorsal n.
Lateral pectoral n.

A Structure of the brachial plexus.

B Division of the cords into terminal branches.

C Course of the brachial plexus, stretched for clarity.

Supraclavicular Branches & Posterior Cord

Fig. 24.12 **Supraclavicular branches**
Right shoulder.

The supraclavicular branches of the brachial plexus arise directly from the plexus roots (anterior rami of the spinal nerves) or from the plexus trunks in the lateral cervical triangle.

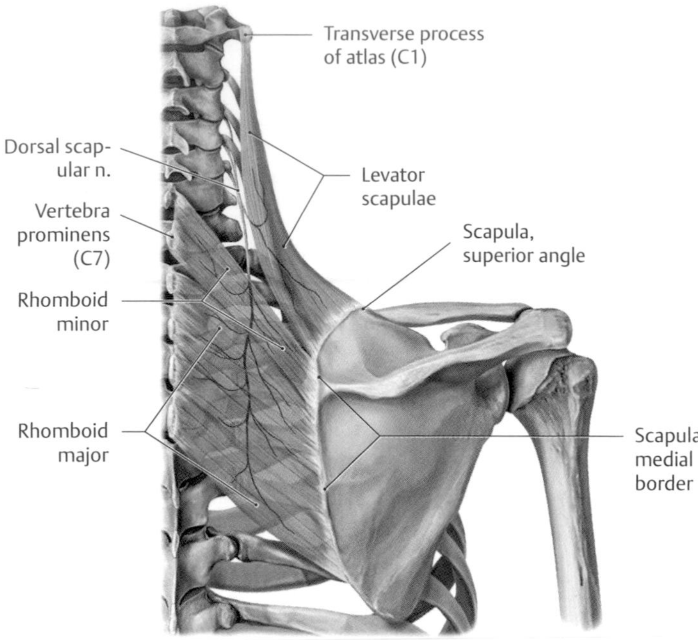
Transverse process
of atlas (C1)
Dorsal scap-
ular n.
Levator
scapulae
Vertebra
prominens
(C7)
Scapula,
superior angle
Rhomboid
minor
Rhomboid
major
Scapula,
medial
border

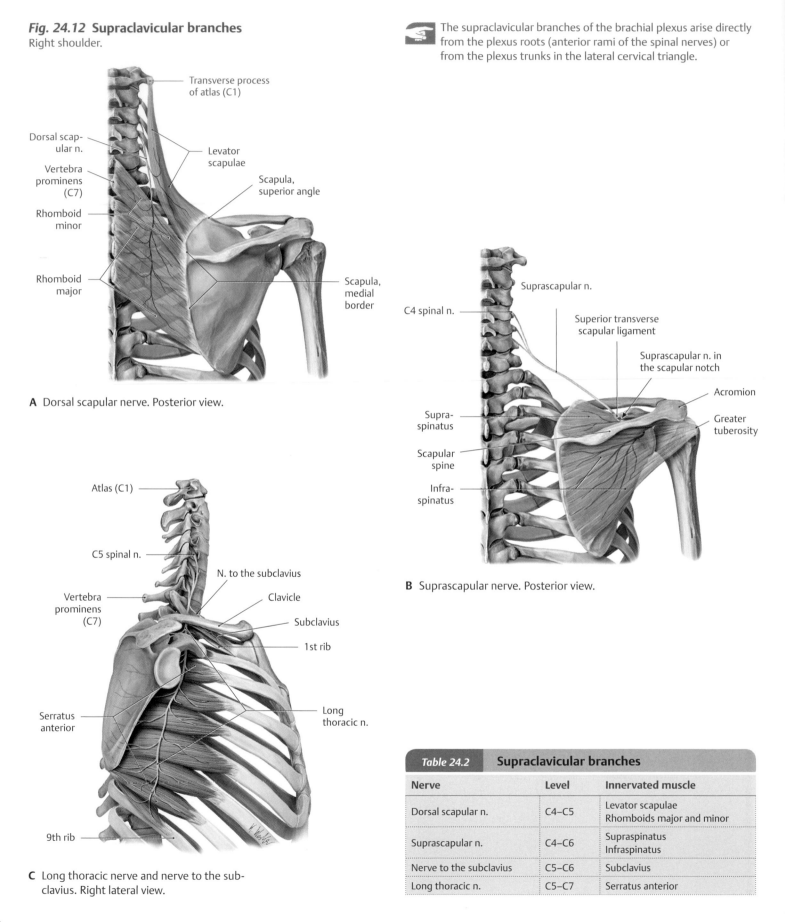

A Dorsal scapular nerve. Posterior view.

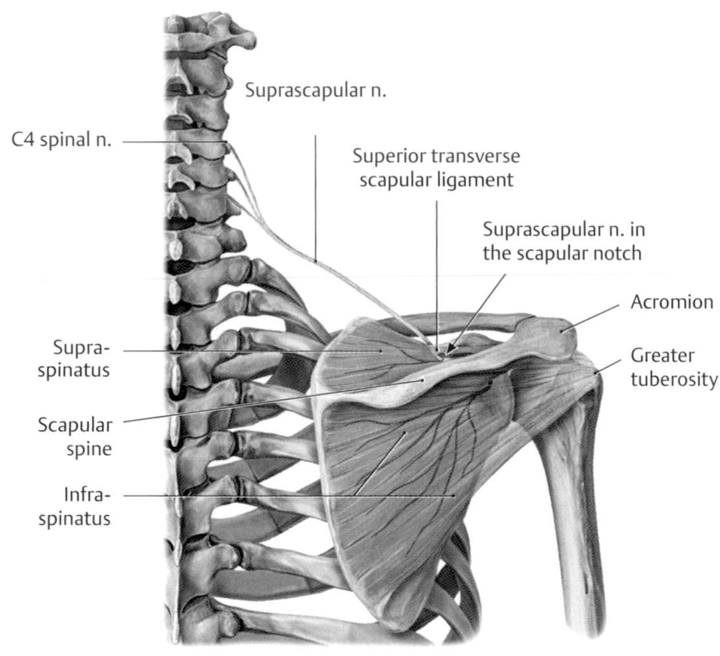
Suprascapular n.
C4 spinal n.
Superior transverse
scapular ligament
Suprascapular n. in
the scapular notch
Acromion
Supra-
spinatus
Greater
tuberosity
Scapular
spine
Infra-
spinatus

B Suprascapular nerve. Posterior view.

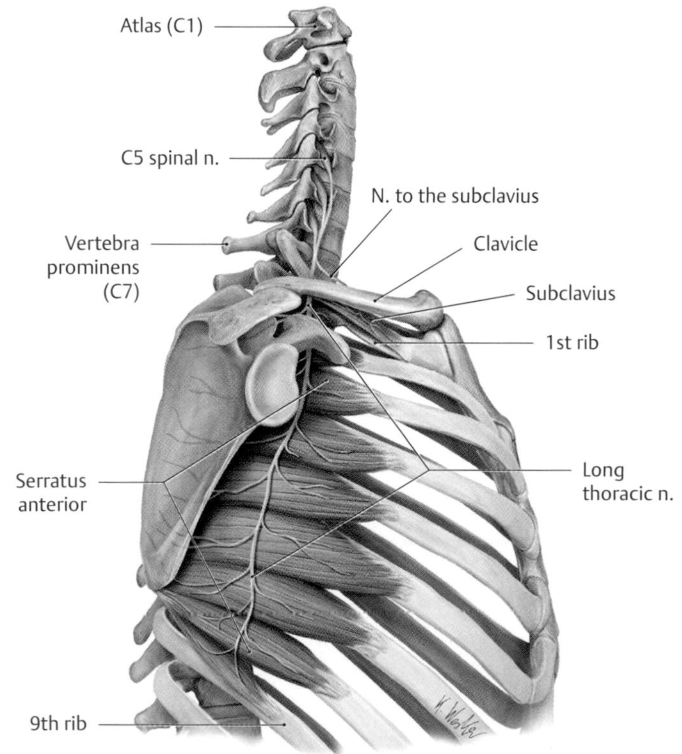
Atlas (C1)
C5 spinal n.
N. to the subclavius
Vertebra
prominens
(C7)
Clavicle
Subclavius
1st rib
Serratus
anterior
Long
thoracic n.
9th rib

C Long thoracic nerve and nerve to the subclavius. Right lateral view.

Table 24.2 **Supraclavicular branches**		
Nerve	**Level**	**Innervated muscle**
Dorsal scapular n.	C4–C5	Levator scapulae Rhomboids major and minor
Suprascapular n.	C4–C6	Supraspinatus Infraspinatus
Nerve to the subclavius	C5–C6	Subclavius
Long thoracic n.	C5–C7	Serratus anterior

Fig. 24.13 Posterior cord: Short branches

Right shoulder.

The posterior cord gives off three short branches (arising at the level of the plexus cords) and two long branches (terminal nerves, see pp. 352–353).

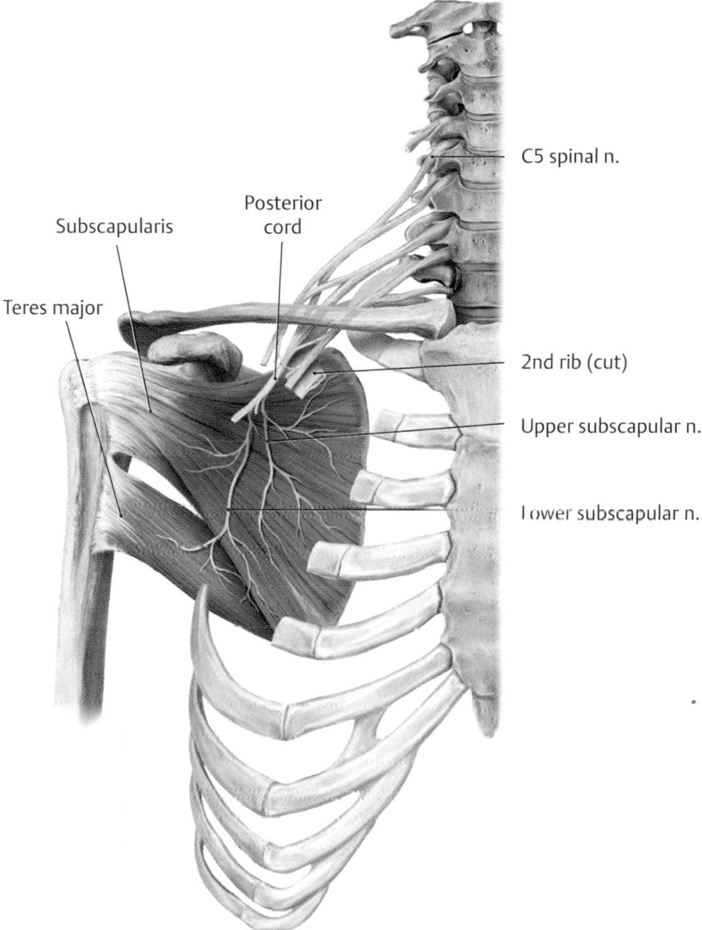
C5 spinal n.
Posterior cord
Subscapularis
Teres major
2nd rib (cut)
Upper subscapular n.
Lower subscapular n.

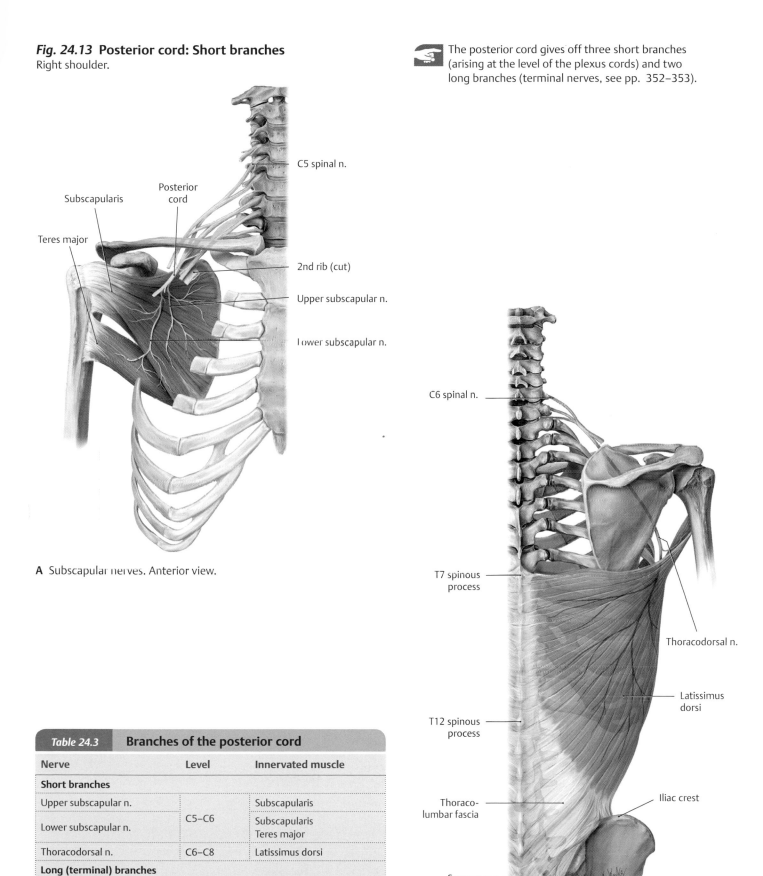

A Subscapular nerves. Anterior view.

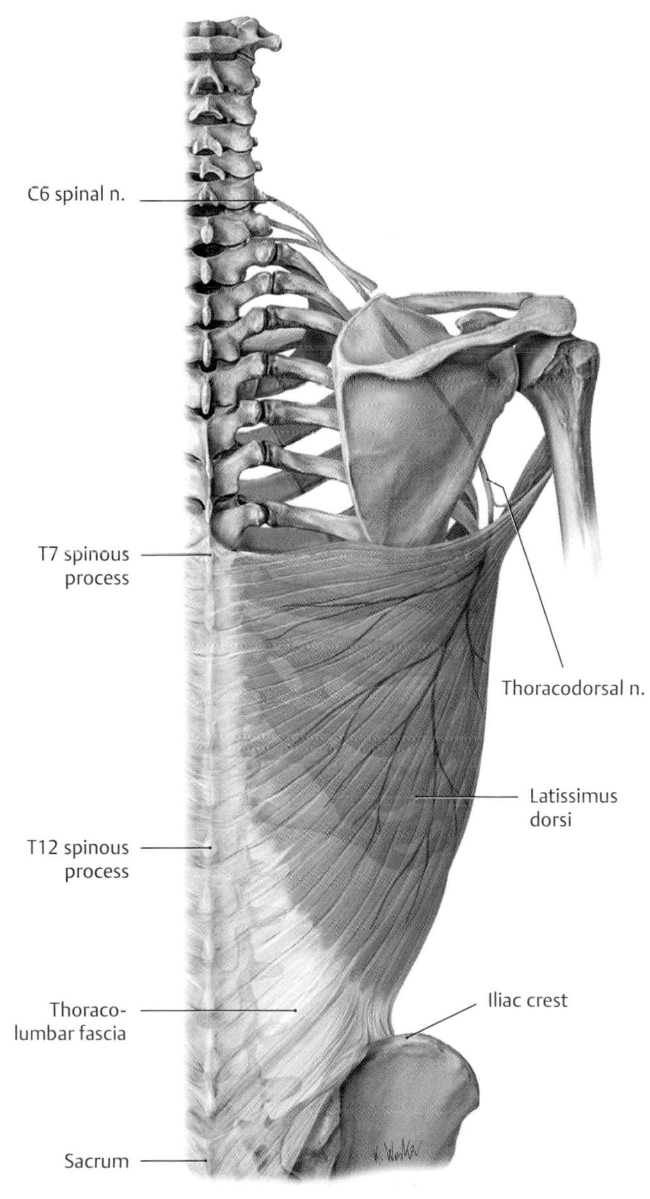
C6 spinal n.
T7 spinous process
Thoracodorsal n.
Latissimus dorsi
T12 spinous process
Iliac crest
Thoraco-lumbar fascia
Sacrum

B Thoracodorsal nerve. Posterior view.

Table 24.3 Branches of the posterior cord

Nerve	Level	Innervated muscle
Short branches		
Upper subscapular n.	C5–C6	Subscapularis
Lower subscapular n.		Subscapularis Teres major
Thoracodorsal n.	C6–C8	Latissimus dorsi
Long (terminal) branches		
Axillary n.	C5–C6	See p. 352
Radial n.	C5–T1	See p. 353

Posterior Cord: Axillary & Radial Nerves

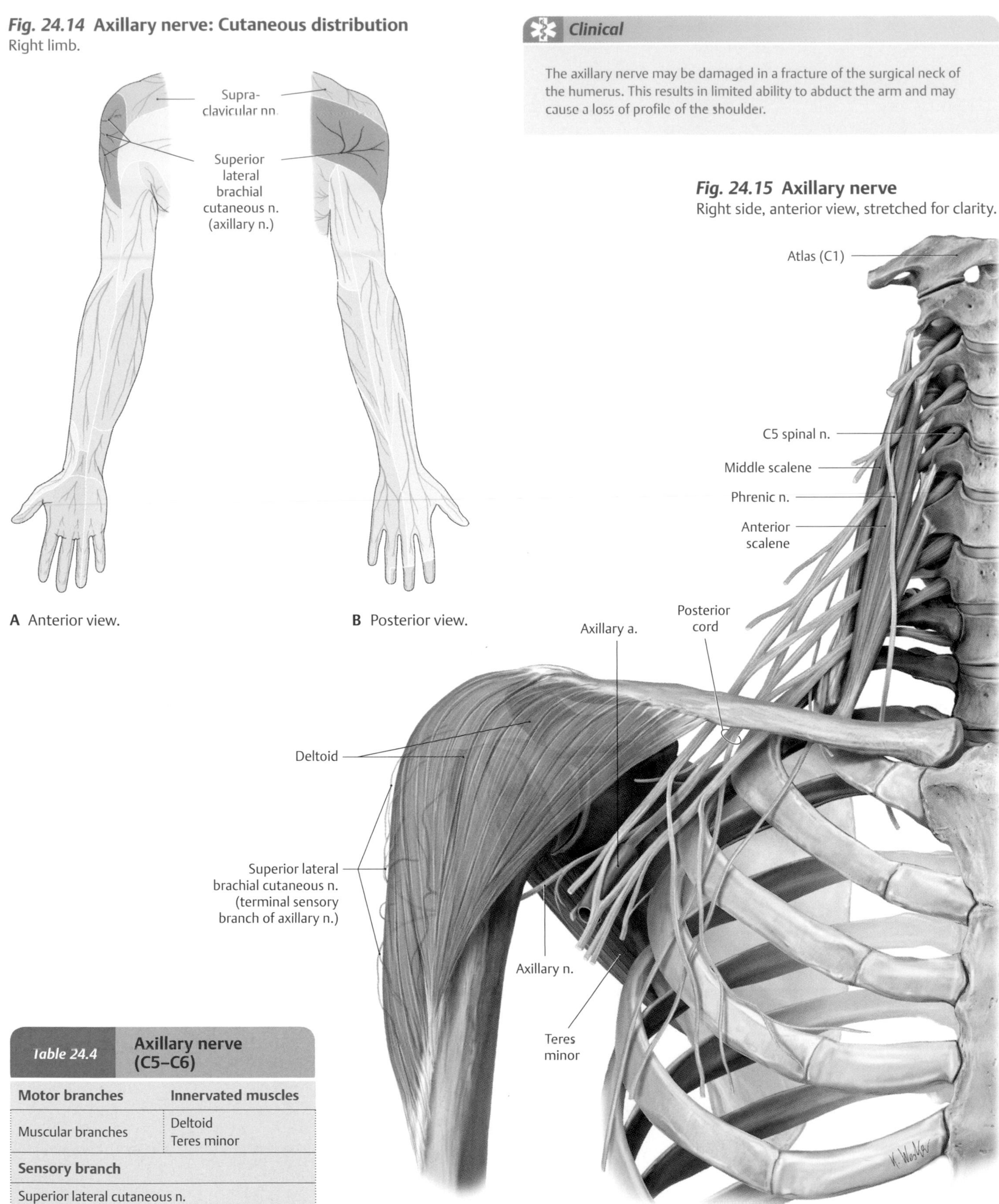
Supra-
clavicular nn.
Superior
lateral
brachial
cutaneous n.
(axillary n.)
Atlas (C1)
C5 spinal n.
Middle scalene
Phrenic n.
Anterior
scalene
Posterior
cord
Axillary a.
Deltoid
Superior lateral
brachial cutaneous n.
(terminal sensory
branch of axillary n.)
Axillary n.
Teres
minor

Fig. 24.14 **Axillary nerve: Cutaneous distribution**
Right limb.

A Anterior view.

B Posterior view.

Clinical

The axillary nerve may be damaged in a fracture of the surgical neck of the humerus. This results in limited ability to abduct the arm and may cause a loss of profile of the shoulder.

Fig. 24.15 **Axillary nerve**
Right side, anterior view, stretched for clarity.

Table 24.4 Axillary nerve (C5–C6)

Motor branches	Innervated muscles
Muscular branches	Deltoid Teres minor
Sensory branch	
Superior lateral cutaneous n.	

Fig. 24.16 Radial nerve: Cutaneous distribution

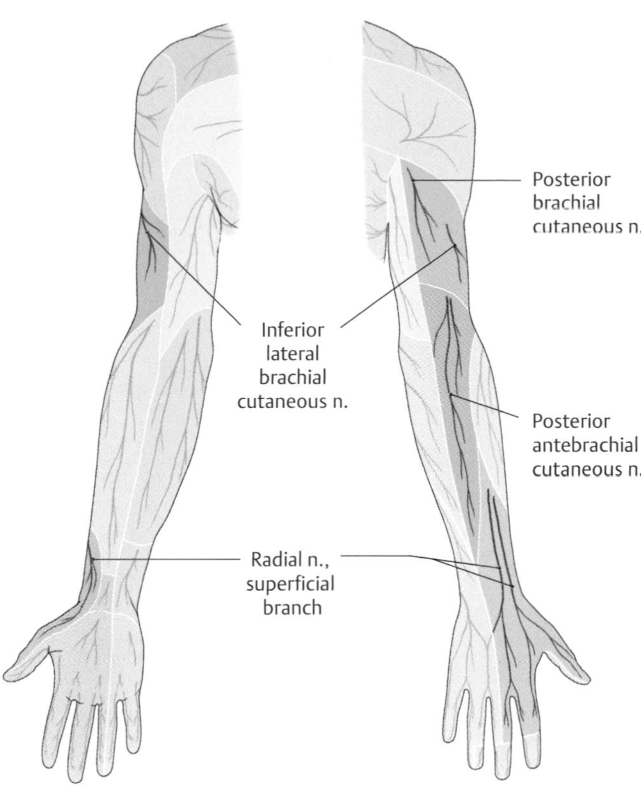
Posterior brachial cutaneous n.
Inferior lateral brachial cutaneous n.
Posterior antebrachial cutaneous n.
Radial n., superficial branch

A Anterior view.

B Posterior view.

Fig. 24.17 Radial nerve

Right limb, anterior view with forearm pronated.

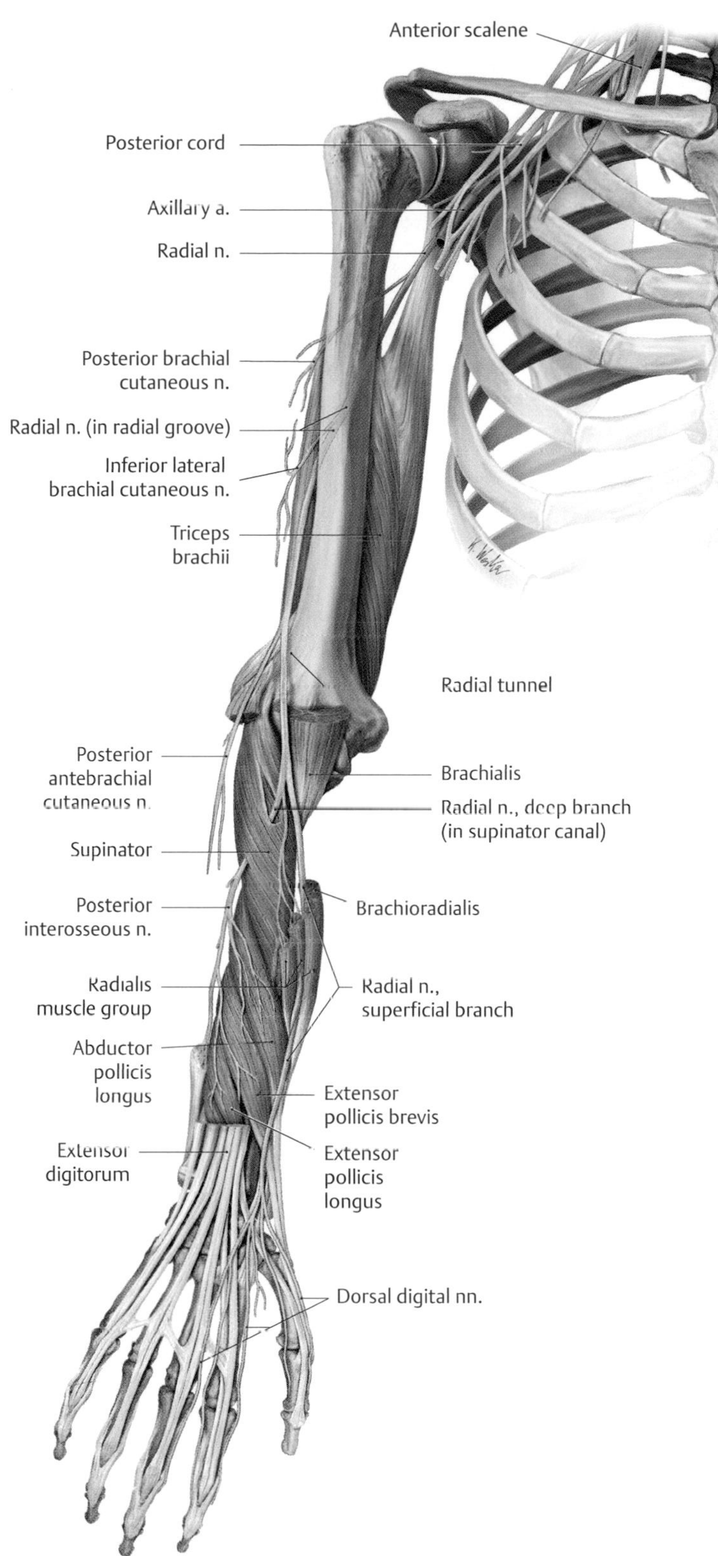
Anterior scalene
Posterior cord
Axillary a.
Radial n.
Posterior brachial cutaneous n.
Radial n. (in radial groove)
Inferior lateral brachial cutaneous n.
Triceps brachii
Radial tunnel
Posterior antebrachial cutaneous n.
Brachialis
Radial n., deep branch (in supinator canal)
Supinator
Posterior interosseous n.
Brachioradialis
Radialis muscle group
Radial n., superficial branch
Abductor pollicis longus
Extensor pollicis brevis
Extensor digitorum
Extensor pollicis longus
Dorsal digital nn.

Table 24.5 Radial nerve (C5–T1)

Motor branches	Innervated muscles
Muscular branches	Brachialis (partial)
	Triceps brachii
	Anconeus
	Brachioradialis
	Extensors carpi radialis longus and brevis
Deep branch (terminal branch: posterior interosseous n.)	Supinator
	Extensor digitorum
	Extensor digiti minimi
	Extensor carpi ulnaris
	Extensors pollicis brevis and longus
	Extensor indicis
	Abductor pollicis longus
Sensory branches	
Articular branches from radial n.: Capsule of the shoulder joint	
Articular branches from posterior interosseous n.: Joint capsule of the wrist and four radial metacarpophalangeal joints	
Posterior brachial cutaneous n.	
Inferior lateral brachial cutaneous n.	
Posterior antebrachial cutaneous n.	
Superficial branches	Dorsal digital nn.
	Ulnar communicating branch

Clinical

Chronic radial nerve compression in the axilla (e.g., due to extended/improper crutch use) may cause loss of sensation or motor function in the hand, forearm, and posterior arm. More distal injuries (e.g., during anesthesia) affect fewer muscles, potentially resulting in wrist drop with intact triceps brachii function.

Medial & Lateral Cords

The medial and lateral cords give off four short branches. The intercostobrachial nerves are included with the short branches of the brachial plexus, although they are actually the cutaneous branches of the 2nd and 3rd intercostal nerves.

Table 24.6 Branches of the medial and lateral cords

Nerve	Level	Cord	Innervated muscle
Short branches			
Lateral pectoral n.	C5–C7	Lateral cord	Pectoralis major
Medial pectoral n.	C8–T1	Medial cord	Pectoralis major and minor
Medial brachial cutaneous n.	T1		– (sensory branches, do not innervate any muscles)
Medial antebrachial cutaneous n.	C8–T1		
Intercostobrachial nn.	T2–T3		
Long (terminal) branches			
Musculocutaneous n.	C5–C7	Lateral cord	Coracobrachialis Biceps brachii Brachialis
Median n.	C6–T1		See p. 356
Ulnar n.	C7–T1	Medial cord	See p. 357

Fig. 24.18 **Medial and lateral cords: Short branches**
Right side, anterior view.

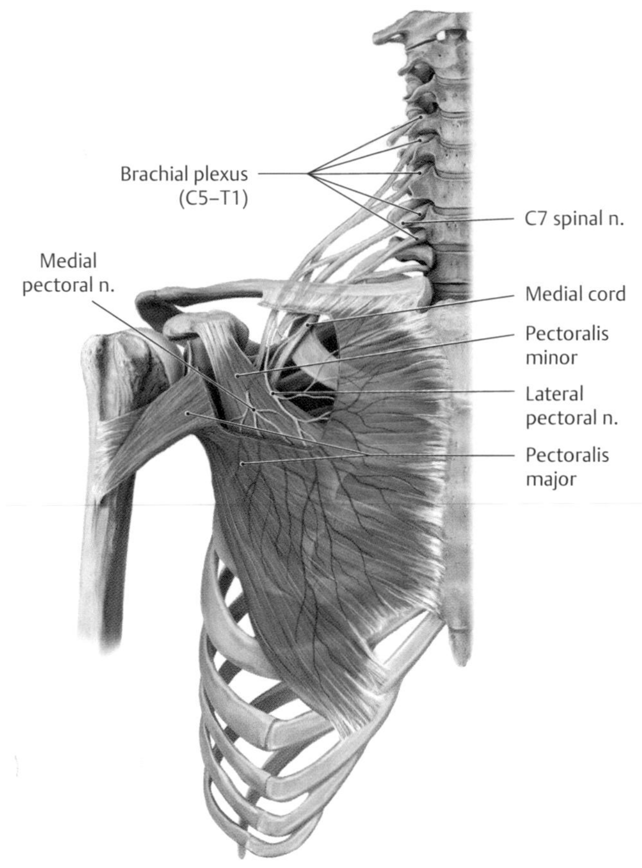
Brachial plexus (C5–T1)
C7 spinal n.
Medial pectoral n.
Medial cord
Pectoralis minor
Lateral pectoral n.
Pectoralis major

A Medial and lateral pectoral nerves.

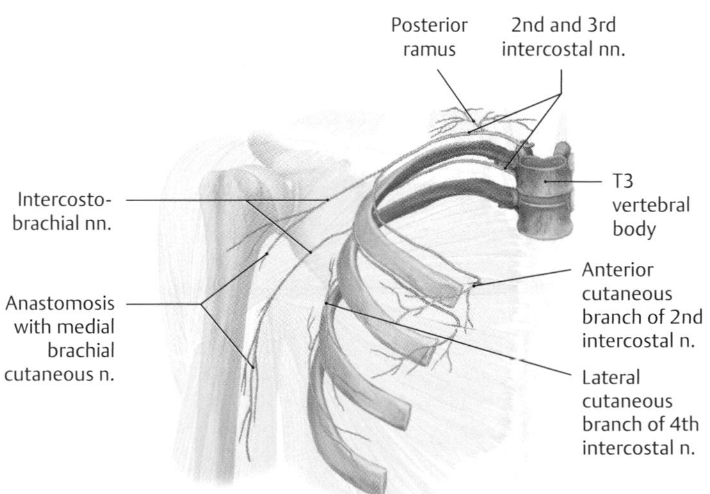
Posterior ramus
2nd and 3rd intercostal nn.
T3 vertebral body
Intercosto-brachial nn.
Anterior cutaneous branch of 2nd intercostal n.
Anastomosis with medial brachial cutaneous n.
Lateral cutaneous branch of 4th intercostal n.

B Intercostobrachial nerves.

Fig. 24.19 **Short branches of medial and lateral chords: Cutaneous distribution**

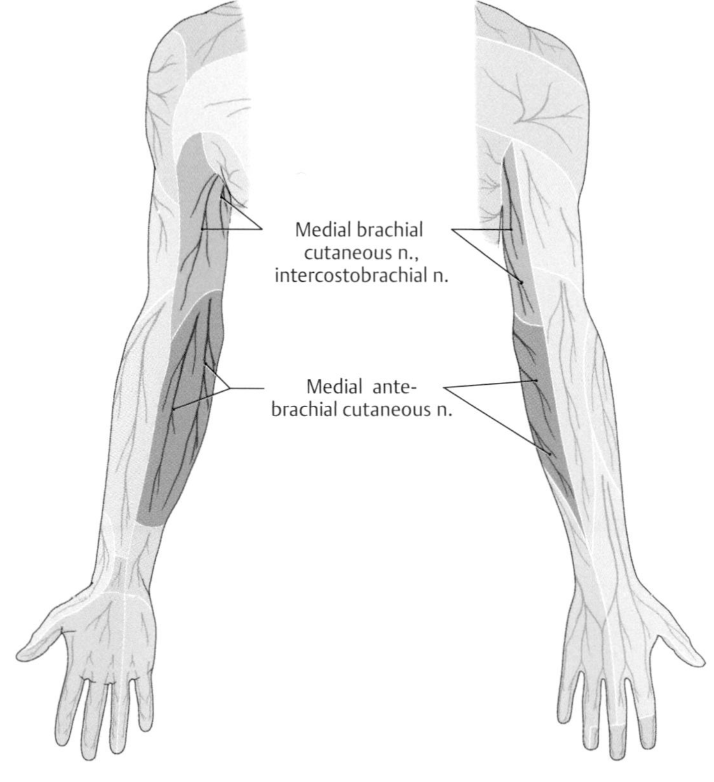
Medial brachial cutaneous n., intercostobrachial n.
Medial ante-brachial cutaneous n.

A Anterior view.

B Posterior view.

Fig. 24.20 **Musculocutaneous nerve**
Right limb, anterior view.

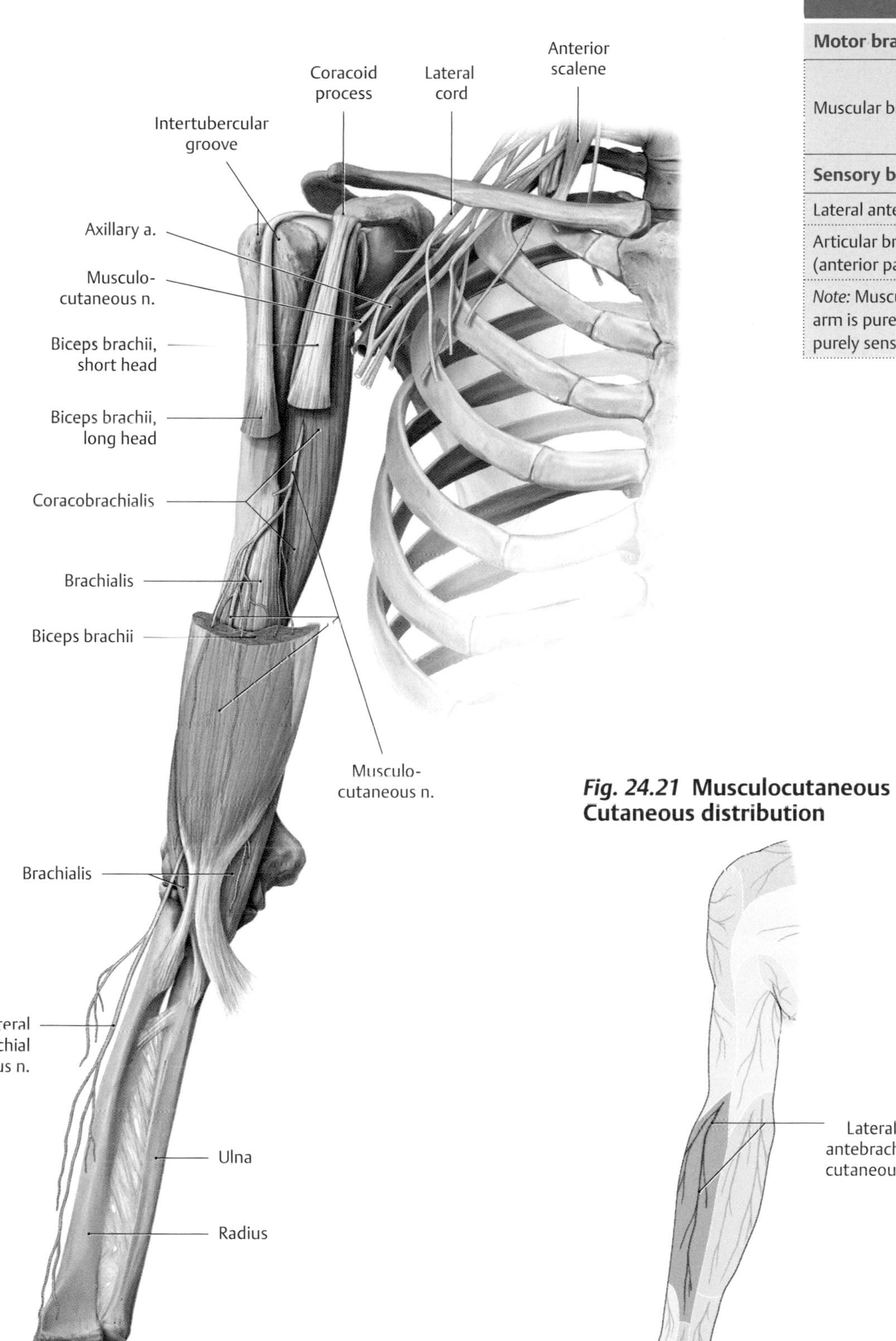
Coracoid process
Lateral cord
Anterior scalene
Intertubercular groove
Axillary a.
Musculo-cutaneous n.
Biceps brachii, short head
Biceps brachii, long head
Coracobrachialis
Brachialis
Biceps brachii
Musculo-cutaneous n.
Brachialis
Lateral antebrachial cutaneous n.
Ulna
Radius

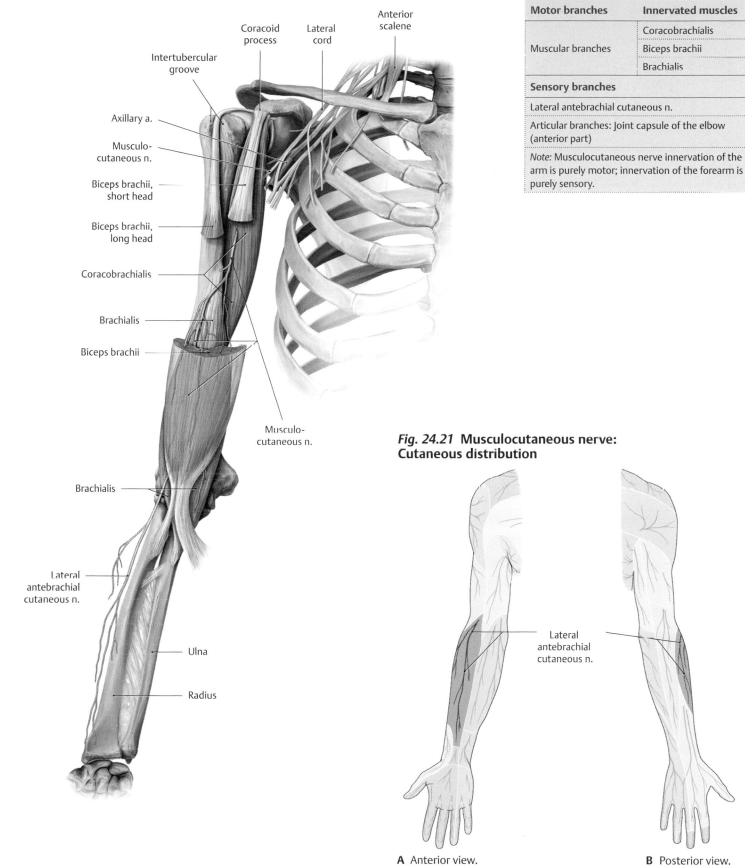

Table 24.7	**Musculocutaneous nerve (C5–C7)**
Motor branches	**Innervated muscles**
Muscular branches	Coracobrachialis
	Biceps brachii
	Brachialis
Sensory branches	
Lateral antebrachial cutaneous n.	
Articular branches: Joint capsule of the elbow (anterior part)	
Note: Musculocutaneous nerve innervation of the arm is purely motor; innervation of the forearm is purely sensory.	

Fig. 24.21 **Musculocutaneous nerve: Cutaneous distribution**

Lateral antebrachial cutaneous n.

A Anterior view.

B Posterior view.

Median & Ulnar Nerves

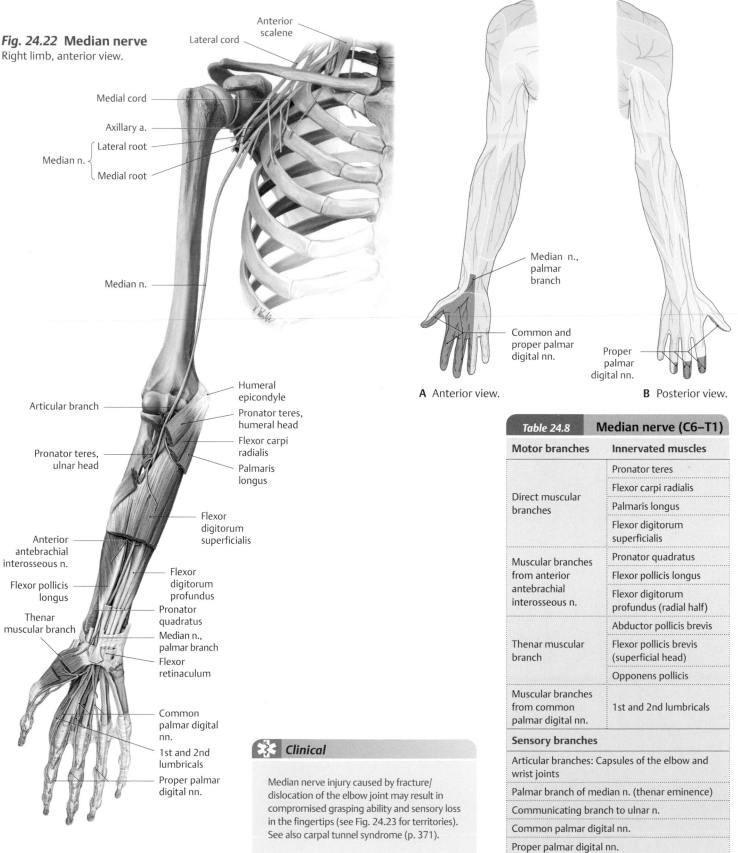

The median nerve is a terminal branch arising from both the medial and the lateral cords. The ulnar nerve arises exclusively from the medial cord.

Fig. 24.22 **Median nerve**
Right limb, anterior view.

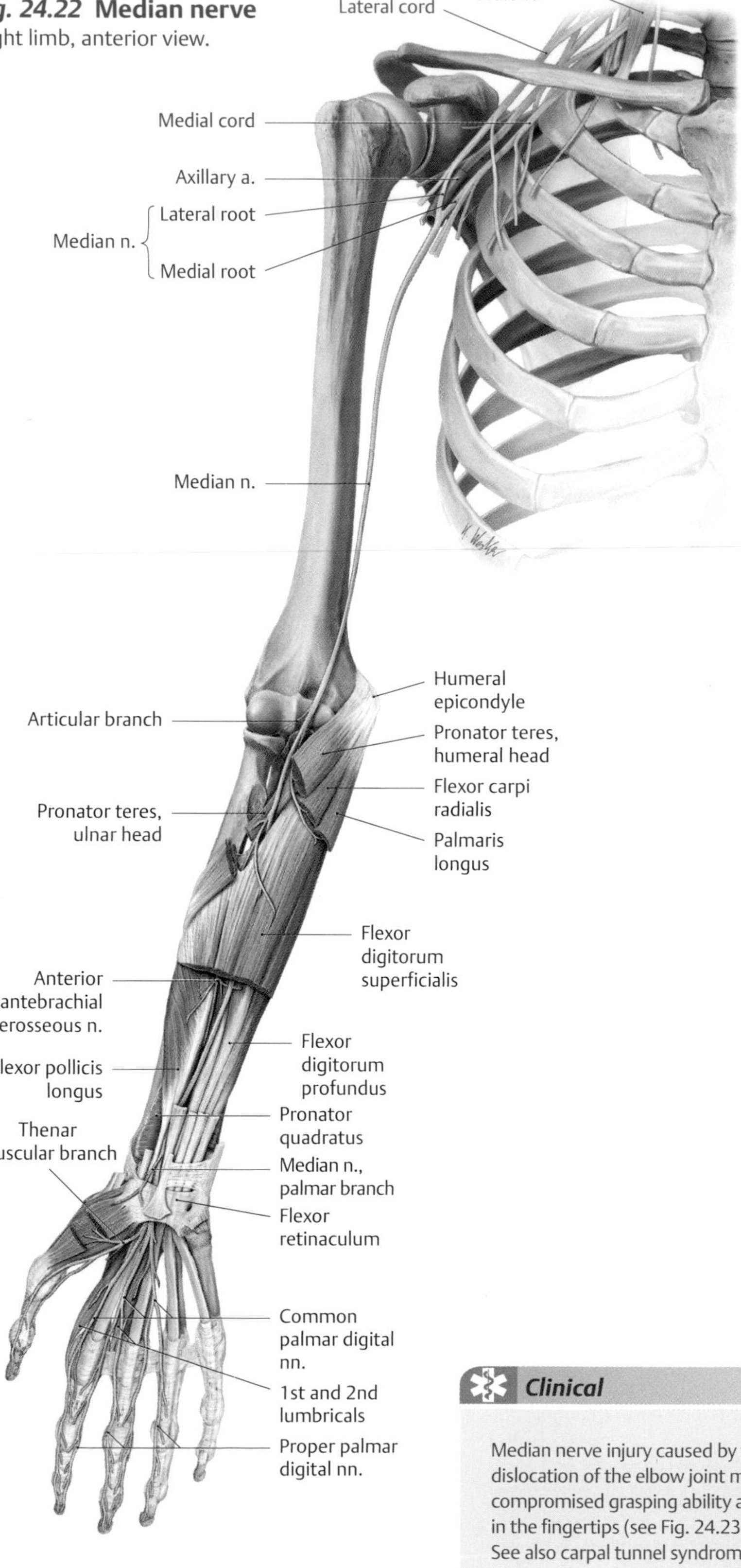

Anterior scalene
Lateral cord
Medial cord
Axillary a.
Median n. { Lateral root, Medial root }
Median n.
Humeral epicondyle
Articular branch
Pronator teres, humeral head
Flexor carpi radialis
Pronator teres, ulnar head
Palmaris longus
Flexor digitorum superficialis
Anterior antebrachial interosseous n.
Flexor digitorum profundus
Flexor pollicis longus
Pronator quadratus
Thenar muscular branch
Median n., palmar branch
Flexor retinaculum
Common palmar digital nn.
1st and 2nd lumbricals
Proper palmar digital nn.

Fig. 24.23 **Median nerve: Cutaneous distribution**

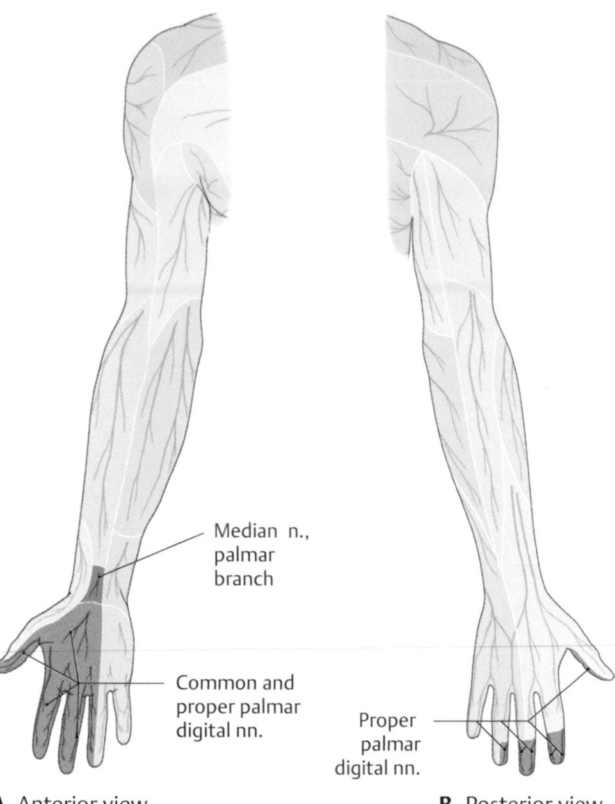
Median n., palmar branch
Common and proper palmar digital nn.
Proper palmar digital nn.

A Anterior view. **B** Posterior view.

Table 24.8	**Median nerve (C6–T1)**
Motor branches	**Innervated muscles**
Direct muscular branches	Pronator teres
	Flexor carpi radialis
	Palmaris longus
	Flexor digitorum superficialis
Muscular branches from anterior antebrachial interosseous n.	Pronator quadratus
	Flexor pollicis longus
	Flexor digitorum profundus (radial half)
Thenar muscular branch	Abductor pollicis brevis
	Flexor pollicis brevis (superficial head)
	Opponens pollicis
Muscular branches from common palmar digital nn.	1st and 2nd lumbricals
Sensory branches	
Articular branches: Capsules of the elbow and wrist joints	
Palmar branch of median n. (thenar eminence)	
Communicating branch to ulnar n.	
Common palmar digital nn.	
Proper palmar digital nn.	

Clinical

Median nerve injury caused by fracture/dislocation of the elbow joint may result in compromised grasping ability and sensory loss in the fingertips (see Fig. 24.23 for territories). See also carpal tunnel syndrome (p. 371).

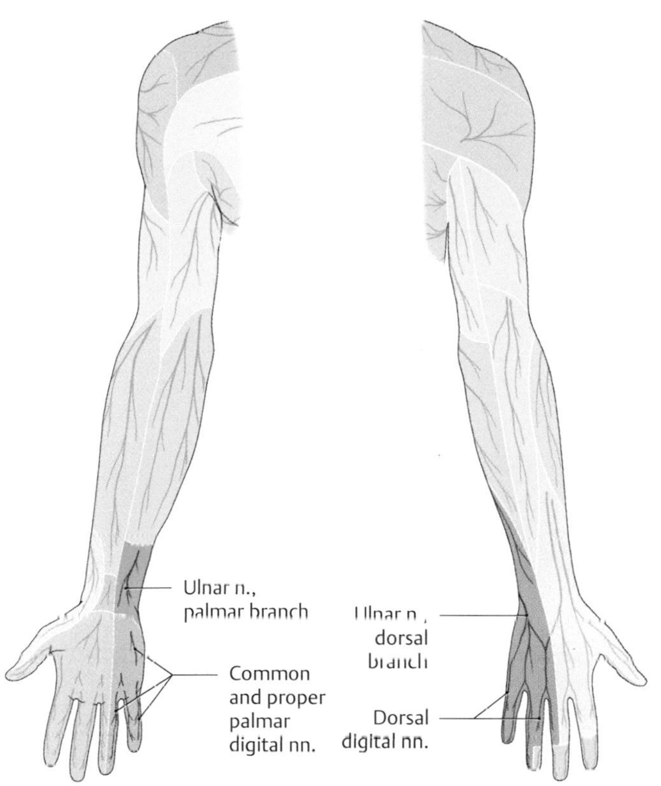
Ulnar n., palmar branch
Common and proper palmar digital nn.
Ulnar n., dorsal branch
Dorsal digital nn.

Fig. 24.24 **Ulnar nerve: Cutaneous distribution**

A Anterior view. **B** Posterior view.

Table 24.9	**Ulnar nerve (C7–T1)**
Motor branches	**Innervated muscles**
Direct muscular branches	Flexor carpi ulnaris
	Flexor digitorum profundus (ulnar half)
Muscular branch from superior ulnar n.	Palmaris brevis
Muscular branches from deep ulnar n.	Abductor digiti minimi
	Flexor digiti minimi
	Opponens digiti minimi
	3rd and 4th lumbricals
	Palmar and dorsal interosseous muscles
	Adductor pollicis
	Flexor pollicis brevis (deep head)
Sensory branches	
Articular branches: Capsules of the elbow, carpal, and metacarpophalangeal joints	
Dorsal branch (terminal branches: dorsal digital nn.)	
Palmar branch	
Proper palmar digital n. (from superficial branch)	
Common palmar digital n. (from superficial branch; terminal branches: proper palmar digital nn.)	

Fig. 24.25 **Ulnar nerve**
Right limb, anterior view.

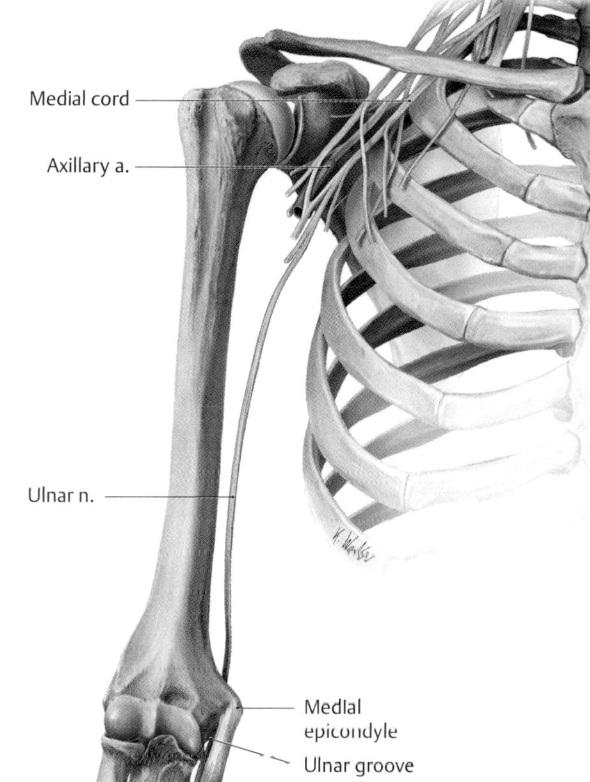
Medial cord
Axillary a.
Ulnar n.
Medial epicondyle
Ulnar groove
Flexor digitorum profundus
Flexor carpi ulnaris
Flexor retinaculum
Dorsal branch
Palmar branch
Superficial branch
Deep branch
4th common palmar digital n.
Interossei
Proper palmar digital nn.

Clinical

Ulnar nerve palsy is the most common peripheral nerve damage. The ulnar nerve is most vulnerable to trauma or chronic compression in the elbow joint and ulnar tunnel (see p. 371). Nerve damage causes "clawing" of the hand and atrophy of the interossei. Sensory losses are often limited to the 5th digit.

Superficial Veins & Nerves of the Upper Limb

Fig. 24.26 **Superficial cutaneous veins and nerves of the upper limb**

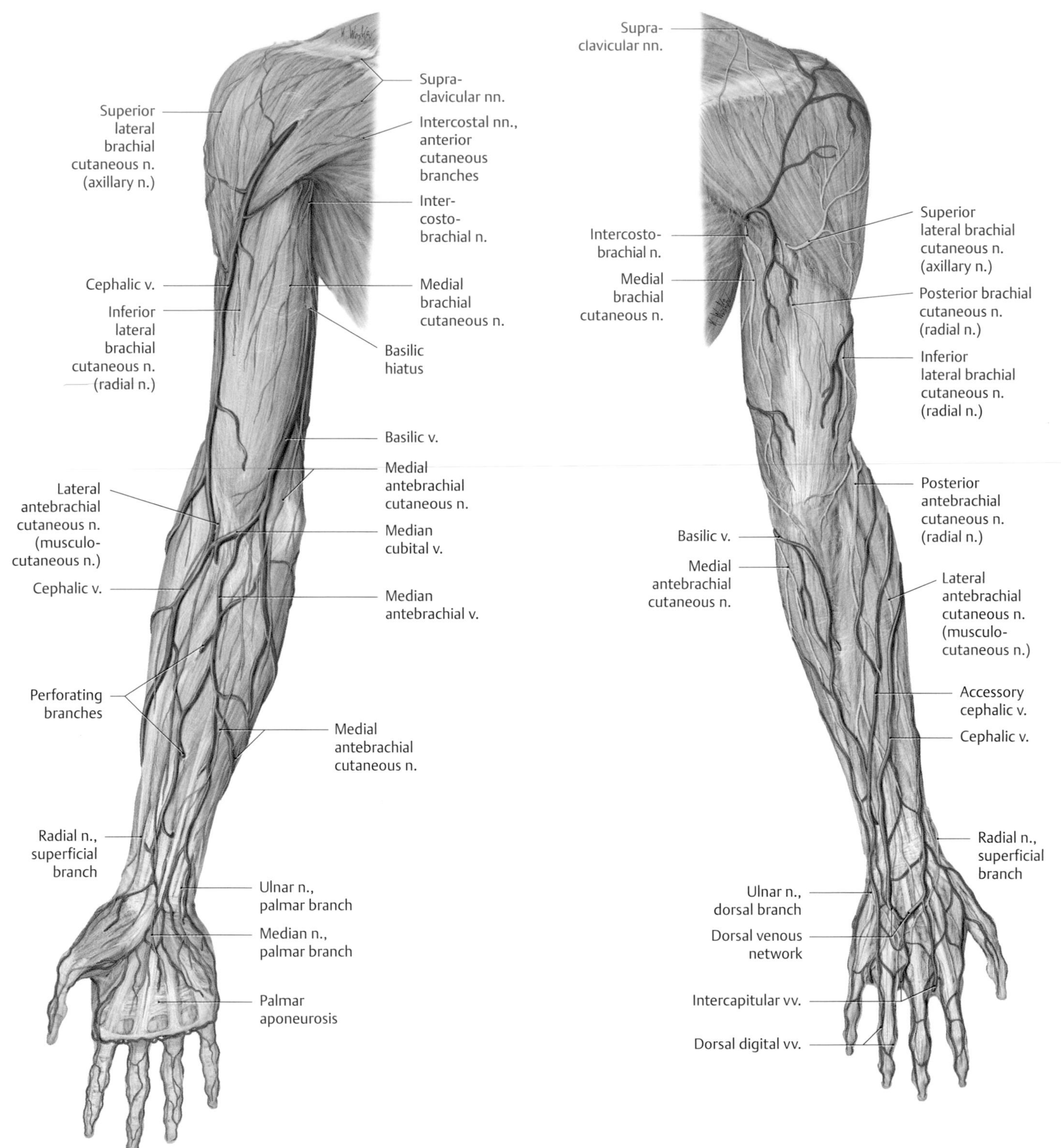
Superior lateral brachial cutaneous n. (axillary n.)
Supra-clavicular nn.
Intercostal nn., anterior cutaneous branches
Inter-costo-brachial n.
Cephalic v.
Inferior lateral brachial cutaneous n. (radial n.)
Medial brachial cutaneous n.
Basilic hiatus
Basilic v.
Medial antebrachial cutaneous n.
Lateral antebrachial cutaneous n. (musculo-cutaneous n.)
Median cubital v.
Cephalic v.
Median antebrachial v.
Perforating branches
Medial antebrachial cutaneous n.
Radial n., superficial branch
Ulnar n., palmar branch
Median n., palmar branch
Palmar aponeurosis
Supra-clavicular nn.
Intercosto-brachial n.
Medial brachial cutaneous n.
Superior lateral brachial cutaneous n. (axillary n.)
Posterior brachial cutaneous n. (radial n.)
Inferior lateral brachial cutaneous n. (radial n.)
Posterior antebrachial cutaneous n. (radial n.)
Basilic v.
Medial antebrachial cutaneous n.
Lateral antebrachial cutaneous n. (musculo-cutaneous n.)
Accessory cephalic v.
Cephalic v.
Radial n., superficial branch
Ulnar n., dorsal branch
Dorsal venous network
Intercapitular vv.
Dorsal digital vv.

A Anterior view. See pp. 372–373 for nerves of the palm.

B Posterior view. See pp. 374–375 for nerves of the dorsum.

Fig. 24.27 **Cutaneous innervation of the upper limb**

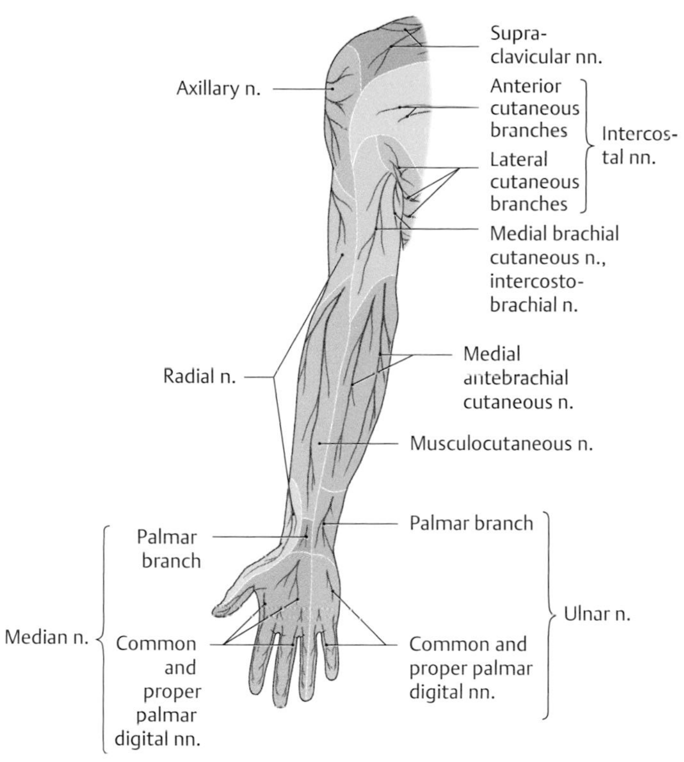
Supra-
clavicular nn.
Axillary n.
Anterior
cutaneous
branches
Intercos-
tal nn.
Lateral
cutaneous
branches
Medial brachial
cutaneous n.,
intercosto-
brachial n.
Radial n.
Medial
antebrachial
cutaneous n.
Musculocutaneous n.
Palmar
branch
Palmar branch
Ulnar n.
Median n.
Common
and
proper
palmar
digital nn.
Common and
proper palmar
digital nn.

A Anterior view.

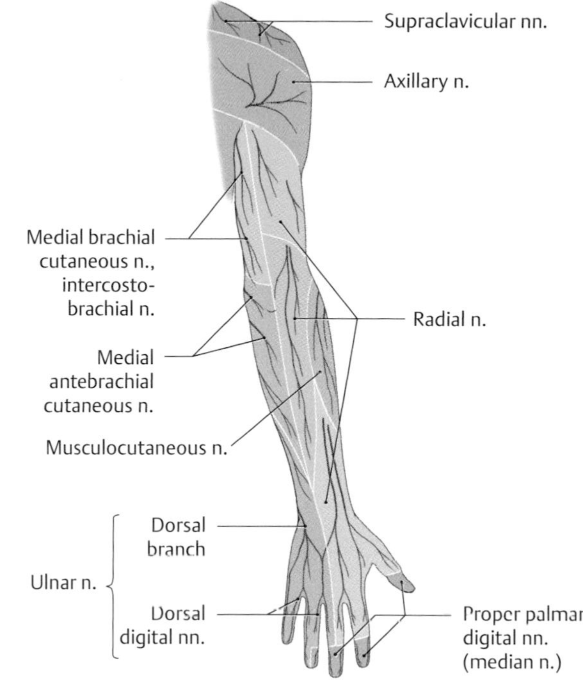
Supraclavicular nn.
Axillary n.
Medial brachial
cutaneous n.,
intercosto-
brachial n.
Radial n.
Medial
antebrachial
cutaneous n.
Musculocutaneous n.
Dorsal
branch
Ulnar n.
Dorsal
digital nn.
Proper palmar
digital nn.
(median n.)

B Posterior view.

Fig. 24.28 **Dermatomes of the upper limb**

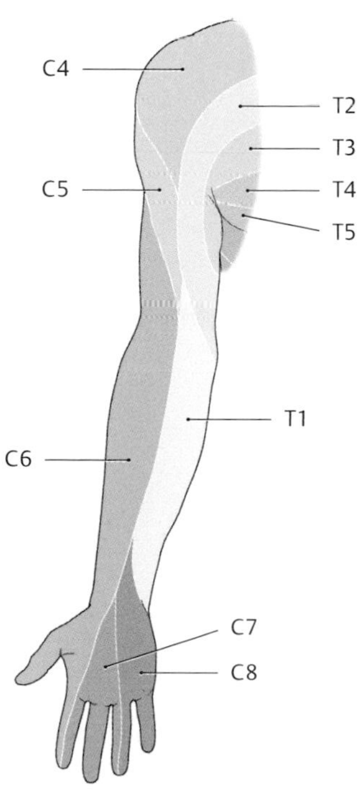
C4
T2
T3
C5
T4
T5
T1
C6
C7
C8

A Anterior view.

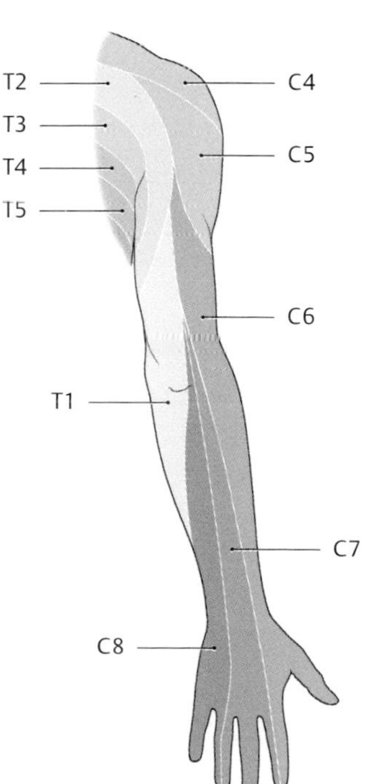
T2
C4
T3
C5
T4
T5
C6
T1
C7
C8

B Posterior view.

Posterior Shoulder & Axilla

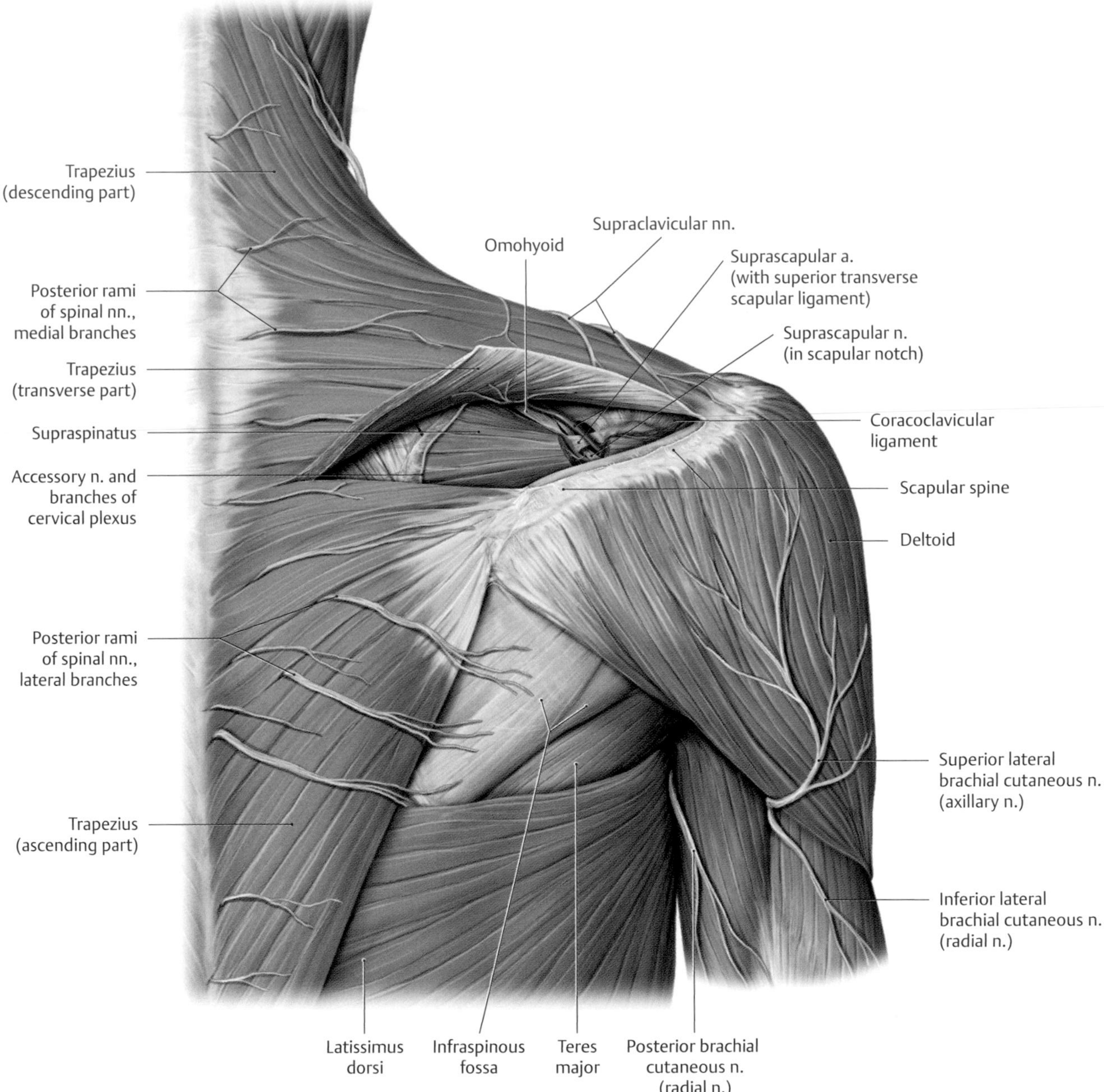
Trapezius (descending part)
Posterior rami of spinal nn., medial branches
Trapezius (transverse part)
Supraspinatus
Accessory n. and branches of cervical plexus
Posterior rami of spinal nn., lateral branches
Trapezius (ascending part)
Omohyoid
Supraclavicular nn.
Suprascapular a. (with superior transverse scapular ligament)
Suprascapular n. (in scapular notch)
Coracoclavicular ligament
Scapular spine
Deltoid
Superior lateral brachial cutaneous n. (axillary n.)
Inferior lateral brachial cutaneous n. (radial n.)
Latissimus dorsi
Infraspinous fossa
Teres major
Posterior brachial cutaneous n. (radial n.)

Fig. 24.29 **Posterior shoulder**
Right shoulder, posterior view. *Raised:* Trapezius (transverse part). *Windowed:* Supraspinatus. *Revealed:* Suprascapular region.

Table 24.10 Neurovascular tracts of the scapula

	Passageway	Boundaries	Transmitted structures
①	Scapular notch	Superior transverse ligament of scapula, scapula	Suprascapular a. and n.
②	Medial border	Scapula	Dorsal scapular a. and n.
③	Triangular space	Teres major and minor	Circumflex scapular a.
④	Triceps hiatus	Triceps brachii, humerus, teres major	Deep a. of arm and radial n.
⑤	Quadrangular space	Teres major and minor, triceps brachii, humerus	Posterior circumflex humeral a. and axillary n.

①
②
③
④
⑤
Superior transverse ligament of scapula
Inferior transverse ligament of scapula

Fig. 24.30 Axilla: Triangular and quadrangular spaces

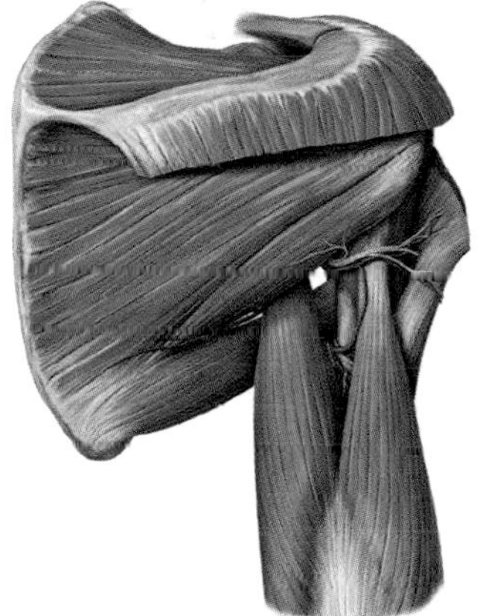

A Right shoulder, posterior view. *Windowed:* Deltoid.

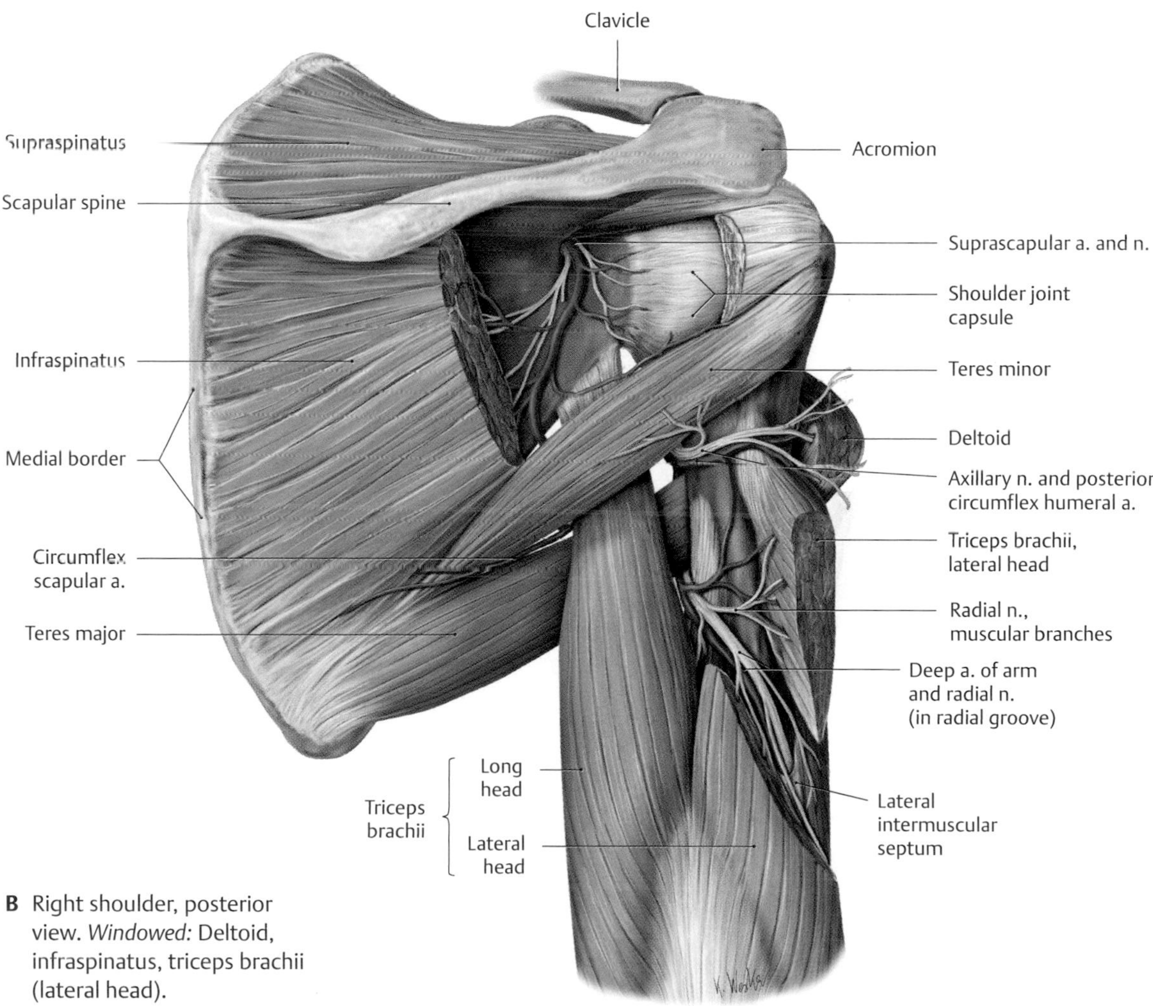
Clavicle
Supraspinatus
Acromion
Scapular spine
Suprascapular a. and n.
Shoulder joint capsule
Infraspinatus
Teres minor
Deltoid
Medial border
Axillary n. and posterior circumflex humeral a.
Circumflex scapular a.
Triceps brachii, lateral head
Teres major
Radial n., muscular branches
Deep a. of arm and radial n. (in radial groove)
Triceps brachii
Long head
Lateral head
Lateral intermuscular septum

B Right shoulder, posterior view. *Windowed:* Deltoid, infraspinatus, triceps brachii (lateral head).

Anterior Shoulder

Fig. 24.31 **Anterior shoulder: Superficial dissection**
Right shoulder.

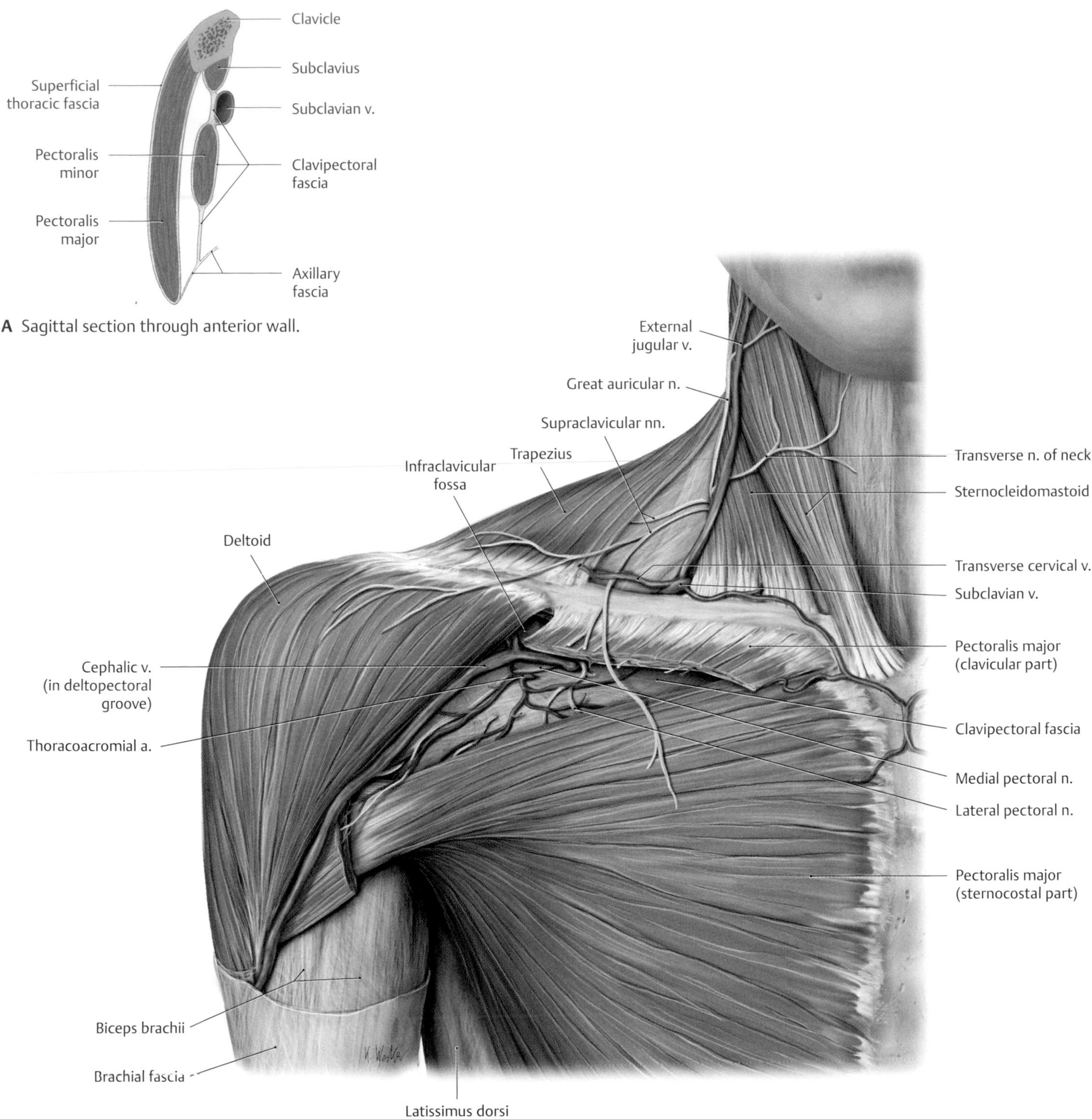
Clavicle
Subclavius
Superficial thoracic fascia
Subclavian v.
Pectoralis minor
Clavipectoral fascia
Pectoralis major
Axillary fascia
External jugular v.
Great auricular n.
Supraclavicular nn.
Trapezius
Infraclavicular fossa
Transverse n. of neck
Sternocleidomastoid
Deltoid
Transverse cervical v.
Subclavian v.
Pectoralis major (clavicular part)
Cephalic v. (in deltopectoral groove)
Clavipectoral fascia
Thoracoacromial a.
Medial pectoral n.
Lateral pectoral n.
Pectoralis major (sternocostal part)
Biceps brachii
Brachial fascia
Latissimus dorsi

A Sagittal section through anterior wall.

B Anterior view. *Removed:* Platysma, muscle fasciae, superficial layer of cervical fascia, and pectoralis major (clavicular part). *Revealed:* Clavipectoral triangle.

Fig. 24.32 Shoulder: Transverse section

Right shoulder, inferior view.

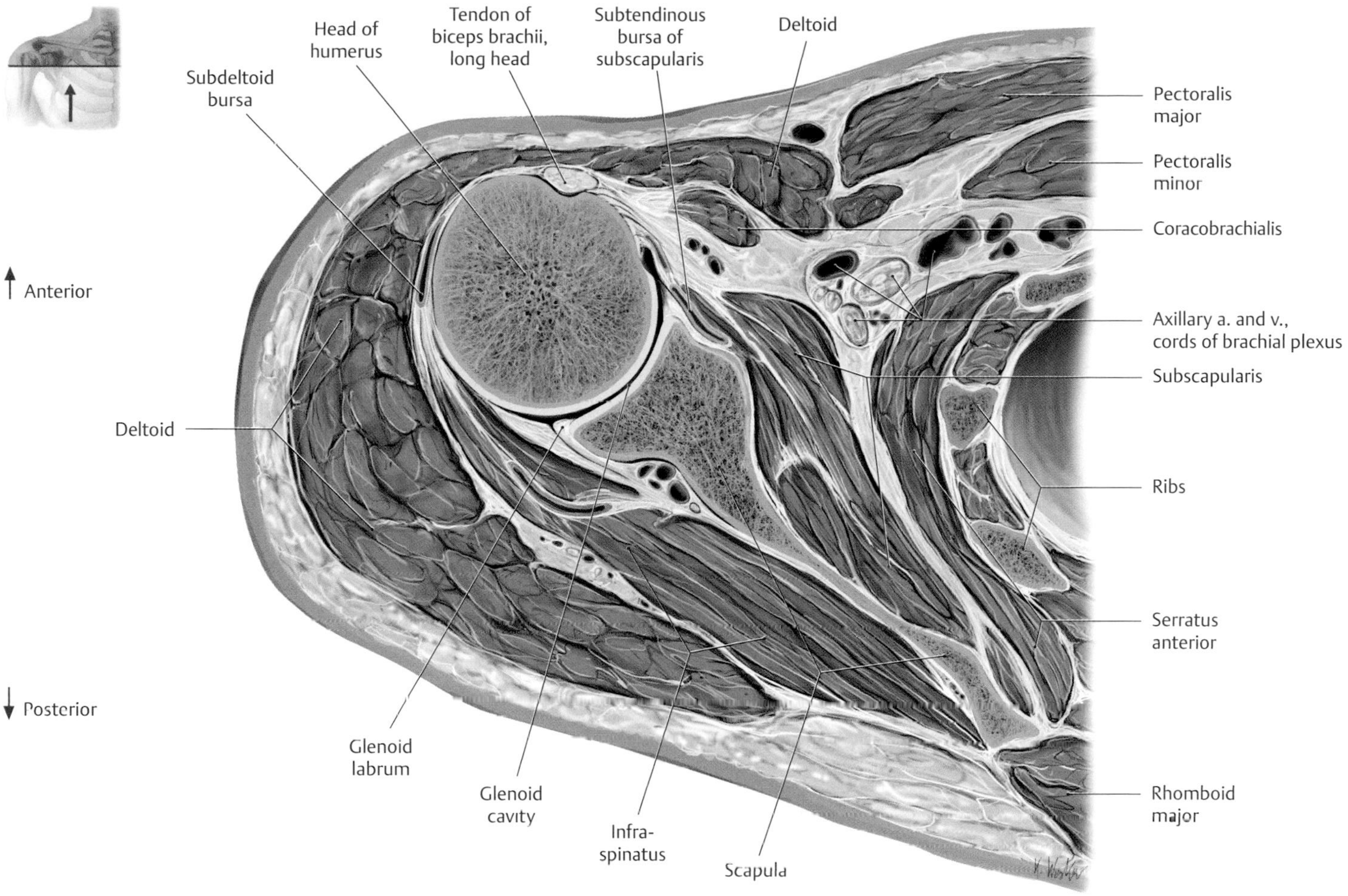

Anterior
Posterior
Subdeltoid bursa
Head of humerus
Tendon of biceps brachii, long head
Subtendinous bursa of subscapularis
Deltoid
Pectoralis major
Pectoralis minor
Coracobrachialis
Axillary a. and v., cords of brachial plexus
Subscapularis
Ribs
Serratus anterior
Rhomboid major
Deltoid
Glenoid labrum
Glenoid cavity
Infra-spinatus
Scapula

Fig. 24.33 Anterior shoulder: Deep dissection

Right limb, anterior view. *Removed:* Sternocleidomastoid, omohyoid, and pectoralis major. This dissection reveals the neurovascular contents of the lateral cervical triangle (see p. 610) and axilla (see pp. 364–365).

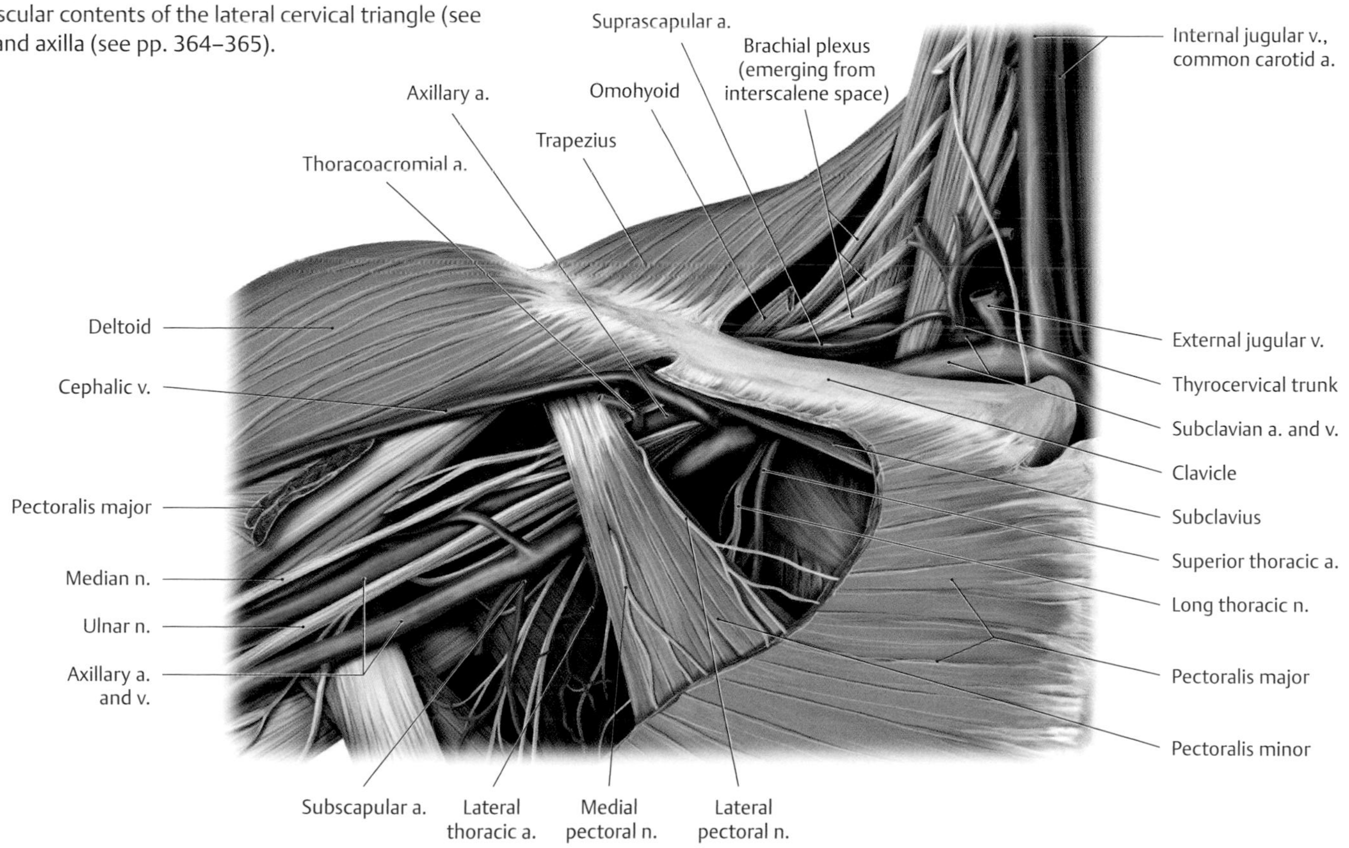

Suprascapular a.
Brachial plexus (emerging from interscalene space)
Internal jugular v., common carotid a.
Axillary a.
Omohyoid
Trapezius
Thoracoacromial a.
Deltoid
Cephalic v.
Pectoralis major
Median n.
Ulnar n.
Axillary a. and v.
External jugular v.
Thyrocervical trunk
Subclavian a. and v.
Clavicle
Subclavius
Superior thoracic a.
Long thoracic n.
Pectoralis major
Pectoralis minor
Subscapular a.
Lateral thoracic a.
Medial pectoral n.
Lateral pectoral n.

Topography of the Axilla

Fig. 24.34 **Axilla: Dissection**
Right shoulder, anterior view.

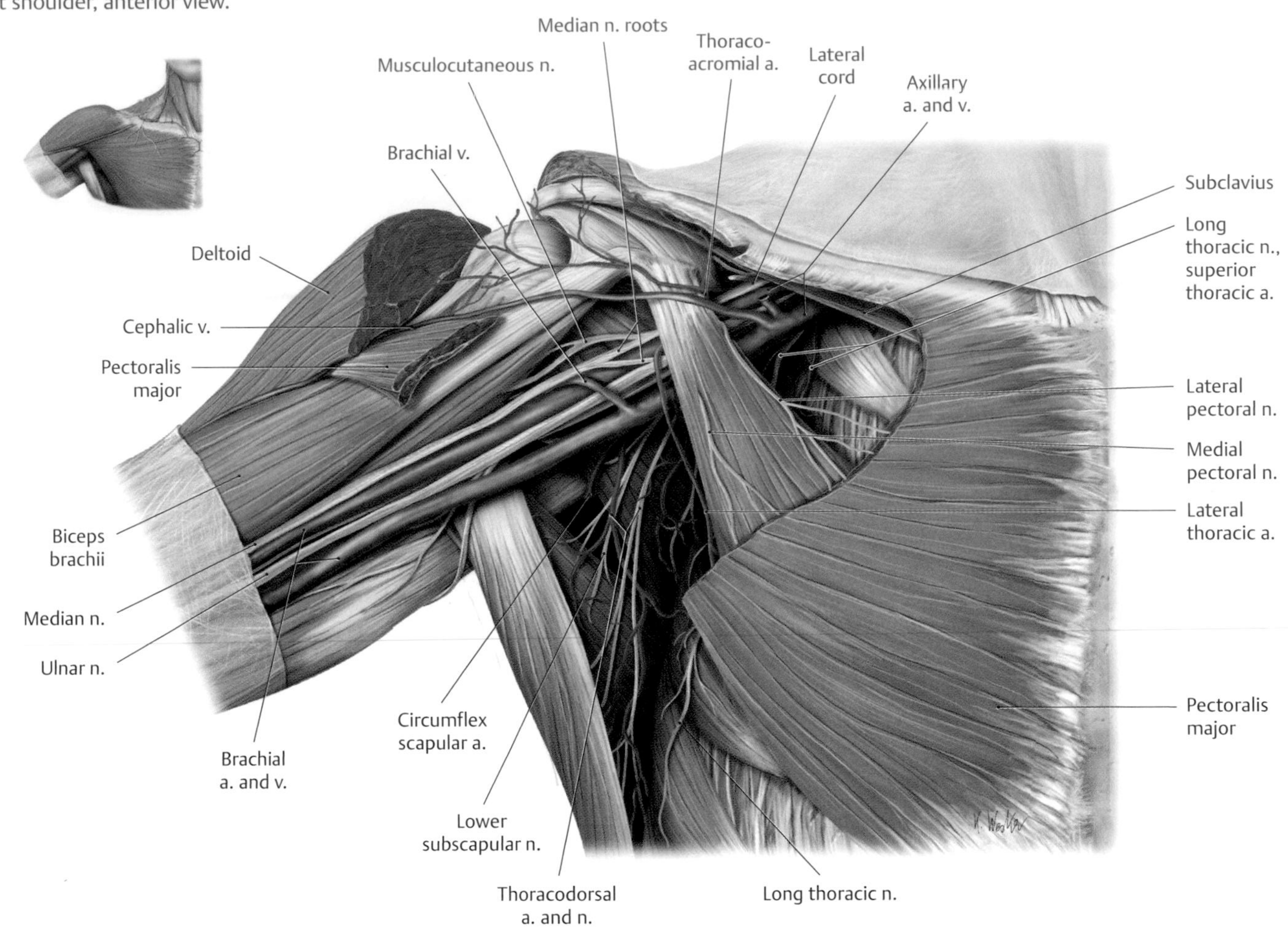
Median n. roots
Thoraco-
acromial a.
Lateral
cord
Musculocutaneous n.
Axillary
a. and v.
Brachial v.
Subclavius
Long
thoracic n.,
superior
thoracic a.
Deltoid
Cephalic v.
Pectoralis
major
Lateral
pectoral n.
Medial
pectoral n.
Lateral
thoracic a.
Biceps
brachii
Median n.
Ulnar n.
Pectoralis
major
Circumflex
scapular a.
Brachial
a. and v.
Lower
subscapular n.
Thoracodorsal
a. and n.
Long thoracic n.

A *Removed:* Pectoralis major and clavipectoral fascia.

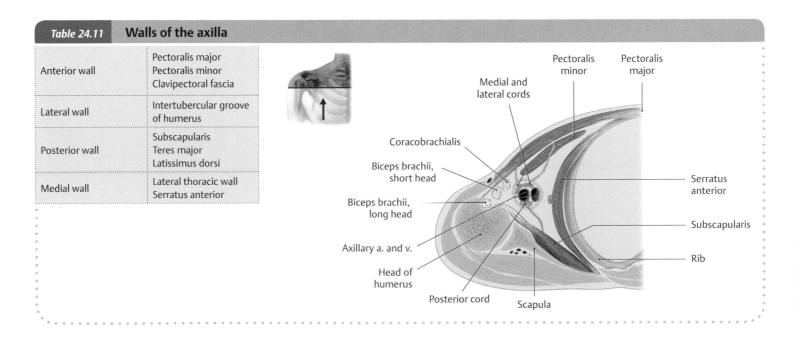

Table 24.11	**Walls of the axilla**
Anterior wall	Pectoralis major Pectoralis minor Clavipectoral fascia
Lateral wall	Intertubercular groove of humerus
Posterior wall	Subscapularis Teres major Latissimus dorsi
Medial wall	Lateral thoracic wall Serratus anterior

Pectoralis
minor
Pectoralis
major
Medial and
lateral cords
Coracobrachialis
Biceps brachii,
short head
Serratus
anterior
Biceps brachii,
long head
Subscapularis
Axillary a. and v.
Rib
Head of
humerus
Posterior cord
Scapula

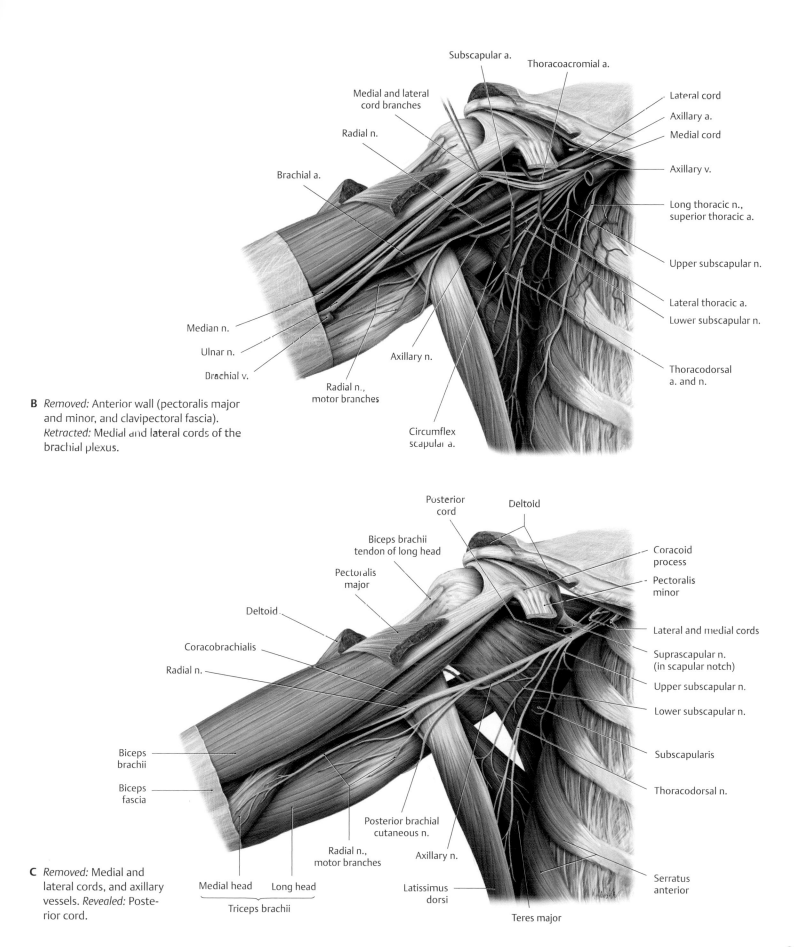

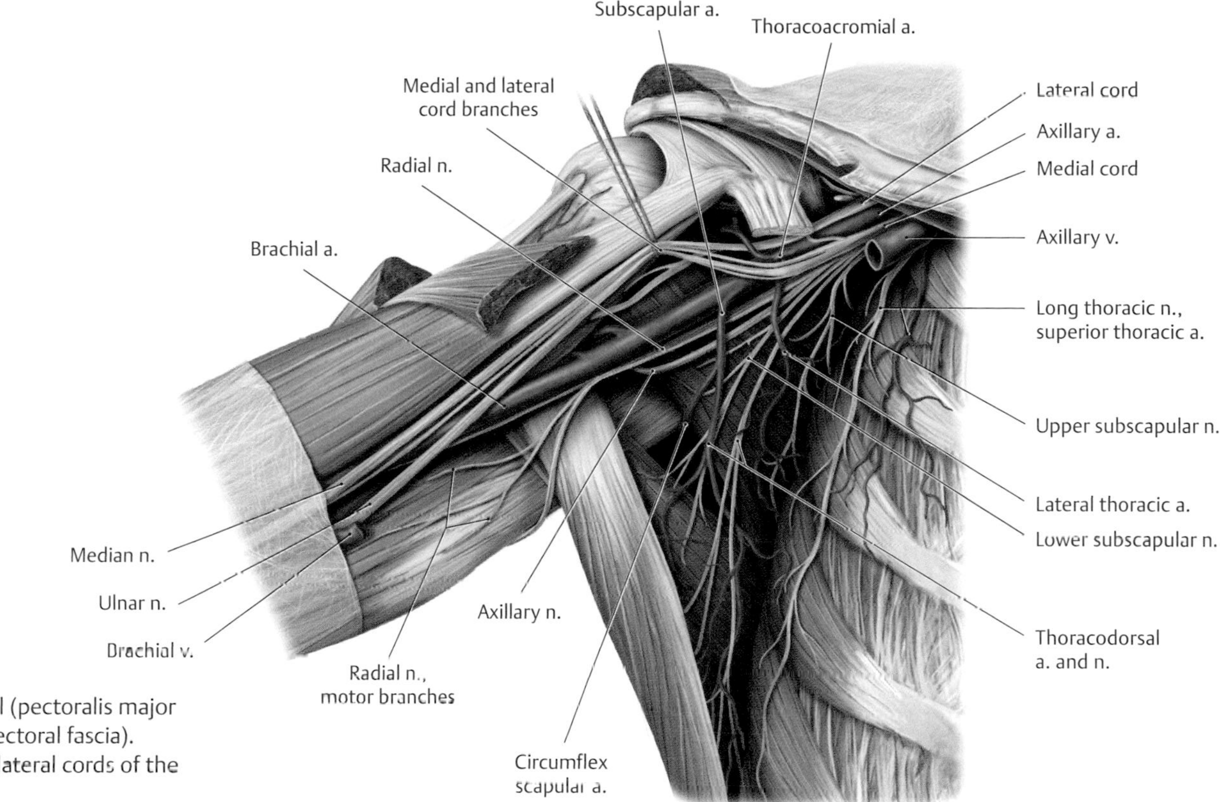
Subscapular a.
Thoracoacromial a.
Medial and lateral cord branches
Radial n.
Brachial a.
Lateral cord
Axillary a.
Medial cord
Axillary v.
Long thoracic n., superior thoracic a.
Upper subscapular n.
Lateral thoracic a.
Lower subscapular n.
Thoracodorsal a. and n.
Median n.
Ulnar n.
Brachial v.
Radial n., motor branches
Axillary n.
Circumflex scapular a.

B *Removed:* Anterior wall (pectoralis major and minor, and clavipectoral fascia). *Retracted:* Medial and lateral cords of the brachial plexus.

Posterior cord
Deltoid
Biceps brachii tendon of long head
Pectoralis major
Deltoid
Coracobrachialis
Radial n.
Coracoid process
Pectoralis minor
Lateral and medial cords
Suprascapular n. (in scapular notch)
Upper subscapular n.
Lower subscapular n.
Subscapularis
Thoracodorsal n.
Biceps brachii
Biceps fascia
Posterior brachial cutaneous n.
Radial n., motor branches
Axillary n.
Medial head
Long head
Triceps brachii
Latissimus dorsi
Teres major
Serratus anterior

C *Removed:* Medial and lateral cords, and axillary vessels. *Revealed:* Posterior cord.

Topography of the Brachial & Cubital Regions

Fig. 24.35 **Brachial region**
Right arm, anterior view. *Removed:* Deltoid, pectoralis major and minor. *Revealed:* Medial bicipital groove.

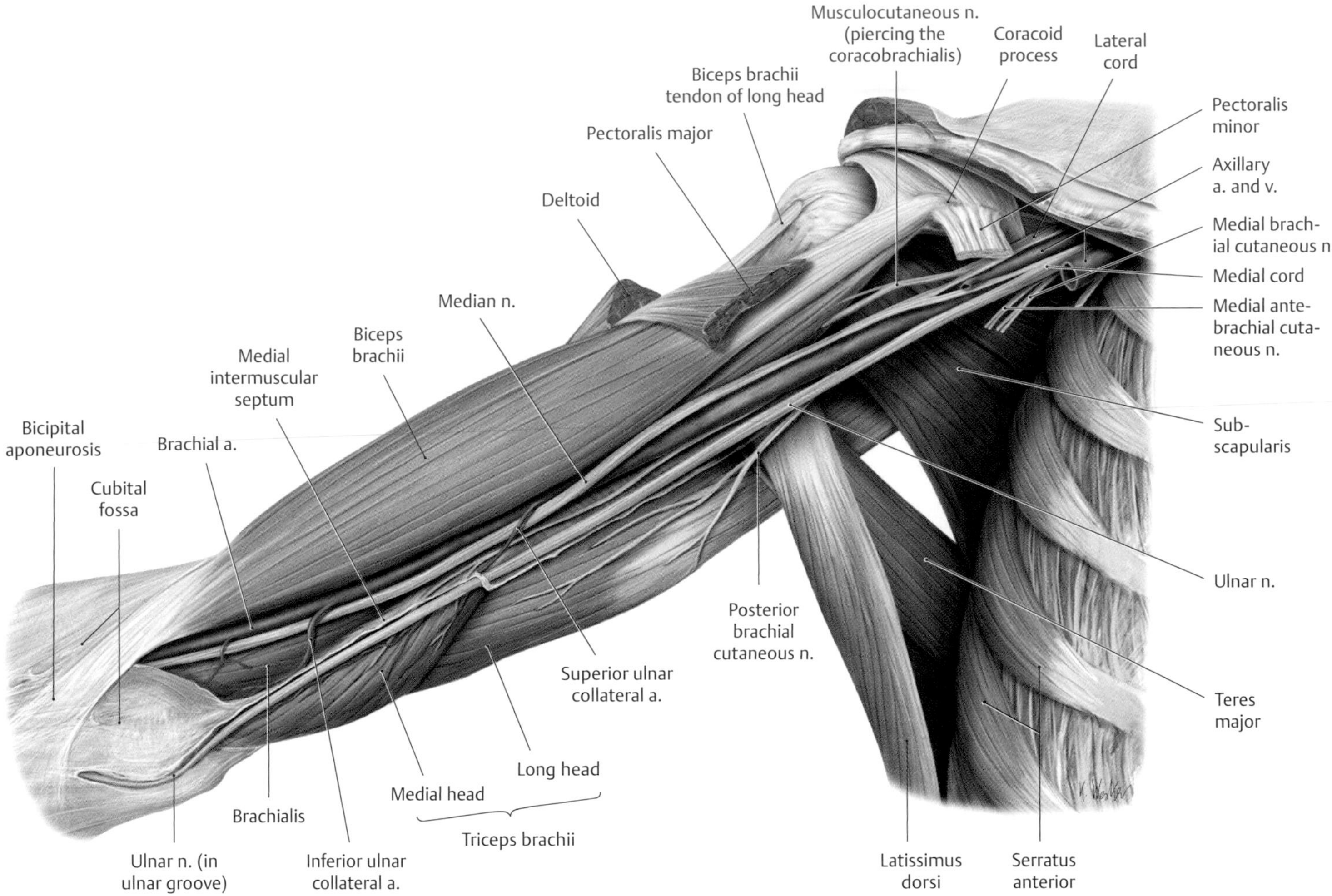

Musculocutaneous n. (piercing the coracobrachialis)
Coracoid process
Lateral cord
Biceps brachii tendon of long head
Pectoralis major
Pectoralis minor
Axillary a. and v.
Deltoid
Medial brachial cutaneous n.
Medial cord
Medial antebrachial cutaneous n.
Median n.
Biceps brachii
Medial intermuscular septum
Sub-scapularis
Bicipital aponeurosis
Brachial a.
Cubital fossa
Ulnar n.
Posterior brachial cutaneous n.
Superior ulnar collateral a.
Teres major
Long head
Medial head
Triceps brachii
Brachialis
Ulnar n. (in ulnar groove)
Inferior ulnar collateral a.
Latissimus dorsi
Serratus anterior

Fig. 24.36 Cubital region

Right elbow, anterior view.

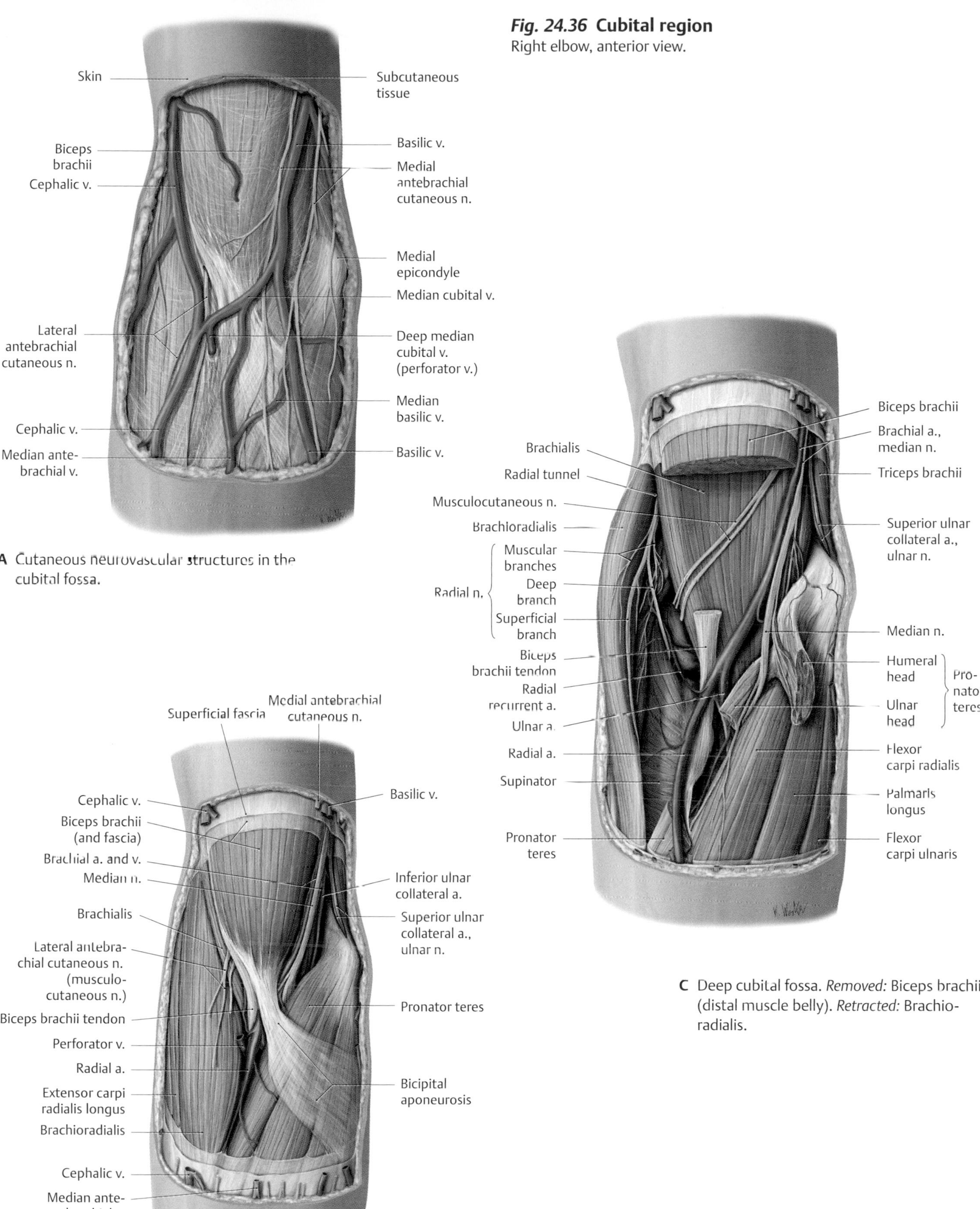

Skin
Subcutaneous tissue
Biceps brachii
Cephalic v.
Basilic v.
Medial antebrachial cutaneous n.
Medial epicondyle
Median cubital v.
Lateral antebrachial cutaneous n.
Deep median cubital v. (perforator v.)
Median basilic v.
Cephalic v.
Median antebrachial v.
Basilic v.
Superficial fascia
Medial antebrachial cutaneous n.
Cephalic v.
Basilic v.
Biceps brachii (and fascia)
Brachial a. and v.
Median n.
Inferior ulnar collateral a.
Brachialis
Superior ulnar collateral a., ulnar n.
Lateral antebrachial cutaneous n. (musculocutaneous n.)
Pronator teres
Biceps brachii tendon
Perforator v.
Radial a.
Bicipital aponeurosis
Extensor carpi radialis longus
Brachioradialis
Cephalic v.
Median antebrachial v.
Biceps brachii
Brachial a., median n.
Brachialis
Radial tunnel
Triceps brachii
Musculocutaneous n.
Brachioradialis
Superior ulnar collateral a., ulnar n.
Radial n.
Muscular branches
Deep branch
Superficial branch
Median n.
Biceps brachii tendon
Humeral head
Pronator teres
Radial recurrent a.
Ulnar head
Ulnar a.
Radial a.
Flexor carpi radialis
Supinator
Palmaris longus
Pronator teres
Flexor carpi ulnaris

A Cutaneous neurovascular structures in the cubital fossa.

B Superficial cubital fossa. *Removed:* Fasciae and epifascial neurovascular structures.

C Deep cubital fossa. *Removed:* Biceps brachii (distal muscle belly). *Retracted:* Brachioradialis.

Topography of the Forearm

Fig. 24.37 Anterior forearm
Right forearm, anterior view.

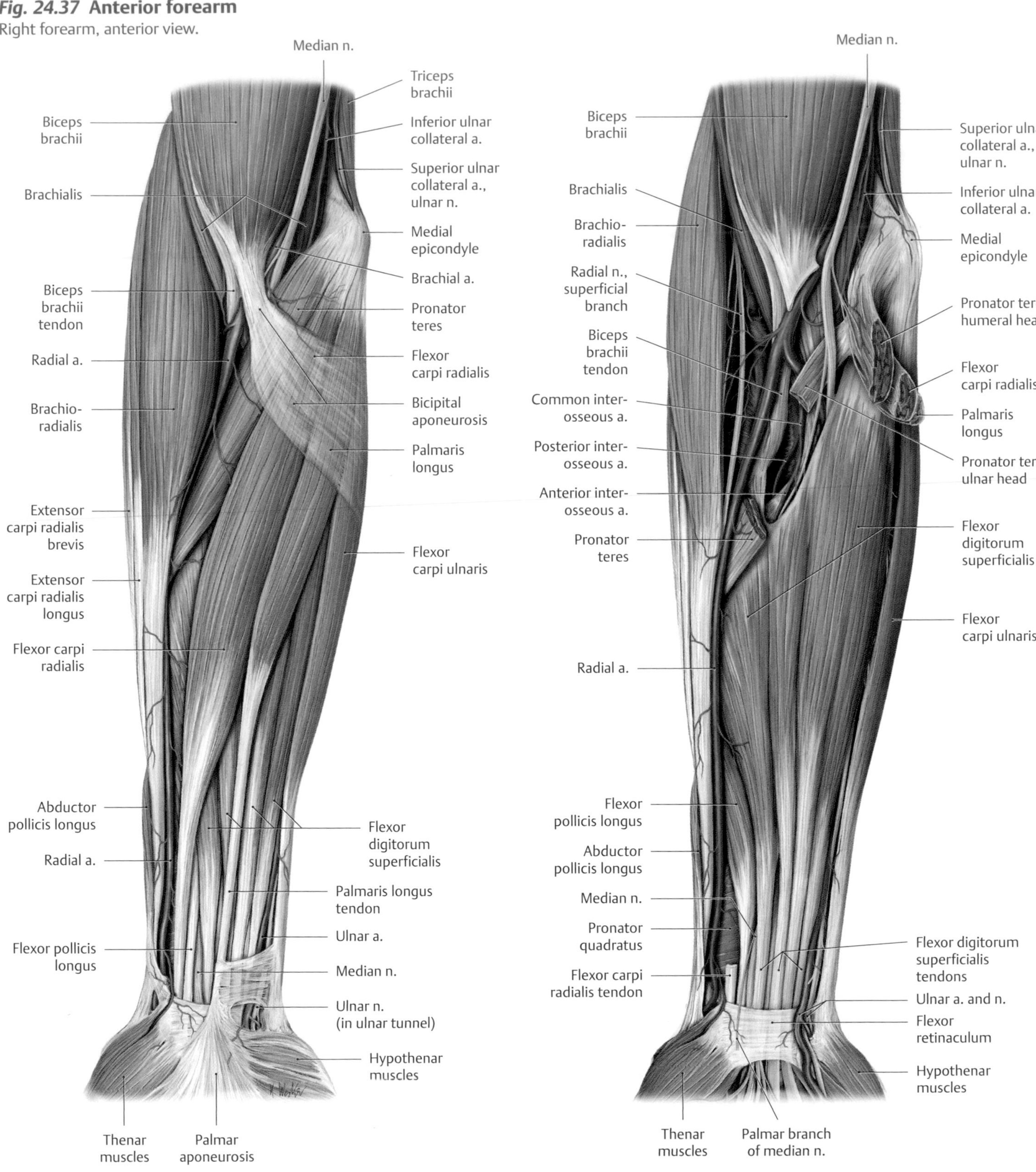
Median n.
Triceps brachii
Biceps brachii
Inferior ulnar collateral a.
Superior ulnar collateral a., ulnar n.
Brachialis
Medial epicondyle
Brachial a.
Biceps brachii tendon
Pronator teres
Radial a.
Flexor carpi radialis
Brachio-radialis
Bicipital aponeurosis
Palmaris longus
Extensor carpi radialis brevis
Flexor carpi ulnaris
Extensor carpi radialis longus
Flexor carpi radialis
Abductor pollicis longus
Flexor digitorum superficialis
Radial a.
Palmaris longus tendon
Ulnar a.
Flexor pollicis longus
Median n.
Ulnar n. (in ulnar tunnel)
Hypothenar muscles
Thenar muscles
Palmar aponeurosis
Median n.
Biceps brachii
Superior ulnar collateral a., ulnar n.
Brachialis
Inferior ulnar collateral a.
Brachio-radialis
Medial epicondyle
Radial n., superficial branch
Pronator teres, humeral head
Biceps brachii tendon
Flexor carpi radialis
Common inter-osseous a.
Palmaris longus
Posterior inter-osseous a.
Pronator teres, ulnar head
Anterior inter-osseous a.
Flexor digitorum superficialis
Pronator teres
Flexor carpi ulnaris
Radial a.
Flexor pollicis longus
Abductor pollicis longus
Median n.
Pronator quadratus
Flexor digitorum superficialis tendons
Flexor carpi radialis tendon
Ulnar a. and n.
Flexor retinaculum
Hypothenar muscles
Thenar muscles
Palmar branch of median n.

A Superficial layer. *Removed:* Fasciae and superficial neurovasculature.

B Middle layer. *Partially removed:* Superficial flexors (pronator teres, flexor digitorum superficialis, palmaris longus, and flexor carpi radialis).

Fig. 24.38 Posterior forearm

Right forearm, anterior view during pronation. *Reflected:* Anconeus and triceps brachii. *Resected:* Extensor carpi ulnaris and extensor digitorum.

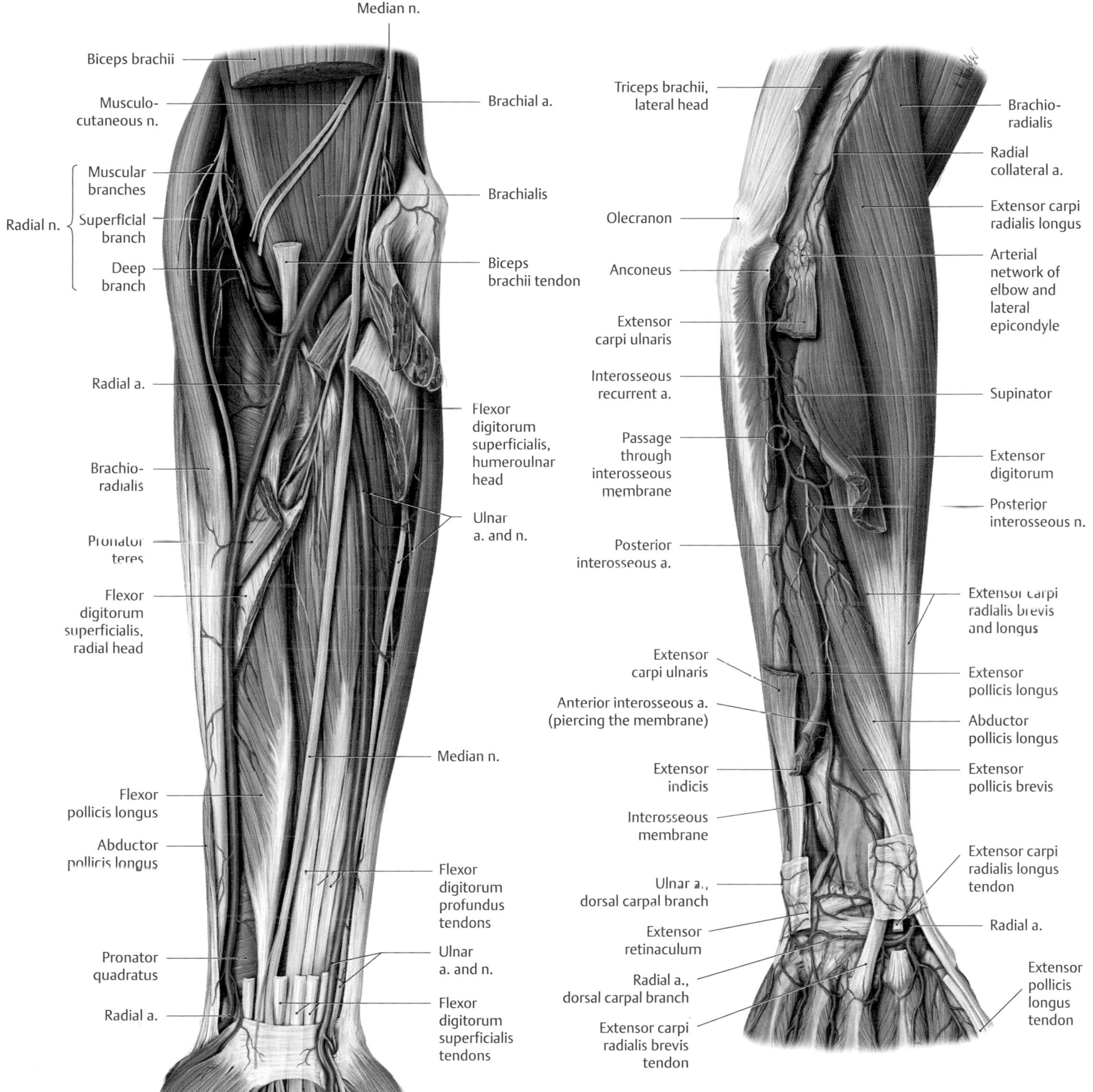
Median n.
Biceps brachii
Musculo-cutaneous n.
Brachial a.
Radial n.
Muscular branches
Superficial branch
Deep branch
Brachialis
Biceps brachii tendon
Radial a.
Flexor digitorum superficialis, humeroulnar head
Brachio-radialis
Ulnar a. and n.
Pronator teres
Flexor digitorum superficialis, radial head
Median n.
Flexor pollicis longus
Abductor pollicis longus
Flexor digitorum profundus tendons
Pronator quadratus
Ulnar a. and n.
Radial a.
Flexor digitorum superficialis tendons
Triceps brachii, lateral head
Brachio-radialis
Radial collateral a.
Olecranon
Extensor carpi radialis longus
Anconeus
Arterial network of elbow and lateral epicondyle
Extensor carpi ulnaris
Interosseous recurrent a.
Supinator
Passage through interosseous membrane
Extensor digitorum
Posterior interosseous n.
Posterior interosseous a.
Extensor carpi radialis brevis and longus
Extensor carpi ulnaris
Extensor pollicis longus
Anterior interosseous a. (piercing the membrane)
Abductor pollicis longus
Extensor indicis
Extensor pollicis brevis
Interosseous membrane
Extensor carpi radialis longus tendon
Ulnar a., dorsal carpal branch
Radial a.
Extensor retinaculum
Radial a., dorsal carpal branch
Extensor pollicis longus tendon
Extensor carpi radialis brevis tendon

C Deep layer. *Removed:* Deep flexors.

Topography of the Carpal Region

Fig. 24.39 Anterior carpal region
Right hand, anterior (palmar) view.

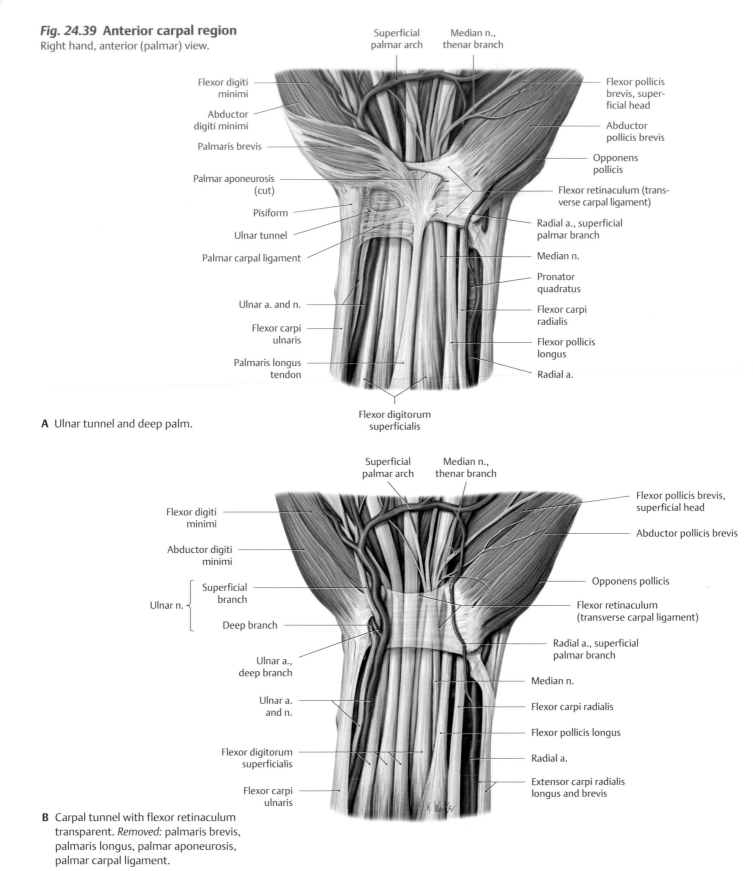

Superficial palmar arch
Median n., thenar branch
Flexor digiti minimi
Abductor digiti minimi
Palmaris brevis
Palmar aponeurosis (cut)
Pisiform
Ulnar tunnel
Palmar carpal ligament
Ulnar a. and n.
Flexor carpi ulnaris
Palmaris longus tendon
Flexor digitorum superficialis
Flexor pollicis brevis, superficial head
Abductor pollicis brevis
Opponens pollicis
Flexor retinaculum (transverse carpal ligament)
Radial a., superficial palmar branch
Median n.
Pronator quadratus
Flexor carpi radialis
Flexor pollicis longus
Radial a.

A Ulnar tunnel and deep palm.

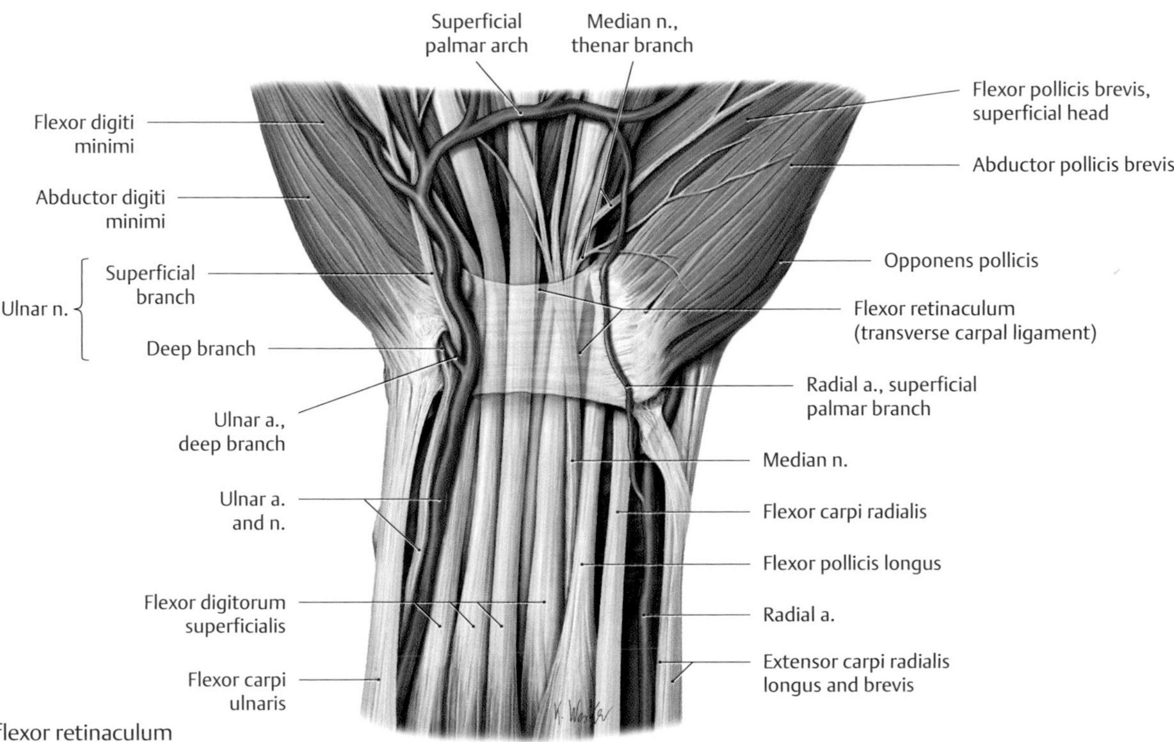
Superficial palmar arch
Median n., thenar branch
Flexor digiti minimi
Abductor digiti minimi
Ulnar n.
Superficial branch
Deep branch
Ulnar a., deep branch
Ulnar a. and n.
Flexor digitorum superficialis
Flexor carpi ulnaris
Flexor pollicis brevis, superficial head
Abductor pollicis brevis
Opponens pollicis
Flexor retinaculum (transverse carpal ligament)
Radial a., superficial palmar branch
Median n.
Flexor carpi radialis
Flexor pollicis longus
Radial a.
Extensor carpi radialis longus and brevis

B Carpal tunnel with flexor retinaculum transparent. *Removed:* palmaris brevis, palmaris longus, palmar aponeurosis, palmar carpal ligament.

Fig. 24.40 **Ulnar tunnel**
Right hand, anterior (palmar) view.

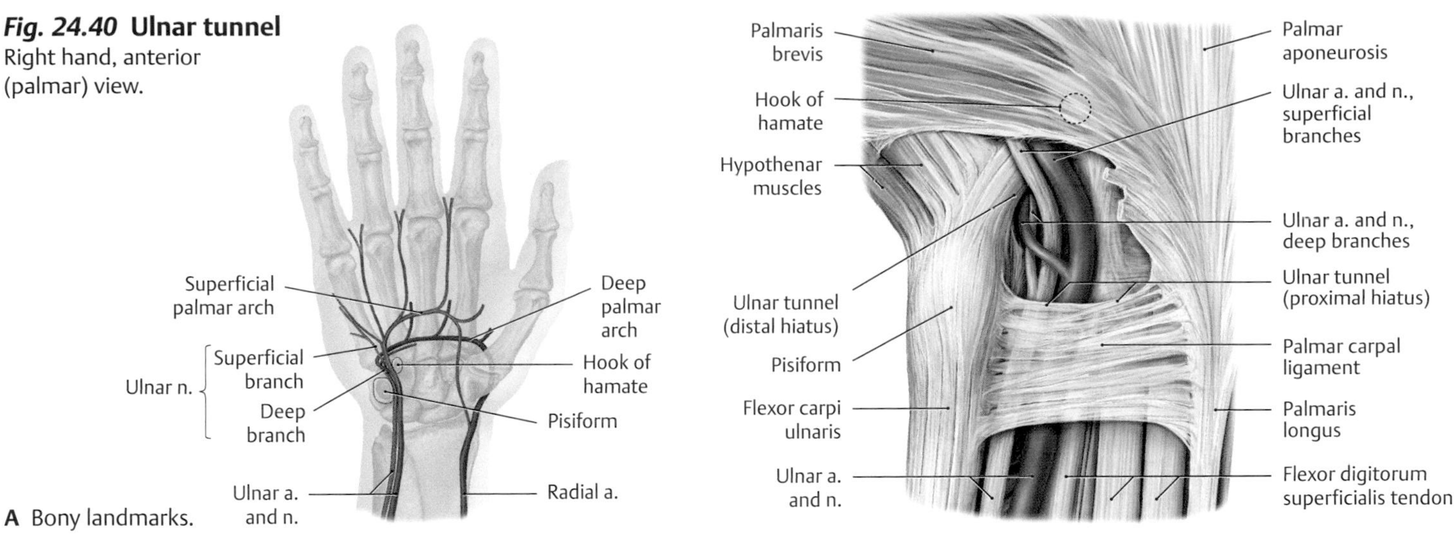
Superficial palmar arch
Deep palmar arch
Ulnar n.
Superficial branch
Deep branch
Hook of hamate
Pisiform
Ulnar a. and n.
Radial a.
Palmaris brevis
Hook of hamate
Hypothenar muscles
Ulnar tunnel (distal hiatus)
Pisiform
Flexor carpi ulnaris
Ulnar a. and n.
Palmar aponeurosis
Ulnar a. and n., superficial branches
Ulnar a. and n., deep branches
Ulnar tunnel (proximal hiatus)
Palmar carpal ligament
Palmaris longus
Flexor digitorum superficialis tendons

A Bony landmarks.

B Apertures and walls of the ulnar tunnel.

Fig. 24.41 **Carpal tunnel: Cross section**
Right hand, proximal view. The tight fit of sensitive neurovascular structures with closely apposed, frequently moving tendons in the carpal tunnel often causes problems (carpal tunnel syndrome) when any of the structures swell or degenerate.

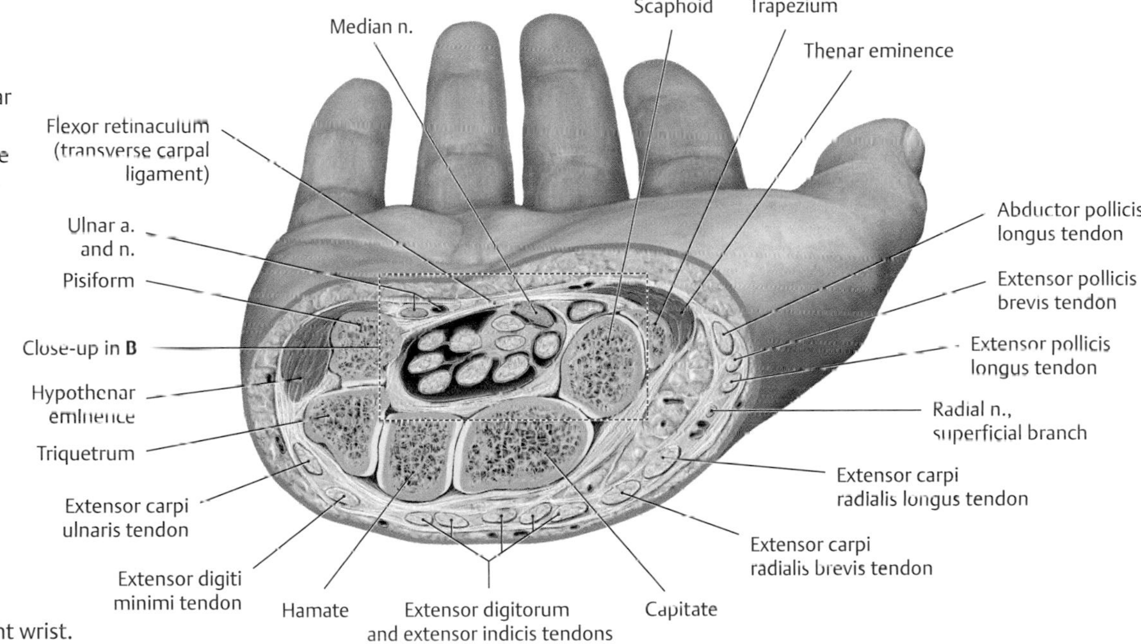
Median n.
Scaphoid
Trapezium
Thenar eminence
Flexor retinaculum (transverse carpal ligament)
Ulnar a. and n.
Pisiform
Close-up in B
Hypothenar eminence
Triquetrum
Extensor carpi ulnaris tendon
Extensor digiti minimi tendon
Hamate
Extensor digitorum and extensor indicis tendons
Capitate
Abductor pollicis longus tendon
Extensor pollicis brevis tendon
Extensor pollicis longus tendon
Radial n., superficial branch
Extensor carpi radialis longus tendon
Extensor carpi radialis brevis tendon

A Cross section through the right wrist.

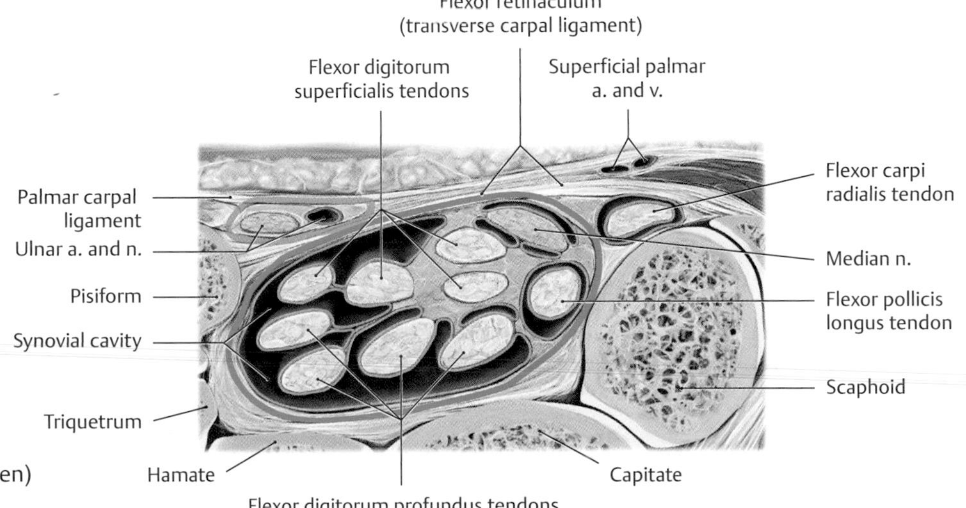
Flexor retinaculum (transverse carpal ligament)
Flexor digitorum superficialis tendons
Superficial palmar a. and v.
Palmar carpal ligament
Ulnar a. and n.
Pisiform
Synovial cavity
Triquetrum
Hamate
Flexor digitorum profundus tendons
Capitate
Flexor carpi radialis tendon
Median n.
Flexor pollicis longus tendon
Scaphoid

B Structures in the ulnar tunnel (green) and carpal tunnel (blue).

Topography of the Palm of the Hand

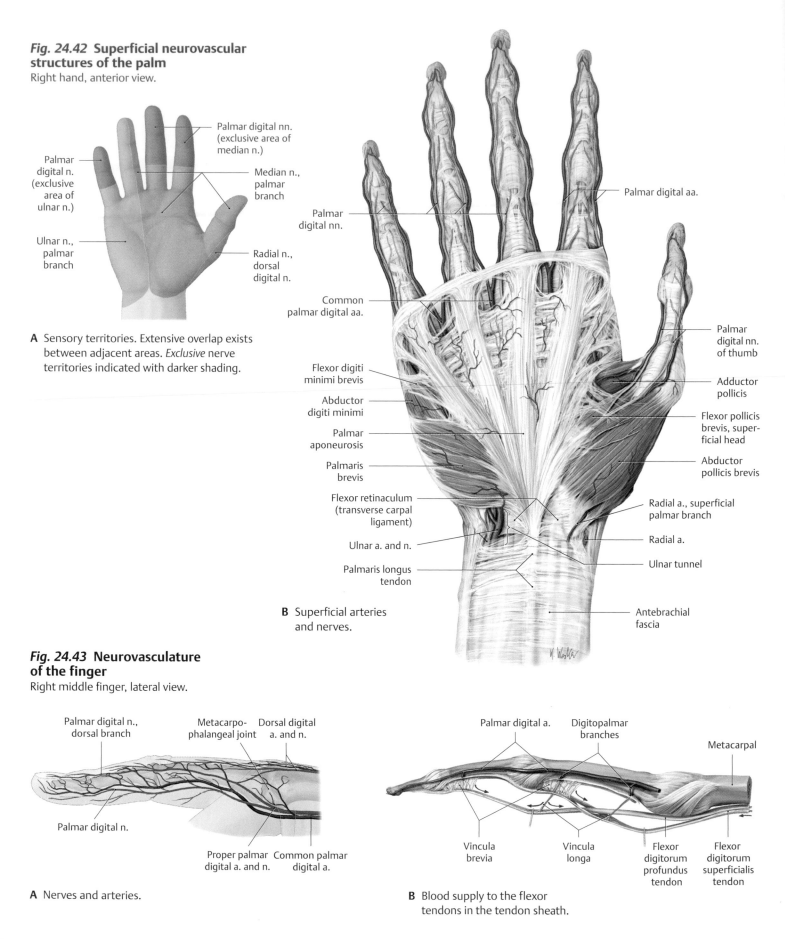

Fig. 24.42 Superficial neurovascular structures of the palm

Right hand, anterior view.

Palmar digital nn. (exclusive area of median n.)
Palmar digital n. (exclusive area of ulnar n.)
Median n., palmar branch
Ulnar n., palmar branch
Radial n., dorsal digital n.

A Sensory territories. Extensive overlap exists between adjacent areas. *Exclusive* nerve territories indicated with darker shading.

Palmar digital aa.
Palmar digital nn.
Common palmar digital aa.
Palmar digital nn. of thumb
Flexor digiti minimi brevis
Adductor pollicis
Abductor digiti minimi
Flexor pollicis brevis, superficial head
Palmar aponeurosis
Abductor pollicis brevis
Palmaris brevis
Flexor retinaculum (transverse carpal ligament)
Radial a., superficial palmar branch
Radial a.
Ulnar a. and n.
Ulnar tunnel
Palmaris longus tendon
Antebrachial fascia

B Superficial arteries and nerves.

Fig. 24.43 Neurovasculature of the finger

Right middle finger, lateral view.

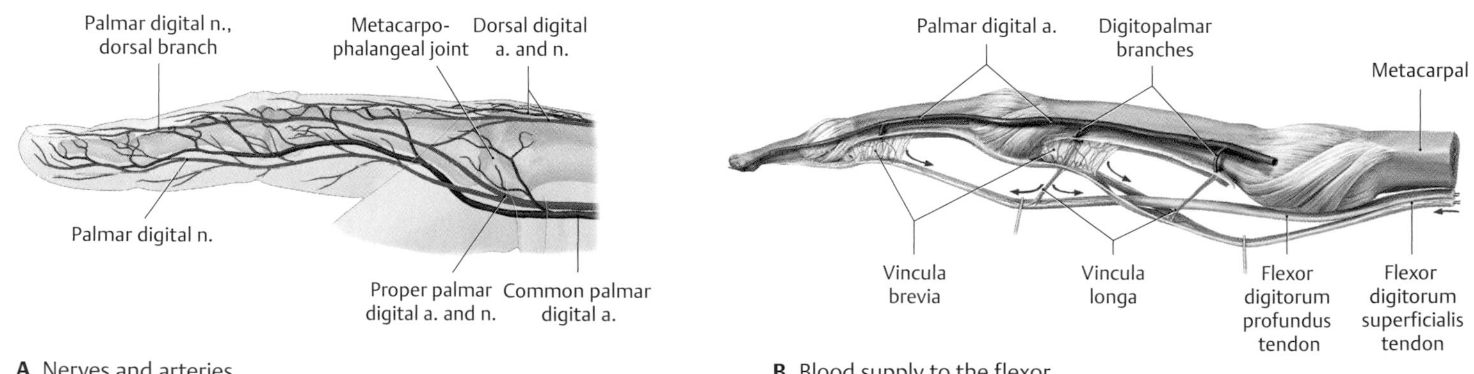
Palmar digital n., dorsal branch
Metacarpo-phalangeal joint
Dorsal digital a. and n.
Palmar digital n.
Proper palmar digital a. and n.
Common palmar digital a.
Palmar digital a.
Digitopalmar branches
Metacarpal
Vincula brevia
Vincula longa
Flexor digitorum profundus tendon
Flexor digitorum superficialis tendon

A Nerves and arteries.

B Blood supply to the flexor tendons in the tendon sheath.

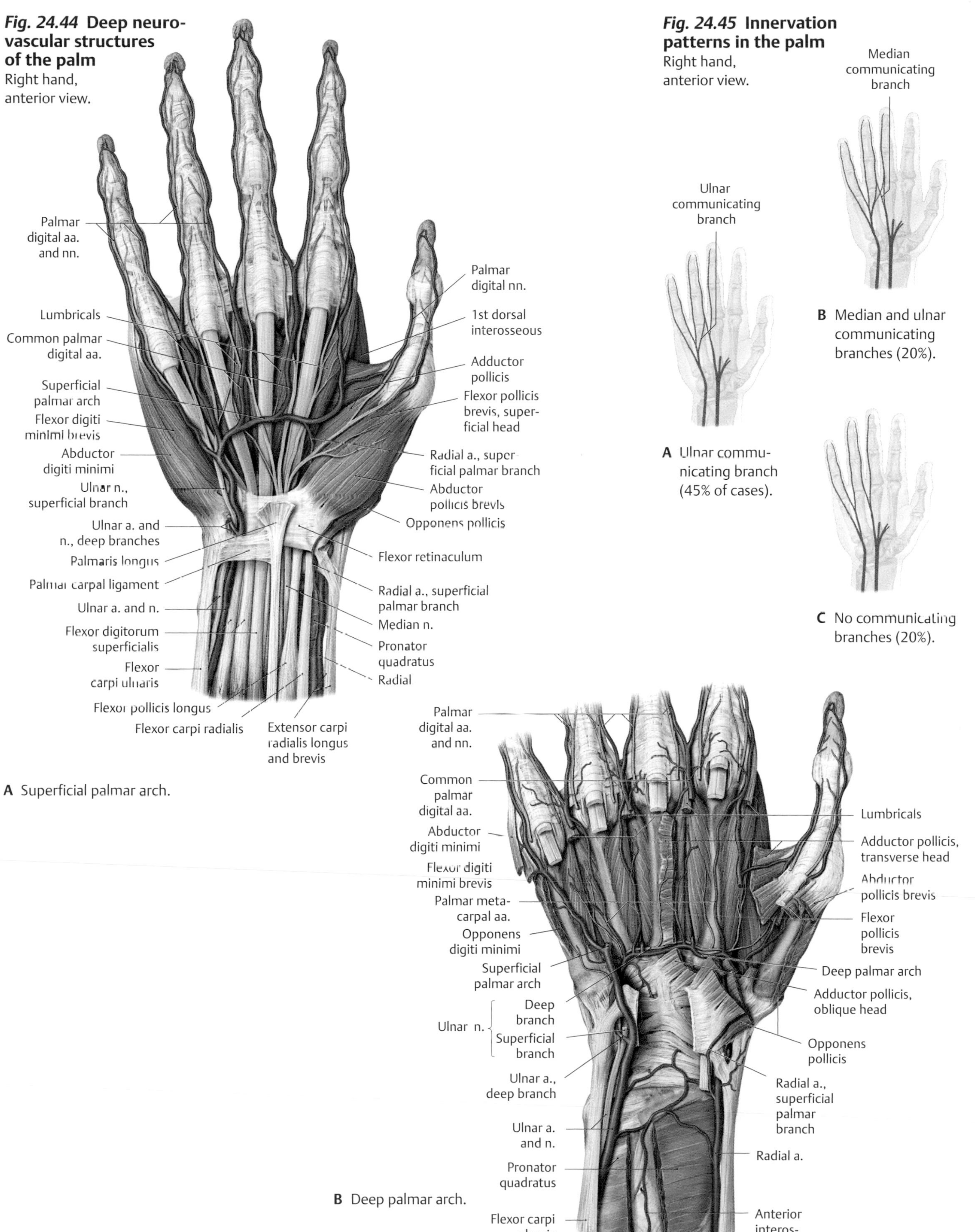

Palmar digital aa. and nn.
Lumbricals
Common palmar digital aa.
Superficial palmar arch
Flexor digiti minimi brevis
Abductor digiti minimi
Ulnar n., superficial branch
Ulnar a. and n., deep branches
Palmaris longus
Palmar carpal ligament
Ulnar a. and n.
Flexor digitorum superficialis
Flexor carpi ulnaris
Flexor pollicis longus
Flexor carpi radialis
Extensor carpi radialis longus and brevis
Palmar digital nn.
1st dorsal interosseous
Adductor pollicis
Flexor pollicis brevis, superficial head
Radial a., superficial palmar branch
Abductor pollicis brevis
Opponens pollicis
Flexor retinaculum
Radial a., superficial palmar branch
Median n.
Pronator quadratus
Radial
Median communicating branch
Ulnar communicating branch
Palmar digital aa. and nn.
Common palmar digital aa.
Abductor digiti minimi
Flexor digiti minimi brevis
Palmar metacarpal aa.
Opponens digiti minimi
Superficial palmar arch
Ulnar n.
Deep branch
Superficial branch
Ulnar a., deep branch
Ulnar a. and n.
Pronator quadratus
Flexor carpi ulnaris
Lumbricals
Adductor pollicis, transverse head
Abductor pollicis brevis
Flexor pollicis brevis
Deep palmar arch
Adductor pollicis, oblique head
Opponens pollicis
Radial a., superficial palmar branch
Radial a.
Anterior interosseous a.

Fig. 24.44 **Deep neurovascular structures of the palm**
Right hand, anterior view.

A Superficial palmar arch.

B Deep palmar arch.

Fig. 24.45 **Innervation patterns in the palm**
Right hand, anterior view.

A Ulnar communicating branch (45% of cases).

B Median and ulnar communicating branches (20%).

C No communicating branches (20%).

Topography of the Dorsum of the Hand

Fig. 24.46 Cutaneous innervation of the dorsum
Right hand, posterior view.

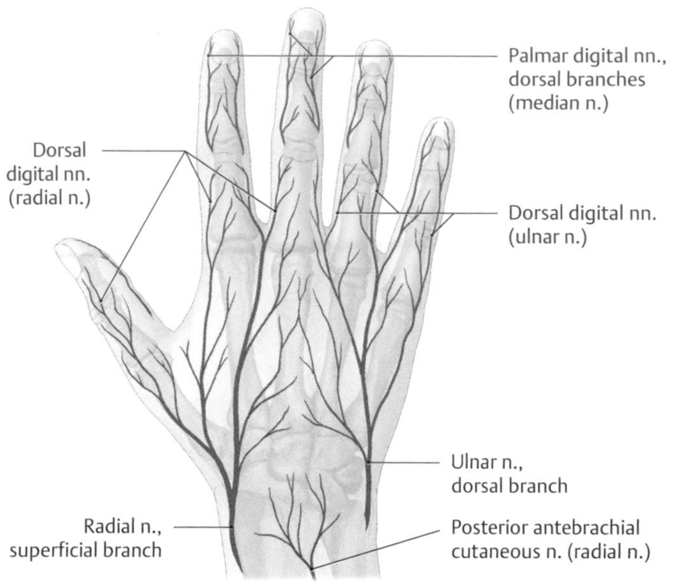
Palmar digital nn., dorsal branches (median n.)
Dorsal digital nn. (radial n.)
Dorsal digital nn. (ulnar n.)
Ulnar n., dorsal branch
Radial n., superficial branch
Posterior antebrachial cutaneous n. (radial n.)

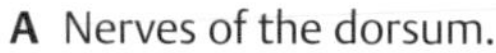

A Nerves of the dorsum.

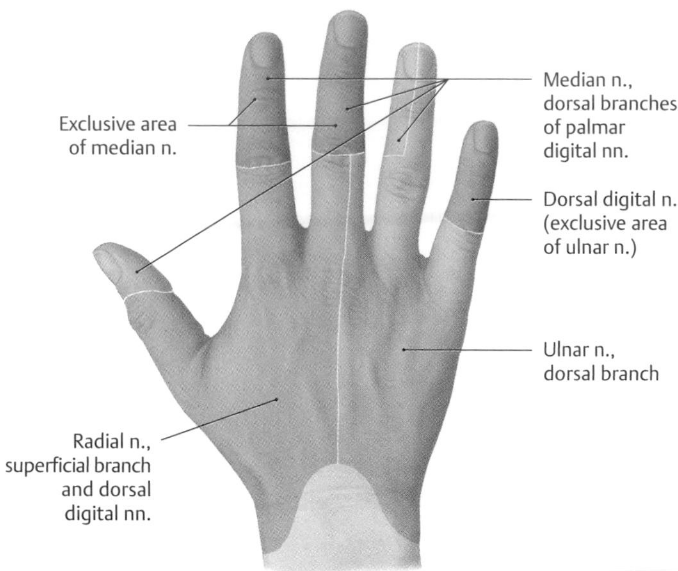
Exclusive area of median n.
Median n., dorsal branches of palmar digital nn.
Dorsal digital n. (exclusive area of ulnar n.)
Ulnar n., dorsal branch
Radial n., superficial branch and dorsal digital nn.

B Sensory territories. Extensive overlap exists between adjacent areas. *Exclusive* nerve territories indicated with darker shading.

Fig. 24.47 Anatomic snuffbox
Right hand, radial view. The three-sided "anatomic snuffbox" is bounded by the tendons of insertion of the abductor pollicis longus and extensors pollicis brevis and longus.

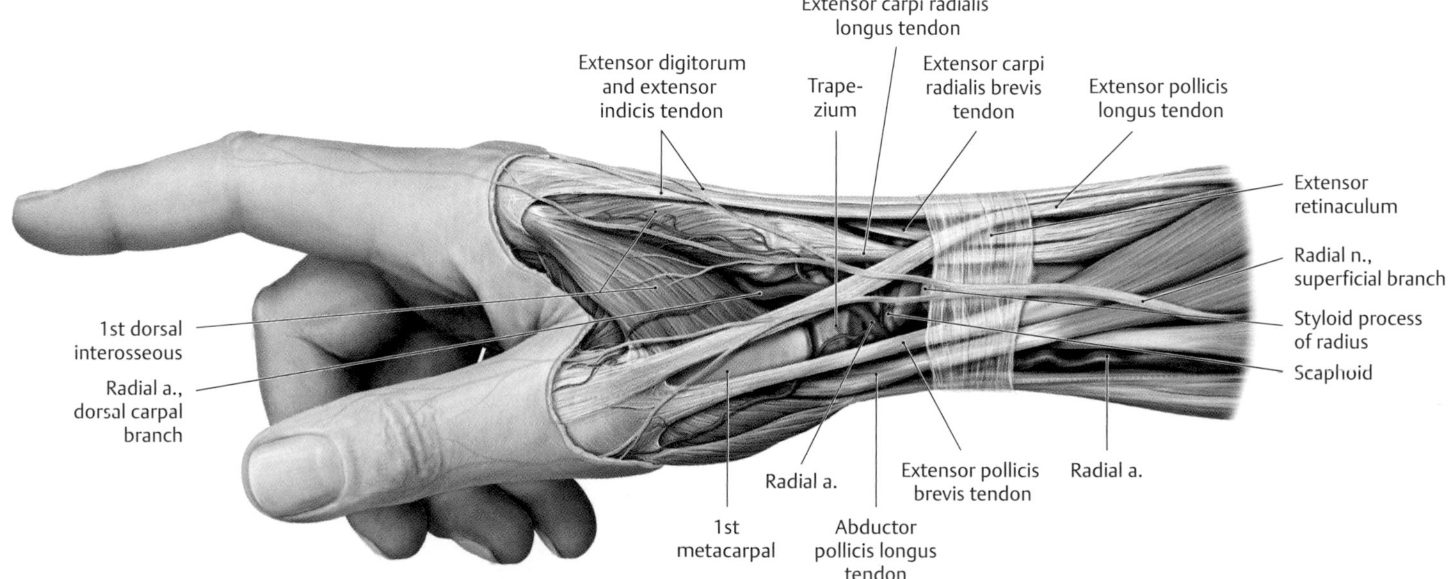
Extensor carpi radialis longus tendon
Extensor digitorum and extensor indicis tendon
Trape-zium
Extensor carpi radialis brevis tendon
Extensor pollicis longus tendon
Extensor retinaculum
Radial n., superficial branch
Styloid process of radius
Scaphoid
1st dorsal interosseous
Radial a., dorsal carpal branch
Radial a.
Extensor pollicis brevis tendon
Radial a.
1st metacarpal
Abductor pollicis longus tendon

Fig. 24.48 **Neurovascular structures of the dorsum**

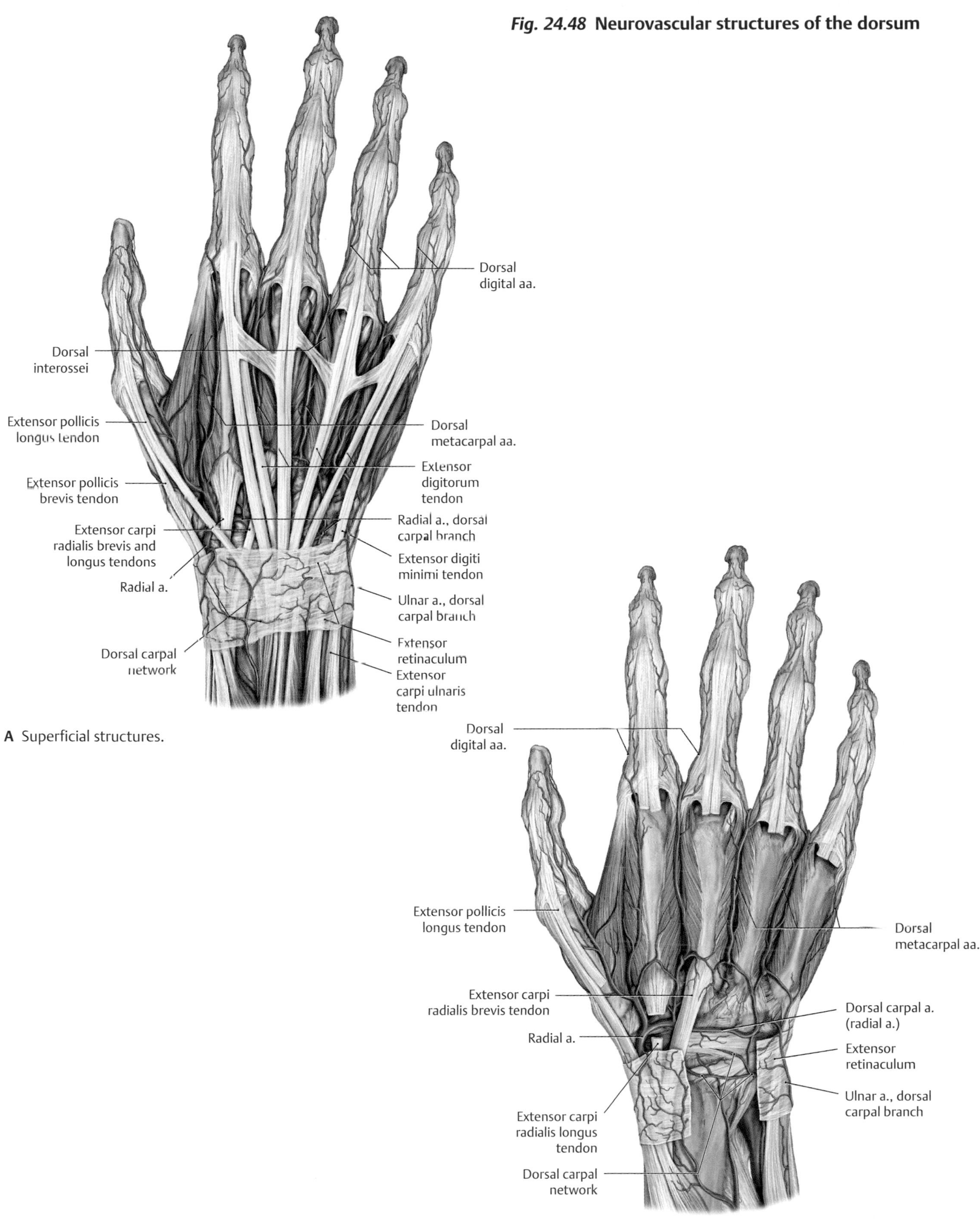
Dorsal digital aa.
Dorsal interossei
Extensor pollicis longus tendon
Dorsal metacarpal aa.
Extensor digitorum tendon
Extensor pollicis brevis tendon
Extensor carpi radialis brevis and longus tendons
Radial a., dorsal carpal branch
Extensor digiti minimi tendon
Radial a.
Ulnar a., dorsal carpal branch
Dorsal carpal network
Extensor retinaculum
Extensor carpi ulnaris tendon
Dorsal digital aa.
Extensor pollicis longus tendon
Dorsal metacarpal aa.
Extensor carpi radialis brevis tendon
Dorsal carpal a. (radial a.)
Radial a.
Extensor retinaculum
Ulnar a., dorsal carpal branch
Extensor carpi radialis longus tendon
Dorsal carpal network

A Superficial structures.

B Deep structures.

Sectional Anatomy of the Upper Limb

Fig. 24.49 **Upper limb: Windowed dissection**
Right limb, anterior view.

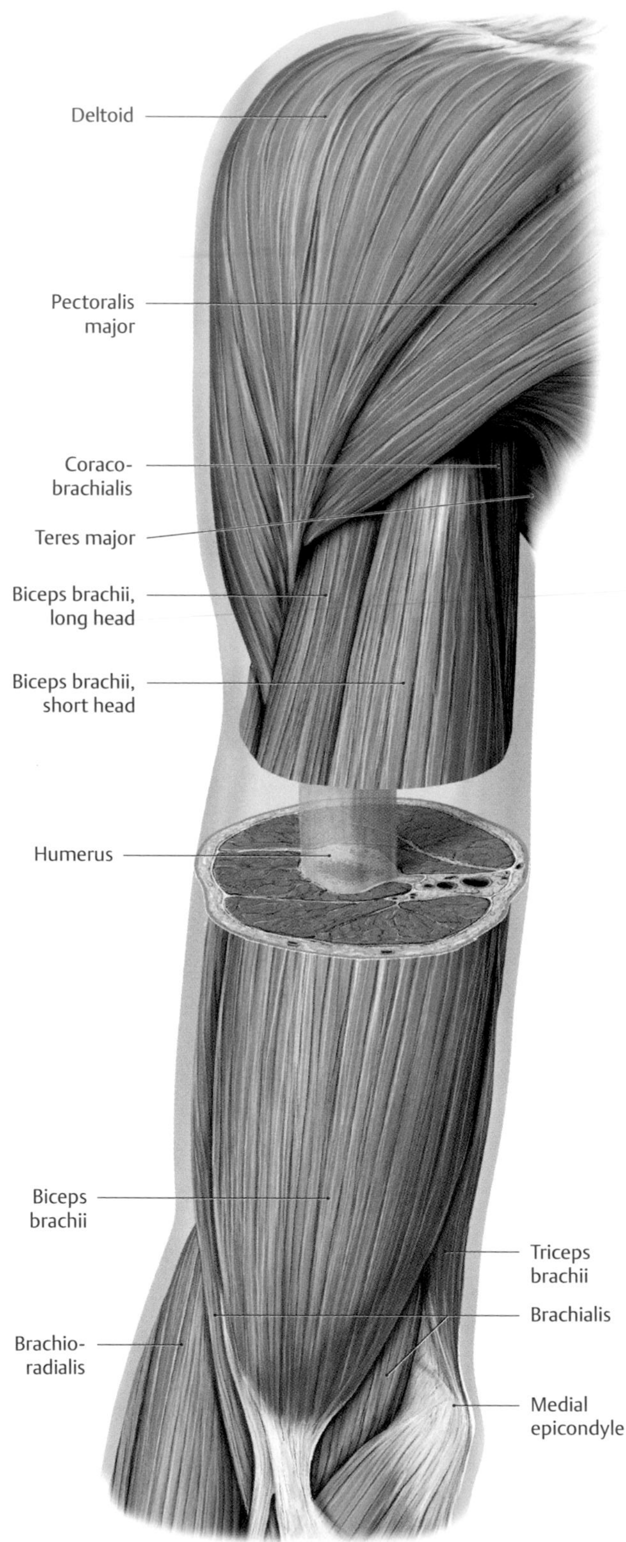
Deltoid
Pectoralis major
Coraco-brachialis
Teres major
Biceps brachii, long head
Biceps brachii, short head
Humerus
Biceps brachii
Brachio-radialis
Triceps brachii
Brachialis
Medial epicondyle

A Dissection of the arm.

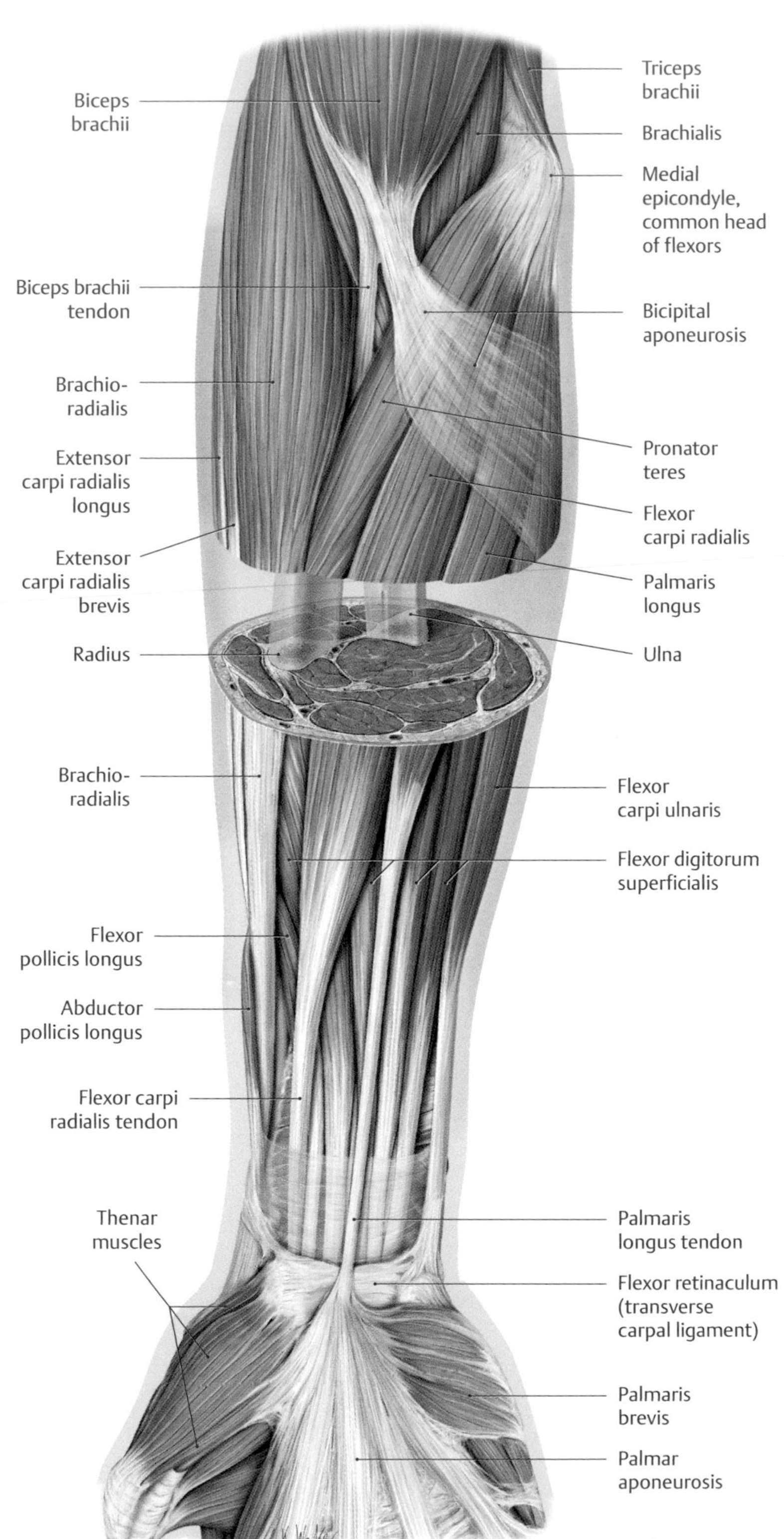
Biceps brachii
Biceps brachii tendon
Brachio-radialis
Extensor carpi radialis longus
Extensor carpi radialis brevis
Radius
Brachio-radialis
Flexor pollicis longus
Abductor pollicis longus
Flexor carpi radialis tendon
Thenar muscles
Triceps brachii
Brachialis
Medial epicondyle, common head of flexors
Bicipital aponeurosis
Pronator teres
Flexor carpi radialis
Palmaris longus
Ulna
Flexor carpi ulnaris
Flexor digitorum superficialis
Palmaris longus tendon
Flexor retinaculum (transverse carpal ligament)
Palmaris brevis
Palmar aponeurosis

B Dissection of the forearm.

***Fig. 24.50* Upper limb: Transverse sections**
Right limb, proximal (superior) view.

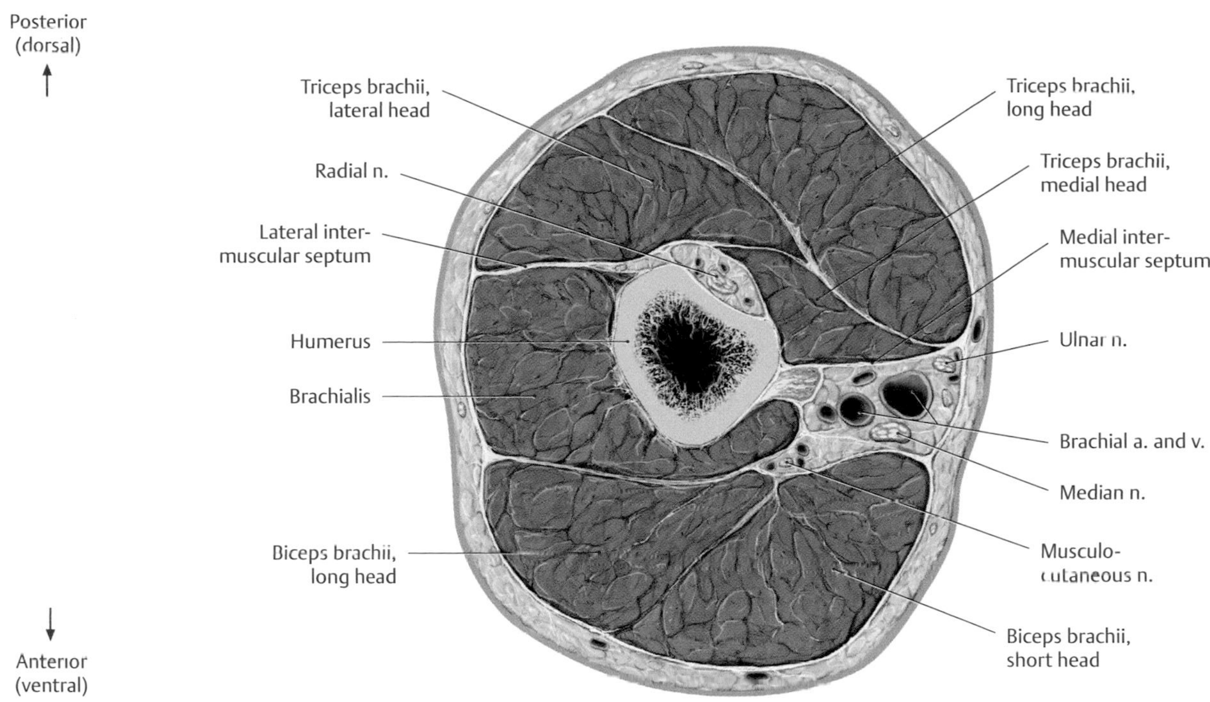
Posterior (dorsal)
Triceps brachii, lateral head
Radial n.
Lateral inter-muscular septum
Humerus
Brachialis
Biceps brachii, long head
Anterior (ventral)
Triceps brachii, long head
Triceps brachii, medial head
Medial inter-muscular septum
Ulnar n.
Brachial a. and v.
Median n.
Musculo-cutaneous n.
Biceps brachii, short head

A Arm (plane of section in Fig. 24.49A).

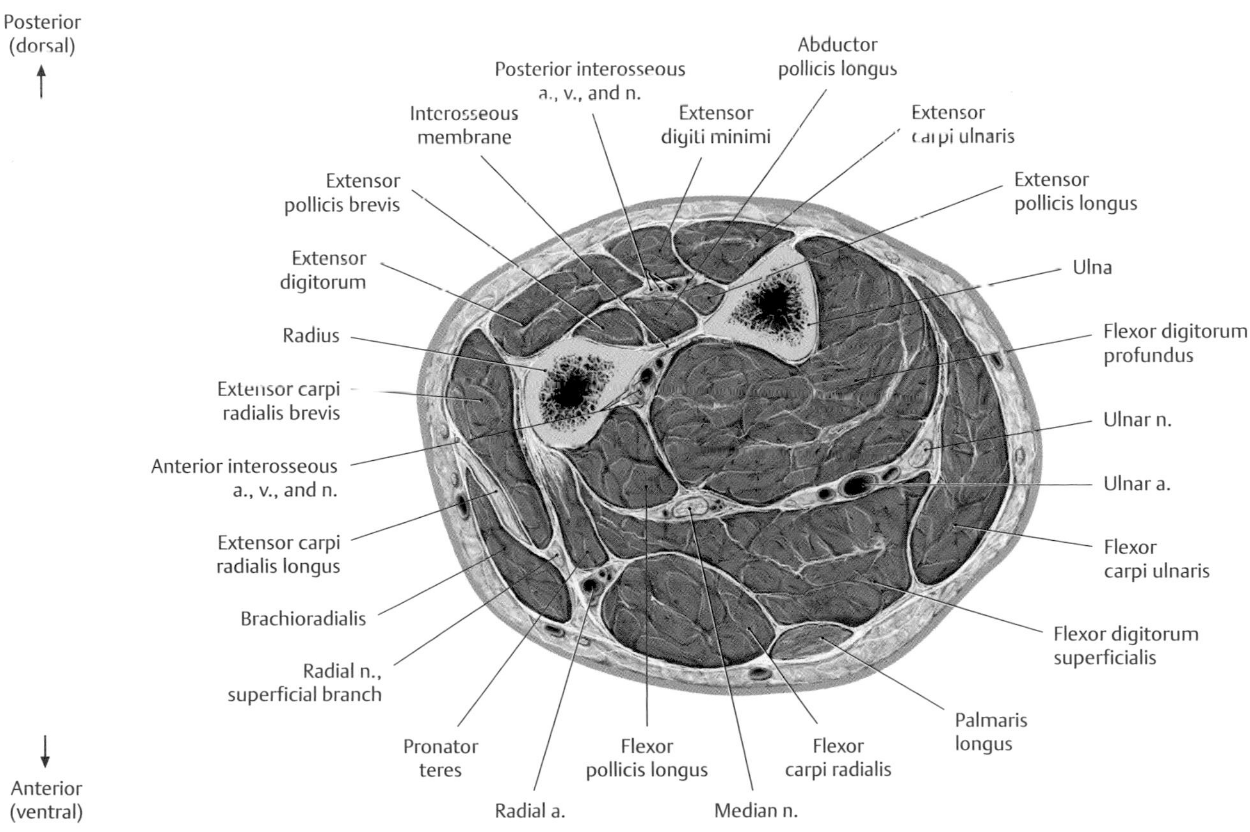
Posterior (dorsal)
Posterior interosseous a., v., and n.
Abductor pollicis longus
Interosseous membrane
Extensor digiti minimi
Extensor carpi ulnaris
Extensor pollicis brevis
Extensor pollicis longus
Extensor digitorum
Ulna
Radius
Flexor digitorum profundus
Extensor carpi radialis brevis
Ulnar n.
Anterior interosseous a., v., and n.
Ulnar a.
Extensor carpi radialis longus
Flexor carpi ulnaris
Brachioradialis
Flexor digitorum superficialis
Radial n., superficial branch
Palmaris longus
Pronator teres
Flexor pollicis longus
Flexor carpi radialis
Anterior (ventral)
Radial a.
Median n.

B Forearm (plane of section in Fig. 24.49B).

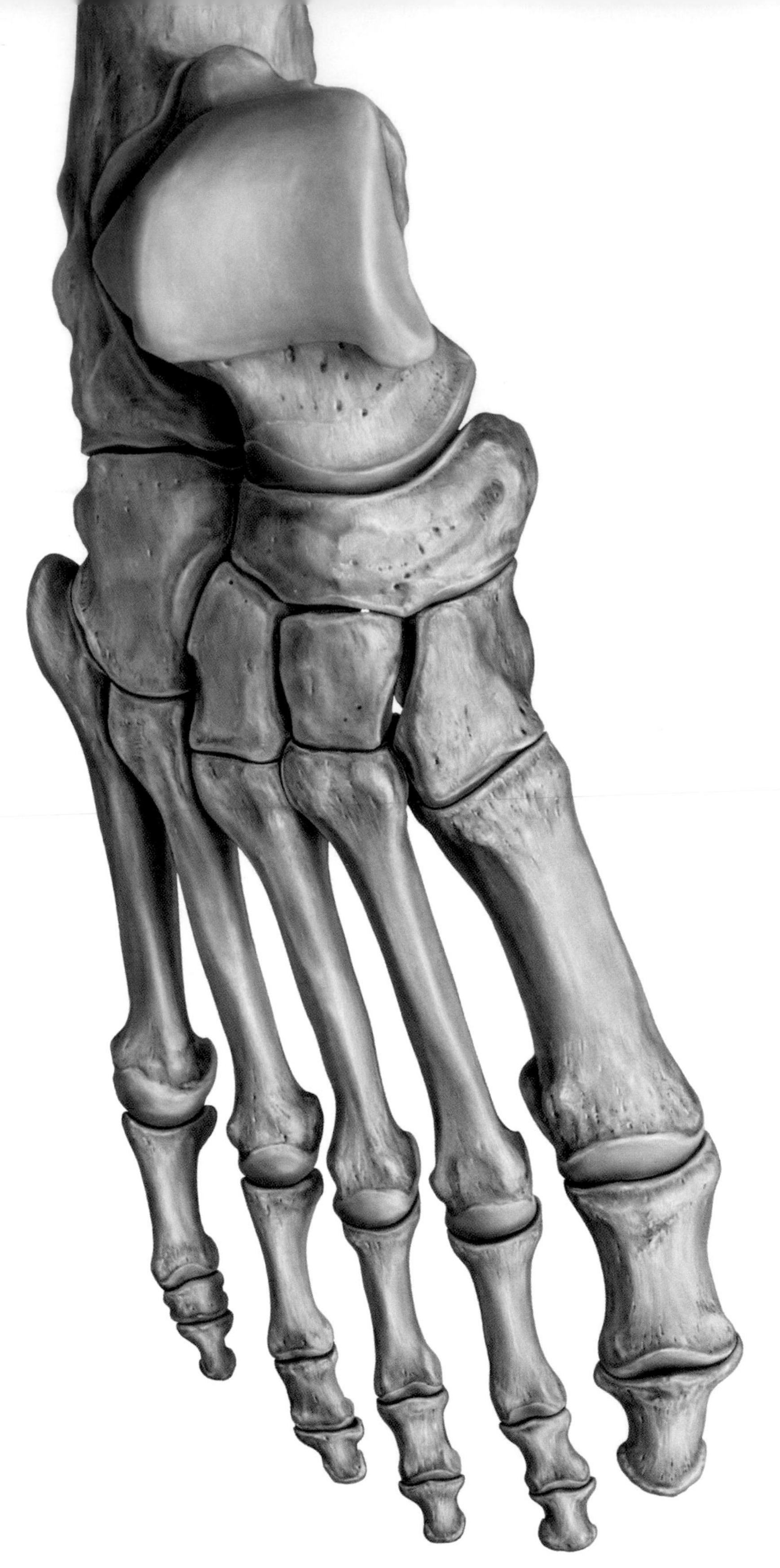

Lower Limb

25 Surface Anatomy

Surface Anatomy 380

26 Hip & Thigh

Bones of the Lower Limb 382
Femur 384
Hip Joint: Overview 386
Hip Joint: Ligaments & Capsule 388
Anterior Muscles of the Hip, Thigh & Gluteal Region (I) . . . 390
Anterior Muscles of the Hip, Thigh & Gluteal Region (II) . . 392
Posterior Muscles of the Hip, Thigh & Gluteal Region (I) . . 394
Posterior Muscles of the Hip, Thigh & Gluteal Region (II) . . 396
Muscle Facts (I) 398
Muscle Facts (II) 400
Muscle Facts (III) 402

27 Knee & Leg

Tibia & Fibula 404
Knee Joint: Overview 406
Knee Joint: Capsule, Ligaments & Bursae 408
Knee Joint: Ligaments & Menisci 410
Cruciate Ligaments 412
Knee Joint Cavity 414
Muscles of the Leg: Anterior & Lateral Compartments 416
Muscles of the Leg: Posterior Compartment 418
Muscle Facts (I) 420
Muscle Facts (II) 422

28 Ankle & Foot

Bones of the Foot 424
Joints of the Foot (I) 426
Joints of the Foot (II) 428
Joints of the Foot (III) 430
Ligaments of the Ankle & Foot 432
Plantar Vault & Arches of the Foot 434
Muscles of the Sole of the Foot 436
Muscles & Tendon Sheaths of the Foot 438
Muscle Facts (I) 440
Muscle Facts (II) 442

29 Neurovasculature

Arteries of the Lower Limb 444
Veins & Lymphatics of the Lower Limb 446
Lumbosacral Plexus 448
Nerves of the Lumbar Plexus 450
Nerves of the Lumbar Plexus: Obturator & Femoral Nerves . 452
Nerves of the Sacral Plexus 454
Nerves of the Sacral Plexus: Sciatic Nerve 456
Superficial Nerves & Vessels of the Lower Limb 458
Topography of the Inguinal Region 460
Topography of the Gluteal Region 462
Topography of the Anterior, Medial & Posterior Thigh 464
Topography of the Posterior Compartment of the Leg & Foot 466
Topography of the Lateral & Anterior Compartments of the Leg 468
Topography of the Sole of the Foot 470
Sectional Anatomy of the Thigh & Leg 472

Surface Anatomy

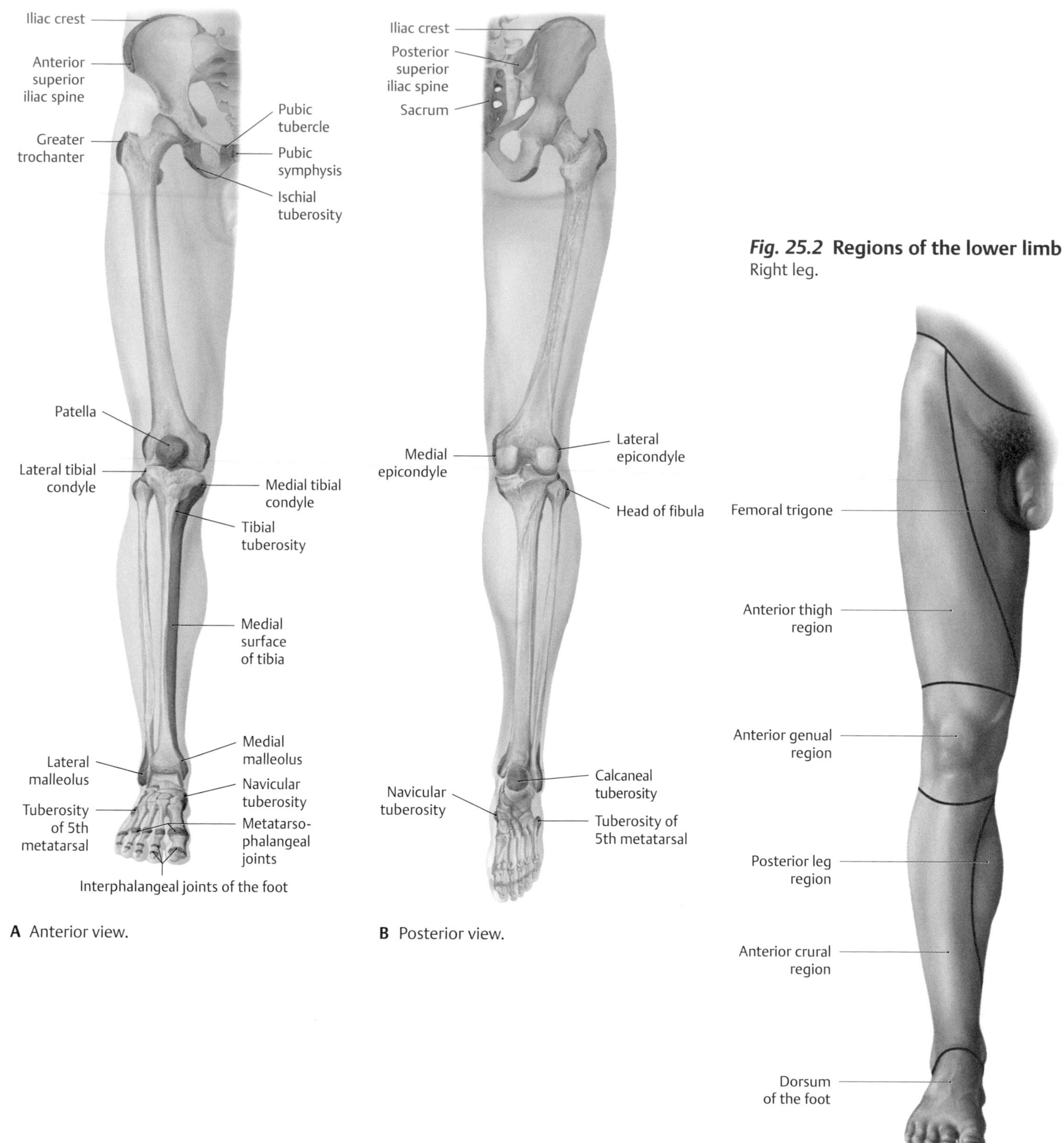
Iliac crest
Anterior superior iliac spine
Greater trochanter
Pubic tubercle
Pubic symphysis
Ischial tuberosity
Patella
Lateral tibial condyle
Medial tibial condyle
Tibial tuberosity
Medial surface of tibia
Lateral malleolus
Medial malleolus
Navicular tuberosity
Tuberosity of 5th metatarsal
Metatarso-phalangeal joints
Interphalangeal joints of the foot
Iliac crest
Posterior superior iliac spine
Sacrum
Medial epicondyle
Lateral epicondyle
Head of fibula
Navicular tuberosity
Calcaneal tuberosity
Tuberosity of 5th metatarsal
Femoral trigone
Anterior thigh region
Anterior genual region
Posterior leg region
Anterior crural region
Dorsum of the foot

Fig. 25.1 **Palpable bony prominences of the lower limb**
Right limb.

A Anterior view.

B Posterior view.

Fig. 25.2 **Regions of the lower limb**
Right leg.

A Anterior view.

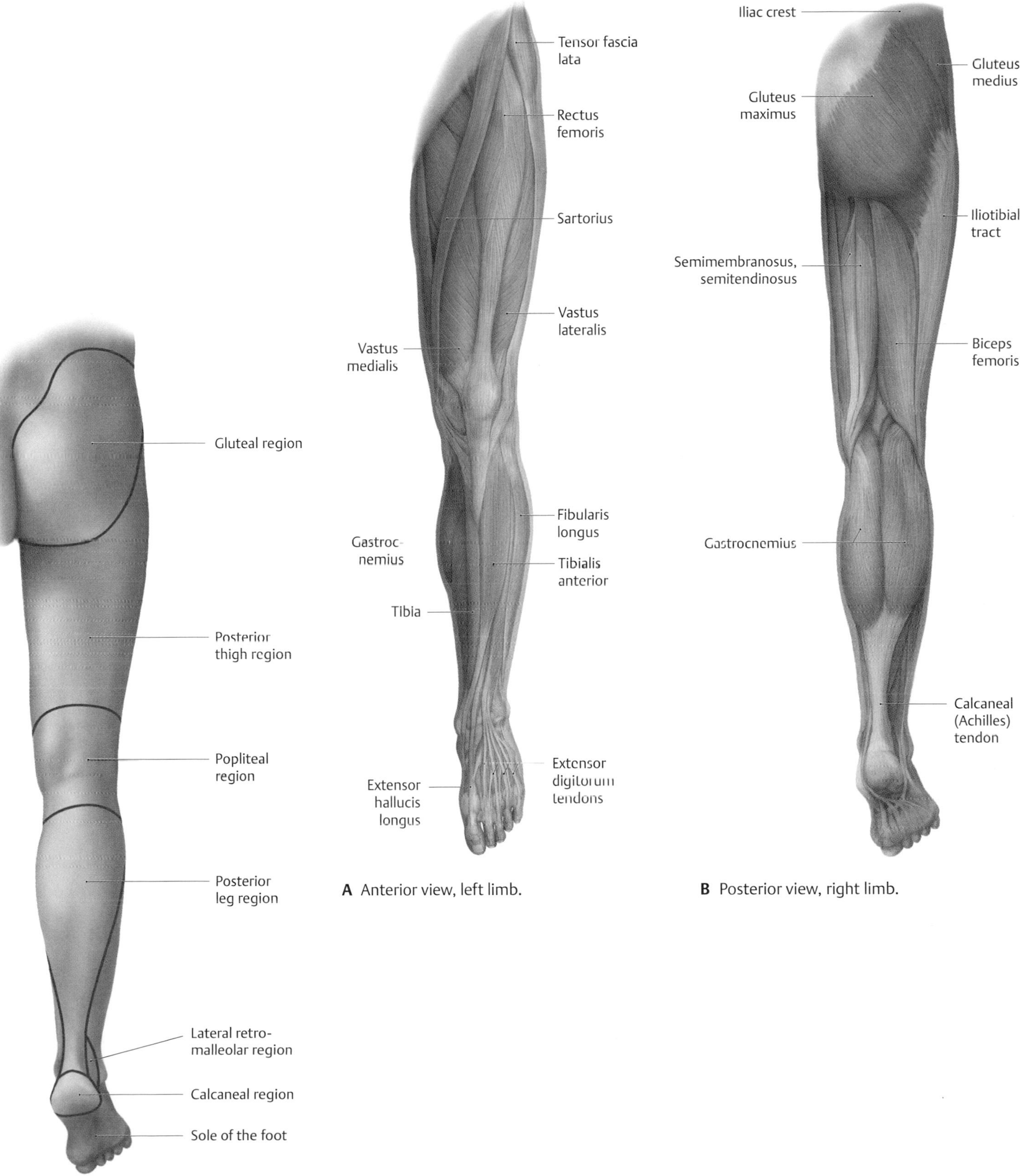
Gluteal region
Posterior thigh region
Popliteal region
Posterior leg region
Lateral retro-malleolar region
Calcaneal region
Sole of the foot

B Posterior view.

Fig. 25.3 **Palpable musculature of the lower limb**

Tensor fascia lata
Rectus femoris
Sartorius
Vastus lateralis
Vastus medialis
Fibularis longus
Gastrocnemius
Tibialis anterior
Tibia
Extensor digitorum tendons
Extensor hallucis longus
Iliac crest
Gluteus medius
Gluteus maximus
Iliotibial tract
Semimembranosus, semitendinosus
Biceps femoris
Gastrocnemius
Calcaneal (Achilles) tendon

A Anterior view, left limb.

B Posterior view, right limb.

Bones of the Lower Limb

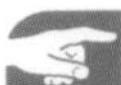

The skeleton of the lower limb consists of a hip bone and a free limb. The paired hip bones attach to the trunk at the sacroiliac joint to form the pelvic girdle (see p. 216), and the free limb, divided into a thigh, leg, and foot, attaches to the pelvic girdle at the hip joint. Stability of the pelvic girdle is important in the distribution of weight from the upper body to the lower limbs.

Fig. 26.1 Bones of the lower limb

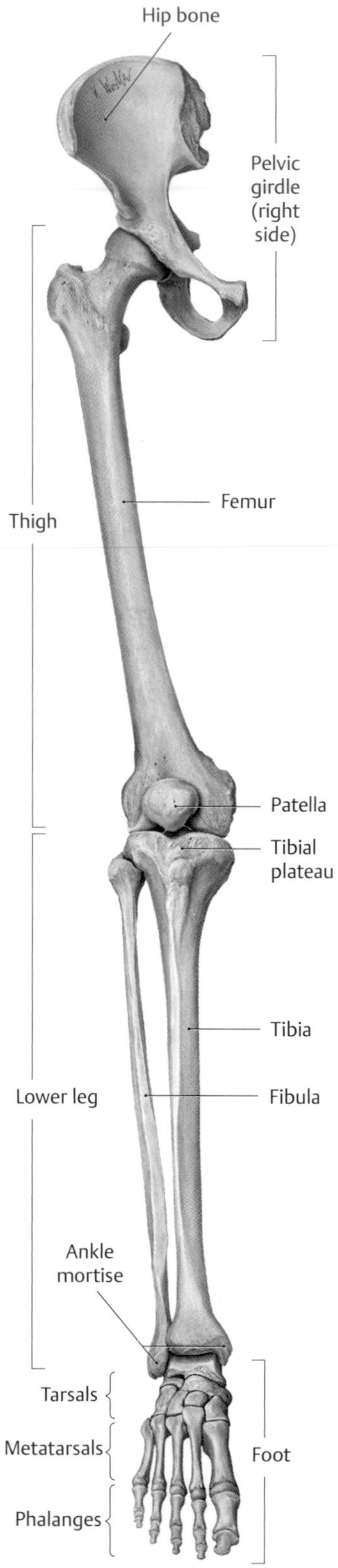

Hip bone
Pelvic girdle (right side)
Thigh
Femur
Patella
Tibial plateau
Tibia
Lower leg
Fibula
Ankle mortise
Tarsals
Metatarsals
Phalanges
Foot

A Anterior view.

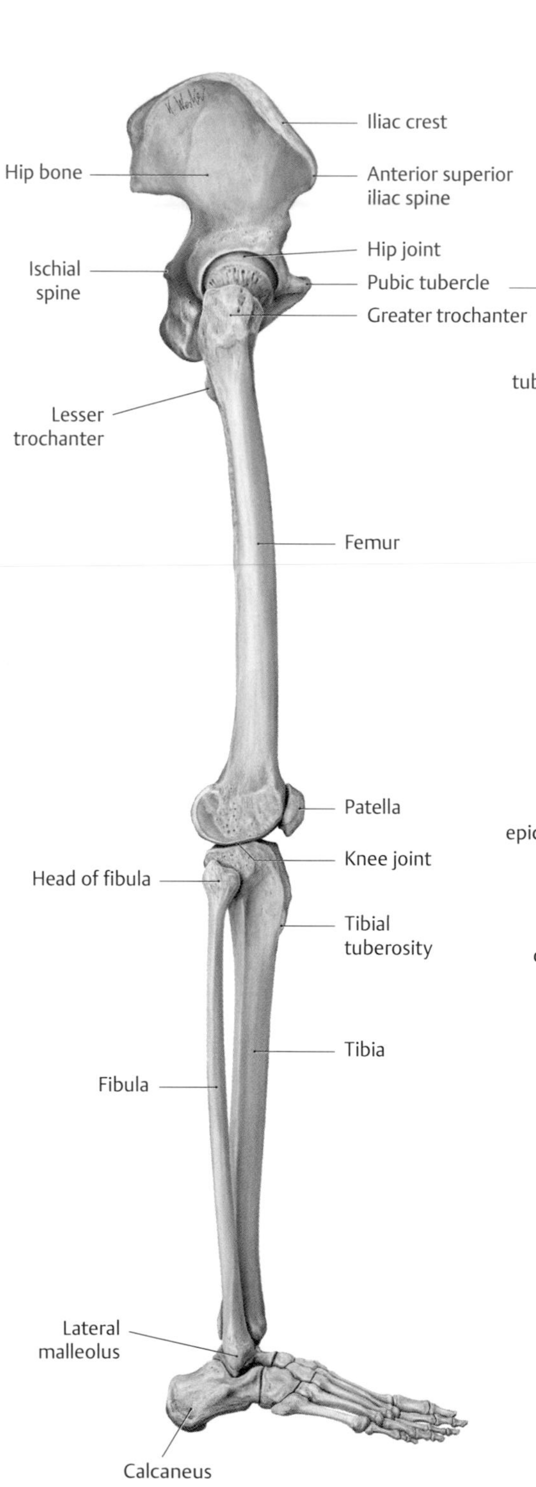

Iliac crest
Hip bone
Anterior superior iliac spine
Ischial spine
Hip joint
Pubic tubercle
Greater trochanter
Lesser trochanter
Femur
Patella
Knee joint
Head of fibula
Tibial tuberosity
Tibia
Fibula
Lateral malleolus
Calcaneus

B Right lateral view.

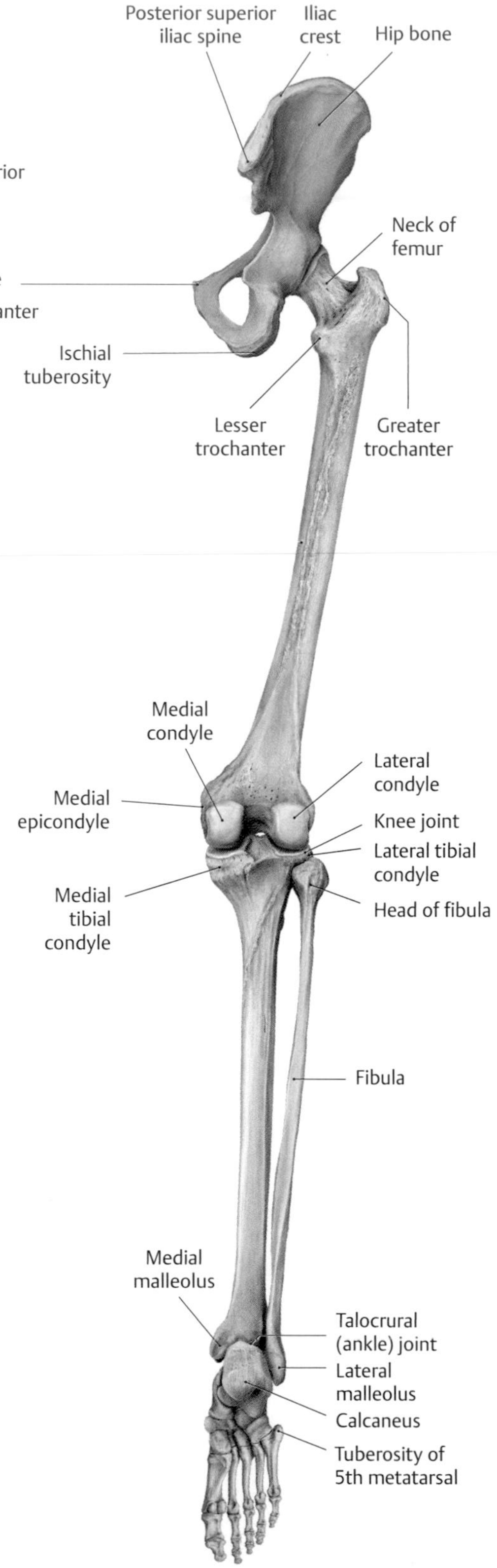

Posterior superior iliac spine
Iliac crest
Hip bone
Neck of femur
Ischial tuberosity
Lesser trochanter
Greater trochanter
Medial condyle
Lateral condyle
Medial epicondyle
Knee joint
Lateral tibial condyle
Medial tibial condyle
Head of fibula
Fibula
Medial malleolus
Talocrural (ankle) joint
Lateral malleolus
Calcaneus
Tuberosity of 5th metatarsal

C Posterior view.

Fig. 26.2 **Line of gravity**
Right lateral view. The line of gravity runs vertically from the whole-body center of gravity to the ground with characteristic points of intersection.

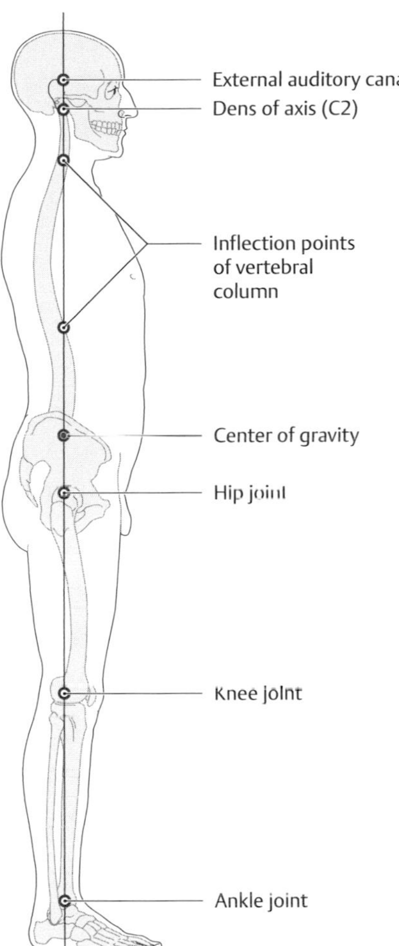
External auditory canal
Dens of axis (C2)
Inflection points of vertebral column
Center of gravity
Hip joint
Knee joint
Ankle joint

Fig. 26.3 **The hip bones and their relation to bones of the trunk.**
The paired hip bones and sacrum form the pelvic girdle (see p. 216).

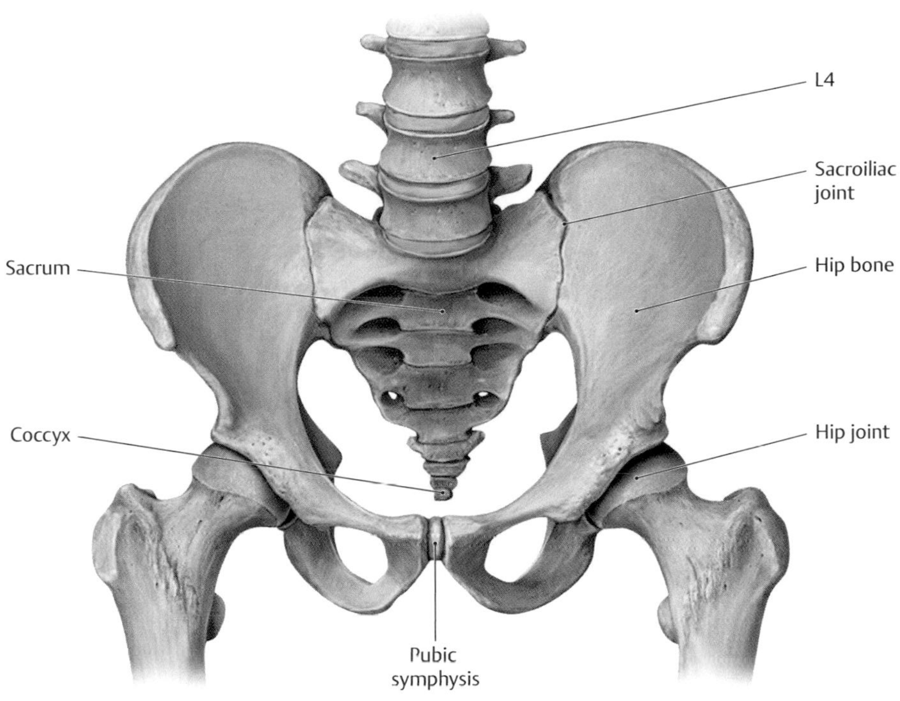
L4
Sacroiliac joint
Hip bone
Sacrum
Coccyx
Hip joint
Pubic symphysis

A Anterior view.

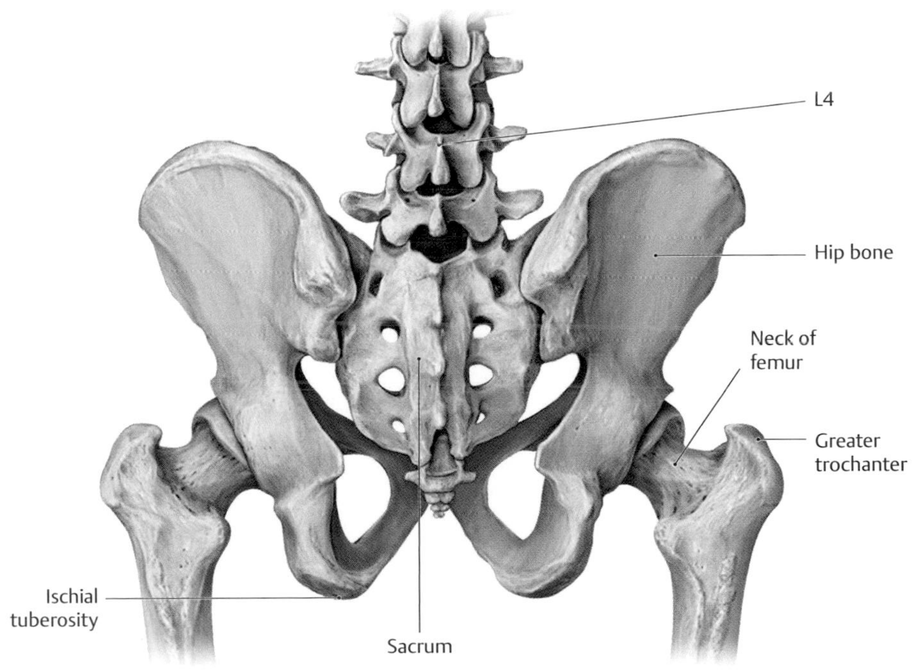
L4
Hip bone
Neck of femur
Greater trochanter
Ischial tuberosity
Sacrum

B Posterior view.

Femur

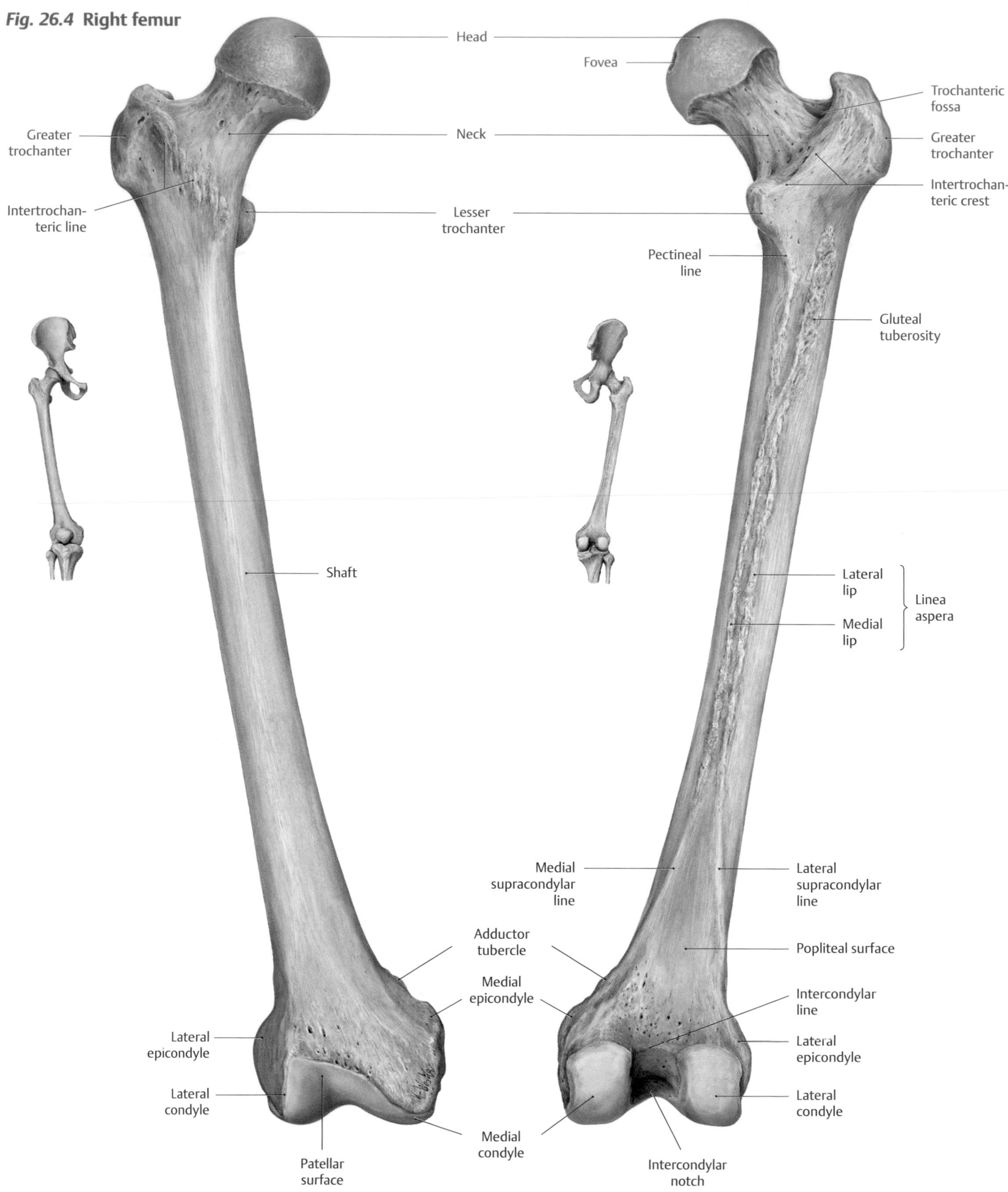

Head
Fovea
Trochanteric fossa
Greater trochanter
Neck
Greater trochanter
Intertrochanteric line
Intertrochanteric crest
Lesser trochanter
Pectineal line
Gluteal tuberosity
Shaft
Lateral lip
Medial lip
Linea aspera
Medial supracondylar line
Lateral supracondylar line
Adductor tubercle
Popliteal surface
Medial epicondyle
Intercondylar line
Lateral epicondyle
Lateral epicondyle
Lateral condyle
Lateral condyle
Medial condyle
Patellar surface
Intercondylar notch

Fig. 26.4 **Right femur**

A Anterior view.

B Posterior view.

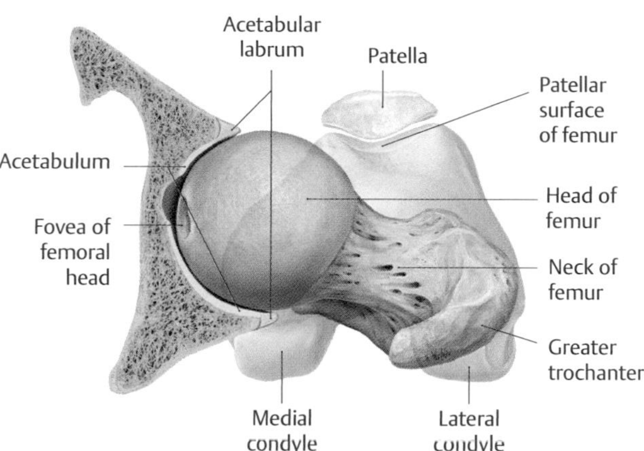
Acetabular
labrum
Patella
Patellar
surface
of femur
Acetabulum
Head of
femur
Fovea of
femoral
head
Neck of
femur
Greater
trochanter
Medial
condyle
Lateral
condyle

C Proximal view. The acetabulum has been sectioned in the horizontal plane.

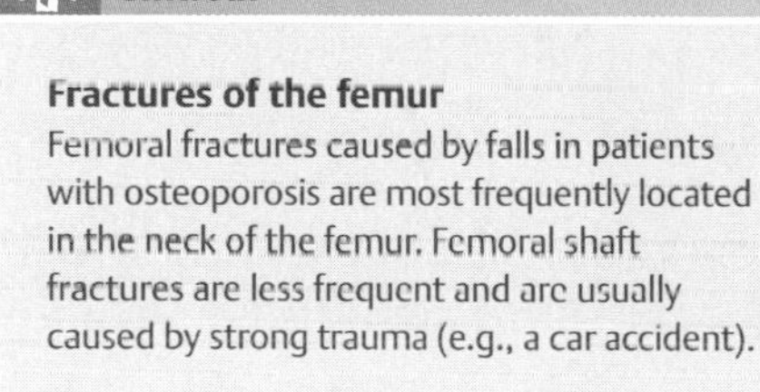

Clinical

Fractures of the femur

Femoral fractures caused by falls in patients with osteoporosis are most frequently located in the neck of the femur. Femoral shaft fractures are less frequent and are usually caused by strong trauma (e.g., a car accident).

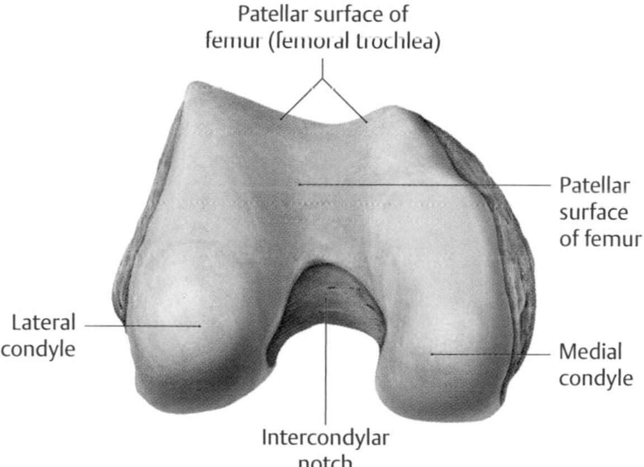
Patellar surface of
femur (femoral trochlea)
Patellar
surface
of femur
Lateral
condyle
Medial
condyle
Intercondylar
notch

D Distal view. See pp. 406–407 for the knee joint.

***Fig. 26.5* Head of femur in the hip joint**
Right hip joint, superior view.

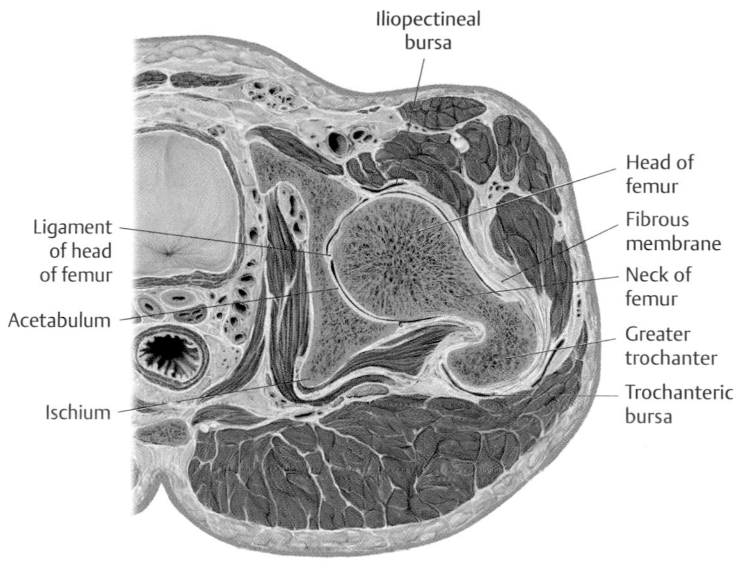
Iliopectineal
bursa
Head of
femur
Fibrous
membrane
Ligament
of head
of femur
Neck of
femur
Acetabulum
Greater
trochanter
Ischium
Trochanteric
bursa

A Transverse section.

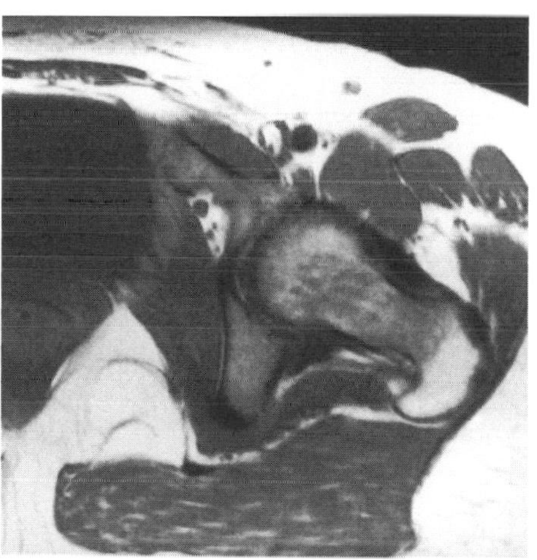

B T1-weighted MRI.

Hip Joint: Overview

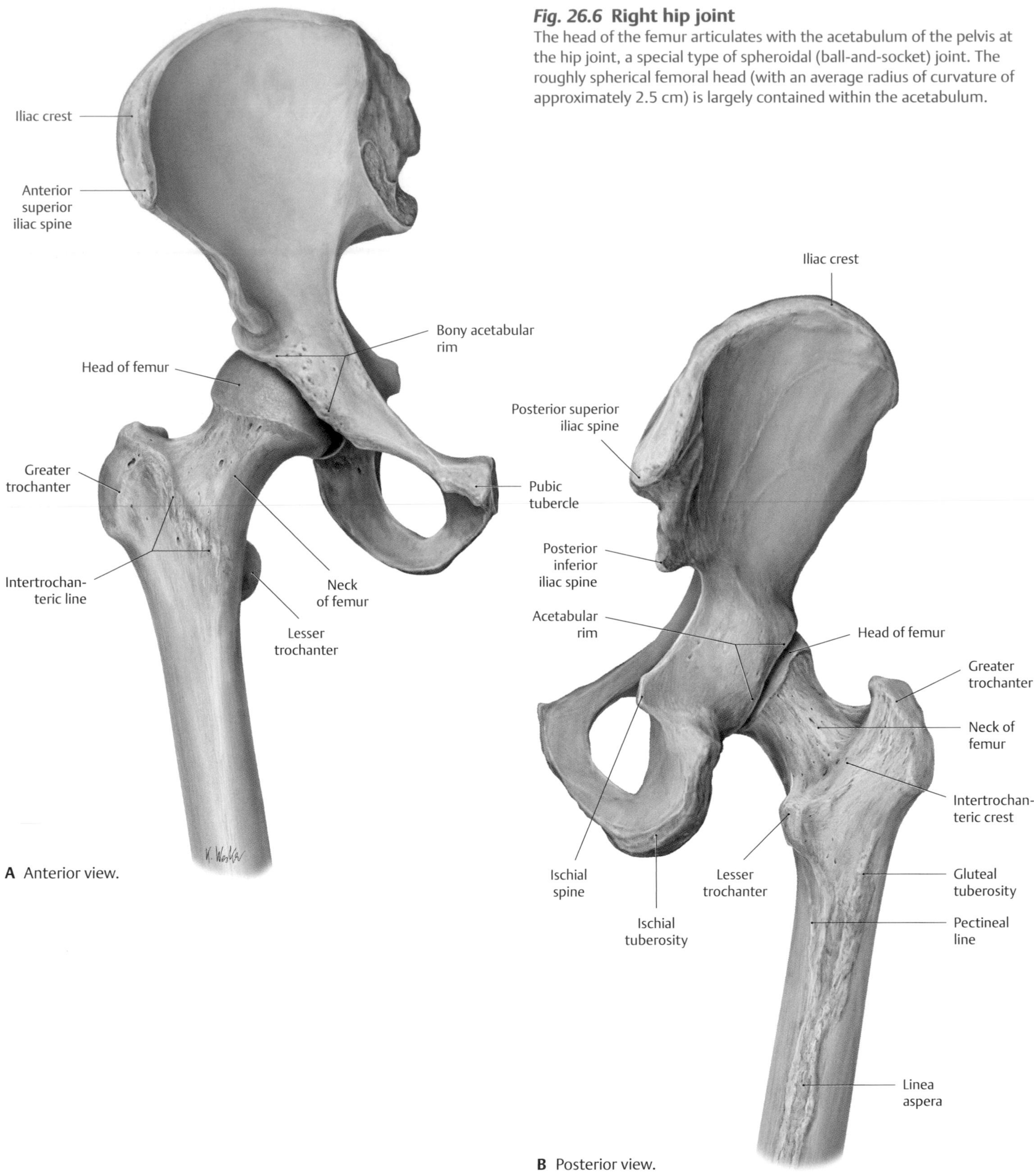
Iliac crest
Anterior superior iliac spine
Bony acetabular rim
Head of femur
Greater trochanter
Pubic tubercle
Intertrochan-teric line
Neck of femur
Lesser trochanter
Iliac crest
Posterior superior iliac spine
Posterior inferior iliac spine
Acetabular rim
Head of femur
Greater trochanter
Neck of femur
Intertrochan-teric crest
Ischial spine
Lesser trochanter
Gluteal tuberosity
Ischial tuberosity
Pectineal line
Linea aspera

A Anterior view.

B Posterior view.

Fig. 26.6 **Right hip joint**
The head of the femur articulates with the acetabulum of the pelvis at the hip joint, a special type of spheroidal (ball-and-socket) joint. The roughly spherical femoral head (with an average radius of curvature of approximately 2.5 cm) is largely contained within the acetabulum.

Fig. 26.7 Hip joint: Coronal section
Right hip joint, anterior view.

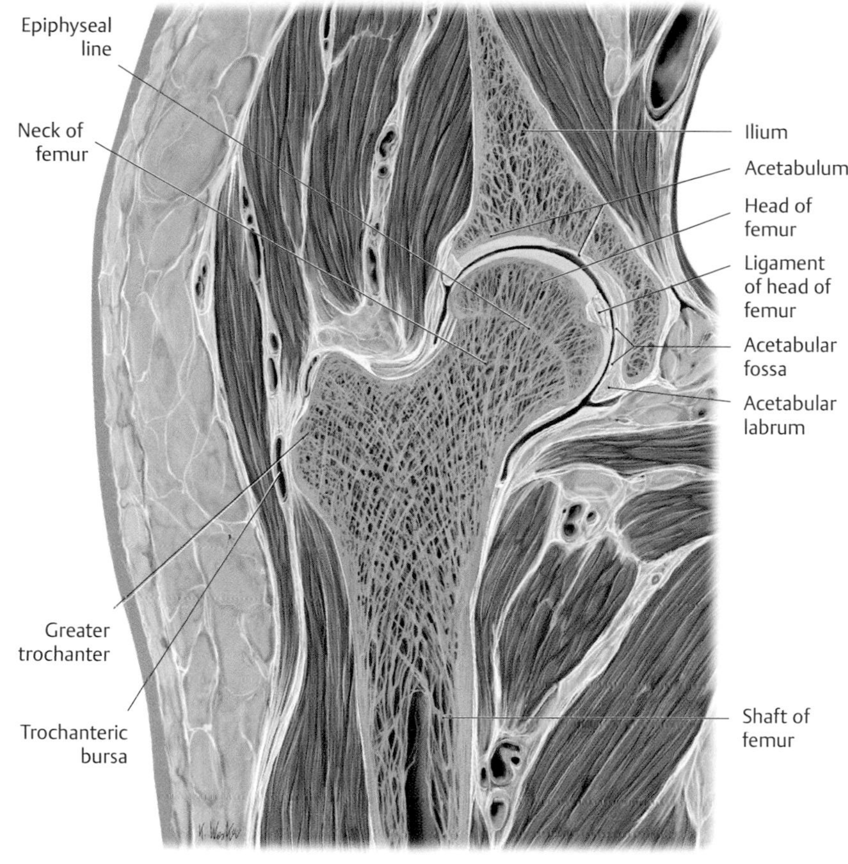
Epiphyseal line
Neck of femur
Greater trochanter
Trochanteric bursa
Ilium
Acetabulum
Head of femur
Ligament of head of femur
Acetabular fossa
Acetabular labrum
Shaft of femur

A Coronal section.

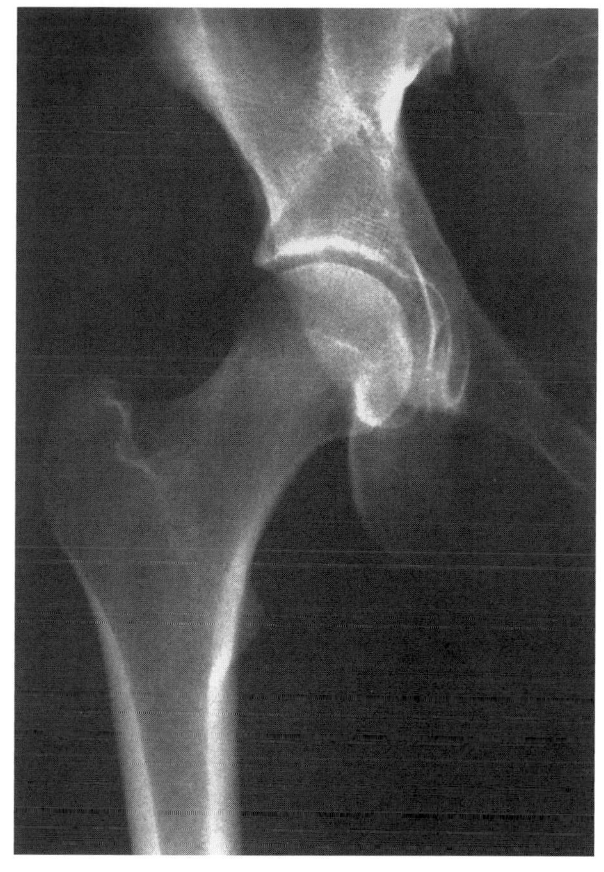

B Radiograph.

Clinical

Diagnosing hip dysplasia and dislocation

Ultrasonography, the most important imaging method for screening the infant hip, is used to identify morphological changes such as hip dysplasia and dislocation. Clinically, hip dislocation presents with instability and limited abduction of the hip joint, and leg shortening with asymmetry of the gluteal folds.

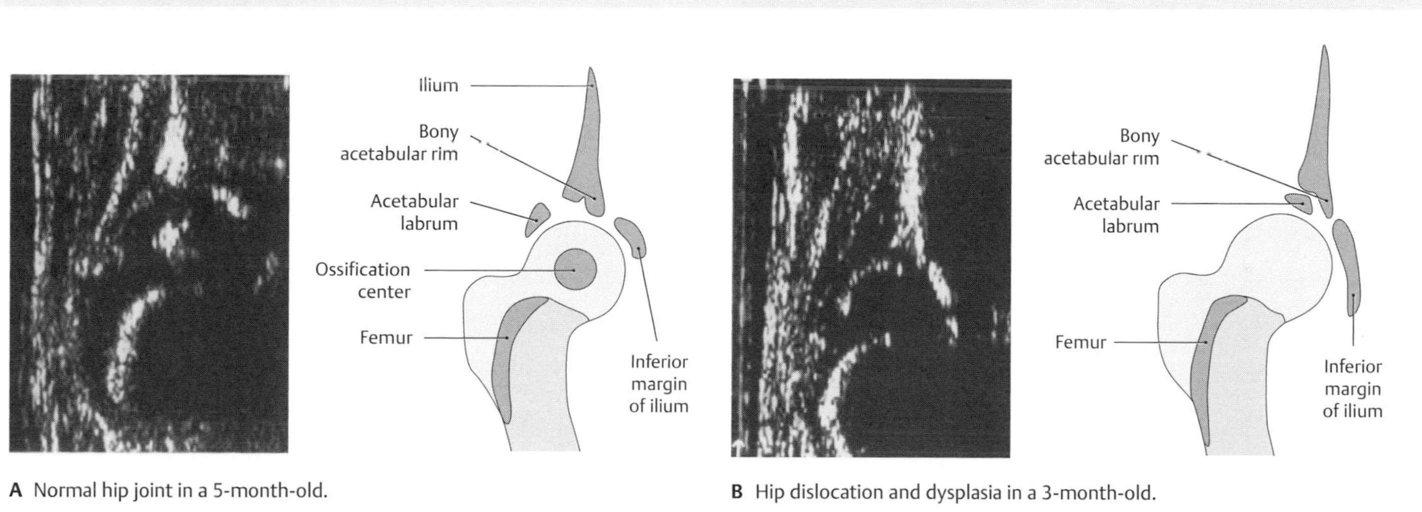
Ilium
Bony acetabular rim
Acetabular labrum
Ossification center
Femur
Inferior margin of ilium
Bony acetabular rim
Acetabular labrum
Femur
Inferior margin of ilium

A Normal hip joint in a 5-month-old.

B Hip dislocation and dysplasia in a 3-month-old.

Hip Joint: Ligaments & Capsule

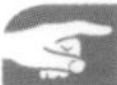

The hip joint has three major ligaments: iliofemoral, pubofemoral, and ischiofemoral. The zona orbicularis (annular ligament) is not visible externally and encircles the femoral neck like a buttonhole.

Fig. 26.8 **Hip joint: Lateral view**
Right hip joint.

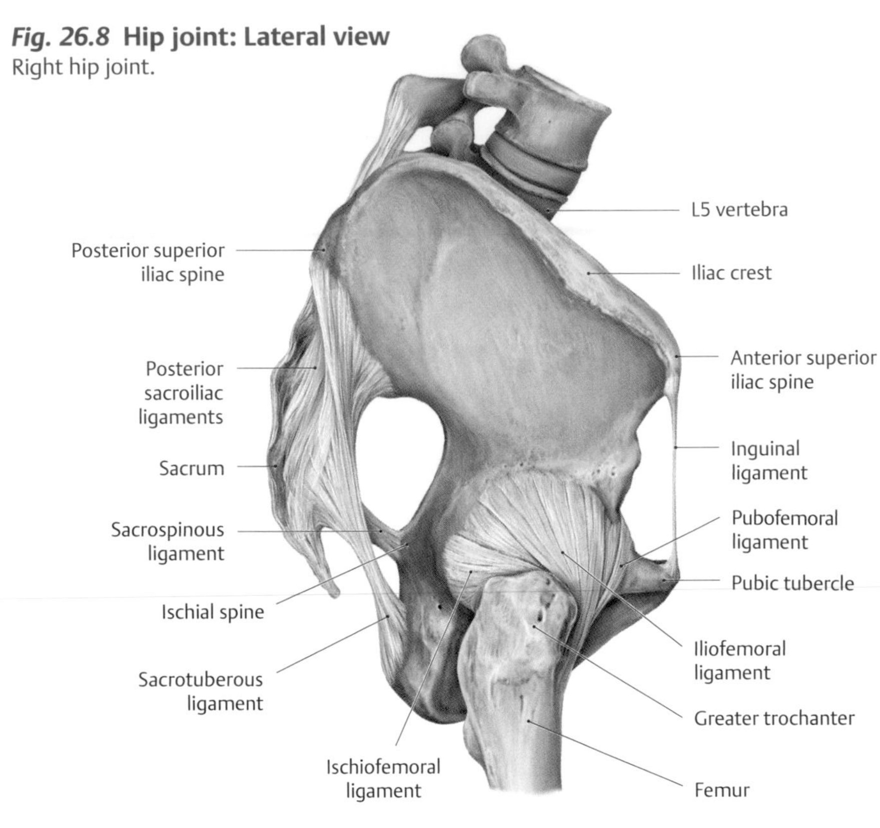
L5 vertebra
Posterior superior iliac spine
Iliac crest
Anterior superior iliac spine
Posterior sacroiliac ligaments
Sacrum
Inguinal ligament
Sacrospinous ligament
Pubofemoral ligament
Pubic tubercle
Ischial spine
Iliofemoral ligament
Sacrotuberous ligament
Greater trochanter
Ischiofemoral ligament
Femur

A Ligaments of the hip joint.

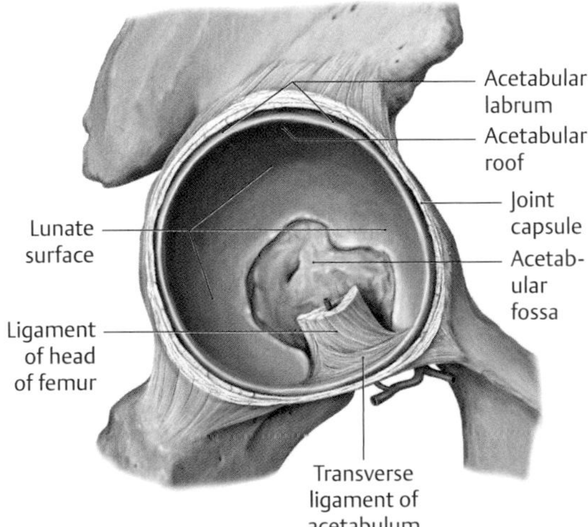
Acetabular labrum
Acetabular roof
Joint capsule
Lunate surface
Acetabular fossa
Ligament of head of femur
Transverse ligament of acetabulum

C Acetabulum of hip joint. *Note:* The ligament of the femoral head (cut) transmits branches from the obturator artery that nourish the femoral head (see p. 445).

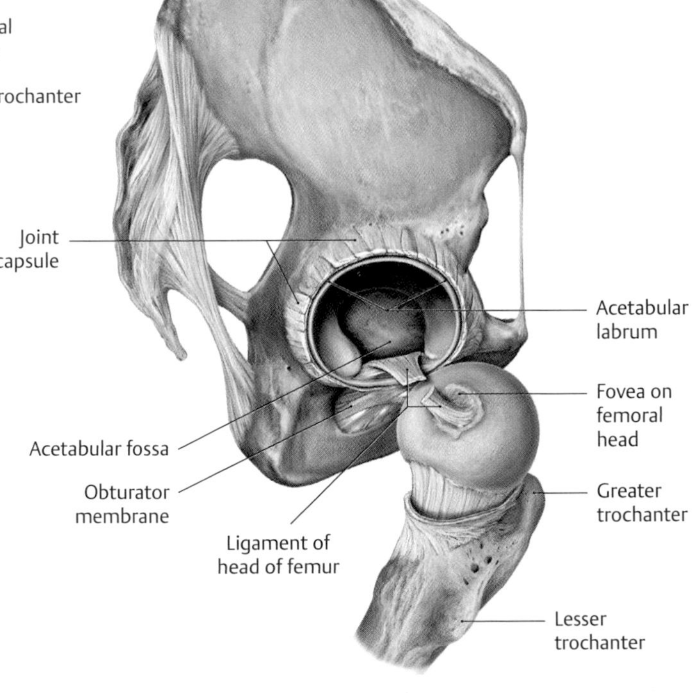
Joint capsule
Acetabular labrum
Fovea on femoral head
Acetabular fossa
Obturator membrane
Greater trochanter
Ligament of head of femur
Lesser trochanter

B Joint capsule. The capsule has been divided and the femoral head dislocated to expose the cut ligament of the head of the femur.

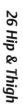

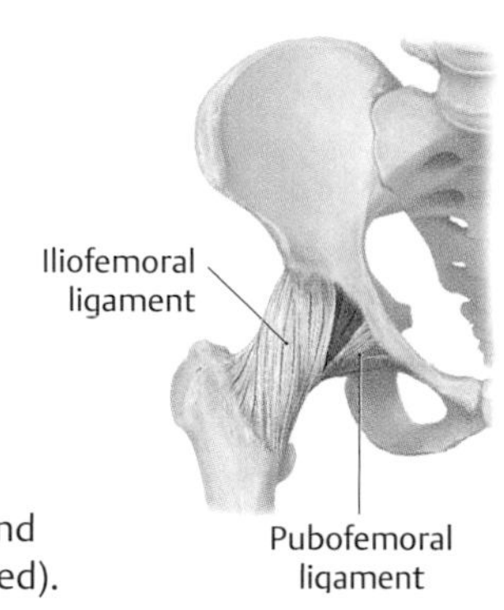
Iliofemoral ligament
Pubofemoral ligament

A Ligaments and weak spot (red).

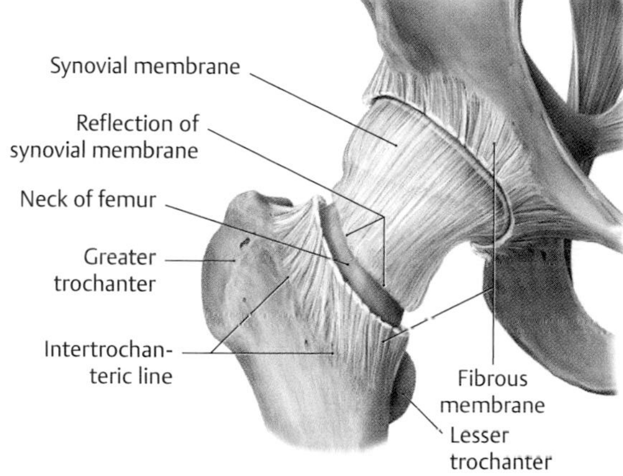
Synovial membrane
Reflection of synovial membrane
Neck of femur
Greater trochanter
Intertrochan-teric line
Fibrous membrane
Lesser trochanter

C Joint capsule. *Removed:* Fibrous membrane (at level of femoral neck). *Exposed:* Synovial membrane.

Fig. 26.9 **Hip joint: Anterior view**
Right hip joint.

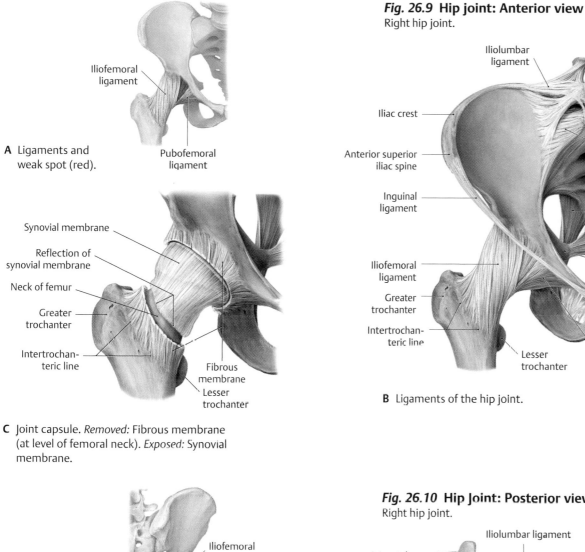

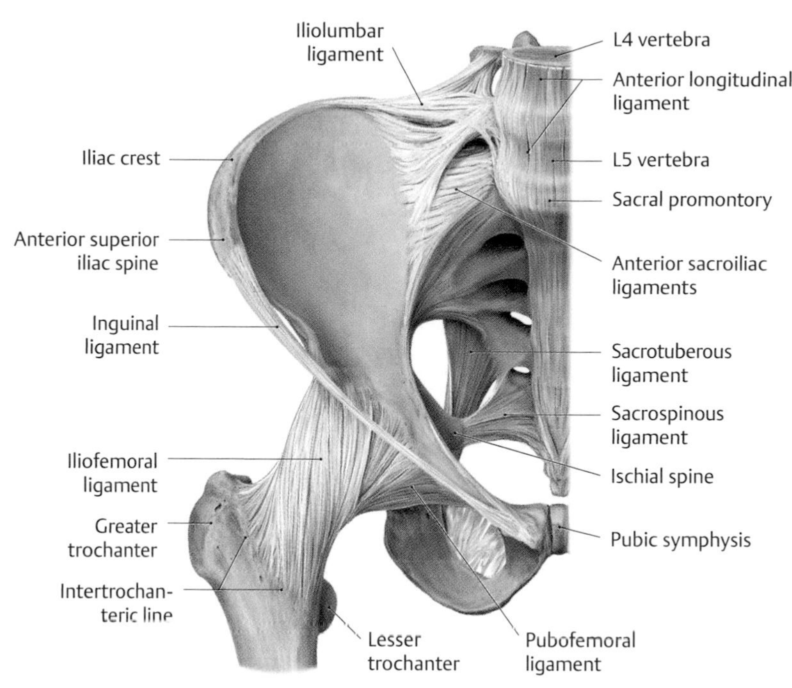
Iliolumbar ligament
L4 vertebra
Anterior longitudinal ligament
Iliac crest
L5 vertebra
Sacral promontory
Anterior superior iliac spine
Anterior sacroiliac ligaments
Inguinal ligament
Sacrotuberous ligament
Sacrospinous ligament
Iliofemoral ligament
Ischial spine
Greater trochanter
Pubic symphysis
Intertrochan-teric line
Lesser trochanter
Pubofemoral ligament

B Ligaments of the hip joint.

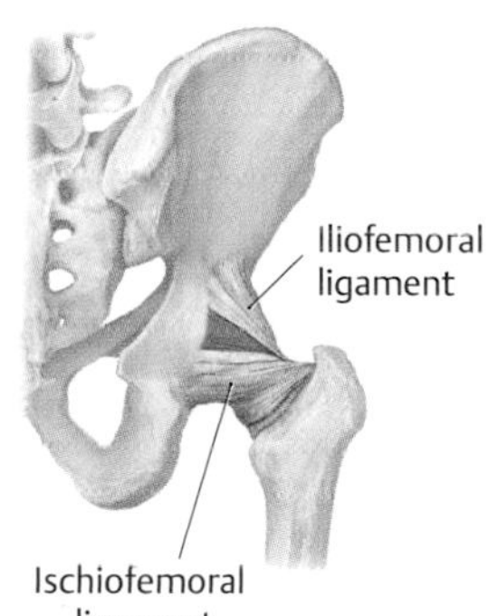
Iliofemoral ligament
Ischiofemoral ligament

A Ligaments and weak spot (red).

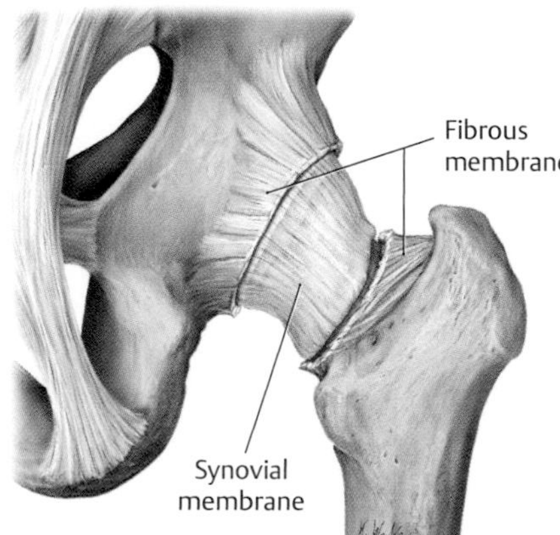
Fibrous membrane
Synovial membrane

C Joint capsule.

Fig. 26.10 **Hip Joint: Posterior view**
Right hip joint.

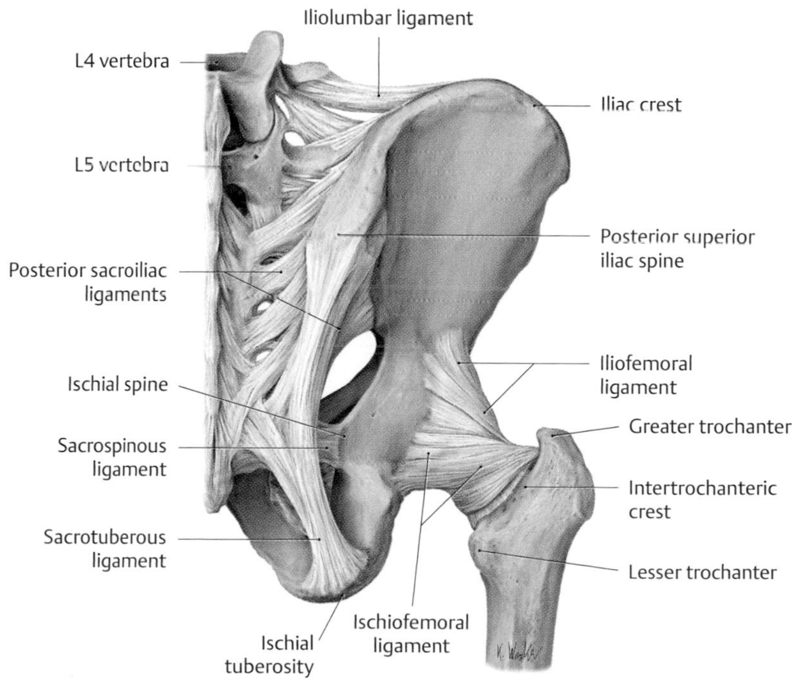
Iliolumbar ligament
L4 vertebra
Iliac crest
L5 vertebra
Posterior superior iliac spine
Posterior sacroiliac ligaments
Iliofemoral ligament
Ischial spine
Greater trochanter
Sacrospinous ligament
Intertrochanteric crest
Sacrotuberous ligament
Lesser trochanter
Ischial tuberosity
Ischiofemoral ligament

B Ligaments of the hip joint.

Anterior Muscles of the Hip, Thigh & Gluteal Region (I)

Fig. 26.11 **Anterior muscles of the hip and thigh (I)**
Right limb. Muscle origins are shown in red, insertions in blue.

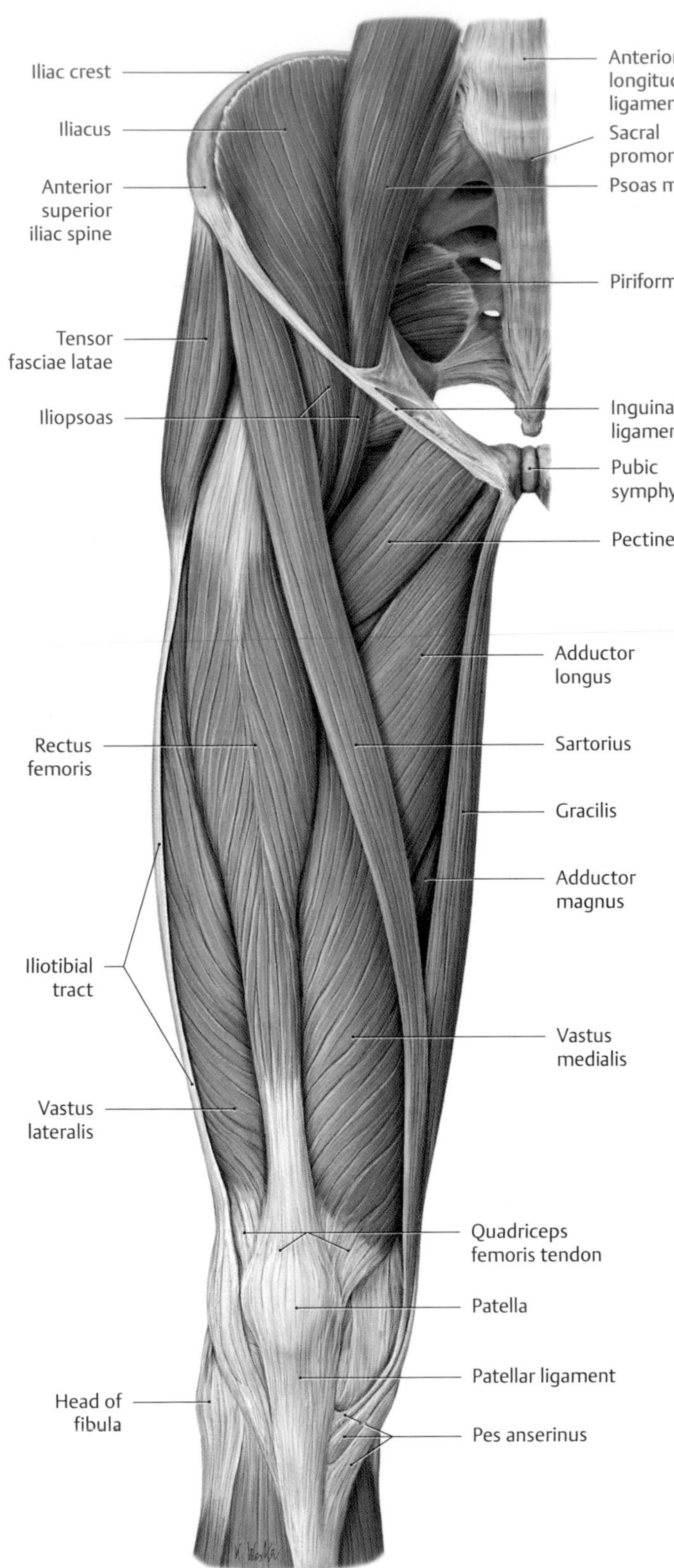
Iliac crest
Iliacus
Anterior superior iliac spine
Tensor fasciae latae
Iliopsoas
Rectus femoris
Iliotibial tract
Vastus lateralis
Head of fibula
Anterior longitudinal ligament
Sacral promontory
Psoas major
Piriformis
Inguinal ligament
Pubic symphysis
Pectineus
Adductor longus
Sartorius
Gracilis
Adductor magnus
Vastus medialis
Quadriceps femoris tendon
Patella
Patellar ligament
Pes anserinus

A *Removed:* Fascia lata of thigh (to the lateral iliotibial tract).

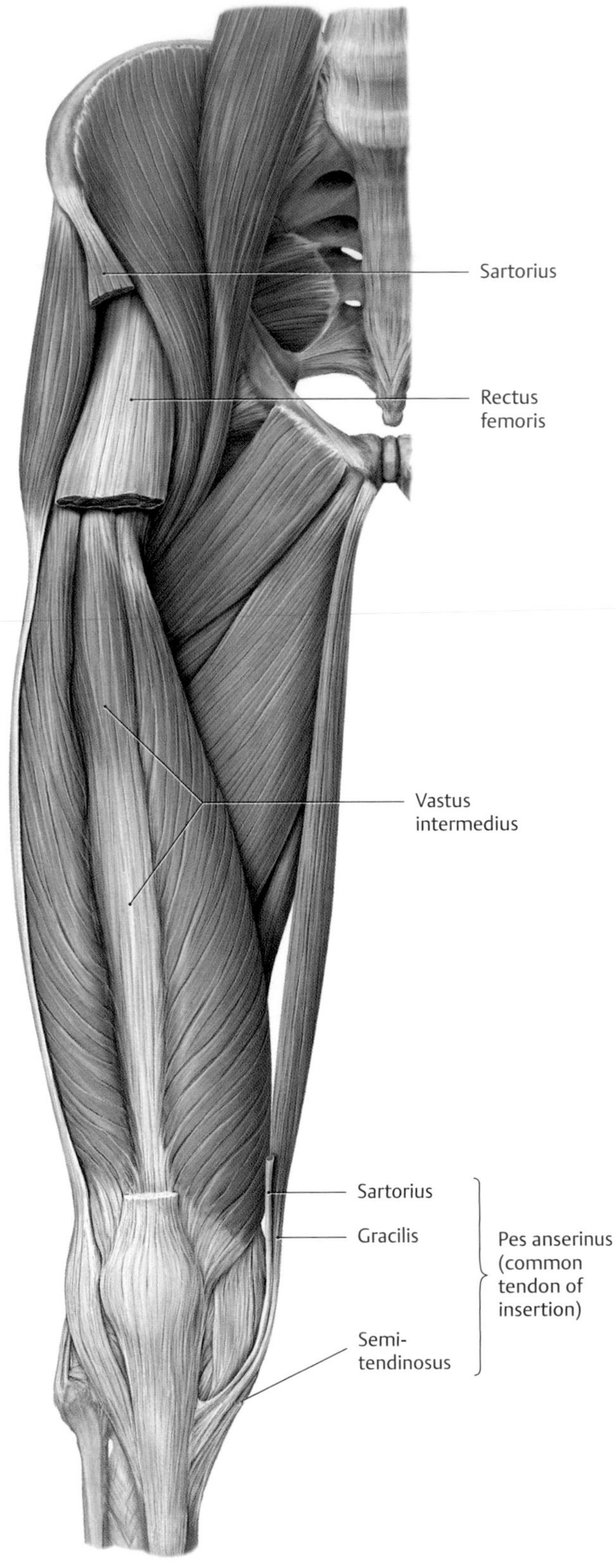
Sartorius
Rectus femoris
Vastus intermedius
Sartorius
Gracilis
Semi-tendinosus
Pes anserinus (common tendon of insertion)

B *Removed:* Sartorius and rectus femoris.

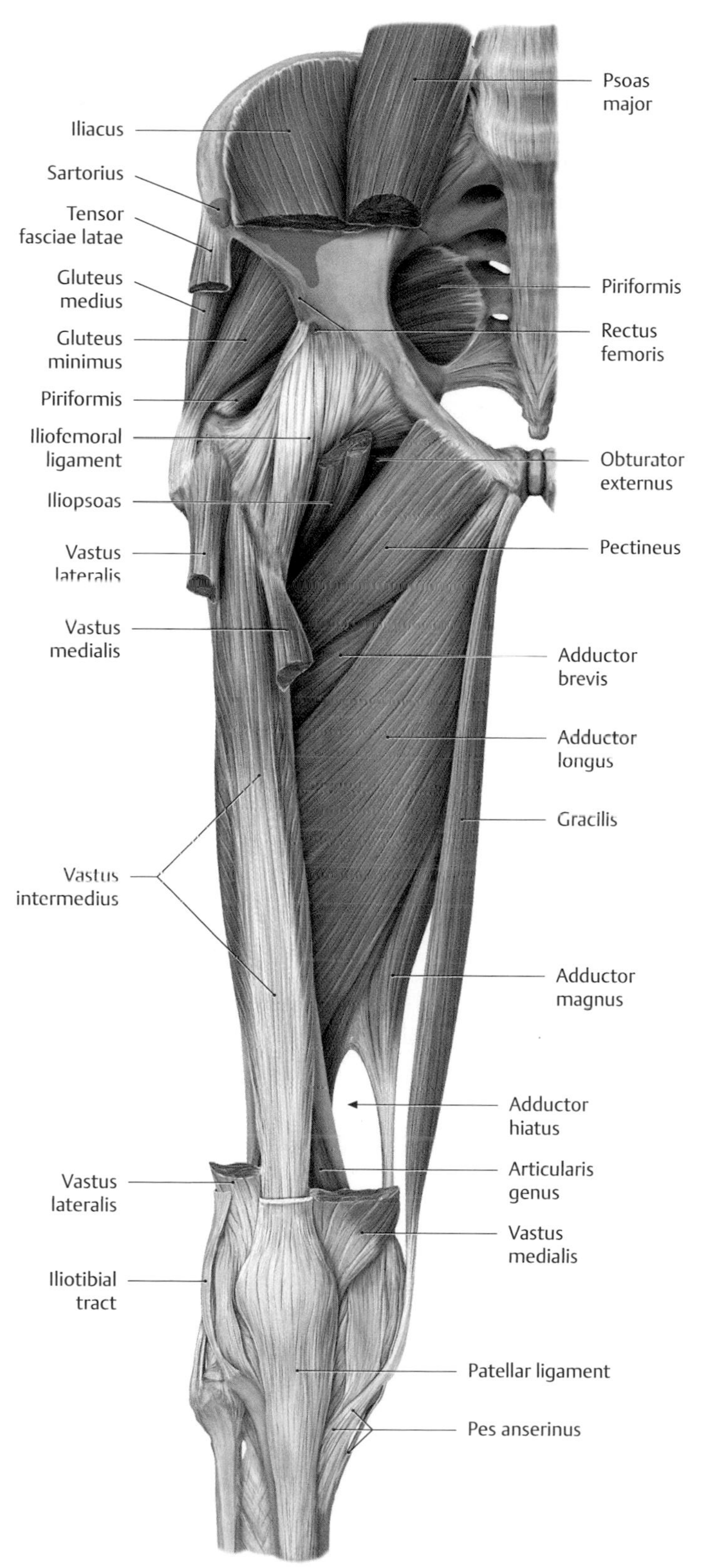
Psoas major
Iliacus
Sartorius
Tensor fasciae latae
Gluteus medius
Gluteus minimus
Piriformis
Rectus femoris
Piriformis
Iliofemoral ligament
Obturator externus
Iliopsoas
Pectineus
Vastus lateralis
Vastus medialis
Adductor brevis
Adductor longus
Gracilis
Vastus intermedius
Adductor magnus
Adductor hiatus
Articularis genus
Vastus lateralis
Vastus medialis
Iliotibial tract
Patellar ligament
Pes anserinus

C *Removed:* Rectus femoris (completely), vastus lateralis, vastus medialis, iliopsoas, and tensor fasciae latae.

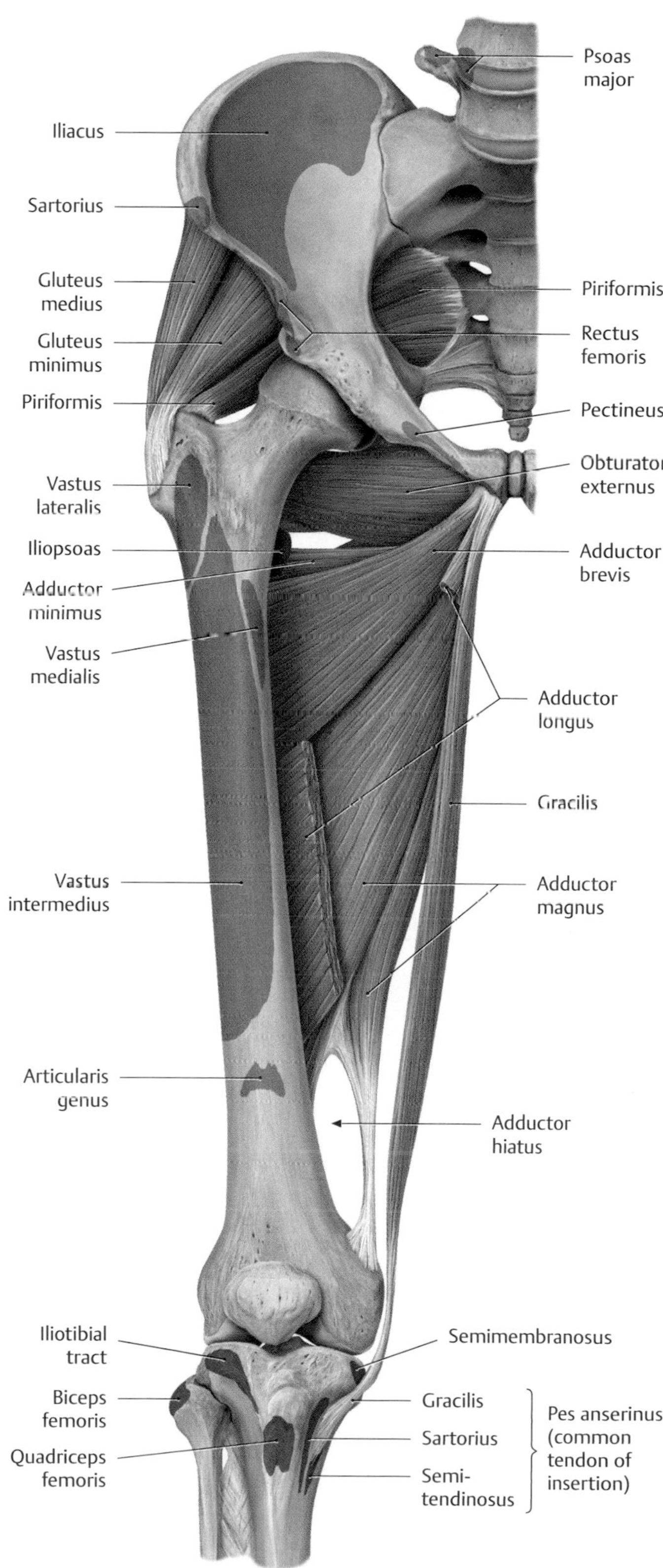
Psoas major
Iliacus
Sartorius
Gluteus medius
Piriformis
Gluteus minimus
Rectus femoris
Piriformis
Pectineus
Vastus lateralis
Obturator externus
Iliopsoas
Adductor brevis
Adductor minimus
Vastus medialis
Adductor longus
Gracilis
Vastus intermedius
Adductor magnus
Articularis genus
Adductor hiatus
Iliotibial tract
Semimembranosus
Biceps femoris
Gracilis
Sartorius
Quadriceps femoris
Semi-tendinosus
Pes anserinus (common tendon of insertion)

D *Removed:* Quadriceps femoris (rectus femoris, vastus lateralis, vastus medialis, vastus intermedius), iliopsoas, tensor fasciae latae, pectineus, and midportion of adductor longus.

Anterior Muscles of the Hip, Thigh & Gluteal Region (II)

Fig. 26.12 **Anterior muscles of the hip and thigh (II)**
Right limb. Muscle origins are shown in red, insertions in blue.

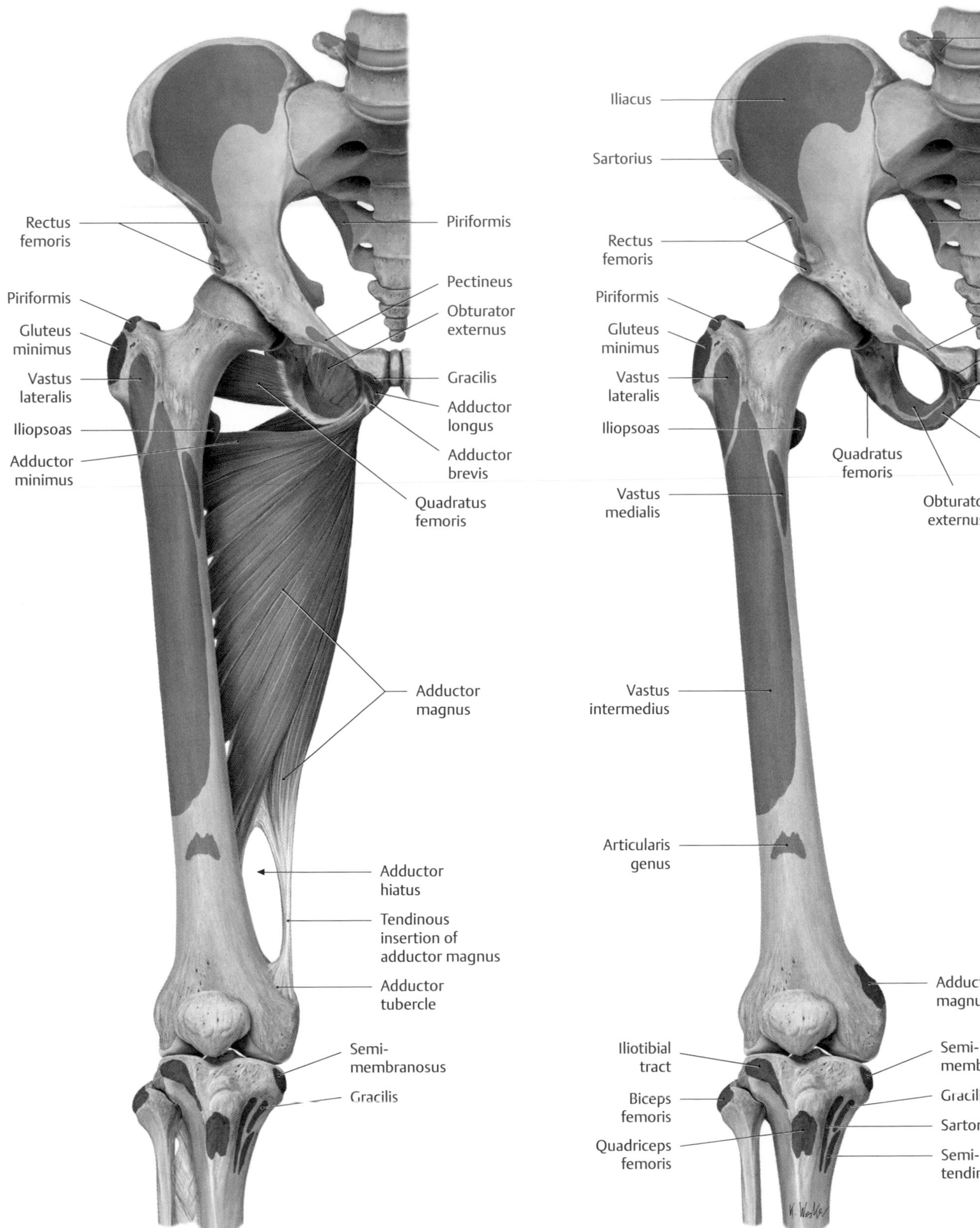
Rectus femoris
Piriformis
Gluteus minimus
Vastus lateralis
Iliopsoas
Adductor minimus
Piriformis
Pectineus
Obturator externus
Gracilis
Adductor longus
Adductor brevis
Quadratus femoris
Adductor magnus
Adductor hiatus
Tendinous insertion of adductor magnus
Adductor tubercle
Semi-membranosus
Gracilis
Iliacus
Sartorius
Rectus femoris
Piriformis
Gluteus minimus
Vastus lateralis
Iliopsoas
Vastus medialis
Vastus intermedius
Articularis genus
Iliotibial tract
Biceps femoris
Quadriceps femoris
Psoas major
Piriformis
Pectineus
Gracilis
Adductor longus
Adductor brevis
Adductor magnus
Quadratus femoris
Obturator externus
Adductor magnus
Semi-membranosus
Gracilis
Sartorius
Semi-tendinosus

A *Removed:* Gluteus medius and minimus, piriformis, obturator externus, adductor brevis and longus, and gracilis.

B *Removed:* All muscles.

***Fig. 26.13* Medial muscles of the hip, thigh, and gluteal region**
Midsagittal section.

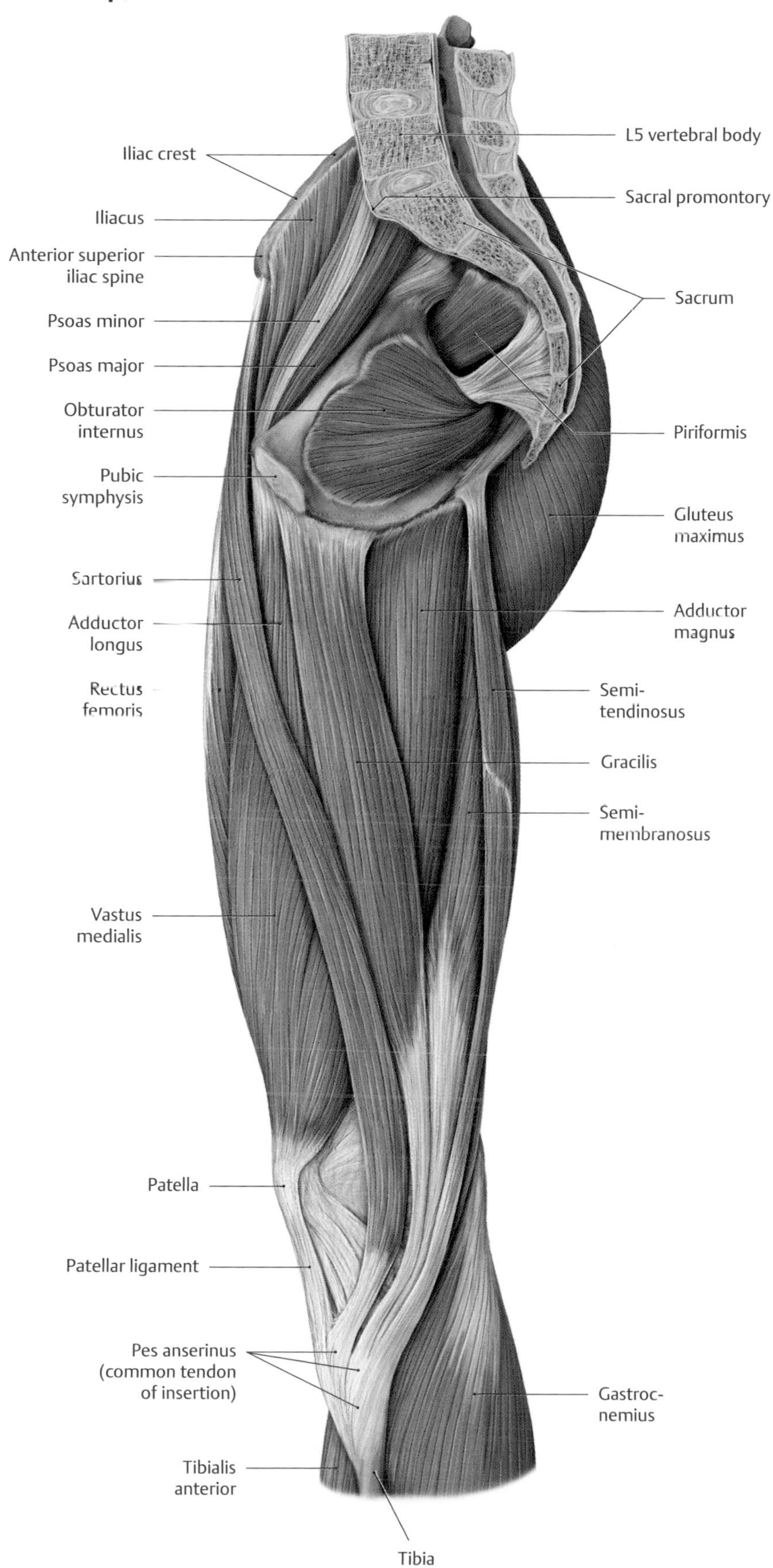
Iliac crest
Iliacus
Anterior superior iliac spine
Psoas minor
Psoas major
Obturator internus
Pubic symphysis
Sartorius
Adductor longus
Rectus femoris
Vastus medialis
Patella
Patellar ligament
Pes anserinus (common tendon of insertion)
Tibialis anterior
Tibia
L5 vertebral body
Sacral promontory
Sacrum
Piriformis
Gluteus maximus
Adductor magnus
Semi-tendinosus
Gracilis
Semi-membranosus
Gastroc-nemius

Posterior Muscles of the Hip, Thigh & Gluteal Region (I)

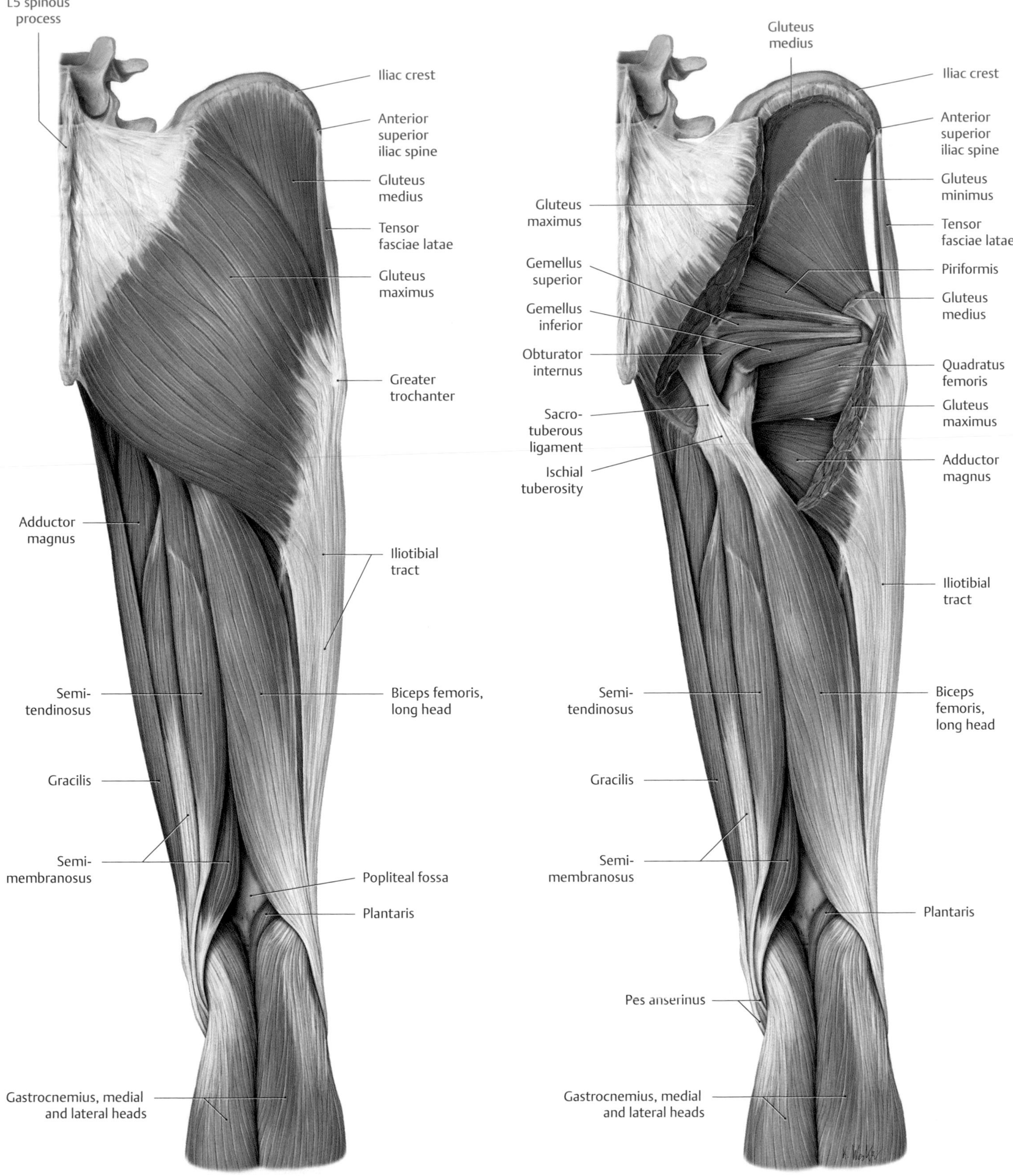
L5 spinous process
Iliac crest
Anterior superior iliac spine
Gluteus medius
Tensor fasciae latae
Gluteus maximus
Greater trochanter
Adductor magnus
Iliotibial tract
Semi-tendinosus
Biceps femoris, long head
Gracilis
Semi-membranosus
Popliteal fossa
Plantaris
Gastrocnemius, medial and lateral heads
Gluteus medius
Iliac crest
Anterior superior iliac spine
Gluteus maximus
Gluteus minimus
Tensor fasciae latae
Gemellus superior
Piriformis
Gluteus medius
Gemellus inferior
Obturator internus
Quadratus femoris
Sacro-tuberous ligament
Gluteus maximus
Ischial tuberosity
Adductor magnus
Iliotibial tract
Semi-tendinosus
Biceps femoris, long head
Gracilis
Semi-membranosus
Plantaris
Pes anserinus
Gastrocnemius, medial and lateral heads

Fig. 26.14 **Posterior muscles of the hip, thigh, and gluteal region (I)**
Right limb. Muscle origins are shown in red, insertions in blue.

A *Removed:* Fascia lata (to iliotibial tract).

B *Partially removed:* Gluteus maximus and medius.

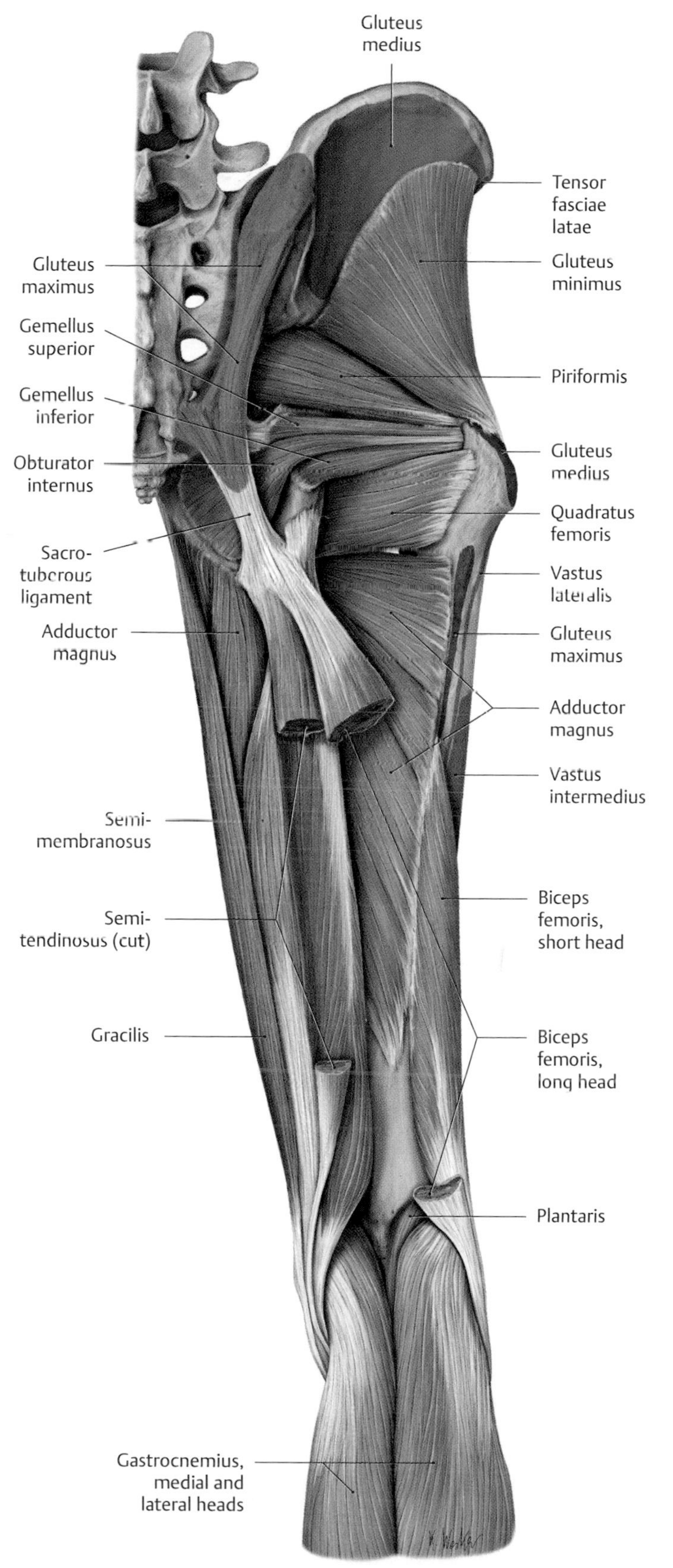
Gluteus
medius
Tensor
fasciae
latae
Gluteus
maximus
Gluteus
minimus
Gemellus
superior
Piriformis
Gemellus
inferior
Gluteus
medius
Obturator
internus
Quadratus
femoris
Sacro-
tuberous
ligament
Vastus
lateralis
Adductor
magnus
Gluteus
maximus
Adductor
magnus
Vastus
intermedius
Semi-
membranosus
Biceps
femoris,
short head
Semi-
tendinosus (cut)
Gracilis
Biceps
femoris,
long head
Plantaris
Gastrocnemius,
medial and
lateral heads

C *Removed:* Semitendinosus and biceps femoris (partially); gluteus maximus and medius (completely).

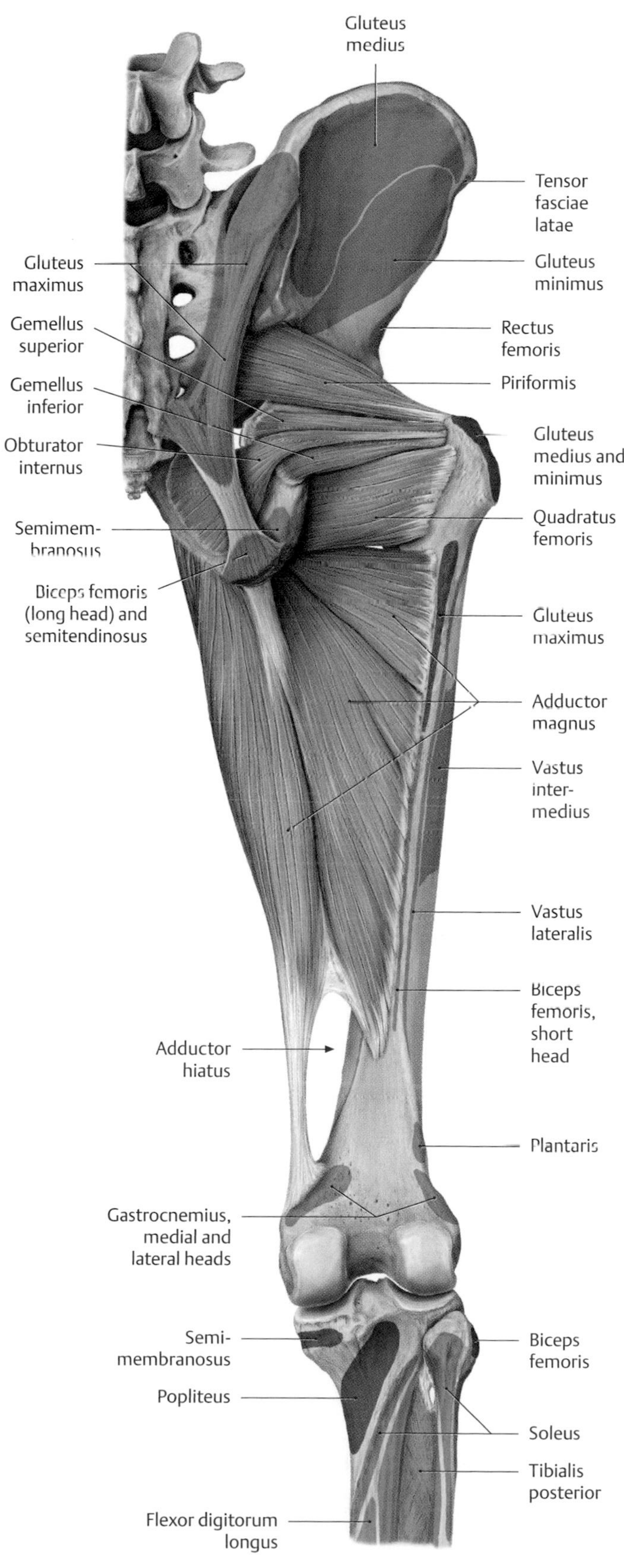
Gluteus
medius
Tensor
fasciae
latae
Gluteus
maximus
Gluteus
minimus
Gemellus
superior
Rectus
femoris
Piriformis
Gemellus
inferior
Obturator
internus
Gluteus
medius and
minimus
Quadratus
femoris
Semimem-
branosus
Biceps femoris
(long head) and
semitendinosus
Gluteus
maximus
Adductor
magnus
Vastus
inter-
medius
Vastus
lateralis
Biceps
femoris,
short
head
Adductor
hiatus
Plantaris
Gastrocnemius,
medial and
lateral heads
Semi-
membranosus
Biceps
femoris
Popliteus
Soleus
Tibialis
posterior
Flexor digitorum
longus

D *Removed:* Hamstrings (semitendinosus, semimembranosus, and biceps femoris), gluteus minimus, gastrocnemius, and muscles of the leg.

Posterior Muscles of the Hip, Thigh & Gluteal Region (II)

Fig. 26.15 **Posterior muscles of the hip, thigh, and gluteal region (II)**
Right limb. Muscle origins are shown in red, insertions in blue.

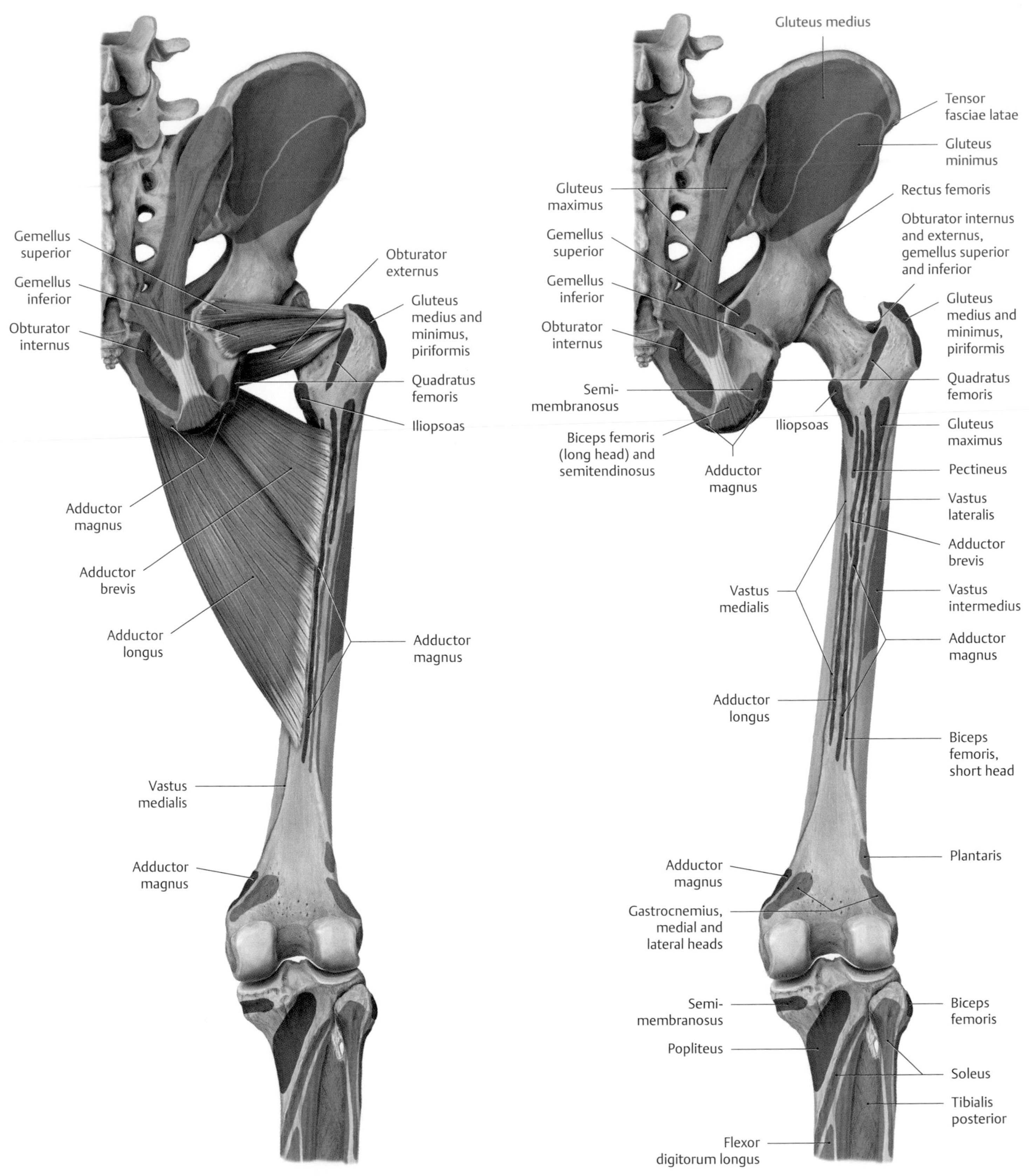
Gemellus superior
Gemellus inferior
Obturator internus
Obturator externus
Gluteus medius and minimus, piriformis
Quadratus femoris
Iliopsoas
Adductor magnus
Adductor brevis
Adductor longus
Adductor magnus
Vastus medialis
Adductor magnus
Gluteus medius
Tensor fasciae latae
Gluteus minimus
Gluteus maximus
Rectus femoris
Obturator internus and externus, gemellus superior and inferior
Gemellus superior
Gemellus inferior
Gluteus medius and minimus, piriformis
Obturator internus
Quadratus femoris
Semi-membranosus
Iliopsoas
Biceps femoris (long head) and semitendinosus
Gluteus maximus
Adductor magnus
Pectineus
Vastus lateralis
Adductor brevis
Vastus medialis
Vastus intermedius
Adductor magnus
Adductor longus
Biceps femoris, short head
Plantaris
Adductor magnus
Gastrocnemius, medial and lateral heads
Semi-membranosus
Biceps femoris
Popliteus
Soleus
Tibialis posterior
Flexor digitorum longus

A *Removed:* Piriformis, obturator internus, quadratus femoris, and adductor magnus.

B *Removed:* All muscles.

Fig. 26.16 Lateral muscles of the hip, thigh, and gluteal region
Note: The iliotibial tract (the thickened band of fascia lata) functions as a tension band to reduce the bending loads on the proximal femur.

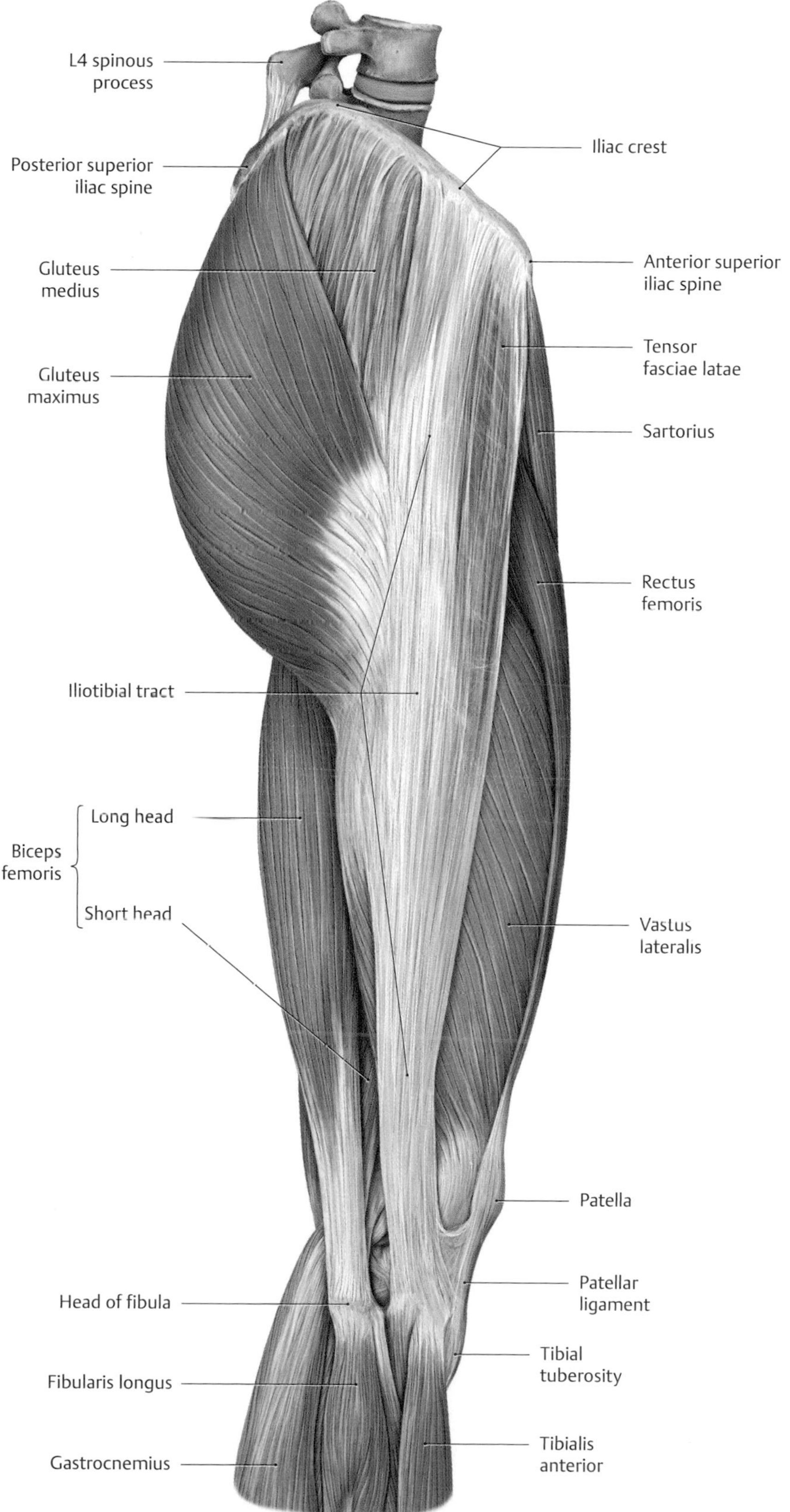
L4 spinous process
Posterior superior iliac spine
Iliac crest
Gluteus medius
Anterior superior iliac spine
Tensor fasciae latae
Gluteus maximus
Sartorius
Rectus femoris
Iliotibial tract
Biceps femoris
Long head
Short head
Vastus lateralis
Patella
Patellar ligament
Head of fibula
Tibial tuberosity
Fibularis longus
Gastrocnemius
Tibialis anterior

Muscle Facts (I)

Table 26.1 Iliopsoas muscle

Muscles		Origin	Insertion	Innervation	Action
③ Iliopsoas	① Psoas major*	*Superficial:* T12–L4 and associated intervertebral disks (lateral surfaces) *Deep:* L1–L5 vertebrae (transverse processes)	Lesser trochanter	Direct branches from the lumbar plexus (psoas) (L2–L4)	• Hip joint: flexion and external rotation • Lumbar spine: *unilateral* contraction (with the femur fixed) bends the trunk laterally to the same side; *bilateral* contraction raises the trunk from the supine position
	② Iliacus	Iliac fossa		Femoral n. (L2–L4)	

* The psoas minor, present in approximately 50% of the population, is often found on the superficial surface of the psoas major (see Fig. 26.17). It is not a muscle of the lower limb. It originates, inserts, and exerts its action on the abdomen (see Table 11.2, p. 140).

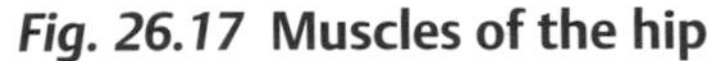

Fig. 26.17 **Muscles of the hip**
Right side, schematic.

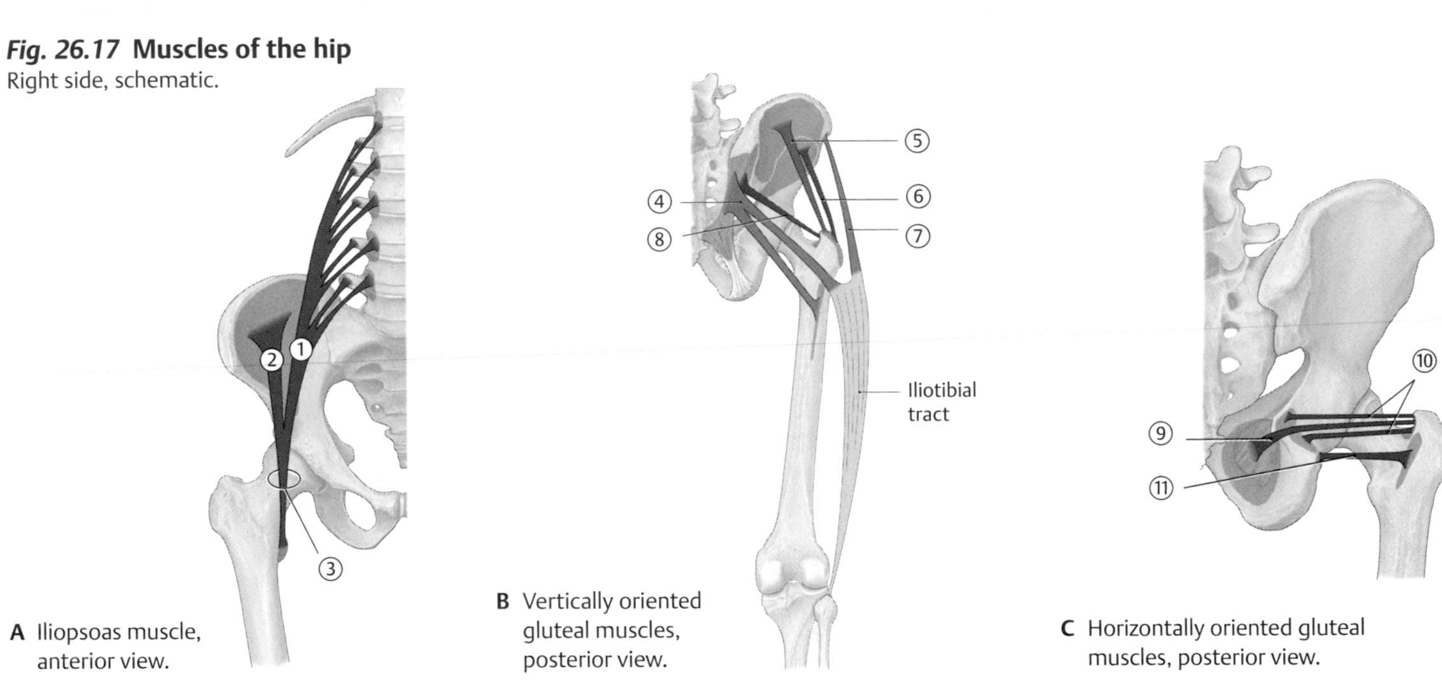

①
②
③
④
⑤
⑥
⑦
⑧
Iliotibial tract
⑨
⑩
⑪

A Iliopsoas muscle, anterior view.

B Vertically oriented gluteal muscles, posterior view.

C Horizontally oriented gluteal muscles, posterior view.

Table 26.2 Gluteal muscles

Muscle	Origin	Insertion	Innervation	Action
④ Gluteus maximus	Sacrum (dorsal surface, lateral part), ilium (gluteal surface, posterior part), thoracolumbar fascia, sacrotuberous ligament	• Upper fibers: iliotibial tract • Lower fibers: gluteal tuberosity	Inferior gluteal n. (L5–S2)	• Entire muscle: extends and externally rotates the hip in sagittal and coronal planes • Upper fibers: abduction • Lower fibers: adduction
⑤ Gluteus medius	Ilium (gluteal surface below the iliac crest between the anterior and posterior gluteal line)	Greater trochanter of the femur (lateral surface)	Superior gluteal n. (L4–S1)	• Entire muscle: abducts the hip, stabilizes the pelvis in the coronal plane • Anterior part: flexion and internal rotation • Posterior part: extension and external rotation
⑥ Gluteus minimus	Ilium (gluteal surface below the origin of gluteus medius)	Greater trochanter of the femur (anterolateral surface)		
⑦ Tensor fasciae latae	Anterior superior iliac spine	Iliotibial tract		• Tenses the fascia lata • Hip joint: abduction, flexion, and internal rotation
⑧ Piriformis	Pelvic surface of the sacrum	Apex of the greater trochanter of the femur	Direct branches from the sacral plexus (S1–S2)	• External rotation, abduction, and extension of the hip joint • Stabilizes the hip joint
⑨ Obturator internus	Inner surface of the obturator membrane and its bony boundaries	Medial surface of the greater trochanter	Direct branches from the sacral plexus (L5, S1)	External rotation, adduction, and extension of the hip joint (also active in abduction, depending on the joint's position)
⑩ Gemelli	• Gemellus superior: ischial spine • Gemellus inferior: ischial tuberosity	Jointly with obturator internus tendon (medial surface, greater trochanter)		
⑪ Quadratus femoris	Lateral border of the ischial tuberosity	Intertrochanteric crest of the femur		External rotation and adduction of the hip joint

Fig. 26.18 Psoas and iliacus muscles
Right side, anterior view.

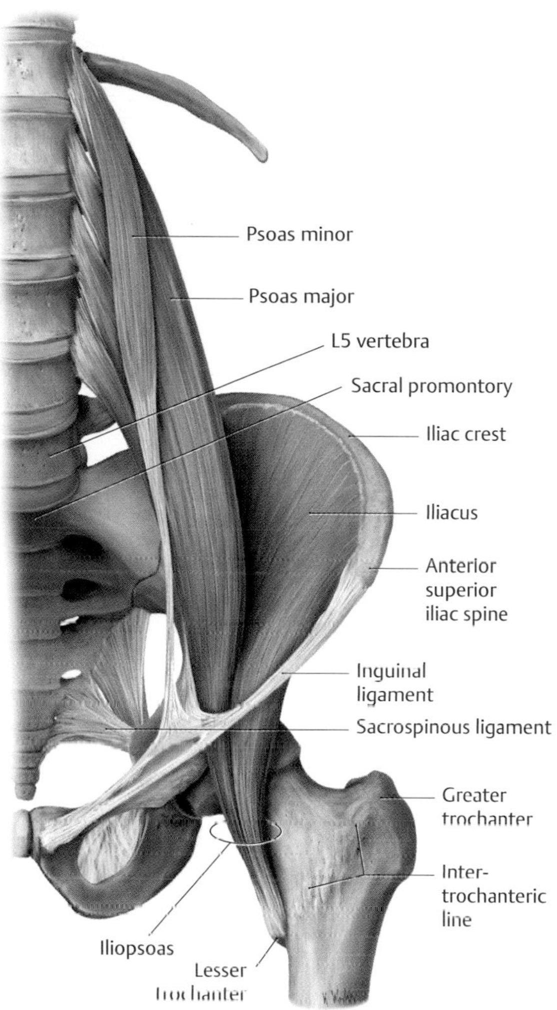
Psoas minor
Psoas major
L5 vertebra
Sacral promontory
Iliac crest
Iliacus
Anterior superior iliac spine
Inguinal ligament
Sacrospinous ligament
Greater trochanter
Inter-trochanteric line
Iliopsoas
Lesser trochanter

Fig. 26.19 Superficial muscles of the gluteal region
Right side, posterior view.

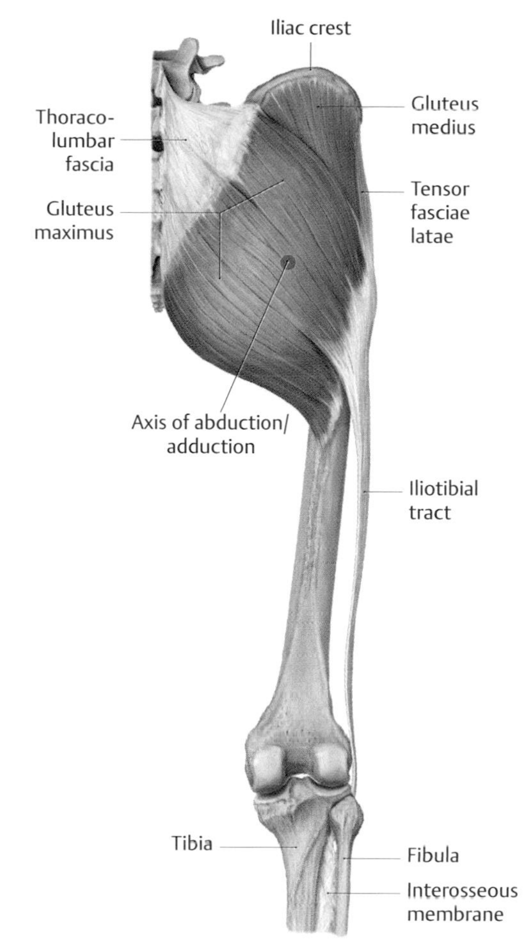
Iliac crest
Thoraco-lumbar fascia
Gluteus medius
Tensor fasciae latae
Gluteus maximus
Axis of abduction/ adduction
Iliotibial tract
Tibia
Fibula
Interosseous membrane

Fig. 26.20 Deep muscles of the gluteal region

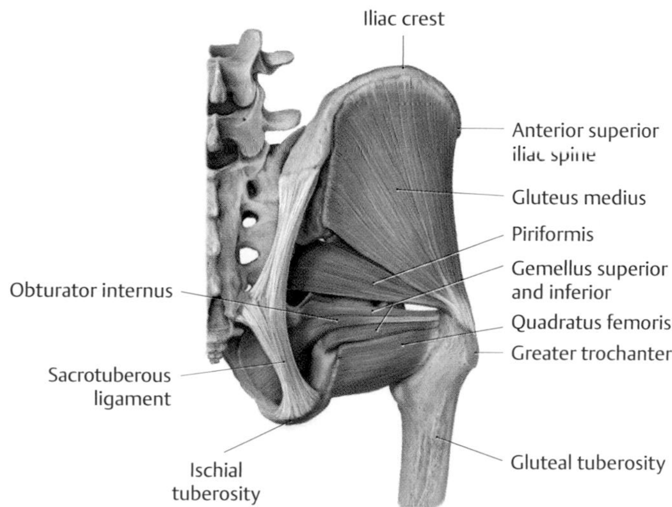
Iliac crest
Anterior superior iliac spine
Gluteus medius
Piriformis
Gemellus superior and inferior
Quadratus femoris
Greater trochanter
Obturator internus
Sacrotuberous ligament
Ischial tuberosity
Gluteal tuberosity

A Deep layer with gluteus maximus removed.

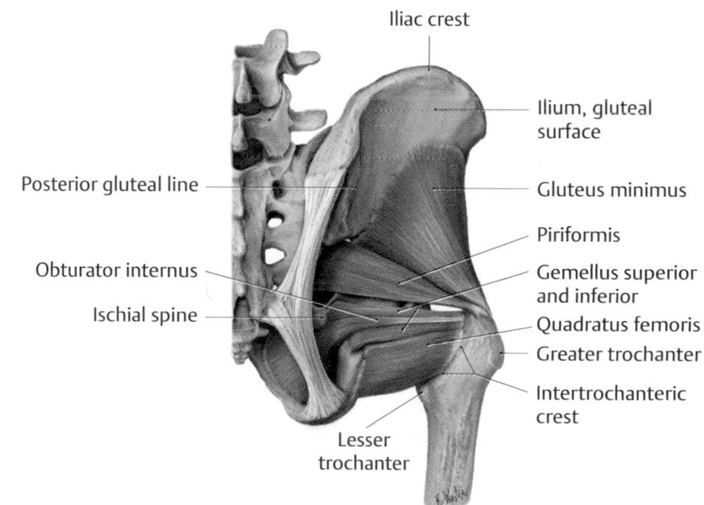
Iliac crest
Ilium, gluteal surface
Posterior gluteal line
Gluteus minimus
Piriformis
Obturator internus
Gemellus superior and inferior
Ischial spine
Quadratus femoris
Greater trochanter
Intertrochanteric crest
Lesser trochanter

B Deep layer with gluteus medius removed.

Muscle Facts (II)

Functionally, the medial thigh muscles are considered the adductors of the hip.

Fig. 26.21 Medial thigh muscles: Superficial layer
Right side, anterior view.

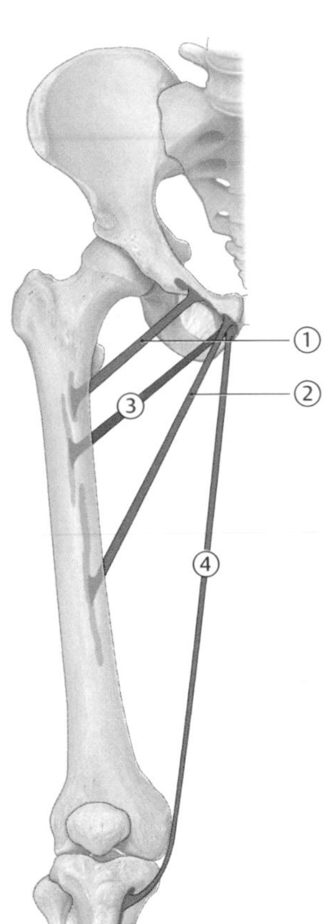
①
②
③
④

A Schematic.

Promontory
Iliac crest
Superior pubic ramus
Greater trochanter
Lesser trochanter
Pectineus
Adductor brevis
Adductor longus
Femur
Gracilis
Patella
Gracilis tendon of insertion
Fibula
Tibia

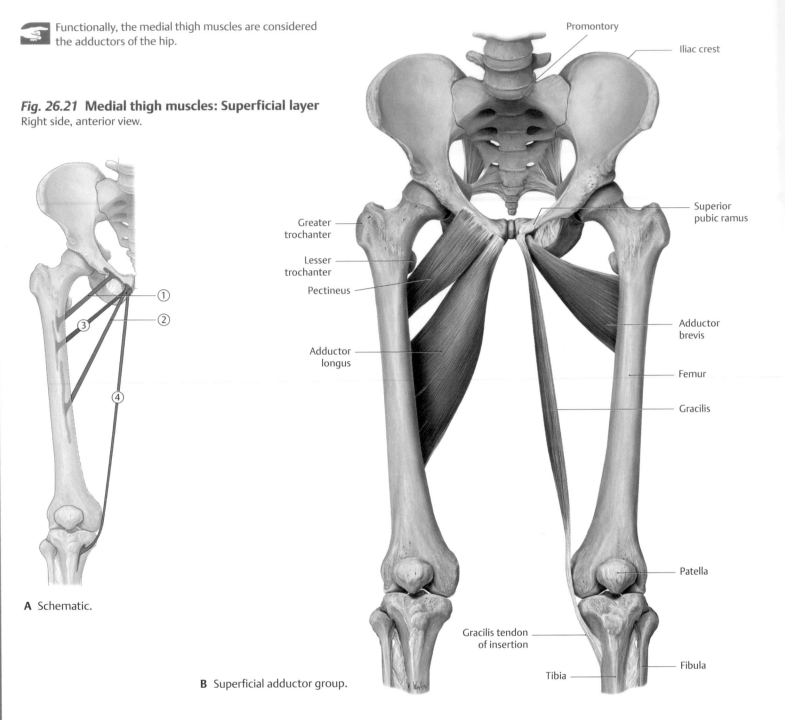

B Superficial adductor group.

Table 26.3 Medial thigh muscles: Superficial layer

Muscle	Origin	Insertion	Innervation	Action
① Pectineus	Pecten pubis	Femur (pectineal line and the proximal linea aspera)	Femoral n., obturator n. (L2, L3)	• Hip joint: adduction, external rotation, and slight flexion • Stabilizes the pelvis in the coronal and sagittal planes
② Adductor longus	Superior pubic ramus and anterior side of the pubic symphysis	Femur (linea aspera, medial lip in the middle third of the femur)	Obturator n. (L2–L4)	• Hip joint: adduction and flexion (up to 70 degrees); extension (past 80 degrees of flexion) • Stabilizes the pelvis in the coronal and sagittal planes
③ Adductor brevis	Inferior pubic ramus		Obturator n. (L2, L3)	
④ Gracilis	Inferior pubic ramus below the pubic symphysis	Tibia (medial border of the tuberosity, along with the tendons of sartorius and semitendinosus)		• Hip joint: adduction and flexion • Knee joint: flexion and internal rotation

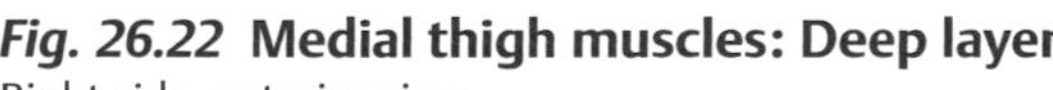
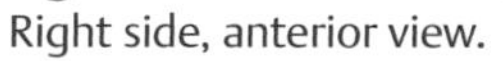

Fig. 26.22 **Medial thigh muscles: Deep layer**
Right side, anterior view.

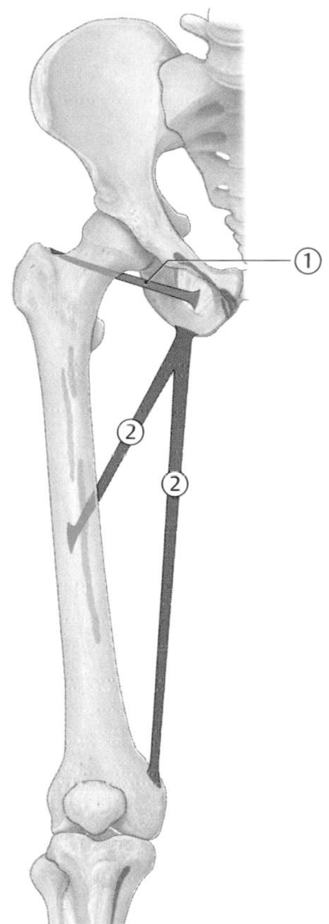
①
②
②

A Schematic.

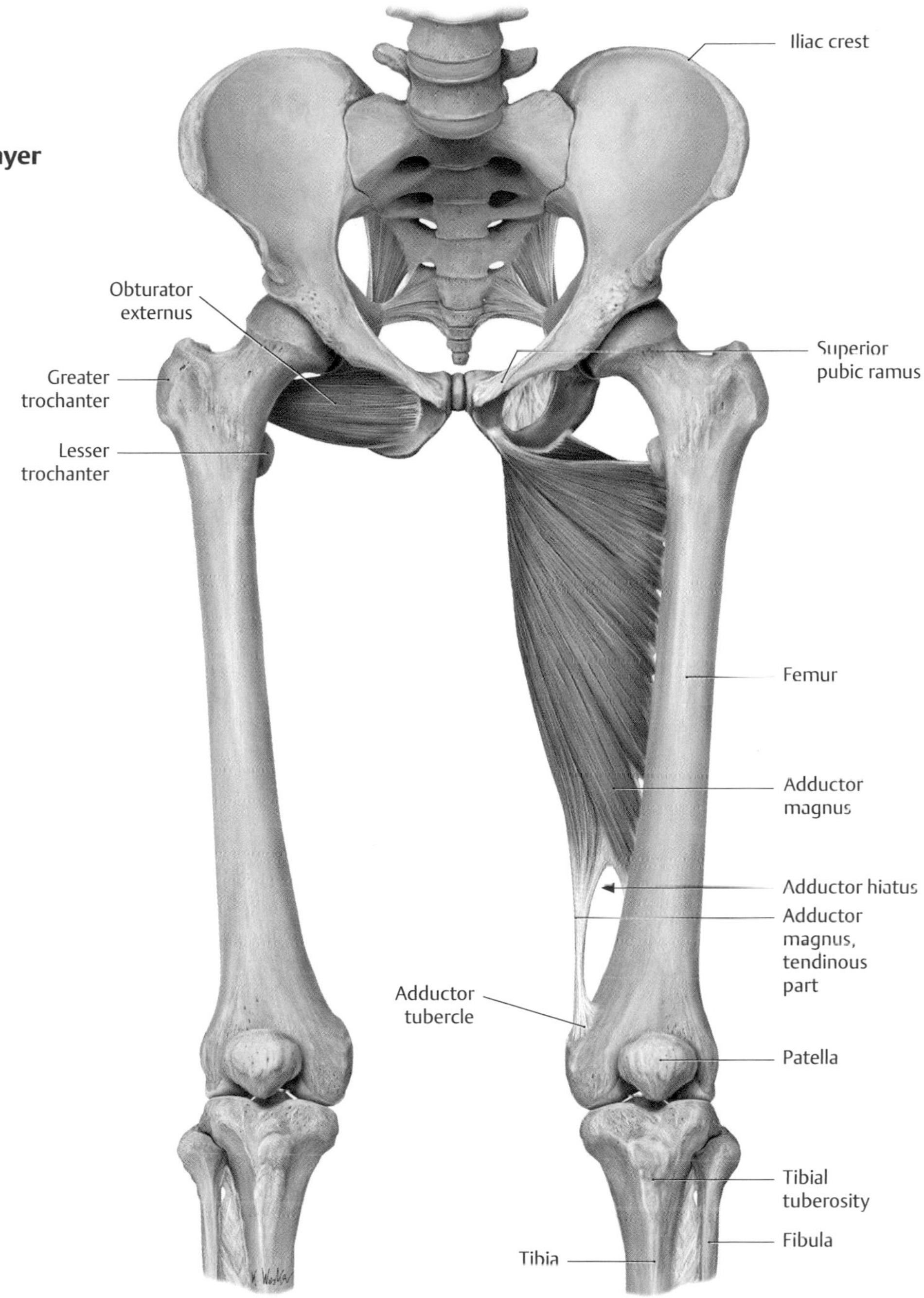

Iliac crest
Obturator externus
Superior pubic ramus
Greater trochanter
Lesser trochanter
Femur
Adductor magnus
Adductor hiatus
Adductor magnus, tendinous part
Adductor tubercle
Patella
Tibial tuberosity
Fibula
Tibia

B Deep adductor group.

Table 26.4 **Medial thigh muscles: Deep layer**

Muscle	Origin	Insertion	Innervation	Action
① Obturator externus	Outer surface of the obturator membrane and its bony boundaries	Trochanteric fossa of the femur	Obturator n. (L3, L4)	• Hip joint: adduction and external rotation • Stabilizes the pelvis in the sagittal plane
② Adductor magnus	Inferior pubic ramus, ischial ramus, and ischial tuberosity	• Deep part ("fleshy insertion"): medial lip of the linea aspera • Superficial part ("tendinous insertion"): adductor tubercle of the femur	• Deep part: obturator n. (L2–L4) • Superficial part: tibial n. (L4)	• Hip joint: adduction, extention, and slight flexion (the tendinous insertion is also active in internal rotation) • Stabilizes the pelvis in the coronal and sagittal plane

Muscle Facts (III)

The anterior and posterior muscles of the thigh can be classified as extensors and flexors, respectively, with regard to the knee joint.

Fig. 26.23 Anterior thigh muscles

Right side, anterior view.

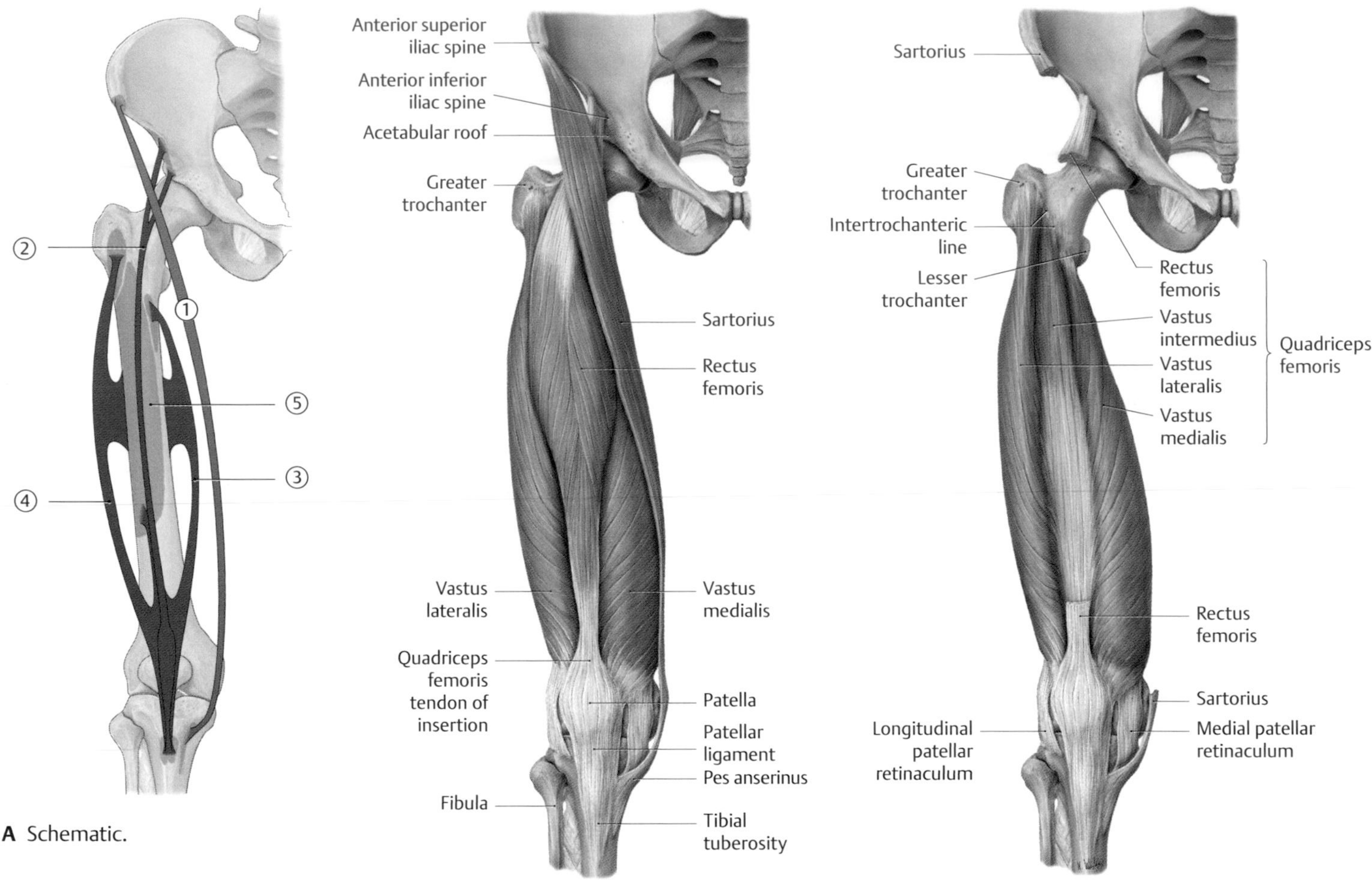

②
①
⑤
③
④
Anterior superior iliac spine
Anterior inferior iliac spine
Acetabular roof
Greater trochanter
Sartorius
Rectus femoris
Vastus lateralis
Vastus medialis
Quadriceps femoris tendon of insertion
Patella
Patellar ligament
Pes anserinus
Fibula
Tibial tuberosity
Sartorius
Greater trochanter
Intertrochanteric line
Lesser trochanter
Rectus femoris
Vastus intermedius
Vastus lateralis
Vastus medialis
Quadriceps femoris
Rectus femoris
Sartorius
Longitudinal patellar retinaculum
Medial patellar retinaculum

A Schematic.

B Superficial group.

C Deep group. *Removed:* Sartorius and rectus femoris.

Table 26.5 Anterior thigh muscles

Muscle		Origin	Insertion	Innervation	Action
① Sartorius		Anterior superior iliac spine	Medial to the tibial tuberosity (together with gracilis and semitendinosus)	Femoral n. (L2, L3)	• Hip joint: flexion, abduction, and external rotation • Knee joint: flexion and internal rotation
Quadriceps femoris*	② Rectus femoris	Anterior inferior iliac spine, acetabular roof of hip joint	Tibial tuberosity (via patellar ligament)	Femoral n. (L2–L4)	• Hip joint: flexion • Knee joint: extension
	③ Vastus medialis	Linea aspera (medial lip), intertrochanteric line (distal part)	Both sides of tuberosity on the medial and lateral condyles (via the medial and longitudinal patellar retinacula)		Knee joint: extension
	④ Vastus lateralis	Linea aspera (lateral lip), greater trochanter (lateral surface)			
	⑤ Vastus intermedius	Femoral shaft (anterior side)	Tibial tuberosity (via patellar ligament)		
	Articularis genus (distal fibers of vastus intermedius)	Anterior side of femoral shaft at level of the suprapatellar recess	Suprapatellar recess of knee joint capsule		Knee joint: extension; prevents entrapment of capsule

*The entire muscle inserts on the tibial tuberosity via the patellar ligament.

Fig. 26.24 **Posterior thigh muscles**
Right side, posterior view.

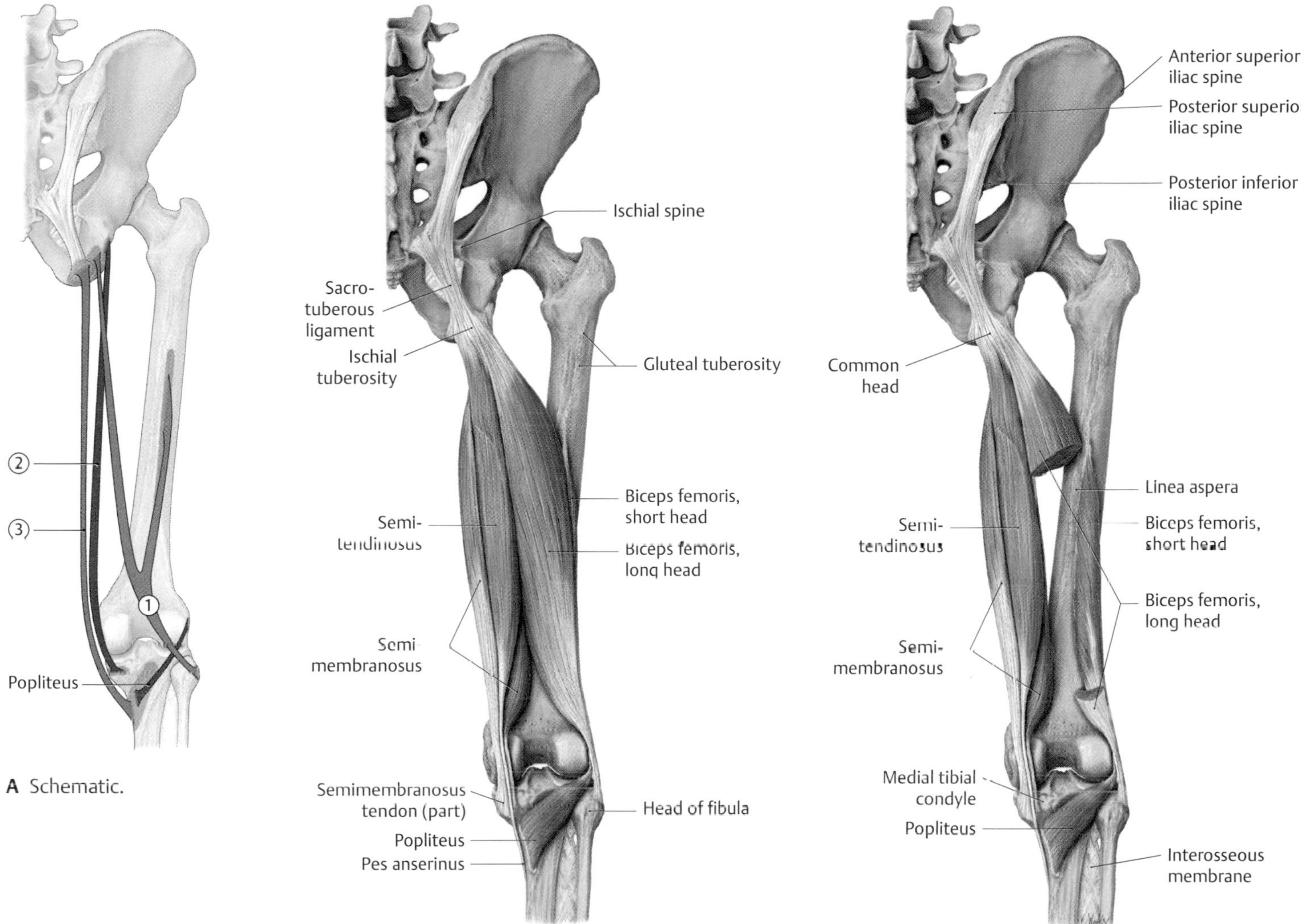
②
③
①
Popliteus
Ischial spine
Sacro-tuberous ligament
Ischial tuberosity
Gluteal tuberosity
Semi-tendinosus
Biceps femoris, short head
Biceps femoris, long head
Semi membranosus
Semimembranosus tendon (part)
Popliteus
Pes anserinus
Head of fibula
Anterior superior iliac spine
Posterior superior iliac spine
Posterior inferior iliac spine
Common head
Linea aspera
Semi-tendinosus
Biceps femoris, short head
Biceps femoris, long head
Semi-membranosus
Medial tibial condyle
Popliteus
Interosseous membrane

A Schematic.

B Superficial group.

C Deep group. *Removed:* Biceps femoris (long head).

Table 26.6 Posterior thigh muscles

Muscle	Origin	Insertion	Innervation	Action
① Biceps femoris	Long head: ischial tuberosity, sacrotuberous ligament (common head with semitendinosus)	Head of fibula	Tibial n. (L5–S2)	• Hip joint (long head): extends the hip, stabilizes the pelvis in the sagittal plane • Knee joint: flexion and external rotation
	Short head: lateral lip of the linea aspera in the middle third of the femur		Common fibular n. (L5–S2)	Knee joint: flexion and external rotation
② Semimembranosus	Ischial tuberosity	Medial tibial condyle, oblique popliteal ligament, popliteus fascia	Tibial n. (L5–S2)	• Hip joint: extends the hip, stabilizes the pelvis in the sagittal plane • Knee joint: flexion and internal rotation
③ Semitendinosus	Ischial tuberosity and sacrotuberous ligament (common head with long head of biceps femoris)	Medial to the tibial tuberosity in the pes anserinus (along with the tendons of gracilis and sartorius)		

See p. 423 for the popliteus.

Tibia & Fibula

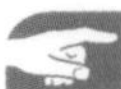

The tibia and fibula articulate at two joints, allowing limited motion (rotation). The crural interosseous membrane is a sheet of tough connective tissue that serves as an origin for several muscles in the leg. It also acts with the tibiofibular syndesmosis to stabilize the ankle joint.

Fig. 27.1 **Tibia and fibula**
Right leg.

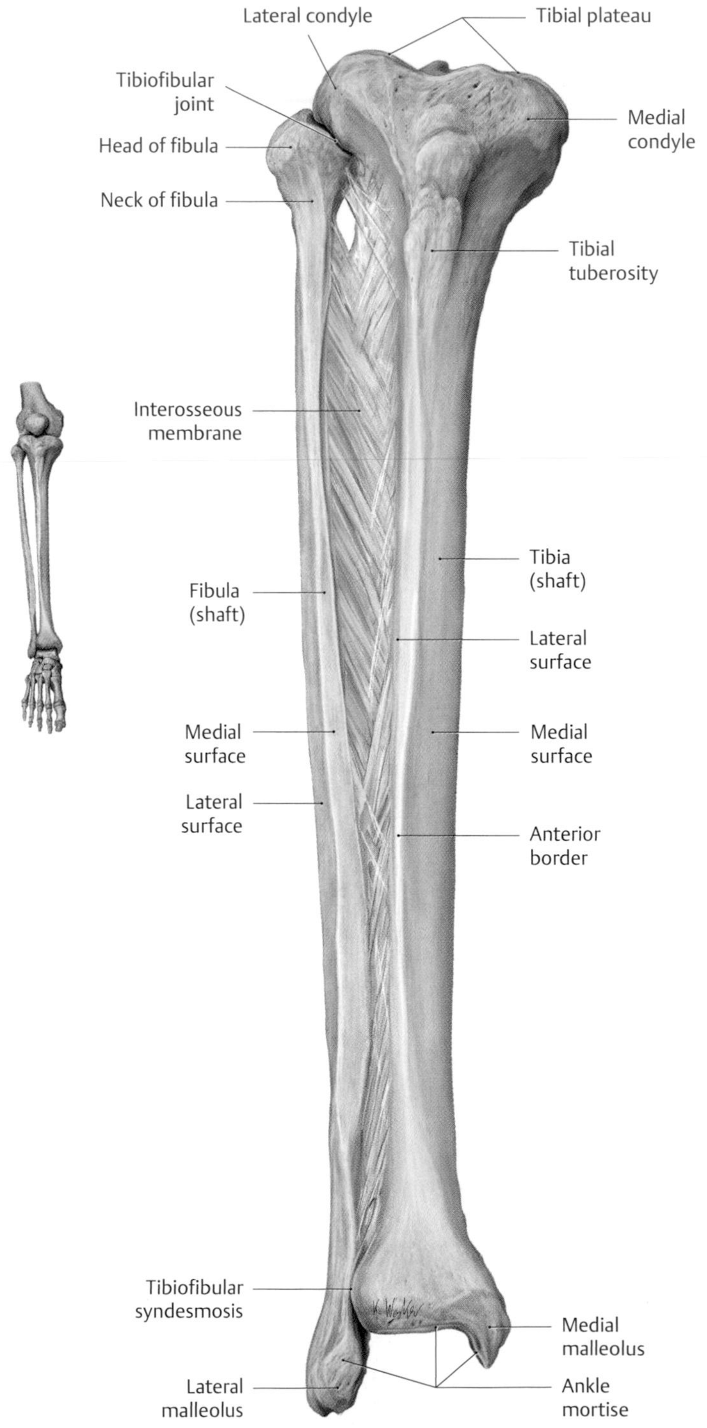

Lateral condyle
Tibial plateau
Tibiofibular joint
Head of fibula
Neck of fibula
Medial condyle
Tibial tuberosity
Interosseous membrane
Fibula (shaft)
Tibia (shaft)
Lateral surface
Medial surface
Medial surface
Lateral surface
Anterior border
Tibiofibular syndesmosis
Medial malleolus
Lateral malleolus
Ankle mortise

A Anterior view.

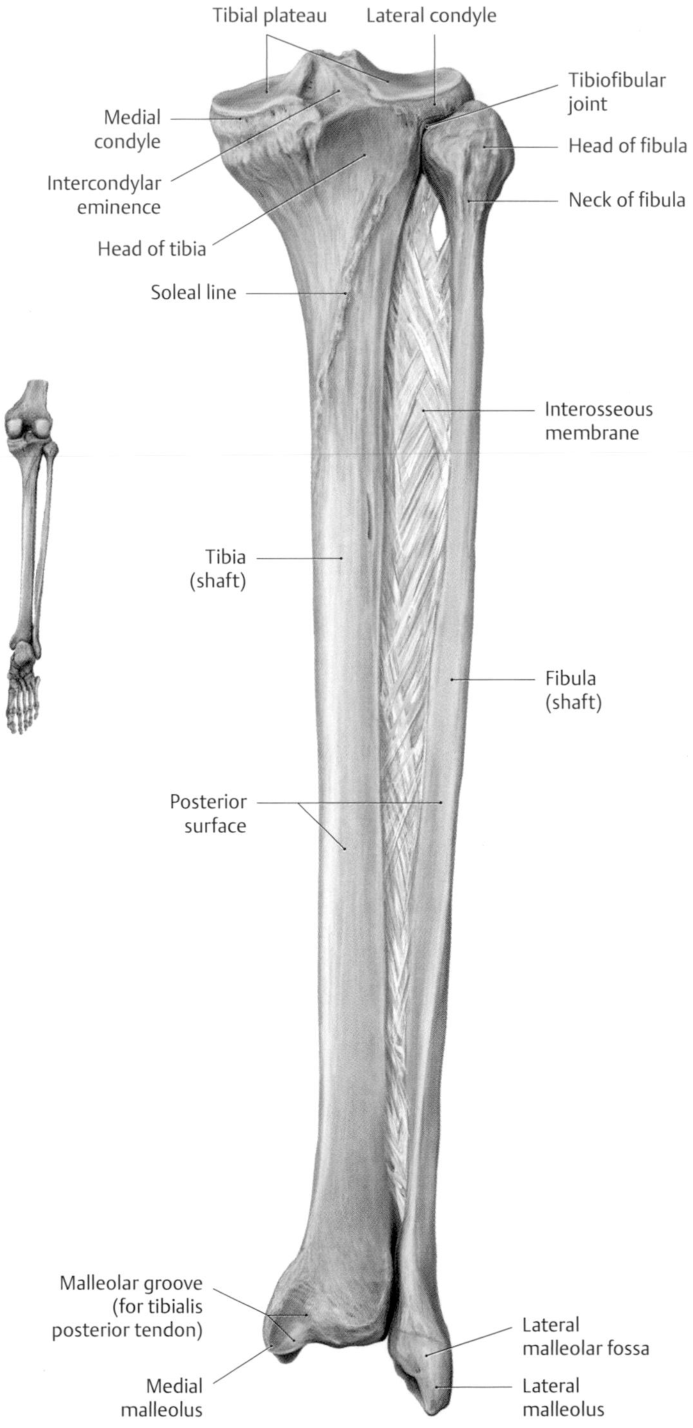

Tibial plateau
Lateral condyle
Tibiofibular joint
Medial condyle
Head of fibula
Intercondylar eminence
Neck of fibula
Head of tibia
Soleal line
Interosseous membrane
Tibia (shaft)
Fibula (shaft)
Posterior surface
Malleolar groove (for tibialis posterior tendon)
Lateral malleolar fossa
Medial malleolus
Lateral malleolus

B Posterior view.

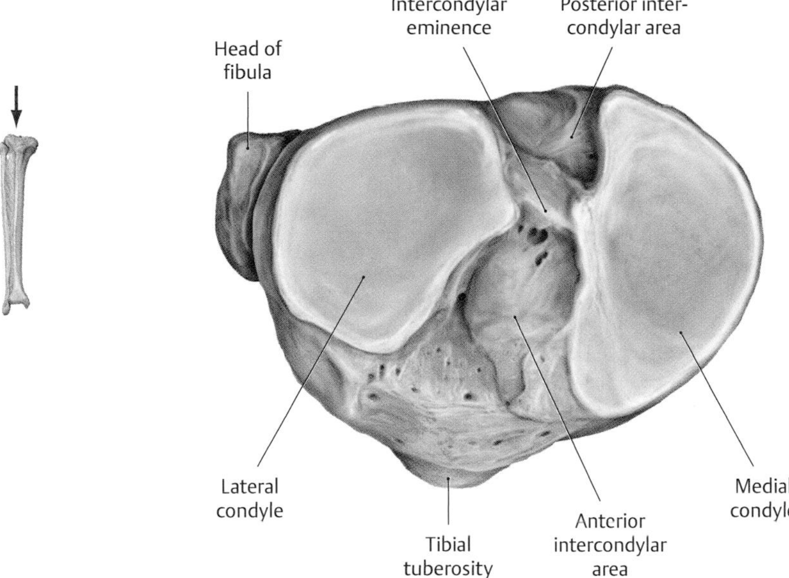
Intercondylar eminence
Posterior intercondylar area
Head of fibula
Lateral condyle
Tibial tuberosity
Anterior intercondylar area
Medial condyle

C Proximal view.

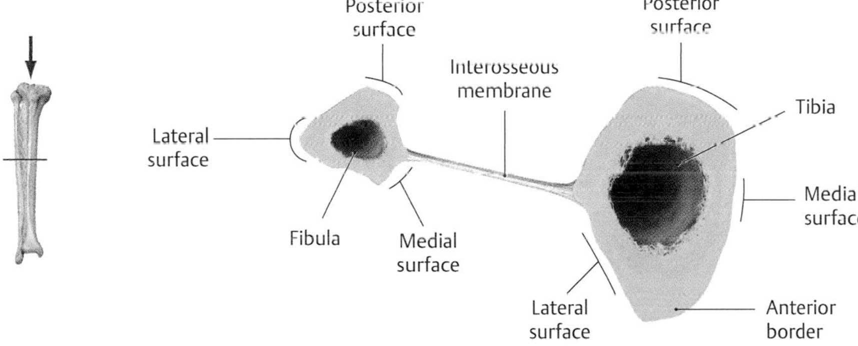
Posterior surface
Interosseous membrane
Posterior surface
Tibia
Lateral surface
Medial surface
Fibula
Medial surface
Lateral surface
Anterior border

D Transverse section, proximal view.

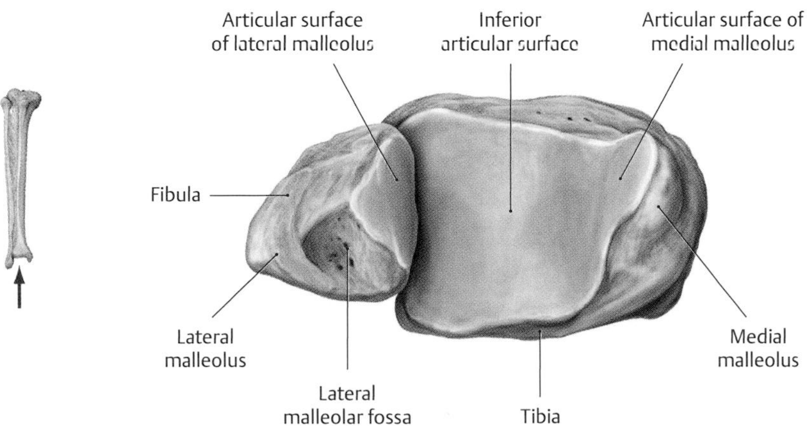
Articular surface of lateral malleolus
Inferior articular surface
Articular surface of medial malleolus
Fibula
Lateral malleolus
Lateral malleolar fossa
Tibia
Medial malleolus

E Distal view.

Clinical

Fibular fracture

When diagnosing a fibular fracture, it is important to determine whether the tibiofibular syndesmosis (see p. 404) is disrupted. Fibular fractures may occur distal to, level with, or proximal to the tibiofibular syndesmosis; the latter two frequently involve tearing of the syndesmosis.

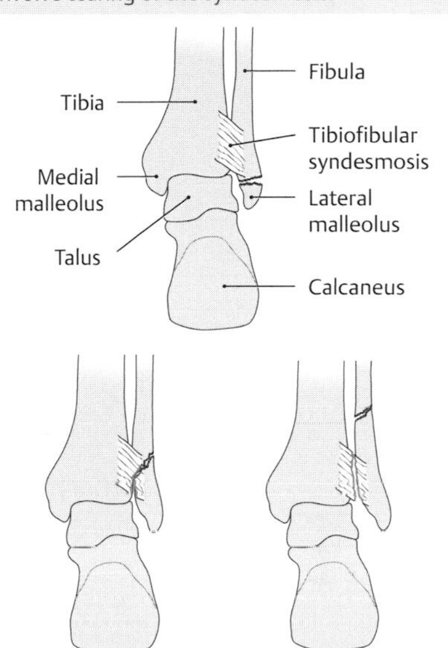
Fibula
Tibia
Tibiofibular syndesmosis
Medial malleolus
Lateral malleolus
Talus
Calcaneus

In this fracture located proximal to the syndesmosis (*arrow*), the syndesmosis is torn, as indicated by the widened medial joint space of the upper ankle joint (see pp. 428–429).

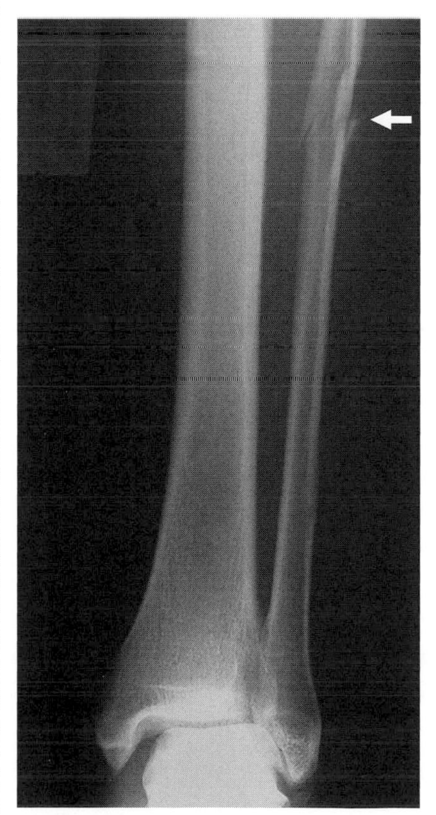

Knee Joint: Overview

In the knee joint, the femur articulates with the tibia and patella. Both joints are contained within a common capsule and have communicating articular cavities. *Note:* The fibula is not included in the knee joint (contrast to the humerus in the elbow; see p. 306). Instead, it forms a separate rigid articulation with the tibia.

Fig. 27.2 **Right knee joint**

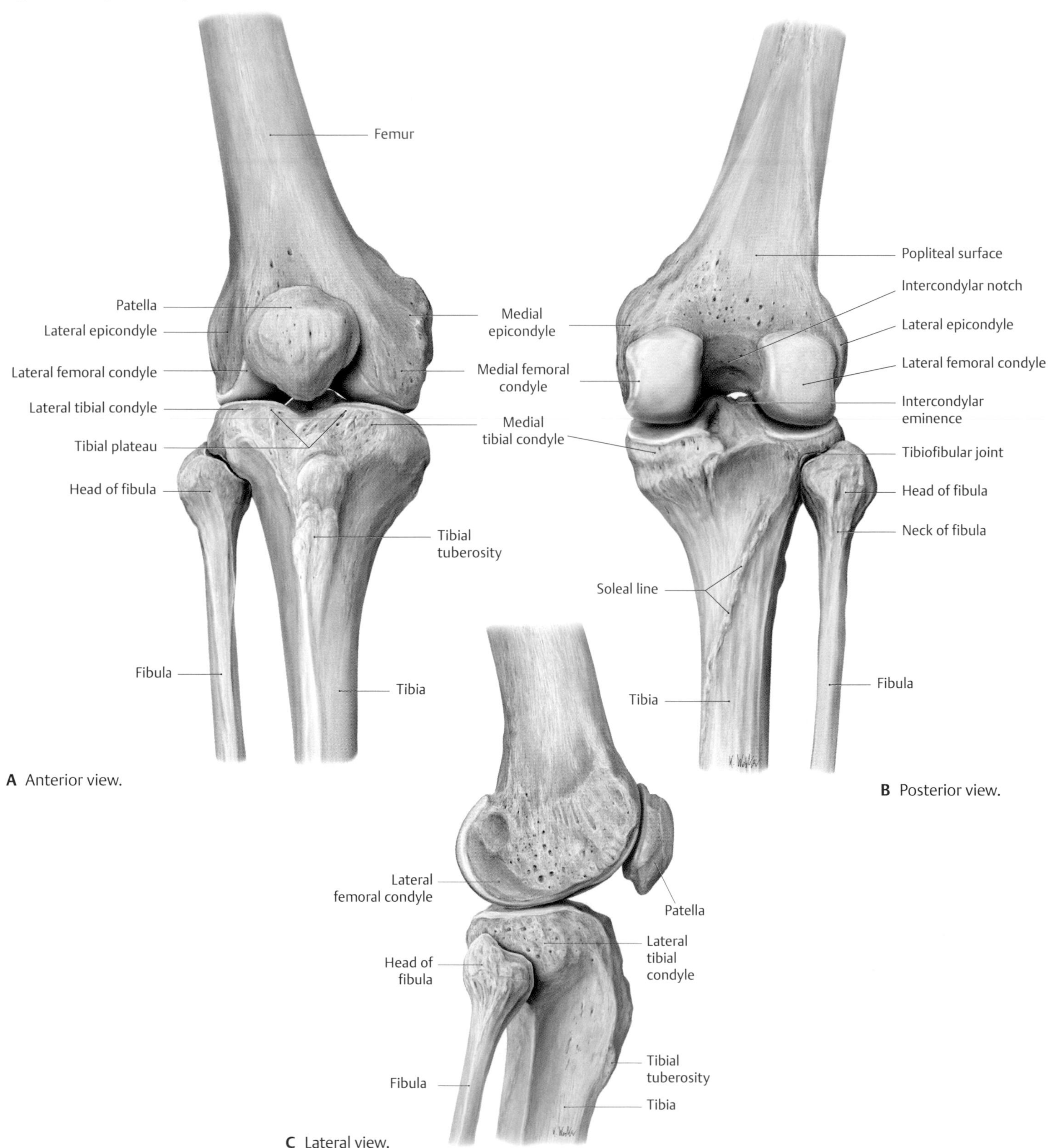
Femur
Patella
Lateral epicondyle
Lateral femoral condyle
Lateral tibial condyle
Tibial plateau
Head of fibula
Medial epicondyle
Medial femoral condyle
Medial tibial condyle
Tibial tuberosity
Fibula
Tibia
Popliteal surface
Intercondylar notch
Lateral epicondyle
Lateral femoral condyle
Intercondylar eminence
Tibiofibular joint
Head of fibula
Neck of fibula
Soleal line
Tibia
Fibula
Lateral femoral condyle
Patella
Head of fibula
Lateral tibial condyle
Fibula
Tibial tuberosity
Tibia

A Anterior view.

B Posterior view.

C Lateral view.

Fig. 27.3 Knee joint: Radiographs

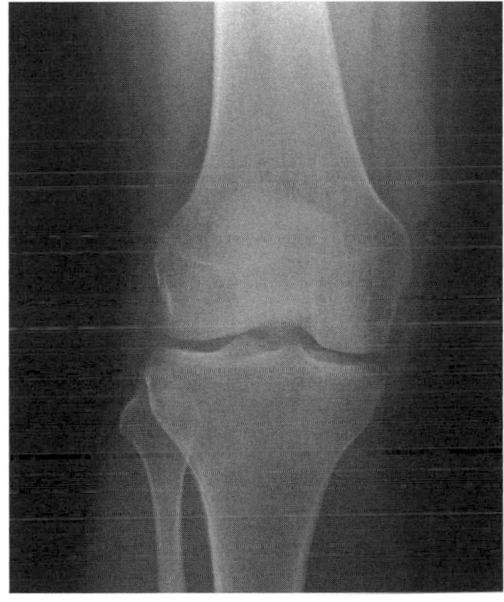

A Anteroposterior projection.

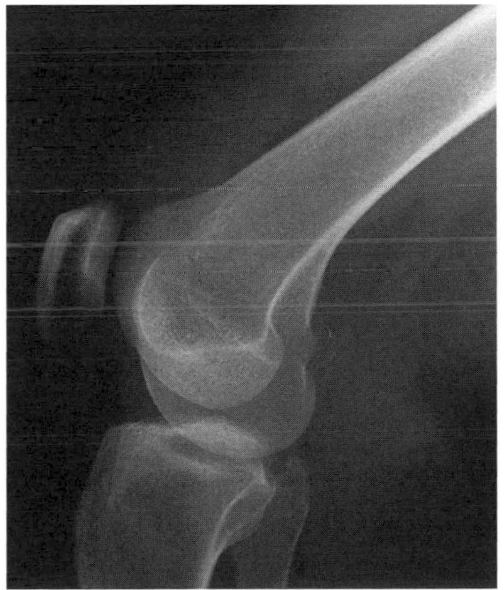

B Lateral projection.

Fig. 27.4 Patella

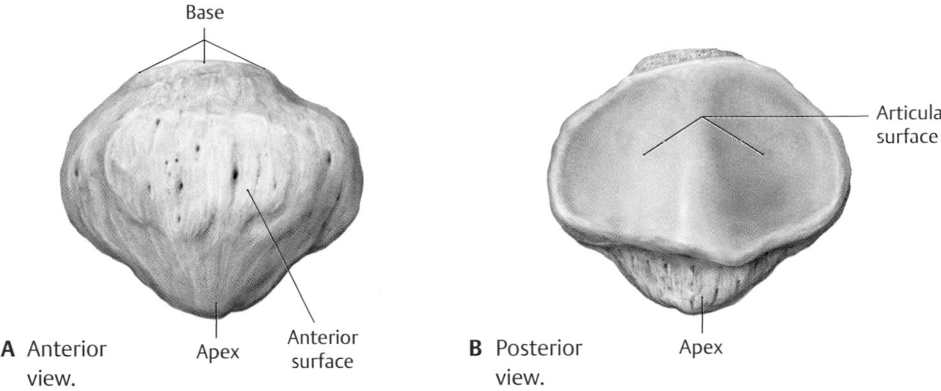
Base
Apex
Anterior surface
Articular surface
Apex

A Anterior view.

B Posterior view.

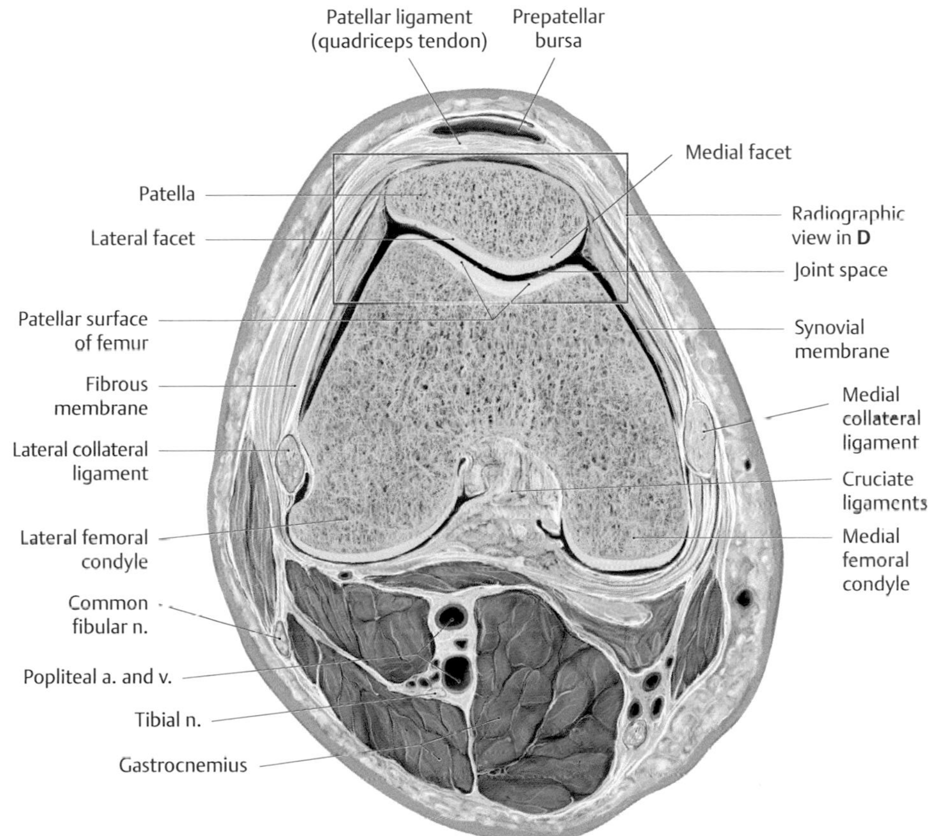
Patellar ligament (quadriceps tendon)
Prepatellar bursa
Medial facet
Patella
Lateral facet
Radiographic view in D
Joint space
Patellar surface of femur
Synovial membrane
Fibrous membrane
Medial collateral ligament
Lateral collateral ligament
Cruciate ligaments
Lateral femoral condyle
Medial femoral condyle
Common fibular n.
Popliteal a. and v.
Tibial n.
Gastrocnemius

C Transverse section through femoropatellar joint. Distal view with right knee in slight flexion.

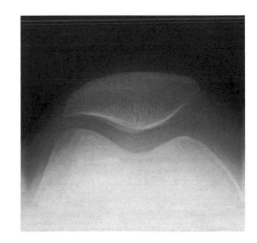

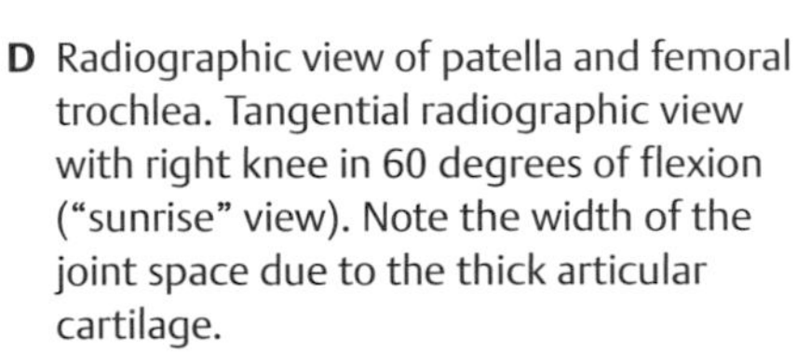

D Radiographic view of patella and femoral trochlea. Tangential radiographic view with right knee in 60 degrees of flexion ("sunrise" view). Note the width of the joint space due to the thick articular cartilage.

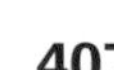

Knee Joint: Capsule, Ligaments & Bursae

Table 27.1	**Ligaments of the knee joint**
Extrinsic ligaments	
Anterior side	Patellar ligament
	Medial longitudinal patellar retinaculum
	Lateral longitudinal patellar retinaculum
	Medial transverse patellar retinaculum
	Lateral transverse patellar retinaculum
Medial and lateral sides	Medial (tibial) collateral ligament
	Lateral (fibular) collateral ligament
Posterior side	Oblique popliteal ligament
	Arcuate popliteal ligament
Intrinsic ligaments	
Anterior cruciate ligament	
Posterior cruciate ligament	
Transverse ligament of knee	
Posterior meniscofemoral ligament	

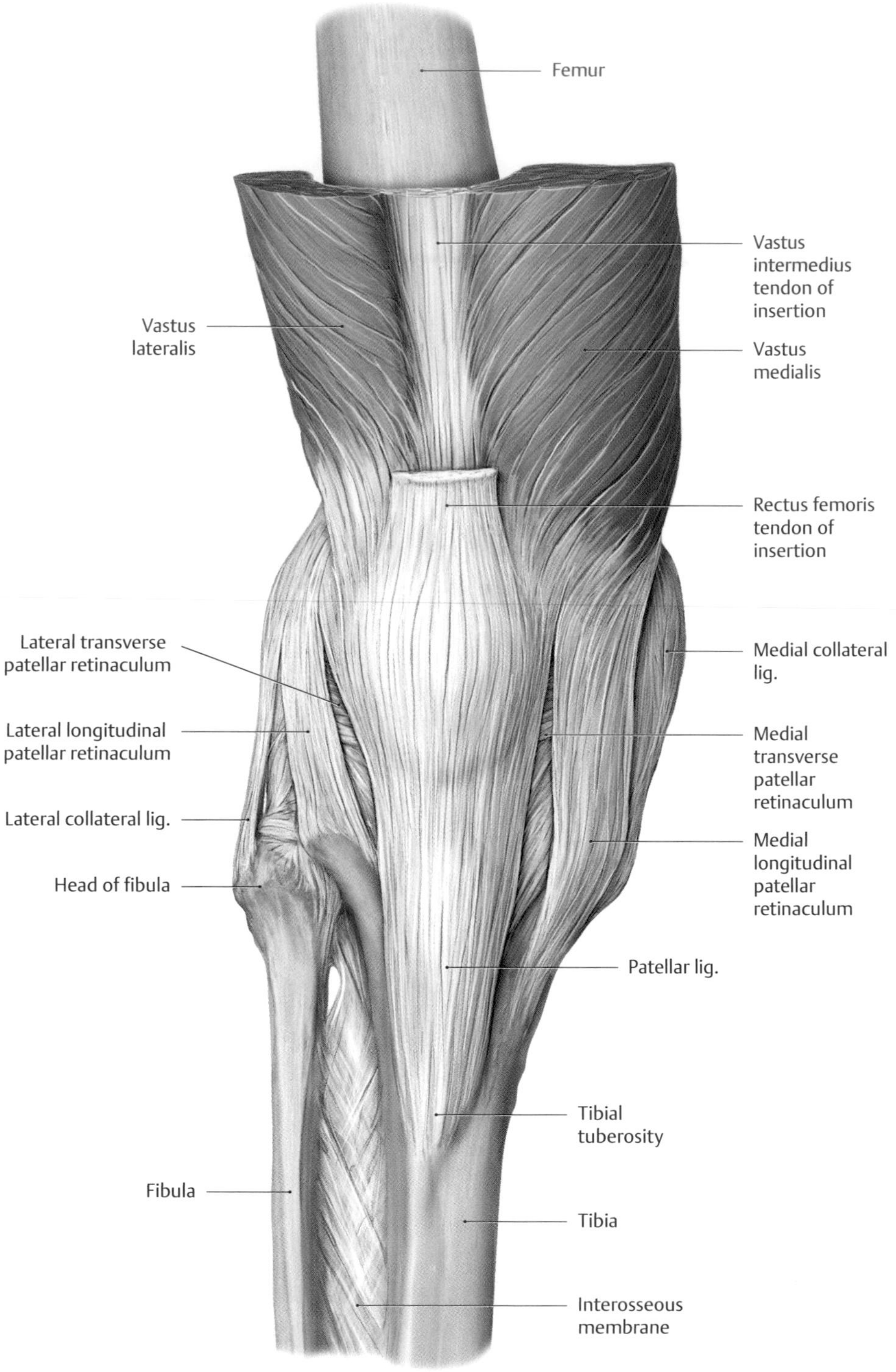

Fig. 27.5 **Ligaments of the knee joint**
Anterior view of right knee.

Femur
Vastus intermedius tendon of insertion
Vastus lateralis
Vastus medialis
Rectus femoris tendon of insertion
Lateral transverse patellar retinaculum
Medial collateral lig.
Lateral longitudinal patellar retinaculum
Medial transverse patellar retinaculum
Lateral collateral lig.
Medial longitudinal patellar retinaculum
Head of fibula
Patellar lig.
Tibial tuberosity
Fibula
Tibia
Interosseous membrane

Fig. 27.6 **Capsule, ligaments, and periarticular bursae**
Posterior view of right knee. The joint cavity communicates with periarticular bursae at the subpopliteal recess, semimembranosus bursa, and medial subtendinous bursa of the gastrocnemius.

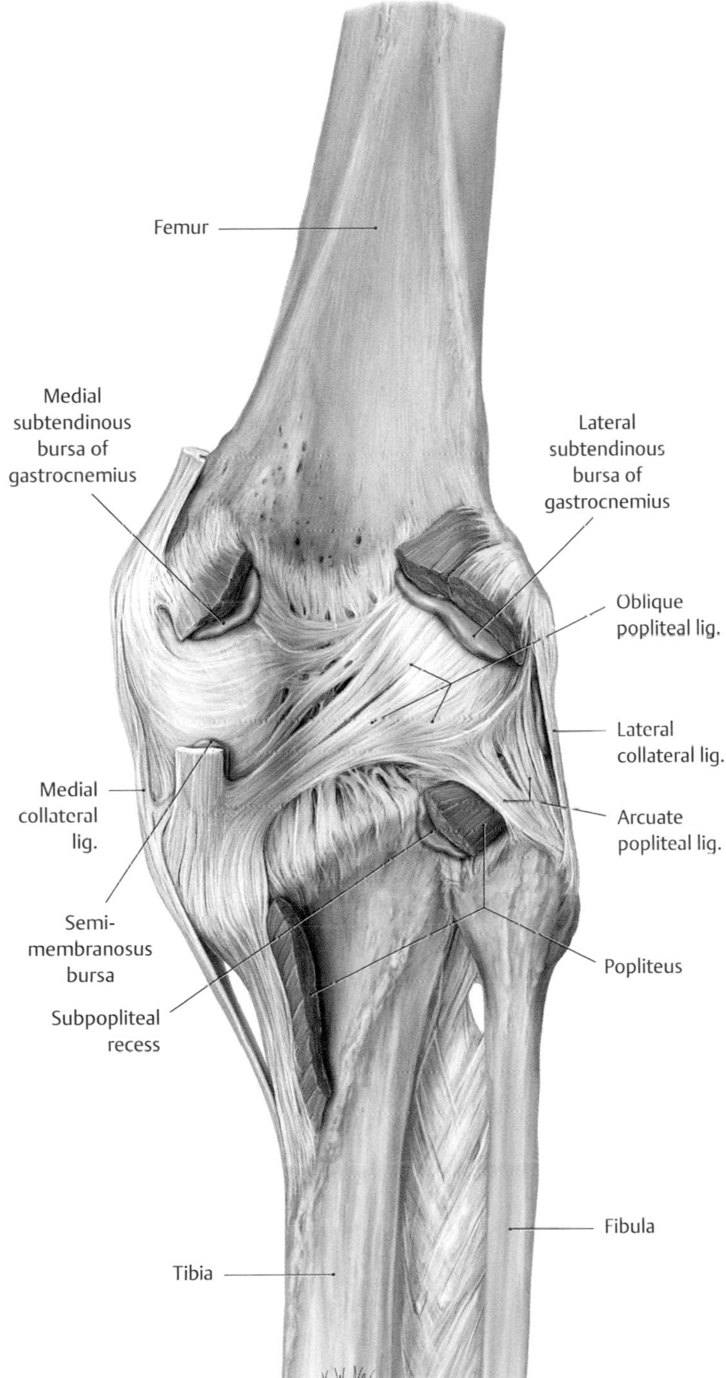

Femur
Medial subtendinous bursa of gastrocnemius
Lateral subtendinous bursa of gastrocnemius
Oblique popliteal lig.
Lateral collateral lig.
Medial collateral lig.
Arcuate popliteal lig.
Semimembranosus bursa
Popliteus
Subpopliteal recess
Fibula
Tibia

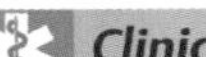

Clinical

Gastrocnemio-semimembranosus bursa (Baker's cyst)
Painful swelling behind the knee may be caused by a cystic outpouching of the joint capsule (synovial popliteal cyst). This frequently results from an increase in intra-articular pressure (e.g., in rheumatoid arthritis).

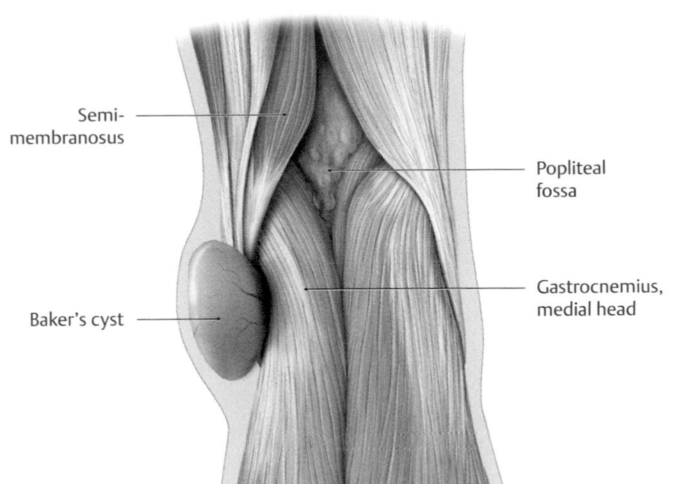

Semimembranosus
Popliteal fossa
Gastrocnemius, medial head
Baker's cyst

A Baker's cyst in the right popliteal fossa. Baker's cysts often occur in the medial part of the popliteal fossa between the semimembranosus tendon and the medial head of the gastrocnemius at the level of the posteromedial femoral condyle.

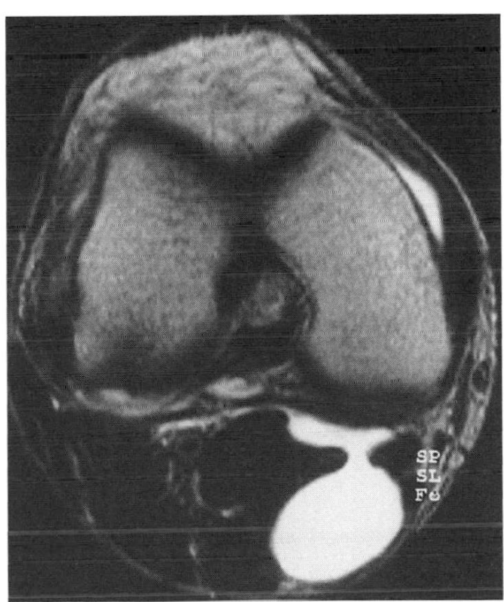

B Axial MRI of a Baker's cyst in the popliteal fossa, inferior view.

Knee Joint: Ligaments & Menisci

***Fig. 27.7* Collateral and patellar ligaments of the knee joint**
Right knee joint. Each knee joint has medial and lateral collateral ligaments. The medial collateral ligament is attached to both the capsule and the medial meniscus, whereas the lateral collateral ligament has no direct contact with either the capsule or the lateral meniscus. Both collateral ligaments are taut when the knee is in extension and stabilize the joint in the coronal plane.

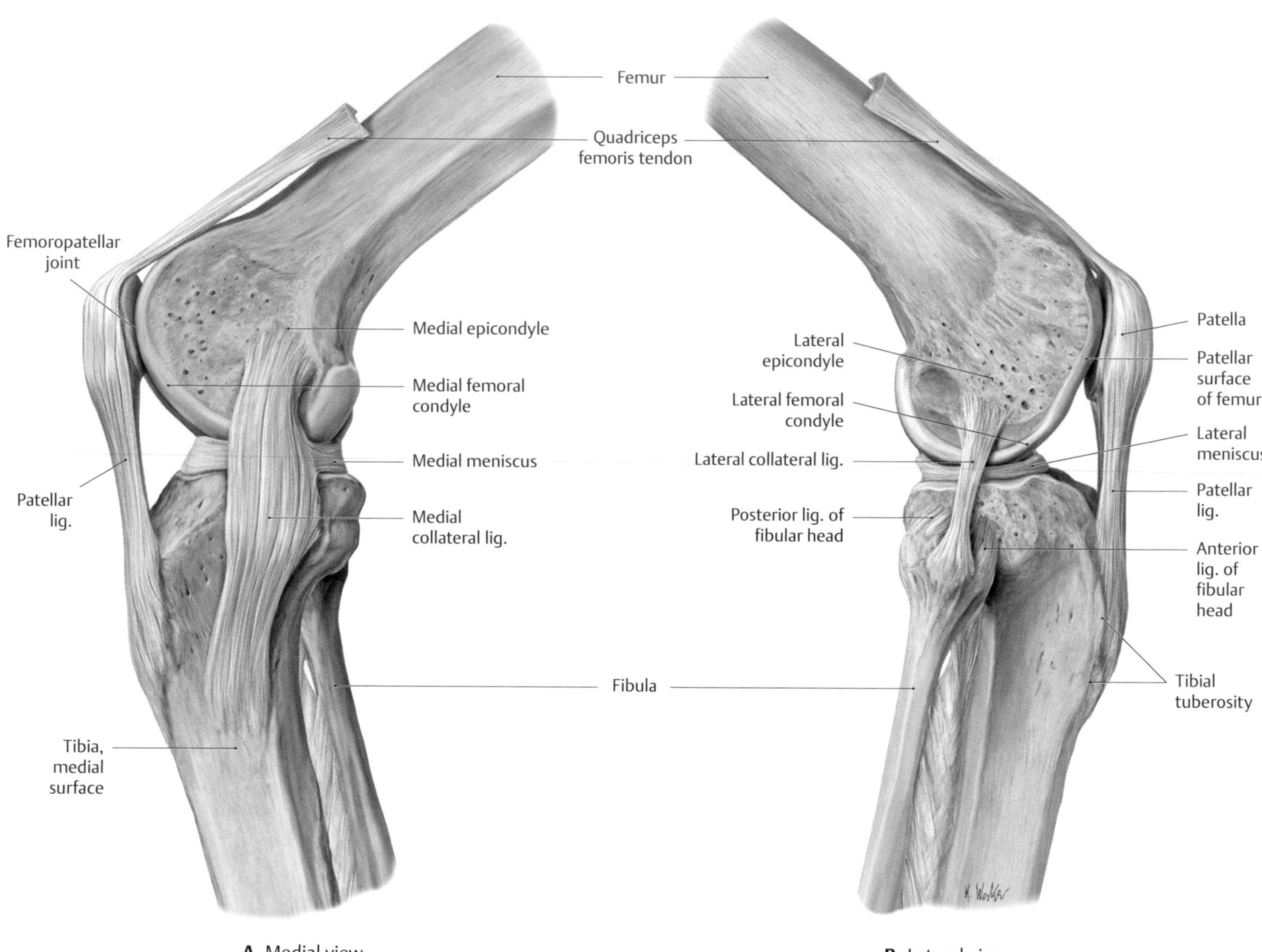
Femur
Quadriceps femoris tendon
Femoropatellar joint
Medial epicondyle
Medial femoral condyle
Medial meniscus
Patellar lig.
Medial collateral lig.
Fibula
Tibia, medial surface
Patella
Lateral epicondyle
Patellar surface of femur
Lateral femoral condyle
Lateral meniscus
Lateral collateral lig.
Patellar lig.
Posterior lig. of fibular head
Anterior lig. of fibular head
Tibial tuberosity

A Medial view.

B Lateral view.

Fig. 27.8 Menisci in the knee joint

Right tibial plateau, proximal view.

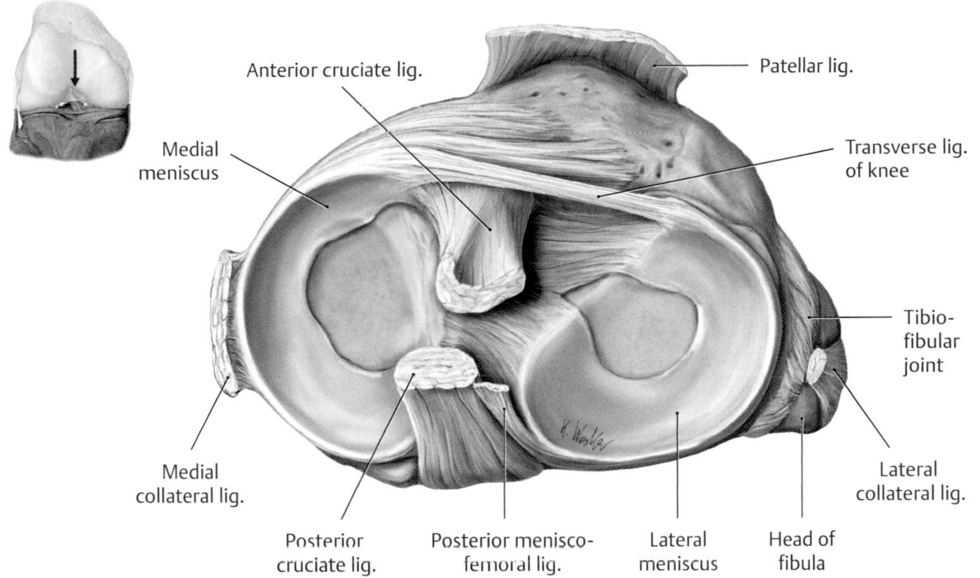

Anterior cruciate lig.
Patellar lig.
Medial meniscus
Transverse lig. of knee
Tibio-fibular joint
Medial collateral lig.
Lateral collateral lig.
Posterior cruciate lig.
Posterior menisco-femoral lig.
Lateral meniscus
Head of fibula

A Right tibial plateau with cruciate, patellar, and collateral ligaments divided.

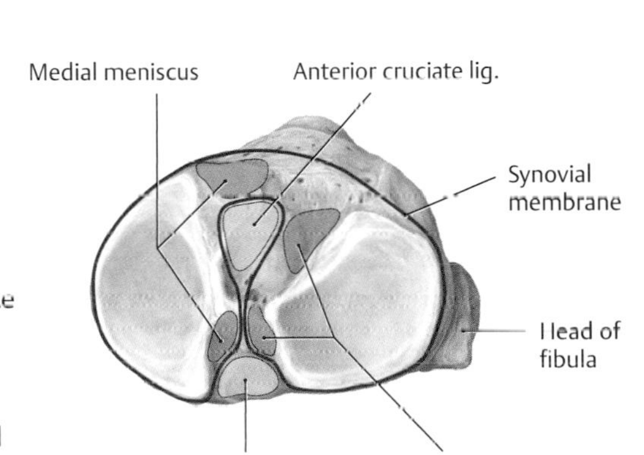
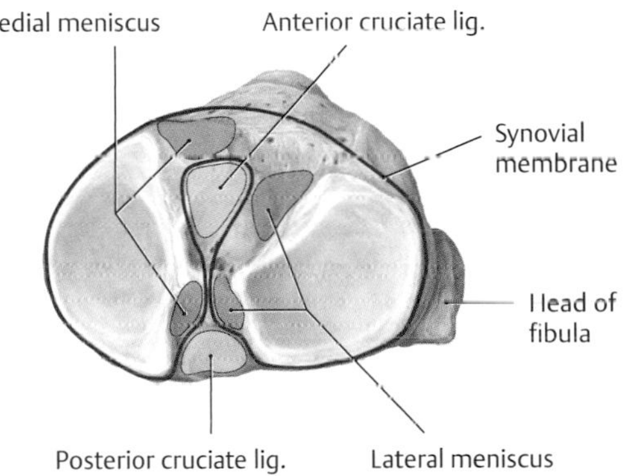

Medial meniscus
Anterior cruciate lig.
Synovial membrane
Head of fibula
Posterior cruciate lig.
Lateral meniscus

B Attachment sites of menisci and cruciate ligaments. Red line indicates the tibial attachment of the synovial membrane that covers the cruciate ligaments. The cruciate ligaments lie in the subsynovial connective tissue.

Clinical

Injury to the menisci

The less mobile medial meniscus is more susceptible to injury than the lateral meniscus. Trauma generally results from sudden extension or rotation of the flexed knee while the leg is fixed.

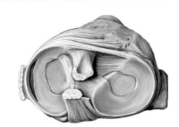

A Bucket-handle tear.

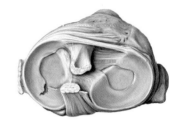

B Radial tear of posterior horn.

Fig. 27.9 Movements of the menisci

Right knee joint.

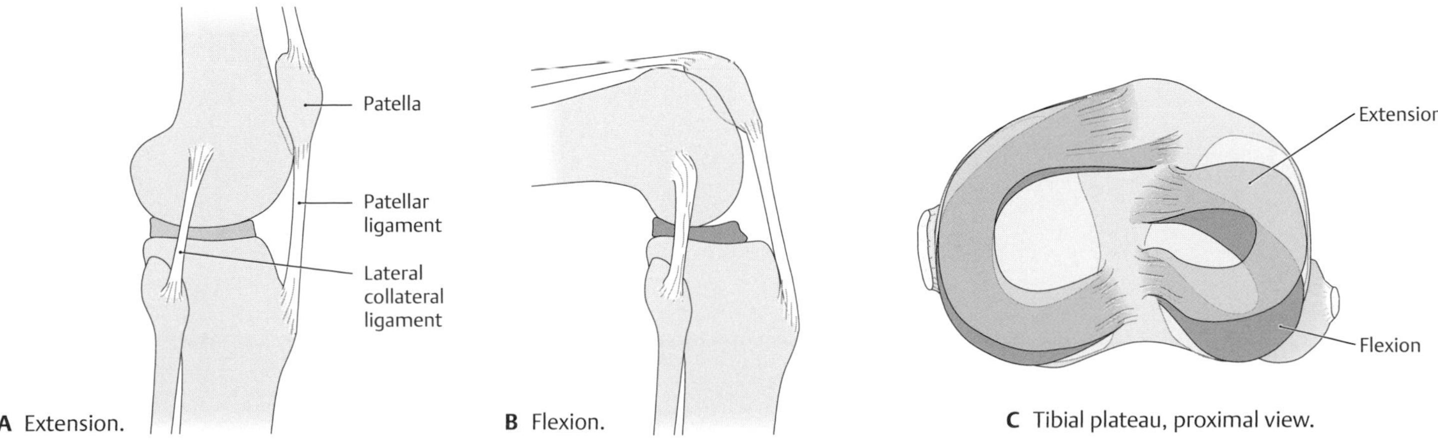

Patella
Patellar ligament
Lateral collateral ligament
Extension
Flexion

A Extension. **B** Flexion. **C** Tibial plateau, proximal view.

Cruciate Ligaments

Fig. 27.10 **Cruciate and collateral ligaments**

Right knee joint. The cruciate ligaments keep the articular surfaces of the femur and tibia in contact, while stabilizing the knee joint primarily in the sagittal plane. Portions of the cruciate ligaments are taut in every joint position.

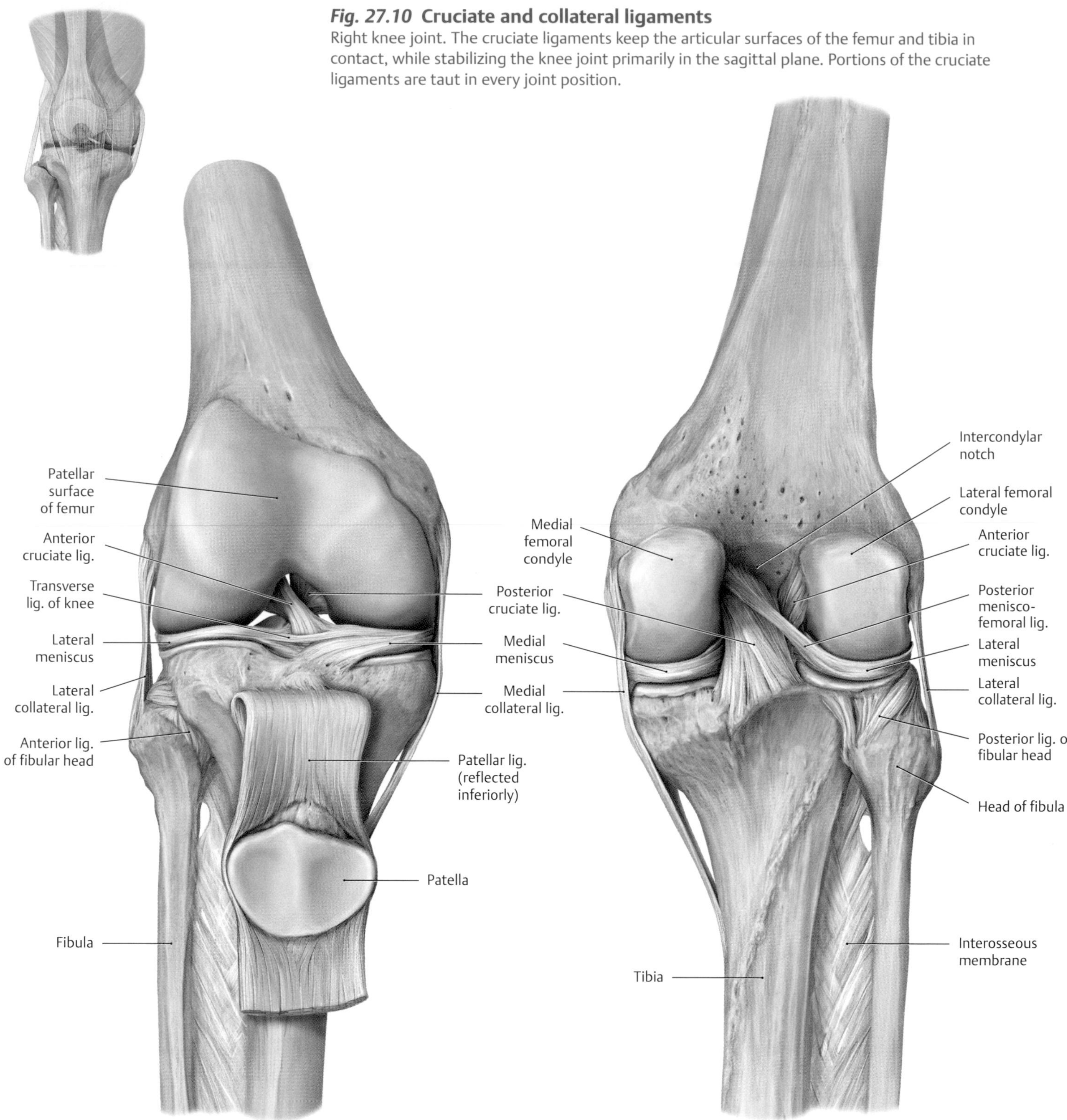
Patellar surface of femur
Anterior cruciate lig.
Transverse lig. of knee
Lateral meniscus
Lateral collateral lig.
Anterior lig. of fibular head
Fibula
Posterior cruciate lig.
Medial meniscus
Medial collateral lig.
Patellar lig. (reflected inferiorly)
Patella
Medial femoral condyle
Posterior cruciate lig.
Medial meniscus
Medial collateral lig.
Tibia
Intercondylar notch
Lateral femoral condyle
Anterior cruciate lig.
Posterior menisco-femoral lig.
Lateral meniscus
Lateral collateral lig.
Posterior lig. of fibular head
Head of fibula
Interosseous membrane

A Anterior view.

B Posterior view.

Fig. 27.11 Right knee joint in flexion
Anterior view with joint capsule and patella removed.

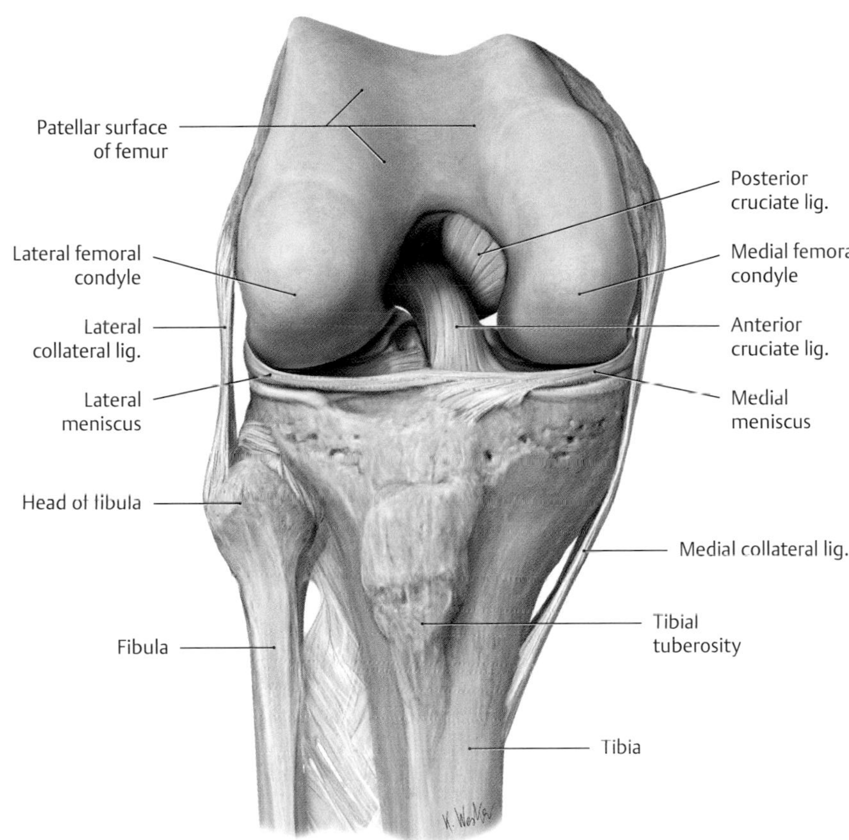
Patellar surface of femur
Posterior cruciate lig.
Lateral femoral condyle
Medial femoral condyle
Lateral collateral lig.
Anterior cruciate lig.
Lateral meniscus
Medial meniscus
Head of fibula
Medial collateral lig.
Fibula
Tibial tuberosity
Tibia

Fig. 27.12 Cruciate and collateral ligaments in flexion and extension
Right knee, anterior view. Taut ligament fibers in red.

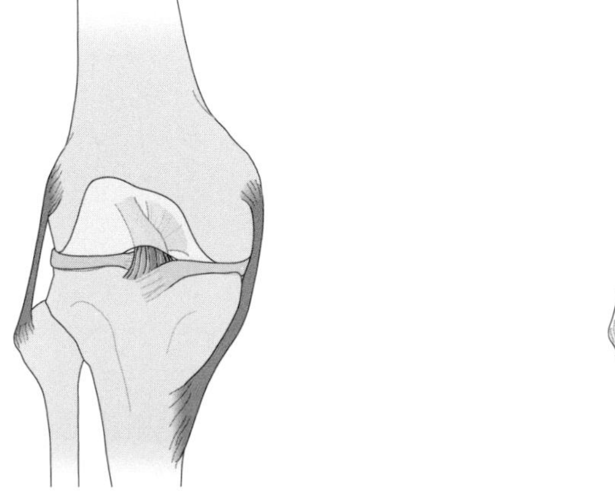

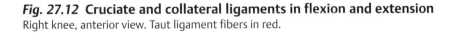

A Extension.

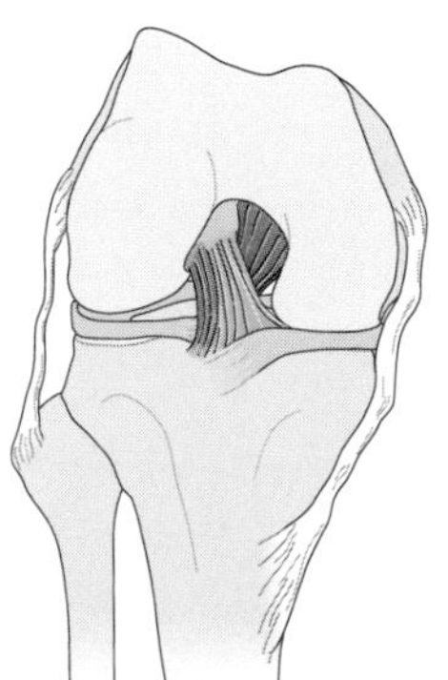

B Flexion.

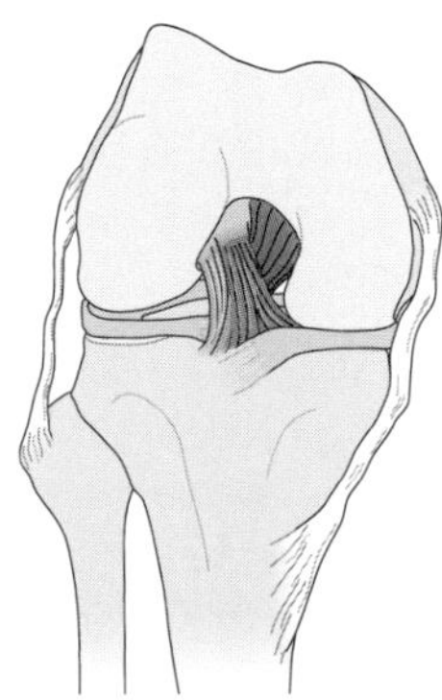

C Flexion and internal rotation.

Clinical

Rupture of cruciate ligaments
Cruciate ligament rupture destabilizes the knee joint, allowing the tibia to move forward (anterior "drawer sign") or backward (posterior "drawer sign") relative to the femur. *Anterior* cruciate ligament ruptures are approximately 10 times more common than posterior ligament ruptures. The most common mechanism of injury is an internal rotation trauma with the leg fixed. A lateral blow to the fully extended knee with the foot planted tends to cause concomitant rupture of the anterior cruciate and medial collateral ligaments, as well as tearing of the attached medial meniscus.

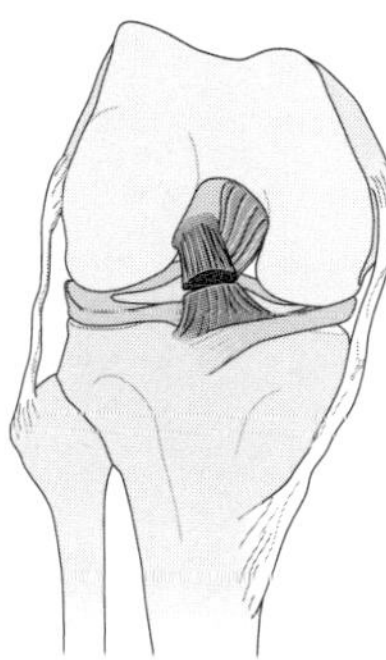

A Right knee in flexion, rupture of anterior cruciate ligament, anterior view.

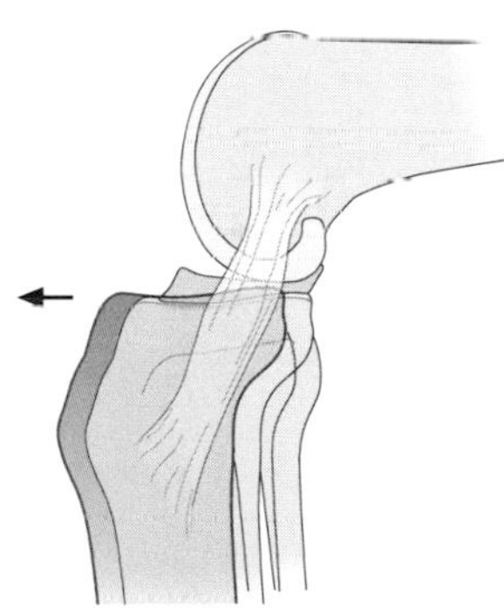

B Right knee in flexion, "anterior drawer sign," medial view. During examination of the flexed knee, the tibia can be pulled forward.

Knee Joint Cavity

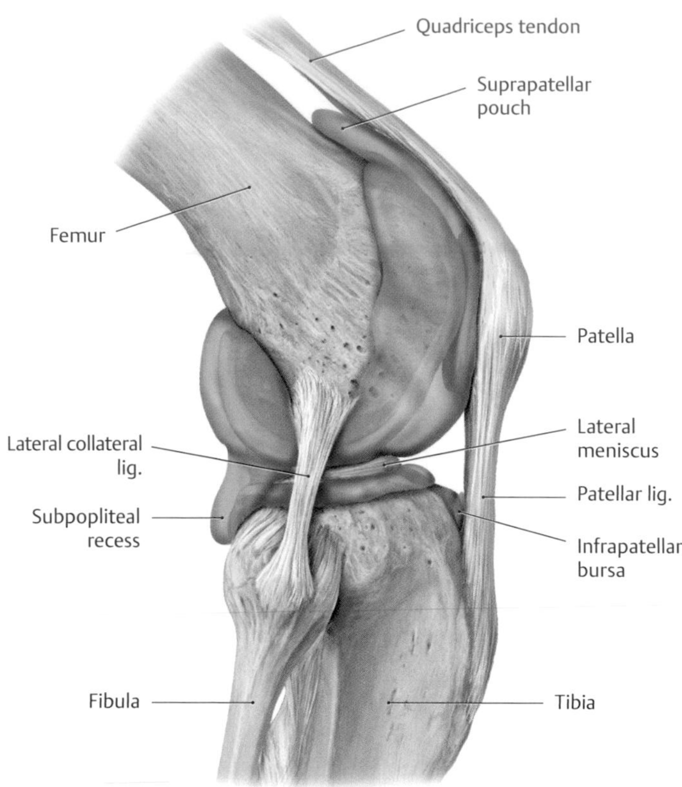
Quadriceps tendon
Suprapatellar pouch
Femur
Patella
Lateral collateral lig.
Lateral meniscus
Patellar lig.
Subpopliteal recess
Infrapatellar bursa
Fibula
Tibia

Fig. 27.13 **Joint cavity**
Right knee, lateral view. The joint cavity was demonstrated by injecting liquid plastic into the knee joint and later removing the capsule.

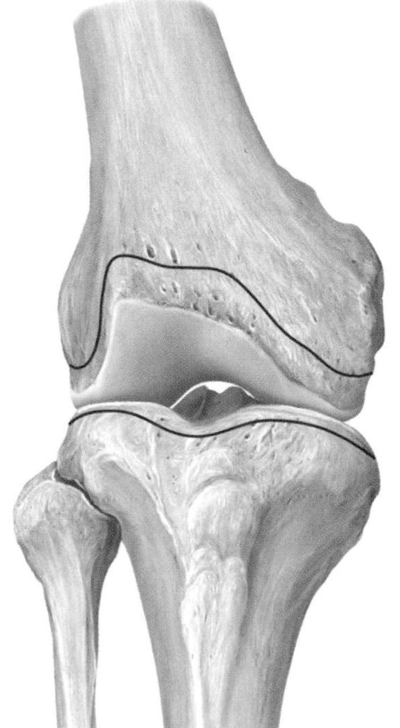

Fig. 27.15 **Attachments of the joint capsule**
Right knee joint, anterior view.

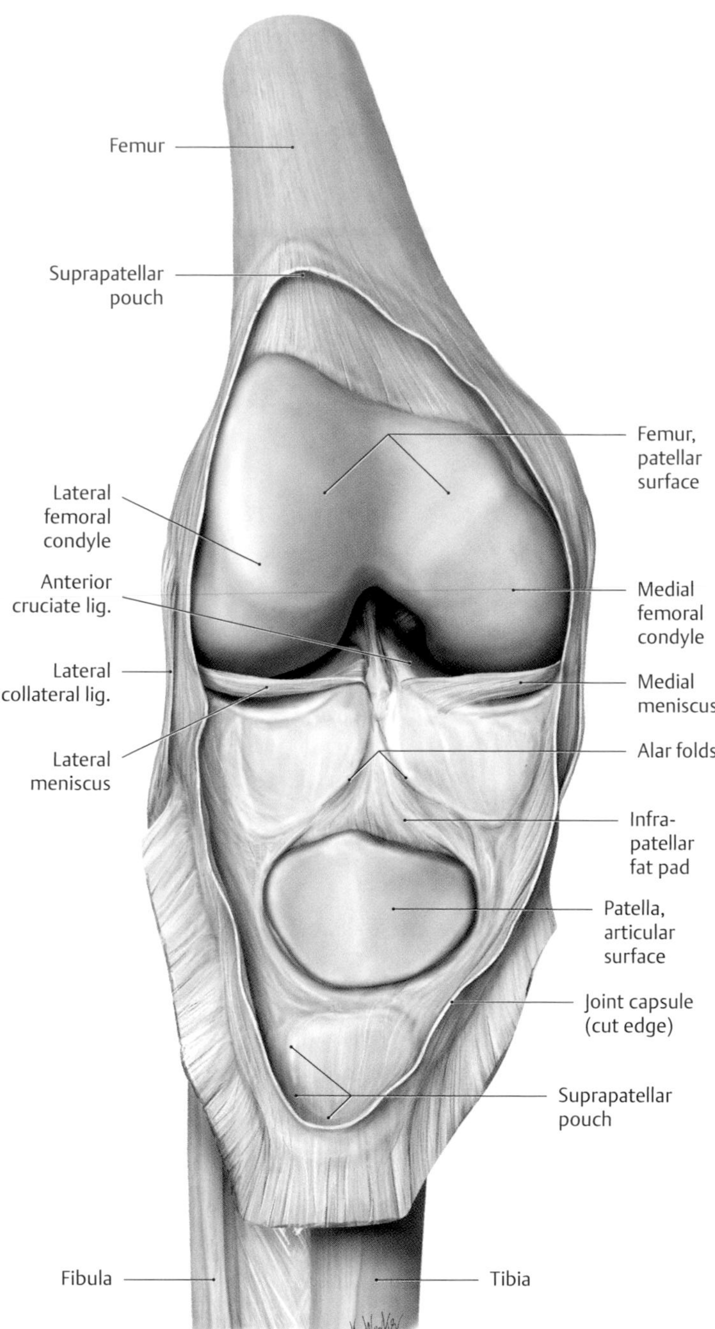
Femur
Suprapatellar pouch
Femur, patellar surface
Lateral femoral condyle
Anterior cruciate lig.
Medial femoral condyle
Lateral collateral lig.
Medial meniscus
Lateral meniscus
Alar folds
Infra-patellar fat pad
Patella, articular surface
Joint capsule (cut edge)
Suprapatellar pouch
Fibula
Tibia

Fig. 27.14 **Opened joint capsule**
Right knee, anterior view with patella reflected downward.

Fig. 27.16 Suprapatellar pouch during flexion
Right knee joint, medial view.

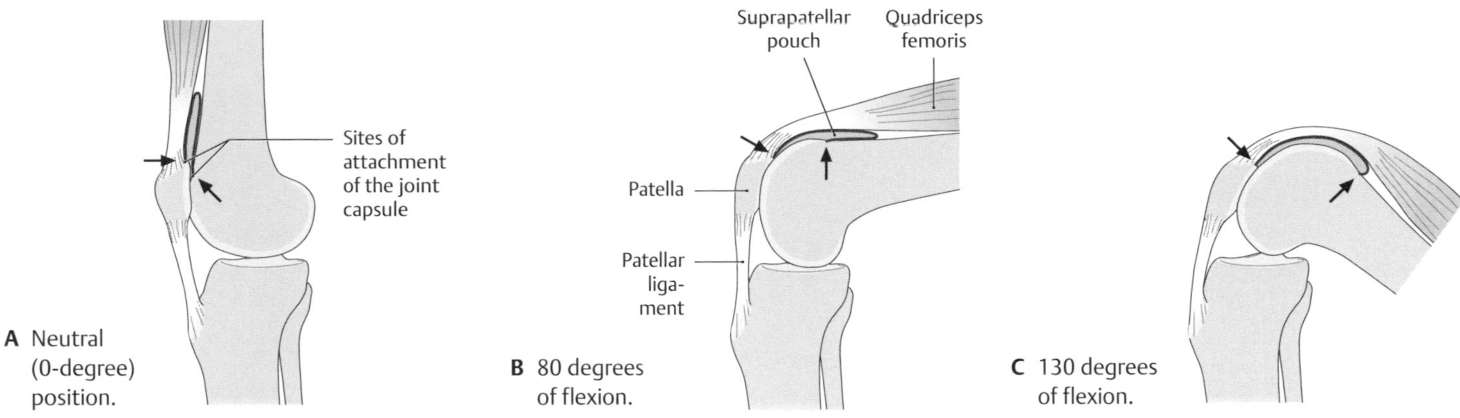
Sites of attachment of the joint capsule
Suprapatellar pouch
Quadriceps femoris
Patella
Patellar liga- ment
A Neutral (0-degree) position.
B 80 degrees of flexion.
C 130 degrees of flexion.

Fig. 27.17 Right knee joint: Midsagittal section

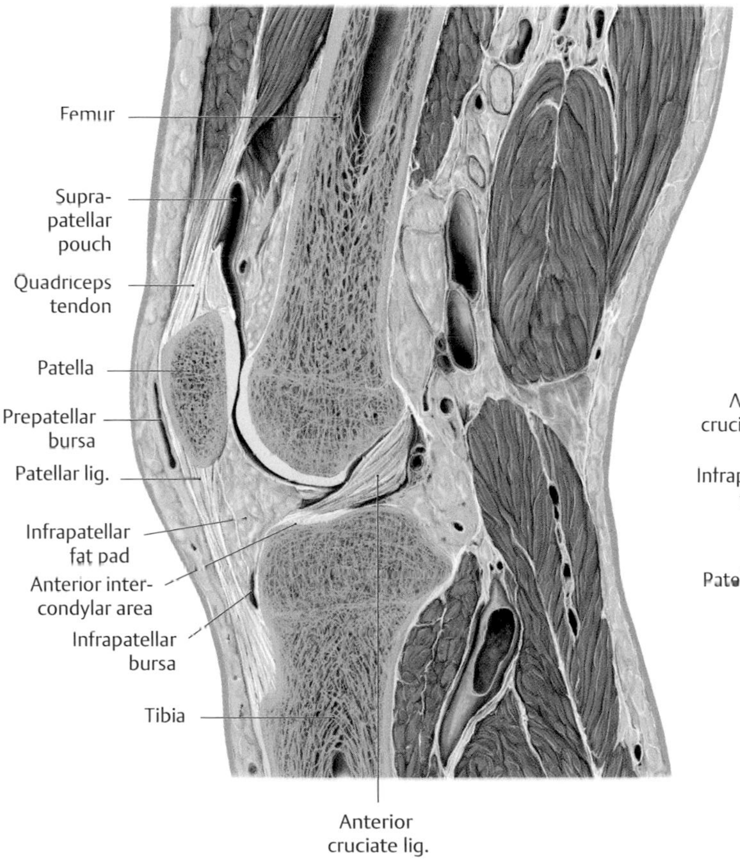

Femur
Supra- patellar pouch
Quadriceps tendon
Patella
Prepatellar bursa
Patellar lig.
Infrapatellar fat pad
Anterior inter- condylar area
Infrapatellar bursa
Tibia
Anterior cruciate lig.

Fig. 27.18 MRI of knee joint
Sagittal T2-weighted MRI.

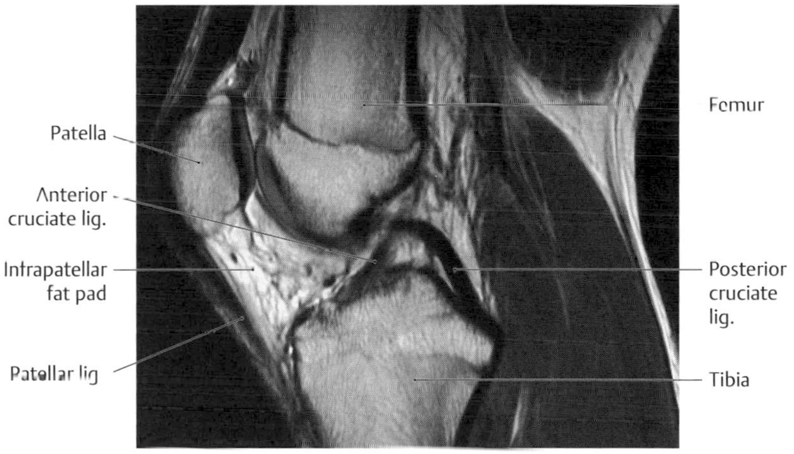

Patella
Anterior cruciate lig.
Infrapatellar fat pad
Patellar lig
Femur
Posterior cruciate lig.
Tibia

Muscles of the Leg: Anterior & Lateral Compartments

Fig. 27.19 **Muscles of the anterior compartment of the leg**
Right leg. Muscle origins shown in red, insertions in blue.

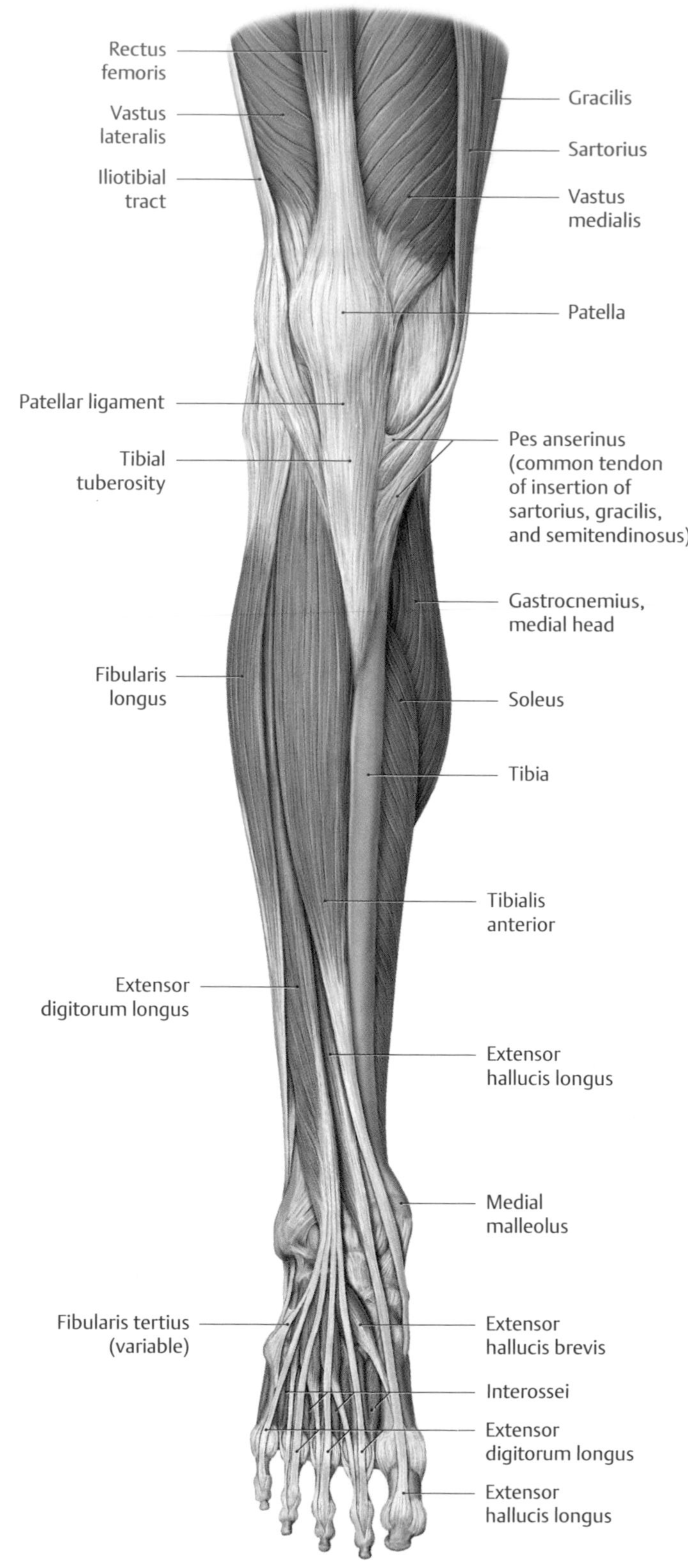
Rectus femoris
Vastus lateralis
Iliotibial tract
Gracilis
Sartorius
Vastus medialis
Patella
Patellar ligament
Tibial tuberosity
Pes anserinus (common tendon of insertion of sartorius, gracilis, and semitendinosus)
Gastrocnemius, medial head
Fibularis longus
Soleus
Tibia
Tibialis anterior
Extensor digitorum longus
Extensor hallucis longus
Medial malleolus
Fibularis tertius (variable)
Extensor hallucis brevis
Interossei
Extensor digitorum longus
Extensor hallucis longus

A All muscles shown.

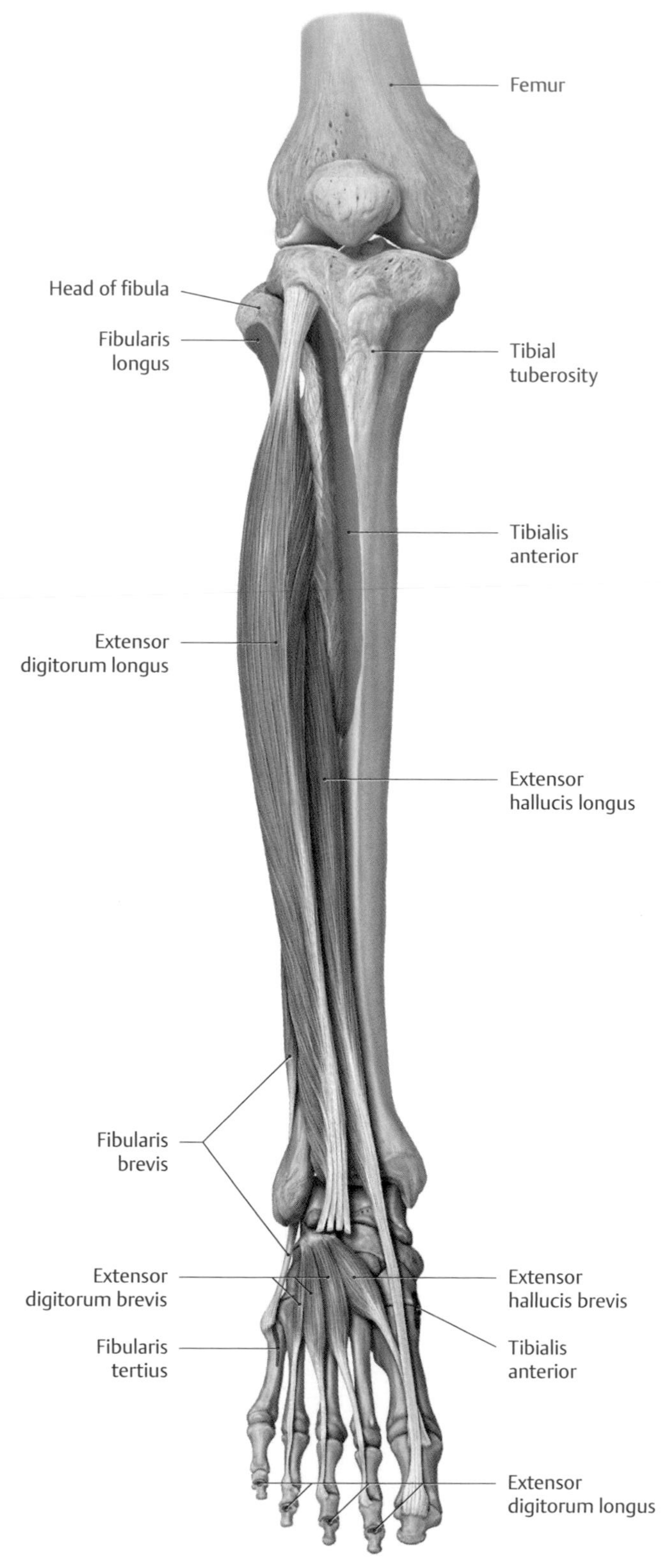
Femur
Head of fibula
Fibularis longus
Tibial tuberosity
Tibialis anterior
Extensor digitorum longus
Extensor hallucis longus
Fibularis brevis
Extensor digitorum brevis
Extensor hallucis brevis
Fibularis tertius
Tibialis anterior
Extensor digitorum longus

B *Removed:* Tibialis anterior and fibularis longus; extensor digitorum longus tendons (distal portions). *Note*: The fibularis tertius is a division of the extensor digitorum longus.

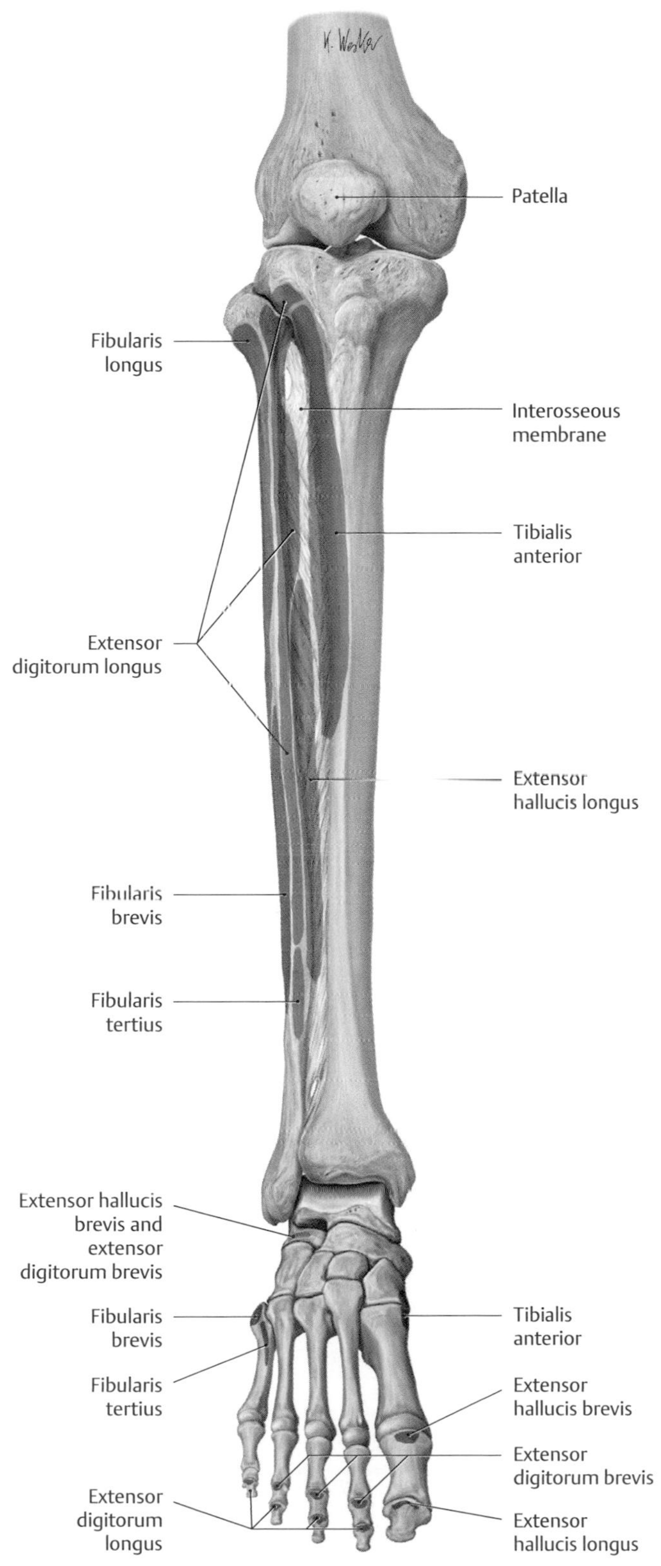
Patella
Fibularis longus
Interosseous membrane
Tibialis anterior
Extensor digitorum longus
Extensor hallucis longus
Fibularis brevis
Fibularis tertius
Extensor hallucis brevis and extensor digitorum brevis
Fibularis brevis
Tibialis anterior
Fibularis tertius
Extensor hallucis brevis
Extensor digitorum brevis
Extensor digitorum longus
Extensor hallucis longus

C *Removed:* All muscles.

Fig. 27.20 **Muscles of the lateral compartment of the leg**
Right leg.

Biceps femoris, long head
Rectus femoris
Vastus lateralis
Biceps femoris, short head
Iliotibial tract
Patella
Biceps femoris common tendon
Patellar ligament
Head of fibula
Lateral tibial condyle
Gastrocnemius, lateral head
Fibularis longus
Tibialis anterior
Soleus
Extensor digitorum longus
Triceps surae
Fibularis brevis
Extensor hallucis longus
Lateral malleolus, fibula
Extensor digitorum brevis
Calcaneal (Achilles') tendon
Fibularis tertius (variable)
Calcaneus
Fibularis longus
Fibularis brevis
Extensor digitorum longus

Muscles of the Leg: Posterior Compartment

Fig. 27.21 Muscles of posterior compartment of the leg
Right leg. Muscle origins shown in red, insertions in blue.

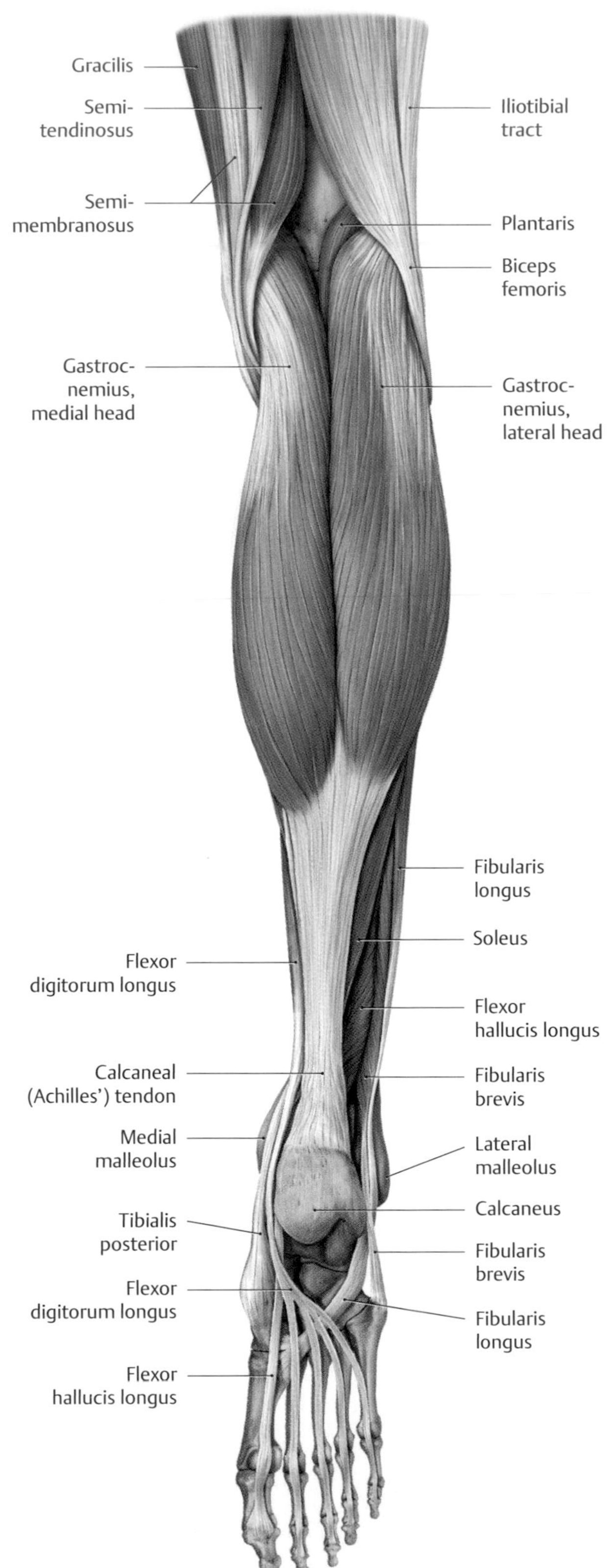
Gracilis
Semi-
tendinosus
Semi-
membranosus
Iliotibial
tract
Plantaris
Biceps
femoris
Gastroc-
nemius,
medial head
Gastroc-
nemius,
lateral head
Fibularis
longus
Soleus
Flexor
digitorum longus
Flexor
hallucis longus
Calcaneal
(Achilles') tendon
Fibularis
brevis
Medial
malleolus
Lateral
malleolus
Calcaneus
Tibialis
posterior
Fibularis
brevis
Flexor
digitorum longus
Fibularis
longus
Flexor
hallucis longus

A *Note:* The bulge of the calf is produced mainly by the triceps surae (soleus and the two heads of the gastrocnemius).

Gastrocnemius,
medial head
Gastrocnemius,
lateral head
Plantaris
Biceps femoris
Popliteus
Fibularis
longus
Soleus
Plantaris
tendon
Fibularis longus
Calcaneal
(Achilles') tendon
Flexor
digitorum longus
Flexor
hallucis longus
Fibularis brevis
Tibialis
posterior
Calcaneus
Fibularis
brevis
Flexor
digitorum longus
Fibularis
longus
Flexor
hallucis longus

B *Removed:* Gastrocnemius (both heads).

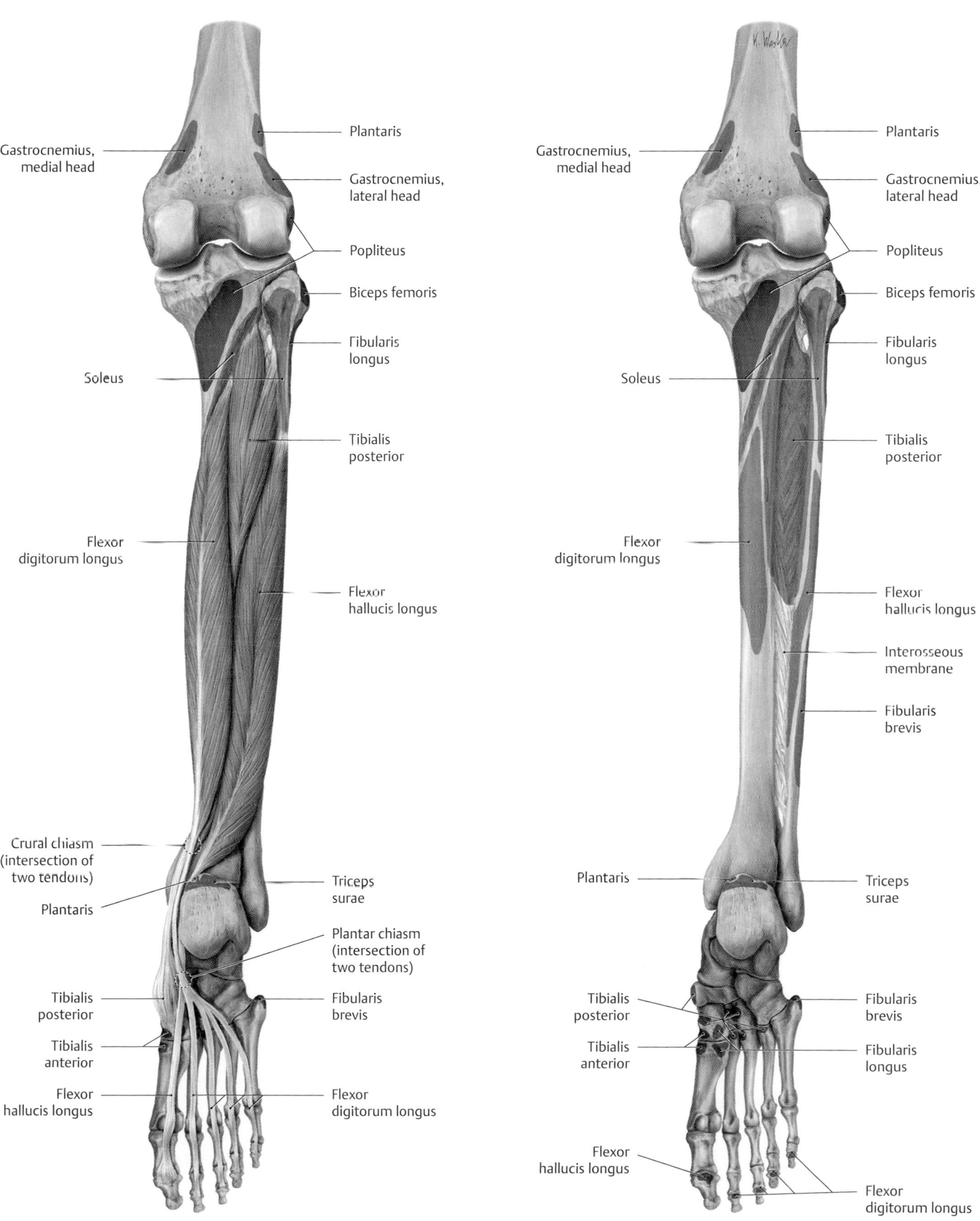
Gastrocnemius, medial head
Plantaris
Gastrocnemius, lateral head
Popliteus
Biceps femoris
Fibularis longus
Soleus
Tibialis posterior
Flexor digitorum longus
Flexor hallucis longus
Crural chiasm (intersection of two tendons)
Plantaris
Triceps surae
Plantar chiasm (intersection of two tendons)
Tibialis posterior
Fibularis brevis
Tibialis anterior
Flexor hallucis longus
Flexor digitorum longus
Gastrocnemius, medial head
Plantaris
Gastrocnemius, lateral head
Popliteus
Biceps femoris
Fibularis longus
Soleus
Tibialis posterior
Flexor digitorum longus
Flexor hallucis longus
Interosseous membrane
Fibularis brevis
Plantaris
Triceps surae
Tibialis posterior
Fibularis brevis
Tibialis anterior
Fibularis longus
Flexor hallucis longus
Flexor digitorum longus

C *Removed:* Triceps surae, plantaris, popliteus, fibularis longus, and fibularis brevis muscles.

D *Removed:* All muscles.

Muscle Facts (I)

The muscles of the leg control the flexion/extension and inversion/eversion of the foot, which provide stability to the lower limb during movements at the knee and hip joint.

Fig. 27.22 Muscles of lateral compartment of the leg
Right leg and foot.

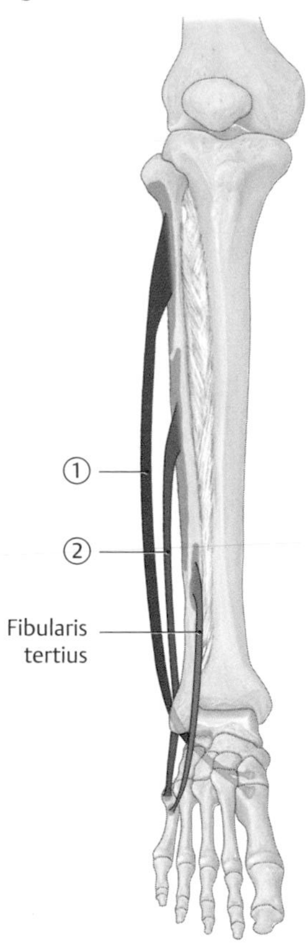

①
②
Fibularis tertius

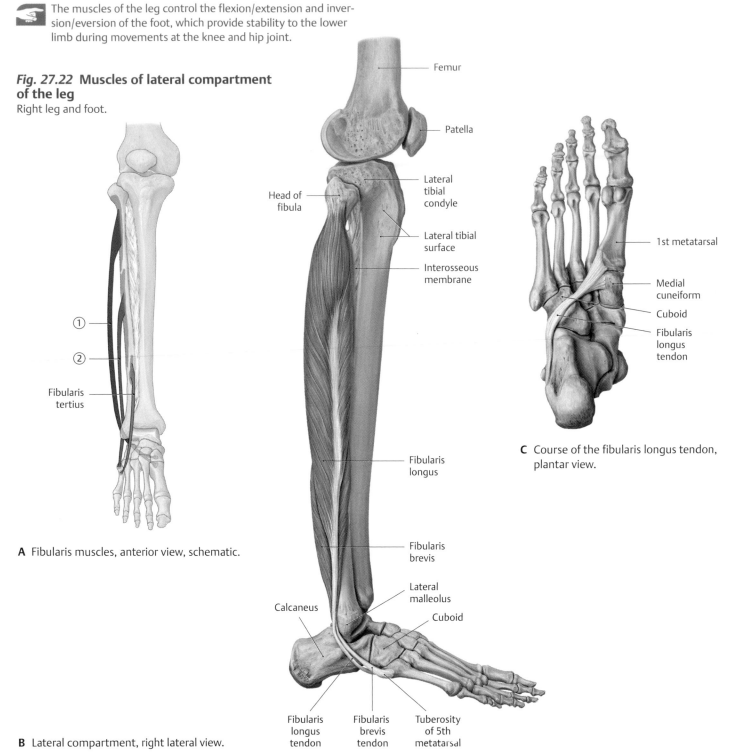

A Fibularis muscles, anterior view, schematic.

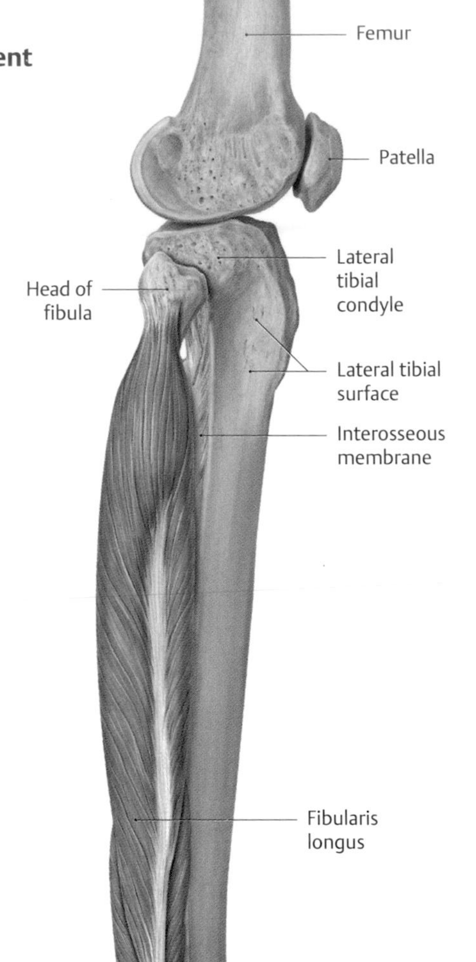

Femur
Patella
Lateral tibial condyle
Head of fibula
Lateral tibial surface
Interosseous membrane
Fibularis longus
Fibularis brevis
Lateral malleolus
Calcaneus
Cuboid
Fibularis longus tendon
Fibularis brevis tendon
Tuberosity of 5th metatarsal

B Lateral compartment, right lateral view.

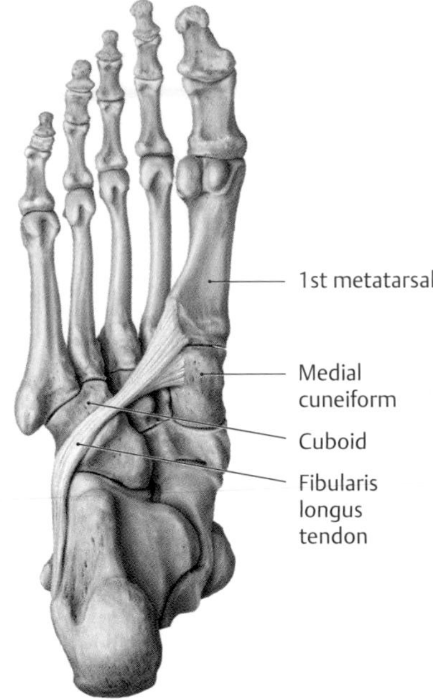

1st metatarsal
Medial cuneiform
Cuboid
Fibularis longus tendon

C Course of the fibularis longus tendon, plantar view.

Table 27.2 Lateral compartment

Muscle	Origin	Insertion	Innervation	Action
① Fibularis longus	Fibula (head and proximal two thirds of the lateral surface, arising partly from the intermuscular septa)	Medial cuneiform (plantar side), 1st metatarsal (base)	Superficial fibular n. (L5, S1)	• Talocrural joint: plantar flexion • Subtalar joint: eversion (pronation) • Supports the transverse arch of the foot
② Fibularis brevis	Fibula (distal half of the lateral surface), intermuscular septa	5th metatarsal (tuberosity at the base, with an occasional division to the dorsal aponeurosis of the 5th toe)		• Talocrural joint: plantar flexion • Subtalar joint: eversion (pronation)

Fig. 27.23 Muscles of anterior compartment of the leg

Right leg, anterior view.

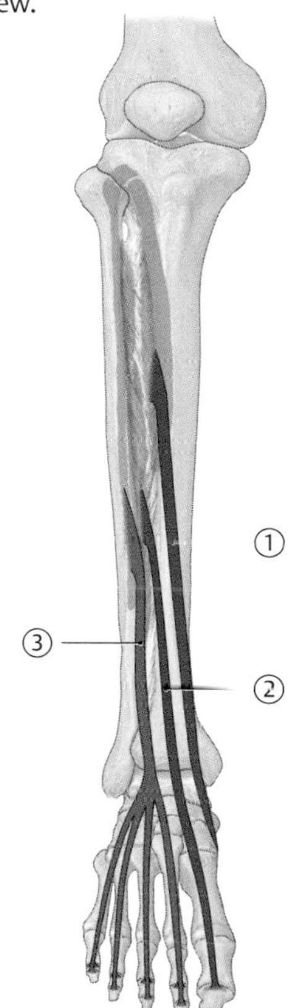

①
③
②

A Schematic.

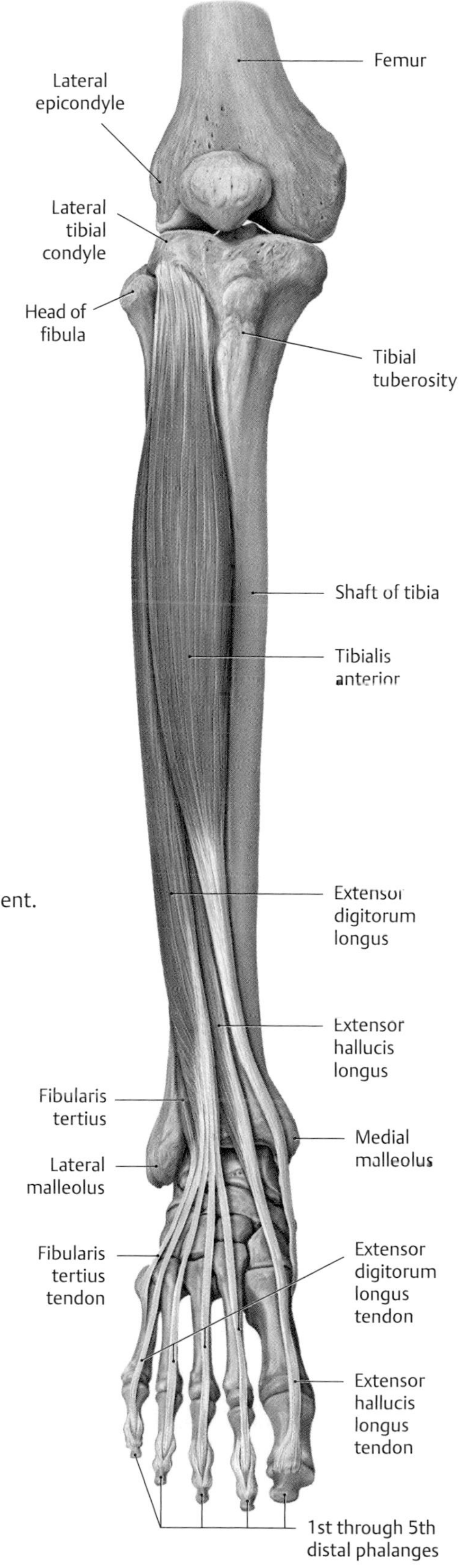

Femur
Lateral epicondyle
Lateral tibial condyle
Head of fibula
Tibial tuberosity
Shaft of tibia
Tibialis anterior
Extensor digitorum longus
Extensor hallucis longus
Fibularis tertius
Medial malleolus
Lateral malleolus
Fibularis tertius tendon
Extensor digitorum longus tendon
Extensor hallucis longus tendon
1st through 5th distal phalanges

B Anterior compartment.

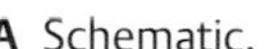

Table 27.3 Anterior compartment

Muscle	Origin	Insertion	Innervation	Action
① Tibialis anterior	Tibia (upper two thirds of the lateral surface), interosseous membrane, and superficial crural fascia (highest part)	Medial cuneiform (medial and plantar surface), first metatarsal (medial base)	Deep fibular n. (L4, L5)	• Talocrural joint: dorsiflexion • Subtalar joint: inversion (supination)
② Extensor hallucis longus	Fibula (middle third of the medial surface) interosseous membrane	1st toe (at the dorsal aponeurosis and the base of its distal phalanx)	Deep fibular n. (L4, L5)	• Talocrural joint: dorsiflexion • Subtalar joint: active in both eversion and inversion (pronation/supination), depending on the initial position of the foot • Extends the MTP and IP joints of the big toe
③ Extensor digitorum longus	Fibula (head and medial surface), tibia (lateral condyle), and interosseous membrane	2nd to 5th toes (at the dorsal aponeuroses at the bases of the distal phalanges)	Deep fibular n. (L4, L5)	• Talocrural joint: dorsiflexion • Subtalar joint: eversion (pronation) • Extends the MTP and IP joints of the 2nd to 5th toes
Fibularis tertius (see Fig. 25.22A)	Distal fibula (anterior border)	5th metatarsal (base)	Deep fibular n. (L4, L5)	• Talocrural joint: dorsiflexion • Subtalar joint: eversion (pronation)

IP, interphalangeal; MTP, metatarsophalangeal.

Muscle Facts (II)

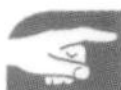

The muscles of the posterior compartment are divided into two groups: the superficial and deep flexors. These groups are separated by the transverse intermuscular septum.

Fig. 27.24 **Posterior compartment of the leg: Superficial flexors**
Right leg, posterior view.

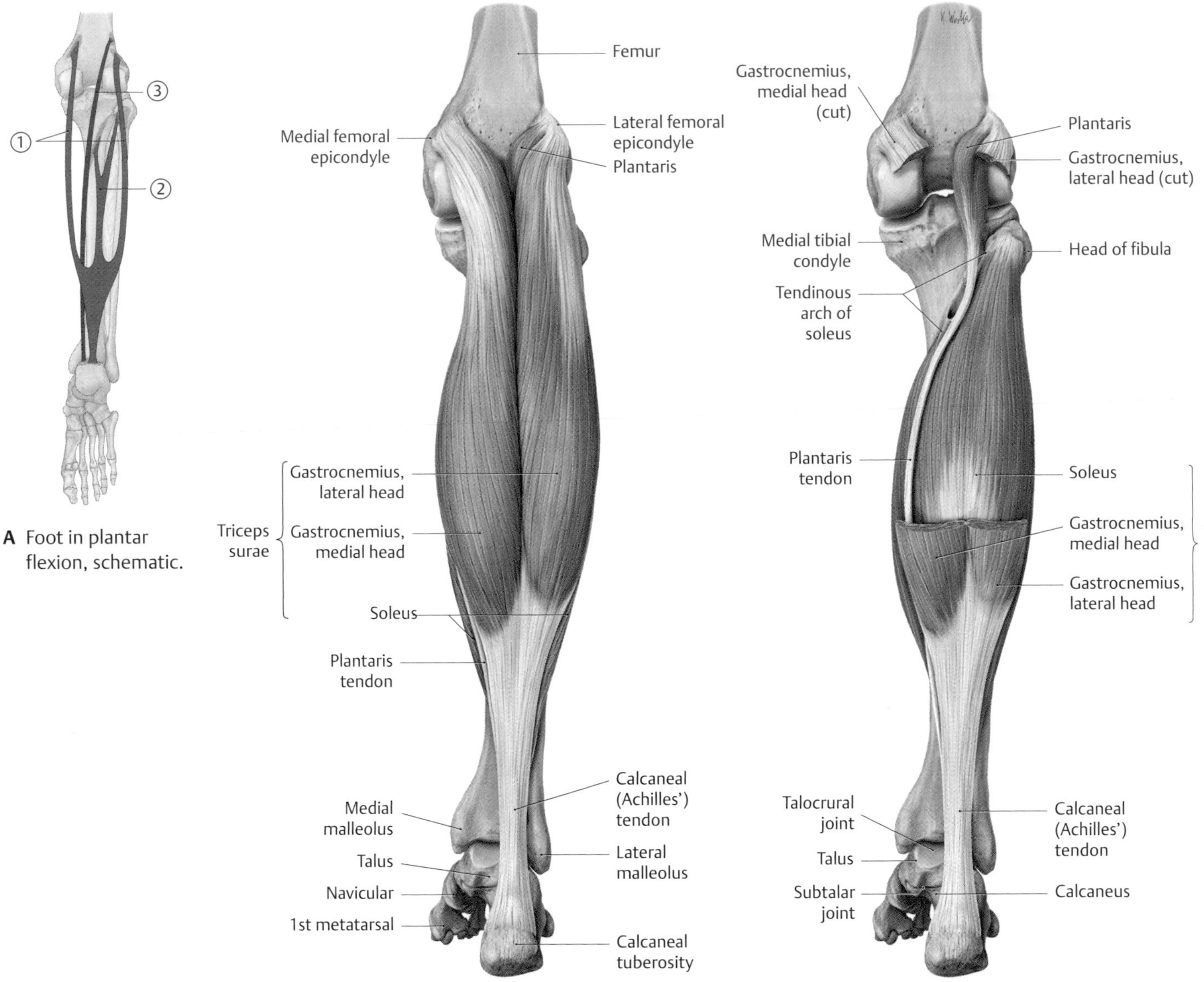

A Foot in plantar flexion, schematic.

B Superficial flexors.

C Superficial flexors with gastrocnemius removed (portions of medial and lateral heads).

Table 27.4	**Superficial flexors of the posterior compartment**				
Muscle		**Origin**	**Insertion**	**Innervation**	**Action**
Triceps surae	① Gastrocnemius	Femur (medial and lateral epicondyles)	Calcaneal tuberosity via the calcaneal (Achilles') tendon	Tibial n. (S1, S2)	• Talocrural joint: plantar flexion • Knee joint: flexion (gastrocnemius)
	② Soleus	Fibula (head and neck, posterior surface), tibia (soleal line via a tendinous arch)			
③ Plantaris		Femur (lateral epicondyle, proximal to lateral head of gastrocnemius)	Calcaneal tuberosity		Negligible; may prevent compression of posterior leg musculature during knee flexion

***Fig. 27.25* Posterior compartment of the leg: Deep flexors**
Right leg with foot in plantar flexion, posterior view.

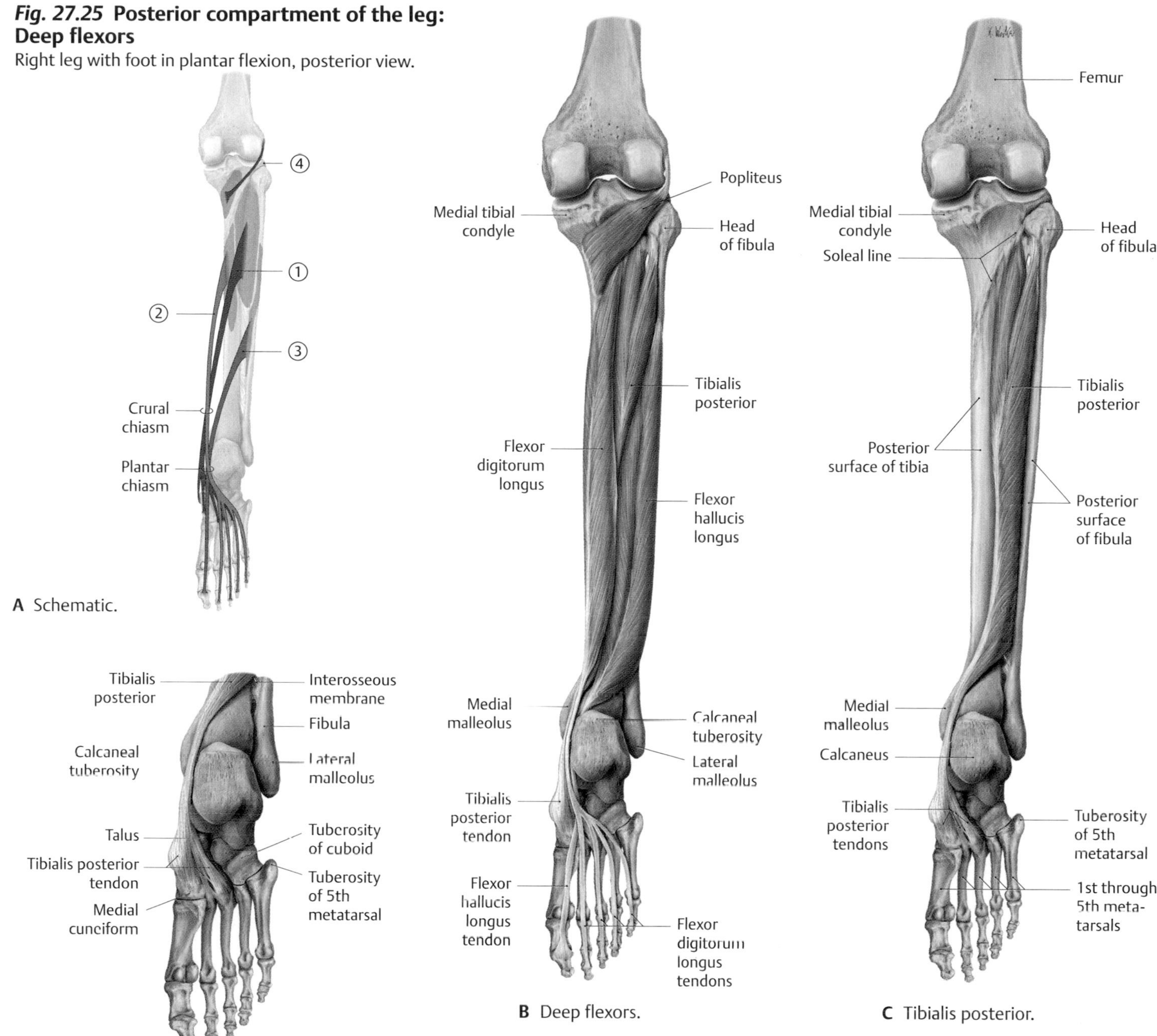
④
①
②
③
Crural chiasm
Plantar chiasm
Popliteus
Medial tibial condyle
Head of fibula
Tibialis posterior
Flexor digitorum longus
Flexor hallucis longus
Medial malleolus
Calcaneal tuberosity
Lateral malleolus
Tibialis posterior tendon
Flexor hallucis longus tendon
Flexor digitorum longus tendons
Femur
Medial tibial condyle
Soleal line
Head of fibula
Tibialis posterior
Posterior surface of tibia
Posterior surface of fibula
Medial malleolus
Calcaneus
Tibialis posterior tendons
Tuberosity of 5th metatarsal
1st through 5th meta-tarsals
Tibialis posterior
Interosseous membrane
Fibula
Calcaneal tuberosity
Lateral malleolus
Talus
Tuberosity of cuboid
Tibialis posterior tendon
Tuberosity of 5th metatarsal
Medial cuneiform

A Schematic.

B Deep flexors.

C Tibialis posterior.

D Insertion of the tibialis posterior.

***Table 27.5* Deep flexors of the posterior compartment**

Muscle	Origin	Insertion	Innervation	Action
① Tibialis posterior	Interosseous membrane, adjacent borders of tibia and fibula	Navicular tuberosity; cuneiforms (medial, intermediate, and lateral); 2nd to 4th metatarsals (bases)	Tibial n. (L4, L5)	• Talocrural joint: plantar flexion • Subtalar joint: inversion (supination) • Supports the longitudinal and transverse arches
② Flexor digitorum longus	Tibia (middle third of posterior surface)	2nd to 5th distal phalanges (bases)	Tibial n. (L5–S2)	• Talocrural joint: plantar flexion • Subtalar joint: inversion (supination) • MTP and IP joints of the 2nd to 5th toes: plantar flexion
③ Flexor hallucis longus	Fibula (distal two thirds of posterior surface), adjacent interosseous membrane	1st distal phalanx (base)		• Talocrural joint: plantar flexion • Subtalar joint: inversion (supination) • MTP and IP joints of the 1st toe: plantar flexion • Supports the medial longitudinal arch
④ Popliteus	Lateral femoral condyle, posterior horn of the lateral meniscus	Posterior tibial surface (above the origin at the soleus)	Tibial n. (L4–S1)	Knee joint: flexion and internal rotation (stabilizes the knee)

IP, interphalangeal; MTP, metatarsophalangeal.

Bones of the Foot

Fig. 28.1 **Subdivisions of the pedal skeleton**
Right foot, dorsal view. Descriptive anatomy divides the skeletal elements of the foot into the tarsus, metatarsus, and forefoot (antetarsus). Functional and clinical criteria divide the pedal skeleton into hindfoot, midfoot, and forefoot.

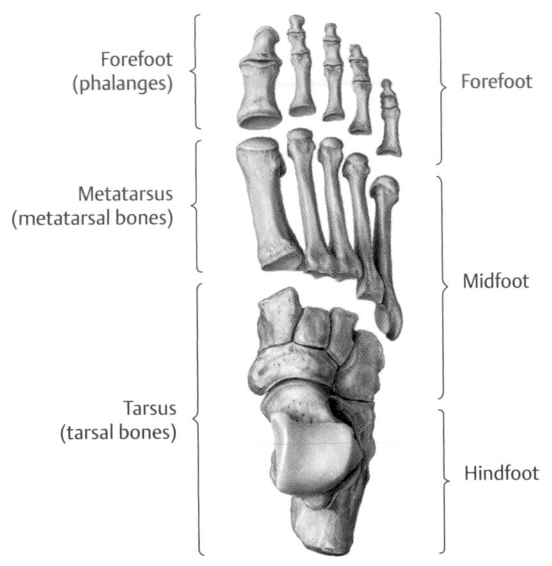

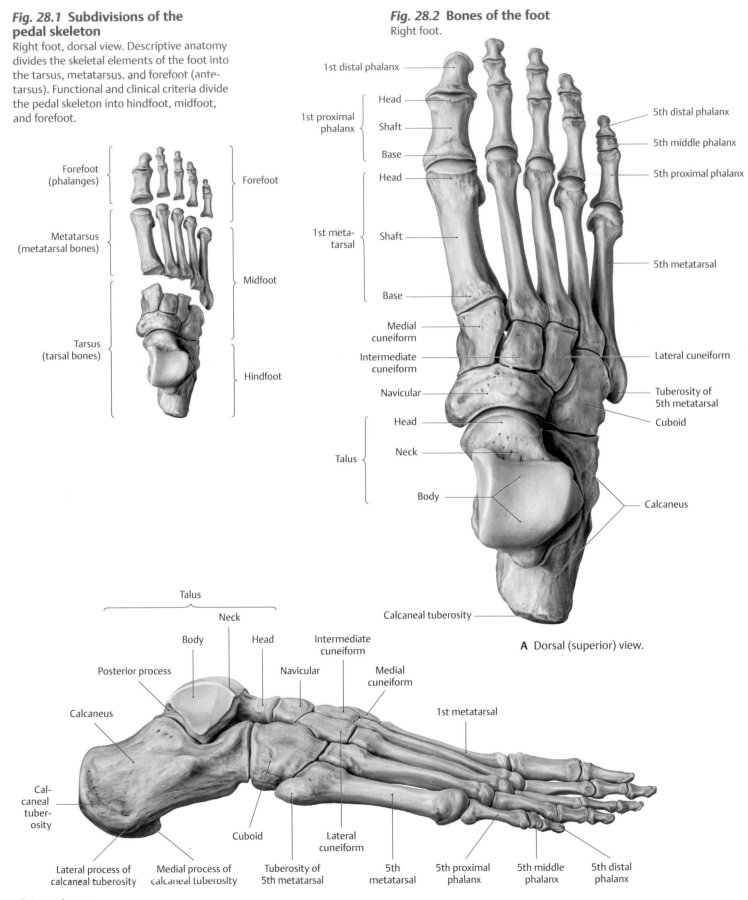

Forefoot (phalanges)
Metatarsus (metatarsal bones)
Tarsus (tarsal bones)
Forefoot
Midfoot
Hindfoot

Fig. 28.2 **Bones of the foot**
Right foot.

1st distal phalanx
1st proximal phalanx
Head
Shaft
Base
1st metatarsal
Head
Shaft
Base
Medial cuneiform
Intermediate cuneiform
Navicular
Talus
Head
Neck
Body
Calcaneal tuberosity
5th distal phalanx
5th middle phalanx
5th proximal phalanx
5th metatarsal
Lateral cuneiform
Tuberosity of 5th metatarsal
Cuboid
Calcaneus

A Dorsal (superior) view.

Talus
Neck
Body
Head
Posterior process
Navicular
Intermediate cuneiform
Medial cuneiform
1st metatarsal
Calcaneus
Calcaneal tuberosity
Cuboid
Lateral cuneiform
Lateral process of calcaneal tuberosity
Medial process of calcaneal tuberosity
Tuberosity of 5th metatarsal
5th metatarsal
5th proximal phalanx
5th middle phalanx
5th distal phalanx

C Lateral view.

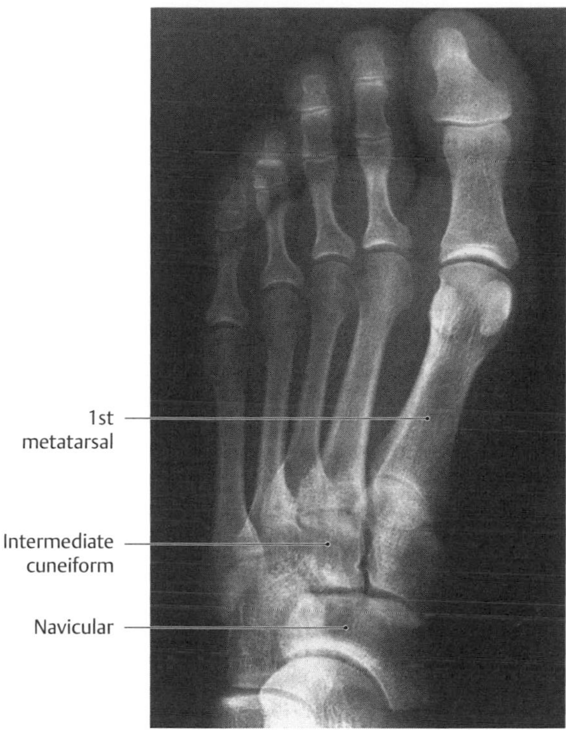
1st metatarsal
Intermediate cuneiform
Navicular

B Radiograph, anterior–posterior view of the left forefoot.

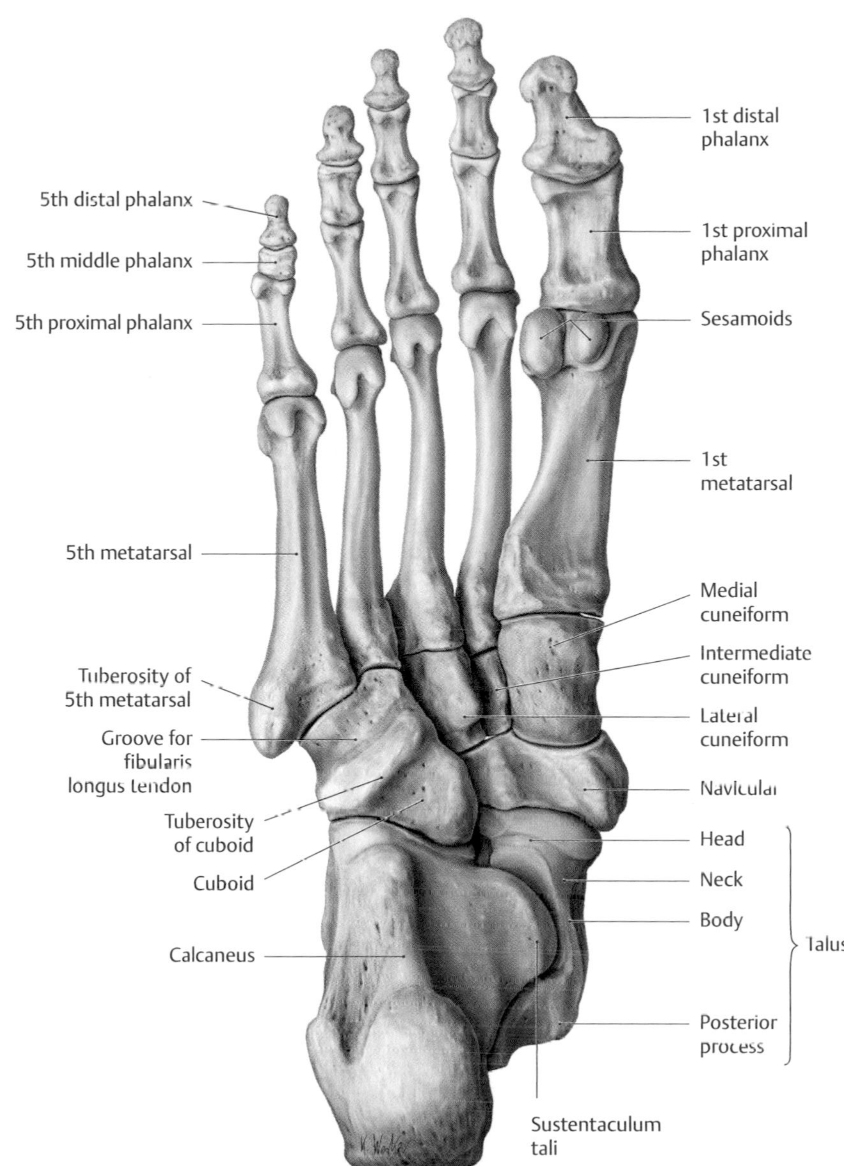
1st distal phalanx
5th distal phalanx
5th middle phalanx
1st proximal phalanx
5th proximal phalanx
Sesamoids
1st metatarsal
5th metatarsal
Medial cuneiform
Intermediate cuneiform
Tuberosity of 5th metatarsal
Lateral cuneiform
Groove for fibularis longus tendon
Navicular
Tuberosity of cuboid
Head
Cuboid
Neck
Body
Talus
Calcaneus
Posterior process
Sustentaculum tali

D Plantar (inferior) view.

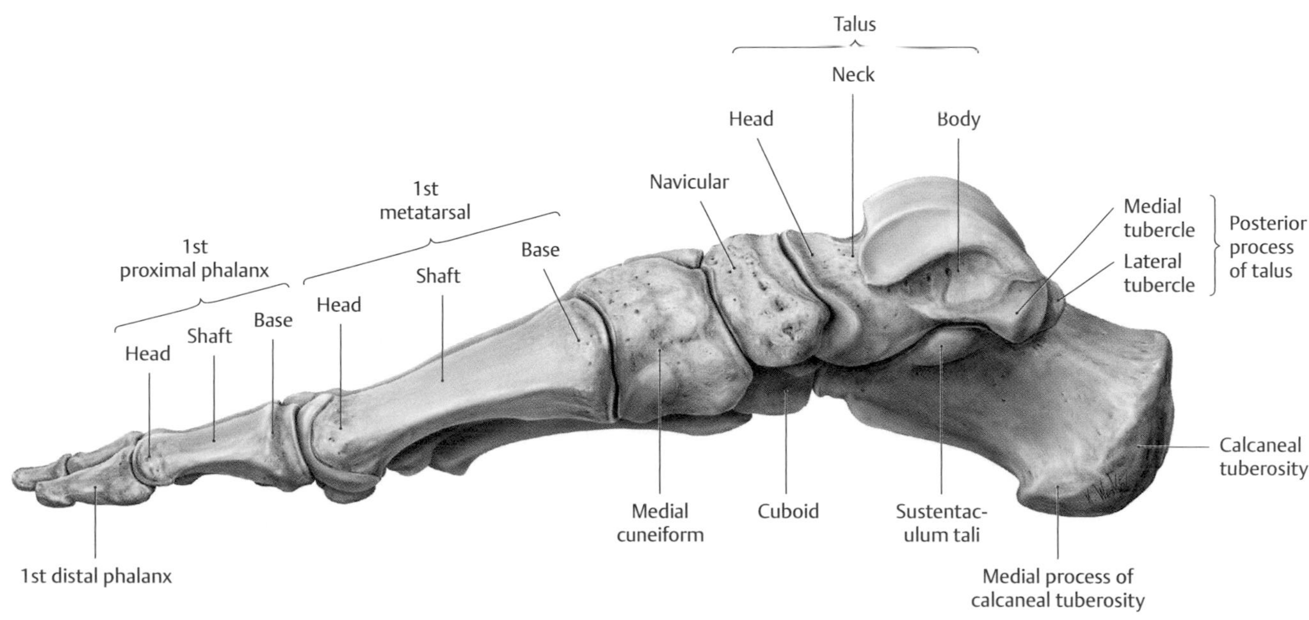
Talus
Neck
Head
Body
Navicular
1st metatarsal
Medial tubercle
Posterior process of talus
Lateral tubercle
1st proximal phalanx
Base
Shaft
Head
Base
Shaft
Head
Calcaneal tuberosity
Medial cuneiform
Cuboid
Sustentaculum tali
1st distal phalanx
Medial process of calcaneal tuberosity

E Medial view.

Joints of the Foot (I)

Fig. 28.3 Joints of the foot
Right foot with talocrural joint in plantar flexion.

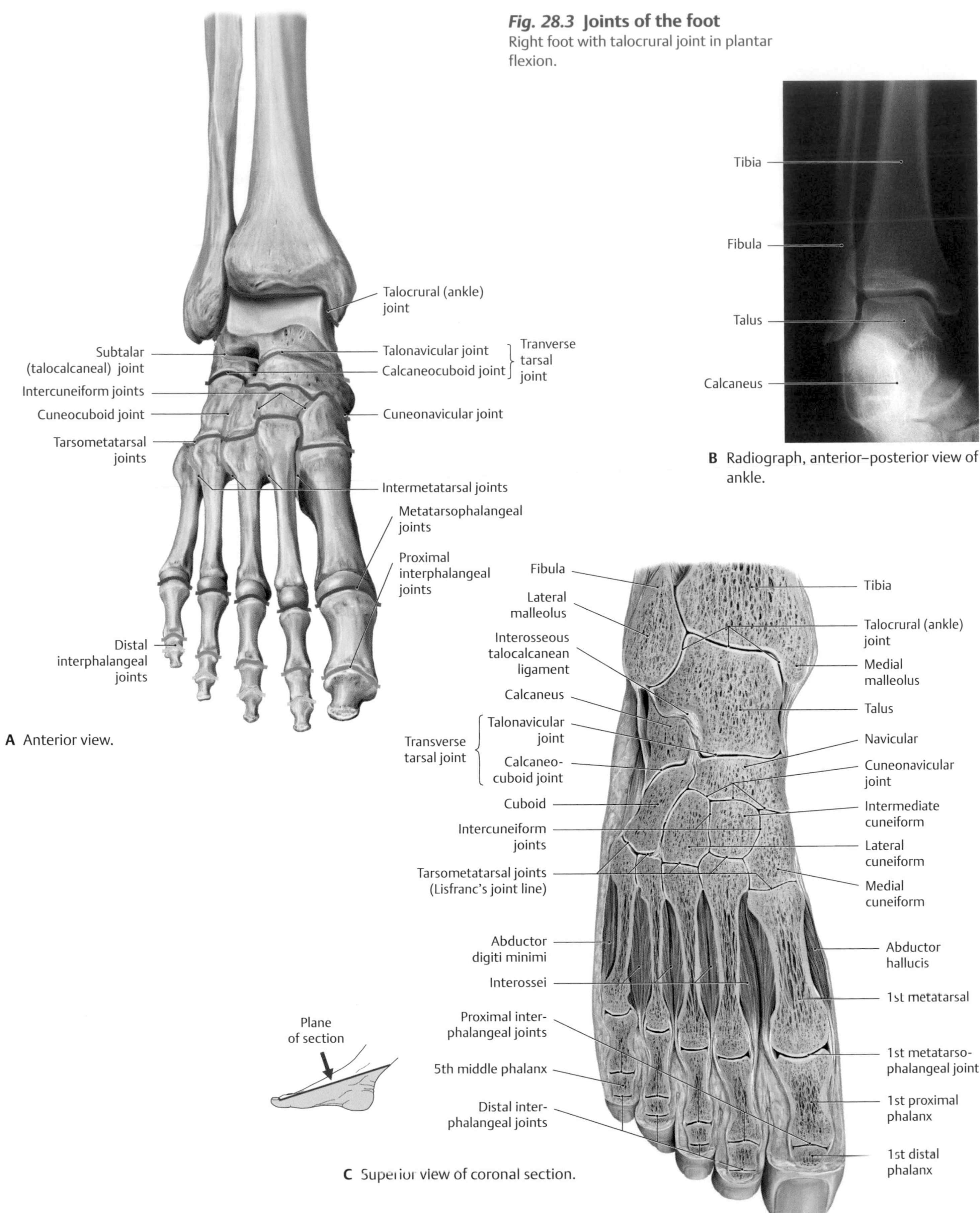
Talocrural (ankle) joint
Subtalar (talocalcaneal) joint
Talonavicular joint
Calcaneocuboid joint
Tranverse tarsal joint
Intercuneiform joints
Cuneocuboid joint
Cuneonavicular joint
Tarsometatarsal joints
Intermetatarsal joints
Metatarsophalangeal joints
Proximal interphalangeal joints
Distal interphalangeal joints
Tibia
Fibula
Talus
Calcaneus
Fibula
Lateral malleolus
Interosseous talocalcanean ligament
Calcaneus
Transverse tarsal joint
Talonavicular joint
Calcaneo-cuboid joint
Cuboid
Intercuneiform joints
Tarsometatarsal joints (Lisfranc's joint line)
Abductor digiti minimi
Interossei
Proximal inter-phalangeal joints
5th middle phalanx
Distal inter-phalangeal joints
Tibia
Talocrural (ankle) joint
Medial malleolus
Talus
Navicular
Cuneonavicular joint
Intermediate cuneiform
Lateral cuneiform
Medial cuneiform
Abductor hallucis
1st metatarsal
1st metatarso-phalangeal joint
1st proximal phalanx
1st distal phalanx
Plane of section

A Anterior view.

B Radiograph, anterior–posterior view of ankle.

C Superior view of coronal section.

Fig. 28.4 Proximal articular surfaces

Right foot, proximal view.

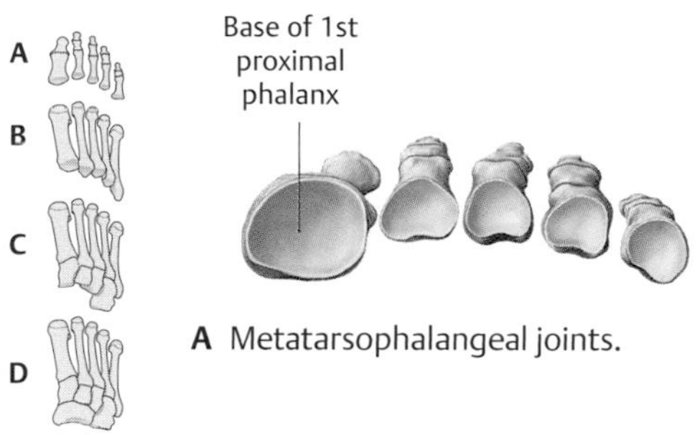
A
B
C
D
Base of 1st proximal phalanx

A Metatarsophalangeal joints.

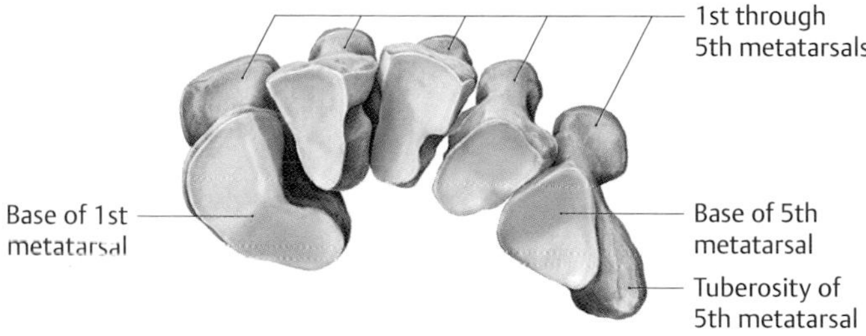
1st through 5th metatarsals
Base of 1st metatarsal
Base of 5th metatarsal
Tuberosity of 5th metatarsal

B Tarsometatarsal joints.

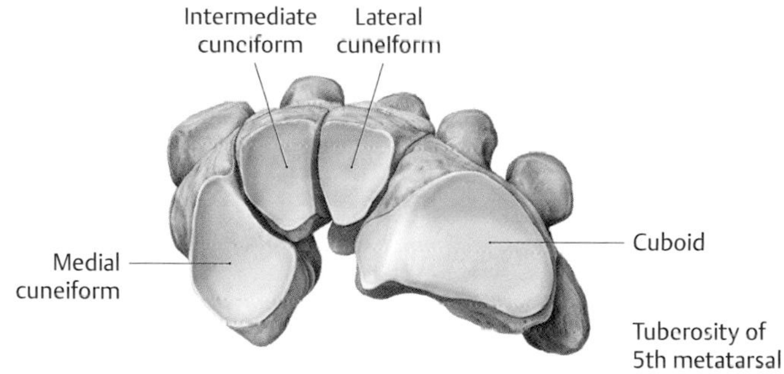
Intermediate cuneiform
Lateral cuneiform
Medial cuneiform
Cuboid
Tuberosity of 5th metatarsal

C Cuneonavicular and calcaneocuboid joints.

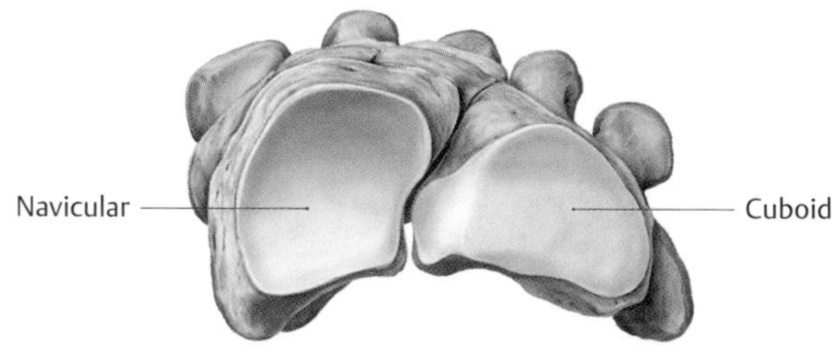
Navicular
Cuboid

D Talonavicular and calcaneocuboid joints.

Fig. 28.5 Distal articular surfaces

Right foot, distal view.

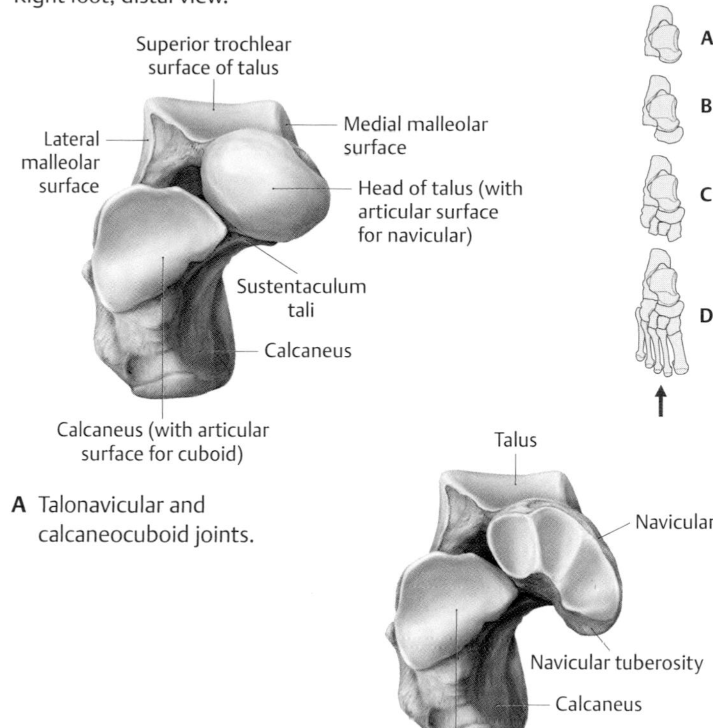
Superior trochlear surface of talus
Lateral malleolar surface
Medial malleolar surface
Head of talus (with articular surface for navicular)
Sustentaculum tali
Calcaneus
Calcaneus (with articular surface for cuboid)
A
B
C
D
Talus
Navicular
Navicular tuberosity
Calcaneus
Calcaneus (with articular surface for cuboid)

A Talonavicular and calcaneocuboid joints.

B Cuneonavicular and calcaneocuboid joints.

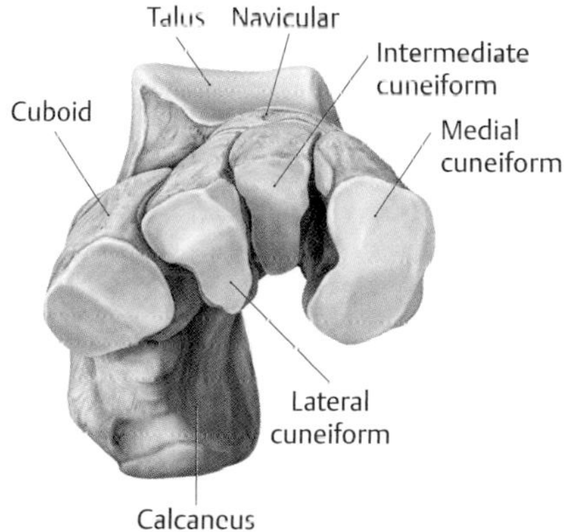
Talus
Navicular
Intermediate cuneiform
Cuboid
Medial cuneiform
Lateral cuneiform
Calcaneus

C Tarsometatarsal joints.

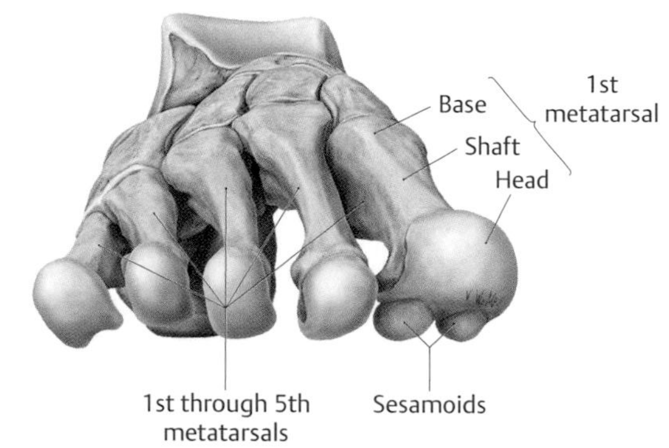
Base
Shaft
Head
1st metatarsal
1st through 5th metatarsals
Sesamoids

D Metatarsophalangeal joints.

Joints of the Foot (II)

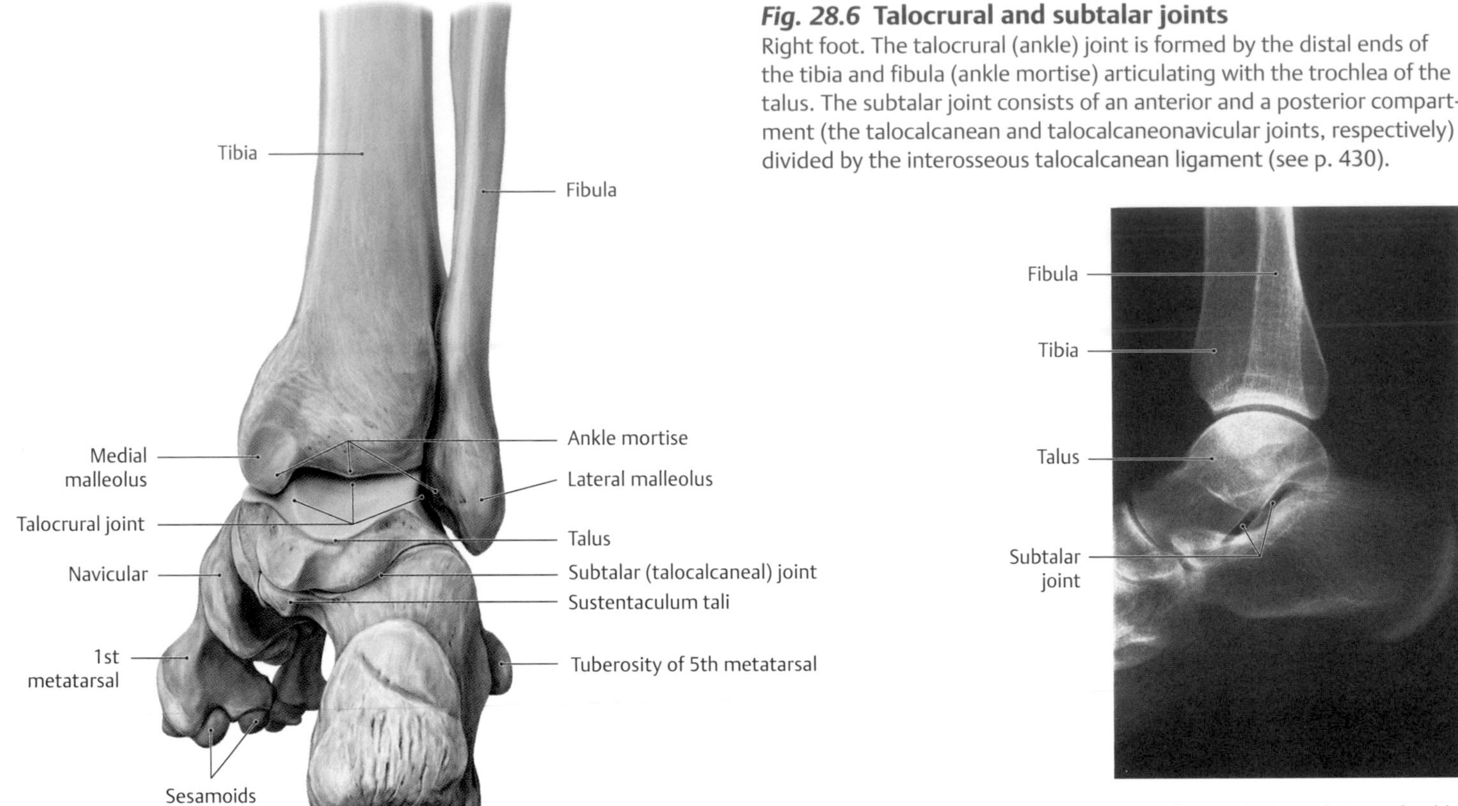
Tibia
Fibula
Medial malleolus
Ankle mortise
Lateral malleolus
Talocrural joint
Talus
Navicular
Subtalar (talocalcaneal) joint
Sustentaculum tali
1st metatarsal
Tuberosity of 5th metatarsal
Sesamoids
Calcaneal tuberosity
Fibula
Tibia
Talus
Subtalar joint

Fig. 28.6 Talocrural and subtalar joints
Right foot. The talocrural (ankle) joint is formed by the distal ends of the tibia and fibula (ankle mortise) articulating with the trochlea of the talus. The subtalar joint consists of an anterior and a posterior compartment (the talocalcanean and talocalcaneonavicular joints, respectively) divided by the interosseous talocalcanean ligament (see p. 430).

A Posterior view with foot in neutral (0-degree) position.

B Radiograph, lateral view of ankle.

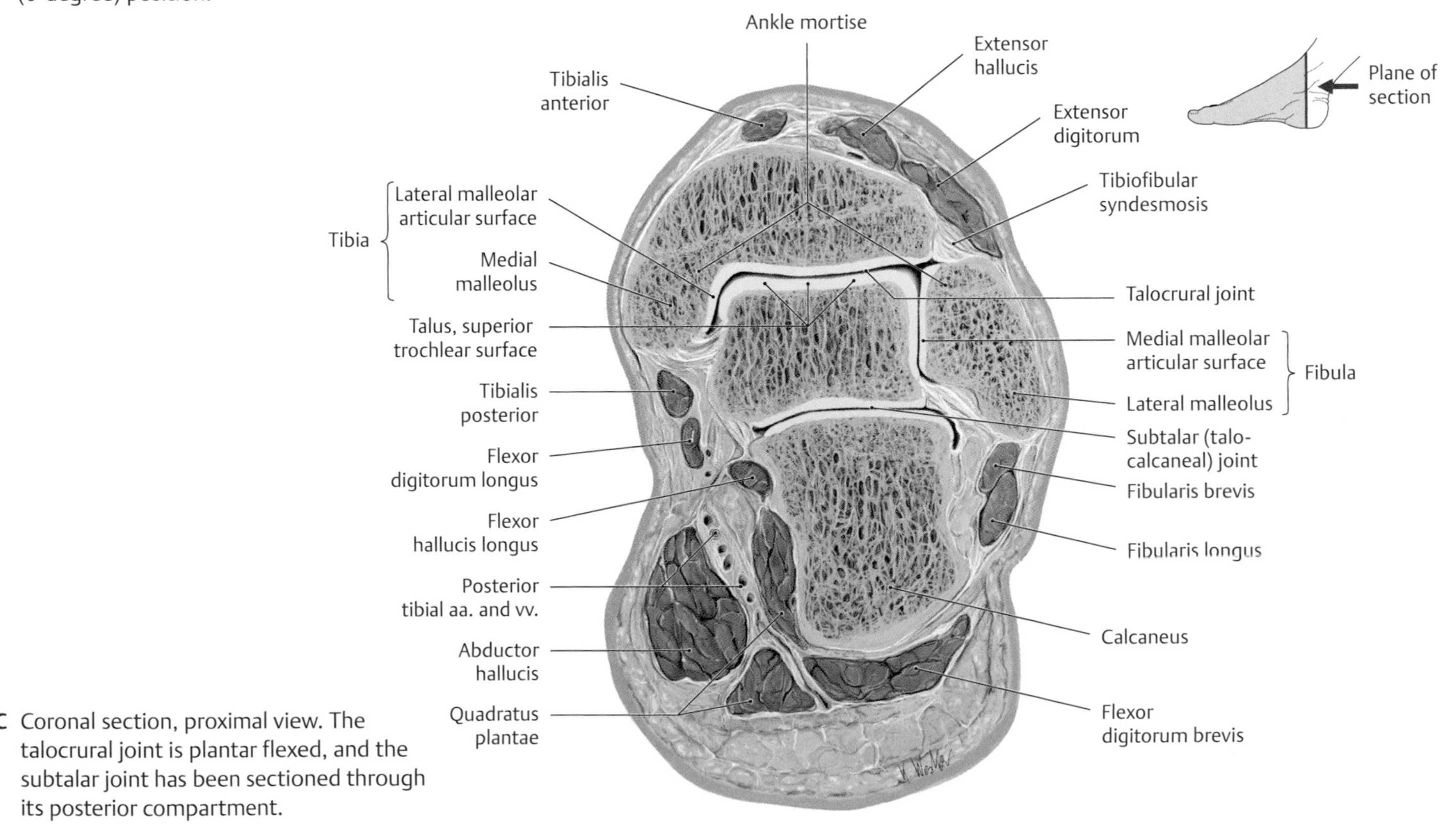
Ankle mortise
Tibialis anterior
Extensor hallucis
Extensor digitorum
Plane of section
Tibia
Lateral malleolar articular surface
Medial malleolus
Tibiofibular syndesmosis
Talocrural joint
Talus, superior trochlear surface
Medial malleolar articular surface
Fibula
Lateral malleolus
Tibialis posterior
Subtalar (talo-calcaneal) joint
Flexor digitorum longus
Fibularis brevis
Flexor hallucis longus
Fibularis longus
Posterior tibial aa. and vv.
Calcaneus
Abductor hallucis
Quadratus plantae
Flexor digitorum brevis

C Coronal section, proximal view. The talocrural joint is plantar flexed, and the subtalar joint has been sectioned through its posterior compartment.

Fig. 28.7 **Talocrural and subtalar joints: Sagittal section**
Right foot, medial view.

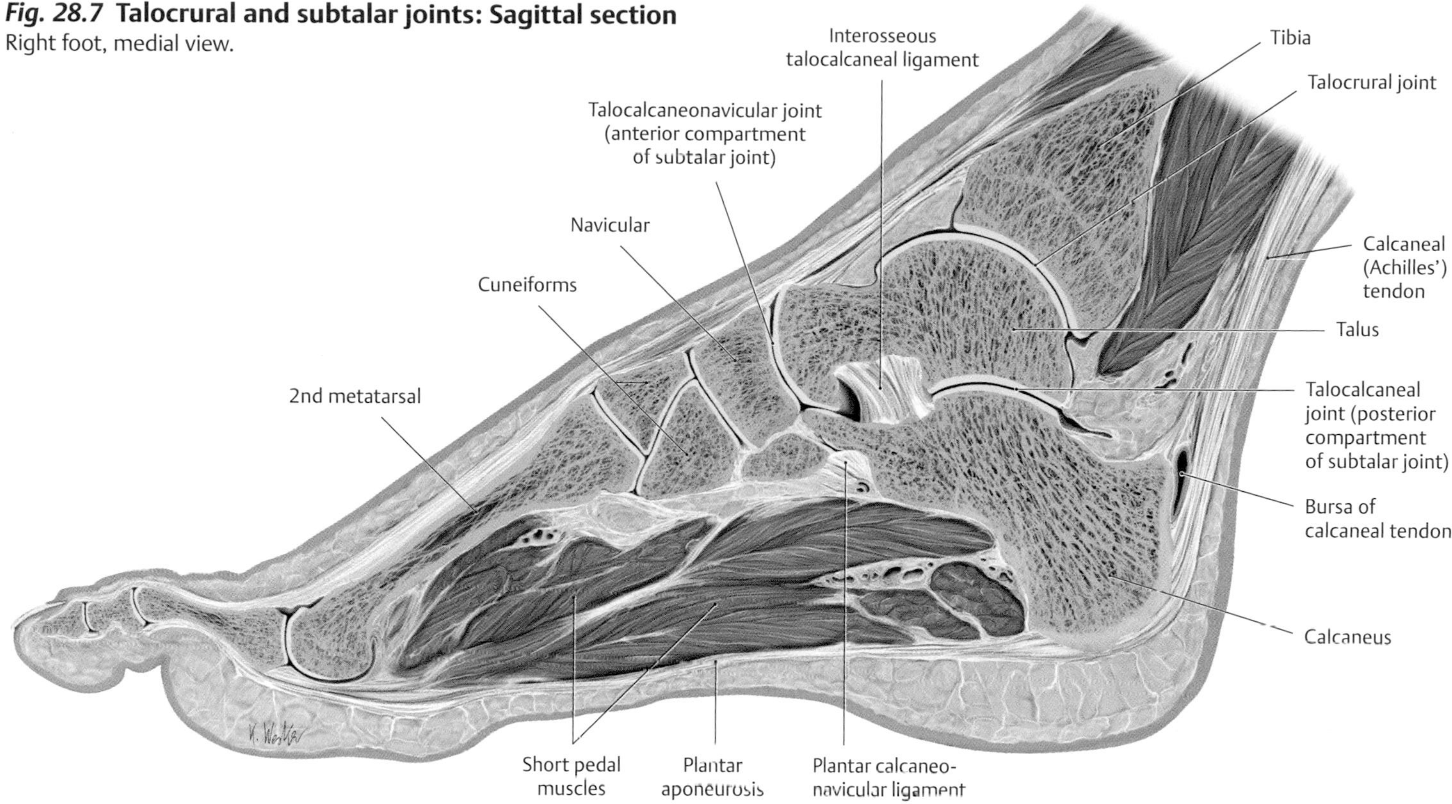
Interosseous talocalcaneal ligament
Tibia
Talocrural joint
Talocalcaneonavicular joint (anterior compartment of subtalar joint)
Navicular
Cuneiforms
2nd metatarsal
Calcaneal (Achilles') tendon
Talus
Talocalcaneal joint (posterior compartment of subtalar joint)
Bursa of calcaneal tendon
Calcaneus
Short pedal muscles
Plantar aponeurosis
Plantar calcaneo-navicular ligament

Fig. 28.8 **Talocrural joint**
Right foot.

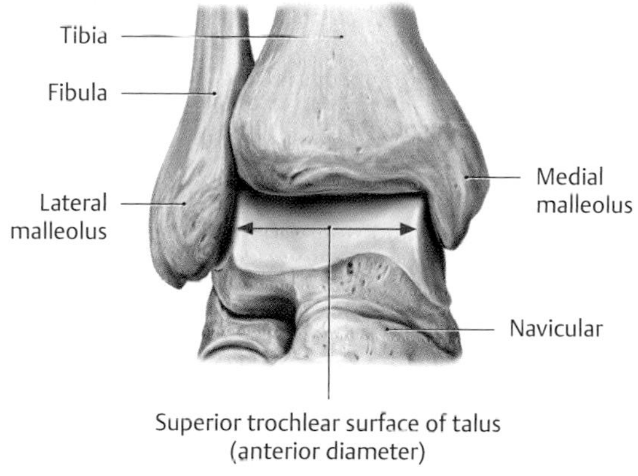
Tibia
Fibula
Lateral malleolus
Medial malleolus
Navicular
Superior trochlear surface of talus (anterior diameter)

A Anterior view.

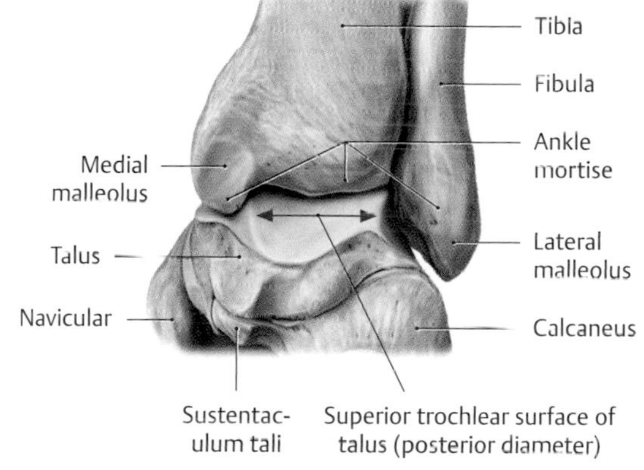
Tibia
Fibula
Medial malleolus
Ankle mortise
Talus
Lateral malleolus
Navicular
Calcaneus
Sustentac-ulum tali
Superior trochlear surface of talus (posterior diameter)

B Posterior view.

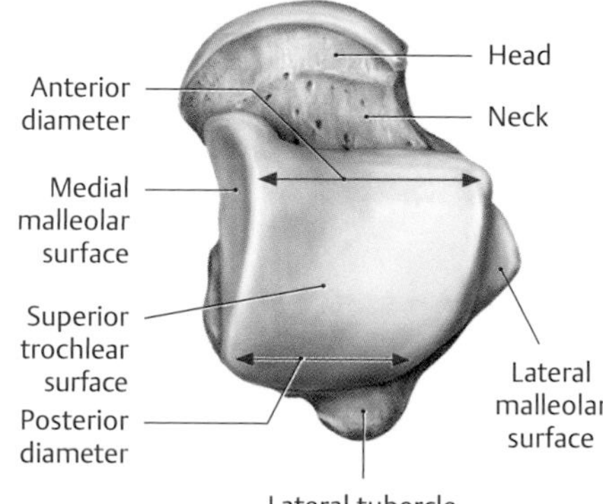
Head
Anterior diameter
Neck
Medial malleolar surface
Superior trochlear surface
Posterior diameter
Lateral malleolar surface
Lateral tubercle

C Proximal (superior) view of talus.

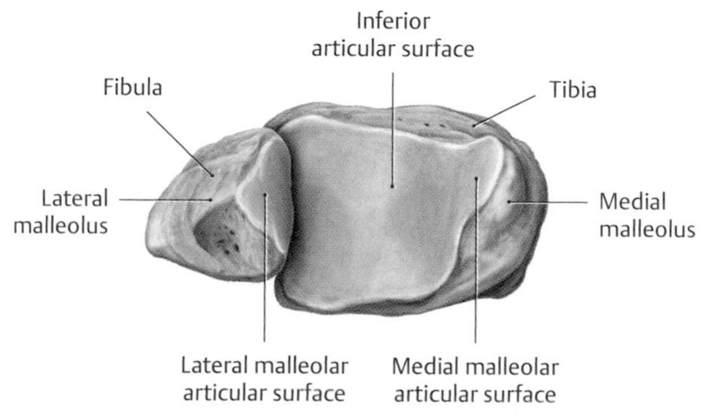
Inferior articular surface
Fibula
Tibia
Lateral malleolus
Medial malleolus
Lateral malleolar articular surface
Medial malleolar articular surface

D Distal (inferior) view of ankle mortise.

Joints of the Foot (III)

Fig. 28.9 **Subtalar joint and ligaments**

Right foot with opened subtalar joint. The subtalar joint consists of two distinct articulations separated by the interosseous talocalcaneal ligament: the posterior compartment (talocalcaneal joint) and the anterior compartment (talocalcaneonavicular joint).

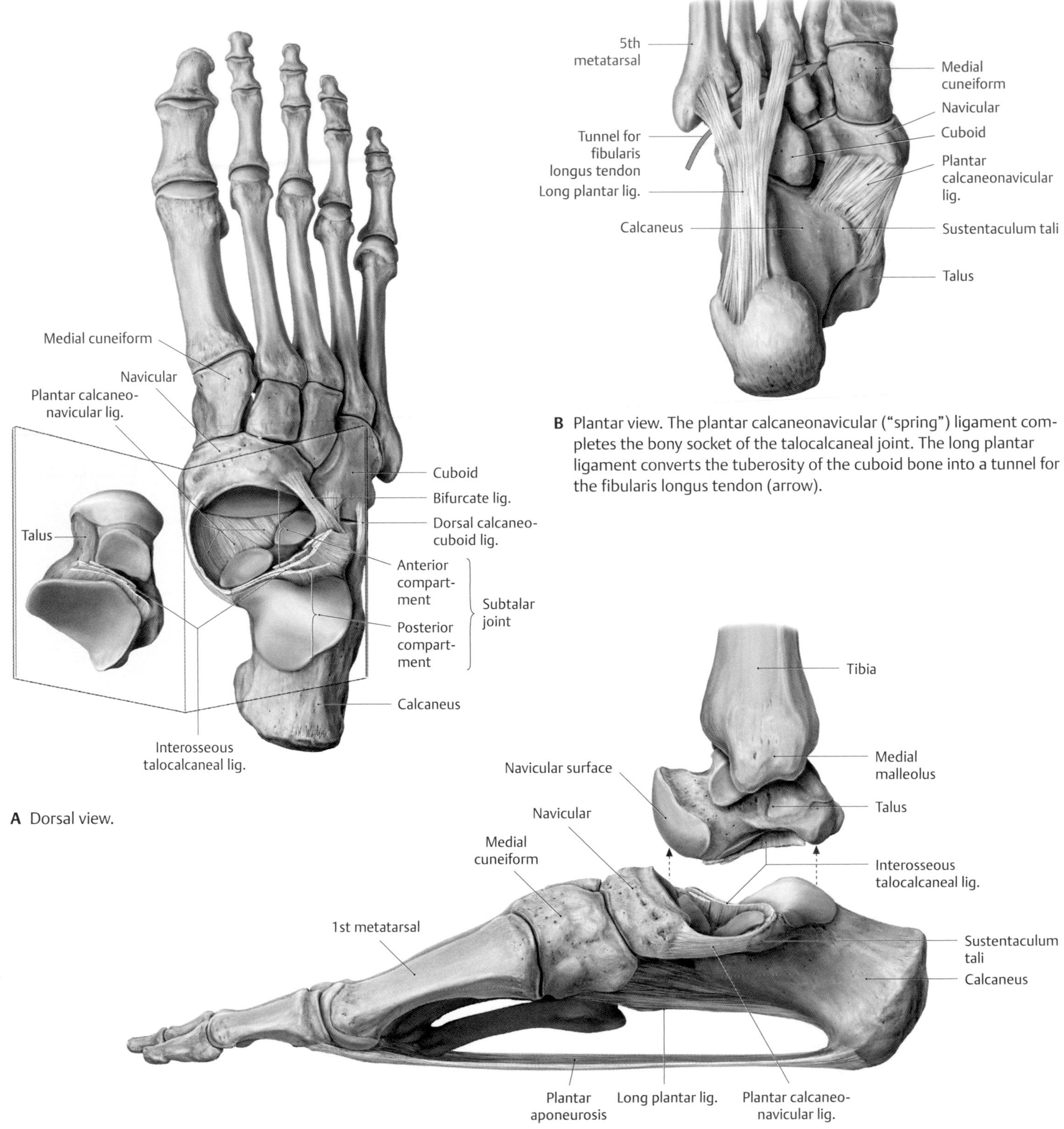

5th metatarsal
Medial cuneiform
Navicular
Cuboid
Tunnel for fibularis longus tendon
Plantar calcaneonavicular lig.
Long plantar lig.
Calcaneus
Sustentaculum tali
Talus
Medial cuneiform
Navicular
Plantar calcaneo-navicular lig.
Talus
Cuboid
Bifurcate lig.
Dorsal calcaneo-cuboid lig.
Anterior compart-ment
Posterior compart-ment
Subtalar joint
Calcaneus
Interosseous talocalcaneal lig.
Tibia
Medial malleolus
Navicular surface
Talus
Navicular
Medial cuneiform
Interosseous talocalcaneal lig.
1st metatarsal
Sustentaculum tali
Calcaneus
Plantar aponeurosis
Long plantar lig.
Plantar calcaneo-navicular lig.

A Dorsal view.

B Plantar view. The plantar calcaneonavicular ("spring") ligament completes the bony socket of the talocalcaneal joint. The long plantar ligament converts the tuberosity of the cuboid bone into a tunnel for the fibularis longus tendon (arrow).

C Medial view. The interosseous talocalcaneal ligament has been divided and the talus displaced upward. Note the course of the plantar calcaneonavicular ligament, which functions with the long plantar ligament and plantar aponeurosis to support the longitudinal arch of the foot.

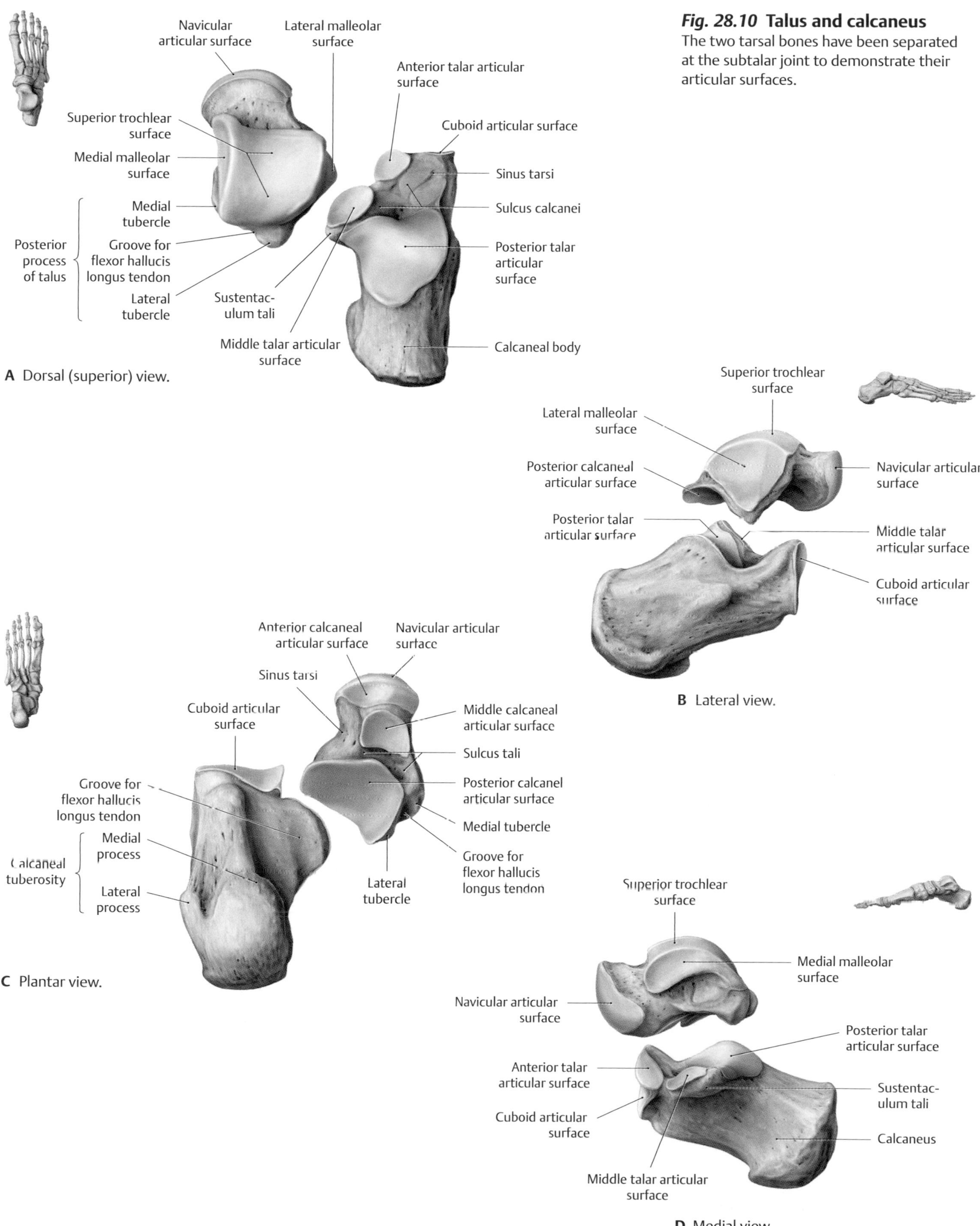
Navicular articular surface
Lateral malleolar surface
Anterior talar articular surface
Cuboid articular surface
Superior trochlear surface
Medial malleolar surface
Sinus tarsi
Medial tubercle
Sulcus calcanei
Posterior process of talus
Groove for flexor hallucis longus tendon
Posterior talar articular surface
Lateral tubercle
Sustentaculum tali
Middle talar articular surface
Calcaneal body
A Dorsal (superior) view.
Superior trochlear surface
Lateral malleolar surface
Posterior calcaneal articular surface
Navicular articular surface
Posterior talar articular surface
Middle talar articular surface
Cuboid articular surface
B Lateral view.
Anterior calcaneal articular surface
Navicular articular surface
Sinus tarsi
Cuboid articular surface
Middle calcaneal articular surface
Sulcus tali
Groove for flexor hallucis longus tendon
Posterior calcanel articular surface
Medial tubercle
Calcaneal tuberosity
Medial process
Lateral process
Groove for flexor hallucis longus tendon
Lateral tubercle
C Plantar view.
Superior trochlear surface
Medial malleolar surface
Navicular articular surface
Posterior talar articular surface
Anterior talar articular surface
Sustentaculum tali
Cuboid articular surface
Calcaneus
Middle talar articular surface
D Medial view.

Fig. 28.10 **Talus and calcaneus**
The two tarsal bones have been separated at the subtalar joint to demonstrate their articular surfaces.

Ligaments of the Ankle & Foot

The ligaments of the foot are classified as belonging to the talocrural joint, subtalar joint, metatarsus, forefoot, or sole of the foot. The medial and lateral collateral ligaments, along with the syndesmotic ligaments, are of major importance in the stabilization of the subtalar joint.

Fig. 28.11 Ligaments of the ankle and foot
Right foot. See p. 430 for inferior view.

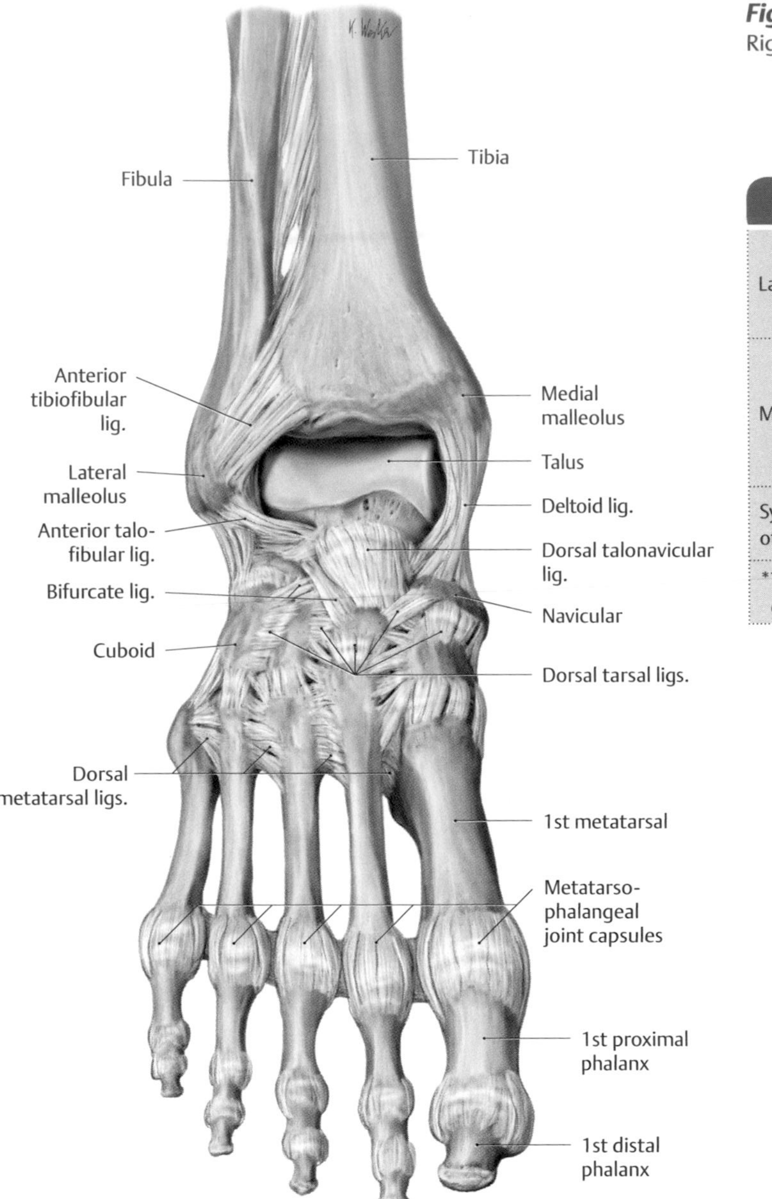
Tibia
Fibula
Anterior tibiofibular lig.
Medial malleolus
Lateral malleolus
Talus
Deltoid lig.
Anterior talofibular lig.
Dorsal talonavicular lig.
Bifurcate lig.
Navicular
Cuboid
Dorsal tarsal ligs.
Dorsal metatarsal ligs.
1st metatarsal
Metatarsophalangeal joint capsules
1st proximal phalanx
1st distal phalanx

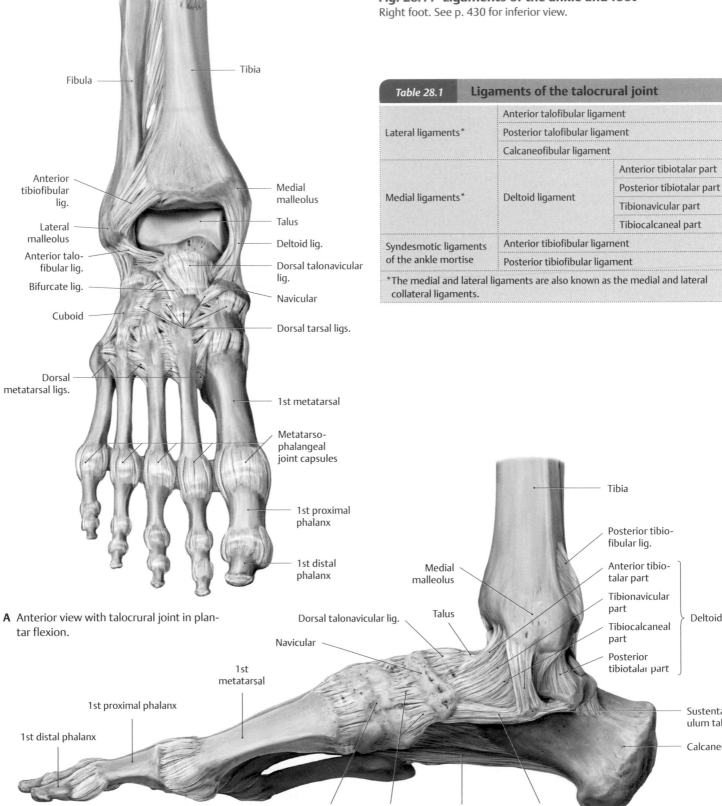

A Anterior view with talocrural joint in plantar flexion.

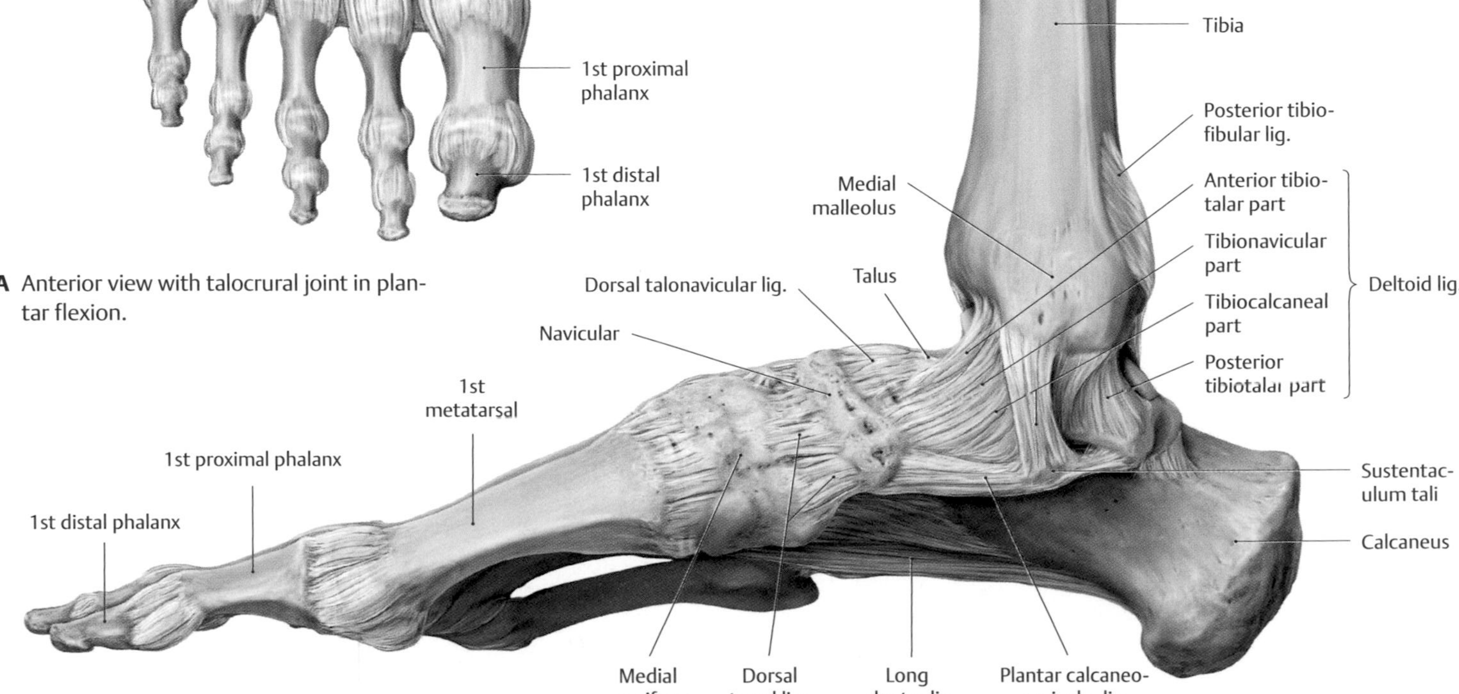
Tibia
Posterior tibiofibular lig.
Medial malleolus
Anterior tibiotalar part
Tibionavicular part
Deltoid lig.
Tibiocalcaneal part
Posterior tibiotalar part
Talus
Dorsal talonavicular lig.
Navicular
1st metatarsal
1st proximal phalanx
1st distal phalanx
Sustentaculum tali
Calcaneus
Medial cuneiform
Dorsal tarsal ligs.
Long plantar lig.
Plantar calcaneonavicular lig.

B Medial view.

Table 28.1 Ligaments of the talocrural joint

Lateral ligaments*	Anterior talofibular ligament	
	Posterior talofibular ligament	
	Calcaneofibular ligament	
Medial ligaments*	Deltoid ligament	Anterior tibiotalar part
		Posterior tibiotalar part
		Tibionavicular part
		Tibiocalcaneal part
Syndesmotic ligaments of the ankle mortise	Anterior tibiofibular ligament	
	Posterior tibiofibular ligament	

*The medial and lateral ligaments are also known as the medial and lateral collateral ligaments.

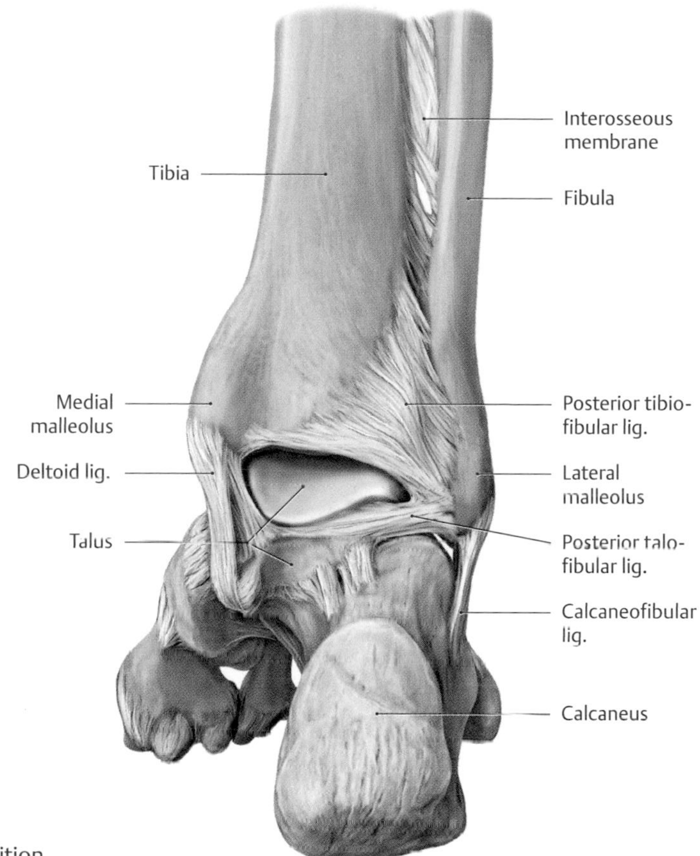
Interosseous
membrane
Tibia
Fibula
Medial
malleolus
Posterior tibio-
fibular lig.
Deltoid lig.
Lateral
malleolus
Talus
Posterior talo-
fibular lig.
Calcaneofibular
lig.
Calcaneus

C Posterior view in plantigrade foot position.

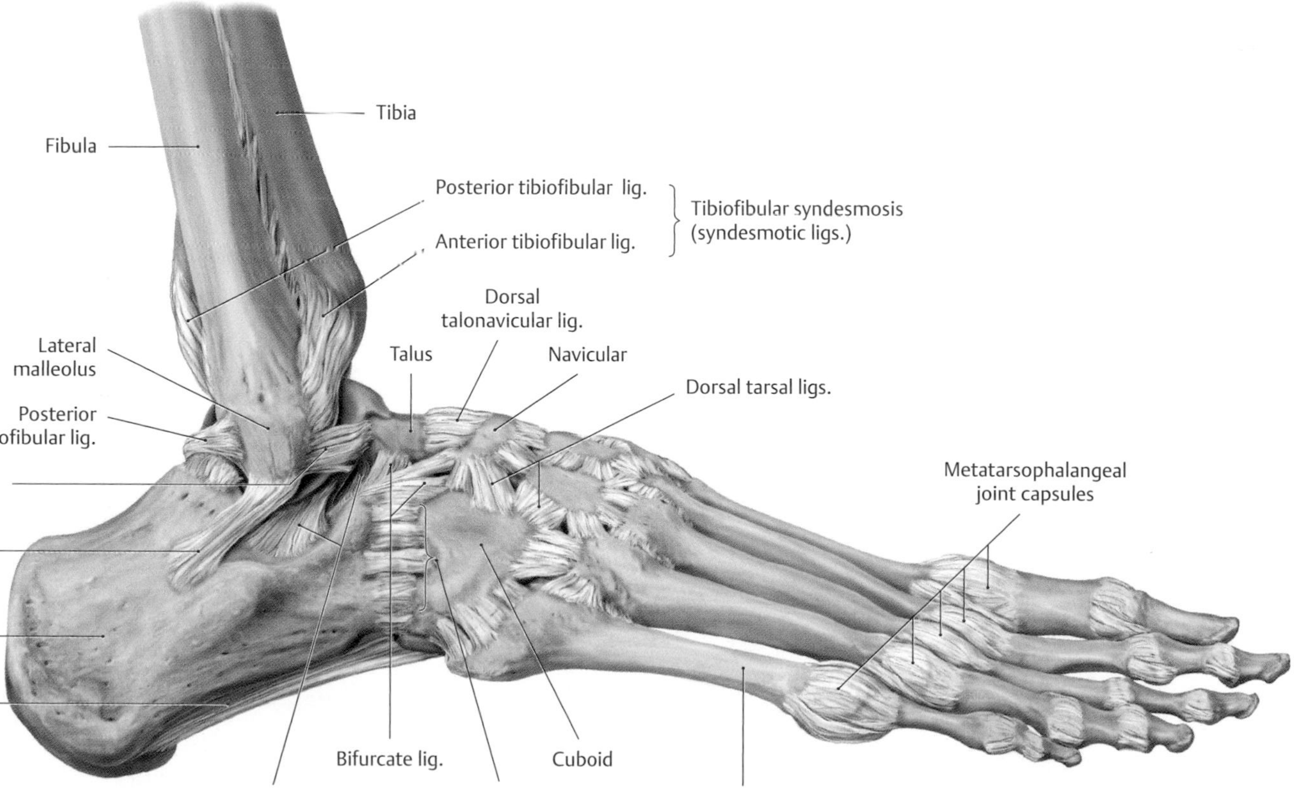

Tibia
Fibula
Posterior tibiofibular lig.
Anterior tibiofibular lig.
Tibiofibular syndesmosis
(syndesmotic ligs.)
Dorsal
talonavicular lig.
Lateral
malleolus
Talus
Navicular
Dorsal tarsal ligs.
Posterior
talofibular lig.
Anterior talo-
fibular ligament
Metatarsophalangeal
joint capsules
Calcaneo-
fibular lig.
Calcaneus
Long plantar lig.
Bifurcate lig.
Cuboid
Interosseous
talocalcaneal lig.
Dorsal calcaneocuboid ligs.
5th metatarsal

D Lateral view.

Plantar Vault & Arches of the Foot

Fig. 28.12 Plantar vault

Right foot. The forces of the foot are distributed among two lateral (fibular) and three medial (tibial) rays. The arrangement of these rays creates a longitudinal and a transverse arch in the sole of the foot, helping the foot absorb vertical loads.

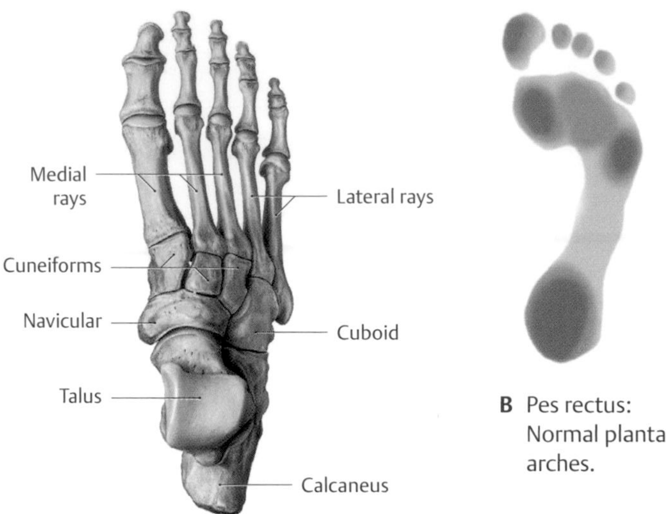

Medial rays
Lateral rays
Cuneiforms
Navicular
Cuboid
Talus
Calcaneus

A Plantar vault, superior view. Lateral rays in green, medial rays in red.

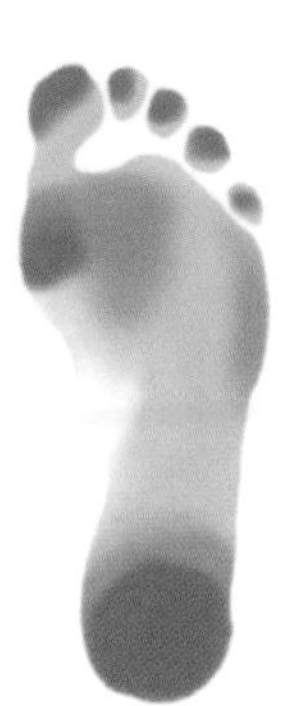
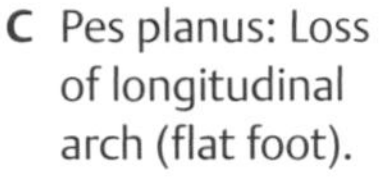

B Pes rectus: Normal plantar arches.

C Pes planus: Loss of longitudinal arch (flat foot).

D Pes cavus: Increased height of longitudinal arch.

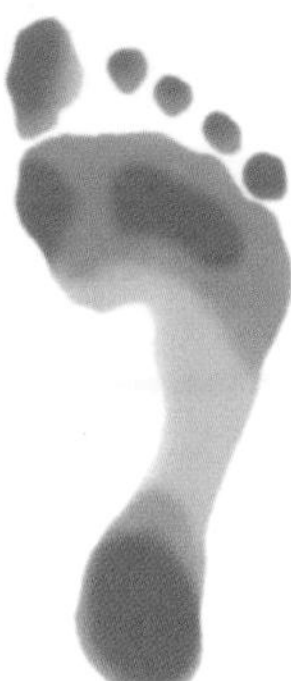

E Pes transverso-planus: Loss of transverse arch (splayfoot).

Fig. 28.13 Stabilizers of the transverse arch

Right foot. The transverse pedal arch is supported by both active and passive stabilizing structures (muscles and ligaments, respectively).

Note: The arch of the forefoot has only passive stabilizers, whereas the arches of the metatarsus and tarsus have only active stabilizers.

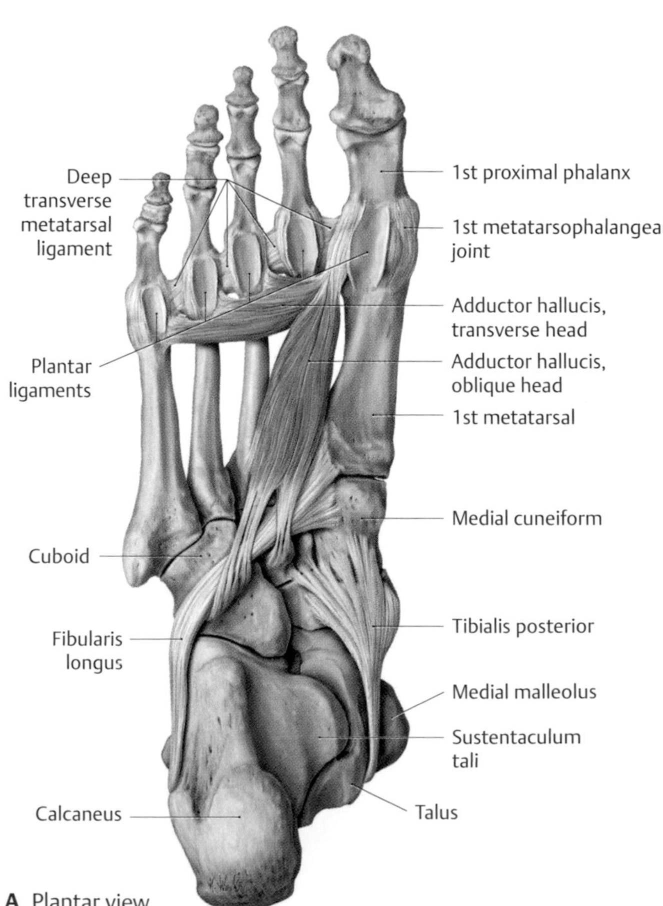

Deep transverse metatarsal ligament
1st proximal phalanx
1st metatarsophalangeal joint
Adductor hallucis, transverse head
Plantar ligaments
Adductor hallucis, oblique head
1st metatarsal
Medial cuneiform
Cuboid
Tibialis posterior
Fibularis longus
Medial malleolus
Sustentaculum tali
Calcaneus
Talus

A Plantar view.

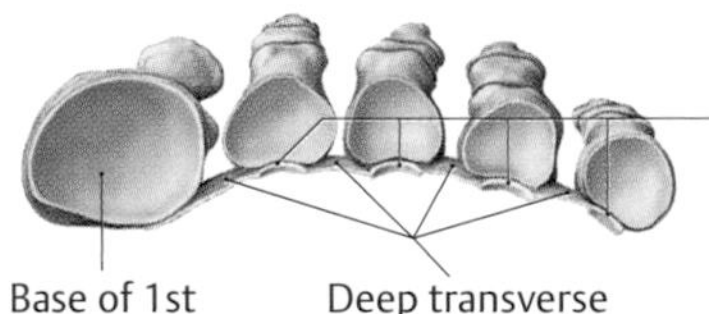

Plantar ligaments
Base of 1st proximal phalanx
Deep transverse metatarsal ligament

B Anterior arch (forefoot), proximal view.

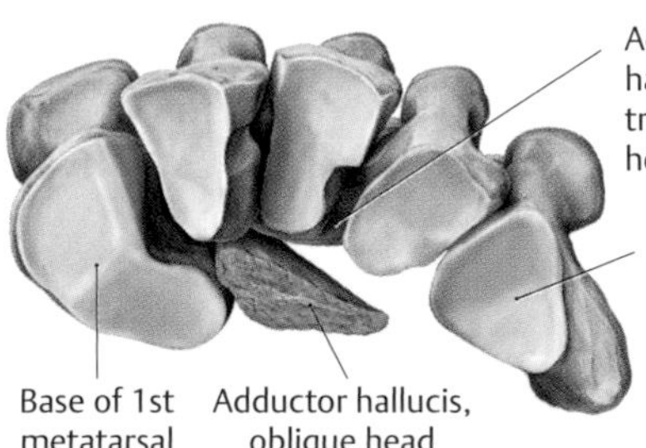

Adductor hallucis, transverse head
Base of 5th meta-tarsal
Base of 1st metatarsal
Adductor hallucis, oblique head

C Metatarsal arch, proximal view.

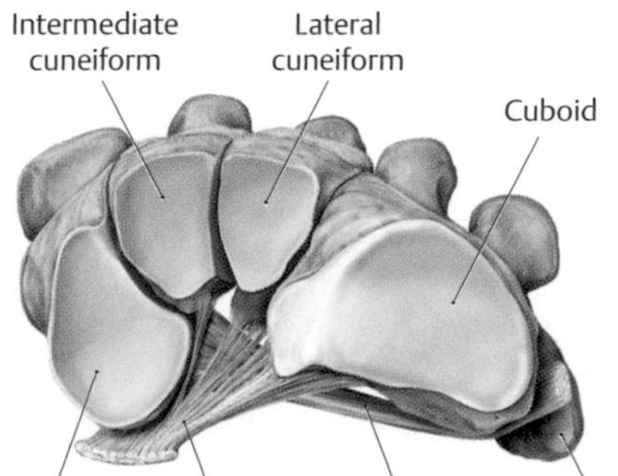

Intermediate cuneiform
Lateral cuneiform
Cuboid
Medial cuneiform
Tibialis posterior
Fibularis longus
Tuberosity of 5th metatarsal

D Tarsal region, proximal view.

Fig. 28.14 Stabilizers of the longitudinal arch
Right foot, medial view.

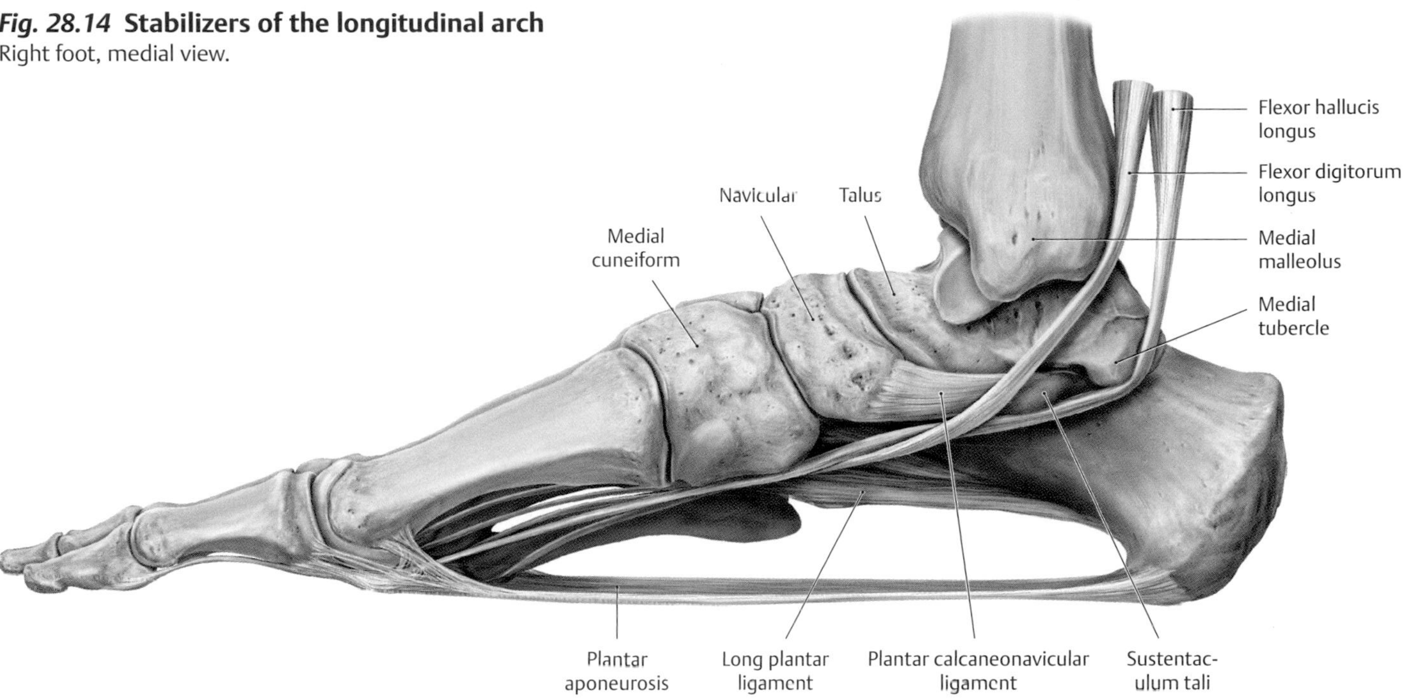
Flexor hallucis longus
Flexor digitorum longus
Navicular
Talus
Medial cuneiform
Medial malleolus
Medial tubercle
Plantar aponeurosis
Long plantar ligament
Plantar calcaneonavicular ligament
Sustentac-ulum tali

A Passive stabilizers of the longitudinal arch. The main passive stabilizers of the longitudinal arch are the plantar aponeurosis (most important), the long plantar ligament, and the plantar calcaneonavicular ligament (weakest component).

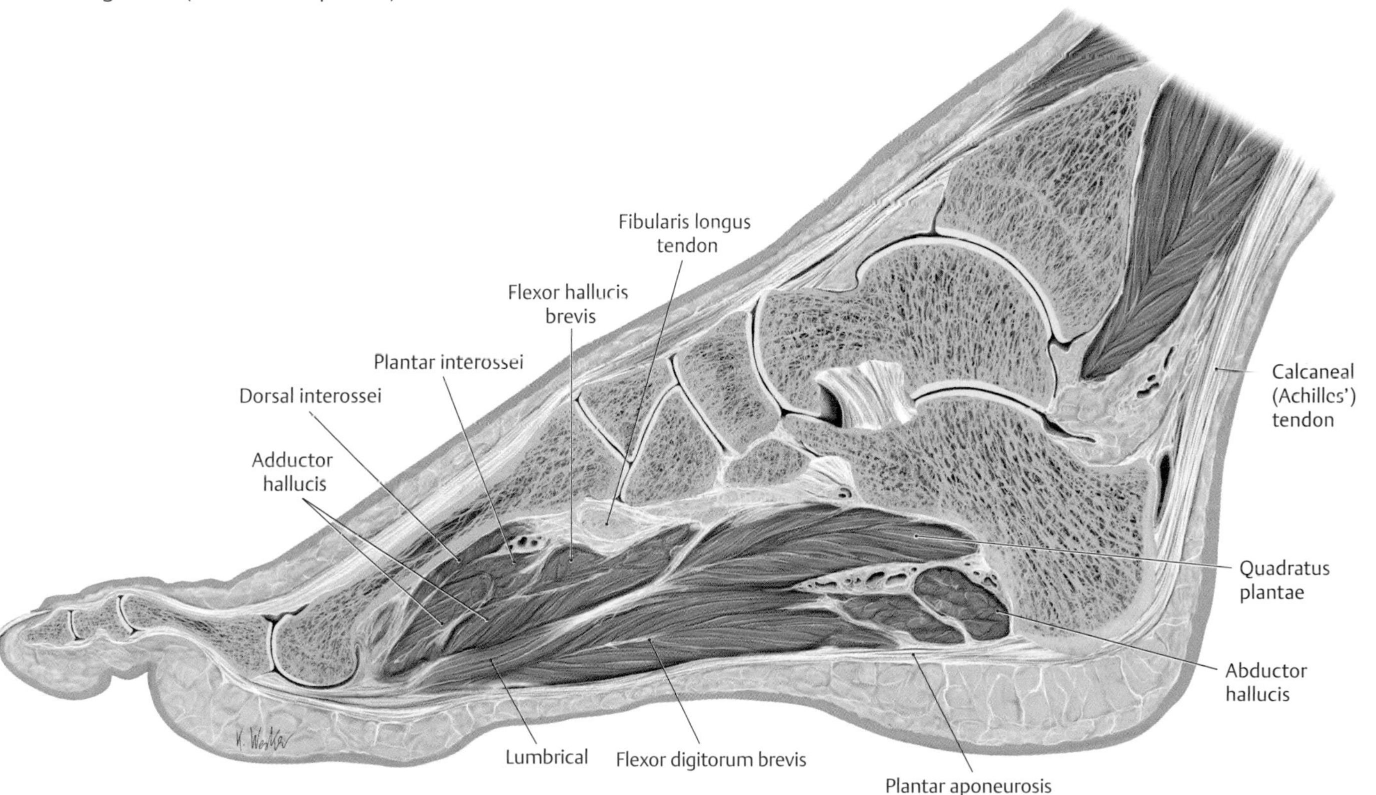
Fibularis longus tendon
Flexor hallucis brevis
Plantar interossei
Dorsal interossei
Adductor hallucis
Calcaneal (Achilles') tendon
Quadratus plantae
Abductor hallucis
Lumbrical
Flexor digitorum brevis
Plantar aponeurosis

B Active stabilizers of the longitudinal arch. Sagittal section at the level of the second ray. The major active stabilizers of the foot are the abductor hallucis, flexor hallucis brevis, flexor digitorum brevis, quadratus plantae, and abductor digiti minimi.

Muscles of the Sole of the Foot

Fig. 28.15 Plantar aponeurosis
Right foot, plantar view. The plantar aponeurosis is a tough aponeurotic sheet, thickest at the center, that blends with the dorsal fascia (not shown) at the borders of the foot.

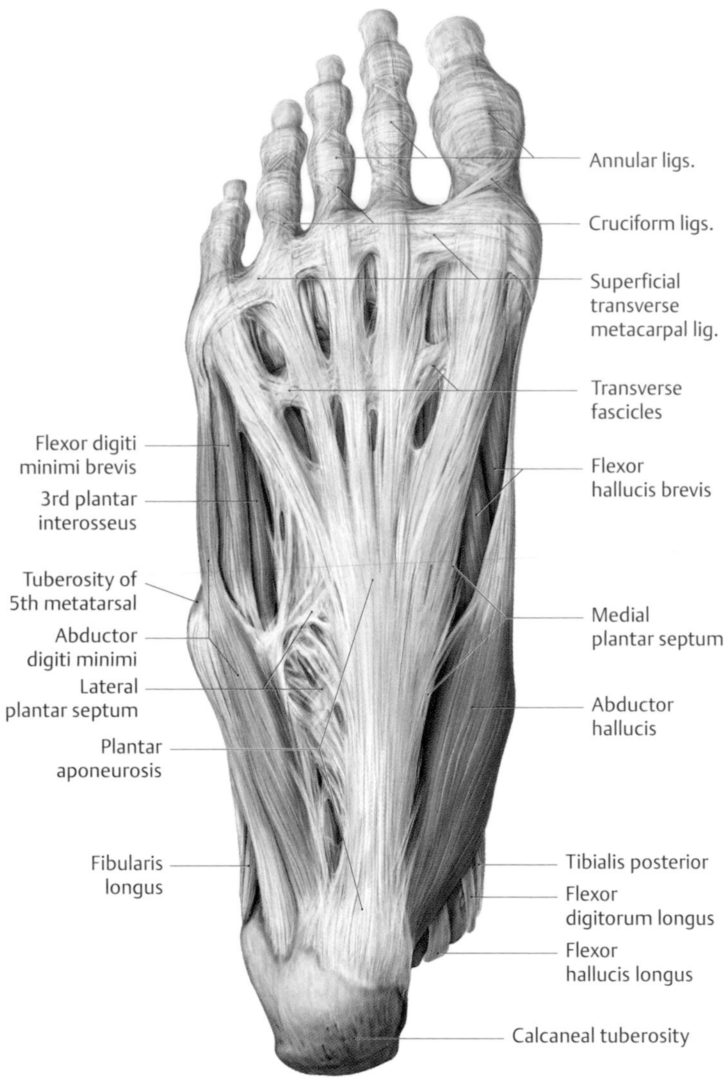
Annular ligs.
Cruciform ligs.
Superficial transverse metacarpal lig.
Transverse fascicles
Flexor hallucis brevis
Medial plantar septum
Abductor hallucis
Tibialis posterior
Flexor digitorum longus
Flexor hallucis longus
Calcaneal tuberosity
Flexor digiti minimi brevis
3rd plantar interosseus
Tuberosity of 5th metatarsal
Abductor digiti minimi
Lateral plantar septum
Plantar aponeurosis
Fibularis longus

Fig. 28.16 Intrinsic muscles of the sole of the foot
Right foot, plantar view.

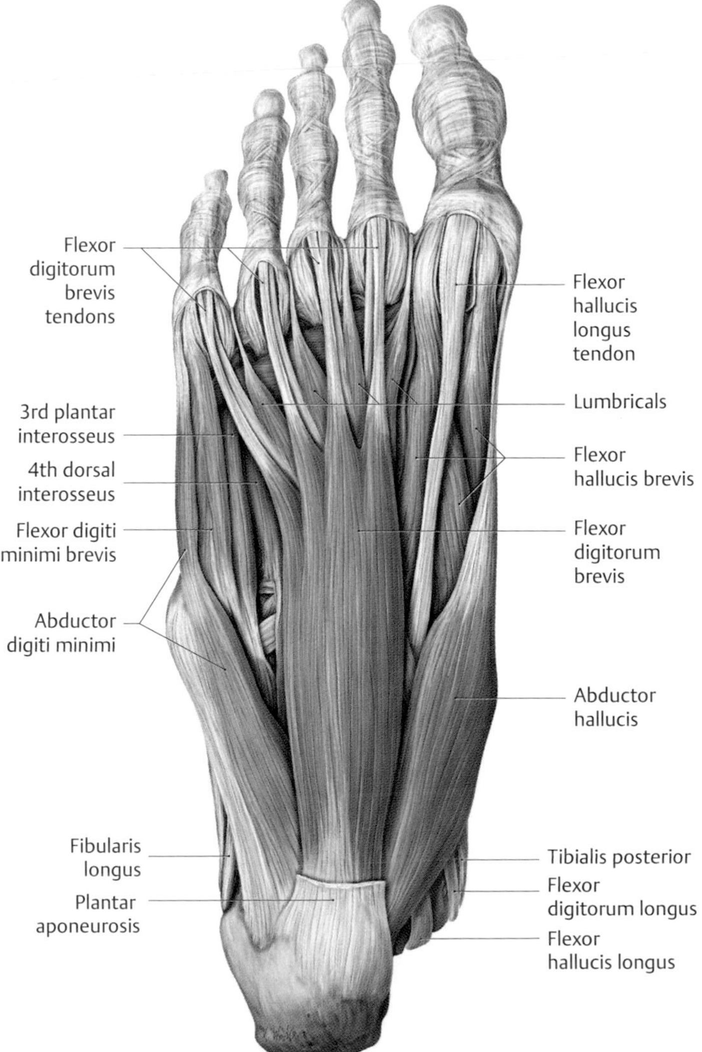
Flexor digitorum brevis tendons
3rd plantar interosseus
4th dorsal interosseus
Flexor digiti minimi brevis
Abductor digiti minimi
Fibularis longus
Plantar aponeurosis
Flexor hallucis longus tendon
Lumbricals
Flexor hallucis brevis
Flexor digitorum brevis
Abductor hallucis
Tibialis posterior
Flexor digitorum longus
Flexor hallucis longus

A Superficial (first) layer. *Removed:* Plantar aponeurosis, including the superficial transverse metacarpal ligament.

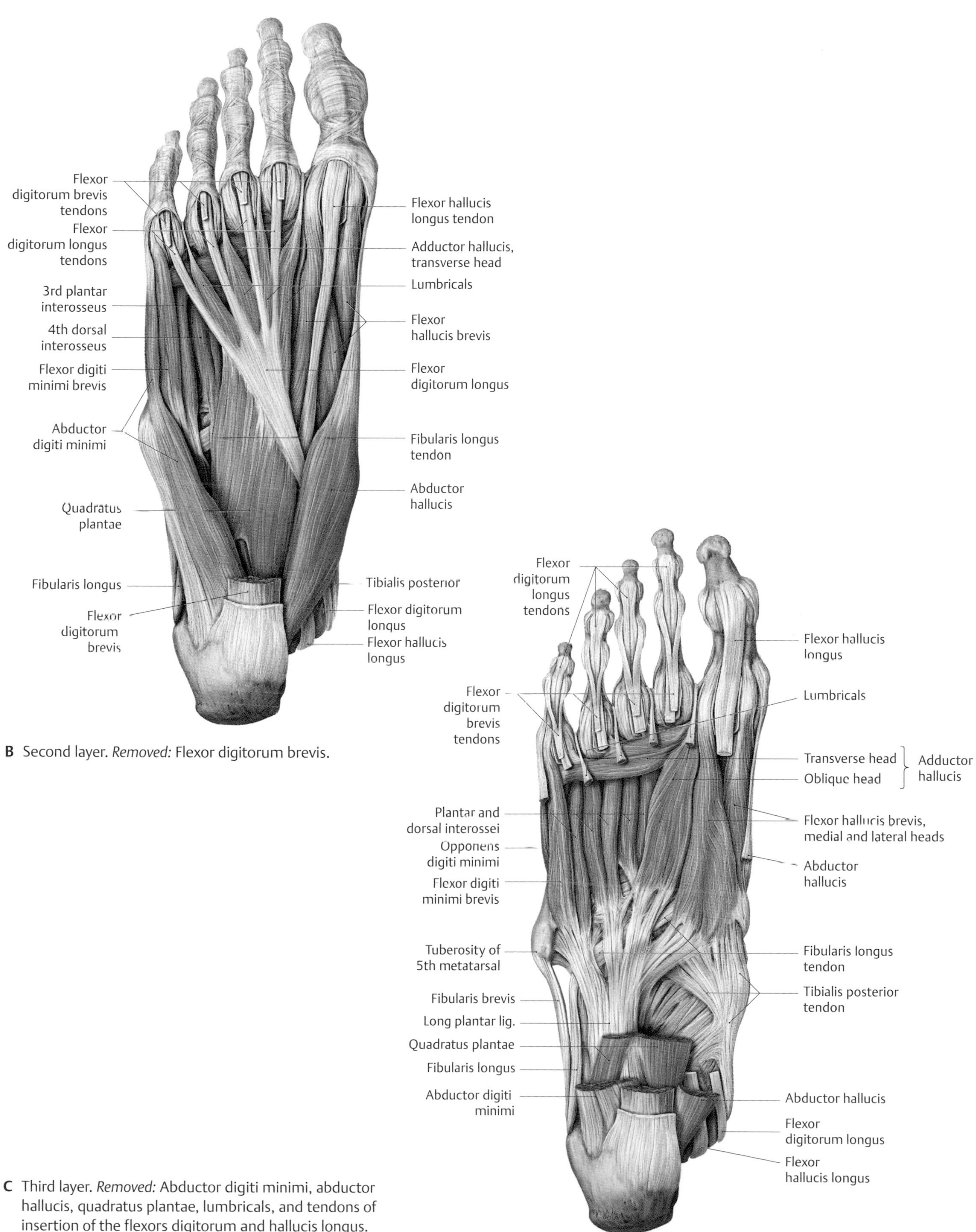
Flexor digitorum brevis tendons
Flexor digitorum longus tendons
3rd plantar interosseus
4th dorsal interosseus
Flexor digiti minimi brevis
Abductor digiti minimi
Quadratus plantae
Fibularis longus
Flexor digitorum brevis
Flexor hallucis longus tendon
Adductor hallucis, transverse head
Lumbricals
Flexor hallucis brevis
Flexor digitorum longus
Fibularis longus tendon
Abductor hallucis
Tibialis posterior
Flexor digitorum longus
Flexor hallucis longus
Flexor digitorum longus tendons
Flexor digitorum brevis tendons
Plantar and dorsal interossei
Opponens digiti minimi
Flexor digiti minimi brevis
Tuberosity of 5th metatarsal
Fibularis brevis
Long plantar lig.
Quadratus plantae
Fibularis longus
Abductor digiti minimi
Flexor hallucis longus
Lumbricals
Transverse head
Oblique head
Adductor hallucis
Flexor hallucis brevis, medial and lateral heads
Abductor hallucis
Fibularis longus tendon
Tibialis posterior tendon
Abductor hallucis
Flexor digitorum longus
Flexor hallucis longus

B Second layer. *Removed:* Flexor digitorum brevis.

C Third layer. *Removed:* Abductor digiti minimi, abductor hallucis, quadratus plantae, lumbricals, and tendons of insertion of the flexors digitorum and hallucis longus.

Muscles & Tendon Sheaths of the Foot

Fig. 28.17 **Deep intrinsic muscles of the sole of the foot**
Right foot, plantar view.

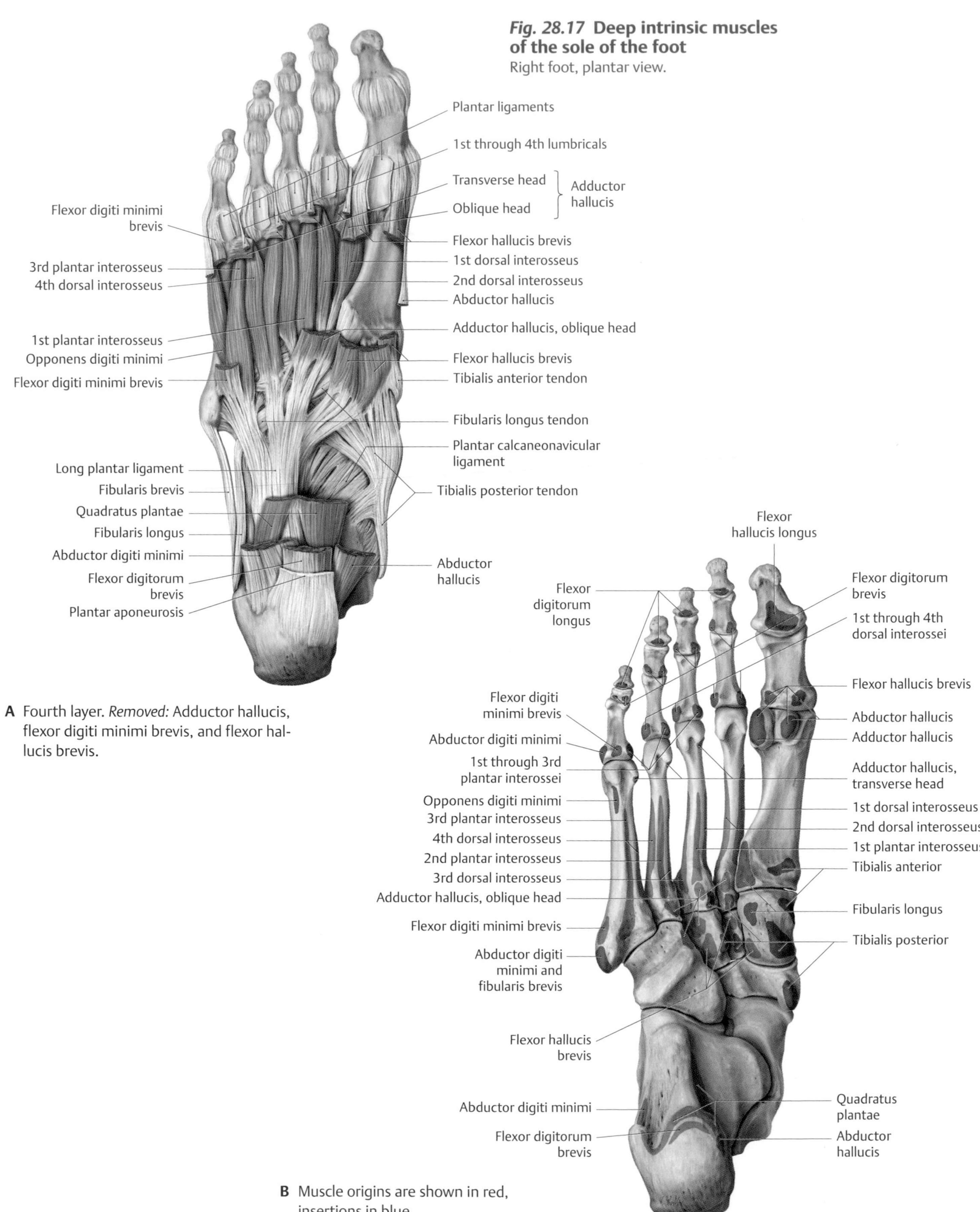

Plantar ligaments
1st through 4th lumbricals
Transverse head
Oblique head
Adductor hallucis
Flexor digiti minimi brevis
Flexor hallucis brevis
3rd plantar interosseus
4th dorsal interosseus
1st dorsal interosseus
2nd dorsal interosseus
Abductor hallucis
Adductor hallucis, oblique head
1st plantar interosseus
Opponens digiti minimi
Flexor hallucis brevis
Flexor digiti minimi brevis
Tibialis anterior tendon
Fibularis longus tendon
Plantar calcaneonavicular ligament
Long plantar ligament
Fibularis brevis
Tibialis posterior tendon
Quadratus plantae
Fibularis longus
Abductor digiti minimi
Abductor hallucis
Flexor digitorum brevis
Plantar aponeurosis
Flexor hallucis longus
Flexor digitorum longus
Flexor digitorum brevis
1st through 4th dorsal interossei
Flexor hallucis brevis
Flexor digiti minimi brevis
Abductor hallucis
Abductor digiti minimi
Adductor hallucis
1st through 3rd plantar interossei
Adductor hallucis, transverse head
Opponens digiti minimi
3rd plantar interosseus
1st dorsal interosseus
4th dorsal interosseus
2nd dorsal interosseus
2nd plantar interosseus
1st plantar interosseus
3rd dorsal interosseus
Tibialis anterior
Adductor hallucis, oblique head
Fibularis longus
Flexor digiti minimi brevis
Tibialis posterior
Abductor digiti minimi and fibularis brevis
Flexor hallucis brevis
Abductor digiti minimi
Quadratus plantae
Flexor digitorum brevis
Abductor hallucis

A Fourth layer. *Removed:* Adductor hallucis, flexor digiti minimi brevis, and flexor hallucis brevis.

B Muscle origins are shown in red, insertions in blue.

Fig. 28.18 **Tendon sheaths and retinacula of the ankle**
Right foot. The superior and inferior extensor retinacula retain the long extensor tendons, the fibularis retinacula hold the fibular muscle tendons in place, and the flexor retinaculum retains the long flexor tendons.

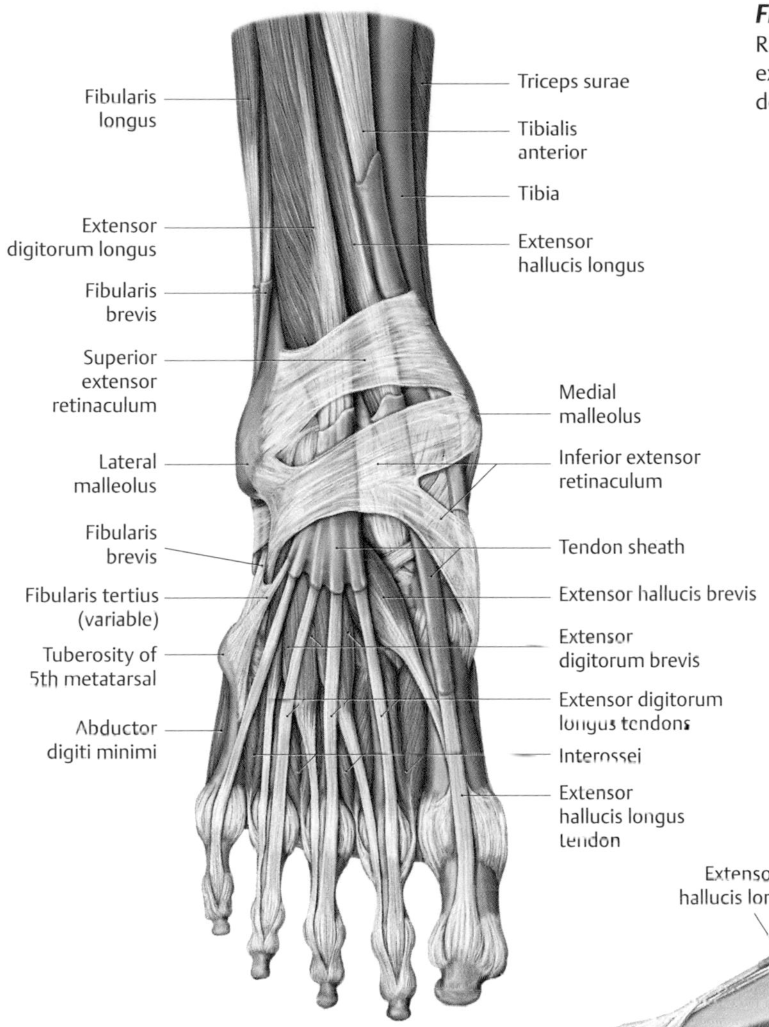

Fibularis longus
Triceps surae
Tibialis anterior
Tibia
Extensor digitorum longus
Extensor hallucis longus
Fibularis brevis
Superior extensor retinaculum
Medial malleolus
Lateral malleolus
Inferior extensor retinaculum
Fibularis brevis
Tendon sheath
Fibularis tertius (variable)
Extensor hallucis brevis
Tuberosity of 5th metatarsal
Extensor digitorum brevis
Extensor digitorum longus tendons
Abductor digiti minimi
Interossei
Extensor hallucis longus tendon

A Anterior view with talocrural joint in plantar flexion.

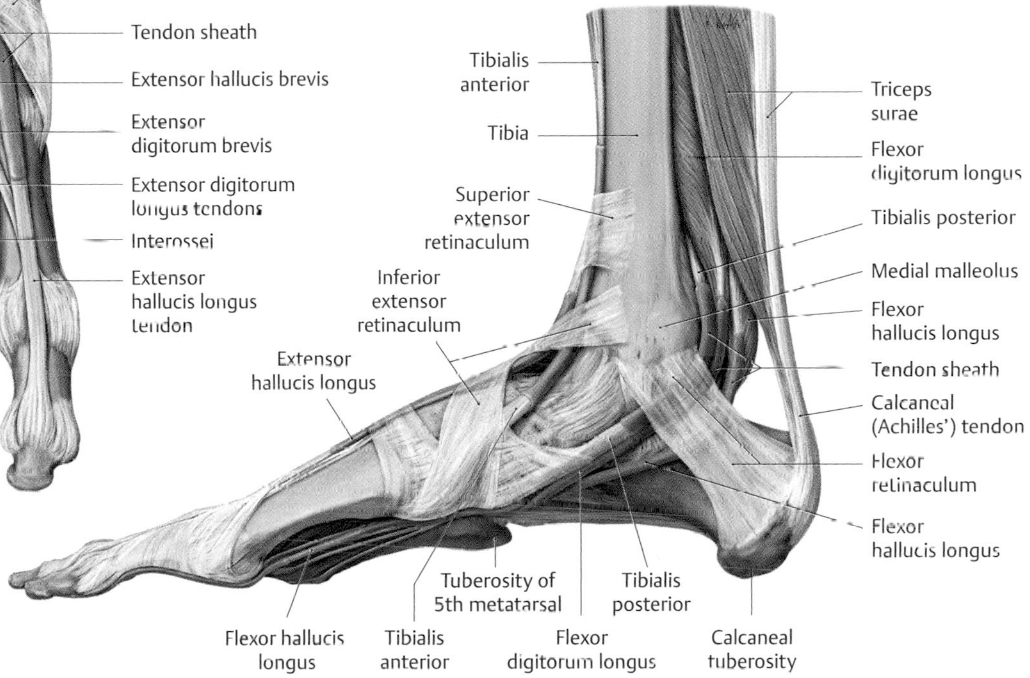

Tibialis anterior
Triceps surae
Tibia
Flexor digitorum longus
Superior extensor retinaculum
Tibialis posterior
Medial malleolus
Inferior extensor retinaculum
Flexor hallucis longus
Extensor hallucis longus
Tendon sheath
Calcaneal (Achilles') tendon
Flexor retinaculum
Flexor hallucis longus
Tuberosity of 5th metatarsal
Tibialis posterior
Flexor hallucis longus
Tibialis anterior
Flexor digitorum longus
Calcaneal tuberosity

B Medial view.

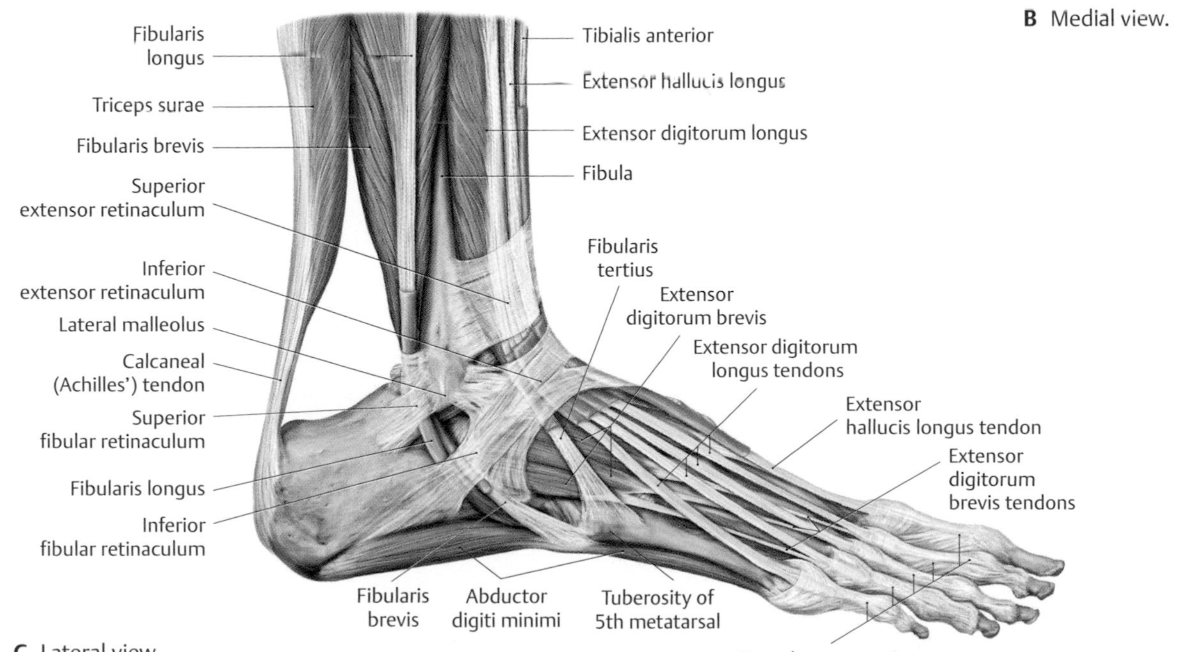
Fibularis longus
Tibialis anterior
Extensor hallucis longus
Triceps surae
Fibularis brevis
Extensor digitorum longus
Fibula
Superior extensor retinaculum
Fibularis tertius
Inferior extensor retinaculum
Extensor digitorum brevis
Lateral malleolus
Extensor digitorum longus tendons
Calcaneal (Achilles') tendon
Superior fibular retinaculum
Extensor hallucis longus tendon
Extensor digitorum brevis tendons
Fibularis longus
Inferior fibular retinaculum
Fibularis brevis
Abductor digiti minimi
Tuberosity of 5th metatarsal
Dorsal aponeurosis

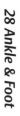

C Lateral view.

Muscle Facts (I)

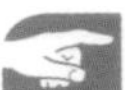

The dorsal surface (dorsum) of the foot contains only two muscles, the extensor digitorum brevis and the extensor hallucis brevis. The sole of the foot, however, is composed of four complex layers that maintain the arches of the foot.

Fig. 28.19 **Intrinsic muscles of the dorsum of the foot**
Right foot, dorsal view.

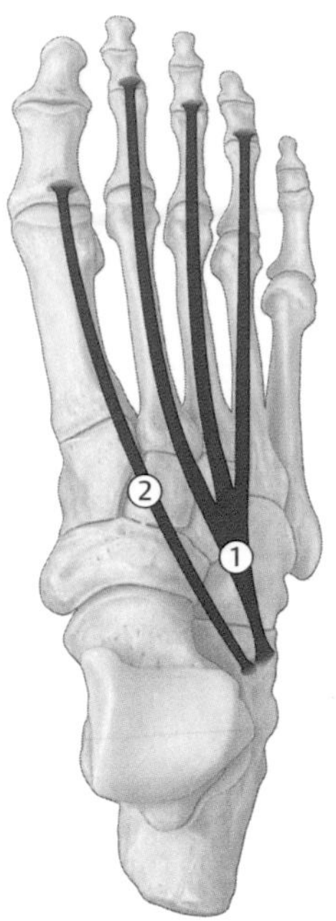

2
1

A Schematic.

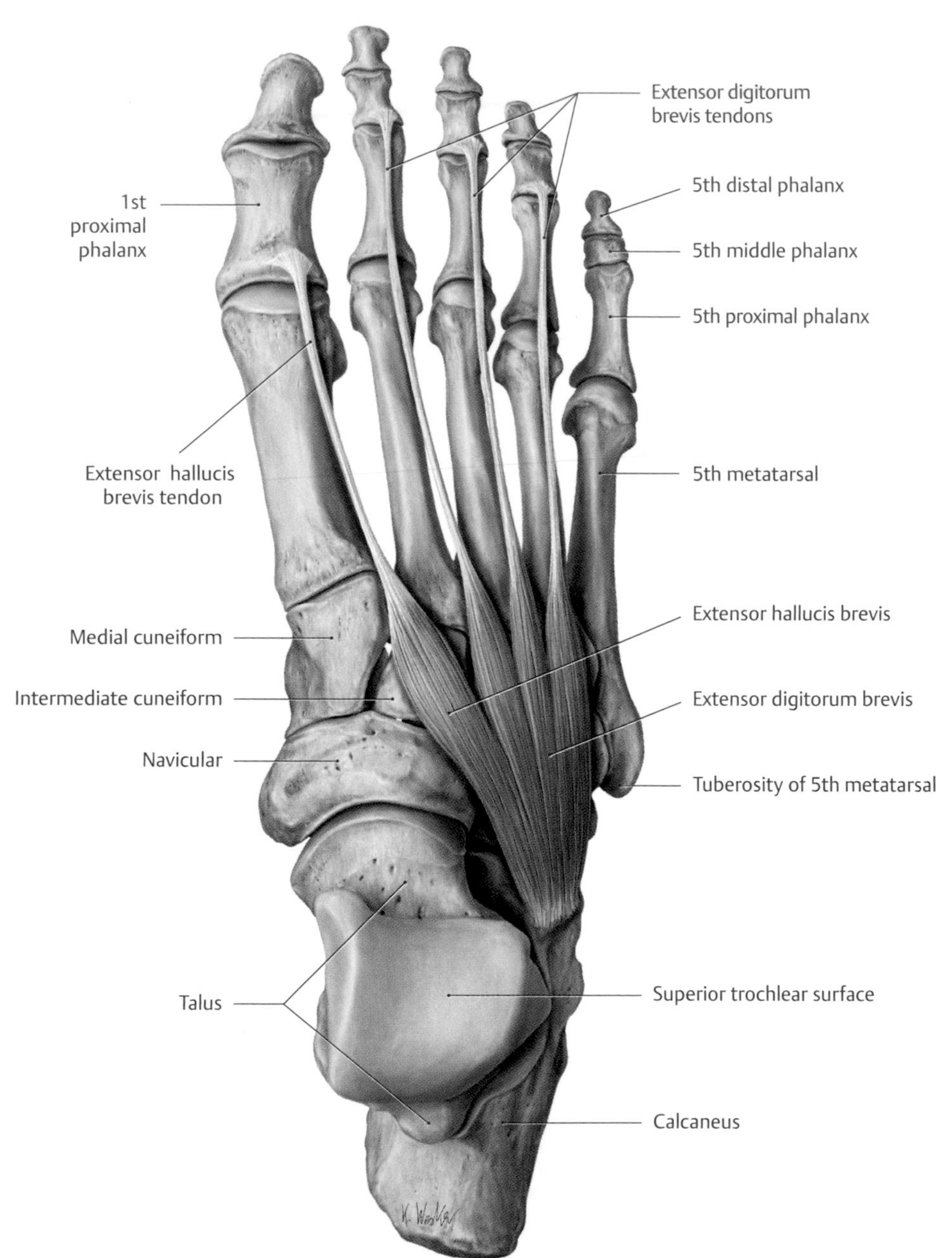

Extensor digitorum brevis tendons
5th distal phalanx
5th middle phalanx
5th proximal phalanx
1st proximal phalanx
Extensor hallucis brevis tendon
5th metatarsal
Extensor hallucis brevis
Medial cuneiform
Intermediate cuneiform
Extensor digitorum brevis
Navicular
Tuberosity of 5th metatarsal
Talus
Superior trochlear surface
Calcaneus

B Dorsal muscles of the foot.

Table 28.2 **Intrinsic muscles of the dorsum of the foot**				
Muscle	**Origin**	**Insertion**	**Innervation**	**Action**
① Extensor digitorum brevis	Calcaneus (dorsal surface)	2nd to 4th toes (at dorsal aponeuroses and bases of the middle phalanges)	Deep fibular n. (L5, S1)	Extension of the MTP and PIP joints of the 2nd to 4th toes
② Extensor hallucis brevis		1st toe (at dorsal aponeurosis and proximal phalanx)		Extension of the MTP joints of the 1st toe
MTP, metatarsophalangeal; PIP, proximal interphalangeal.				

Fig. 28.20 **Superficial intrinsic muscles of the sole of the foot**
Right foot, plantar view.

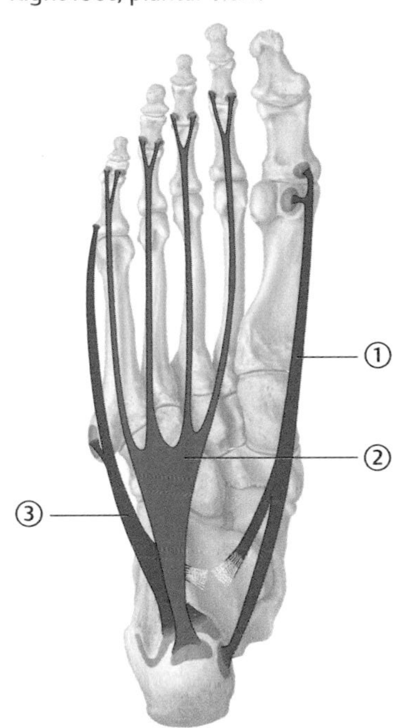
①
②
③

A First layer, schematic.

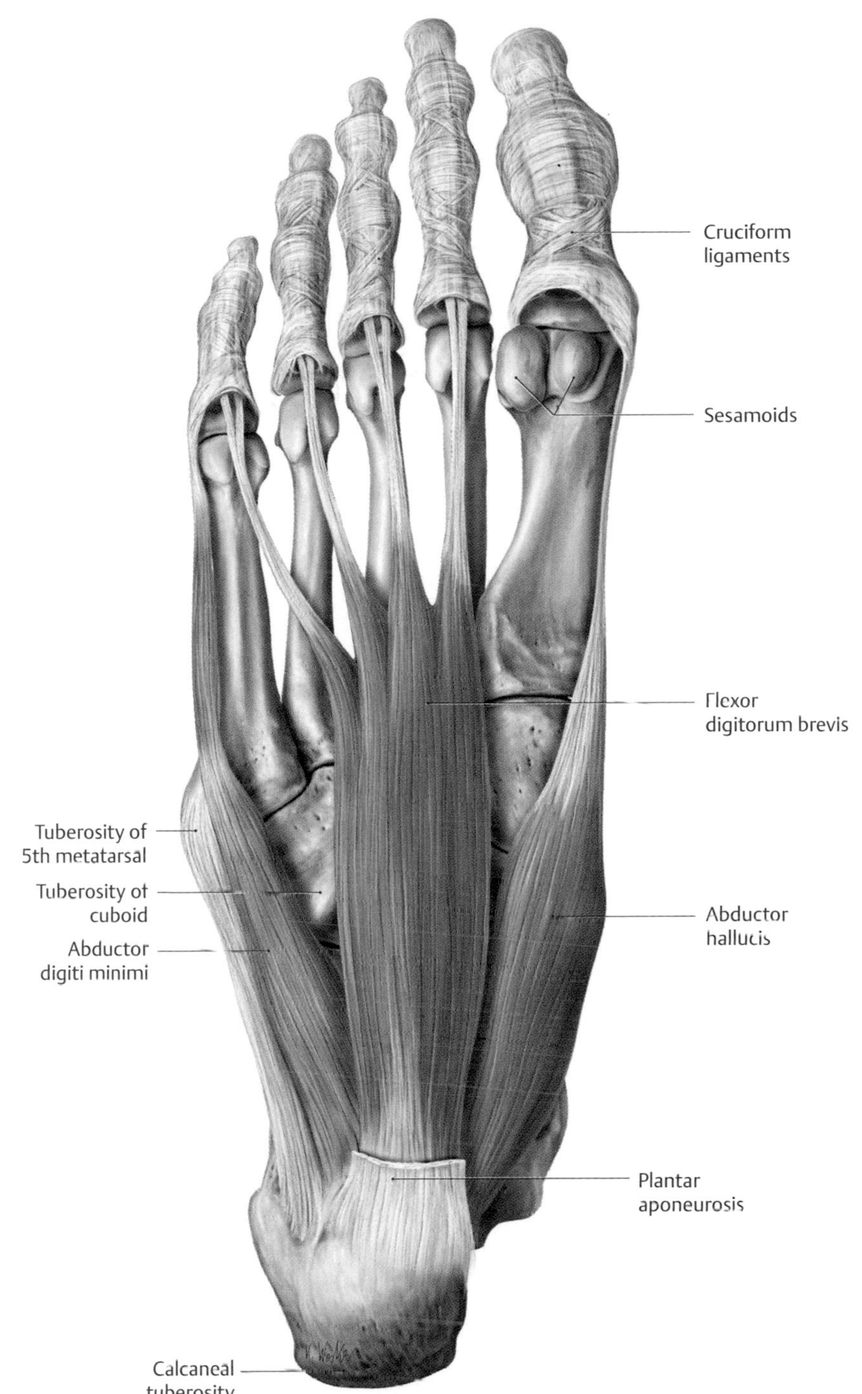
Cruciform ligaments
Sesamoids
Flexor digitorum brevis
Tuberosity of 5th metatarsal
Tuberosity of cuboid
Abductor digiti minimi
Abductor hallucis
Plantar aponeurosis
Calcaneal tuberosity

B Intrinsic muscles of the sole, first layer.

Table 28.3 **Superficial intrinsic muscles of the sole of the foot**

Muscle	Origin	Insertion	Innervation	Action
① Abductor hallucis	Calcaneal tuberosity (medial process)	1st toe (base of proximal phalanx via the medial sesamoid)	Medial plantar n. (S1, S2)	• 1st MTP joint: flexion and abduction of the 1st toe • Supports the longitudinal arch
② Flexor digitorum brevis	Calcaneal tuberosity (medial tubercle), plantar aponeurosis	2nd to 5th toes (sides of middle phalanges)		• Flexes the MTP and PIP joints of the 2nd to 5th toes • Supports the longitudinal arch
③ Abductor digiti minimi		5th toe (base of proximal phalanx), 5th metatarsal (at tuberosity)	Lateral plantar n. (S1–S3)	• Flexes the MTP joint of the 5th toe • Abducts the 5th toe • Supports the longitudinal arch

MTP, metatarsophalangeal; PIP, proximal interphalangeal.

Muscle Facts (II)

Fig. 28.21 **Deep intrinsic muscles of the sole of the foot**
Right foot, plantar view, schematics.

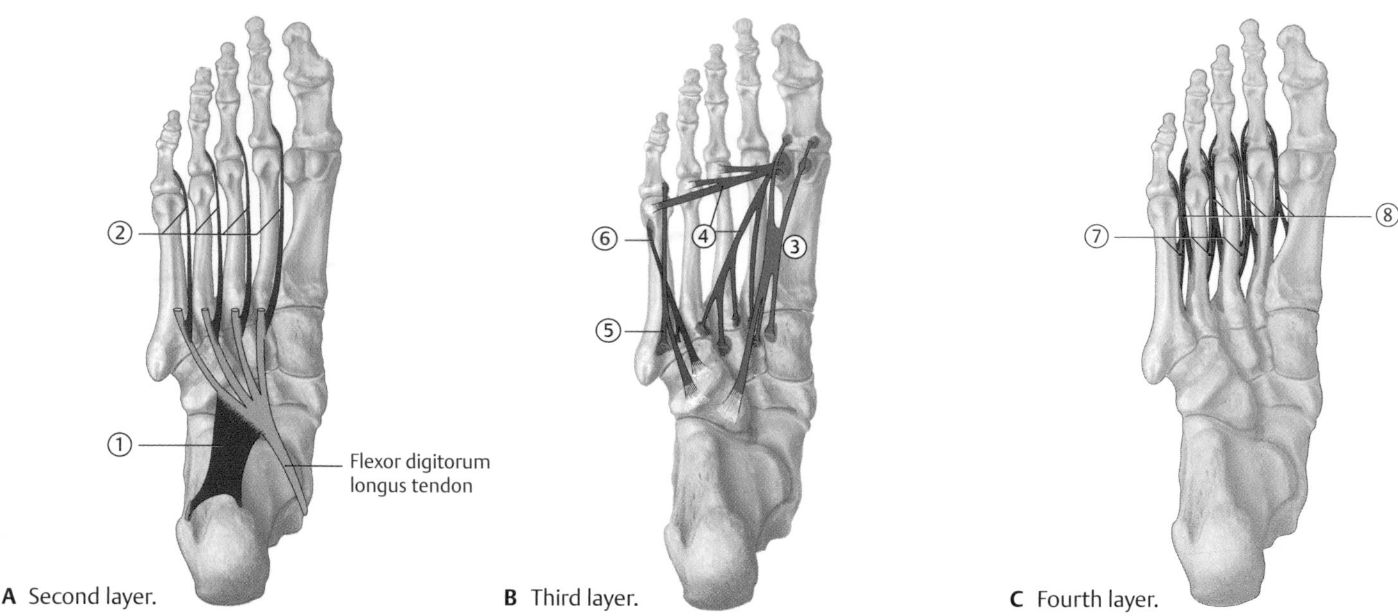

②
①
Flexor digitorum longus tendon
⑥
④
③
⑤
⑦
⑧

A Second layer. **B** Third layer. **C** Fourth layer.

Table 28.4 Deep intrinsic muscles of the sole

Muscle	Origin	Insertion	Innervation	Action
① Quadratus plantae	Calcaneal tuberosity (medial and plantar borders on plantar side)	Flexor digitorum longus tendon (lateral border)	Lateral plantar n. (S1–S3)	Redirects and augments the pull of flexor digitorum longus
② Lumbricals (four muscles)	Flexor digitorum longus tendons (medial borders)	2nd to 5th toes (at dorsal aponeuroses)	1st lumbrical: medial plantar n. (S2, S3) 2nd to 4th lumbrical: lateral plantar n. (S2, S3)	• Flexes the MTP joints of 2nd to 5th toes • Extension of IP joints of 2nd to 5th toes • Adducts 2nd to 5th toes toward the big toe
③ Flexor hallucis brevis	Cuboid, lateral cuneiforms, and plantar calcaneocuboid ligament	1st toe (at base of proximal phalanx via medial and lateral sesamoids)	Medial head: medial plantar n. (S1, S2) Lateral head: lateral plantar n. (S1, S2)	• Flexes the first MTP joint • Supports the longitudinal arch
④ Adductor hallucis	Oblique head: 2nd to 4th metatarsals (at bases) Transverse head: MTPs of 3rd to 5th toes, deep transverse metatarsal ligament	1st proximal phalanx (at base, by a common tendon via the lateral sesamoid)	Lateral plantar n., deep branch (S2, S3)	• Flexes the first MTP joint • Adducts big toe • Transverse head: supports transverse arch • Oblique head: supports longitudinal arch
⑤ Flexor digiti minimi brevis	5th metatarsal (base), long plantar ligament	5th toe (base of proximal phalanx)	Lateral plantar n., superficial branch (S2, S3)	Flexes the MTP joint of the little toe
⑥ Opponens digiti minimi*	Long plantar ligament; fibularis longus (at plantar tendon sheath)	5th metatarsal		Pulls 5th metatarsal in plantar and medial direction
⑦ Plantar interossei (three muscles)	3rd to 5th metatarsals (medial border)	3rd to 5th toes (medial base of proximal phalanx)	Lateral plantar n. (S2, S3)	• Flexes the MTP joints of 3rd to 5th toes • Extension of IP joints of 3rd to 5th toes • Adducts 3rd to 5th toes toward 2nd toe
⑧ Dorsal interossei (four muscles)	1st to 5th metatarsals (by two heads on opposing sides)	1st interosseus: 2nd proximal phalanx (medial base) 2nd to 4th interossei: 2nd to 4th proximal phalanges (lateral base), 2nd to 4th toes (at dorsal aponeuroses)		• Flexes the MTP joints of 2nd to 4th toes • Extension of IP joints of 2nd to 4th toes • Abducts 3rd and 4th toes from 2nd toe

IP, interphalangeal; MTP, metatarsophalangeal. *May be absent.

Fig. 28.22 **Deep intrinsic muscles of the sole of the foot**
Right foot, plantar view.

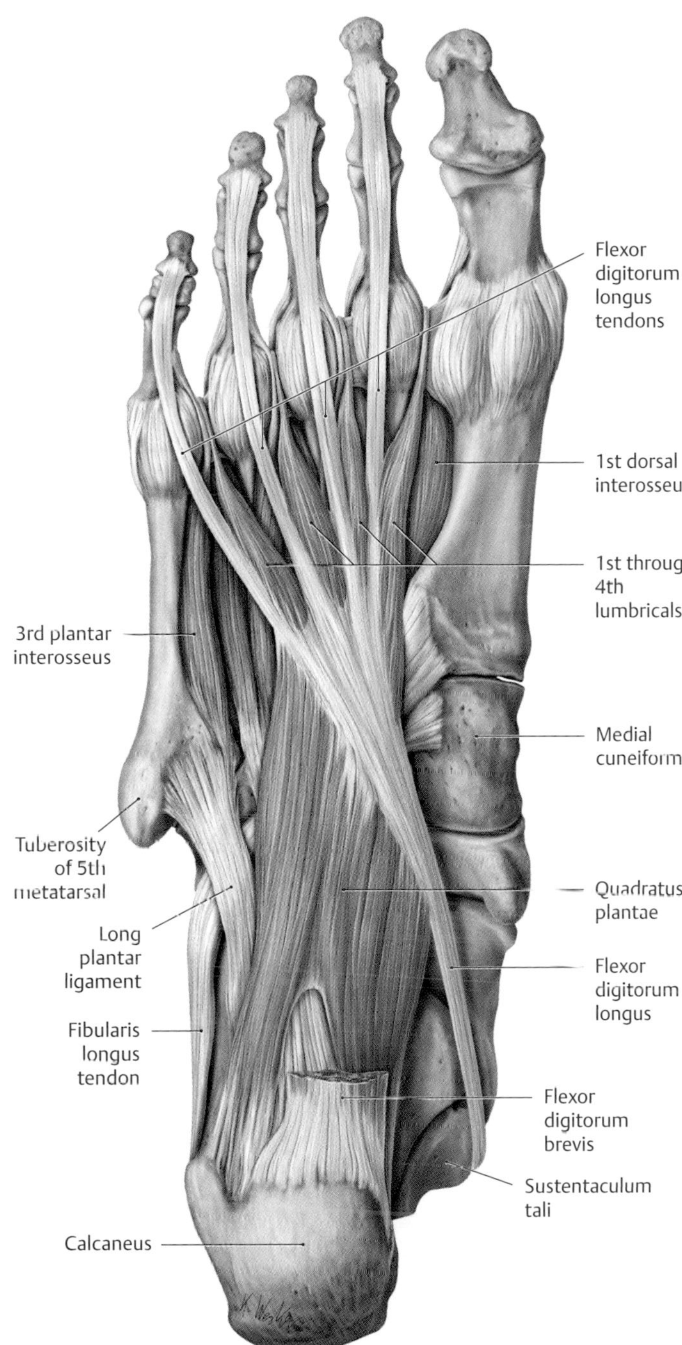
Flexor digitorum longus tendons
1st dorsal interosseus
1st through 4th lumbricals
3rd plantar interosseus
Medial cuneiform
Tuberosity of 5th metatarsal
Quadratus plantae
Long plantar ligament
Flexor digitorum longus
Fibularis longus tendon
Flexor digitorum brevis
Sustentaculum tali
Calcaneus

A Intrinsic muscles of the sole, second and fourth layers.

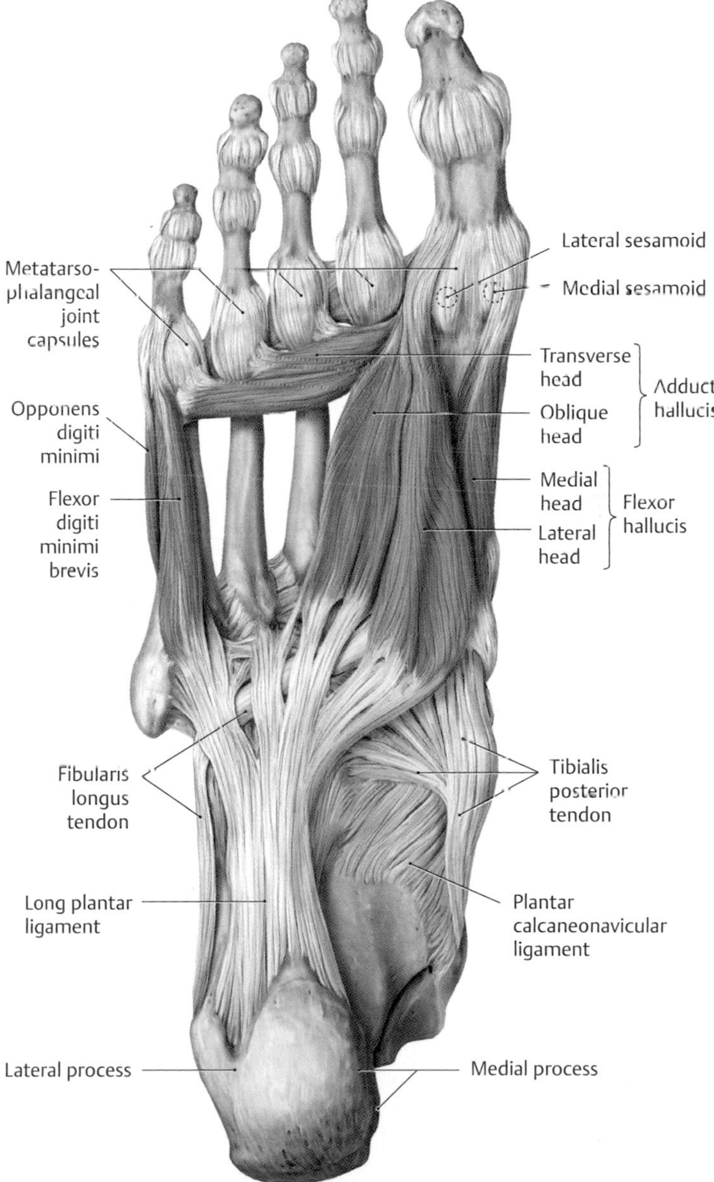
Lateral sesamoid
Medial sesamoid
Metatarso-phalangeal joint capsules
Transverse head
Oblique head
Adductor hallucis
Opponens digiti minimi
Medial head
Lateral head
Flexor hallucis
Flexor digiti minimi brevis
Fibularis longus tendon
Tibialis posterior tendon
Long plantar ligament
Plantar calcaneonavicular ligament
Lateral process
Medial process

B Intrinsic muscles of the sole, third layer.

Arteries of the Lower Limb

Fig. 29.1 **Arteries of the lower limb and the sole of the foot**

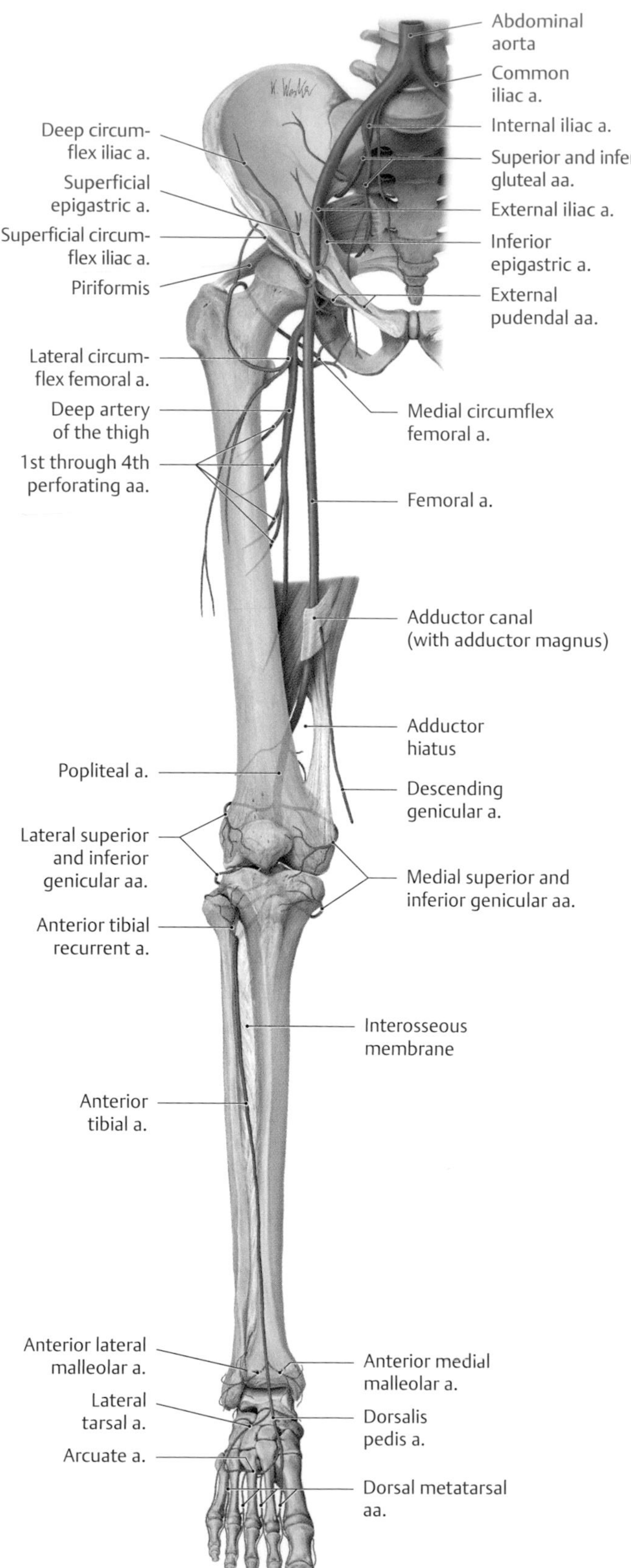
Abdominal aorta
Common iliac a.
Internal iliac a.
Superior and inferior gluteal aa.
External iliac a.
Inferior epigastric a.
External pudendal aa.
Deep circumflex iliac a.
Superficial epigastric a.
Superficial circumflex iliac a.
Piriformis
Lateral circumflex femoral a.
Deep artery of the thigh
1st through 4th perforating aa.
Medial circumflex femoral a.
Femoral a.
Adductor canal (with adductor magnus)
Adductor hiatus
Popliteal a.
Descending genicular a.
Lateral superior and inferior genicular aa.
Medial superior and inferior genicular aa.
Anterior tibial recurrent a.
Interosseous membrane
Anterior tibial a.
Anterior lateral malleolar a.
Anterior medial malleolar a.
Lateral tarsal a.
Dorsalis pedis a.
Arcuate a.
Dorsal metatarsal aa.

A Right leg, anterior view.

Adductor hiatus
Popliteal a.
Adductor magnus
Lateral superior genicular a.
Medial superior genicular a.
Sural aa.
Middle genicular a.
Lateral inferior genicular a.
Medial inferior genicular a.
Posterior tibial recurrent a.
Anterior tibial a.
Anterior tibial recurrent a.
Posterior tibial a.
Fibular a.
Muscular branches
Communicating branch
Perforating branch
Medial malleolar branches
Lateral malleolar branches
Medial plantar a.
Calcaneal branches

B Right leg, posterior view.

Proper plantar digital aa.
Common plantar digital aa.
Plantar metatarsal aa.
Superficial branch
Deep branch
Medial plantar a.
Deep plantar arch
Abductor hallucis
Lateral plantar a.
Medial plantar a.
Posterior tibial a.

C Sole of right foot, plantar view.

Fig. 29.2 Segments of the femoral artery

The blood supply to the lower limbs originates from the femoral artery. Color is used to identify the named distal segments of this vessel.

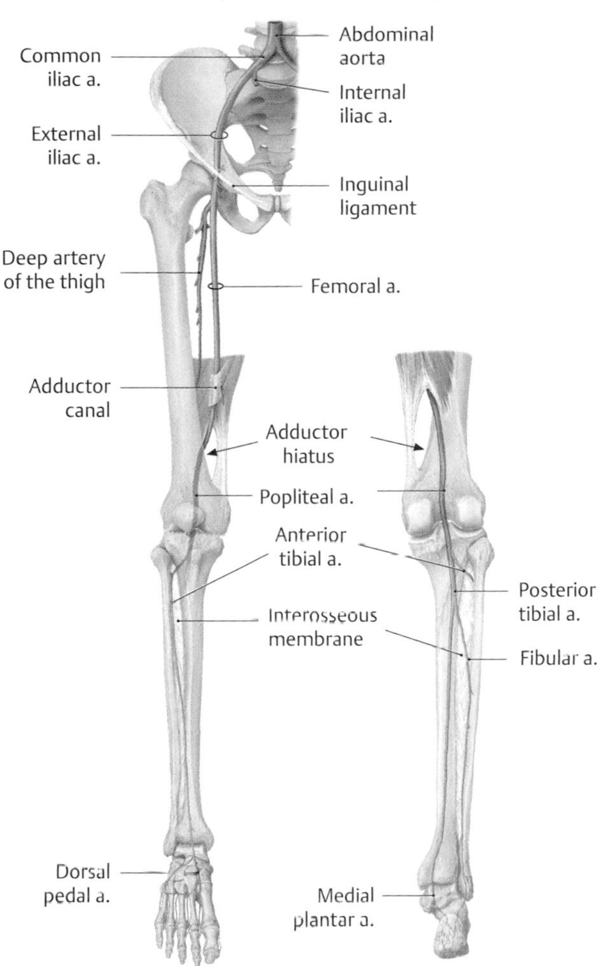
Common iliac a.
Abdominal aorta
Internal iliac a.
External iliac a.
Inguinal ligament
Deep artery of the thigh
Femoral a.
Adductor canal
Adductor hiatus
Popliteal a.
Anterior tibial a.
Posterior tibial a.
Interosseous membrane
Fibular a.
Dorsal pedal a.
Medial plantar a.

Fig. 29.3 Deep artery of the thigh

Right leg. The artery passes posteriorly through the adductor muscles of the medial thigh to supply the muscles of the posterior compartment via 3 to 5 perforating branches. Ligation of the femoral artery proximal to the origin of the deep artery of the thigh (*left*) is well tolerated owing to the collateral blood supply (*arrows*) from branches of the internal iliac artery that anastomose with the perforating branches.

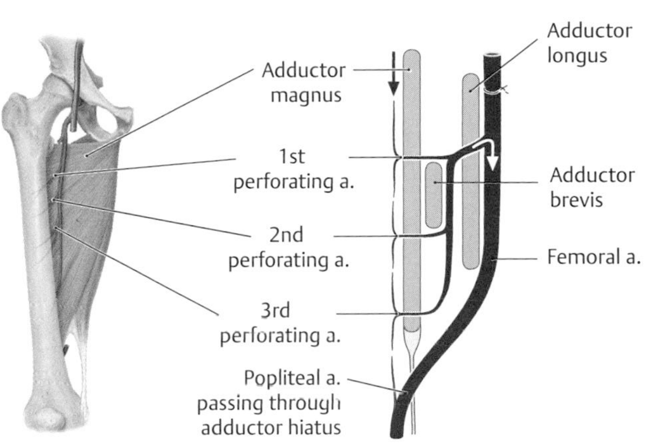
Adductor longus
Adductor magnus
1st perforating a.
Adductor brevis
2nd perforating a.
Femoral a.
3rd perforating a.
Popliteal a. passing through adductor hiatus

Clinical

Femoral head necrosis

Dislocation or fracture of the femoral head (e.g., in patients with osteoporosis) may tear the femoral neck vessels, resulting in femoral head necrosis.

Fig. 29.4 Arteries of the femoral head

Anterior view.

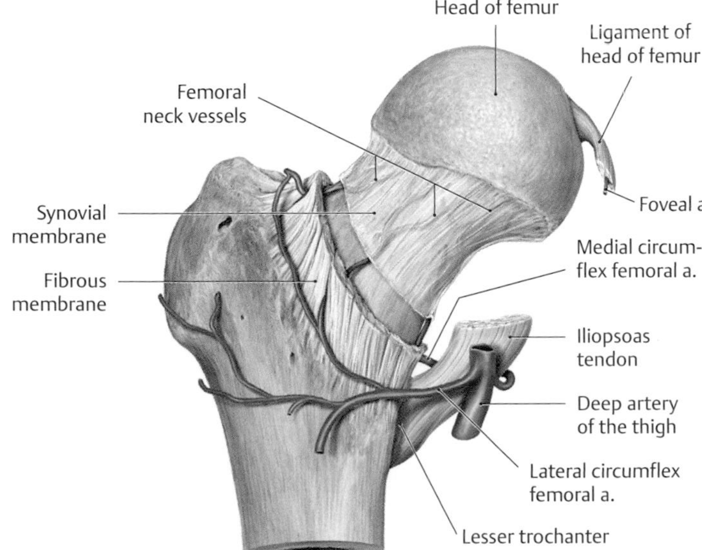
Head of femur
Ligament of head of femur
Femoral neck vessels
Synovial membrane
Foveal a.
Medial circumflex femoral a.
Fibrous membrane
Iliopsoas tendon
Deep artery of the thigh
Lateral circumflex femoral a.
Lesser trochanter

A Right femur.

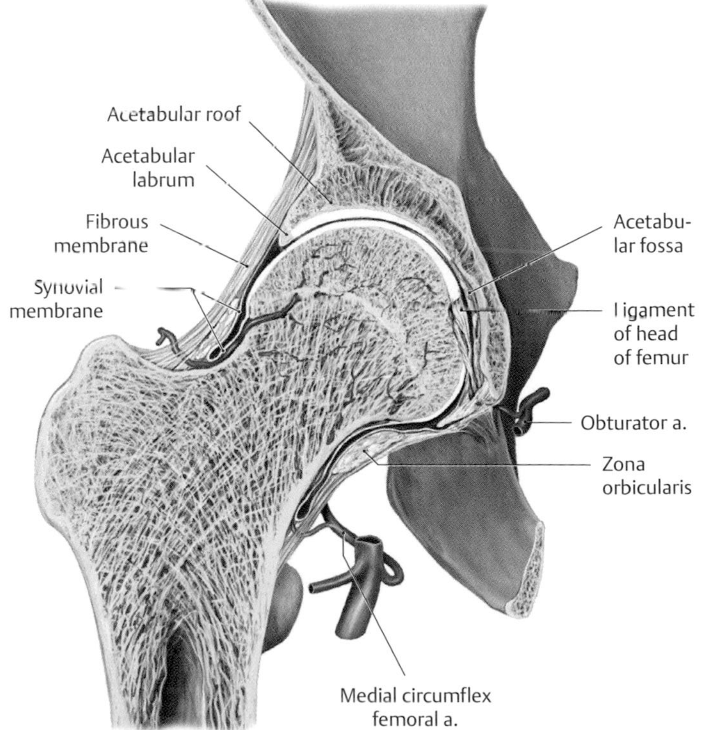
Acetabular roof
Acetabular labrum
Fibrous membrane
Acetabular fossa
Synovial membrane
Ligament of head of femur
Obturator a.
Zona orbicularis
Medial circumflex femoral a.

B Right femur, coronal section.

Veins & Lymphatics of the Lower Limb

Fig. 29.5 **Superficial (epifascial) veins of the lower limb**

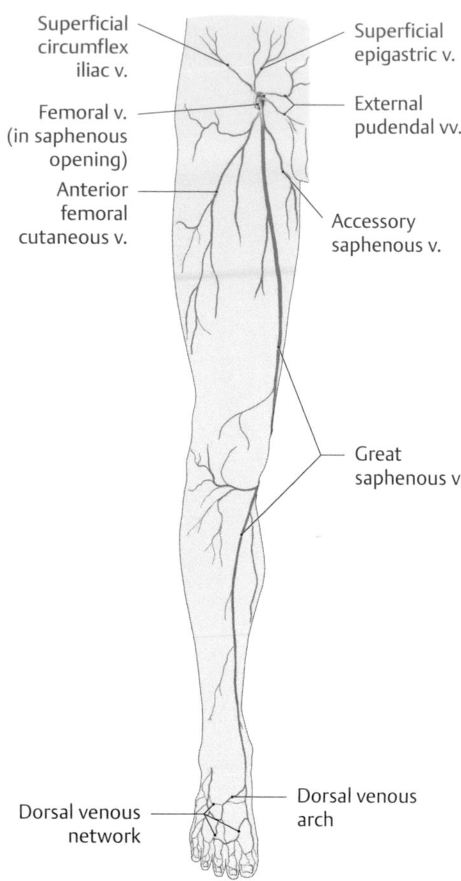
Superficial circumflex iliac v.
Superficial epigastric v.
Femoral v. (in saphenous opening)
External pudendal vv.
Anterior femoral cutaneous v.
Accessory saphenous v.
Great saphenous v.
Dorsal venous network
Dorsal venous arch

A Right limb, anterior view.

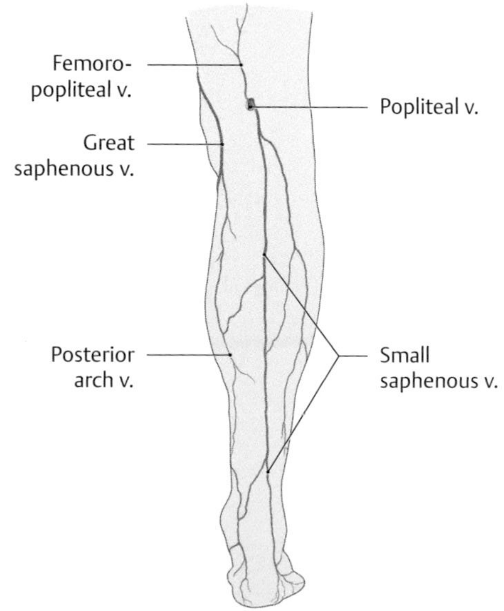
Femoro-popliteal v.
Popliteal v.
Great saphenous v.
Posterior arch v.
Small saphenous v.

B Right limb, posterior view.

Fig. 29.6 **Deep veins of the lower limb**

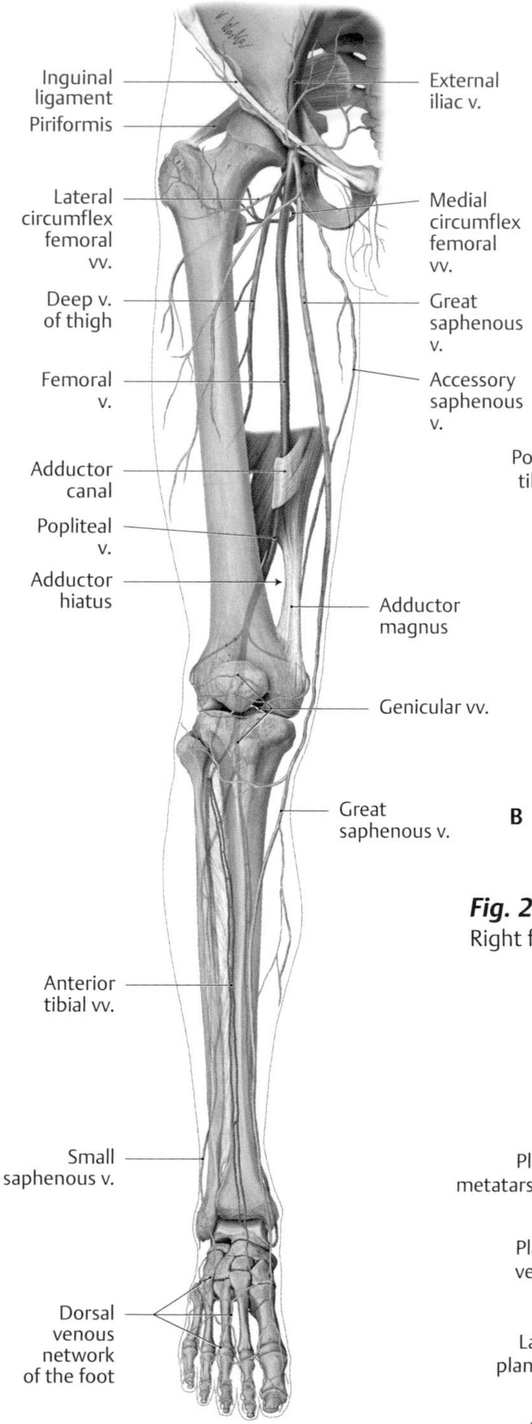

Inguinal ligament
Piriformis
Lateral circumflex femoral vv.
Deep v. of thigh
Femoral v.
Adductor canal
Popliteal v.
Adductor hiatus
Anterior tibial vv.
Small saphenous v.
Dorsal venous network of the foot
External iliac v.
Medial circumflex femoral vv.
Great saphenous v.
Accessory saphenous v.
Adductor magnus
Genicular vv.
Great saphenous v.

A Right limb, anterior view.

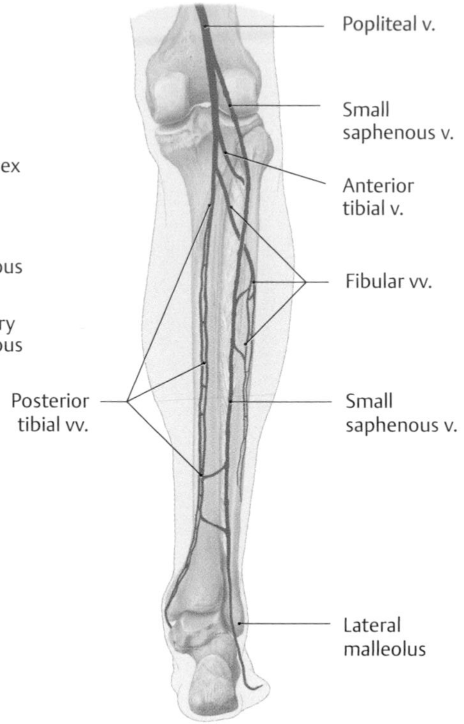

Popliteal v.
Small saphenous v.
Anterior tibial v.
Fibular vv.
Posterior tibial vv.
Small saphenous v.
Lateral malleolus

B Right limb, posterior view.

Fig. 29.7 **Veins of the sole of the foot**

Right foot, plantar view.

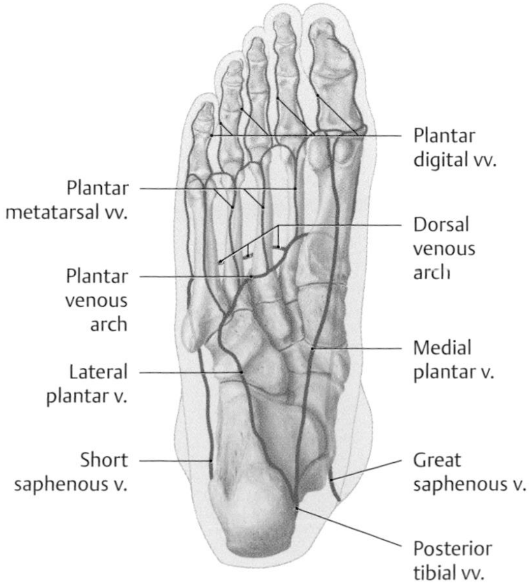

Plantar metatarsal vv.
Plantar venous arch
Lateral plantar v.
Short saphenous v.
Plantar digital vv.
Dorsal venous arch
Medial plantar v.
Great saphenous v.
Posterior tibial vv.

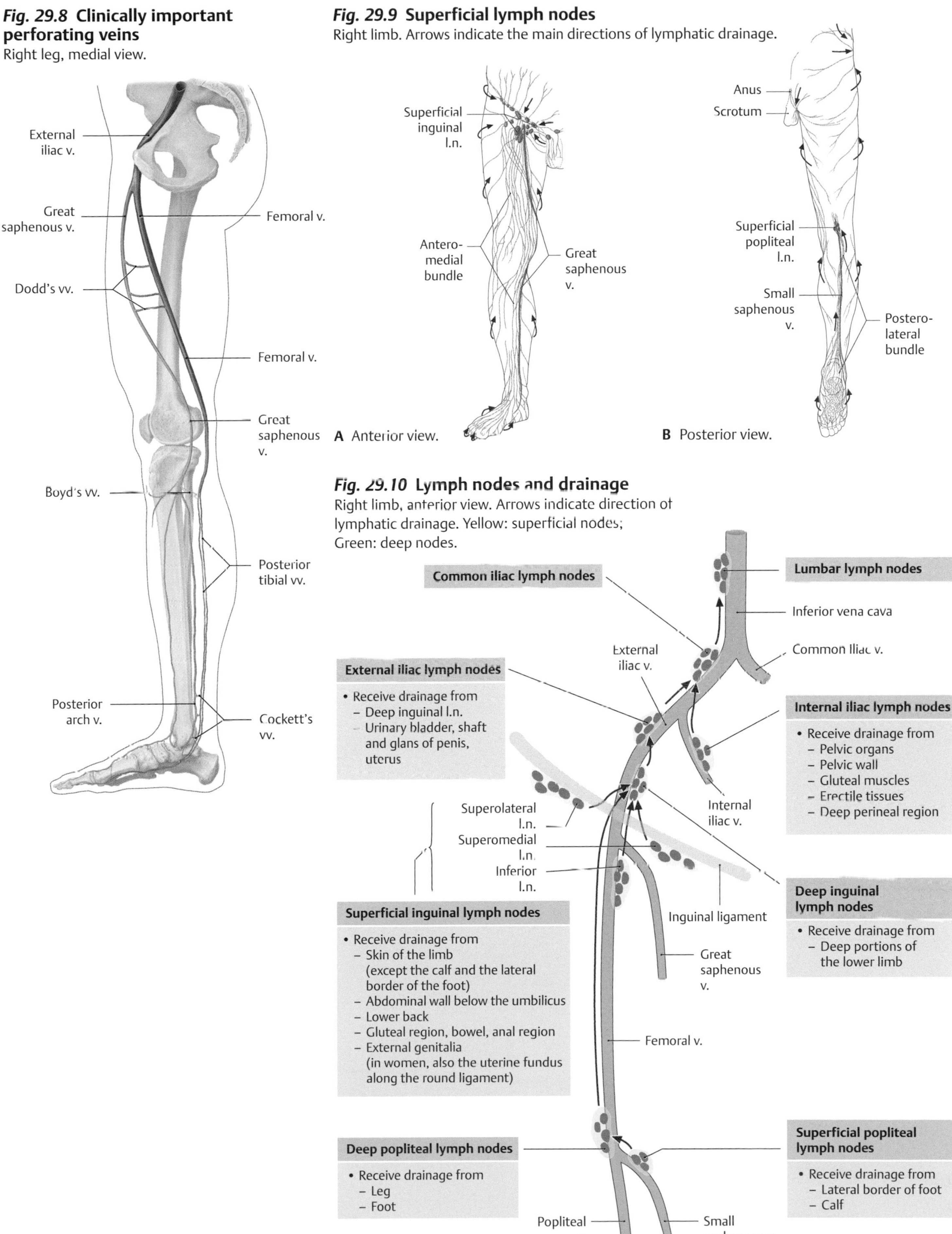

External iliac v.
Great saphenous v.
Femoral v.
Dodd's vv.
Femoral v.
Great saphenous v.
Boyd's vv.
Posterior tibial vv.
Posterior arch v.
Cockett's vv.
Superficial inguinal l.n.
Antero-medial bundle
Great saphenous v.
Anus
Scrotum
Superficial popliteal l.n.
Small saphenous v.
Postero-lateral bundle
Common iliac lymph nodes
Lumbar lymph nodes
Inferior vena cava
External iliac v.
Common Iliac v.
External iliac lymph nodes
• Receive drainage from
– Deep inguinal l.n.
– Urinary bladder, shaft and glans of penis, uterus
Internal iliac lymph nodes
• Receive drainage from
– Pelvic organs
– Pelvic wall
– Gluteal muscles
– Erectile tissues
– Deep perineal region
Superolateral l.n.
Superomedial l.n.
Inferior l.n.
Internal iliac v.
Deep inguinal lymph nodes
• Receive drainage from
– Deep portions of the lower limb
Inguinal ligament
Superficial inguinal lymph nodes
• Receive drainage from
– Skin of the limb (except the calf and the lateral border of the foot)
– Abdominal wall below the umbilicus
– Lower back
– Gluteal region, bowel, anal region
– External genitalia (in women, also the uterine fundus along the round ligament)
Great saphenous v.
Femoral v.
Deep popliteal lymph nodes
• Receive drainage from
– Leg
– Foot
Superficial popliteal lymph nodes
• Receive drainage from
– Lateral border of foot
– Calf
Popliteal v.
Small saphenous v.

Fig. 29.8 **Clinically important perforating veins**
Right leg, medial view.

Fig. 29.9 **Superficial lymph nodes**
Right limb. Arrows indicate the main directions of lymphatic drainage.

A Anterior view.

B Posterior view.

Fig. 29.10 **Lymph nodes and drainage**
Right limb, anterior view. Arrows indicate direction of lymphatic drainage. Yellow: superficial nodes; Green: deep nodes.

Lumbosacral Plexus

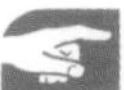

The lumbosacral plexus supplies sensory and motor innervation to the lower limb. It is formed by the anterior (ventral) rami of the lumbar and sacral spinal nerves, with contributions from the subcostal nerve (T12) and coccygeal nerve (Co1).

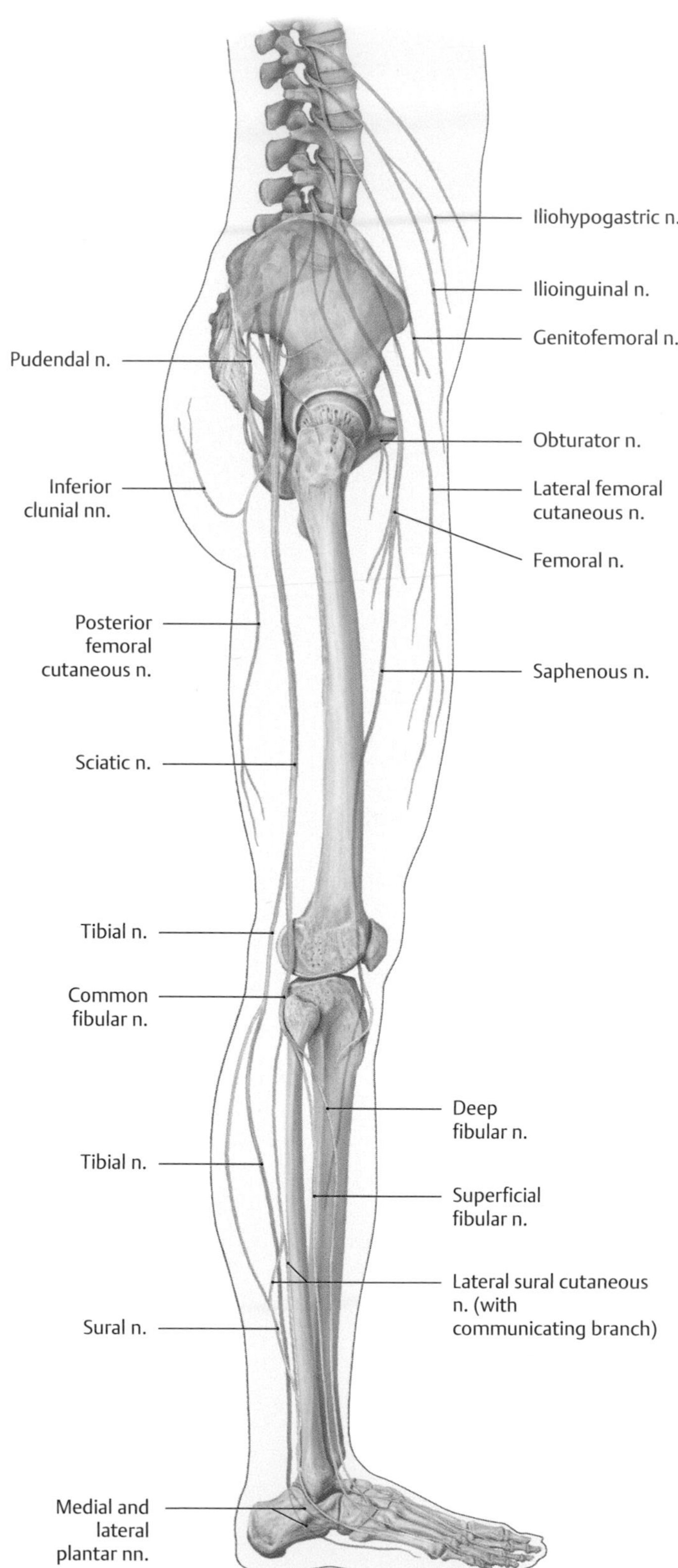
Iliohypogastric n.
Ilioinguinal n.
Genitofemoral n.
Pudendal n.
Obturator n.
Inferior clunial nn.
Lateral femoral cutaneous n.
Femoral n.
Posterior femoral cutaneous n.
Saphenous n.
Sciatic n.
Tibial n.
Common fibular n.
Deep fibular n.
Tibial n.
Superficial fibular n.
Lateral sural cutaneous n. (with communicating branch)
Sural n.
Medial and lateral plantar nn.

Table 29.1 Nerves of the lumbosacral plexus

Lumbar plexus			
Iliohypogastric n.		(T12) L1	p. 451
Ilioinguinal n.		L1	
Genitofemoral n.		L1–L2	
Lateral femoral cutaneous n.		L2–L3	
Obturator n.		L2–L4	p. 452
Femoral n.			p. 453
Sacral plexus			
Superior gluteal n.		L4–S1	p. 455
Inferior gluteal n.		L5–S2	
Posterior femoral cutaneous n.		S1–S3	p. 454
Sciatic n.	Common fibular n.	L4–S2	p. 456
	Tibial n.	L4–S3	p. 457
Pudendal n.		S2–S4	pp. 266, 268

Fig. 29.11 Lumbosacral plexus
Right side, anterior view.

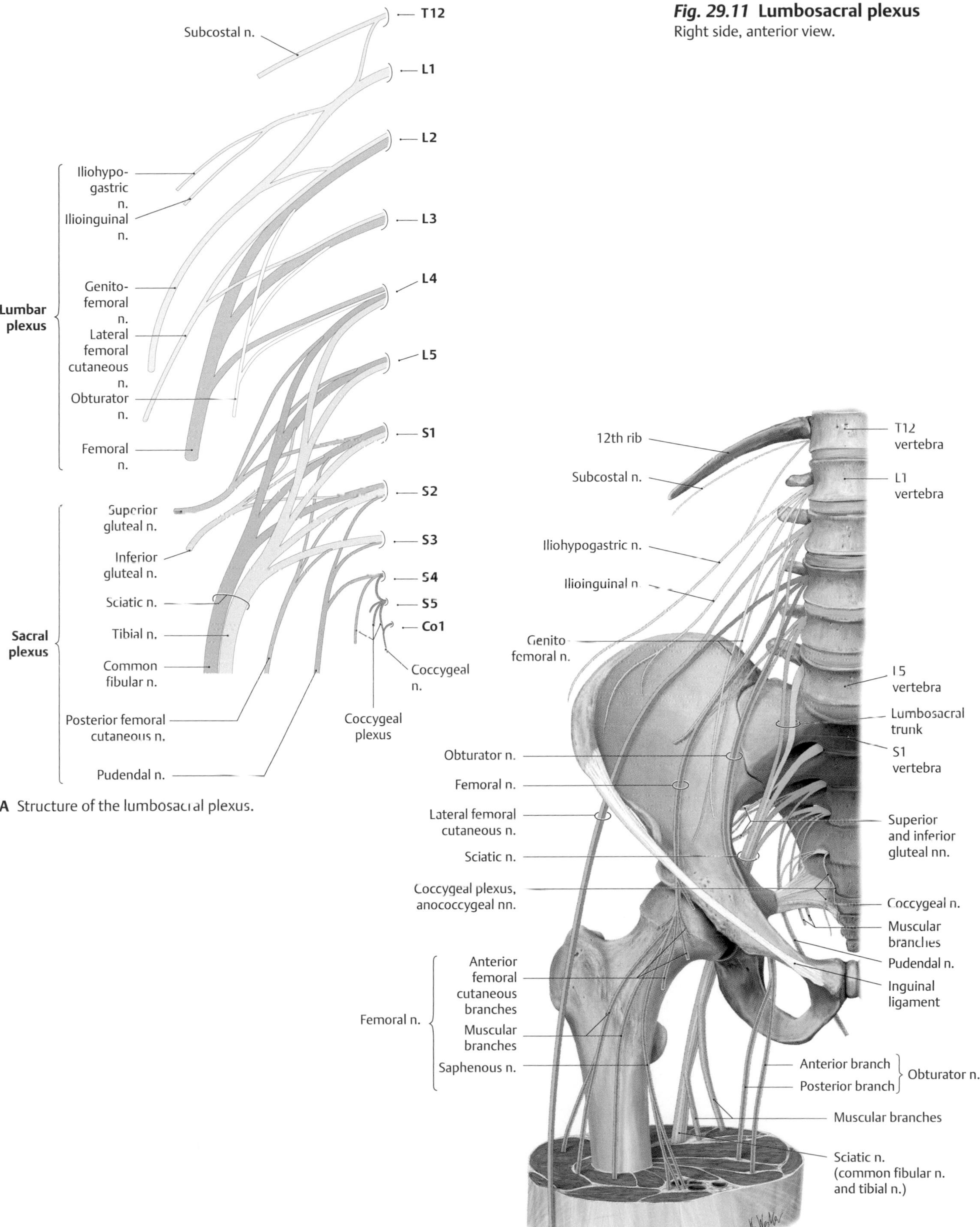

T12
L1
L2
L3
L4
L5
S1
S2
S3
S4
S5
Co1
Subcostal n.
Lumbar plexus
Iliohypogastric n.
Ilioinguinal n.
Genitofemoral n.
Lateral femoral cutaneous n.
Obturator n.
Femoral n.
Sacral plexus
Superior gluteal n.
Inferior gluteal n.
Sciatic n.
Tibial n.
Common fibular n.
Posterior femoral cutaneous n.
Pudendal n.
Coccygeal n.
Coccygeal plexus
12th rib
Subcostal n.
Iliohypogastric n.
Ilioinguinal n.
Genitofemoral n.
T12 vertebra
L1 vertebra
L5 vertebra
Lumbosacral trunk
S1 vertebra
Obturator n.
Femoral n.
Lateral femoral cutaneous n.
Sciatic n.
Coccygeal plexus, anococcygeal nn.
Superior and inferior gluteal nn.
Coccygeal n.
Muscular branches
Pudendal n.
Inguinal ligament
Femoral n.
Anterior femoral cutaneous branches
Muscular branches
Saphenous n.
Anterior branch
Posterior branch
Obturator n.
Muscular branches
Sciatic n. (common fibular n. and tibial n.)

A Structure of the lumbosacral plexus.

B Course of the lumbosacral plexus.

Nerves of the Lumbar Plexus

Table 29.2 Nerves of the lumbar plexus

Nerve	Level	Innervated muscle	Cutaneous branches
Iliohypogastric n.	T12–L1	Transversus abdominis and internal oblique (inferior portions)	Anterior and lateral cutaneous branches
Ilioinguinal n.	L1		♂: Anterior scrotal nn. ♀: Anterior labial nn.
Genitofemoral n.	L1–L2	♂: Cremaster (genital branch)	Genital branch Femoral branch
Lateral femoral cutaneous n.	L2–L3	–	Lateral femoral cutaneous n.
Obturator n.	L2–L4	See p. 452	
Femoral n.	L2–L4	See p. 453	
Short, direct muscular branches	T12–L4	Psoas major Quadratus lumborum Iliacus Intertransversarii lumborum	–

Fig. 29.12 **Cutaneous innervation of the inguinal region**
Right male inguinal region, anterior view.

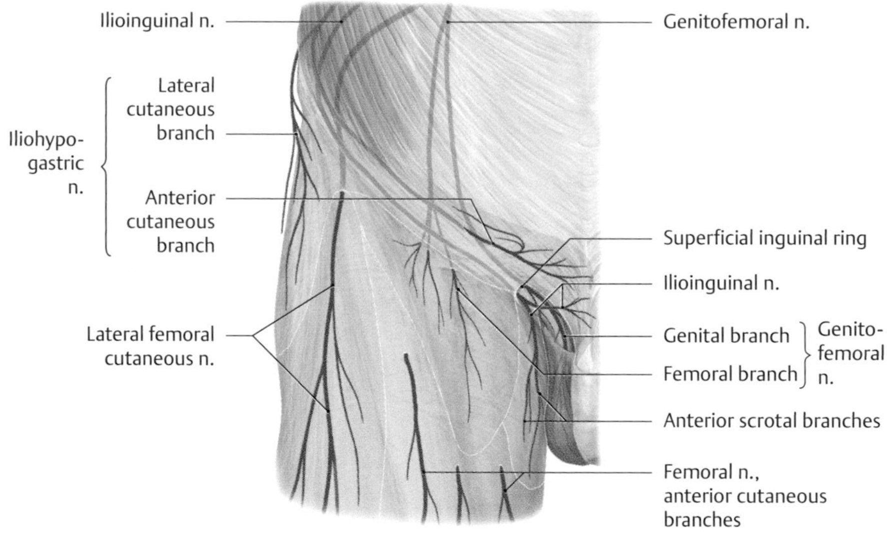

Ilioinguinal n.
Genitofemoral n.
Iliohypo-gastric n.
Lateral cutaneous branch
Anterior cutaneous branch
Superficial inguinal ring
Ilioinguinal n.
Lateral femoral cutaneous n.
Genital branch
Femoral branch
Genito-femoral n.
Anterior scrotal branches
Femoral n., anterior cutaneous branches

Clinical

Entrapment of the lateral femoral cutaneous nerve (meralgia paresthetica)

Ischemia (diminished blood flow) of the lateral femoral cutaneous nerve can result when the nerve is stretched or entrapped by the inguinal ligament (see Figure 29.11B) during hyperextension of the hip or with increased lordosis (curvature) of the lumbar spine, as often occurs during pregnancy. This results in pain, numbness, or paresthesia (tingling or burning) on the outer aspect of the thigh. It is most commonly found in obese or diabetic individuals and in pregnant women.

Fig. 29.13 Nerves of the lumbar plexus

Right side, anterior view with the anterior abdominal wall removed.

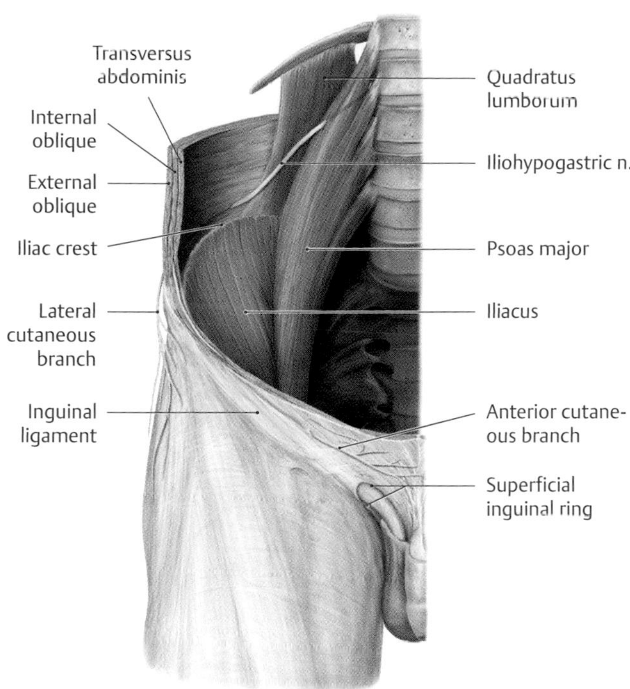

Transversus abdominis
Internal oblique
External oblique
Iliac crest
Lateral cutaneous branch
Inguinal ligament
Quadratus lumborum
Iliohypogastric n.
Psoas major
Iliacus
Anterior cutaneous branch
Superficial inguinal ring

A Iliohypogastric nerve.

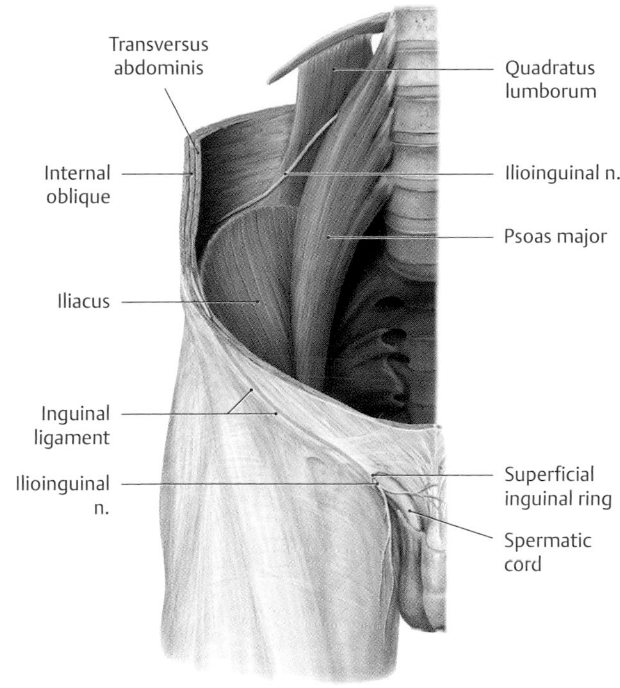

Transversus abdominis
Internal oblique
Iliacus
Inguinal ligament
Ilioinguinal n.
Quadratus lumborum
Ilioinguinal n.
Psoas major
Superficial inguinal ring
Spermatic cord

B Ilioinguinal nerve.

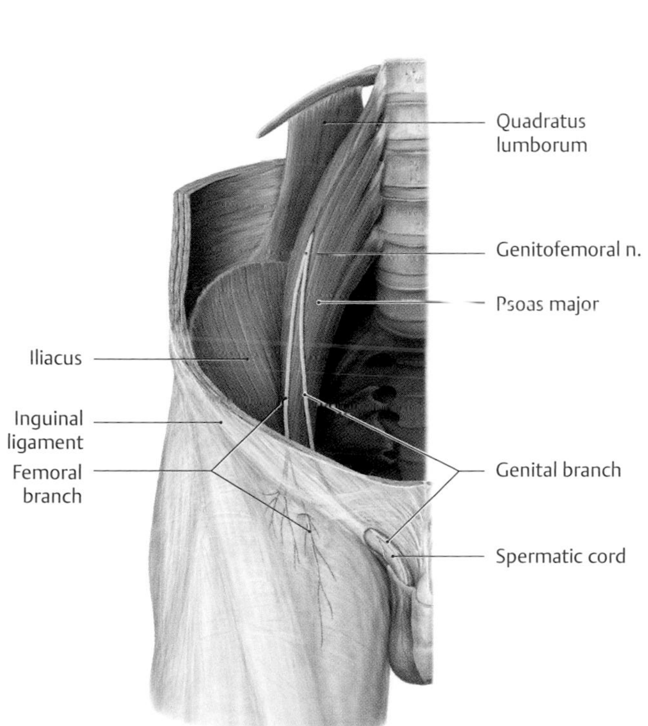

Iliacus
Inguinal ligament
Femoral branch
Quadratus lumborum
Genitofemoral n.
Psoas major
Genital branch
Spermatic cord

C Genitofemoral nerve.

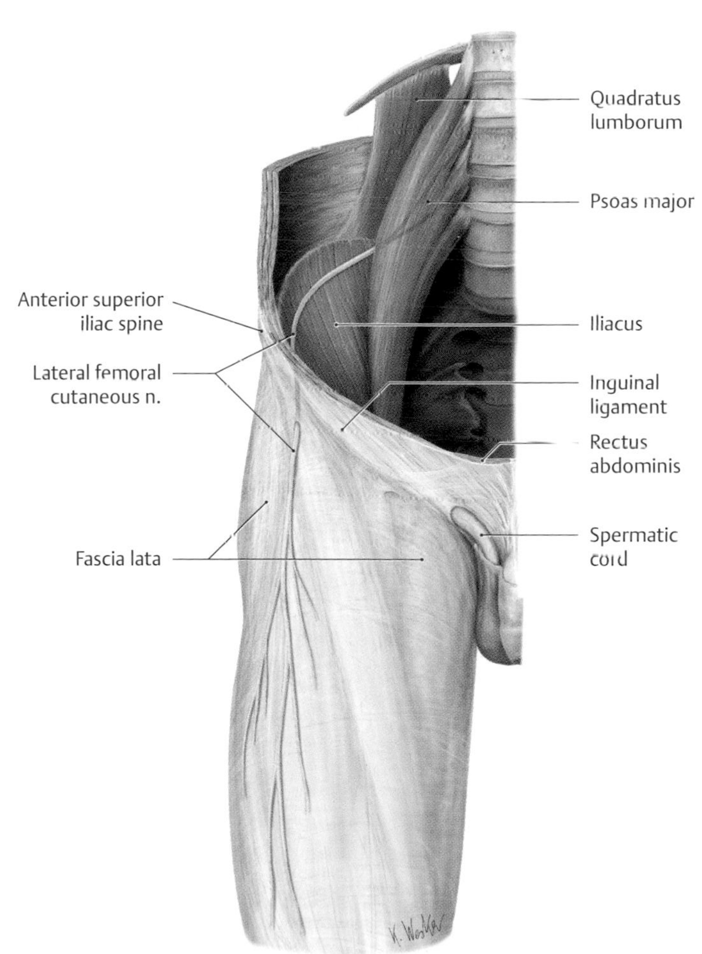

Anterior superior iliac spine
Lateral femoral cutaneous n.
Fascia lata
Quadratus lumborum
Psoas major
Iliacus
Inguinal ligament
Rectus abdominis
Spermatic cord

D Lateral femoral cutaneous nerve.

Nerves of the Lumbar Plexus: Obturator & Femoral Nerves

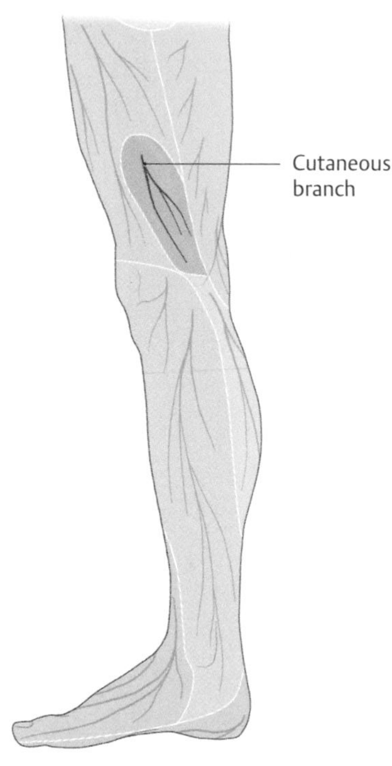
Cutaneous
branch

Fig. 29.14 **Obturator nerve: Cutaneous distribution**
Right leg, medial view.

Table 29.3	**Obturator nerve (L2–L4)**
Motor branches	**Innervated muscles**
Direct branch	Obturator externus
Anterior branch	Adductor longus
	Adductor brevis
	Gracilis
	Pectineus
Posterior branch	Adductor magnus
Sensory branches	
Cutaneous branch	

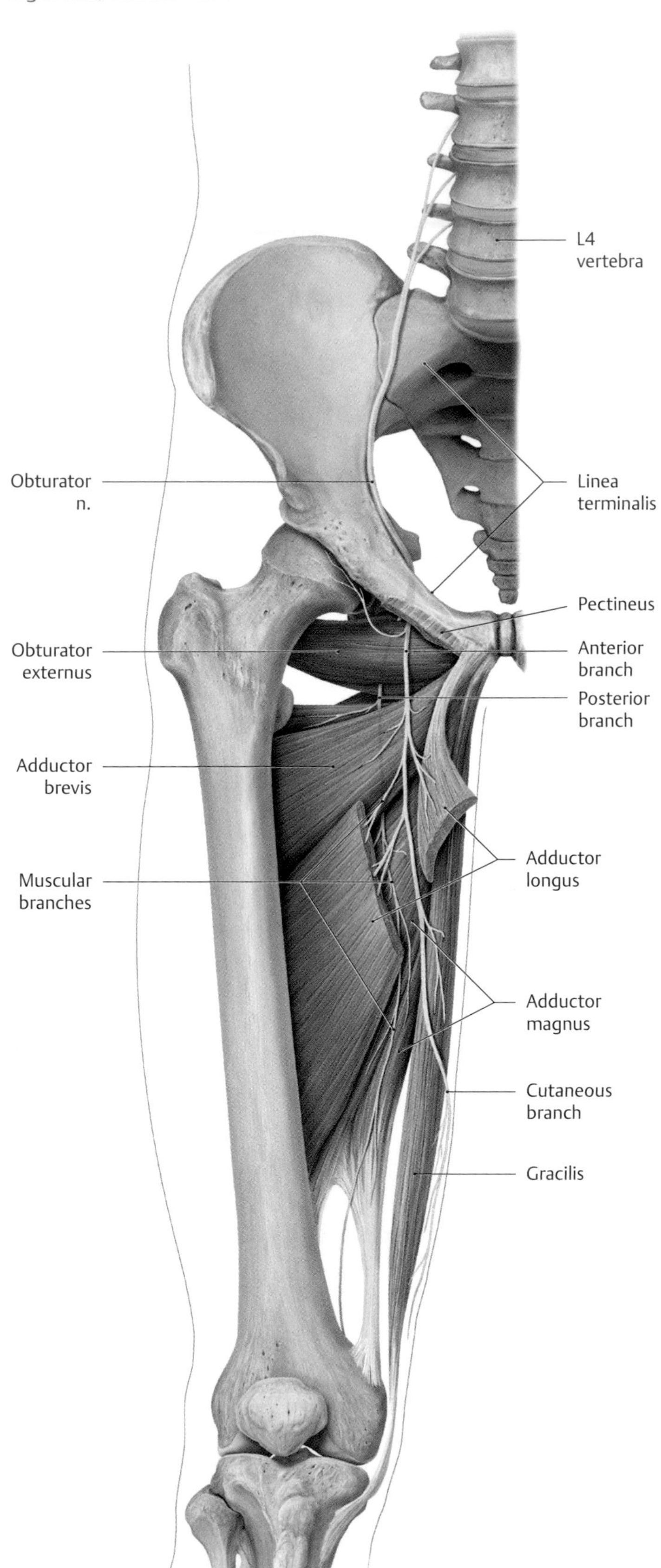
L4
vertebra
Obturator
n.
Linea
terminalis
Pectineus
Obturator
externus
Anterior
branch
Posterior
branch
Adductor
brevis
Adductor
longus
Muscular
branches
Adductor
magnus
Cutaneous
branch
Gracilis

Fig. 29.15 **Obturator nerve**
Right side, anterior view.

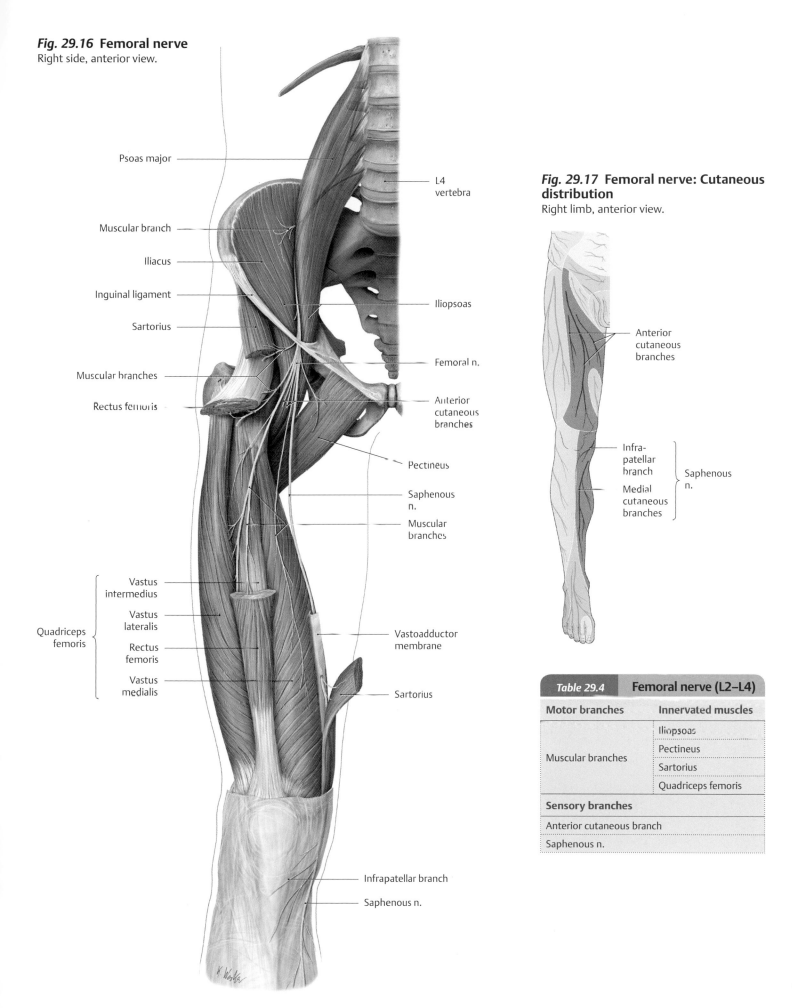

Fig. 29.16 Femoral nerve
Right side, anterior view.

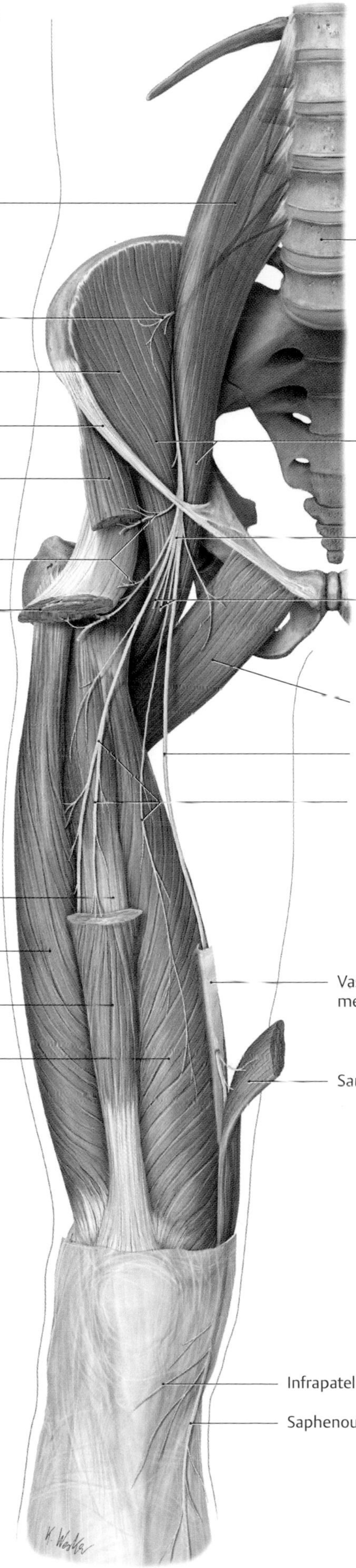

Psoas major
L4 vertebra
Muscular branch
Iliacus
Inguinal ligament
Iliopsoas
Sartorius
Femoral n.
Muscular branches
Rectus femoris
Anterior cutaneous branches
Pectineus
Saphenous n.
Muscular branches
Quadriceps femoris
Vastus intermedius
Vastus lateralis
Rectus femoris
Vastus medialis
Vastoadductor membrane
Sartorius
Infrapatellar branch
Saphenous n.

Fig. 29.17 Femoral nerve: Cutaneous distribution
Right limb, anterior view.

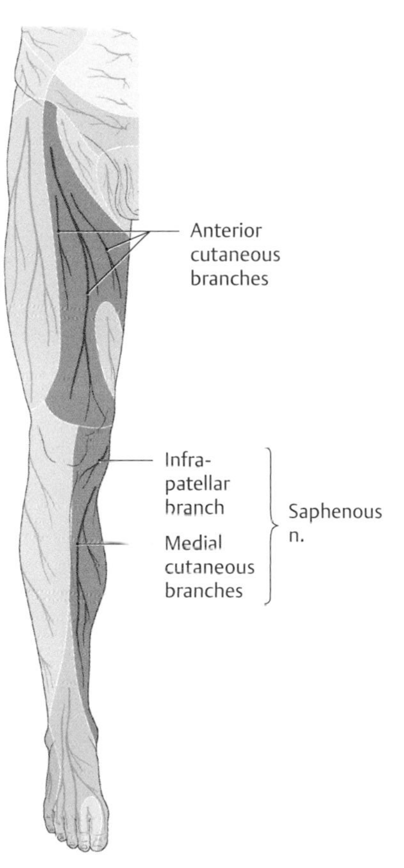
Anterior cutaneous branches
Infra-patellar branch
Medial cutaneous branches
Saphenous n.

Table 29.4	**Femoral nerve (L2–L4)**
Motor branches	**Innervated muscles**
Muscular branches	Iliopsoas
	Pectineus
	Sartorius
	Quadriceps femoris
Sensory branches	
Anterior cutaneous branch	
Saphenous n.	

Nerves of the Sacral Plexus

Table 29.5 Nerves of the sacral plexus

Nerve		Level	Innervated muscle	Cutaneous branches	
Superior gluteal n.		L4–S1	Gluteus medius Gluteus minimus Tensor fasciae latae	—	
Inferior gluteal n.		L5–S2	Gluteus maximus	—	
Posterior femoral cutaneous n.		S1–S3	—	Posterior femoral cutaneous n.	Inferior clunial nn.
					Perineal branches
Direct branches	N. of piriformis	S1–S2	Piriformis	—	
	N. of obturator internus	L5–S1	Obturator internus Gemelli	—	
	N. of quadratus femoris		Quadratus femoris	—	
Sciatic n.	Common fibular n.	L4–S2	See p. 456		
	Tibial n.	L4–S3	See p. 457		
Pudenal n.		S2–S4	See pp. 266, 268		

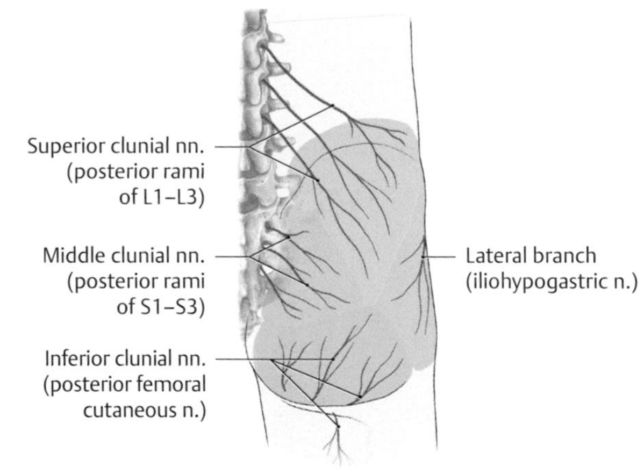
Superior clunial nn.
(posterior rami
of L1–L3)
Middle clunial nn.
(posterior rami
of S1–S3)
Inferior clunial nn.
(posterior femoral
cutaneous n.)
Lateral branch
(iliohypogastric n.)

Fig. 29.18 **Cutaneous innervation of the gluteal region**
Right limb, posterior view.

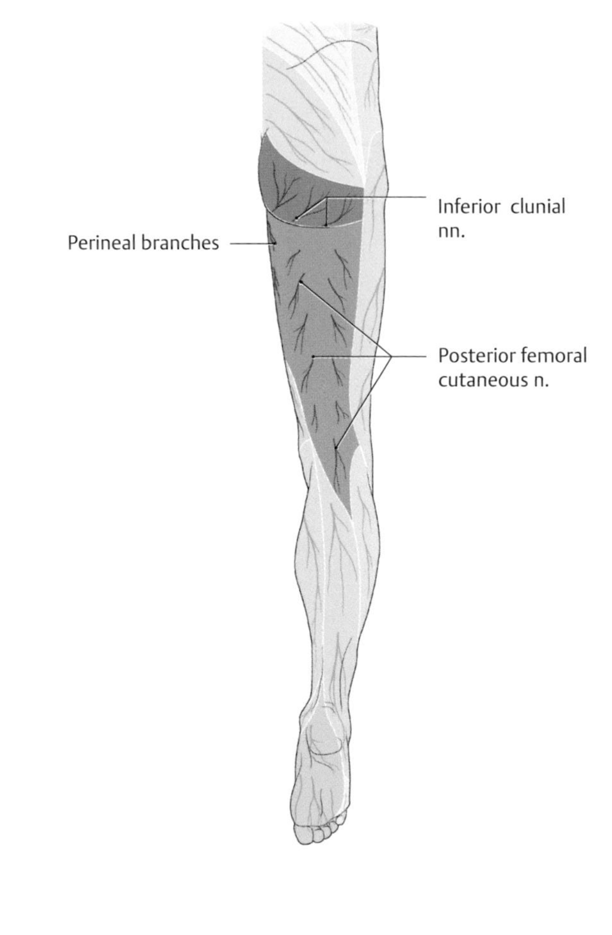
Perineal branches
Inferior clunial
nn.
Posterior femoral
cutaneous n.

Fig. 29.19 **Posterior femoral cutaneous nerve: Cutaneous distribution**
Right limb, posterior view.

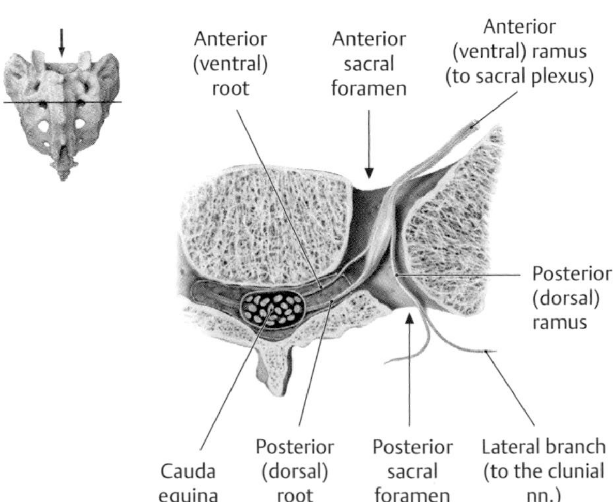
Anterior
(ventral)
root
Anterior
sacral
foramen
Anterior
(ventral) ramus
(to sacral plexus)
Posterior
(dorsal)
ramus
Cauda
equina
Posterior
(dorsal)
root
Posterior
sacral
foramen
Lateral branch
(to the clunial
nn.)

Fig. 29.20 **Emerging spinal nerve**
Horizontal section, superior view.

Fig. 29.21 Nerves of the sacral plexus

Right limb.

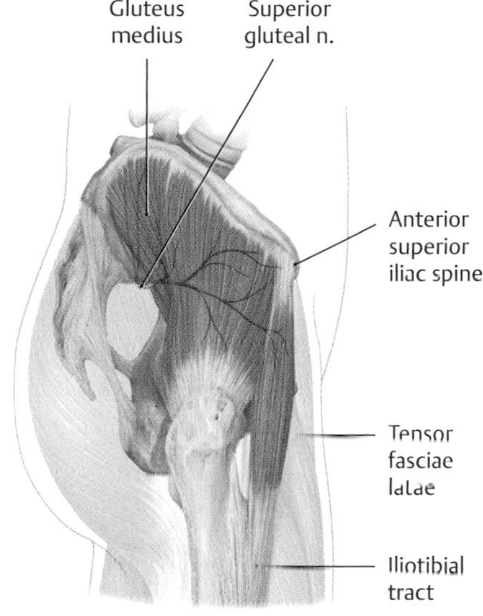
Gluteus medius
Superior gluteal n.
Anterior superior iliac spine
Tensor fasciae latae
Iliotibial tract

A Superior gluteal nerve. Lateral view.

Clinical

Small gluteal muscle weakness

The small gluteal muscles on the stance side stabilize the pelvis in the coronal plane (**A**). Weakness or paralysis of the small gluteal muscles from damage to the superior gluteal nerve (e.g., due to a faulty intramuscular injection) is manifested by weak abduction of the affected hip joint. In a positive Trendelenburg's test, the pelvis sags toward the normal, unsupported side (**B**). Tilting the upper body toward the affected side shifts the center of gravity onto the stance side, thereby elevating the pelvis on the swing side (Duchenne's limp) (**C**). With bilateral loss of the small gluteals, the patient exhibits a typical waddling gait.

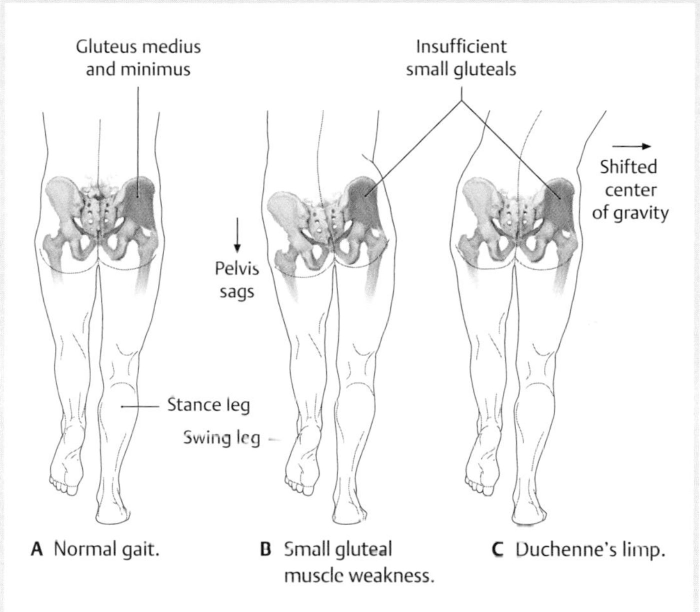
Gluteus medius and minimus
Insufficient small gluteals
Shifted center of gravity
Pelvis sags
Stance leg
Swing leg

A Normal gait. **B** Small gluteal muscle weakness. **C** Duchenne's limp.

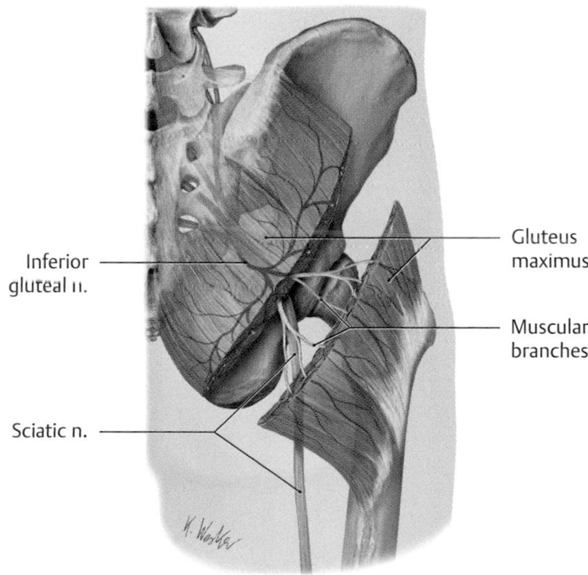
Inferior gluteal n.
Gluteus maximus
Muscular branches
Sciatic n.

B Inferior gluteal nerve. Posterior view.

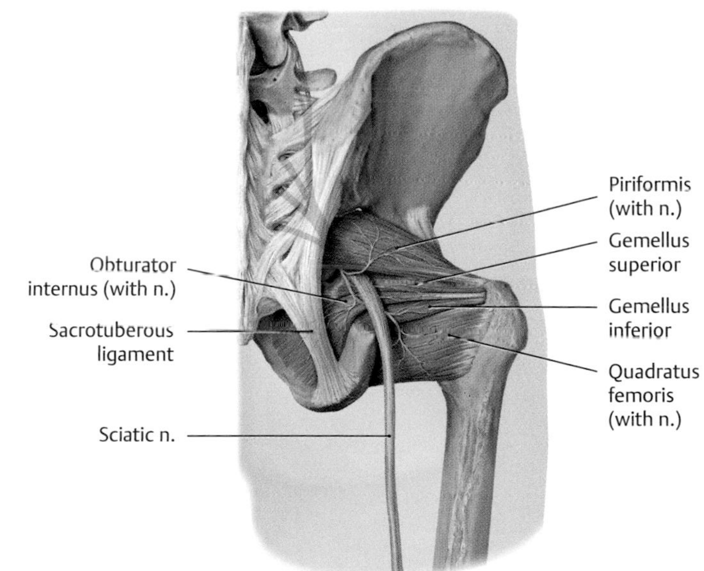
Piriformis (with n.)
Gemellus superior
Obturator internus (with n.)
Gemellus inferior
Sacrotuberous ligament
Quadratus femoris (with n.)
Sciatic n.

C Direct branches. Posterior view.

Nerves of the Sacral Plexus: Sciatic Nerve

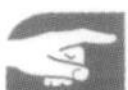

The sciatic nerve gives off several direct muscular branches before dividing into the tibial and common fibular nerves proximal to the popliteal fossa.

Fig. 29.22 Common fibular nerve: Cutaneous distribution

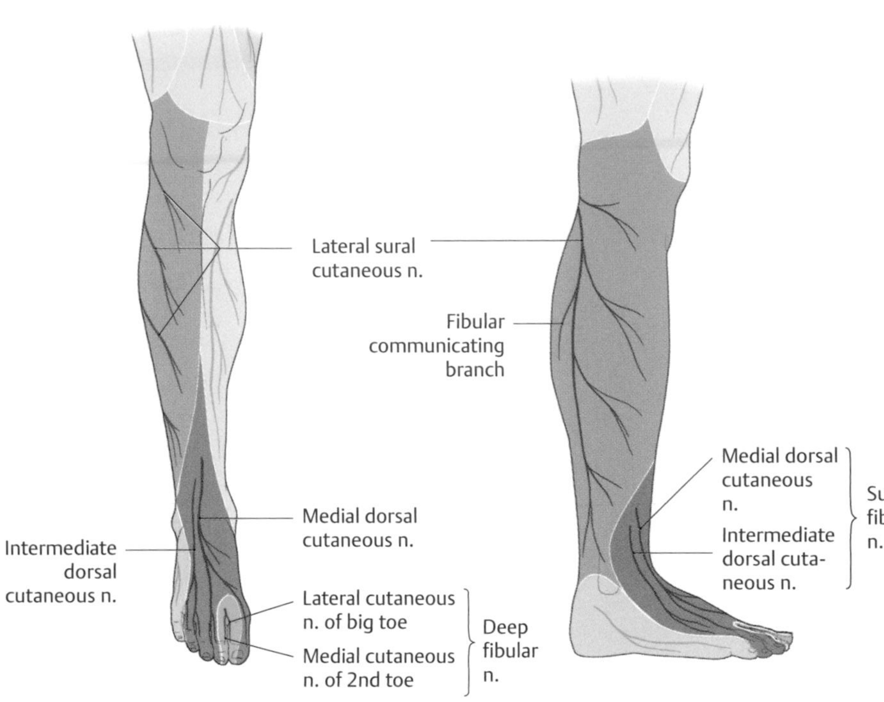
Lateral sural cutaneous n.
Fibular communicating branch
Medial dorsal cutaneous n.
Intermediate dorsal cutaneous n.
Lateral cutaneous n. of big toe
Medial cutaneous n. of 2nd toe
Deep fibular n.
Medial dorsal cutaneous n.
Intermediate dorsal cutaneous n.
Superficial fibular n.

A Right leg, anterior view.

B Right leg, lateral view.

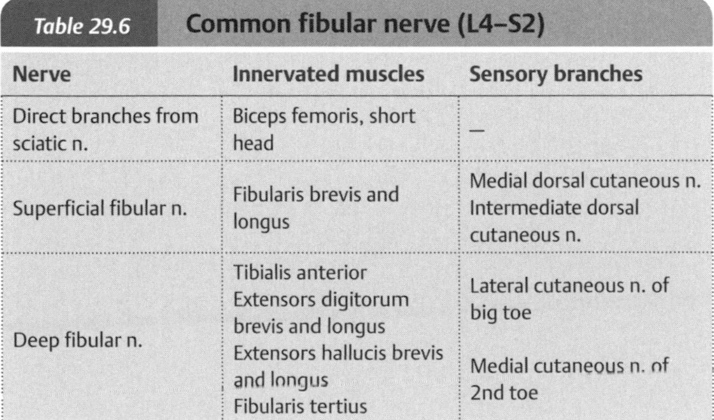

Table 29.6 Common fibular nerve (L4–S2)		
Nerve	**Innervated muscles**	**Sensory branches**
Direct branches from sciatic n.	Biceps femoris, short head	–
Superficial fibular n.	Fibularis brevis and longus	Medial dorsal cutaneous n. Intermediate dorsal cutaneous n.
Deep fibular n.	Tibialis anterior Extensors digitorum brevis and longus Extensors hallucis brevis and longus Fibularis tertius	Lateral cutaneous n. of big toe Medial cutaneous n. of 2nd toe

Fig. 29.23 Common fibular nerve
Right limb, lateral view.

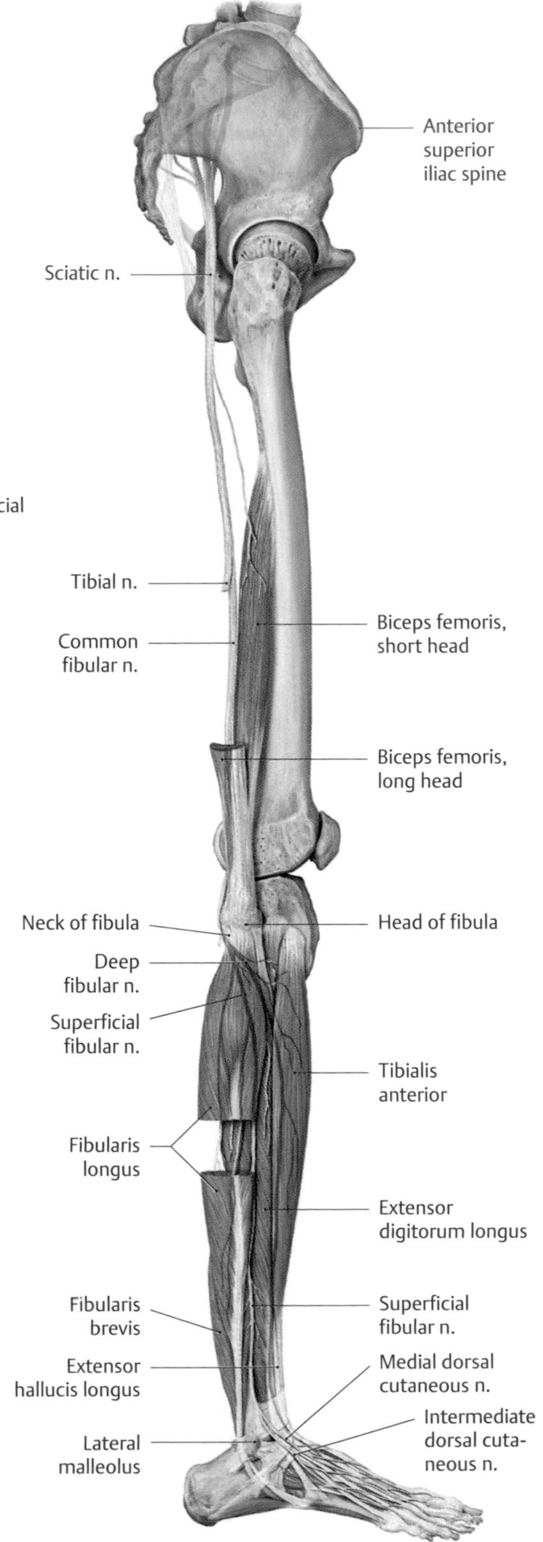
Anterior superior iliac spine
Sciatic n.
Tibial n.
Common fibular n.
Biceps femoris, short head
Biceps femoris, long head
Neck of fibula
Head of fibula
Deep fibular n.
Superficial fibular n.
Tibialis anterior
Fibularis longus
Extensor digitorum longus
Fibularis brevis
Superficial fibular n.
Extensor hallucis longus
Medial dorsal cutaneous n.
Intermediate dorsal cutaneous n.
Lateral malleolus

Fig. 29.24 Tibial nerve
Right limb.

Fig. 29.25 Tibial nerve: Cutaneous distribution
Right lower limb, posterior view.

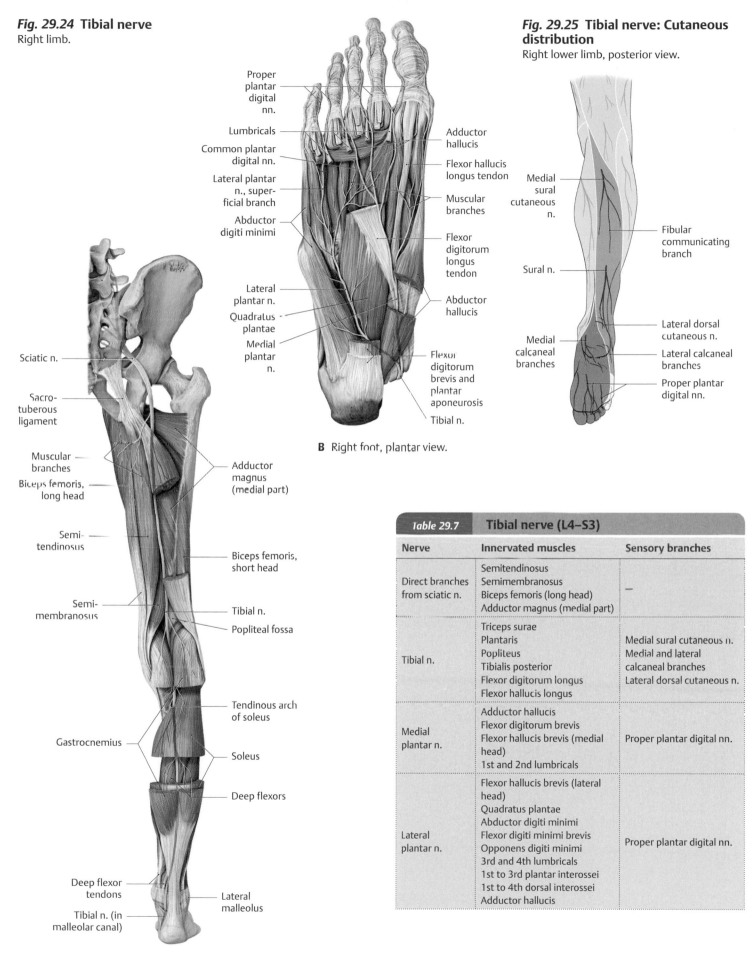

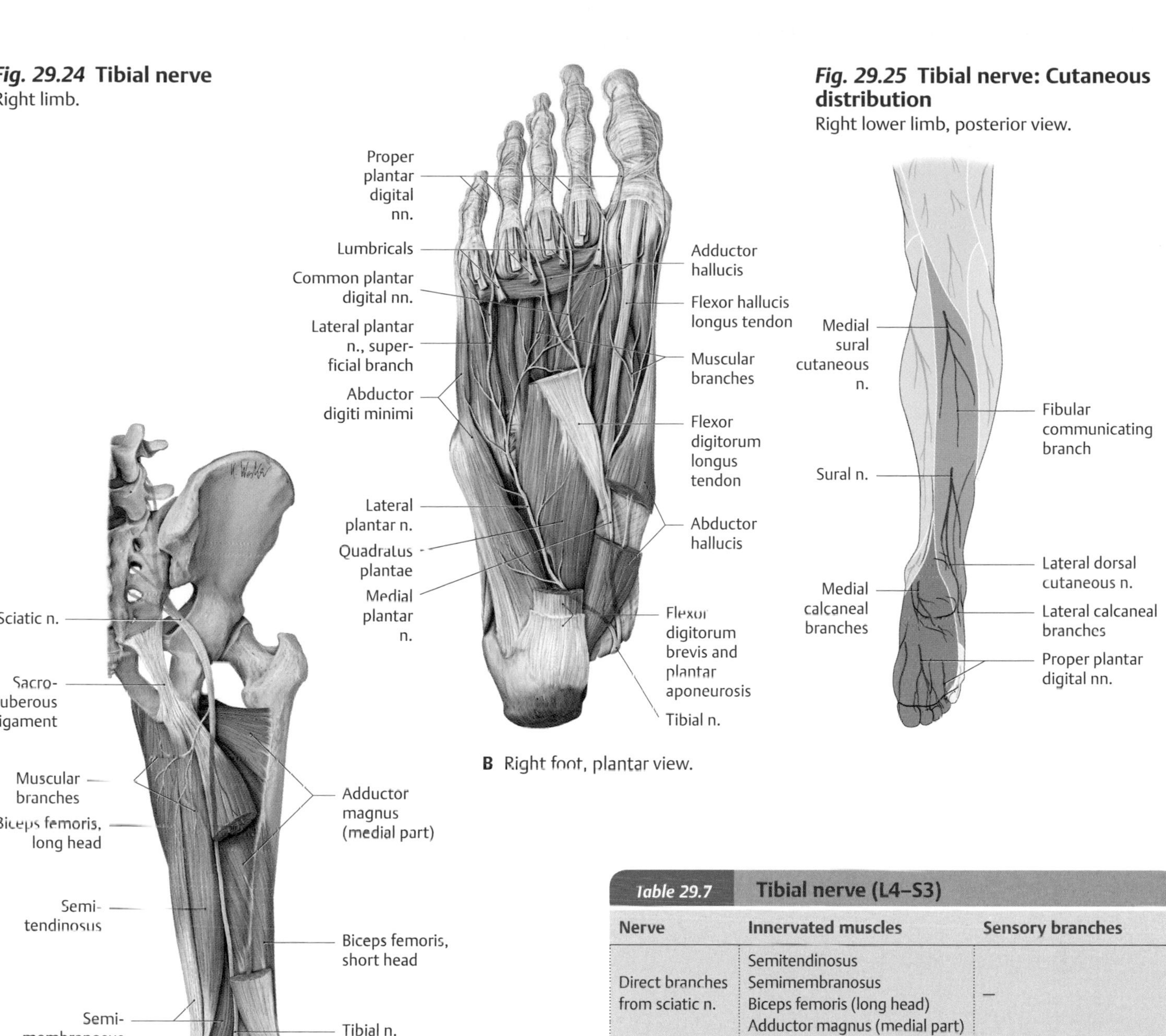
Proper plantar digital nn.
Lumbricals
Common plantar digital nn.
Lateral plantar n., superficial branch
Abductor digiti minimi
Lateral plantar n.
Quadratus plantae
Medial plantar n.
Adductor hallucis
Flexor hallucis longus tendon
Muscular branches
Flexor digitorum longus tendon
Abductor hallucis
Flexor digitorum brevis and plantar aponeurosis
Tibial n.
Sciatic n.
Sacrotuberous ligament
Muscular branches
Biceps femoris, long head
Semitendinosus
Semimembranosus
Gastrocnemius
Deep flexor tendons
Tibial n. (in malleolar canal)
Adductor magnus (medial part)
Biceps femoris, short head
Tibial n.
Popliteal fossa
Tendinous arch of soleus
Soleus
Deep flexors
Lateral malleolus
Medial sural cutaneous n.
Sural n.
Medial calcaneal branches
Fibular communicating branch
Lateral dorsal cutaneous n.
Lateral calcaneal branches
Proper plantar digital nn.

B Right foot, plantar view.

A Posterior view.

Table 29.7 Tibial nerve (L4–S3)

Nerve	Innervated muscles	Sensory branches
Direct branches from sciatic n.	Semitendinosus Semimembranosus Biceps femoris (long head) Adductor magnus (medial part)	–
Tibial n.	Triceps surae Plantaris Popliteus Tibialis posterior Flexor digitorum longus Flexor hallucis longus	Medial sural cutaneous n. Medial and lateral calcaneal branches Lateral dorsal cutaneous n.
Medial plantar n.	Adductor hallucis Flexor digitorum brevis Flexor hallucis brevis (medial head) 1st and 2nd lumbricals	Proper plantar digital nn.
Lateral plantar n.	Flexor hallucis brevis (lateral head) Quadratus plantae Abductor digiti minimi Flexor digiti minimi brevis Opponens digiti minimi 3rd and 4th lumbricals 1st to 3rd plantar interossei 1st to 4th dorsal interossei Adductor hallucis	Proper plantar digital nn.

Superficial Nerves & Vessels of the Lower Limb

Fig. 29.26 Superficial cutaneous veins and nerves of right lower limb

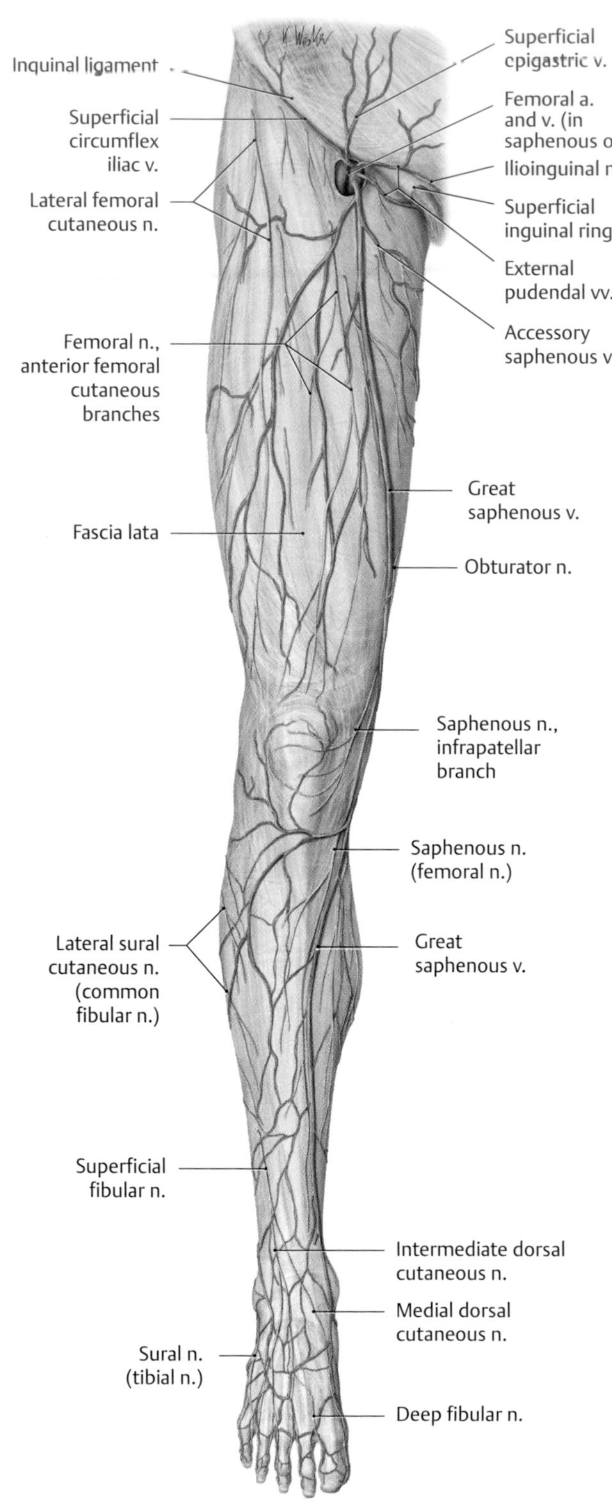
Inguinal ligament
Superficial circumflex iliac v.
Lateral femoral cutaneous n.
Femoral n., anterior femoral cutaneous branches
Fascia lata
Lateral sural cutaneous n. (common fibular n.)
Superficial fibular n.
Sural n. (tibial n.)
Superficial epigastric v.
Femoral a. and v. (in saphenous opening)
Ilioinguinal n.
Superficial inguinal ring
External pudendal vv.
Accessory saphenous v.
Great saphenous v.
Obturator n.
Saphenous n., infrapatellar branch
Saphenous n. (femoral n.)
Great saphenous v.
Intermediate dorsal cutaneous n.
Medial dorsal cutaneous n.
Deep fibular n.

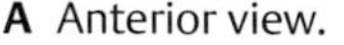

A Anterior view.

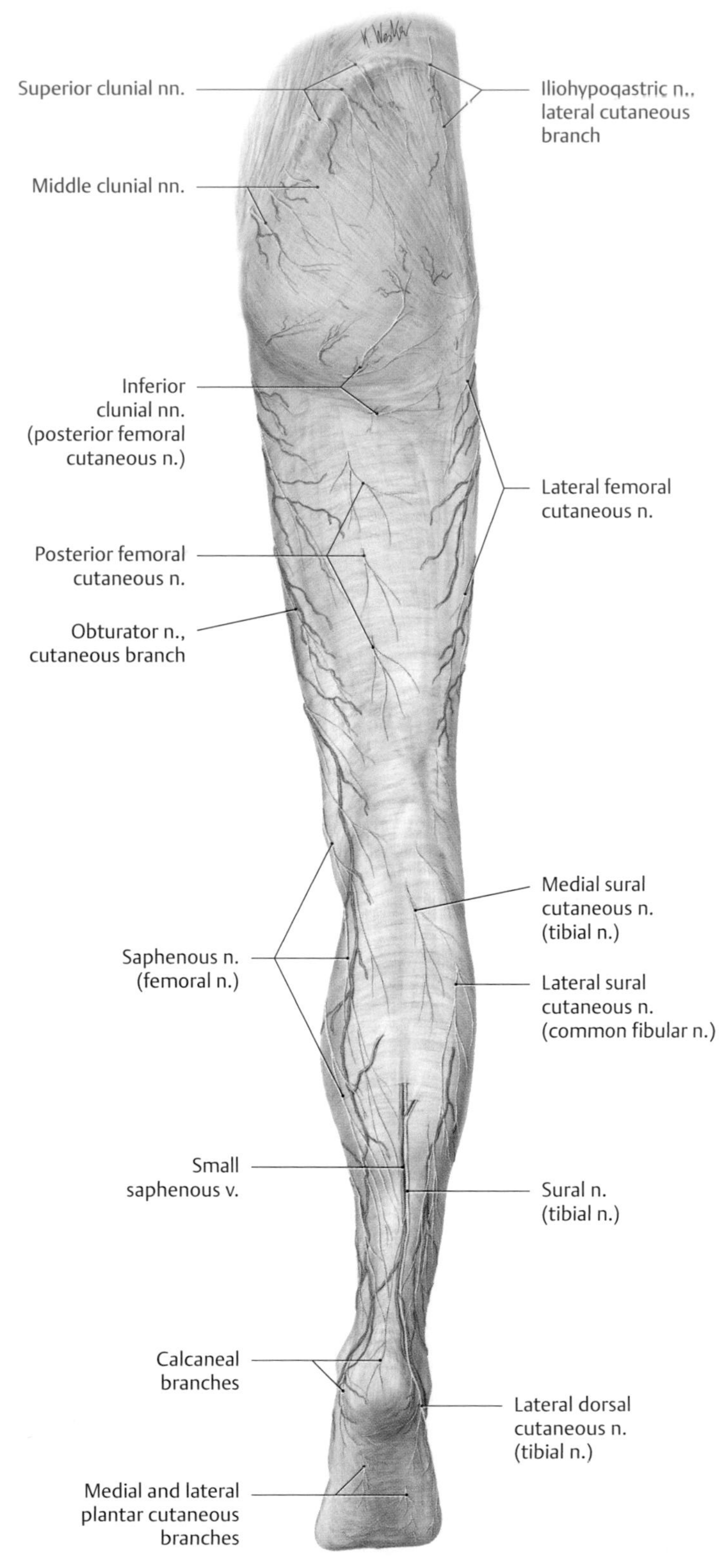
Superior clunial nn.
Middle clunial nn.
Inferior clunial nn. (posterior femoral cutaneous n.)
Posterior femoral cutaneous n.
Obturator n., cutaneous branch
Saphenous n. (femoral n.)
Small saphenous v.
Calcaneal branches
Medial and lateral plantar cutaneous branches
Iliohypogastric n., lateral cutaneous branch
Lateral femoral cutaneous n.
Medial sural cutaneous n. (tibial n.)
Lateral sural cutaneous n. (common fibular n.)
Sural n. (tibial n.)
Lateral dorsal cutaneous n. (tibial n.)

B Posterior view.

Fig. 29.27 Cutaneous innervation of the lower limb

Right lower limb.

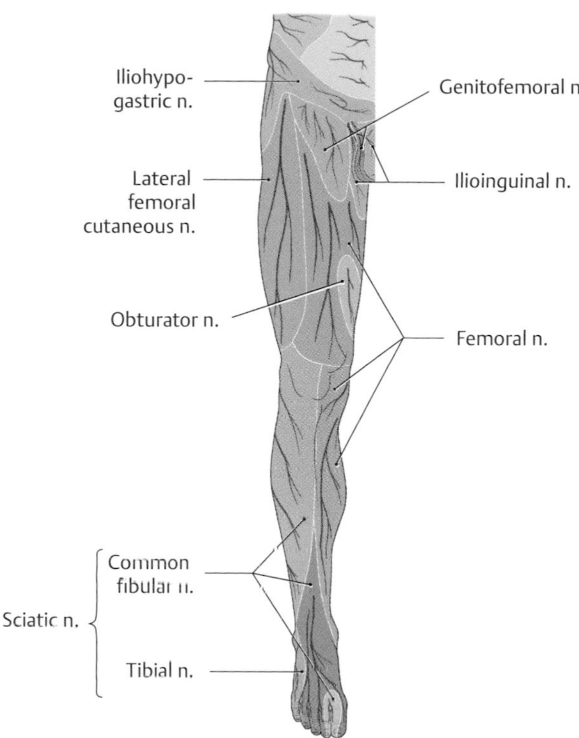
Iliohypo-
gastric n.
Genitofemoral n.
Lateral
femoral
cutaneous n.
Ilioinguinal n.
Obturator n.
Femoral n.
Common
fibular n.
Sciatic n.
Tibial n.

A Anterior view.

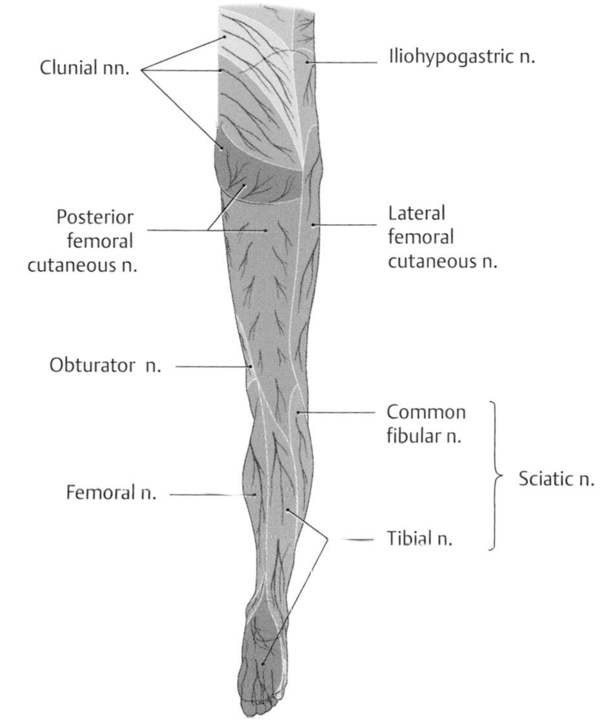
Clunial nn.
Iliohypogastric n.
Posterior
femoral
cutaneous n.
Lateral
femoral
cutaneous n.
Obturator n.
Common
fibular n.
Sciatic n.
Femoral n.
Tibial n.

B Posterior view.

Fig. 29.28 Dermatomes of the lower limb

Right lower limb.

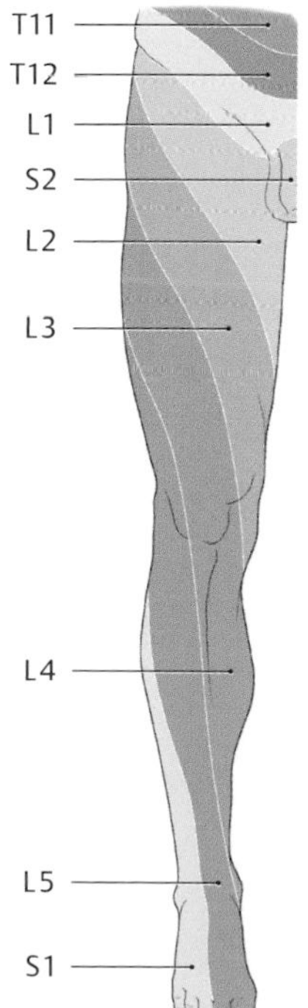
T11
T12
L1
S2
L2
L3
L4
L5
S1

A Anterior view.

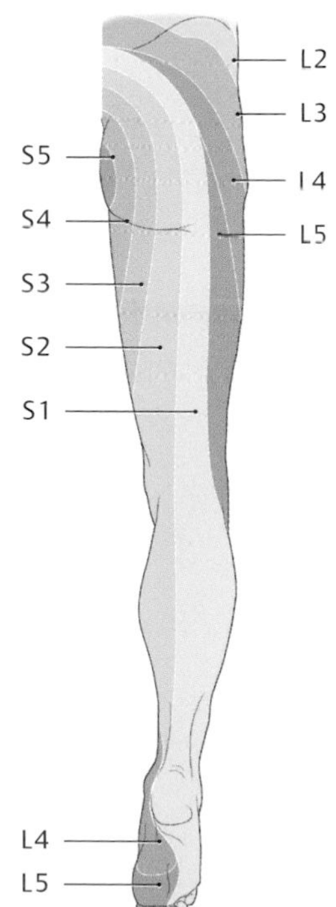
L2
L3
S5
L4
S4
L5
S3
S2
S1
L4
L5

B Posterior view.

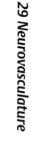

Topography of the Inguinal Region

Fig. 29.29 **Superficial veins and lymph nodes**
Right male inguinal region, anterior view. *Removed:* Cribriform fascia about the saphenous hiatus.

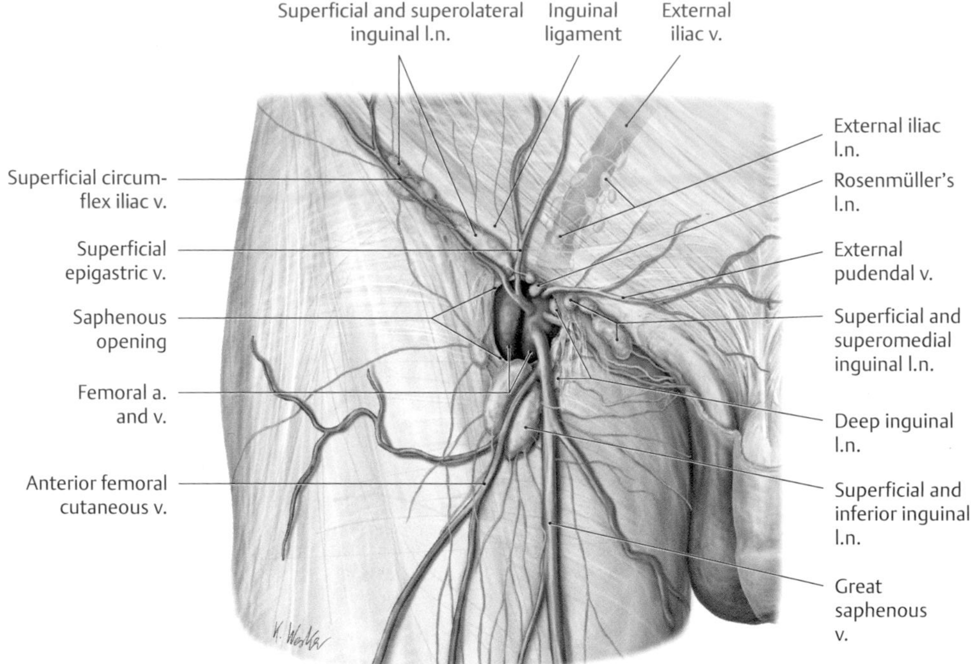

Superficial and superolateral inguinal l.n.
Inguinal ligament
External iliac v.
Superficial circumflex iliac v.
Superficial epigastric v.
Saphenous opening
Femoral a. and v.
Anterior femoral cutaneous v.
External iliac l.n.
Rosenmüller's l.n.
External pudendal v.
Superficial and superomedial inguinal l.n.
Deep inguinal l.n.
Superficial and inferior inguinal l.n.
Great saphenous v.

Fig. 29.30 **Inguinal region**
Right male inguinal region, anterior view.

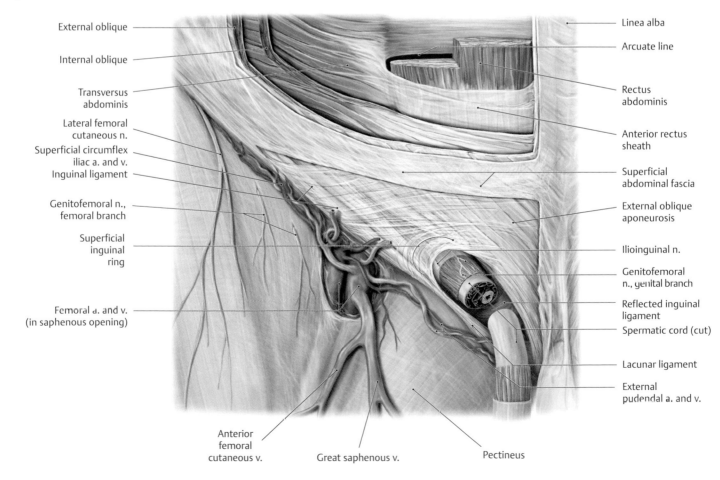

External oblique
Internal oblique
Transversus abdominis
Lateral femoral cutaneous n.
Superficial circumflex iliac a. and v.
Inguinal ligament
Genitofemoral n., femoral branch
Superficial inguinal ring
Femoral a. and v. (in saphenous opening)
Linea alba
Arcuate line
Rectus abdominis
Anterior rectus sheath
Superficial abdominal fascia
External oblique aponeurosis
Ilioinguinal n.
Genitofemoral n., genital branch
Reflected inguinal ligament
Spermatic cord (cut)
Lacunar ligament
External pudendal a. and v.
Anterior femoral cutaneous v.
Great saphenous v.
Pectineus

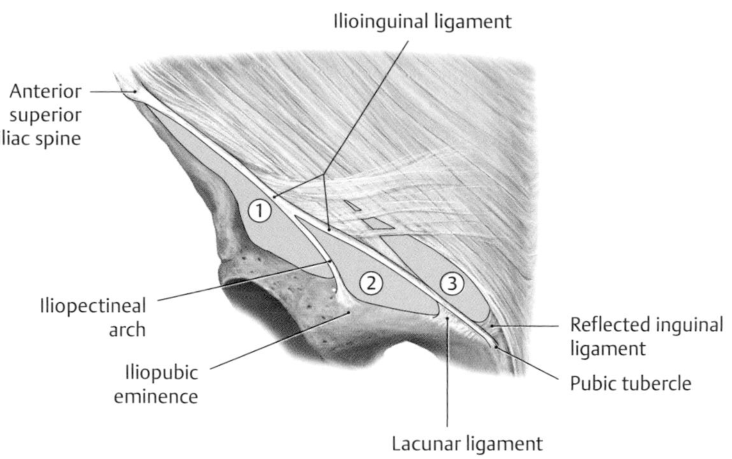
Ilioinguinal ligament
Anterior superior iliac spine
Iliopectineal arch
Iliopubic eminence
Lacunar ligament
Reflected inguinal ligament
Pubic tubercle
①
②
③

Table 29.8 Structures in the inguinal region

Region	Boundaries	Contents
Retro-inguinal space		
① Muscular compartment	Anterior superior iliac spine Inguinal lig. Iliopectineal arch	Femoral n. Lateral femoral cutaneous n. Iliacus Psoas major
② Vascular compartment	Inguinal lig. Iliopectineal arch Lacunar lig.	Femoral a. and v. Genitofemoral n., femoral branch Rosenmüller's lymph node
Inguinal canal		
③ Superficial inguinal ring	Medial crus Lateral crus Reflected inguinal lig.	Ilioinguinal n. Genitofemoral n., genital branch Spermatic cord

Fig. 29.31 **Retro-inguinal space: Muscular and vascular compartments**
Right inguinal region, anterior view.

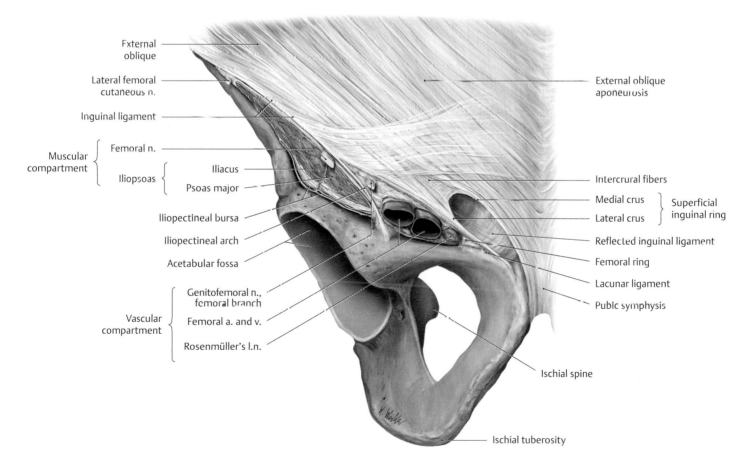

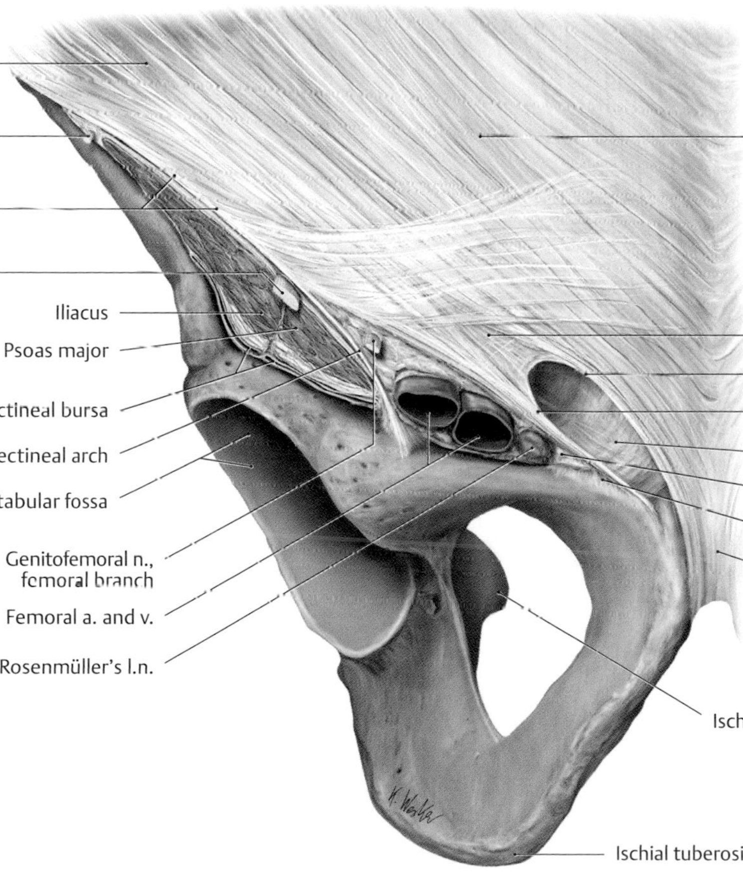

External oblique
Lateral femoral cutaneous n.
Inguinal ligament
Muscular compartment
Femoral n.
Iliopsoas
Iliacus
Psoas major
Iliopectineal bursa
Iliopectineal arch
Acetabular fossa
Vascular compartment
Genitofemoral n., femoral branch
Femoral a. and v.
Rosenmüller's l.n.
External oblique aponeurosis
Intercrural fibers
Medial crus
Lateral crus
Superficial inguinal ring
Reflected inguinal ligament
Femoral ring
Lacunar ligament
Pubic symphysis
Ischial spine
Ischial tuberosity

Topography of the Gluteal Region

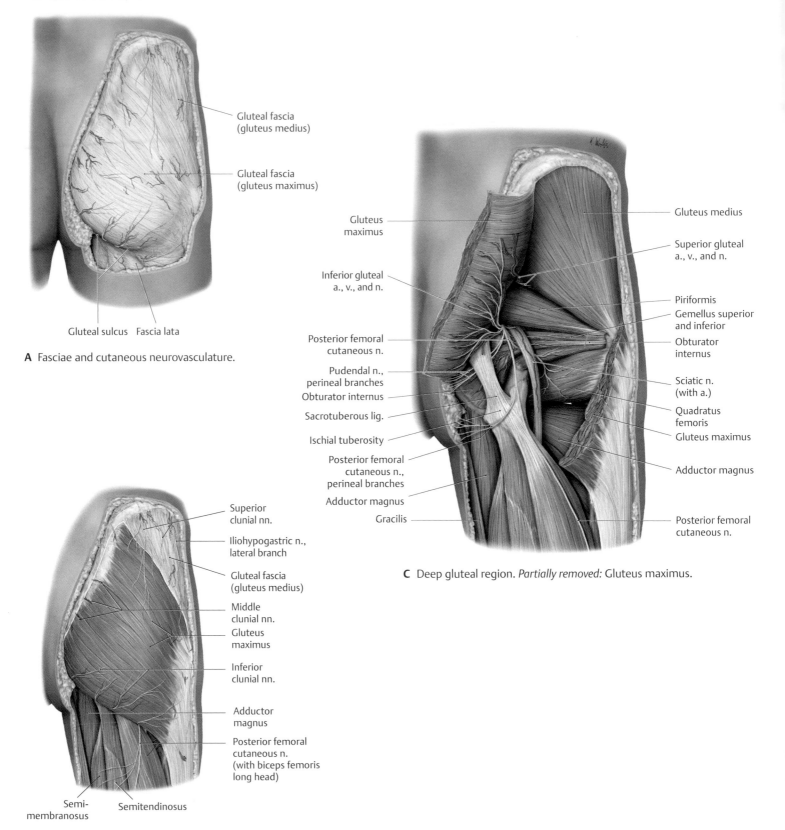

Fig. 29.32 Gluteal region
Right gluteal region, posterior view.

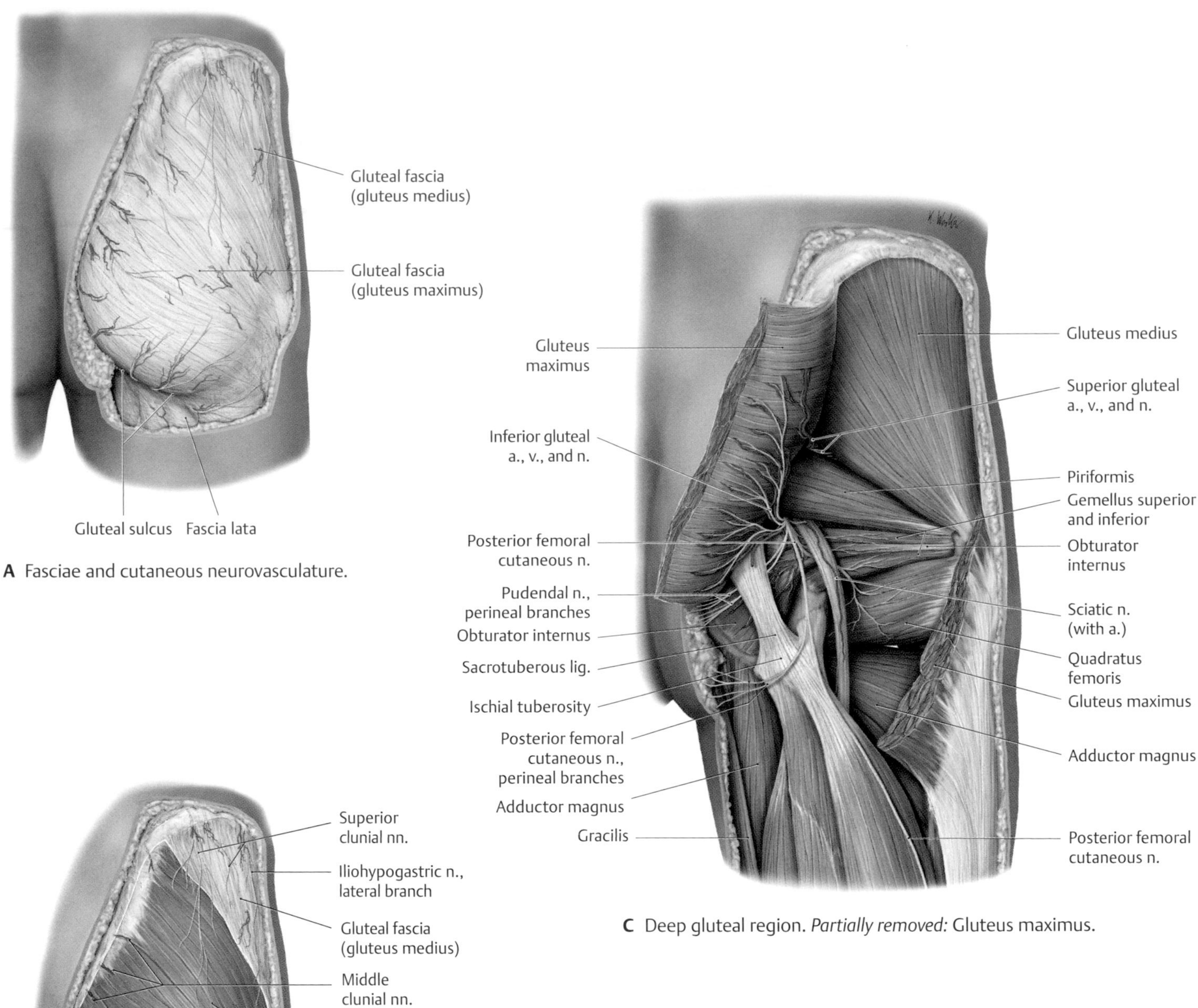
Gluteal fascia
(gluteus medius)
Gluteal fascia
(gluteus maximus)
Gluteal sulcus
Fascia lata
Gluteus
maximus
Inferior gluteal
a., v., and n.
Posterior femoral
cutaneous n.
Pudendal n.,
perineal branches
Obturator internus
Sacrotuberous lig.
Ischial tuberosity
Posterior femoral
cutaneous n.,
perineal branches
Adductor magnus
Gracilis
Gluteus medius
Superior gluteal
a., v., and n.
Piriformis
Gemellus superior
and inferior
Obturator
internus
Sciatic n.
(with a.)
Quadratus
femoris
Gluteus maximus
Adductor magnus
Posterior femoral
cutaneous n.
Superior
clunial nn.
Iliohypogastric n.,
lateral branch
Gluteal fascia
(gluteus medius)
Middle
clunial nn.
Gluteus
maximus
Inferior
clunial nn.
Adductor
magnus
Posterior femoral
cutaneous n.
(with biceps femoris
long head)
Semi-
membranosus
Semitendinosus

A Fasciae and cutaneous neurovasculature.

C Deep gluteal region. *Partially removed:* Gluteus maximus.

B Gluteal region. *Removed:* Fascia lata.

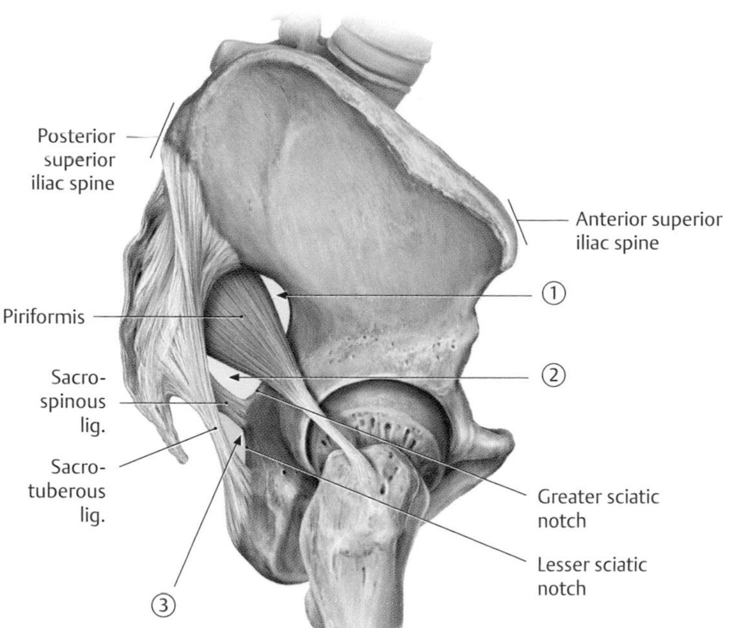

Posterior superior iliac spine
Anterior superior iliac spine
Piriformis
①
②
Sacro-spinous lig.
Sacro-tuberous lig.
Greater sciatic notch
Lesser sciatic notch
③

Table 29.9 Sciatic foramina			
Foramen		**Transmitted structures**	**Boundaries**
Greater sciatic foramen	① Suprapiriform portion	Superior gluteal a., v., and n.	Greater sciatic notch Sacrospinous lig. Sacrum
	② Infrapiriform portion	Inferior gluteal a., v., and n. Internal pudendal a. and v. Pudendal n. Sciatic n. Posterior femoral cutaneous n.	
③ Lesser sciatic foramen		Internal pudendal a. and v. Pudendal n. Obturator internus	Lesser sciatic notch Sacrospinous lig. Sacrotuberous lig.

Fig. 29.33 **Gluteal region and ischioanal fossa**
Right gluteal region, posterior view.
Removed: Gluteus maximus and medius.

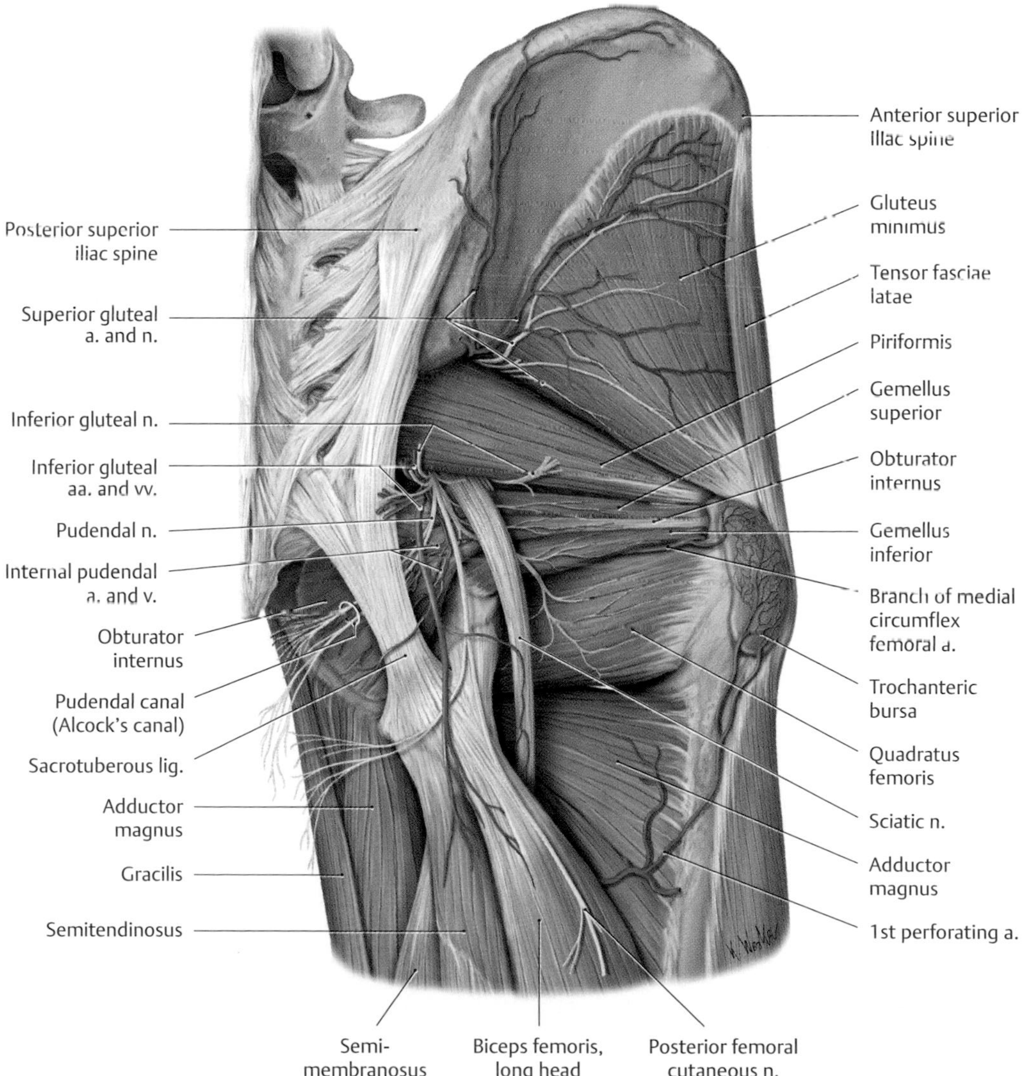

Anterior superior iliac spine
Gluteus minimus
Tensor fasciae latae
Piriformis
Gemellus superior
Obturator internus
Gemellus inferior
Branch of medial circumflex femoral a.
Trochanteric bursa
Quadratus femoris
Sciatic n.
Adductor magnus
1st perforating a.
Posterior superior iliac spine
Superior gluteal a. and n.
Inferior gluteal n.
Inferior gluteal aa. and vv.
Pudendal n.
Internal pudendal a. and v.
Obturator internus
Pudendal canal (Alcock's canal)
Sacrotuberous lig.
Adductor magnus
Gracilis
Semitendinosus
Semi-membranosus
Biceps femoris, long head
Posterior femoral cutaneous n.

Topography of the Anterior, Medial & Posterior Thigh

Fig. 29.34 Anterior and medial thigh
Right thigh, anterior view.

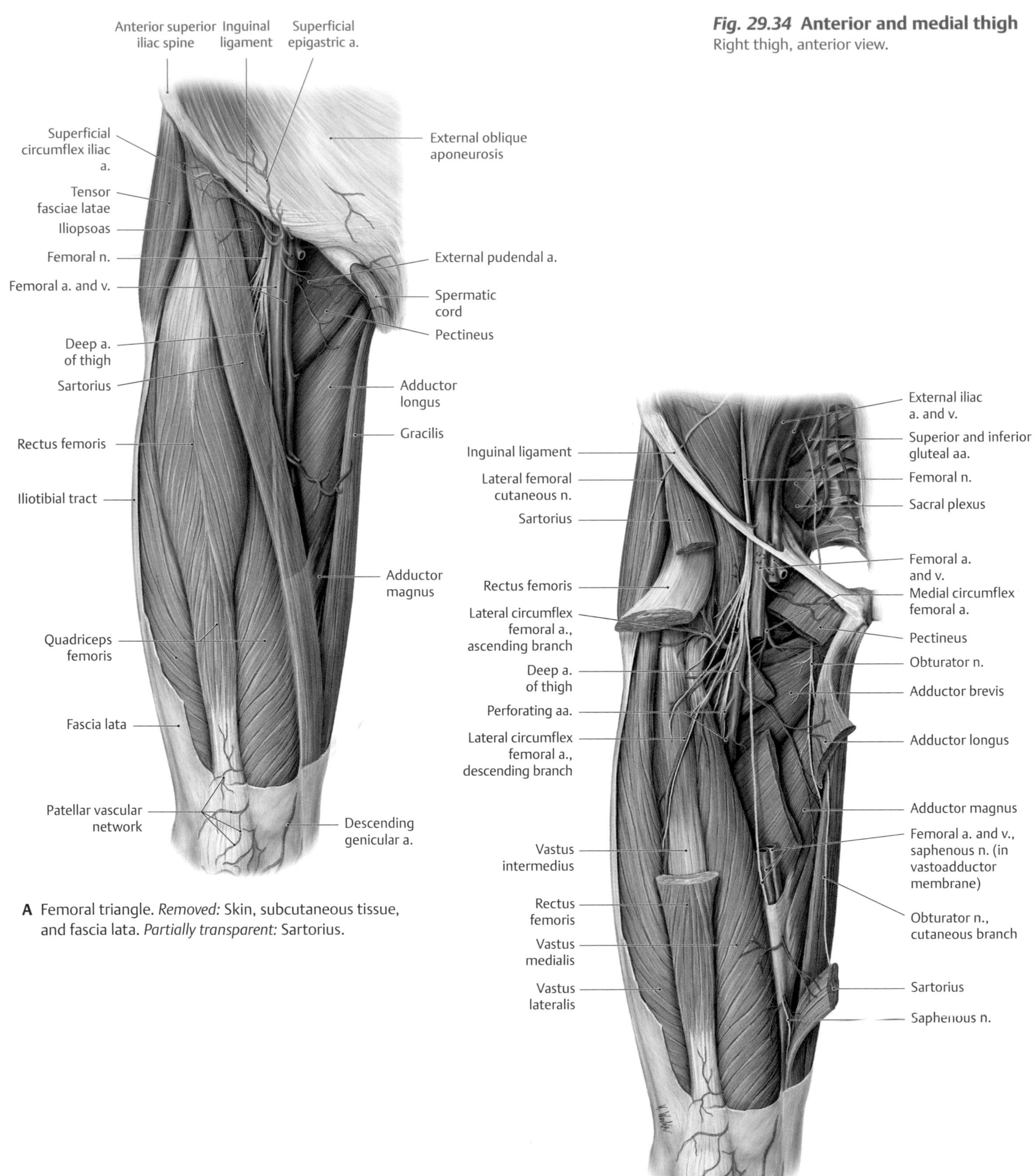
Anterior superior iliac spine
Inguinal ligament
Superficial epigastric a.
Superficial circumflex iliac a.
External oblique aponeurosis
Tensor fasciae latae
Iliopsoas
Femoral n.
External pudendal a.
Femoral a. and v.
Spermatic cord
Pectineus
Deep a. of thigh
Sartorius
Adductor longus
Gracilis
Rectus femoris
Iliotibial tract
Adductor magnus
Quadriceps femoris
Fascia lata
Patellar vascular network
Descending genicular a.
External iliac a. and v.
Superior and inferior gluteal aa.
Inguinal ligament
Femoral n.
Lateral femoral cutaneous n.
Sacral plexus
Sartorius
Femoral a. and v.
Rectus femoris
Medial circumflex femoral a.
Lateral circumflex femoral a., ascending branch
Pectineus
Obturator n.
Deep a. of thigh
Adductor brevis
Perforating aa.
Lateral circumflex femoral a., descending branch
Adductor longus
Adductor magnus
Vastus intermedius
Femoral a. and v., saphenous n. (in vastoadductor membrane)
Rectus femoris
Obturator n., cutaneous branch
Vastus medialis
Vastus lateralis
Sartorius
Saphenous n.

A Femoral triangle. *Removed:* Skin, subcutaneous tissue, and fascia lata. *Partially transparent:* Sartorius.

B Neurovasculature of the anterior thigh. *Removed:* Anterior abdominal wall. *Partially removed:* Sartorius, rectus femoris, adductor longus, and pectineus.

Fig. 29.35 Posterior thigh
Right thigh, posterior view.

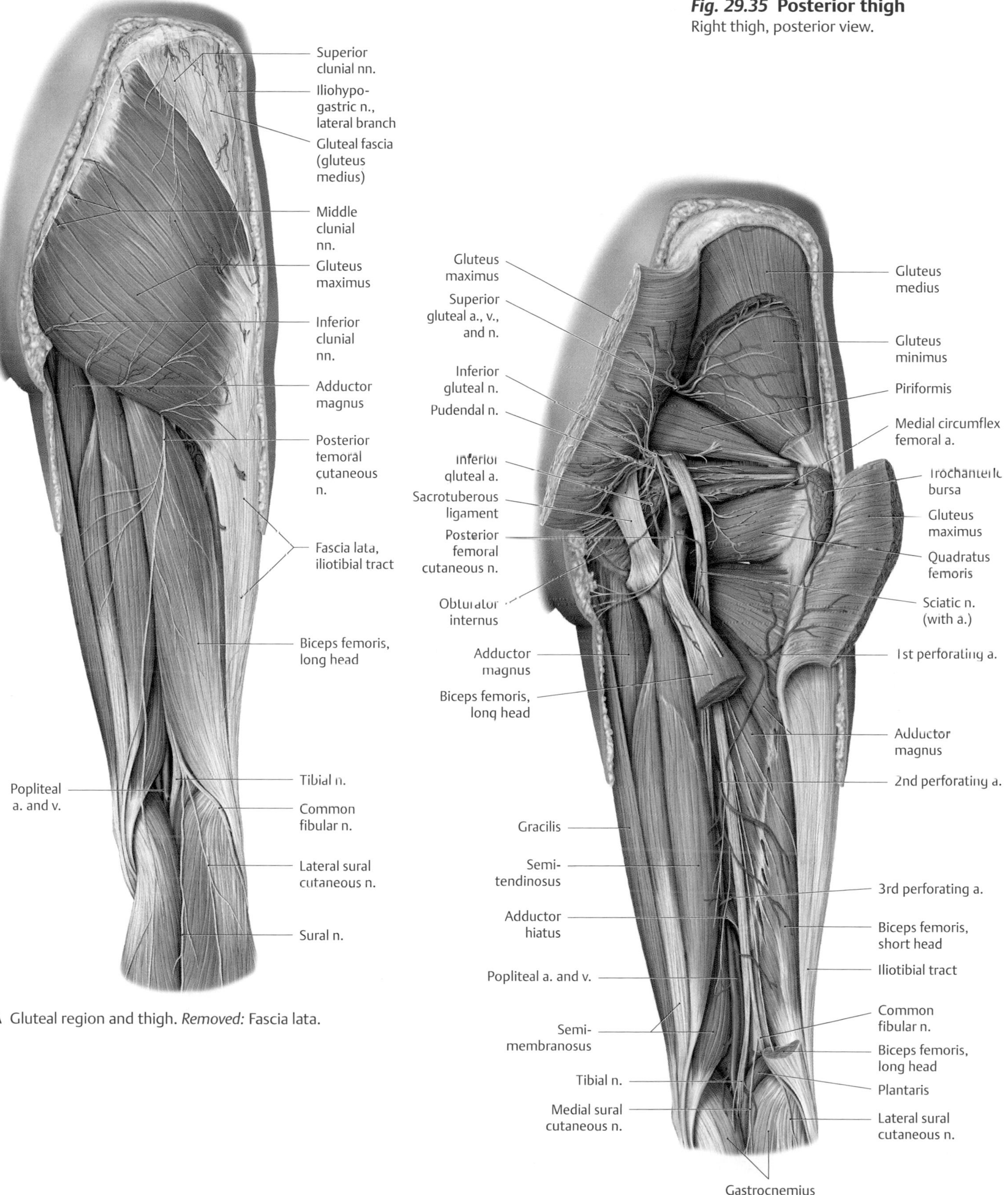
Superior
clunial nn.
Iliohypo-
gastric n.,
lateral branch
Gluteal fascia
(gluteus
medius)
Middle
clunial
nn.
Gluteus
maximus
Inferior
clunial
nn.
Adductor
magnus
Posterior
temoral
cutaneous
n.
Fascia lata,
iliotibial tract
Biceps femoris,
long head
Popliteal
a. and v.
Tibial n.
Common
fibular n.
Lateral sural
cutaneous n.
Sural n.
Gluteus
maximus
Superior
gluteal a., v.,
and n.
Inferior
gluteal n.
Pudendal n.
Inferior
gluteal a.
Sacrotuberous
ligament
Posterior
femoral
cutaneous n.
Obturator
internus
Adductor
magnus
Biceps femoris,
long head
Gracilis
Semi-
tendinosus
Adductor
hiatus
Popliteal a. and v.
Semi-
membranosus
Tibial n.
Medial sural
cutaneous n.
Gastrocnemius
Gluteus
medius
Gluteus
minimus
Piriformis
Medial circumflex
femoral a.
Trochanteric
bursa
Gluteus
maximus
Quadratus
femoris
Sciatic n.
(with a.)
1st perforating a.
Adductor
magnus
2nd perforating a.
3rd perforating a.
Biceps femoris,
short head
Iliotibial tract
Common
fibular n.
Biceps femoris,
long head
Plantaris
Lateral sural
cutaneous n.

A Gluteal region and thigh. *Removed:* Fascia lata.

B Neurovasculature of the posterior thigh. *Partially removed:* Gluteus maximus, gluteus medius, and biceps femoris. *Retracted:* Semimembranosus.

Topography of the Posterior Compartment of the Leg & Foot

Fig. 29.36 Posterior compartment of leg
Right leg, posterior view.

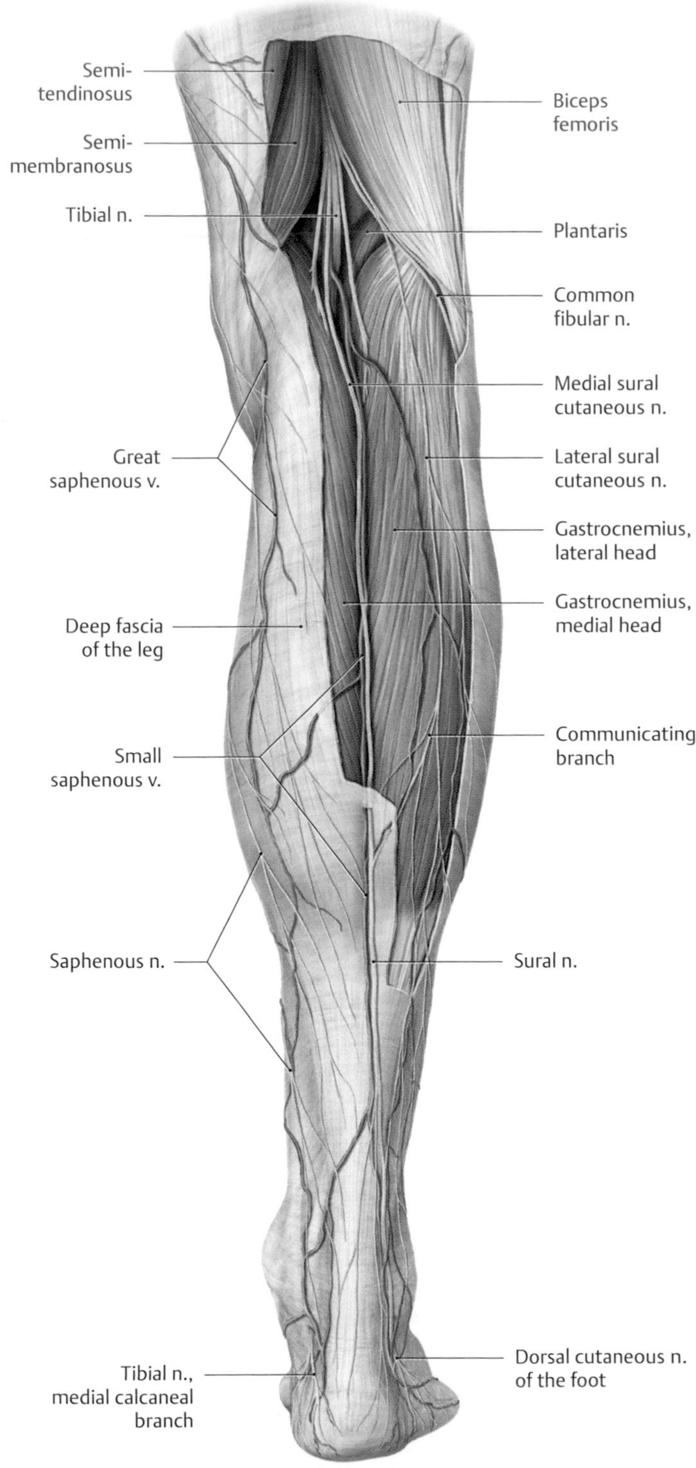
Semi-
tendinosus
Semi-
membranosus
Tibial n.
Great
saphenous v.
Deep fascia
of the leg
Small
saphenous v.
Saphenous n.
Tibial n.,
medial calcaneal
branch
Biceps
femoris
Plantaris
Common
fibular n.
Medial sural
cutaneous n.
Lateral sural
cutaneous n.
Gastrocnemius,
lateral head
Gastrocnemius,
medial head
Communicating
branch
Sural n.
Dorsal cutaneous n.
of the foot

A Superficial neurovascular structures.

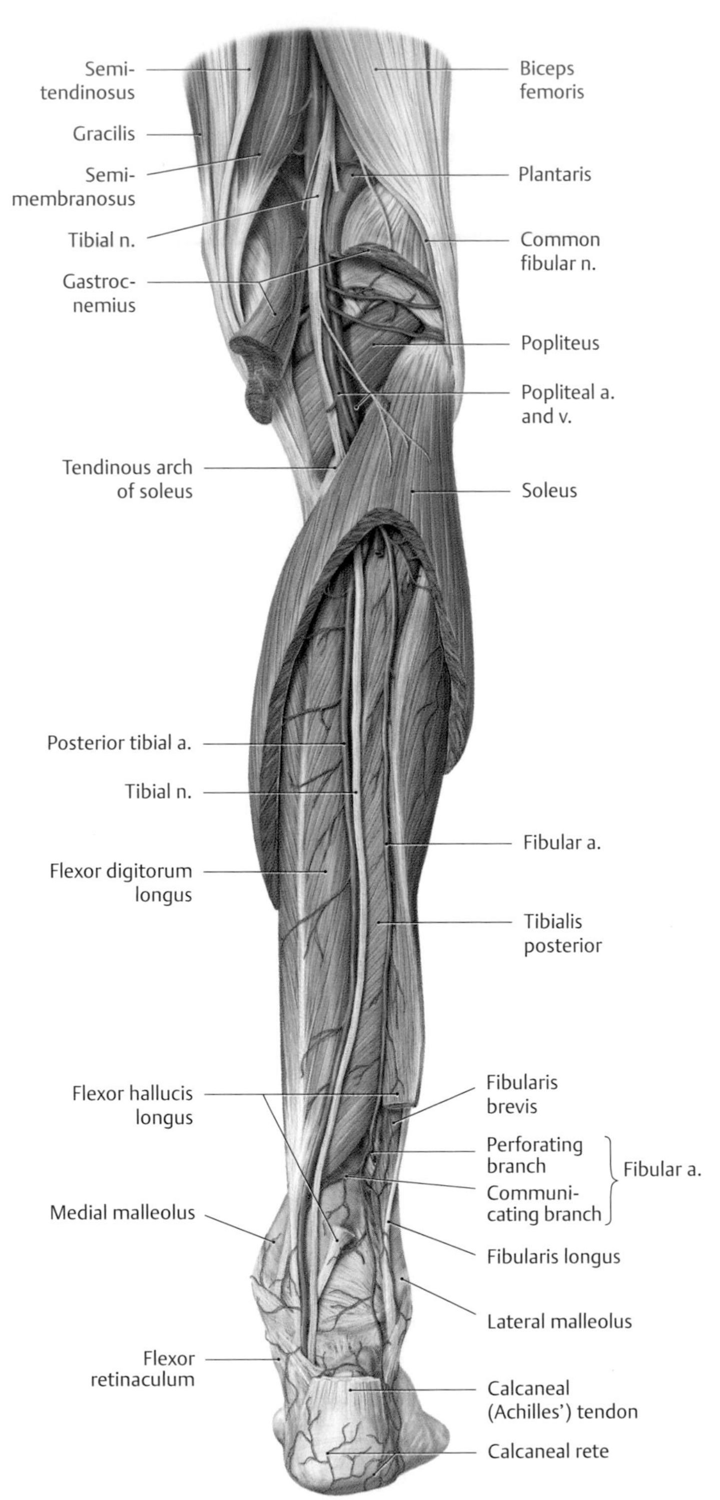
Semi-
tendinosus
Gracilis
Semi-
membranosus
Tibial n.
Gastroc-
nemius
Tendinous arch
of soleus
Posterior tibial a.
Tibial n.
Flexor digitorum
longus
Flexor hallucis
longus
Medial malleolus
Flexor
retinaculum
Biceps
femoris
Plantaris
Common
fibular n.
Popliteus
Popliteal a.
and v.
Soleus
Fibular a.
Tibialis
posterior
Fibularis
brevis
Perforating
branch
Communi-
cating branch
Fibular a.
Fibularis longus
Lateral malleolus
Calcaneal
(Achilles') tendon
Calcaneal rete

B Deep neurovascular structures. *Removed:* Gastrocnemius. *Windowed:* Soleus.

Fig. 29.37 Popliteal region

Right leg, posterior view.

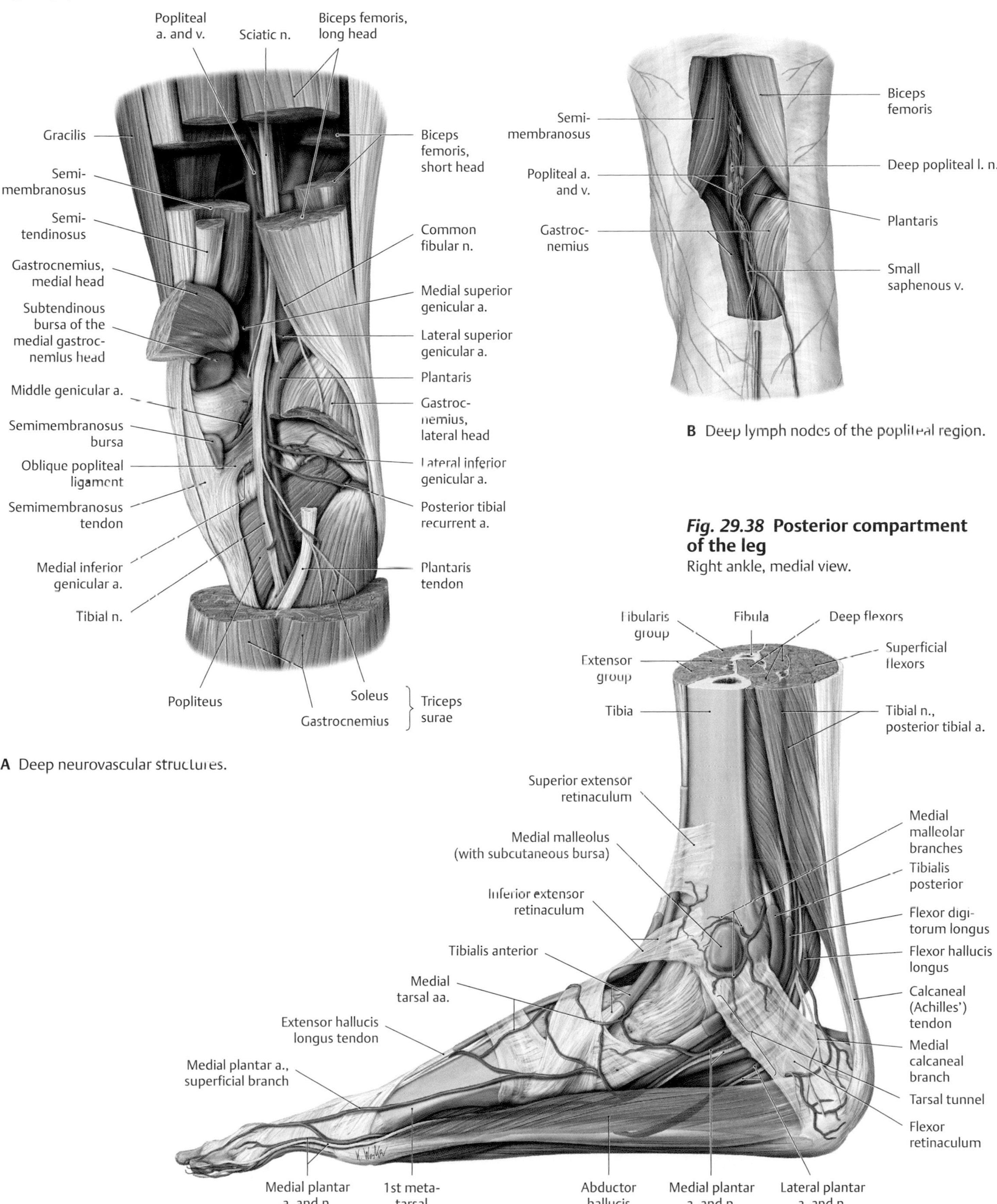
Popliteal a. and v.
Sciatic n.
Biceps femoris, long head
Gracilis
Semi-membranosus
Semi-tendinosus
Gastrocnemius, medial head
Subtendinous bursa of the medial gastrocnemius head
Middle genicular a.
Semimembranosus bursa
Oblique popliteal ligament
Semimembranosus tendon
Medial inferior genicular a.
Tibial n.
Biceps femoris, short head
Common fibular n.
Medial superior genicular a.
Lateral superior genicular a.
Plantaris
Gastroc-nemius, lateral head
Lateral inferior genicular a.
Posterior tibial recurrent a.
Plantaris tendon
Popliteus
Soleus
Gastrocnemius
Triceps surae
Semi-membranosus
Popliteal a. and v.
Gastroc-nemius
Biceps femoris
Deep popliteal l. n.
Plantaris
Small saphenous v.
Fibularis group
Fibula
Deep flexors
Superficial flexors
Extensor group
Tibia
Tibial n., posterior tibial a.
Superior extensor retinaculum
Medial malleolus (with subcutaneous bursa)
Inferior extensor retinaculum
Tibialis anterior
Medial tarsal aa.
Extensor hallucis longus tendon
Medial plantar a., superficial branch
Medial plantar a. and n.
1st meta-tarsal
Abductor hallucis
Medial plantar a. and n.
Lateral plantar a. and n.
Medial malleolar branches
Tibialis posterior
Flexor digi-torum longus
Flexor hallucis longus
Calcaneal (Achilles') tendon
Medial calcaneal branch
Tarsal tunnel
Flexor retinaculum

A Deep neurovascular structures.

B Deep lymph nodes of the popliteal region.

Fig. 29.38 Posterior compartment of the leg

Right ankle, medial view.

Topography of the Lateral & Anterior Compartments of the Leg

Fig. 29.39 **Neurovasculature of the lateral compartment of the leg**
Right limb. *Removed:* Origins of the fibularis longus and extensor digitorum longus.

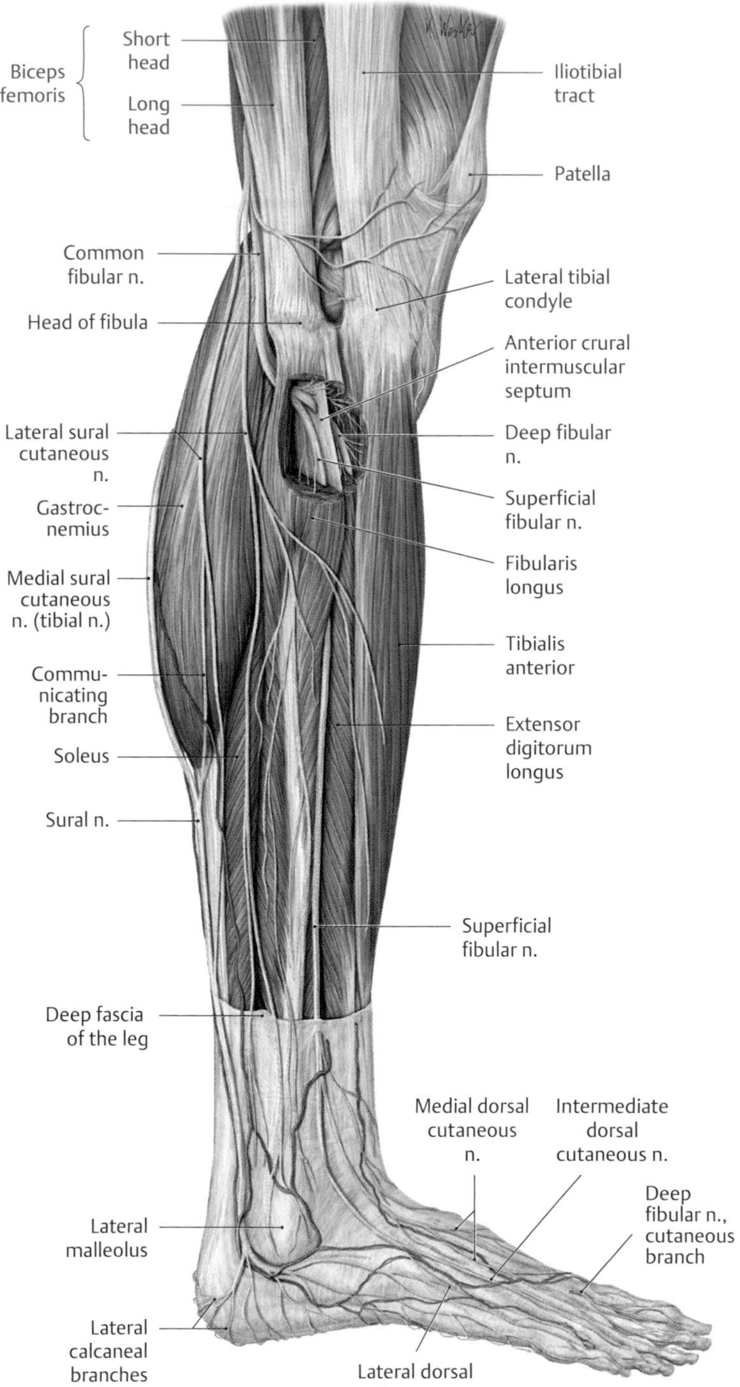

Biceps femoris
Short head
Long head
Iliotibial tract
Patella
Common fibular n.
Head of fibula
Lateral tibial condyle
Anterior crural intermuscular septum
Lateral sural cutaneous n.
Deep fibular n.
Gastroc-nemius
Superficial fibular n.
Fibularis longus
Medial sural cutaneous n. (tibial n.)
Tibialis anterior
Commu-nicating branch
Extensor digitorum longus
Soleus
Sural n.
Superficial fibular n.
Deep fascia of the leg
Medial dorsal cutaneous n.
Intermediate dorsal cutaneous n.
Deep fibular n., cutaneous branch
Lateral malleolus
Lateral calcaneal branches
Lateral dorsal cutaneous n.

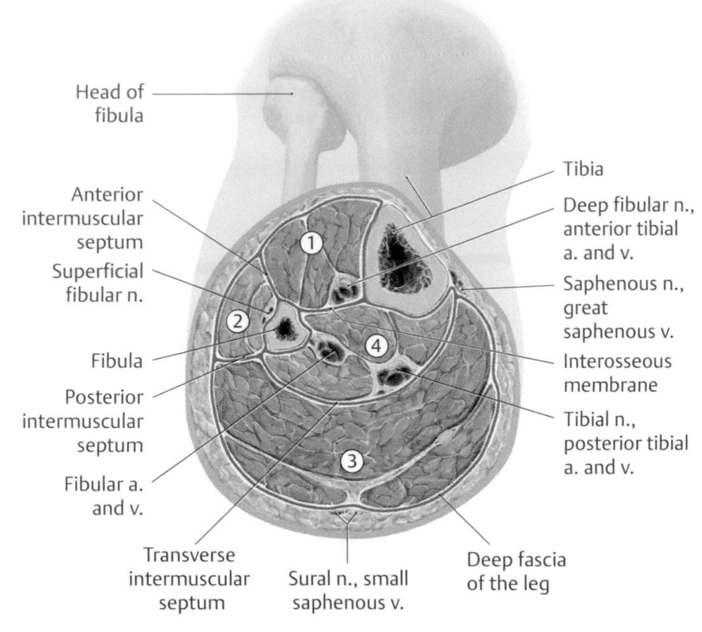

Head of fibula
Tibia
Anterior intermuscular septum
Deep fibular n., anterior tibial a. and v.
Superficial fibular n.
Saphenous n., great saphenous v.
Fibula
Interosseous membrane
Posterior intermuscular septum
Tibial n., posterior tibial a. and v.
Fibular a. and v.
Transverse intermuscular septum
Sural n., small saphenous v.
Deep fascia of the leg
①
②
③
④

Table 29.10 **Compartments of the leg**

Compartment		Muscular contents	Neurovascular contents
① Anterior compartment		Tibialis anterior	Deep fibular n. Anterior tibial a. and v.
		Extensor digitorum longus	
		Extensor hallucis longus	
		Fibularis tertius	
② Lateral compartment		Fibularis longus	Superficial fibular n.
		Fibularis brevis	
Posterior compartment	③ Superficial part	Triceps surae (gastroc-nemius and soleus)	–
		Plantaris	
	④ Deep part	Tibialis posterior	Tibial n. Posterior tibial a. and v. Fibular a. and v.
		Flexor digitorum longus	
		Flexor hallucis longus	

Clinical

Compartment syndrome
Muscle edema or hematoma can lead to a rise in tissue fluid pressure in the compartments of the leg. Subsequent compression of neurovascular structures due to this increased pressure may cause ischemia and irreversible muscle and nerve damage. Patients with *anterior* compartment syndrome, the most common form, suffer excruciating pain and cannot dorsiflex the toes. Emergency incision of the fascia of the leg may be performed to relieve compression.

Fig. 29.40 Neurovasculature of the anterior compartment of the leg and foot

Right limb with foot in plantar flexion.

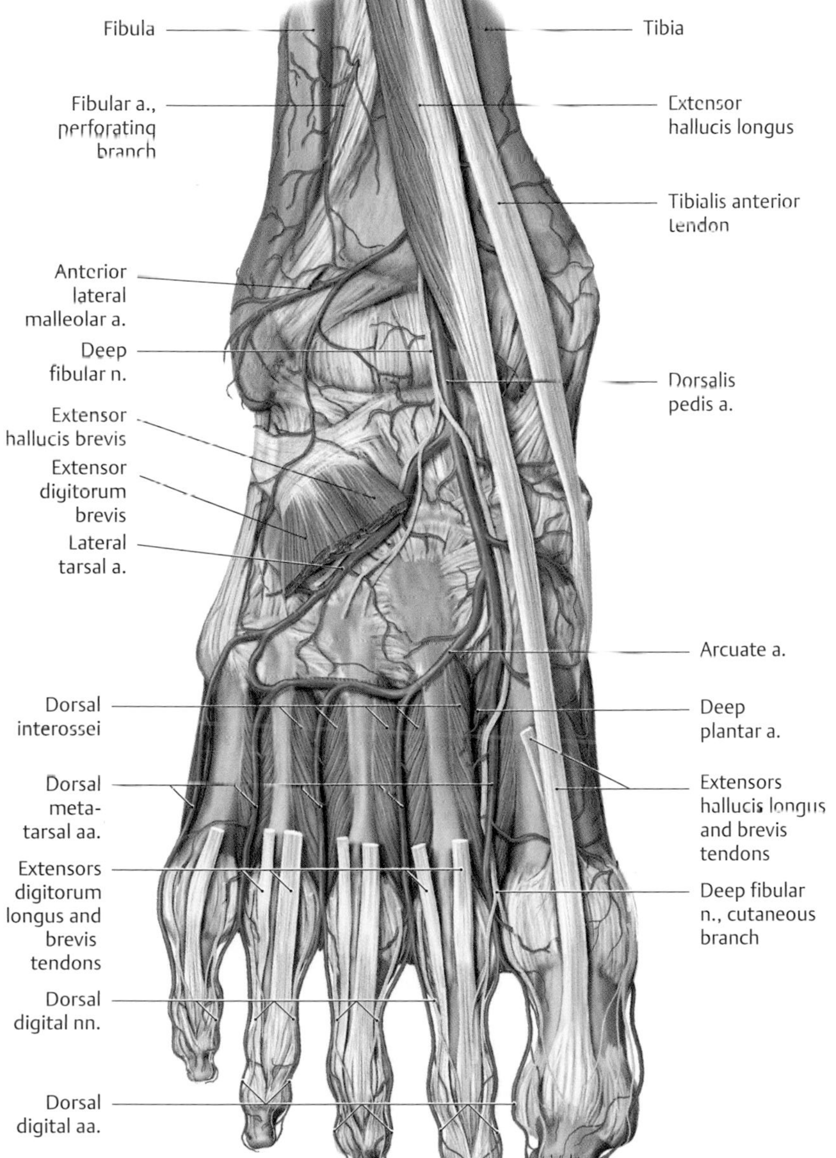
Fibula
Tibia
Fibular a., perforating branch
Extensor hallucis longus
Tibialis anterior tendon
Anterior lateral malleolar a.
Deep fibular n.
Dorsalis pedis a.
Extensor hallucis brevis
Extensor digitorum brevis
Lateral tarsal a.
Arcuate a.
Dorsal interossei
Deep plantar a.
Dorsal meta-tarsal aa.
Extensors hallucis longus and brevis tendons
Extensors digitorum longus and brevis tendons
Deep fibular n., cutaneous branch
Dorsal digital nn.
Dorsal digital aa.

A Neurovasculature of the dorsum.

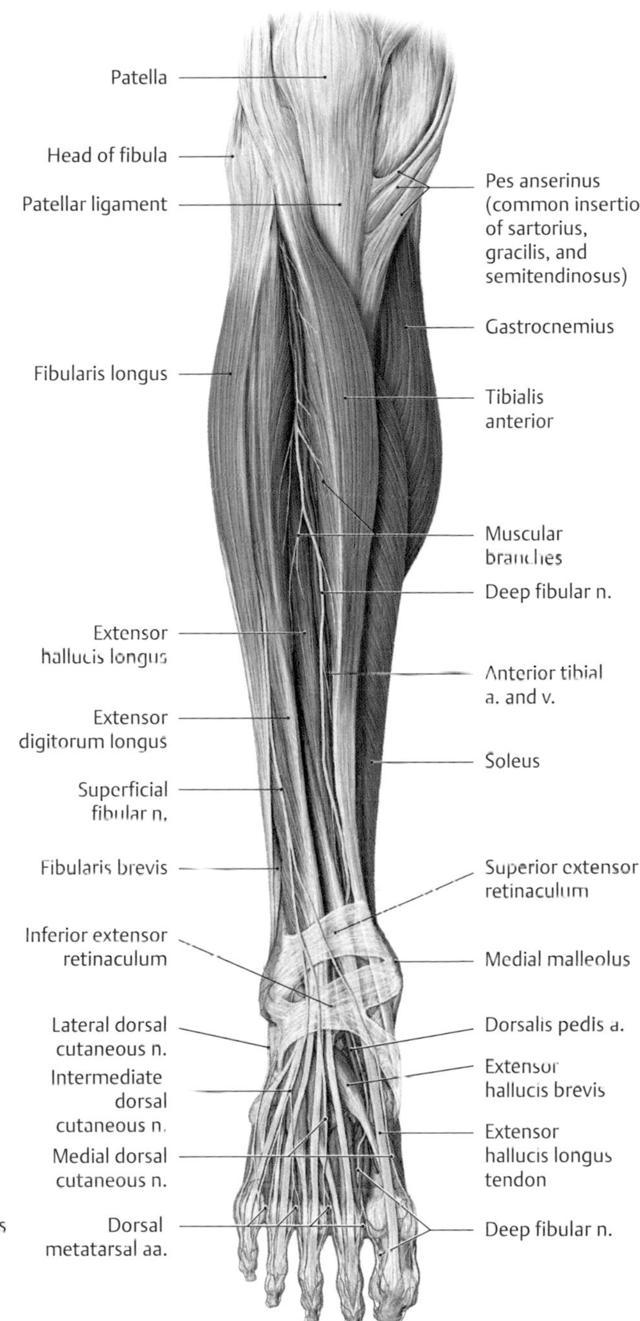
Patella
Head of fibula
Patellar ligament
Pes anserinus (common insertion of sartorius, gracilis, and semitendinosus)
Gastrocnemius
Fibularis longus
Tibialis anterior
Muscular branches
Deep fibular n.
Extensor hallucis longus
Anterior tibial a. and v.
Extensor digitorum longus
Soleus
Superficial fibular n.
Fibularis brevis
Superior extensor retinaculum
Inferior extensor retinaculum
Medial malleolus
Lateral dorsal cutaneous n.
Dorsalis pedis a.
Intermediate dorsal cutaneous n.
Extensor hallucis brevis
Medial dorsal cutaneous n.
Extensor hallucis longus tendon
Dorsal metatarsal aa.
Deep fibular n.

B Neurovasculature of the leg. *Removed:* Skin, subcutaneous tissue, and fasciae. *Retracted:* Tibialis anterior and extensor hallucis longus.

Topography of the Sole of the Foot

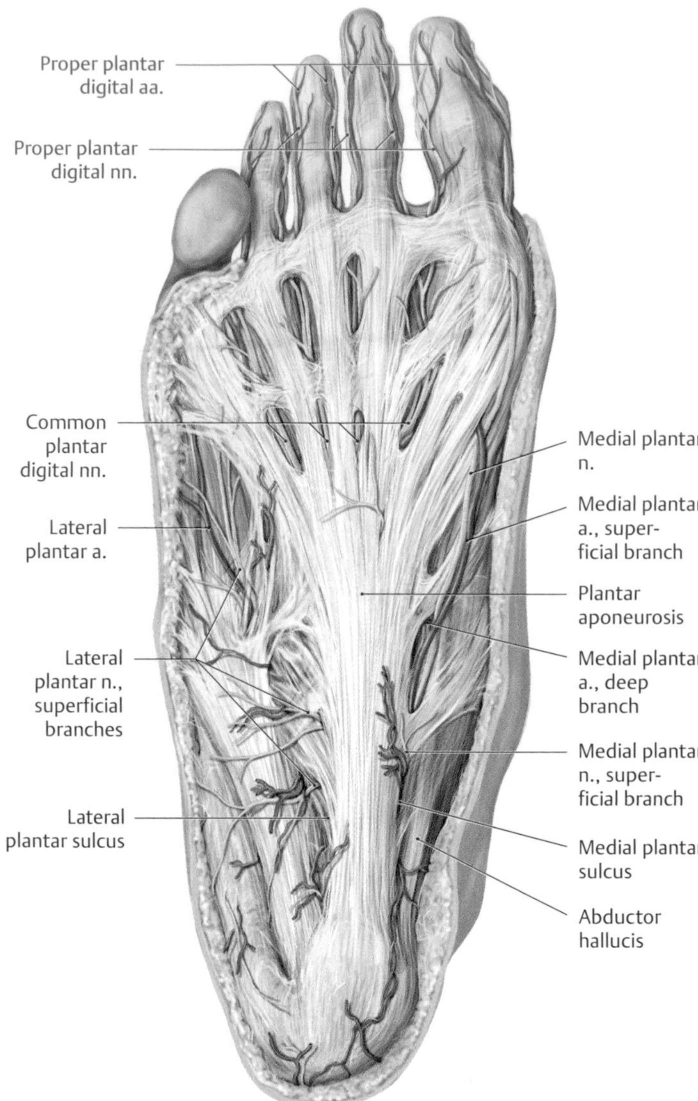
Proper plantar digital aa.
Proper plantar digital nn.
Common plantar digital nn.
Lateral plantar a.
Lateral plantar n., superficial branches
Lateral plantar sulcus
Medial plantar n.
Medial plantar a., superficial branch
Plantar aponeurosis
Medial plantar a., deep branch
Medial plantar n., superficial branch
Medial plantar sulcus
Abductor hallucis

A Superficial layer. *Removed:* Skin, subcutaneous tissue, and fascia.

Fig. 29.41 **Neurovasculature of the sole of the foot**
Right foot, plantar view.

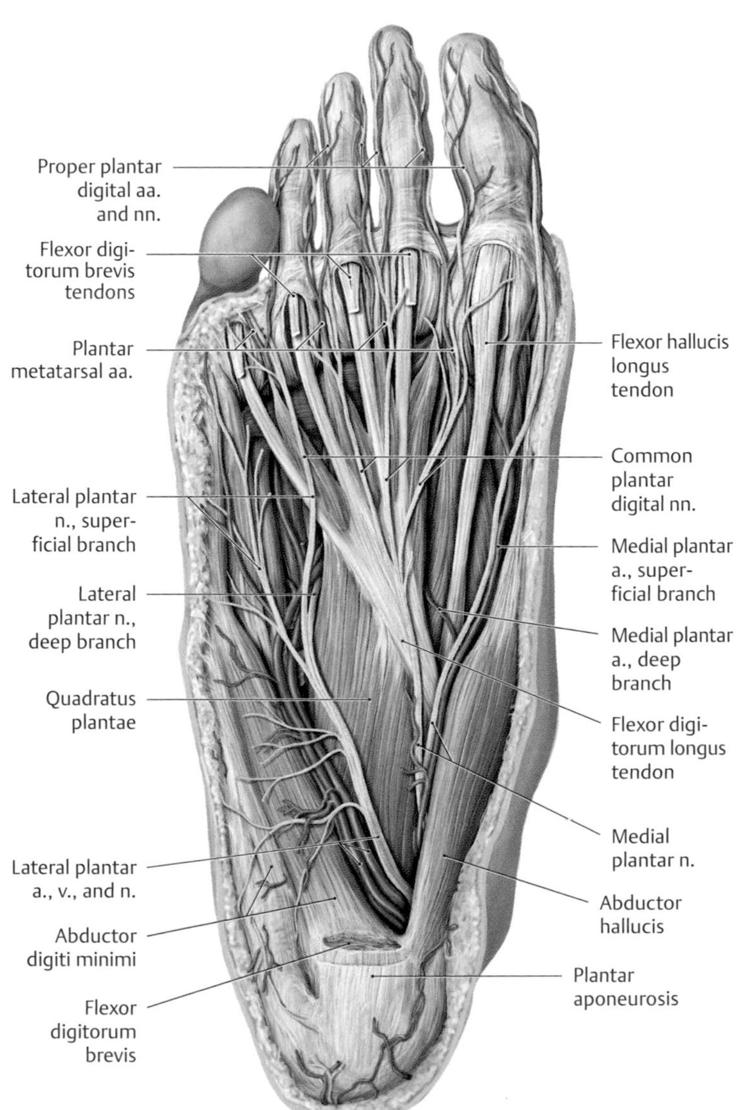
Proper plantar digital aa. and nn.
Flexor digitorum brevis tendons
Plantar metatarsal aa.
Lateral plantar n., superficial branch
Lateral plantar n., deep branch
Quadratus plantae
Lateral plantar a., v., and n.
Abductor digiti minimi
Flexor digitorum brevis
Flexor hallucis longus tendon
Common plantar digital nn.
Medial plantar a., superficial branch
Medial plantar a., deep branch
Flexor digitorum longus tendon
Medial plantar n.
Abductor hallucis
Plantar aponeurosis

B Middle layer. *Removed:* Plantar aponeurosis and flexor digitorum brevis.

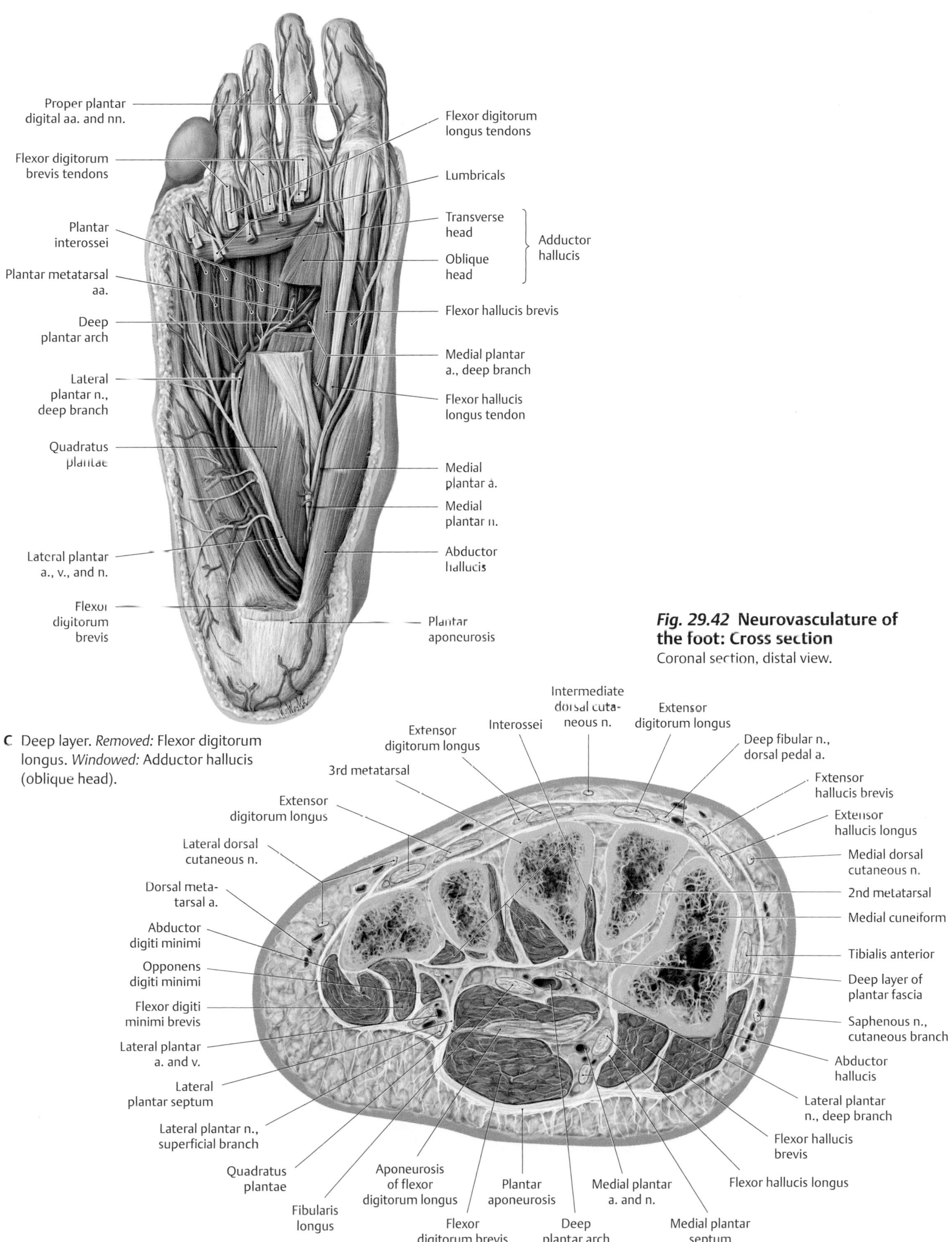

Proper plantar digital aa. and nn.
Flexor digitorum brevis tendons
Plantar interossei
Plantar metatarsal aa.
Deep plantar arch
Lateral plantar n., deep branch
Quadratus plantae
Lateral plantar a., v., and n.
Flexor digitorum brevis
Flexor digitorum longus tendons
Lumbricals
Transverse head
Oblique head
Adductor hallucis
Flexor hallucis brevis
Medial plantar a., deep branch
Flexor hallucis longus tendon
Medial plantar a.
Medial plantar n.
Abductor hallucis
Plantar aponeurosis

C Deep layer. *Removed:* Flexor digitorum longus. *Windowed:* Adductor hallucis (oblique head).

Fig. 29.42 Neurovasculature of the foot: Cross section
Coronal section, distal view.

Intermediate dorsal cutaneous n.
Interossei
Extensor digitorum longus
Extensor digitorum longus
Deep fibular n., dorsal pedal a.
3rd metatarsal
Extensor hallucis brevis
Extensor digitorum longus
Extensor hallucis longus
Lateral dorsal cutaneous n.
Medial dorsal cutaneous n.
Dorsal metatarsal a.
2nd metatarsal
Medial cuneiform
Abductor digiti minimi
Tibialis anterior
Opponens digiti minimi
Deep layer of plantar fascia
Flexor digiti minimi brevis
Saphenous n., cutaneous branch
Lateral plantar a. and v.
Abductor hallucis
Lateral plantar septum
Lateral plantar n., deep branch
Lateral plantar n., superficial branch
Flexor hallucis brevis
Quadratus plantae
Aponeurosis of flexor digitorum longus
Plantar aponeurosis
Medial plantar a. and n.
Flexor hallucis longus
Fibularis longus
Flexor digitorum brevis
Deep plantar arch
Medial plantar septum

Sectional Anatomy of the Thigh & Leg

Fig. 29.43 **Thigh and Leg: Windowed dissection**
Right lower limb, posterior view.

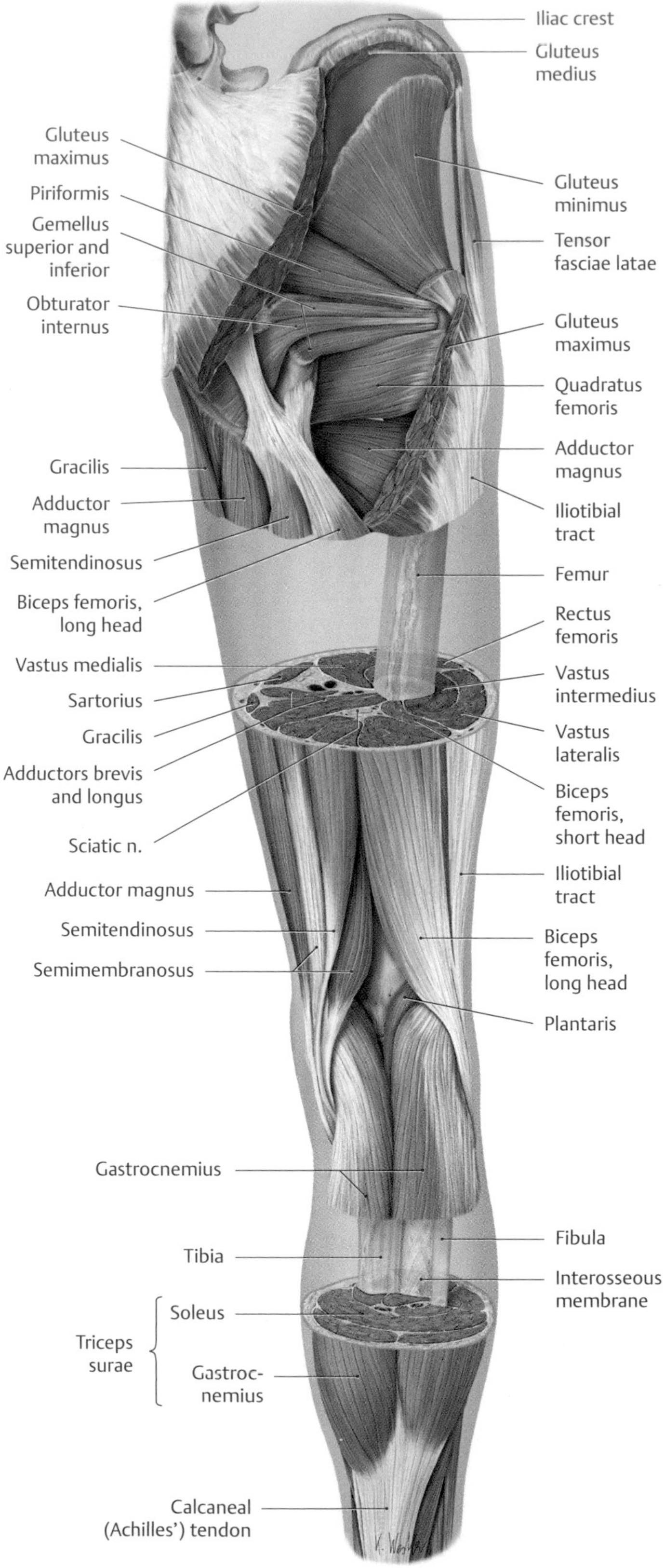

Iliac crest
Gluteus medius
Gluteus maximus
Piriformis
Gemellus superior and inferior
Obturator internus
Gluteus minimus
Tensor fasciae latae
Gluteus maximus
Quadratus femoris
Adductor magnus
Gracilis
Adductor magnus
Iliotibial tract
Semitendinosus
Femur
Biceps femoris, long head
Rectus femoris
Vastus medialis
Vastus intermedius
Sartorius
Gracilis
Vastus lateralis
Adductors brevis and longus
Biceps femoris, short head
Sciatic n.
Iliotibial tract
Adductor magnus
Semitendinosus
Biceps femoris, long head
Semimembranosus
Plantaris
Gastrocnemius
Fibula
Tibia
Interosseous membrane
Triceps surae: Soleus, Gastrocnemius
Calcaneal (Achilles') tendon

Fig. 29.44 **Lower limb: Transverse sections**
Right limb, proximal (superior) view.

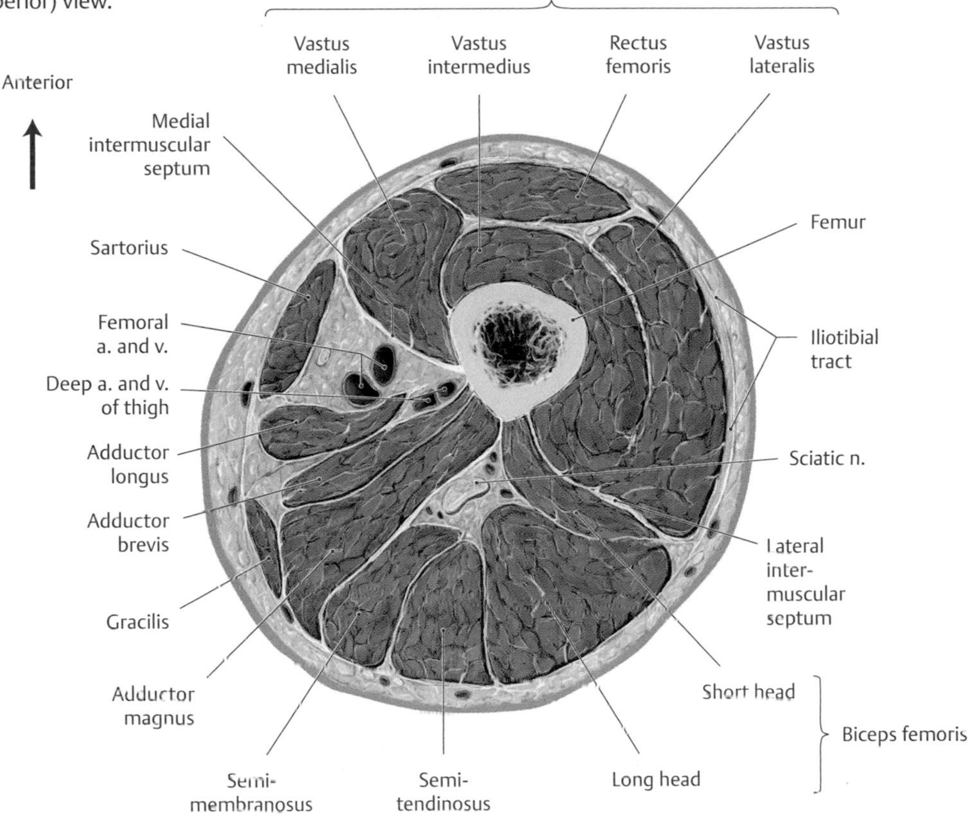
Quadriceps femoris
Vastus medialis
Vastus intermedius
Rectus femoris
Vastus lateralis
Anterior
Medial intermuscular septum
Sartorius
Femoral a. and v.
Deep a. and v. of thigh
Adductor longus
Adductor brevis
Gracilis
Adductor magnus
Femur
Iliotibial tract
Sciatic n.
Lateral inter-muscular septum
Short head
Biceps femoris
Long head
Semi-membranosus
Semi-tendinosus

A Thigh (plane of upper section in Fig. 29.43)

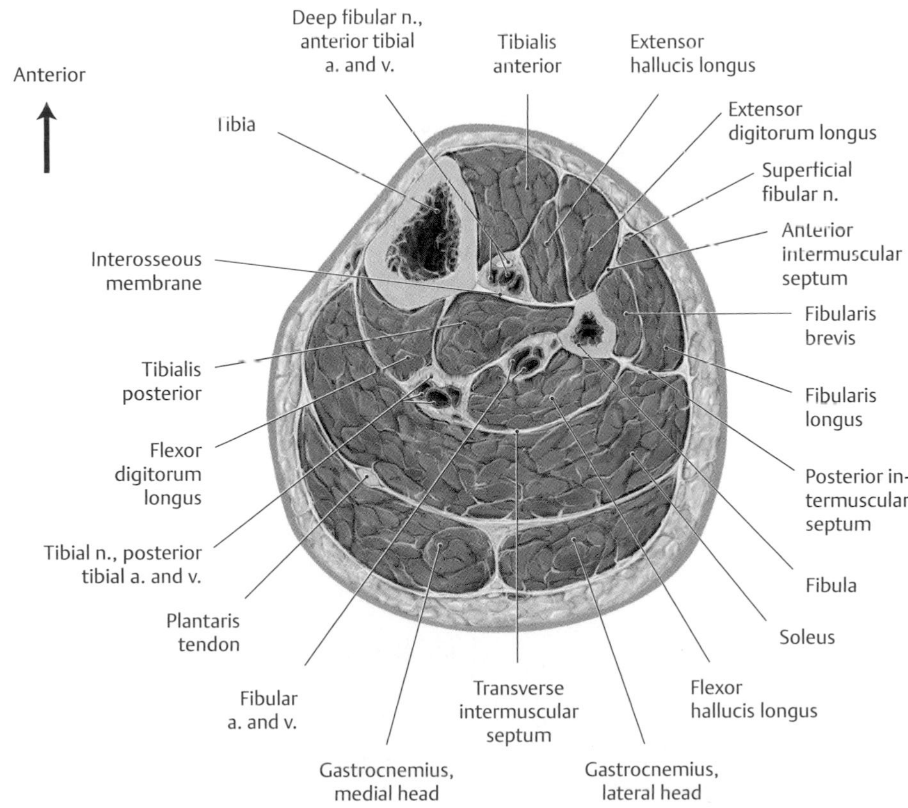
Deep fibular n., anterior tibial a. and v.
Tibialis anterior
Extensor hallucis longus
Anterior
Tibia
Extensor digitorum longus
Superficial fibular n.
Anterior intermuscular septum
Interosseous membrane
Fibularis brevis
Tibialis posterior
Fibularis longus
Flexor digitorum longus
Posterior in-termuscular septum
Tibial n., posterior tibial a. and v.
Fibula
Plantaris tendon
Soleus
Fibular a. and v.
Transverse intermuscular septum
Flexor hallucis longus
Gastrocnemius, medial head
Gastrocnemius, lateral head

B Leg (plane of lower section in Fig. 29.43).

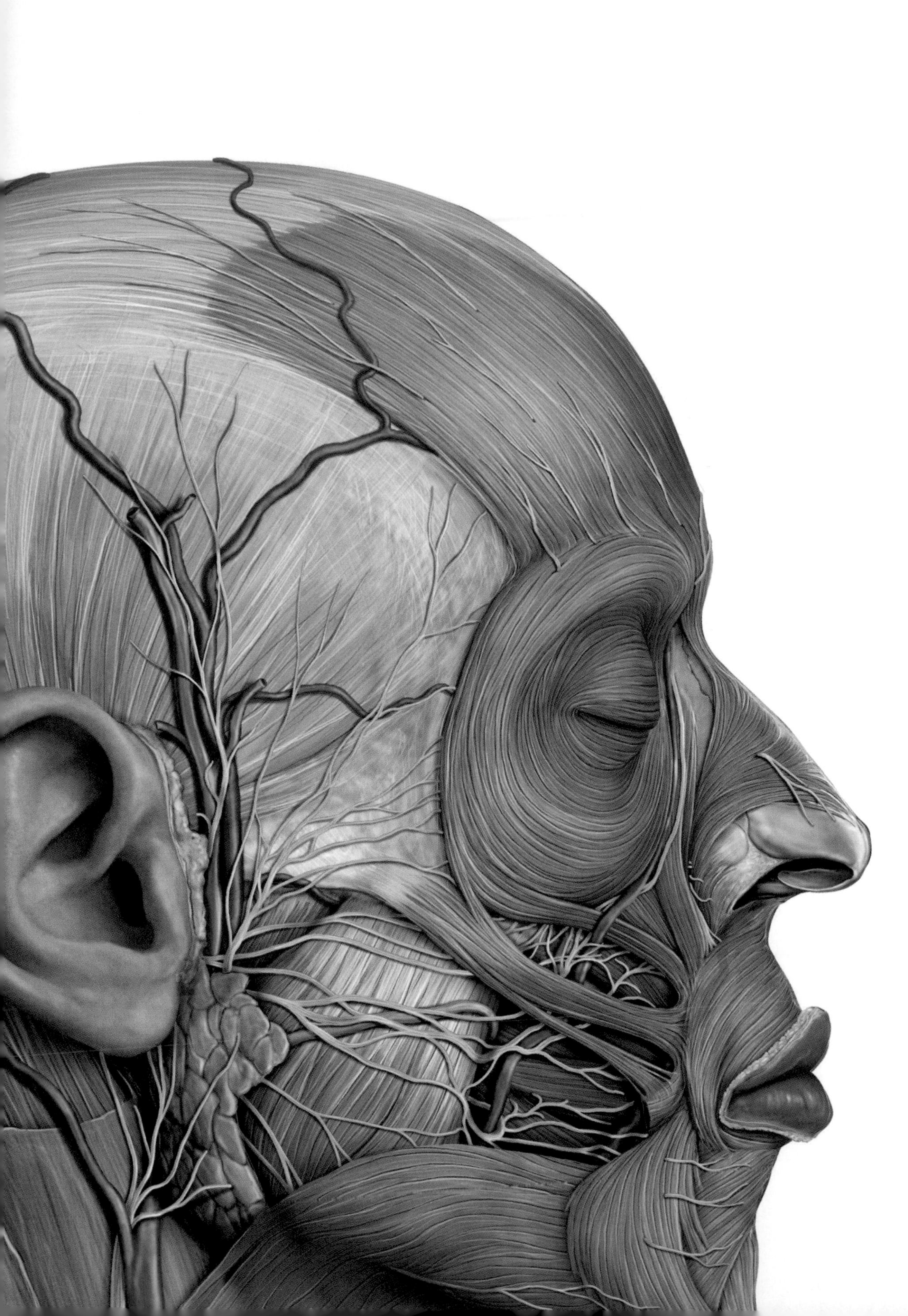

Head & Neck

30 Surface Anatomy

Surface Anatomy 476

31 Bones of the Head

Anterior & Lateral Skull 478
Posterior Skull & Calvaria 480
Base of the Skull 482
Neurovascular Pathways Exiting or Entering the Cranial Cavity 484
Ethmoid & Sphenoid Bones 486

32 Muscles of the Skull & Face

Muscles of Facial Expression & of Mastication 488
Muscle Origins & Insertions on the Skull 490
Muscle Facts (I) 492
Muscle Facts (II) 494

33 Cranial Nerves

Cranial Nerves: Overview 496
CN I & II: Olfactory & Optic Nerves 498
CN III, IV & VI:
Oculomotor, Trochlear & Abducent Nerves 500
CN V: Trigeminal Nerve 502
CN VII: Facial Nerve 504
CN VIII: Vestibulocochlear Nerve 506
CN IX: Glossopharyngeal Nerve 508
CN X: Vagus Nerve 510
CN XI & XII: Accessory & Hypoglossal Nerves 512

34 Neurovasculature of the Skull & Face

Innervation of the Face 514
Arteries of the Head & Neck 516
External Carotid Artery:
Anterior, Medial & Posterior Branches 518
External Carotid Artery: Terminal Branches 520
Veins of the Head & Neck 522
Meninges 524
Dural Sinuses 526
Topography of the Superficial Face 528
Topography of the Parotid Region & Temporal Fossa 530
Topography of the Infratemporal Fossa 532
Topography of the Pterygopalatine Fossa 534

35 Orbit & Eye

Bones of the Orbit 536
Muscles of the Orbit 538
Neurovasculature of the Orbit 540
Topography of the Orbit 542
Orbit & Eyelid 544
Eyeball 546
Cornea, Iris & Lens 548

36 Nasal Cavity & Nose

Bones of the Nasal Cavity 550
Paranasal Air Sinuses 552
Neurovasculature of the Nasal Cavity 554

37 Temporal Bone & Ear

Temporal Bone 556
External Ear & Auditory Canal 558
Middle Ear: Tympanic Cavity 560
Middle Ear: Ossicular Chain & Tympanic Membrane 562
Arteries of the Middle Ear 564
Inner Ear 566

38 Oral Cavity & Pharynx

Bones of the Oral Cavity 568
Temporomandibular Joint 570
Teeth 572
Oral Cavity Muscle Facts 574
Innervation of the Oral Cavity 576
Tongue 578
Topography of the Oral Cavity & Salivary Glands 580
Tonsils & Pharynx 582
Pharyngeal Muscles 584
Neurovasculature of the Pharynx 586

39 Neck

Muscle Facts (I) 588
Muscle Facts (II) 590
Muscle Facts (III) 592
Arteries & Veins of the Neck 594
Innervation of the Neck 596
Larynx: Cartilage & Structure 598
Larynx: Muscles & Levels 600
Neurovasculature of the Larynx, Thyroid & Parathyroids 602
Topography of the Neck: Regions & Fascia 604
Topography of the Anterior Cervical Region 606
Topography of the Anterior & Lateral Cervical Regions 608
Topography of the Lateral Cervical Region 610
Topography of the Posterior Cervical Region 612
Lymphatics of the Neck 614
Coronal Sections of the Head 616
Transverse Sections of the Head & Neck 618
Sagittal Sections of the Head 620

Surface Anatomy

Fig. 30.1 Regions of the head and neck

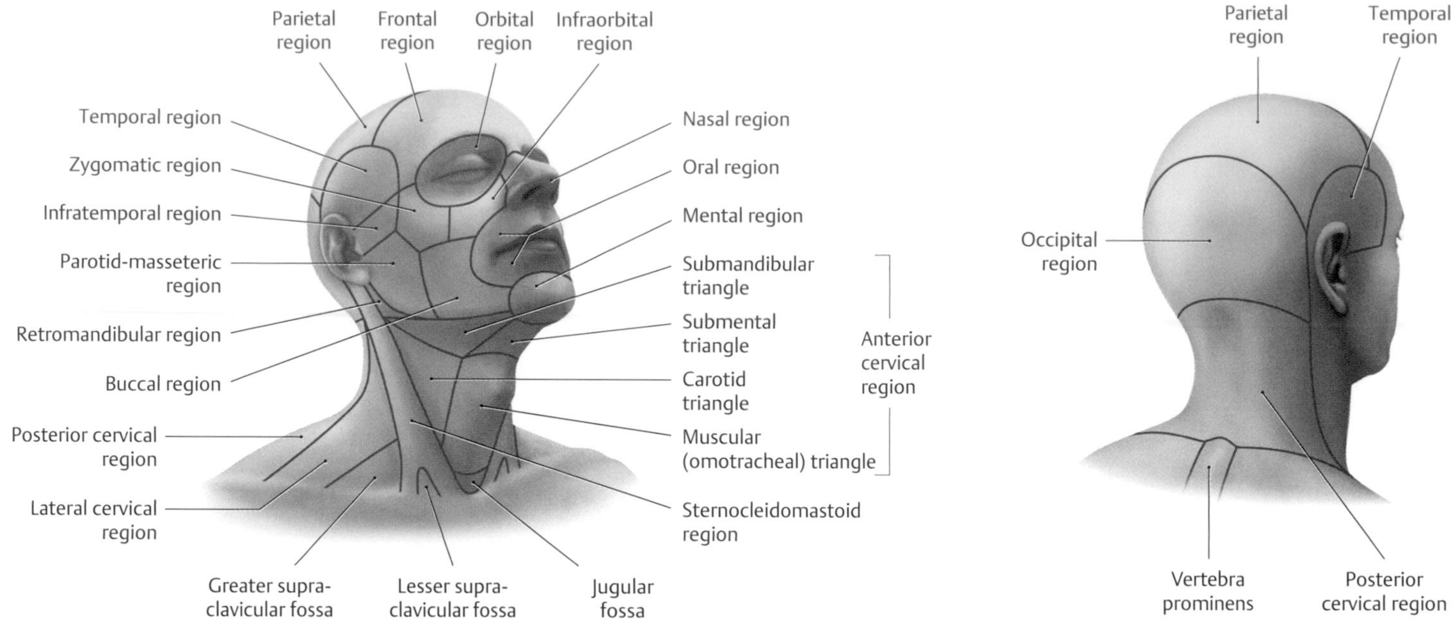
Parietal region
Frontal region
Orbital region
Infraorbital region
Temporal region
Zygomatic region
Infratemporal region
Parotid-masseteric region
Retromandibular region
Buccal region
Posterior cervical region
Lateral cervical region
Greater supra-clavicular fossa
Lesser supra-clavicular fossa
Jugular fossa
Nasal region
Oral region
Mental region
Submandibular triangle
Submental triangle
Carotid triangle
Muscular (omotracheal) triangle
Anterior cervical region
Sternocleidomastoid region
Parietal region
Temporal region
Occipital region
Vertebra prominens
Posterior cervical region

A Right anterolateral view.

B Right posterolateral view.

Fig. 30.2 Surface anatomy of the head and neck

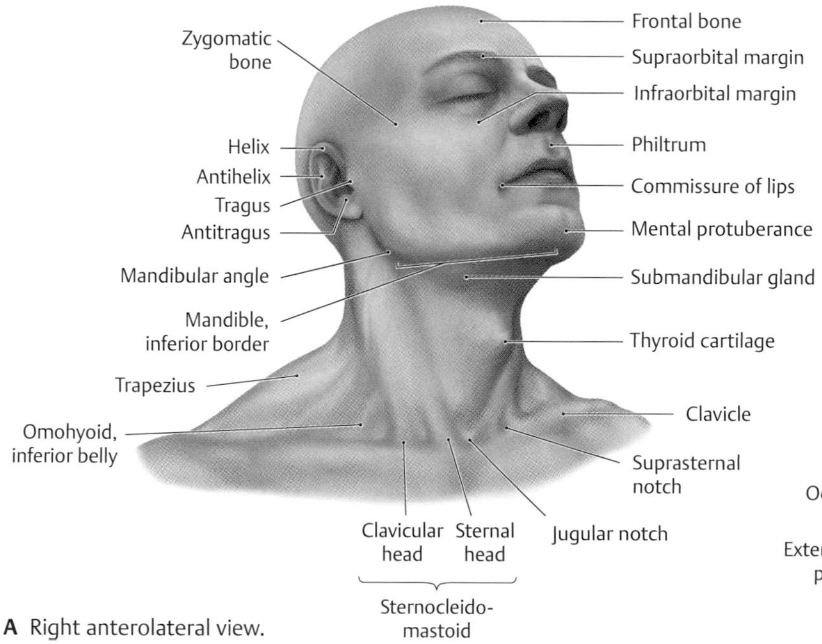

Zygomatic bone
Helix
Antihelix
Tragus
Antitragus
Mandibular angle
Mandible, inferior border
Trapezius
Omohyoid, inferior belly
Frontal bone
Supraorbital margin
Infraorbital margin
Philtrum
Commissure of lips
Mental protuberance
Submandibular gland
Thyroid cartilage
Clavicle
Suprasternal notch
Jugular notch
Clavicular head
Sternal head
Sternocleido-mastoid

A Right anterolateral view.

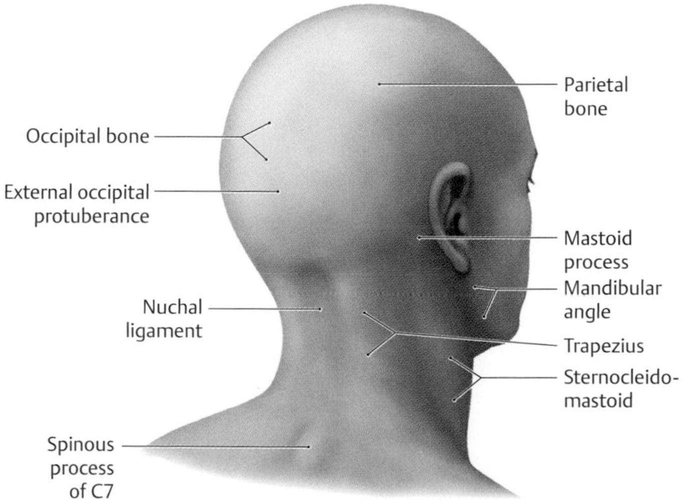

Occipital bone
External occipital protuberance
Nuchal ligament
Spinous process of C7
Parietal bone
Mastoid process
Mandibular angle
Trapezius
Sternocleido-mastoid

B Right posterolateral view.

Fig. 30.3 **Palpable bony prominences of the head and neck**

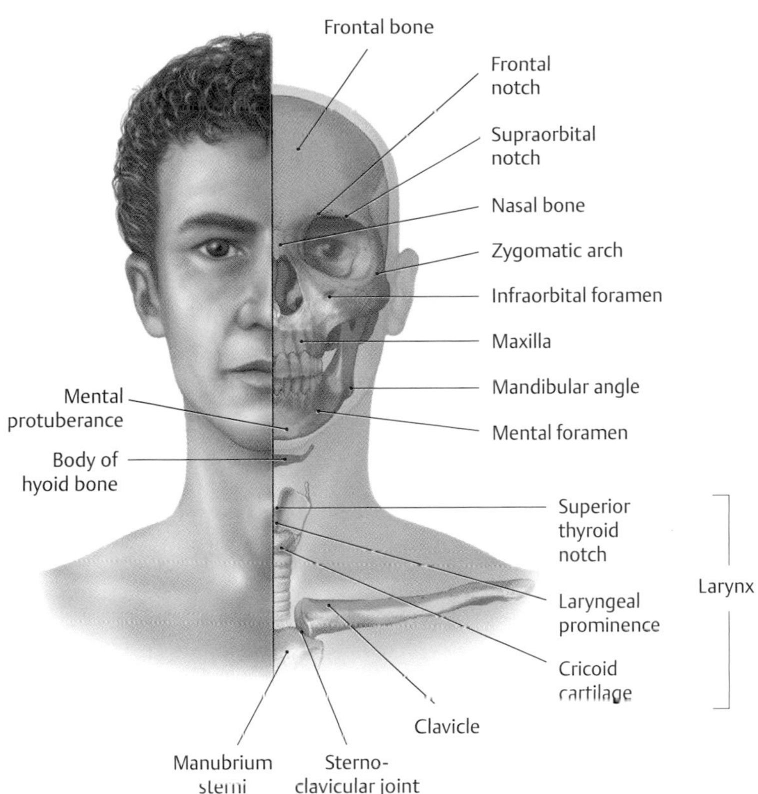
Frontal bone
Frontal notch
Supraorbital notch
Nasal bone
Zygomatic arch
Infraorbital foramen
Maxilla
Mandibular angle
Mental foramen
Mental protuberance
Body of hyoid bone
Superior thyroid notch
Laryngeal prominence
Cricoid cartilage
Larynx
Clavicle
Manubrium sterni
Sterno-clavicular joint

A Anterior view.

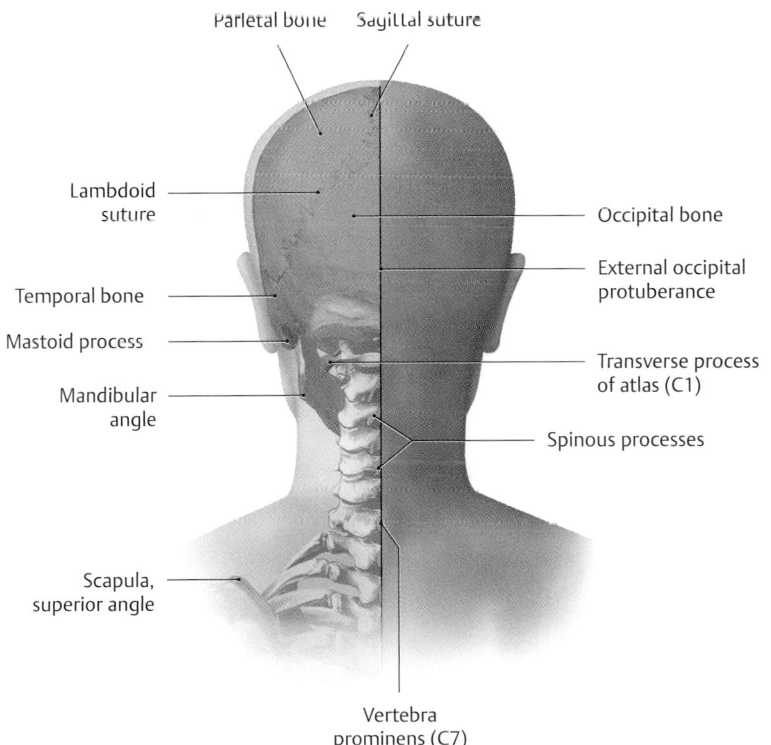
Parietal bone
Sagittal suture
Lambdoid suture
Occipital bone
External occipital protuberance
Temporal bone
Mastoid process
Transverse process of atlas (C1)
Mandibular angle
Spinous processes
Scapula, superior angle
Vertebra prominens (C7)

B Posterior view.

Anterior & Lateral Skull

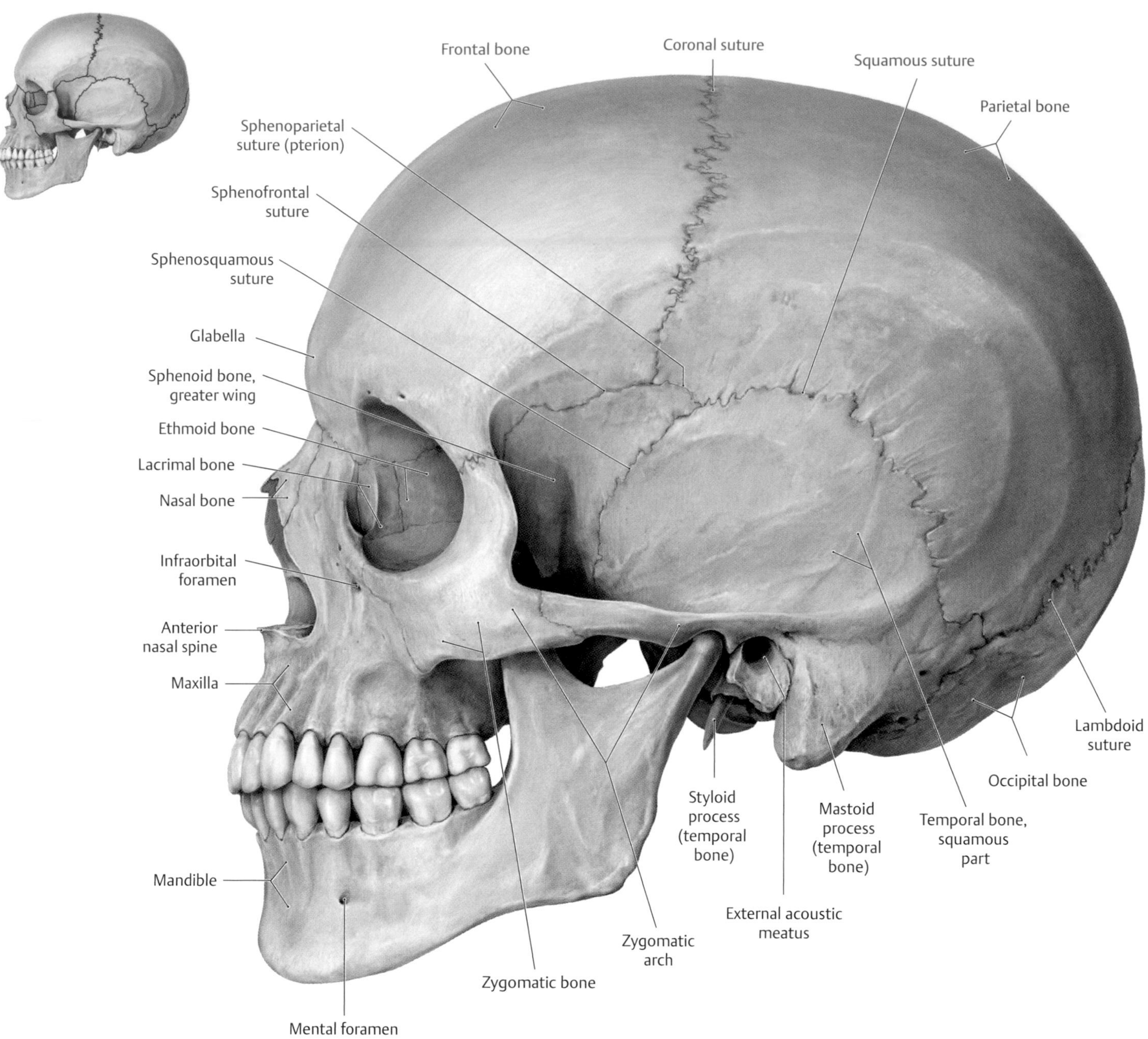

Frontal bone
Coronal suture
Squamous suture
Parietal bone
Sphenoparietal suture (pterion)
Sphenofrontal suture
Sphenosquamous suture
Glabella
Sphenoid bone, greater wing
Ethmoid bone
Lacrimal bone
Nasal bone
Infraorbital foramen
Anterior nasal spine
Maxilla
Mandible
Mental foramen
Zygomatic bone
Zygomatic arch
External acoustic meatus
Styloid process (temporal bone)
Mastoid process (temporal bone)
Temporal bone, squamous part
Occipital bone
Lambdoid suture

Fig. 31.1 **Lateral skull**
Left lateral view.

Table 31.1 Bones of the skull

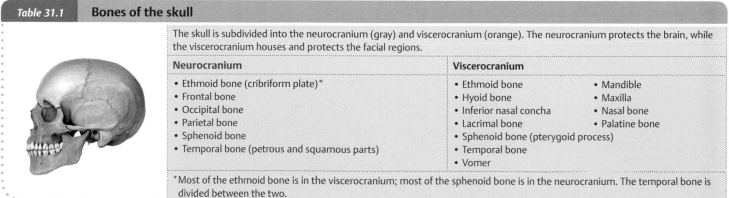

The skull is subdivided into the neurocranium (gray) and viscerocranium (orange). The neurocranium protects the brain, while the viscerocranium houses and protects the facial regions.

Neurocranium	Viscerocranium	
• Ethmoid bone (cribriform plate)*	• Ethmoid bone	• Mandible
• Frontal bone	• Hyoid bone	• Maxilla
• Occipital bone	• Inferior nasal concha	• Nasal bone
• Parietal bone	• Lacrimal bone	• Palatine bone
• Sphenoid bone	• Sphenoid bone (pterygoid process)	
• Temporal bone (petrous and squamous parts)	• Temporal bone	
	• Vomer	

*Most of the ethmoid bone is in the viscerocranium; most of the sphenoid bone is in the neurocranium. The temporal bone is divided between the two.

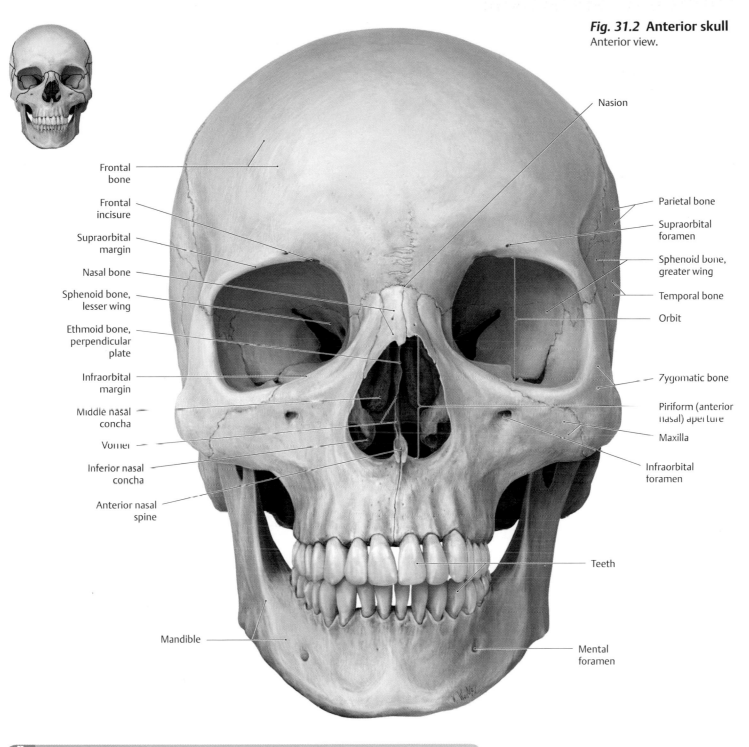

Fig. 31.2 Anterior skull
Anterior view.

Nasion
Frontal bone
Frontal incisure
Supraorbital margin
Nasal bone
Sphenoid bone, lesser wing
Ethmoid bone, perpendicular plate
Infraorbital margin
Middle nasal concha
Vomer
Inferior nasal concha
Anterior nasal spine
Parietal bone
Supraorbital foramen
Sphenoid bone, greater wing
Temporal bone
Orbit
Zygomatic bone
Piriform (anterior nasal) aperture
Maxilla
Infraorbital foramen
Teeth
Mandible
Mental foramen

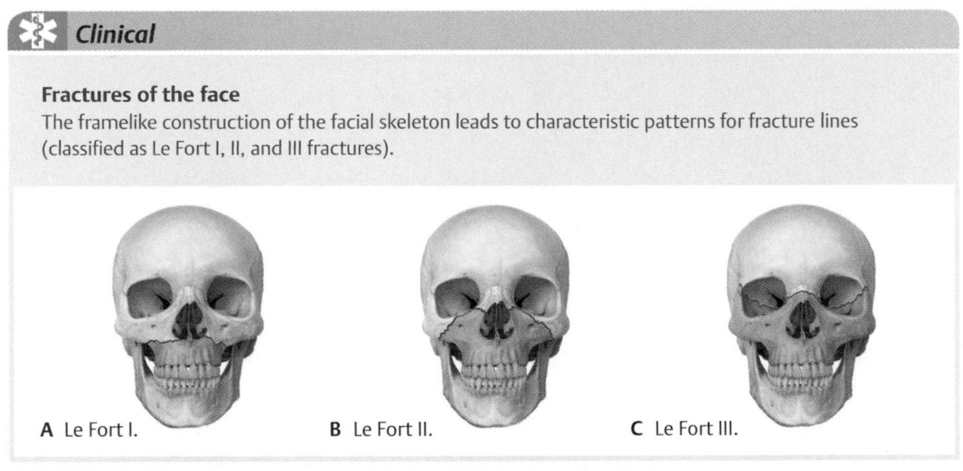

Clinical

Fractures of the face

The framelike construction of the facial skeleton leads to characteristic patterns for fracture lines (classified as Le Fort I, II, and III fractures).

A Le Fort I. **B** Le Fort II. **C** Le Fort III.

Posterior Skull & Calvaria

Fig. 31.3 **Posterior skull**
Posterior view.

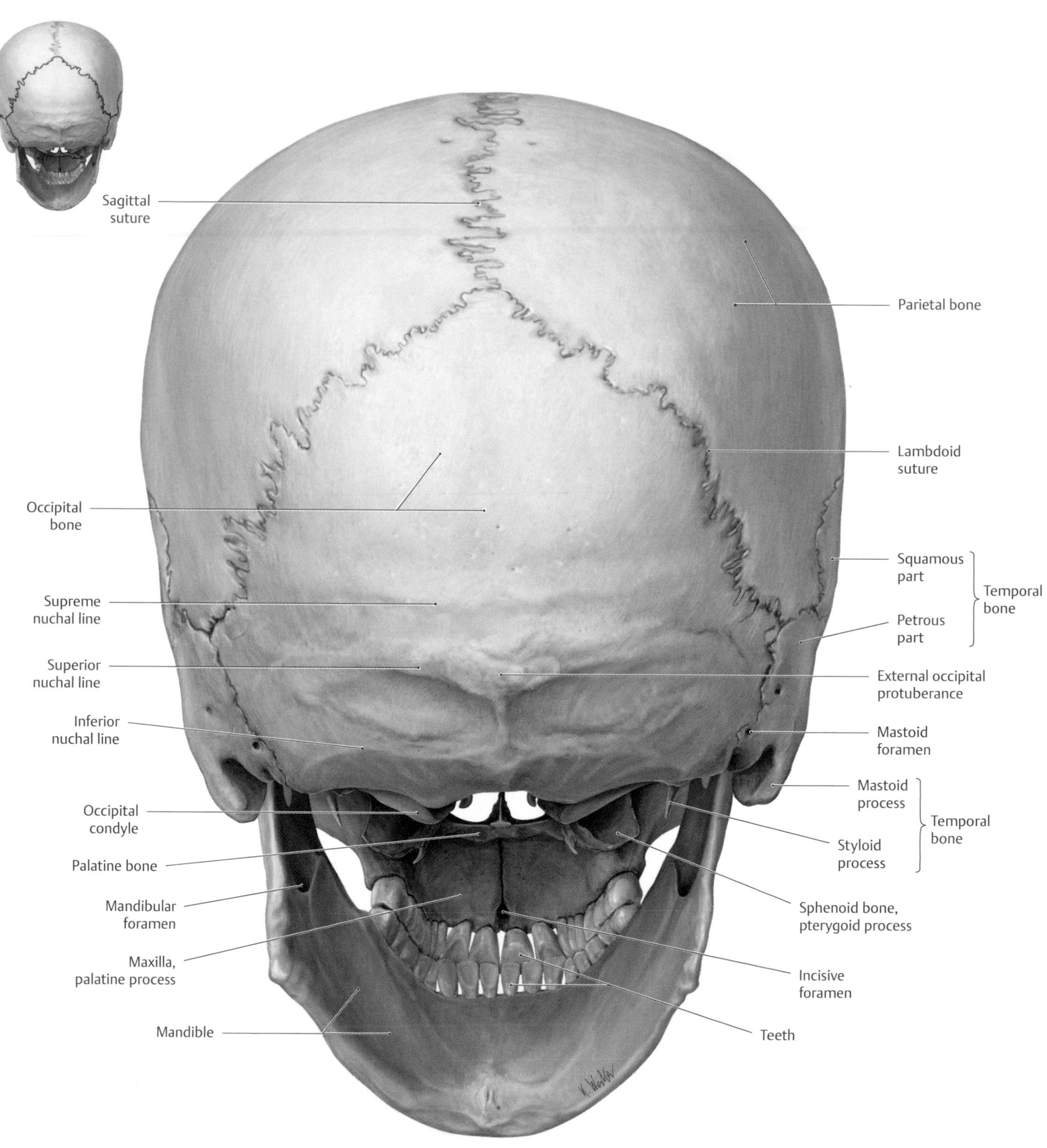
Sagittal suture
Parietal bone
Lambdoid suture
Occipital bone
Squamous part
Petrous part
Temporal bone
Supreme nuchal line
Superior nuchal line
External occipital protuberance
Inferior nuchal line
Mastoid foramen
Mastoid process
Temporal bone
Occipital condyle
Styloid process
Palatine bone
Mandibular foramen
Sphenoid bone, pterygoid process
Maxilla, palatine process
Incisive foramen
Mandible
Teeth

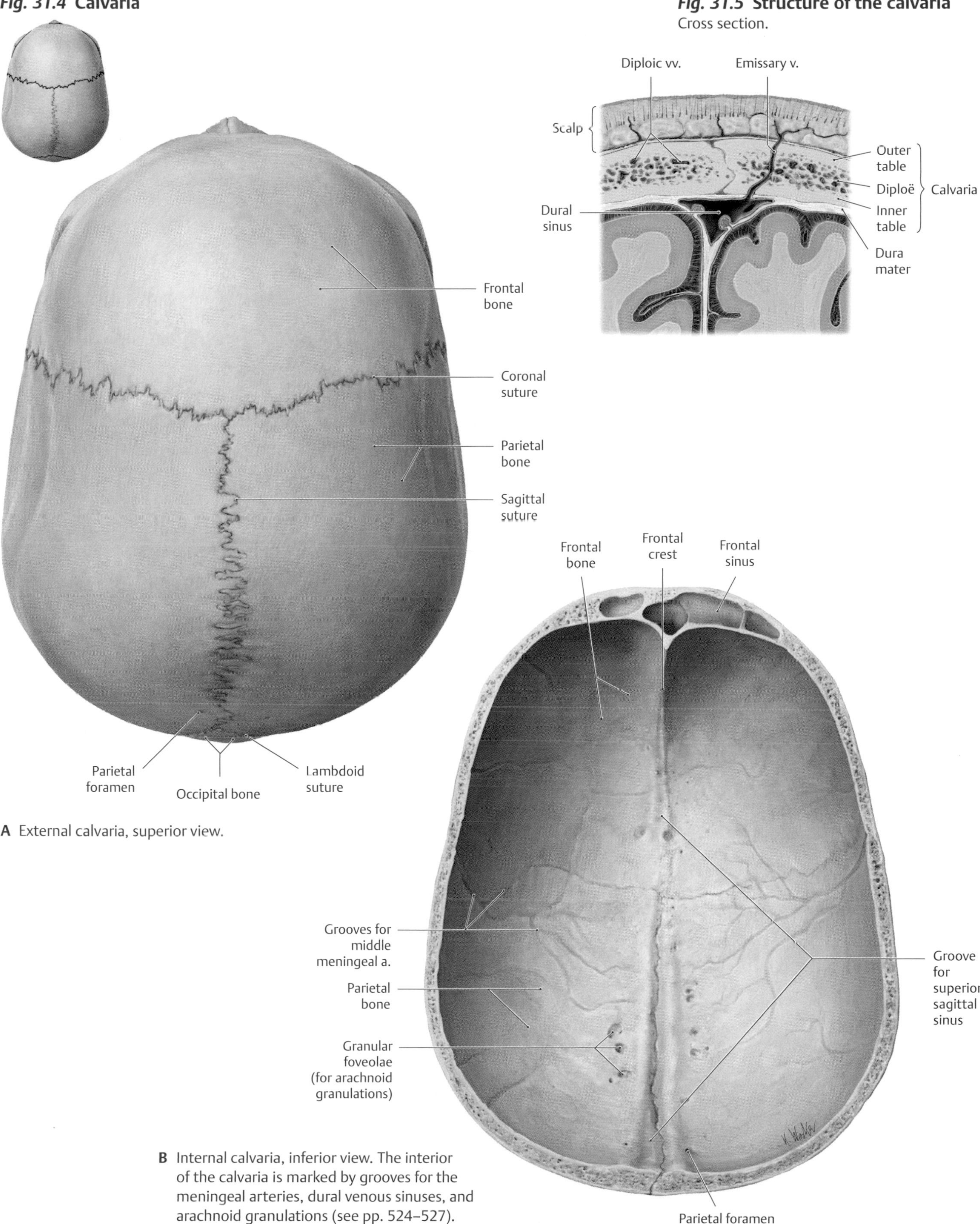

Fig. 31.4 Calvaria
Frontal bone
Coronal suture
Parietal bone
Sagittal suture
Parietal foramen
Occipital bone
Lambdoid suture
Fig. 31.5 Structure of the calvaria
Cross section.
Diploic vv.
Emissary v.
Scalp
Outer table
Diploë
Calvaria
Inner table
Dural sinus
Dura mater
Frontal bone
Frontal crest
Frontal sinus
Grooves for middle meningeal a.
Parietal bone
Granular foveolae (for arachnoid granulations)
Groove for superior sagittal sinus
Parietal foramen

A External calvaria, superior view.

B Internal calvaria, inferior view. The interior of the calvaria is marked by grooves for the meningeal arteries, dural venous sinuses, and arachnoid granulations (see pp. 524–527).

Base of the Skull

Fig. 31.6 Base of the skull: Exterior
Inferior view. *Revealed:* Foramina and canals for blood vessels (see p. 516) and cranial nerves. *Note:* This view allows visual access into the posterior region of the nasal cavity.

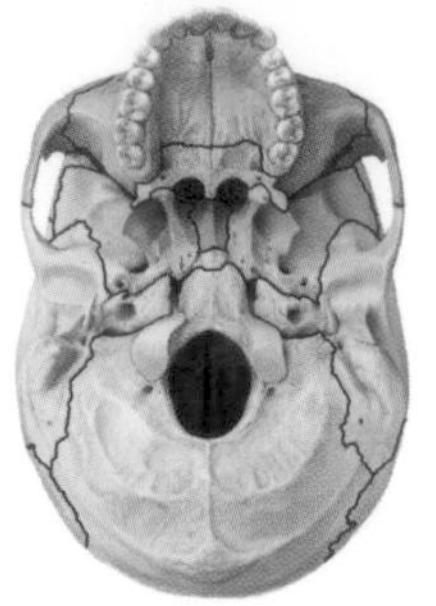

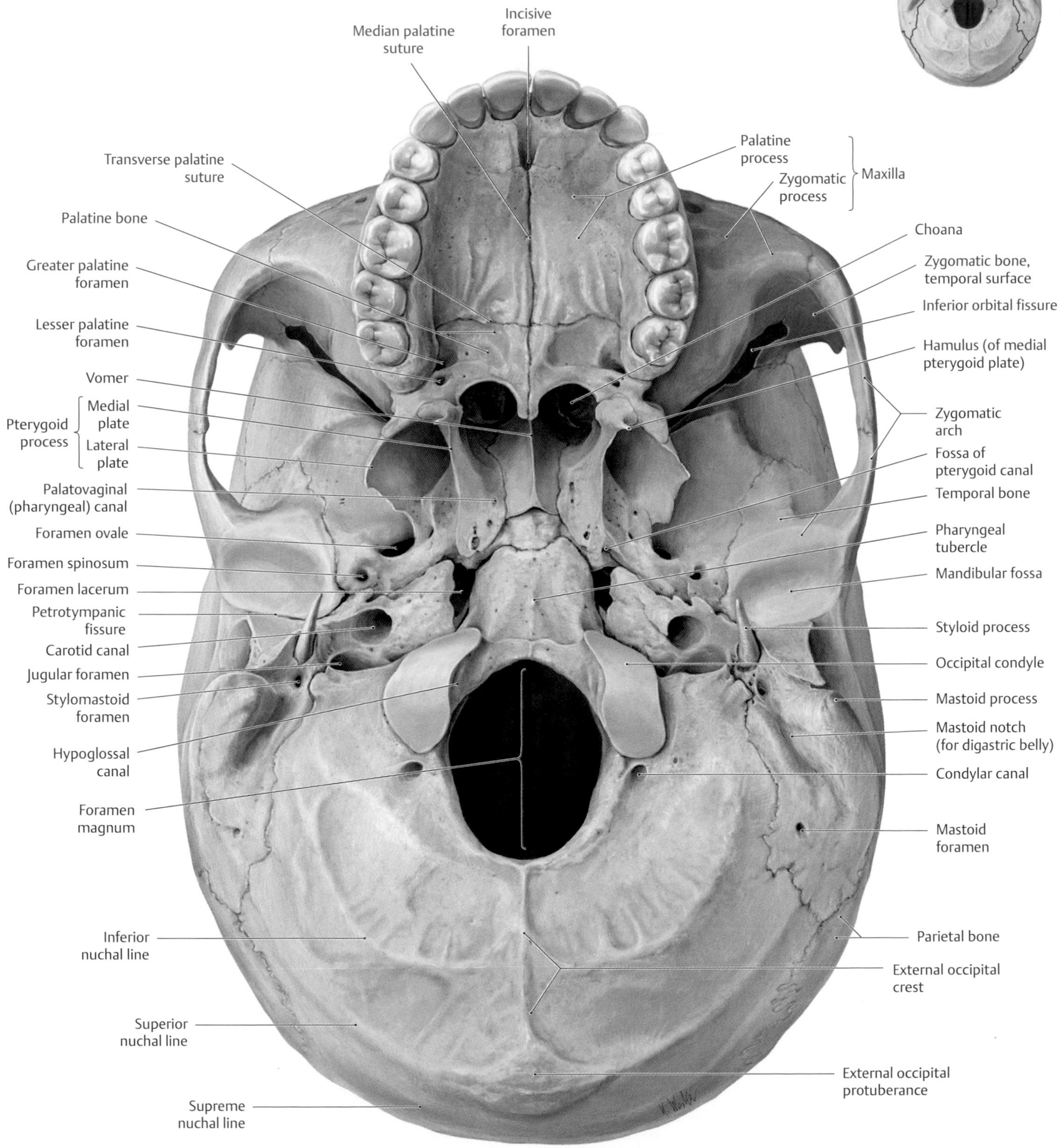

Median palatine suture
Incisive foramen
Transverse palatine suture
Palatine bone
Greater palatine foramen
Lesser palatine foramen
Vomer
Pterygoid process
Medial plate
Lateral plate
Palatovaginal (pharyngeal) canal
Foramen ovale
Foramen spinosum
Foramen lacerum
Petrotympanic fissure
Carotid canal
Jugular foramen
Stylomastoid foramen
Hypoglossal canal
Foramen magnum
Inferior nuchal line
Superior nuchal line
Supreme nuchal line
Palatine process
Zygomatic process
Maxilla
Choana
Zygomatic bone, temporal surface
Inferior orbital fissure
Hamulus (of medial pterygoid plate)
Zygomatic arch
Fossa of pterygoid canal
Temporal bone
Pharyngeal tubercle
Mandibular fossa
Styloid process
Occipital condyle
Mastoid process
Mastoid notch (for digastric belly)
Condylar canal
Mastoid foramen
Parietal bone
External occipital crest
External occipital protuberance

Fig. 31.7 **Cranial fossae**
The interior of the skull base consists of three successive fossae that become progressively deeper in the frontal-to-occipital direction.

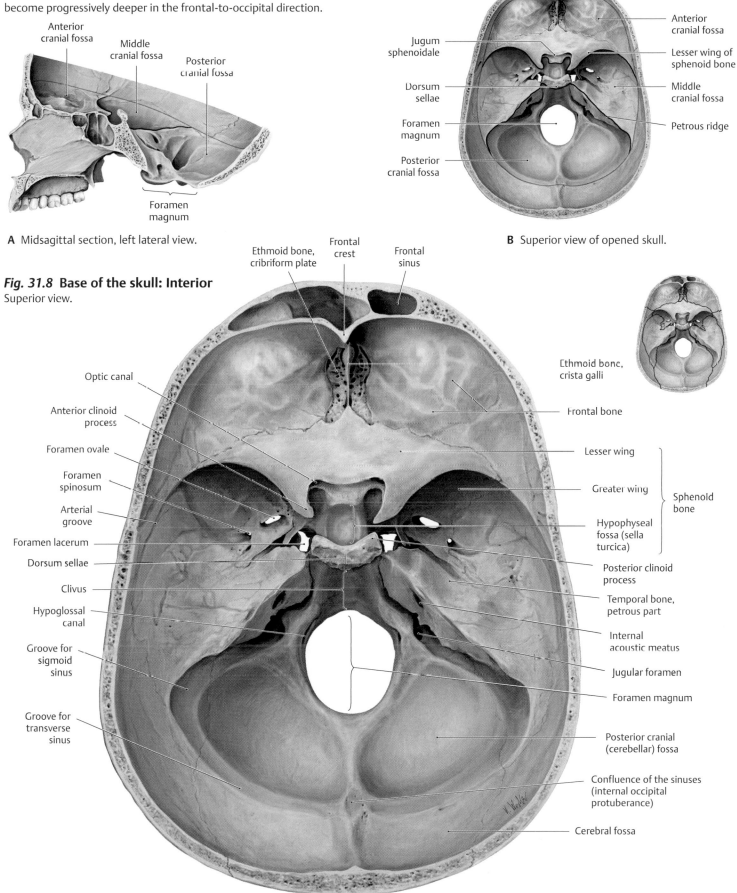

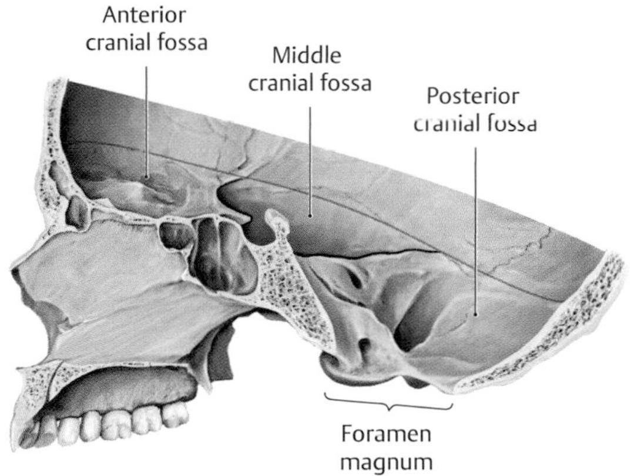
Anterior cranial fossa
Middle cranial fossa
Posterior cranial fossa
Foramen magnum

A Midsagittal section, left lateral view.

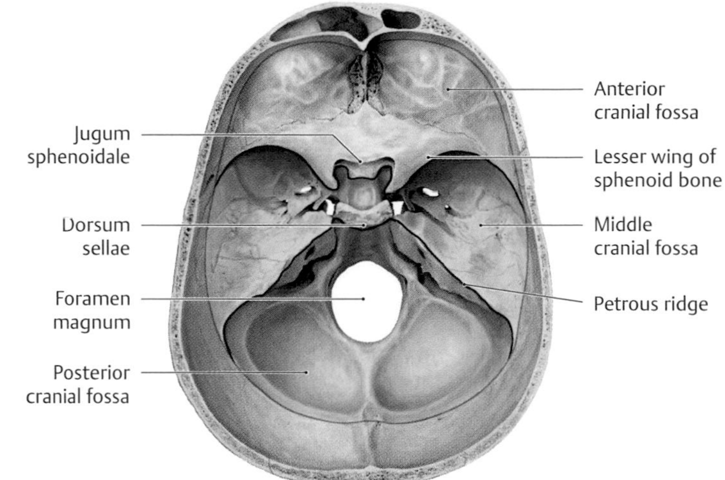
Jugum sphenoidale
Dorsum sellae
Foramen magnum
Posterior cranial fossa
Anterior cranial fossa
Lesser wing of sphenoid bone
Middle cranial fossa
Petrous ridge

B Superior view of opened skull.

Fig. 31.8 **Base of the skull: Interior**
Superior view.

Ethmoid bone, cribriform plate
Frontal crest
Frontal sinus
Ethmoid bone, crista galli
Optic canal
Anterior clinoid process
Foramen ovale
Foramen spinosum
Arterial groove
Foramen lacerum
Dorsum sellae
Clivus
Hypoglossal canal
Groove for sigmoid sinus
Groove for transverse sinus
Frontal bone
Lesser wing
Greater wing
Hypophyseal fossa (sella turcica)
Sphenoid bone
Posterior clinoid process
Temporal bone, petrous part
Internal acoustic meatus
Jugular foramen
Foramen magnum
Posterior cranial (cerebellar) fossa
Confluence of the sinuses (internal occipital protuberance)
Cerebral fossa

Neurovascular Pathways Exiting or Entering the Cranial Cavity

Fig. 31.9 **Summary of the neurovascular structures exiting or entering the cranial cavity**

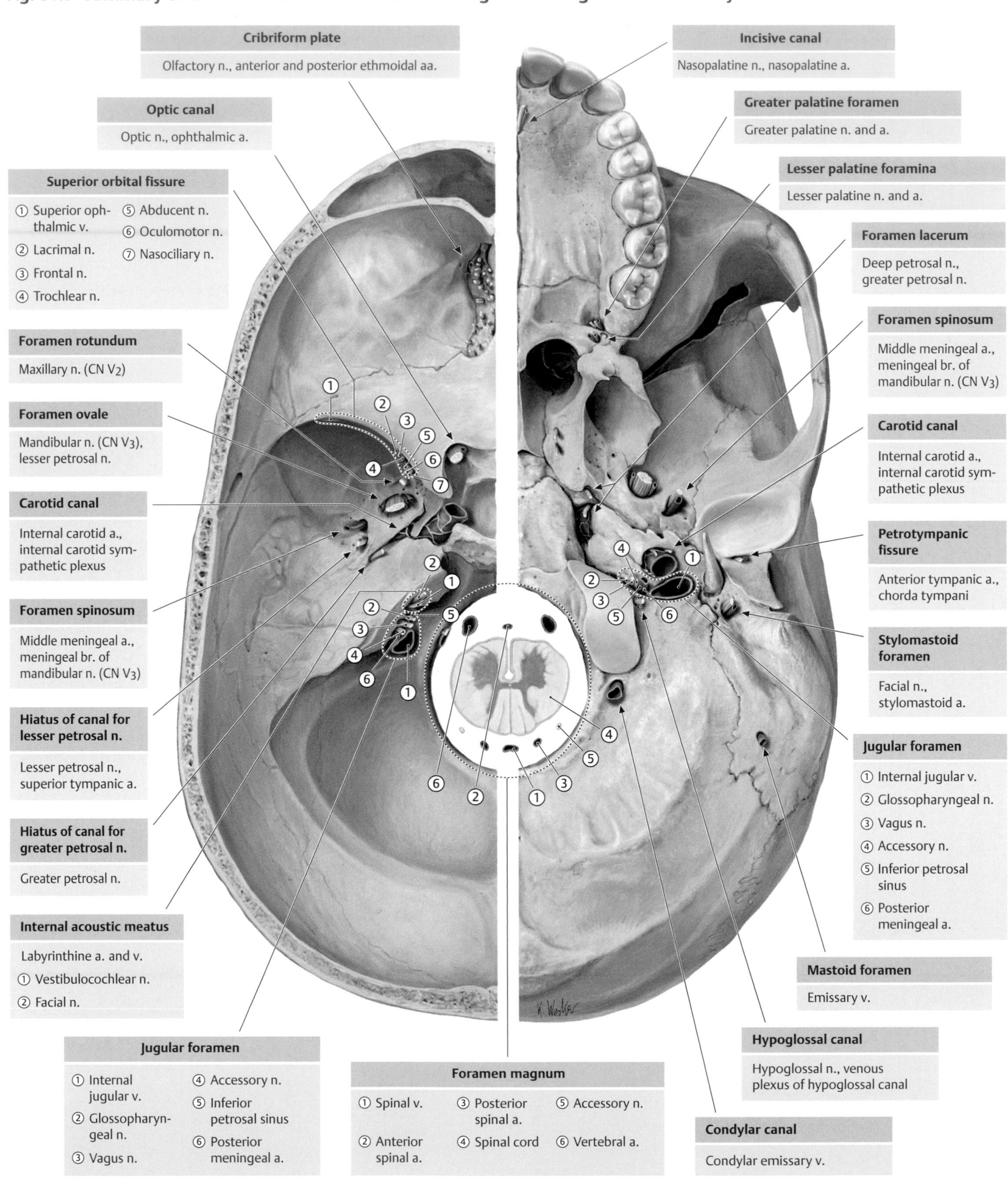
Cribriform plate
Olfactory n., anterior and posterior ethmoidal aa.
Optic canal
Optic n., ophthalmic a.
Superior orbital fissure
① Superior ophthalmic v.
② Lacrimal n.
③ Frontal n.
④ Trochlear n.
⑤ Abducent n.
⑥ Oculomotor n.
⑦ Nasociliary n.
Foramen rotundum
Maxillary n. (CN V2)
Foramen ovale
Mandibular n. (CN V3), lesser petrosal n.
Carotid canal
Internal carotid a., internal carotid sympathetic plexus
Foramen spinosum
Middle meningeal a., meningeal br. of mandibular n. (CN V3)
Hiatus of canal for lesser petrosal n.
Lesser petrosal n., superior tympanic a.
Hiatus of canal for greater petrosal n.
Greater petrosal n.
Internal acoustic meatus
Labyrinthine a. and v.
① Vestibulocochlear n.
② Facial n.
Jugular foramen
① Internal jugular v.
② Glossopharyngeal n.
③ Vagus n.
④ Accessory n.
⑤ Inferior petrosal sinus
⑥ Posterior meningeal a.
Foramen magnum
① Spinal v.
② Anterior spinal a.
③ Posterior spinal a.
④ Spinal cord
⑤ Accessory n.
⑥ Vertebral a.
Incisive canal
Nasopalatine n., nasopalatine a.
Greater palatine foramen
Greater palatine n. and a.
Lesser palatine foramina
Lesser palatine n. and a.
Foramen lacerum
Deep petrosal n., greater petrosal n.
Foramen spinosum
Middle meningeal a., meningeal br. of mandibular n. (CN V3)
Carotid canal
Internal carotid a., internal carotid sympathetic plexus
Petrotympanic fissure
Anterior tympanic a., chorda tympani
Stylomastoid foramen
Facial n., stylomastoid a.
Jugular foramen
① Internal jugular v.
② Glossopharyngeal n.
③ Vagus n.
④ Accessory n.
⑤ Inferior petrosal sinus
⑥ Posterior meningeal a.
Mastoid foramen
Emissary v.
Hypoglossal canal
Hypoglossal n., venous plexus of hypoglossal canal
Condylar canal
Condylar emissary v.

A Cranial cavity (interior of skull base), left side, superior view.

B Exterior of skull base, left side, inferior view

Fig. 31.10 **Cranial nerves exiting the cranial cavity**
Cranial cavity (interior of skull base), left side, superior view. *Removed:* Brain and tentorium cerebelli. The ends of the cranial nerves have been cut to reveal the fissures, fossa, or dural cave where they pass through the cranial fossa.

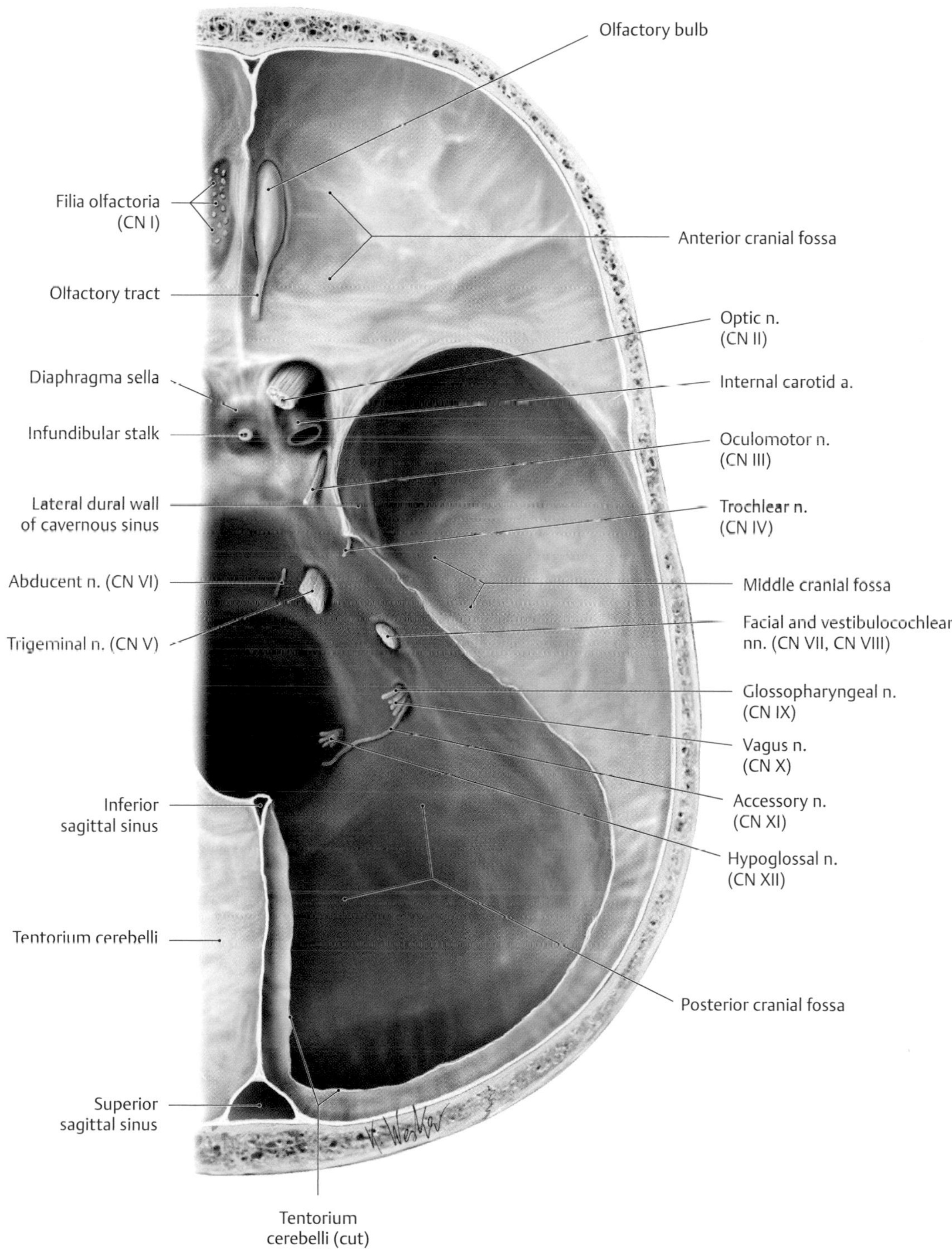
Olfactory bulb
Filia olfactoria (CN I)
Anterior cranial fossa
Olfactory tract
Optic n. (CN II)
Diaphragma sella
Internal carotid a.
Infundibular stalk
Oculomotor n. (CN III)
Lateral dural wall of cavernous sinus
Trochlear n. (CN IV)
Abducent n. (CN VI)
Middle cranial fossa
Trigeminal n. (CN V)
Facial and vestibulocochlear nn. (CN VII, CN VIII)
Glossopharyngeal n. (CN IX)
Vagus n. (CN X)
Accessory n. (CN XI)
Inferior sagittal sinus
Hypoglossal n. (CN XII)
Tentorium cerebelli
Posterior cranial fossa
Superior sagittal sinus
Tentorium cerebelli (cut)

Ethmoid & Sphenoid Bones

The structurally complex ethmoid and sphenoid bones are shown here in isolation. The other bones of the skull are shown in their respective regions: orbit (see pp. 536–537), nasal cavity (see pp. 550–551), oral cavity (see pp. 568–569), and ear (see pp. 556–557).

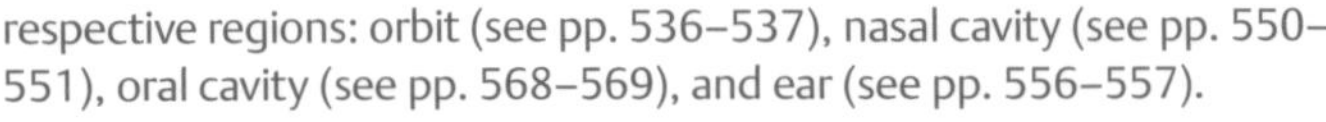

Fig. 31.11 Ethmoid bone

The ethmoid bone is the central bone of the nose and paranasal air sinuses (see pp. 550–553).

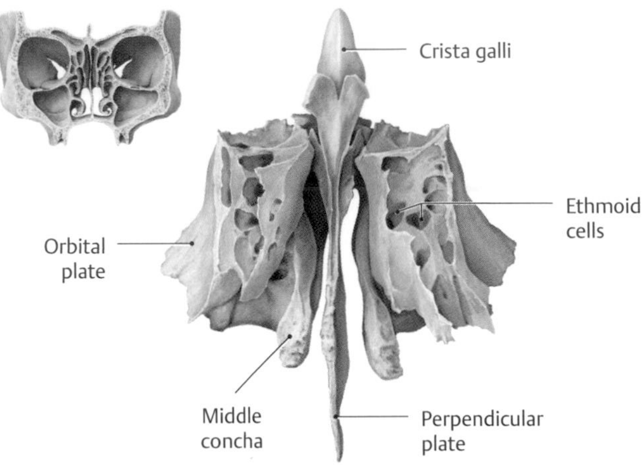
Crista galli
Ethmoid cells
Orbital plate
Middle concha
Perpendicular plate

A Anterior view.

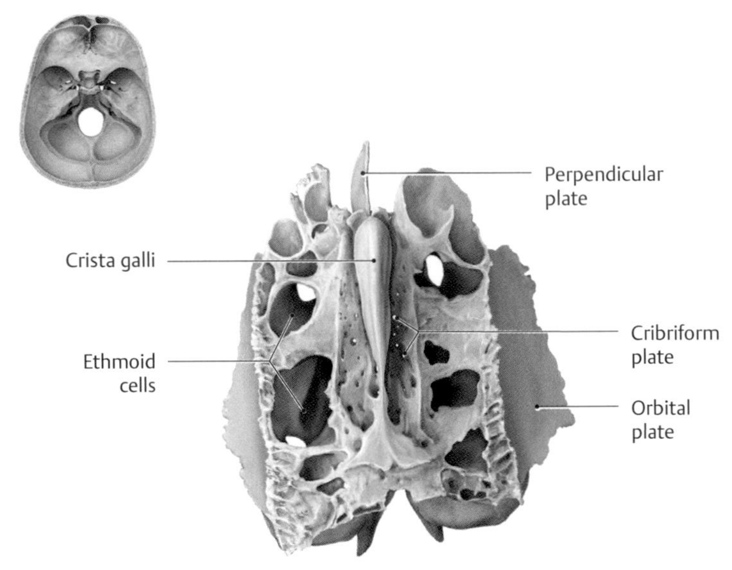
Perpendicular plate
Crista galli
Ethmoid cells
Cribriform plate
Orbital plate

B Superior view.

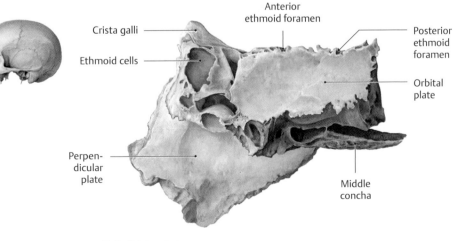

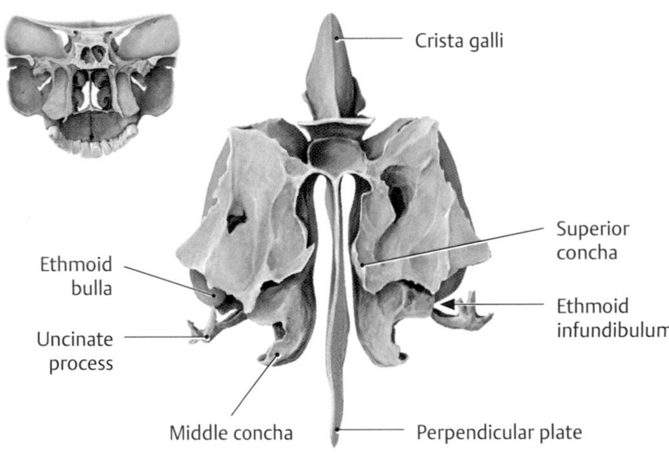
Crista galli
Ethmoid bulla
Uncinate process
Middle concha
Superior concha
Ethmoid infundibulum
Perpendicular plate

C Posterior view.

Crista galli
Ethmoid cells
Anterior ethmoid foramen
Posterior ethmoid foramen
Orbital plate
Perpen-dicular plate
Middle concha

D Left lateral view.

Fig. 31.12 Sphenoid bone

The sphenoid bone is the most structurally complex bone in the human body.

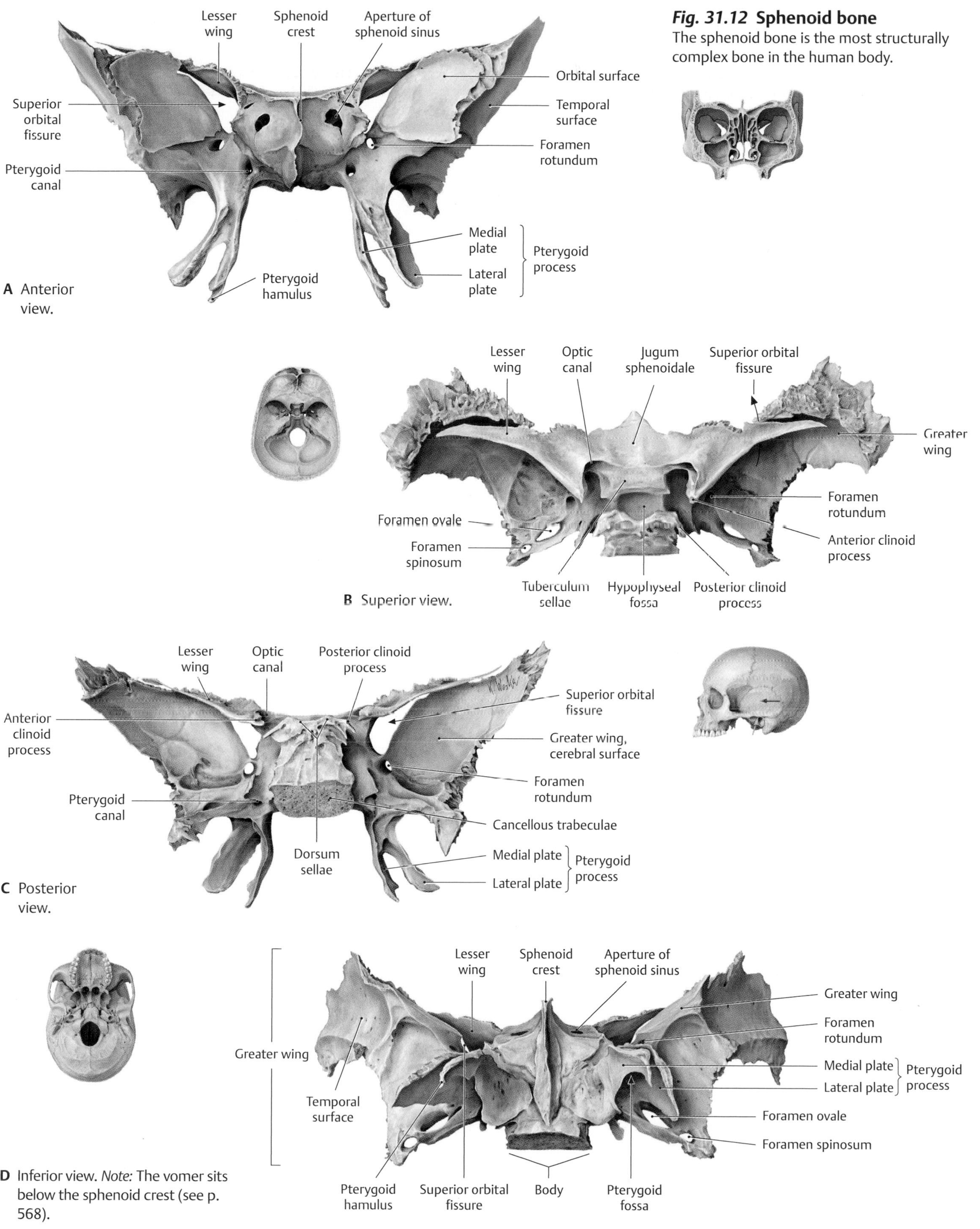

Lesser wing
Sphenoid crest
Aperture of sphenoid sinus
Orbital surface
Superior orbital fissure
Temporal surface
Foramen rotundum
Pterygoid canal
Medial plate
Lateral plate
Pterygoid process
Pterygoid hamulus
Lesser wing
Optic canal
Jugum sphenoidale
Superior orbital fissure
Greater wing
Foramen rotundum
Anterior clinoid process
Foramen ovale
Foramen spinosum
Tuberculum sellae
Hypophyseal fossa
Posterior clinoid process
Lesser wing
Optic canal
Posterior clinoid process
Anterior clinoid process
Superior orbital fissure
Greater wing, cerebral surface
Foramen rotundum
Pterygoid canal
Cancellous trabeculae
Dorsum sellae
Medial plate
Lateral plate
Pterygoid process
Lesser wing
Sphenoid crest
Aperture of sphenoid sinus
Greater wing
Foramen rotundum
Greater wing
Medial plate
Lateral plate
Pterygoid process
Temporal surface
Foramen ovale
Foramen spinosum
Pterygoid hamulus
Superior orbital fissure
Body
Pterygoid fossa

A Anterior view.

B Superior view.

C Posterior view.

D Inferior view. *Note:* The vomer sits below the sphenoid crest (see p. 568).

Muscles of Facial Expression & of Mastication

The muscles of the skull and face are divided into two groups. The muscles of facial expression make up the superficial muscle layer in the face. The muscles of mastication are responsible for the movement of the mandible during mastication (chewing).

Fig. 32.1 Muscles of facial expression

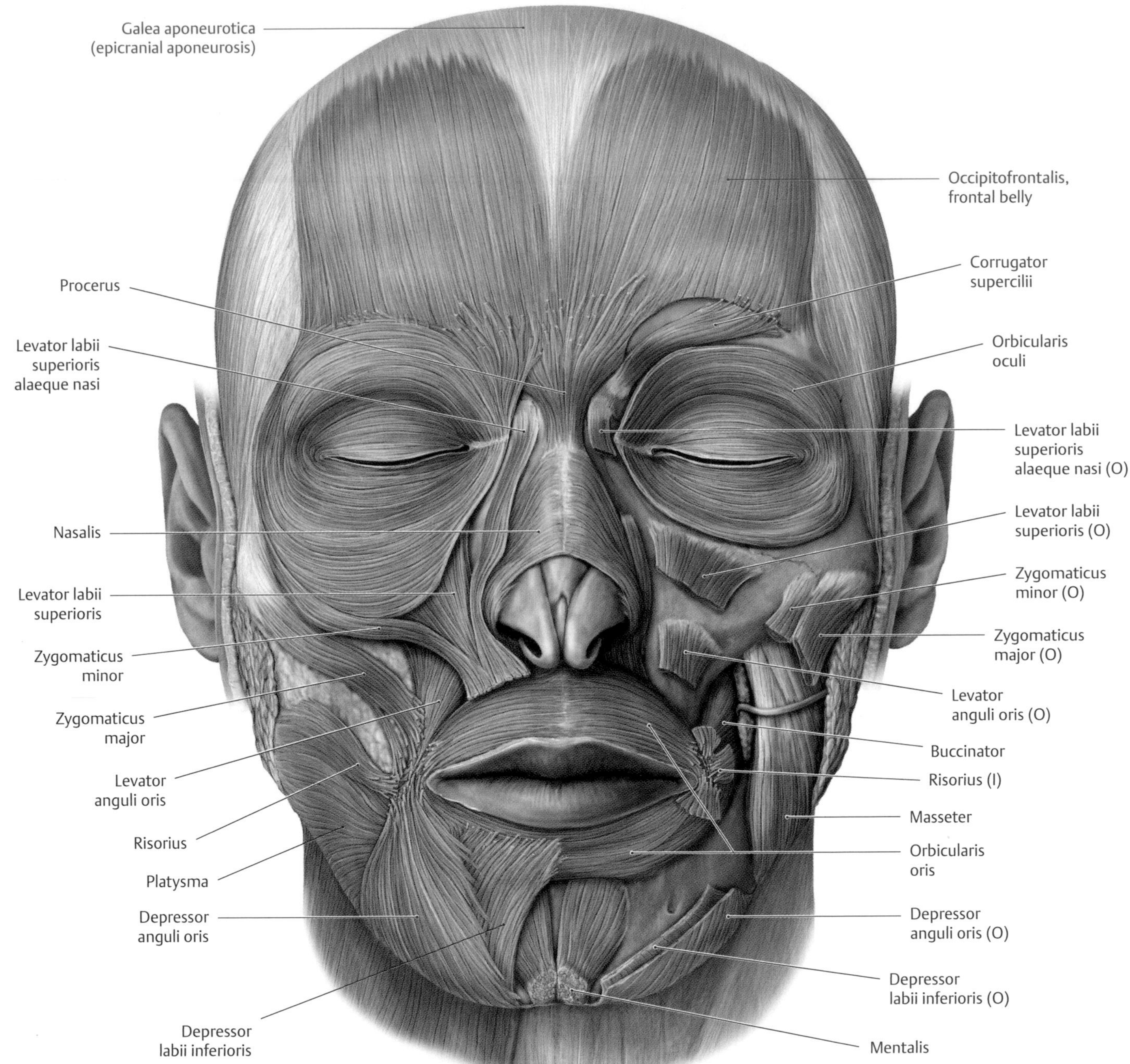

Galea aponeurotica
(epicranial aponeurosis)
Occipitofrontalis,
frontal belly
Procerus
Corrugator
supercilii
Levator labii
superioris
alaeque nasi
Orbicularis
oculi
Levator labii
superioris
alaeque nasi (O)
Nasalis
Levator labii
superioris (O)
Levator labii
superioris
Zygomaticus
minor (O)
Zygomaticus
minor
Zygomaticus
major (O)
Zygomaticus
major
Levator
anguli oris (O)
Buccinator
Levator
anguli oris
Risorius (I)
Masseter
Risorius
Orbicularis
oris
Platysma
Depressor
anguli oris
Depressor
anguli oris (O)
Depressor
labii inferioris (O)
Depressor
labii inferioris
Mentalis

A Anterior view. Muscle origins (O) and insertions (I) indicated on left side of face.

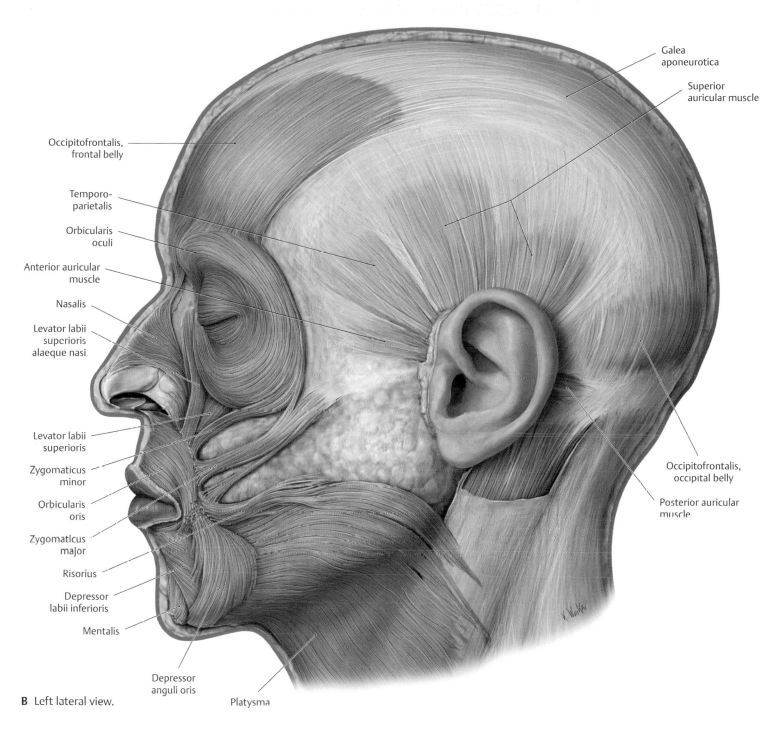

Galea aponeurotica
Superior auricular muscle
Occipitofrontalis, frontal belly
Temporoparietalis
Orbicularis oculi
Anterior auricular muscle
Nasalis
Levator labii superioris alaeque nasi
Levator labii superioris
Zygomaticus minor
Orbicularis oris
Zygomaticus major
Risorius
Depressor labii inferioris
Mentalis
Depressor anguli oris
Platysma
Occipitofrontalis, occipital belly
Posterior auricular muscle

B Left lateral view.

Fig. 32.2 Muscles of mastication

Left lateral view.

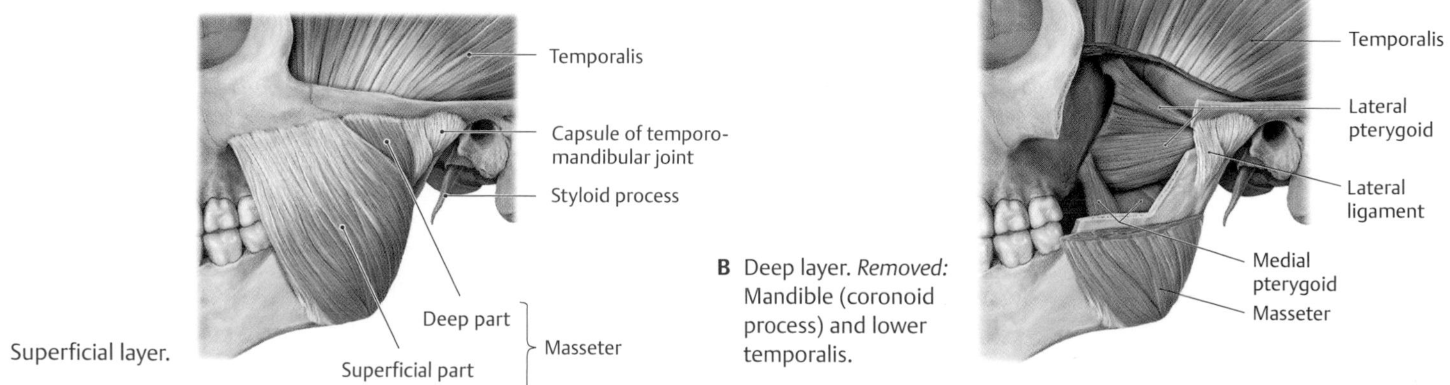

Temporalis
Capsule of temporomandibular joint
Styloid process
Deep part
Superficial part
Masseter
Temporalis
Lateral pterygoid
Lateral ligament
Medial pterygoid
Masseter

A Superficial layer.

B Deep layer. *Removed:* Mandible (coronoid process) and lower temporalis.

Muscle Origins & Insertions on the Skull

Fig. 32.3 **Lateral skull: Origins and insertions**
Left lateral view. Muscle origins are shown in red, insertions in blue. *Note*: There are generally no bony insertions for the muscles of facial expression. These muscles insert into skin and other muscles of facial expression.

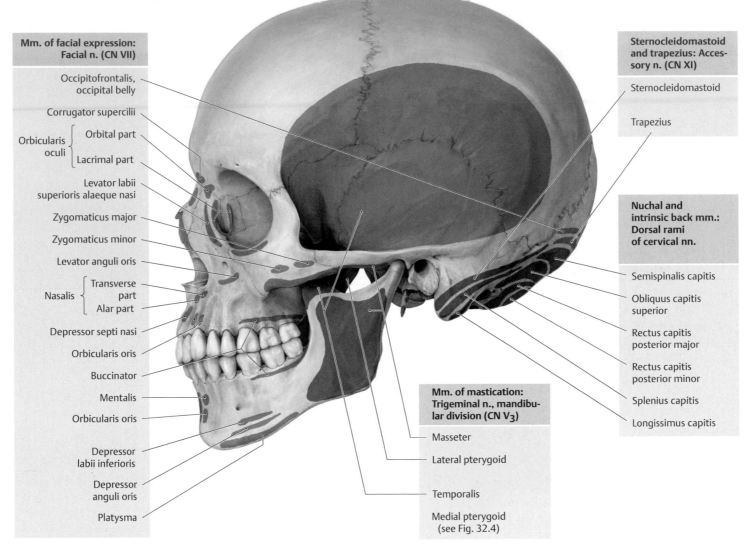

Mm. of facial expression: Facial n. (CN VII)

- Occipitofrontalis, occipital belly
- Corrugator supercilii
- Orbicularis oculi
  - Orbital part
  - Lacrimal part
- Levator labii superioris alaeque nasi
- Zygomaticus major
- Zygomaticus minor
- Levator anguli oris
- Nasalis
  - Transverse part
  - Alar part
- Depressor septi nasi
- Orbicularis oris
- Buccinator
- Mentalis
- Orbicularis oris
- Depressor labii inferioris
- Depressor anguli oris
- Platysma

Sternocleidomastoid and trapezius: Accessory n. (CN XI)

- Sternocleidomastoid
- Trapezius

Nuchal and intrinsic back mm.: Dorsal rami of cervical nn.

- Semispinalis capitis
- Obliquus capitis superior
- Rectus capitis posterior major
- Rectus capitis posterior minor
- Splenius capitis
- Longissimus capitis

Mm. of mastication: Trigeminal n., mandibular division (CN V_3)

- Masseter
- Lateral pterygoid
- Temporalis
- Medial pterygoid (see Fig. 32.4)

Fig. 32.4 **Mandible: Origins and insertions**
Medial view of right hemimandible (inner surface). Muscle origins are shown in red, insertions in blue.

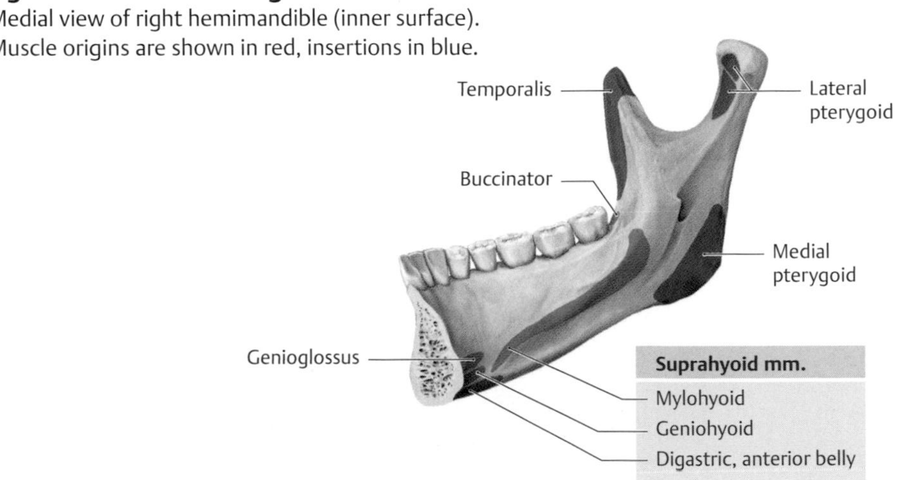
Temporalis
Lateral pterygoid
Buccinator
Medial pterygoid
Genioglossus
Suprahyoid mm.
Mylohyoid
Geniohyoid
Digastric, anterior belly

Fig. 32.5 Skull base: Origins and insertions

Inferior view of external skull.
Muscle origins are shown in red, insertions in blue.

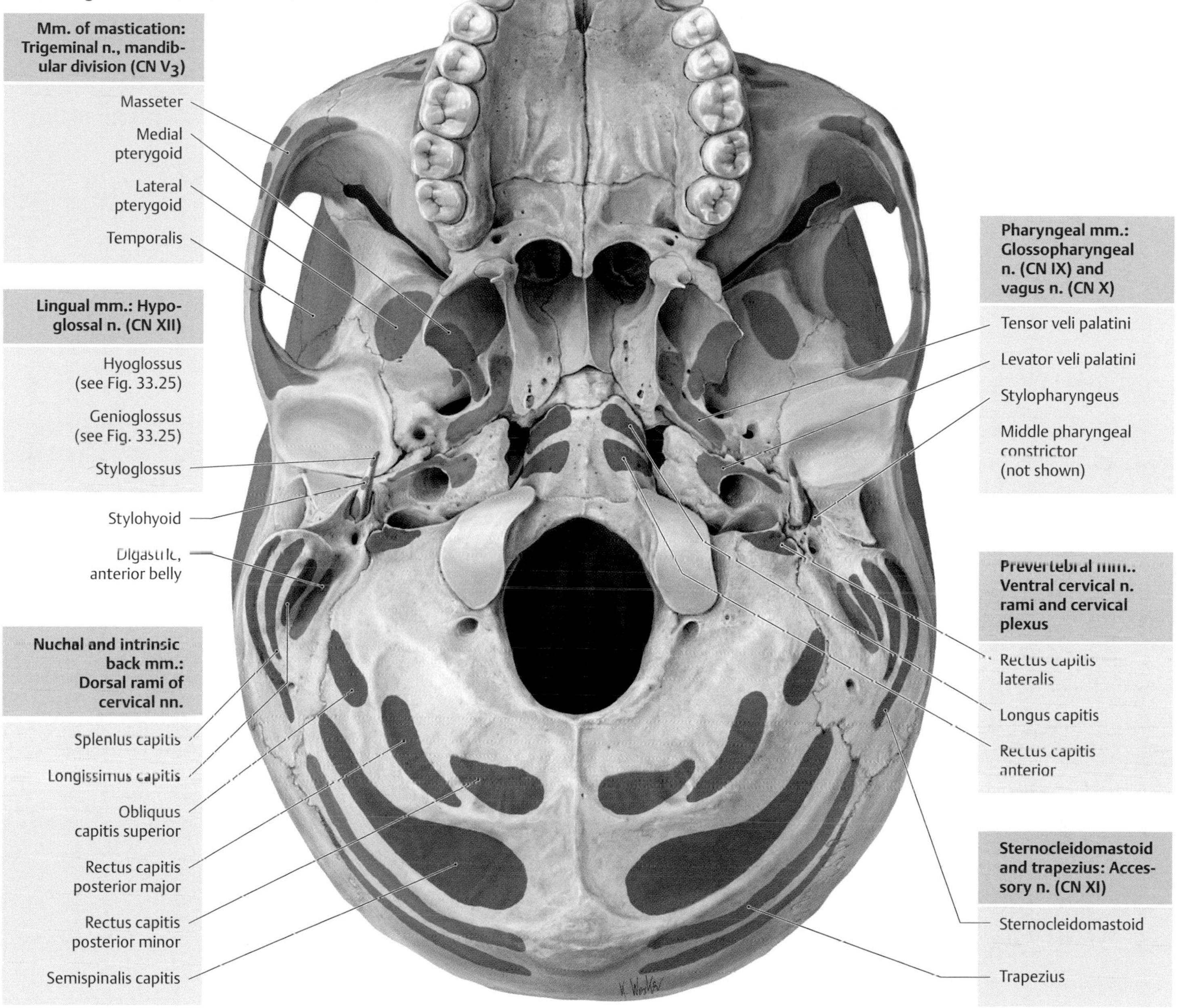

Mm. of mastication: Trigeminal n., mandibular division (CN V_3)

Masseter
Medial pterygoid
Lateral pterygoid
Temporalis

Lingual mm.: Hypoglossal n. (CN XII)

Hyoglossus (see Fig. 33.25)
Genioglossus (see Fig. 33.25)
Styloglossus

Stylohyoid
Digastric, anterior belly

Nuchal and intrinsic back mm.: Dorsal rami of cervical nn.

Splenius capitis
Longissimus capitis
Obliquus capitis superior
Rectus capitis posterior major
Rectus capitis posterior minor
Semispinalis capitis

Pharyngeal mm.: Glossopharyngeal n. (CN IX) and vagus n. (CN X)

Tensor veli palatini
Levator veli palatini
Stylopharyngeus
Middle pharyngeal constrictor (not shown)

Prevertebral mm.: Ventral cervical n. rami and cervical plexus

Rectus capitis lateralis
Longus capitis
Rectus capitis anterior

Sternocleidomastoid and trapezius: Accessory n. (CN XI)

Sternocleidomastoid
Trapezius

Fig. 32.6 Hyoid bone: Origins and insertions

The larynx is suspended from the hyoid bone, primarily by the thyrohyoid membrane. The hyoid bone is the site for attachment for the suprahyoid and infrahyoid muscles. Muscle insertions are shown in blue.

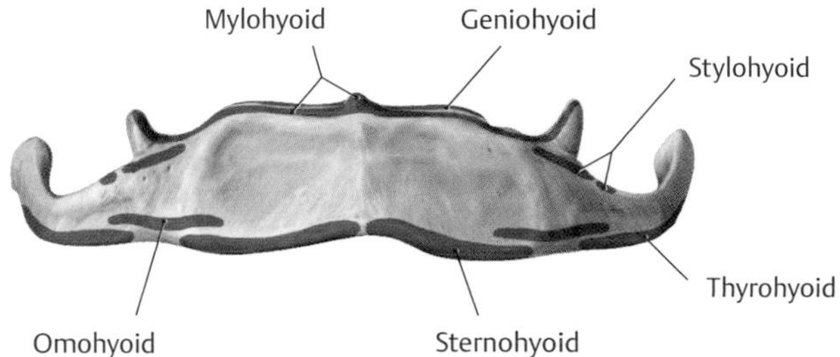
Mylohyoid
Geniohyoid
Stylohyoid
Thyrohyoid
Omohyoid
Sternohyoid

A Anterior view.

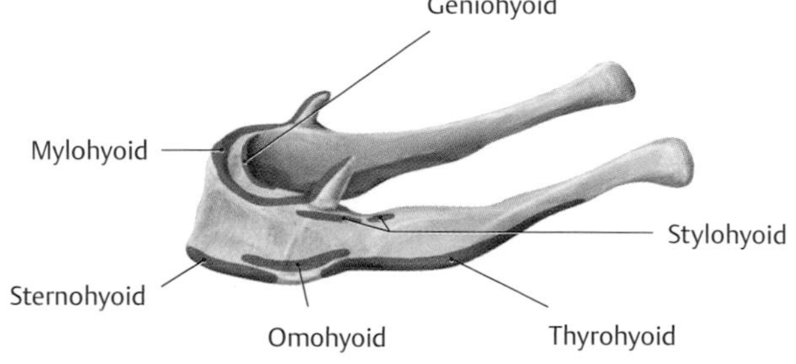
Geniohyoid
Mylohyoid
Stylohyoid
Sternohyoid
Omohyoid
Thyrohyoid

B Oblique left lateral view.

Muscle Facts (I)

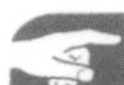

The muscles of facial expression originate on bone and/or fascia and insert into the subcutaneous tissue of the face. This allows them to produce their effects by pulling on the skin.

Fig. 32.7 Occipitofrontalis
Anterior view.

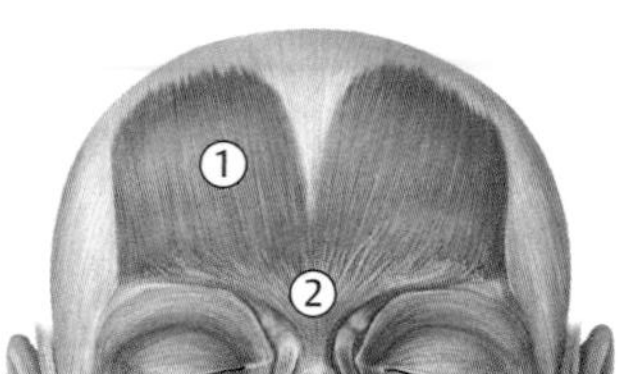
①
②

Fig. 32.8 Muscles of the palpebral fissure and nose
Anterior view.

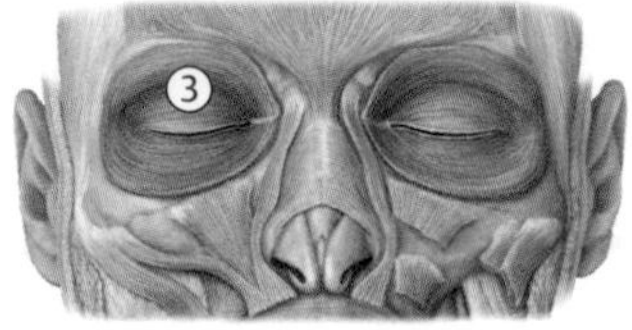
③

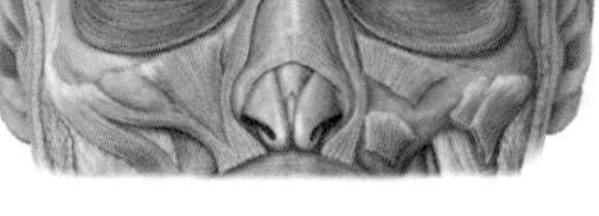

A Orbicularis oculi.

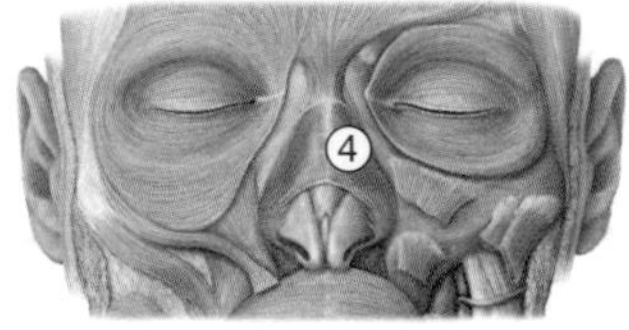
④

B Nasalis.

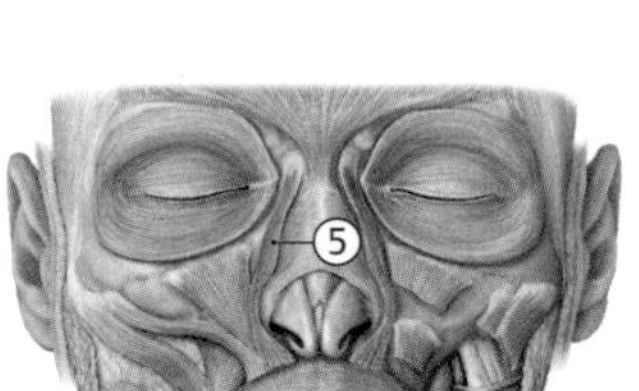
⑤

C Levator labii superioris alaeque nasi.

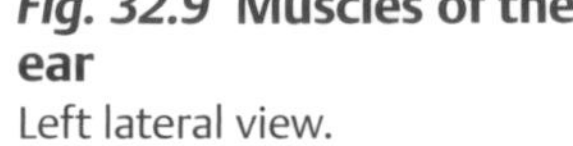

Fig. 32.9 Muscles of the ear
Left lateral view.

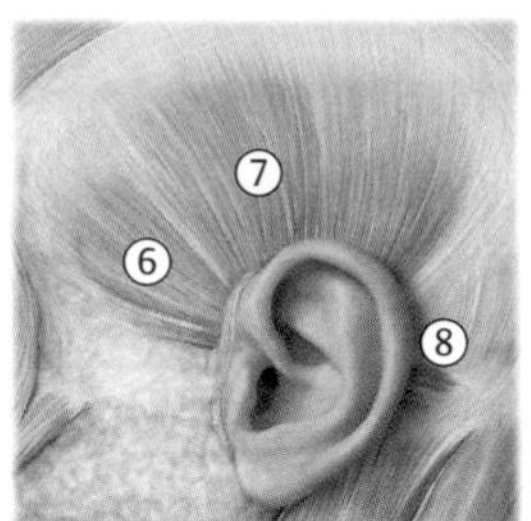
⑦
⑥
⑧

Table 32.1 Muscles of facial expression: Forehead, nose, and ear

Muscle	Origin	Insertion*	Main action(s)**
Calvaria			
① Occipitofrontalis (frontal belly)	Epicranial aponeurosis	Skin and subcutaneous tissue of eyebrows and forehead	Elevates eyebrows, wrinkles skin of forehead
Palpebral fissure and nose			
② Procerus	Nasal bone, lateral nasal cartilage (upper part)	Skin of lower forehead between eyebrows	Pulls medial angle of eyebrows inferiorly, producing transverse wrinkles over bridge of nose
③ Orbicularis oculi	Medial orbital margin, medial palpebral ligament; lacrimal bone	Skin around margin of orbit, superior and inferior tarsal plates	Acts as orbital sphincter (closes eyelids) • Palpebral portion gently closes • Orbital portion tightly closes (as in winking)
④ Nasalis	Maxilla (superior region of canine ridge)	Nasal cartilages	Flares nostrils by drawing ala (side) of nose toward nasal septum
⑤ Levator labii superioris alaeque nasi	Maxilla (frontal process)	Alar cartilage of nose and upper lip	Elevates upper lip, opens nostril
Ear			
⑥ Anterior auricular muscles	Temporal fascia (anterior portion)	Helix of the ear	Pull ear superiorly and anteriorly
⑦ Superior auricular muscles	Epicranial aponeurosis on side of head	Upper portion of auricle	Elevate ear
⑧ Posterior auricular muscles	Mastoid process	Convexity of concha of ear	Pull ear superiorly and posteriorly

*There are no bony insertions for the muscles of facial expression.
**All muscles of facial expression are innervated by the facial nerve (CN VII) via temporal, zygomatic, buccal, mandibular, or cervical branches arising from the parotid plexus (see pp. 504–505).

Fig. 32.10 **Muscles of the mouth**
Left lateral view.

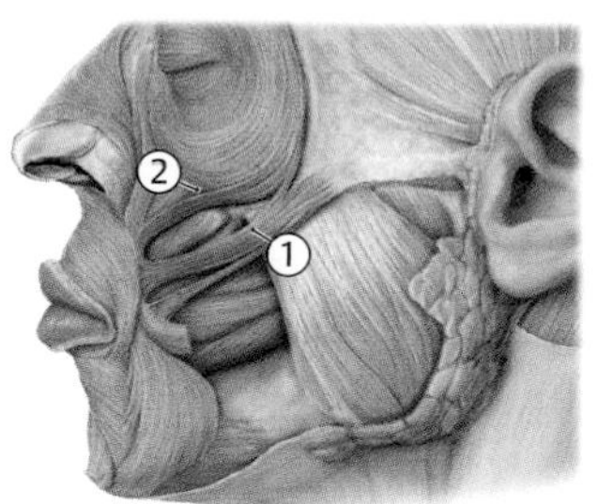

2
1

A Zygomaticus major and minor.

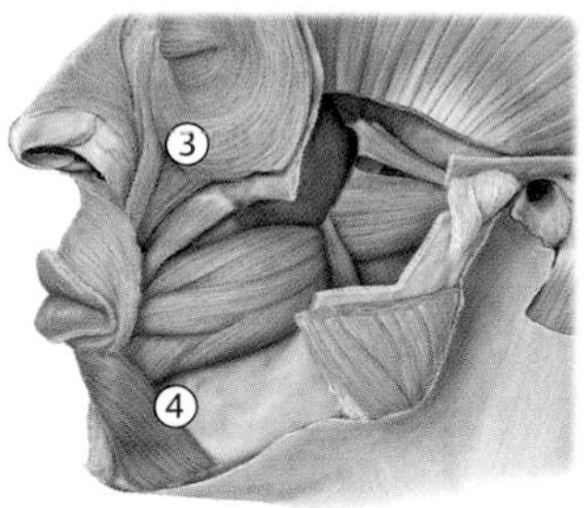

3
4

B Levator labii superioris and depressor labii inferioris.

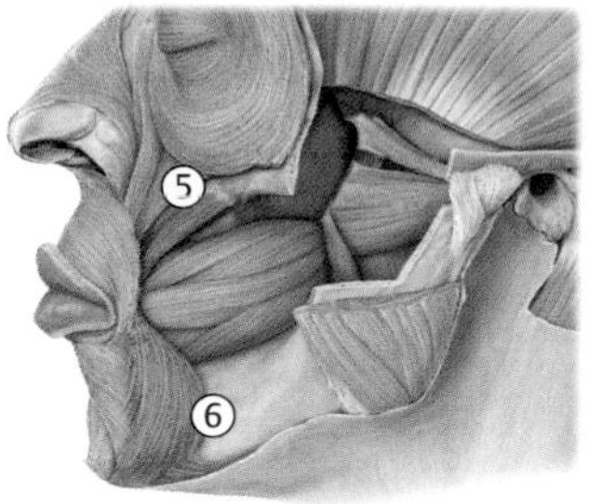

5
6

C Levator and depressor anguli oris.

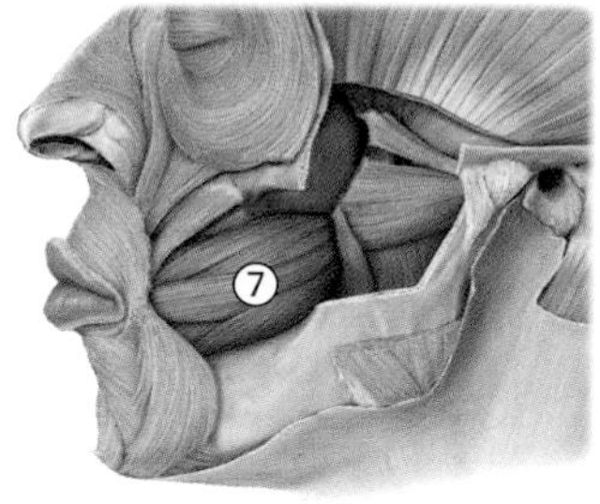

7

D Buccinator.

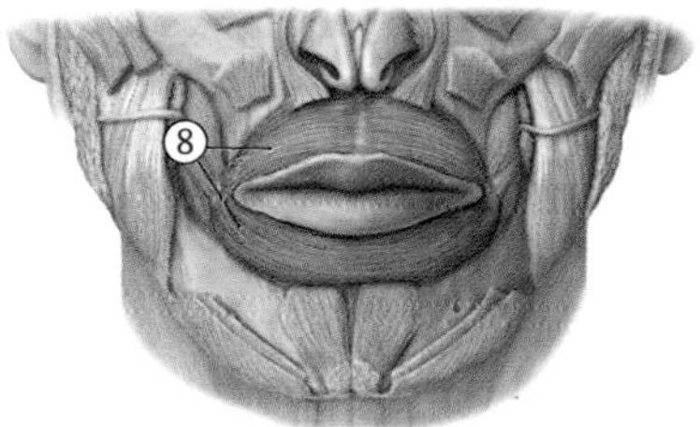

8

E Orbicularis oris, anterior view.

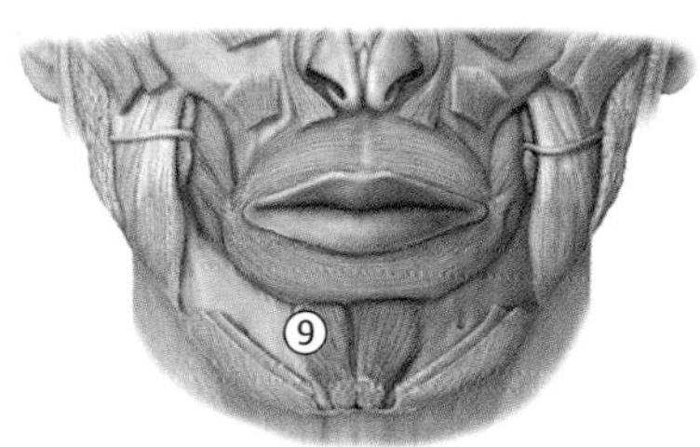

9

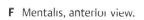

F Mentalis, anterior view.

Table 32.2 **Muscles of facial expression: Mouth and neck**

Muscle	Origin	Insertion*	Main action(s)**
Mouth			
① Zygomaticus major	Zygomatic bone (lateral surface, posterior part)	Skin at corner of the mouth	Pulls corner of mouth superiorly and laterally
② Zygomaticus minor		Upper lip just medial to corner of the mouth	Pulls upper lip superiorly
Levator labii superioris alaeque nasi (see Fig. 32.8C)	Maxilla (frontal process)	Alar cartilage of nose and upper lip	Elevates upper lip, opens nostril
③ Levator labii superioris	Maxilla (frontal process) and infraorbital region	Skin of upper lip, alar cartilages of nose	Elevates upper lip, dilates nostril, raises angle of the mouth
④ Depressor labii inferioris	Mandible (anterior portion of oblique line)	Lower lip at midline; blends with muscle from opposite side	Pulls lower lip inferiorly and laterally
⑤ Levator anguli oris	Maxilla (below infraorbital foramen)	Skin at corner of the mouth	Raises angle of mouth, helps form nasolabial furrow
⑥ Depressor anguli oris	Mandible (oblique line below canine, premolar, and first molar teeth)	Skin at corner of the mouth; blends with orbicularis oris	Pulls angle of mouth inferiorly and laterally
⑦ Buccinator	Mandible, alveolar processes of maxilla and mandible, pterygo-mandibular raphe	Angle of mouth, orbicularis oris	Presses cheek against molar teeth, working with tongue to keep food between occlusal surfaces and out of oral vestibule; expels air from oral cavity/resists distension when blowing *Unilateral:* Draws mouth to one side
⑧ Orbicularis oris	Deep surface of skin Superiorly: maxilla (median plane) Inferiorly: mandible	Mucous membrane of lips	Acts as oral sphincter • Compresses and protrudes lips (e.g., when whistling, sucking, and kissing) • Resists distension (when blowing)
Risorius (see pp. 488–489)	Fascia over masseter	Skin of corner of the mouth	Retracts corner of mouth as in grimacing
⑨ Mentalis	Mandible (incisive fossa)	Skin of chin	Elevates and protrudes lower lip
Neck			
Platysma (see pp. 488–489)	Skin over lower neck and upper lateral thorax	Mandible (inferior border), skin over lower face, angle of mouth	Depresses and wrinkles skin of lower face and mouth; tenses skin of neck; aids in forced depression of the mandible

*There are no bony insertions for the muscles of facial expression.
**All muscles of facial expression are innervated by the facial nerve (CN VII) via temporal, zygomatic, buccal, mandibular, or cervical branches arising from its parotid plexus.

Muscle Facts (II)

The muscles of mastication are located at various depths in the parotid and infratemporal regions of the face. They attach to the mandible and receive their motor innervation from the mandibular division of the trigeminal nerve (CN V_3). The muscles of the oral floor that aid in opening the mouth are found on p. 590.

Table 32.3 Muscles of mastication: Masseter and temporalis

Muscle	Origin	Insertion	Innervation	Action
① Masseter	Superficial head: zygomatic arch (anterior two thirds) Deep head: zygomatic arch (posterior one third)	Mandibular angle (masseteric tuberosity)	Mandibular n. (CN V_3) via masseteric n.	Elevates (adducts) and protrudes mandible
② Temporalis	Temporal fossa (inferior temporal line)	Coronoid process of mandible (apex and medial surface)	Mandibular n. (CN V_3) via deep temporal nn.	*Vertical fibers:* Elevate (adduct) mandible *Horizontal fibers:* Retract (retrude) mandible *Unilateral:* Lateral movement of mandible (chewing)

Fig. 32.11 **Masseter muscle**
Left lateral view.

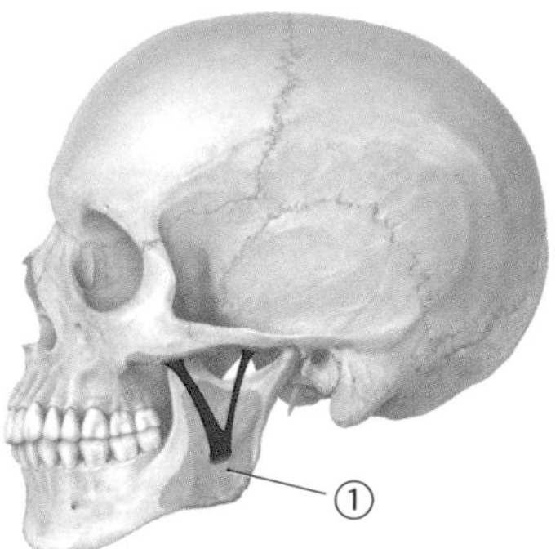
①

A Schematic.

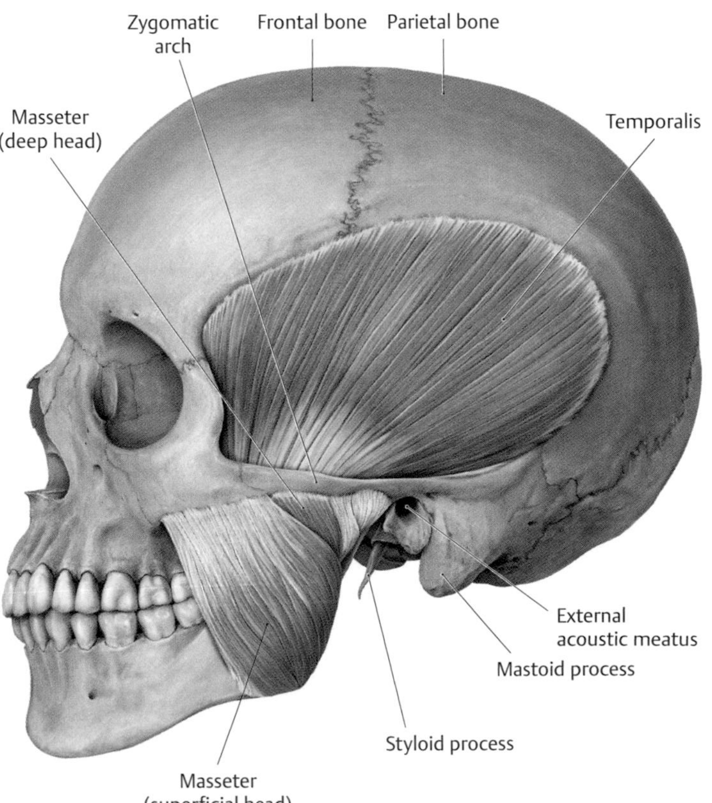
Zygomatic arch
Frontal bone
Parietal bone
Masseter (deep head)
Temporalis
External acoustic meatus
Mastoid process
Styloid process
Masseter (superficial head)

B Masseter with temporalis muscle.

Fig. 32.12 **Temporalis muscle**
Left lateral view.

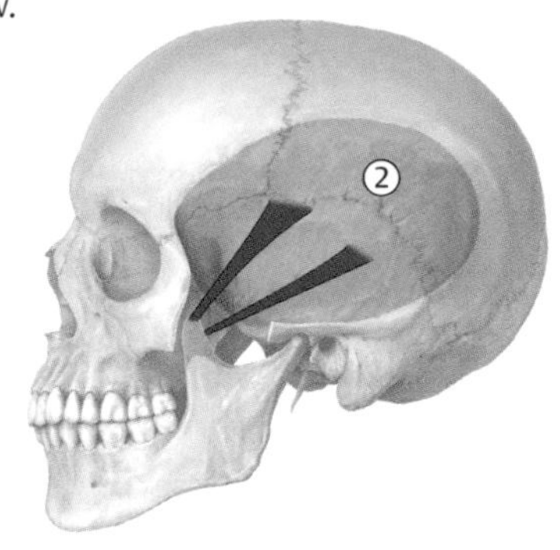
②

A Schematic.

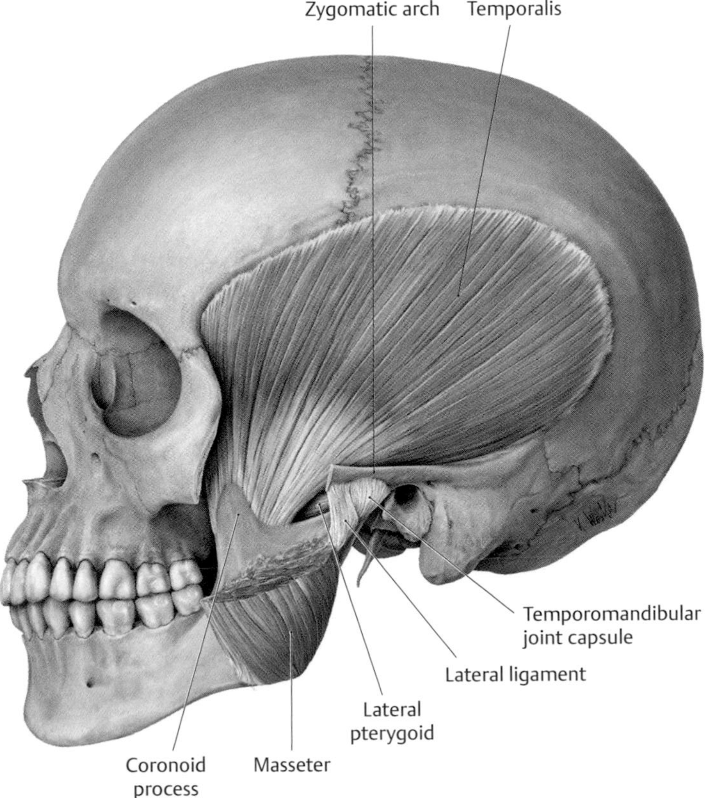
Zygomatic arch
Temporalis
Temporomandibular joint capsule
Lateral ligament
Lateral pterygoid
Coronoid process
Masseter

B Temporalis muscle. *Removed:* Masseter and zygomatic arch.

Table 32.4 Muscles of mastication: Pterygoid muscles

Muscle		Origin	Insertion	Innervation	Action
Lateral pterygoid	③ Superior head	Greater wing of sphenoid bone (infratemporal crest)	Temporomandibular joint (articular disk)	Mandibular n. (CN V_3) via lateral pterygoid n.	*Bilateral:* Protrudes mandible (pulls articular disk forward) *Unilateral:* Lateral movements of mandible (chewing)
	④ Inferior head	Lateral pterygoid plate (lateral surface)	Mandible (condylar process)		
Medial pterygoid	⑤ Superficial head	Maxilla (tuberosity)	Pterygoid tuberosity on medial surface of the mandibular angle	Mandibular n. (CN V_3) via medial pterygoid n.	Elevates (adducts) mandible
	⑥ Deep head	Medial surface of lateral pterygoid plate and pterygoid fossa			

Fig. 32.13 Lateral pterygoid muscle

Left lateral view.

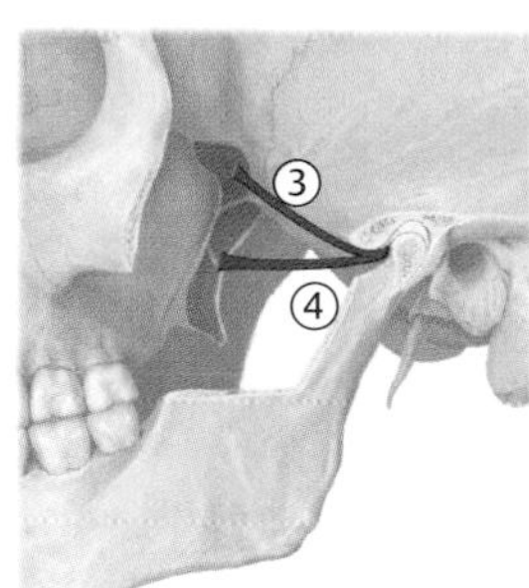
③
④

A Schematic.

Superior head
Inferior head
Lateral pterygoid
Zygomatic arch (cut)
Articular disk
Condylar head
Styloid process
Coronoid process (cut)

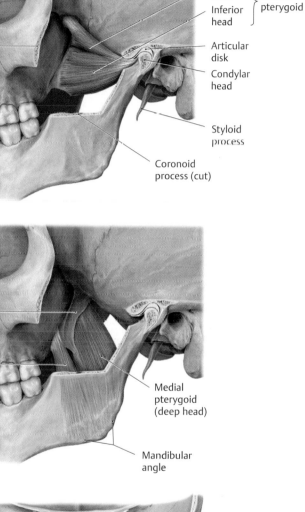

B Left lateral pterygoid muscle. *Removed:* Coronoid process of mandible.

Fig. 32.14 Medial pterygoid muscle

Left lateral view.

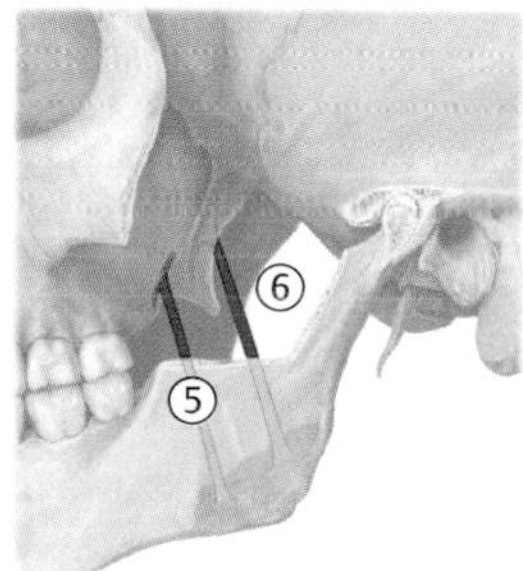
⑥
⑤

A Schematic.

Pterygoid process, lateral plate
Medial pterygoid (superficial head)
Medial pterygoid (deep head)
Mandibular angle

B Left medial pterygoid muscle. *Removed:* Coronoid process of mandible.

Fig. 32.15 Masticatory muscle sling

Oblique posterior view.

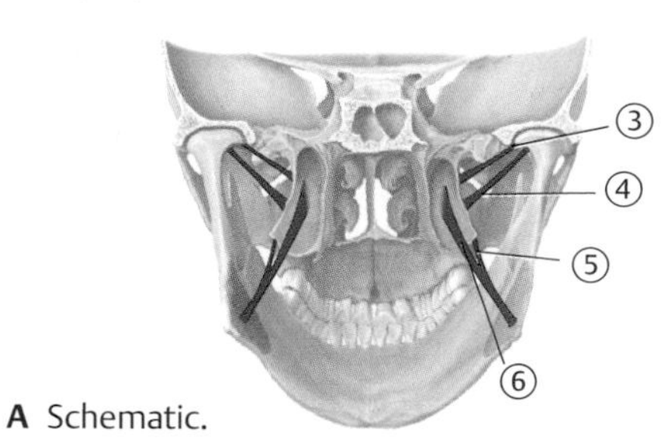
③
④
⑤
⑥

A Schematic.

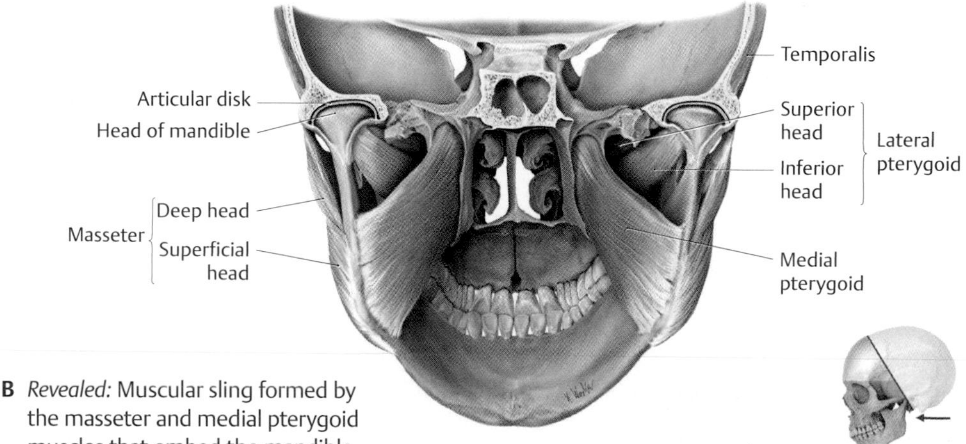
Temporalis
Articular disk
Head of mandible
Superior head
Inferior head
Lateral pterygoid
Masseter
Deep head
Superficial head
Medial pterygoid

B *Revealed:* Muscular sling formed by the masseter and medial pterygoid muscles that embed the mandible.

Cranial Nerves: Overview

Fig. 33.1 **Cranial nerves**
Inferior (basal) view. The 12 pairs of cranial nerves (CN) are numbered according to the order of their emergence from the brainstem. *Note:* The sensory and motor fibers of the cranial nerves enter and exit the brainstem at the same sites (in contrast to spinal nerves, whose sensory and motor fibers enter and leave through posterior and anterior roots, respectively).

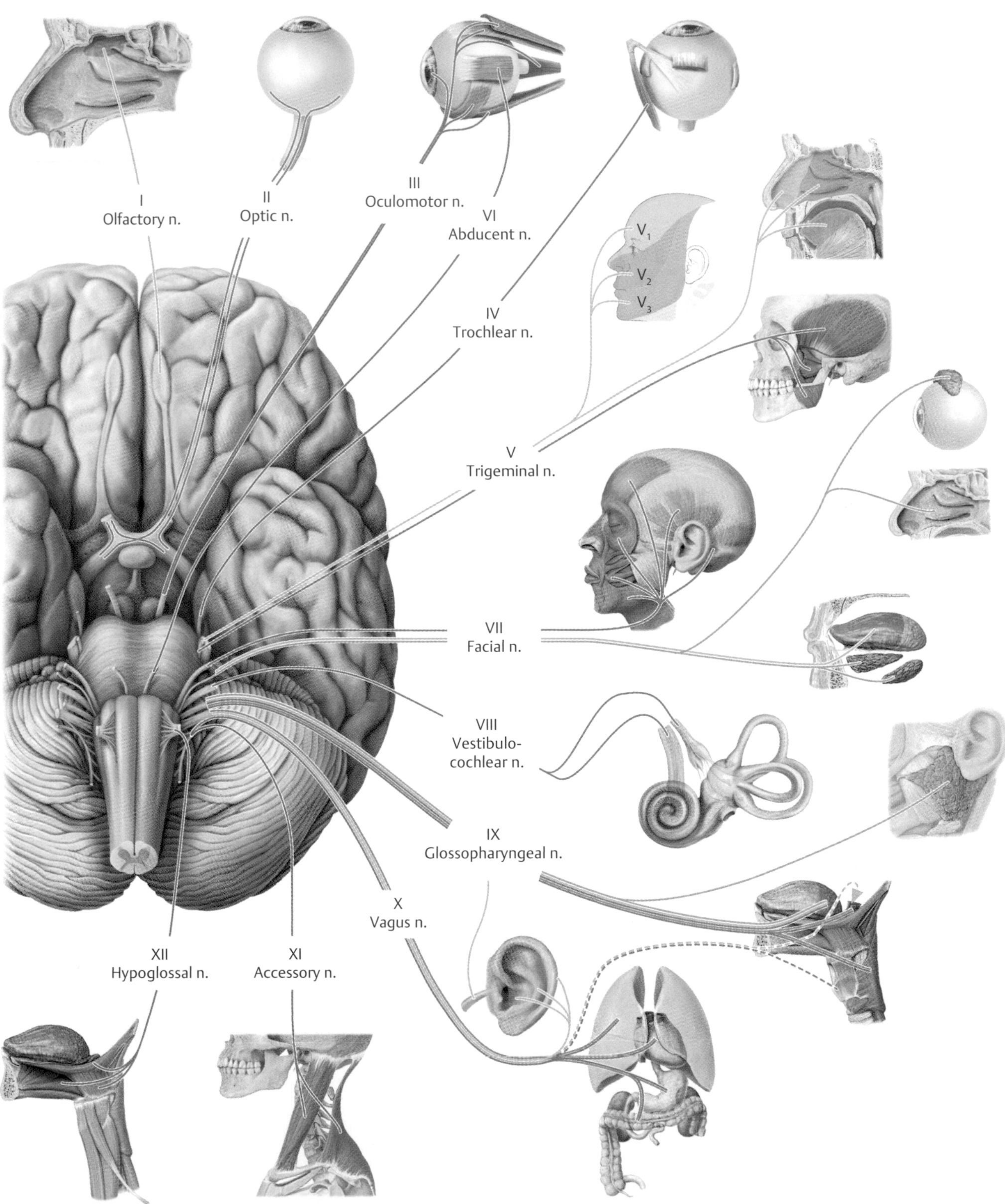

I
Olfactory n.
II
Optic n.
III
Oculomotor n.
VI
Abducent n.
IV
Trochlear n.
V_1
V_2
V_3
V
Trigeminal n.
VII
Facial n.
VIII
Vestibulo-
cochlear n.
IX
Glossopharyngeal n.
X
Vagus n.
XII
Hypoglossal n.
XI
Accessory n.

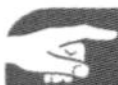

The cranial nerves contain both afferent (sensory) and efferent (motor) axons that belong to either the somatic or the autonomic (visceral) nervous system (see pp. 648–649). The somatic fibers allow interaction with the environment, whereas the visceral fibers regulate the autonomic activity of internal organs.

In addition to the general fiber types, the cranial nerves may contain special fiber types associated with particular structures (e.g., auditory apparatus and taste buds). The cranial nerve fibers originate or terminate at specific nuclei, which are similarly classified as either general or special, somatic or visceral, and afferent or efferent.

Table 33.1 Classification of cranial nerve fibers and nuclei

This color coding is used in subsequent chapters to indicate fiber and nuclei classifications.

	Fiber type	Example		Fiber type	Example
	General somatic efferent (somatomotor function)	Innervate skeletal muscles		General somatic afferent (somatic sensation)	Conduct impulses from skin, skeletal muscle spindles
	General visceral efferent (visceromotor function)	Innervate smooth muscle of the viscera, intraocular muscles, heart, salivary glands, etc.		Special somatic afferent	Conduct impulses from retina, auditory and vestibular apparatuses
	Special visceral efferent	Innervate skeletal muscles derived from branchial arches		General visceral afferent (visceral sensation)	Conduct impulses from viscera, blood vessels
				Special visceral afferent	Conduct impulses from taste buds, olfactory mucosa

Fig. 33.2 Cranial nerve nuclei

The sensory and motor fibers of cranial nerves III to XII originate and terminate in the brainstem at specific nuclei.

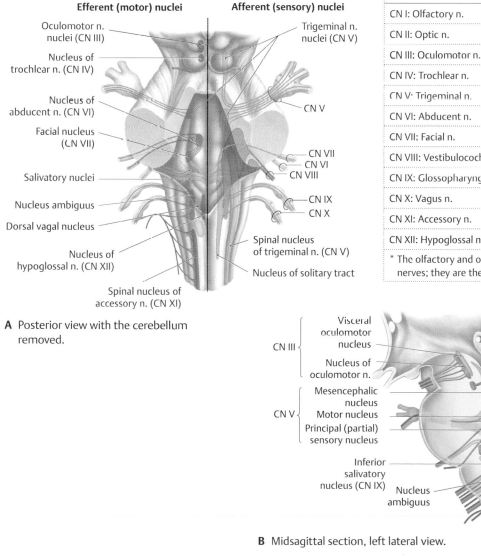

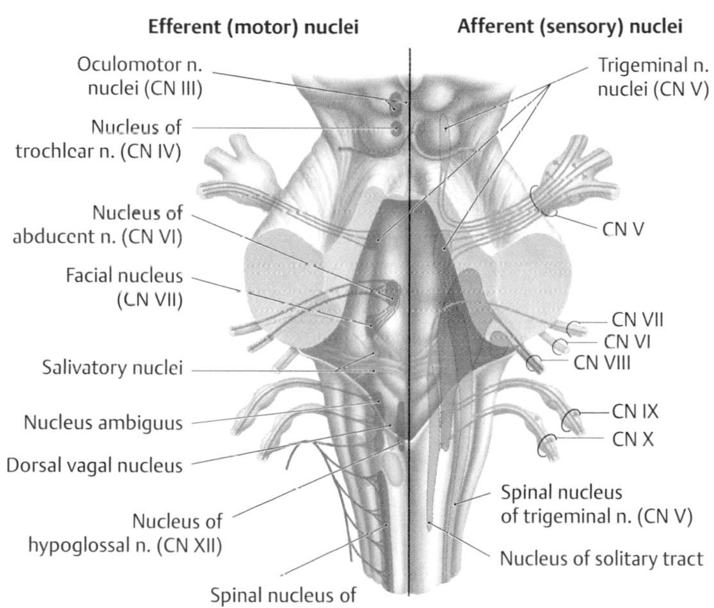

Efferent (motor) nuclei
Afferent (sensory) nuclei
Oculomotor n. nuclei (CN III)
Nucleus of trochlear n. (CN IV)
Nucleus of abducent n. (CN VI)
Facial nucleus (CN VII)
Salivatory nuclei
Nucleus ambiguus
Dorsal vagal nucleus
Nucleus of hypoglossal n. (CN XII)
Spinal nucleus of accessory n. (CN XI)
Trigeminal n. nuclei (CN V)
CN V
CN VII
CN VI
CN VIII
CN IX
CN X
Spinal nucleus of trigeminal n. (CN V)
Nucleus of solitary tract

A Posterior view with the cerebellum removed.

Table 33.2 Cranial nerves

Cranial nerve	Origin	Functional fiber types
CN I: Olfactory n.	Telencephalon*	●
CN II: Optic n.	Diencephalon*	●
CN III: Oculomotor n.	Mesencephalon	● ●
CN IV: Trochlear n.		●
CN V: Trigeminal n.	Pons	● ●
CN VI: Abducent n.		●
CN VII: Facial n.		● ● ● ●
CN VIII: Vestibulocochlear n.	Medulla oblongata	●
CN IX: Glossopharyngeal n.		● ● ● ● ●
CN X: Vagus n.		● ● ● ● ●
CN XI: Accessory n.		● ●
CN XII: Hypoglossal n.		●

* The olfactory and optic nerves are extensions of the brain rather than true nerves; they are therefore not associated with nuclei in the brainstem.

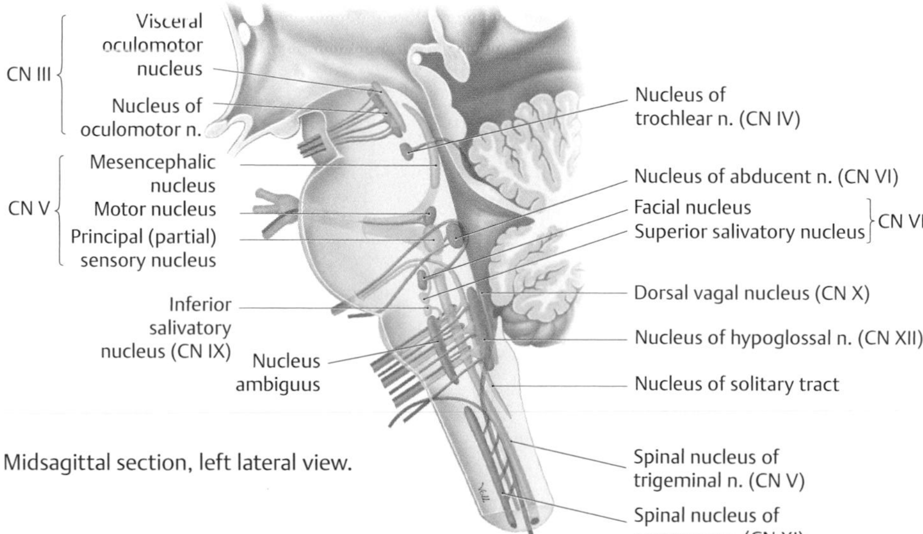

CN III
Visceral oculomotor nucleus
Nucleus of oculomotor n.
CN V
Mesencephalic nucleus
Motor nucleus
Principal (partial) sensory nucleus
Inferior salivatory nucleus (CN IX)
Nucleus ambiguus
Nucleus of trochlear n. (CN IV)
Nucleus of abducent n. (CN VI)
Facial nucleus
Superior salivatory nucleus
CN VII
Dorsal vagal nucleus (CN X)
Nucleus of hypoglossal n. (CN XII)
Nucleus of solitary tract
Spinal nucleus of trigeminal n. (CN V)
Spinal nucleus of accessory n. (CN XI)

B Midsagittal section, left lateral view.

CN I & II: Olfactory & Optic Nerves

The olfactory and optic nerves are not true peripheral nerves but extensions (tracts) of the telencephalon and diencephalon, respectively. They are therefore not associated with cranial nerve nuclei in the brainstem.

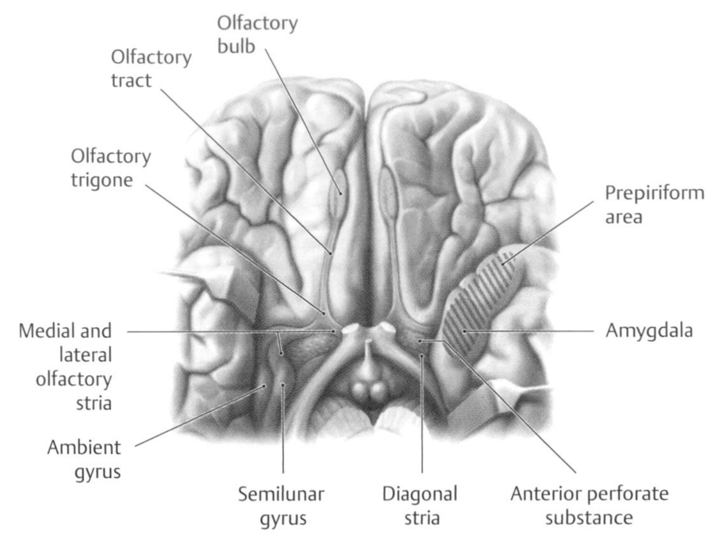
Olfactory bulb
Olfactory tract
Olfactory trigone
Prepiriform area
Medial and lateral olfactory stria
Amygdala
Ambient gyrus
Semilunar gyrus
Diagonal stria
Anterior perforate substance

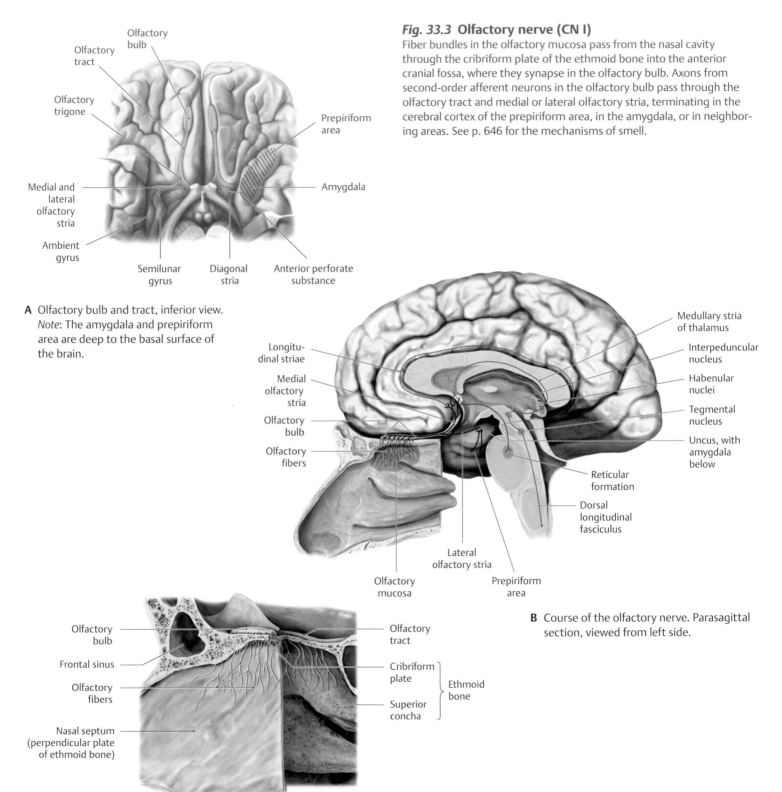

A Olfactory bulb and tract, inferior view. *Note*: The amygdala and prepiriform area are deep to the basal surface of the brain.

Fig. 33.3 Olfactory nerve (CN I)

Fiber bundles in the olfactory mucosa pass from the nasal cavity through the cribriform plate of the ethmoid bone into the anterior cranial fossa, where they synapse in the olfactory bulb. Axons from second-order afferent neurons in the olfactory bulb pass through the olfactory tract and medial or lateral olfactory stria, terminating in the cerebral cortex of the prepiriform area, in the amygdala, or in neighboring areas. See p. 646 for the mechanisms of smell.

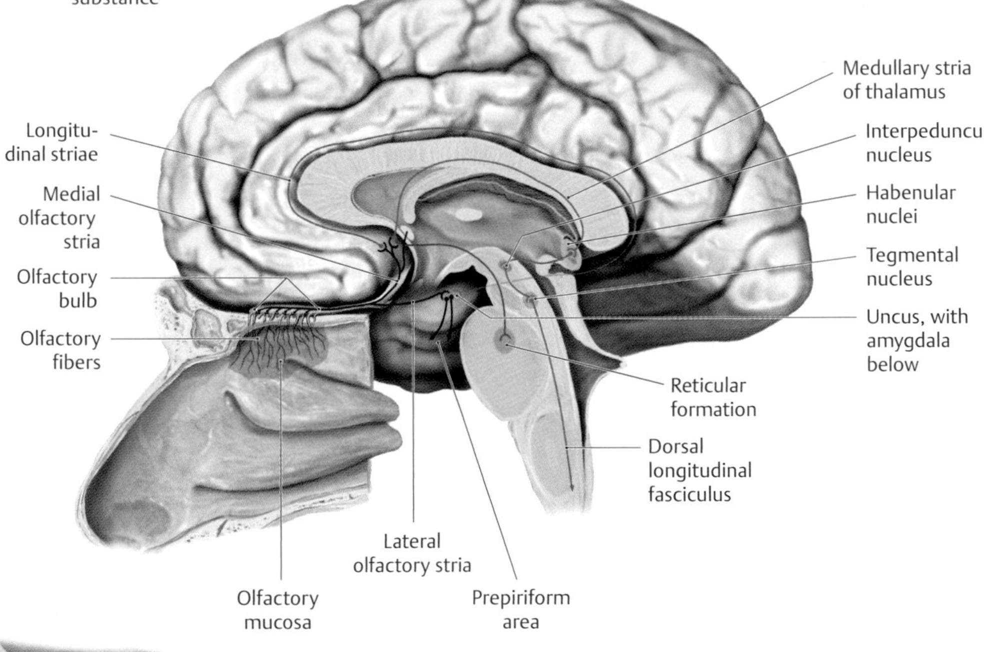
Longitu-dinal striae
Medial olfactory stria
Olfactory bulb
Olfactory fibers
Medullary stria of thalamus
Interpeduncular nucleus
Habenular nuclei
Tegmental nucleus
Uncus, with amygdala below
Reticular formation
Dorsal longitudinal fasciculus
Lateral olfactory stria
Olfactory mucosa
Prepiriform area

B Course of the olfactory nerve. Parasagittal section, viewed from left side.

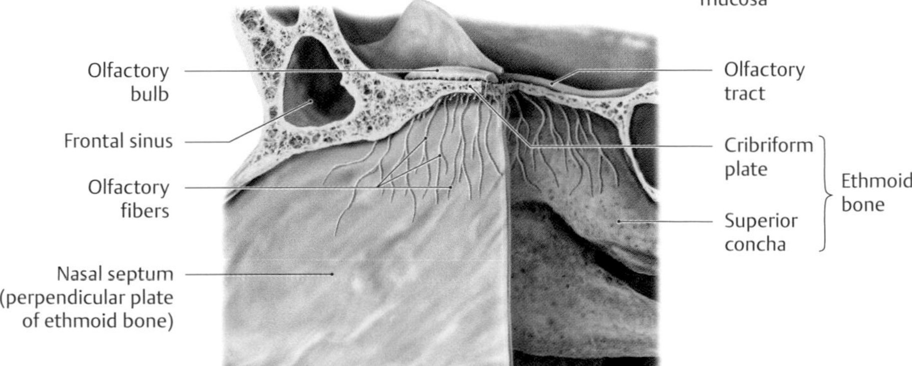
Olfactory bulb
Frontal sinus
Olfactory fibers
Nasal septum (perpendicular plate of ethmoid bone)
Olfactory tract
Cribriform plate
Superior concha
Ethmoid bone

C Olfactory fibers. Portion of left nasal septum and lateral wall of right nasal cavity, left lateral view.

Fig. 33.4 Optic nerve (CN II)

The optic nerve passes from the eyeball through the optic canal into the middle cranial fossa. The two optic nerves join below the base of the diencephalon to form the optic chiasm, before dividing into the two optic tracts. Each of these tracts divides into a lateral and medial root. Many retinal cell ganglion axons cross the midline to the contralateral side of the brain in the optic chiasm. See p. 642 for the mechanisms of sight.

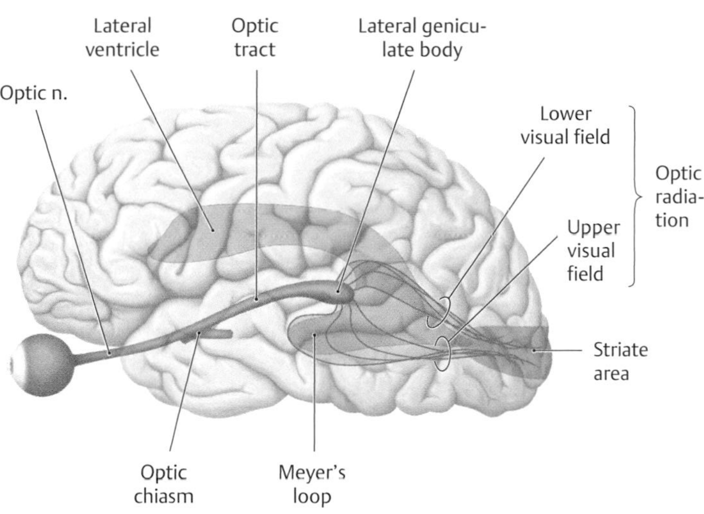
Lateral ventricle
Optic tract
Lateral geniculate body
Optic n.
Lower visual field
Optic radiation
Upper visual field
Striate area
Optic chiasm
Meyer's loop

A Optic nerve in the geniculate visual pathway, left lateral view.

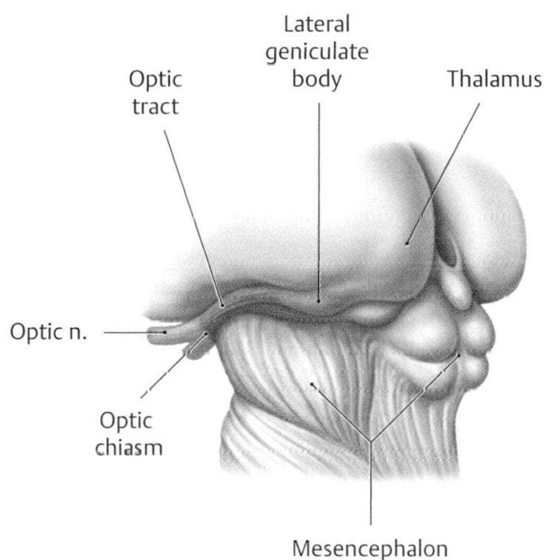
Lateral geniculate body
Optic tract
Thalamus
Optic n.
Optic chiasm
Mesencephalon

B Termination of the optic tract, left posterolateral view of the brainstem. The optic nerve contains the axons of retinal ganglion cells, which terminate mainly in the lateral geniculate body of the diencephalon and in the mesencephalon (superior colliculus).

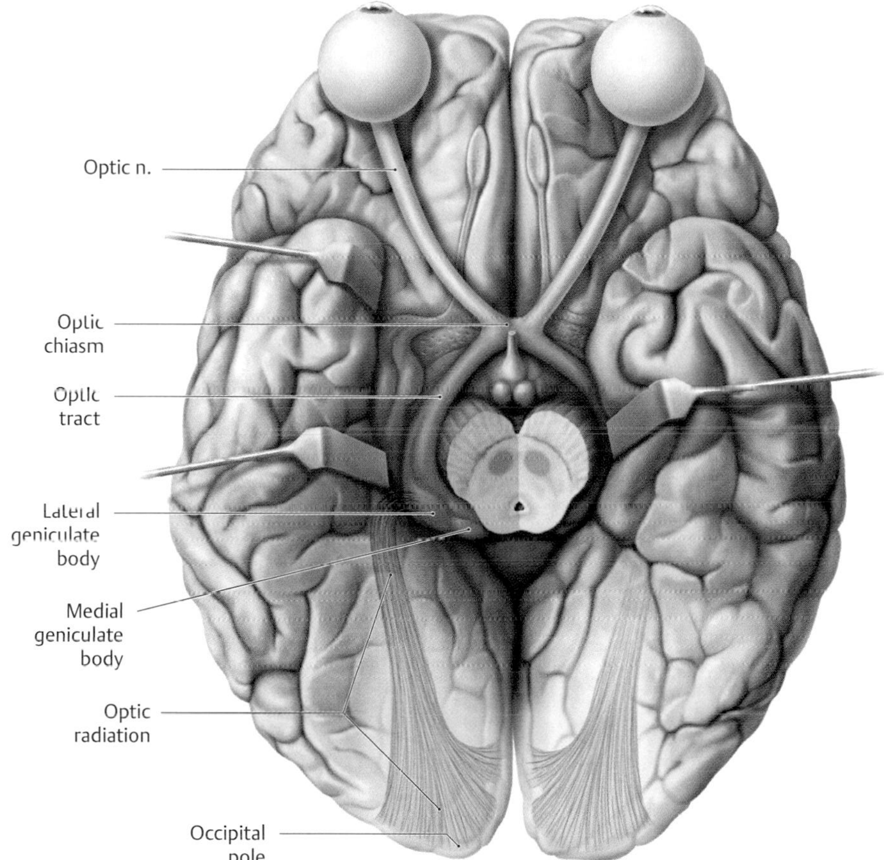
Optic n.
Optic chiasm
Optic tract
Lateral geniculate body
Medial geniculate body
Optic radiation
Occipital pole

C Course of the optic nerve, inferior (basal) view.

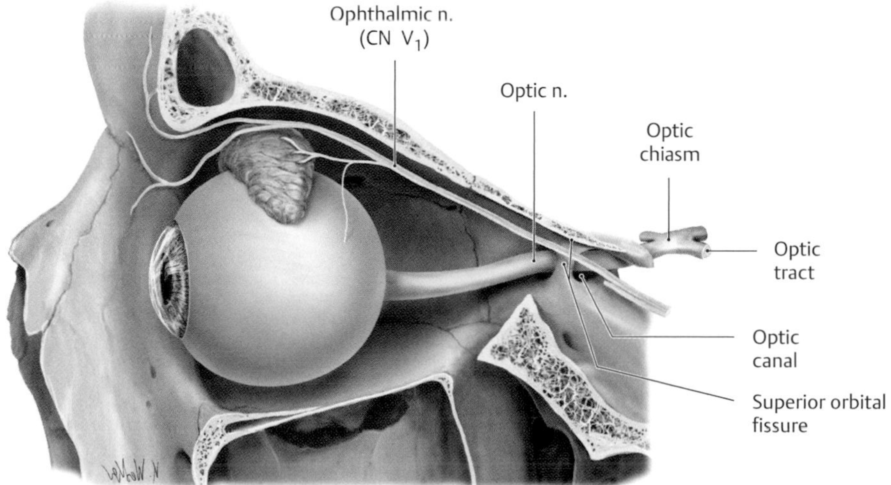
Ophthalmic n. (CN V_1)
Optic n.
Optic chiasm
Optic tract
Optic canal
Superior orbital fissure

D Optic nerve in the left orbit, lateral view. The optic nerve exits the orbit via the optic canal. *Note*: The other cranial nerves entering the orbit do so via the superior orbital fissure.

CN III, IV & VI: Oculomotor, Trochlear & Abducent Nerves

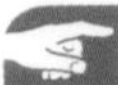

Cranial nerves III, IV, and VI innervate the extraocular muscles (see p. 539). Of the three, only the oculomotor nerve (CN III) contains both somatic and visceral efferent fibers; it is also the only cranial nerve of the extraocular muscles to innervate multiple extra- and intraocular muscles.

Fig. 33.5 Nuclei of the oculomotor, trochlear, and abducent nerves

The trochlear nerve (CN IV) is the only cranial nerve in which all the fibers cross to the opposite side. It is also the only cranial nerve to emerge from the dorsal side of the brainstem and, consequently, has the longest intradural (intracranial) course of any cranial nerve.

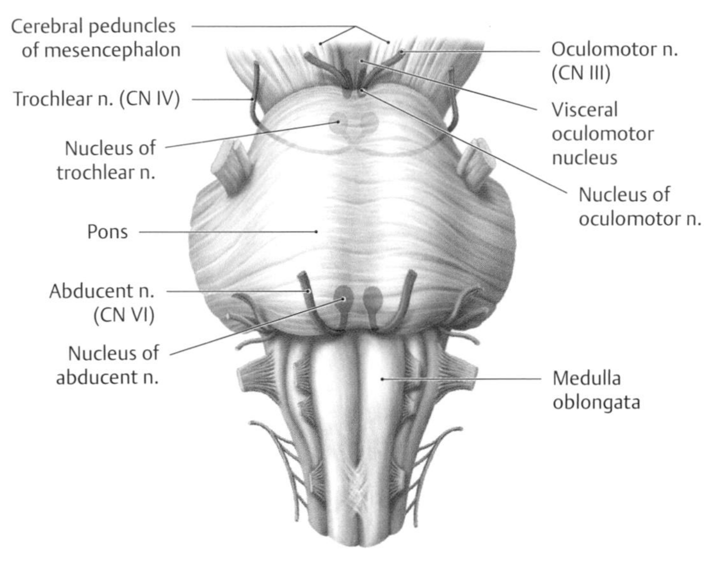
Cerebral peduncles of mesencephalon
Trochlear n. (CN IV)
Nucleus of trochlear n.
Pons
Abducent n. (CN VI)
Nucleus of abducent n.
Oculomotor n. (CN III)
Visceral oculomotor nucleus
Nucleus of oculomotor n.
Medulla oblongata

A Emergence of the cranial nerves of the extraocular muscles. Anterior view of the brainstem.

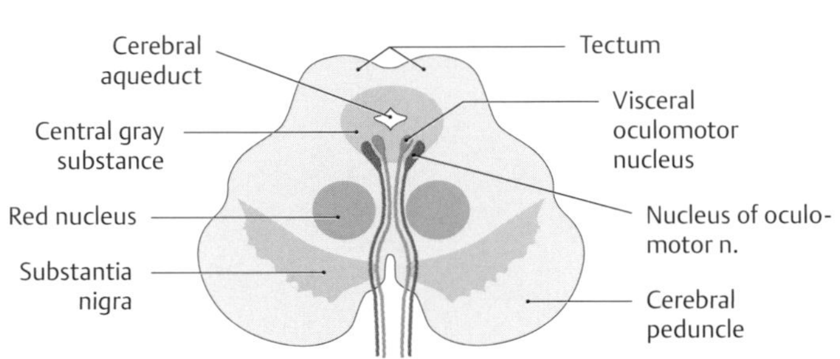
Cerebral aqueduct
Central gray substance
Red nucleus
Substantia nigra
Tectum
Visceral oculomotor nucleus
Nucleus of oculomotor n.
Cerebral peduncle

B Oculomotor nerve nuclei. Transverse section, superior view.

Table 33.3 Cranial nerves of the extraocular muscles

Course*	Fibers	Nuclei	Function	Effects of nerve injury
Oculomotor nerve (CN III)				
Runs anteriorly from mesencephalon	Somatic efferent	Oculomotor nucleus	Innervates: • Levator palpebrae superioris • Superior, medial, and inferior rectus • Inferior oblique	Complete oculomotor palsy (paralysis of extra- and intraocular muscles): • Ptosis (drooping of eyelid) • Downward and lateral gaze deviation • Diplopia (double vision) • Mydriasis (pupil dilation) • Accommodation difficulties (ciliary paralysis)
	Visceral efferent	Visceral oculomotor (Edinger-Westphal) nucleus	Synapse with neurons in ciliary ganglia. Innervates: • Pupillary sphincter • Ciliary muscle	
Trochlear nerve (CN IV)				
Emerges from posterior surface of brainstem near midline, courses anteriorly around the cerebral peduncle	Somatic efferent	Nucleus of the trochlear n.	Innervates: • Superior oblique	• Diplopia • Affected eye is higher and deviated medially (dominance of inferior oblique)
Abducent nerve (CN VI)				
Follows a long extradural path**	Somatic efferent	Nucleus of the abducent n.	Innervates: • Lateral rectus	• Diplopia • Medial strabismas (due to unopposed action of medial rectus)

* All three nerves enter the orbit through the superior orbital fissure; CN III and CN VI pass through the common tendinous ring of the extraocular muscles.
** The abducent nerve follows an extradural course; abducent nerve palsy may therefore develop in association with meningitis and subarachnoid hemorrhage.

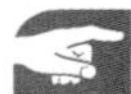

Note: The oculomotor nerve supplies parasympathetic innervation to the intraocular muscles and somatic motor innervation to most of the extraocular muscles (also the levator palpebrae superioris). Its parasympathetic fibers synapse in the ciliary ganglion. Oculomotor nerve palsy may affect exclusively the parasympathetic or somatic fibers, or both concurrently.

***Fig. 33.6* Course of the nerves innervating the extraocular muscles**
Right orbit.

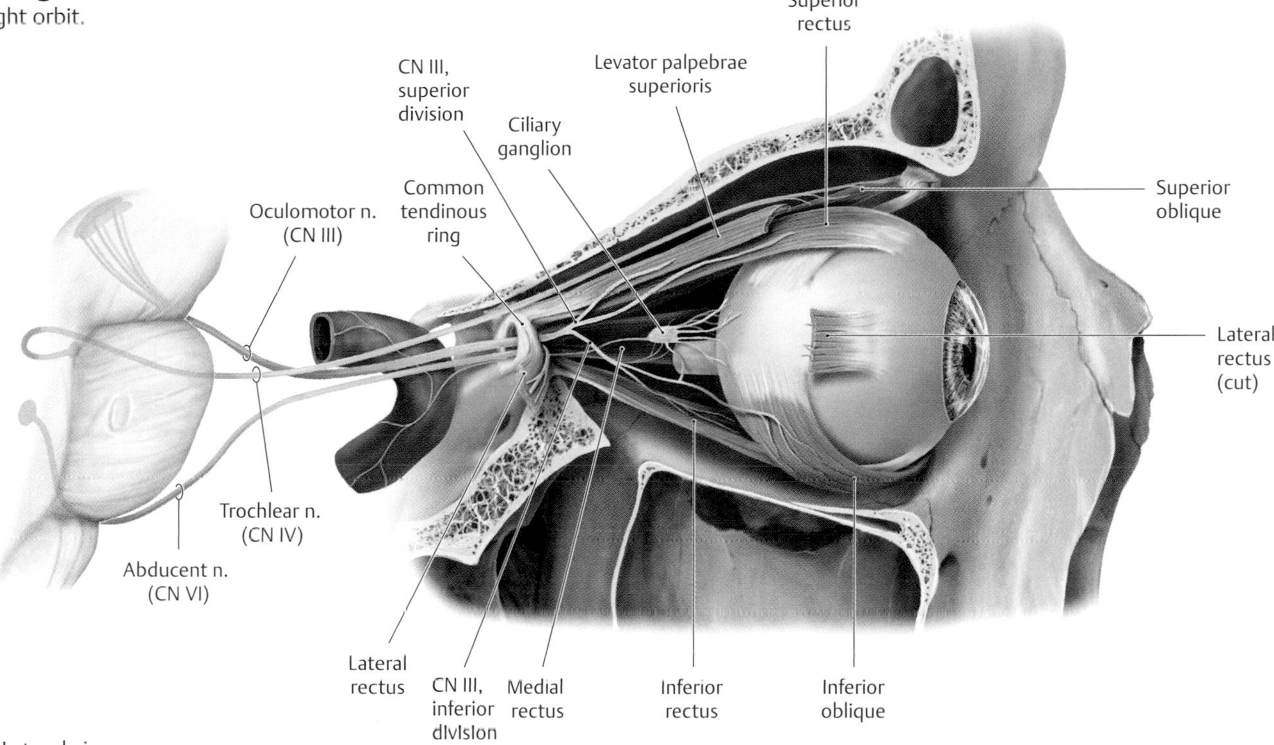
Superior rectus
CN III, superior division
Levator palpebrae superioris
Ciliary ganglion
Common tendinous ring
Oculomotor n. (CN III)
Superior oblique
Lateral rectus (cut)
Trochlear n. (CN IV)
Abducent n. (CN VI)
Lateral rectus
CN III, inferior division
Medial rectus
Inferior rectus
Inferior oblique

A Lateral view.

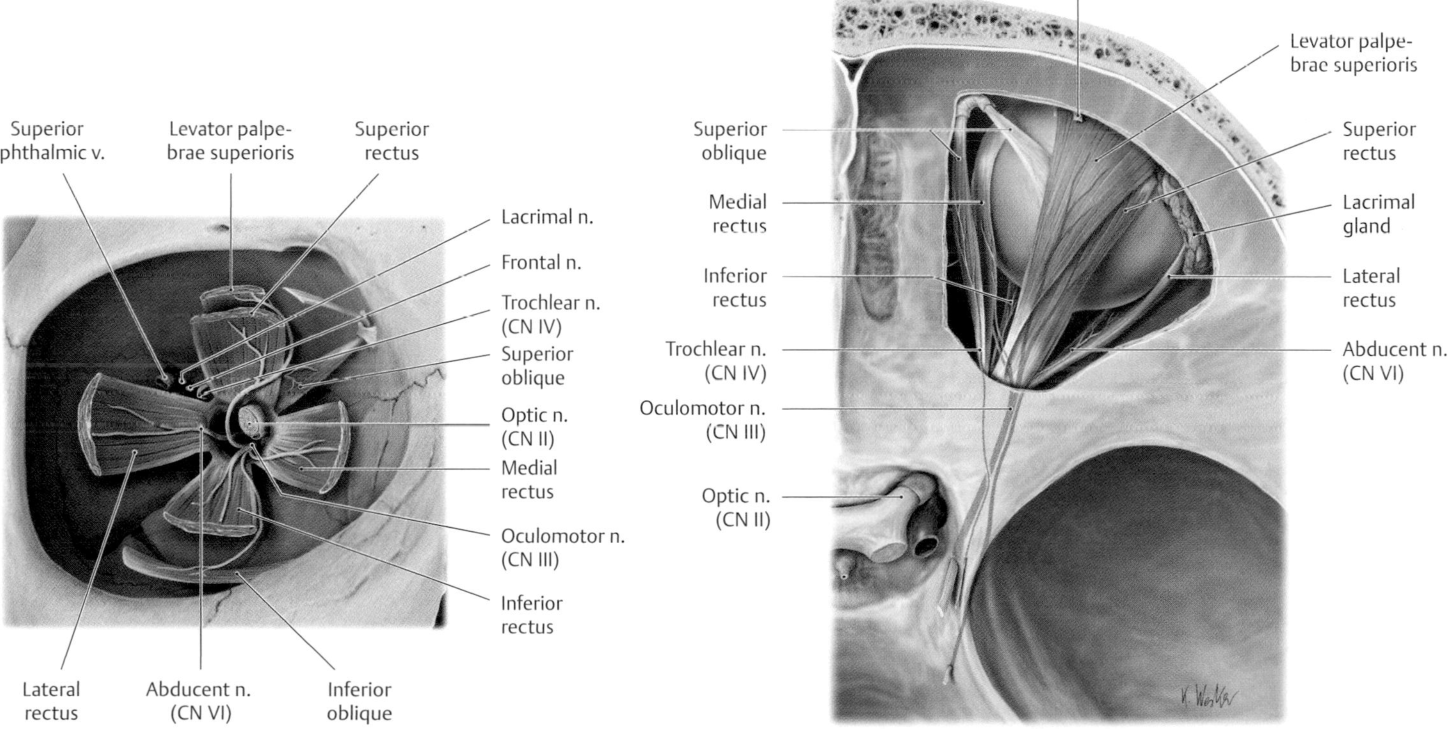
Superior ophthalmic v.
Levator palpebrae superioris
Superior rectus
Lacrimal n.
Frontal n.
Trochlear n. (CN IV)
Superior oblique
Optic n. (CN II)
Medial rectus
Oculomotor n. (CN III)
Inferior rectus
Lateral rectus
Abducent n. (CN VI)
Inferior oblique
Supraorbital n.
Levator palpebrae superioris
Superior oblique
Superior rectus
Medial rectus
Lacrimal gland
Inferior rectus
Lateral rectus
Trochlear n. (CN IV)
Abducent n. (CN VI)
Oculomotor n. (CN III)
Optic n. (CN II)

B Anterior view. CN II exits the orbit via the optic canal, which lies medial to the superior orbital fissure (site of emergence of CN III, IV, and VI).

C Superior view of the opened orbit. Note the relationship between the optic canal and the superior orbital fissure.

CN V: Trigeminal Nerve

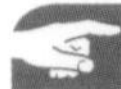

The trigeminal nerve, the sensory nerve of the head, has three somatic afferent nuclei: the mesencephalic nucleus, which receives proprioceptive fibers from the muscles of mastication; the principal (pontine) sensory nucleus, which chiefly mediates

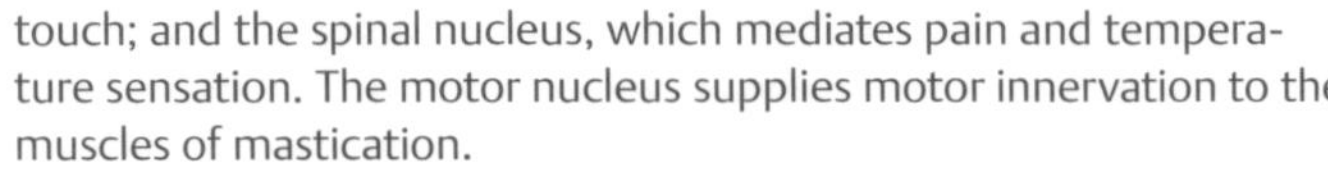

touch; and the spinal nucleus, which mediates pain and temperature sensation. The motor nucleus supplies motor innervation to the muscles of mastication.

Fig. 33.7 Trigeminal nerve nuclei

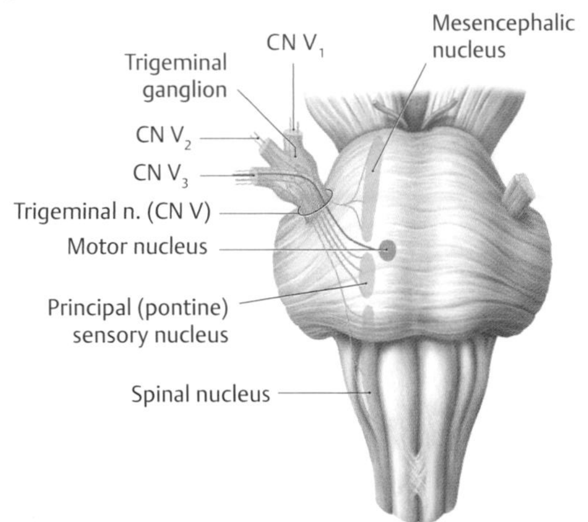

CN V₁
Mesencephalic nucleus
Trigeminal ganglion
CN V₂
CN V₃
Trigeminal n. (CN V)
Motor nucleus
Principal (pontine) sensory nucleus
Spinal nucleus

A Anterior view of the brainstem.

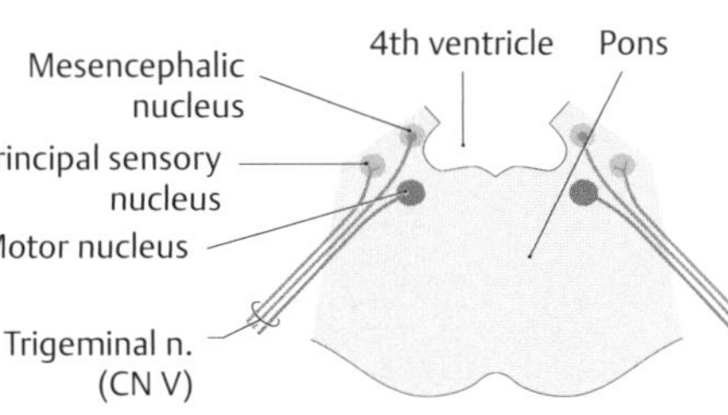

4th ventricle
Pons
Mesencephalic nucleus
Principal sensory nucleus
Motor nucleus
Trigeminal n. (CN V)

B Cross section through the pons, superior view.

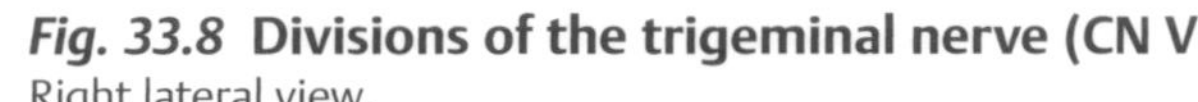

Fig. 33.8 Divisions of the trigeminal nerve (CN V)

Right lateral view.

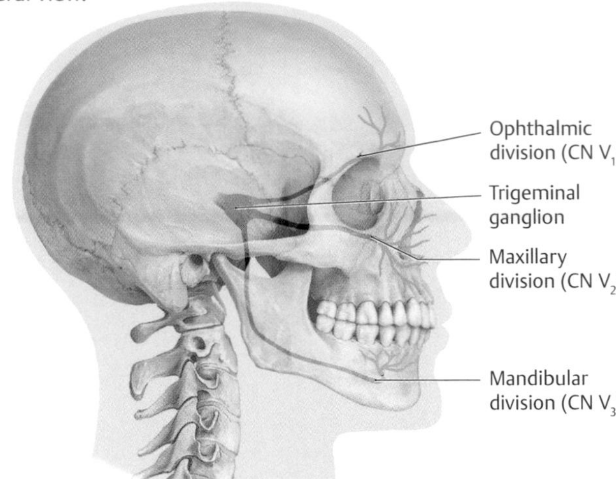

Ophthalmic division (CN V₁)
Trigeminal ganglion
Maxillary division (CN V₂)
Mandibular division (CN V₃)

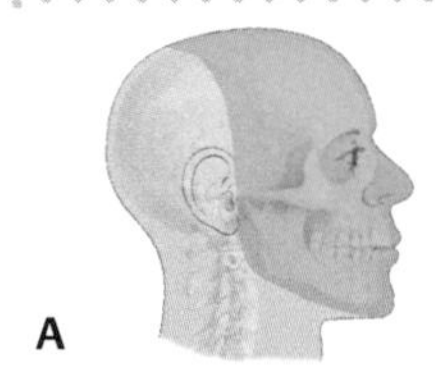

A

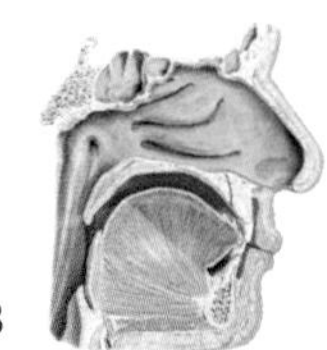

B

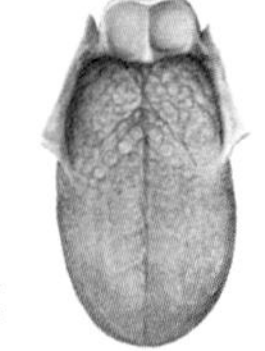

C

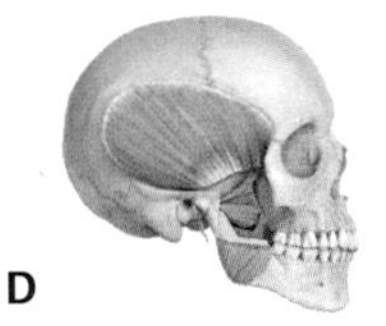

D

Table 33.4 Trigeminal nerve (CN V)

Course	Fibers	Nuclei	Function	Effects of nerve injury
Exits from the middle cranial fossa. **Ophthalmic division ($CN\ V_1$):** Enters orbit through superior orbital fissure **Maxillary division ($CN\ V_2$):** Enters pterygopalatine fossa through foramen rotundum **Mandibular division ($CN\ V_3$):** Passes through foramen ovale into infratemporal fossa	Somatic afferent	• Principal (pontine) sensory nucleus of the trigeminal n. • Mesencephalic nucleus of the trigeminal n. • Spinal nucleus of the trigeminal n.	Innervates: • Facial skin (**A**) • Nasopharyngeal mucosa (**B**) • Tongue (anterior two thirds) (**C**) Involved in the corneal reflex (reflex closure of eyelid)	• Sensory loss (traumatic nerve lesions) • Herpes zoster ophthalmicus (varicella-zoster virus); herpes zoster of the face
	Special visceral efferent	Motor nucleus of the trigeminal n.	Innervates (via $CN\ V_3$): • Muscles of mastication (temporalis, masseter, medial and lateral pterygoids (**D**)) • Oral floor muscles (mylohyoid, anterior digastric) • Tensor tympani • Tensor veli palatini	
	Visceral efferent pathway*	• Lacrimal n. ($CN\ V_1$) conveys parasympathetic fibers from CN VII along the zygomatic n. ($CN\ V_2$) to the lacrimal gland • Lingual n. ($CN\ V_3$) conveys parasympathetic fibers from CN VII (via the chorda tympani) to the submandibular and sublingual glands • Auriculotemporal n. ($CN\ V_3$) conveys parasympathetic fibers from CN IX to the parotid gland		
	Visceral afferent pathway*	Gustatory (taste) fibers from CN VII (via chorda tympani) travel with the lingual n. ($CN\ V_3$) to the anterior two thirds of the tongue		

* Fibers of certain cranial nerves adhere to divisions or branches of the trigeminal nerve, by which they travel to their destination.

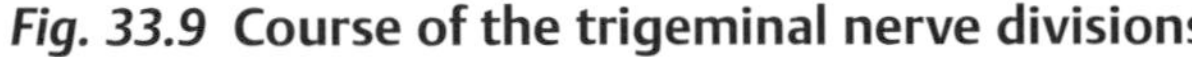

Fig. 33.9 **Course of the trigeminal nerve divisions**

Right lateral view.

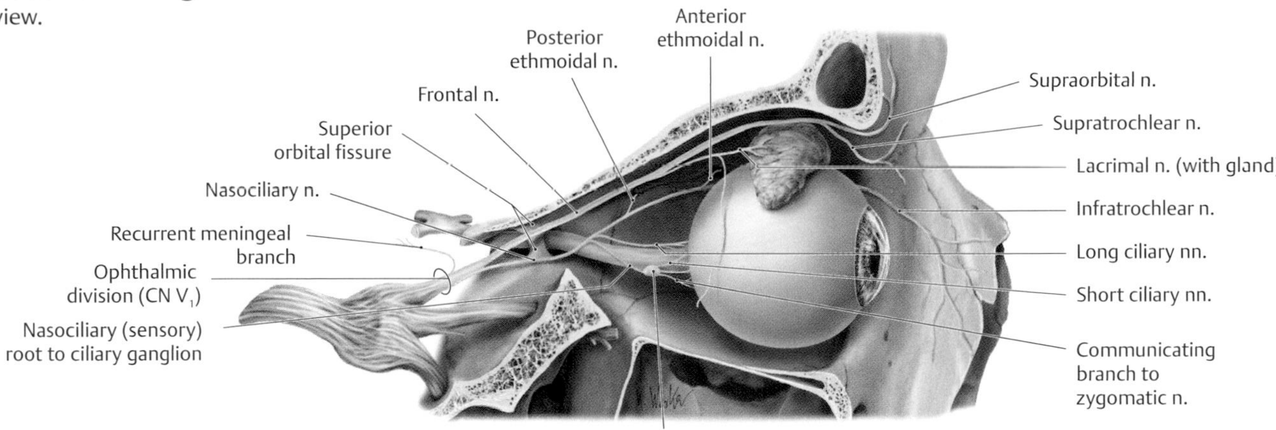

Anterior ethmoidal n.
Posterior ethmoidal n.
Frontal n.
Superior orbital fissure
Nasociliary n.
Recurrent meningeal branch
Ophthalmic division (CN V1)
Nasociliary (sensory) root to ciliary ganglion
Supraorbital n.
Supratrochlear n.
Lacrimal n. (with gland)
Infratrochlear n.
Long ciliary nn.
Short ciliary nn.
Communicating branch to zygomatic n.
Ciliary ganglion

A Ophthalmic division (CN V_1). Partially opened right orbit.

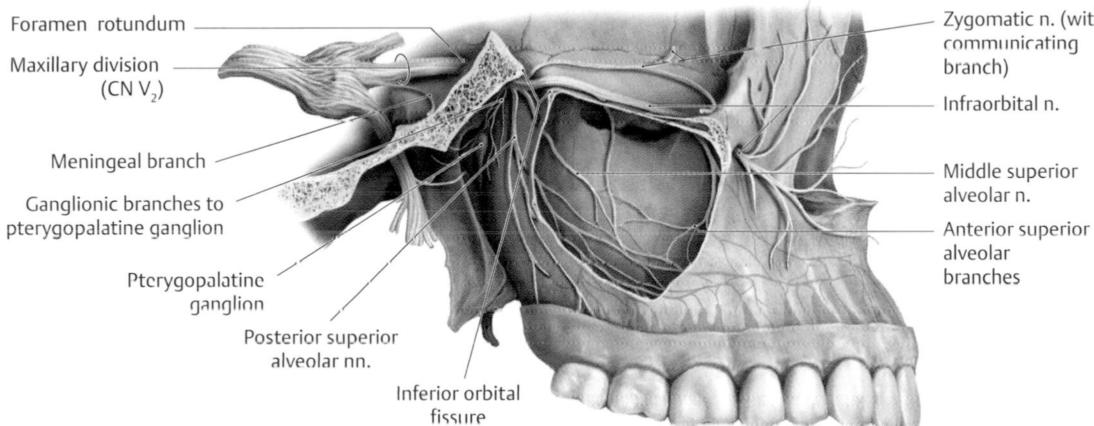

Foramen rotundum
Maxillary division (CN V2)
Meningeal branch
Ganglionic branches to pterygopalatine ganglion
Pterygopalatine ganglion
Posterior superior alveolar nn.
Inferior orbital fissure
Zygomatic n. (with communicating branch)
Infraorbital n.
Middle superior alveolar n.
Anterior superior alveolar branches

B Maxillary division (CN V_2). Partially opened right maxillary sinus with the zygomatic arch removed.

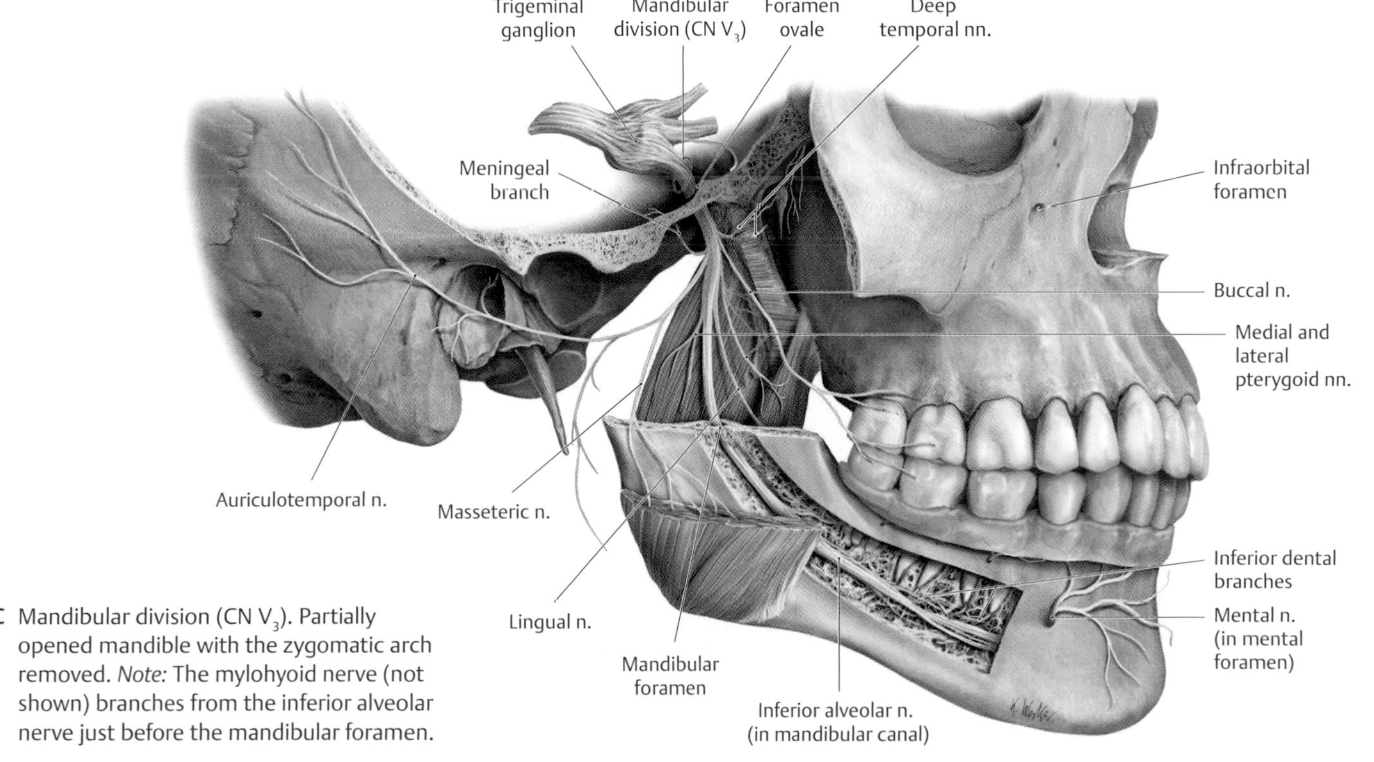

Trigeminal ganglion
Mandibular division (CN V3)
Foramen ovale
Deep temporal nn.
Meningeal branch
Infraorbital foramen
Buccal n.
Medial and lateral pterygoid nn.
Auriculotemporal n.
Masseteric n.
Lingual n.
Mandibular foramen
Inferior alveolar n. (in mandibular canal)
Inferior dental branches
Mental n. (in mental foramen)

C Mandibular division (CN V_3). Partially opened mandible with the zygomatic arch removed. *Note:* The mylohyoid nerve (not shown) branches from the inferior alveolar nerve just before the mandibular foramen.

CN VII: Facial Nerve

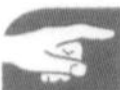

The facial nerve mainly conveys special visceral efferent (branchiogenic) fibers from the facial nerve nucleus to the muscles of facial expression. The other visceral efferent (parasympathetic) fibers from the superior salivatory nucleus are grouped with the visceral afferent (gustatory) fibers to form the nervus intermedius.

Fig. 33.10 Facial nerve nuclei

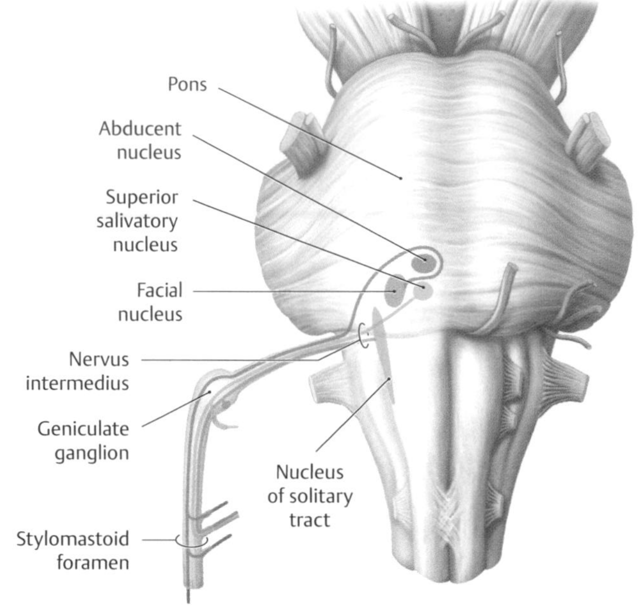
Pons
Abducent nucleus
Superior salivatory nucleus
Facial nucleus
Nervus intermedius
Geniculate ganglion
Nucleus of solitary tract
Stylomastoid foramen

A Anterior view of the brainstem.

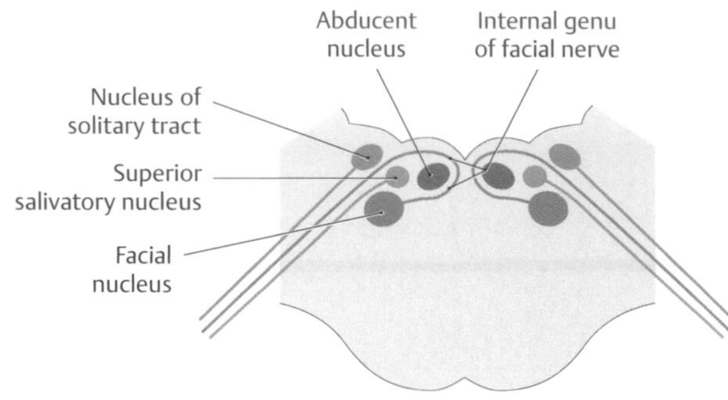
Abducent nucleus
Internal genu of facial nerve
Nucleus of solitary tract
Superior salivatory nucleus
Facial nucleus

B Cross section through the pons, superior view.

Fig. 33.11 Branches of the facial nerve

Right lateral view.

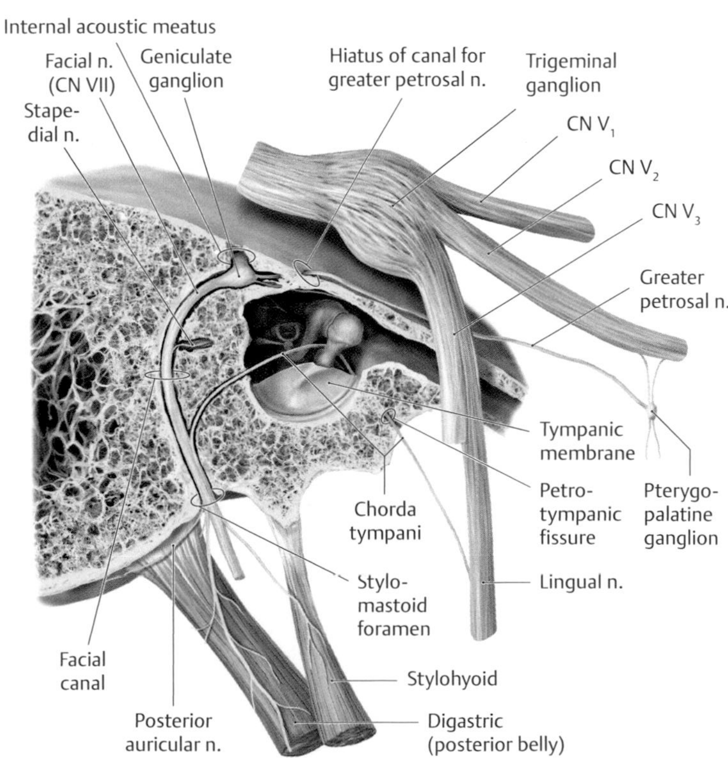
Internal acoustic meatus
Facial n. (CN VII)
Geniculate ganglion
Stapedial n.
Hiatus of canal for greater petrosal n.
Trigeminal ganglion
CN V1
CN V2
CN V3
Greater petrosal n.
Tympanic membrane
Chorda tympani
Petro-tympanic fissure
Pterygo-palatine ganglion
Stylo-mastoid foramen
Lingual n.
Facial canal
Stylohyoid
Posterior auricular n.
Digastric (posterior belly)

A Facial nerve in the temporal bone.

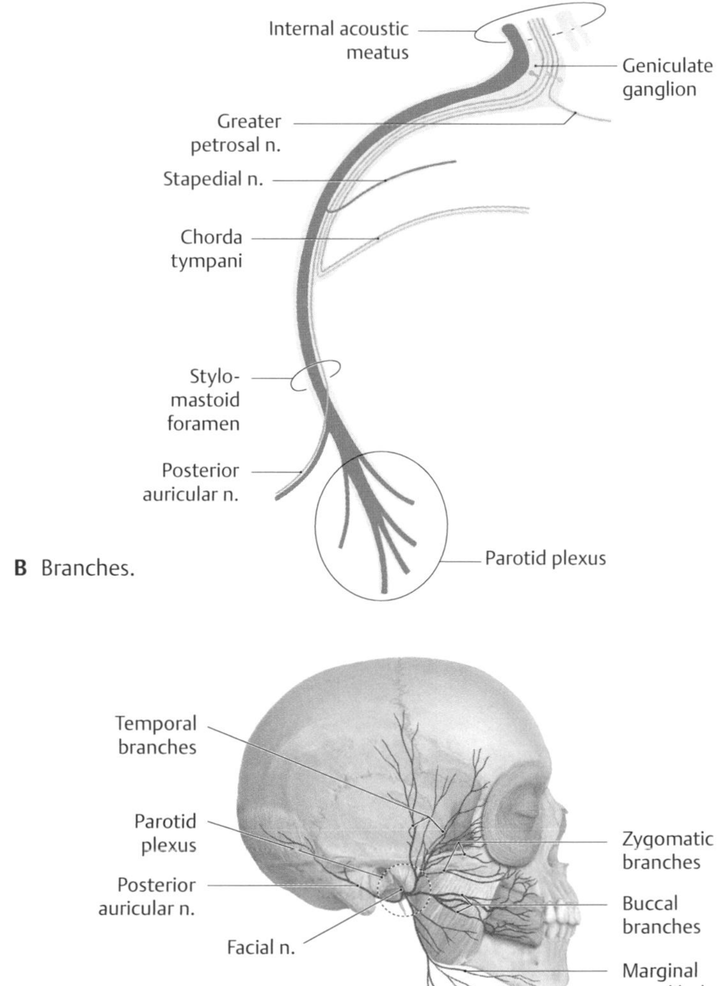
Internal acoustic meatus
Geniculate ganglion
Greater petrosal n.
Stapedial n.
Chorda tympani
Stylo-mastoid foramen
Posterior auricular n.
Parotid plexus
Temporal branches
Parotid plexus
Posterior auricular n.
Facial n.
Zygomatic branches
Buccal branches
Marginal mandibular branch
Cervical branch

B Branches.

C Parotid plexus.

Table 33.5 Facial nerve (CN VII)

Course	Fibers	Nuclei	Function	Effects of nerve injury
Emerges in the cerebellopontine angle between the pons and olive; passes through the internal acoustic meatus into the temporal bone (petrous part), where it divides into: • Greater petrosal nerve • Stapedial nerve • Chorda tympani Certain special visceral efferent fibers pass through the stylomastoid foramen to the skull base, forming the intraparotid plexus	Special visceral afferent	Facial nucleus	Innervate: • Muscles of facial expression • Stylohyoid • Digastric (posterior belly) • Stapedius	Peripheral facial nerve injury: paralysis of muscles of facial expression on affected side Associated disturbances of taste, lacrimation, salivation, hyperacusis, etc.
	Visceral efferent (parasympathetic)*	Superior salivatory nucleus	Synapse with neurons in the pterygopalatine or submandibular ganglion. Innervate: • Lacrimal gland • Small glands of nasal mucosa, hard and soft palate • Submandibular gland • Sublingual gland • Small salivary glands of tongue (dorsum)	
	Special visceral afferent*	Nucleus of the solitary tract	Peripheral processes of fibers from geniculate ganglion form the chorda tympani (gustatory fibers from tongue)	
	Somatic afferent	Sensory fibers from the auricle, skin of the auditory canal, and outer surface of the tympanic membrane travel via CN VII to the principal sensory nucleus of the trigeminal nerve		

* Grouped to form nervus intermedius, which aggregates with the visceral efferent fibers from the facial nerve nucleus.

***Fig. 33.12* Course of the facial nerve**
Right lateral view. Visceral efferent (parasympathetic) and special visceral afferent (taste) fibers shown in black.

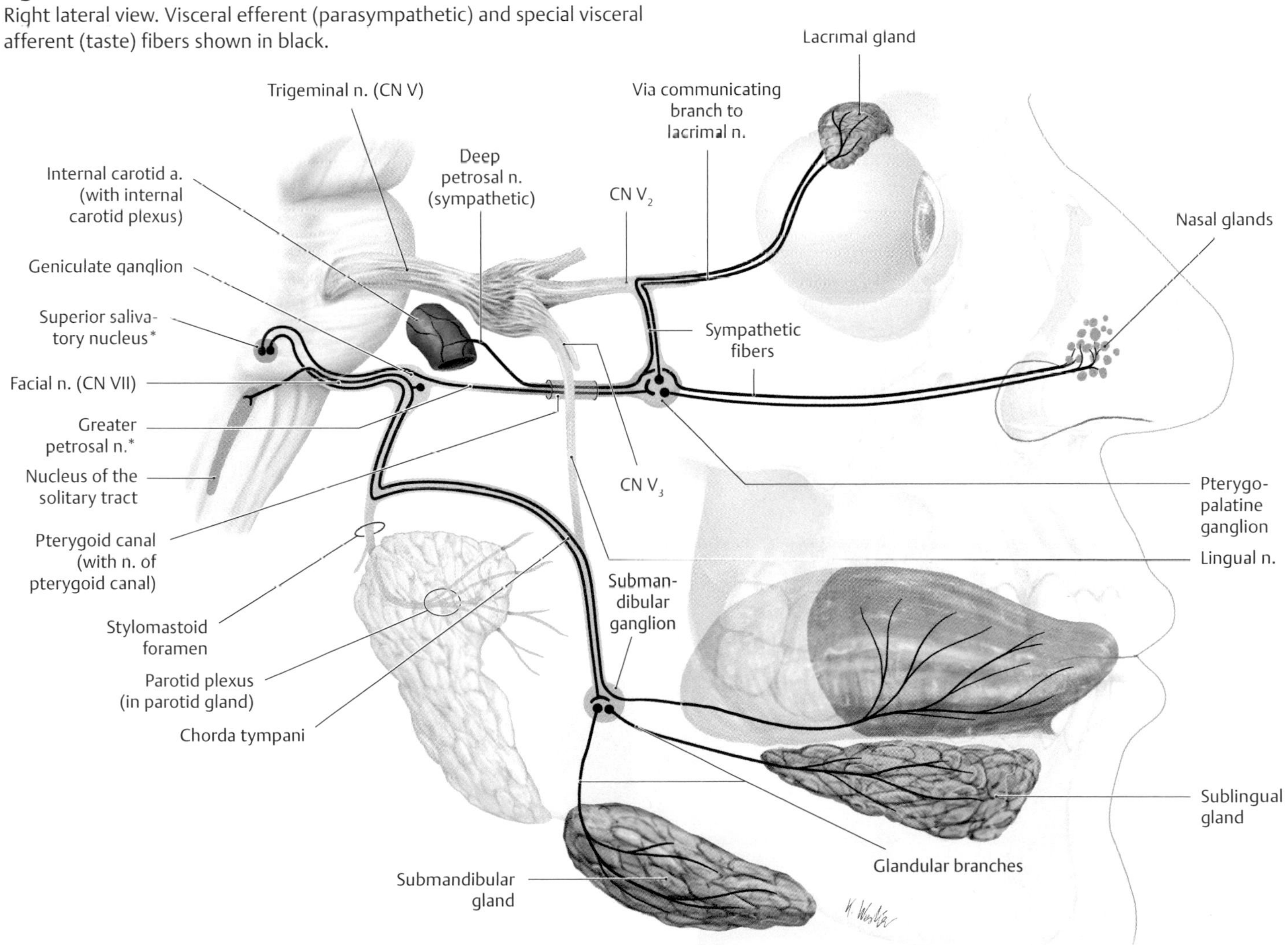

Lacrimal gland
Trigeminal n. (CN V)
Via communicating branch to lacrimal n.
Deep petrosal n. (sympathetic)
CN V_2
Internal carotid a. (with internal carotid plexus)
Nasal glands
Geniculate ganglion
Sympathetic fibers
Superior salivatory nucleus*
Facial n. (CN VII)
Greater petrosal n.*
Nucleus of the solitary tract
CN V_3
Pterygopalatine ganglion
Pterygoid canal (with n. of pterygoid canal)
Lingual n.
Submandibular ganglion
Stylomastoid foramen
Parotid plexus (in parotid gland)
Chorda tympani
Sublingual gland
Glandular branches
Submandibular gland

*Parasympathetic

CN VIII: Vestibulocochlear Nerve

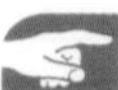

The vestibulochochlear nerve is a special somatic afferent nerve that consists of two roots. The vestibular root transmits impulses from the vestibular apparatus (balance, see p. 644); the cochlear root transmits impulses from the auditory apparatus (hearing, see p. 645).

Fig. 33.13 Vestibulocochlear nerve: Vestibular part

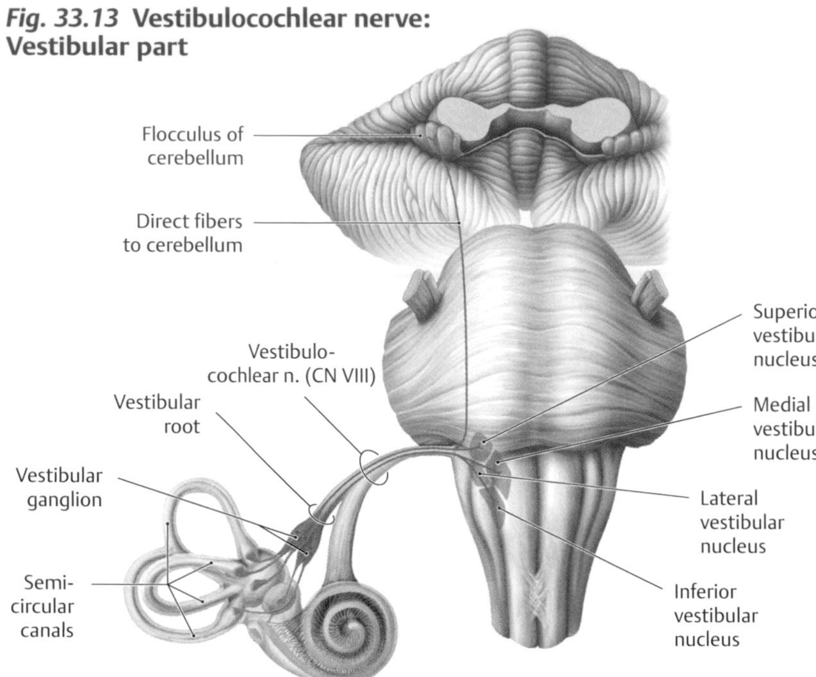

Flocculus of cerebellum
Direct fibers to cerebellum
Vestibulo-cochlear n. (CN VIII)
Vestibular root
Vestibular ganglion
Semi-circular canals
Superior vestibular nucleus
Medial vestibular nucleus
Lateral vestibular nucleus
Inferior vestibular nucleus

A Anterior view of the medulla oblongata and pons with cerebellum.

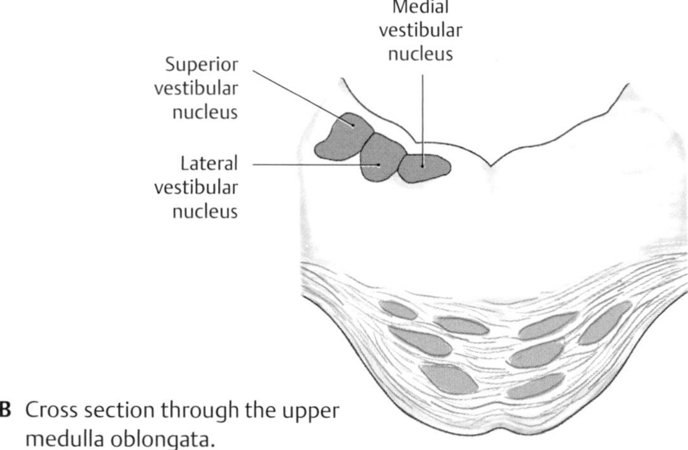

Medial vestibular nucleus
Superior vestibular nucleus
Lateral vestibular nucleus

B Cross section through the upper medulla oblongata.

Fig. 33.14 Vestibulocochlear nerve: Cochlear part

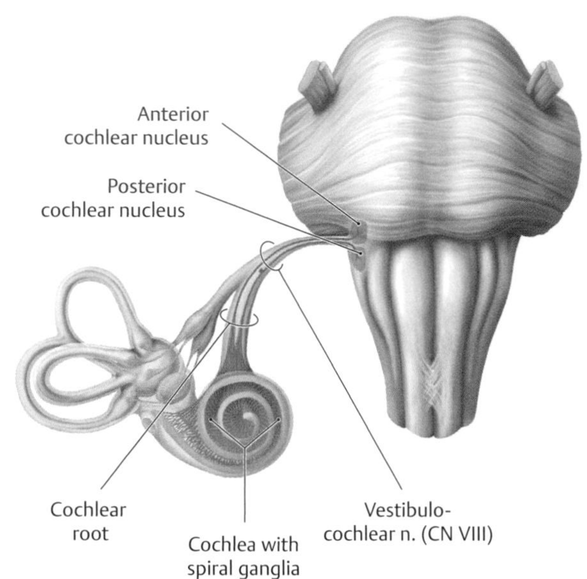

Anterior cochlear nucleus
Posterior cochlear nucleus
Cochlear root
Cochlea with spiral ganglia
Vestibulo-cochlear n. (CN VIII)

A Anterior view of the medulla oblongata and pons.

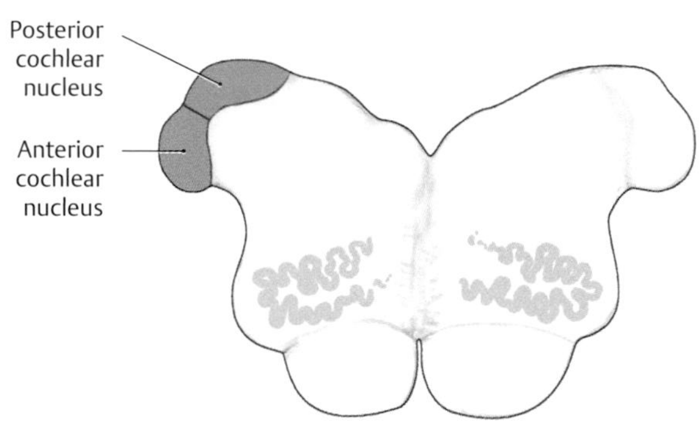

Posterior cochlear nucleus
Anterior cochlear nucleus

B Cross section through the upper medulla oblongata.

Table 33.6 **Vestibulocochlear nerve (CN VIII)**

Part	Course	Fibers	Nuclei	Function	Effects of nerve injury
Vestibular part	Pass from the inner ear through the internal acoustic meatus to the cerebellopontine angle, where they enter the brain	Special somatic afferent	Superior, lateral, medial, and inferior vestibular nuclei	Peripheral processes from the semicircular canals, saccule, and utricle pass to the vestibular ganglion and then to the four vestibular nuclei	Dizziness
Cochlear part			Anterior and posterior cochlear nuclei	Peripheral processes beginning at the hair cells of the organ of Corti pass to the spiral ganglion and then to the two cochlear nuclei	Hearing loss

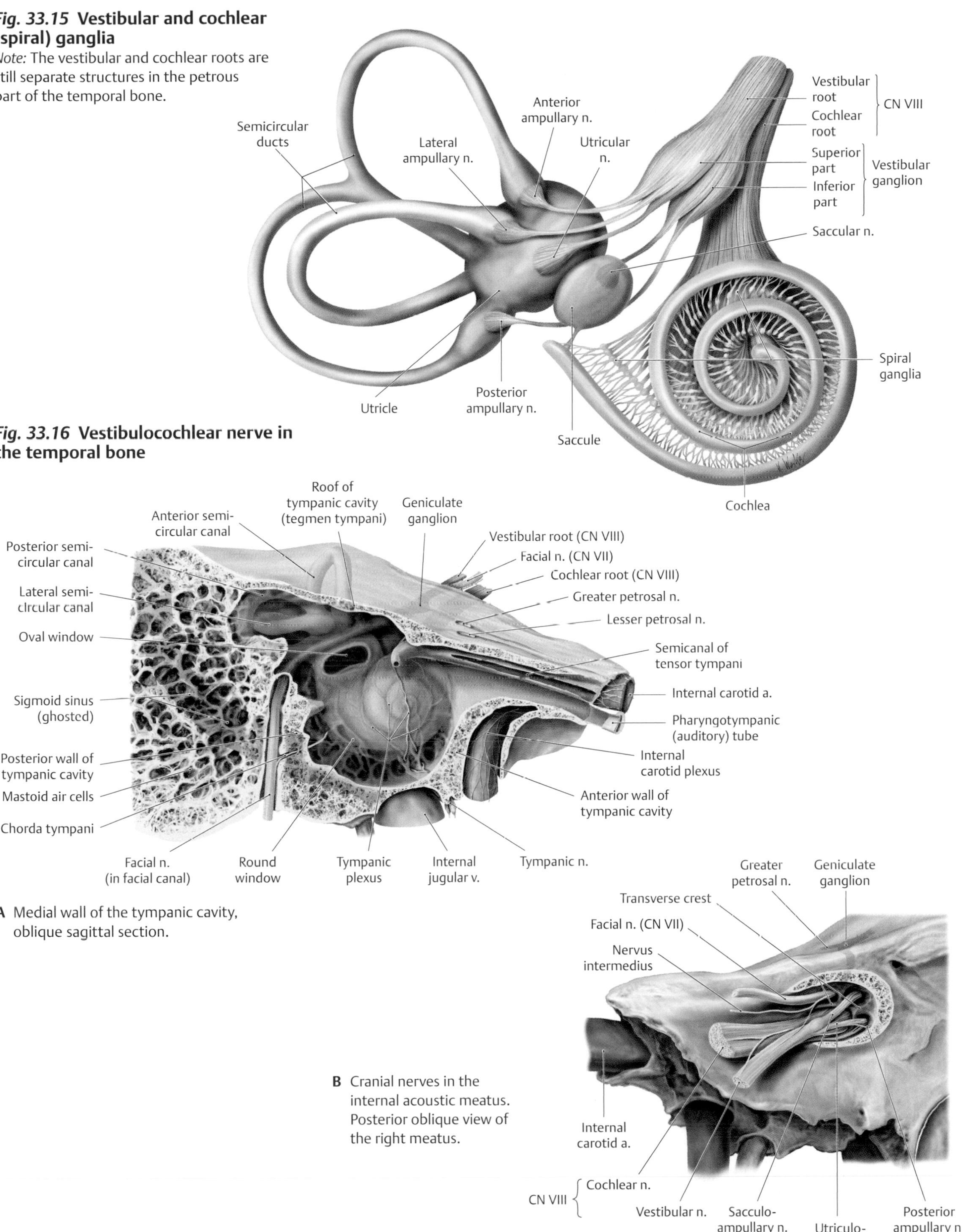
Semicircular ducts
Anterior ampullary n.
Lateral ampullary n.
Utricular n.
Vestibular root
Cochlear root
CN VIII
Superior part
Inferior part
Vestibular ganglion
Saccular n.
Spiral ganglia
Utricle
Posterior ampullary n.
Saccule
Cochlea
Roof of tympanic cavity (tegmen tympani)
Geniculate ganglion
Anterior semi-circular canal
Posterior semi-circular canal
Lateral semi-circular canal
Oval window
Sigmoid sinus (ghosted)
Posterior wall of tympanic cavity
Mastoid air cells
Chorda tympani
Vestibular root (CN VIII)
Facial n. (CN VII)
Cochlear root (CN VIII)
Greater petrosal n.
Lesser petrosal n.
Semicanal of tensor tympani
Internal carotid a.
Pharyngotympanic (auditory) tube
Internal carotid plexus
Anterior wall of tympanic cavity
Facial n. (in facial canal)
Round window
Tympanic plexus
Internal jugular v.
Tympanic n.
Greater petrosal n.
Geniculate ganglion
Transverse crest
Facial n. (CN VII)
Nervus intermedius
Internal carotid a.
CN VIII
Cochlear n.
Vestibular n.
Sacculo-ampullary n.
Utriculo-ampullary n.
Posterior ampullary n.

Fig. 33.15 **Vestibular and cochlear (spiral) ganglia**

Note: The vestibular and cochlear roots are still separate structures in the petrous part of the temporal bone.

Fig. 33.16 **Vestibulocochlear nerve in the temporal bone**

A Medial wall of the tympanic cavity, oblique sagittal section.

B Cranial nerves in the internal acoustic meatus. Posterior oblique view of the right meatus.

CN IX: Glossopharyngeal Nerve

Fig. 33.17 Glossopharyngeal nerve nuclei

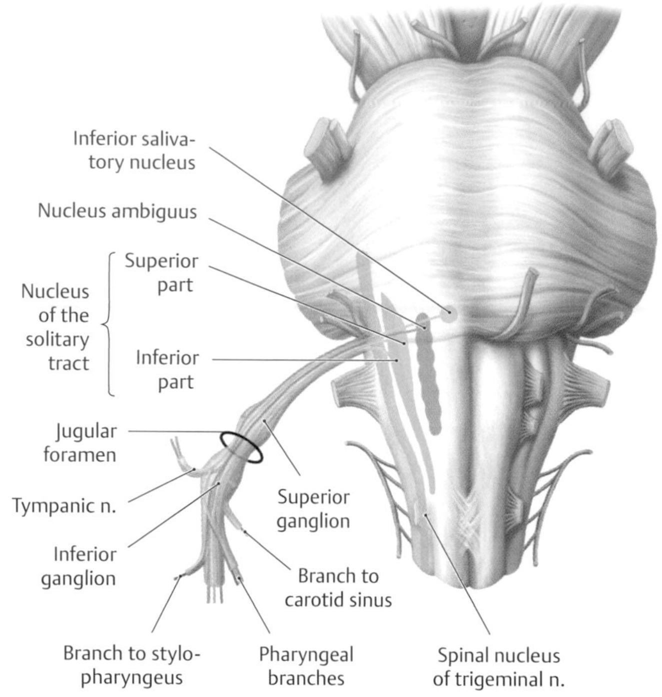
Inferior salivatory nucleus
Nucleus ambiguus
Nucleus of the solitary tract
Superior part
Inferior part
Jugular foramen
Tympanic n.
Inferior ganglion
Superior ganglion
Branch to carotid sinus
Branch to stylopharyngeus
Pharyngeal branches
Spinal nucleus of trigeminal n.

A Anterior view of the medulla oblongata.

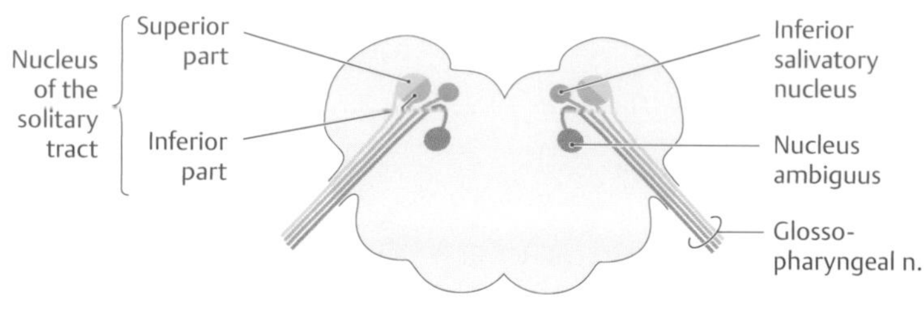
Nucleus of the solitary tract
Superior part
Inferior part
Inferior salivatory nucleus
Nucleus ambiguus
Glosso-pharyngeal n.

B Cross section through the medulla oblongata, superior view. *Not shown:* Nuclei of the trigeminal nerve.

Fig. 33.18 Course of the glossopharyngeal nerve

Left lateral view. *Note:* Fibers from the vagus nerve (CN X) combine with fibers from CN IX to form the pharyngeal plexus and supply the carotid sinus.

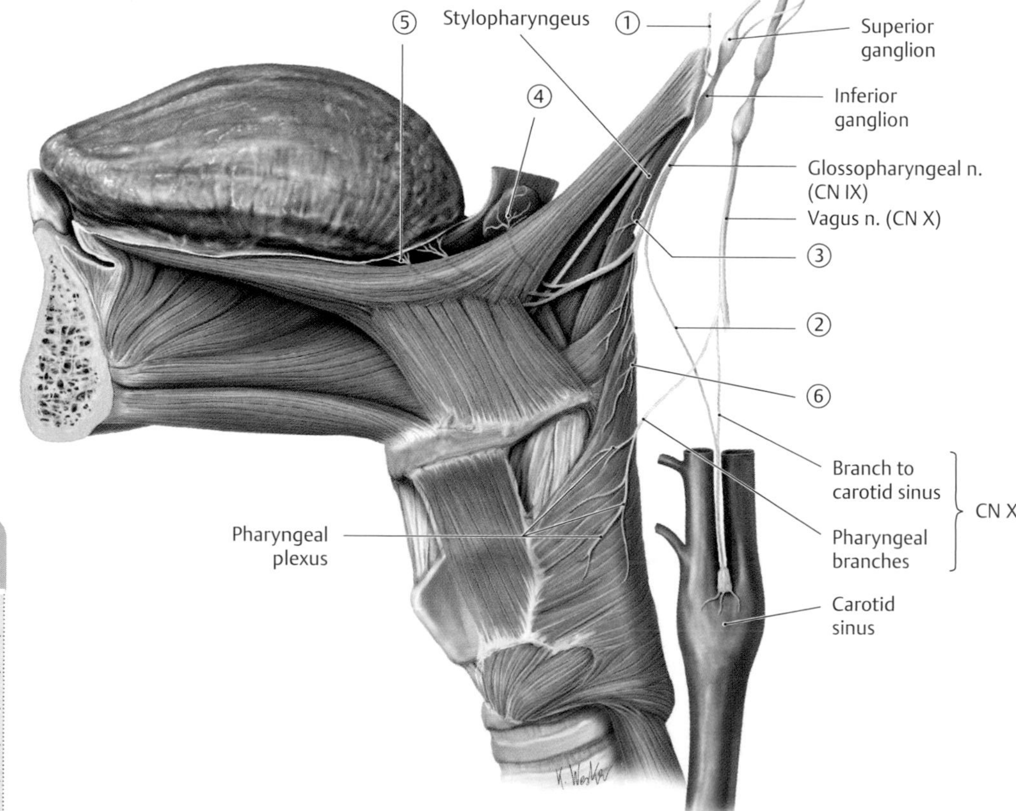
⑤
Stylopharyngeus
①
④
Superior ganglion
Inferior ganglion
Glossopharyngeal n. (CN IX)
Vagus n. (CN X)
③
②
⑥
Branch to carotid sinus
Pharyngeal branches
CN X
Pharyngeal plexus
Carotid sinus

Table 33.7	Glossopharyngeal nerve branches
①	Tympanic n.
②	Branch to carotid sinus
③	Branch to stylopharyngeus muscle
④	Tonsillar branches
⑤	Lingual branches
⑥	Pharyngeal branches

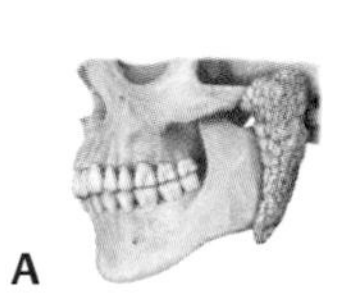
A

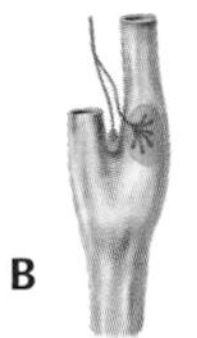
B

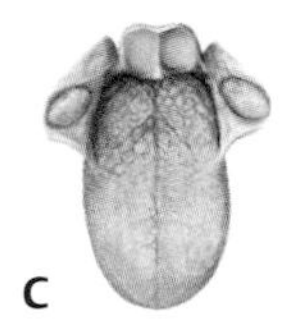
C

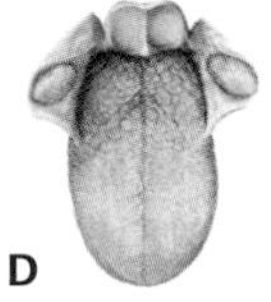
D

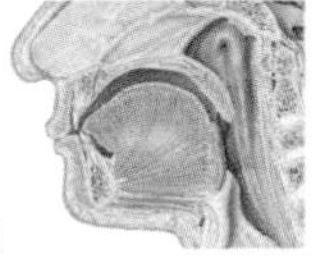
E

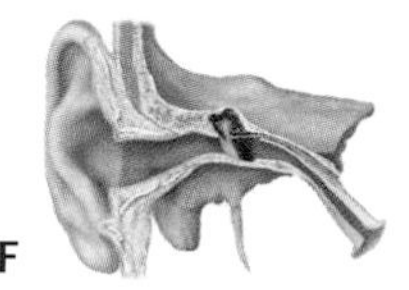
F

Table 33.8 **Glossopharyngeal nerve (CN IX)**

Course	Fibers	Nuclei	Function	Effects of nerve injury
Emerges from the medulla oblongata; leaves cranial cavity through the jugular foramen	Visceral efferent (parasympathetic)	Inferior salivatory nucleus	Parasympathetic presynaptic fibers are sent to the otic ganglion; postsynaptic fibers are distributed to • Parotid gland (**A**) • Buccal gland • Labial gland	Isolated lesions of CN IX are rare. Lesions are generally accompanied by lesions of CN X and CN XI (cranial part), as all three emerge jointly from the jugular foramen and are susceptible to injury in basal skull fractures.
	Special visceral efferent (branchiogenic)	Nucleus ambiguus	Innervate: • Constrictor muscles of the pharynx (pharyngeal branches join with the vagus nerve to form the pharyngeal plexus) • Stylopharyngeus	
	Visceral afferent	Nucleus of the solitary tract (inferior part)	Receive sensory information from • Chemoreceptors in the carotid body (**B**) • Pressure receptors in the carotid sinus	
	Special visceral afferent	Nucleus of the solitary tract (superior part)	Receives sensory information from the posterior third of the tongue (via the inferior ganglion) (**C**)	
	Somatic afferent	Spinal nucleus of trigeminal nerve	Peripheral processes of the intracranial superior ganglion or the extracranial inferior ganglion arise from • Tongue, soft palate, pharyngeal mucosa, and tonsils (**D,E**) • Mucosa of the tympanic cavity, internal surface of the tympanic membrane, pharyngotympanic tube (tympanic plexus) (**F**) • Skin of the external ear and auditory canal (blends with the vagus nerve)	

Fig. 33.19 **Glossopharyngeal nerve in the tympanic cavity**
Left anterolateral view. The tympanic nerve contains visceral efferent (presynaptic parasympathetic) fibers for the otic ganglion, as well as somatic afferent fibers for the tympanic cavity and pharyngotympanic tube. It joins with sympathetic fibers from the internal carotid plexus (via the caroticotympanic nerve) to form the tympanic plexus.

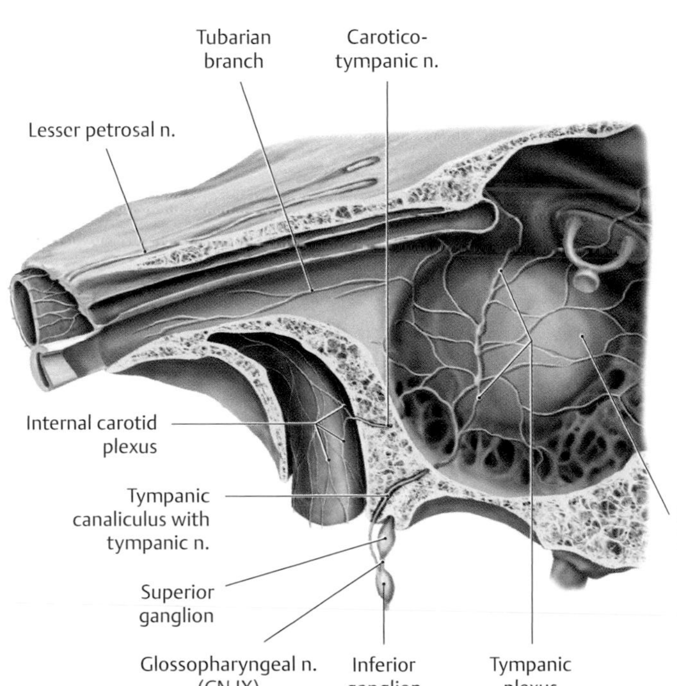
Tubarian branch
Carotico-tympanic n.
Lesser petrosal n.
Internal carotid plexus
Tympanic canaliculus with tympanic n.
Superior ganglion
Glossopharyngeal n. (CN IX)
Inferior ganglion
Tympanic plexus
Promontory of labyrinthine wall

Fig. 33.20 **Visceral efferent (parasympathetic) fibers of CN IX**

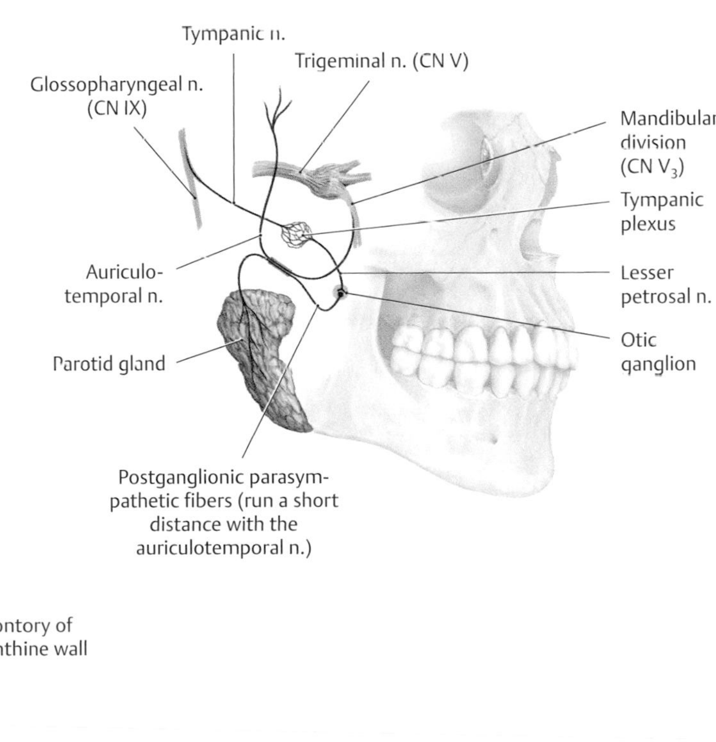
Tympanic n.
Trigeminal n. (CN V)
Glossopharyngeal n. (CN IX)
Mandibular division (CN V_3)
Tympanic plexus
Auriculo-temporal n.
Lesser petrosal n.
Otic ganglion
Parotid gland
Postganglionic parasympathetic fibers (run a short distance with the auriculotemporal n.)

CN X: Vagus Nerve

Fig. 33.21 **Vagus nerve nuclei**

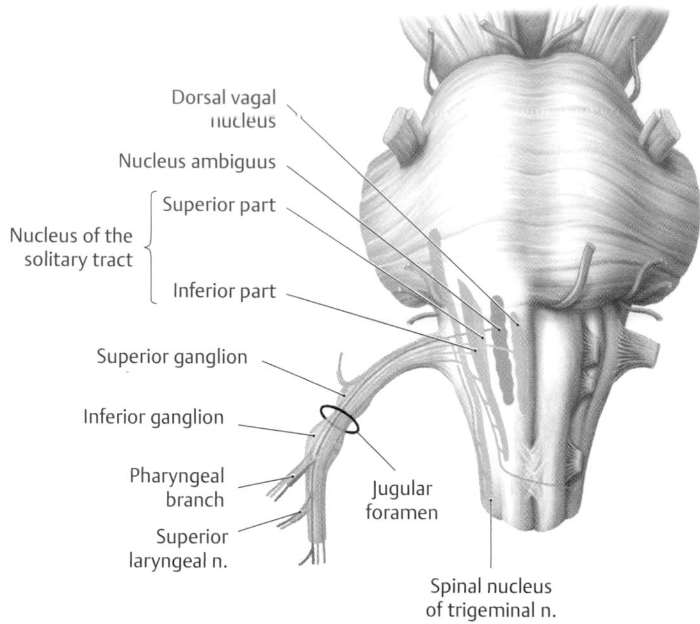
Dorsal vagal nucleus
Nucleus ambiguus
Nucleus of the solitary tract
Superior part
Inferior part
Superior ganglion
Inferior ganglion
Pharyngeal branch
Superior laryngeal n.
Jugular foramen
Spinal nucleus of trigeminal n.

A Anterior view of the medulla oblongata.

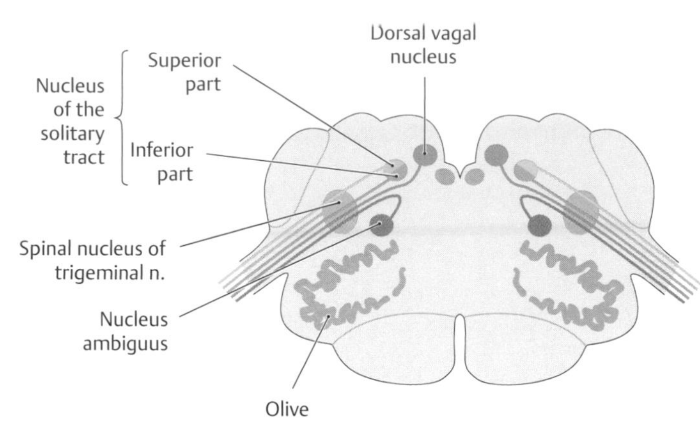
Nucleus of the solitary tract
Superior part
Inferior part
Dorsal vagal nucleus
Spinal nucleus of trigeminal n.
Nucleus ambiguus
Olive

B Cross section through the medulla oblongata, superior view.

Table 33.9 Vagus nerve (CN X)

Course	Fibers	Nuclei	Function	Effects of nerve injury
Emerges from the medulla oblongata; leaves the cranial cavity through the jugular foramen. CN X has the most extensive distribution of all the cranial nerves (vagus = "vagabond"), consisting of cranial, cervical, thoracic (see p. 82), and abdominal (see p. 203) parts.	Special visceral efferent (branchiogenic)	Nucleus ambiguus	Innervate: • Pharyngeal muscles (via pharyngeal plexus with CN IX) • Muscles of the soft palate • Laryngeal muscles (superior laryngeal n. supplies the cricothyroid; inferior laryngeal n. supplies all other laryngeal muscles)	The recurrent laryngeal nerve supplies visceromotor innervation to the only muscle abducting the vocal cords, the posterior cricoarytenoid. Unilateral destruction of this nerve leads to hoarseness; bilateral destruction leads to respiratory distress (dyspnea).
	Visceral efferent (parasympathetic)	Dorsal vagal nucleus	Synapse in prevertebral or intramural ganglia. Innervate smooth muscle and glands of • Thoracic viscera (**A**) • Abdominal viscera (**A**)	
	Somatic afferent	Spinal nucleus of trigeminal nerve	Superior (jugular) ganglion receives peripheral fibers from • Dura in posterior cranial fossa (**C**) • Skin of ear (**D**), external auditory canal (**E**)	
	Special visceral afferent	Nucleus of solitary tract (superior part)	Inferior nodose ganglion receives peripheral processes from • Taste buds on the epiglottis (**F**)	
	Visceral afferent	Nucleus of solitary tract (inferior part)	Inferior ganglion receives peripheral processes from • Mucosa of lower pharynx at its esophageal junction (**G**) • Laryngeal mucosa above (superior laryngeal n.) and below (inferior laryngeal n.) the vocal fold (**G**) • Pressure receptors in the aortic arch (**B**) • Chemoreceptors in the para-aortic body (**B**) • Thoracic and abdominal viscera (**A**)	

Fig. 33.22 Course of the vagus nerve
The vagus nerve gives off four major branches in the neck. The inferior laryngeal nerves are the terminal branches of the recurrent laryngeal nerves. *Note:* The left recurrent laryngeal nerve hooks around the aortic arch, while the right nerve hooks around the subclavian artery.

Table 33.10	Vagus nerve branches in the neck
①	Pharyngeal branches
②	Superior laryngeal n.
3R	Right recurrent laryngeal n.
3L	Left recurrent laryngeal n.
④	Cervical cardiac branches

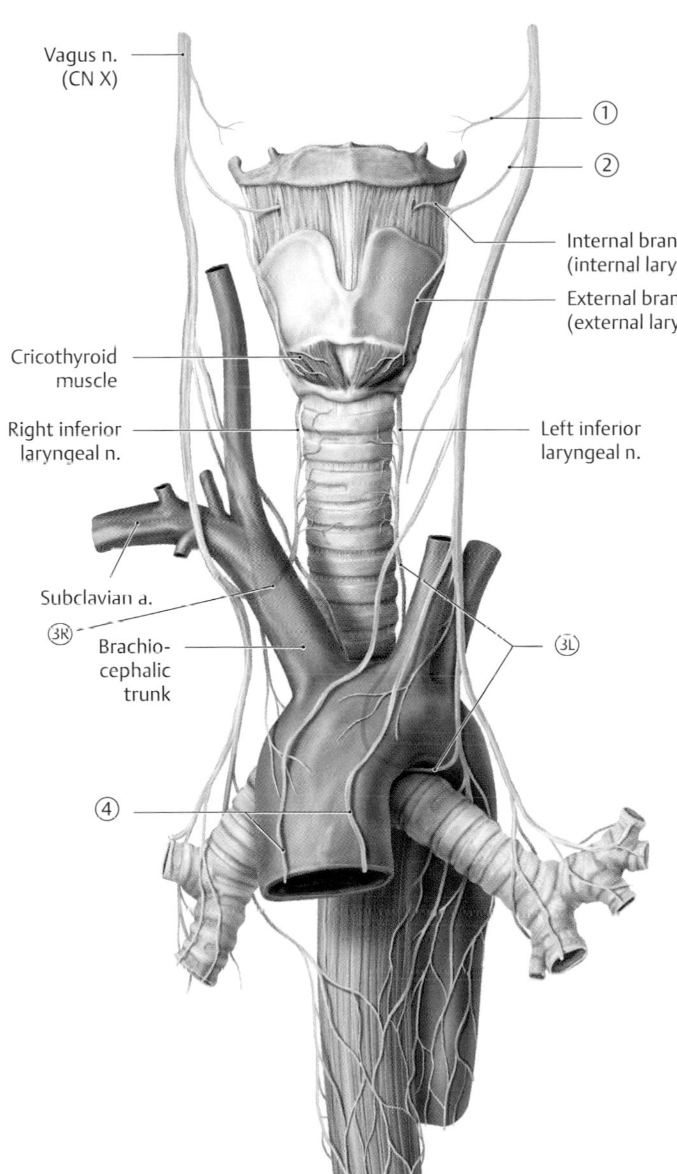
Vagus n. (CN X)
①
②
Internal branch (internal laryngeal n.)
External branch (external laryngeal n.)
Cricothyroid muscle
Right inferior laryngeal n.
Left inferior laryngeal n.
Subclavian a.
3R
Brachio-cephalic trunk
3L
④

A Branches of the vagus nerve in the neck. Anterior view.

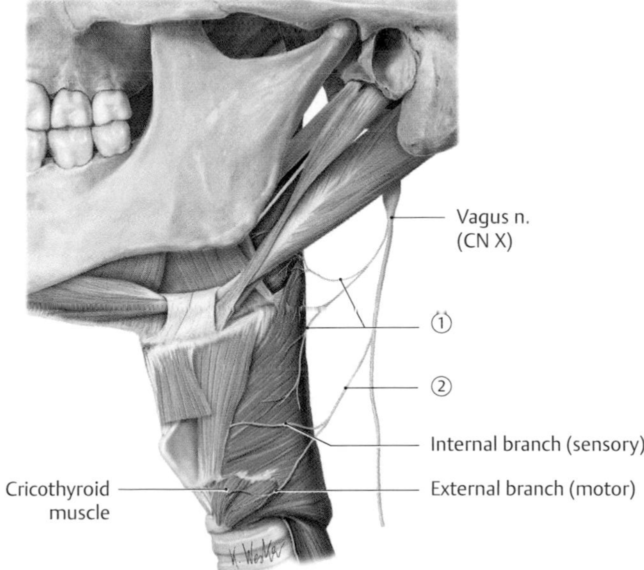
Vagus n. (CN X)
①
②
Internal branch (sensory)
External branch (motor)
Cricothyroid muscle

B Innervation of the pharyngeal and laryngeal muscles. Left lateral view.

CN XI & XII: Accessory & Hypoglossal Nerves

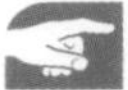

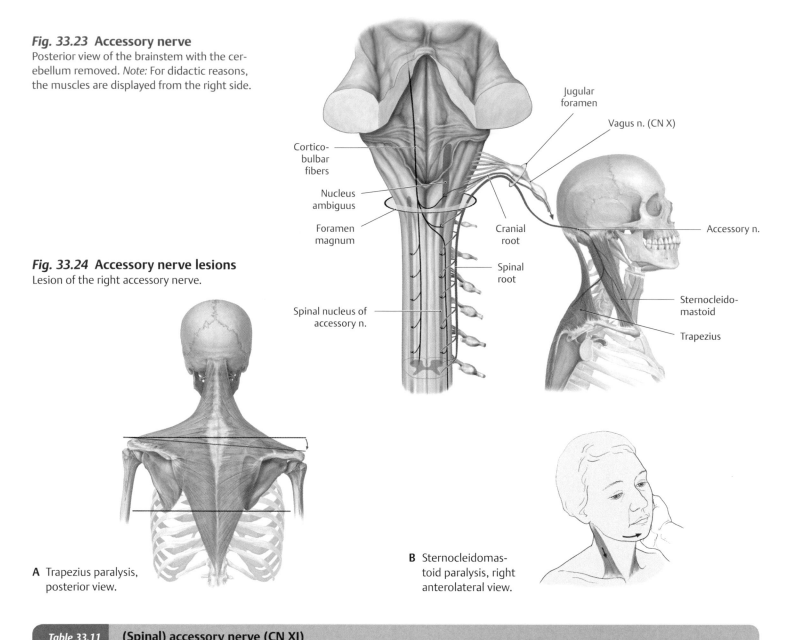

The traditional "cranial root" of the accessory nerve (CN XI) is now considered a part of the vagus nerve (CN X) that travels with the spinal root for a short distance before splitting. The cranial fibers are distributed via the vagus nerve while the spinal root fibers continue on as the accessory nerve (CN XI).

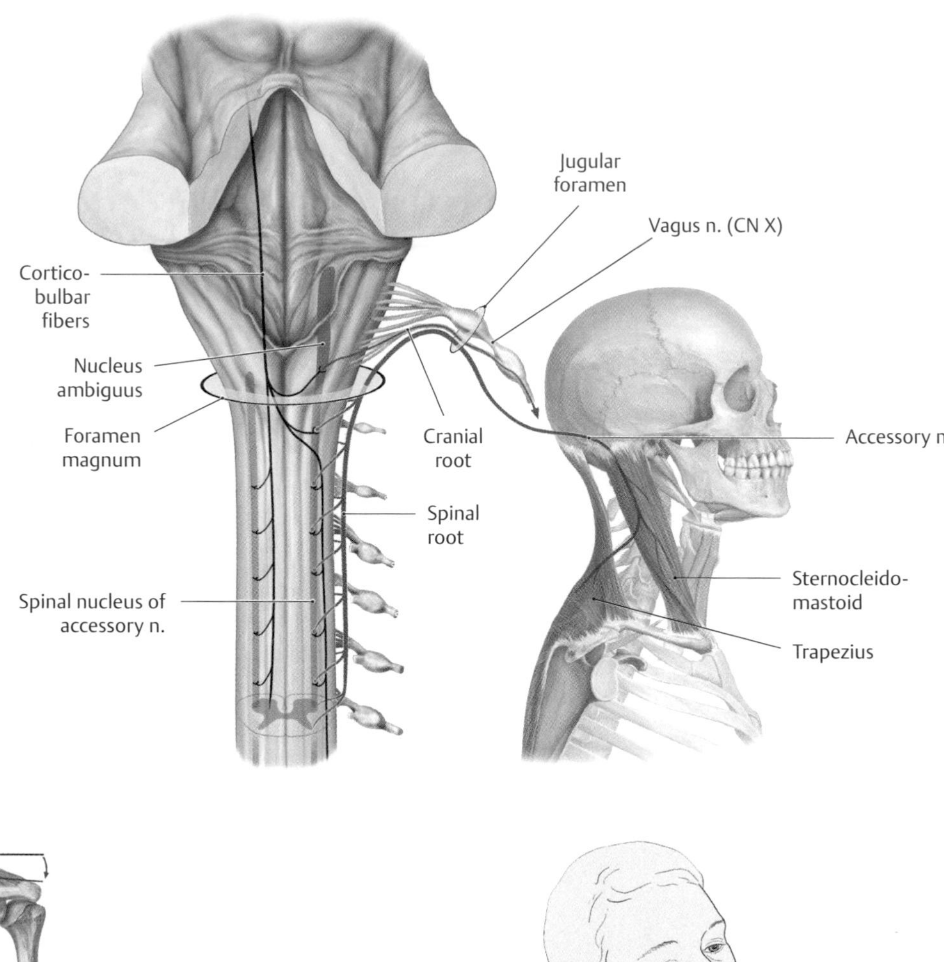

Cortico-
bulbar
fibers
Nucleus
ambiguus
Foramen
magnum
Spinal nucleus of
accessory n.
Jugular
foramen
Vagus n. (CN X)
Cranial
root
Spinal
root
Accessory n.
Sternocleido-
mastoid
Trapezius

Fig. 33.23 **Accessory nerve**
Posterior view of the brainstem with the cerebellum removed. *Note:* For didactic reasons, the muscles are displayed from the right side.

Fig. 33.24 **Accessory nerve lesions**
Lesion of the right accessory nerve.

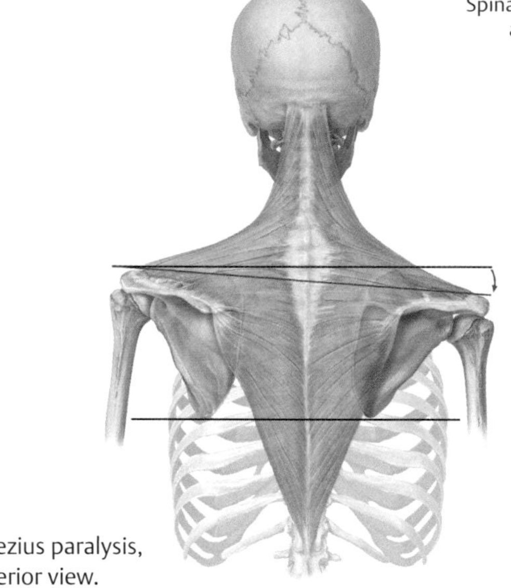

A Trapezius paralysis, posterior view.

B Sternocleidomastoid paralysis, right anterolateral view.

Table 33.11 **(Spinal) accessory nerve (CN XI)**

Course	Fibers	Nuclei	Function	Effects of nerve injury
The spinal root emerges from the spinal cord (at the level of C1–C5/6), passes superiorly, and enters the skull through the foramen magnum, where it joins with the cranial root from the medulla oblongata. Both roots leave the skull through the jugular foramen. Within the jugular foramen, fibers from the cranial root pass to the vagus nerve (internal branch). The spinal portion descends to the nuchal region as the external branch.	Special visceral efferent	Nucleus ambiguus (caudal part)	Join CN X and are distributed with the recurrent laryngeal nerve. Innervate: • All laryngeal muscles (except cricothyroid)	*Trapezius paralysis:* drooping of shoulder on affected side and difficulty raising arm above horizontal plane. This paralysis is a concern during neck operations (e.g., lymph node biopsies). An injury of the accessory nerve will not result in complete trapezius paralysis (the muscle is also innervated by segments C3 and C4/5). *Sternocleidomastoid paralysis:* torticollis (wry neck, i.e., difficulty turning head). Unilateral lesions cause flaccid paralysis (the muscle is supplied exclusively by the accessory nerve). Bilateral lesions make it difficult to hold the head upright.
	Somatic efferent	Spinal nucleus of accessory n.	Form the external branch of the accessory nerve. Innervate: • Trapezius • Sternocleidomastoid	

Fig. 33.25 **Hypoglossal nerve**
Posterior view of the brainstem with the cerebellum removed. *Note:* C1, which innervates the thyrohyoid and geniohyoid, runs briefly with the hypoglossal nerve.

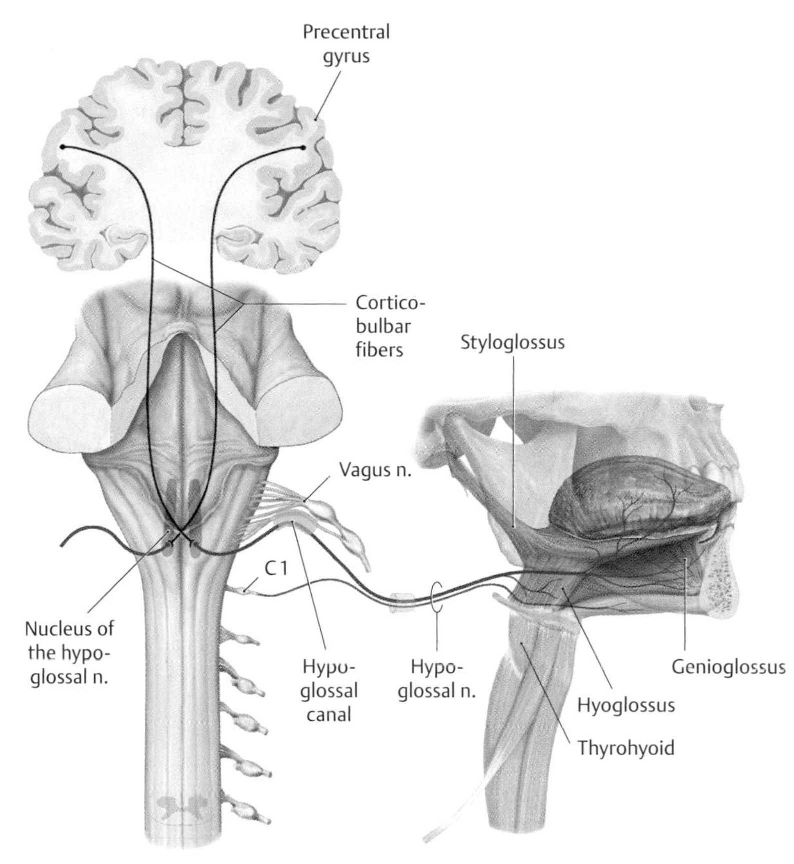
Precentral gyrus
Cortico-bulbar fibers
Styloglossus
Vagus n.
C1
Nucleus of the hypo-glossal n.
Hypo-glossal canal
Hypo-glossal n.
Genioglossus
Hyoglossus
Thyrohyoid

Fig. 33.26 **Hypoglossal nerve nuclei**
Note: The nucleus of the hypoglossal nerve is innervated by cortical neurons from the contralateral side.

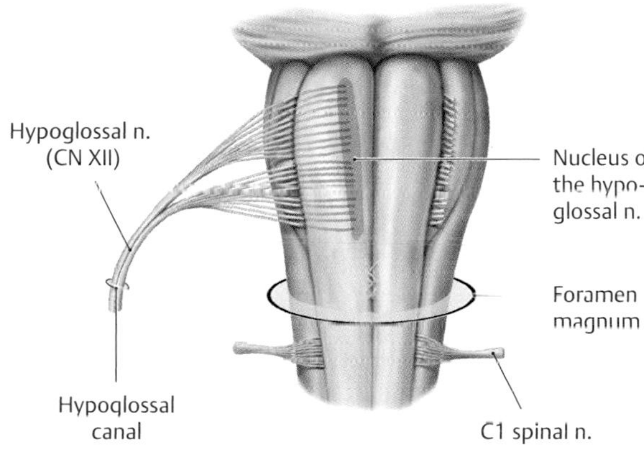
Hypoglossal n. (CN XII)
Nucleus of the hypo-glossal n.
Foramen magnum
Hypoglossal canal
C1 spinal n.

A Anterior view.

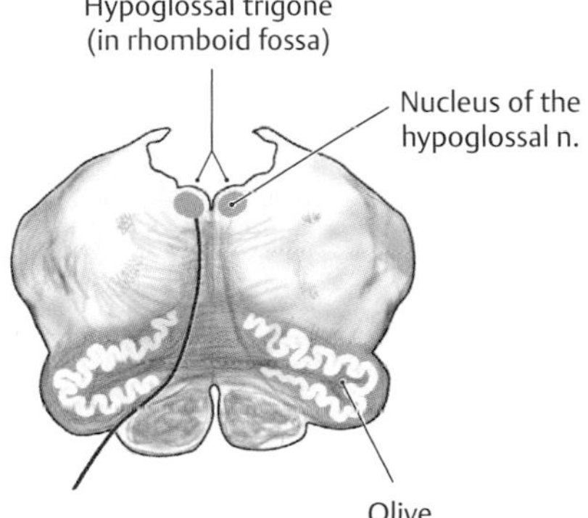
Hypoglossal trigone (in rhomboid fossa)
Nucleus of the hypoglossal n.
Olive

B Cross section through the medulla oblongata.

Fig. 33.27 **Hypoglossal nerve lesions**
Superior view.

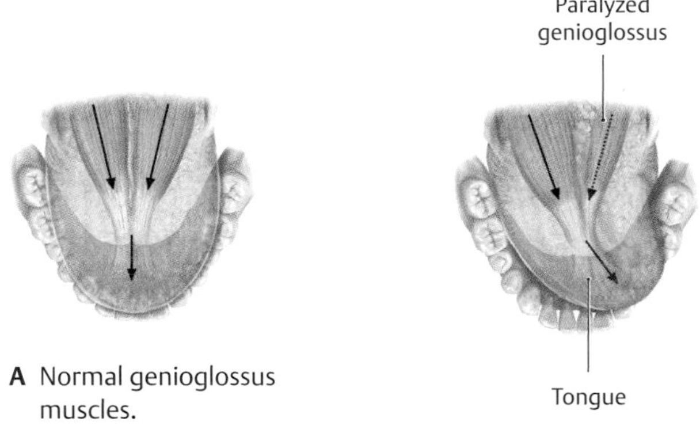
Paralyzed genioglossus
Tongue

A Normal genioglossus muscles.

B Unilateral nuclear or peripheral lesion.

Table 33.12 **Hypoglossal nerve (CN XII)**

Course	Fibers	Nuclei	Function	Effects of nerve injury
Emerges from the medulla oblongata, leaves the cranial cavity through the hypoglossal canal, and descends laterally to the vagus nerve. CN XII enters the root of the tongue above the hyoid bone.	Somatic efferent	Nucleus of the hypo-glossal n.	Innervates: • Intrinsic and extrinsic muscles of the tongue (except the palatoglossus, supplied by CN X)	Central hypoglossal paralysis (supranuclear): tongue deviates *away* from the side of the lesion Nuclear or peripheral paralysis: tongue deviates *toward* the affected side (due to preponderance of muscle on healthy side) Flaccid paralysis: both nuclei injured; tongue cannot be protruded

Innervation of the Face

Fig. 34.1 Motor innervation of the face
Left lateral view. Five branches of the facial nerve (CN VII) provide motor innervation to the muscles of facial expression. The mandibular division of the trigeminal nerve (CN V_3) supplies motor innervation to the muscles of mastication.

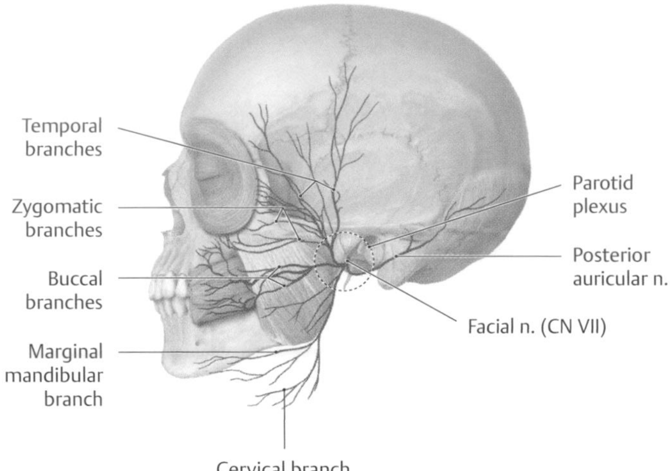
Temporal branches
Zygomatic branches
Buccal branches
Marginal mandibular branch
Cervical branch
Parotid plexus
Posterior auricular n.
Facial n. (CN VII)

A Motor innervation of the muscles of facial expression.

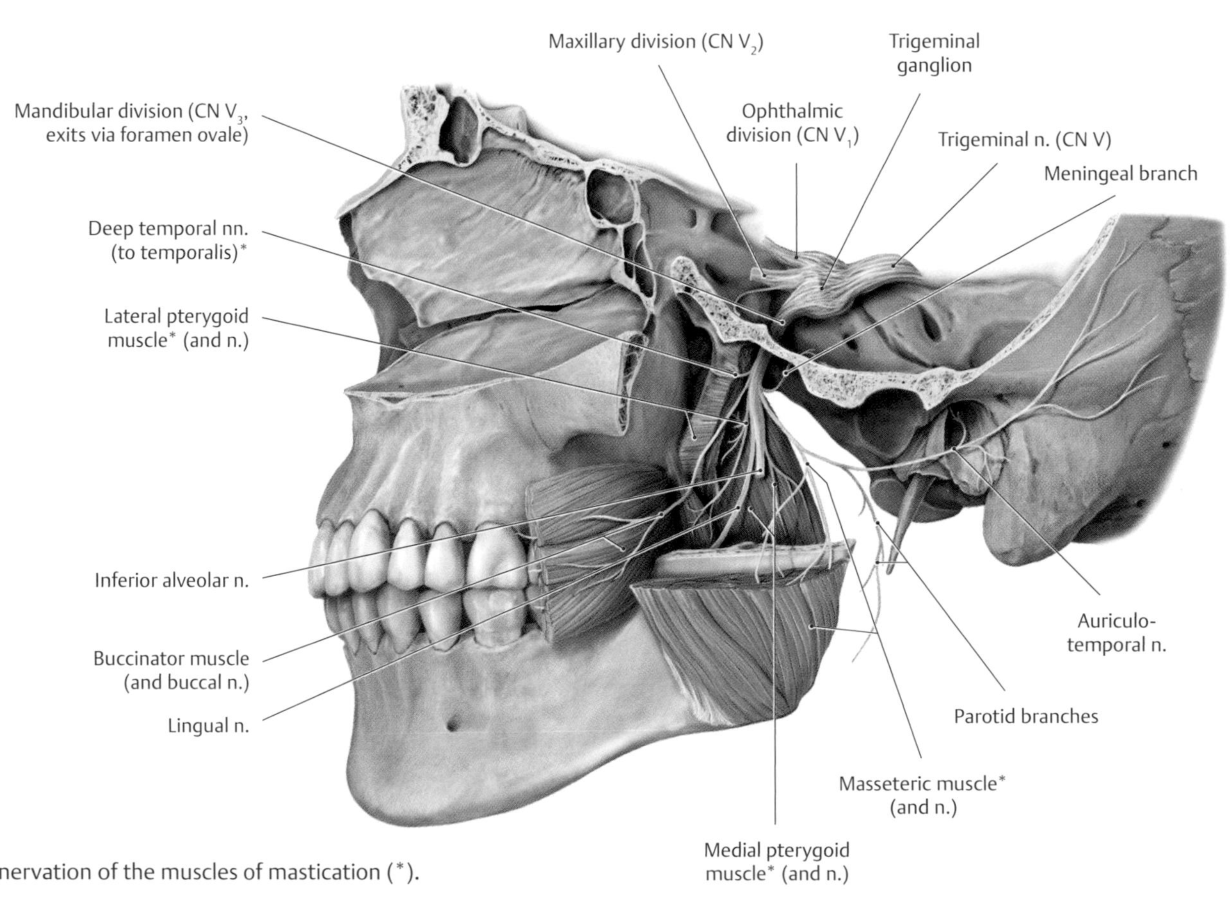
Maxillary division (CN V_2)
Trigeminal ganglion
Mandibular division (CN V_3, exits via foramen ovale)
Ophthalmic division (CN V_1)
Trigeminal n. (CN V)
Meningeal branch
Deep temporal nn. (to temporalis)*
Lateral pterygoid muscle* (and n.)
Inferior alveolar n.
Buccinator muscle (and buccal n.)
Lingual n.
Auriculo-temporal n.
Parotid branches
Masseteric muscle* (and n.)
Medial pterygoid muscle* (and n.)

B Motor innervation of the muscles of mastication (*).

Fig. 34.2 **Sensory innervation of the face**

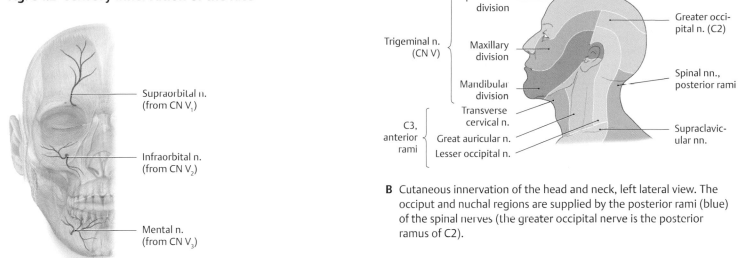

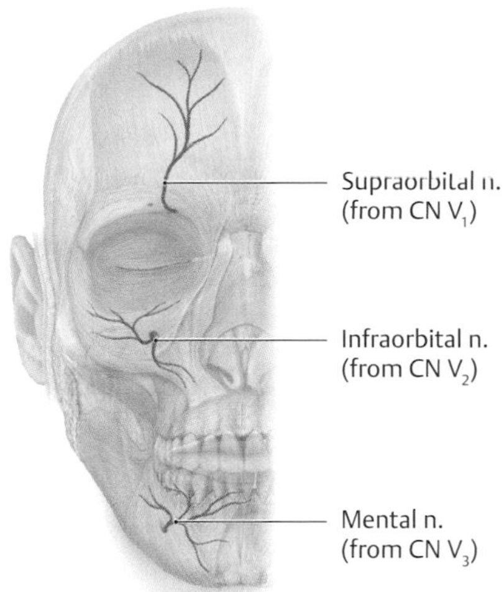

Supraorbital n.
(from CN V_1)
Infraorbital n.
(from CN V_2)
Mental n.
(from CN V_3)

A Sensory branches of the trigeminal nerve, anterior view. The sensory branches of the three divisions emerge from the supraorbital, infraorbital, and mental foramina, respectively.

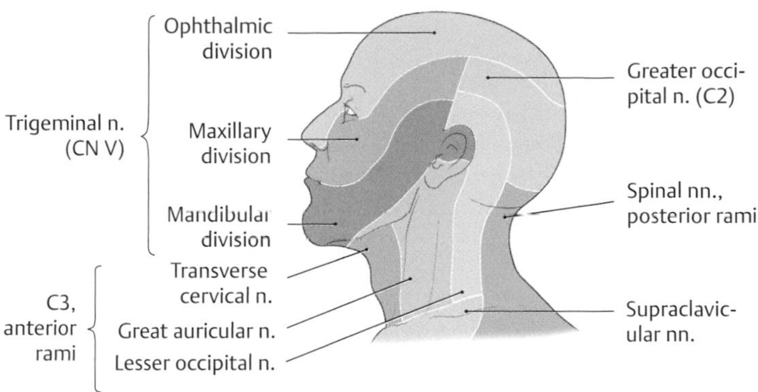

Trigeminal n.
(CN V)
Ophthalmic division
Maxillary division
Mandibular division
C3,
anterior rami
Transverse cervical n.
Great auricular n.
Lesser occipital n.
Greater occipital n. (C2)
Spinal nn., posterior rami
Supraclavicular nn.

B Cutaneous innervation of the head and neck, left lateral view. The occiput and nuchal regions are supplied by the posterior rami (blue) of the spinal nerves (the greater occipital nerve is the posterior ramus of C2).

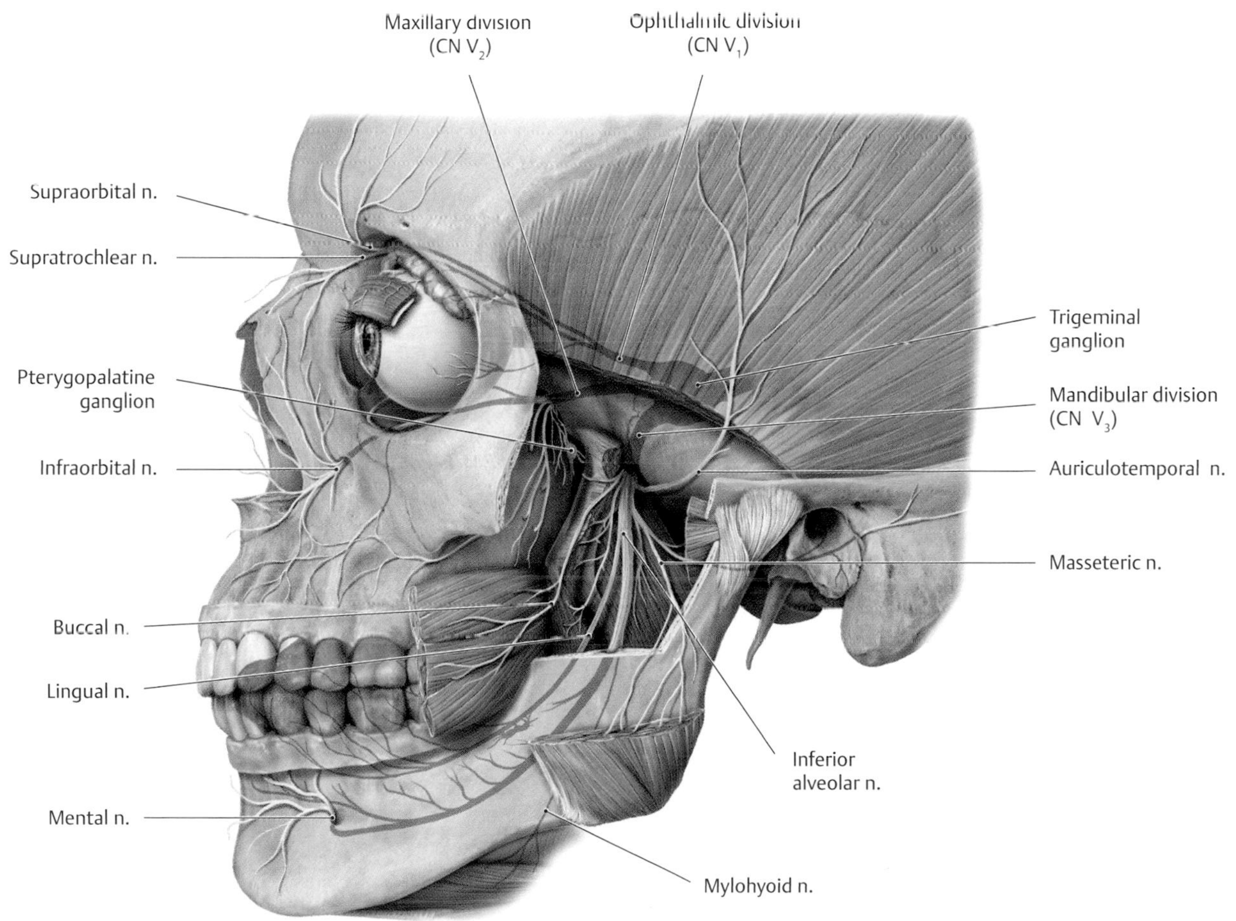

Maxillary division
(CN V_2)
Ophthalmic division
(CN V_1)
Supraorbital n.
Supratrochlear n.
Pterygopalatine ganglion
Infraorbital n.
Buccal n.
Lingual n.
Mental n.
Trigeminal ganglion
Mandibular division
(CN V_3)
Auriculotemporal n.
Masseteric n.
Inferior alveolar n.
Mylohyoid n.

C Divisions of the trigeminal nerve, left lateral view.

Arteries of the Head & Neck

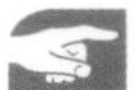

The head and neck are supplied by branches of the common carotid artery. The common carotid splits at the carotid bifurcation into two branches: the internal and external carotid arteries. The internal carotid chiefly supplies the brain (p. 634), although its branches anastomose with the external carotid in the orbit and nasal septum. The external carotid is the major supplier of structures of the head and neck.

Fig. 34.3 Internal carotid artery
Left lateral view. The most important extra-cerebral branch of the internal carotid artery is the ophthalmic artery, which supplies the upper nasal septum (p. 554) and the orbit (p. 542). See pp. 634–635 for the arteries of the brain.

Ophthalmic a.
Angular a.
Facial a.
Common carotid a.
Internal carotid a.
External carotid a.
Vertebral a.
Subclavian a.

A Schematic.

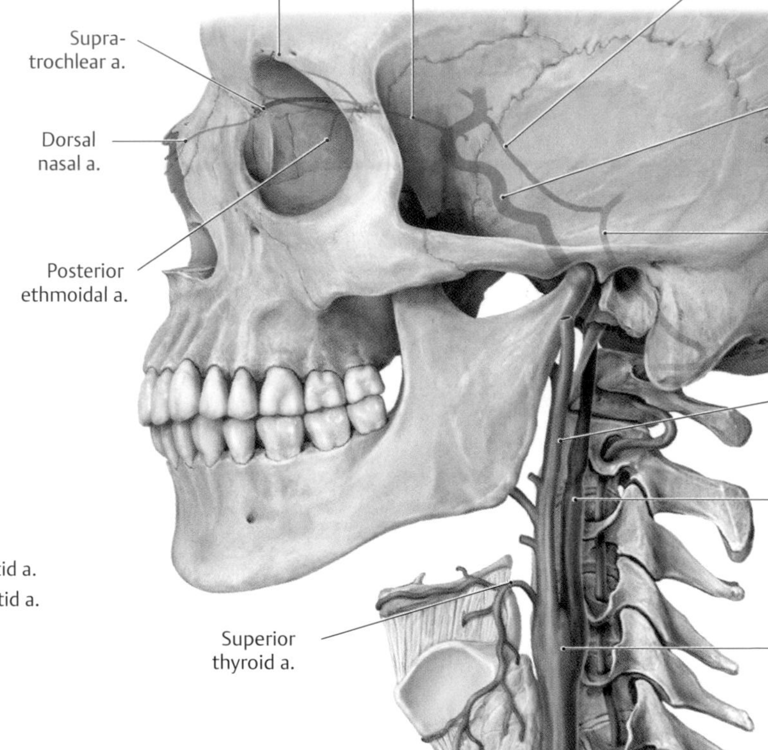

Supraorbital a.
Ophthalmic a.
Posterior communicating a.
Supra-trochlear a.
Internal carotid a.
Dorsal nasal a.
Basilar a.
Posterior ethmoidal a.
External carotid a.
Internal carotid a.
Superior thyroid a.
Carotid bifurcation
Vertebral a.
Subclavian a.

C Course of the internal carotid artery.

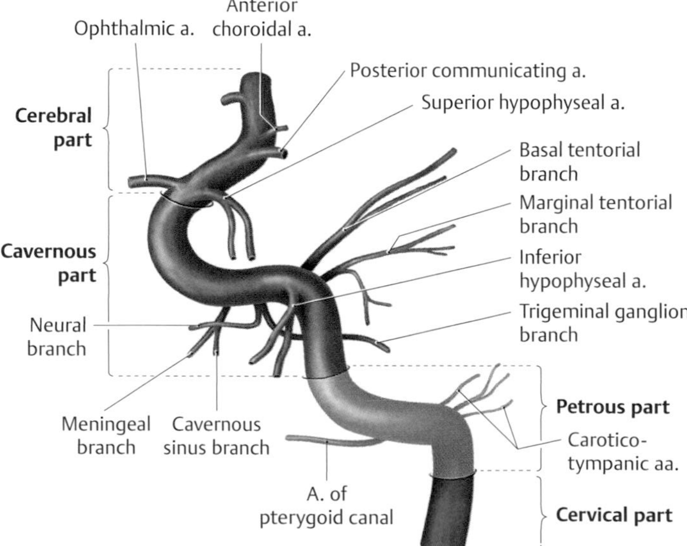

Ophthalmic a.
Anterior choroidal a.
Posterior communicating a.
Superior hypophyseal a.
Cerebral part
Basal tentorial branch
Marginal tentorial branch
Cavernous part
Inferior hypophyseal a.
Trigeminal ganglion branch
Neural branch
Petrous part
Meningeal branch
Cavernous sinus branch
Carotico-tympanic aa.
A. of pterygoid canal
Cervical part

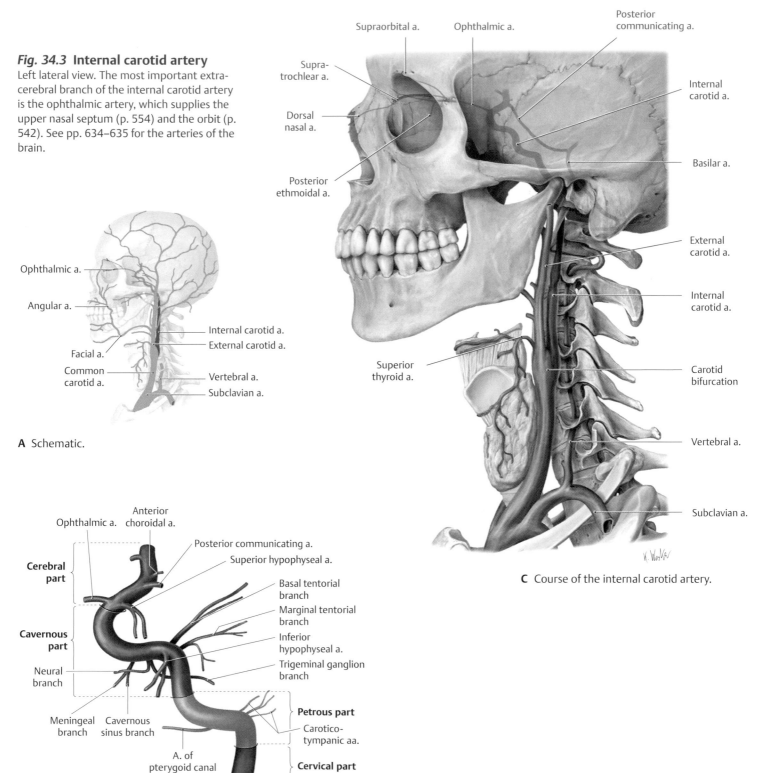

B Parts and branches of the internal carotid artery.

Clinical

Carotid artery atherosclerosis

The carotid artery is often affected by atherosclerosis, a hardening of arterial walls due to plaque formation. The examiner can determine the status of the arteries using ultrasound. *Note:* The absence of atherosclerosis in the carotid artery does not preclude coronary heart disease or atherosclerotic changes in other locations.

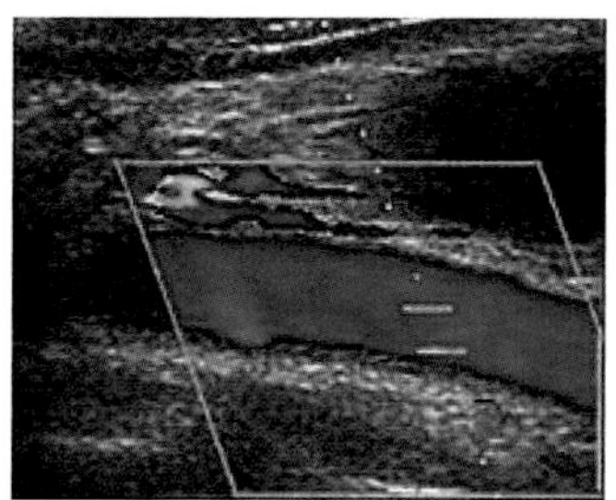

A Common carotid artery with "normal" flow.

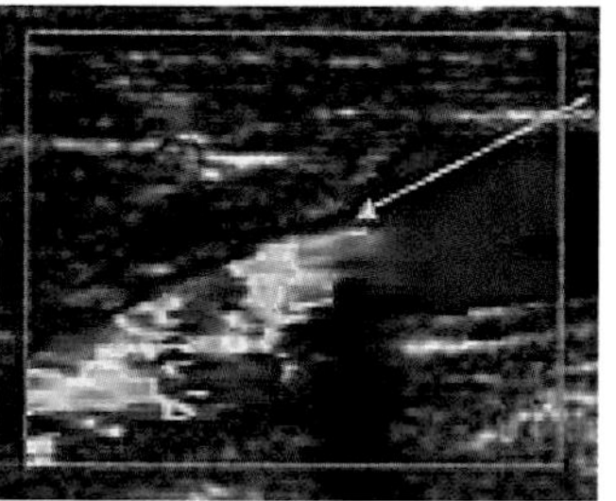

B Calcified plaque in the carotid bulb.

Fig. 34.4 External carotid artery: Overview

Left lateral view.

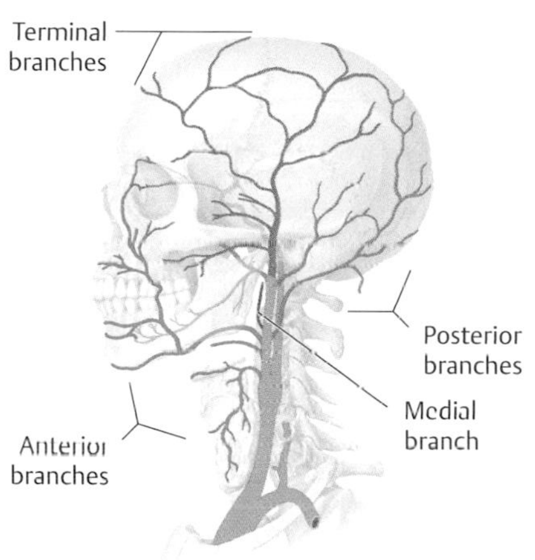
Terminal branches
Posterior branches
Medial branch
Anterior branches

A Schematic of the external carotid artery.

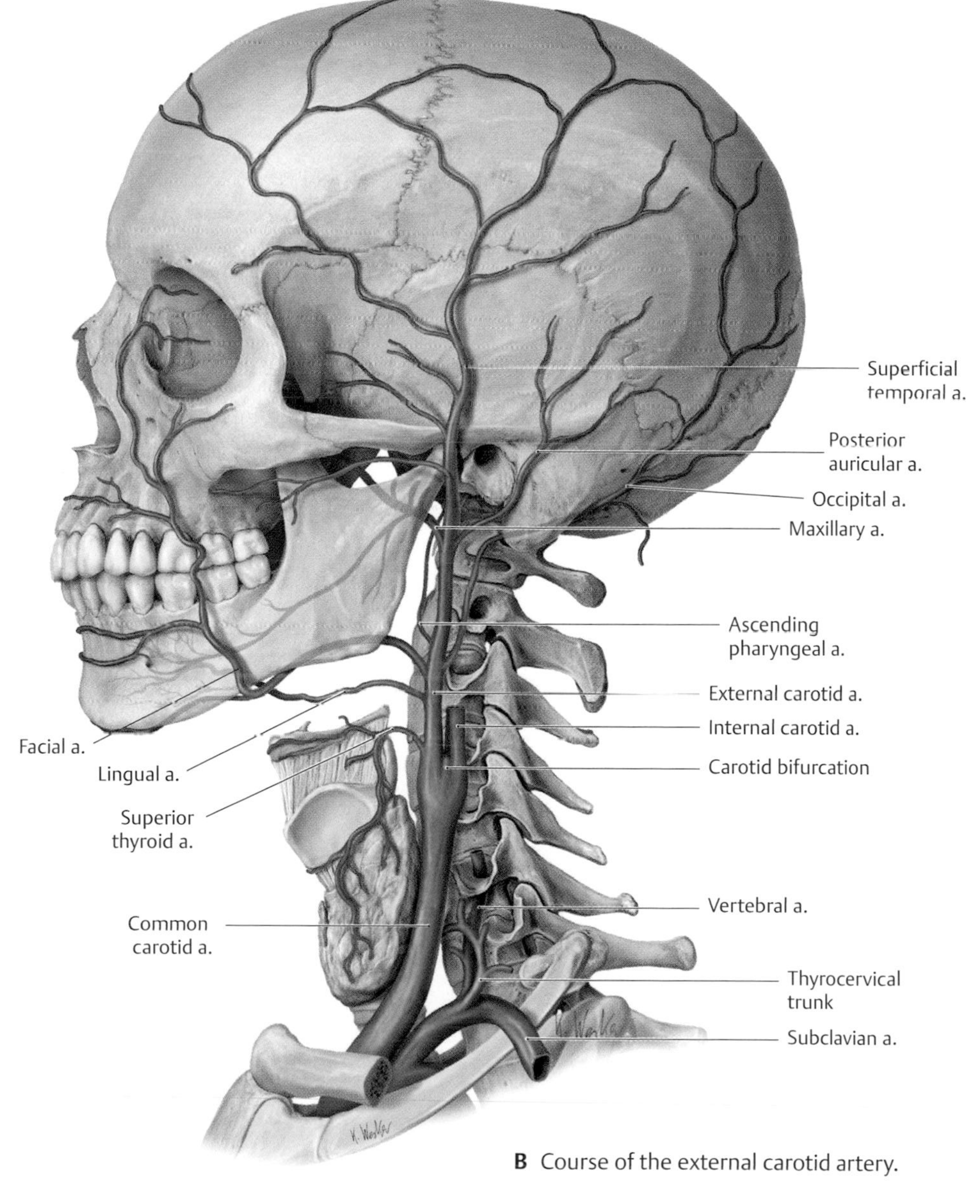
Superficial temporal a.
Posterior auricular a.
Occipital a.
Maxillary a.
Ascending pharyngeal a.
External carotid a.
Internal carotid a.
Carotid bifurcation
Facial a.
Lingual a.
Superior thyroid a.
Common carotid a.
Vertebral a.
Thyrocervical trunk
Subclavian a.

B Course of the external carotid artery.

Table 34.1 **Branches of the external carotid artery**

Group	Artery
Anterior (p. 518)	Superior thyroid a.
	Lingual a.
	Facial a.
Medial (p. 518)	Ascending pharyngeal a.
Posterior (p. 519)	Occipital a.
	Posterior auricular a.
Terminal (p. 520)	Maxillary a.
	Superficial temporal a.

External Carotid Artery: Anterior, Medial & Posterior Branches

Fig. 34.5 Anterior and medial branches
Left lateral view. The arteries of the anterior aspect supply the anterior structures of the head and neck, including the orbit (p. 540), ear (p. 564), larynx (p. 603), pharynx (p. 586), and oral cavity. *Note:* The angular artery anastomoses with the dorsal nasal artery of the internal carotid (via the ophthalmic artery).

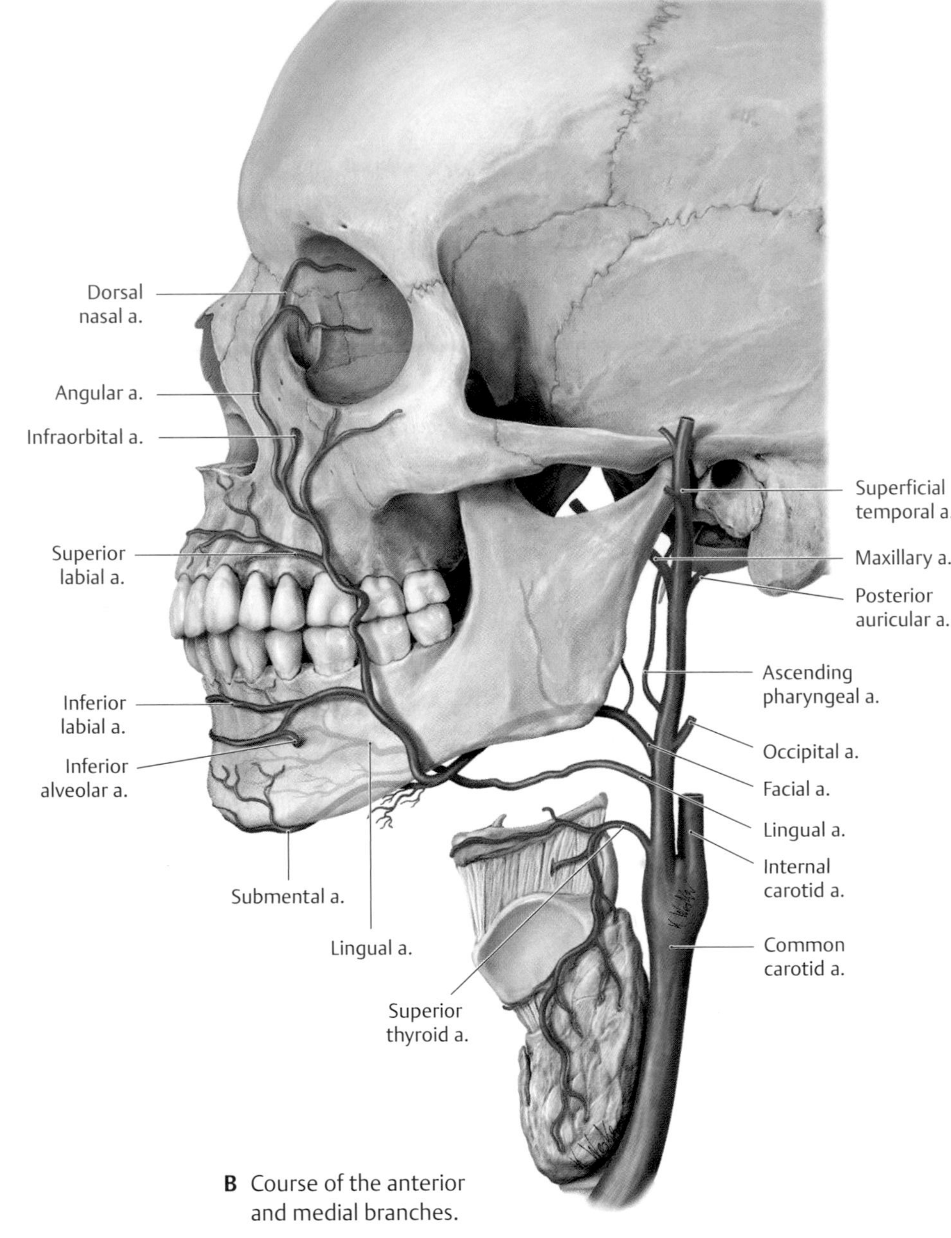
Dorsal nasal a.
Angular a.
Infraorbital a.
Superior labial a.
Inferior labial a.
Inferior alveolar a.
Submental a.
Lingual a.
Superior thyroid a.
Superficial temporal a.
Maxillary a.
Posterior auricular a.
Ascending pharyngeal a.
Occipital a.
Facial a.
Lingual a.
Internal carotid a.
Common carotid a.

B Course of the anterior and medial branches.

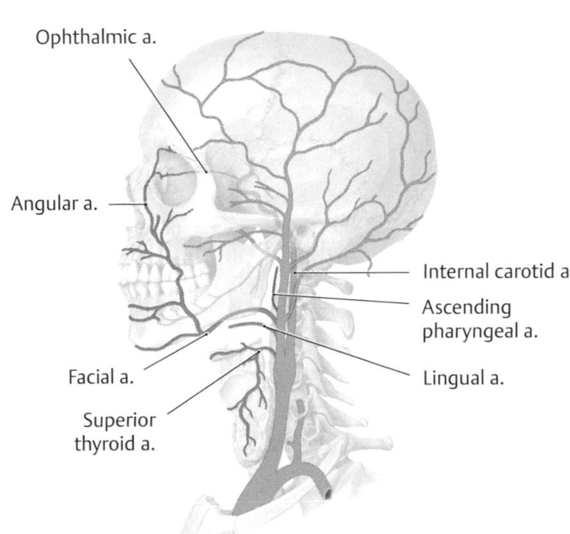
Ophthalmic a.
Angular a.
Internal carotid a.
Ascending pharyngeal a.
Facial a.
Lingual a.
Superior thyroid a.

A Arteries of the anterior and medial branches. The copious blood supply to the face makes facial injuries bleed profusely but heal quickly. There are extensive anastomoses between branches of the external carotid and between the external carotid artery and branches of the ophthalmic artery.

***Fig. 34.6* Posterior branches**
Left lateral view. The posterior branches of the external carotid artery supply the ear (p. 564), posterior skull (p. 529), and posterior neck muscles (p. 613).

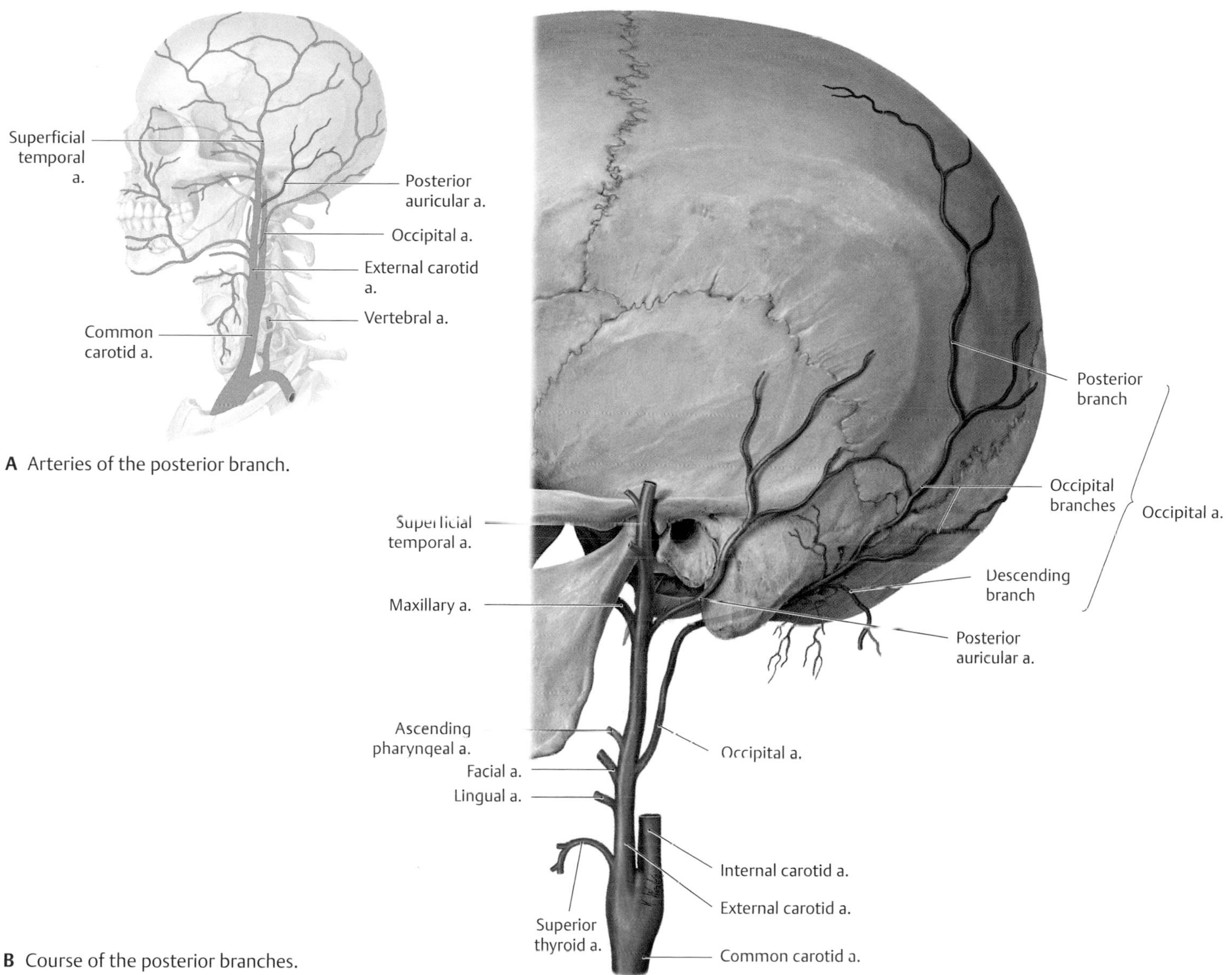
Superficial temporal a.
Posterior auricular a.
Occipital a.
External carotid a.
Vertebral a.
Common carotid a.
Superficial temporal a.
Maxillary a.
Ascending pharyngeal a.
Facial a.
Lingual a.
Posterior branch
Occipital branches
Occipital a.
Descending branch
Posterior auricular a.
Occipital a.
Internal carotid a.
External carotid a.
Superior thyroid a.
Common carotid a.

A Arteries of the posterior branch.

B Course of the posterior branches.

Table 34.2 **Anterior, medial, and posterior branches of the external carotid artery**

Branch	Artery	Divisions and distribution
Anterior branch	Superior thyroid a.	Glandular branch (to thyroid gland); superior laryngeal a.; sternocleidomastoid branch
	Lingual a.	Dorsal lingual branches (to base of tongue, epiglottis); sublingual a. (to sublingual gland, tongue, oral floor, oral cavity)
	Facial a.	Ascending palatine a. (to pharyngeal wall, soft palate, pharyngotympanic tube); tonsillar branch (to palatine tonsils); submental a. (to oral floor, submandibular gland); labial aa.; angular a. (to nasal root)
Medial branch	Ascending pharyngeal a.	Pharyngeal branches; interior tympanic a. (to mucosa of inner ear); posterior meningeal a.
Posterior branches	Occipital a.	Occipital branches; descending branch (to posterior neck muscles)
	Posterior auricular a.	Stylomastoid a. (to facial nerve in facial canal); posterior tympanic a.; auricular branch; occipital branch; parotid branch
For terminal branches, see Table 34.3.		

External Carotid Artery: Terminal Branches

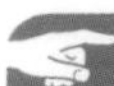

The terminal branches of the external carotid artery consist of two major arteries: superficial temporal and maxillary. The superficial temporal artery supplies the lateral skull. The maxillary artery is a major artery for internal structures of the face.

Fig. 34.7 **Superficial temporal artery**
Left lateral view. Inflammation of the superficial temporal artery due to temporal arteritis can cause severe headaches. The course of the frontal branch of the artery can often be seen superficially under the skin of elderly patients.

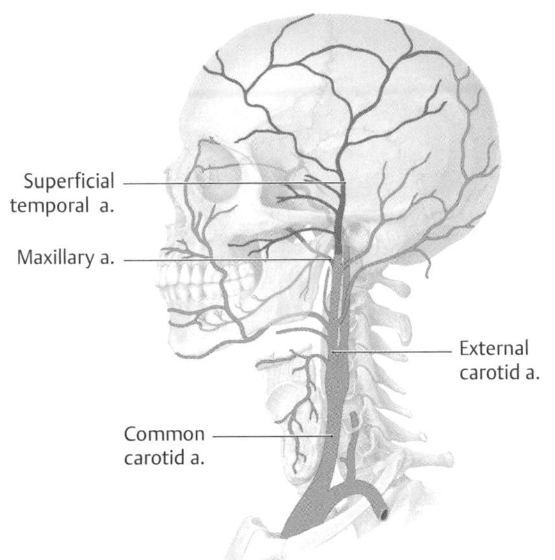
Superficial temporal a.
Maxillary a.
External carotid a.
Common carotid a.

A Arteries of the terminal branch.

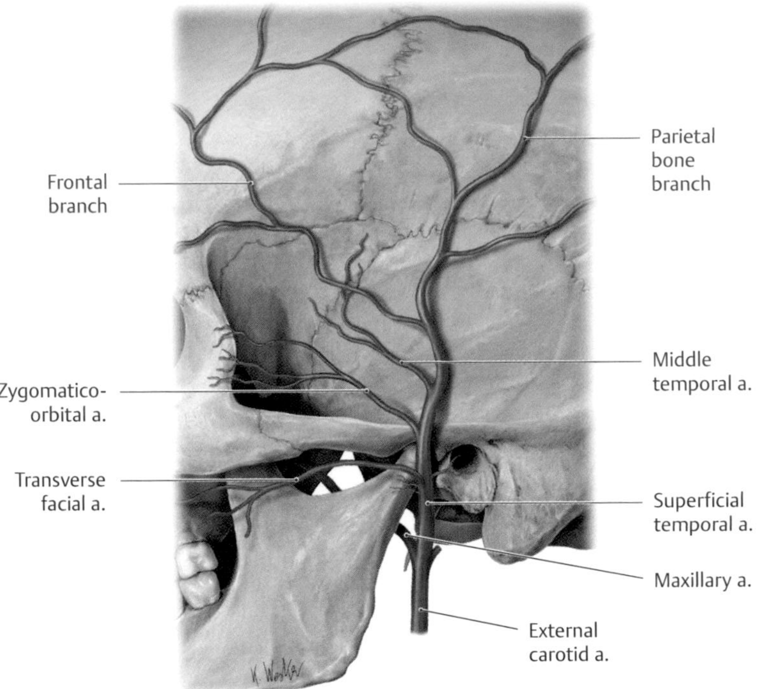
Frontal branch
Parietal bone branch
Middle temporal a.
Zygomatico-orbital a.
Transverse facial a.
Superficial temporal a.
Maxillary a.
External carotid a.

B Course of the superficial temporal artery.

Table 34.3 Terminal branches of the external carotid artery

Branch	Artery		Divisions and distribution	
Terminal branches	Superficial temporal a.		Transverse facial a. (to soft tissues below the zygomatic arch); frontal branches; parietal branches; zygomatico-orbital a. (to lateral orbital wall)	
	Maxillary a.	Mandibular part	Inferior alveolar a. (to mandible, teeth, gingiva); middle meningeal a.; deep auricular a. (to temporomandibular joint, external auditory canal); anterior tympanic a.	
		Pterygoid part	Masseteric a.; deep temporal branches; pterygoid branches; buccal a.	
		Pterygopalatine part	Posterosuperior alveolar a. (to maxillary molars, maxillary sinus, gingiva); infraorbital a. (to maxillary alveoli)	
			Descending palatine a.	Greater palatine a. (to hard palate)
				Lesser palatine a. (to soft palate, palatine tonsil, pharyngeal wall)
			Sphenopalatine a.	Lateral posterior nasal aa. (to lateral wall of nasal cavity, conchae)
				Posterior septal branches (to nasal septum)

Fig. 34.8 Maxillary artery

Left lateral view. The maxillary artery consists of three parts: mandibular (blue), pterygoid (green), and pterygopalatine (yellow).

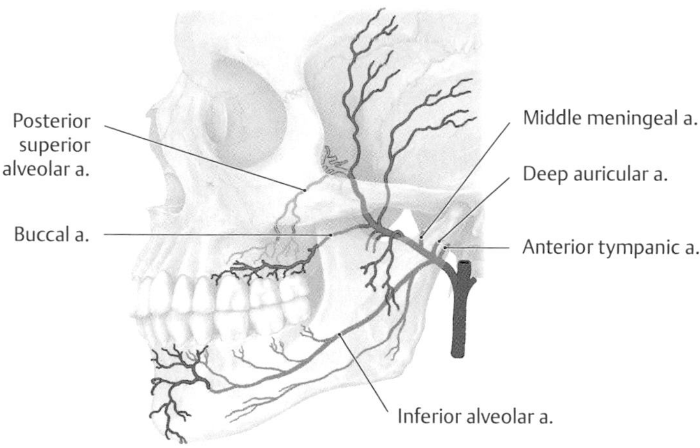

Posterior superior alveolar a.
Buccal a.
Middle meningeal a.
Deep auricular a.
Anterior tympanic a.
Inferior alveolar a.

A Divisions of the maxillary artery.

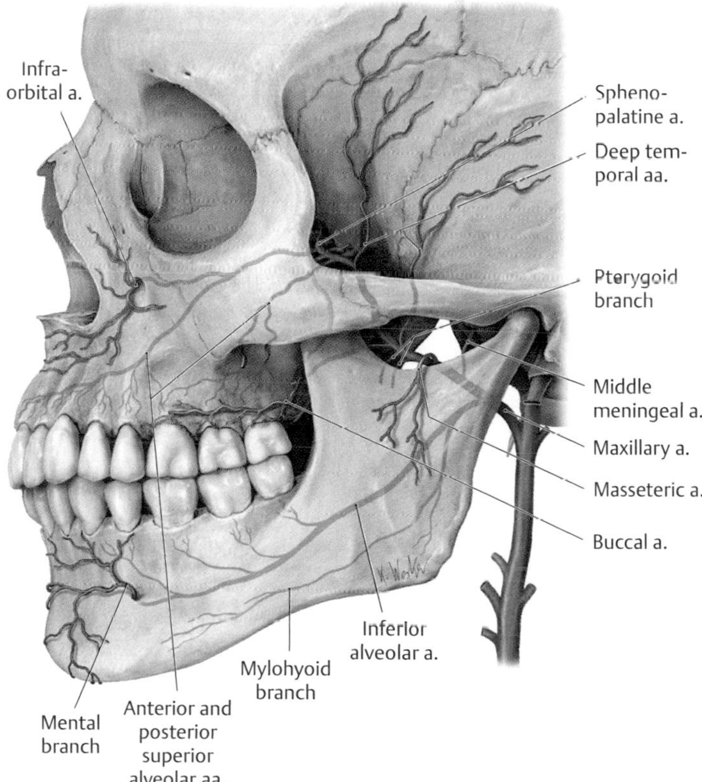

Infra-orbital a.
Spheno-palatine a.
Deep temporal aa.
Pterygoid branch
Middle meningeal a.
Maxillary a.
Masseteric a.
Buccal a.
Inferior alveolar a.
Mylohyoid branch
Mental branch
Anterior and posterior superior alveolar aa.

B Course of the maxillary artery.

Clinical

Middle meningeal artery

The middle meningeal artery supplies the meninges and overlying calvaria. Rupture of the artery (generally due to head trauma) results in an epidural hematoma.

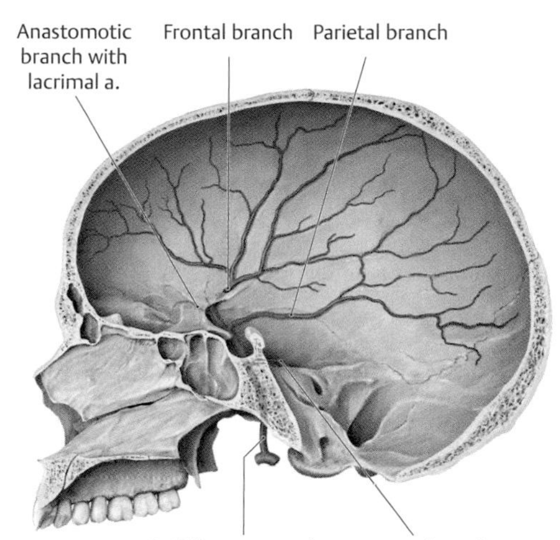

Anastomotic branch with lacrimal a.
Frontal branch
Parietal branch
Middle meningeal a.
Petrous branch

A Right middle meningeal artery, medial view of opened skull.

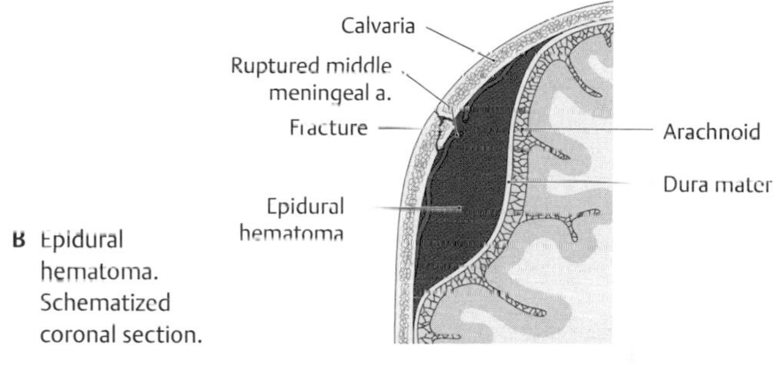

Calvaria
Ruptured middle meningeal a.
Fracture
Epidural hematoma
Arachnoid
Dura mater

B Epidural hematoma. Schematized coronal section.

Sphenopalatine artery

The sphenopalatine artery supplies the wall of the nasal cavity. Excessive nasopharyngeal bleeding from the branches of the sphenopalatine artery may necessitate ligation of the maxillary artery in the pterygopalatine fossa.

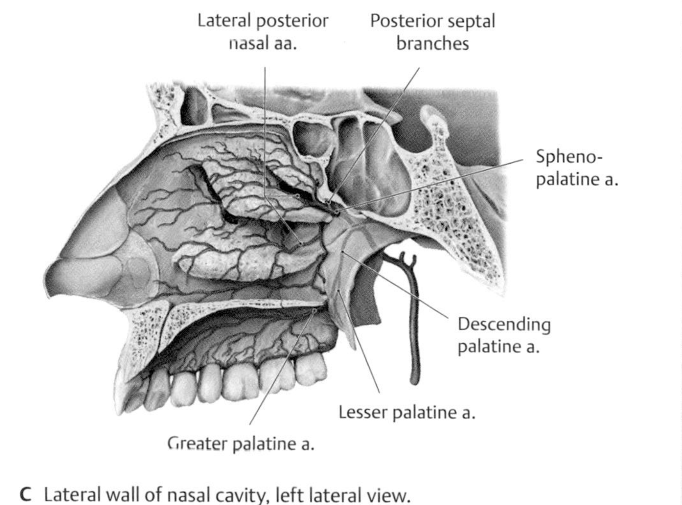

Lateral posterior nasal aa.
Posterior septal branches
Spheno-palatine a.
Descending palatine a.
Lesser palatine a.
Greater palatine a.

C Lateral wall of nasal cavity, left lateral view.

Veins of the Head & Neck

Fig. 34.9 Veins of the head and neck

Left lateral view. The veins of the head and neck drain into the brachiocephalic vein. *Note:* The left and right brachiocephalic veins are not symmetrical.

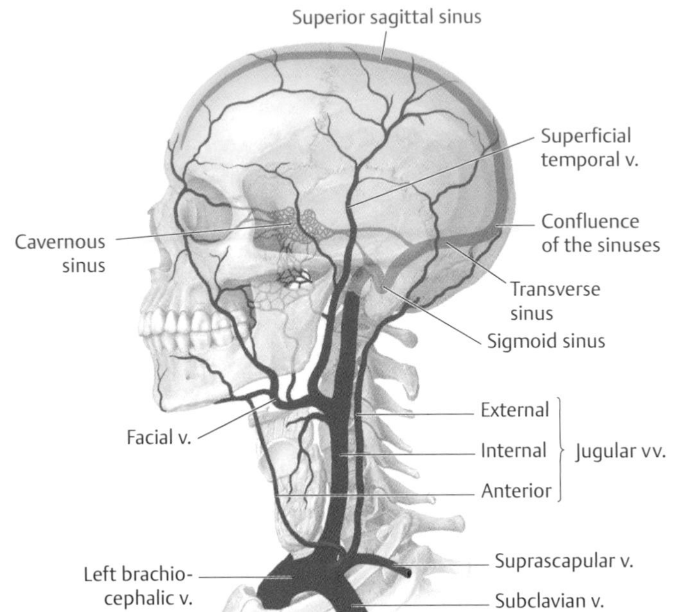
Superior sagittal sinus
Superficial temporal v.
Cavernous sinus
Confluence of the sinuses
Transverse sinus
Sigmoid sinus
External
Internal
Anterior
Jugular vv.
Facial v.
Suprascapular v.
Left brachio-cephalic v.
Subclavian v.

A Principal veins of the head and neck.

Table 34.4	**Principal superficial veins**	
Vein	**Region drained**	**Location**
Internal jugular v.	Interior of skull (including brain)	Within carotid sheath
External jugular v.	Superficial head	Within superficial cervical fascia
Anterior jugular v.	Neck, portions of head	

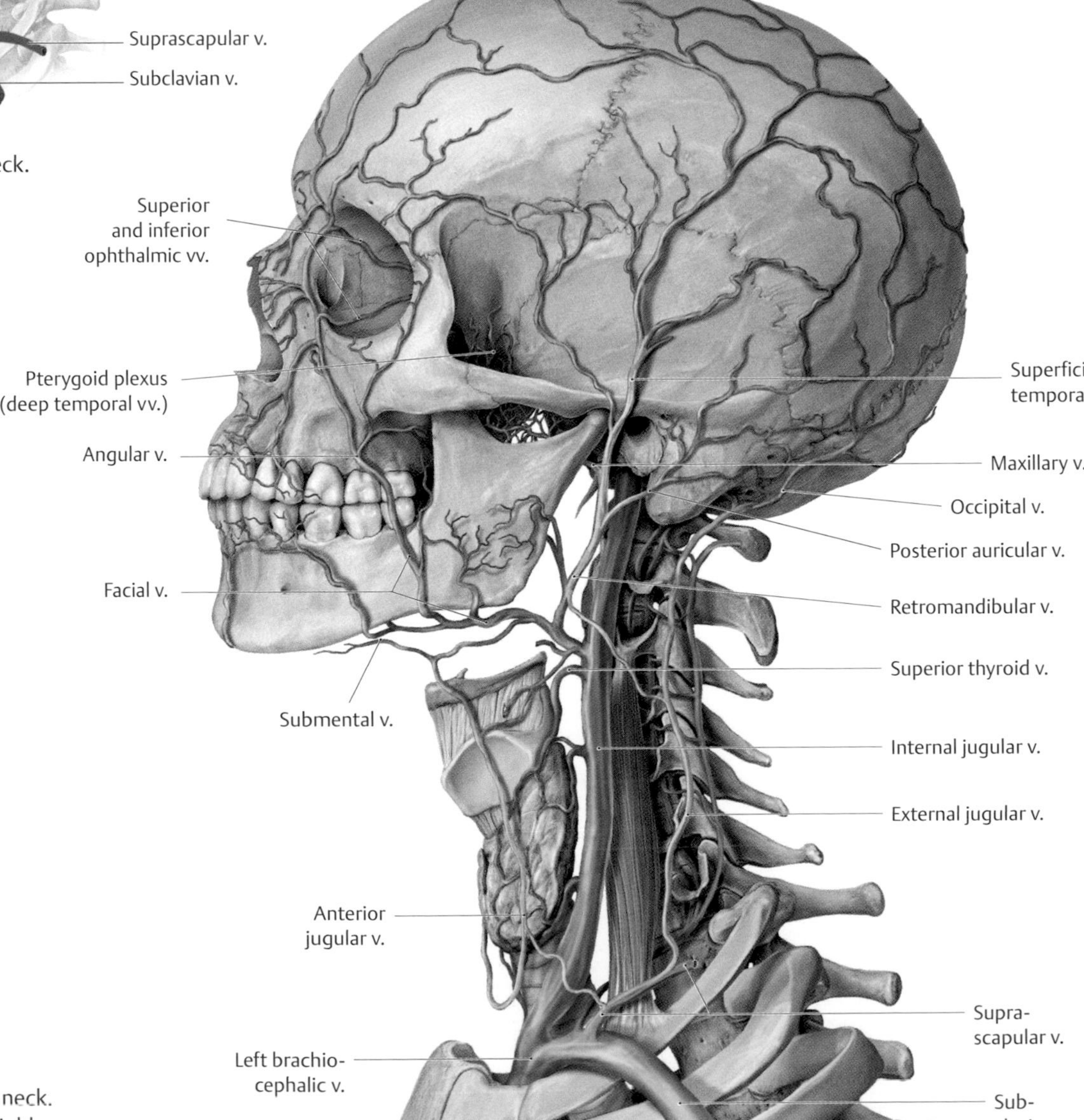
Superior and inferior ophthalmic vv.
Pterygoid plexus (deep temporal vv.)
Angular v.
Facial v.
Submental v.
Anterior jugular v.
Left brachio-cephalic v.
Superficial temporal v.
Maxillary v.
Occipital v.
Posterior auricular v.
Retromandibular v.
Superior thyroid v.
Internal jugular v.
External jugular v.
Supra-scapular v.
Sub-clavian v.

B Superficial veins of the head and neck. *Note*: The course of the veins is highly variable.

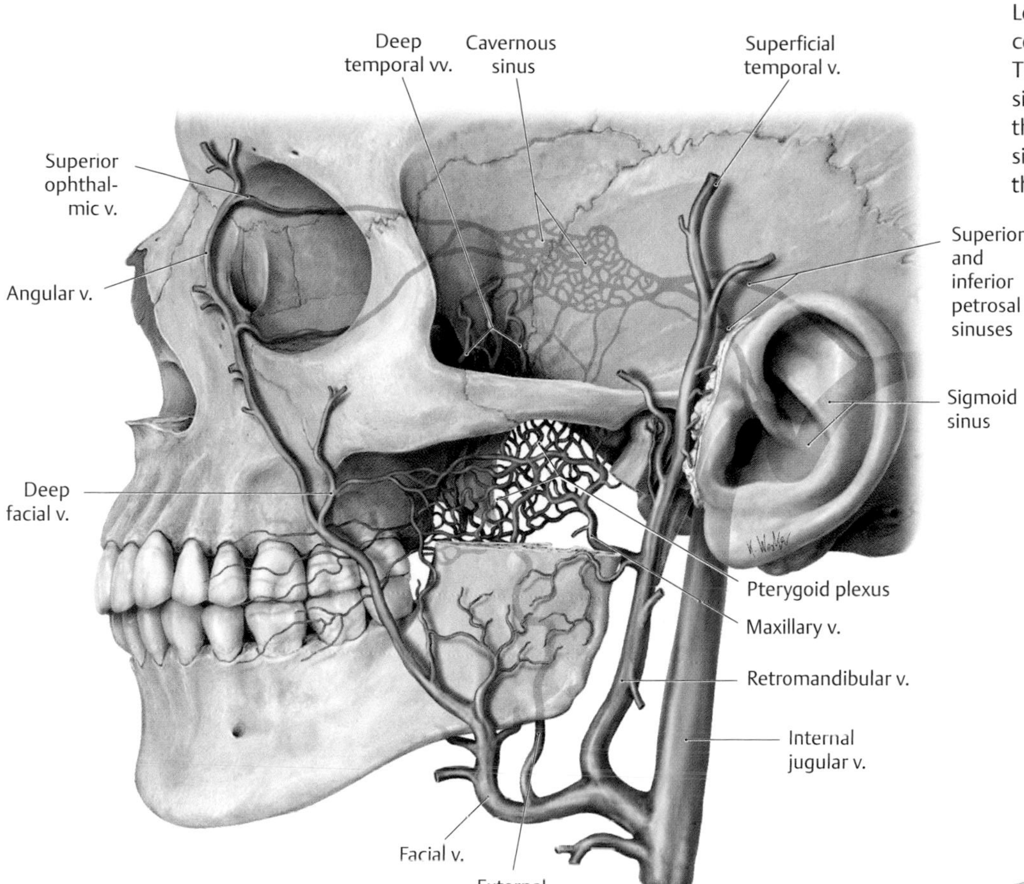
Deep temporal vv.
Cavernous sinus
Superficial temporal v.
Superior ophthalmic v.
Angular v.
Superior and inferior petrosal sinuses
Sigmoid sinus
Deep facial v.
Pterygoid plexus
Maxillary v.
Retromandibular v.
Internal jugular v.
Facial v.
External palatine v.

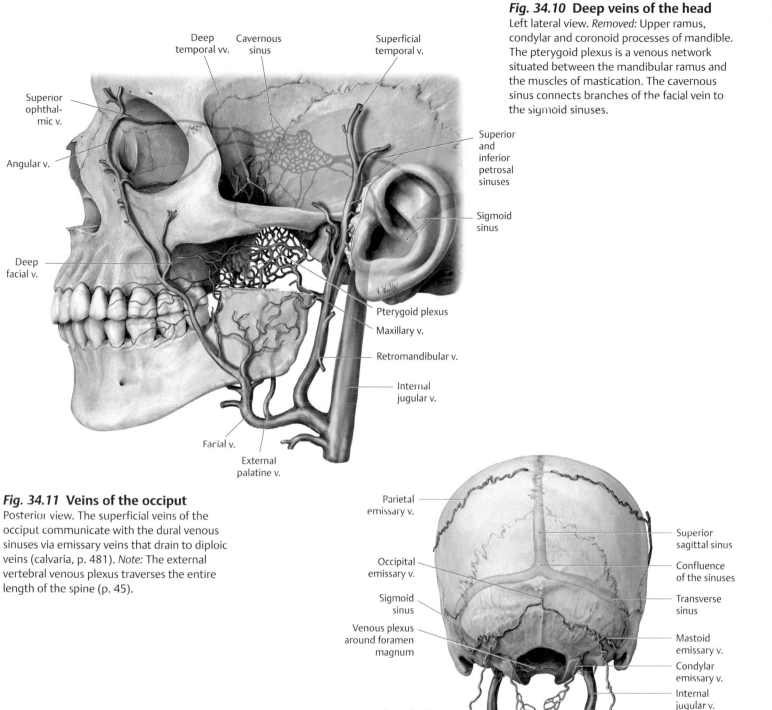

Fig. 34.10 Deep veins of the head
Left lateral view. *Removed:* Upper ramus, condylar and coronoid processes of mandible. The pterygoid plexus is a venous network situated between the mandibular ramus and the muscles of mastication. The cavernous sinus connects branches of the facial vein to the sigmoid sinuses.

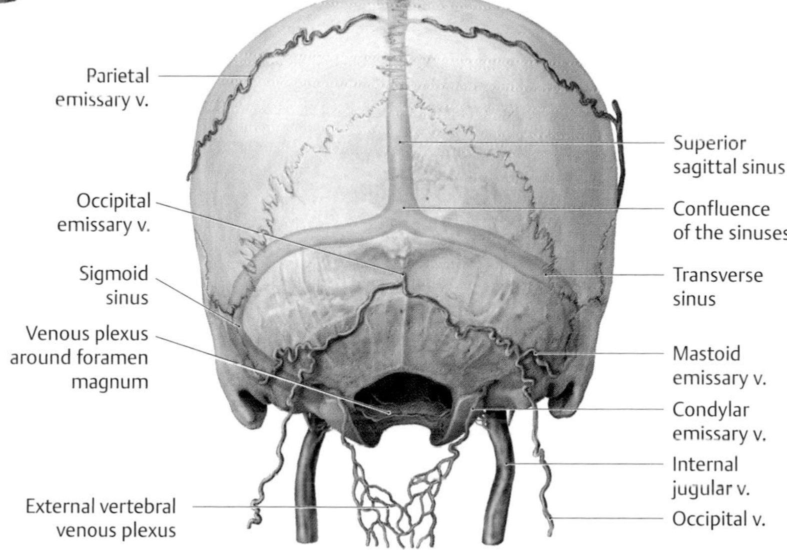
Parietal emissary v.
Superior sagittal sinus
Occipital emissary v.
Confluence of the sinuses
Sigmoid sinus
Transverse sinus
Venous plexus around foramen magnum
Mastoid emissary v.
Condylar emissary v.
Internal jugular v.
External vertebral venous plexus
Occipital v.

Fig. 34.11 Veins of the occiput
Posterior view. The superficial veins of the occiput communicate with the dural venous sinuses via emissary veins that drain to diploic veins (calvaria, p. 481). *Note:* The external vertebral venous plexus traverses the entire length of the spine (p. 45).

Table 34.5 Venous anastomoses

The extensive venous anastomoses in this region provide routes for the spread of infections.

Extracranial vein	Connecting vein	Venous sinus
Angular v.	Superior and inferior ophthalmic vv.	Cavernous sinus*
Vv. of palatine tonsil	Pterygoid plexus; inferior ophthalmic v.	
Superficial temporal v.	Parietal emissary vv.	Superior sagittal sinus
Occipital v.	Occipital emissary v.	Transverse sinus, confluence of the sinuses
Posterior auricular v.	Mastoid emissary v.	Sigmoid sinus
External vertebral venous plexus	Condylar emissary v.	

*Deep spread of bacterial infection from the facial region may result in cavernous sinus thrombosis.

Meninges

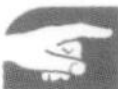

The brain and spinal cord are covered by membranes called meninges. The meninges are composed of three layers: dura mater (dura), arachnoid (arachnoid membrane), and pia mater.

The subarachnoid space, located between the arachnoid and pia, contains cerebrospinal fluid (CSF, see p. 632). See p. 40 for the coverings of the spinal cord.

Fig. 34.12 Layers of the meninges

See pp. 636–637 for the veins of the brain.

Diploic vv.
Epidural hematoma
Cranial bone
Neurothelium
Dura mater
Arachnoid
Subdural hemorrhage
Arachnoid trabeculae
Cerebral cortex
Pia mater
Cerebral a.
Subarachnoid space
Cerebral v.

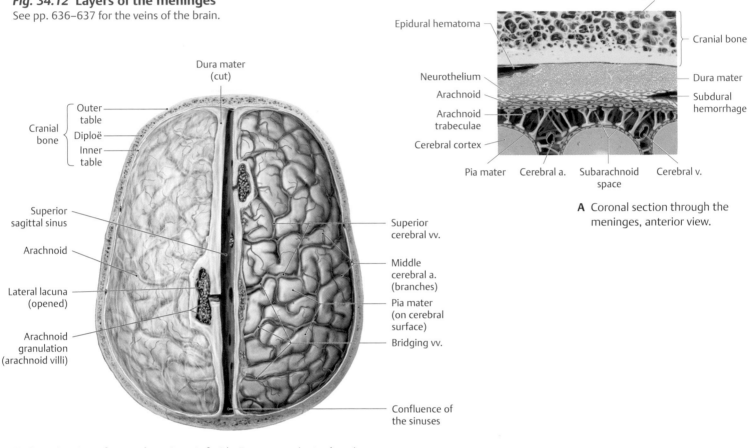

A Coronal section through the meninges, anterior view.

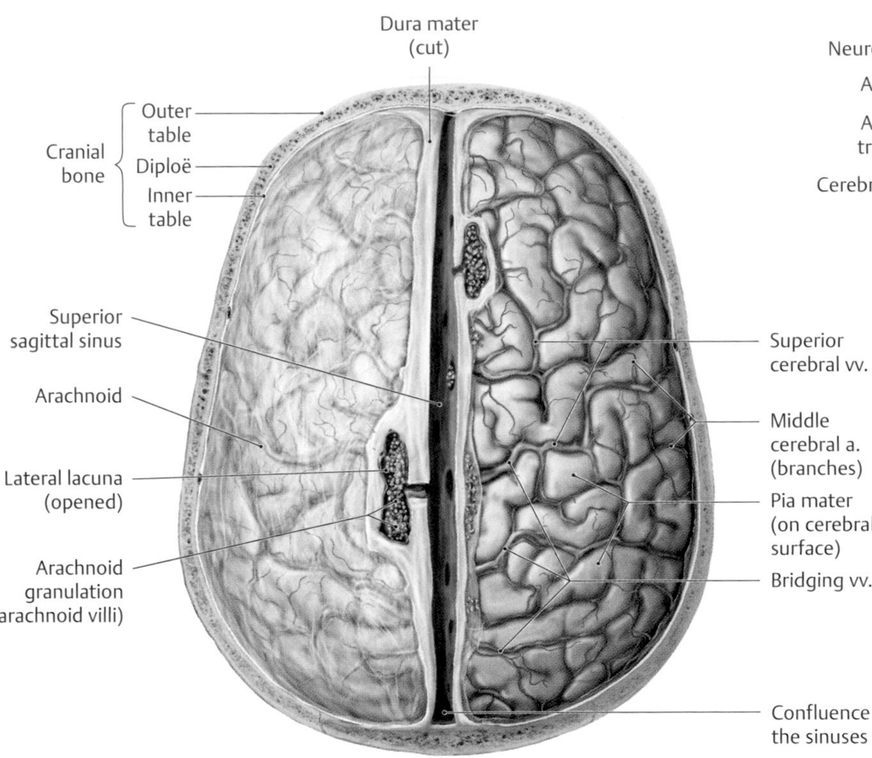

Dura mater (cut)
Cranial bone
Outer table
Diploë
Inner table
Superior sagittal sinus
Arachnoid
Lateral lacuna (opened)
Arachnoid granulation (arachnoid villi)
Superior cerebral vv.
Middle cerebral a. (branches)
Pia mater (on cerebral surface)
Bridging vv.
Confluence of the sinuses

B Superior view of opened cranium. *Left side:* Dura mater (outer layer) cut to reveal arachnoid (middle layer). *Right side:* Dura mater and arachnoid removed to reveal pia mater (inner layer) lining the surface of the brain. *Note:* Arachnoid granulations, sites for loss of cerebrospinal fluid into the venous blood, are protrusions of the arachnoid layer of the meninges into the venous sinus system.

Fig. 34.13 Dural septa (folds)

Left anterior oblique view. Two layers of meningeal dura come together, after separating from the periosteal dura during formation of a dural (venous) sinus, to form a dural fold or septa. These include the falx cerebri (separating right and left cerebral hemispheres); the tentorium cerebelli (supporting the cerebrum to keep it from crushing the underlying cerebellum); the falx cerebelli (not shown, that separates right and left cerebellar lobes under the tentorium); and the diaphragma sellae (forms the roof over the hypophyseal fossa and is invaginated by the hypophysis).

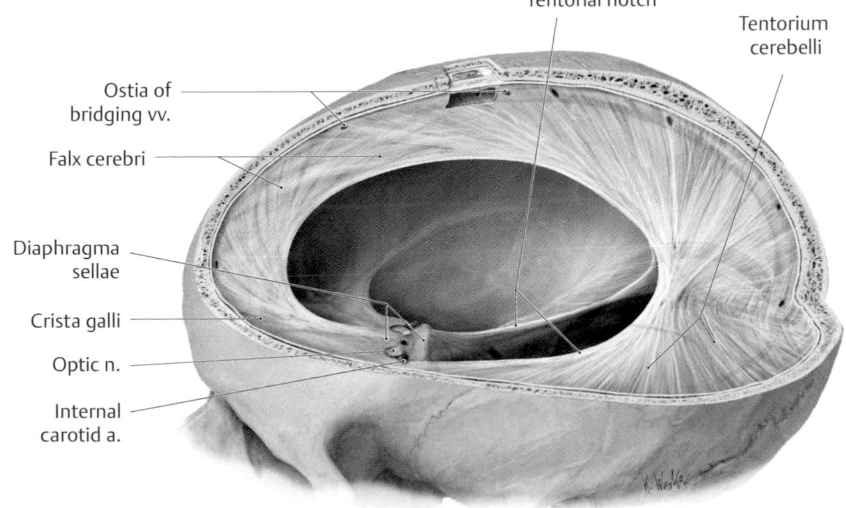

Tentorial notch
Tentorium cerebelli
Ostia of bridging vv.
Falx cerebri
Diaphragma sellae
Crista galli
Optic n.
Internal carotid a.

Clinical

Extracerebral hemorrhages

Bleeding between the bony calvarium and the soft tissue of the brain (extracerebral hemorrhage) exerts pressure on the brain. A rise of intracranial pressure may damage brain tissue both at the bleeding site and in more remote brain areas. Three types of intracranial hemorrhage are distinguished based on the relationship to the dura mater. See pp. 634–635 for the arteries of the brain.

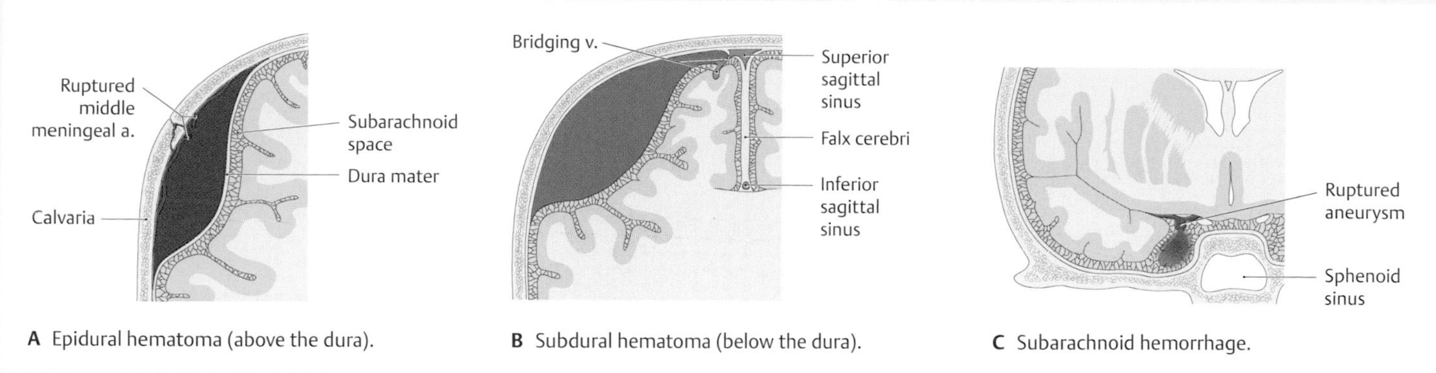

Ruptured middle meningeal a.
Subarachnoid space
Dura mater
Calvaria
Bridging v.
Superior sagittal sinus
Falx cerebri
Inferior sagittal sinus
Ruptured aneurysm
Sphenoid sinus

A Epidural hematoma (above the dura).

B Subdural hematoma (below the dura).

C Subarachnoid hemorrhage.

Fig. 34.14 **Arteries of the dura mater**
Midsagittal section, left lateral view. See pp. 634–635 for the arteries of the brain.

Middle meningeal a. (frontal branch)
Middle meningeal a. (parietal branch)
Occipital a. (mastoid branch)
Middle meningeal a. (via foramen spinosum)
Vertebral a. (branches)

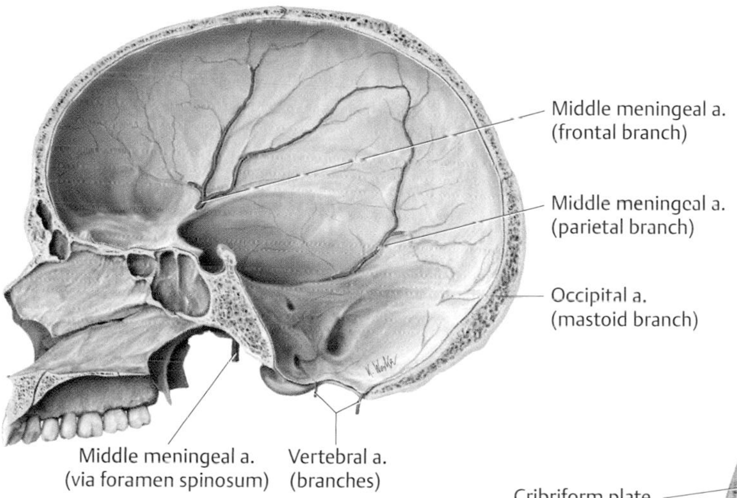

Fig. 34.15 **Innervation of the dura mater**
Superior view. *Removed:* Tentorium cerebelli (right side).

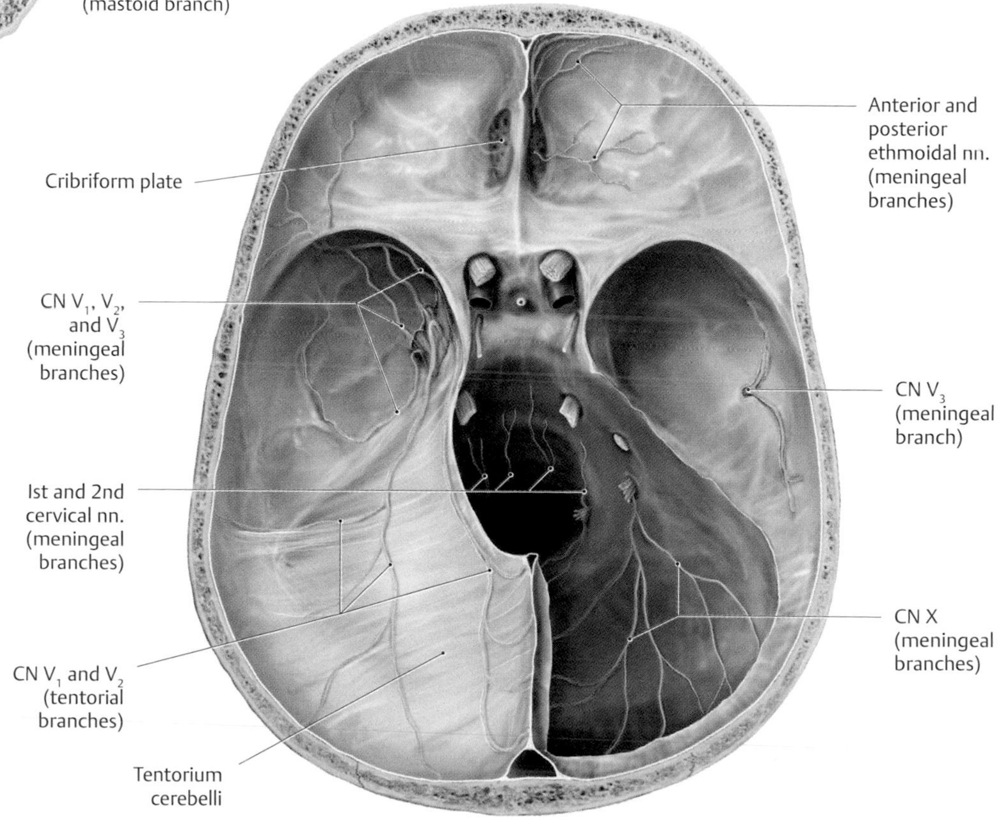

Anterior and posterior ethmoidal nn. (meningeal branches)
Cribriform plate
CN V_1, V_2, and V_3 (meningeal branches)
CN V_3 (meningeal branch)
Ist and 2nd cervical nn. (meningeal branches)
CN X (meningeal branches)
CN V_1 and V_2 (tentorial branches)
Tentorium cerebelli

Dural Sinuses

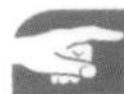

The dura mater is composed of two layers that separate in the region of a venous sinus into an outer periosteal layer, which lines the calvarium and an inner meningeal layer, which forms the unattached boundaries of the sinus. In the region of a sinus, the two meningeal dural layers come together after forming the sinus to create a dural fold, or septa (see Fig. 34.13, p. 524). The network of venous sinuses collect blood from the scalp, the calvarial bones, and the brain and eventually drain into the internal jugular vein at the jugular foramen.

Fig. 34.16 Dural sinus

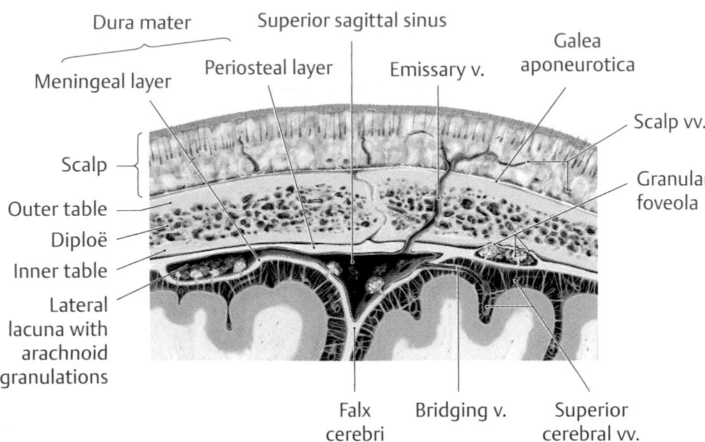

Dura mater
Superior sagittal sinus
Meningeal layer
Periosteal layer
Emissary v.
Galea aponeurotica
Scalp vv.
Scalp
Granular foveola
Outer table
Diploë
Inner table
Lateral lacuna with arachnoid granulations
Falx cerebri
Bridging v.
Superior cerebral vv.

A Structure of a dural sinus. Superior sagittal sinus, coronal section, anterior view.

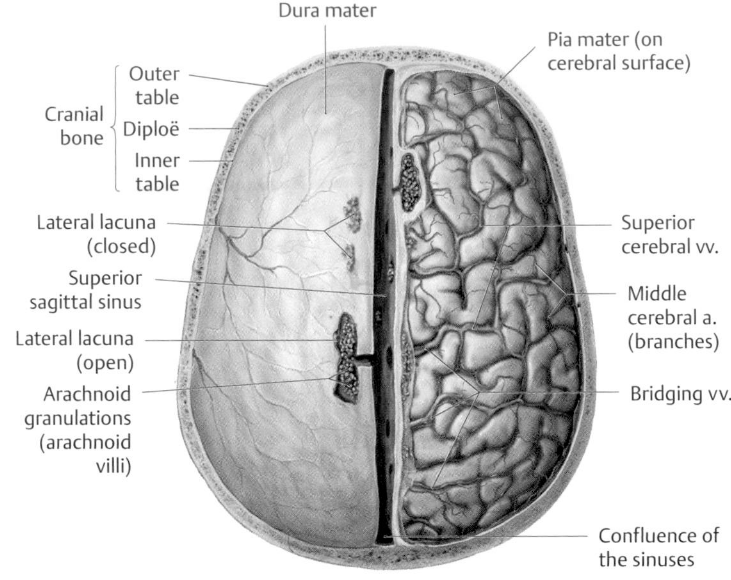

Dura mater
Pia mater (on cerebral surface)
Cranial bone
Outer table
Diploë
Inner table
Lateral lacuna (closed)
Superior sagittal sinus
Lateral lacuna (open)
Arachnoid granulations (arachnoid villi)
Superior cerebral vv.
Middle cerebral a. (branches)
Bridging vv.
Confluence of the sinuses

B Superior sagittal sinus in situ. Superior view of opened cranial cavity. The roof of the sinus (the periosteal layer of the dura attached to the calvarium) is removed. *Left side:* Areas of dura mater removed to show arachnoid granulations (protrusions of the arachnoid layer of the meninges) in the sinus. *Right side:* Dura mater and arachnoid layers removed to reveal pia mater adhering to the cerebral cortex.

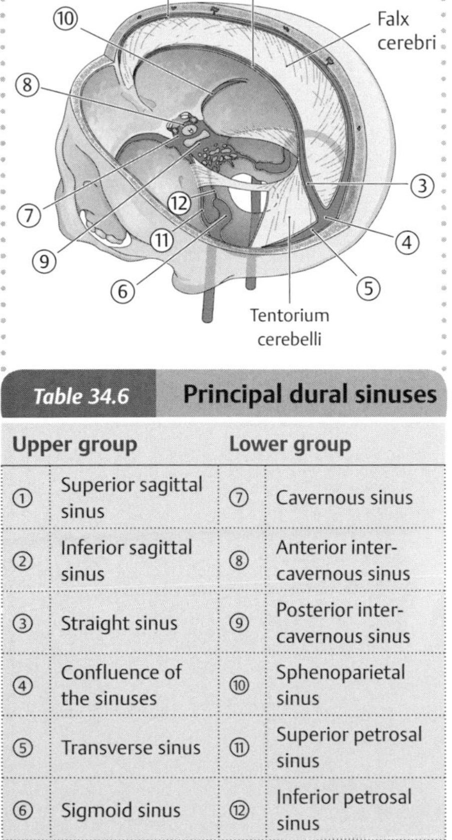

①
②
⑩
Falx cerebri
⑧
③
⑦
⑫
⑪
④
⑨
⑥
⑤
Tentorium cerebelli

Table 34.6	**Principal dural sinuses**		
Upper group		**Lower group**	
①	Superior sagittal sinus	⑦	Cavernous sinus
②	Inferior sagittal sinus	⑧	Anterior intercavernous sinus
③	Straight sinus	⑨	Posterior intercavernous sinus
④	Confluence of the sinuses	⑩	Sphenoparietal sinus
⑤	Transverse sinus	⑪	Superior petrosal sinus
⑥	Sigmoid sinus	⑫	Inferior petrosal sinus
The occipital sinus is also included in the upper group (see Fig. 41.1, p. 636).			

Fig. 34.17 Dural sinuses in the cranial cavity

Superior view of opened cranial cavity, dural sinus system ghosted in blue. *Removed:* Tentorium cerebelli (right side).

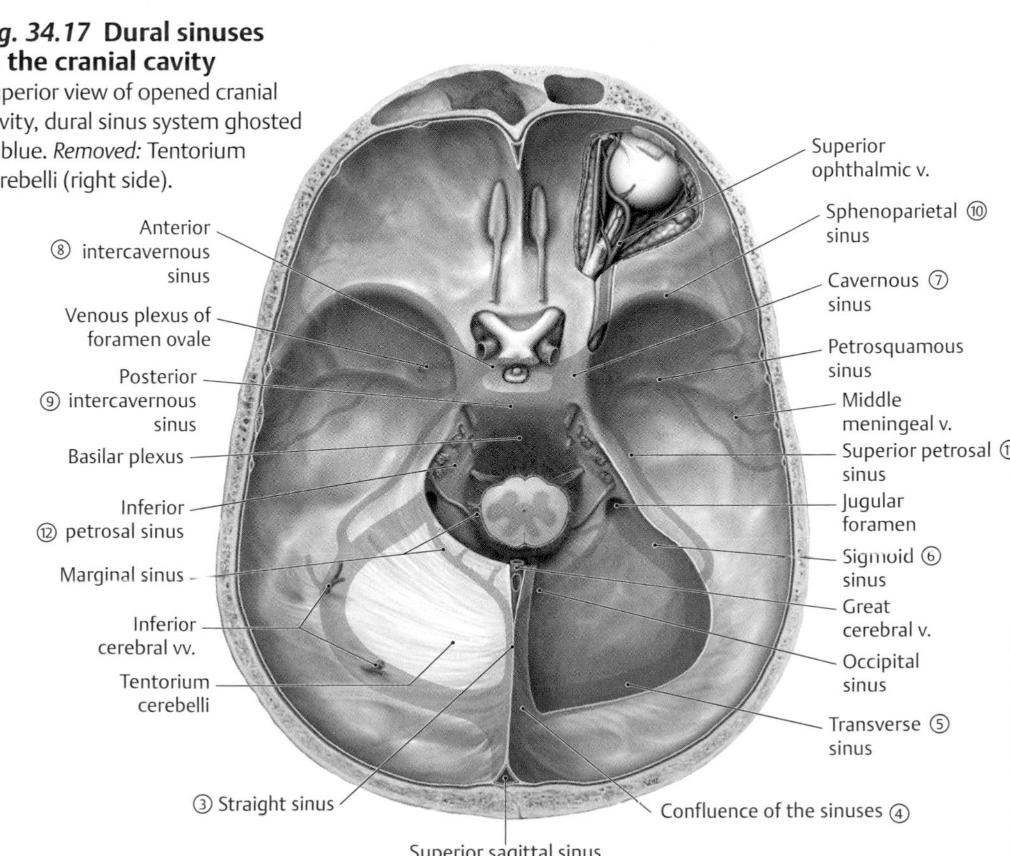

Superior ophthalmic v.
Sphenoparietal ⑩ sinus
Anterior ⑧ intercavernous sinus
Cavernous ⑦ sinus
Venous plexus of foramen ovale
Petrosquamous sinus
Posterior ⑨ intercavernous sinus
Middle meningeal v.
Basilar plexus
Superior petrosal ⑪ sinus
Inferior ⑫ petrosal sinus
Jugular foramen
Marginal sinus
Sigmoid ⑥ sinus
Inferior cerebral vv.
Great cerebral v.
Occipital sinus
Tentorium cerebelli
Transverse ⑤ sinus
③ Straight sinus
Confluence of the sinuses ④
Superior sagittal sinus ①

Fig. 34.18 Cavernous sinus and cranial nerves
Superior view of the left anterior and middle cranial fossae. *Removed:* Lateral dural wall and roof of the cavernous sinus. The trigeminal ganglion is cut and retracted laterally following removal of its dural covering

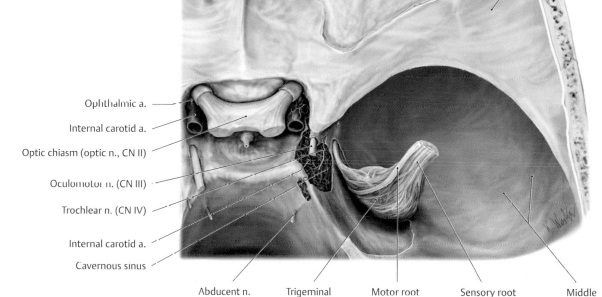

Periorbita (periosteum of the orbit)
Supratrochlear n.
Supraorbital n.
Adipose tissue of the orbit
Frontal n.
Anterior cranial fossa
Ophthalmic a.
Internal carotid a.
Optic chiasm (optic n., CN II)
Oculomotor n. (CN III)
Trochlear n. (CN IV)
Internal carotid a.
Cavernous sinus
Abducent n. (CN VI)
Trigeminal ganglion
Motor root
Sensory root
Trigeminal nerve (CN V)
Middle cranial fossa

Fig. 34.19 Cavernous sinus, coronal section through middle cranial fossa
Anterior view. The right and left cavernous sinuses connect via the intercavernous sinuses that pass around the hypophysis, which sits in the hypophyseal fossa after invaginating the diaphragma sellae. On each side, this coronal section cuts through the internal carotid artery twice due to the presence of the carotid siphon, a 180 degree bend in the cavernous part of the artery. Of the five cranial nerves, or their divisions, associated with the sinus only the abducent nerve (CN VI) is not embedded in the lateral dural wall.

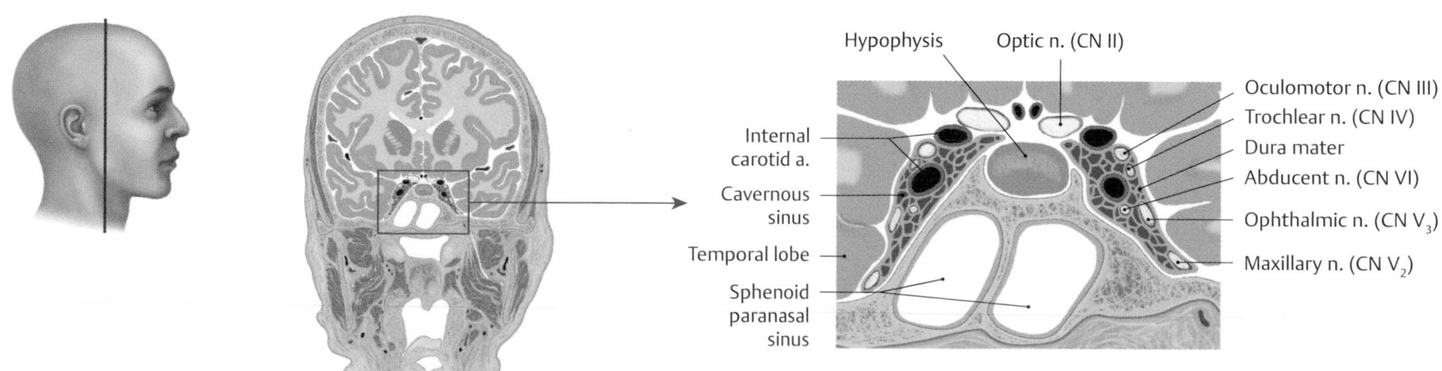
Hypophysis
Optic n. (CN II)
Internal carotid a.
Cavernous sinus
Temporal lobe
Sphenoid paranasal sinus
Oculomotor n. (CN III)
Trochlear n. (CN IV)
Dura mater
Abducent n. (CN VI)
Ophthalmic n. (CN V_1)
Maxillary n. (CN V_2)

Topography of the Superficial Face

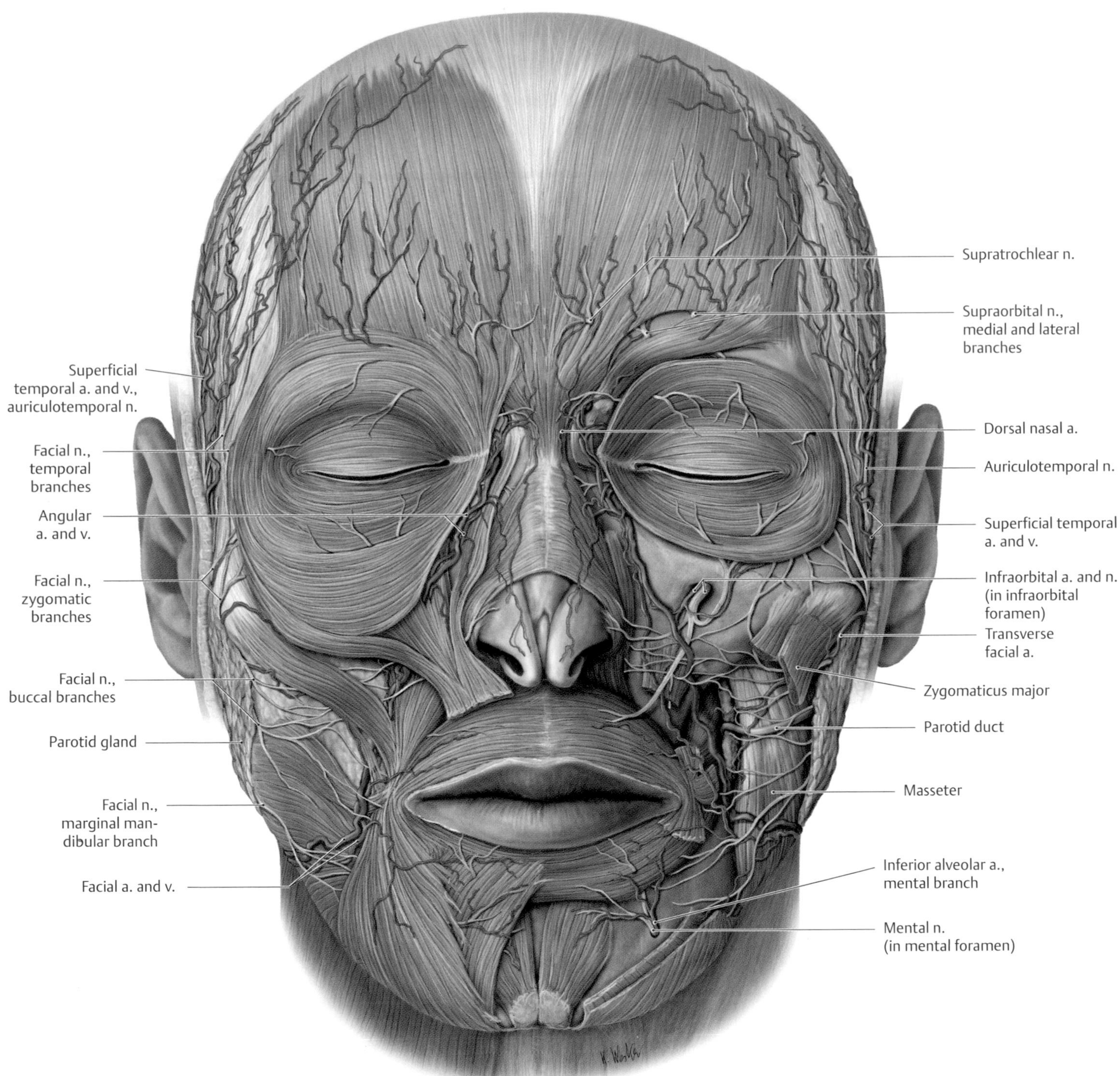

Supratrochlear n.
Supraorbital n., medial and lateral branches
Superficial temporal a. and v., auriculotemporal n.
Dorsal nasal a.
Facial n., temporal branches
Auriculotemporal n.
Angular a. and v.
Superficial temporal a. and v.
Facial n., zygomatic branches
Infraorbital a. and n. (in infraorbital foramen)
Transverse facial a.
Facial n., buccal branches
Zygomaticus major
Parotid duct
Parotid gland
Masseter
Facial n., marginal mandibular branch
Inferior alveolar a., mental branch
Facial a. and v.
Mental n. (in mental foramen)

Fig. 34.20 Superficial neurovasculature of the face
Anterior view. *Removed:* Skin and fatty subcutaneous tissue; muscles of facial expression (left side).

Fig. 34.21 **Superficial neurovasculature of the head**
Left lateral view.

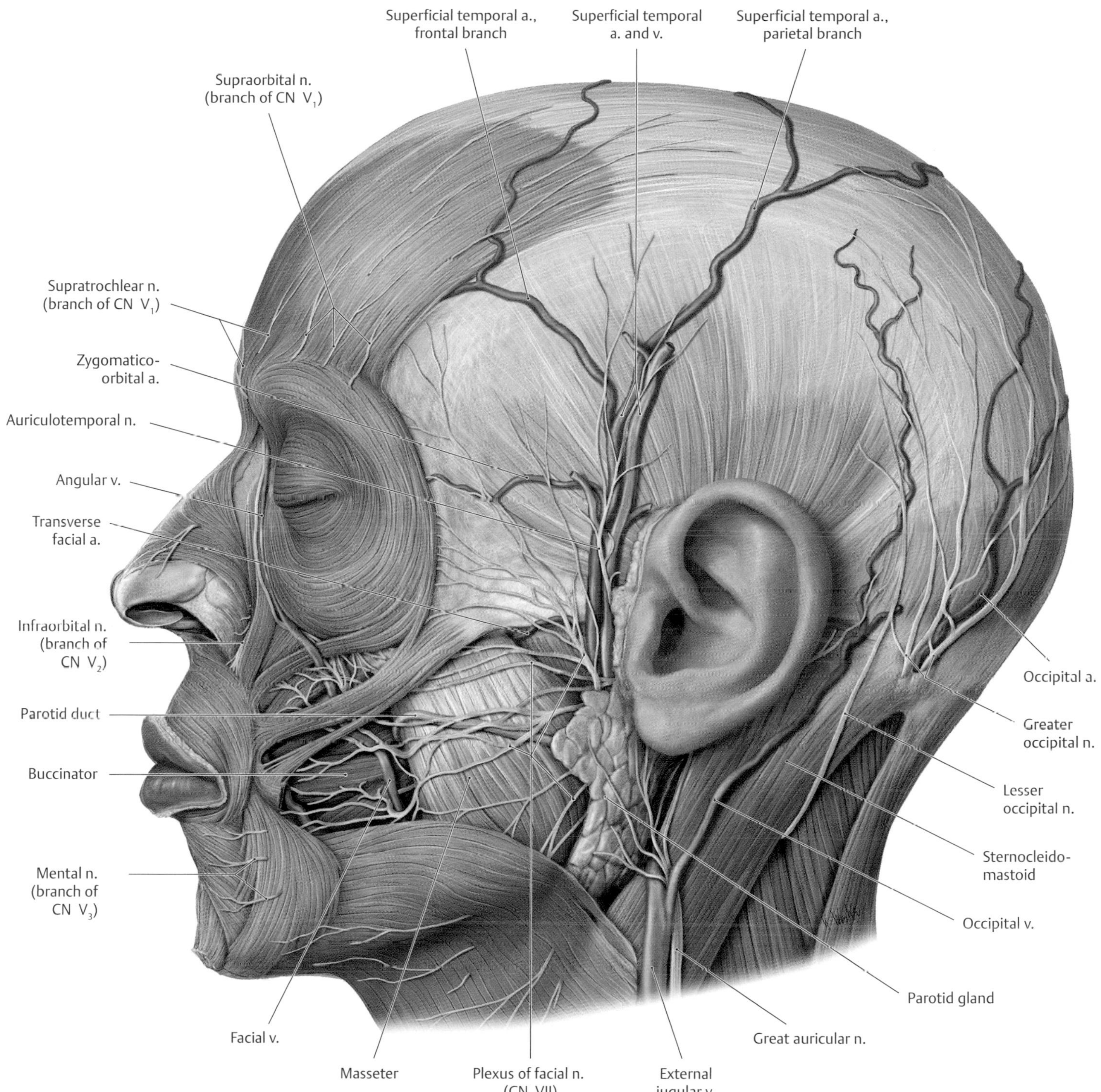

Superficial temporal a., frontal branch
Superficial temporal a. and v.
Superficial temporal a., parietal branch
Supraorbital n. (branch of CN V_1)
Supratrochlear n. (branch of CN V_1)
Zygomatico-orbital a.
Auriculotemporal n.
Angular v.
Transverse facial a.
Infraorbital n. (branch of CN V_2)
Parotid duct
Buccinator
Mental n. (branch of CN V_3)
Facial v.
Masseter
Plexus of facial n. (CN VII)
External jugular v.
Great auricular n.
Parotid gland
Occipital v.
Sternocleido-mastoid
Lesser occipital n.
Greater occipital n.
Occipital a.

Topography of the Parotid Region & Temporal Fossa

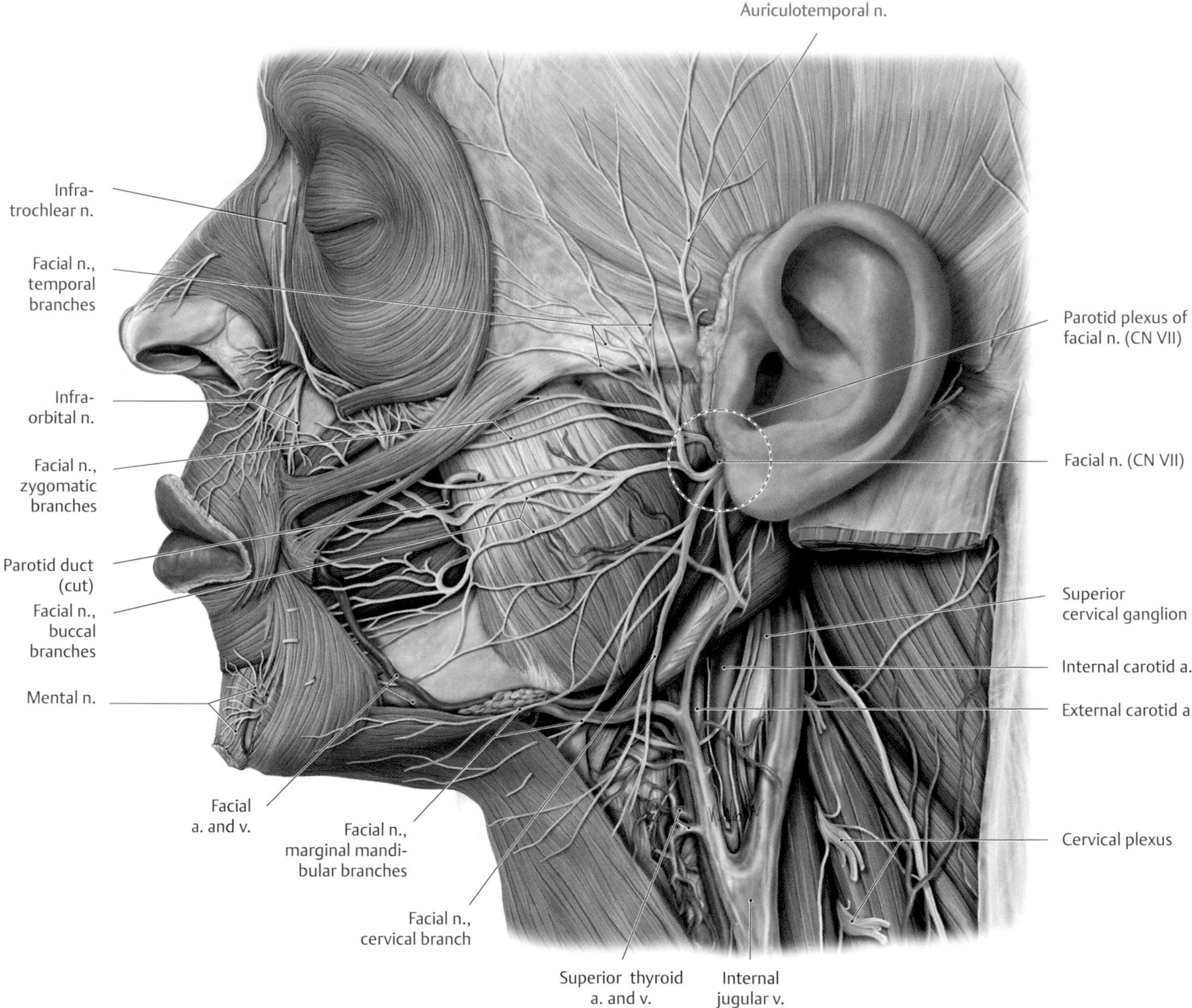
Auriculotemporal n.
Infra-
trochlear n.
Facial n.,
temporal
branches
Infra-
orbital n.
Facial n.,
zygomatic
branches
Parotid duct
(cut)
Facial n.,
buccal
branches
Mental n.
Facial
a. and v.
Facial n.,
marginal mandi-
bular branches
Facial n.,
cervical branch
Superior thyroid
a. and v.
Internal
jugular v.
Parotid plexus of
facial n. (CN VII)
Facial n. (CN VII)
Superior
cervical ganglion
Internal carotid a.
External carotid a.
Cervical plexus

Fig. 34.22 **Parotid region**
Left lateral view. *Removed:* Parotid gland, sternocleidomastoid, and veins of the head. *Revealed:* Parotid bed and carotid triangle.

Fig. 34.23 **Temporal fossa**
Left lateral view. *Removed:* Sternocleidomastoid and masseter. *Revealed:* Temporal fossa and temporomandibular joint (p. 570).

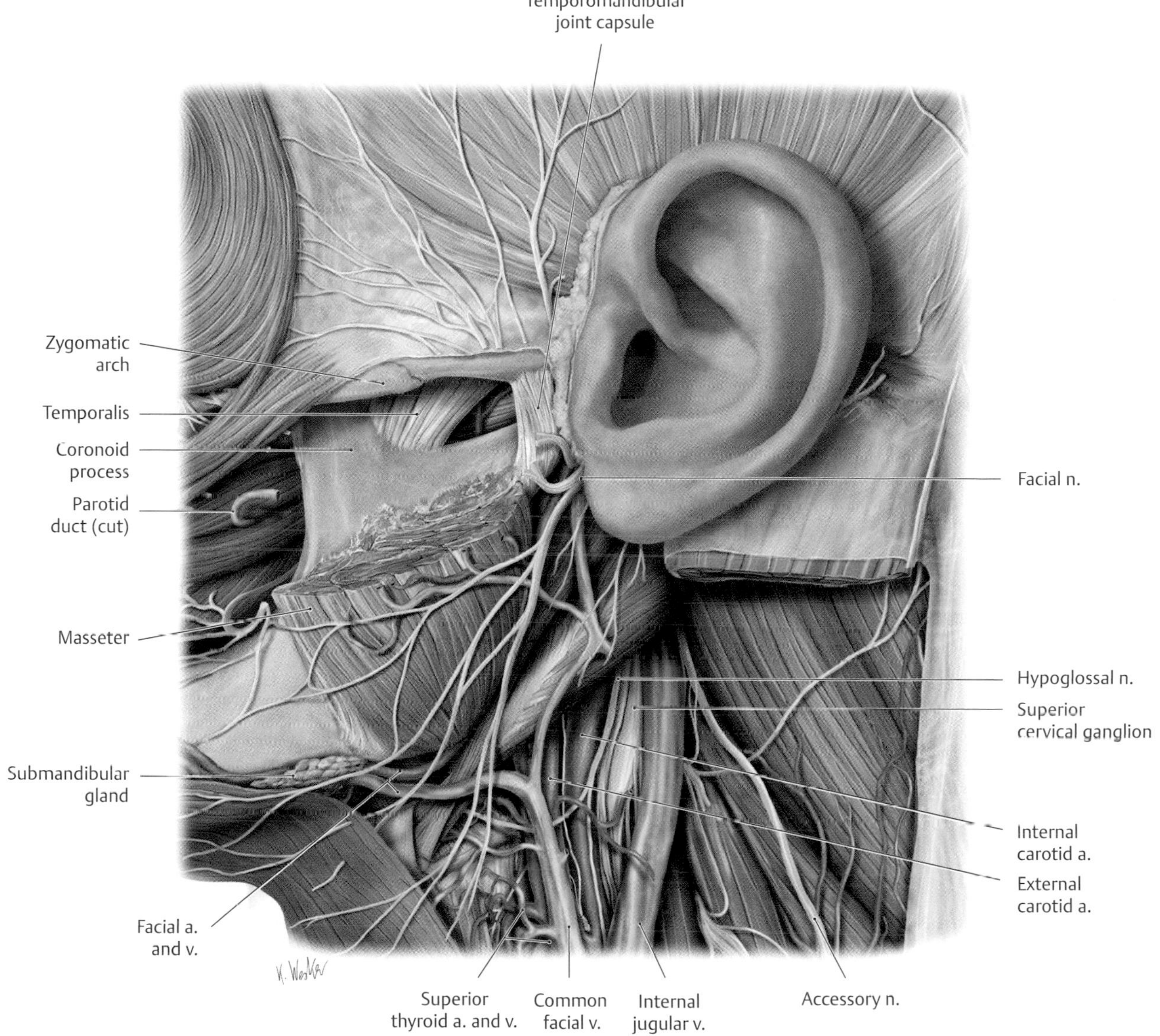
Temporomandibular joint capsule
Zygomatic arch
Temporalis
Coronoid process
Parotid duct (cut)
Masseter
Submandibular gland
Facial a. and v.
Superior thyroid a. and v.
Common facial v.
Internal jugular v.
Accessory n.
Facial n.
Hypoglossal n.
Superior cervical ganglion
Internal carotid a.
External carotid a.

Topography of the Infratemporal Fossa

Fig. 34.24 Infratemporal fossa: Superficial layer

Left lateral view. *Removed:* Ramus of mandible. *Note:* The mylohyoid nerve (see Fig. 38.17 and 38.19A) branches from the inferior alveolar nerve just before the mandibular foramen.

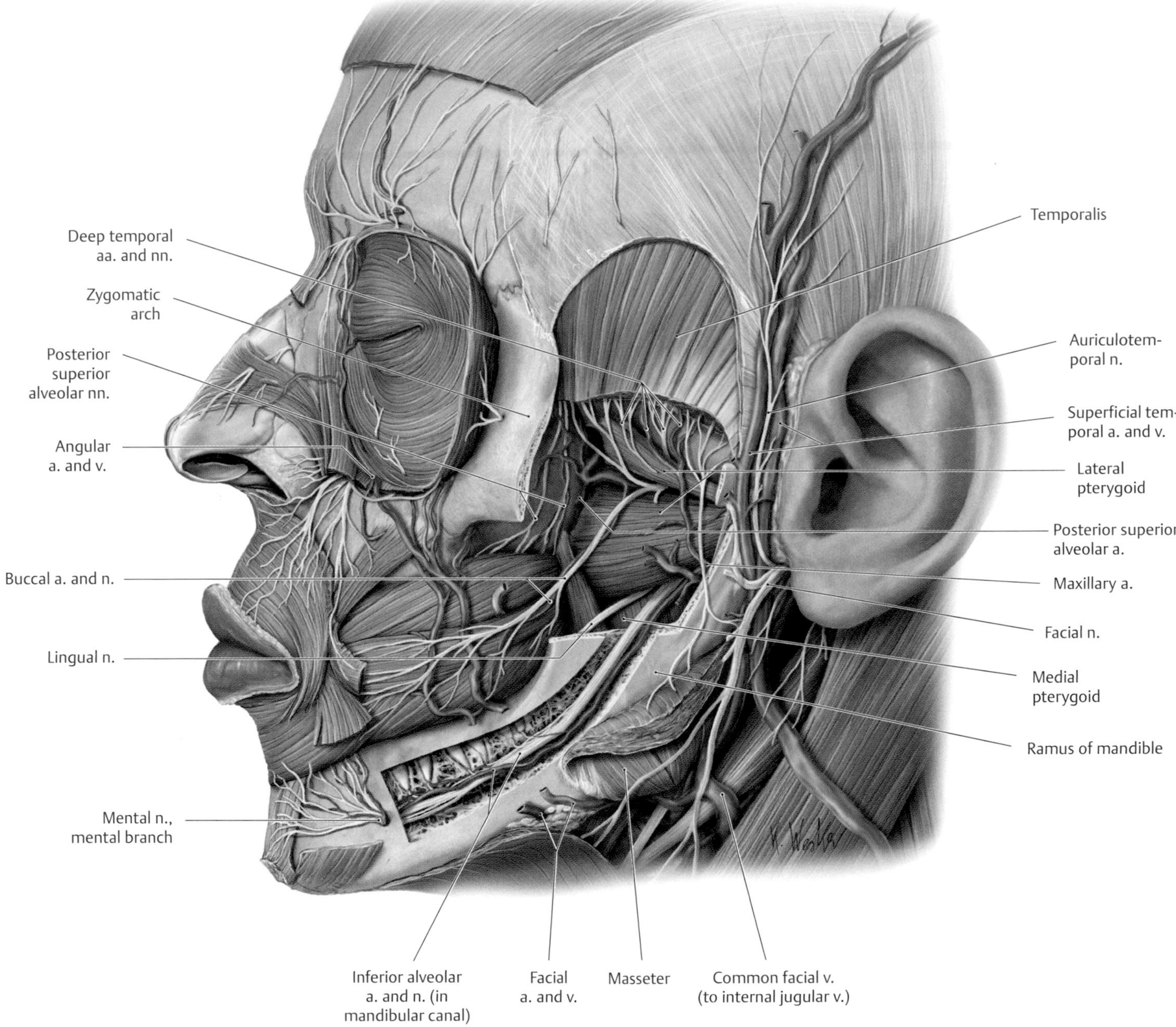
Deep temporal
aa. and nn.
Zygomatic
arch
Posterior
superior
alveolar nn.
Angular
a. and v.
Buccal a. and n.
Lingual n.
Mental n.,
mental branch
Temporalis
Auriculotem-
poral n.
Superficial tem-
poral a. and v.
Lateral
pterygoid
Posterior superior
alveolar a.
Maxillary a.
Facial n.
Medial
pterygoid
Ramus of mandible
Inferior alveolar
a. and n. (in
mandibular canal)
Facial
a. and v.
Masseter
Common facial v.
(to internal jugular v.)

Fig. 34.25 Deep layer

Left lateral view. *Removed:* Lateral pterygoid muscle (both heads). *Revealed:* Deep infratemporal fossa and mandibular nerve as it enters the mandibular canal via the foramen ovale in the roof of the fossa.

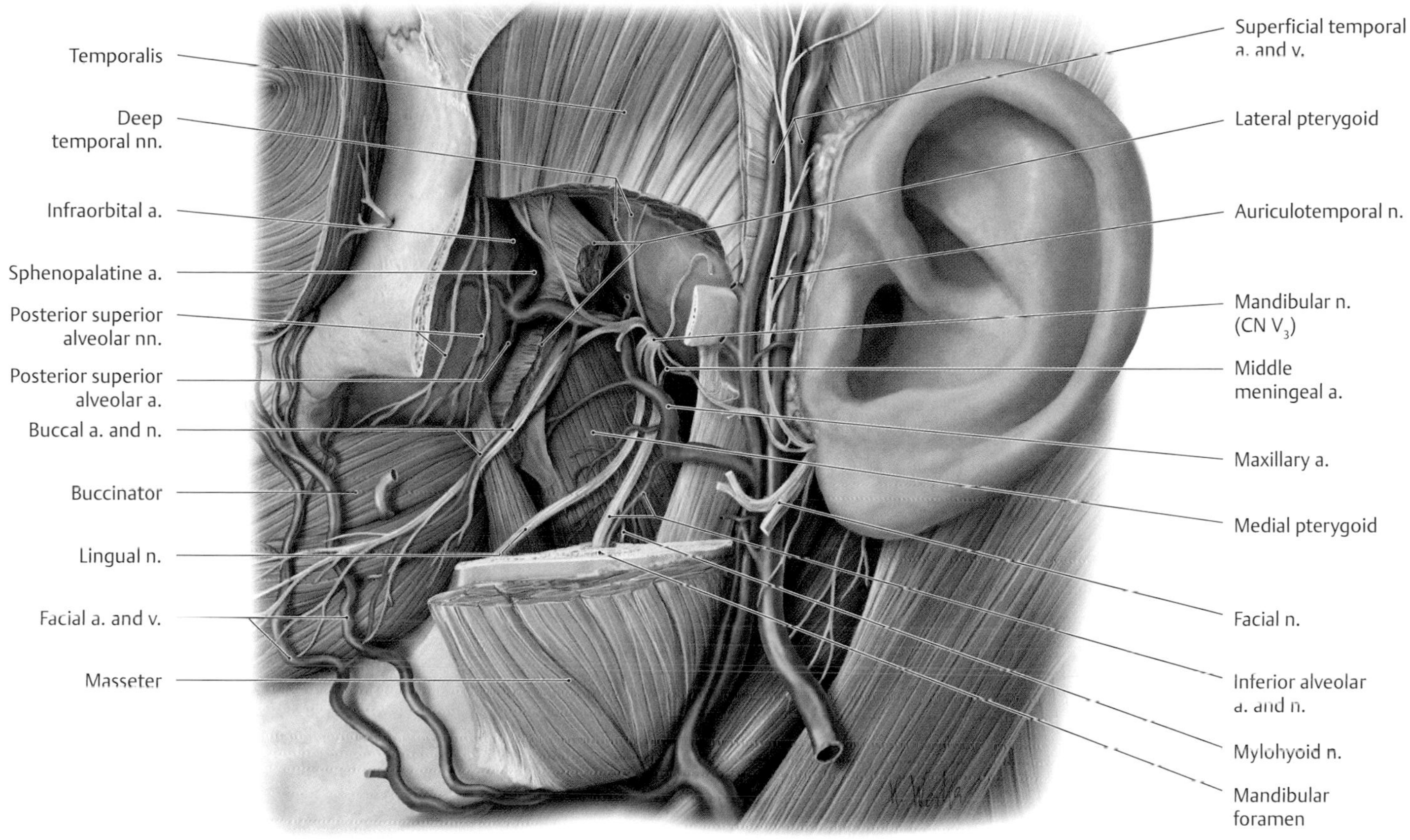
Temporalis
Deep temporal nn.
Infraorbital a.
Sphenopalatine a.
Posterior superior alveolar nn.
Posterior superior alveolar a.
Buccal a. and n.
Buccinator
Lingual n.
Facial a. and v.
Masseter
Superficial temporal a. and v.
Lateral pterygoid
Auriculotemporal n.
Mandibular n. (CN V_3)
Middle meningeal a.
Maxillary a.
Medial pterygoid
Facial n.
Inferior alveolar a. and n.
Mylohyoid n.
Mandibular foramen

Fig. 34.26 Mandibular nerve (CN V_3) in the infratemporal fossa

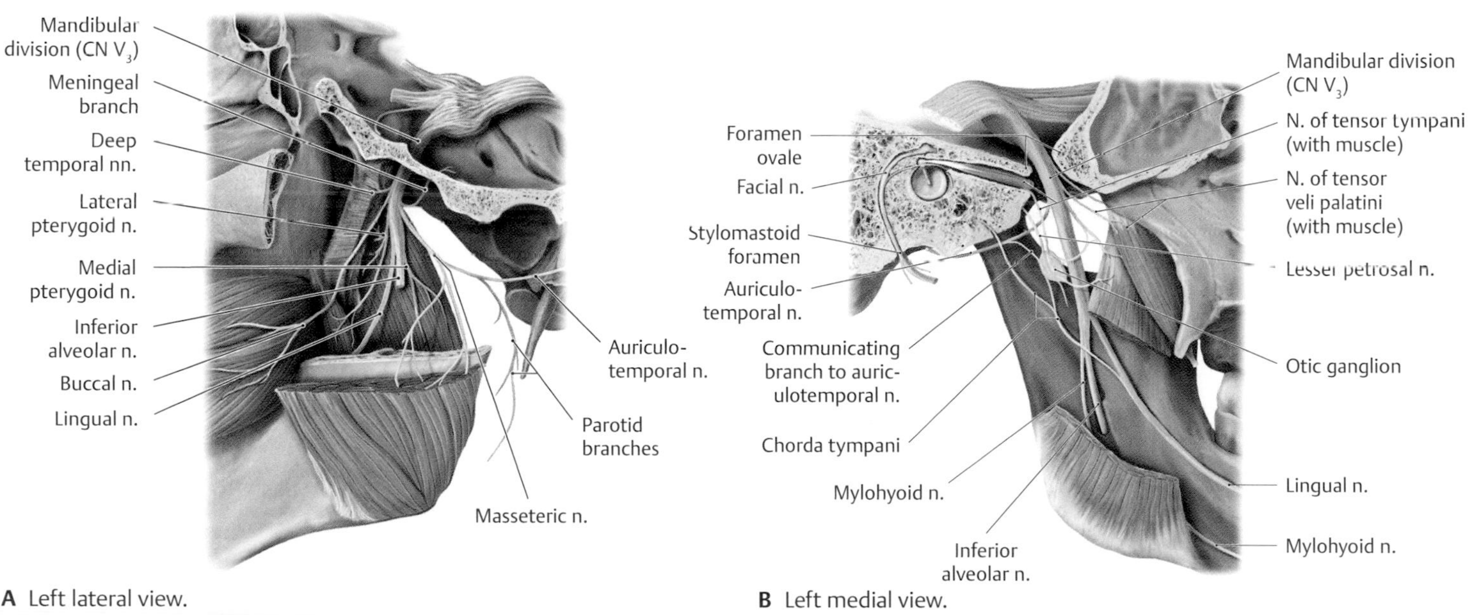
Mandibular division (CN V_3)
Meningeal branch
Deep temporal nn.
Lateral pterygoid n.
Medial pterygoid n.
Inferior alveolar n.
Buccal n.
Lingual n.
Masseteric n.
Auriculo-temporal n.
Parotid branches
Foramen ovale
Facial n.
Stylomastoid foramen
Auriculo-temporal n.
Communicating branch to auric-ulotemporal n.
Chorda tympani
Mylohyoid n.
Inferior alveolar n.
Mandibular division (CN V_3)
N. of tensor tympani (with muscle)
N. of tensor veli palatini (with muscle)
Lesser petrosal n.
Otic ganglion
Lingual n.
Mylohyoid n.

A Left lateral view.

B Left medial view.

Topography of the Pterygopalatine Fossa

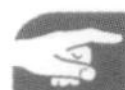

The pterygopalatine fossa is a small pyramidal space just inferior to the apex of the orbit. It is continuous with the infratemporal fossa laterally through the pterygomaxillary fissure.

The pterygopalatine fossa is a crossroads for neurovascular structures traveling between the middle cranial fossa, orbit, nasal cavity, and oral cavity.

Table 34.7 Borders of the pterygopalatine fossa

Direction	Boundaries	Direction	Boundaries
Superior	Sphenoid bone (greater wing), junction with inferior orbital fissure	Posterior	Pterygoid process (lateral plate)
Anterior	Maxillary tuberosity	Lateral	Communicates with the infratemporal fossa via the pterygomaxillary fissure
Medial	Palatine bone (perpendicular plate)	Inferior	None; opens into the retropharyngeal space

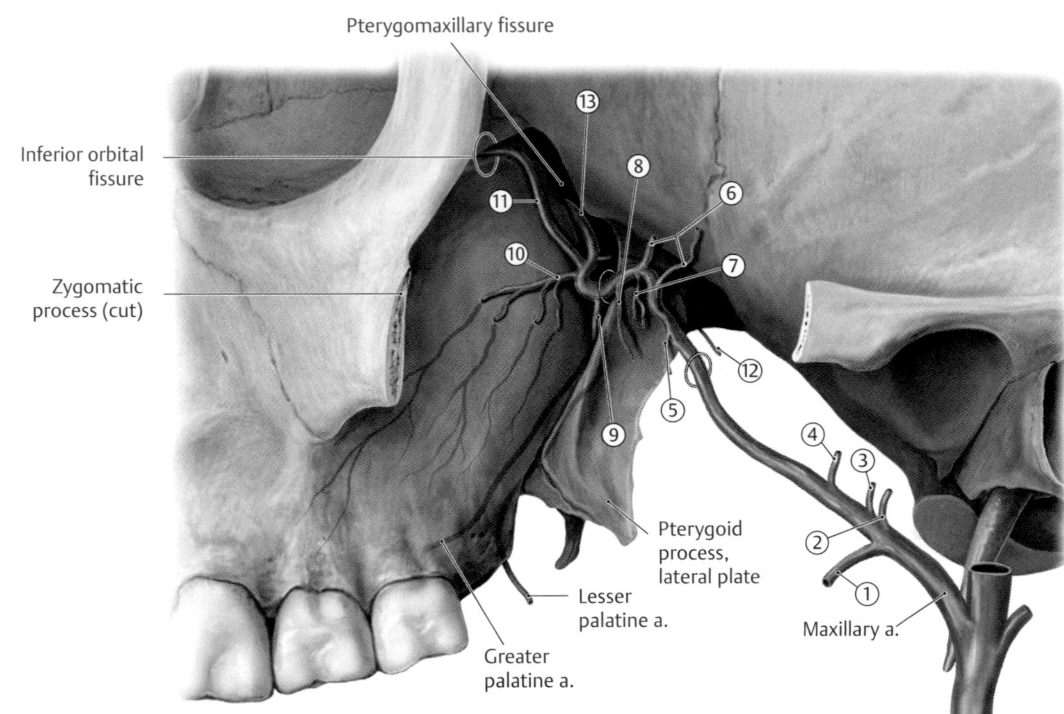

Pterygomaxillary fissure
Inferior orbital fissure
Zygomatic process (cut)
Pterygoid process, lateral plate
Lesser palatine a.
Greater palatine a.
Maxillary a.
①
②
③
④
⑤
⑥
⑦
⑧
⑨
⑩
⑪
⑫
⑬

Fig. 34.27 **Arteries in the pterygopalatine fossa**
Left lateral view into area. The maxillary artery passes either superficial or deep to the lateral pterygoid in the infratemporal fossa (see Fig. 34.24) and enters the pterygopalatine fossa through the pterygomaxillary fissure.

Table 34.8 Branches of the maxillary artery

Part	Artery		Distribution
Mandibular part (between the origin and the first circle around artery)	① Inferior alveolar a.		Mandible, teeth, gingiva
	② Anterior tympanic a.		Tympanic cavity
	③ Deep auricular a.		Temporomandibular joint, external auditory canal
	④ Middle meningeal a.		Calvaria, dura, anterior and middle cranial fossae
Pterygoid part (between circles around the artery)	⑤ Masseteric a.		Masseter muscle
	⑥ Deep temporal aa.		Temporalis muscle
	⑦ Pterygoid branches		Pterygoid muscles
	⑧ Buccal a.		Buccal mucosa
Pterygopalatine part (from second circle through the pterygomaxillary fissure)	⑨ Descending palatine a.	Greater palatine a.	Hard palate
		Lesser palatine a.	Soft palate, palatine tonsil, pharyngeal wall
	⑩ Posterior superior alveolar a.		Maxillary molars, maxillary sinus, gingiva
	⑪ Infraorbital a.		Maxillary alveoli
	⑫ A. of pterygoid canal		
	⑬ Sphenopalatine a.	Lateral posterior nasal aa.	Lateral wall of nasal cavity, choanae
		Posterior septal branches	Nasal septum

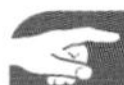

The maxillary division of the trigeminal nerve (CN V_2, see p. 503) passes from the middle cranial fossa through the foramen rotundum into the pterygopalatine fossa. The parasympathetic pterygopalatine ganglion receives presynaptic fibers from the greater petrosal nerve (the parasympathetic root of the nervus intermedius branch of the facial nerve). The preganglionic fibers of the pterygopalatine ganglion synapse with ganglion cells that innervate the lacrimal, small palatal, and small nasal glands. The sympathetic fibers of the deep petrosal nerve (sympathetic root) and sensory fibers of the maxillary nerve (sensory root) pass through the pterygopalatine ganglion without synapsing.
The pterygopalatine structures can be seen from the medial view in Fig. 36.8B, p. 555.

Fig. 34.28 **Nerves in the pterygopalatine fossa**
Left lateral view.

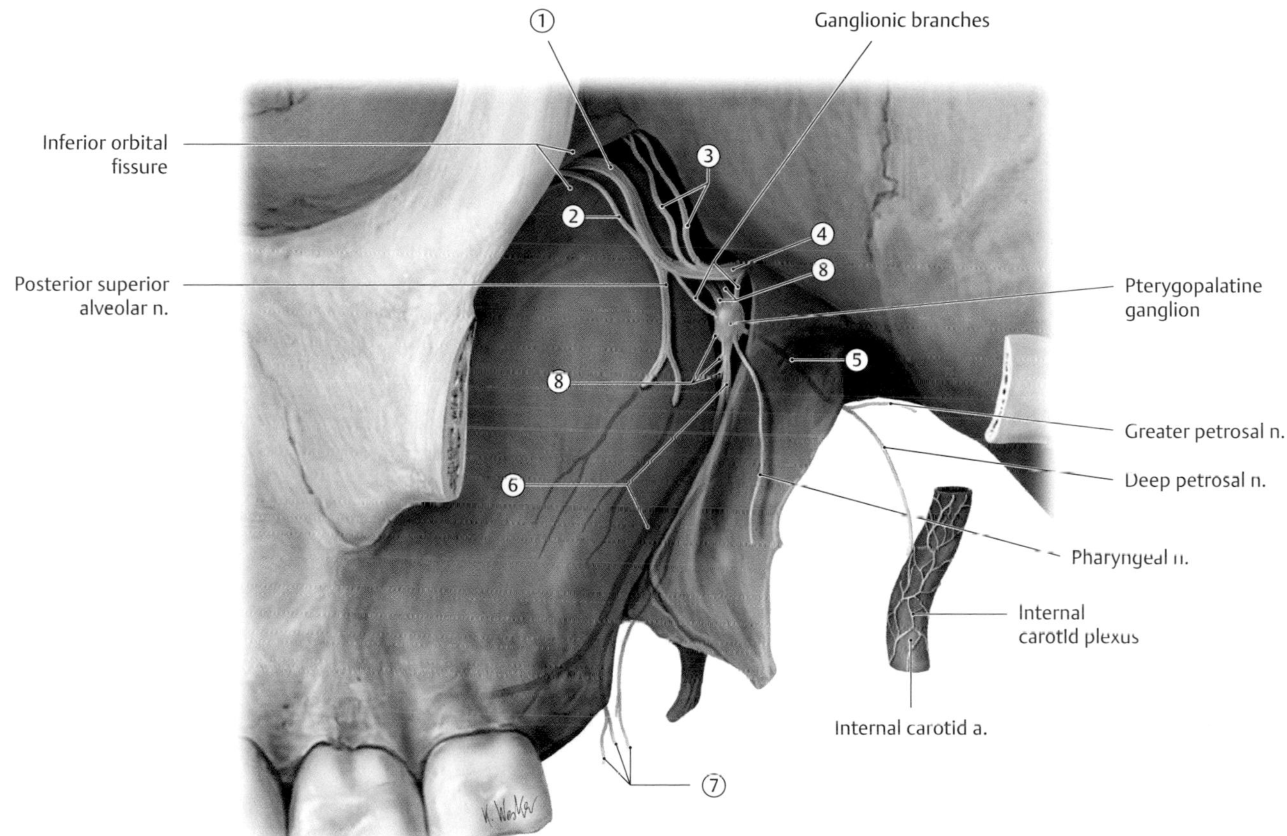

①
Ganglionic branches
Inferior orbital fissure
③
②
④
⑧
Posterior superior alveolar n.
Pterygopalatine ganglion
⑤
⑧
Greater petrosal n.
Deep petrosal n.
⑥
Pharyngeal n.
Internal carotid plexus
Internal carotid a.
⑦

Table 34.9 Passage of neurovascular structures into pterygopalatine fossa

Origin of structures	Passageway	Transmitted nerves	Transmitted vessels
Orbit	Inferior orbital fissure	① Infraorbital n.	Infraorbital a. (and accompanying vv.)
		② Zygomatic n.	Inferior ophthalmic v.
		③ Orbital branches (from CN V_2)	
Middle cranial fossa	Foramen rotundum	④ Maxillary n. (CN V_2)	
Base of skull	Pterygoid canal	⑤ N. of pterygoid canal (greater and deep petrosal nn.)	A. of pterygoid canal (with accompanying vv.)
Palate	Greater palatine canal	⑥ Greater palatine n.	Descending palatine a.
			Greater palatine a.
	Lesser palatine canals	⑦ Lesser palatine nn.	Lesser palatine aa. (terminal branches of descending palatine a.)
Nasal cavity	Sphenopalatine foramen	⑧ Medial and lateral posterior superior and posterior inferior nasal branches (from nasopalatine n., CN V_2)	Sphenopalatine a. (with accompanying vv.)

Bones of the Orbit

Fig. 35.1 **Bones of the orbit**

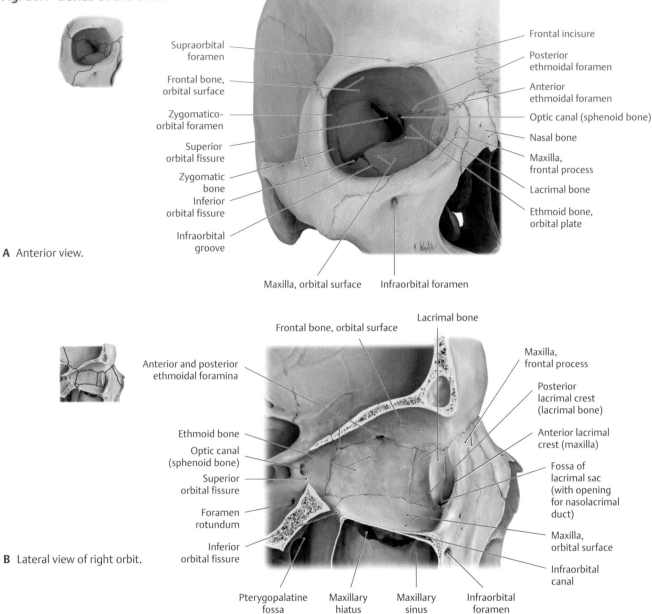

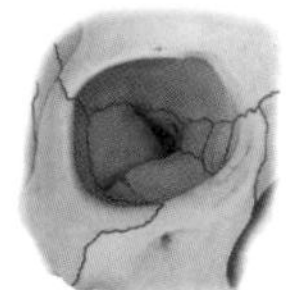
Supraorbital foramen
Frontal bone, orbital surface
Zygomatico-orbital foramen
Superior orbital fissure
Zygomatic bone
Inferior orbital fissure
Infraorbital groove
Maxilla, orbital surface
Infraorbital foramen
Frontal incisure
Posterior ethmoidal foramen
Anterior ethmoidal foramen
Optic canal (sphenoid bone)
Nasal bone
Maxilla, frontal process
Lacrimal bone
Ethmoid bone, orbital plate

A Anterior view.

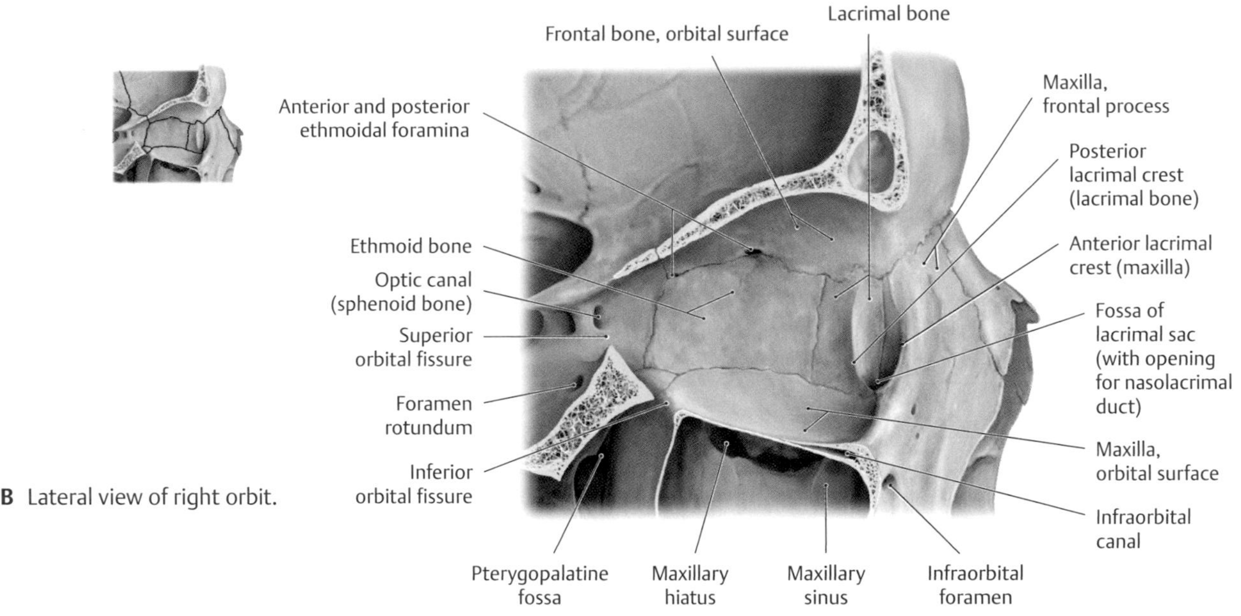
Frontal bone, orbital surface
Lacrimal bone
Anterior and posterior ethmoidal foramina
Ethmoid bone
Optic canal (sphenoid bone)
Superior orbital fissure
Foramen rotundum
Inferior orbital fissure
Maxilla, frontal process
Posterior lacrimal crest (lacrimal bone)
Anterior lacrimal crest (maxilla)
Fossa of lacrimal sac (with opening for nasolacrimal duct)
Maxilla, orbital surface
Infraorbital canal
Pterygopalatine fossa
Maxillary hiatus
Maxillary sinus
Infraorbital foramen

B Lateral view of right orbit.

Table 35.1 Openings in the orbit for neurovascular structures

Opening*	Nerves		Vessels
Optic canal	Optic n. (CN II)		Ophthalmic a.
Superior orbital fissure	Oculomotor n. (CN III) Trochlear n. (CN IV) Abducent n. (CN VI)	Trigeminal n., ophthalmic division (CN V_1) • Lacrimal n. • Frontal n. • Nasociliary n.	Superior ophthalmic v.
Inferior orbital fissure	Infraorbital n. (CN V_2) Zygomatic n. (CN V_2)		Infraorbital a. and v., inferior ophthalmic v.
Infraorbital canal	Infraorbital n. (CN V_2), a., and v.		
Supraorbital foramen	Supraorbital n. (lateral branch)		Supraorbital a.
Frontal incisure	Supraorbital n. (medial branch)		Supratrochlear a.
Anterior ethmoidal foramen	Anterior ethmoidal n., a., and v.		
Posterior ethmoidal foramen	Posterior ethmoidal n., a., and v.		

* The nasolacrimal canal transmits the nasolacrimal duct.

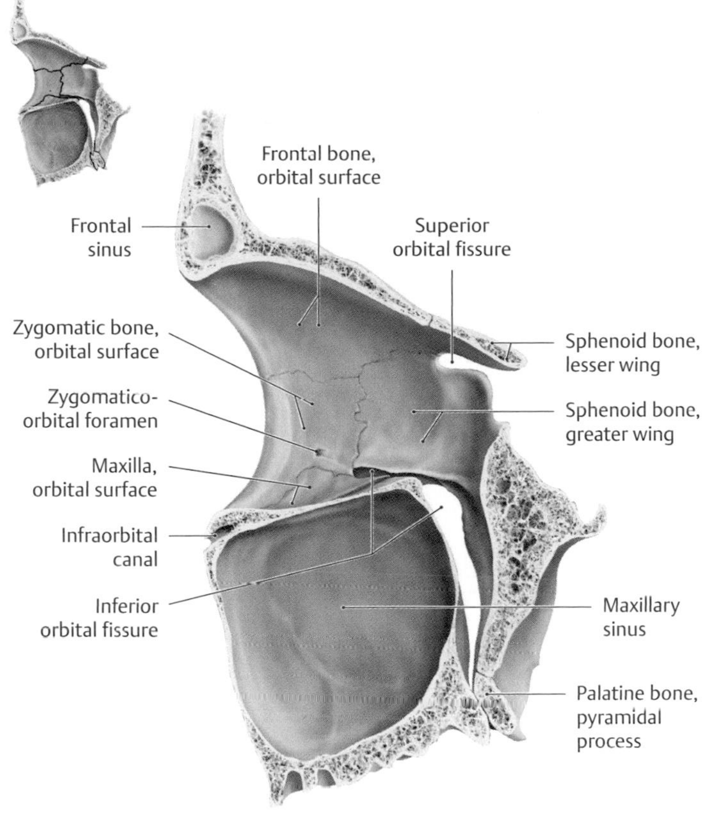
Frontal bone, orbital surface
Frontal sinus
Superior orbital fissure
Zygomatic bone, orbital surface
Sphenoid bone, lesser wing
Zygomatico-orbital foramen
Sphenoid bone, greater wing
Maxilla, orbital surface
Infraorbital canal
Inferior orbital fissure
Maxillary sinus
Palatine bone, pyramidal process

C Medial view of right orbit.

Table 35.2	**Structures surrounding the orbit**
Direction	**Bordering structure**
Superior	Frontal sinus
	Anterior cranial fossa
Medial	Ethmoid sinus
Inferior	Maxillary sinus
Certain deeper structures also have a clinically important relationship to the orbit:	
Sphenoid sinus	Hypophysis (pituitary)
Middle cranial fossa	Cavernous sinus
Optic chiasm	Pterygopalatine fossa

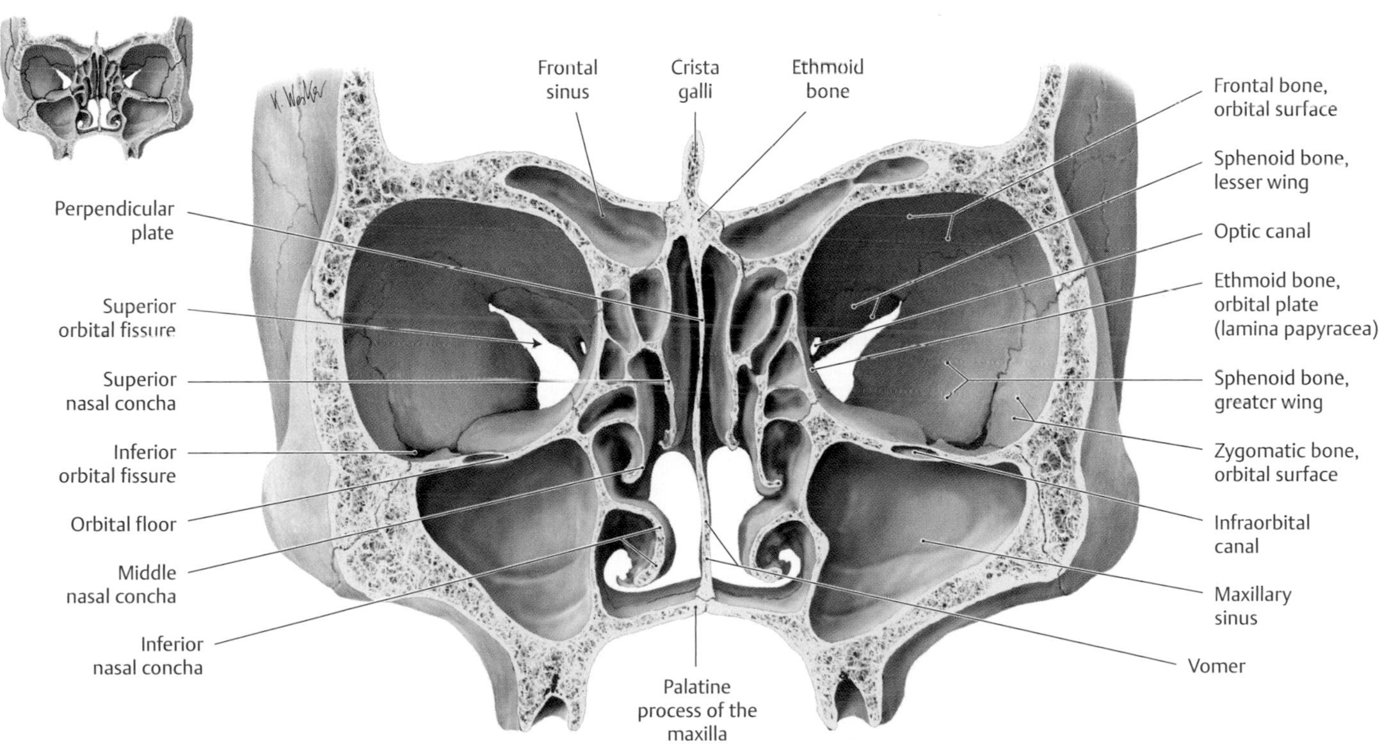
Frontal sinus
Crista galli
Ethmoid bone
Frontal bone, orbital surface
Perpendicular plate
Sphenoid bone, lesser wing
Optic canal
Superior orbital fissure
Ethmoid bone, orbital plate (lamina papyracea)
Superior nasal concha
Sphenoid bone, greater wing
Inferior orbital fissure
Zygomatic bone, orbital surface
Orbital floor
Infraorbital canal
Middle nasal concha
Maxillary sinus
Inferior nasal concha
Vomer
Palatine process of the maxilla

D Coronal section, anterior view.

Muscles of the Orbit

Fig. 35.2 Extraocular muscles

The eyeball is moved by six extrinsic muscles: four rectus (superior, inferior, medial, and lateral) and two oblique (superior and inferior).

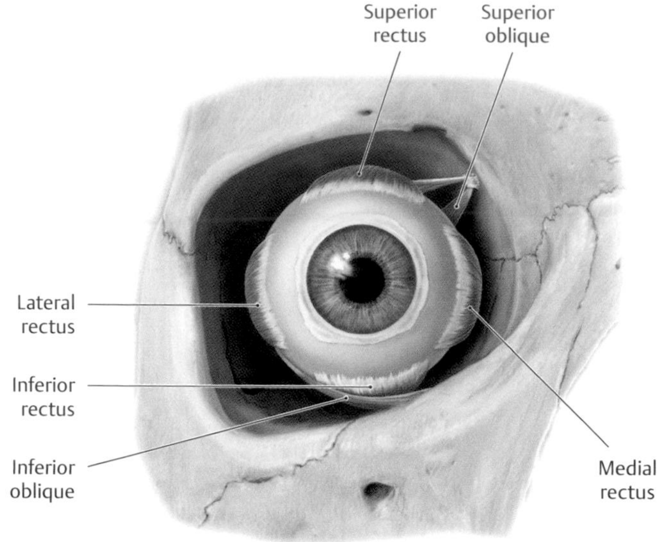
Superior rectus
Superior oblique
Lateral rectus
Inferior rectus
Inferior oblique
Medial rectus

A Right eye, anterior view.

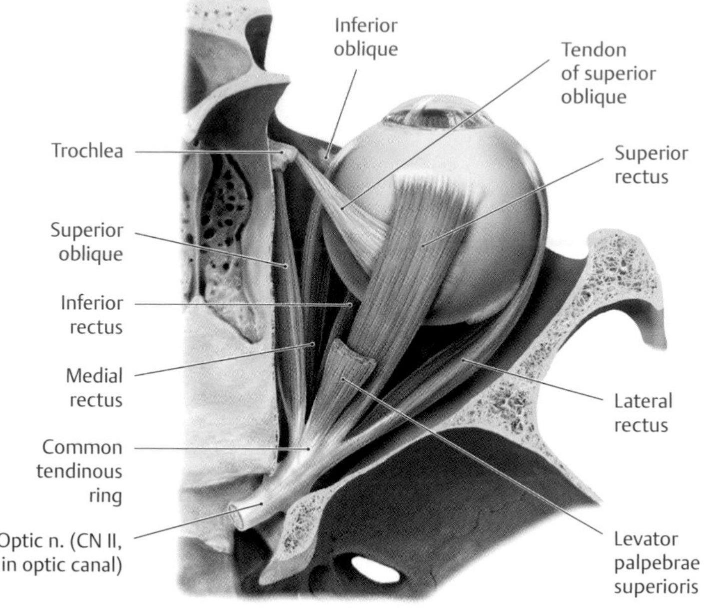
Inferior oblique
Tendon of superior oblique
Trochlea
Superior rectus
Superior oblique
Inferior rectus
Medial rectus
Common tendinous ring
Lateral rectus
Optic n. (CN II, in optic canal)
Levator palpebrae superioris

B Right eye, superior view of opened orbit.

Fig. 35.3 Actions of the extraocular muscles

Superior view of opened orbit. Vertical axis, red circle; horizontal axis, black; anteroposterior axis, blue.

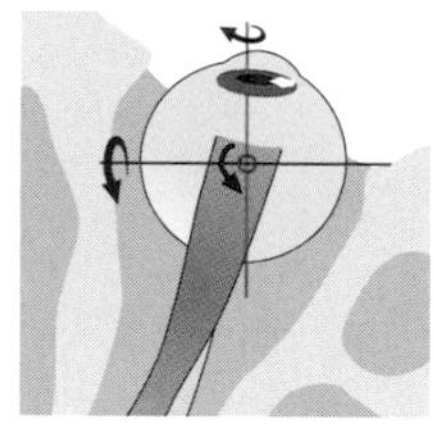

A Superior rectus.

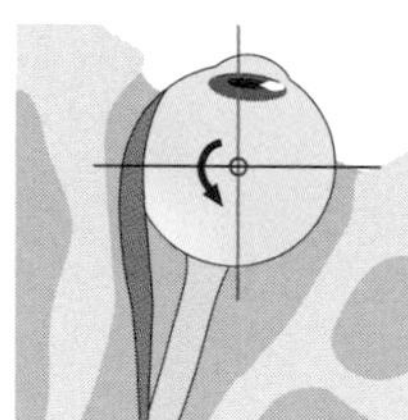

B Medial rectus.

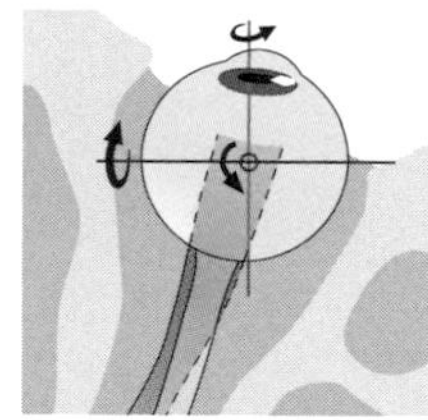

C Inferior rectus.

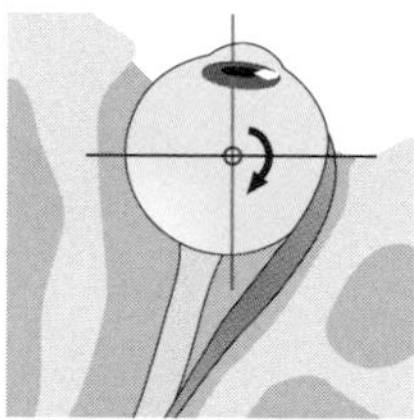

D Lateral rectus.

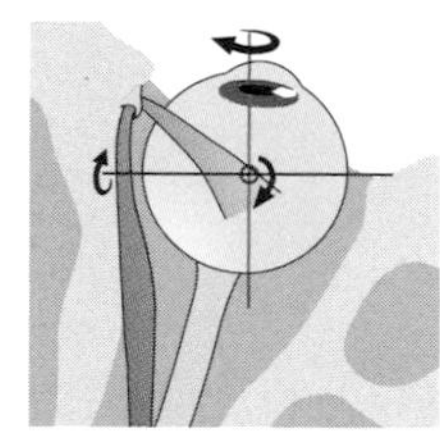

E Superior oblique.

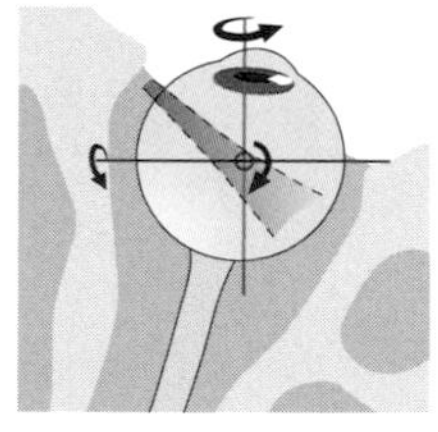

F Inferior oblique.

Table 35.3 Extraocular muscles

Muscle	Origin	Insertion	Action (see Fig. 35.3)* Vertical axis (red)	Horizontal axis (black)	Anteroposterior axis (blue)	Innervation
Superior rectus	Common tendinous ring (common annular tendon)	Sclera of the eye	Elevates	Adducts	Rotates medially	Oculomotor n. (CN III), superior branch
Medial rectus			—	Adducts	—	Oculomotor n. (CN III), inferior branch
Inferior rectus			Depresses	Adducts	Rotates laterally	
Lateral rectus			—	Abducts	—	Abducent n. (CN VI)
Superior oblique	Sphenoid bone⁺		Depresses	Abducts	Rotates medially	Trochlear n. (CN IV)
Inferior oblique	Medial orbital margin		Elevates	Abducts	Rotates laterally	Oculomotor n. (CN III), inferior branch

* Starting from gaze directed anteriorly

⁺ The tendon of insertion of the superior oblique passes through a tendinous loop (trochlea) attached to the superomedial orbital margin.

Fig. 35.4 Testing the extraocular muscles

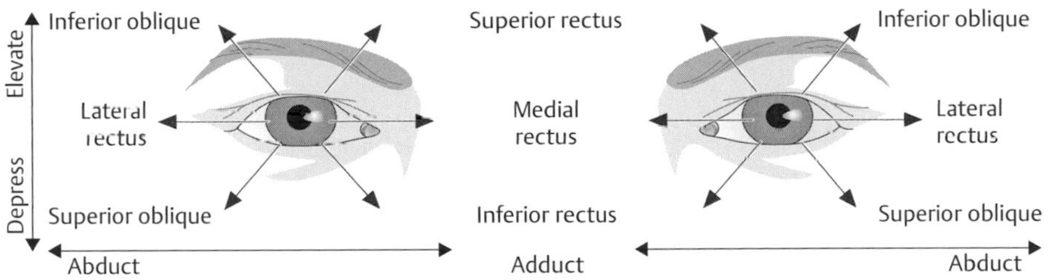
Elevate
Depress
Inferior oblique
Lateral rectus
Superior oblique
Abduct
Superior rectus
Medial rectus
Inferior rectus
Adduct
Inferior oblique
Lateral rectus
Superior oblique
Abduct

A Starting with the eyes directed anteriorly, movement to any of the cardinal directions of gaze (*arrows*) requires activation of two extraocular muscles, each of which is innervated by a different cranial nerve, thus testing the function of those pairs of muscles.

Superior rectus
Inferior oblique
Inferior rectus
Superior oblique
Abduct
Adduct

B Starting with the eyes adducted or abducted, elevating or lowering the eyes activates only the oblique or the rectus muscles, respectively, allowing for testing of the function of individual muscles.

Fig. 35.5 Innervation of the extraocular muscles

Right eye, lateral view with the temporal wall of the orbit removed.

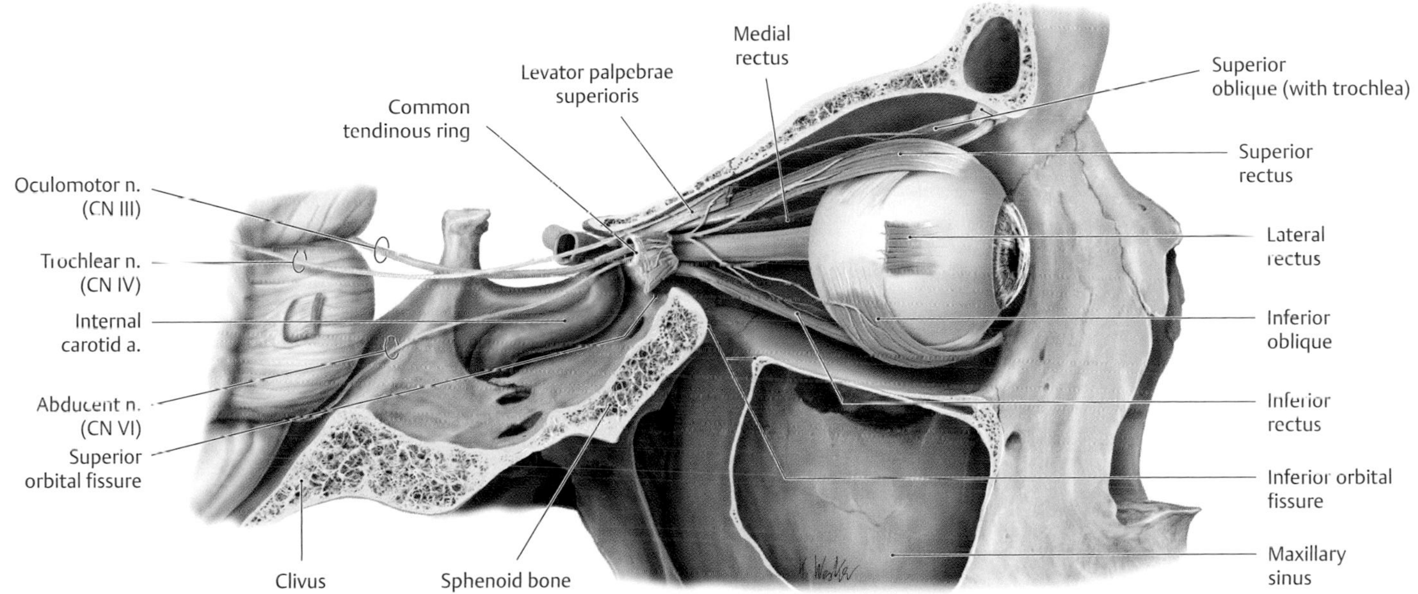
Medial rectus
Levator palpebrae superioris
Common tendinous ring
Oculomotor n. (CN III)
Trochlear n. (CN IV)
Internal carotid a.
Abducent n. (CN VI)
Superior orbital fissure
Clivus
Sphenoid bone
Superior oblique (with trochlea)
Superior rectus
Lateral rectus
Inferior oblique
Inferior rectus
Inferior orbital fissure
Maxillary sinus

Clinical

Oculomotor palsies

Oculomotor palsies may result from a lesion involving an eye muscle or its associated cranial nerve (at the nucleus or along the course of the nerve). If one extraocular muscle is weak or paralyzed, deviation of the eye will be noted.

Impairment of the coordinated actions of the extraocular muscles may cause the visual axis of one eye to deviate from its normal position. The patient will therefore perceive a double image (diplopia).

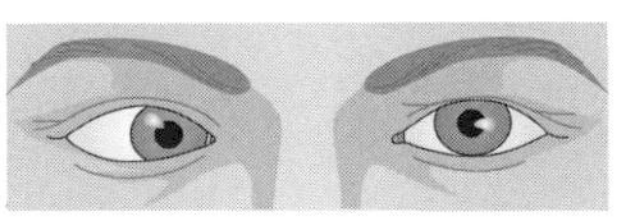
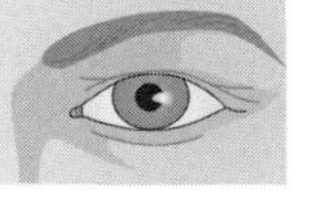

A Abducent nerve palsy. *Disabled:* Lateral rectus.

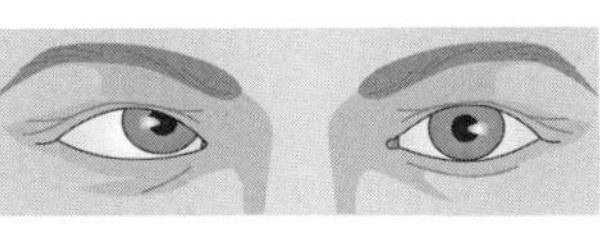

B Trochlear nerve palsy. *Disabled:* Superior oblique.

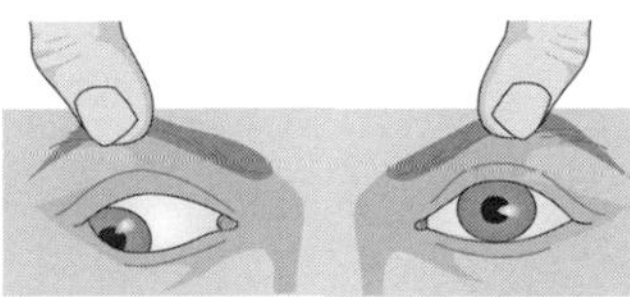

C Complete oculomotor palsy. *Disabled:* Superior, inferior, and medial recti and inferior oblique.

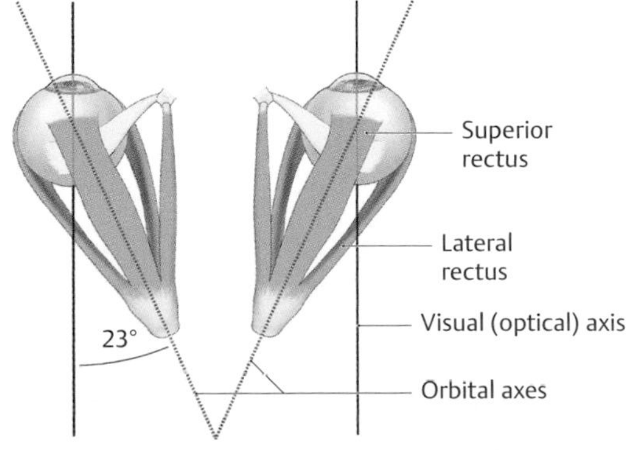
Superior rectus
Lateral rectus
Visual (optical) axis
Orbital axes
23°

D Normal visual and orbital axes.

Neurovasculature of the Orbit

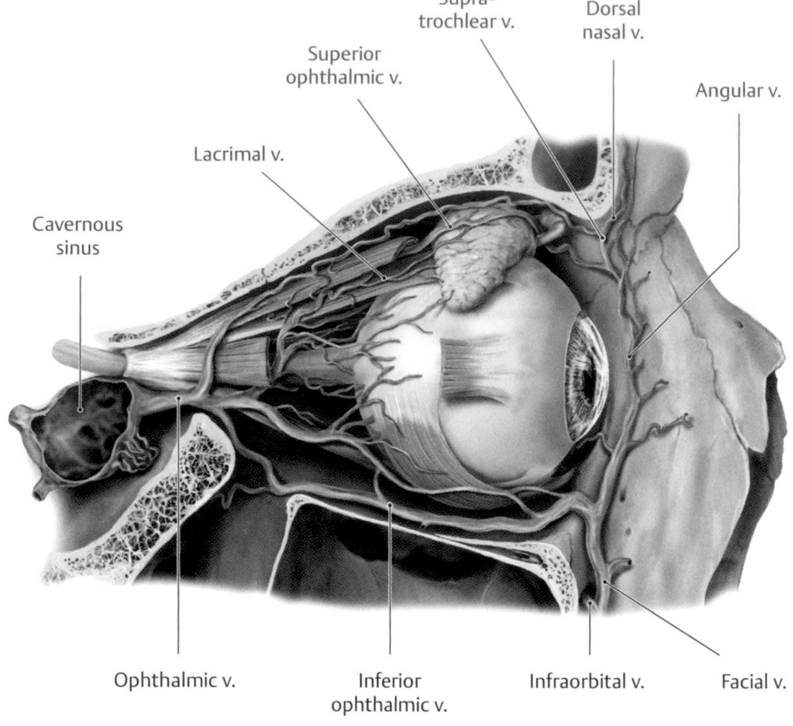
Supra-
trochlear v.
Dorsal
nasal v.
Superior
ophthalmic v.
Angular v.
Lacrimal v.
Cavernous
sinus
Ophthalmic v.
Inferior
ophthalmic v.
Infraorbital v.
Facial v.

Fig. 35.6 **Veins of the orbit**
Lateral view of the right orbit. *Removed:* Lateral orbital wall. *Opened:* Maxillary sinus.

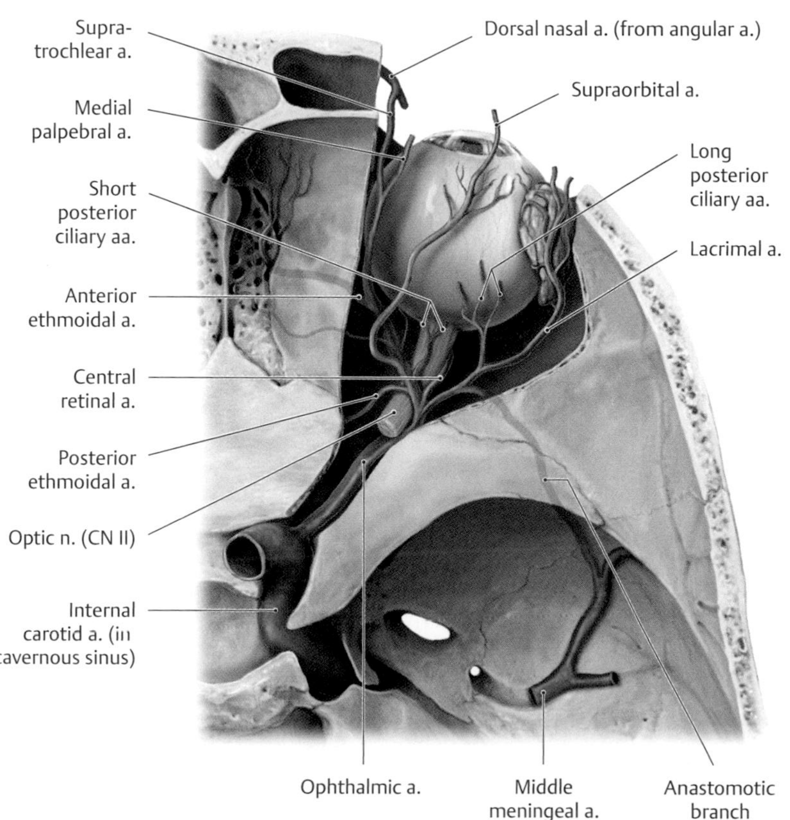
Supra-
trochlear a.
Medial
palpebral a.
Short
posterior
ciliary aa.
Anterior
ethmoidal a.
Central
retinal a.
Posterior
ethmoidal a.
Optic n. (CN II)
Internal
carotid a. (in
cavernous sinus)
Dorsal nasal a. (from angular a.)
Supraorbital a.
Long
posterior
ciliary aa.
Lacrimal a.
Ophthalmic a.
Middle
meningeal a.
(from maxillary a.)
Anastomotic
branch

Fig. 35.7 **Arteries of the orbit**
Superior view of the right orbit. *Opened:* Optic canal and orbital roof.

Clinical

Cavernous sinus syndrome

Gravity allows venous blood from the danger triangle region of the face (see figure) to drain to the cavernous sinus via the valveless ophthalmic veins. Squeezing a pimple or boil in this facial region can result in infectious thrombi being forced into the venous system and passing back into the cavernous sinus. Cavernous sinus syndrome (CIS) is diagnosed by the loss of eyeball movement due to the various cranial nerves associated with the cavernous sinus becoming infected.

The abducent nerve (CN VI) is bathed in blood within the sinus, the first ocular movement to be affected is lateral deviation of the eyeball. The oculomotor (CN III) and trochlear (CN IV) nerves, embedded in the dural lateral wall of the sinus are also eventually affected as the infection penetrates the dura. The eyeball becomes frozen in the orbit as all nerves activating the extraocular mm. become infected. CN V1 is also in the lateral dural wall so a tingling/parathesia is felt in the sensory region covered (forehead). Occasionally CN V2 may also be involved and this parasthesia may also extend to the skin of the face below the orbit. The intercavernous sinuses allow the infection to spread to the cavernous sinus on the opposite side. If left untreated, death can result however cavernous sinus septic thrombophlebitis mortality has decreased from 100% to 20% with the implementation of improvement in diagnosis and therapeutics

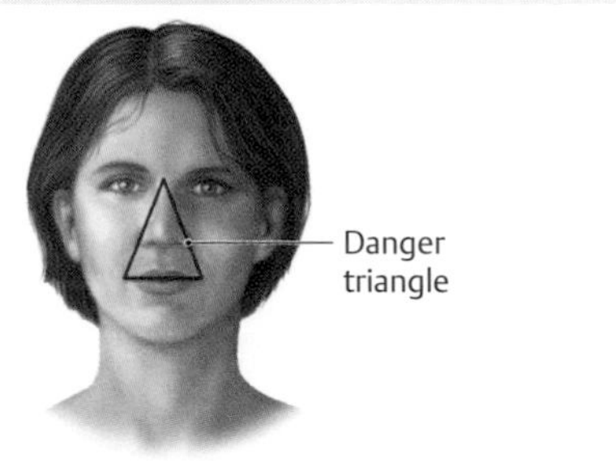
Danger
triangle

Fig. 35.8 **Innervation of the orbit**
Lateral view of the right orbit. *Removed:* Temporal bony wall.

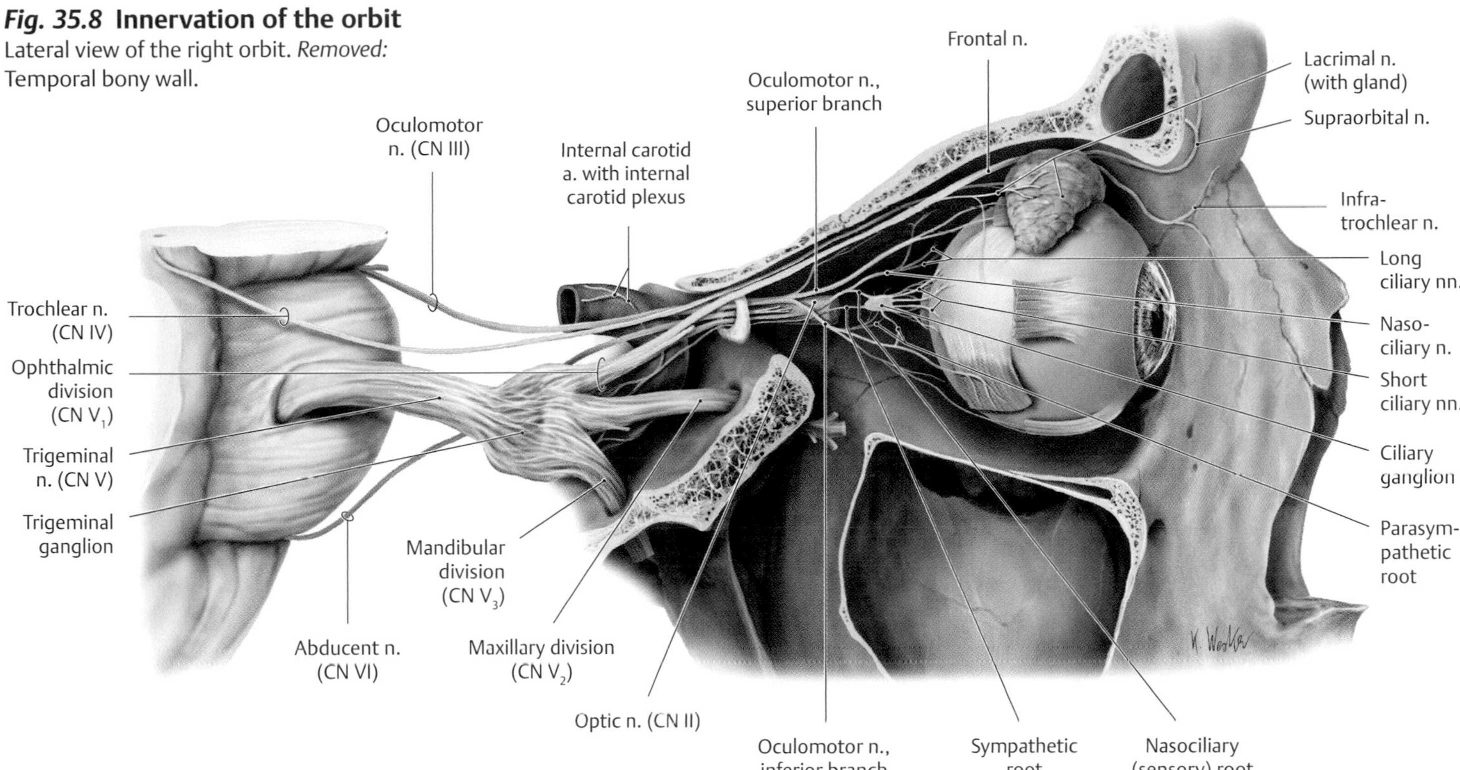
Frontal n.
Oculomotor n., superior branch
Lacrimal n. (with gland)
Supraorbital n.
Oculomotor n. (CN III)
Internal carotid a. with internal carotid plexus
Infra-trochlear n.
Long ciliary nn.
Trochlear n. (CN IV)
Naso-ciliary n.
Ophthalmic division (CN V_1)
Short ciliary nn.
Trigeminal n. (CN V)
Ciliary ganglion
Trigeminal ganglion
Mandibular division (CN V_3)
Parasym-pathetic root
Abducent n. (CN VI)
Maxillary division (CN V_2)
Optic n. (CN II)
Oculomotor n., inferior branch
Sympathetic root
Nasociliary (sensory) root

Fig. 35.9 **Cranial nerves in the orbit**
Superior view of the anterior and middle cranial fossae. *Removed:* Cavernous sinus (lateral and superior walls), orbital roof, and periorbita (portions). The trigeminal ganglion has been retracted laterally.

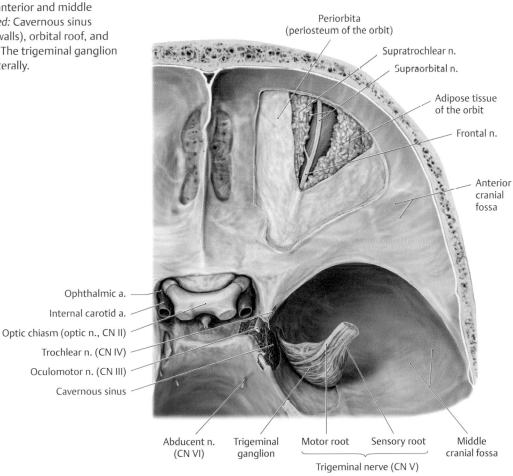

Periorbita (periosteum of the orbit)
Supratrochlear n.
Supraorbital n.
Adipose tissue of the orbit
Frontal n.
Anterior cranial fossa
Ophthalmic a.
Internal carotid a.
Optic chiasm (optic n., CN II)
Trochlear n. (CN IV)
Oculomotor n. (CN III)
Cavernous sinus
Abducent n. (CN VI)
Trigeminal ganglion
Motor root
Sensory root
Trigeminal nerve (CN V)
Middle cranial fossa

Topography of the Orbit

Fig. 35.10 **Neurovascular structures of the orbit**
Anterior view. *Right side:* Orbicularis oculi removed. *Left side:* Orbital septum partially removed.

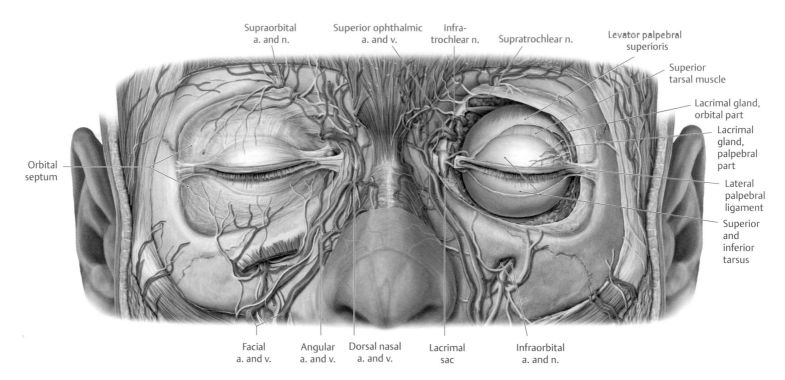

Supraorbital a. and n.
Superior ophthalmic a. and v.
Infra-trochlear n.
Supratrochlear n.
Levator palpebral superioris
Superior tarsal muscle
Lacrimal gland, orbital part
Lacrimal gland, palpebral part
Lateral palpebral ligament
Superior and inferior tarsus
Orbital septum
Facial a. and v.
Angular a. and v.
Dorsal nasal a. and v.
Lacrimal sac
Infraorbital a. and n.

Fig. 35.11 **Passage of neurovascular structures through the orbit**
Anterior view. *Removed:* Orbital contents. *Note:* The optic nerve and ophthalmic artery travel in the optic canal. The remaining structures pass through the superior orbital fissure.

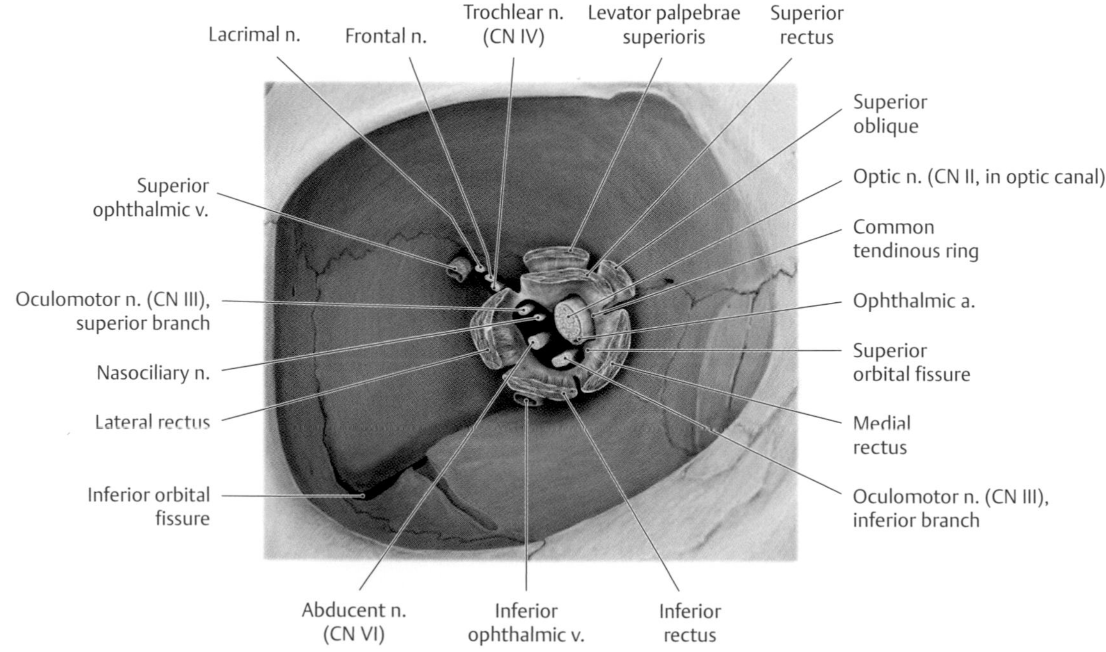
Lacrimal n.
Frontal n.
Trochlear n. (CN IV)
Levator palpebrae superioris
Superior rectus
Superior oblique
Optic n. (CN II, in optic canal)
Common tendinous ring
Ophthalmic a.
Superior orbital fissure
Medial rectus
Oculomotor n. (CN III), inferior branch
Superior ophthalmic v.
Oculomotor n. (CN III), superior branch
Nasociliary n.
Lateral rectus
Inferior orbital fissure
Abducent n. (CN VI)
Inferior ophthalmic v.
Inferior rectus

Fig. 35.12 **Neurovascular contents of the orbit**
Superior view. *Removed:* Bony roof of orbit, peritorbita, and retro-orbital fat.

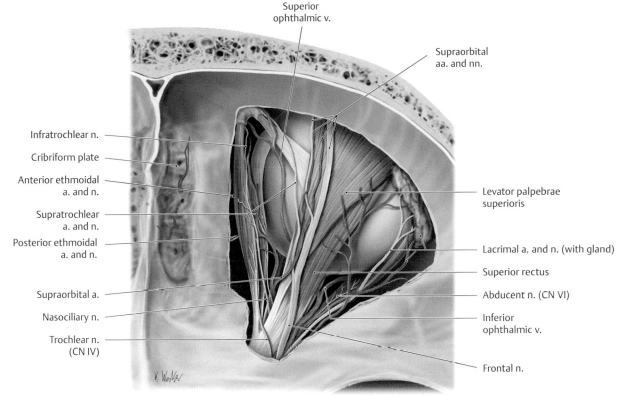

Superior ophthalmic v.
Supraorbital aa. and nn.
Infratrochlear n.
Cribriform plate
Anterior ethmoidal a. and n.
Supratrochlear a. and n.
Posterior ethmoidal a. and n.
Supraorbital a.
Nasociliary n.
Trochlear n. (CN IV)
Levator palpebrae superioris
Lacrimal a. and n. (with gland)
Superior rectus
Abducent n. (CN VI)
Inferior ophthalmic v.
Frontal n.

A Upper level.

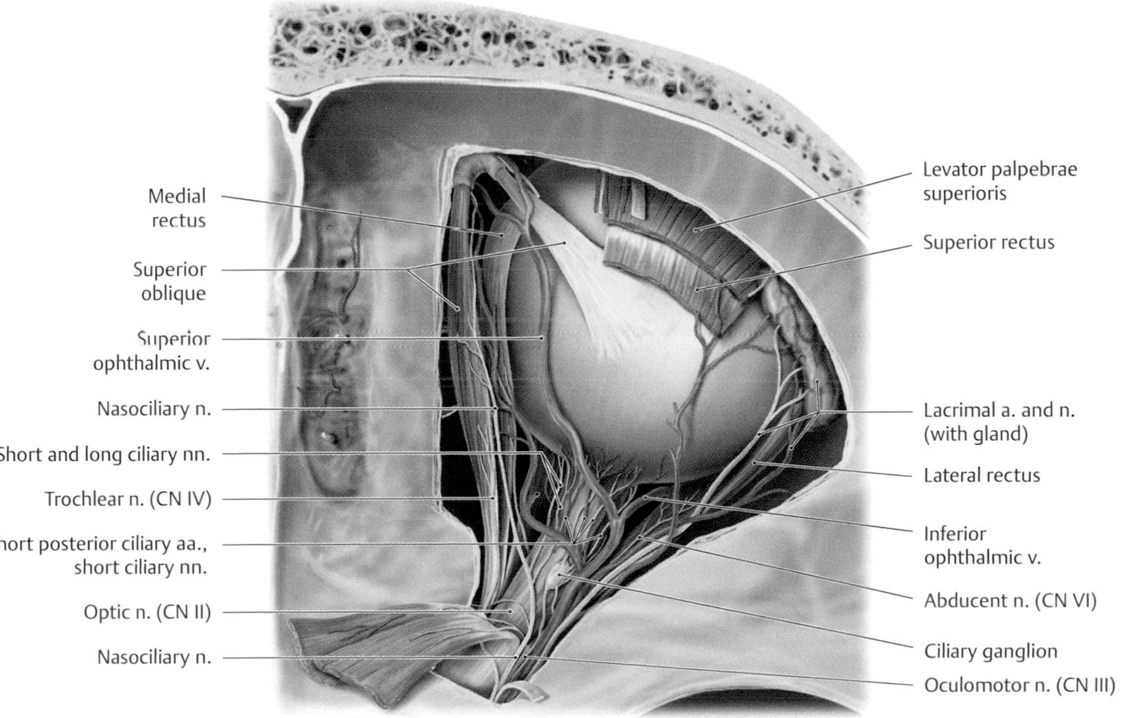

Medial rectus
Superior oblique
Superior ophthalmic v.
Nasociliary n.
Short and long ciliary nn.
Trochlear n. (CN IV)
Short posterior ciliary aa., short ciliary nn.
Optic n. (CN II)
Nasociliary n.
Levator palpebrae superioris
Superior rectus
Lacrimal a. and n. (with gland)
Lateral rectus
Inferior ophthalmic v.
Abducent n. (CN VI)
Ciliary ganglion
Oculomotor n. (CN III)

B Middle level. *Reflected:* Levator palpebrae superioris and superior rectus. *Revealed:* Optic nerve.

Orbit & Eyelid

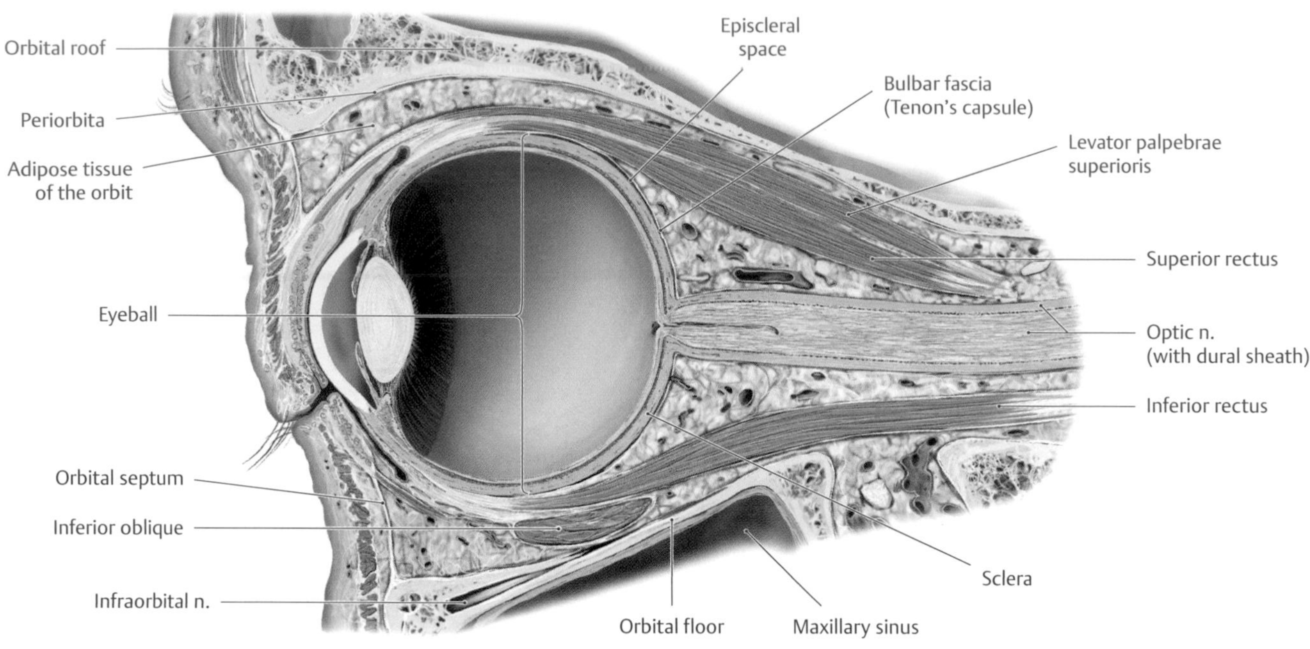
Orbital roof
Periorbita
Adipose tissue of the orbit
Eyeball
Orbital septum
Inferior oblique
Infraorbital n.
Episcleral space
Bulbar fascia (Tenon's capsule)
Levator palpebrae superioris
Superior rectus
Optic n. (with dural sheath)
Inferior rectus
Sclera
Orbital floor
Maxillary sinus

Fig. 35.13 **Topography of the orbit**
Sagittal section through the right orbit, medial view.

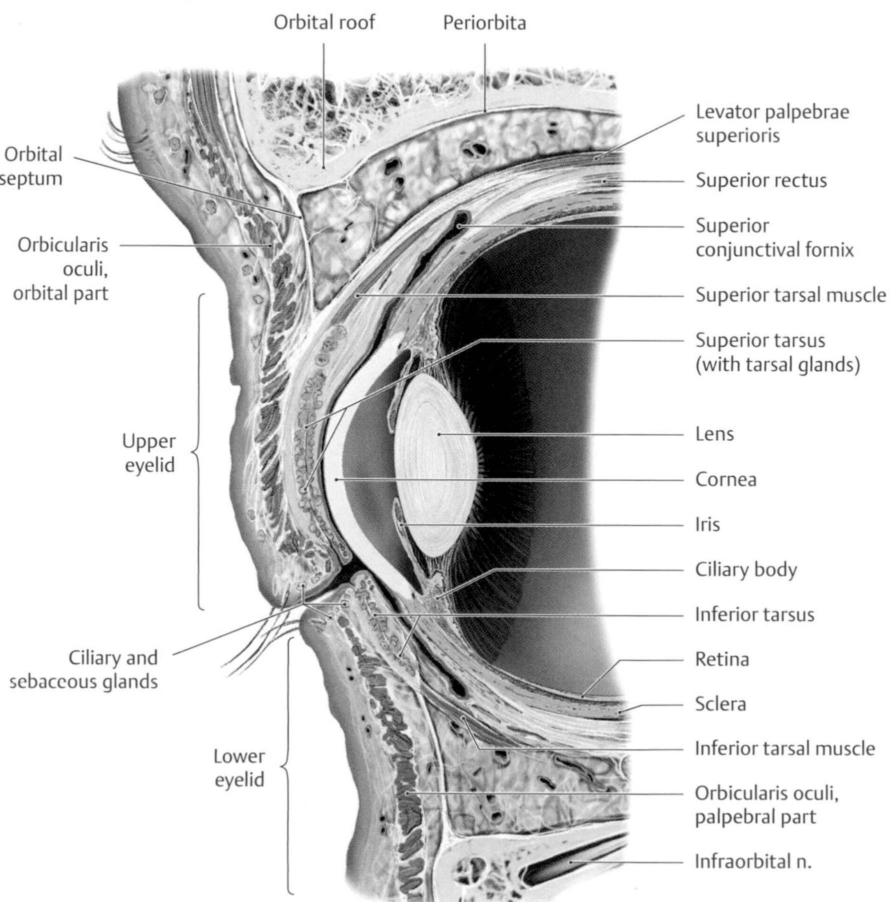
Orbital roof
Periorbita
Orbital septum
Orbicularis oculi, orbital part
Upper eyelid
Ciliary and sebaceous glands
Lower eyelid
Levator palpebrae superioris
Superior rectus
Superior conjunctival fornix
Superior tarsal muscle
Superior tarsus (with tarsal glands)
Lens
Cornea
Iris
Ciliary body
Inferior tarsus
Retina
Sclera
Inferior tarsal muscle
Orbicularis oculi, palpebral part
Infraorbital n.

Fig. 35.14 **Eyelids and conjuctiva**
Sagittal section through the anterior orbital cavity.

Fig. 35.15 Lacrimal apparatus
Right eye, anterior view. *Removed:* Orbital septum (partial). *Divided:* Levator palpebrae superioris (tendon of insertion).

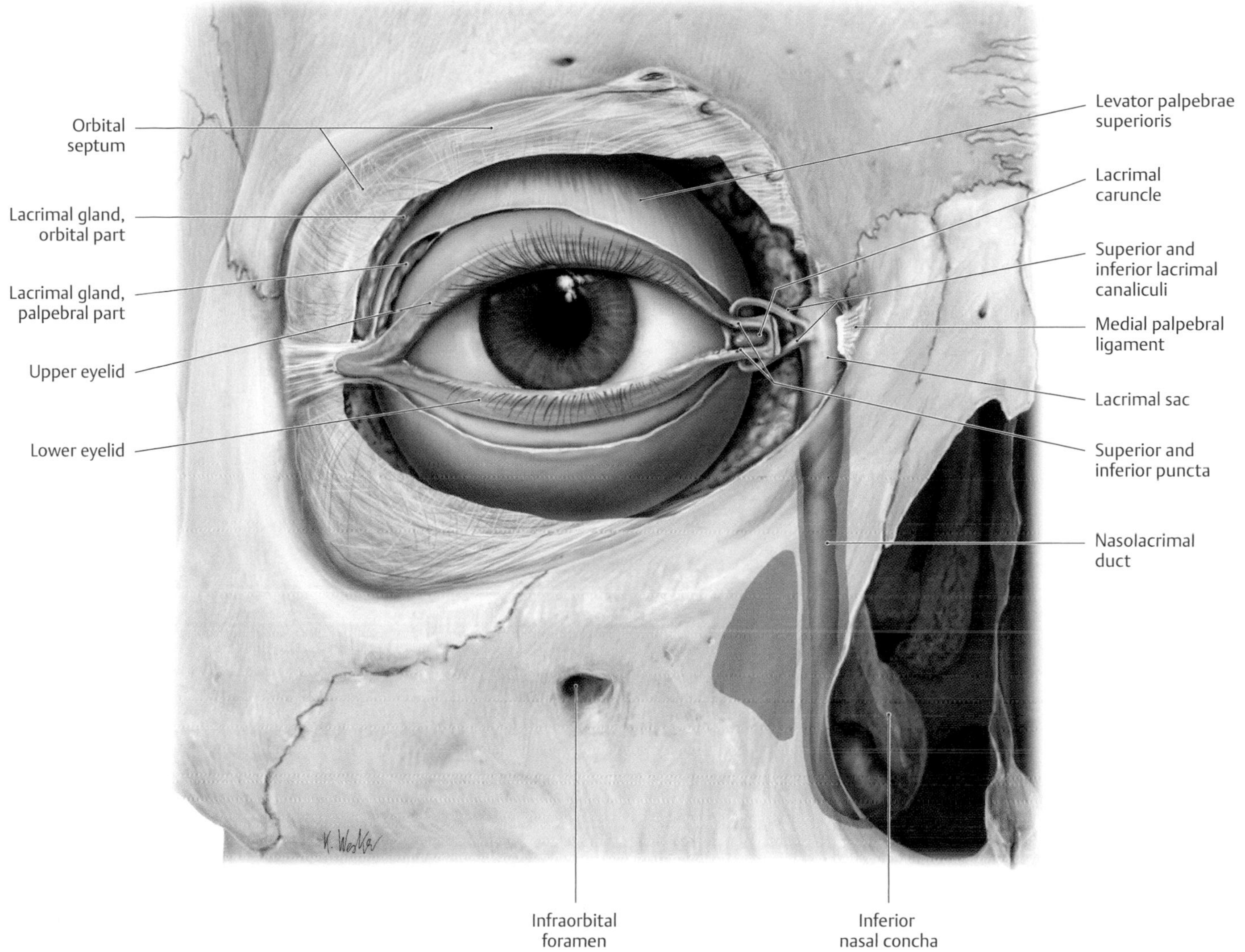

Orbital septum
Lacrimal gland, orbital part
Lacrimal gland, palpebral part
Upper eyelid
Lower eyelid
Levator palpebrae superioris
Lacrimal caruncle
Superior and inferior lacrimal canaliculi
Medial palpebral ligament
Lacrimal sac
Superior and inferior puncta
Nasolacrimal duct
Infraorbital foramen
Inferior nasal concha

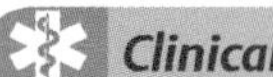 *Clinical*

Lacrimal drainage

Perimenopausal women are frequently subject to chronically dry eyes (*keratoconjunctivitis sicca*), due to insufficient tear production by the lacrimal gland. Acute inflammation of the lacrimal gland (due to bacteria) is less common and characterized by intense inflammation and extreme tenderness to palpation. The upper eyelid shows a characteristic S-curve.

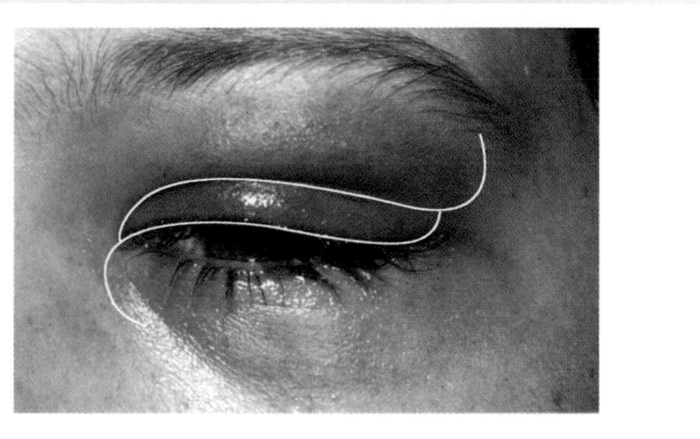

Eyeball

Fig. 35.16 Structure of the eyeball
Transverse section through right eyeball, superior view. *Note:* The orbital axis (running along the optic nerve through the optic disk) deviates from the optical axis (running down the center of the eye to the fovea centralis) by 23 degrees.

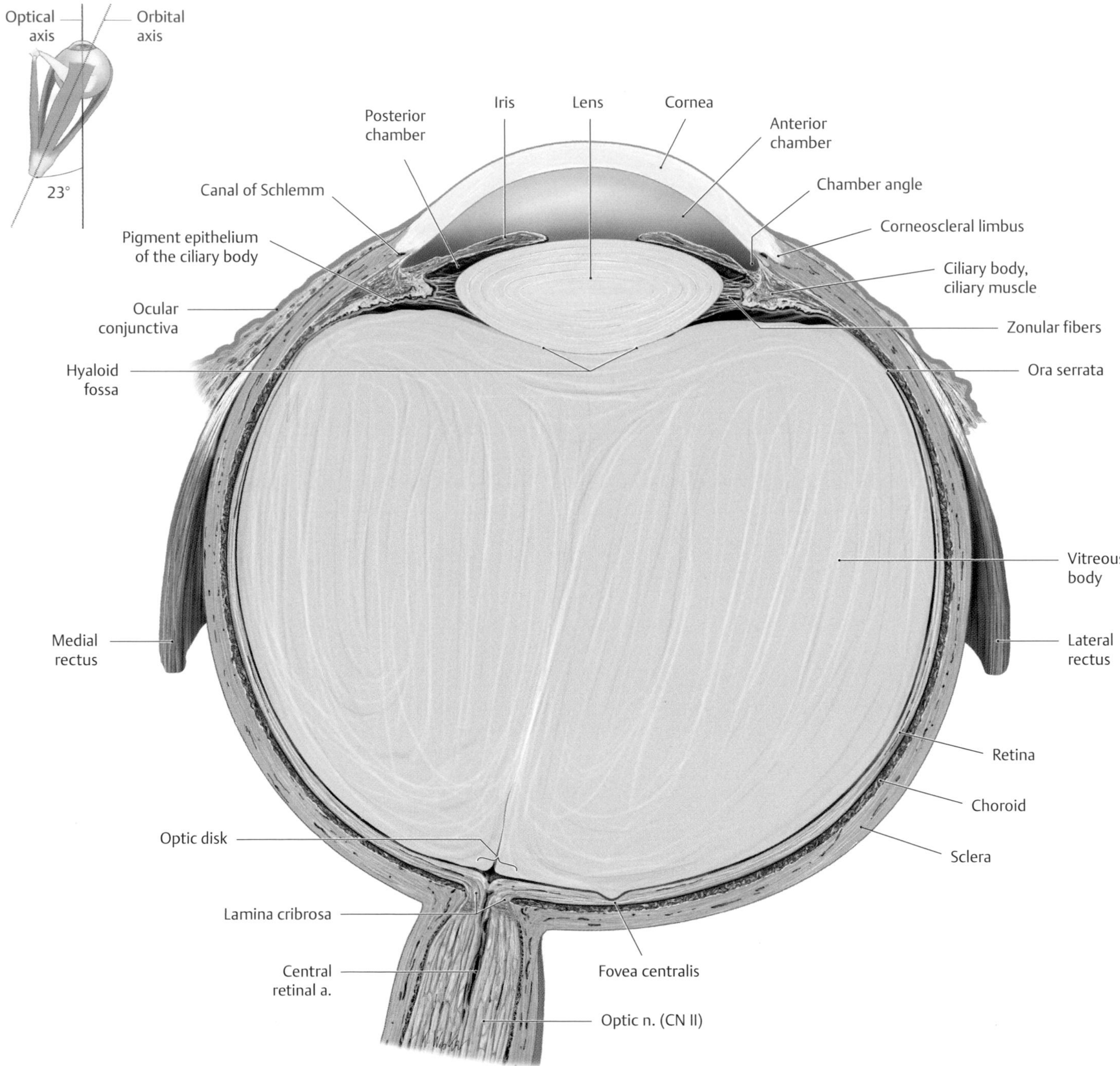
Optical axis
Orbital axis
23°
Iris
Lens
Cornea
Posterior chamber
Anterior chamber
Canal of Schlemm
Chamber angle
Corneoscleral limbus
Pigment epithelium of the ciliary body
Ciliary body, ciliary muscle
Ocular conjunctiva
Zonular fibers
Hyaloid fossa
Ora serrata
Vitreous body
Medial rectus
Lateral rectus
Retina
Choroid
Optic disk
Sclera
Lamina cribrosa
Central retinal a.
Fovea centralis
Optic n. (CN II)

Fig. 35.17 **Blood vessels of the eyeball**
Transverse section through the right eyeball at the level of the optic nerve, superior view. The arteries of the eye arise from the ophthalmic artery, a terminal branch of the internal carotid artery. Blood is drained by four to eight vorticose veins that open into the superior and inferior ophthalmic veins.

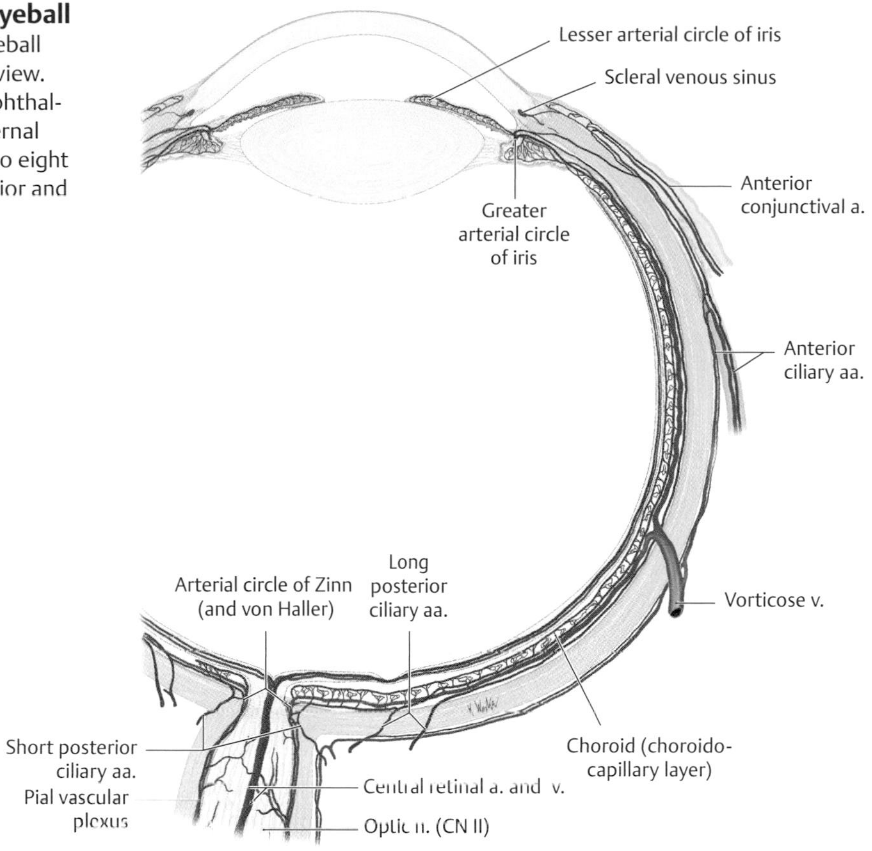

Lesser arterial circle of iris
Scleral venous sinus
Anterior conjunctival a.
Greater arterial circle of iris
Anterior ciliary aa.
Vorticose v.
Long posterior ciliary aa.
Arterial circle of Zinn (and von Haller)
Short posterior ciliary aa.
Pial vascular plexus
Central retinal a. and v.
Optic n. (CN II)
Choroid (choroido-capillary layer)

Clinical

Optic fundus

The optic fundus is the only place in the body where capillaries can be examined directly. Examination of the optic fundus permits observation of vascular changes that may be caused by high blood pressure or diabetes. Examination of the optic disk is important in determining intracranial pressure and diagnosing multiple sclerosis.

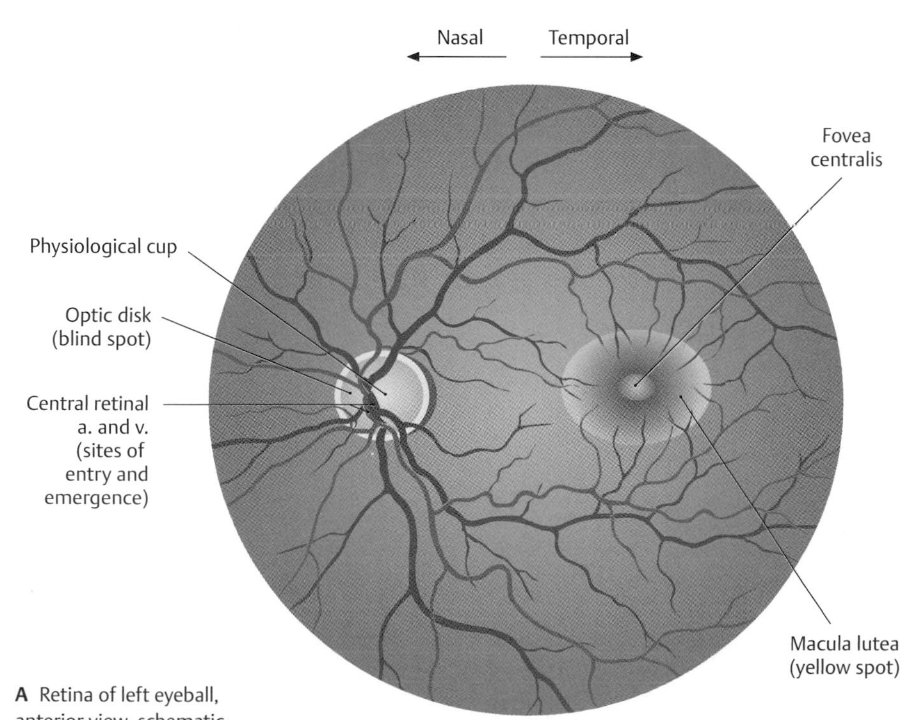

Nasal
Temporal
Fovea centralis
Physiological cup
Optic disk (blind spot)
Central retinal a. and v. (sites of entry and emergence)
Macula lutea (yellow spot)

A Retina of left eyeball, anterior view, schematic.

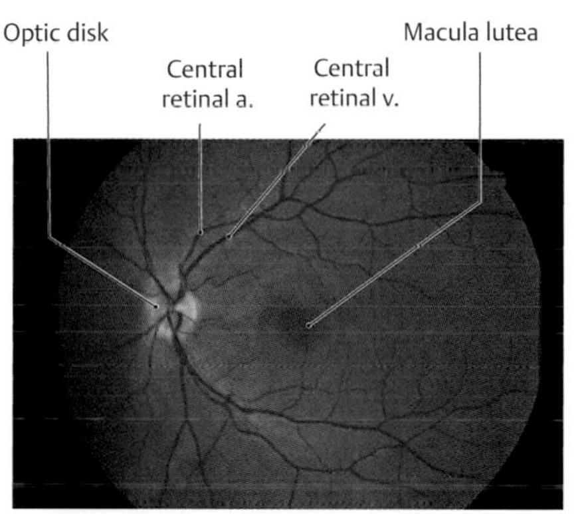

Optic disk
Central retinal a.
Central retinal v.
Macula lutea

B Normal optic fundus in the ophthalmoscopic examination.

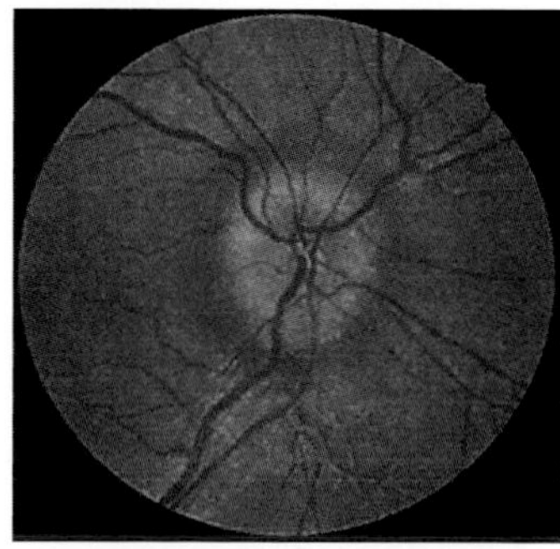

C High intracranial pressure; the edges of the optic disk appear less sharp.

Cornea, Iris & Lens

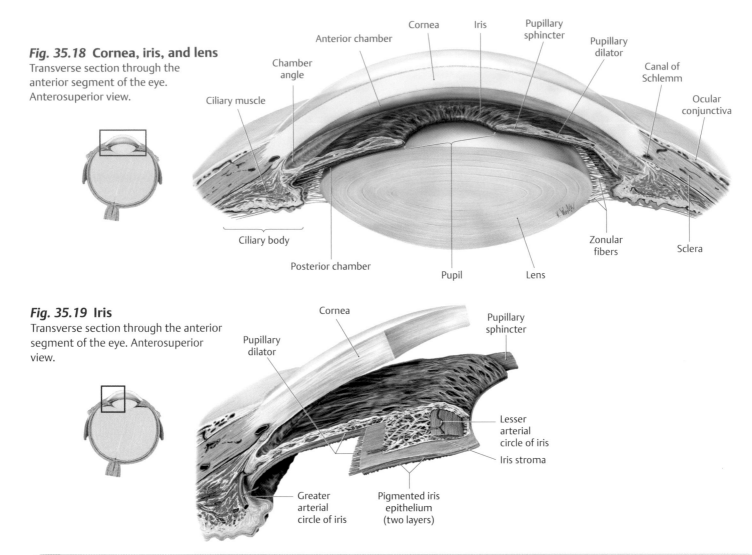

Fig. 35.18 **Cornea, iris, and lens**
Transverse section through the anterior segment of the eye. Anterosuperior view.

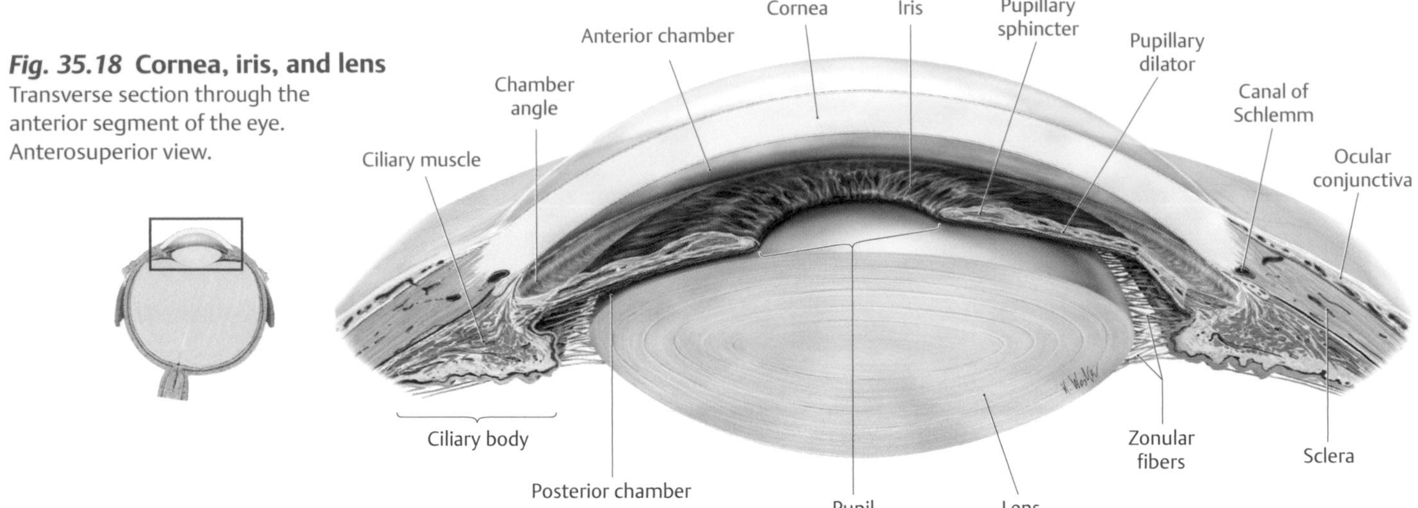

Cornea
Iris
Pupillary sphincter
Anterior chamber
Pupillary dilator
Chamber angle
Canal of Schlemm
Ciliary muscle
Ocular conjunctiva
Ciliary body
Posterior chamber
Pupil
Lens
Zonular fibers
Sclera

Fig. 35.19 **Iris**
Transverse section through the anterior segment of the eye. Anterosuperior view.

Cornea
Pupillary sphincter
Pupillary dilator
Lesser arterial circle of iris
Iris stroma
Greater arterial circle of iris
Pigmented iris epithelium (two layers)

Clinical

Glaucoma

Aqueous humor produced in the posterior chamber passes through the pupil into the anterior chamber. It seeps through the spaces of the trabecular meshwork into the canal of Schlemm and enters the venous sinus of the sclera before passing into the episcleral veins. Obstruction of aqueous humor drainage causes an increase in intraocular pressure (glaucoma), which constricts the optic nerve in the lamina cribrosa. This constriction eventually leads to blindness. The most common glaucoma (approximately 90% of cases) is chronic (open-angle) glaucoma. The more rare acute glaucoma is characterized by red eye, strong headache and/or eye pain, nausea, dilated episcleral veins, and edema of the cornea.

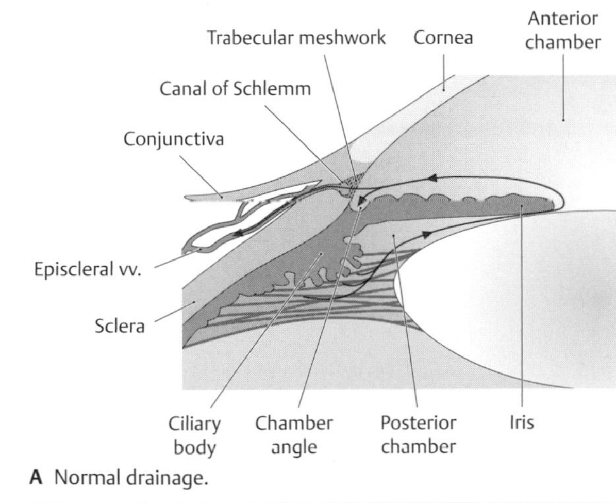

Trabecular meshwork
Cornea
Anterior chamber
Canal of Schlemm
Conjunctiva
Episcleral vv.
Sclera
Ciliary body
Chamber angle
Posterior chamber
Iris

A Normal drainage.

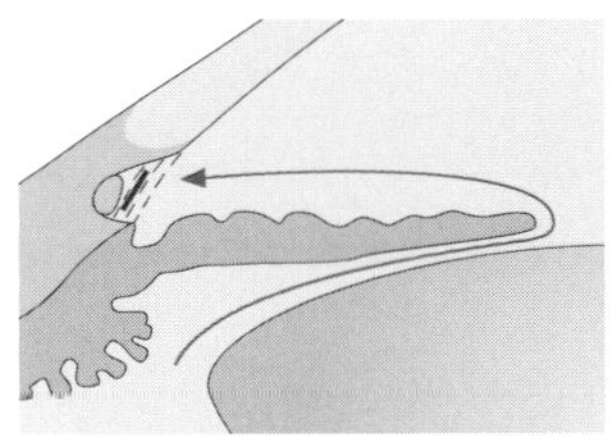

B Chronic (open-angle) glaucoma. Drainage through the trabecular meshwork is impaired.

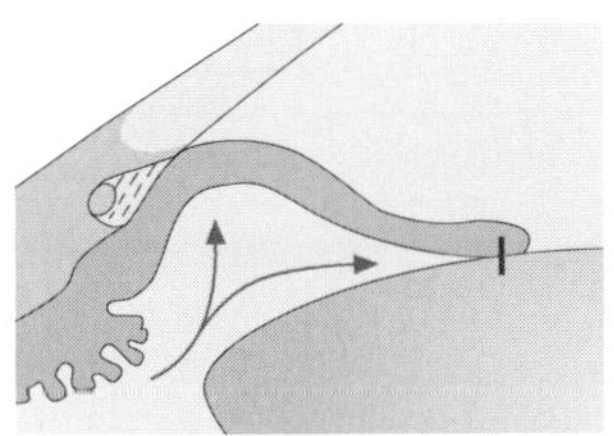

C Acute (angle-closure) glaucoma. The chamber angle is obstructed by iris tissue. Aqueous fluid cannot drain into the anterior chamber, which pushes portions of the iris upward, blocking the chamber angle.

***Fig. 35.20* Pupil**
Pupil size is regulated by two intraocular muscles of the iris: the pupillary sphincter, which narrows the pupil (parasympathetic innervation), and the pupillary dilator, which enlarges it (sympathetic innervation).

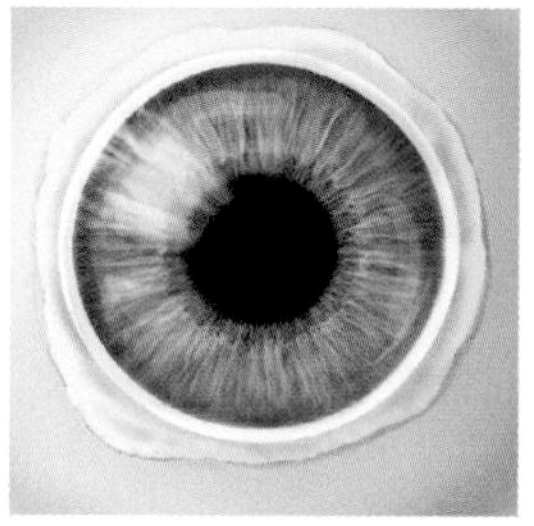

A Normal pupil size.

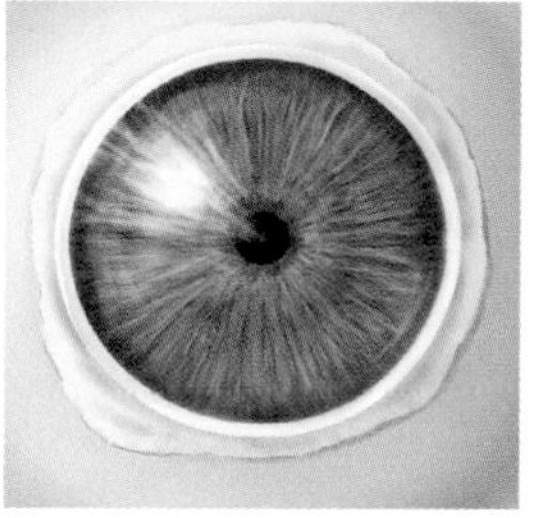

B Maximum constriction (miosis).

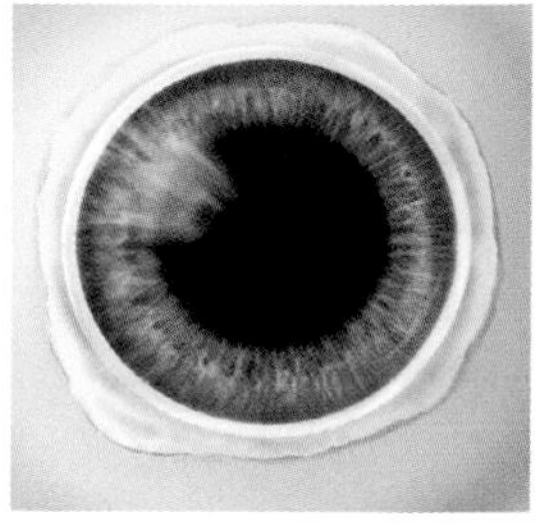

C Maximum dilation (mydriasis).

***Fig. 35.21* Lens and ciliary body**
Posterior view. The curvature of the lens is regulated by the muscle fibers of the annular ciliary body.

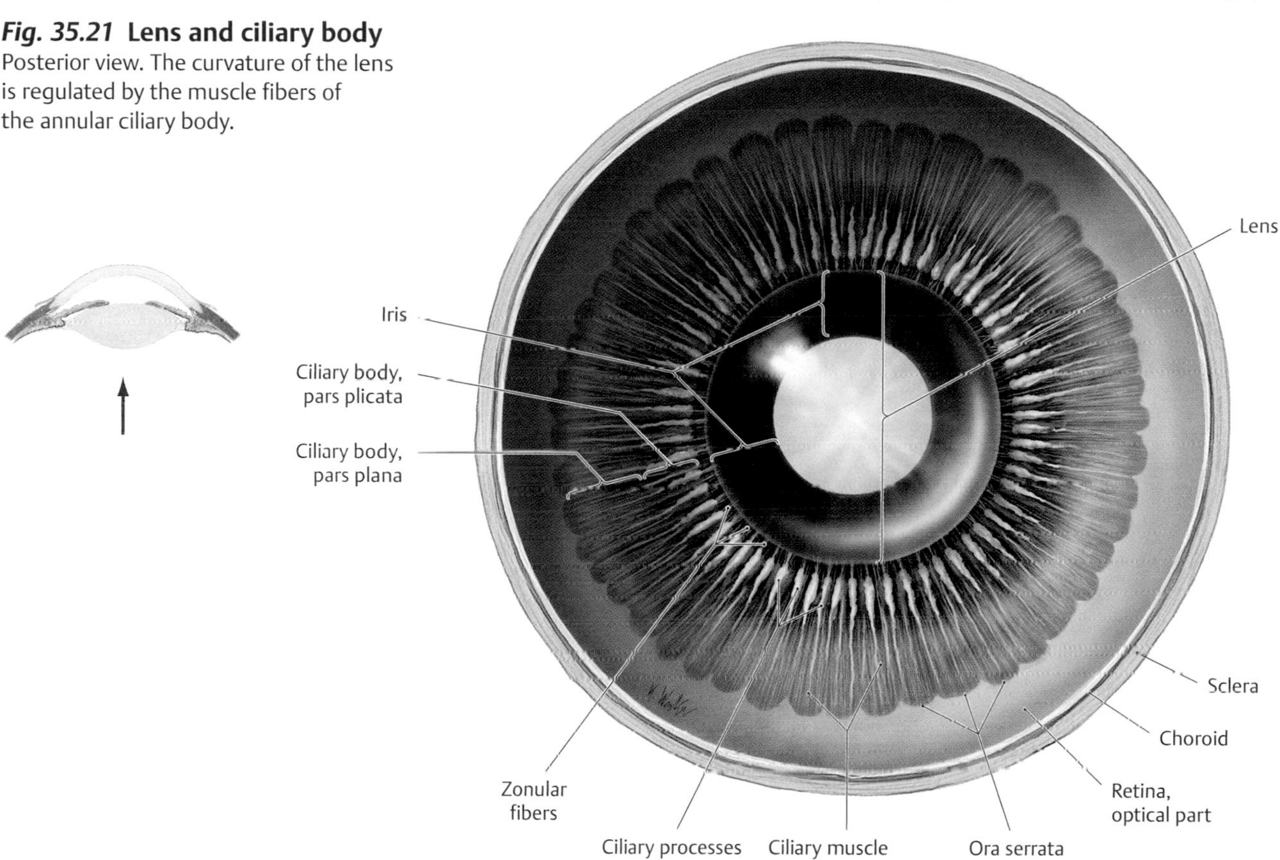
Lens
Iris
Ciliary body, pars plicata
Ciliary body, pars plana
Sclera
Choroid
Retina, optical part
Zonular fibers
Ciliary processes
Ciliary muscle
Ora serrata

***Fig. 35.22* Light refraction by the lens**
Transverse section, superior view. In the normal (emmetropic) eye, light rays are refracted by the lens (and cornea) to a focal point on the retinal surface (fovea centralis). Tensing of the zonular fibers, with ciliary muscle relaxation, flattens the lens in response to parallel rays arriving from a distant source (far vision). Contraction of the ciliary muscle, with zonular fiber relaxation, causes the lens to assume a more rounded shape (near vision).

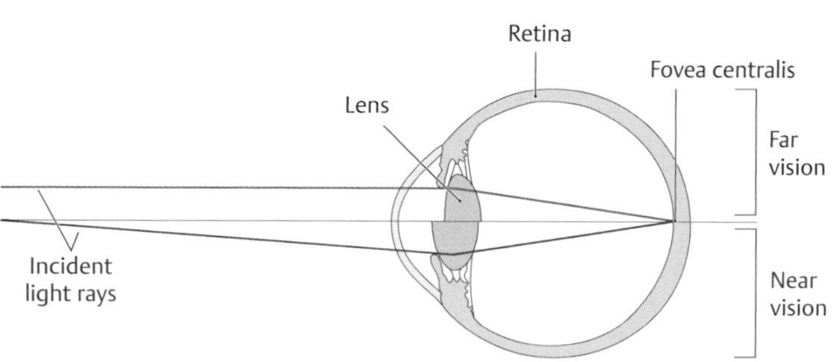
Retina
Fovea centralis
Lens
Far vision
Near vision
Incident light rays

A Normal dynamics of the lens.

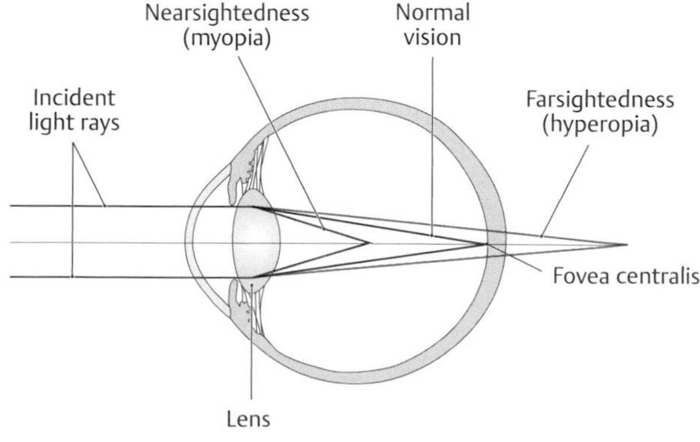
Nearsightedness (myopia)
Normal vision
Incident light rays
Farsightedness (hyperopia)
Fovea centralis
Lens

B Abnormal lens dynamics.

Bones of the Nasal Cavity

Fig. 36.1 Skeleton of the nose

The skeleton of the nose is composed of an upper bony portion and a lower cartilaginous portion. The proximal portions of the nostrils (alae) are composed of connective tissue with small embedded pieces of cartilage.

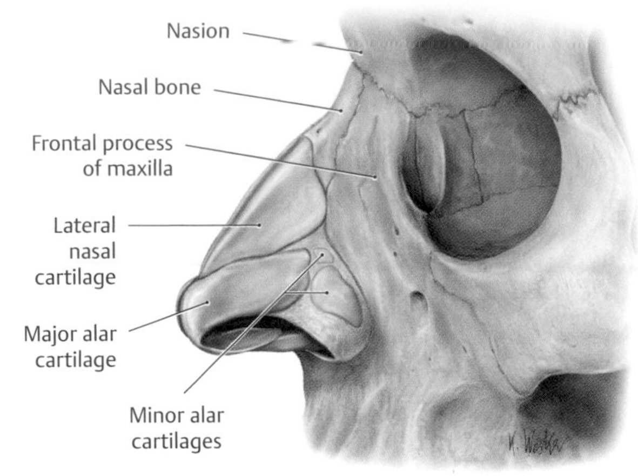
Nasion
Nasal bone
Frontal process of maxilla
Lateral nasal cartilage
Major alar cartilage
Minor alar cartilages

A Left lateral view.

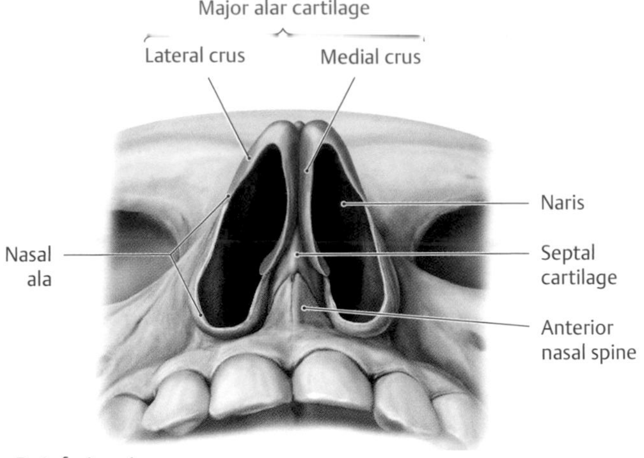
Major alar cartilage
Lateral crus
Medial crus
Naris
Nasal ala
Septal cartilage
Anterior nasal spine

B Inferior view.

Fig. 36.2 Bones of the nasal cavity

The left and right nasal cavities are flanked by lateral walls and separated by the nasal septum. Air enters the nasal cavity through the anterior nasal aperture and travels through three passages: the superior, middle, and inferior meatuses (*arrows*). These passages are separated by the superior, middle, and inferior conchae. Air leaves the nose through the choanae, entering the nasopharynx.

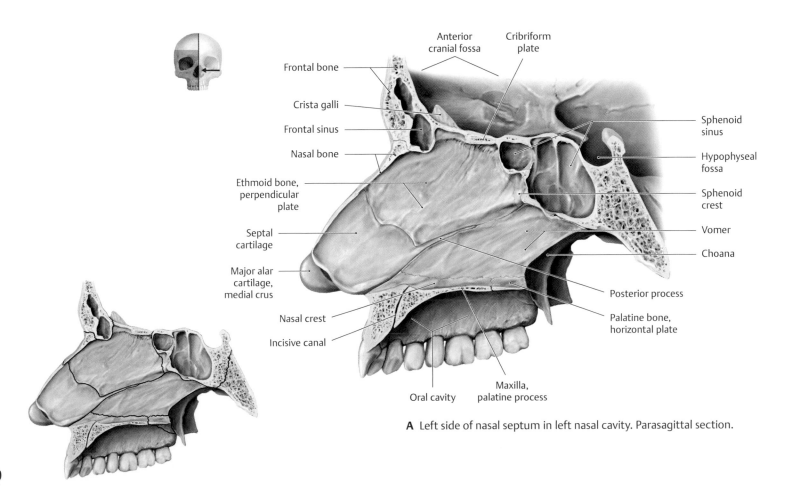

Anterior cranial fossa
Cribriform plate
Frontal bone
Crista galli
Frontal sinus
Nasal bone
Ethmoid bone, perpendicular plate
Septal cartilage
Major alar cartilage, medial crus
Nasal crest
Incisive canal
Oral cavity
Maxilla, palatine process
Sphenoid sinus
Hypophyseal fossa
Sphenoid crest
Vomer
Choana
Posterior process
Palatine bone, horizontal plate

A Left side of nasal septum in left nasal cavity. Parasagittal section.

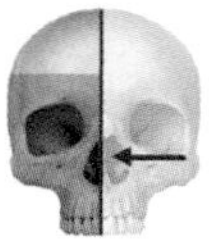

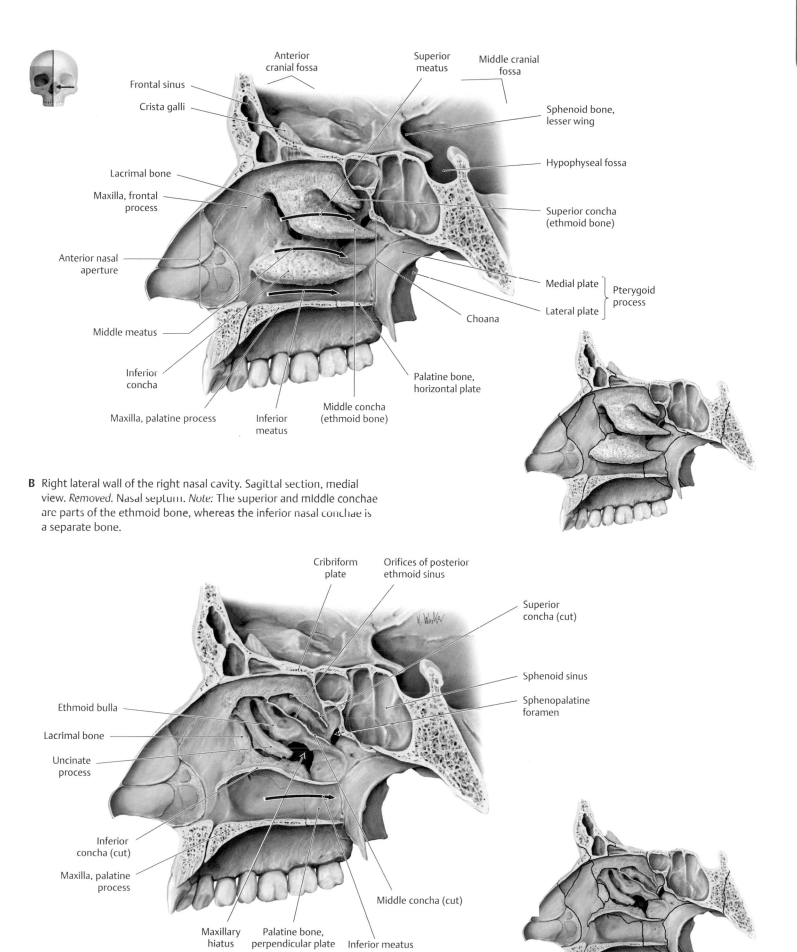

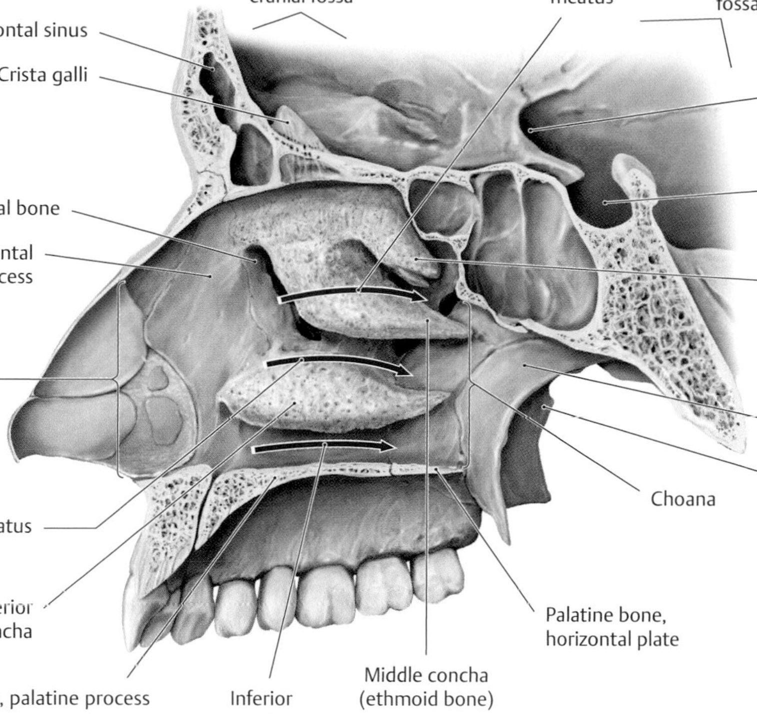

Anterior cranial fossa
Superior meatus
Middle cranial fossa
Frontal sinus
Crista galli
Sphenoid bone, lesser wing
Hypophyseal fossa
Lacrimal bone
Maxilla, frontal process
Superior concha (ethmoid bone)
Anterior nasal aperture
Medial plate
Pterygoid process
Lateral plate
Choana
Middle meatus
Inferior concha
Palatine bone, horizontal plate
Maxilla, palatine process
Inferior meatus
Middle concha (ethmoid bone)

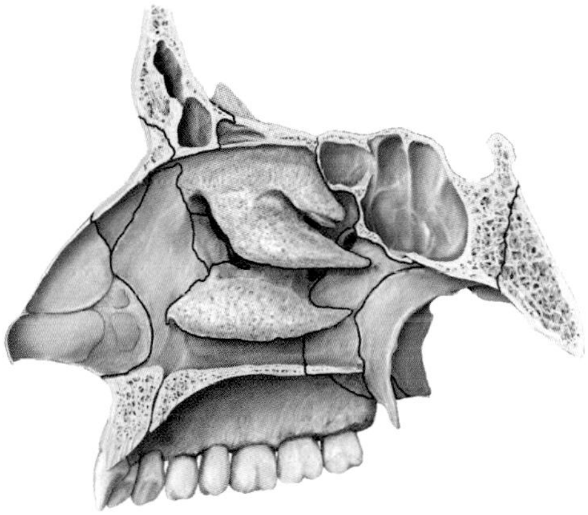

B Right lateral wall of the right nasal cavity. Sagittal section, medial view. *Removed.* Nasal septum. *Note:* The superior and middle conchae are parts of the ethmoid bone, whereas the inferior nasal conchae is a separate bone.

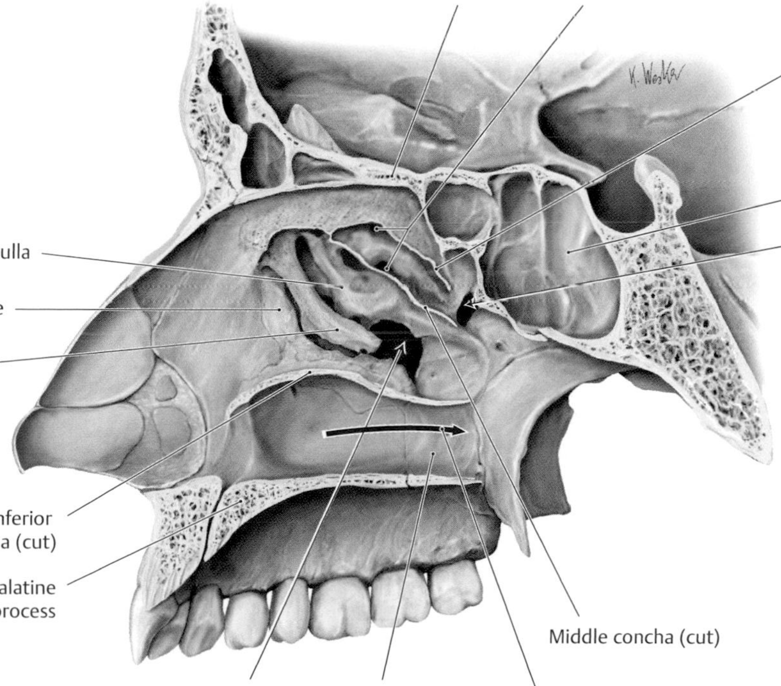

Cribriform plate
Orifices of posterior ethmoid sinus
Superior concha (cut)
Sphenoid sinus
Ethmoid bulla
Sphenopalatine foramen
Lacrimal bone
Uncinate process
Inferior concha (cut)
Maxilla, palatine process
Middle concha (cut)
Maxillary hiatus
Palatine bone, perpendicular plate
Inferior meatus

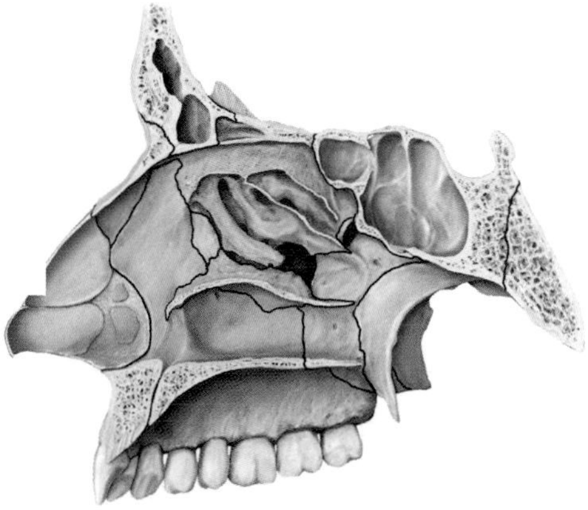

C Lateral wall of the right nasal cavity with the conchae removed. Sagittal section, medial view. *Revealed:* Paranasal sinuses (p. 552).

Paranasal Air Sinuses

Fig. 36.3 Location of the paranasal sinuses

The paranasal sinuses (frontal, ethmoid, maxillary, and sphenoid) are air-filled cavities that reduce the weight of the skull.

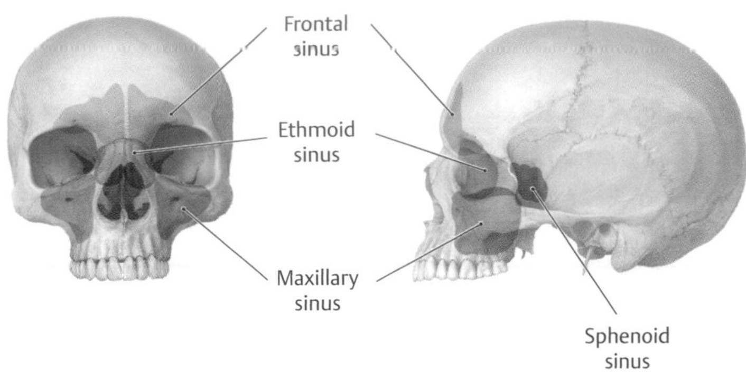
Frontal sinus
Ethmoid sinus
Maxillary sinus
Sphenoid sinus

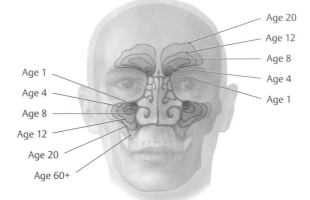

A Anterior view.

B Left lateral view.

C Pneumatization (the formation of air-filled cells and cavities) of the sinuses with age. The frontal (yellow) and maxillary (orange) sinuses develop gradually over the course of cranial growth.

Fig. 36.4 Paranasal sinuses

Arrows indicate the flow of mucosal secretions from the sinuses and the nasolacrimal duct into the nasal cavity.

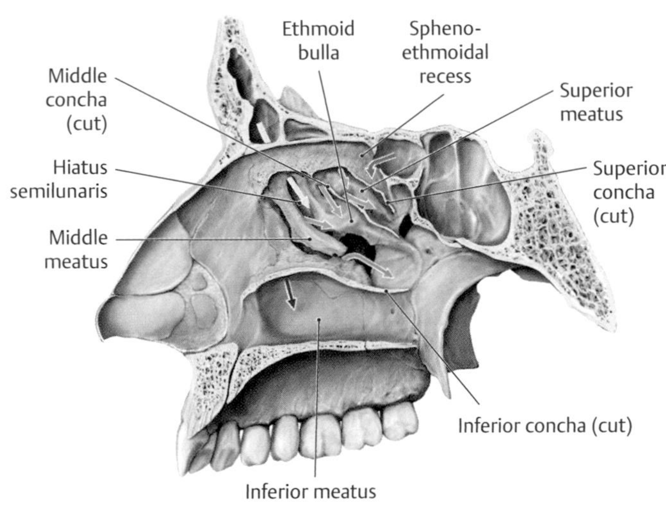
Ethmoid bulla
Spheno-ethmoidal recess
Middle concha (cut)
Superior meatus
Hiatus semilunaris
Superior concha (cut)
Middle meatus
Inferior concha (cut)
Inferior meatus

A Openings of the paranasal sinuses and nasolacrimal duct. Sagittal section, medial view of the right nasal cavity.

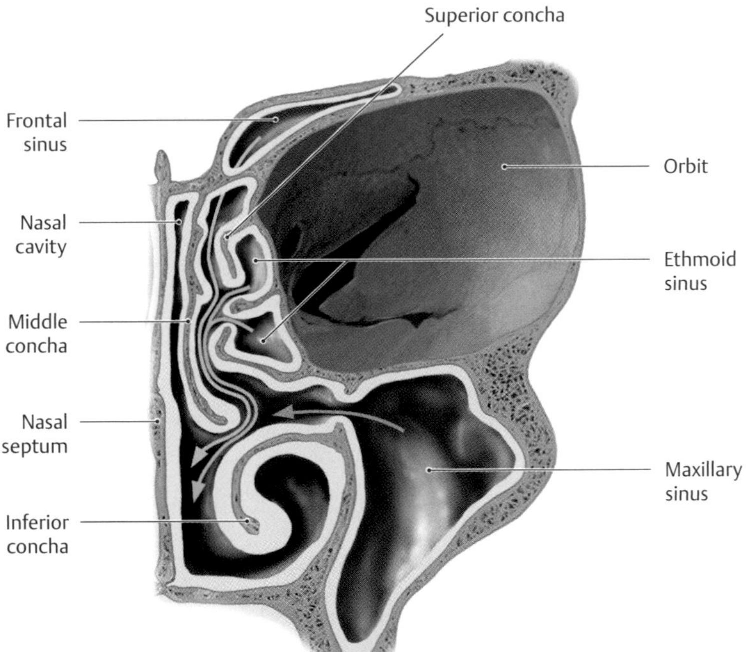
Superior concha
Frontal sinus
Orbit
Nasal cavity
Ethmoid sinus
Middle concha
Nasal septum
Maxillary sinus
Inferior concha

B Paranasal sinuses and osteomeatal unit in the left nasal cavity. Coronal section, anterior view.

Table 36.1 Nasal passages into which sinuses empty

Sinuses/duct		Nasal passage	Via
Sphenoid sinus (blue)		Sphenoethmoidal recess	Direct
Ethmoid sinus (green)	Posterior cells	Superior meatus	Direct
	Anterior and middle cells	Middle meatus	Ethmoid bulla
Frontal sinus (yellow)		Middle meatus	Frontonasal duct into hiatus semilunaris
Maxillary sinus (orange)		Middle meatus	Hiatus semilunaris
Nasolacrimal duct (red)		Inferior meatus	Direct

Fig. 36.5 Bony structure of the paranasal sinuses

Coronal section, anterior view.

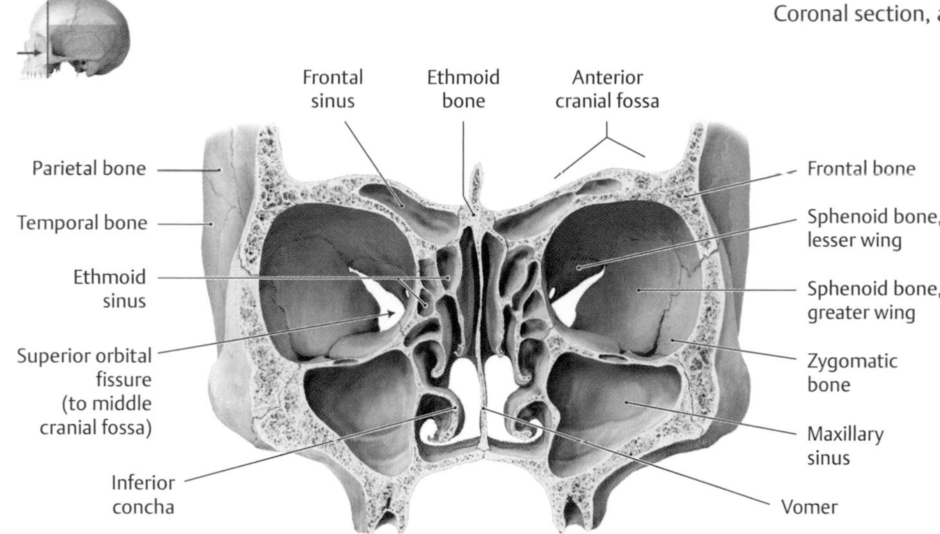

Frontal sinus
Ethmoid bone
Anterior cranial fossa
Parietal bone
Temporal bone
Ethmoid sinus
Superior orbital fissure (to middle cranial fossa)
Inferior concha
Frontal bone
Sphenoid bone, lesser wing
Sphenoid bone, greater wing
Zygomatic bone
Maxillary sinus
Vomer

A Bones of the paranasal sinuses.

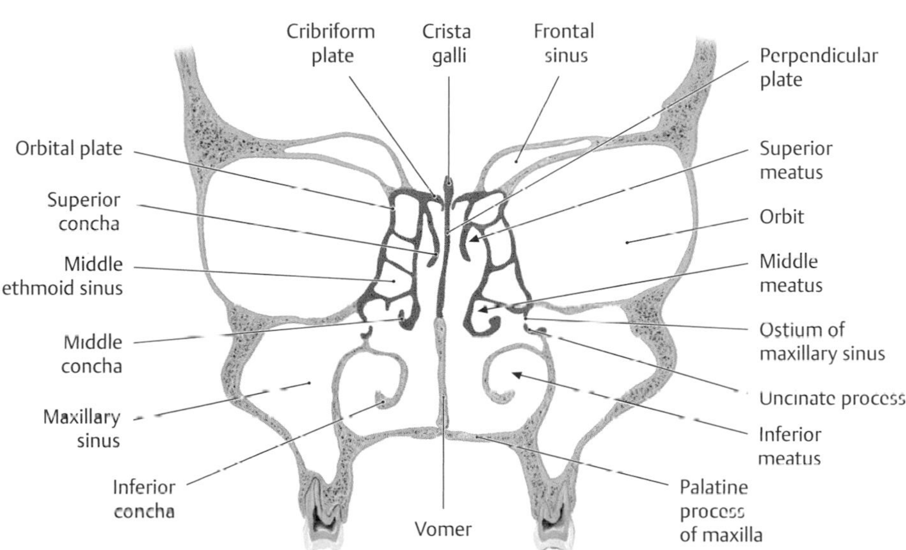

Cribriform plate
Crista galli
Frontal sinus
Perpendicular plate
Orbital plate
Superior concha
Middle ethmoid sinus
Middle concha
Maxillary sinus
Inferior concha
Vomer
Superior meatus
Orbit
Middle meatus
Ostium of maxillary sinus
Uncinate process
Inferior meatus
Palatine process of maxilla

B Ethmoid bone (red) in the paranasal sinuses.

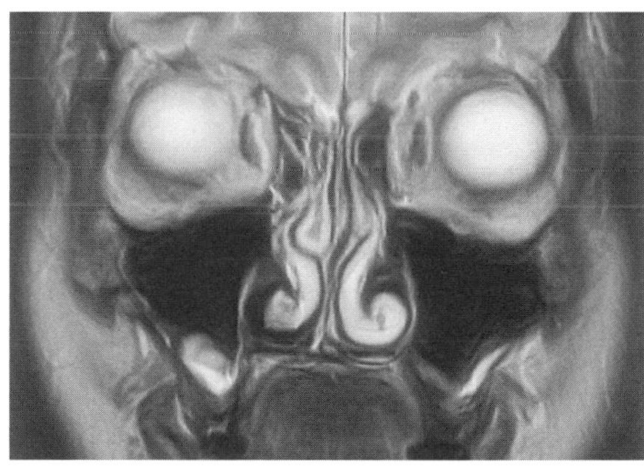

C MRI through the paranasal sinuses.

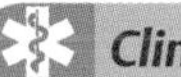

Clinical

Deviated septum

The normal position of the nasal septum creates two roughly symmetrical nasal cavities. Extreme lateral deviation of the septum may result in obstruction of the nasal passages. This may be corrected by removing portions of the cartilage (septoplasty).

Sinusitis

When the mucosa in the ethmoid sinuses becomes swollen due to inflammation (*sinusitis*), it blocks the flow of secretions from the frontal and maxillary sinuses in the osteomeatal unit (see Fig. 36.4). This may cause microorganisms to become trapped, causing secondary inflammations. In patients with chronic sinusitis, the narrow sites can be surgically widened to establish more effective drainage routes.

Neurovasculature of the Nasal Cavity

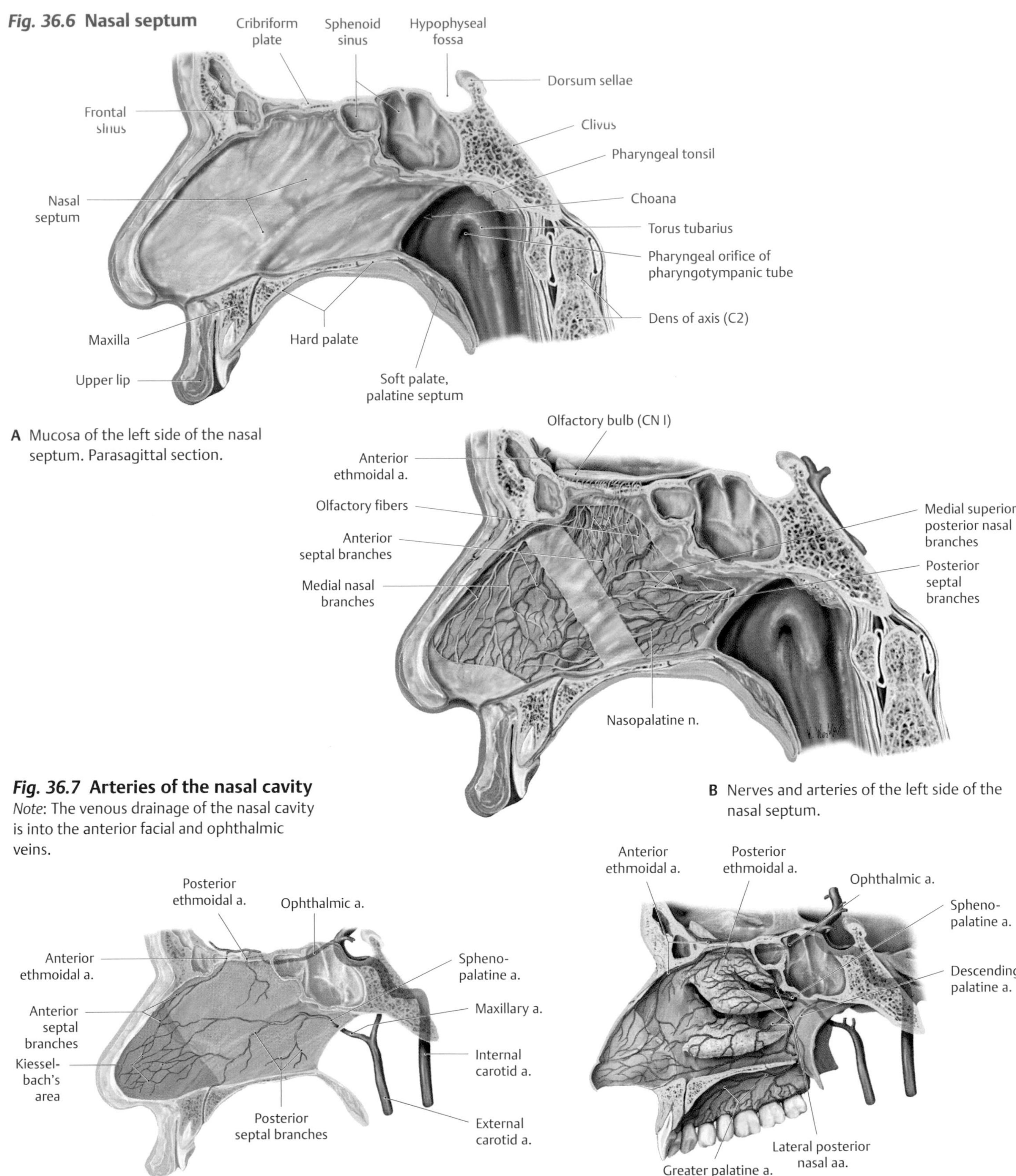

Fig. 36.6 Nasal septum
Cribriform plate
Sphenoid sinus
Hypophyseal fossa
Dorsum sellae
Frontal sinus
Clivus
Pharyngeal tonsil
Nasal septum
Choana
Torus tubarius
Pharyngeal orifice of pharyngotympanic tube
Dens of axis (C2)
Maxilla
Hard palate
Upper lip
Soft palate, palatine septum
Olfactory bulb (CN I)
Anterior ethmoidal a.
Olfactory fibers
Medial superior posterior nasal branches
Anterior septal branches
Posterior septal branches
Medial nasal branches
Nasopalatine n.
Posterior ethmoidal a.
Ophthalmic a.
Anterior ethmoidal a.
Spheno-palatine a.
Maxillary a.
Anterior septal branches
Kiessel-bach's area
Internal carotid a.
Posterior septal branches
External carotid a.
Anterior ethmoidal a.
Posterior ethmoidal a.
Ophthalmic a.
Spheno-palatine a.
Descending palatine a.
Lateral posterior nasal aa.
Greater palatine a.

Fig. 36.6 Nasal septum

A Mucosa of the left side of the nasal septum. Parasagittal section.

B Nerves and arteries of the left side of the nasal septum.

Fig. 36.7 Arteries of the nasal cavity

Note: The venous drainage of the nasal cavity is into the anterior facial and ophthalmic veins.

A Arteries of the left side of the nasal septum.

B Arteries of the right lateral nasal wall.

Fig. 36.8 Lateral nasal wall

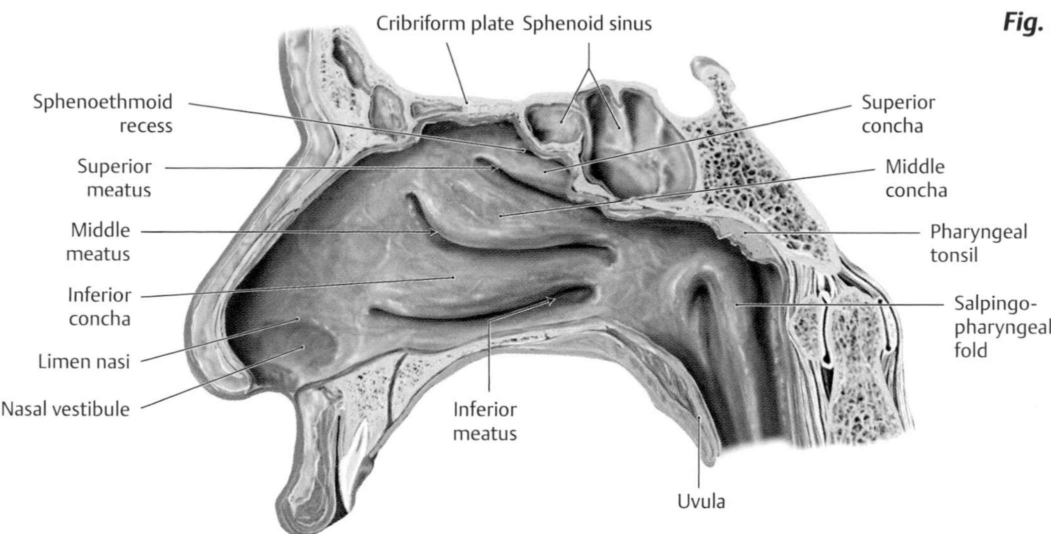
Cribriform plate
Sphenoid sinus
Sphenoethmoid recess
Superior meatus
Middle meatus
Inferior concha
Limen nasi
Nasal vestibule
Inferior meatus
Uvula
Superior concha
Middle concha
Pharyngeal tonsil
Salpingo-pharyngeal fold

A Mucosa of the right lateral nasal wall. Sagittal section.

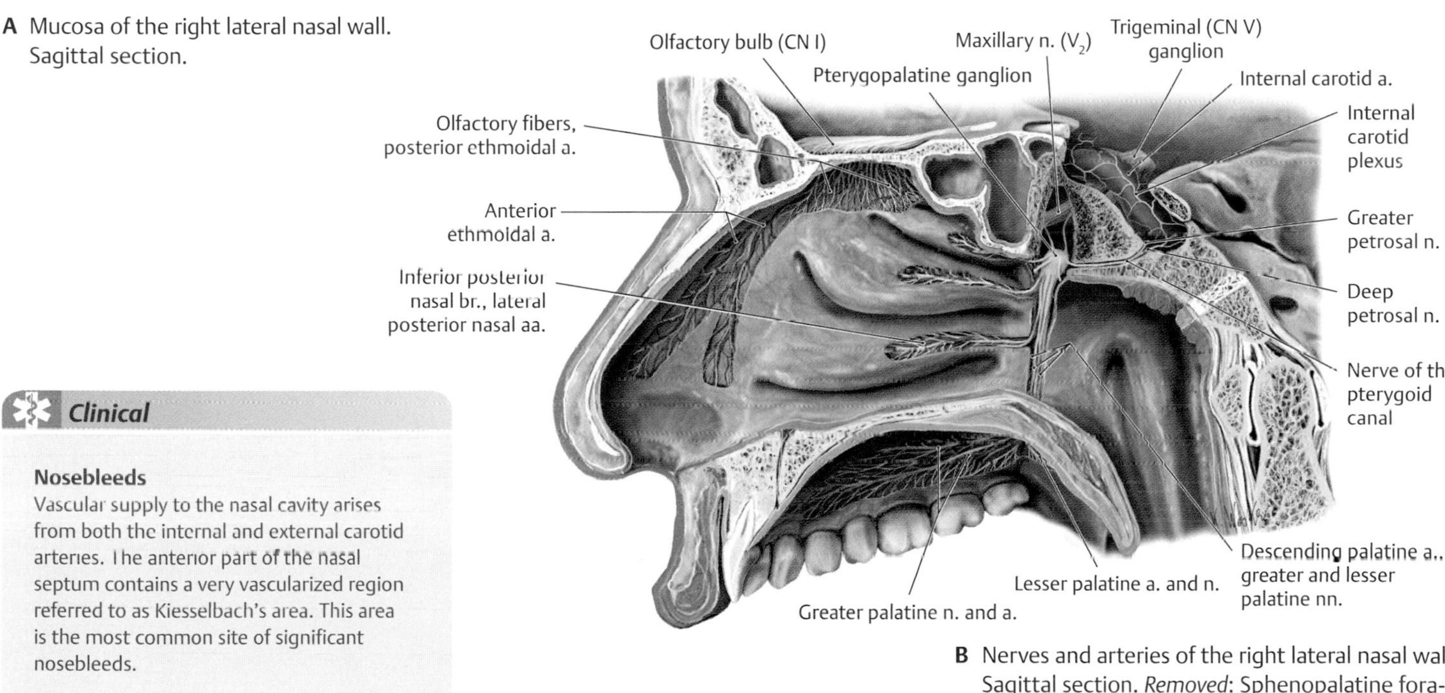
Olfactory bulb (CN I)
Maxillary n. (V_2)
Trigeminal (CN V) ganglion
Pterygopalatine ganglion
Internal carotid a.
Olfactory fibers, posterior ethmoidal a.
Internal carotid plexus
Anterior ethmoidal a.
Greater petrosal n.
Inferior posterior nasal br., lateral posterior nasal aa.
Deep petrosal n.
Nerve of the pterygoid canal
Descending palatine a., greater and lesser palatine nn.
Lesser palatine a. and n.
Greater palatine n. and a.

B Nerves and arteries of the right lateral nasal wall. Sagittal section. *Removed*: Sphenopalatine foramen.

Clinical

Nosebleeds

Vascular supply to the nasal cavity arises from both the internal and external carotid arteries. The anterior part of the nasal septum contains a very vascularized region referred to as Kiesselbach's area. This area is the most common site of significant nosebleeds.

Fig. 36.9 Nerves of the nasal cavity

Left lateral view.

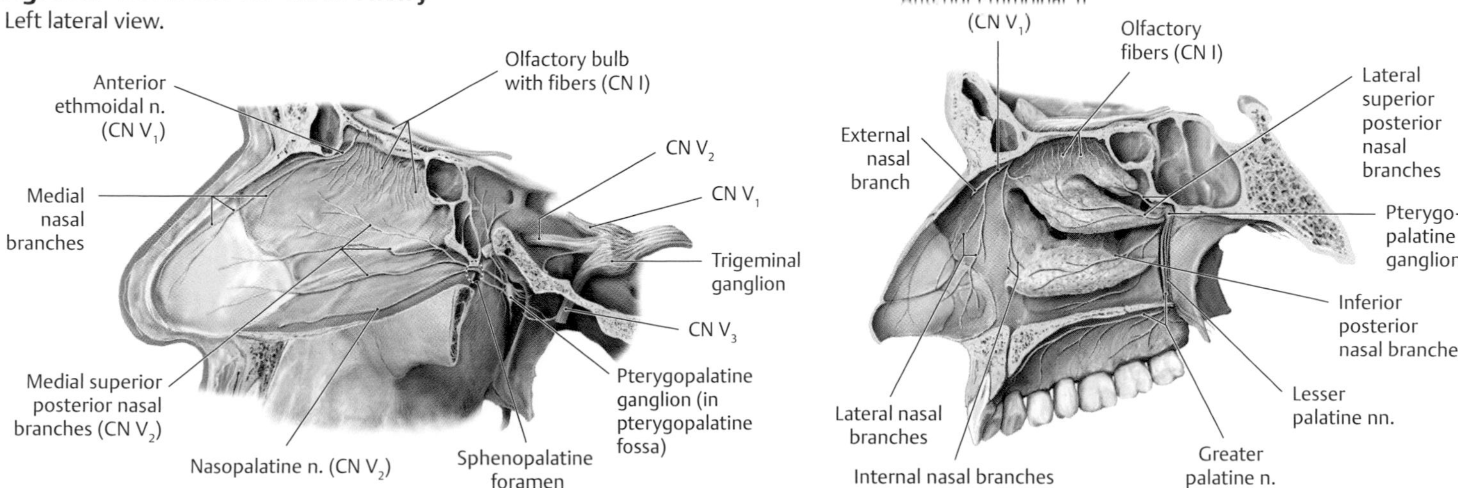
Anterior ethmoidal n. (CN V_1)
Olfactory bulb with fibers (CN I)
Medial nasal branches
CN V_2
CN V_1
Trigeminal ganglion
CN V_3
Medial superior posterior nasal branches (CN V_2)
Pterygopalatine ganglion (in pterygopalatine fossa)
Nasopalatine n. (CN V_2)
Sphenopalatine foramen
Anterior ethmoidal n. (CN V_1)
Olfactory fibers (CN I)
External nasal branch
Lateral superior posterior nasal branches
Pterygo-palatine ganglion
Inferior posterior nasal branches
Lesser palatine nn.
Lateral nasal branches
Internal nasal branches
Greater palatine n.

A Nerves of the left side of the nasal septum.

B Nerves of the right lateral nasal wall.

Temporal Bone

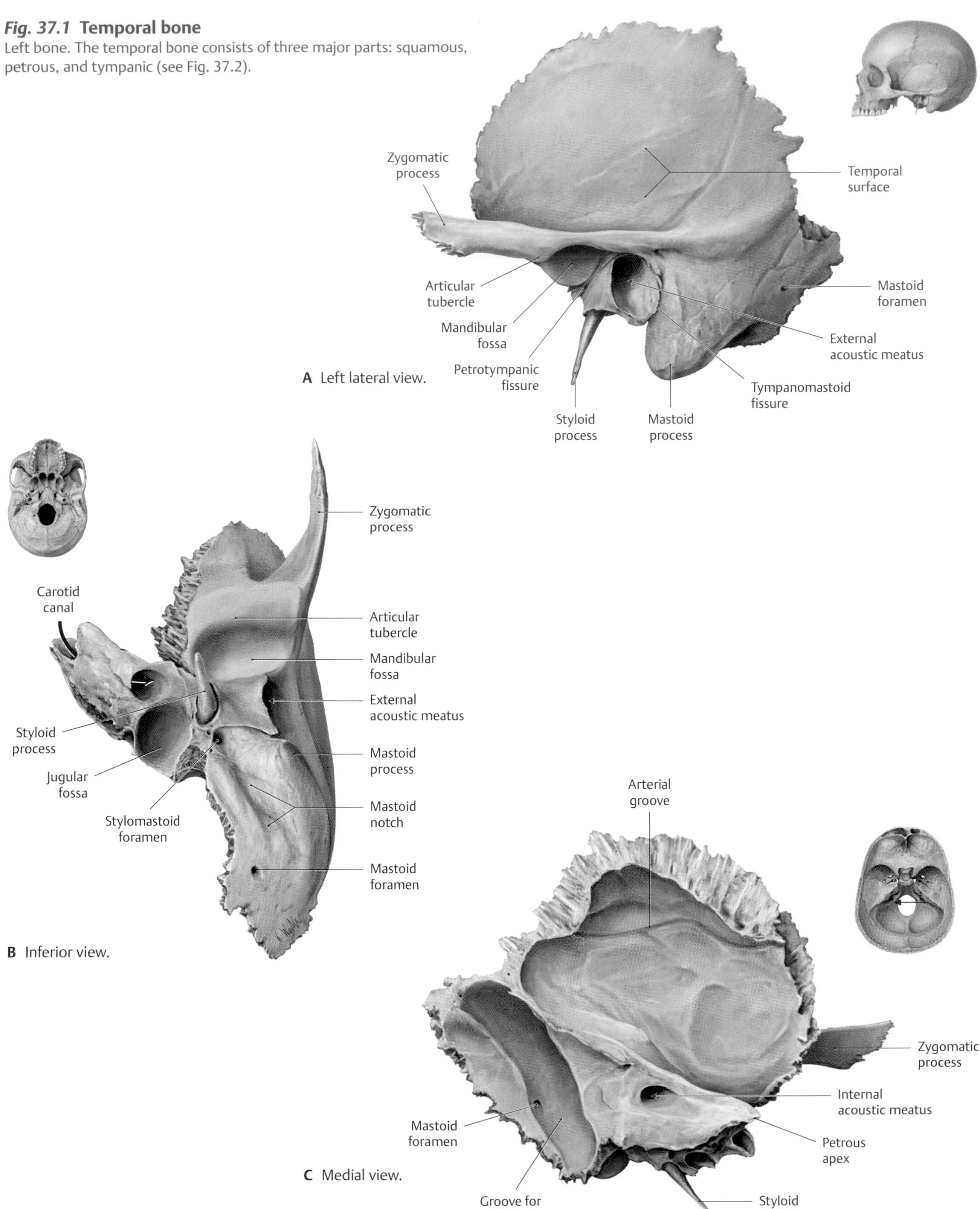
Zygomatic process
Temporal surface
Articular tubercle
Mandibular fossa
Petrotympanic fissure
Mastoid foramen
External acoustic meatus
Tympanomastoid fissure
Styloid process
Mastoid process
A Left lateral view.
Zygomatic process
Carotid canal
Articular tubercle
Mandibular fossa
External acoustic meatus
Styloid process
Mastoid process
Jugular fossa
Mastoid notch
Stylomastoid foramen
Mastoid foramen
B Inferior view.
Arterial groove
Zygomatic process
Internal acoustic meatus
Mastoid foramen
Petrous apex
C Medial view.
Groove for sigmoid sinus
Styloid process

Fig. 37.1 **Temporal bone**
Left bone. The temporal bone consists of three major parts: squamous, petrous, and tympanic (see Fig. 37.2).

Fig. 37.2 Parts of the temporal bone

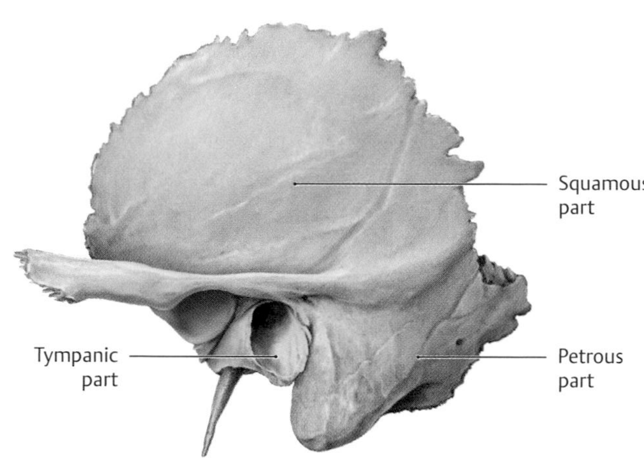
Squamous part
Tympanic part
Petrous part

A Left lateral view.

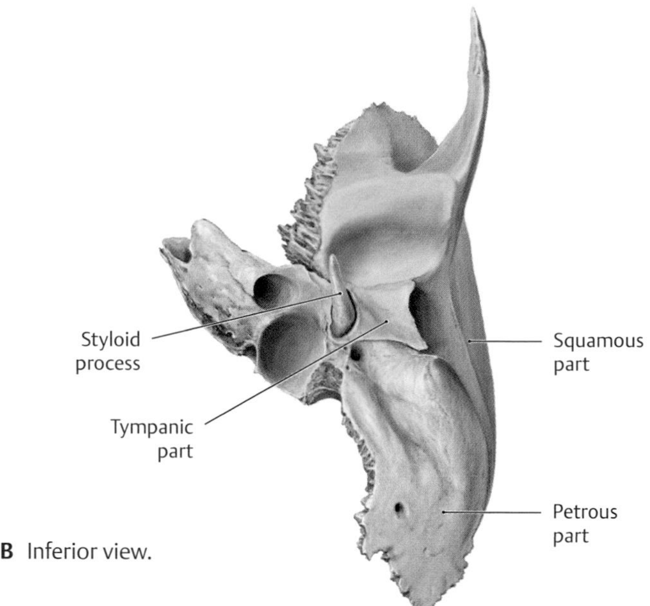
Styloid process
Tympanic part
Squamous part
Petrous part

B Inferior view.

Clinical

Structures in the temporal bone

The mastoid process contains mastoid air cells that communicate with the middle ear; the middle ear in turn communicates with the nasopharynx via the pharyngotympanic (auditory) tube (**A**). Bacteria may use this pathway to move from the nasopharynx into the middle ear. In severe cases, bacteria may pass from the mastoid air cells into the cranial cavity, causing meningitis.

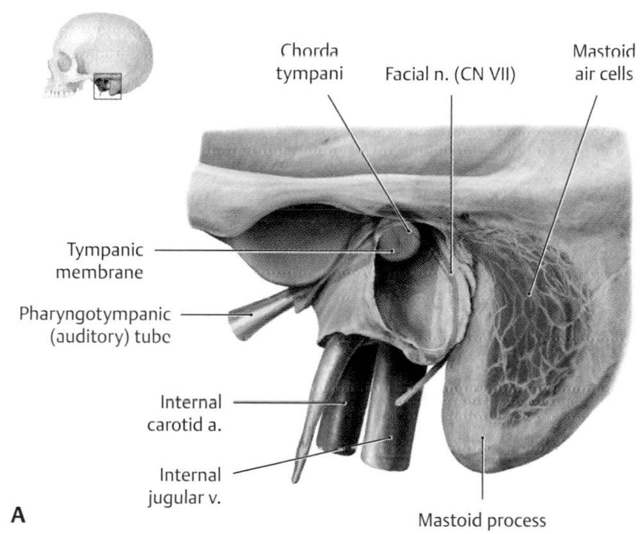
Chorda tympani
Facial n. (CN VII)
Mastoid air cells
Tympanic membrane
Pharyngotympanic (auditory) tube
Internal carotid a.
Internal jugular v.
Mastoid process

A

Irrigation of the auditory canal with warm (44°C) or cool (30°C) water can induce a thermal current in the endolymph of the semicircular canal, causing the patient to manifest vestibular nystagmus (jerky eye movements, vestibulo-ocular reflex). This caloric testing is important in the diagnosis of unexplained vertigo. The patient must be oriented so that the semicircular canal of interest lies in the vertical plane (**C**).

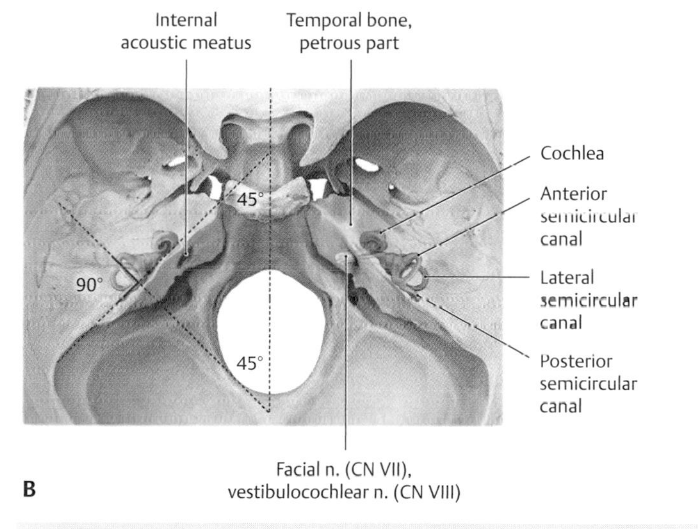
Internal acoustic meatus
Temporal bone, petrous part
45°
90°
45°
Cochlea
Anterior semicircular canal
Lateral semicircular canal
Posterior semicircular canal
Facial n. (CN VII), vestibulocochlear n. (CN VIII)

B

The petrous portion of the temporal bone contains the middle and inner ear as well as the tympanic membrane. The bony semicircular canals are oriented at an approximately 45-degree angle from the coronal, transverse, and sagittal planes (**B**).

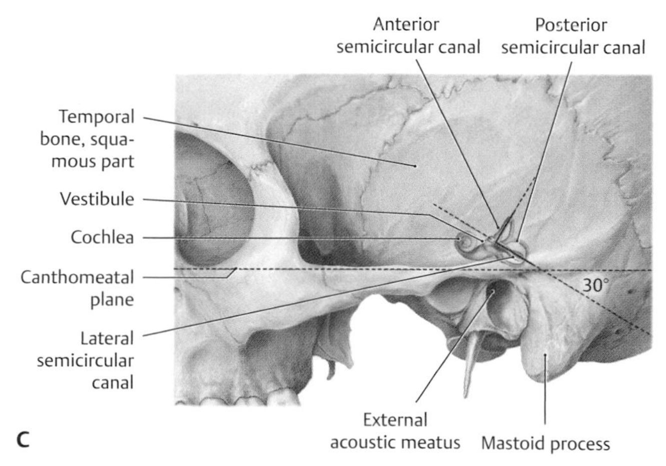
Anterior semicircular canal
Posterior semicircular canal
Temporal bone, squamous part
Vestibule
Cochlea
Canthomeatal plane
30°
Lateral semicircular canal
External acoustic meatus
Mastoid process

C

External Ear & Auditory Canal

The auditory apparatus is divided into three main parts: external, middle, and inner ear. The external and middle ear are part of the sound conduction apparatus, and the inner ear is the actual organ of hearing (see p. 566). The inner ear also contains the vestibular apparatus, the organ of balance (see p. 566).

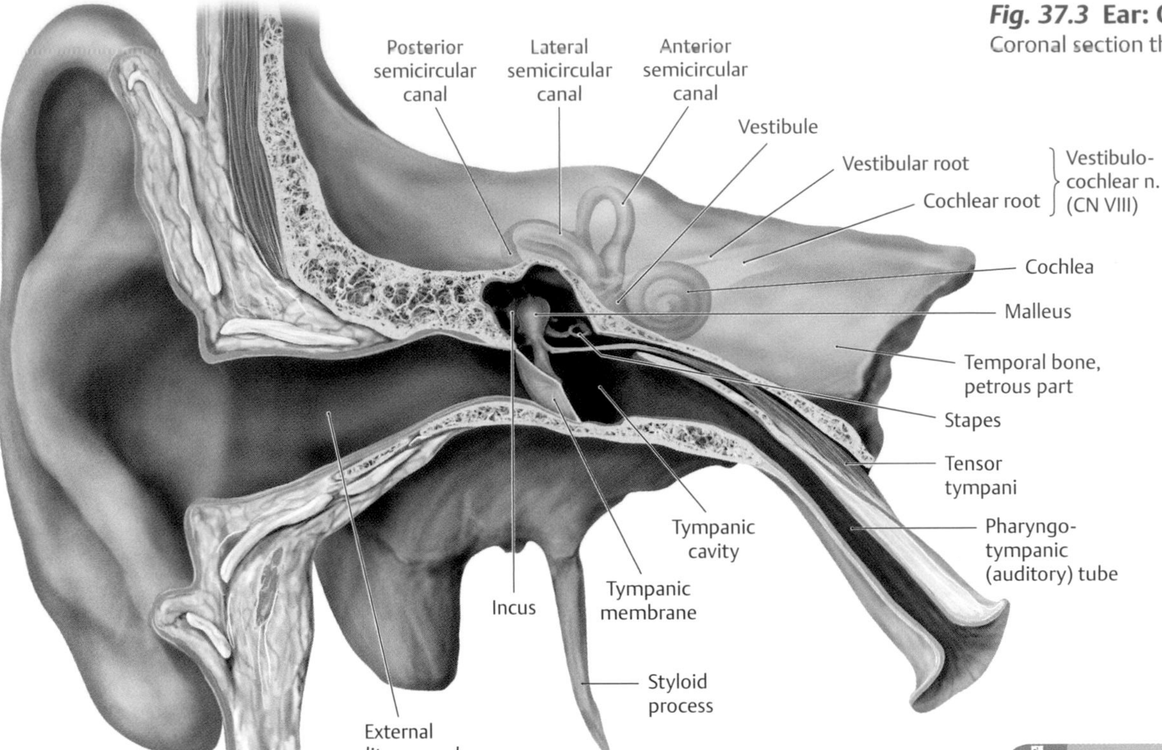
Posterior semicircular canal
Lateral semicircular canal
Anterior semicircular canal
Vestibule
Vestibular root
Cochlear root
Vestibulo-cochlear n. (CN VIII)
Cochlea
Malleus
Temporal bone, petrous part
Stapes
Tensor tympani
Pharyngo-tympanic (auditory) tube
Tympanic cavity
Tympanic membrane
Incus
Styloid process
External auditory canal

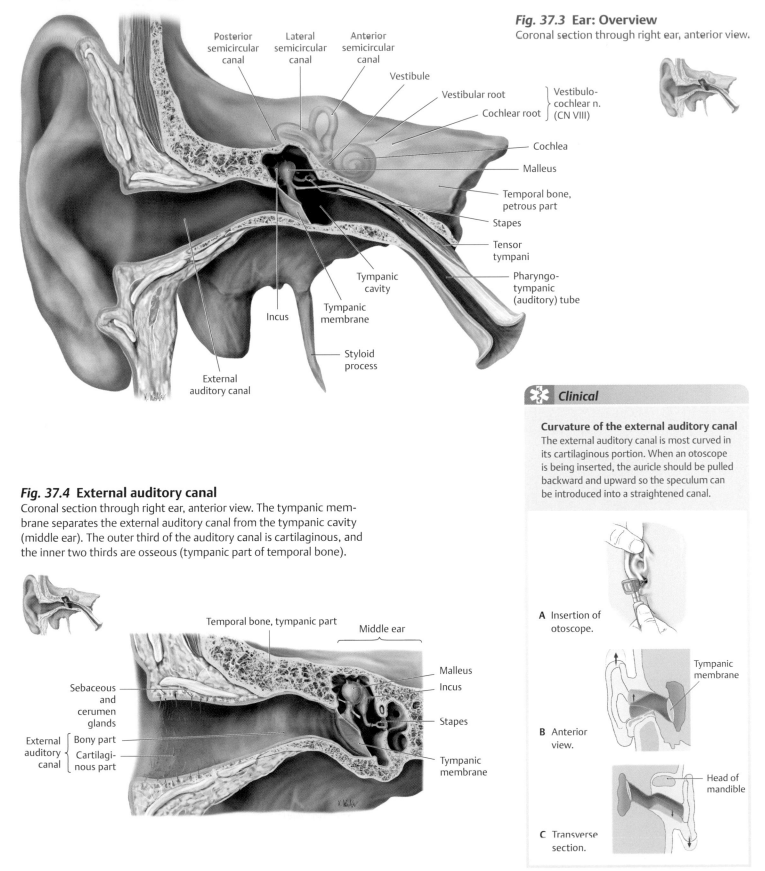

Fig. 37.3 **Ear: Overview**
Coronal section through right ear, anterior view.

Fig. 37.4 **External auditory canal**
Coronal section through right ear, anterior view. The tympanic membrane separates the external auditory canal from the tympanic cavity (middle ear). The outer third of the auditory canal is cartilaginous, and the inner two thirds are osseous (tympanic part of temporal bone).

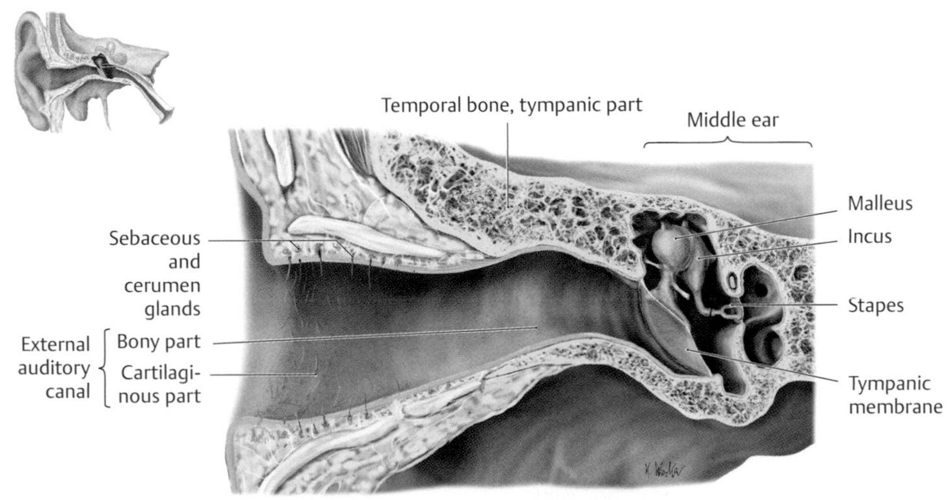
Temporal bone, tympanic part
Middle ear
Malleus
Incus
Stapes
Tympanic membrane
Sebaceous and cerumen glands
External auditory canal
Bony part
Cartilagi-nous part

Clinical

Curvature of the external auditory canal
The external auditory canal is most curved in its cartilaginous portion. When an otoscope is being inserted, the auricle should be pulled backward and upward so the speculum can be introduced into a straightened canal.

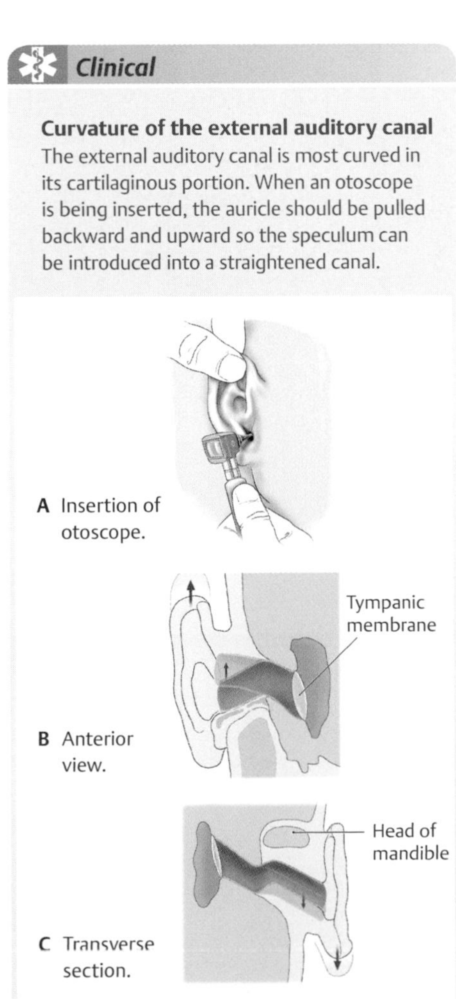
A Insertion of otoscope.
B Anterior view.
Tympanic membrane
Head of mandible
C Transverse section.

Fig. 37.5 Structure of the auricle

The auricle of the ear encloses a cartilaginous framework that forms a funnel-shaped receptor for acoustic vibrations. The muscles of the auricle are considered muscles of facial expression, although they are vestigial in humans.

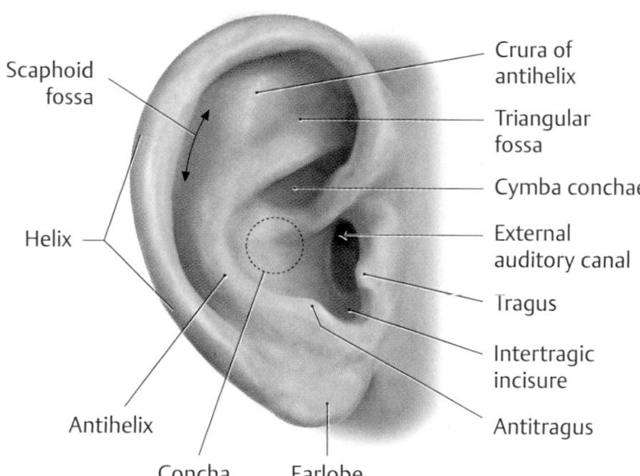

Scaphoid fossa
Helix
Antihelix
Concha
Earlobe
Crura of antihelix
Triangular fossa
Cymba conchae
External auditory canal
Tragus
Intertragic incisure
Antitragus

A Right auricle, right lateral view.

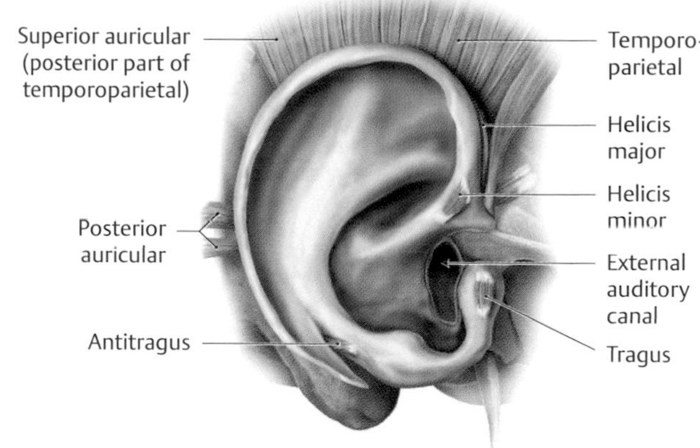

Superior auricular (posterior part of temporoparietal)
Posterior auricular
Antitragus
Temporo-parietal
Helicis major
Helicis minor
External auditory canal
Tragus

B Cartilage and muscles of the right auricle, right lateral view.

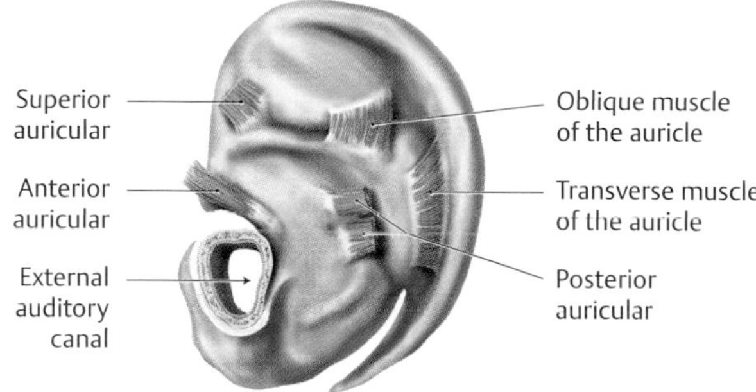

Superior auricular
Anterior auricular
External auditory canal
Oblique muscle of the auricle
Transverse muscle of the auricle
Posterior auricular

C Cartilage and muscles of the right auricle, medial view of posterior surface.

Fig. 37.6 Arteries of the auricle

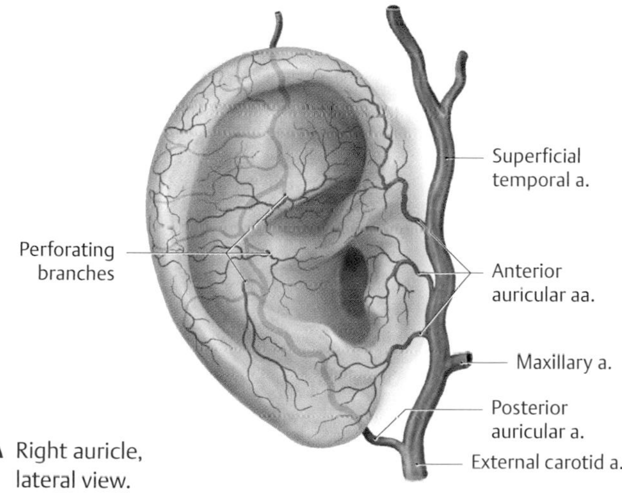

Perforating branches
Superficial temporal a.
Anterior auricular aa.
Maxillary a.
Posterior auricular a.
External carotid a.

A Right auricle, lateral view.

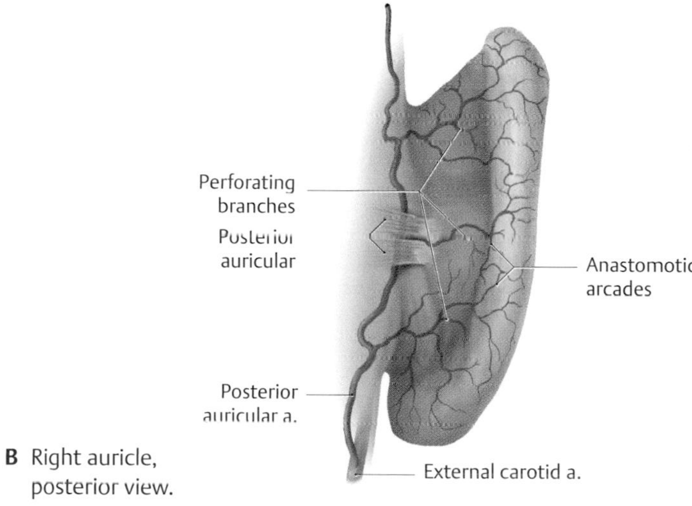

Perforating branches
Posterior auricular
Posterior auricular a.
Anastomotic arcades
External carotid a.

B Right auricle, posterior view.

Fig. 37.7 Innervation of the auricle

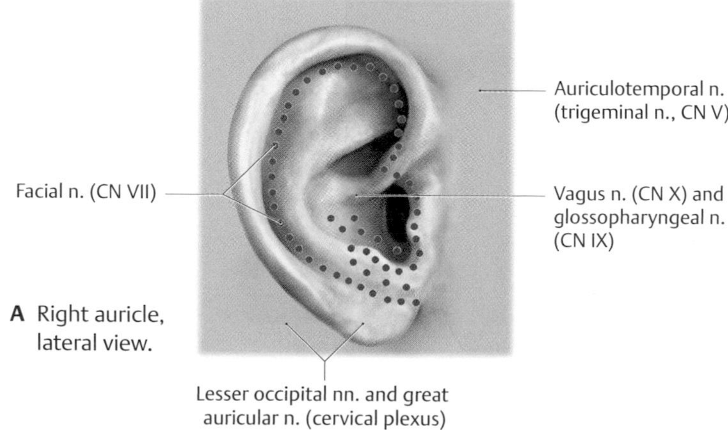

Facial n. (CN VII)
Auriculotemporal n. (trigeminal n., CN V)
Vagus n. (CN X) and glossopharyngeal n. (CN IX)
Lesser occipital nn. and great auricular n. (cervical plexus)

A Right auricle, lateral view.

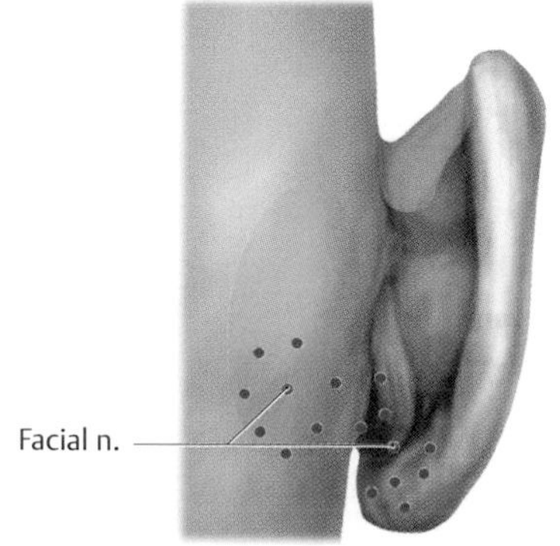

Facial n.

B Right auricle, posterior view.

Middle Ear: Tympanic Cavity

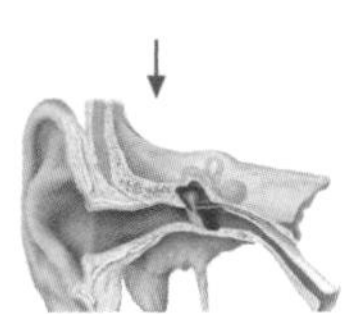

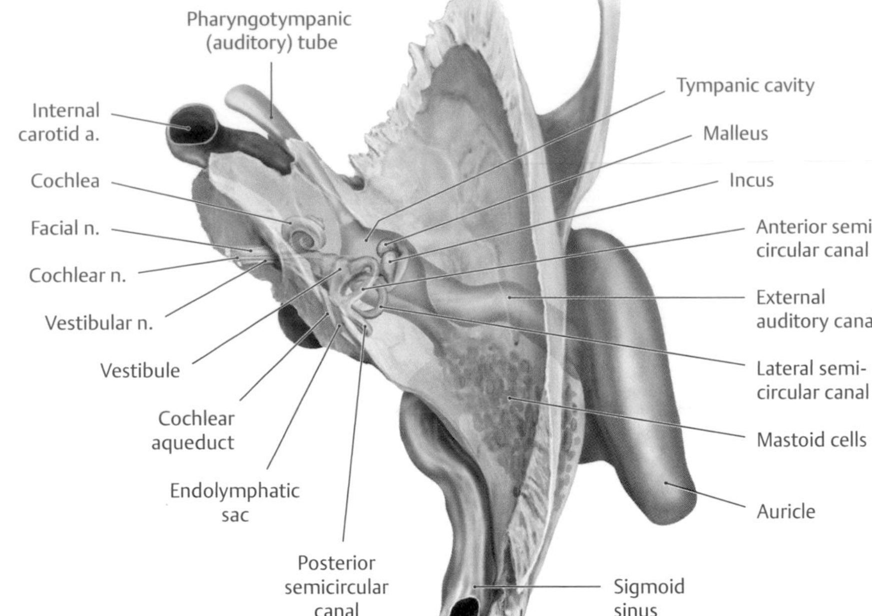
Pharyngotympanic (auditory) tube
Internal carotid a.
Cochlea
Facial n.
Cochlear n.
Vestibular n.
Vestibule
Cochlear aqueduct
Endolymphatic sac
Posterior semicircular canal
Tympanic cavity
Malleus
Incus
Anterior semi-circular canal
External auditory canal
Lateral semi-circular canal
Mastoid cells
Auricle
Sigmoid sinus

Fig. 37.8 **Middle ear**
Right petrous bone, superior view. The tympanic cavity of the middle ear communicates anteriorly with the pharynx via the pharyngotympanic (auditory) tube and posteriorly with the mastoid air cells.

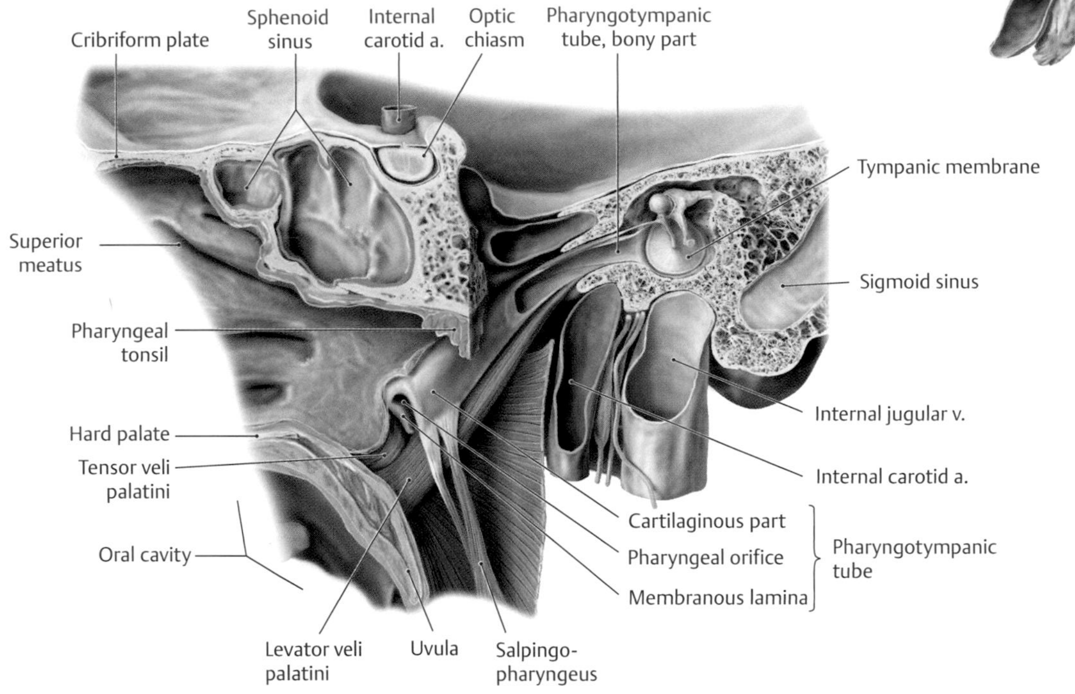
Cribriform plate
Sphenoid sinus
Internal carotid a.
Optic chiasm
Pharyngotympanic tube, bony part
Tympanic membrane
Superior meatus
Sigmoid sinus
Pharyngeal tonsil
Internal jugular v.
Hard palate
Tensor veli palatini
Internal carotid a.
Cartilaginous part
Pharyngeal orifice
Membranous lamina
Pharyngotympanic tube
Oral cavity
Levator veli palatini
Uvula
Salpingo-pharyngeus

Fig. 37.9 **Tympanic cavity and pharyngotympanic tube**
Medial view of opened tympanic cavity.

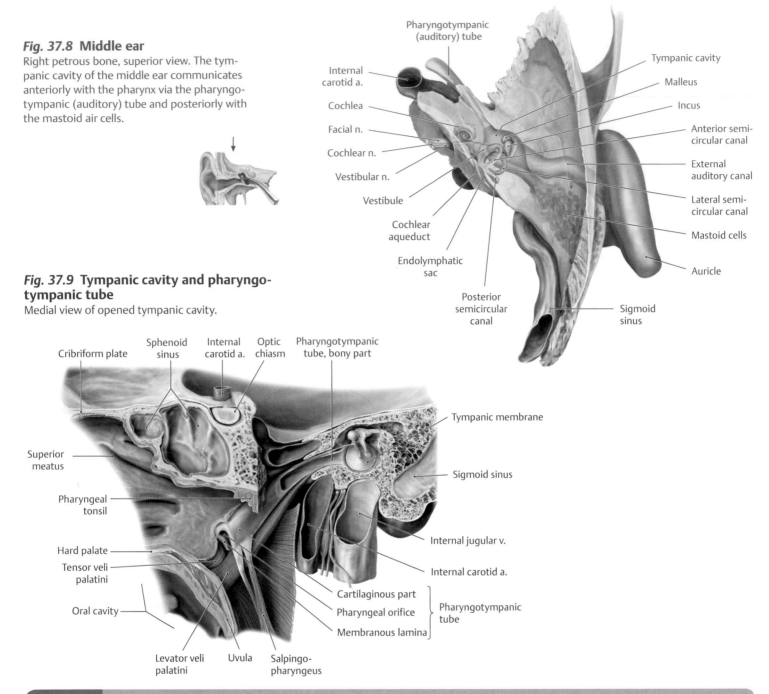

Table 37.1 **Boundaries of the tympanic cavity**

During chronic suppurative otitis media (inflammation of the middle ear), pathogenic bacteria may spread to adjacent regions.

Direction	Wall	Anatomical boundary	Neighboring structures	Infection
Anterior	Carotid	Opening to pharyngotympanic tube	Carotid canal	
Lateral	Membranous	Tympanic membrane	External ear	
Superior	Tegmental	Tegmen tympani	Middle cranial fossa	Meningitis, cerebral abscess (especially of temporal lobe)
Medial	Labyrinthine	Promontory overlying basal turn of cochlea	Inner ear	
			CSF space (via petrous apex)	Abducent paralysis, trigeminal nerve irritation, visual disturbances (Gradenigo's syndrome)
Inferior	Jugular	Temporal bone, tympanic part	Bulb of jugular vein	
			Sigmoid sinus	Sinus thrombosis
Posterior	Mastoid	Aditus to mastoid antrum	Air cells of mastoid process	Mastoiditis
			Facial nerve canal	Facial paralysis

CSF, cerebrospinal fluid.

Fig. 37.10 Tympanic cavity

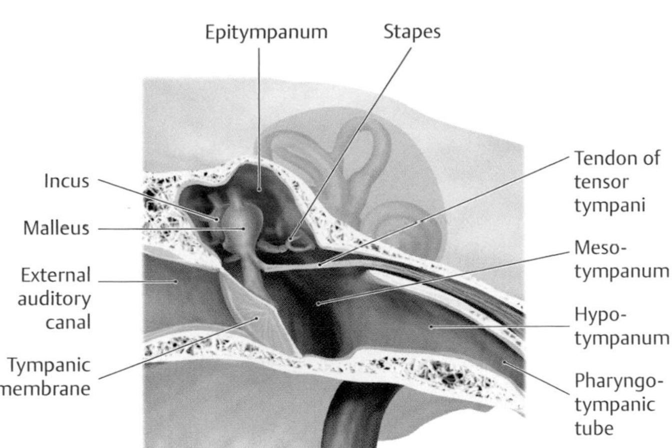
Epitympanum
Stapes
Incus
Malleus
External auditory canal
Tympanic membrane
Tendon of tensor tympani
Meso-tympanum
Hypo-tympanum
Pharyngo-tympanic tube

A Levels of the tympanic cavity. Anterior view. The tympanic cavity is divided into three levels: epi-, meso-, and hypotympanum.

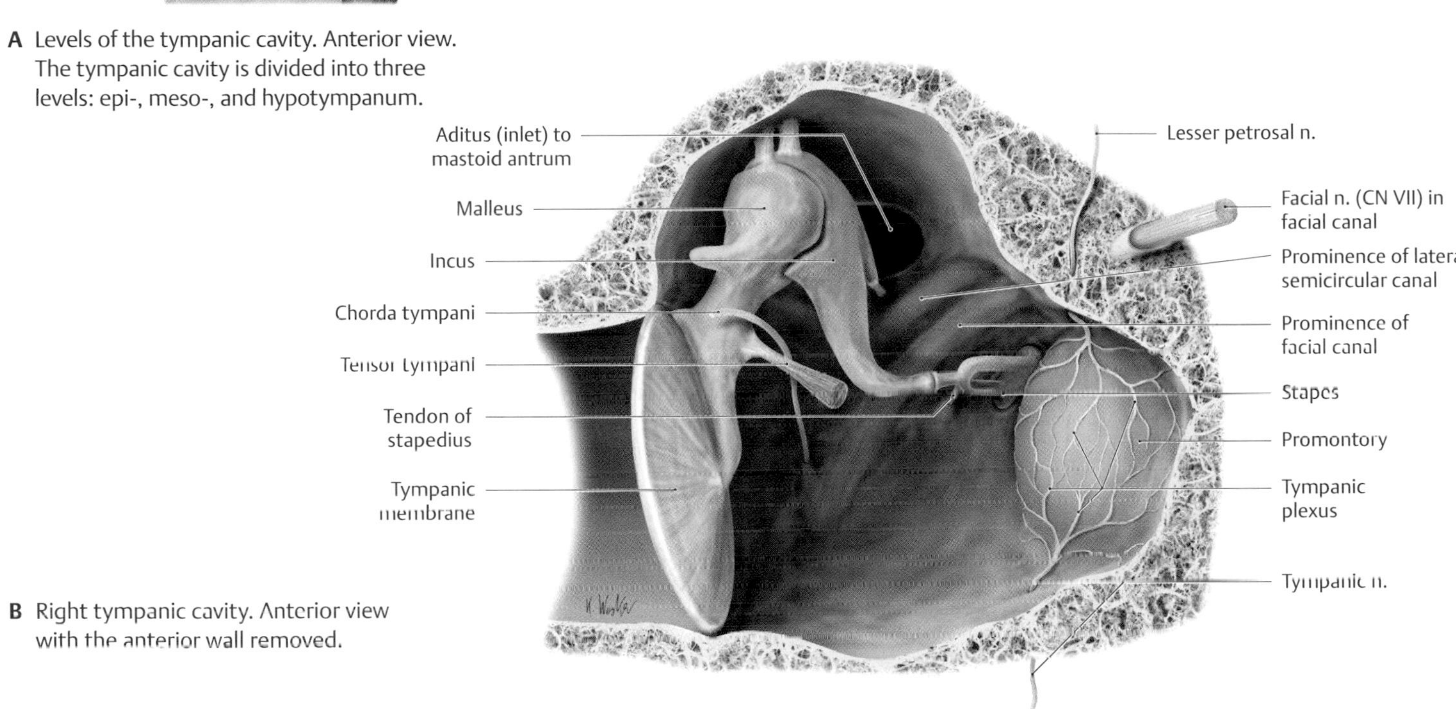
Aditus (inlet) to mastoid antrum
Malleus
Incus
Chorda tympani
Tensor tympani
Tendon of stapedius
Tympanic membrane
Lesser petrosal n.
Facial n. (CN VII) in facial canal
Prominence of lateral semicircular canal
Prominence of facial canal
Stapes
Promontory
Tympanic plexus
Tympanic n.

B Right tympanic cavity. Anterior view with the anterior wall removed.

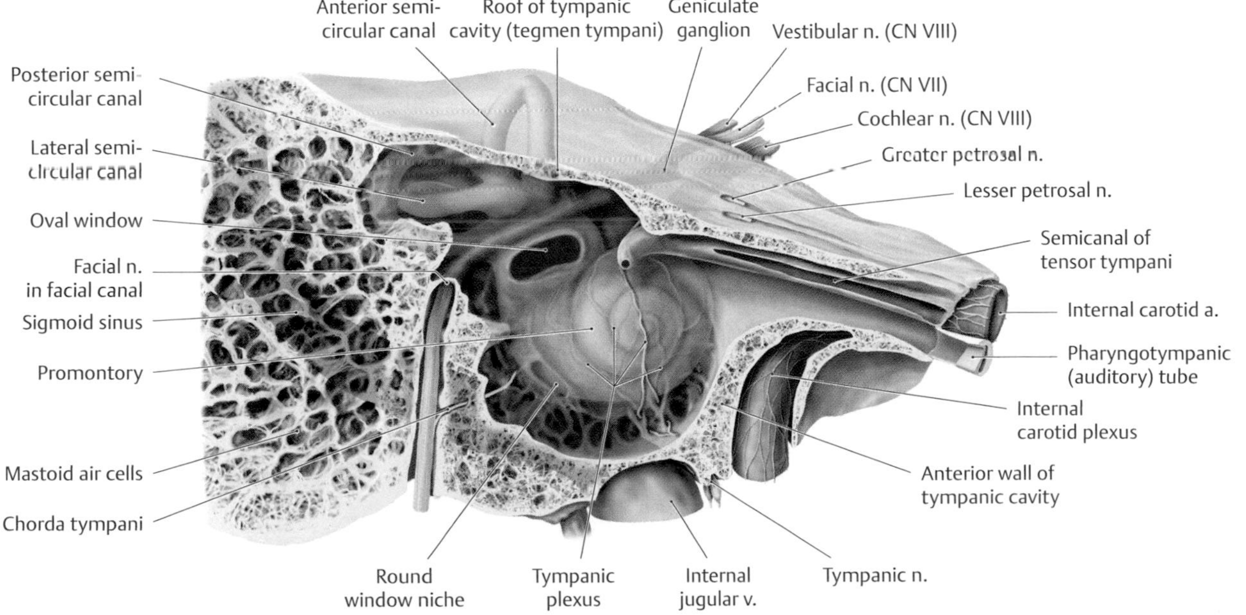
Anterior semi-circular canal
Roof of tympanic cavity (tegmen tympani)
Geniculate ganglion
Vestibular n. (CN VIII)
Facial n. (CN VII)
Cochlear n. (CN VIII)
Greater petrosal n.
Lesser petrosal n.
Semicanal of tensor tympani
Internal carotid a.
Pharyngotympanic (auditory) tube
Internal carotid plexus
Anterior wall of tympanic cavity
Tympanic n.
Internal jugular v.
Tympanic plexus
Round window niche
Posterior semi-circular canal
Lateral semi-circular canal
Oval window
Facial n. in facial canal
Sigmoid sinus
Promontory
Mastoid air cells
Chorda tympani

C Anatomical relationships of the tympanic cavity. Oblique sagittal section showing the medial wall.

Middle Ear: Ossicular Chain & Tympanic Membrane

Fig. 37.11 Auditory ossicles
Left ear. The ossicular chain consists of three small bones that establish an articular connection between the tympanic membrane and the oval window.

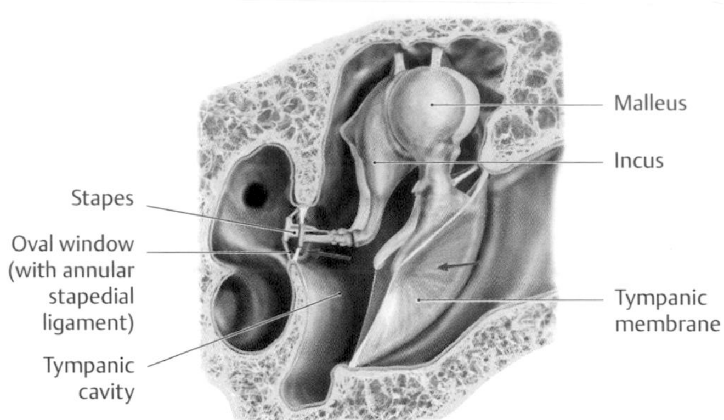
Malleus
Incus
Stapes
Oval window (with annular stapedial ligament)
Tympanic membrane
Tympanic cavity

A Auditory ossicles in the middle ear. Anterior view of the left ear.

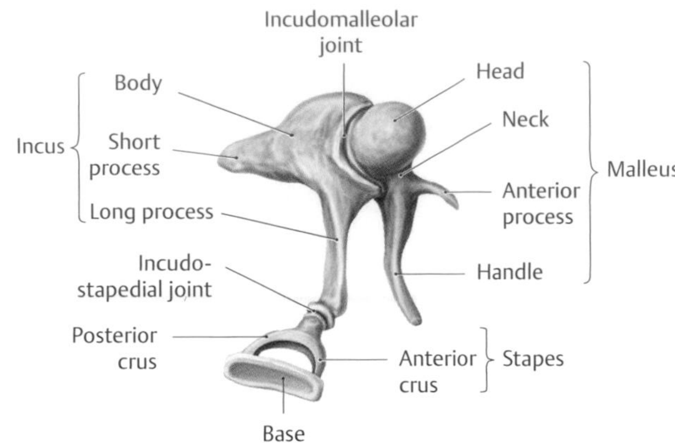
Incudomalleolar joint
Incus
Body
Short process
Long process
Head
Neck
Malleus
Anterior process
Handle
Incudo-stapedial joint
Posterior crus
Anterior crus
Stapes
Base

B Bones of the ossicular chain. Medial view of the left ossicular chain.

Fig. 37.12 Malleus ("hammer")
Left ear.

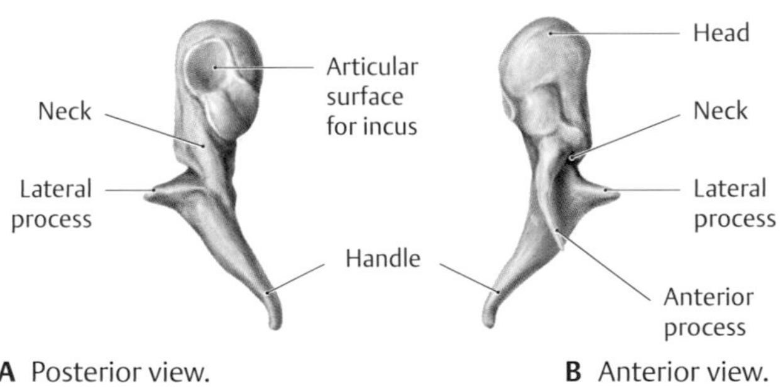
Neck
Articular surface for incus
Lateral process
Handle
Head
Neck
Lateral process
Anterior process

A Posterior view. **B** Anterior view.

Fig. 37.13 Incus ("anvil")
Left ear.

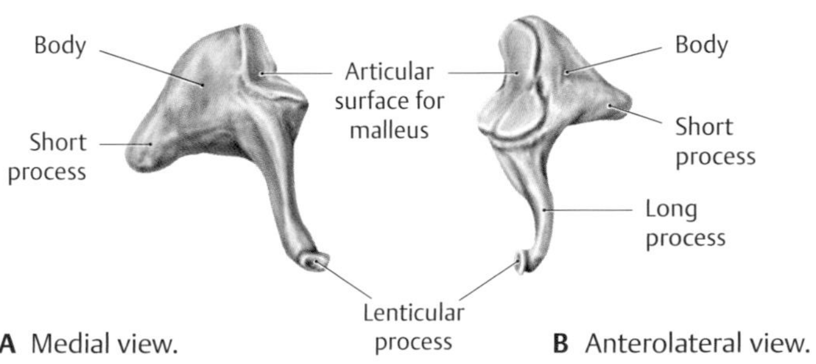
Body
Short process
Articular surface for malleus
Body
Short process
Long process
Lenticular process

A Medial view. **B** Anterolateral view.

Fig. 37.14 Stapes ("stirrup")
Left ear.

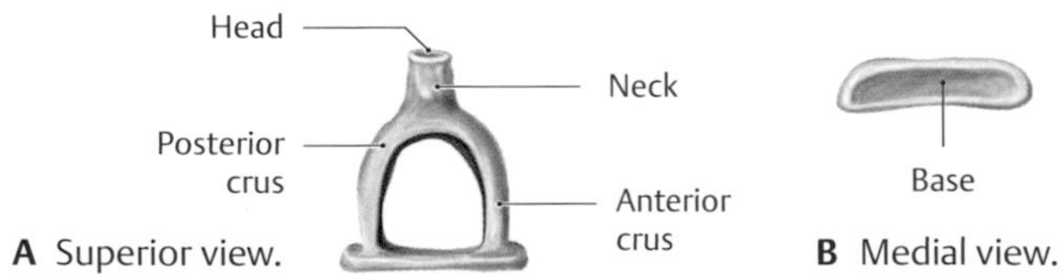
Head
Neck
Posterior crus
Anterior crus
Base

A Superior view. **B** Medial view.

Fig. 37.15 Tympanic membrane
Right tympanic membrane. The tympanic membrane is divided into four quadrants: anterosuperior (I), anteroinferior (II), posteroinferior (III), and posterosuperior (IV).

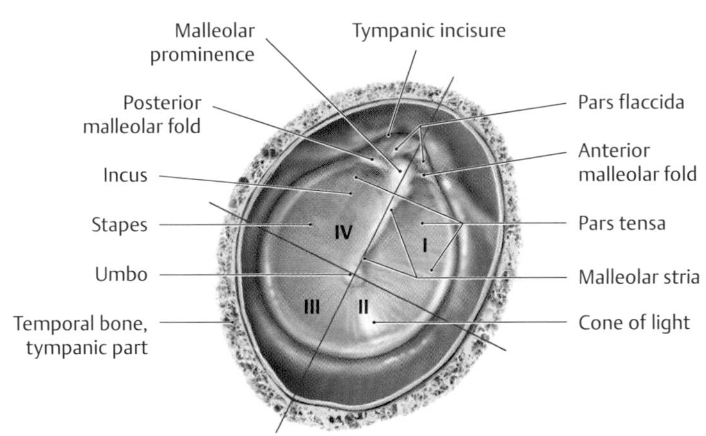
Malleolar prominence
Tympanic incisure
Posterior malleolar fold
Pars flaccida
Anterior malleolar fold
Incus
Stapes
Pars tensa
Umbo
Malleolar stria
Temporal bone, tympanic part
Cone of light
I
II
III
IV

A Lateral view of the right tympanic membrane.

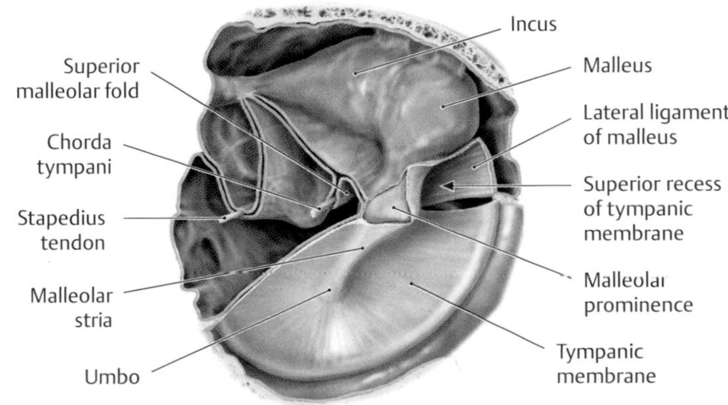
Incus
Superior malleolar fold
Malleus
Lateral ligament of malleus
Chorda tympani
Superior recess of tympanic membrane
Stapedius tendon
Malleolar stria
Malleolar prominence
Umbo
Tympanic membrane

B Mucosal lining of the tympanic cavity. Posterolateral view with the tympanic membrane partially removed.

Fig. 37.16 Ossicular chain in the tympanic cavity
Lateral view of the right ear. *Revealed:* Ligaments of the ossicular chain and muscles of the middle ear (stapedius and tensor tympani).

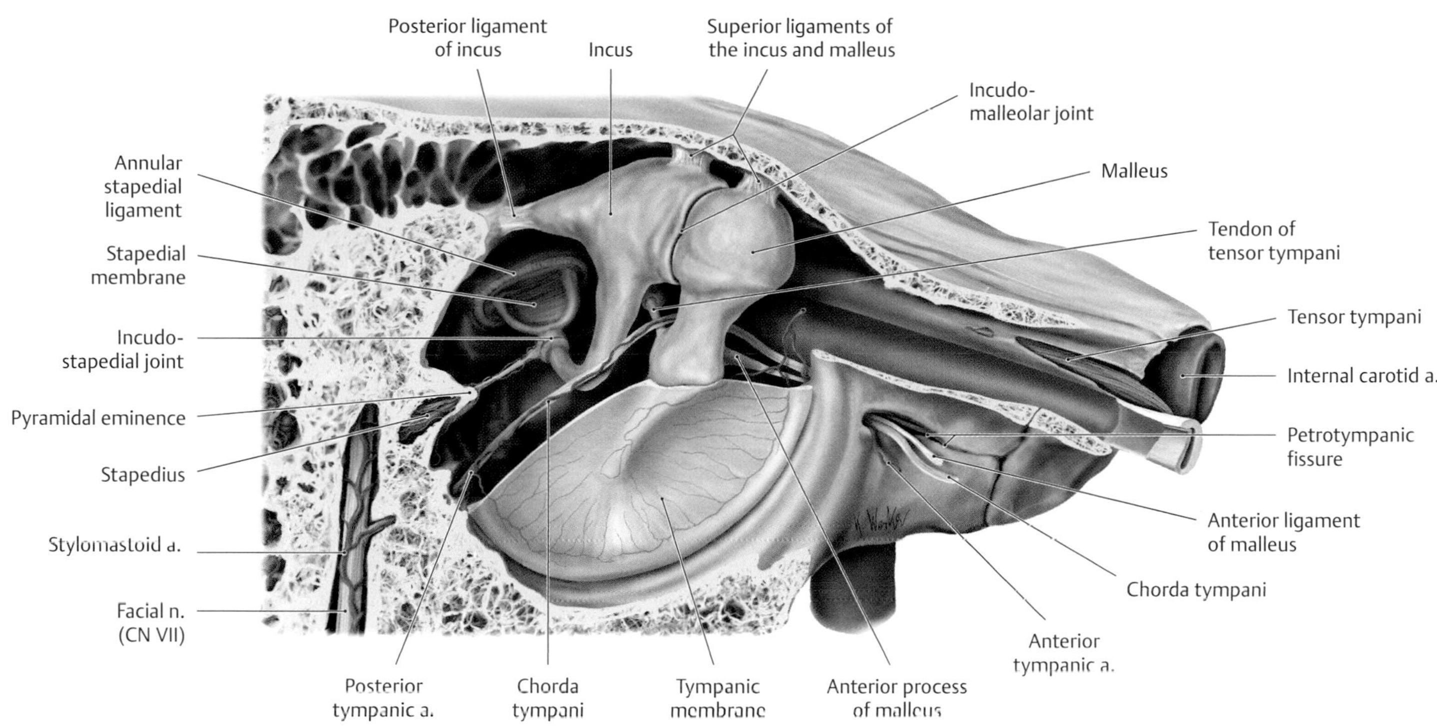
Posterior ligament of incus
Incus
Superior ligaments of the incus and malleus
Incudo-malleolar joint
Malleus
Tendon of tensor tympani
Tensor tympani
Internal carotid a.
Petrotympanic fissure
Anterior ligament of malleus
Chorda tympani
Anterior tympanic a.
Annular stapedial ligament
Stapedial membrane
Incudo-stapedial joint
Pyramidal eminence
Stapedius
Stylomastoid a.
Facial n. (CN VII)
Posterior tympanic a.
Chorda tympani
Tympanic membrane
Anterior process of malleus

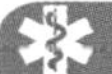

Clinical

Ossicular chain in hearing

Sound waves funneled into the external auditory canal set the tympanic membrane into vibration. The ossicular chain transmits the vibrations to the oval window, which communicates them to the fluid column of the inner ear. Sound waves in fluid meet with higher impedance; they must therefore be amplified in the middle ear. The difference in surface area between the tympanic membrane and the oval window increases the sound pressure 17-fold. A total amplification factor of 22 is achieved through the lever action of the ossicular chain. If the ossicular chain fails to transform the sound pressure between the tympanic membrane and the footplate of the stapes, the patient will experience conductive hearing loss of magnitude 20 dB. See p. 645 for hearing.

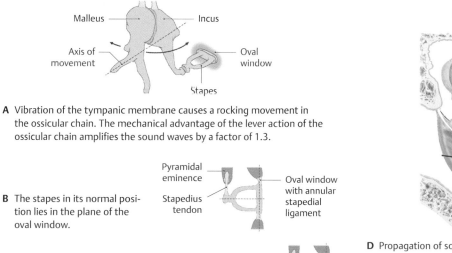

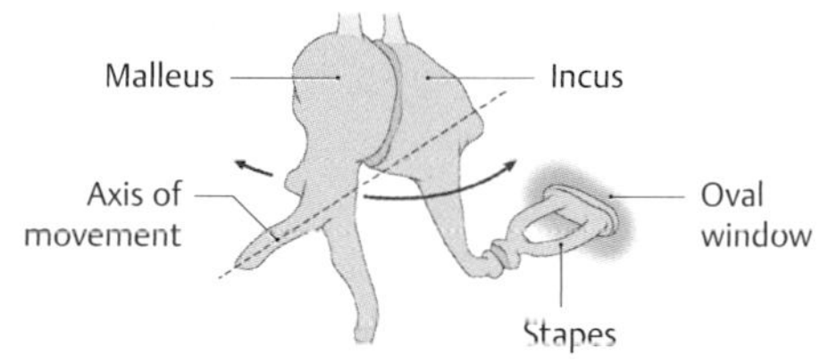
Malleus
Incus
Axis of movement
Oval window
Stapes

A Vibration of the tympanic membrane causes a rocking movement in the ossicular chain. The mechanical advantage of the lever action of the ossicular chain amplifies the sound waves by a factor of 1.3.

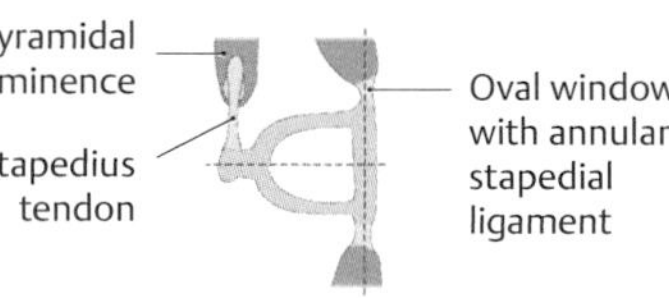
Pyramidal eminence
Stapedius tendon
Oval window with annular stapedial ligament

B The stapes in its normal position lies in the plane of the oval window.

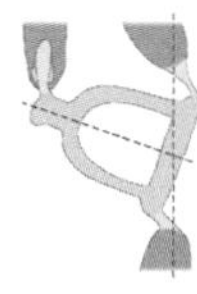

C Rocking of the ossicular chain causes the stapes to tilt. The movement of the stapes base against the membrane of the oval window (stapedial membrane) induces corresponding waves in the fluid column of the inner ear.

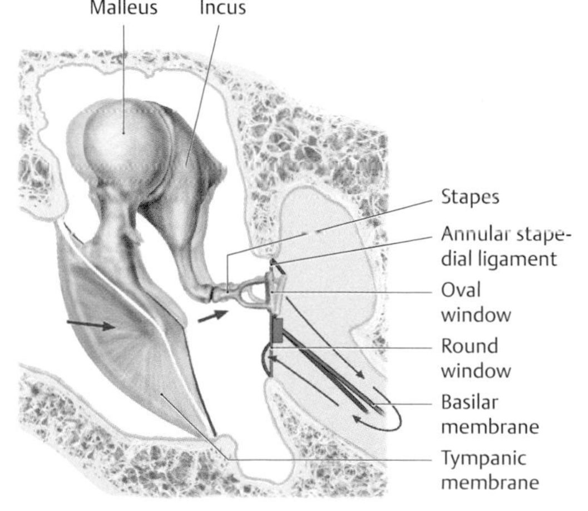
Malleus
Incus
Stapes
Annular stapedial ligament
Oval window
Round window
Basilar membrane
Tympanic membrane

D Propagation of sound waves by the ossicular chain.

Arteries of the Middle Ear

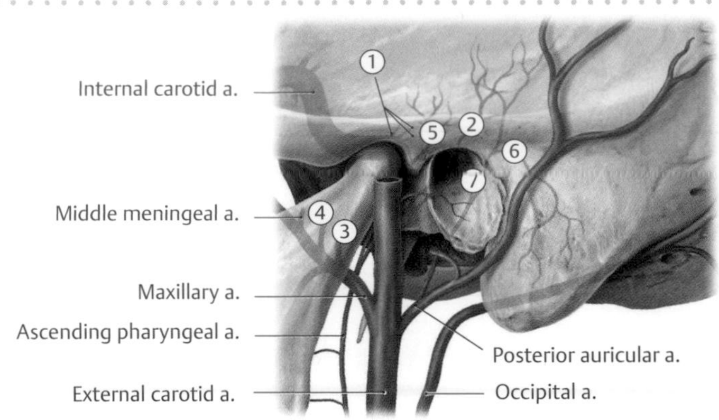
Internal carotid a.
Middle meningeal a.
Maxillary a.
Ascending pharyngeal a.
External carotid a.
Posterior auricular a.
Occipital a.
1
2
3
4
5
6
7

Table 37.2 Principal arteries of the middle ear

Origin	Artery			Distribution
Internal carotid a.	① Caroticotympanic aa.			Tympanic cavity (anterior wall), pharyngotympanic (auditory) tube
External carotid a.	Ascending pharyngeal a. (medial branch)	② Inferior tympanic a.		Tympanic cavity (floor), promontory
	Maxillary a. (terminal branch)	③ Deep auricular a.		Tympanic cavity (floor), tympanic membrane
		④ Anterior tympanic a.		Tympanic membrane, mastoid antrum, malleus, incus
		Middle meningeal a.	⑤ Superior tympanic a.	Tympanic cavity (roof), tensor tympani, stapes
	Posterior auricular a. (posterior branch)	Stylomastoid a.	⑥ Stylomastoid a.	Tympanic cavity (posterior wall), mastoid air cells, stapedius muscle, stapes
			⑦ Posterior tympanic a.	Chorda tympani, tympanic membrane, malleus

Fig. 37.17 **Arteries of the middle ear: Ossicular chain and tympanic membrane**

Medial view of the right tympanic membrane. With inflammation, the arteries of the tympanic membrane may become so dilated that their course can be observed (as shown here).

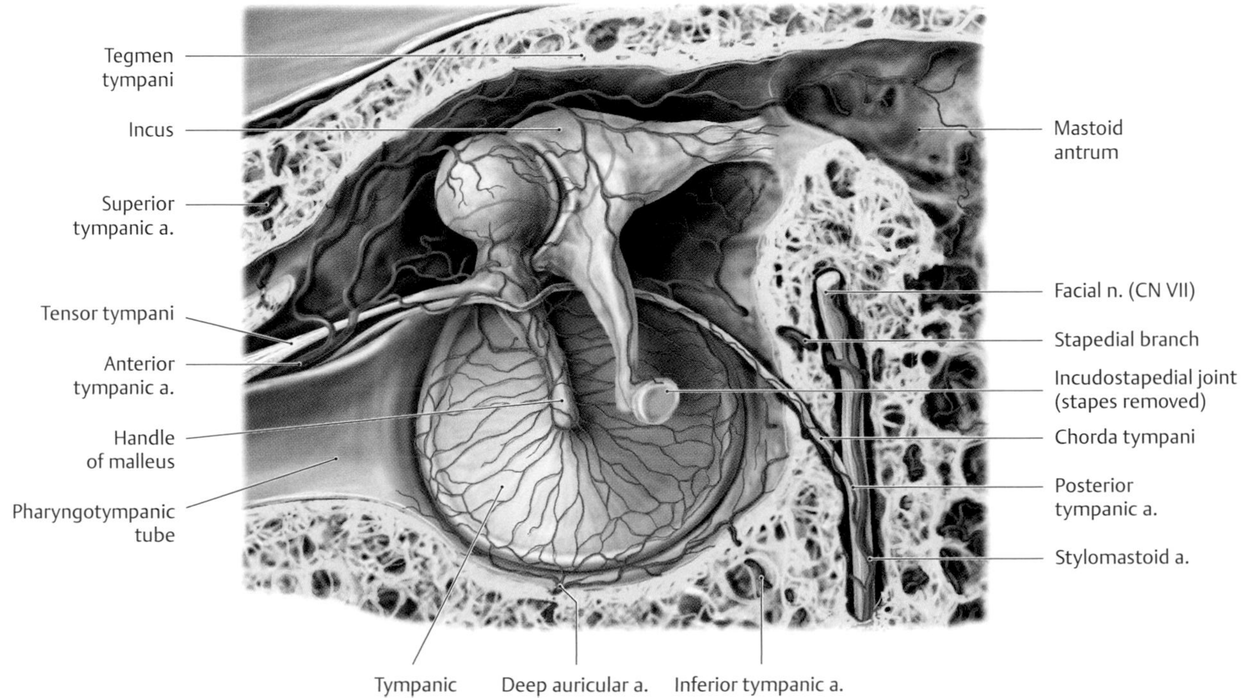
Tegmen tympani
Incus
Superior tympanic a.
Tensor tympani
Anterior tympanic a.
Handle of malleus
Pharyngotympanic tube
Mastoid antrum
Facial n. (CN VII)
Stapedial branch
Incudostapedial joint (stapes removed)
Chorda tympani
Posterior tympanic a.
Stylomastoid a.
Tympanic membrane
Deep auricular a.
Inferior tympanic a.

Fig. 37.18 **Arteries of the middle ear: Tympanic cavity**
Right petrous bone, anterior view. *Removed:* Malleus, incus, portions of chorda tympani, and anterior tympanic artery.

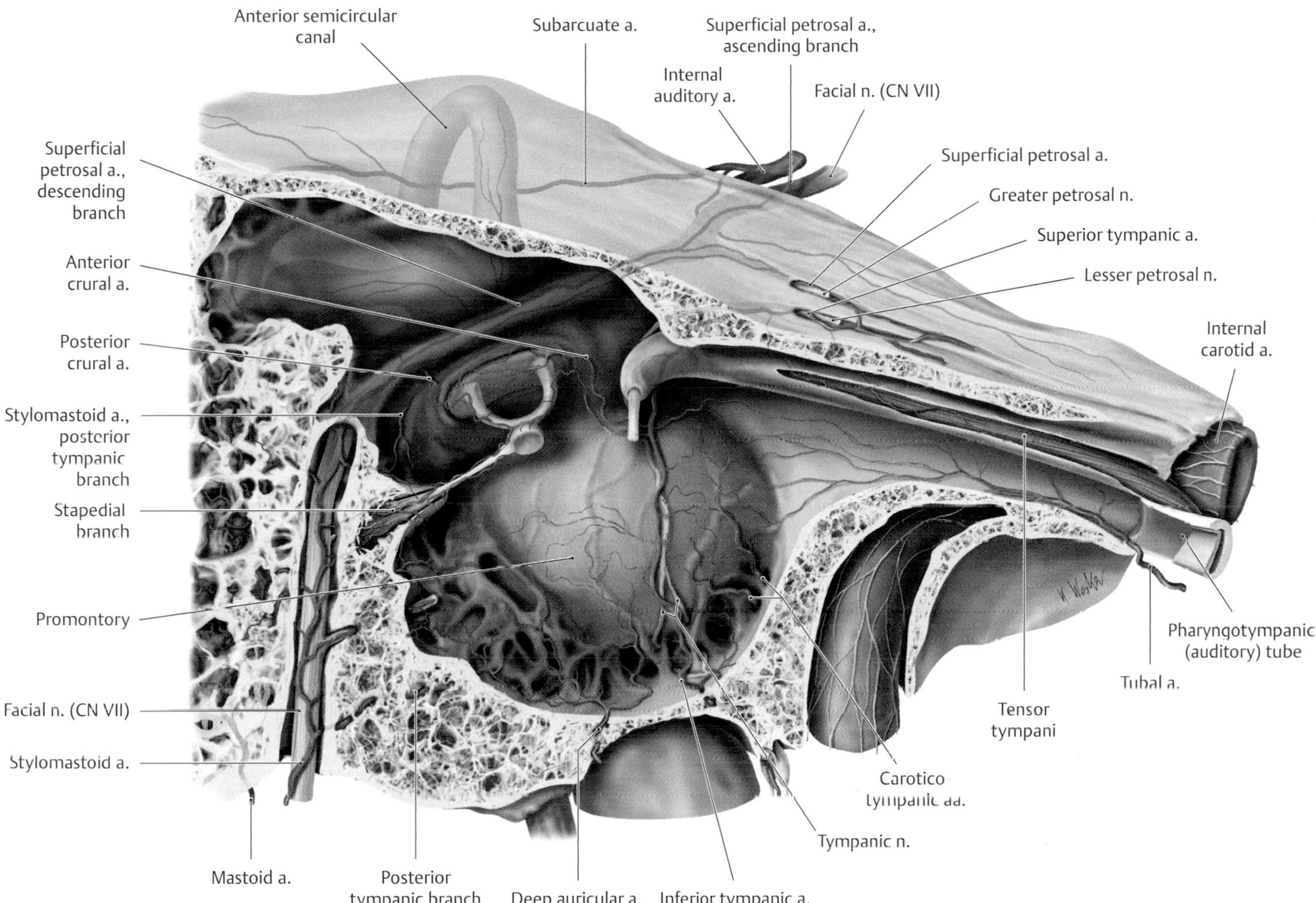
Anterior semicircular canal
Subarcuate a.
Superficial petrosal a., ascending branch
Internal auditory a.
Facial n. (CN VII)
Superficial petrosal a.
Greater petrosal n.
Superior tympanic a.
Lesser petrosal n.
Internal carotid a.
Superficial petrosal a., descending branch
Anterior crural a.
Posterior crural a.
Stylomastoid a., posterior tympanic branch
Stapedial branch
Promontory
Facial n. (CN VII)
Stylomastoid a.
Pharyngotympanic (auditory) tube
Tubal a.
Tensor tympani
Caroticotympanic aa.
Tympanic n.
Mastoid a.
Posterior tympanic branch
Deep auricular a.
Inferior tympanic a.

Inner Ear

The inner ear consists of the vestibular apparatus (for balance) and the auditory apparatus (for hearing). Both are formed by a membranous labyrinth filled with endolymph floating within a bony labyrinth filled with perilymph and embedded in the petrous part of the temporal bone.

Fig. 37.19 Vestibular apparatus

Right lateral view.

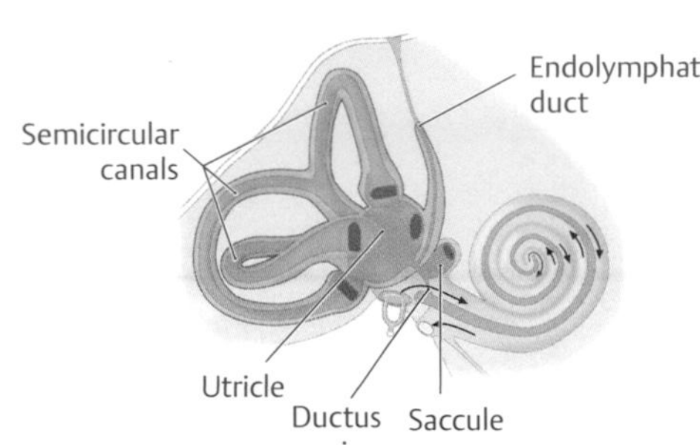
Endolymphatic duct
Semicircular canals
Utricle
Ductus reuniens
Saccule

A Schematic. Ampullary crests and maculae of utricle and saccule shown in red.

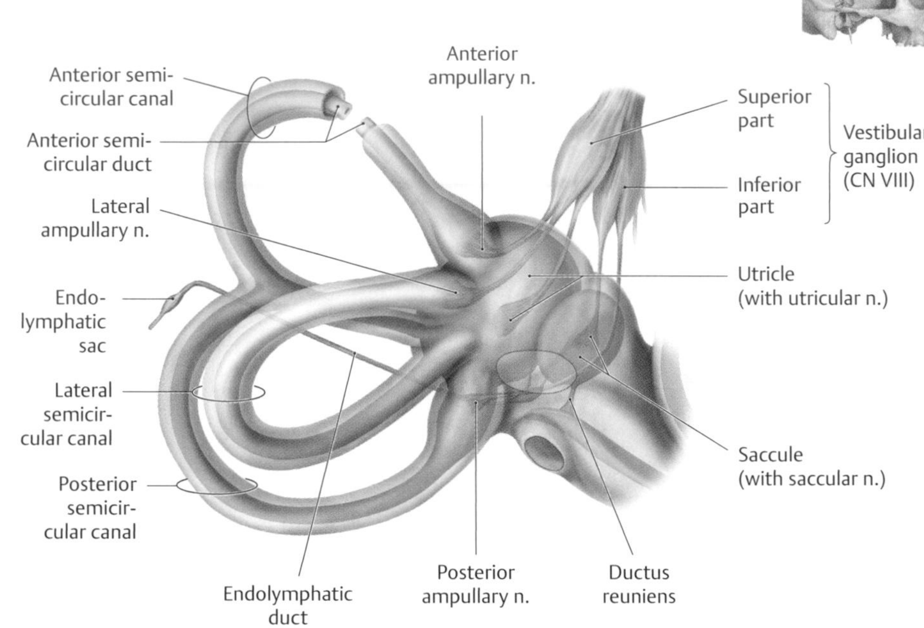
Anterior semi-circular canal
Anterior semi-circular duct
Lateral ampullary n.
Endo-lymphatic sac
Lateral semicir-cular canal
Posterior semicir-cular canal
Endolymphatic duct
Anterior ampullary n.
Posterior ampullary n.
Ductus reuniens
Superior part
Inferior part
Vestibular ganglion (CN VIII)
Utricle (with utricular n.)
Saccule (with saccular n.)

B Structure of the vestibular apparatus.

Fig. 37.20 Auditory apparatus

The cochlear labyrinth and its bony shell form the cochlea, which contains the sensory epithelium of the auditory apparatus (organ of Corti).

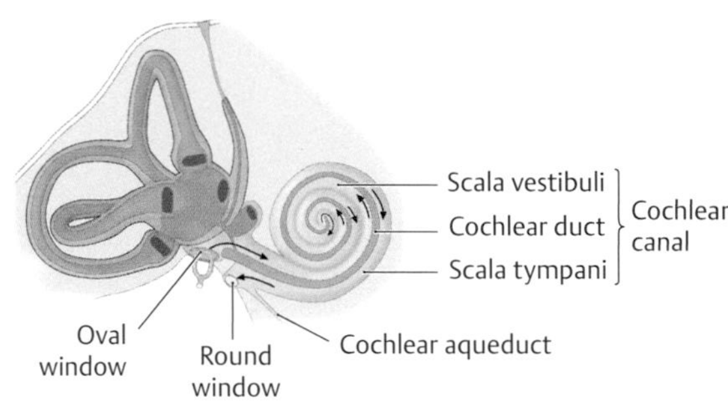
Scala vestibuli
Cochlear duct
Scala tympani
Cochlear canal
Oval window
Round window
Cochlear aqueduct

A Schematic.

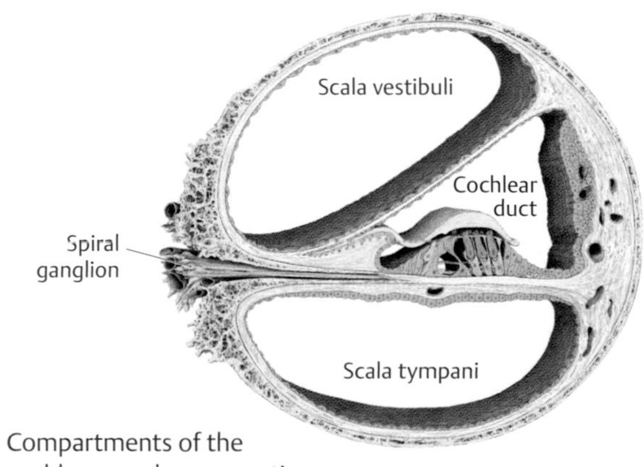
Scala vestibuli
Cochlear duct
Spiral ganglion
Scala tympani

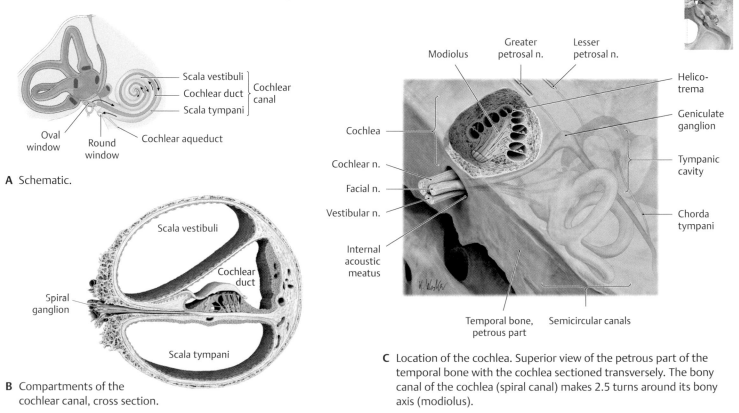

B Compartments of the cochlear canal, cross section.

Modiolus
Greater petrosal n.
Lesser petrosal n.
Helico-trema
Geniculate ganglion
Tympanic cavity
Chorda tympani
Cochlea
Cochlear n.
Facial n.
Vestibular n.
Internal acoustic meatus
Temporal bone, petrous part
Semicircular canals

C Location of the cochlea. Superior view of the petrous part of the temporal bone with the cochlea sectioned transversely. The bony canal of the cochlea (spiral canal) makes 2.5 turns around its bony axis (modiolus).

***Fig. 37.21* Innervation of the membranous labyrinth**

Right ear, anterior view. The vestibulocochlear nerve (CN VIII; see p. 506) transmits afferent impulses from the inner ear to the brainstem through the internal acoustic meatus. The vestibulocochlear nerve is divided into the vestibular and cochlear nerves. *Note:* The sensory organs in the semicircular canals respond to angular acceleration, and the macular organs respond to horizontal and vertical linear acceleration.

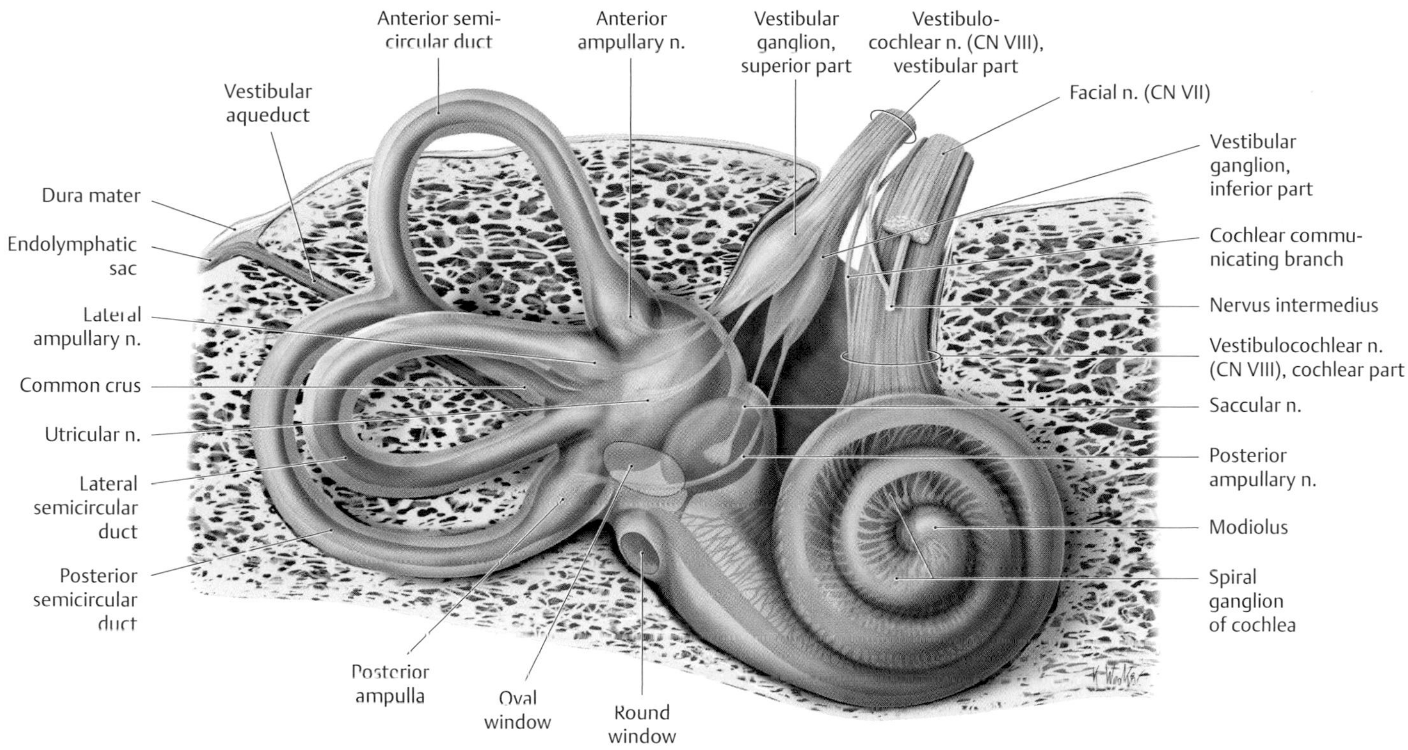
Anterior semicircular duct
Anterior ampullary n.
Vestibular ganglion, superior part
Vestibulocochlear n. (CN VIII), vestibular part
Facial n. (CN VII)
Vestibular aqueduct
Vestibular ganglion, inferior part
Dura mater
Endolymphatic sac
Cochlear communicating branch
Nervus intermedius
Lateral ampullary n.
Vestibulocochlear n. (CN VIII), cochlear part
Common crus
Saccular n.
Utricular n.
Posterior ampullary n.
Lateral semicircular duct
Modiolus
Posterior semicircular duct
Spiral ganglion of cochlea
Posterior ampulla
Oval window
Round window

***Fig. 37.22* Blood vessels of the inner ear**

Right anterior view. The labyrinth receives its blood supply from the internal auditory artery, a branch of the anteroinferior cerebellar artery (see p. 634).

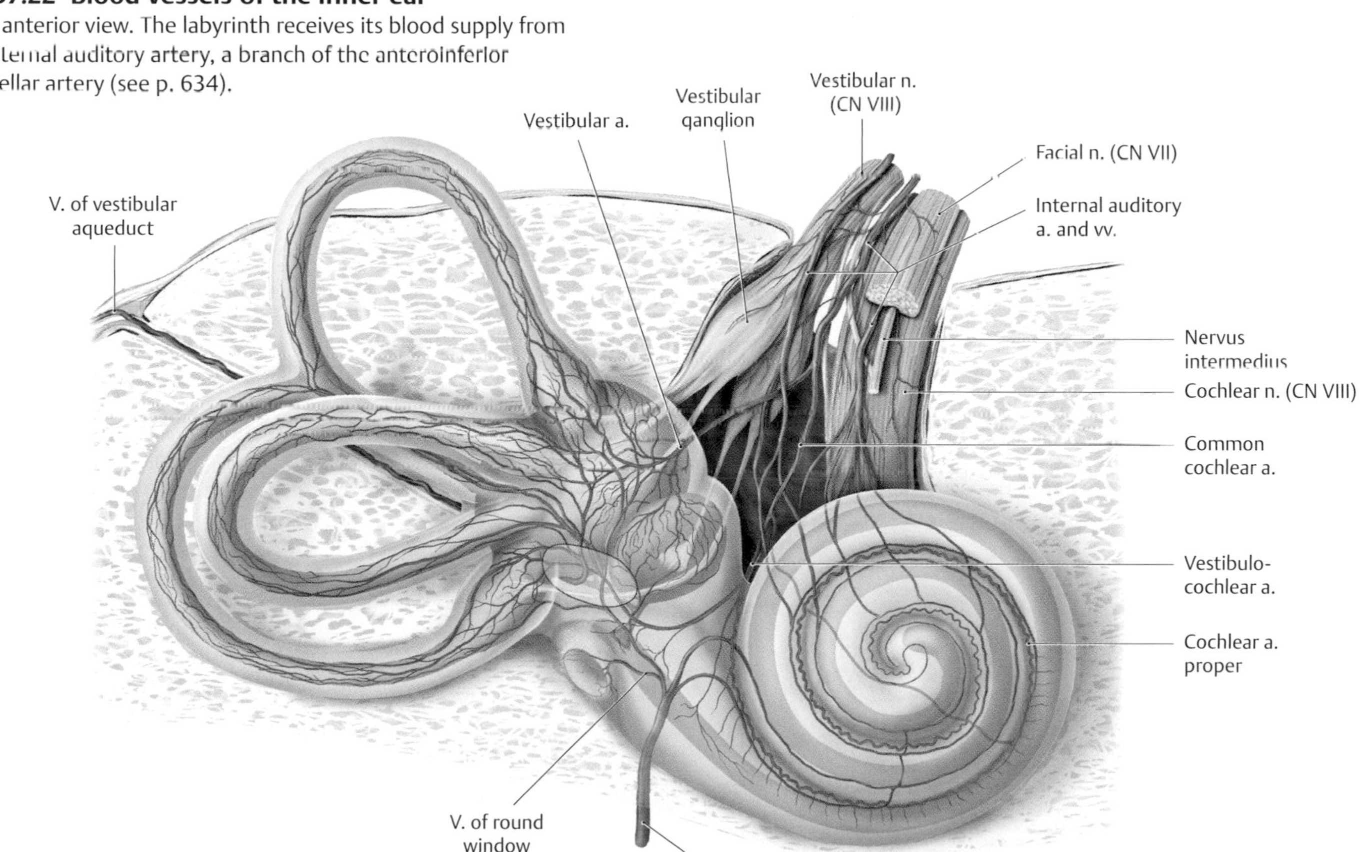
Vestibular n. (CN VIII)
Vestibular ganglion
Vestibular a.
Facial n. (CN VII)
V. of vestibular aqueduct
Internal auditory a. and vv.
Nervus intermedius
Cochlear n. (CN VIII)
Common cochlear a.
Vestibulocochlear a.
Cochlear a. proper
V. of round window
V. of cochlear aqueduct

Bones of the Oral Cavity

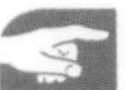

The floor of the nasal cavity (the maxilla and palatine bone) forms the roof of the oral cavity, the hard palate. The two horizontal processes of the maxilla (the palatine processes) grow together during development, eventually fusing at the median palatine suture. Failure to fuse results in a cleft palate.

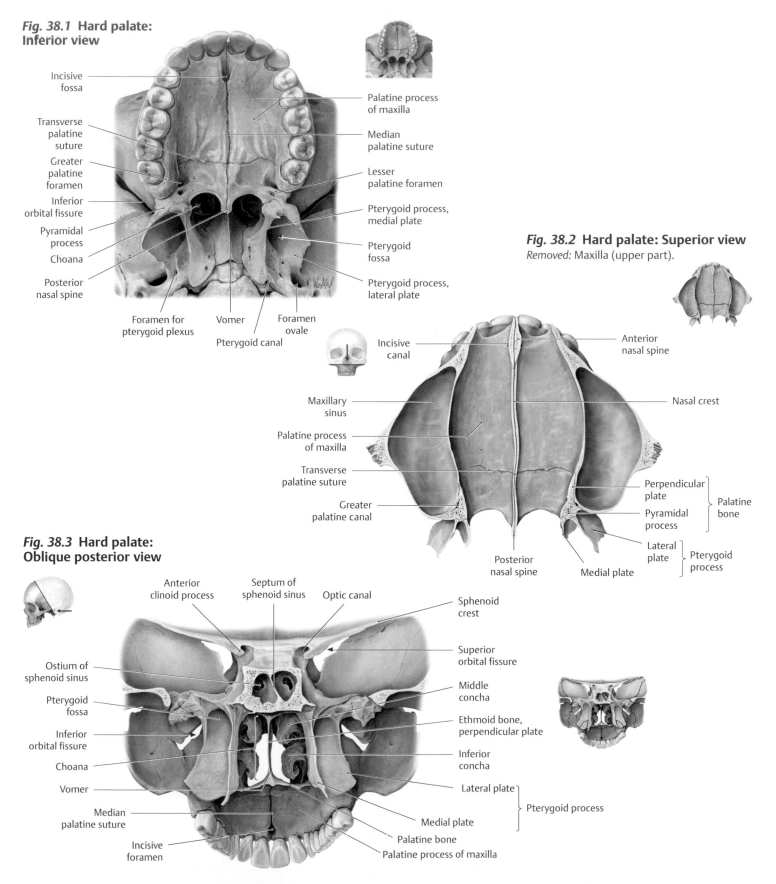

Fig. 38.1 **Hard palate: Inferior view**

Incisive fossa
Transverse palatine suture
Greater palatine foramen
Inferior orbital fissure
Pyramidal process
Choana
Posterior nasal spine
Foramen for pterygoid plexus
Vomer
Foramen ovale
Pterygoid canal
Palatine process of maxilla
Median palatine suture
Lesser palatine foramen
Pterygoid process, medial plate
Pterygoid fossa
Pterygoid process, lateral plate

Fig. 38.2 **Hard palate: Superior view**
Removed: Maxilla (upper part).

Incisive canal
Anterior nasal spine
Maxillary sinus
Nasal crest
Palatine process of maxilla
Transverse palatine suture
Greater palatine canal
Perpendicular plate
Pyramidal process
Palatine bone
Lateral plate
Medial plate
Pterygoid process
Posterior nasal spine

Fig. 38.3 **Hard palate: Oblique posterior view**

Anterior clinoid process
Septum of sphenoid sinus
Optic canal
Sphenoid crest
Superior orbital fissure
Ostium of sphenoid sinus
Pterygoid fossa
Inferior orbital fissure
Choana
Vomer
Median palatine suture
Incisive foramen
Middle concha
Ethmoid bone, perpendicular plate
Inferior concha
Lateral plate
Medial plate
Pterygoid process
Palatine bone
Palatine process of maxilla

Head
Condylar process
Coronoid process
Oblique line
Ramus
Alveolar process
Mental foramen
Alveoli (tooth sockets)
Body
Mental protuberance

A Anterior view.

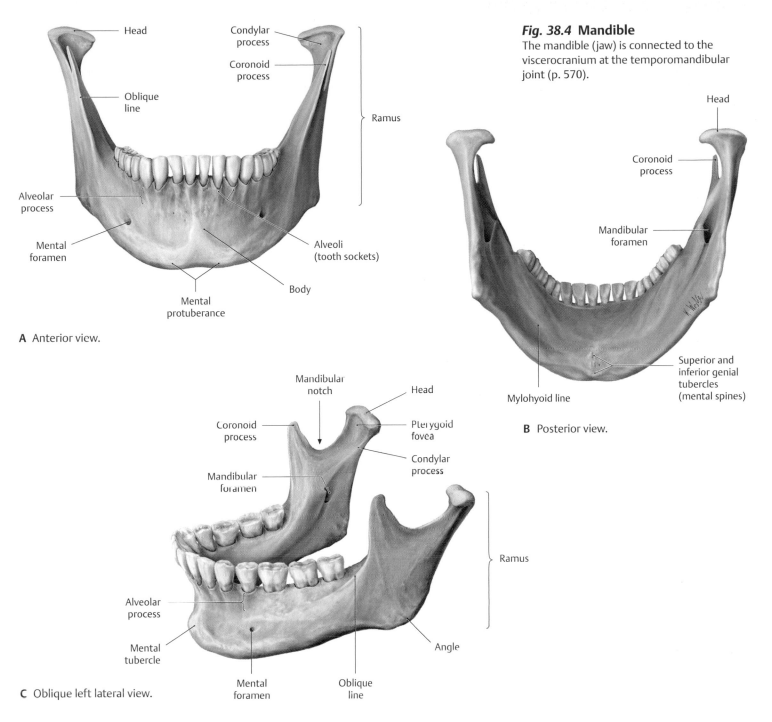

Fig. 38.4 Mandible

The mandible (jaw) is connected to the viscerocranium at the temporomandibular joint (p. 570).

Head
Coronoid process
Mandibular foramen
Superior and inferior genial tubercles (mental spines)
Mylohyoid line

B Posterior view.

Mandibular notch
Head
Coronoid process
Pterygoid fovea
Condylar process
Mandibular foramen
Ramus
Alveolar process
Mental tubercle
Angle
Mental foramen
Oblique line

C Oblique left lateral view.

Fig. 38.5 Hyoid bone

The hyoid bone is suspended in the neck by muscles between the floor of the mouth and the larynx. Although not listed among the cranial bones, the hyoid bone gives attachment to the muscles of the oral floor. The greater horn and body of the hyoid are palpable in the neck.

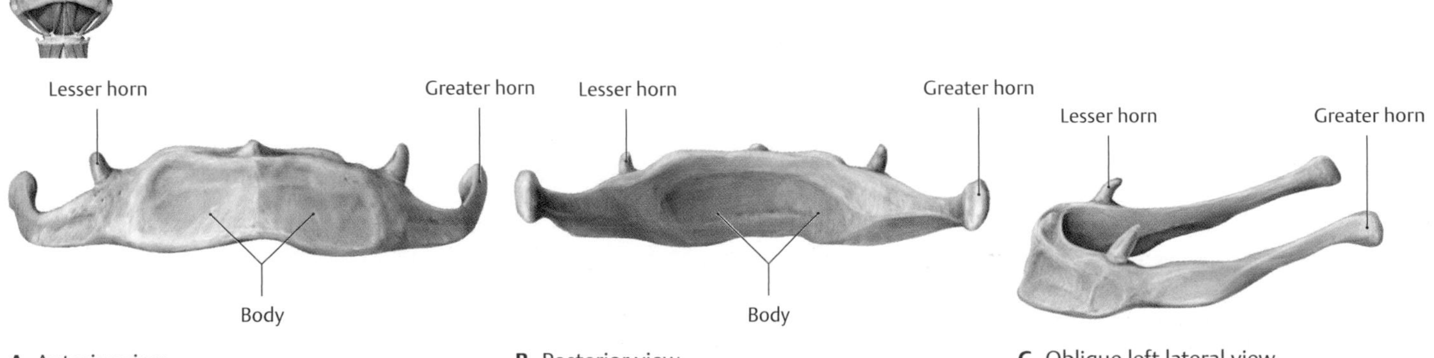
Lesser horn
Greater horn
Body
Lesser horn
Greater horn
Body
Lesser horn
Greater horn

A Anterior view. **B** Posterior view. **C** Oblique left lateral view.

Temporomandibular Joint

Fig. 38.6 Temporomandibular joint

The head of the mandible articulates with the mandibular fossa in the temporomandibular joint.

Articular tubercle
Mandibular fossa
Articular disk
Head of mandible

A Sagittally sectioned temporomandibular joint, left lateral view.

Head of mandible
Pterygoid fovea
Coronoid process
Neck of mandible

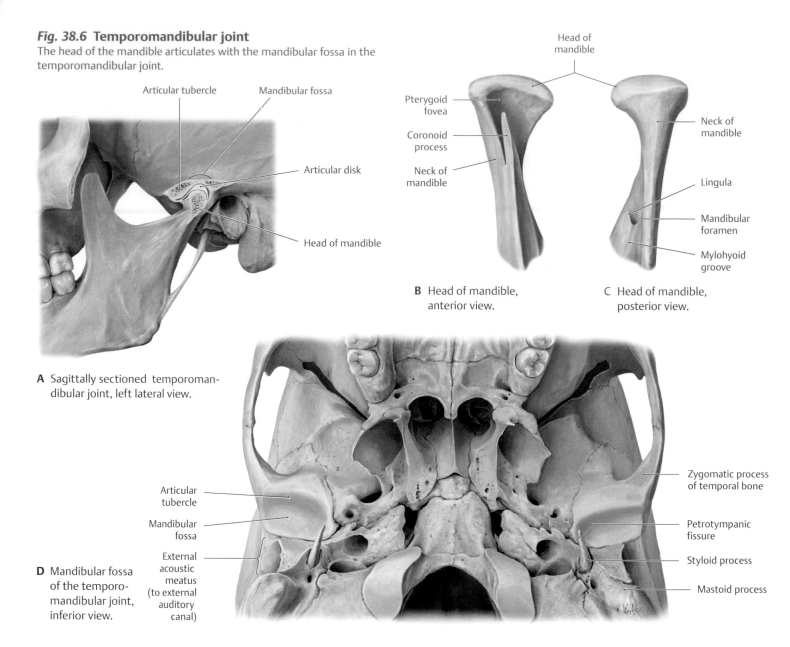

B Head of mandible, anterior view.

Neck of mandible
Lingula
Mandibular foramen
Mylohyoid groove

C Head of mandible, posterior view.

Articular tubercle
Mandibular fossa
External acoustic meatus (to external auditory canal)
Zygomatic process of temporal bone
Petrotympanic fissure
Styloid process
Mastoid process

D Mandibular fossa of the temporomandibular joint, inferior view.

Fig. 38.7 Ligaments of the temporomandibular joint

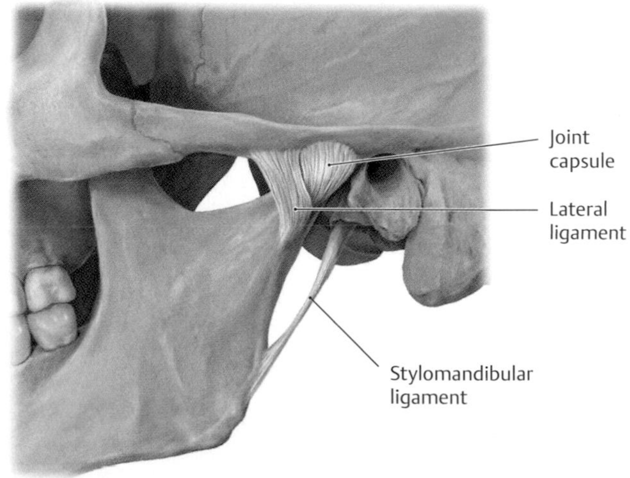
Joint capsule
Lateral ligament
Stylomandibular ligament

A Lateral view of the left temporomandibular joint.

Pterygoid process, lateral plate
Pterygospinous ligament
Sphenomandibular ligament
Stylomandibular ligament
Pterygoid process, medial plate

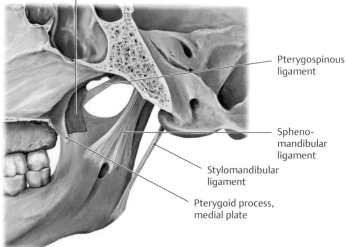

B Medial view of the right temporomandibular joint.

Fig. 38.8 Movement of the temporomandibular joint
Left lateral view. During the first 15 degrees of mandibular depression (opening of the mouth), the head of the mandible remains in the mandibular fossa. Past 15 degrees, the head of the mandible glides forward onto the articular tubercle.

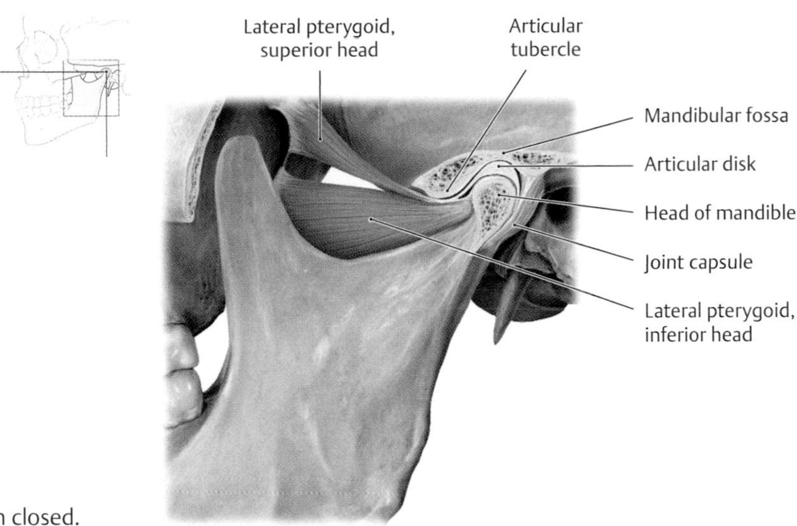
Lateral pterygoid, superior head
Articular tubercle
Mandibular fossa
Articular disk
Head of mandible
Joint capsule
Lateral pterygoid, inferior head

A Mouth closed.

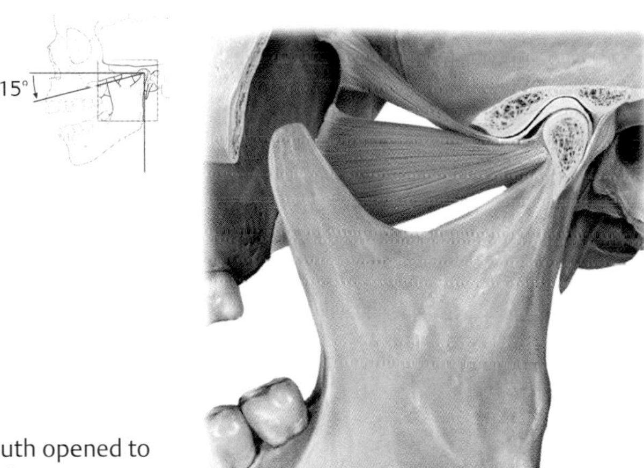
15°

B Mouth opened to 15 degrees.

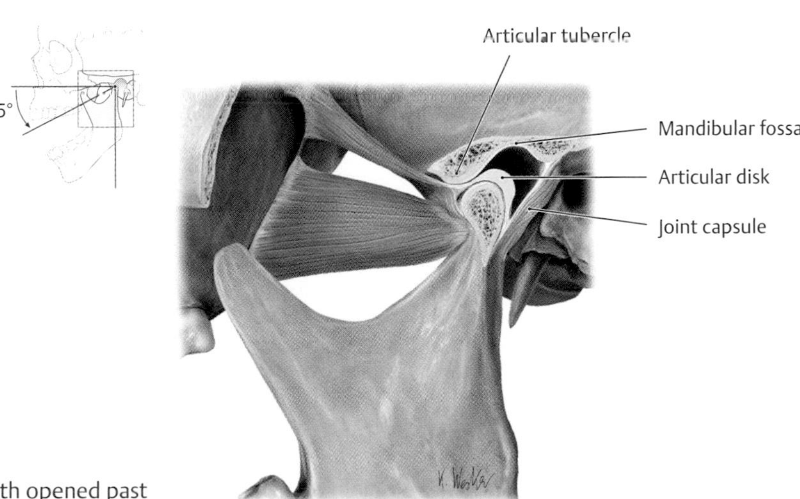
>15°
Articular tubercle
Mandibular fossa
Articular disk
Joint capsule

C Mouth opened past 15 degrees.

Clinical

Dislocation of the temporomandibular joint
Dislocation may occur if the head of the mandible slides past the articular tubercle. The mandible then becomes locked in a protruded position, a condition reduced by pressing on the mandibular row of teeth.

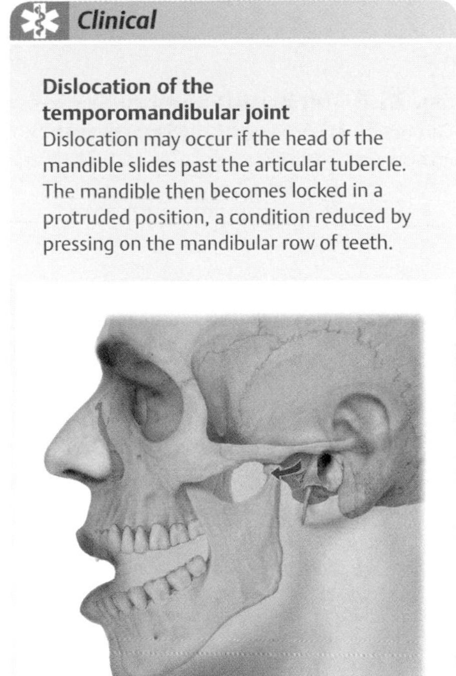

Fig. 38.9 Innervation of the temporomandibular joint capsule
Superior view.

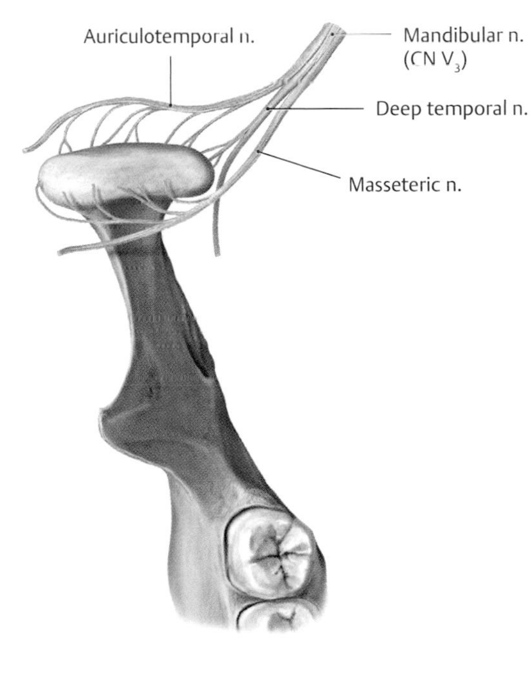
Auriculotemporal n.
Mandibular n. (CN V_3)
Deep temporal n.
Masseteric n.

Teeth

Fig. 38.10 Structure of a tooth
Each tooth consists of hard tissue (enamel, dentin, cementum) and soft tissue (dental pulp) arranged into a crown, neck (cervix), and root.

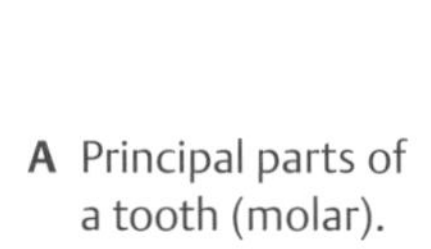

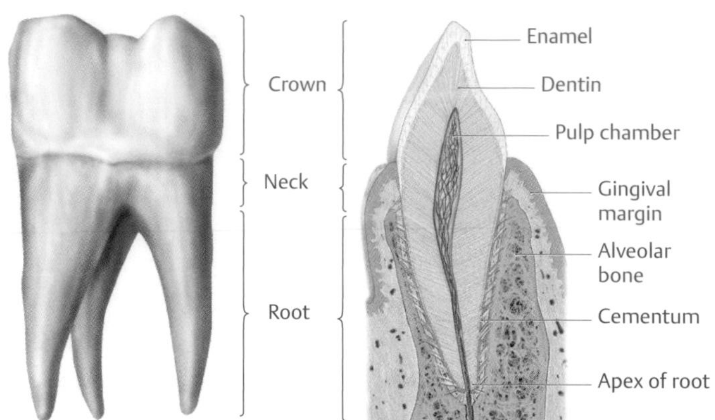
Crown
Neck
Root
Enamel
Dentin
Pulp chamber
Gingival margin
Alveolar bone
Cementum
Apex of root

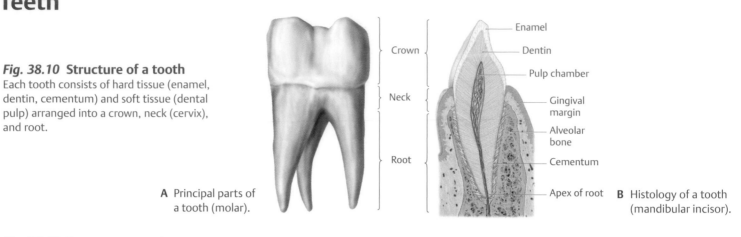

A Principal parts of a tooth (molar).

B Histology of a tooth (mandibular incisor).

Fig. 38.11 Permanent teeth
Each half of the maxilla and mandible contains a set of three anterior teeth (two incisors, one canine) and five posterior (postcanine) teeth (two premolars, three molars).

Incisive fossa
Incisors
Interalveolar septum
Canine
Incisive suture
Premolars
Median palatine suture
Molars
Transverse palatine suture

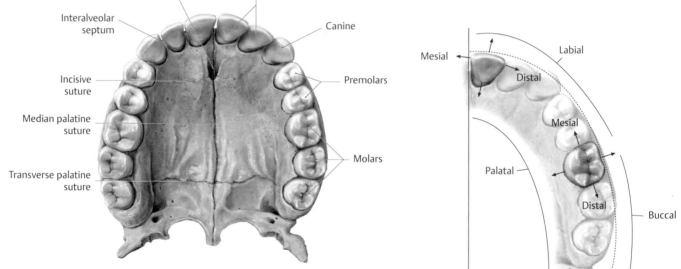

A Maxillary teeth. Inferior view of the maxilla.

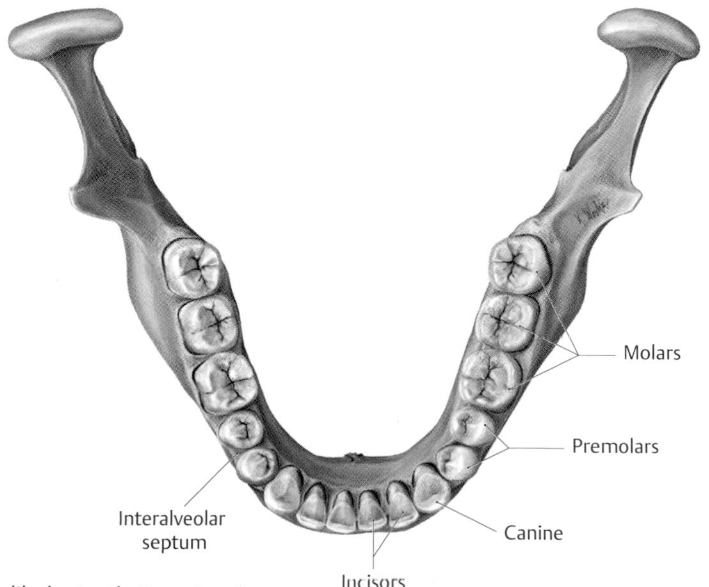
Molars
Premolars
Interalveolar septum
Canine
Incisors

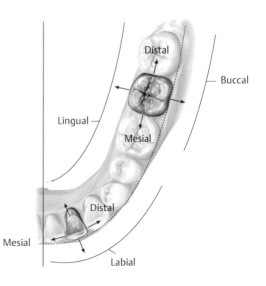

B Mandibular teeth. Superior view of the mandible.

Fig. 38.12 Tooth surfaces
The top of the tooth is known as the occlusal surface.

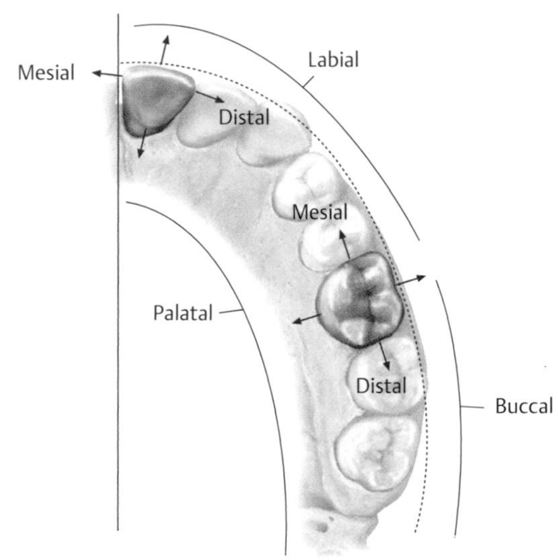
Mesial
Labial
Distal
Mesial
Palatal
Distal
Buccal

Distal
Buccal
Lingual
Mesial
Distal
Mesial
Labial

Fig. 38.13 Coding of the teeth

In the United States, the 32 permanent teeth are numbered sequentially (not assigned to quadrants). *Note*: The 20 deciduous (baby) teeth are coded A to J (upper arch), and K to T in a similar clockwise fashion. The third upper right molar is 1; the second upper right premolar is A.

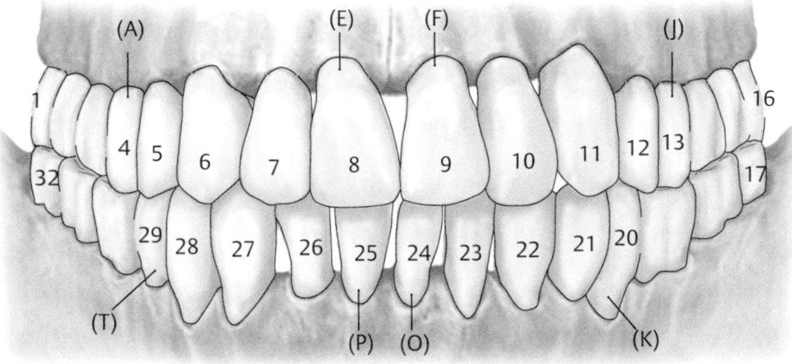
(A)
(E)
(F)
(J)
1
4
5
6
7
8
9
10
11
12
13
16
32
17
29
28
27
26
25
24
23
22
21
20
(T)
(P)
(O)
(K)

Fig. 38.14 Dental panoramic tomogram

The dental panoramic tomogram (DPT) is a survey radiograph that allows preliminary assessment of the temporomandibular joints, maxillary sinuses, maxillomandibular bone, and dental status (carious lesions, location of wisdom teeth, etc.). *DPT courtesy of Dr. U. J. Rother, Director of the Department of Diagnostic Radiology, Center for Dentistry and Oromaxillofacial Surgery, Eppendorf University Medical Center, Hamburg, Germany.*

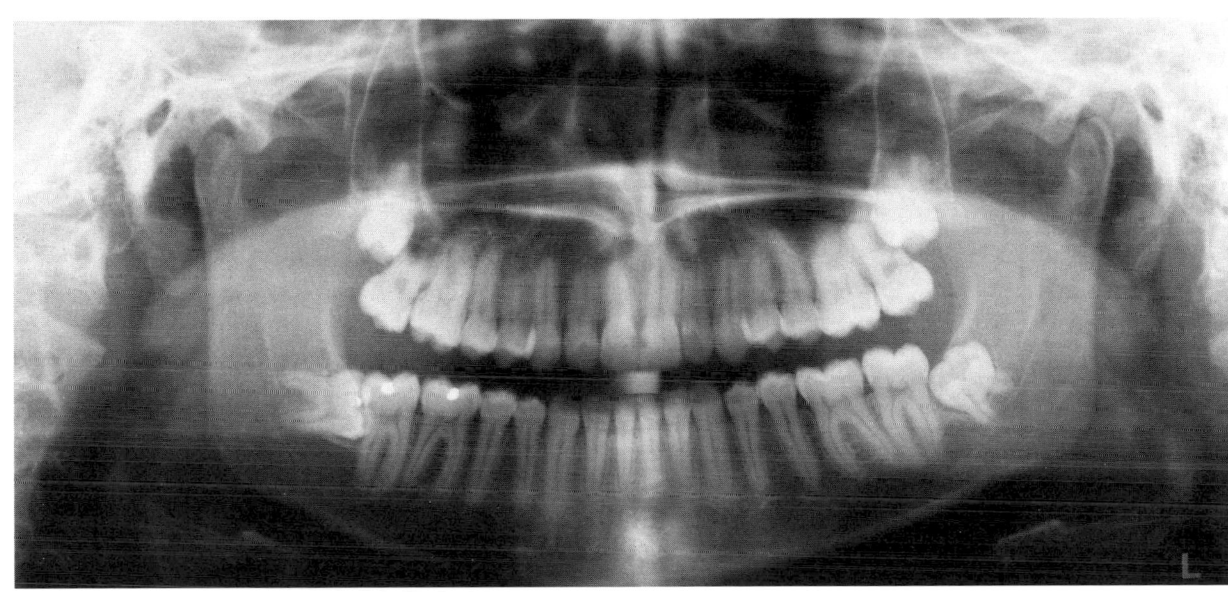

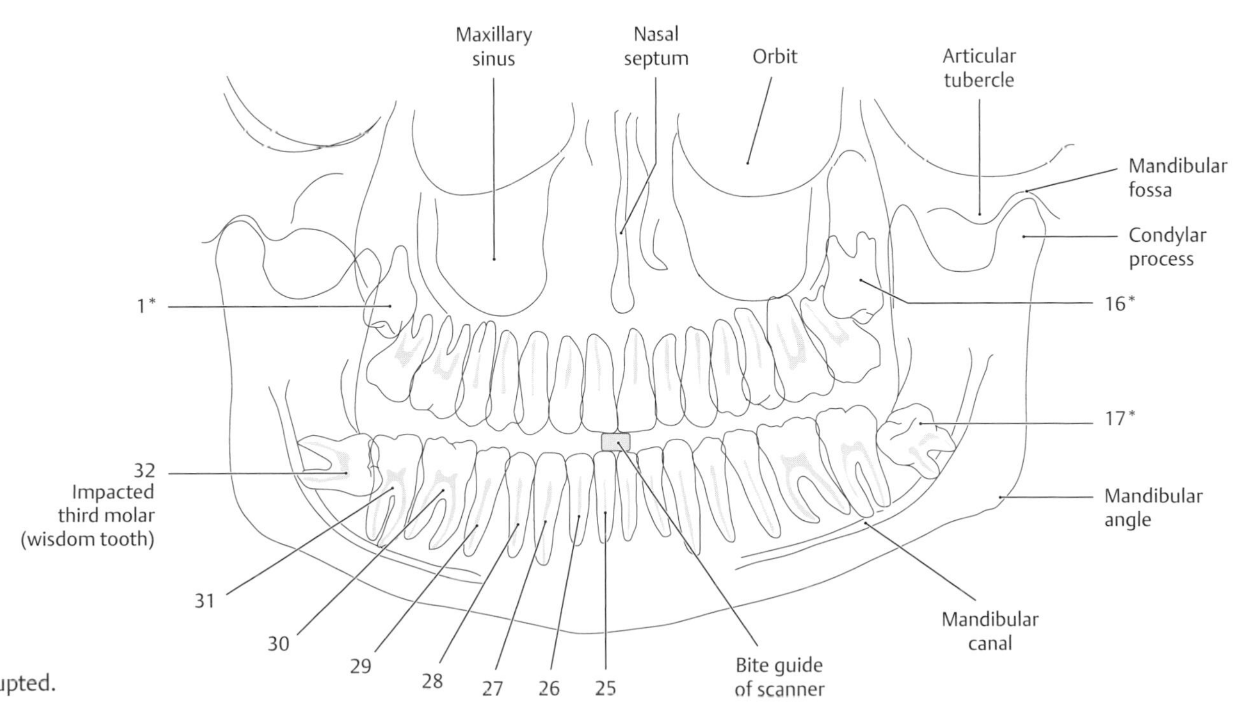
Maxillary sinus
Nasal septum
Orbit
Articular tubercle
Mandibular fossa
Condylar process
1*
16*
17*
32
Impacted third molar (wisdom tooth)
Mandibular angle
31
30
29
28
27
26
25
Bite guide of scanner
Mandibular canal

*Not fully erupted.

Oral Cavity Muscle Facts

Fig. 38.15 **Muscles of the oral floor**
See pp. 590–591 for the infrahyoid muscles.

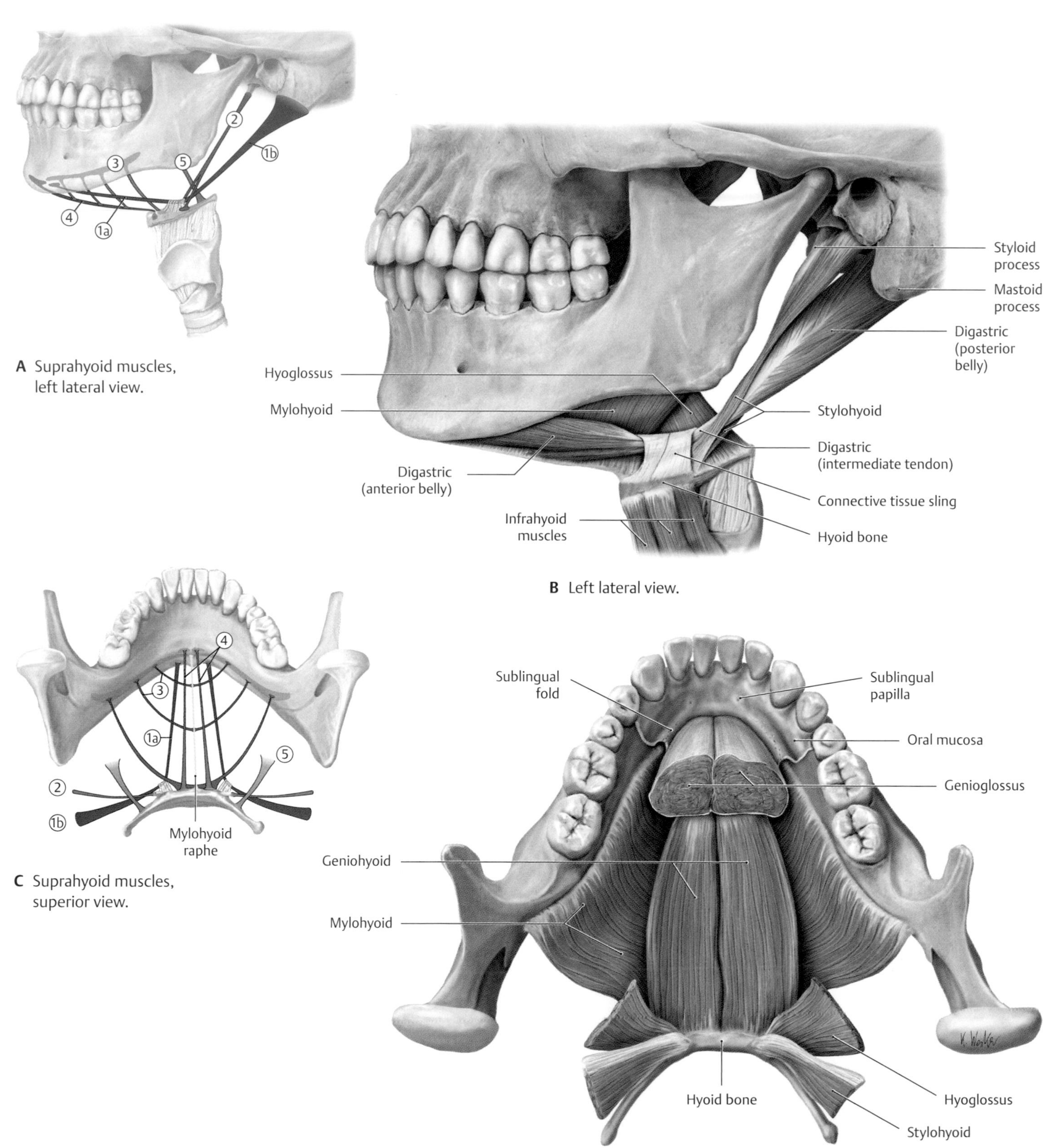

2
1b
3
5
4
1a
Styloid process
Mastoid process
Digastric (posterior belly)
Hyoglossus
Mylohyoid
Stylohyoid
Digastric (intermediate tendon)
Digastric (anterior belly)
Connective tissue sling
Infrahyoid muscles
Hyoid bone
4
3
1a
5
2
1b
Mylohyoid raphe
Sublingual fold
Sublingual papilla
Oral mucosa
Genioglossus
Geniohyoid
Mylohyoid
Hyoid bone
Hyoglossus
Stylohyoid

A Suprahyoid muscles, left lateral view.

B Left lateral view.

C Suprahyoid muscles, superior view.

D Superior view of the mandible and hyoid bone.

Table 38.1 Suprahyoid muscles

Muscle		Origin	Insertion		Innervation	Action
① Digastric	ⓐ Anterior belly	Mandible (digastric fossa)	Hyoid bone (body)	Via an intermediate tendon with a fibrous loop	Mylohyoid n. (from CN V_3)	Elevates hyoid bone (during swallowing), assists in opening mandible
	ⓑ Posterior belly	Temporal bone (mastoid notch, medial to mastoid process)			Facial n. (CN VII)	
② Stylohyoid		Temporal bone (styloid process)		Via a split tendon		
③ Mylohyoid		Mandible (mylohyoid line)		Via median tendon of insertion (mylohyoid raphe)	Mylohyoid n. (from CN V_3)	Tightens and elevates oral floor, draws hyoid bone forward (during swallowing), assists in opening mandible and moving it side to side (mastication)
④ Geniohyoid		Mandible (inferior mental spine)		Body of hyoid bone	Anterior ramus of C1 via hypoglossal n. (CN XII)	Draws hyoid bone forward (during swallowing), assists in opening mandible
⑤ Hyoglossus		Hyoid bone (superior border of greater cornu)	Sides of tongue		Hypoglossal n. (CN XII)	Depresses the tongue

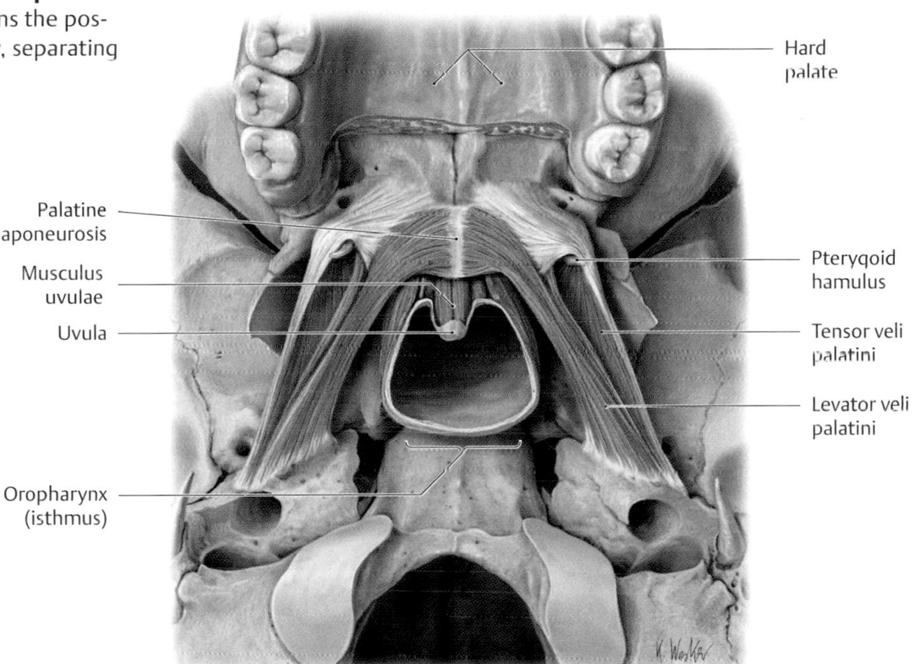
Hard palate
Palatine aponeurosis
Musculus uvulae
Uvula
Oropharynx (isthmus)
Pterygoid hamulus
Tensor veli palatini
Levator veli palatini

Fig. 38.16 **Muscles of the soft palate**
Inferior view. The soft palate forms the posterior boundary of the oral cavity, separating it from the oropharynx.

Table 38.2 Muscles of the soft palate

Muscle	Origin	Insertion	Innervation	Action
Tensor veli palatini	Medial pterygoid plate (scaphoid fossa); sphenoid bone (spine); cartilage of pharyngotympanic tube	Palatine aponeurosis	Medial pterygoid n. (CN V_3 via otic ganglion)	Tightens soft palate; opens inlet to pharyngotympanic tube (during swallowing, yawning)
Levator veli palatini	Cartilage of pharyngotympanic tube; temporal bone (petrous part)		Accessory n. (CN XI, cranial part) via pharyngeal plexus (vagus n., CN X)	Raises soft palate to horizontal position
Musculus uvulae	Uvula (mucosa)	Palatine aponeurosis; posterior nasal spine		Shortens and raises uvula
Palatoglossus*	Tongue (side)	Palatine aponeurosis		Elevates tongue (posterior portion); pulls soft palate onto tongue
Palatopharyngeus*				Tightens soft palate; during swallowing pulls pharyngeal walls superiorly, anteriorly, and medially

*For the palatoglossus, see Figs. 38.20 and 38.21, p. 578; and for the palatopharyngeus, see Fig. 38.31C, p. 585.

Innervation of the Oral Cavity

Fig. 38.17 Trigeminal nerve in the oral cavity
Right lateral view.

Trigeminal n. (CN V)
Maxillary division (CN V_2, via foramen rotundum)
Pterygo-palatine ganglion
Posterior
Middle
Anterior
Superior alveolar nn.
Zygomatic n.
Infraorbital n. (and foramen)
Mandibular division (CN V_3, via foramen ovale)
Buccal n.
Medial and lateral pterygoid nn.
Auriculo-temporal n.
Masseteric n.
Mylohyoid n.
Lingual n.
Inferior alveolar n. (in mandibular canal)
Inferior dental branches
Mental n. (and foramen)

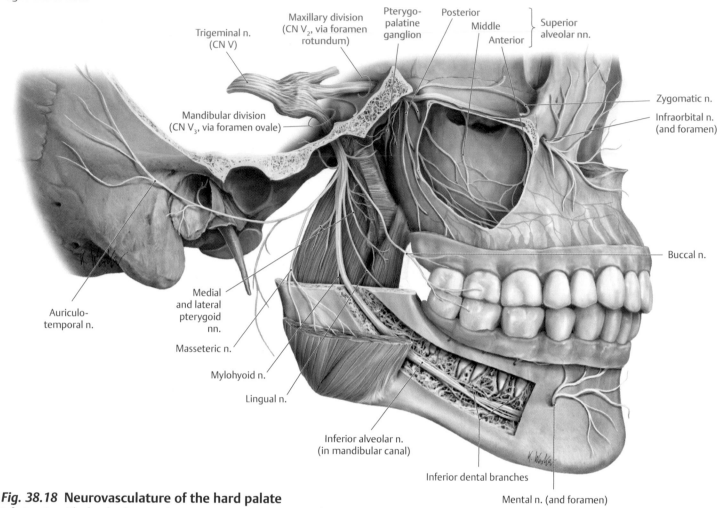

Fig. 38.18 Neurovasculature of the hard palate
Inferior view. The hard palate receives sensory innervation primarily from terminal branches of the maxillary division of the trigeminal nerve (CN V_2). The arteries of the hard palate arise from the maxillary artery.

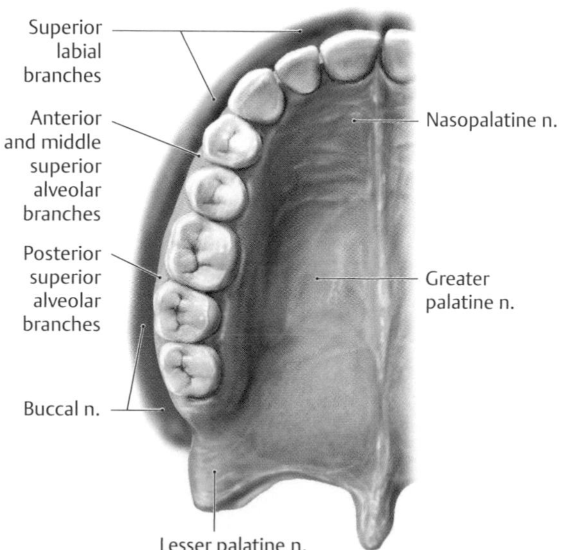
Superior labial branches
Anterior and middle superior alveolar branches
Posterior superior alveolar branches
Buccal n.
Lesser palatine n.
Nasopalatine n.
Greater palatine n.

A Sensory innervation. *Note:* The buccal nerve is a branch of the mandibular division (CN V_3).

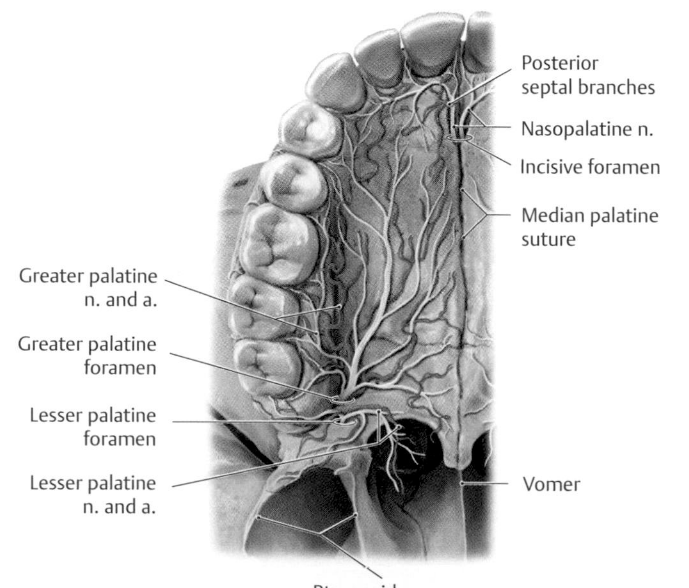
Posterior septal branches
Nasopalatine n.
Incisive foramen
Median palatine suture
Greater palatine n. and a.
Greater palatine foramen
Lesser palatine foramen
Lesser palatine n. and a.
Vomer
Pterygoid process

B Nerves and arteries.

The muscles of the oral floor have a complex nerve supply with contributions from the trigeminal nerve (CN V_3), facial nerve (CN VII), and C1 spinal nerve via the hypoglossal nerve (CN XII).

Fig. 38.19 Innervation of the oral floor muscles

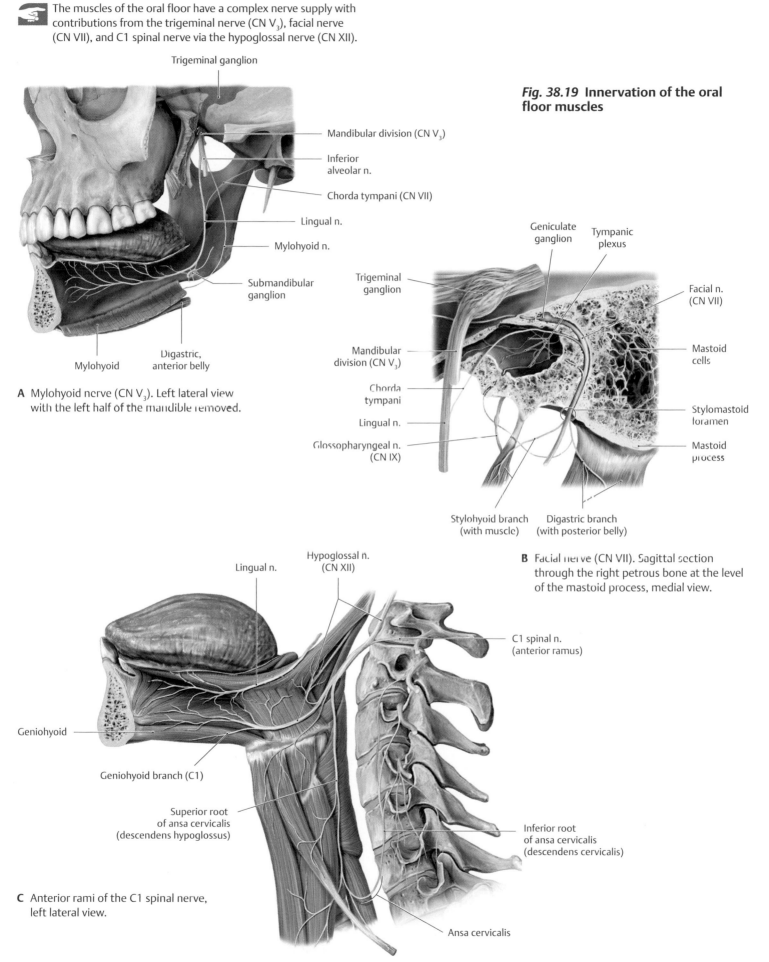

Trigeminal ganglion
Mandibular division (CN V_3)
Inferior alveolar n.
Chorda tympani (CN VII)
Lingual n.
Mylohyoid n.
Submandibular ganglion
Mylohyoid
Digastric, anterior belly

A Mylohyoid nerve (CN V_3). Left lateral view with the left half of the mandible removed.

Geniculate ganglion
Tympanic plexus
Trigeminal ganglion
Facial n. (CN VII)
Mandibular division (CN V_3)
Mastoid cells
Chorda tympani
Stylomastoid foramen
Lingual n.
Glossopharyngeal n. (CN IX)
Mastoid process
Stylohyoid branch (with muscle)
Digastric branch (with posterior belly)

B Facial nerve (CN VII). Sagittal section through the right petrous bone at the level of the mastoid process, medial view.

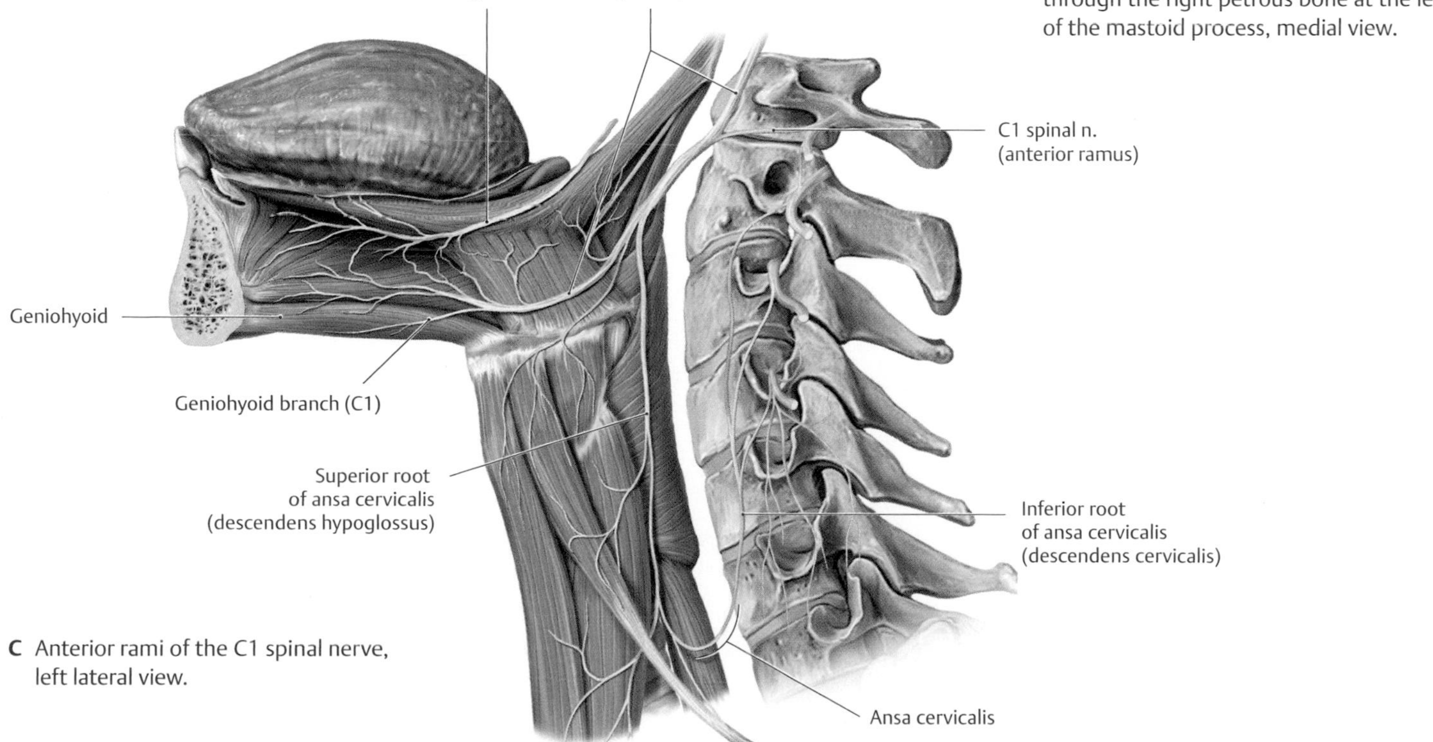
Lingual n.
Hypoglossal n. (CN XII)
C1 spinal n. (anterior ramus)
Geniohyoid
Geniohyoid branch (C1)
Superior root of ansa cervicalis (descendens hypoglossus)
Inferior root of ansa cervicalis (descendens cervicalis)
Ansa cervicalis

C Anterior rami of the C1 spinal nerve, left lateral view.

Tongue

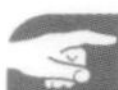

The dorsum of the tongue is covered by a highly specialized mucosa that supports its sensory functions (taste and fine tactile discrimination; see p. 645). The tongue is endowed with a very powerful muscular body to support its motor properties during mastication, swallowing, and speaking.

Fig. 38.20 Structure of the tongue

Superior view. The V-shaped sulcus terminalis divides the tongue into an anterior (oral, presulcal) and a posterior (pharyngeal, postsulcal) part.

Palatopharyngeal arch
Epiglottis
Lingual tonsil
Foramen cecum
Palatine tonsil
Palato-glossal arch
Terminal sulcus
Median furrow
Root of tongue
Body of tongue
Apex of tongue
Dorsum of tongue

Fig. 38.21 Muscles of the tongue

The extrinsic lingual muscles (genioglossus, hyoglossus, palatoglossus, and styloglossus) have bony attachments and move the tongue as a whole. The intrinsic lingual muscles (superior and inferior longitudinal muscles, transverse muscle, and vertical muscle) have no bony attachments and alter the shape of the tongue.

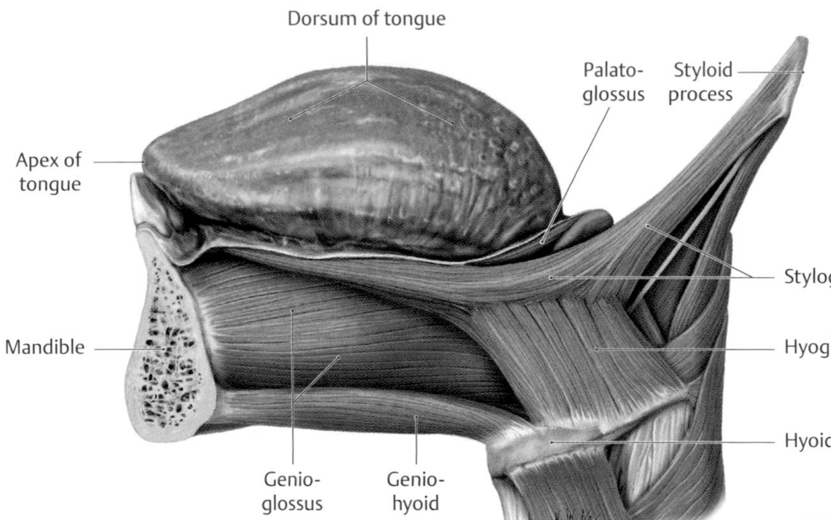
Dorsum of tongue
Palato-glossus
Styloid process
Apex of tongue
Styloglossus
Mandible
Hyoglossus
Hyoid bone
Genio-glossus
Genio-hyoid

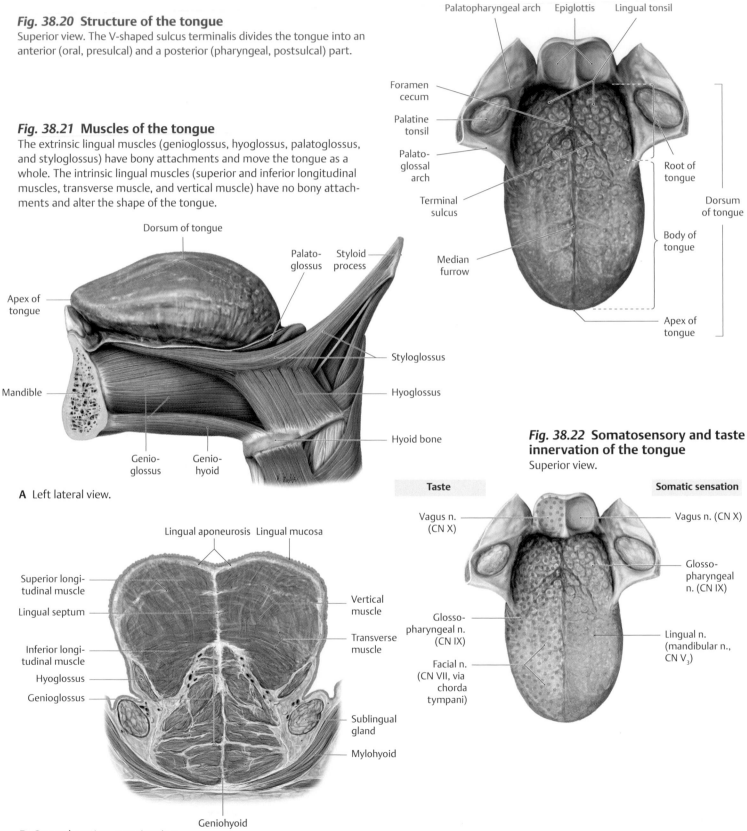

A Left lateral view.

Lingual aponeurosis
Lingual mucosa
Superior longitudinal muscle
Lingual septum
Inferior longitudinal muscle
Hyoglossus
Genioglossus
Vertical muscle
Transverse muscle
Sublingual gland
Mylohyoid
Geniohyoid

B Coronal section, anterior view.

Fig. 38.22 Somatosensory and taste innervation of the tongue

Superior view.

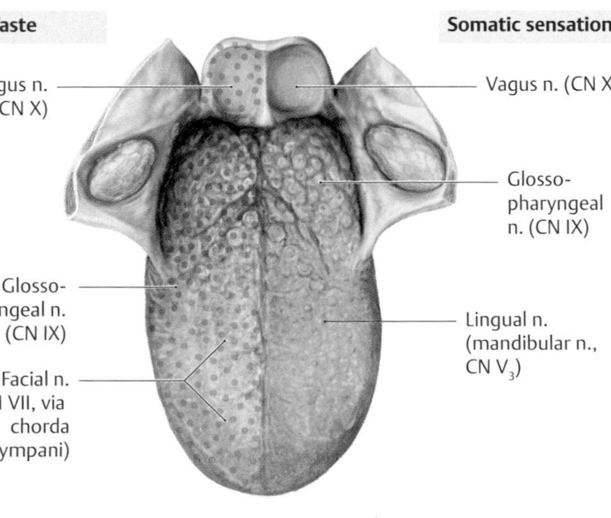
Taste
Somatic sensation
Vagus n. (CN X)
Vagus n. (CN X)
Glosso-pharyngeal n. (CN IX)
Glosso-pharyngeal n. (CN IX)
Lingual n. (mandibular n., CN V_3)
Facial n. (CN VII, via chorda tympani)

Fig. 38.23 Neurovasculature of the tongue

The lingual muscles receive somatomotor innervation from the hypoglossal nerve (CN XII), with the exception of the palatoglossus (supplied by the vagus nerve, CN X).

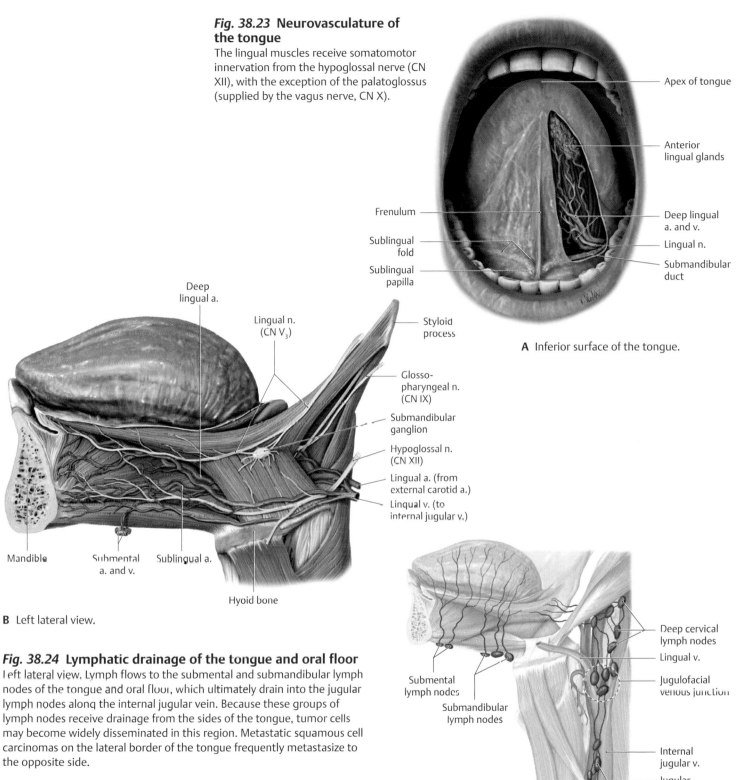

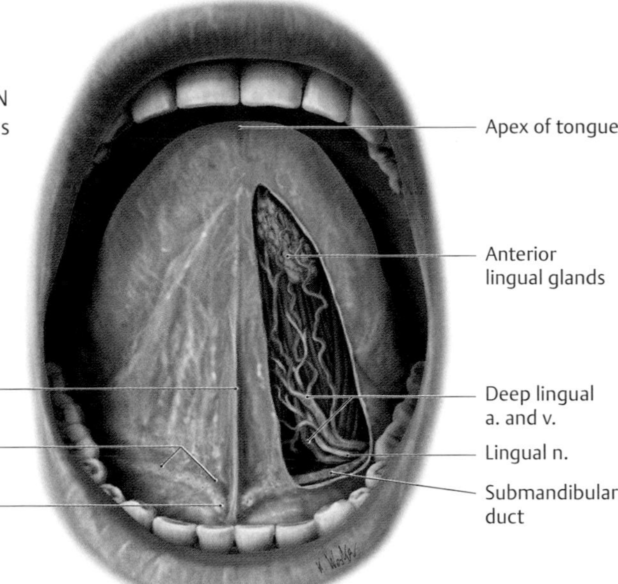
Apex of tongue
Anterior lingual glands
Frenulum
Deep lingual a. and v.
Lingual n.
Sublingual fold
Sublingual papilla
Submandibular duct

A Inferior surface of the tongue.

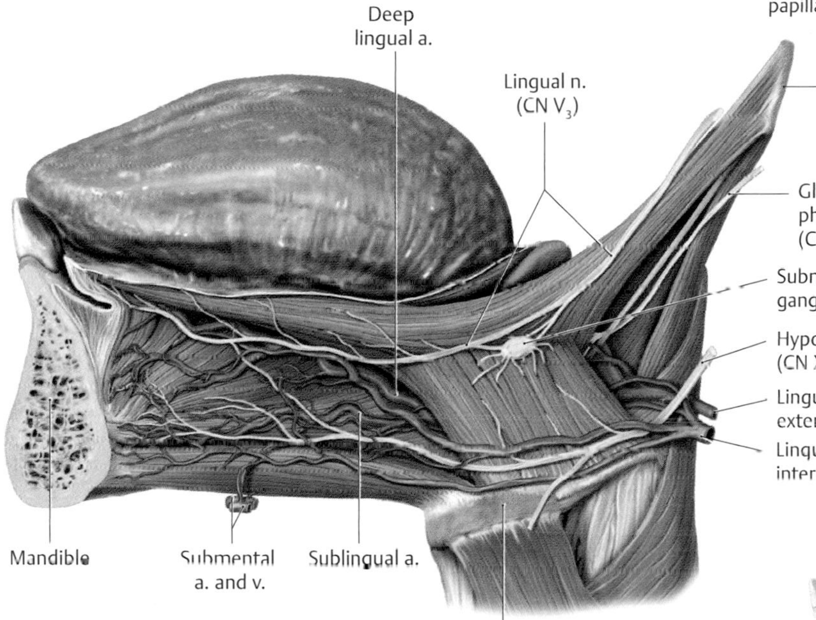
Deep lingual a.
Lingual n. (CN V_3)
Styloid process
Glosso-pharyngeal n. (CN IX)
Submandibular ganglion
Hypoglossal n. (CN XII)
Lingual a. (from external carotid a.)
Lingual v. (to internal jugular v.)
Mandible
Submental a. and v.
Sublingual a.
Hyoid bone

B Left lateral view.

Fig. 38.24 Lymphatic drainage of the tongue and oral floor

Left lateral view. Lymph flows to the submental and submandibular lymph nodes of the tongue and oral floor, which ultimately drain into the jugular lymph nodes along the internal jugular vein. Because these groups of lymph nodes receive drainage from the sides of the tongue, tumor cells may become widely disseminated in this region. Metastatic squamous cell carcinomas on the lateral border of the tongue frequently metastasize to the opposite side.

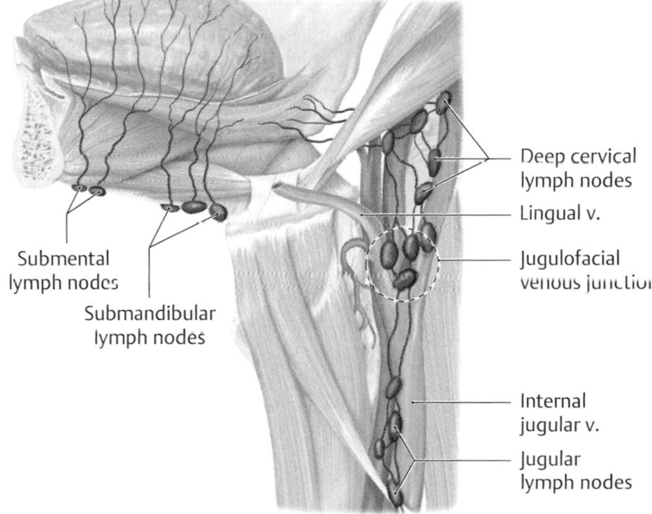
Deep cervical lymph nodes
Lingual v.
Submental lymph nodes
Jugulofacial venous junction
Submandibular lymph nodes
Internal jugular v.
Jugular lymph nodes

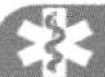 *Clinical*

Unilateral hypoglossal nerve palsy

Damage to the hypoglossal nerve causes paralysis of the genioglossus muscle on the affected side. The healthy (innervated) genioglossus on the unaffected side will therefore dominate. Upon protrusion, the tongue will deviate *toward* the paralyzed side.

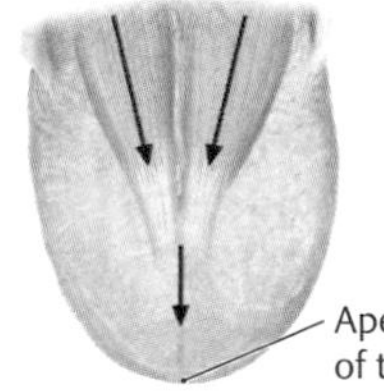
Apex of tongue

A Active protrusion with an intact hypoglossal nerve.

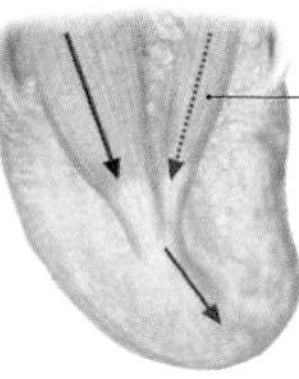
Paralyzed genio-glossus on affected side

B Active protrusion with a unilateral hypoglossal nerve lesion.

Topography of the Oral Cavity & Salivary Glands

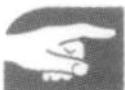

The oral cavity is located below the nasal cavity and anterior to the pharynx. It is bounded by the hard and soft palates, the tongue and muscles of the oral floor, and the uvula.

Airway
Foodway
Naso-pharynx
Oro-pharynx
Laryngo-pharynx

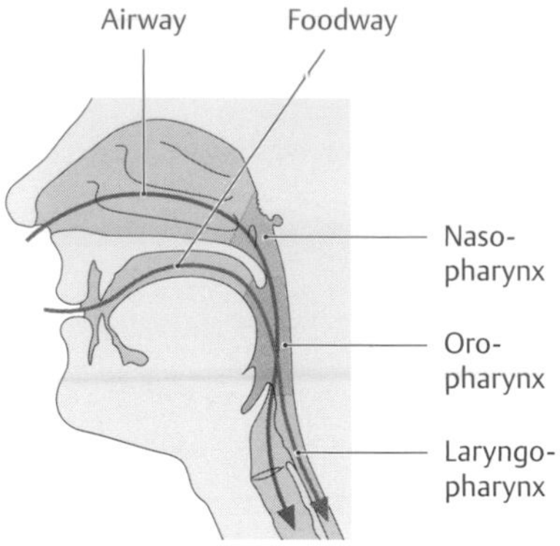

A Organization of the oral cavity.

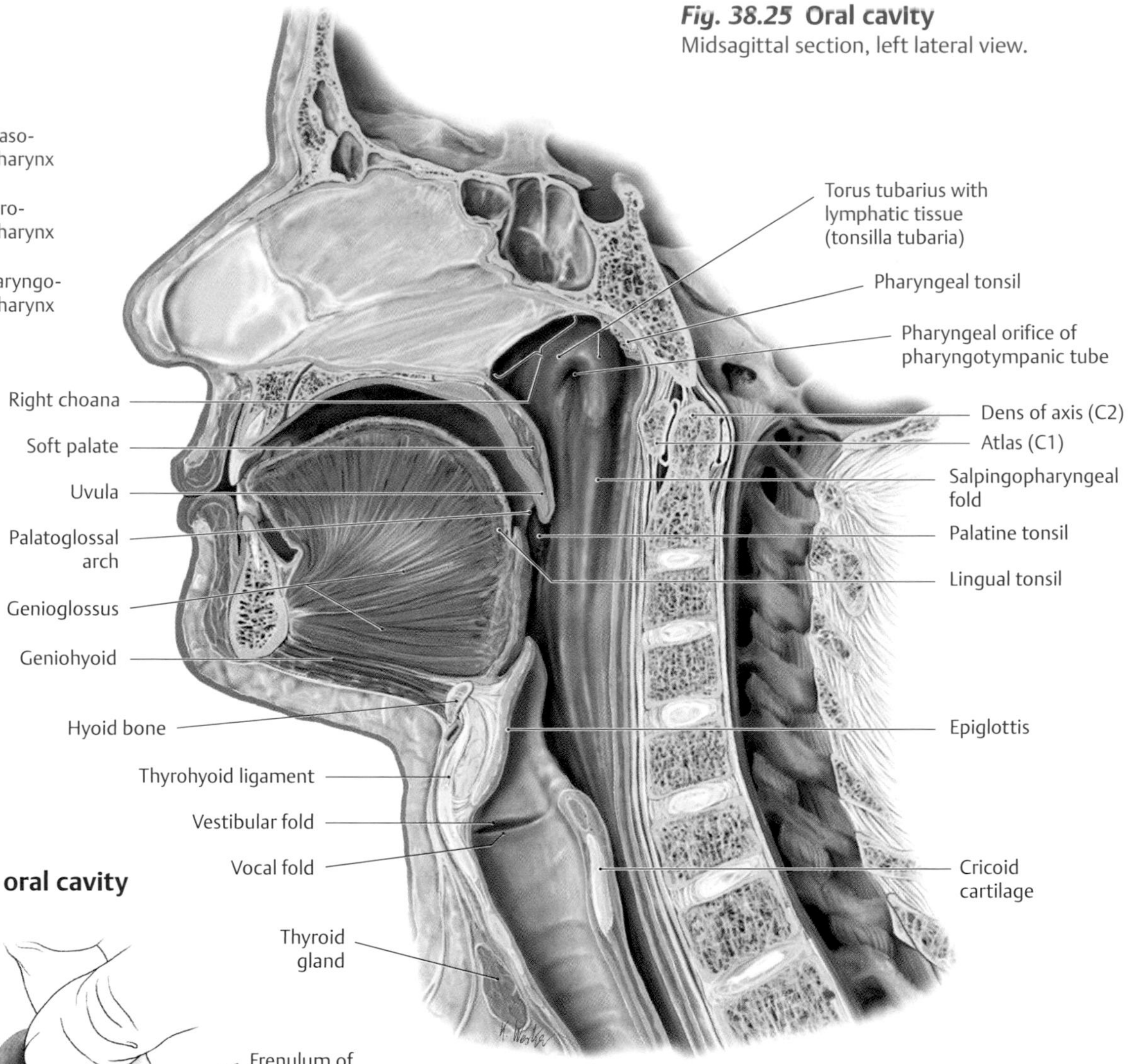

Torus tubarius with lymphatic tissue (tonsilla tubaria)
Pharyngeal tonsil
Pharyngeal orifice of pharyngotympanic tube
Right choana
Dens of axis (C2)
Atlas (C1)
Soft palate
Uvula
Salpingopharyngeal fold
Palatoglossal arch
Palatine tonsil
Lingual tonsil
Genioglossus
Geniohyoid
Hyoid bone
Epiglottis
Thyrohyoid ligament
Vestibular fold
Vocal fold
Cricoid cartilage
Thyroid gland

B Boundaries of the oral cavity.

Fig. 38.25 **Oral cavity**
Midsagittal section, left lateral view.

Fig. 38.26 **Divisions of the oral cavity**
Anterior view.

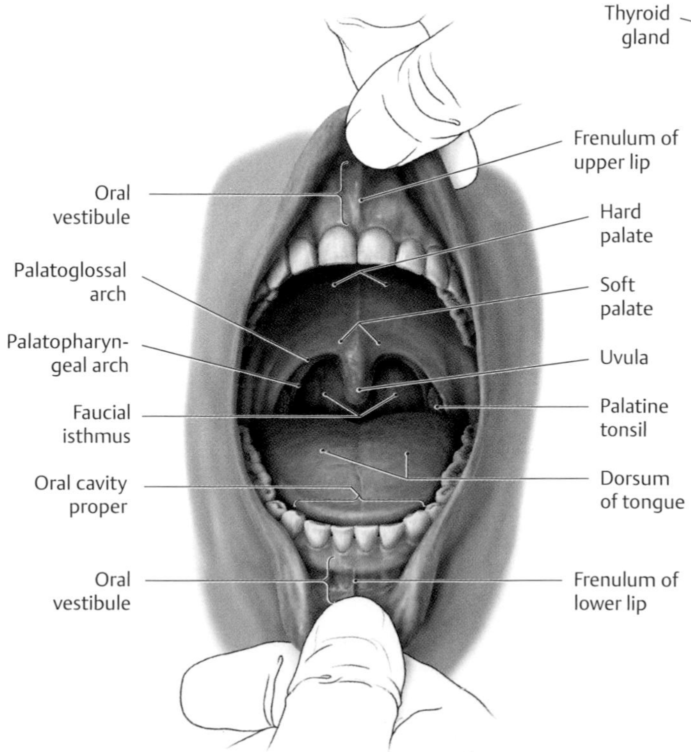

Oral vestibule
Frenulum of upper lip
Hard palate
Palatoglossal arch
Soft palate
Palatopharyn-geal arch
Uvula
Faucial isthmus
Palatine tonsil
Oral cavity proper
Dorsum of tongue
Oral vestibule
Frenulum of lower lip

Table 38.3 **Divisions of the oral cavity**

Part	Anterior boundary	Posterior boundary
Oral vestibule	Lips/cheek	Dental arches
Oral cavity proper	Dental arches	Palatoglossal arch
Fauces (throat)	Palatoglossal arch	Palatopharyngeal arch

The three large, paired salivary glands are the parotid, submandibular, and sublingual glands. The parotid gland is a purely serous (watery) salivary gland. The sublingual gland is predominantly mucous; the submandibular gland is a mixed seromucous gland.

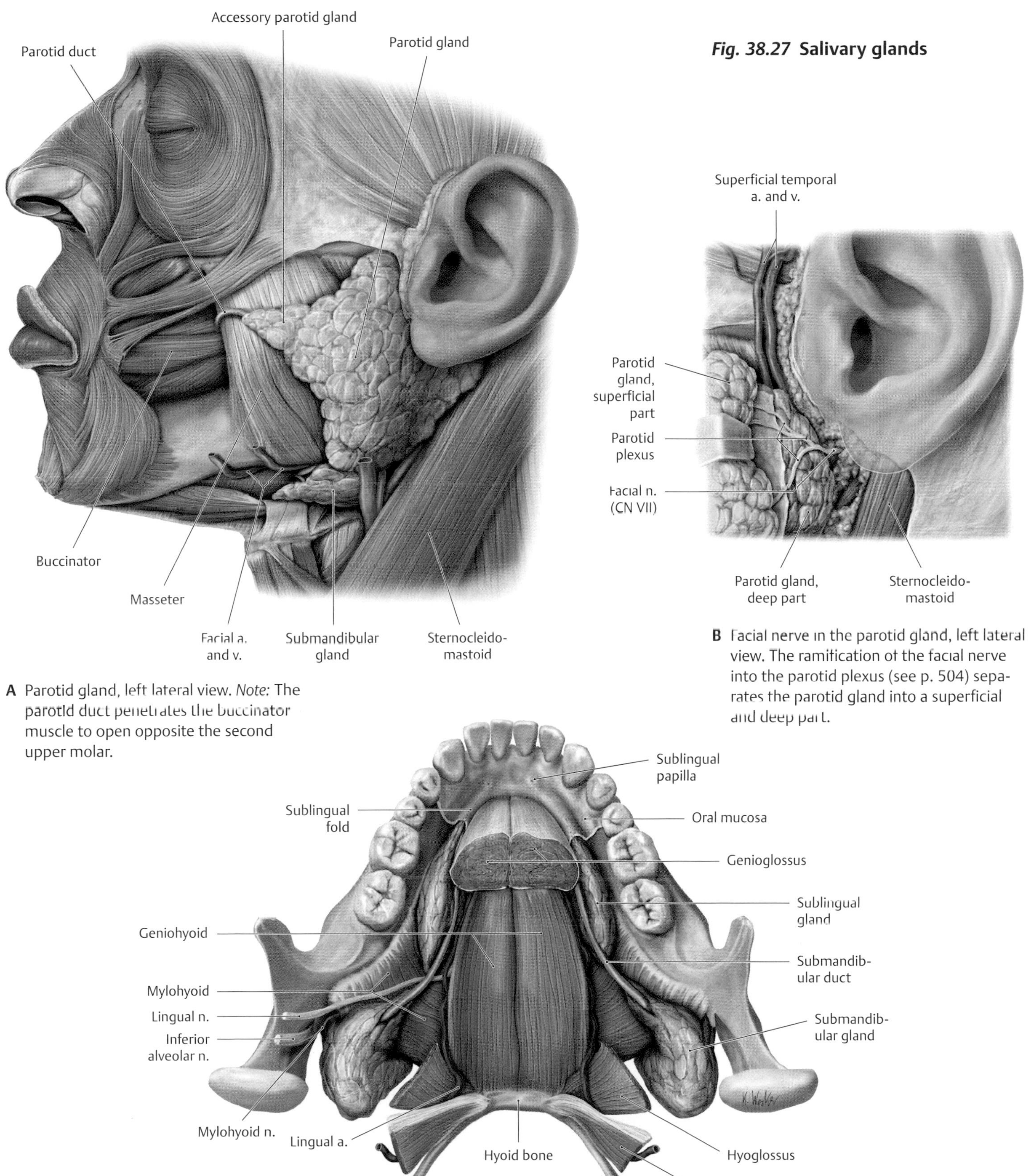

Accessory parotid gland
Parotid duct
Parotid gland
Buccinator
Masseter
Facial a. and v.
Submandibular gland
Sternocleido-mastoid
Superficial temporal a. and v.
Parotid gland, superficial part
Parotid plexus
Facial n. (CN VII)
Parotid gland, deep part
Sternocleido-mastoid
Sublingual papilla
Sublingual fold
Oral mucosa
Genioglossus
Sublingual gland
Geniohyoid
Submandib-ular duct
Mylohyoid
Lingual n.
Inferior alveolar n.
Submandib-ular gland
Mylohyoid n.
Lingual a.
Hyoid bone
Hyoglossus
Stylohyoid

Fig. 38.27 **Salivary glands**

A Parotid gland, left lateral view. *Note:* The parotid duct penetrates the buccinator muscle to open opposite the second upper molar.

B Facial nerve in the parotid gland, left lateral view. The ramification of the facial nerve into the parotid plexus (see p. 504) separates the parotid gland into a superficial and deep part.

C Submandibular and sublingual glands, superior view with tongue removed.

Tonsils & Pharynx

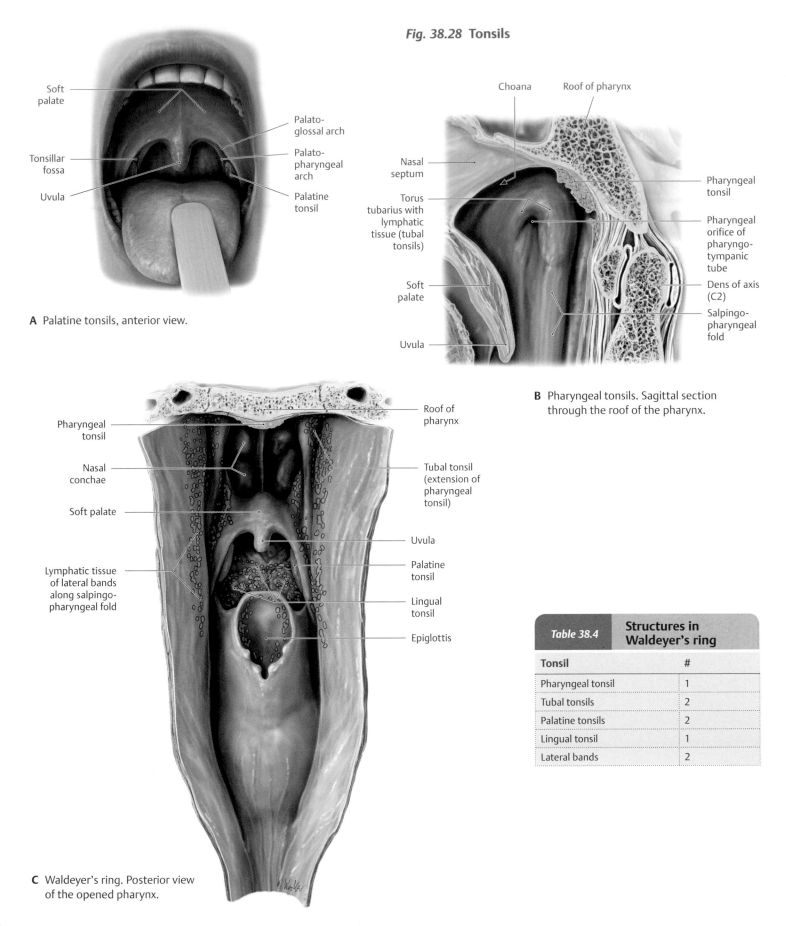

Fig. 38.28 **Tonsils**

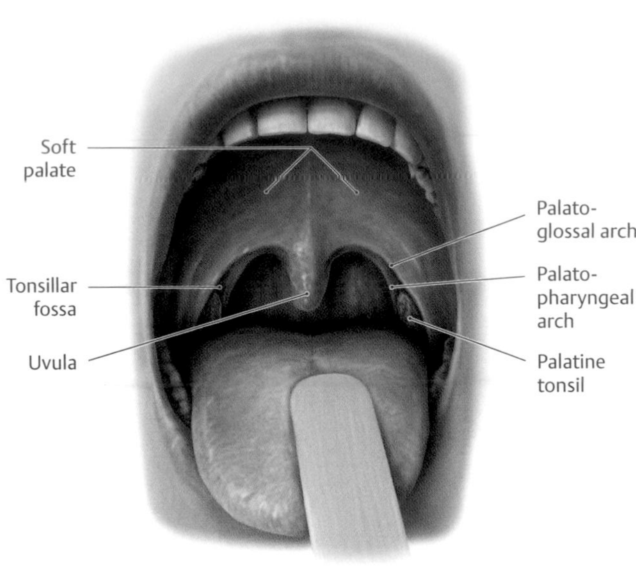
Soft palate
Tonsillar fossa
Uvula
Palato-glossal arch
Palato-pharyngeal arch
Palatine tonsil

A Palatine tonsils, anterior view.

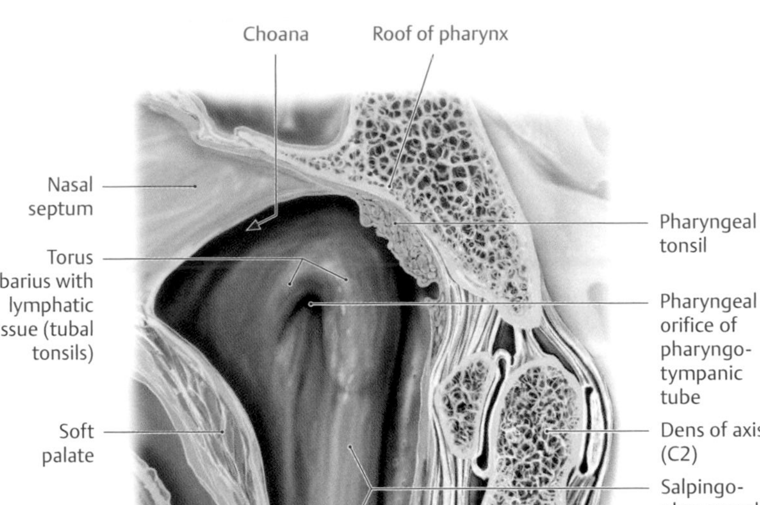
Choana
Roof of pharynx
Nasal septum
Torus tubarius with lymphatic tissue (tubal tonsils)
Soft palate
Uvula
Pharyngeal tonsil
Pharyngeal orifice of pharyngo-tympanic tube
Dens of axis (C2)
Salpingo-pharyngeal fold

B Pharyngeal tonsils. Sagittal section through the roof of the pharynx.

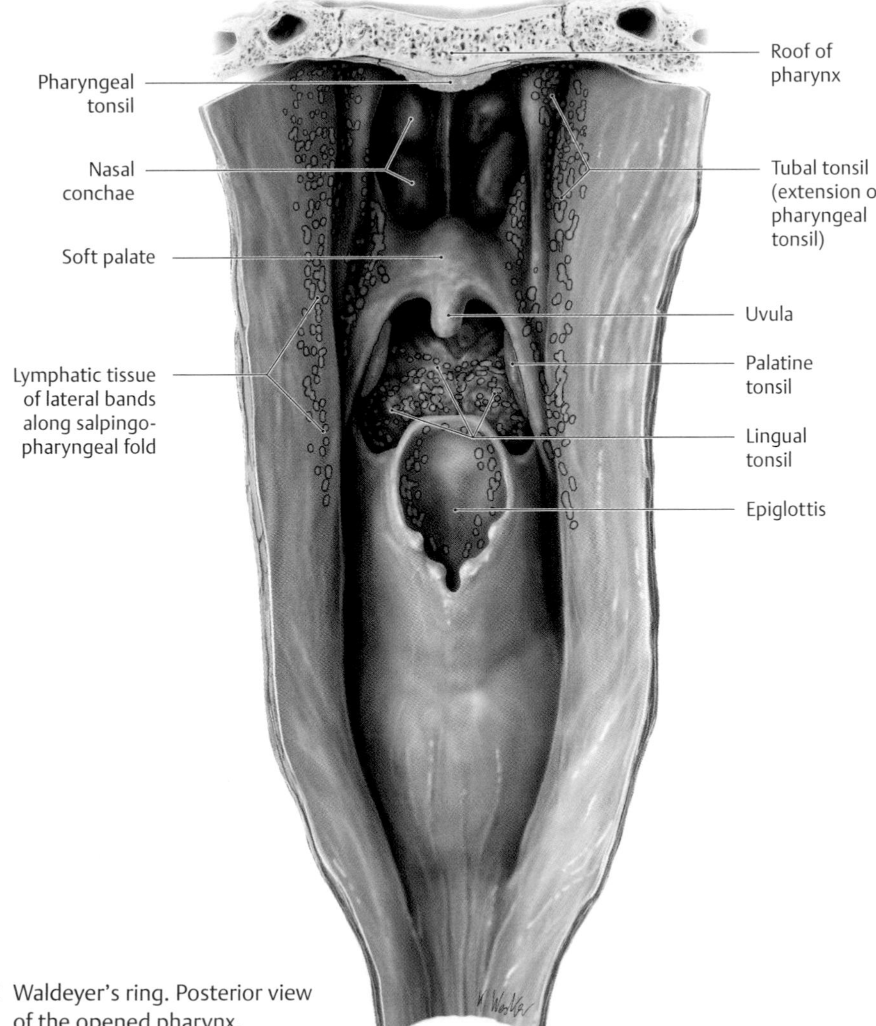
Pharyngeal tonsil
Nasal conchae
Soft palate
Lymphatic tissue of lateral bands along salpingo-pharyngeal fold
Roof of pharynx
Tubal tonsil (extension of pharyngeal tonsil)
Uvula
Palatine tonsil
Lingual tonsil
Epiglottis

C Waldeyer's ring. Posterior view of the opened pharynx.

Table 38.4 **Structures in Waldeyer's ring**

Tonsil	#
Pharyngeal tonsil	1
Tubal tonsils	2
Palatine tonsils	2
Lingual tonsil	1
Lateral bands	2

Clinical

Tonsil infections

Abnormal enlargement of the palatine tonsils due to severe viral or bacterial infection can result in obstruction of the oropharynx, causing difficulty swallowing.

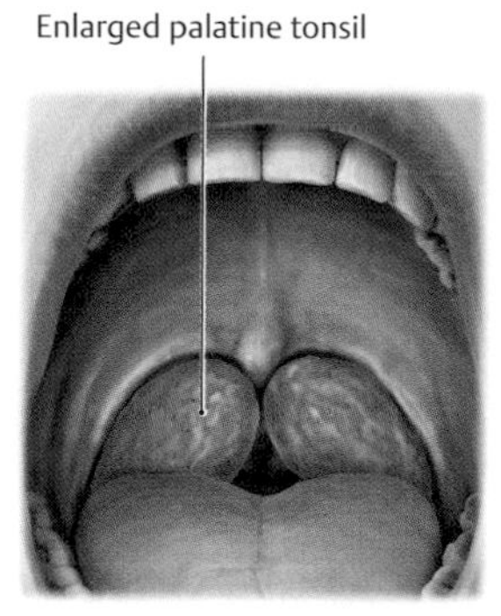
Enlarged palatine tonsil

Particularly well developed in young children, the pharyngeal tonsil begins to regress at 6 to 7 years of age. Abnormal enlargement is common, with the tonsil bulging into the nasopharynx and obstructing air passages, forcing the child to "mouth breathe."

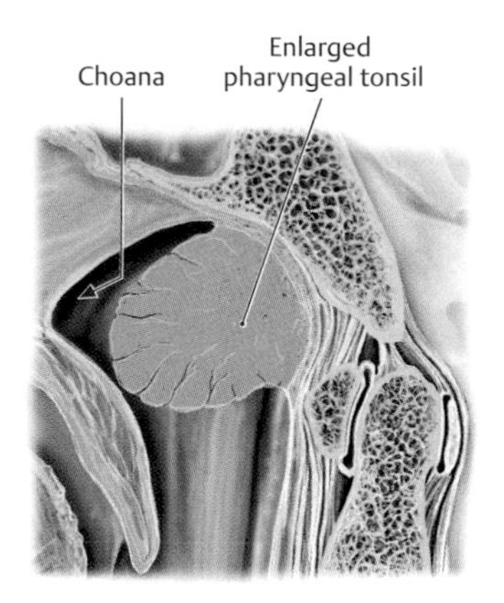
Choana
Enlarged pharyngeal tonsil

Fig. 38.29 **Pharyngeal mucosa**

Posterior view of the opened pharynx. The anterior portion of the muscular tube contains three openings: choanae (to the nasal cavity), faucial isthmus (to the oral cavity), and aditus (to the laryngeal inlet).

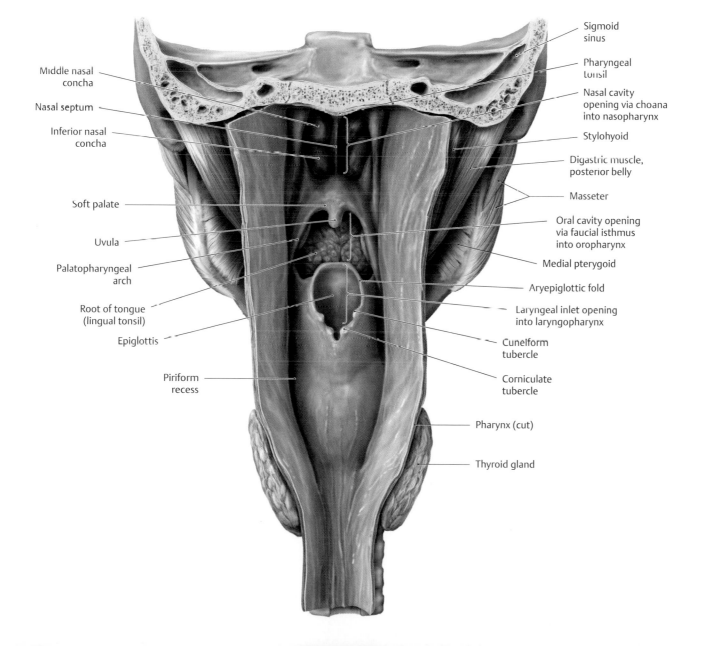

Middle nasal concha
Nasal septum
Inferior nasal concha
Soft palate
Uvula
Palatopharyngeal arch
Root of tongue (lingual tonsil)
Epiglottis
Piriform recess
Sigmoid sinus
Pharyngeal tonsil
Nasal cavity opening via choana into nasopharynx
Stylohyoid
Digastric muscle, posterior belly
Masseter
Oral cavity opening via faucial isthmus into oropharynx
Medial pterygoid
Aryepiglottic fold
Laryngeal inlet opening into laryngopharynx
Cuneiform tubercle
Corniculate tubercle
Pharynx (cut)
Thyroid gland

Pharyngeal Muscles

Fig. 38.30 **Pharyngeal muscles: Left lateral view**

The pharyngeal musculature consists of the pharyngeal constrictors and the relatively weak pharyngeal elevators.

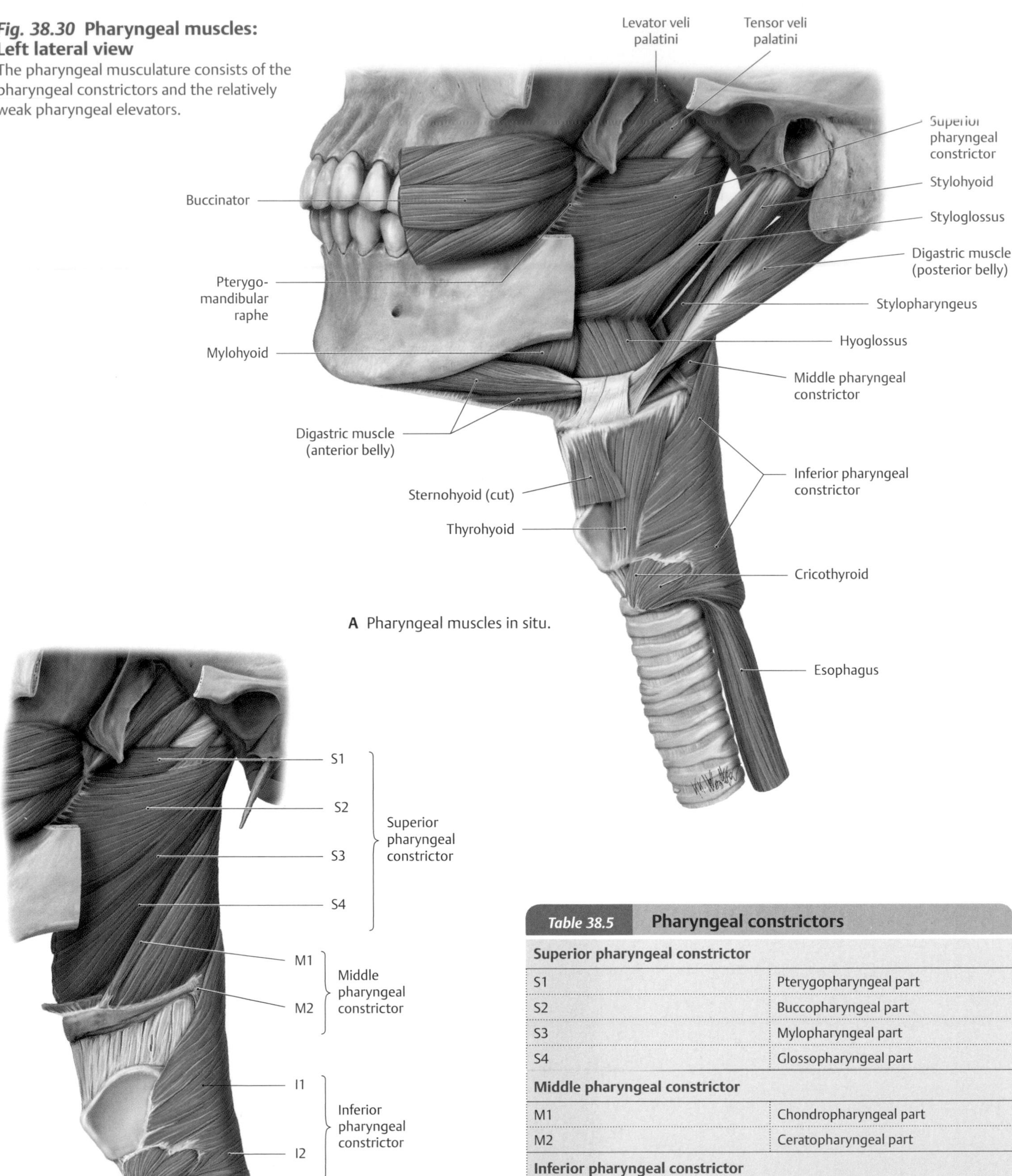

Levator veli palatini
Tensor veli palatini
Superior pharyngeal constrictor
Stylohyoid
Styloglossus
Digastric muscle (posterior belly)
Stylopharyngeus
Hyoglossus
Middle pharyngeal constrictor
Inferior pharyngeal constrictor
Cricothyroid
Esophagus
Buccinator
Pterygo-mandibular raphe
Mylohyoid
Digastric muscle (anterior belly)
Sternohyoid (cut)
Thyrohyoid
S1
S2
S3
S4
Superior pharyngeal constrictor
M1
M2
Middle pharyngeal constrictor
I1
I2
Inferior pharyngeal constrictor

A Pharyngeal muscles in situ.

B Subdivisions of the pharyngeal constrictors.

Table 38.5	**Pharyngeal constrictors**
Superior pharyngeal constrictor	
S1	Pterygopharyngeal part
S2	Buccopharyngeal part
S3	Mylopharyngeal part
S4	Glossopharyngeal part
Middle pharyngeal constrictor	
M1	Chondropharyngeal part
M2	Ceratopharyngeal part
Inferior pharyngeal constrictor	
I1	Thyropharyngeal part
I2	Cricopharyngeal part

Fig. 38.31 Pharyngeal muscles: Posterior view

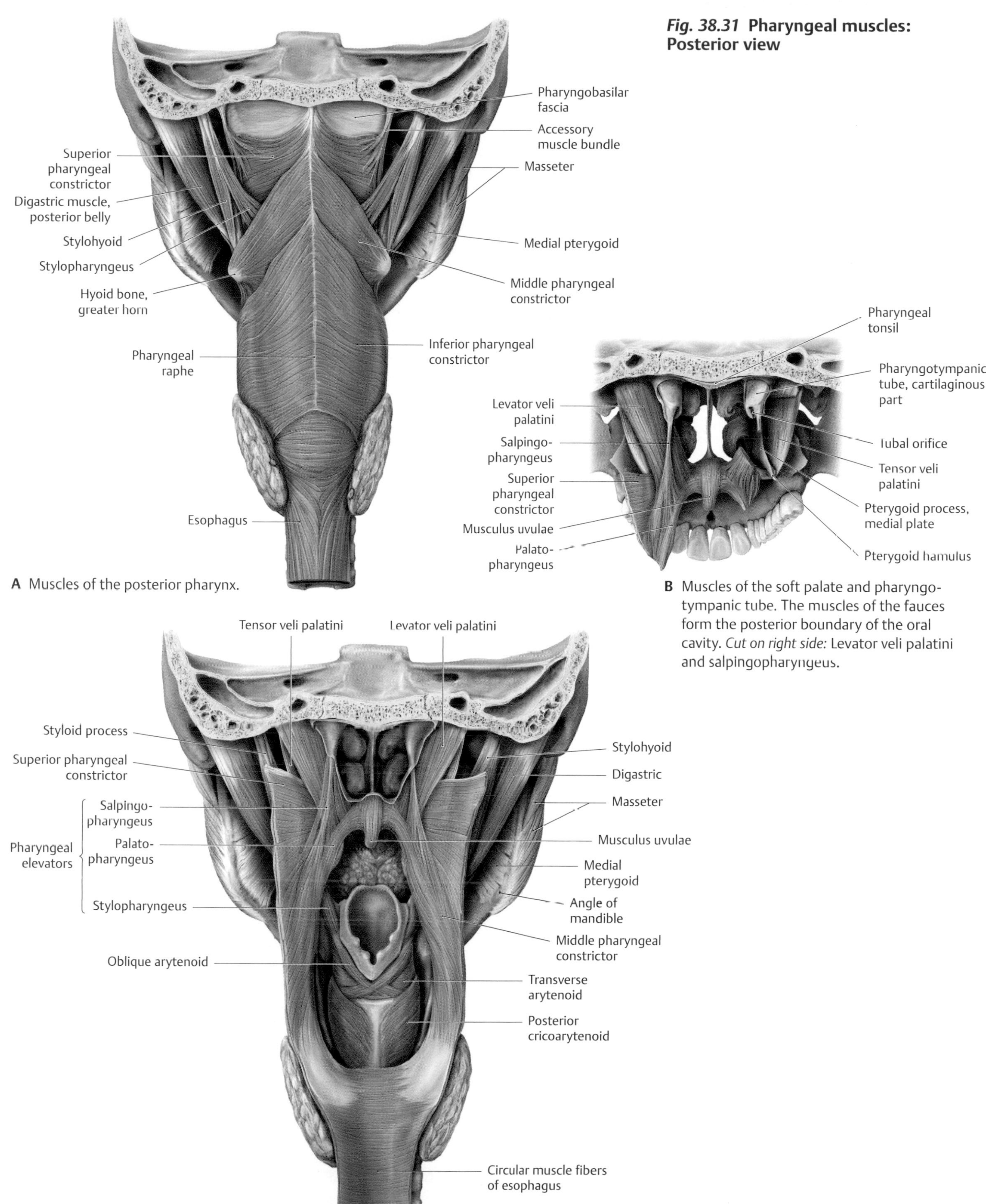

Pharyngobasilar fascia
Accessory muscle bundle
Superior pharyngeal constrictor
Masseter
Digastric muscle, posterior belly
Stylohyoid
Medial pterygoid
Stylopharyngeus
Middle pharyngeal constrictor
Hyoid bone, greater horn
Inferior pharyngeal constrictor
Pharyngeal raphe
Esophagus
Pharyngeal tonsil
Pharyngotympanic tube, cartilaginous part
Levator veli palatini
Salpingo-pharyngeus
Tubal orifice
Tensor veli palatini
Superior pharyngeal constrictor
Pterygoid process, medial plate
Musculus uvulae
Palato-pharyngeus
Pterygoid hamulus
Tensor veli palatini
Levator veli palatini
Styloid process
Stylohyoid
Superior pharyngeal constrictor
Digastric
Salpingo-pharyngeus
Masseter
Pharyngeal elevators
Palato-pharyngeus
Musculus uvulae
Medial pterygoid
Stylopharyngeus
Angle of mandible
Middle pharyngeal constrictor
Oblique arytenoid
Transverse arytenoid
Posterior cricoarytenoid
Circular muscle fibers of esophagus

A Muscles of the posterior pharynx.

B Muscles of the soft palate and pharyngotympanic tube. The muscles of the fauces form the posterior boundary of the oral cavity. *Cut on right side:* Levator veli palatini and salpingopharyngeus.

C Muscles in the opened pharynx.

Neurovasculature of the Pharynx

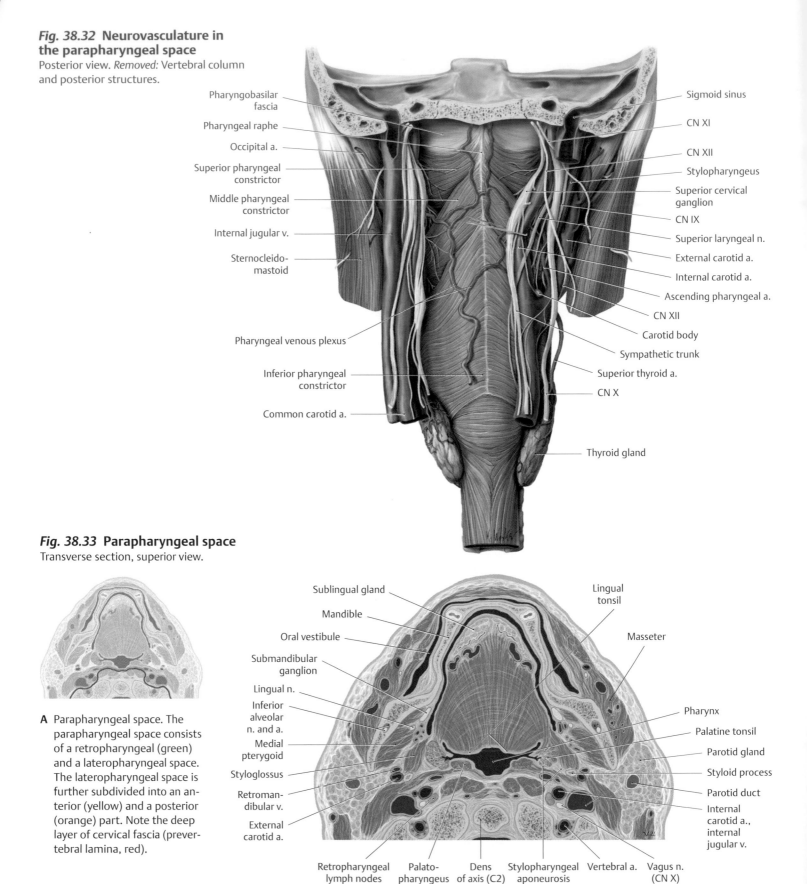

Fig. 38.32 Neurovasculature in the parapharyngeal space
Posterior view. *Removed:* Vertebral column and posterior structures.

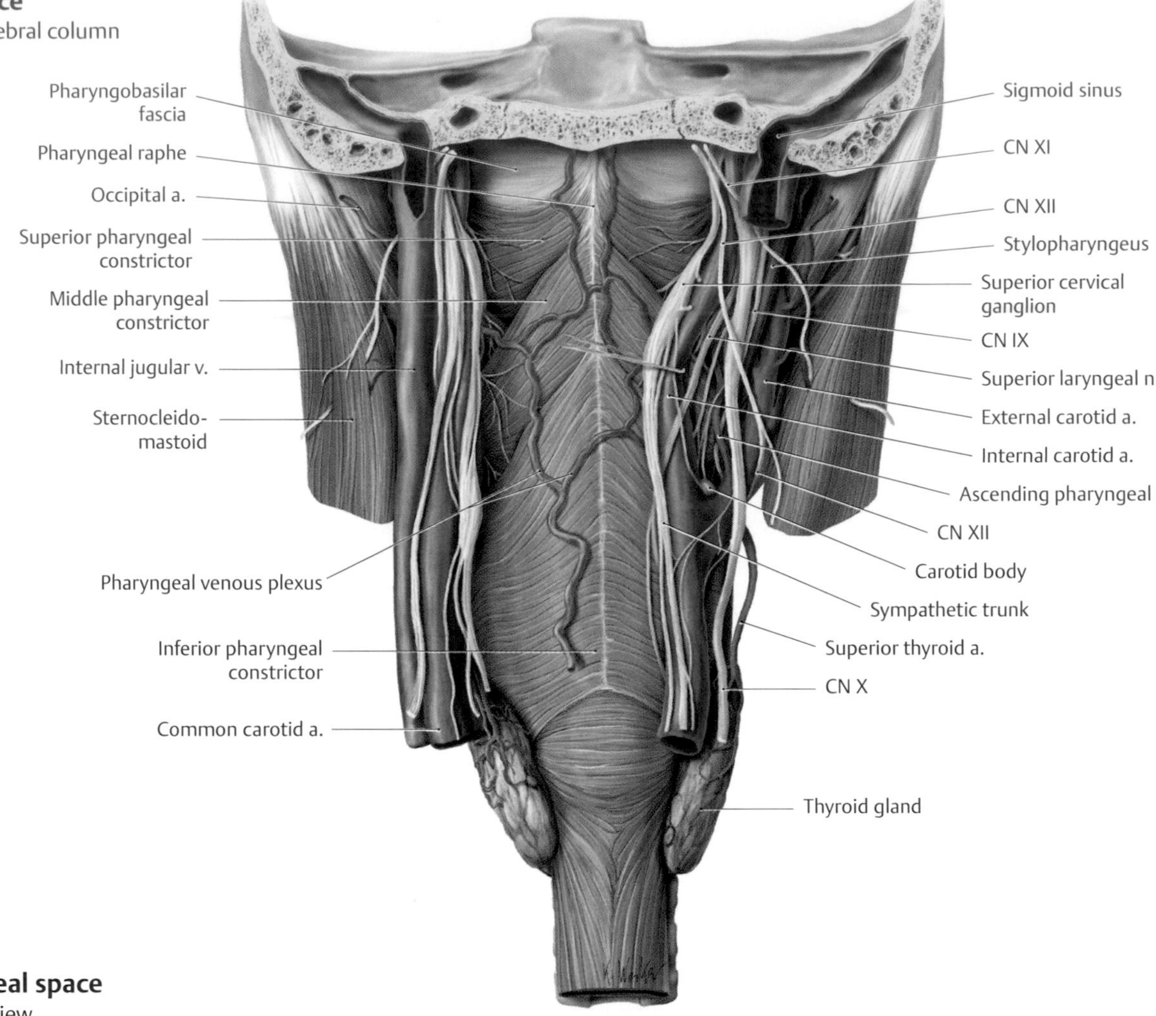
Pharyngobasilar fascia
Pharyngeal raphe
Occipital a.
Superior pharyngeal constrictor
Middle pharyngeal constrictor
Internal jugular v.
Sternocleido-mastoid
Pharyngeal venous plexus
Inferior pharyngeal constrictor
Common carotid a.
Sigmoid sinus
CN XI
CN XII
Stylopharyngeus
Superior cervical ganglion
CN IX
Superior laryngeal n.
External carotid a.
Internal carotid a.
Ascending pharyngeal a.
CN XII
Carotid body
Sympathetic trunk
Superior thyroid a.
CN X
Thyroid gland

Fig. 38.33 Parapharyngeal space
Transverse section, superior view.

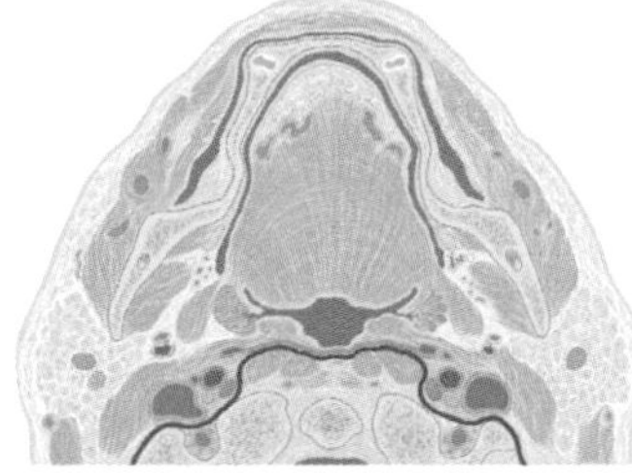

A Parapharyngeal space. The parapharyngeal space consists of a retropharyngeal (green) and a lateropharyngeal space. The lateropharyngeal space is further subdivided into an anterior (yellow) and a posterior (orange) part. Note the deep layer of cervical fascia (prevertebral lamina, red).

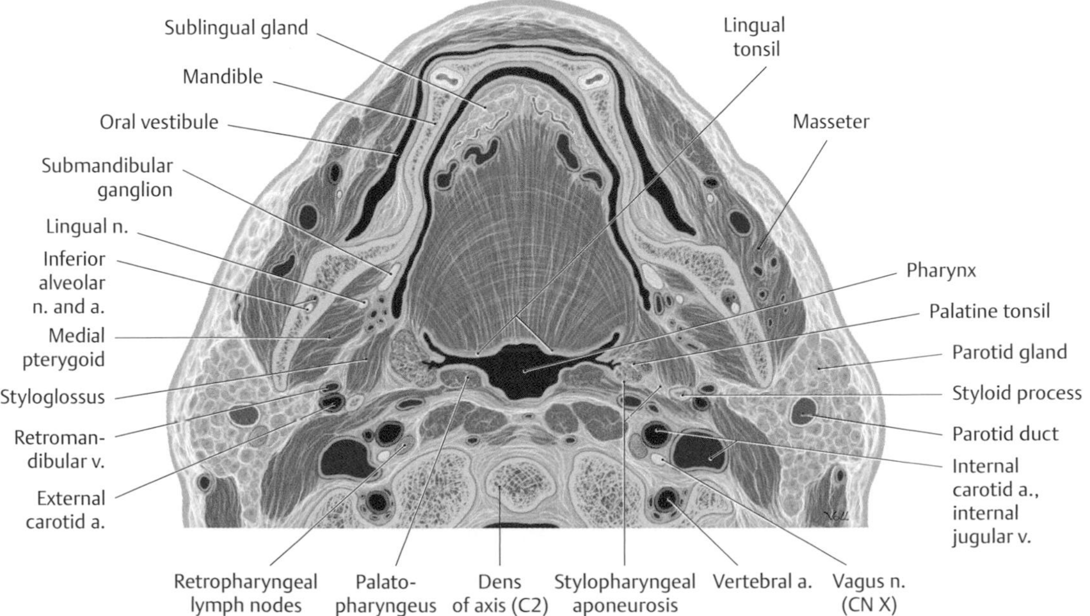
Sublingual gland
Mandible
Oral vestibule
Submandibular ganglion
Lingual n.
Inferior alveolar n. and a.
Medial pterygoid
Styloglossus
Retroman-dibular v.
External carotid a.
Lingual tonsil
Masseter
Pharynx
Palatine tonsil
Parotid gland
Styloid process
Parotid duct
Internal carotid a., internal jugular v.
Retropharyngeal lymph nodes
Palato-pharyngeus
Dens of axis (C2)
Stylopharyngeal aponeurosis
Vertebral a.
Vagus n. (CN X)

B Superior view of the transverse section at the level of the tonsillar fossa.

Fig. 38.34 **Neurovasculature of the opened pharynx**
Posterior view.

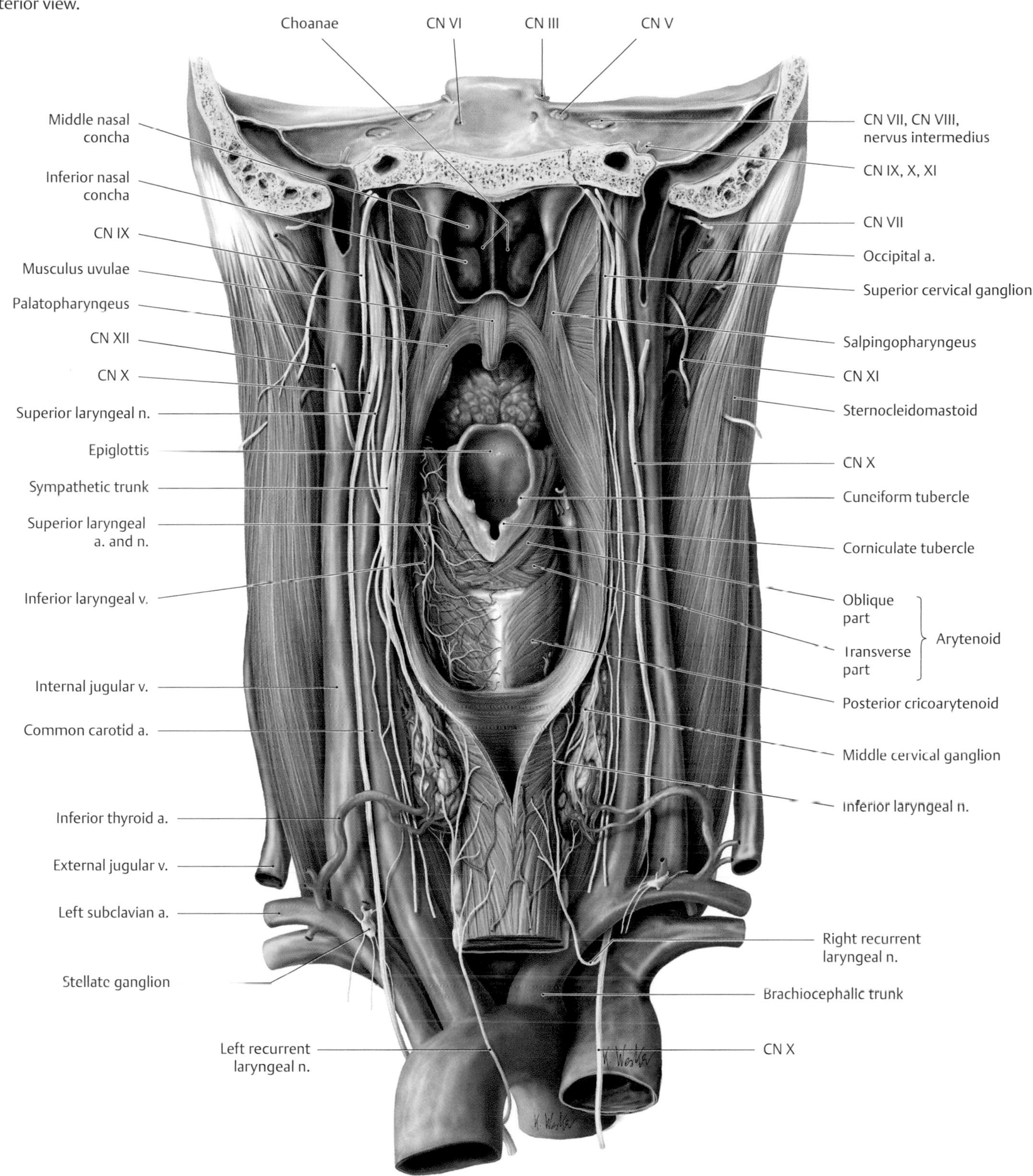
Choanae
CN VI
CN III
CN V
Middle nasal concha
Inferior nasal concha
CN IX
Musculus uvulae
Palatopharyngeus
CN XII
CN X
Superior laryngeal n.
Epiglottis
Sympathetic trunk
Superior laryngeal a. and n.
Inferior laryngeal v.
Internal jugular v.
Common carotid a.
Inferior thyroid a.
External jugular v.
Left subclavian a.
Stellate ganglion
Left recurrent laryngeal n.
CN VII, CN VIII, nervus intermedius
CN IX, X, XI
CN VII
Occipital a.
Superior cervical ganglion
Salpingopharyngeus
CN XI
Sternocleidomastoid
CN X
Cuneiform tubercle
Corniculate tubercle
Oblique part
Transverse part
Arytenoid
Posterior cricoarytenoid
Middle cervical ganglion
Inferior laryngeal n.
Right recurrent laryngeal n.
Brachiocephalic trunk
CN X

CN III, oculomotor n.; CN V, trigeminal n.; CN VI, abducent n.; CN VII, facial n.; CN VIII, vestibulocochlear n.; CN IX, glossopharyngeal n.; CN X, vagus n.; CN XI, accessory n.; CN XII, hypoglossal n..
See Chapter 33 for the cranial nerves.

Muscle Facts (I)

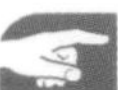

The bones, joints, and ligaments of the neck and the six topographic classes of neck muscles are covered in this or the Back unit (see Table 39.1). However, some muscles in the same topographic class belong in different functional classes; for example, the platysma belongs to the muscles of facial expression; the trapezius, to the muscles of the shoulder girdle; and the nuchal muscles, to the intrinsic back muscles. Note that the suboccipital muscles (short nuchal and craniovertebral muscles) are covered with the lateral (deep) muscles of the neck.

Table 39.1 Bones, joints, ligaments, and muscles of the neck

Bones, joints, and ligaments					
	Bones of the cervical spine	See pp. 8-9		Joints & ligaments of the craniovertebral junction	See pp. 18-19
	Joints & ligaments of the cervical spine	See pp. 16-17, 20-21		Hyoid bone & larynx	Fig. 38.5, Fig. 39.18
Muscles					
I	**Superficial neck muscles**		III	**Suprahyoid muscles**	
	Platysma, ①, ② sternocleidomastoid, ③, ④, ⑤ trapezius	Fig. 39.3		Digastric, geniohyoid, mylohyoid, stylohyoid	Fig. 39.4A
II	**Nuchal muscles (intrinsic back muscles)**		IV	**Infrahyoid muscles**	
	⑥ Semispinalis capitis ⑦ Semispinalis cervicis	See p. 34		Sternohyoid, sternothyroid, thyrohyoid, omohyoid	Fig. 39.4B
	⑧ Splenius capitis ⑨ Splenius cervicis		V	**Prevertebral muscles**	
	⑩ Longissimus capitis ⑪ Longissimus cervicis	See p. 32		Longus capitis, longus coli, rectus capitis anterior and lateralis	See p. 31 Fig. 39.6A
	⑫ Iliocostalis cervicis		VI	**Lateral (deep) neck muscles**	
	Suboccipital muscles (short nuchal and craniovertebral joint muscles)	Fig. 39.6C		Anterior, middle, and posterior scalenes	Fig. 39.6B

Fig. 39.1 **Superficial neck muscles**
See Table 39.2 for details.

②
①

A Sternocleidomastoid.

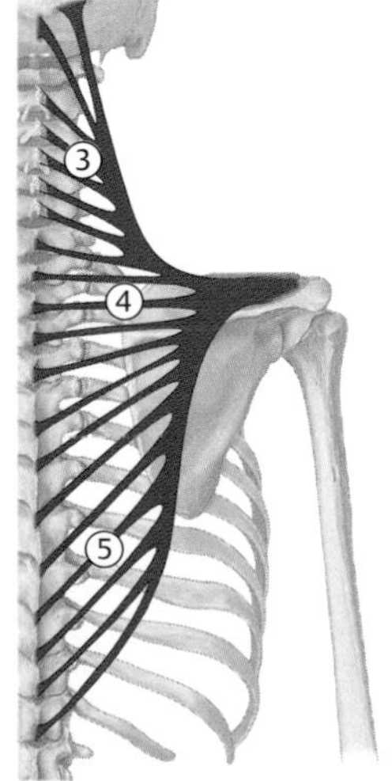

③
④
⑤

B Trapezius.

Fig. 39.2 **Nuchal muscles**

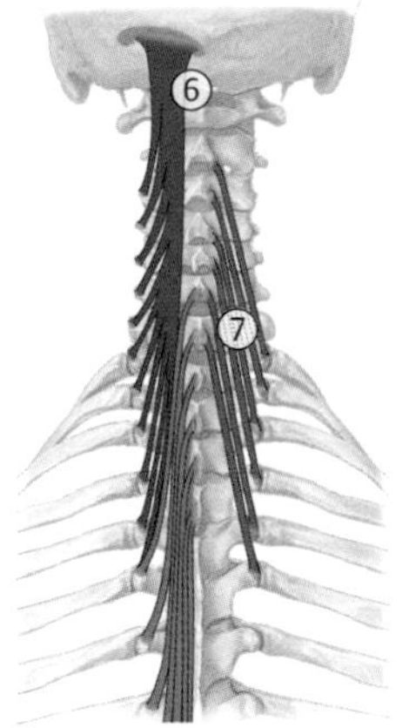

⑥
⑦

A Semispinalis.

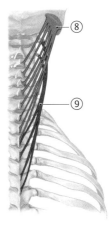

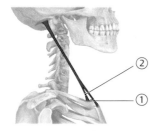

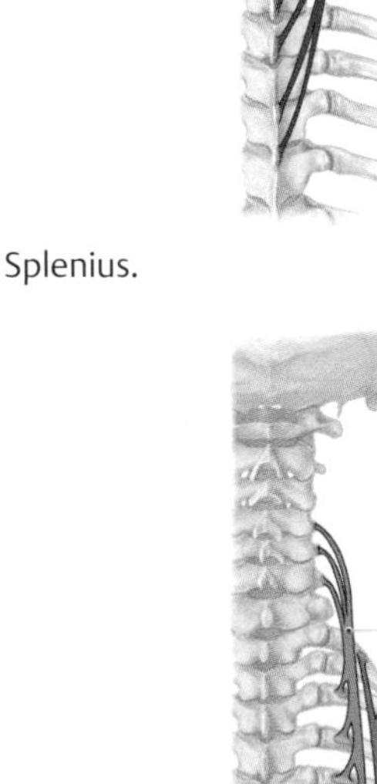

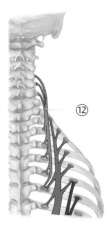

⑧
⑨

B Splenius.

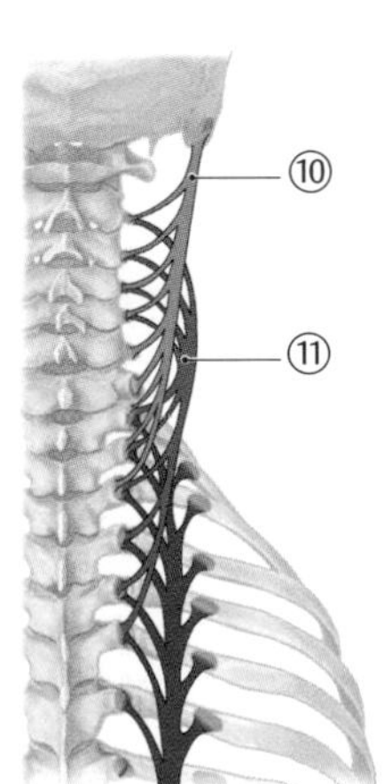

⑩
⑪

C Longissimus.

⑫

D Iliocostalis.

Fig. 39.3 **Superficial musculature of the neck**

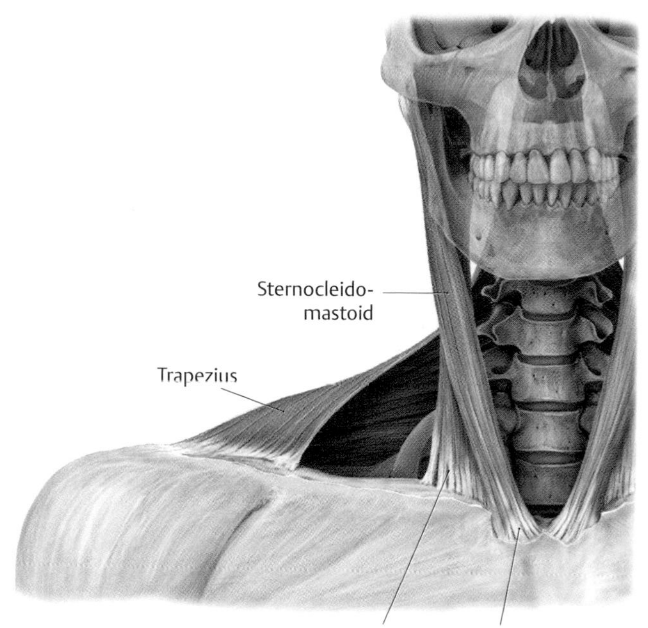
Sternocleido-
mastoid
Trapezius

Clavicular head
Sternal head

A Anterior view.

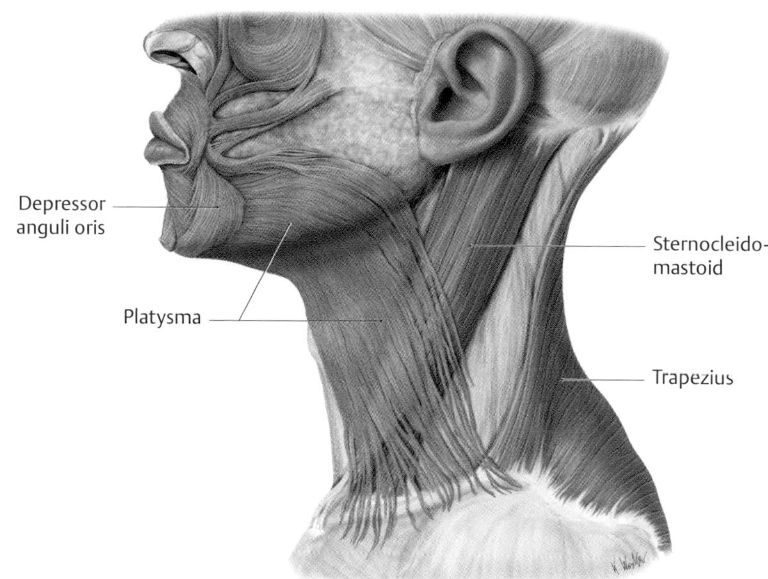
Depressor
anguli oris
Sternocleido-
mastoid
Platysma
Trapezius

B Left lateral view.

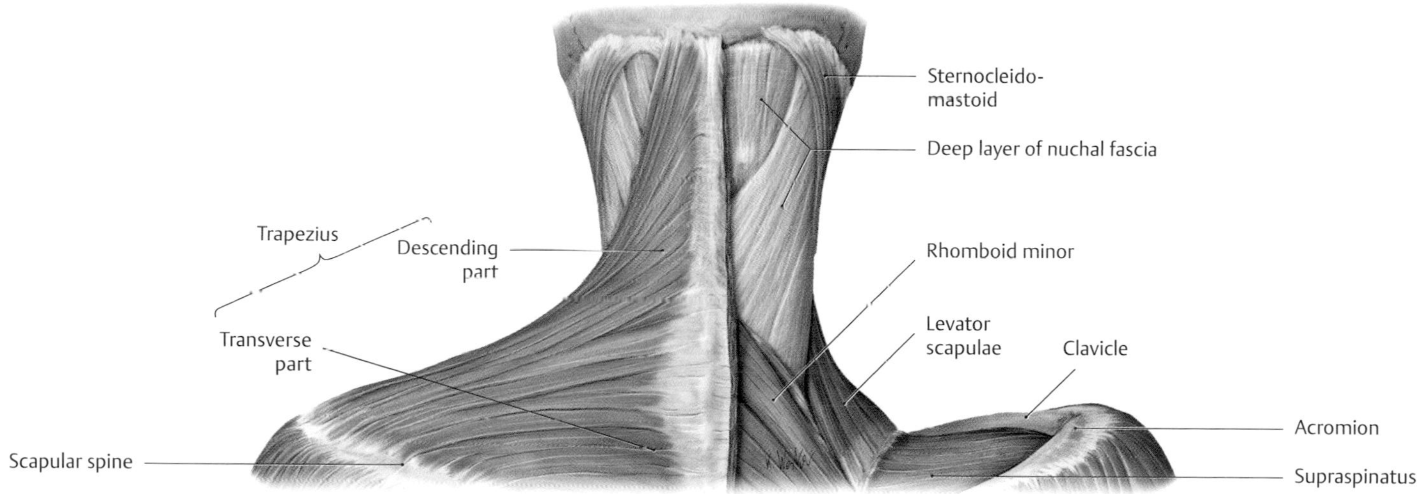
Sternocleido-
mastoid
Deep layer of nuchal fascia
Trapezius
Descending
part
Rhomboid minor
Transverse
part
Levator
scapulae
Clavice
Acromion
Scapular spine
Supraspinatus

C Posterior view. *Removed:* Trapezius (right side)

Table 39.2 Superficial neck muscles

Muscle		Origin	Insertion	Innervation	Action
Platysma		Skin over lower neck and upper lateral thorax	Mandible (inferior border), skin over lower face and angle of mouth	Cervical branch of facial n. (CN VII)	Depresses and wrinkles skin of lower face and mouth, tenses skin of neck, aids forced depression of mandible
Sternocleido-mastoid	① Sternal head	Sternum (manubrium)	Temporal bone (mastoid process), occipital bone (superior nuchal line)	*Motor:* Accessory n. (CN XI) *Pain and proprioception:* Cervical plexus (C2, C3)	*Unilateral:* Tilts head to same side, rotates head to opposite side *Bilateral:* Extends head, aids in respiration when head is fixed
	② Clavicular head	Clavicle (medial one third)			
Trapezius	③ Descending part*	Occipital bone, spinous processes of C1–C7	Clavicle (lateral one third)		Draws scapula obliquely upward, rotates glenoid cavity superiorly

* The transverse ④ and ascending ⑤ parts are described on p. 300.

Muscle Facts (II)

Table 39.3 Suprahyoid muscles

The suprahyoid muscles are also considered accessory muscles of mastication.

Muscle		Origin	Insertion		Innervation	Action
Digastric	1a Anterior belly	Mandible (digastric fossa)	Hyoid bone (body)	Via an intermediate tendon with a fibrous loop	Mylohyoid n. (from CN V_3)	Elevates hyoid bone (during swallowing), assists in opening mandible
	1b Posterior belly	Temporal bone (mastoid notch, medial to mastoid process)			Facial n. (CN VII)	
② Stylohyoid		Temporal bone (styloid process)		Via a split tendon		
③ Mylohyoid		Mandible (mylohyoid line)		Via median tendon of insertion (mylohyoid raphe)	Mylohyoid n. (from CN V_3)	Tightens and elevates oral floor, draws hyoid bone forward (swallowing), assists in opening mandible and moving it side to side (mastication)
④ Geniohyoid		Mandible (inferior mental spine)		Directly	Anterior ramus of C1 via hypoglossal n. (CN XII)	Draws hyoid bone forward (swallowing), assists in opening mandible

Fig. 39.4 **Suprahyoid and infrahyoid muscles**

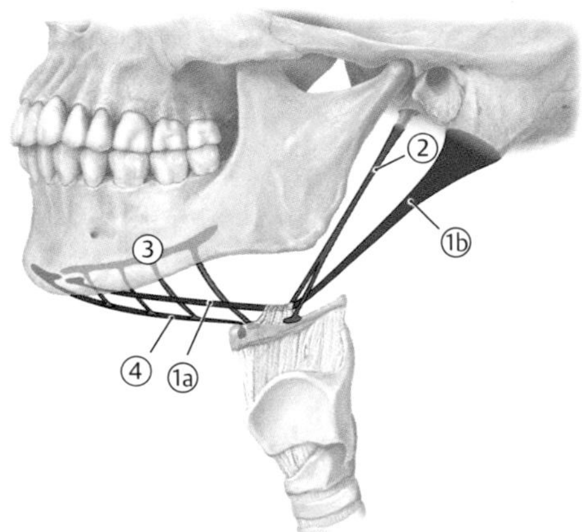

②
③
1b
④
1a

A Suprahyoid muscles, left lateral view.

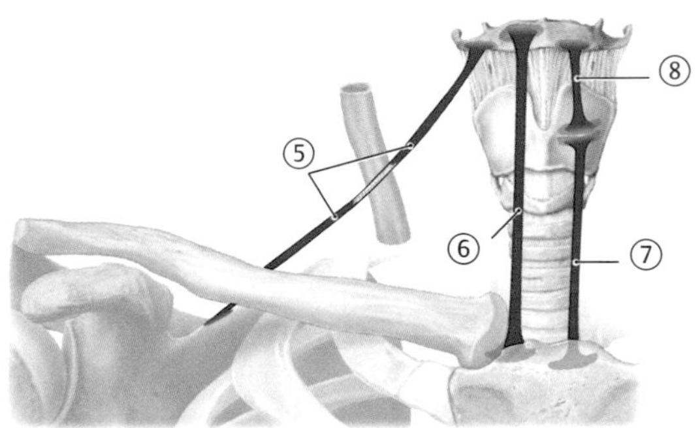

⑧
⑤
⑥
⑦

B Infrahyoid muscles, anterior view.

Table 39.4 Infrahyoid muscles

Muscle	Origin	Insertion	Innervation	Action
⑤ Omohyoid	Scapula (superior border)	Hyoid bone (body)	Ansa cervicalis of cervical plexus (C1–C3)	Depresses (fixes) hyoid, draws larynx and hyoid down for phonation and terminal phases of swallowing*
⑥ Sternohyoid	Manubrium and sternoclavicular joint (posterior surface)			
⑦ Sternothyroid	Manubrium (posterior surface)	Thyroid cartilage (oblique line)	Ansa cervicalis (C2–C3)	
⑧ Thyrohyoid	Thyroid cartilage (oblique line)	Hyoid bone (body)	C1 via hypoglossal n. (CN XII)	Depresses and fixes hyoid, raises the larynx during swallowing

* The omohyoid also tenses the cervical fascia (with an intermediate tendon).

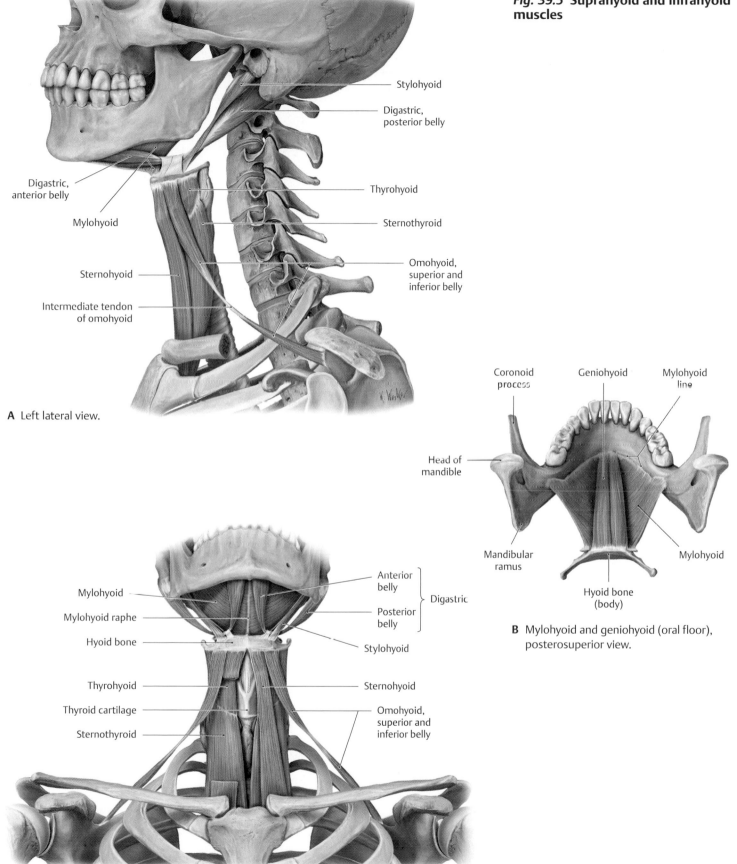

Fig. 39.5 Suprahyoid and infrahyoid muscles

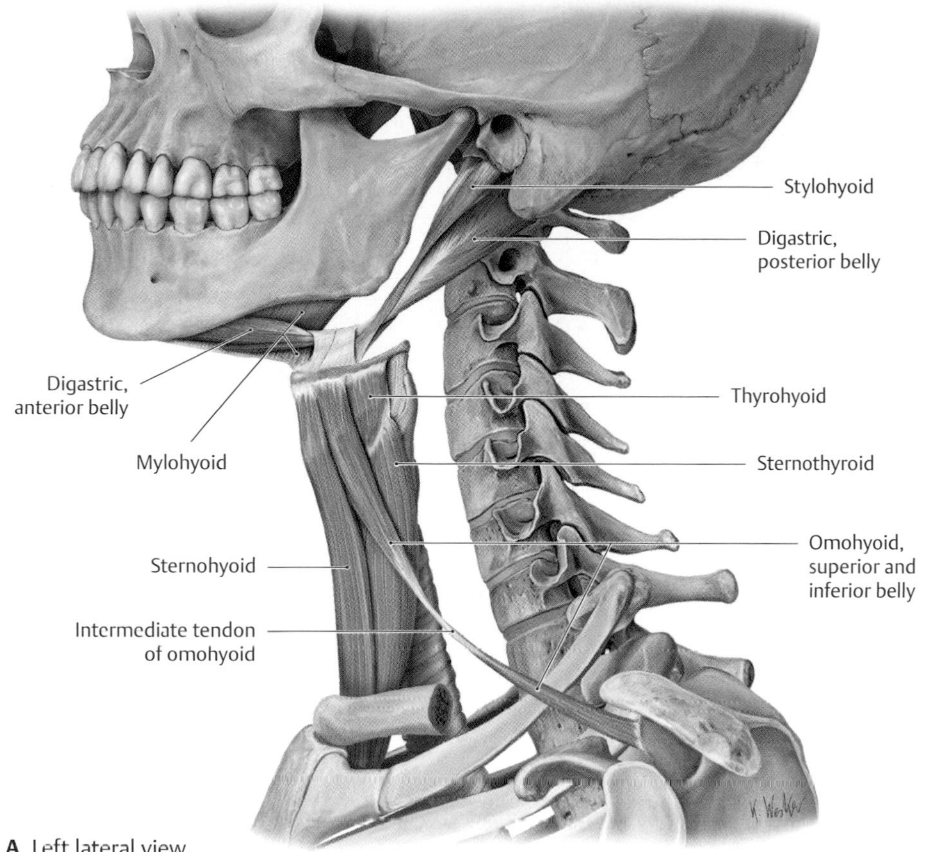
Stylohyoid
Digastric, posterior belly
Digastric, anterior belly
Mylohyoid
Thyrohyoid
Sternothyroid
Sternohyoid
Omohyoid, superior and inferior belly
Intermediate tendon of omohyoid

A Left lateral view.

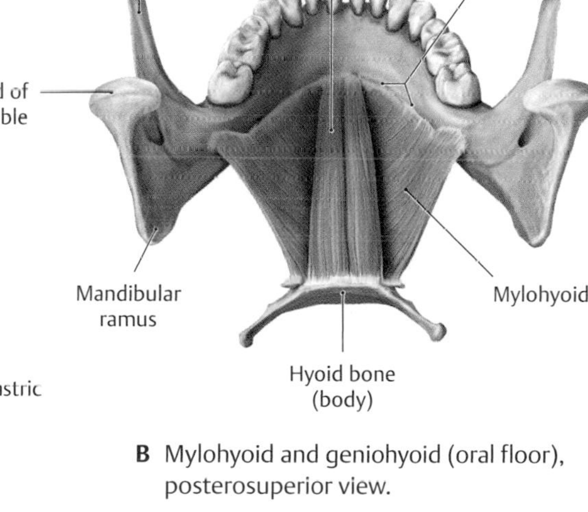
Coronoid process
Geniohyoid
Mylohyoid line
Head of mandible
Mandibular ramus
Mylohyoid
Hyoid bone (body)

B Mylohyoid and geniohyoid (oral floor), posterosuperior view.

Mylohyoid
Mylohyoid raphe
Hyoid bone
Thyrohyoid
Thyroid cartilage
Sternothyroid
Anterior belly
Posterior belly
Digastric
Stylohyoid
Sternohyoid
Omohyoid, superior and inferior belly

C Anterior view. The sternohyoid has been cut (right).

Muscle Facts (III)

Fig. 39.6 **Deep muscles of the neck**

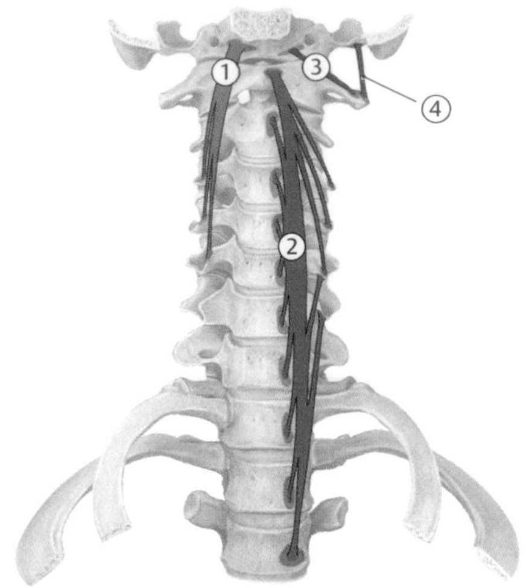

1
2
3
4

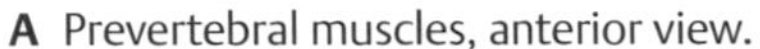

A Prevertebral muscles, anterior view.

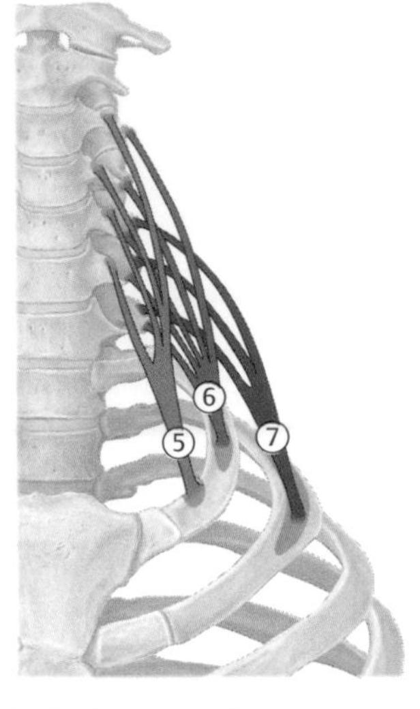

5
6
7

B Scalene muscles, anterior view.

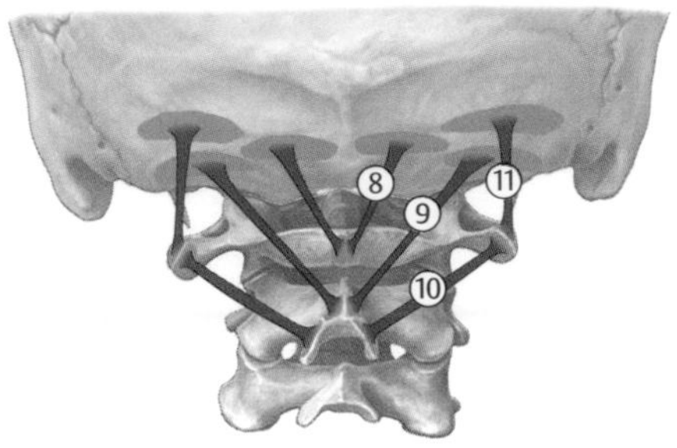

8
9
10
11

C Suboccipital muscles, posterior view.

Table 39.5 **Deep muscles of the neck**

Muscle		Origin	Insertion	Innervation	Action
Prevertebral muscles					
① Longus capitis		C3–C6 (anterior tubercles of transverse processes)	Occipital bone (basilar part)	Direct branches from cervical plexus (C1–C3)	Flexion of head at atlanto-occipital joints
② Longus colli	Vertical (intermediate) part	C5–T3 (anterior surfaces of vertebral bodies)	C2–C4 (anterior surfaces)	Direct branches from cervical plexus (C2–C6)	*Unilateral:* Tilts and rotates cervical spine to opposite side *Bilateral:* Forward flexion of cervical spine
	Superior oblique part	C3–C5 (anterior tubercles of transverse processes)	Atlas (anterior tubercle)		
	Inferior oblique part	T1–T3 (anterior surfaces of vertebral bodies)	C5–C6 (anterior tubercles of transverse processes)		
③ Rectus capitis anterior		C1 (lateral mass)	Occipital bone (basilar part)	Anterior rami of C1 and C2	*Unilateral:* Lateral flexion of the head at the atlanto-occipital joint *Bilateral:* Flexion of the head at the atlanto-occipital joint
④ Rectus capitis lateralis		C1 (transverse process)	Occipital bone (basilar part, lateral to occipital condyles)		
Scalene muscles					
⑤ Anterior scalene		C3–C6 (anterior tubercles of transverse processes)	1st rib (scalene tubercle)	Direct branches from cervical and brachial plexuses (C3–C8)	*With ribs mobile:* Elevates upper ribs (during forced inspiration) *With ribs fixed:* Bends cervical spine to same side (unilateral), flexes neck (bilateral)
⑥ Middle scalene		C1–C2 (transverse processes), C3–C7 (posterior tubercles of transverse processes)	1st rib (posterior to groove for subclavian artery)		
⑦ Posterior scalene		C5–C7 (posterior tubercles of transverse processes)	2nd rib (outer surface)		
Suboccipital muscles (short nuchal and craniovertebral joint muscles)					
⑧ Rectus capitis posterior minor		C1 (posterior tubercle)	Occipital bone (inner third of inferior nuchal line)	Posterior ramus of C1 (suboccipital n.)	*Unilateral:* Rotates head to same side *Bilateral:* Extends head
⑨ Rectus capitis posterior major		C2 (spinous process)	Occipital bone (middle third of inferior nuchal line)		
⑩ Obliquus capitis inferior			C1 (transverse process)		
⑪ Obliquus capitis superior		C1 (transverse process)	Occipital bone (above insertion of rectus capitis posterior major)		*Unilateral:* Tilts head to same side, rotates it to opposite side *Bilateral:* Extends head

Fig. 39.7 **Deep muscles of the neck**

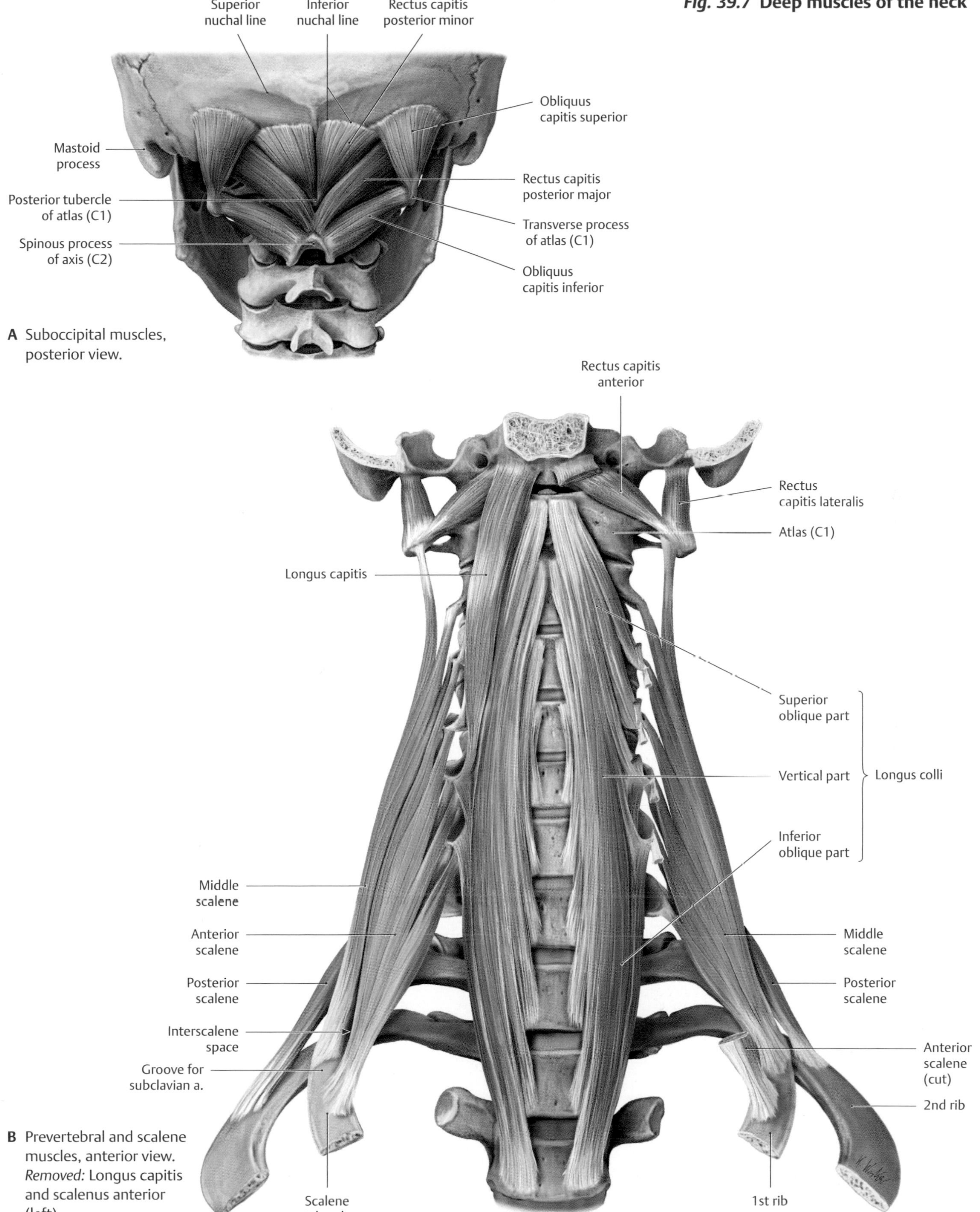
Superior nuchal line
Inferior nuchal line
Rectus capitis posterior minor
Obliquus capitis superior
Mastoid process
Rectus capitis posterior major
Posterior tubercle of atlas (C1)
Transverse process of atlas (C1)
Spinous process of axis (C2)
Obliquus capitis inferior
Rectus capitis anterior
Rectus capitis lateralis
Atlas (C1)
Longus capitis
Superior oblique part
Vertical part
Inferior oblique part
Longus colli
Middle scalene
Anterior scalene
Posterior scalene
Interscalene space
Groove for subclavian a.
Middle scalene
Posterior scalene
Anterior scalene (cut)
2nd rib
Scalene tubercle
1st rib

A Suboccipital muscles, posterior view.

B Prevertebral and scalene muscles, anterior view. *Removed:* Longus capitis and scalenus anterior (left).

Arteries & Veins of the Neck

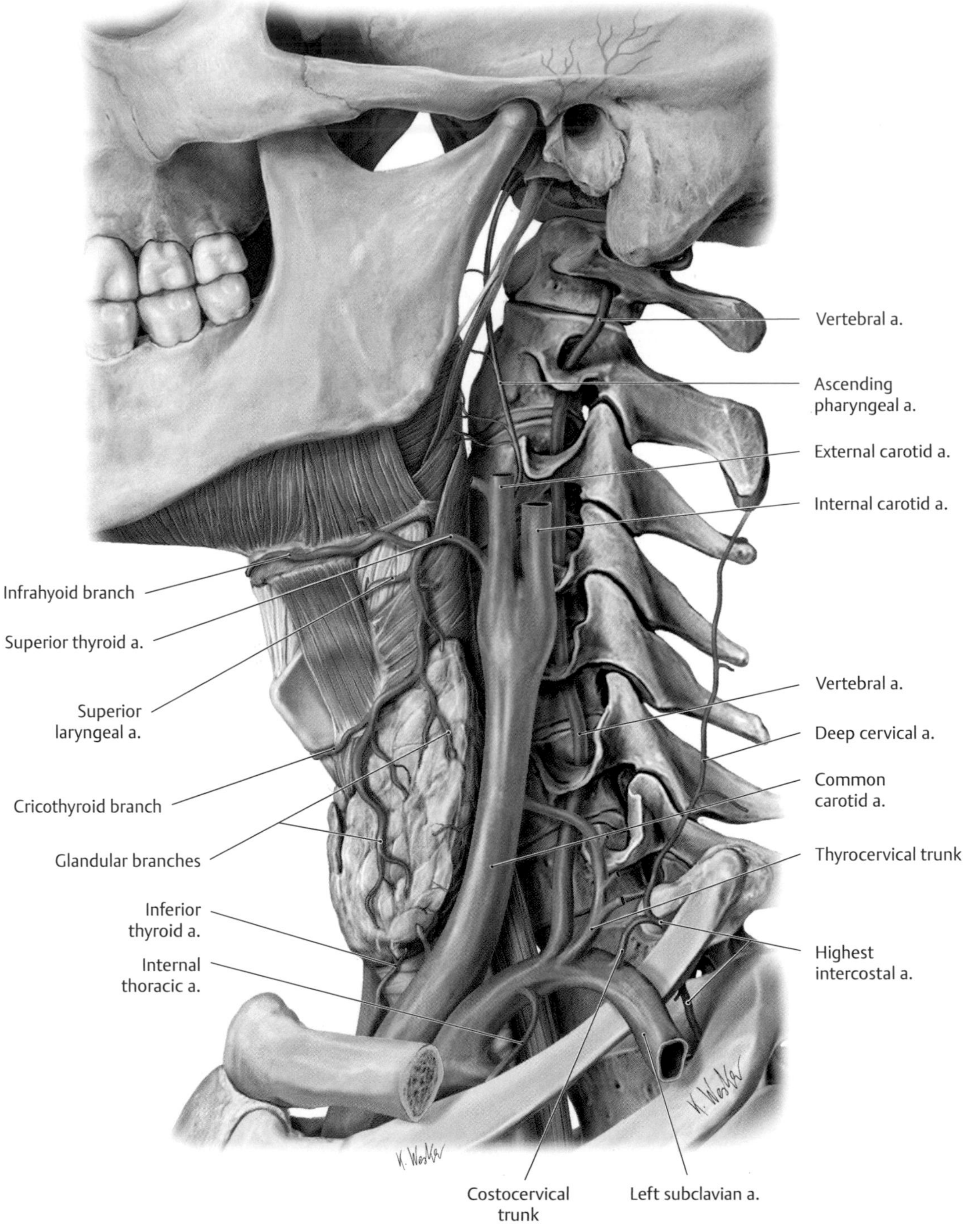
Vertebral a.
Ascending pharyngeal a.
External carotid a.
Internal carotid a.
Infrahyoid branch
Superior thyroid a.
Superior laryngeal a.
Vertebral a.
Deep cervical a.
Common carotid a.
Cricothyroid branch
Glandular branches
Thyrocervical trunk
Inferior thyroid a.
Internal thoracic a.
Highest intercostal a.
Costocervical trunk
Left subclavian a.

Fig. 39.8 **Arteries of the neck**
Left lateral view. The structures of the neck are primarily supplied by the external carotid artery (anterior branches) and the subclavian artery (vertebral artery, thyrocervical trunk, and costocervical trunk).

Fig. 39.9 **Veins of the neck**
Left lateral view. The principal veins of the neck are the internal, external, and anterior jugular veins.

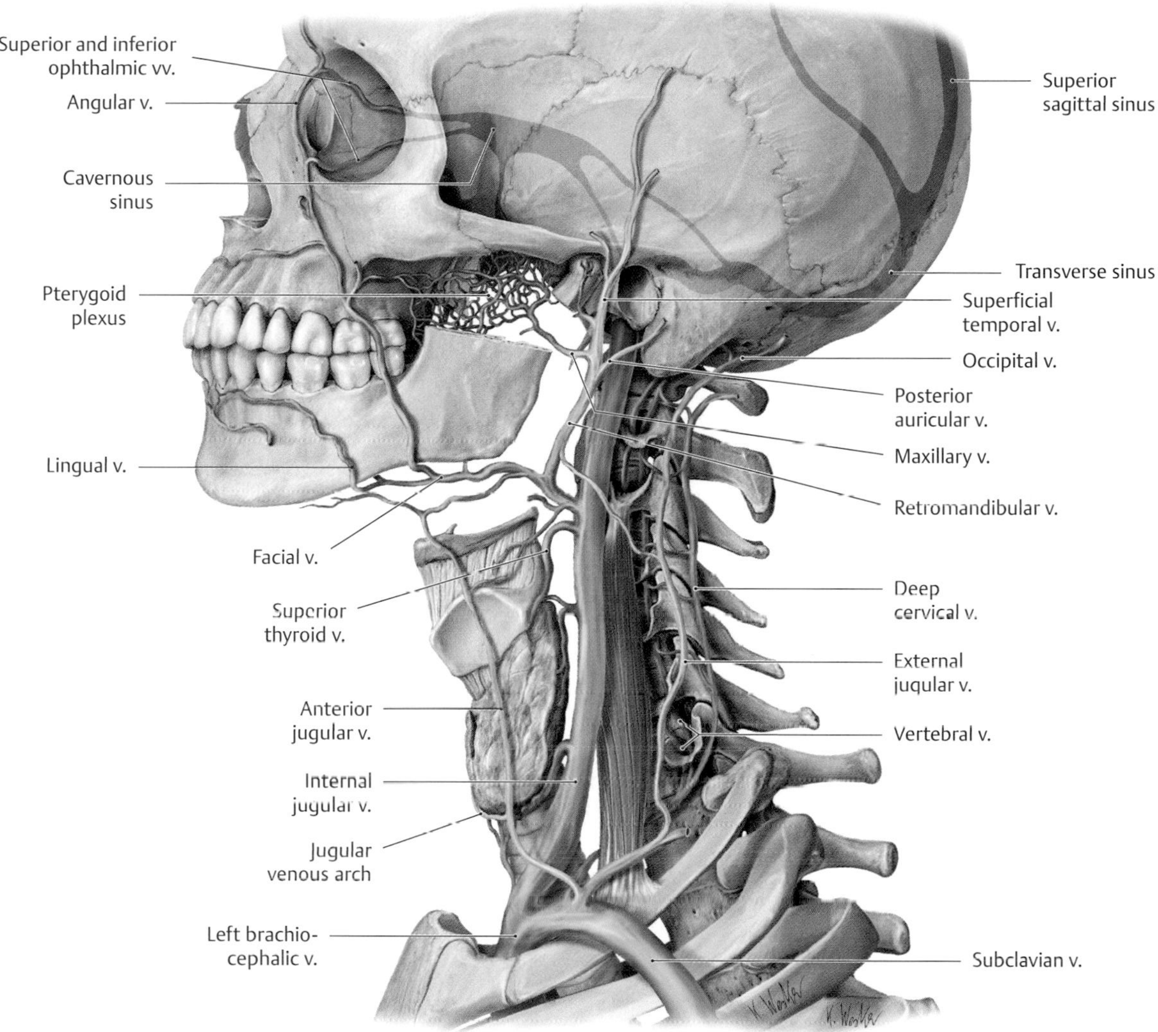
Superior and inferior ophthalmic vv.
Angular v.
Cavernous sinus
Pterygoid plexus
Lingual v.
Facial v.
Superior thyroid v.
Anterior jugular v.
Internal jugular v.
Jugular venous arch
Left brachio-cephalic v.
Superior sagittal sinus
Transverse sinus
Superficial temporal v.
Occipital v.
Posterior auricular v.
Maxillary v.
Retromandibular v.
Deep cervical v.
External jugular v.
Vertebral v.
Subclavian v.

Clinical

Impeded blood flow and veins of the neck
When clinical factors (e.g., chronic lung disease, mediastinal tumors, or infections) impede the flow of blood to the right heart, blood dams up in the superior vena cava and, consequently, the jugular veins (**A**). This causes conspicuous swelling in the jugular (and sometimes more minor) veins (**B**).

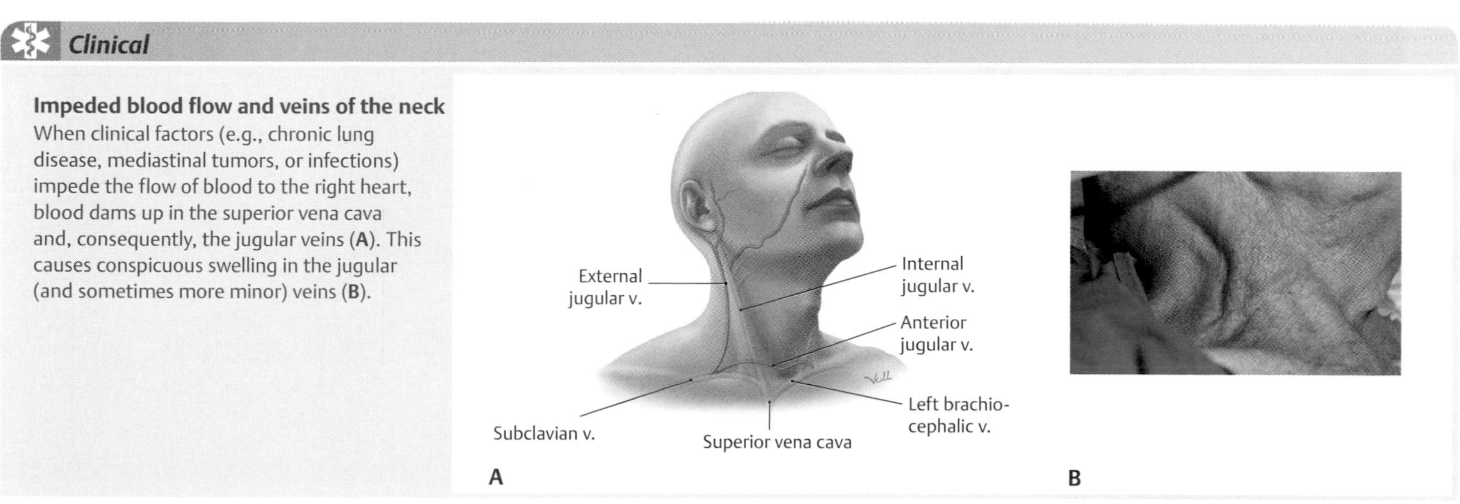
External jugular v.
Internal jugular v.
Anterior jugular v.
Left brachio-cephalic v.
Subclavian v.
Superior vena cava
A
B

Innervation of the Neck

Table 39.6 Branches of the spinal nerves in the neck

Posterior (dorsal) ramus

	Nerve	Sensory function	Motor function
C1	Suboccipital n.	No C1 dermatome	Innervate intrinsic nuchal muscles
C2	Greater occipital n.	Innervate C2 dermatome	
C3	3rd occipital n.	Innervate C3 dermatome	

Anterior (ventral) ramus

	Sensory branches	Sensory function	Motor branches	Motor function
C1	–	–	Form ansa cervicalis (motor part of cervical plexus)	Innervate infrahyoid muscles (except thyrohyoid)
C2	Lesser occipital n.	Form sensory part of cervical plexus, innervate anterior and lateral neck		
C2–C3	Great auricular n.			
	Transverse cervical n.			
C3–C4	Supraclavicular nn.		Contribute to phrenic n.*	Innervate diaphragm and pericardium*

* The anterior roots of C3–C5 combine to form the phrenic nerve (see p. 62).

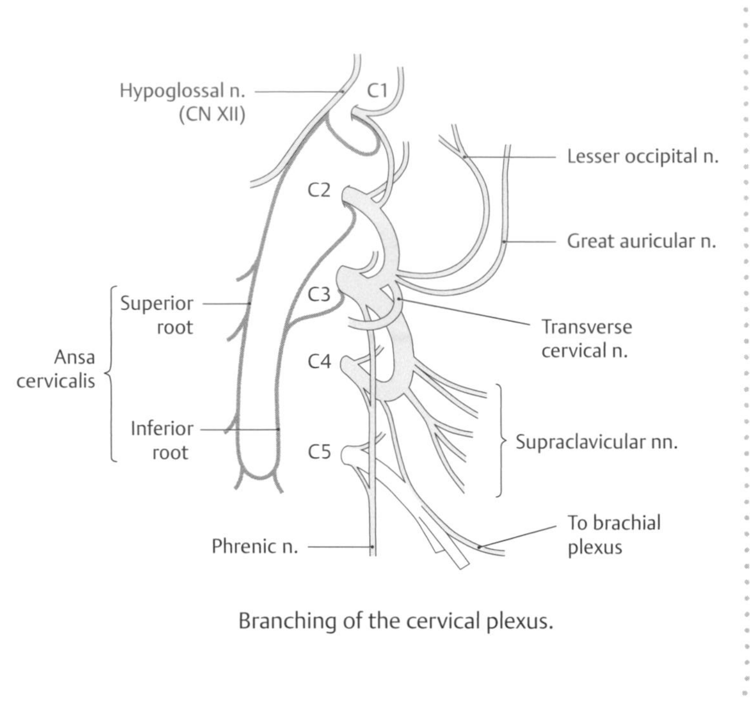

Hypoglossal n. (CN XII)
C1
C2
C3
C4
C5
Lesser occipital n.
Great auricular n.
Transverse cervical n.
Supraclavicular nn.
To brachial plexus
Phrenic n.
Ansa cervicalis
Superior root
Inferior root

Branching of the cervical plexus.

Fig. 39.10 **Sensory innervation of the nuchal region**
Posterior view.

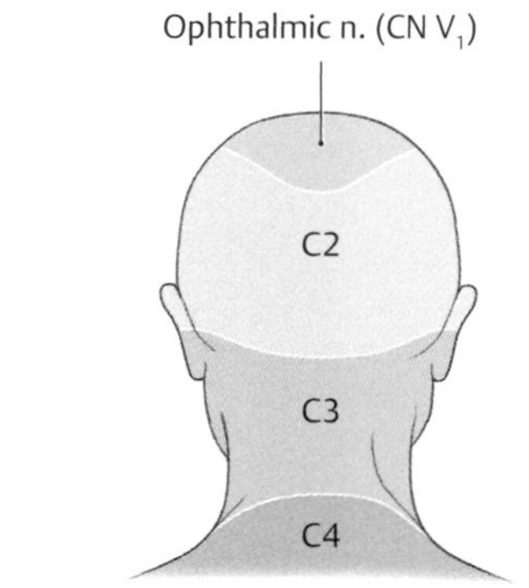

Ophthalmic n. (CN V_1)
C2
C3
C4

A Dermatomes.

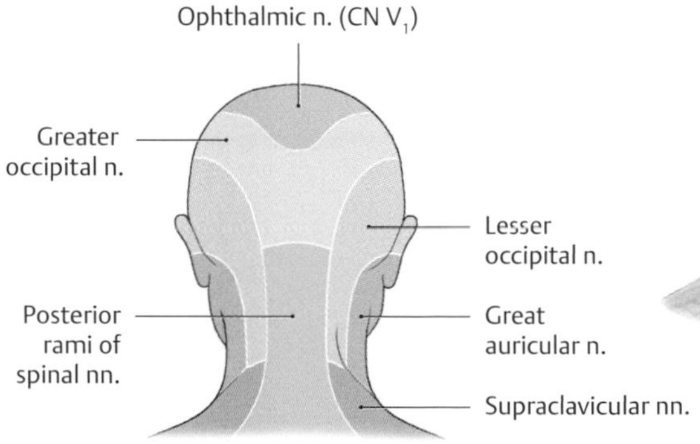

Ophthalmic n. (CN V_1)
Greater occipital n.
Lesser occipital n.
Posterior rami of spinal nn.
Great auricular n.
Supraclavicular nn.

B Cutaneous nerve territories.

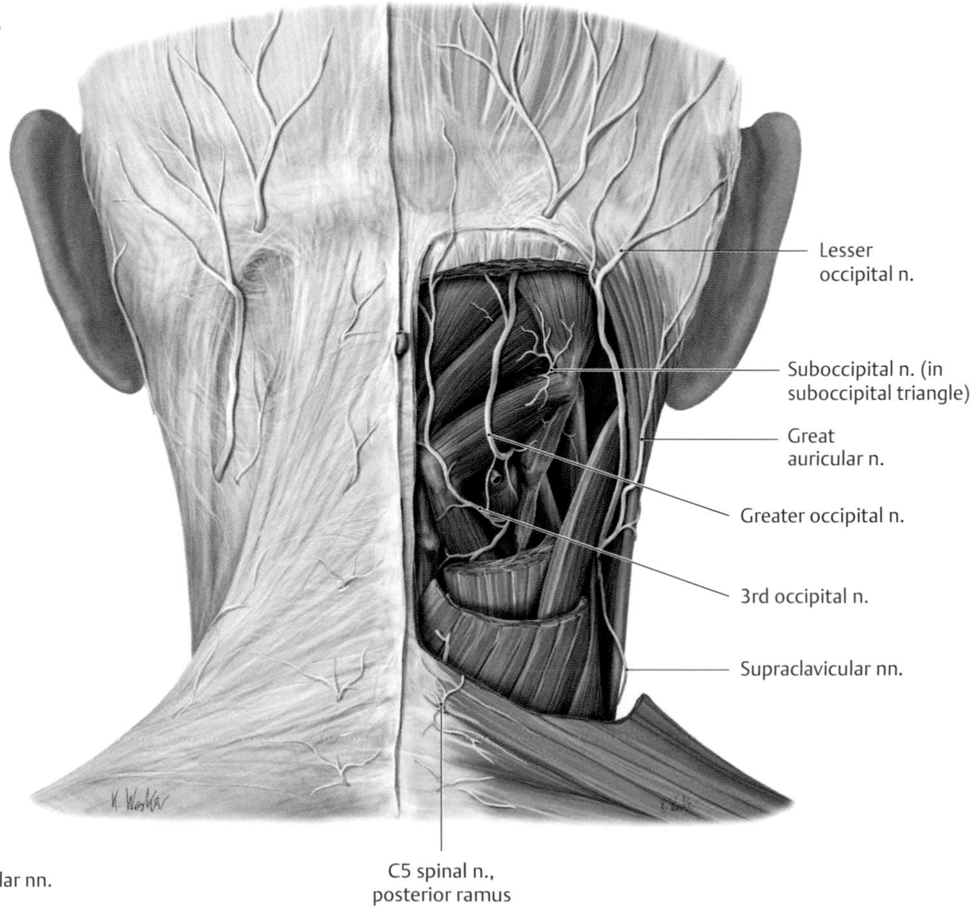

Lesser occipital n.
Suboccipital n. (in suboccipital triangle)
Great auricular n.
Greater occipital n.
3rd occipital n.
Supraclavicular nn.
C5 spinal n., posterior ramus

C Spinal nerve branches.

Fig. 39.11 **Sensory innervation of the anterolateral neck**
Left lateral view.

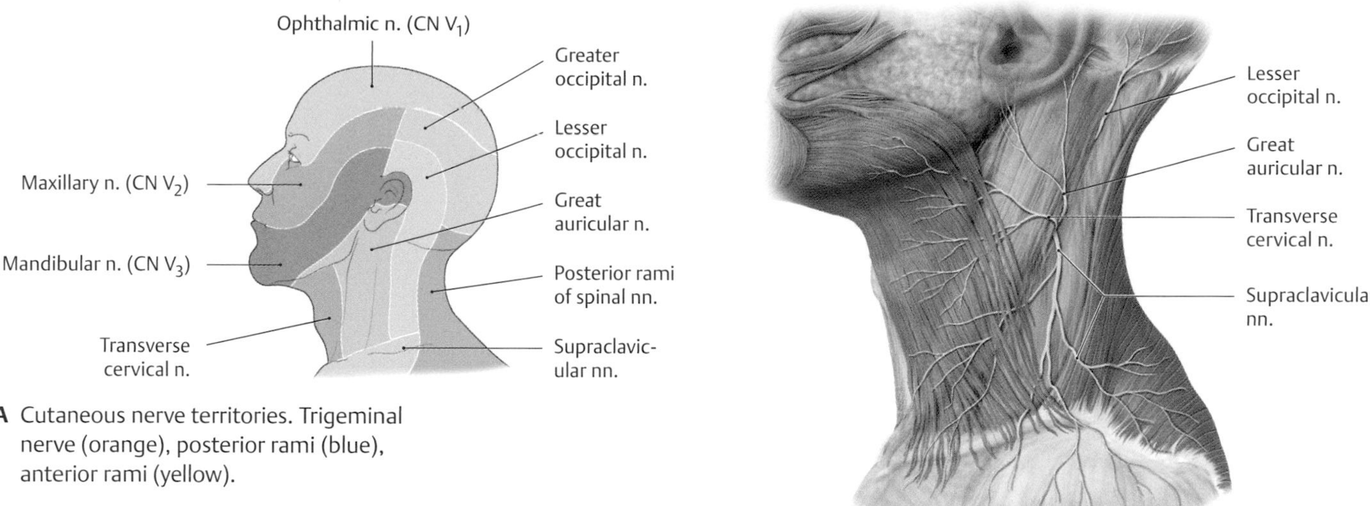
Ophthalmic n. (CN V_1)
Greater occipital n.
Lesser occipital n.
Maxillary n. (CN V_2)
Great auricular n.
Mandibular n. (CN V_3)
Posterior rami of spinal nn.
Transverse cervical n.
Supraclavicular nn.
Lesser occipital n.
Great auricular n.
Transverse cervical n.
Supraclavicular nn.

A Cutaneous nerve territories. Trigeminal nerve (orange), posterior rami (blue), anterior rami (yellow).

B Sensory branches of the cervical plexus.

Fig. 39.12 **Motor innervation of the anterolateral neck**
Left lateral view.

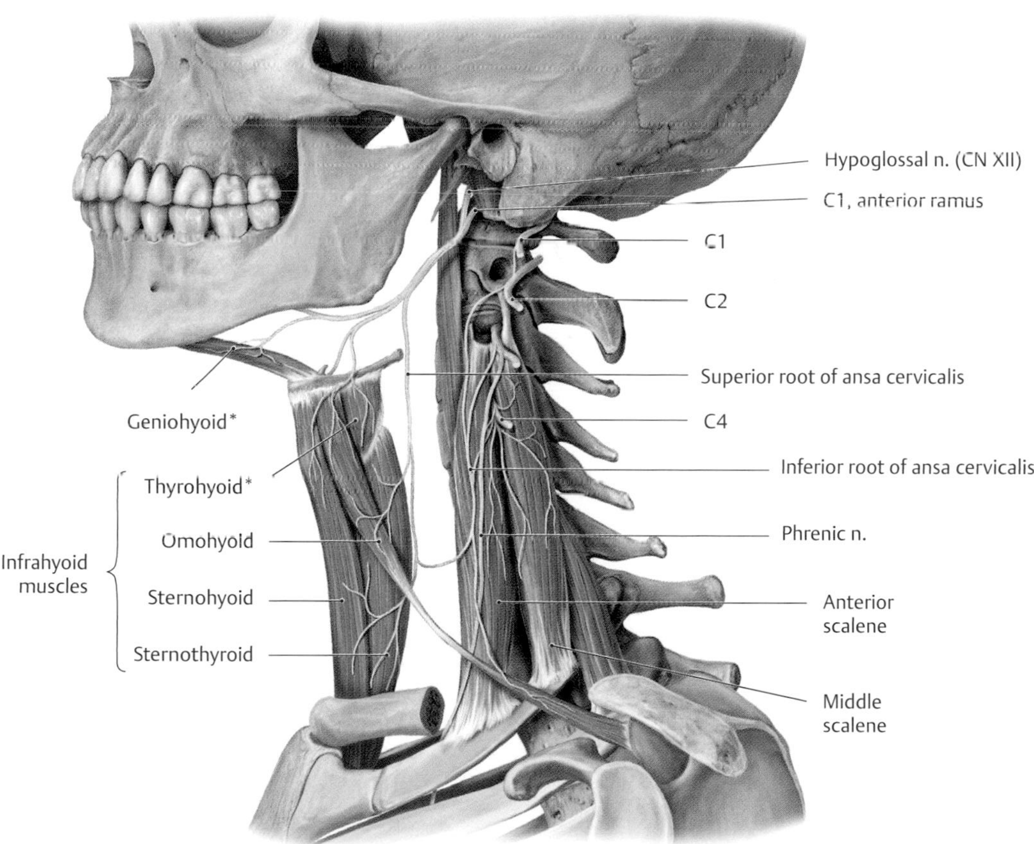
Hypoglossal n. (CN XII)
C1, anterior ramus
C1
C2
Superior root of ansa cervicalis
C4
Inferior root of ansa cervicalis
Phrenic n.
Anterior scalene
Middle scalene
Geniohyoid*
Thyrohyoid*
Omohyoid
Sternohyoid
Sternothyroid
Infrahyoid muscles

* Innervated by the anterior ramus of C1 (distributed by the hypoglossal n.).

Larynx: Cartilage & Structure

Fig. 39.13 **Laryngeal cartilages**
Left lateral view. The larynx consists of five laryngeal cartilages: epiglottic, thyroid, cricoid, and the paired arytenoid and corniculate cartilages. They are connected to each other, the trachea, and the hyoid bone by elastic ligaments.

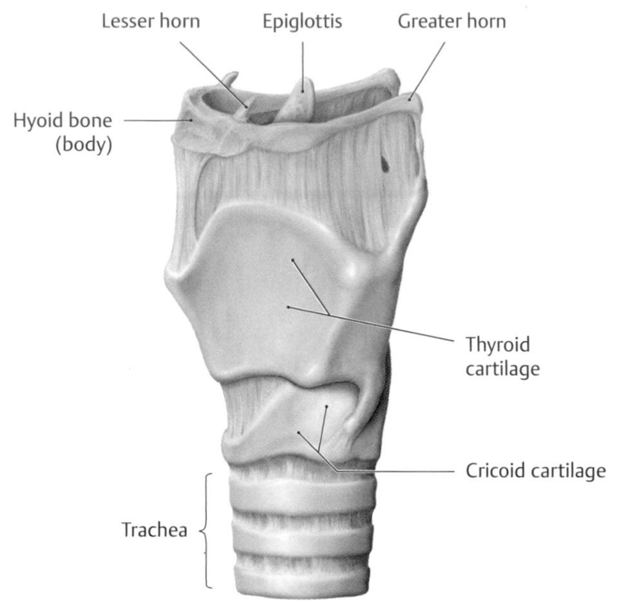

Lesser horn
Epiglottis
Greater horn
Hyoid bone (body)
Thyroid cartilage
Cricoid cartilage
Trachea

Fig. 39.14 **Epiglottic cartilage**
The elastic epiglottic cartilage comprises the internal skeleton of the epiglottis, providing resilience to return it to its initial position after swallowing.

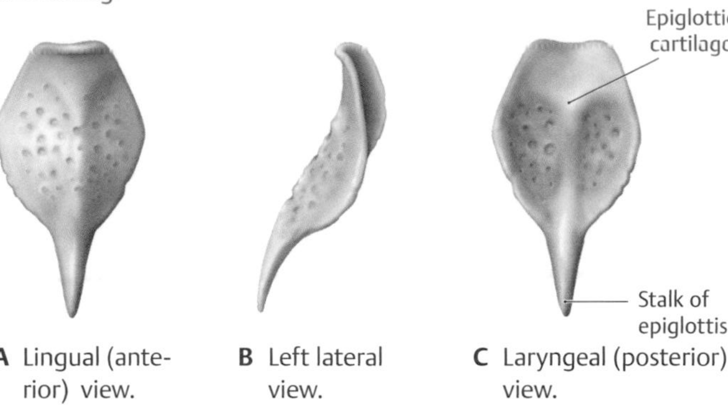

Epiglottic cartilage
Stalk of epiglottis

A Lingual (anterior) view. **B** Left lateral view. **C** Laryngeal (posterior) view.

Fig. 39.15 **Thyroid cartilage**
Left oblique view.

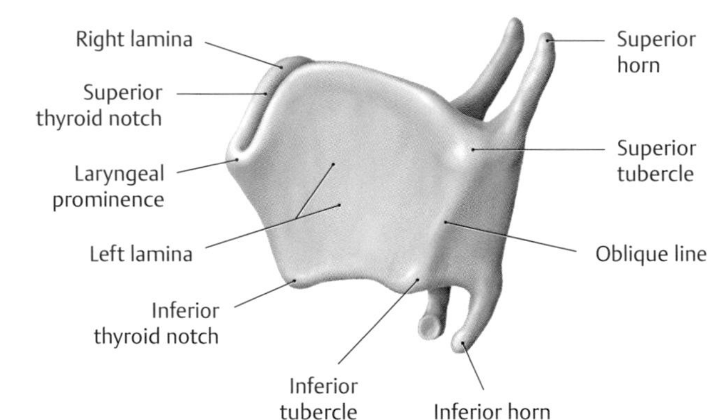

Right lamina
Superior thyroid notch
Laryngeal prominence
Left lamina
Inferior thyroid notch
Inferior tubercle
Inferior horn
Oblique line
Superior tubercle
Superior horn

Fig. 39.16 **Cricoid cartilage**

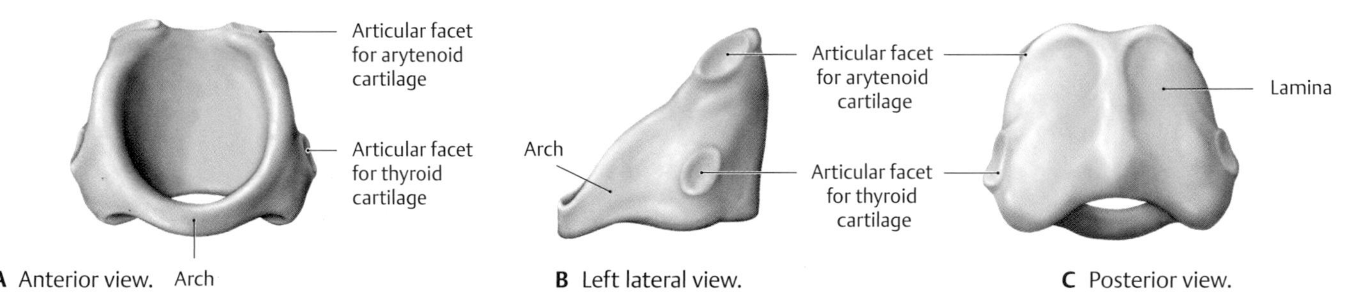

Articular facet for arytenoid cartilage
Articular facet for thyroid cartilage
Arch
Articular facet for arytenoid cartilage
Articular facet for thyroid cartilage
Lamina

A Anterior view. **B** Left lateral view. **C** Posterior view.

Fig. 39.17 **Arytenoid and corniculate cartilages**
Right cartilages.

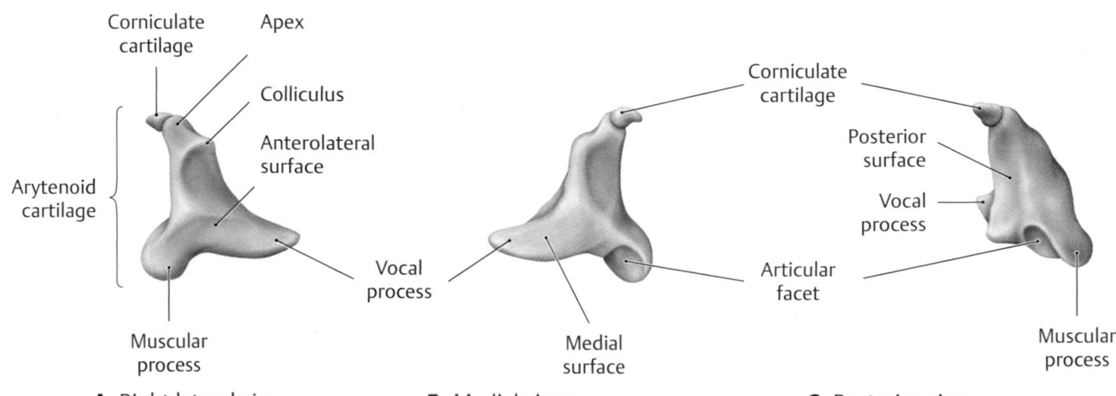

Corniculate cartilage
Apex
Colliculus
Anterolateral surface
Arytenoid cartilage
Muscular process
Vocal process
Medial surface
Corniculate cartilage
Articular facet
Posterior surface
Vocal process
Muscular process

A Right lateral view. **B** Medial view. **C** Posterior view.

***Fig. 39.18* Structure of the larynx**
The larynx is suspended from the hyoid bone, primarily by the thyrohyoid membrane. The hyoid bone provides the sites for attachment of the suprahyoid and infrahyoid muscles.

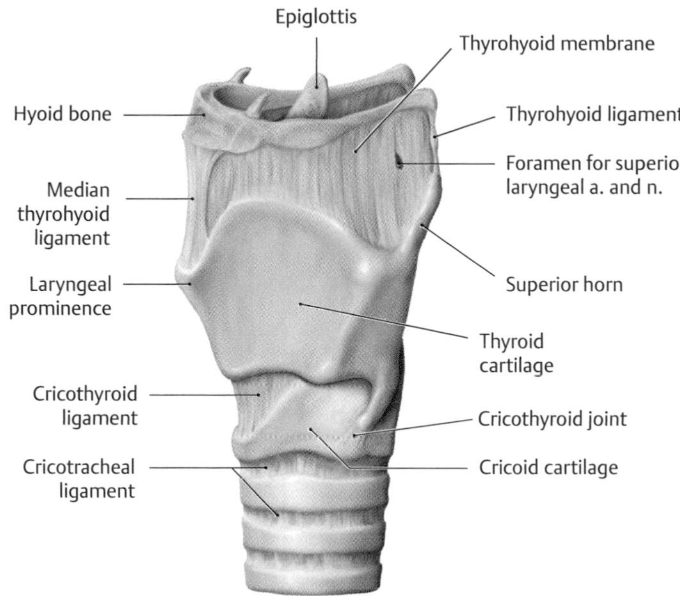
Epiglottis
Thyrohyoid membrane
Hyoid bone
Thyrohyoid ligament
Foramen for superior laryngeal a. and n.
Median thyrohyoid ligament
Laryngeal prominence
Superior horn
Thyroid cartilage
Cricothyroid ligament
Cricothyroid joint
Cricotracheal ligament
Cricoid cartilage

A Left anterior oblique view.

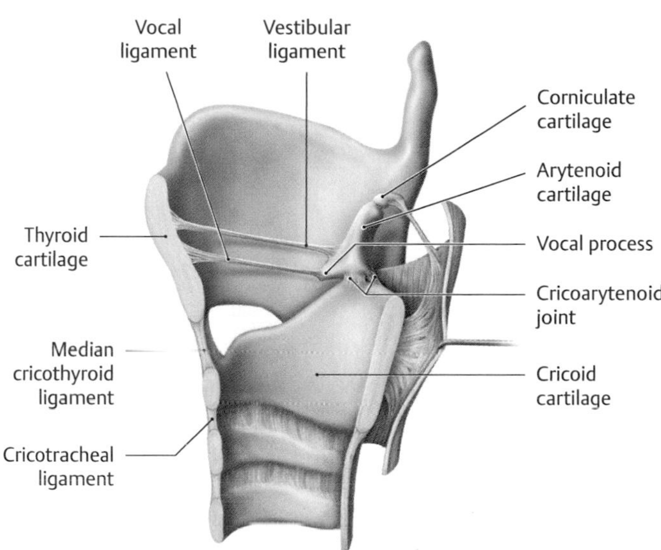
Vocal ligament
Vestibular ligament
Corniculate cartilage
Arytenoid cartilage
Thyroid cartilage
Vocal process
Cricoarytenoid joint
Median cricothyroid ligament
Cricoid cartilage
Cricotracheal ligament

B Sagittal section, viewed from the left medial aspect. The arytenoid cartilage alters the position of the vocal folds during phonation.

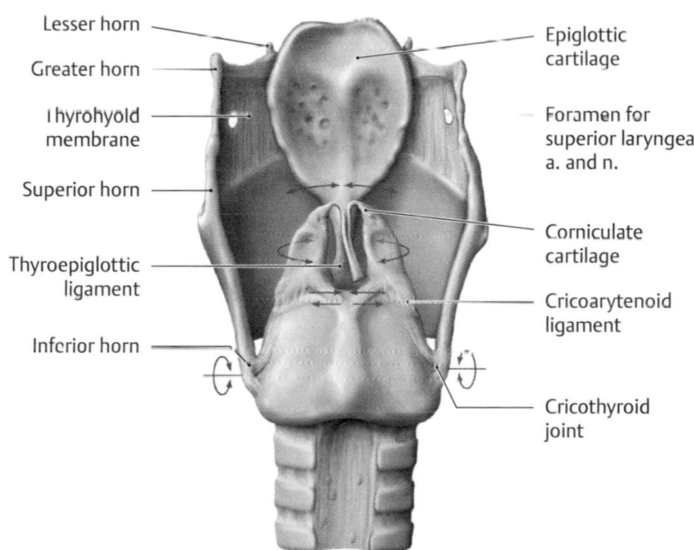
Lesser horn
Greater horn
Thyrohyoid membrane
Superior horn
Thyroepiglottic ligament
Inferior horn
Epiglottic cartilage
Foramen for superior laryngeal a. and n.
Corniculate cartilage
Cricoarytenoid ligament
Cricothyroid joint

C Posterior view. Arrows indicate the directions of movement in the various joints.

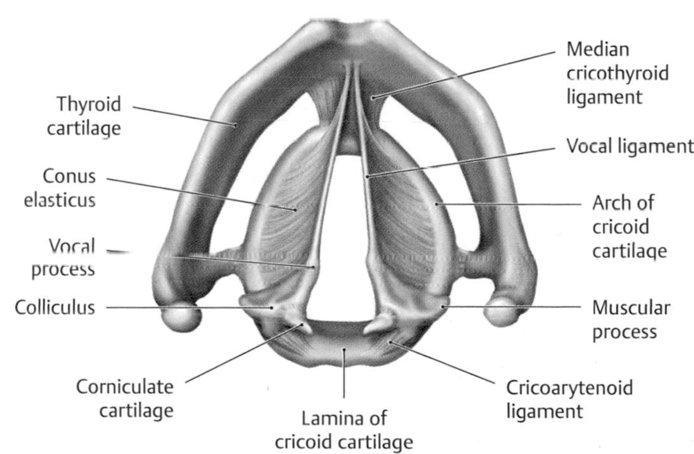
Median cricothyroid ligament
Thyroid cartilage
Vocal ligament
Conus elasticus
Arch of cricoid cartilage
Vocal process
Colliculus
Muscular process
Corniculate cartilage
Lamina of cricoid cartilage
Cricoarytenoid ligament

D Superior view.

Larynx: Muscles & Levels

Fig. 39.19 Laryngeal muscles

The laryngeal muscles move the laryngeal cartilages relative to one another, affecting the tension and/or position of the vocal folds. Muscles that move the larynx as a whole (infra- and suprahyoid muscles) are described on p. 590.

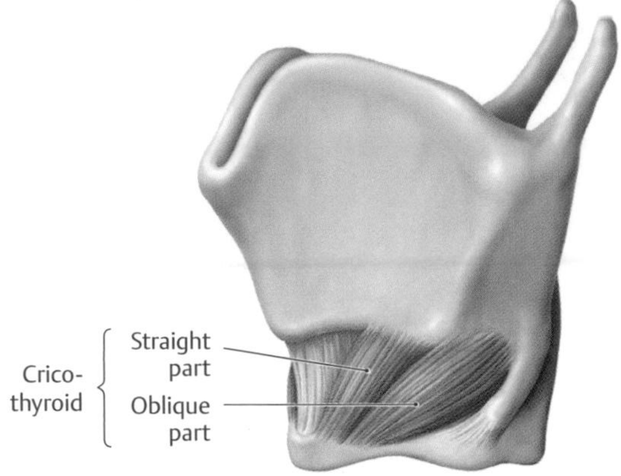
Crico-
thyroid
Straight
part
Oblique
part

A Intrinsic laryngeal muscles, left lateral oblique view.

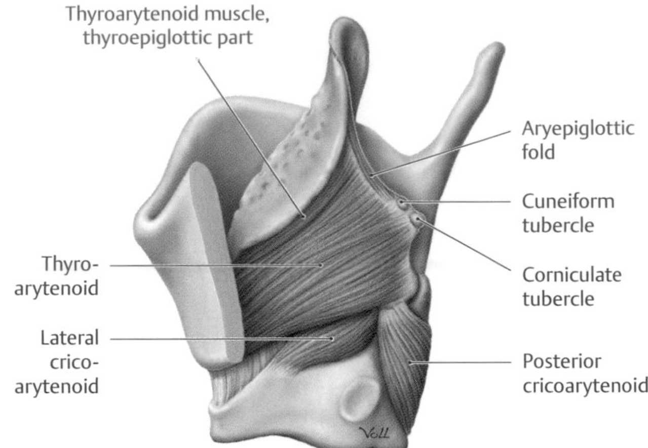
Thyroarytenoid muscle,
thyroepiglottic part
Aryepiglottic
fold
Cuneiform
tubercle
Corniculate
tubercle
Thyro-
arytenoid
Lateral
crico-
arytenoid
Posterior
cricoarytenoid

B Intrinsic laryngeal muscles, left lateral view. *Removed:* Thyroid cartilage (left half). *Revealed:* Epiglottis and external thyroarytenoid muscle.

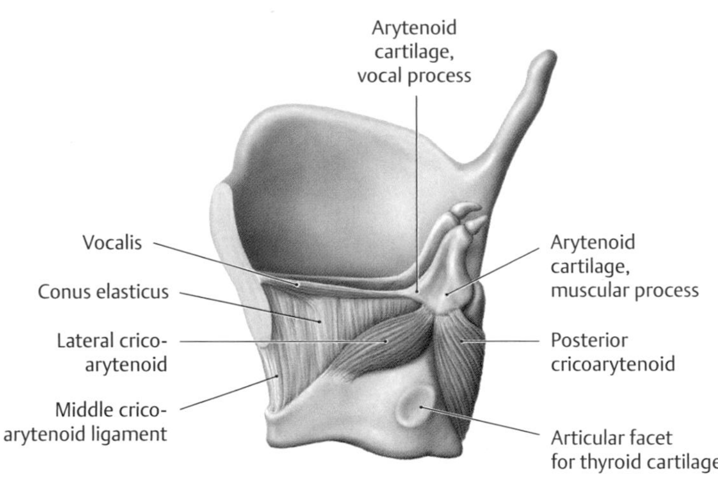
Arytenoid
cartilage,
vocal process
Vocalis
Conus elasticus
Lateral crico-
arytenoid
Middle crico-
arytenoid ligament
Arytenoid
cartilage,
muscular process
Posterior
cricoarytenoid
Articular facet
for thyroid cartilage

C Left lateral view with the epiglottis removed.

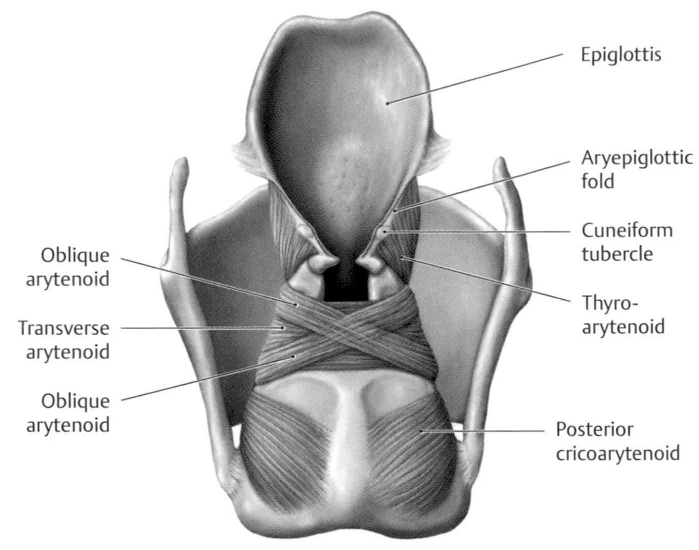
Epiglottis
Aryepiglottic
fold
Cuneiform
tubercle
Thyro-
arytenoid
Oblique
arytenoid
Transverse
arytenoid
Oblique
arytenoid
Posterior
cricoarytenoid

D Posterior view.

① ② ③ ④ ⑤ ⑥

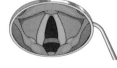

A Laryngeal muscles, superior view.

B Open rima glottidis.

C Closed rima glottidis.

Table 39.7	Actions of the laryngeal muscles	
Muscle	**Action**	**Effect on rima glottidis**
① Cricothyroid m.*	Tightens the vocal folds	None
② Vocalis m.	Tightens the vocal folds	None
③ Thyroarytenoid m.	Adducts the vocal folds	Closes
④ Transverse arytenoid m.	Adducts the vocal folds	Closes
⑤ Posterior cricoarytenoid m.	Abducts the vocal folds	Opens
⑥ Lateral cricoarytenoid m.	Adducts the vocal folds	Closes

* The cricothyroid is innervated by the external laryngeal nerve. All other intrinsic laryngeal muscles are innervated by the recurrent laryngeal nerve.

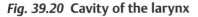

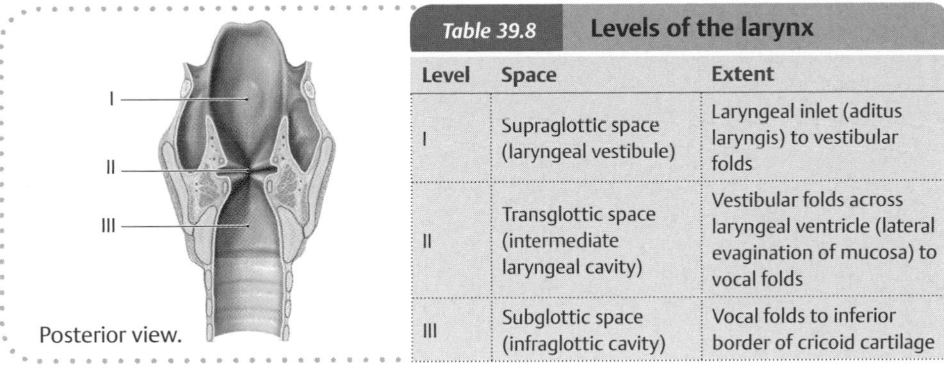

I
II
III
Posterior view.

Table 39.8 Levels of the larynx

Level	Space	Extent
I	Supraglottic space (laryngeal vestibule)	Laryngeal inlet (aditus laryngis) to vestibular folds
II	Transglottic space (intermediate laryngeal cavity)	Vestibular folds across laryngeal ventricle (lateral evagination of mucosa) to vocal folds
III	Subglottic space (infraglottic cavity)	Vocal folds to inferior border of cricoid cartilage

Fig. 39.20 **Cavity of the larynx**

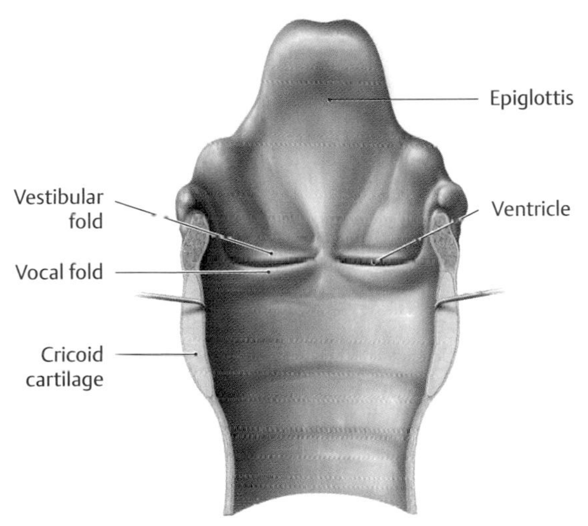

Epiglottis
Vestibular fold
Ventricle
Vocal fold
Cricoid cartilage

A Posterior view with the larynx splayed open.

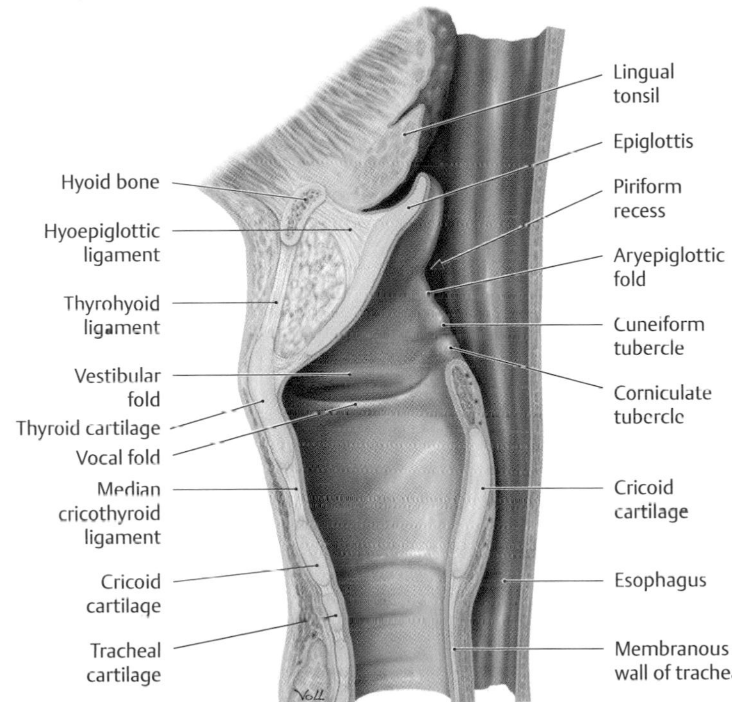

Lingual tonsil
Epiglottis
Hyoid bone
Piriform recess
Hyoepiglottic ligament
Aryepiglottic fold
Thyrohyoid ligament
Cuneiform tubercle
Vestibular fold
Corniculate tubercle
Thyroid cartilage
Vocal fold
Median cricothyroid ligament
Cricoid cartilage
Cricoid cartilage
Esophagus
Tracheal cartilage
Membranous wall of trachea

B Midsagittal section viewed from the left side.

Fig. 39.21 **Vestibular and vocal folds**

Coronal section, superior view.

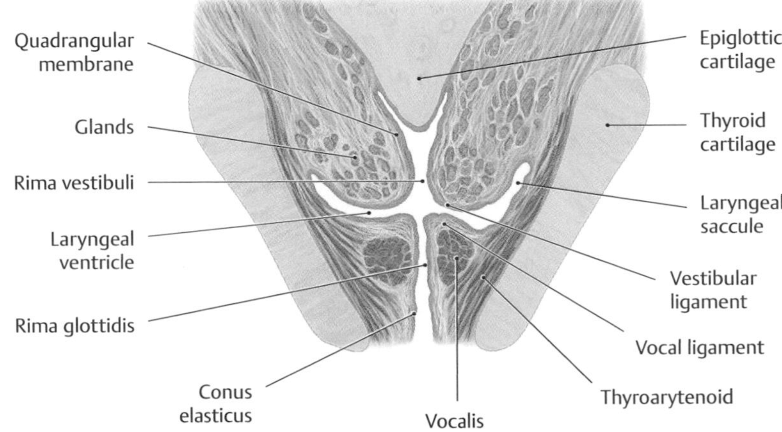

Quadrangular membrane
Epiglottic cartilage
Glands
Thyroid cartilage
Rima vestibuli
Laryngeal saccule
Laryngeal ventricle
Vestibular ligament
Rima glottidis
Vocal ligament
Conus elasticus
Vocalis
Thyroarytenoid

Neurovasculature of the Larynx, Thyroid & Parathyroids

Fig. 39.22 **Thyroid and parathyroid glands**

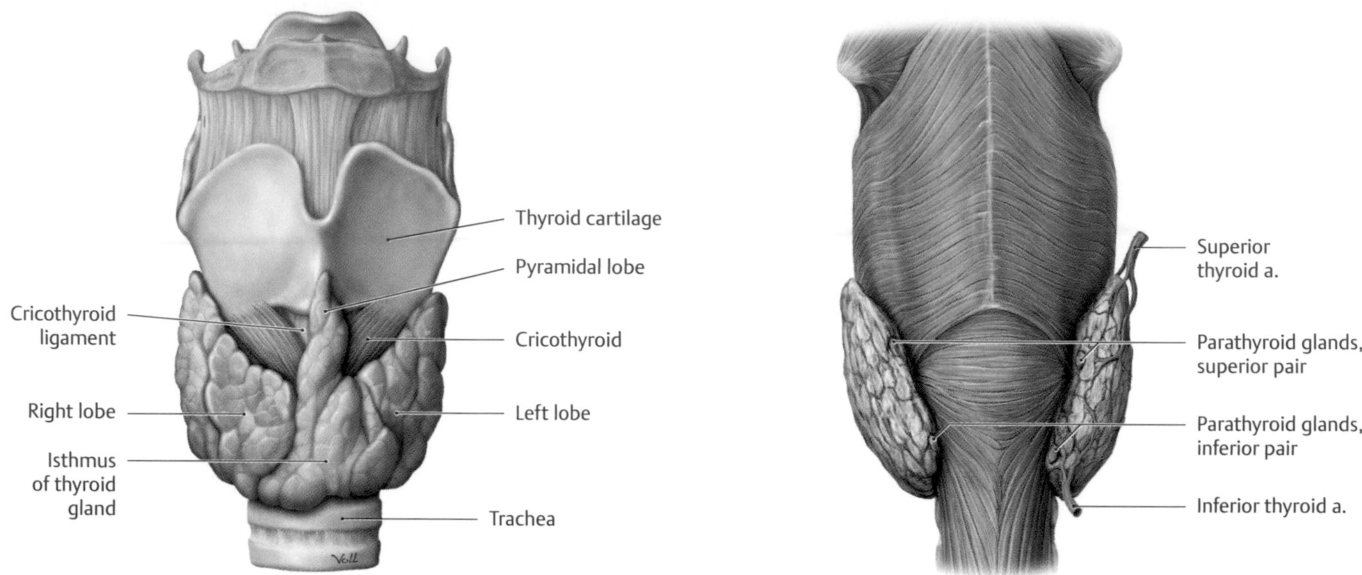
Thyroid cartilage
Pyramidal lobe
Cricothyroid ligament
Cricothyroid
Right lobe
Left lobe
Isthmus of thyroid gland
Trachea
Superior thyroid a.
Parathyroid glands, superior pair
Parathyroid glands, inferior pair
Inferior thyroid a.

A Thyroid gland, anterior view.

B Thyroid and parathyroid glands, posterior view.

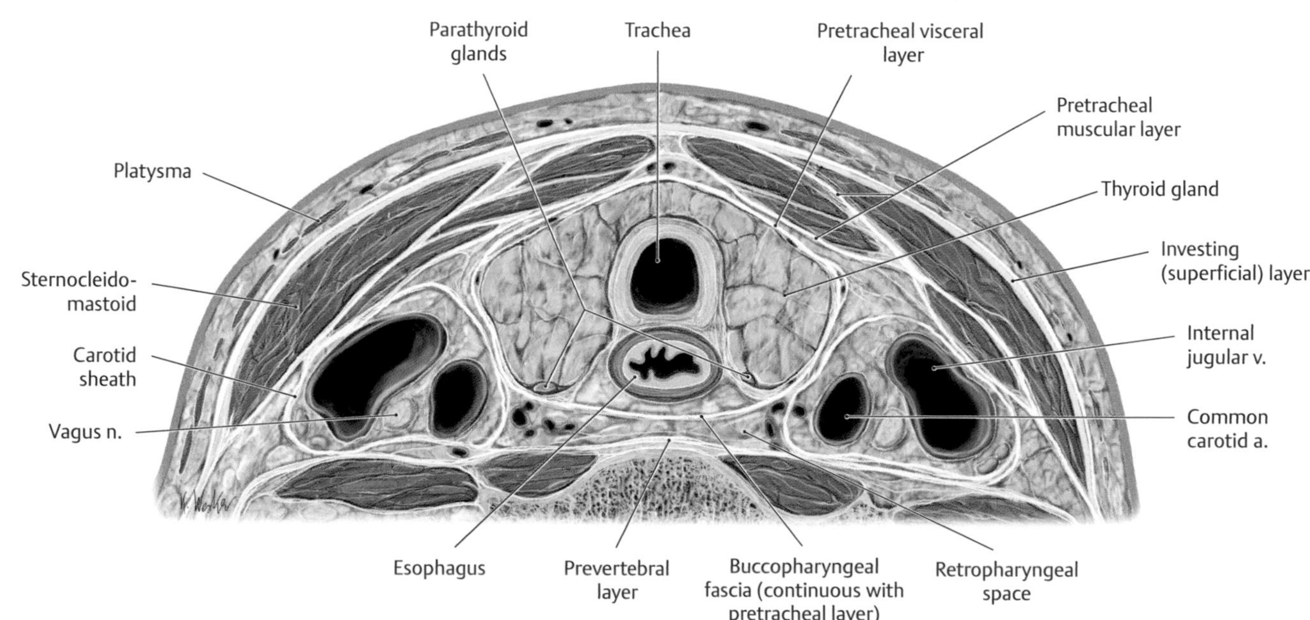
Parathyroid glands
Trachea
Pretracheal visceral layer
Pretracheal muscular layer
Platysma
Thyroid gland
Investing (superficial) layer
Sternocleido-mastoid
Internal jugular v.
Carotid sheath
Vagus n.
Common carotid a.
Esophagus
Prevertebral layer
Buccopharyngeal fascia (continuous with pretracheal layer)
Retropharyngeal space

C Topographical relations of the thyroid and parathyroid glands. See p. 605 for coverage of the layers of the deep cervical fascia, shown here.

Fig. 39.23 Arteries and nerves
Anterior view.

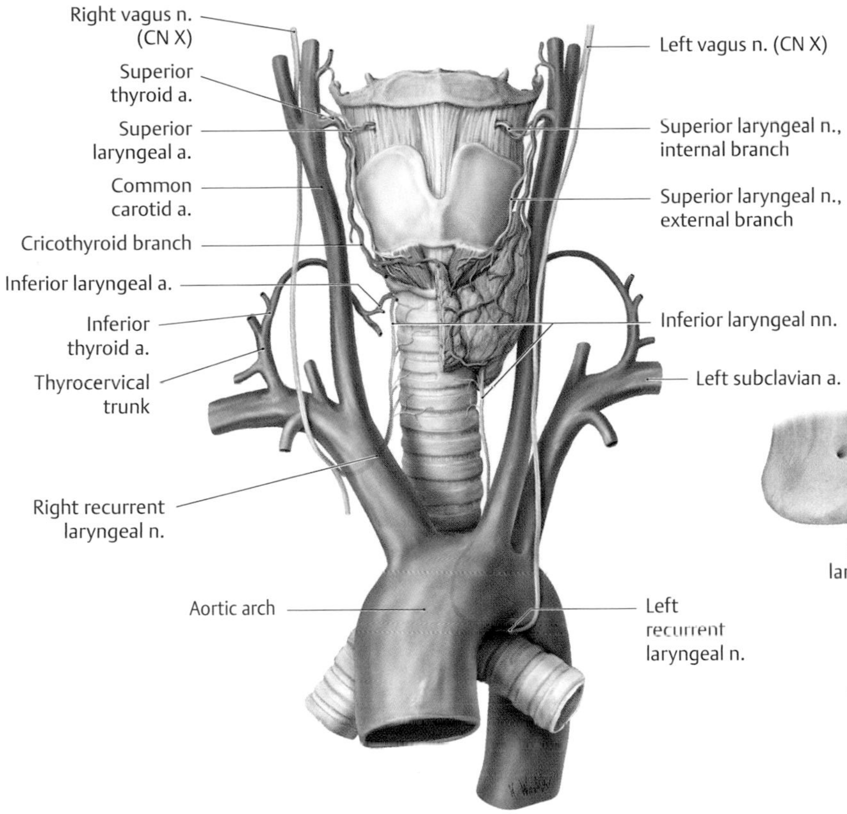

Right vagus n. (CN X)
Superior thyroid a.
Superior laryngeal a.
Common carotid a.
Cricothyroid branch
Inferior laryngeal a.
Inferior thyroid a.
Thyrocervical trunk
Right recurrent laryngeal n.
Aortic arch
Left vagus n. (CN X)
Superior laryngeal n., internal branch
Superior laryngeal n., external branch
Inferior laryngeal nn.
Left subclavian a.
Left recurrent laryngeal n.

Fig. 39.24 Veins
Left lateral view. *Note:* The inferior thyroid vein generally drains into the left brachiocephalic vein.

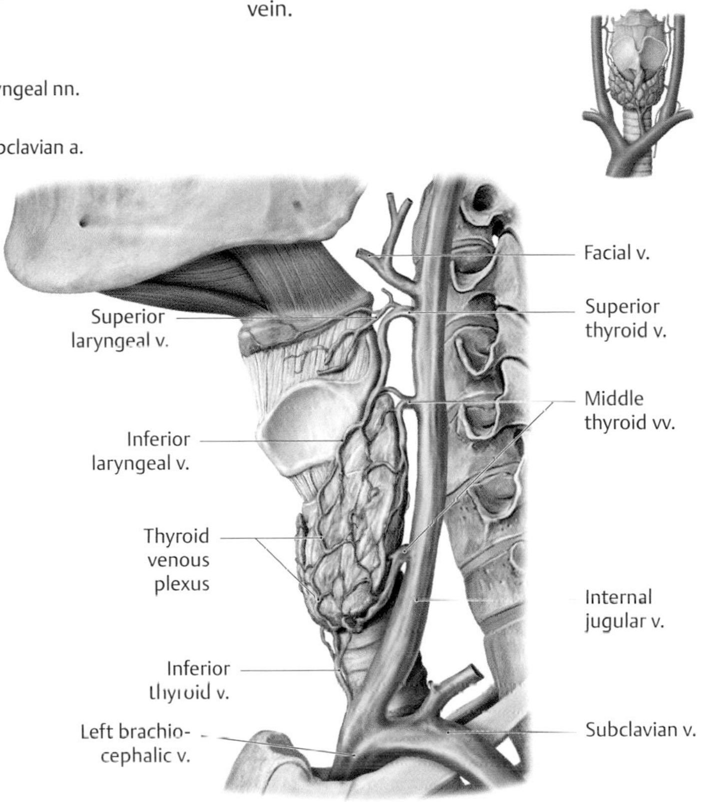

Superior laryngeal v.
Inferior laryngeal v.
Thyroid venous plexus
Inferior thyroid v.
Left brachio-cephalic v.
Facial v.
Superior thyroid v.
Middle thyroid vv.
Internal jugular v.
Subclavian v.

Fig. 39.25 Neurovasculature
Left lateral view.

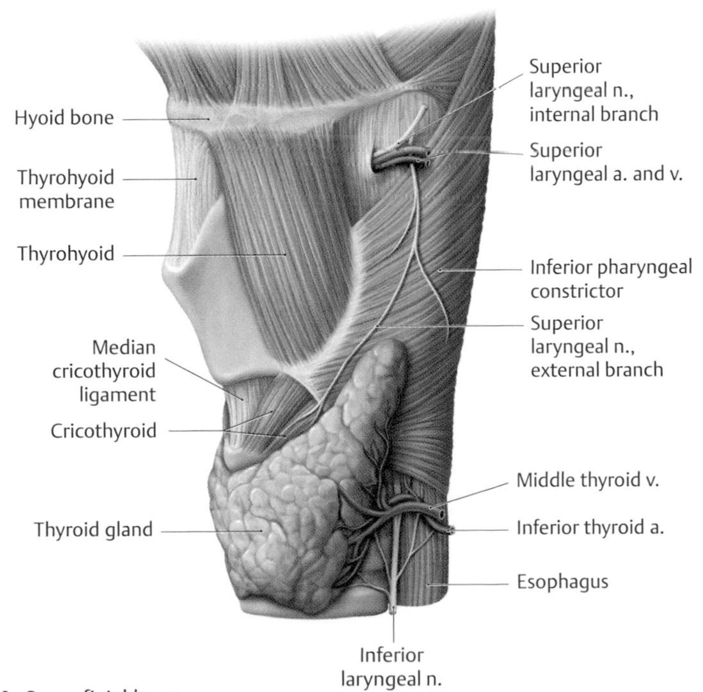
Hyoid bone
Thyrohyoid membrane
Thyrohyoid
Median cricothyroid ligament
Cricothyroid
Thyroid gland
Superior laryngeal n., internal branch
Superior laryngeal a. and v.
Inferior pharyngeal constrictor
Superior laryngeal n., external branch
Middle thyroid v.
Inferior thyroid a.
Esophagus
Inferior laryngeal n.

A Superficial layer.

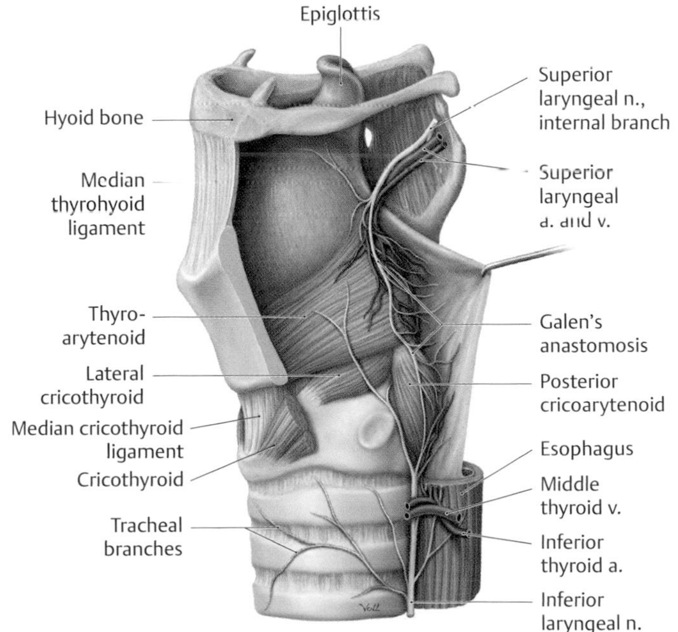
Epiglottis
Hyoid bone
Median thyrohyoid ligament
Thyro-arytenoid
Lateral cricothyroid
Median cricothyroid ligament
Cricothyroid
Tracheal branches
Superior laryngeal n., internal branch
Superior laryngeal a. and v.
Galen's anastomosis
Posterior cricoarytenoid
Esophagus
Middle thyroid v.
Inferior thyroid a.
Inferior laryngeal n.

B Deep layer. *Removed:* Cricothyroid muscle and left lamina of thyroid cartilage. *Retracted:* Pharyngeal mucosa.

Topography of the Neck: Regions & Fascia

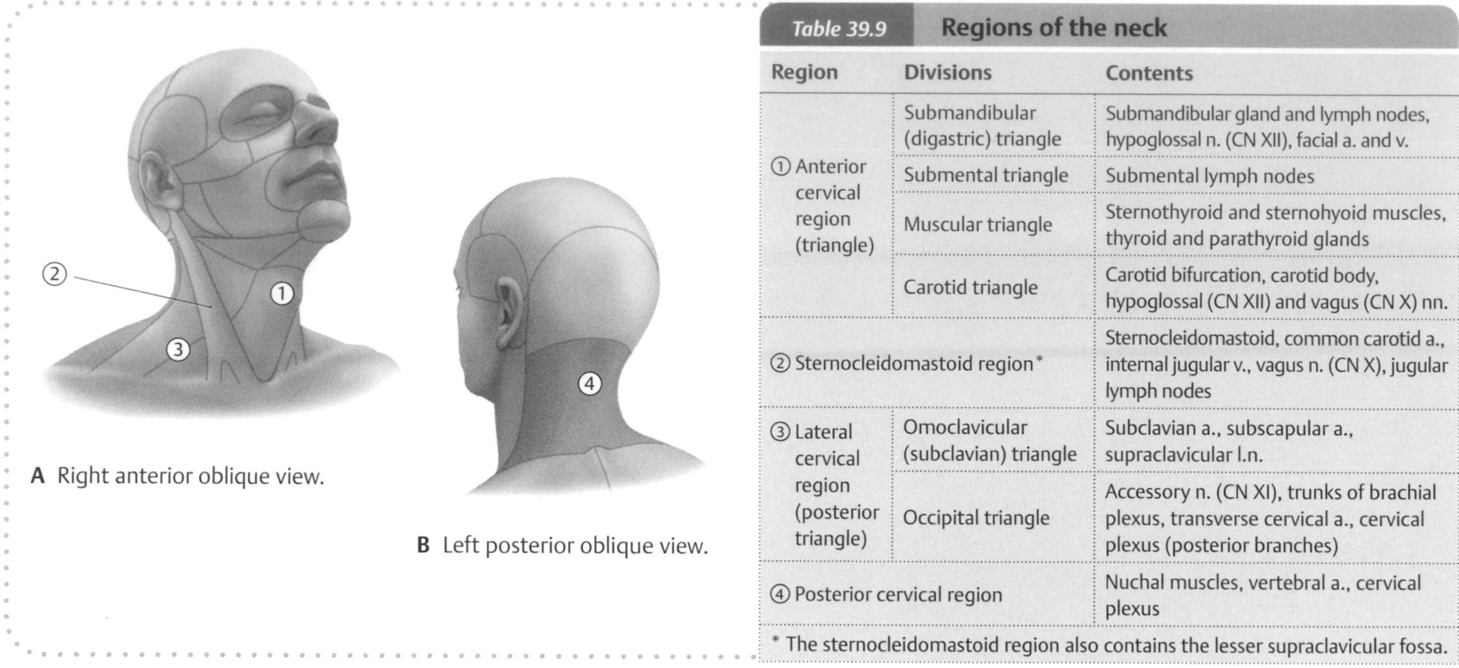

②
①
③
④

A Right anterior oblique view.

B Left posterior oblique view.

Table 39.9 Regions of the neck

Region	Divisions	Contents
① Anterior cervical region (triangle)	Submandibular (digastric) triangle	Submandibular gland and lymph nodes, hypoglossal n. (CN XII), facial a. and v.
	Submental triangle	Submental lymph nodes
	Muscular triangle	Sternothyroid and sternohyoid muscles, thyroid and parathyroid glands
	Carotid triangle	Carotid bifurcation, carotid body, hypoglossal (CN XII) and vagus (CN X) nn.
② Sternocleidomastoid region*		Sternocleidomastoid, common carotid a., internal jugular v., vagus n. (CN X), jugular lymph nodes
③ Lateral cervical region (posterior triangle)	Omoclavicular (subclavian) triangle	Subclavian a., subscapular a., supraclavicular l.n.
	Occipital triangle	Accessory n. (CN XI), trunks of brachial plexus, transverse cervical a., cervical plexus (posterior branches)
④ Posterior cervical region		Nuchal muscles, vertebral a., cervical plexus

* The sternocleidomastoid region also contains the lesser supraclavicular fossa.

Fig. 39.26 **Cervical regions**

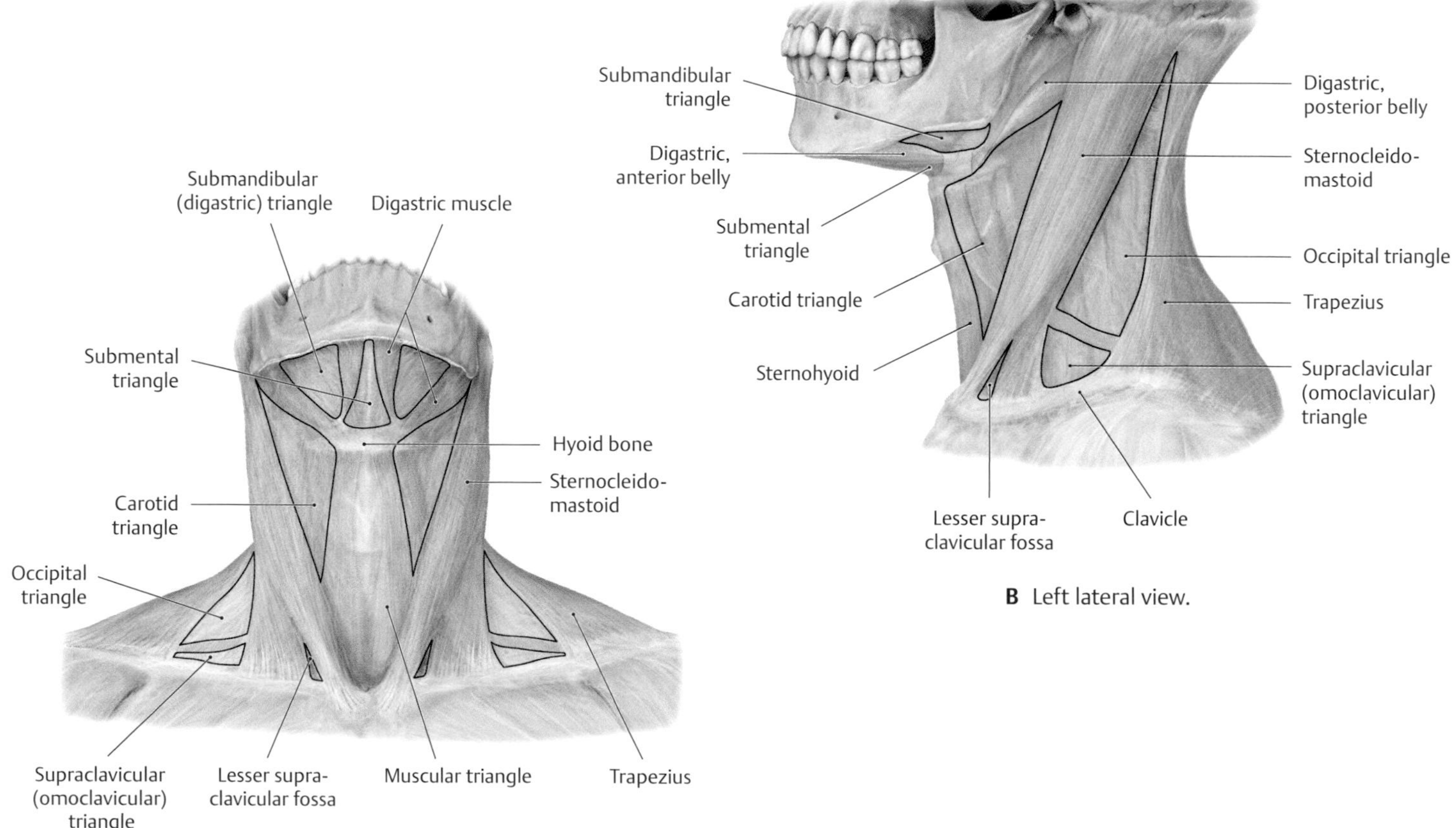

Submandibular (digastric) triangle
Digastric muscle
Submental triangle
Hyoid bone
Sternocleido-mastoid
Carotid triangle
Occipital triangle
Supraclavicular (omoclavicular) triangle
Lesser supra-clavicular fossa
Muscular triangle
Trapezius
Submandibular triangle
Digastric, anterior belly
Submental triangle
Carotid triangle
Sternohyoid
Digastric, posterior belly
Sternocleido-mastoid
Occipital triangle
Trapezius
Supraclavicular (omoclavicular) triangle
Lesser supra-clavicular fossa
Clavicle

A Anterior view.

B Left lateral view.

Table 39.10 Deep cervical fascia

The deep cervical fascia is divided into four layers that enclose the structures of the neck.

Layer	Type of fascia	Description
① Investing (superficial) layer	Muscular	Envelopes entire neck; splits to enclose sternocleidomastoid and trapezius muscles
Pretracheal layer	② Muscular	Encloses infrahyoid muscles
	③ Visceral	Surrounds thyroid gland, larynx, trachea, pharynx, and esophagus
④ Prevertebral layer	Muscular	Surrounds cervical vertebral column and associated muscles
⑤ Carotid sheath	Neurovascular	Encloses common carotid artery, internal jugular vein, and vagus nerve

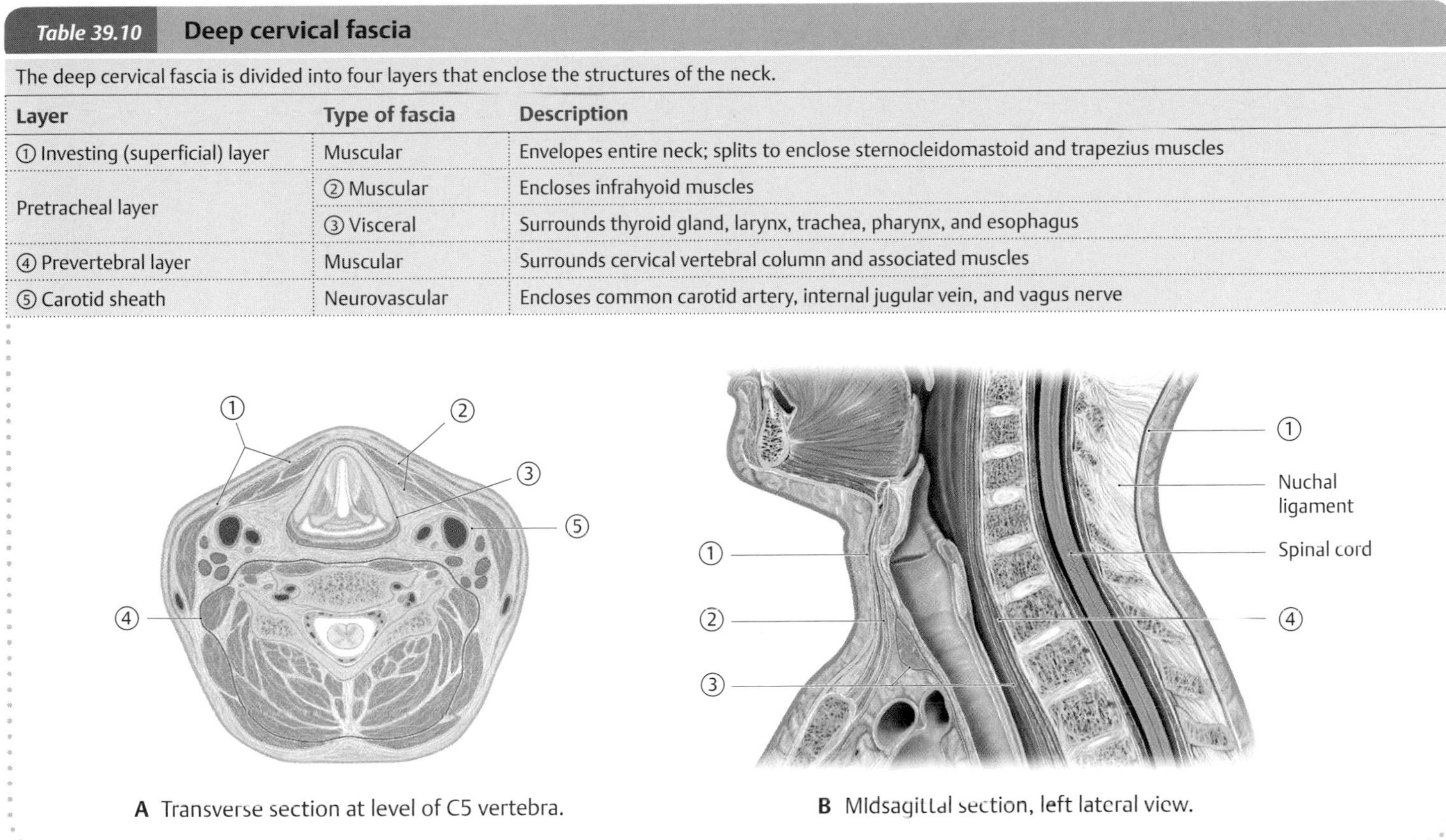
①
②
③
⑤
④
①
②
③
①
Nuchal ligament
Spinal cord
④

A Transverse section at level of C5 vertebra.

B Midsagittal section, left lateral view.

Fig. 39.27 **Deep cervical fascial layers**
Anterior view.

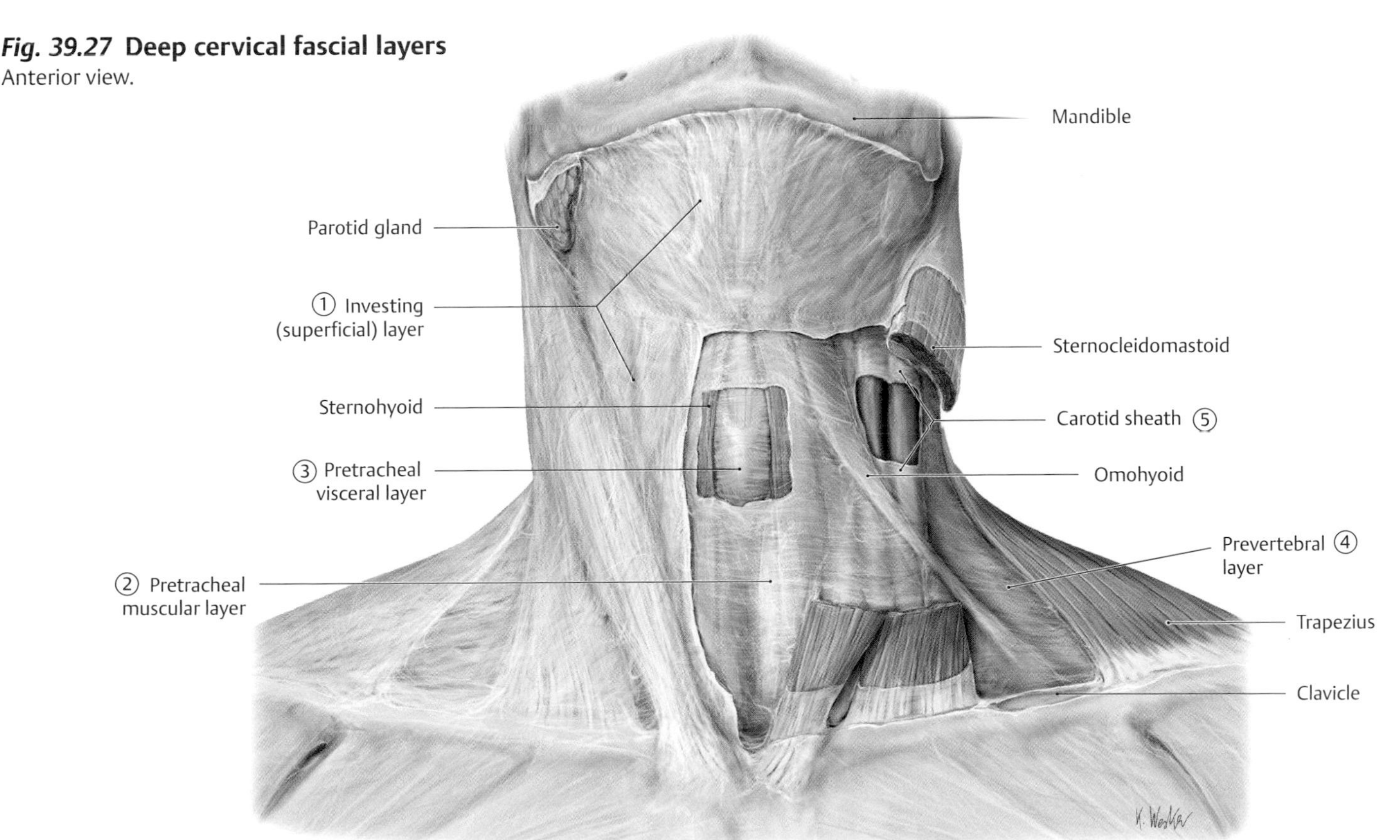
Mandible
Parotid gland
① Investing (superficial) layer
Sternohyoid
③ Pretracheal visceral layer
② Pretracheal muscular layer
Sternocleidomastoid
Carotid sheath ⑤
Omohyoid
Prevertebral ④ layer
Trapezius
Clavicle

Topography of the Anterior Cervical Region

Fig. 39.28 Anterior cervical triangle
Anterior view.

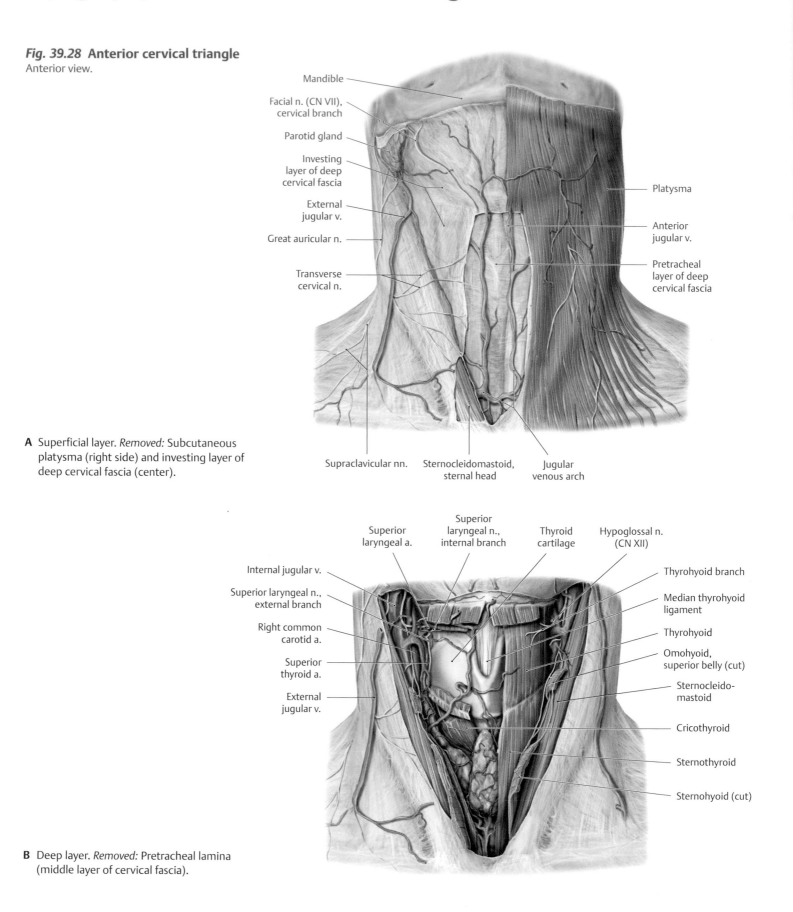

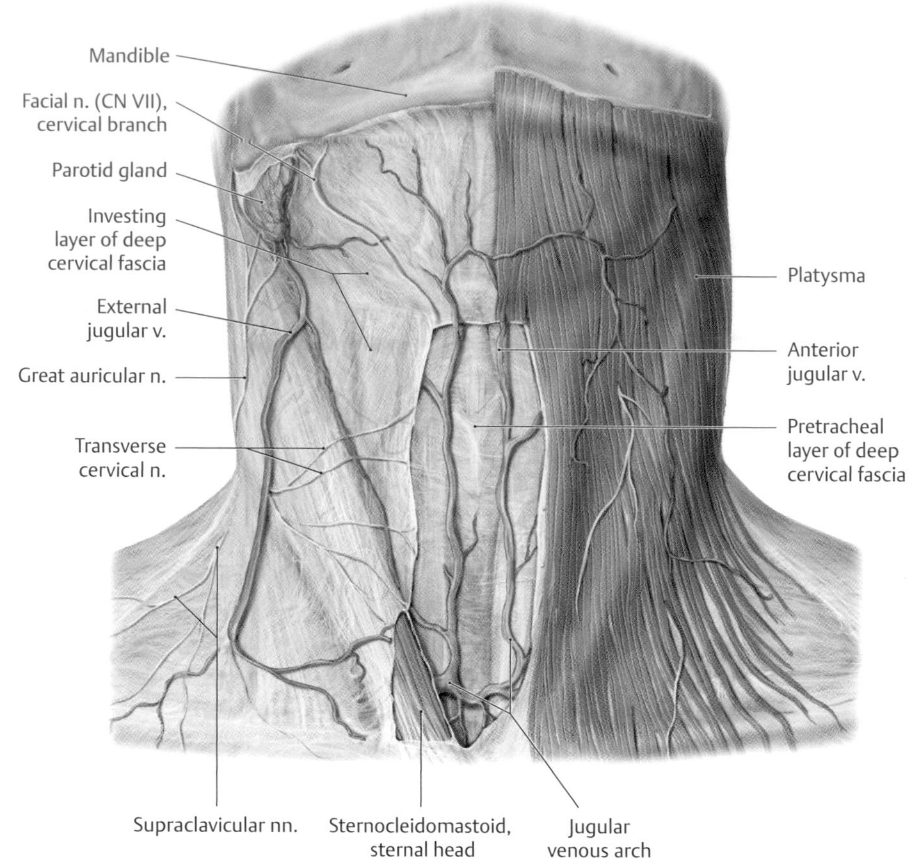
Mandible
Facial n. (CN VII), cervical branch
Parotid gland
Investing layer of deep cervical fascia
External jugular v.
Great auricular n.
Transverse cervical n.
Platysma
Anterior jugular v.
Pretracheal layer of deep cervical fascia
Supraclavicular nn.
Sternocleidomastoid, sternal head
Jugular venous arch

A Superficial layer. *Removed:* Subcutaneous platysma (right side) and investing layer of deep cervical fascia (center).

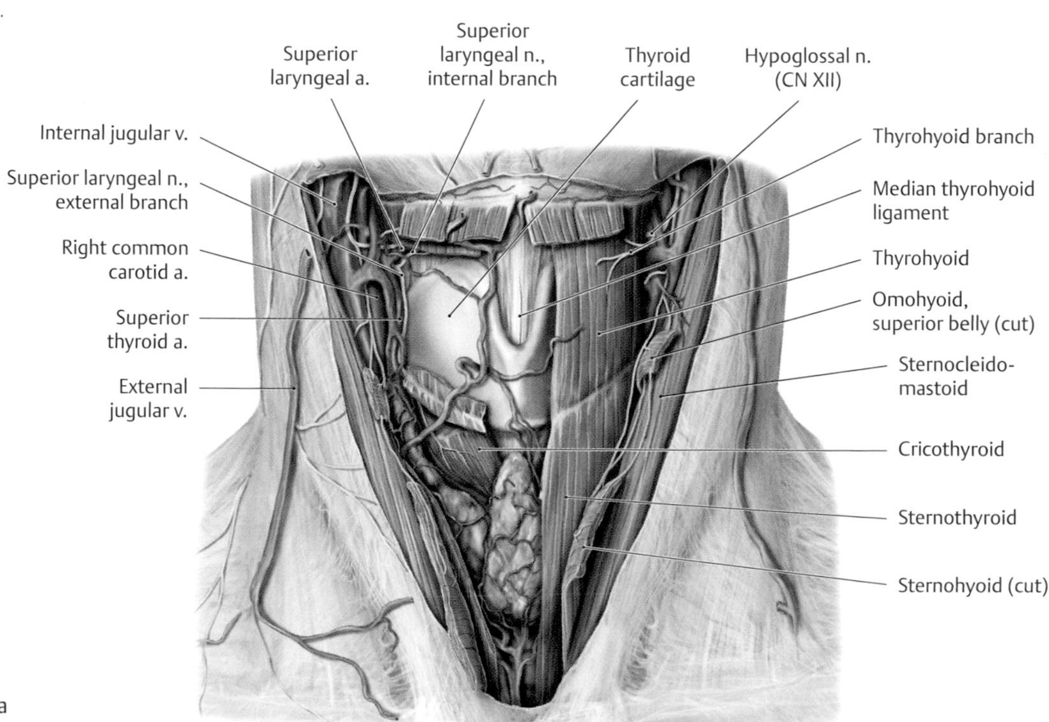
Superior laryngeal a.
Superior laryngeal n., internal branch
Thyroid cartilage
Hypoglossal n. (CN XII)
Internal jugular v.
Superior laryngeal n., external branch
Right common carotid a.
Superior thyroid a.
External jugular v.
Thyrohyoid branch
Median thyrohyoid ligament
Thyrohyoid
Omohyoid, superior belly (cut)
Sternocleido-mastoid
Cricothyroid
Sternothyroid
Sternohyoid (cut)

B Deep layer. *Removed:* Pretracheal lamina (middle layer of cervical fascia).

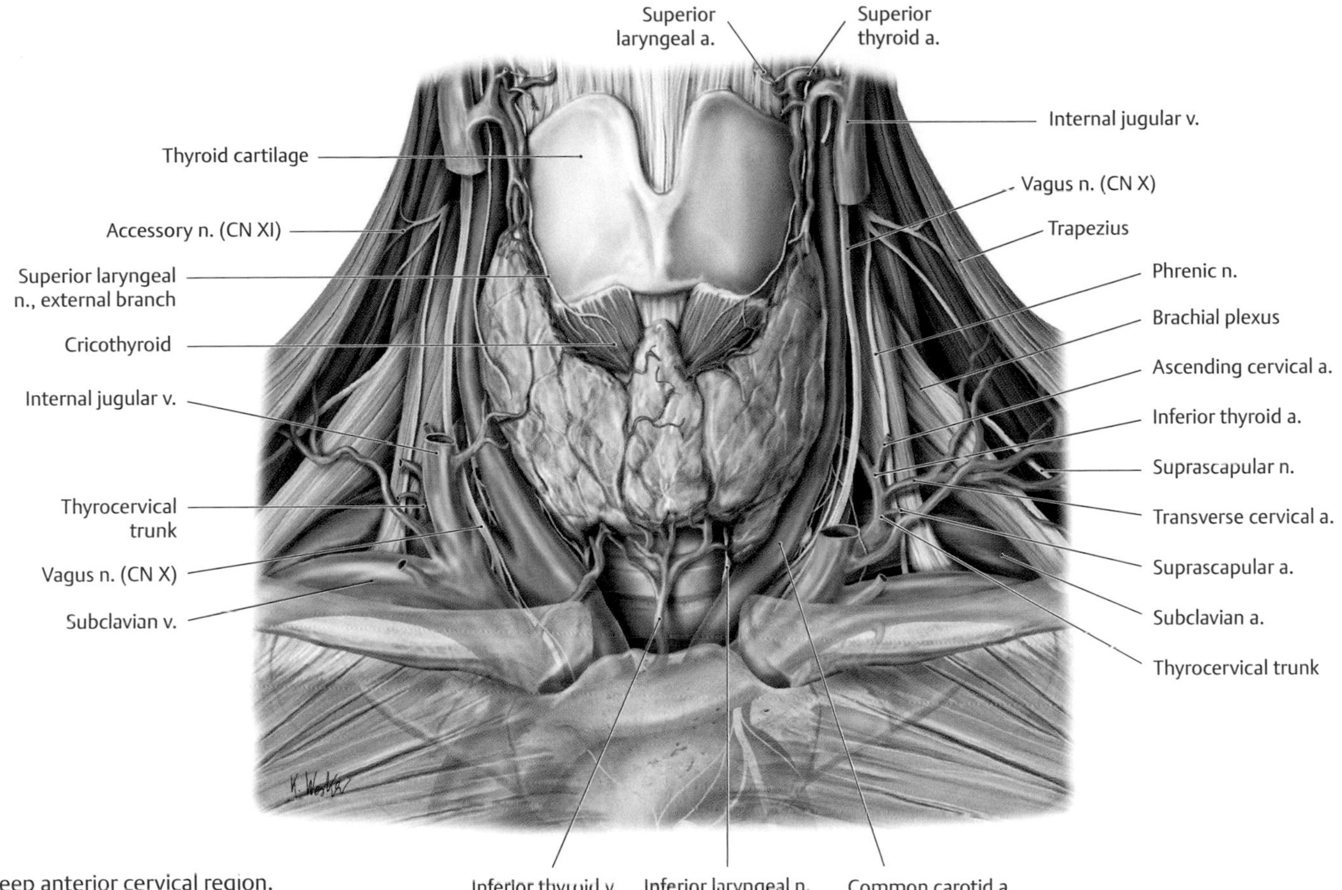
Superior
laryngeal a.
Superior
thyroid a.
Internal jugular v.
Thyroid cartilage
Vagus n. (CN X)
Accessory n. (CN XI)
Trapezius
Superior laryngeal
n., external branch
Phrenic n.
Brachial plexus
Cricothyroid
Ascending cervical a.
Internal jugular v.
Inferior thyroid a.
Suprascapular n.
Thyrocervical
trunk
Transverse cervical a.
Vagus n. (CN X)
Suprascapular a.
Subclavian v.
Subclavian a.
Thyrocervical trunk
Inferior thyroid v.
Inferior laryngeal n.
Common carotid a.

C Deep anterior cervical region.

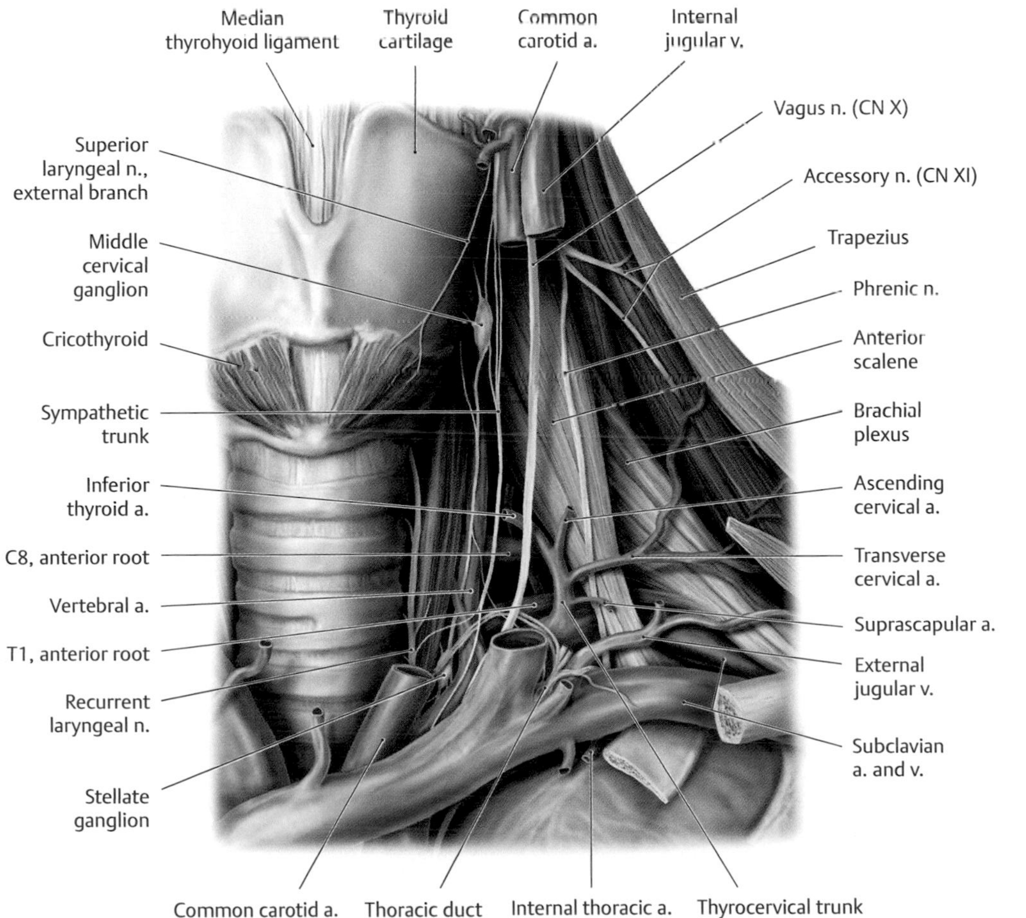
Median
thyrohyoid ligament
Thyroid
cartilage
Common
carotid a.
Internal
jugular v.
Vagus n. (CN X)
Superior
laryngeal n.,
external branch
Accessory n. (CN XI)
Trapezius
Middle
cervical
ganglion
Phrenic n.
Cricothyroid
Anterior
scalene
Sympathetic
trunk
Brachial
plexus
Inferior
thyroid a.
Ascending
cervical a.
C8, anterior root
Transverse
cervical a.
Vertebral a.
Suprascapular a.
T1, anterior root
External
jugular v.
Recurrent
laryngeal n.
Subclavian
a. and v.
Stellate
ganglion
Common carotid a.
Thoracic duct
Internal thoracic a.
Thyrocervical trunk

D Root of the neck.

Topography of the Anterior & Lateral Cervical Regions

Fig. 39.29 **Deep anterior cervical region**
The deep midline viscera of the anterior cervical region are the larynx and thyroid gland. The two lateral neurovascular pathways primarily supply these organs.

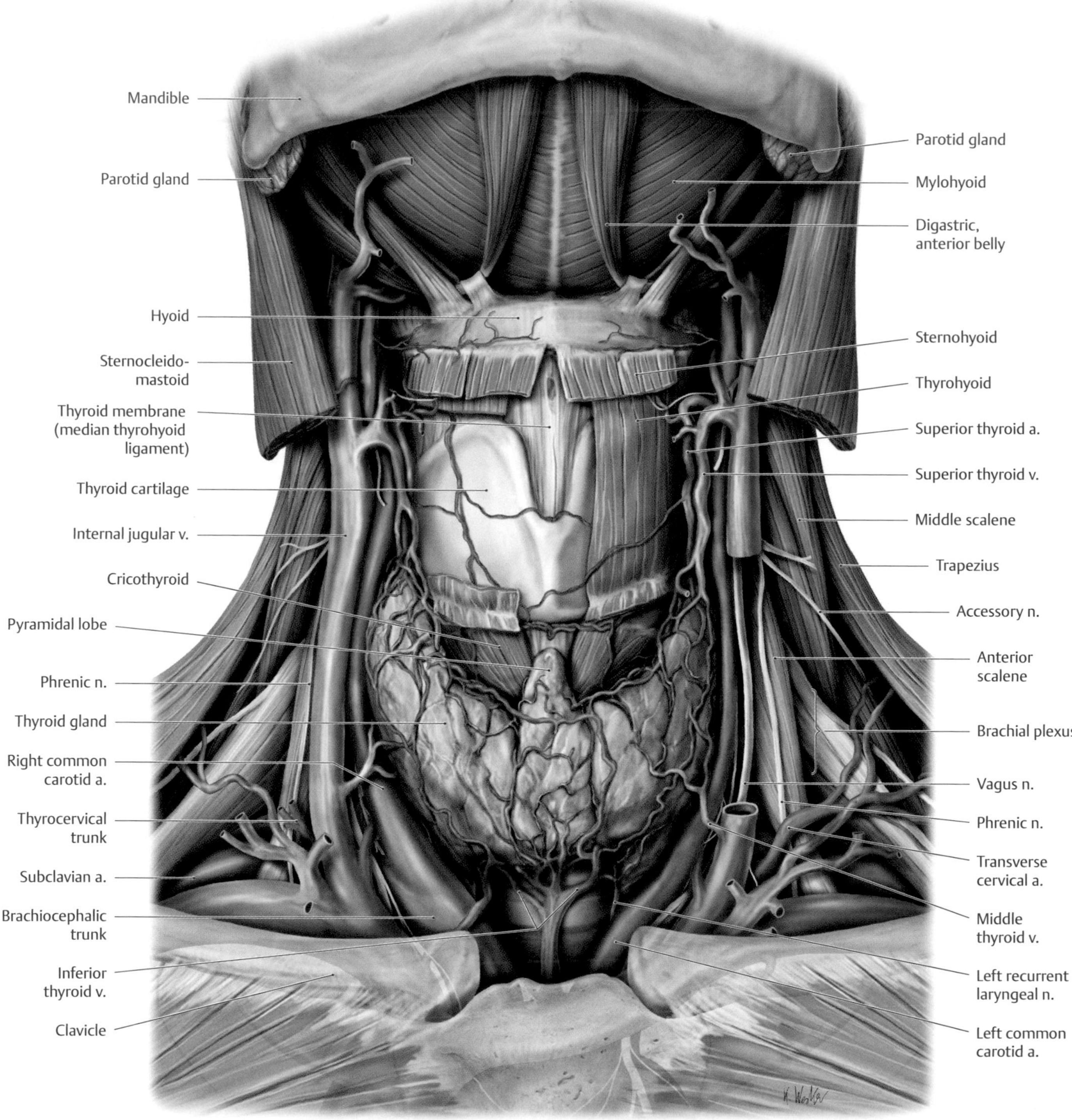
Mandible
Parotid gland
Hyoid
Sternocleido-
mastoid
Thyroid membrane
(median thyrohyoid
ligament)
Thyroid cartilage
Internal jugular v.
Cricothyroid
Pyramidal lobe
Phrenic n.
Thyroid gland
Right common
carotid a.
Thyrocervical
trunk
Subclavian a.
Brachiocephalic
trunk
Inferior
thyroid v.
Clavicle
Parotid gland
Mylohyoid
Digastric,
anterior belly
Sternohyoid
Thyrohyoid
Superior thyroid a.
Superior thyroid v.
Middle scalene
Trapezius
Accessory n.
Anterior
scalene
Brachial plexus
Vagus n.
Phrenic n.
Transverse
cervical a.
Middle
thyroid v.
Left recurrent
laryngeal n.
Left common
carotid a.

Fig. 39.30 Carotid triangle
Right lateral view.

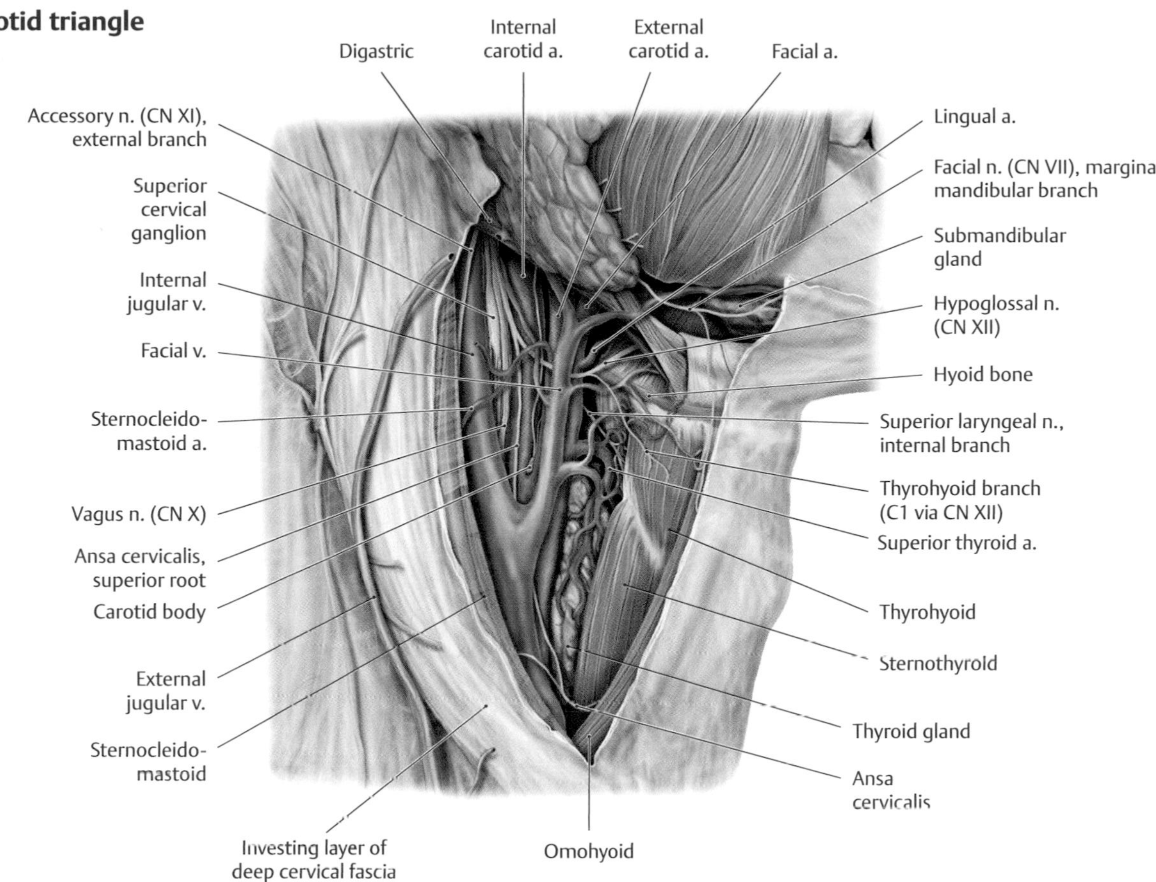
Digastric
Internal carotid a.
External carotid a.
Facial a.
Accessory n. (CN XI), external branch
Superior cervical ganglion
Internal jugular v.
Facial v.
Sternocleido-mastoid a.
Vagus n. (CN X)
Ansa cervicalis, superior root
Carotid body
External jugular v.
Sternocleido-mastoid
Investing layer of deep cervical fascia
Omohyoid
Lingual a.
Facial n. (CN VII), marginal mandibular branch
Submandibular gland
Hypoglossal n. (CN XII)
Hyoid bone
Superior laryngeal n., internal branch
Thyrohyoid branch (C1 via CN XII)
Superior thyroid a.
Thyrohyoid
Sternothyroid
Thyroid gland
Ansa cervicalis

Fig. 39.31 Deep lateral cervical region
Right lateral view with sternocleidomastoid windowed.

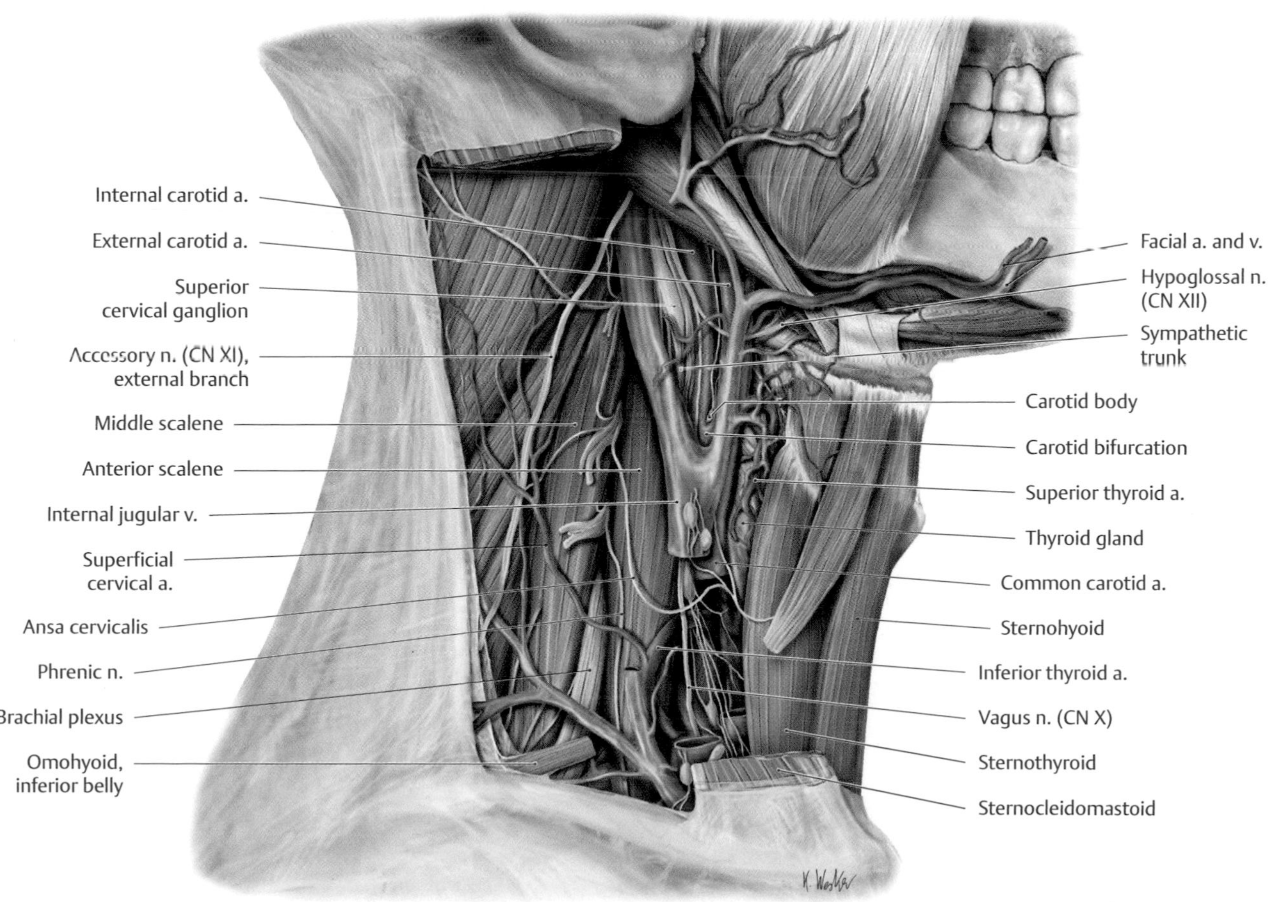
Internal carotid a.
External carotid a.
Superior cervical ganglion
Accessory n. (CN XI), external branch
Middle scalene
Anterior scalene
Internal jugular v.
Superficial cervical a.
Ansa cervicalis
Phrenic n.
Brachial plexus
Omohyoid, inferior belly
Facial a. and v.
Hypoglossal n. (CN XII)
Sympathetic trunk
Carotid body
Carotid bifurcation
Superior thyroid a.
Thyroid gland
Common carotid a.
Sternohyoid
Inferior thyroid a.
Vagus n. (CN X)
Sternothyroid
Sternocleidomastoid

Topography of the Lateral Cervical Region

Fig. 39.32 Lateral cervical region
Right lateral view. The contents of the deep lateral cervical region are found in Fig. 39.31.

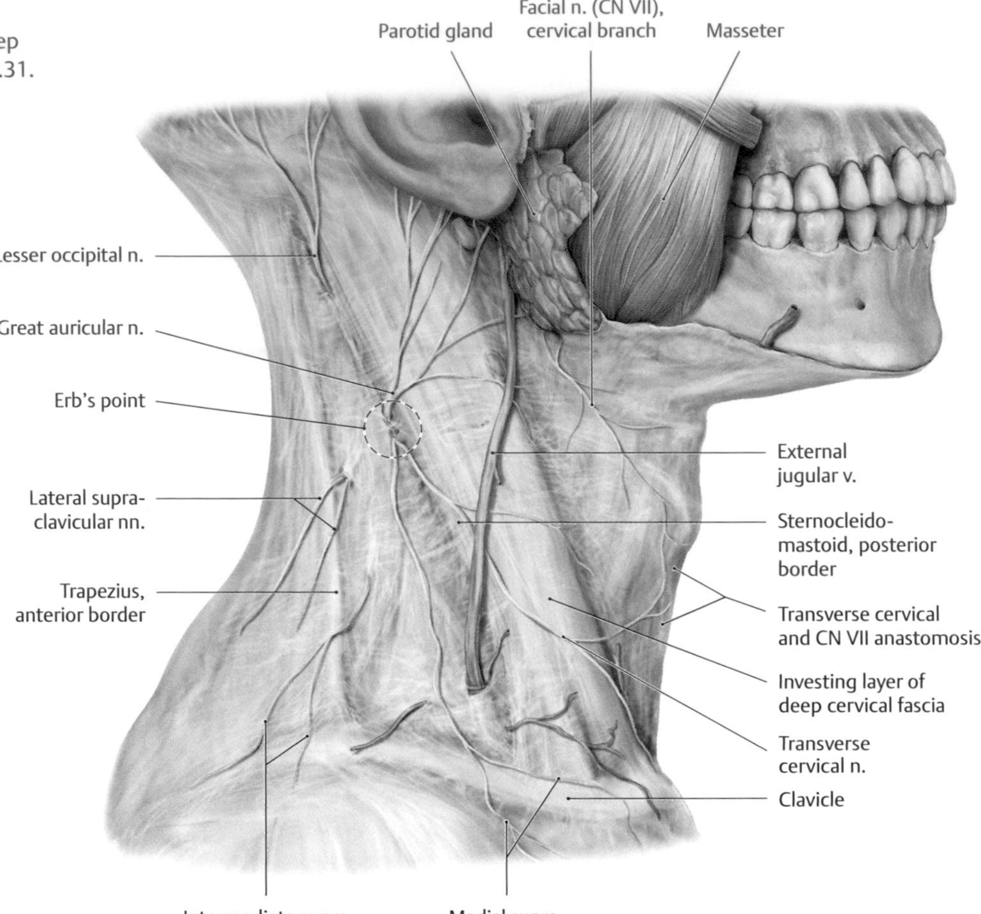

Parotid gland
Facial n. (CN VII), cervical branch
Masseter
Lesser occipital n.
Great auricular n.
Erb's point
Lateral supra-clavicular nn.
Trapezius, anterior border
External jugular v.
Sternocleido-mastoid, posterior border
Transverse cervical and CN VII anastomosis
Investing layer of deep cervical fascia
Transverse cervical n.
Clavicle
Intermediate supra-clavicular nn.
Medial supra-clavicular nn.

A Subcutaneous layer.

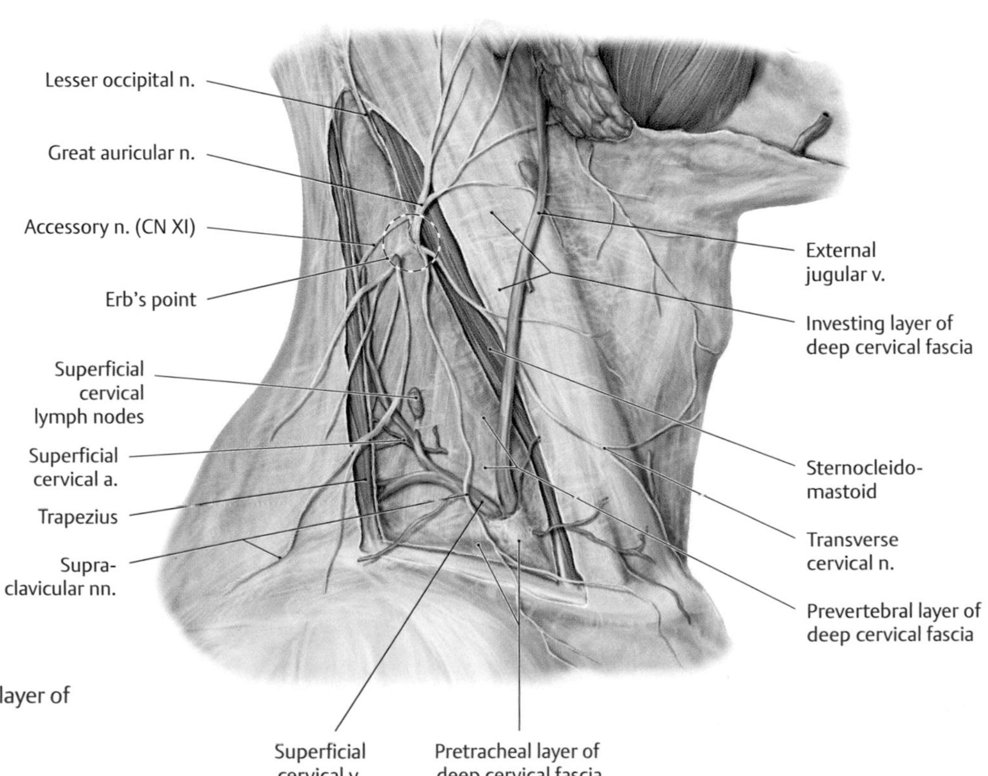

Lesser occipital n.
Great auricular n.
Accessory n. (CN XI)
Erb's point
Superficial cervical lymph nodes
Superficial cervical a.
Trapezius
Supra-clavicular nn.
External jugular v.
Investing layer of deep cervical fascia
Sternocleido-mastoid
Transverse cervical n.
Prevertebral layer of deep cervical fascia
Superficial cervical v.
Pretracheal layer of deep cervical fascia

B Subfascial layer. *Removed:* Investing layer of deep cervical fascia.

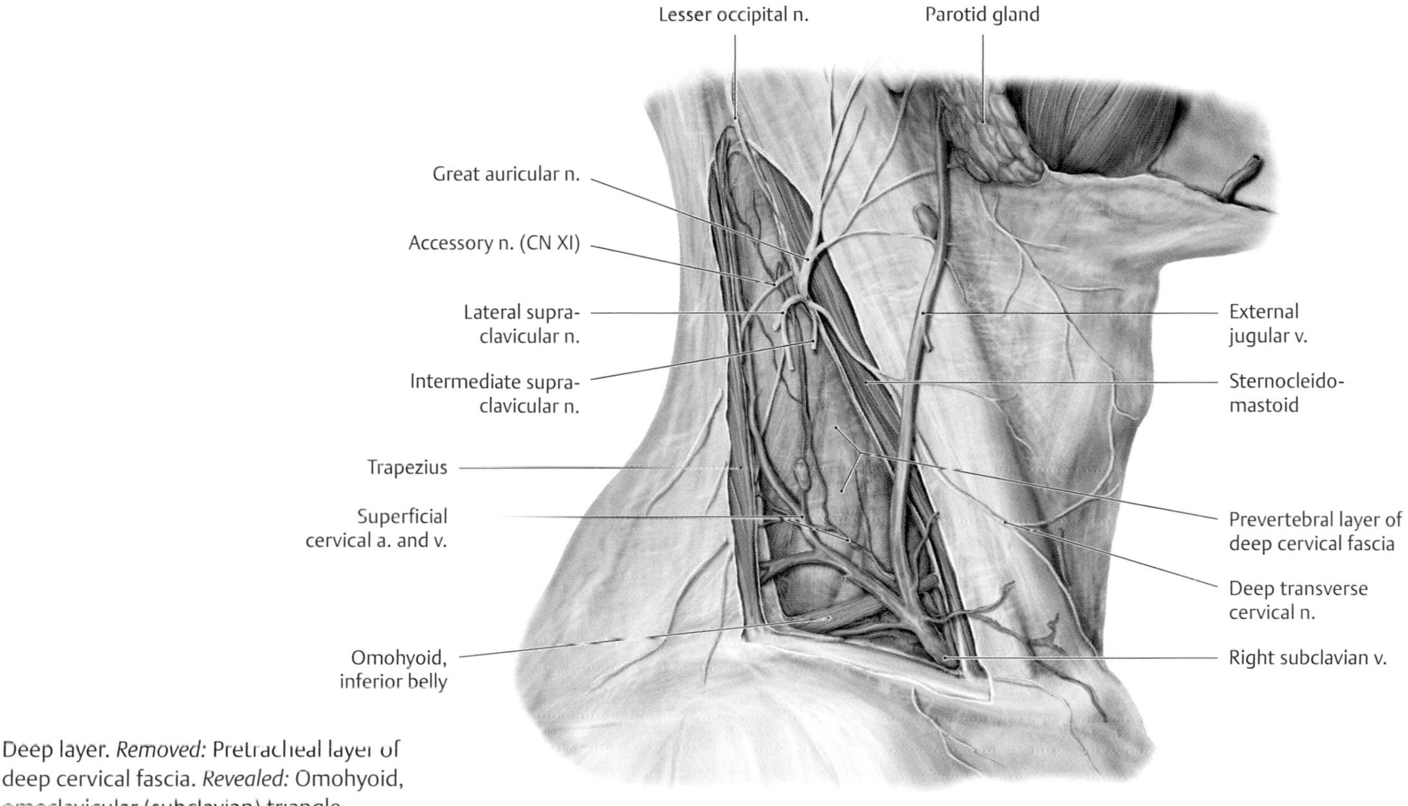
Lesser occipital n.
Parotid gland
Great auricular n.
Accessory n. (CN XI)
Lateral supra-clavicular n.
Intermediate supra-clavicular n.
Trapezius
Superficial cervical a. and v.
Omohyoid, inferior belly
External jugular v.
Sternocleido-mastoid
Prevertebral layer of deep cervical fascia
Deep transverse cervical n.
Right subclavian v.

C Deep layer. *Removed:* Pretracheal layer of deep cervical fascia. *Revealed:* Omohyoid, omoclavicular (subclavian) triangle.

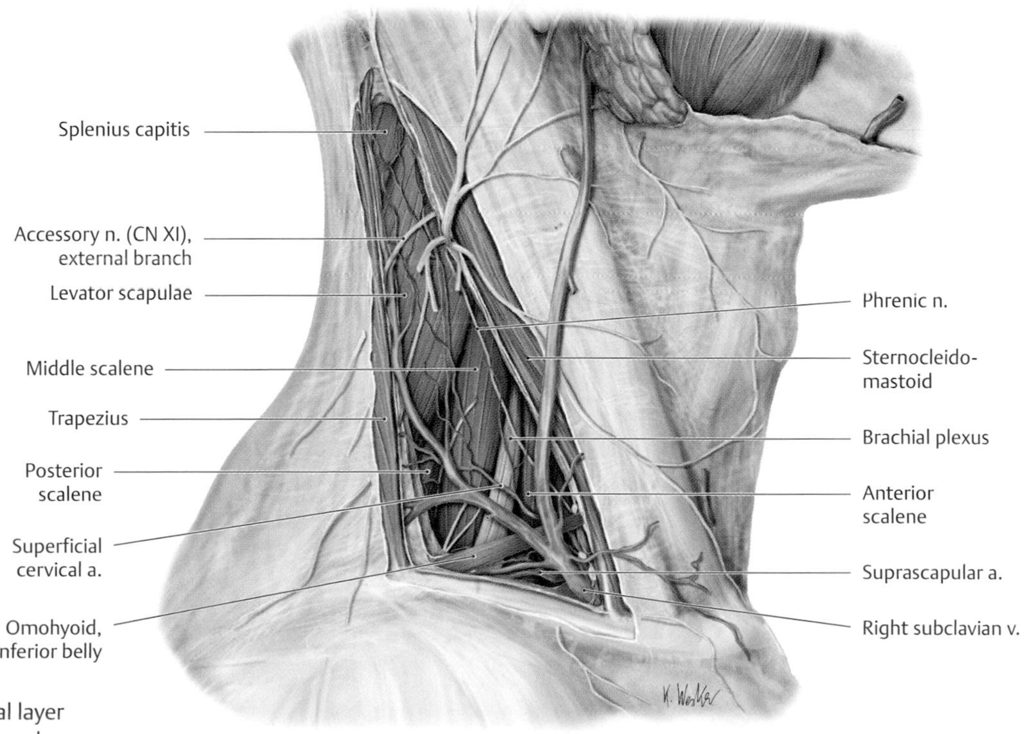
Splenius capitis
Accessory n. (CN XI), external branch
Levator scapulae
Middle scalene
Trapezius
Posterior scalene
Superficial cervical a.
Omohyoid, inferior belly
Phrenic n.
Sternocleido-mastoid
Brachial plexus
Anterior scalene
Suprascapular a.
Right subclavian v.

D Deepest layer. *Removed:* Prevertebral layer of deep cervical fascia. *Revealed:* Muscular floor of posterior triangle, brachial plexus, and phrenic nerve.

Topography of the Posterior Cervical Region

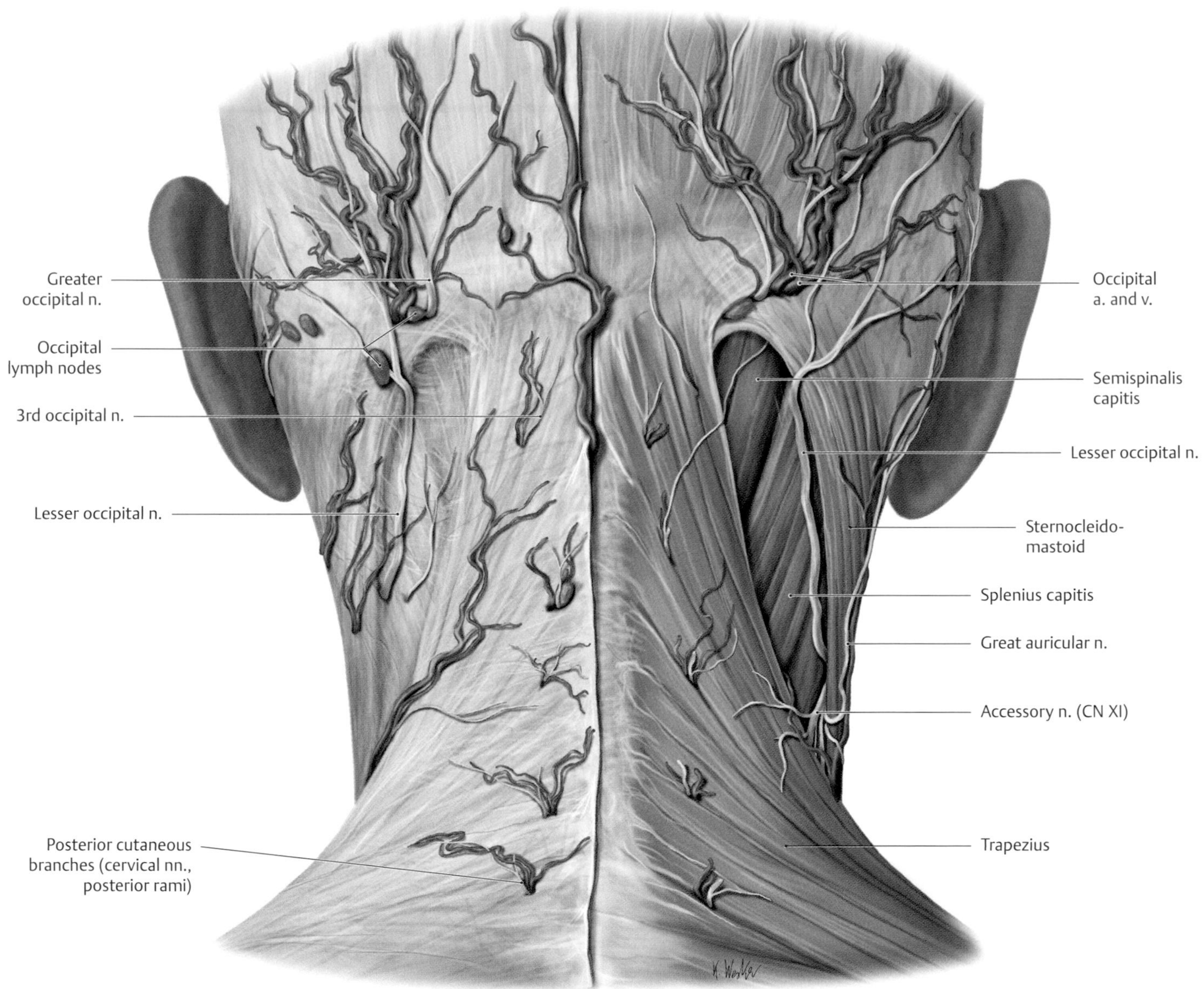
Greater occipital n.
Occipital lymph nodes
3rd occipital n.
Lesser occipital n.
Posterior cutaneous branches (cervical nn., posterior rami)
Occipital a. and v.
Semispinalis capitis
Lesser occipital n.
Sternocleido-mastoid
Splenius capitis
Great auricular n.
Accessory n. (CN XI)
Trapezius

Fig. 39.33 **Occipital and posterior cervical regions**
Posterior view. Subcutaneous layer (left), subfascial layer (right). The occiput is technically a region of the head, but it is included here due to the continuity of the vessels and nerves from the neck. *Removed on right side:* Investing layer of deep cervical fascia.

Fig. 39.34 **Suboccipital triangle**
Right side, posterior view, windowed. The suboccipital triangle is bounded by the suboccipital muscles (rectus capitis posterior major and obliquus capitis superior and inferior) and contains the vertebral artery. The left and right vertebral arteries pass through the atlanto-occipital membrane and combine to form the basilar artery.

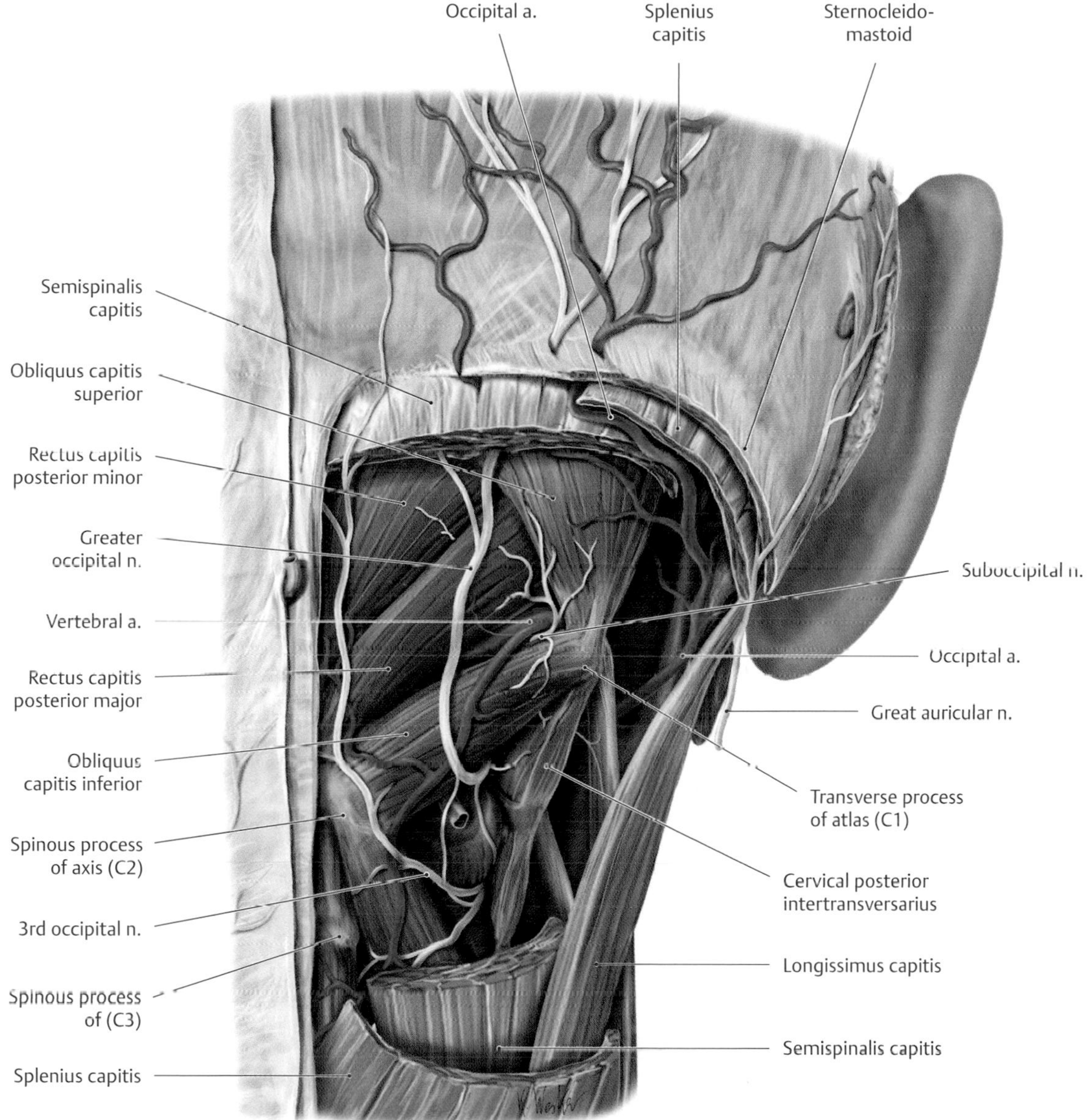
Occipital a.
Splenius capitis
Sternocleido-mastoid
Semispinalis capitis
Obliquus capitis superior
Rectus capitis posterior minor
Greater occipital n.
Vertebral a.
Rectus capitis posterior major
Obliquus capitis inferior
Spinous process of axis (C2)
3rd occipital n.
Spinous process of (C3)
Splenius capitis
Suboccipital n.
Occipital a.
Great auricular n.
Transverse process of atlas (C1)
Cervical posterior intertransversarius
Longissimus capitis
Semispinalis capitis

Lymphatics of the Neck

Fig. 39.35 Lymphatic drainage regions
Right lateral view.

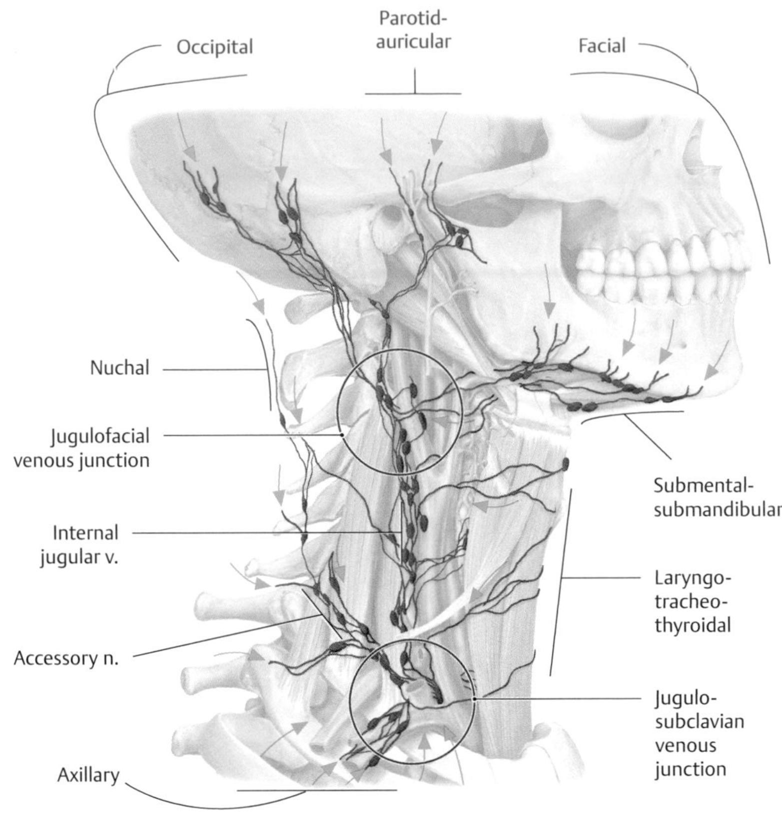
Occipital
Parotid-auricular
Facial
Nuchal
Jugulofacial venous junction
Internal jugular v.
Accessory n.
Axillary
Submental-submandibular
Laryngo-tracheo-thyroidal
Jugulo-subclavian venous junction

Clinical

Tumor metastasis
Lymph from the entire body is channeled to the left and right jugulosubclavian junctions (red circles). Gastric carcinoma may metastasize to the left supraclavicular group of lymph nodes, producing an enlarged *sentinel node* (see p. 73). Systemic lymphomas may also spread to the cervical lymph nodes by this pathway.

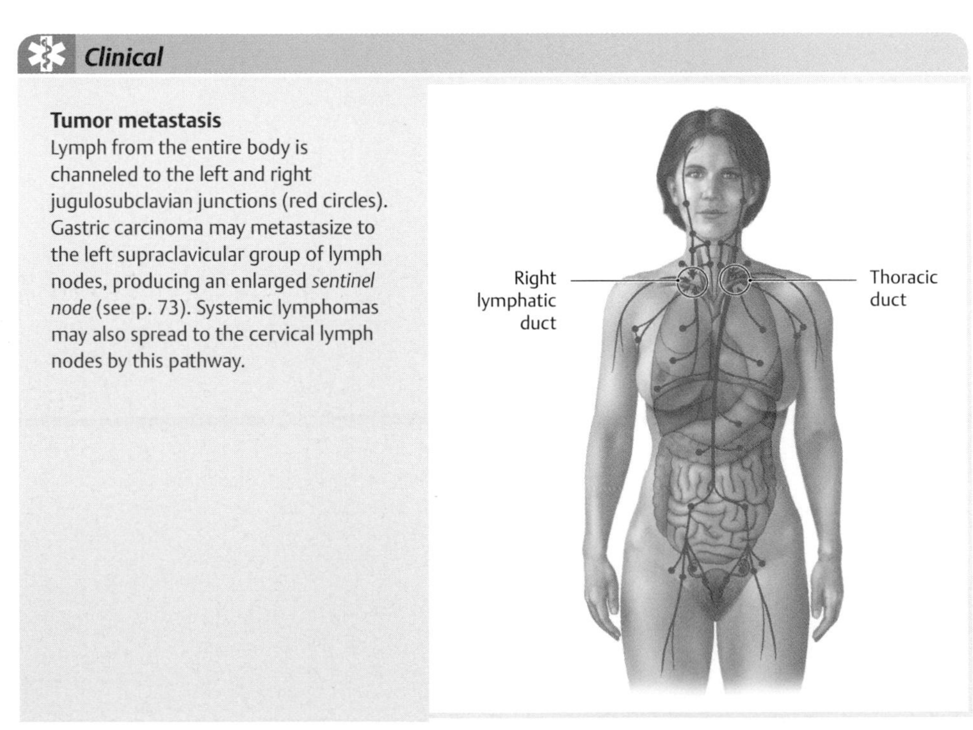
Right lymphatic duct
Thoracic duct

Fig. 39.36 **Superficial cervical lymph nodes**
Right lateral view.

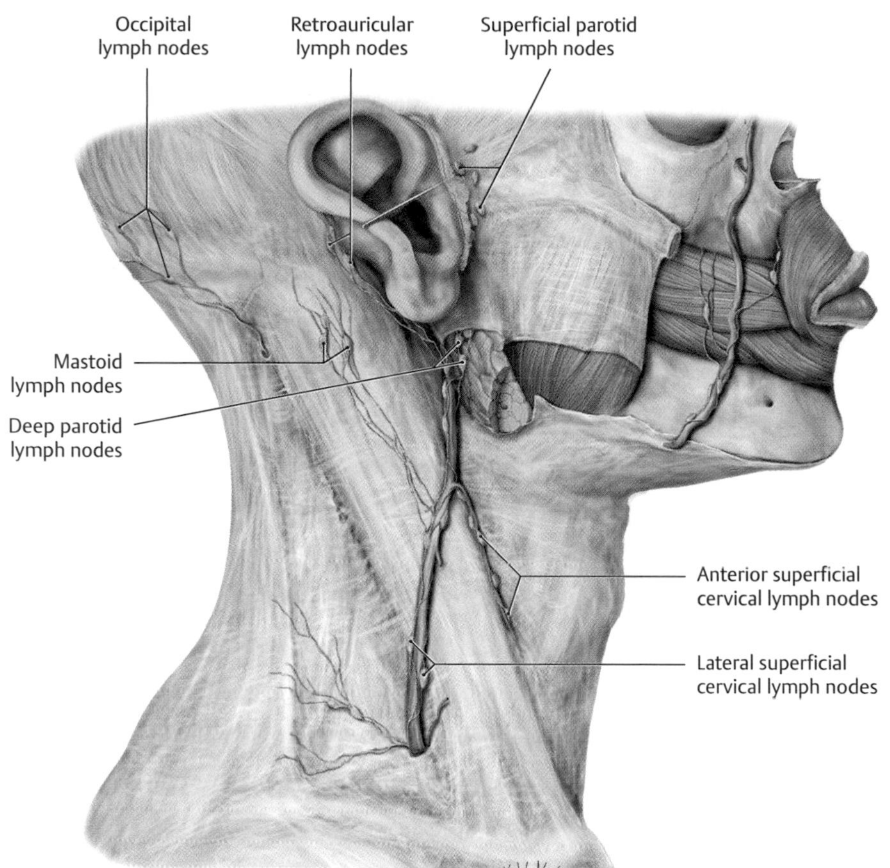
Occipital lymph nodes
Retroauricular lymph nodes
Superficial parotid lymph nodes
Mastoid lymph nodes
Deep parotid lymph nodes
Anterior superficial cervical lymph nodes
Lateral superficial cervical lymph nodes

Table 39.11	Superficial cervical lymph nodes
Lymph nodes (l.n.)	**Drainage region**
Retroauricular l.n.	Occiput
Occipital l.n.	
Mastoid l.n.	
Superficial parotid l.n.	Parotid-auricular region
Deep parotid l.n.	
Anterior superficial cervical l.n.	Sternocleidomastoid region
Lateral superficial cervical l.n.	

Fig. 39.37 **Deep cervical lymph nodes**
Right lateral view.

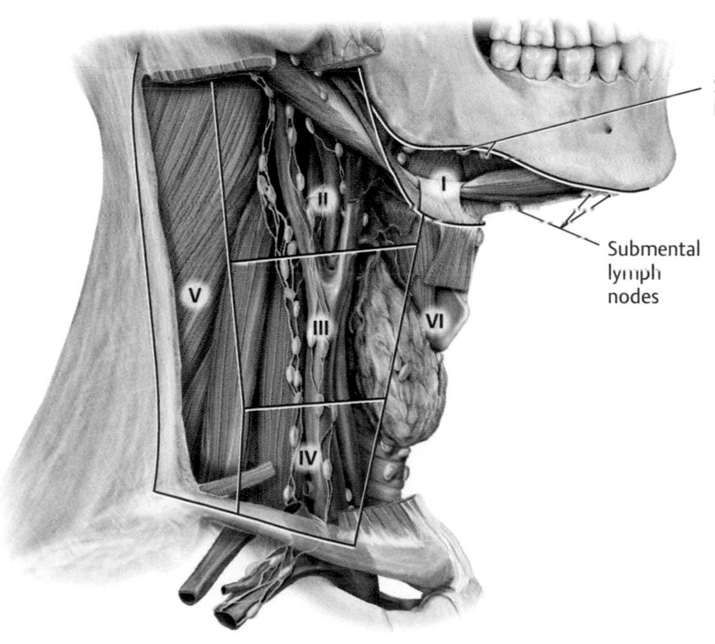
Submandibular lymph nodes
Submental lymph nodes
I
II
III
IV
V
VI

Table 39.12	Deep cervical lymph nodes		
Level	**Lymph nodes (l.n.)**		**Drainage region**
I	Submental l.n.		Face
	Submandibular l.n.		
II	Lateral jugular l.n. group	Upper lateral group	Nuchal region, laryngo-tracheo-thyroidal region
III		Middle lateral group	
IV		Lower lateral group	
V	L.n. in posterior cervical triangle		Nuchal region
VI	Anterior cervical l.n.		Laryngo-tracheo-thyroidal region

Coronal Sections of the Head

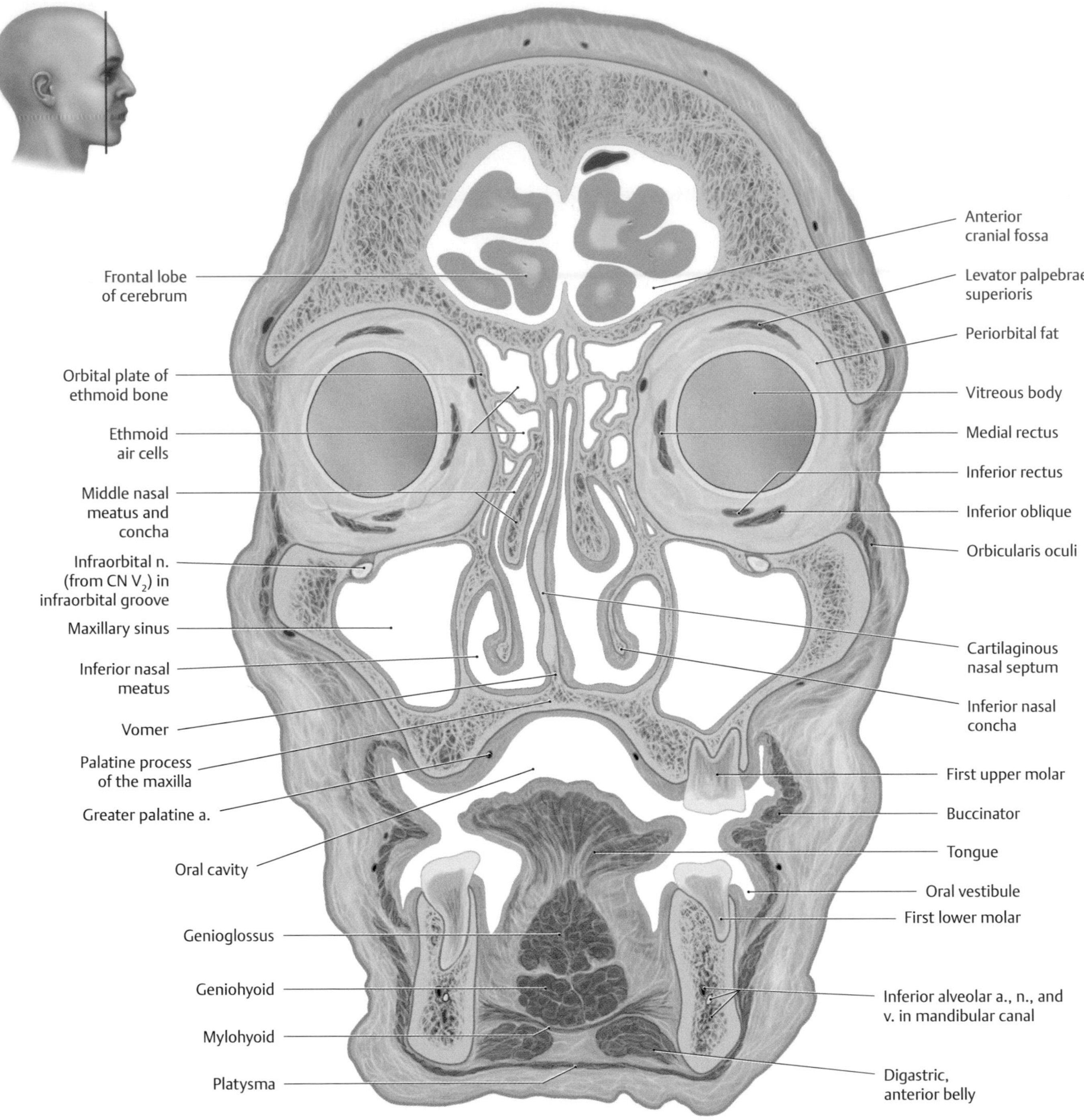
Frontal lobe of cerebrum
Orbital plate of ethmoid bone
Ethmoid air cells
Middle nasal meatus and concha
Infraorbital n. (from CN V_2) in infraorbital groove
Maxillary sinus
Inferior nasal meatus
Vomer
Palatine process of the maxilla
Greater palatine a.
Oral cavity
Genioglossus
Geniohyoid
Mylohyoid
Platysma
Anterior cranial fossa
Levator palpebrae superioris
Periorbital fat
Vitreous body
Medial rectus
Inferior rectus
Inferior oblique
Orbicularis oculi
Cartilaginous nasal septum
Inferior nasal concha
First upper molar
Buccinator
Tongue
Oral vestibule
First lower molar
Inferior alveolar a., n., and v. in mandibular canal
Digastric, anterior belly

Fig. 39.38 **Coronal section through the anterior orbital margin**

Anterior view. This section shows four regions of the head: the oral cavity, the nasal cavity and sinuses, the orbit, and the anterior cranial fossa. Muscles of the oral floor, the apex of the tongue, the hard palate, the neurovascular structures in the mandibular canal, and the first molar are all seen in the region of the oral cavity. This section reinforces the clinical implications of the relationship of the maxillary sinus with the maxillary teeth and the floor of the orbit and with the maxillary nerve in the infraorbital groove. The medial wall of the orbit shares a thin bony wall (orbital plate) with the ethmoid air cells (sinus). The section is enough anterior so that the lateral bony walls of the orbit are not included due to the lateral curvature of the skull.

Fig. 39.39 **Coronal section through the orbital apex**
Anterior view. In this more posterior section than that of Fig. 39.38, the soft palate now separates the oral and nasal cavities. The buccal fat pad is also visible. The section is slightly angled, producing an apparent discontinuity in the mandibular ramus on the left side.

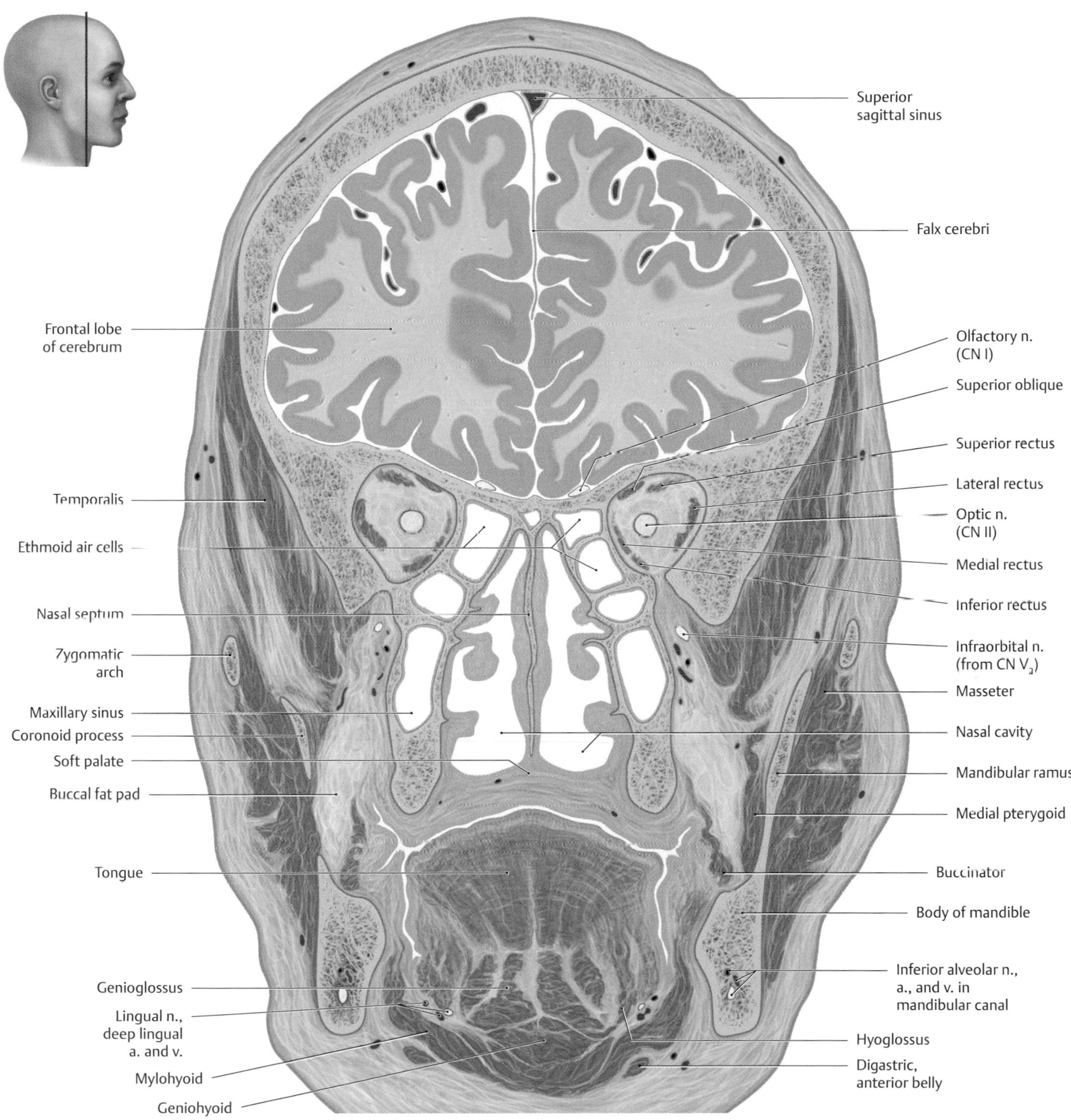
Superior sagittal sinus
Falx cerebri
Frontal lobe of cerebrum
Olfactory n. (CN I)
Superior oblique
Superior rectus
Temporalis
Lateral rectus
Optic n. (CN II)
Ethmoid air cells
Medial rectus
Nasal septum
Inferior rectus
Zygomatic arch
Infraorbital n. (from CN V_2)
Masseter
Maxillary sinus
Coronoid process
Nasal cavity
Soft palate
Mandibular ramus
Buccal fat pad
Medial pterygoid
Tongue
Buccinator
Body of mandible
Inferior alveolar n., a., and v. in mandibular canal
Genioglossus
Lingual n., deep lingual a. and v.
Hyoglossus
Digastric, anterior belly
Mylohyoid
Geniohyoid

Transverse Sections of the Head & Neck

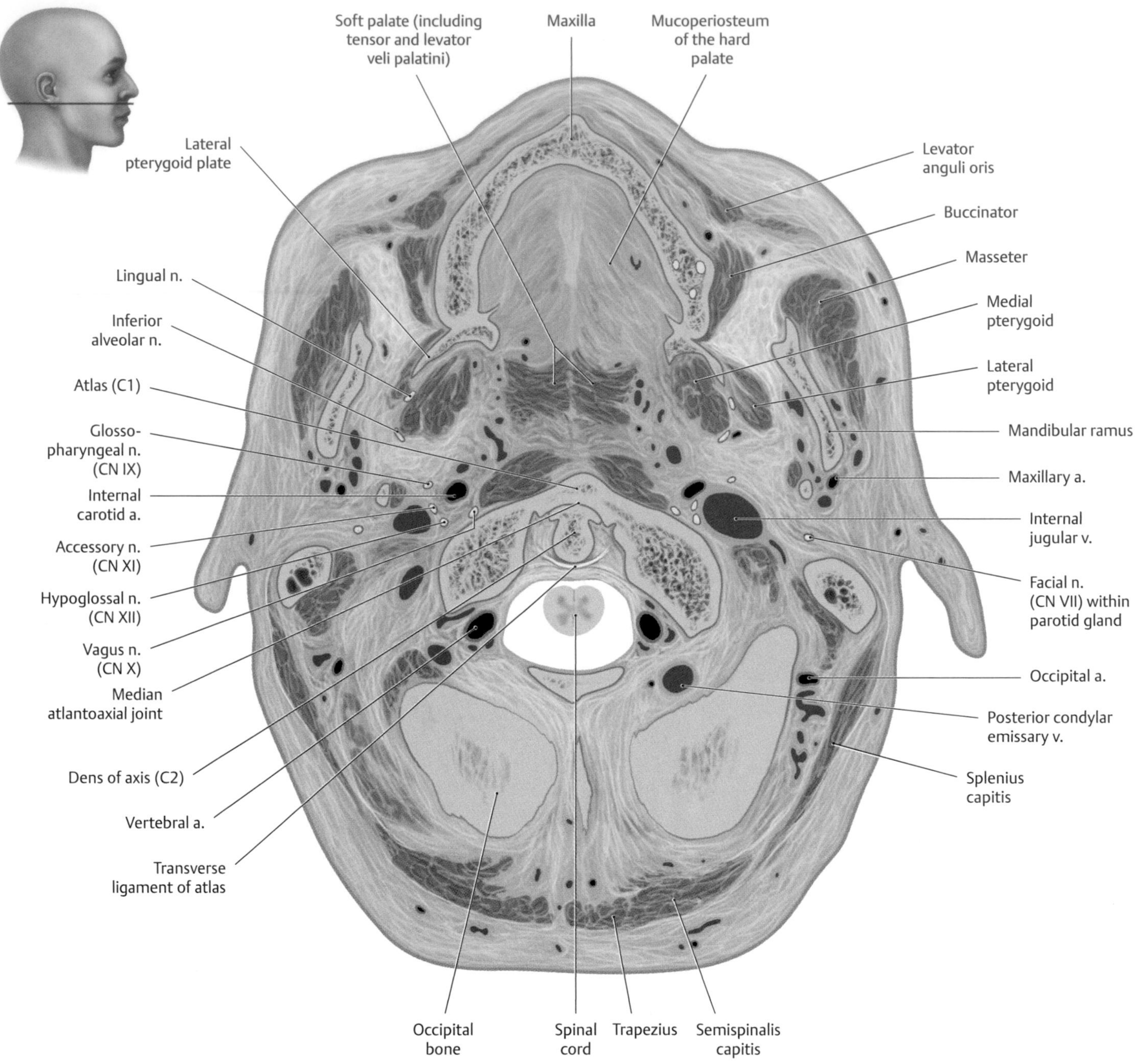
Soft palate (including tensor and levator veli palatini)
Maxilla
Mucoperiosteum of the hard palate
Lateral pterygoid plate
Levator anguli oris
Buccinator
Masseter
Lingual n.
Inferior alveolar n.
Medial pterygoid
Lateral pterygoid
Atlas (C1)
Mandibular ramus
Glosso-pharyngeal n. (CN IX)
Maxillary a.
Internal carotid a.
Internal jugular v.
Accessory n. (CN XI)
Facial n. (CN VII) within parotid gland
Hypoglossal n. (CN XII)
Vagus n. (CN X)
Occipital a.
Median atlantoaxial joint
Posterior condylar emissary v.
Splenius capitis
Dens of axis (C2)
Vertebral a.
Transverse ligament of atlas
Occipital bone
Spinal cord
Trapezius
Semispinalis capitis

Fig. 39.40 **Transverse section of head through the median atlantoaxial joint**

Superior view. This section passes through the soft palate and mucoperiosteum of the hard palate. The articulation of the odontoid process (dens of C2) with the axis (C1) at the median atlantoaxial joint is shown, as well as the carotid sheath, containing the vertical neurovascular elements of the neck. The vertebral artery is sectioned as it prepares to enter the foramen magnum and fuse with its opposite to form the basilar artery.

Fig. 39.41 Transverse section of the neck

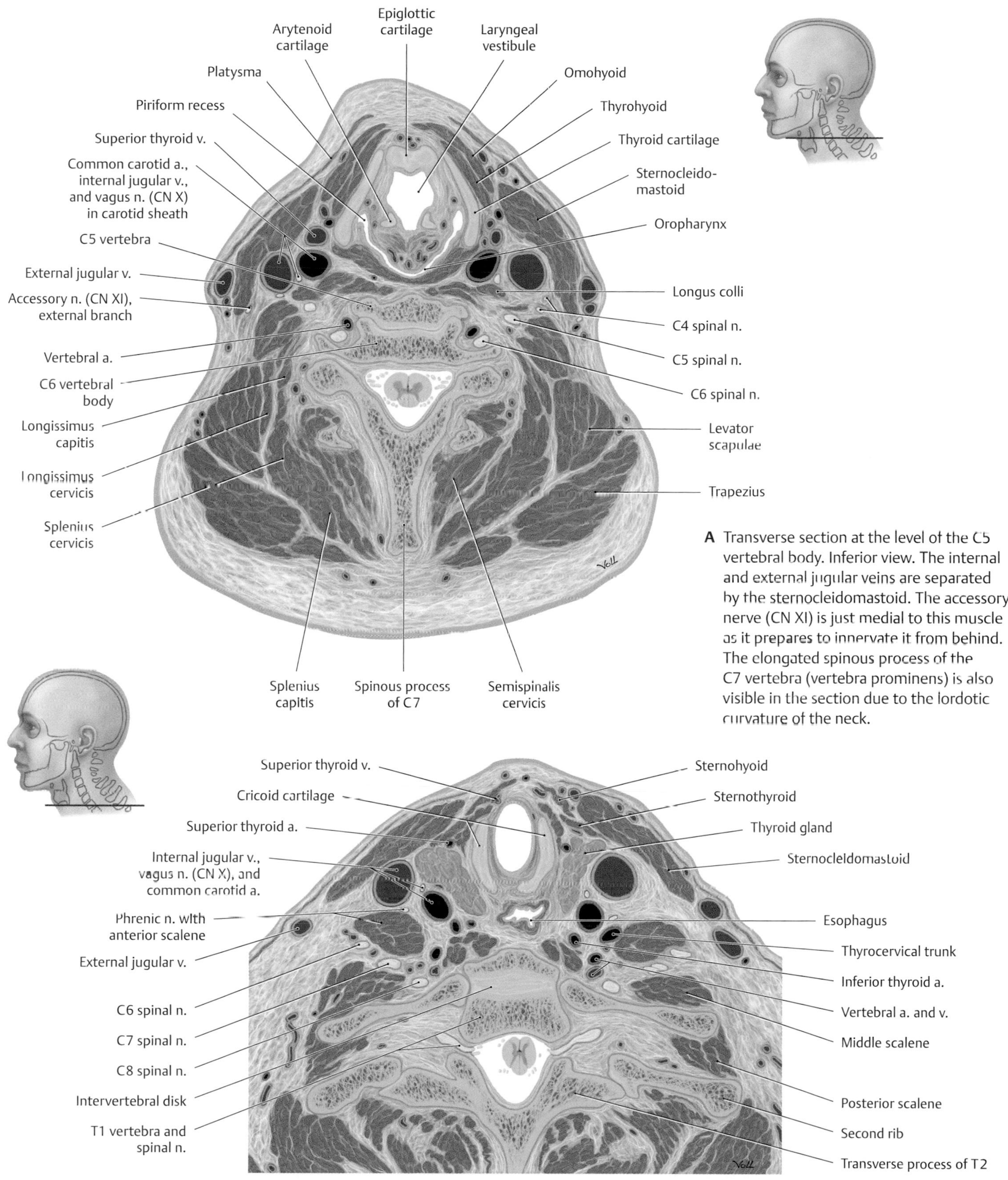
Epiglottic cartilage
Arytenoid cartilage
Laryngeal vestibule
Platysma
Omohyoid
Piriform recess
Thyrohyoid
Superior thyroid v.
Thyroid cartilage
Common carotid a., internal jugular v., and vagus n. (CN X) in carotid sheath
Sternocleido-mastoid
Oropharynx
C5 vertebra
External jugular v.
Longus colli
Accessory n. (CN XI), external branch
C4 spinal n.
C5 spinal n.
Vertebral a.
C6 vertebral body
C6 spinal n.
Longissimus capitis
Levator scapulae
Longissimus cervicis
Trapezius
Splenius cervicis
Splenius capitis
Spinous process of C7
Semispinalis cervicis
Superior thyroid v.
Sternohyoid
Cricoid cartilage
Sternothyroid
Superior thyroid a.
Thyroid gland
Internal jugular v., vagus n. (CN X), and common carotid a.
Sternocleidomastoid
Phrenic n. with anterior scalene
Esophagus
External jugular v.
Thyrocervical trunk
Inferior thyroid a.
C6 spinal n.
Vertebral a. and v.
C7 spinal n.
Middle scalene
C8 spinal n.
Posterior scalene
Intervertebral disk
Second rib
T1 vertebra and spinal n.
Transverse process of T2

A Transverse section at the level of the C5 vertebral body. Inferior view. The internal and external jugular veins are separated by the sternocleidomastoid. The accessory nerve (CN XI) is just medial to this muscle as it prepares to innervate it from behind. The elongated spinous process of the C7 vertebra (vertebra prominens) is also visible in the section due to the lordotic curvature of the neck.

B Transverse section at the level of the C7/T1 vertebral junction. Inferior view. This section reveals the roots of spinal nerves C6 to C8 of the brachial plexus passing between the anterior and middle scalene muscles. The phrenic nerve is on the anterior surface of the anterior scalene and the components of the carotid sheath (internal jugular vein, common carotid artery, and vagus nerve) lie in the interval between this muscle, the sternocleidomastoid, and the thyroid gland.

Sagittal Sections of the Head

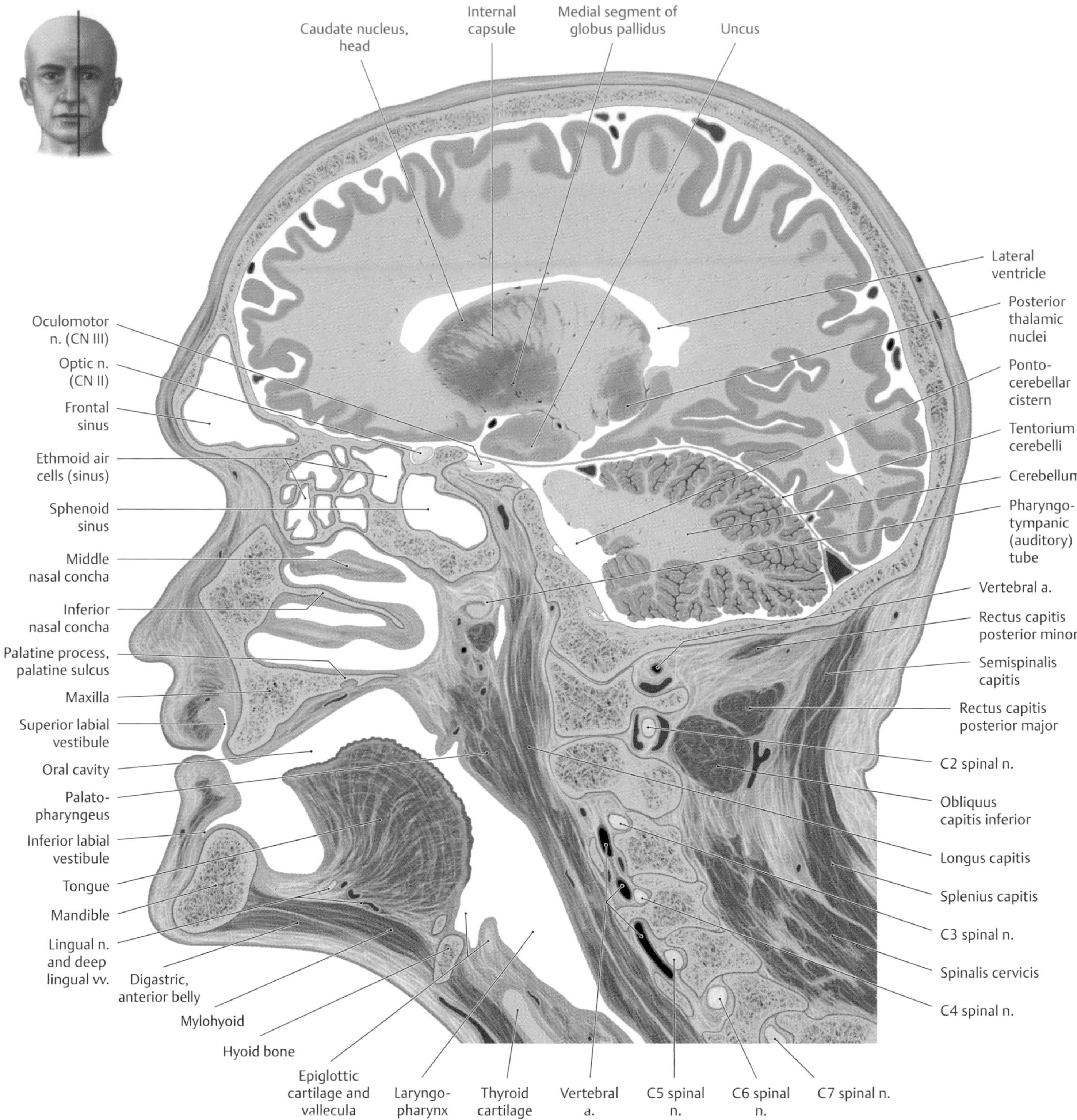
Caudate nucleus, head
Internal capsule
Medial segment of globus pallidus
Uncus
Lateral ventricle
Posterior thalamic nuclei
Ponto-cerebellar cistern
Tentorium cerebelli
Cerebellum
Pharyngo-tympanic (auditory) tube
Vertebral a.
Rectus capitis posterior minor
Semispinalis capitis
Rectus capitis posterior major
C2 spinal n.
Obliquus capitis inferior
Longus capitis
Splenius capitis
C3 spinal n.
Spinalis cervicis
C4 spinal n.
Oculomotor n. (CN III)
Optic n. (CN II)
Frontal sinus
Ethmoid air cells (sinus)
Sphenoid sinus
Middle nasal concha
Inferior nasal concha
Palatine process, palatine sulcus
Maxilla
Superior labial vestibule
Oral cavity
Palato-pharyngeus
Inferior labial vestibule
Tongue
Mandible
Lingual n. and deep lingual vv.
Digastric, anterior belly
Mylohyoid
Hyoid bone
Epiglottic cartilage and vallecula
Laryngo-pharynx
Thyroid cartilage
Vertebral a.
C5 spinal n.
C6 spinal n.
C7 spinal n.

Fig. 39.42 **Sagittal section through the medial orbital wall**

Left lateral view. This section passes through the inferior and middle conchae of the lateral nasal wall. Three of the four paranasal air sinuses (ethmoid, sphenoid, and frontal) are seen in this section and in relation to the nasal cavity into which they drain. In the region of the cervical spine, the vertebral artery is cut at multiple levels. The spinal nerves have been cut just prior to their lateral exit through the intervertebral foramina.

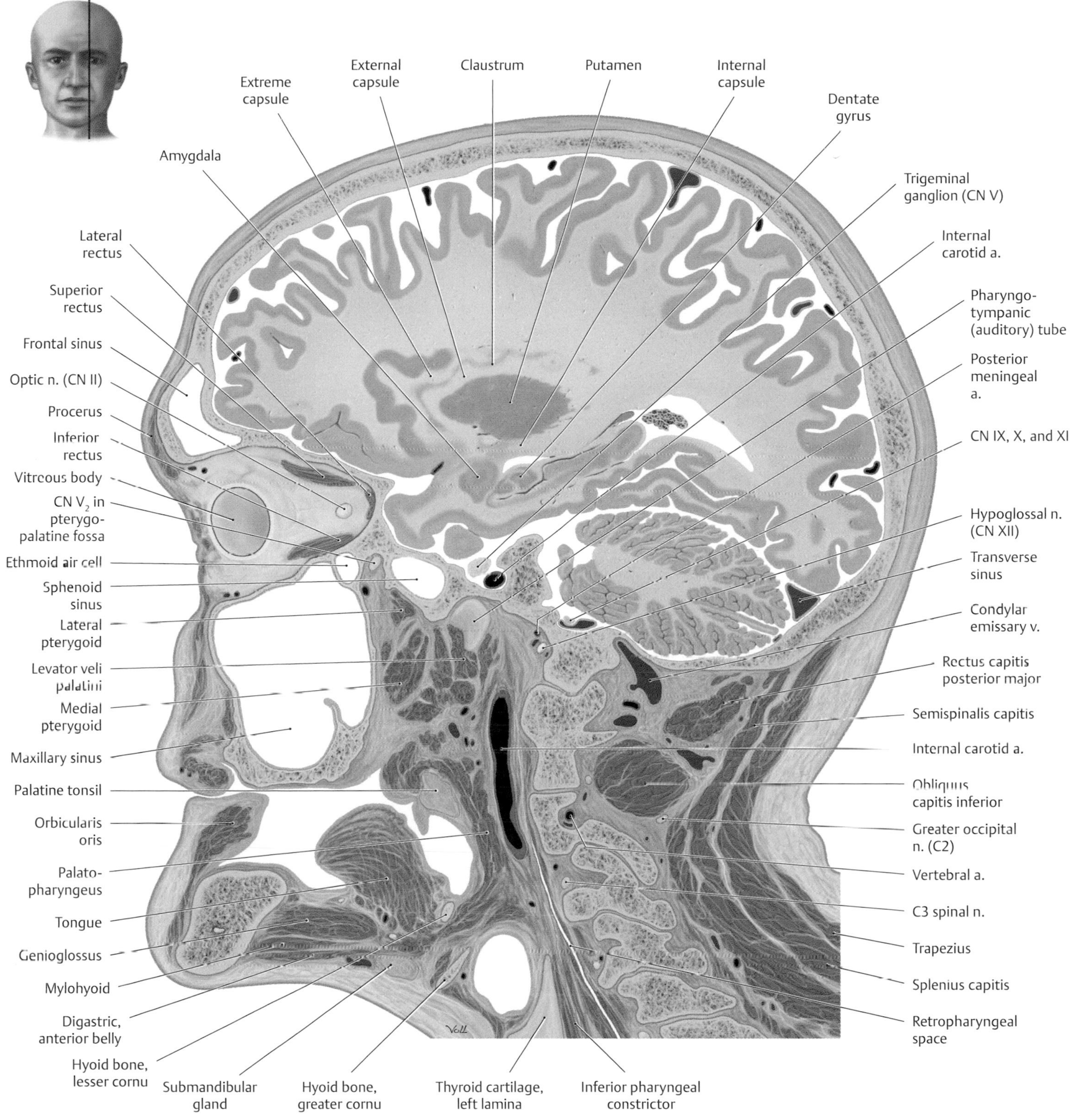

Extreme capsule
External capsule
Claustrum
Putamen
Internal capsule
Dentate gyrus
Amygdala
Trigeminal ganglion (CN V)
Internal carotid a.
Lateral rectus
Superior rectus
Frontal sinus
Optic n. (CN II)
Procerus
Inferior rectus
Vitreous body
CN V₂ in pterygo-palatine fossa
Ethmoid air cell
Sphenoid sinus
Lateral pterygoid
Levator veli palatini
Medial pterygoid
Maxillary sinus
Palatine tonsil
Orbicularis oris
Palato-pharyngeus
Tongue
Genioglossus
Mylohyoid
Digastric, anterior belly
Hyoid bone, lesser cornu
Submandibular gland
Hyoid bone, greater cornu
Thyroid cartilage, left lamina
Inferior pharyngeal constrictor
Pharyngo-tympanic (auditory) tube
Posterior meningeal a.
CN IX, X, and XI
Hypoglossal n. (CN XII)
Transverse sinus
Condylar emissary v.
Rectus capitis posterior major
Semispinalis capitis
Internal carotid a.
Obliquus capitis inferior
Greater occipital n. (C2)
Vertebral a.
C3 spinal n.
Trapezius
Splenius capitis
Retropharyngeal space

Fig. 39.43 **Sagittal section through the inner third of the orbit**

Left lateral view. This section passes through the maxillary, frontal, and sphenoid sinuses and a single ethmoidal air cell. The pharyngeal and masticatory muscles are revealed grouped around the cartilaginous part of the pharnygotympanic (auditory) tube. The palatine tonsil of the oral cavity and medial portion of the submandibular gland below the floor of the mouth are also seen in this section.

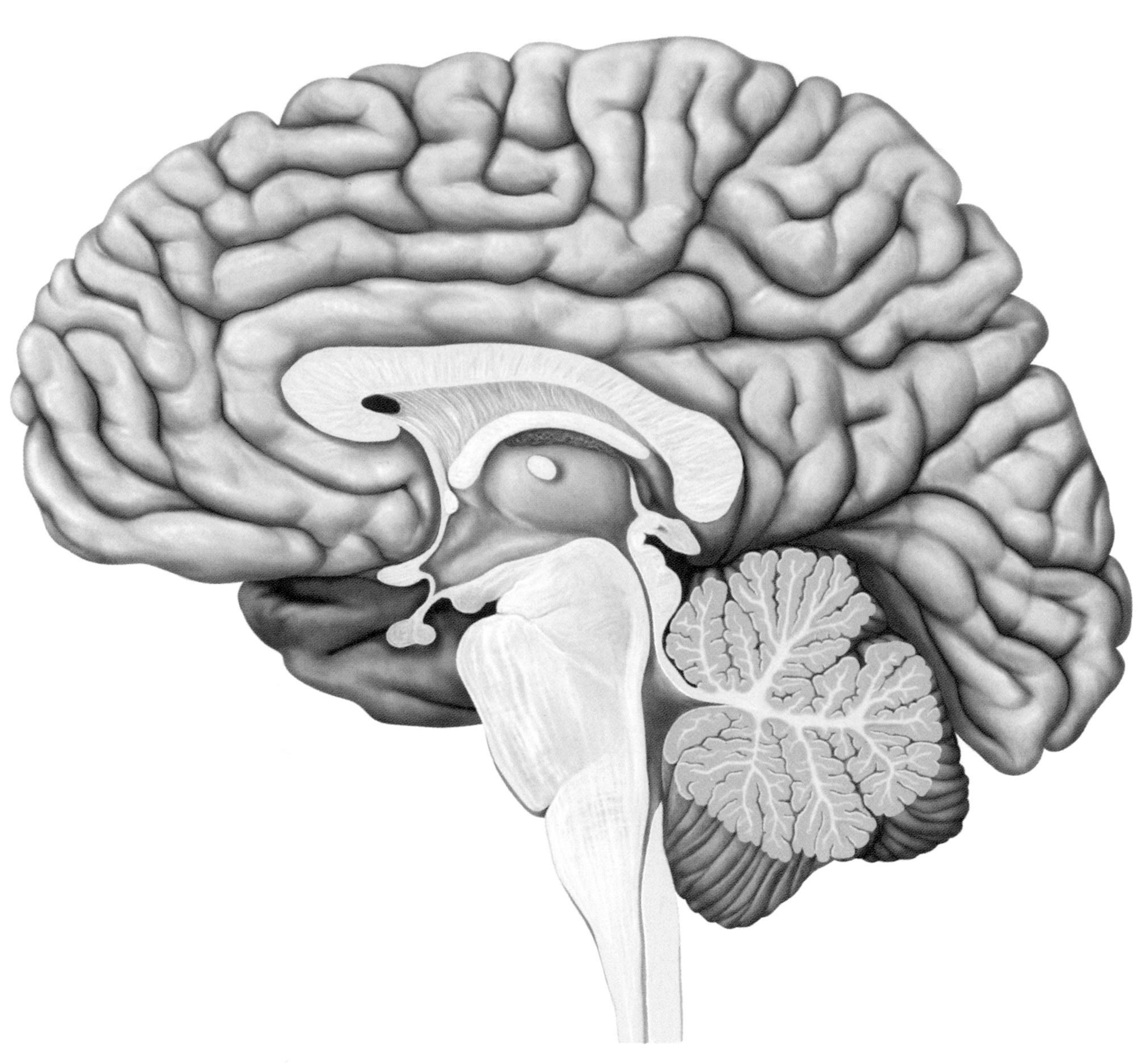

Neuroanatomy

40 Brain

Nervous System: Overview 624
Telencephalon 626
Telencephalon & Diencephalon 628
Diencephalon, Brainstem & Cerebellum 630
Ventricles & CSF Spaces 632

41 Blood Vessels of the Brain

Veins of the Brain 634
Arteries of the Brain 636

42 Functional Systems

Circuitry 638
Sensory & Motor Pathways 640
Sensory Systems (I) 642
Sensory Systems (II) 644
Sensory Systems (III) 646

43 Autonomic Nervous System

Autonomic Nervous System 648

Nervous System: Overview

Fig. 40.1 Central and peripheral nervous systems

The nervous system is divided into the central (CNS) and peripheral (PNS) nervous systems. The CNS consists of the brain and spinal cord, which constitute a functional unit. The PNS consists of the nerves emerging from the brain and spinal cord (cranial and spinal nerves, respectively).

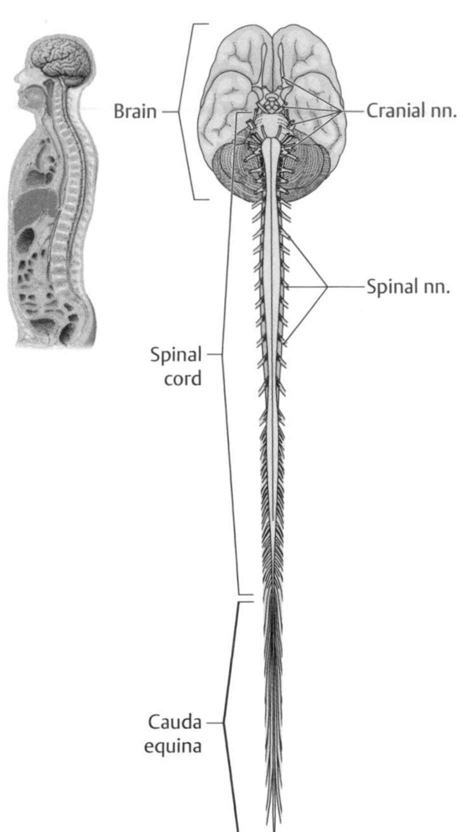

Brain
Cranial nn.
Spinal nn.
Spinal cord
Cauda equina

Fig. 40.2 Neurons (nerve cells)

The nervous system is composed of neurons (nerve cells) and supporting neuroglial cells, which vastly outnumber them (10 to 1). Each neuron contains a cell body (soma) with one axon (projecting segment) and one or more dendrites (receptor segments). The release of neurotransmitters at synapses creates an excitatory or inhibitory postsynaptic potential at the target neuron. If this exceeds the depolarization threshold of the neuron, the axon "fires," initiating the release of a transmitter from its presynaptic knob (bouton).

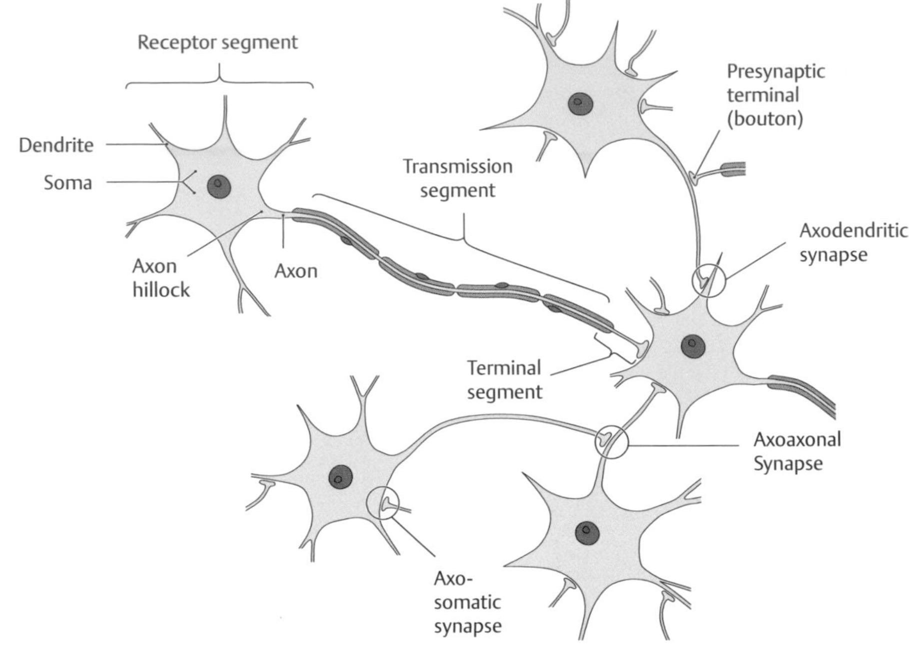

Receptor segment
Dendrite
Soma
Axon hillock
Axon
Transmission segment
Presynaptic terminal (bouton)
Axodendritic synapse
Terminal segment
Axoaxonal Synapse
Axo-somatic synapse

Fig. 40.3 Myelination

Certain glial cells with lipid-rich membranes may myelinate axons (nerve fibers). Myelination electrically insulates axons, thereby increasing impulse conduction speed. In the CNS, one oligodendrocyte myelinates one internode on multiple axons; in the PNS, one Schwann cell myelinates one internode on a single axon.

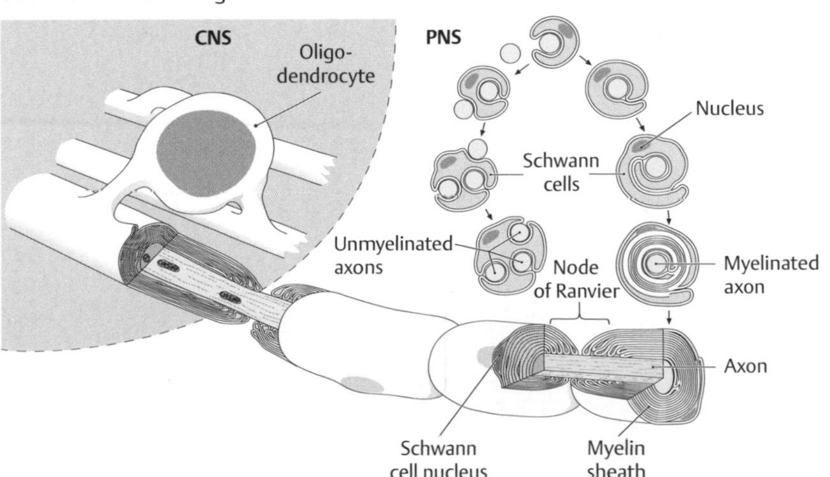

CNS
Oligo-dendrocyte
PNS
Nucleus
Schwann cells
Unmyelinated axons
Node of Ranvier
Myelinated axon
Axon
Schwann cell nucleus
Myelin sheath

Fig. 40.4 Gray and white matter in the CNS

Nerve cell bodies appear gray in gross inspection, whereas nerve cell processes (axons) and their insulating myelin sheaths appear white.

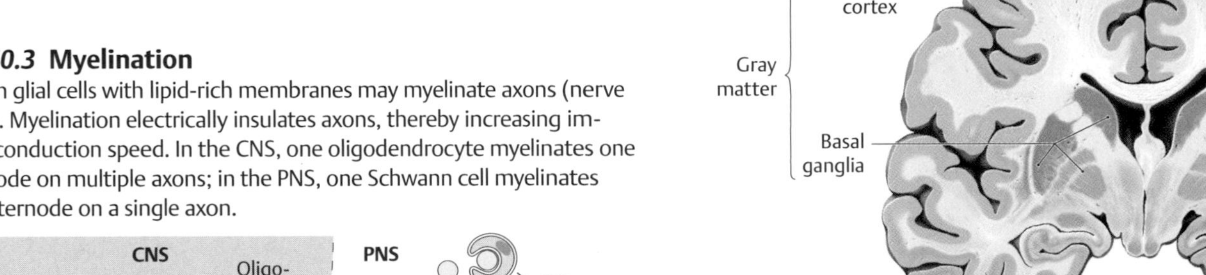

Cerebral cortex
Gray matter
Basal ganglia
White matter

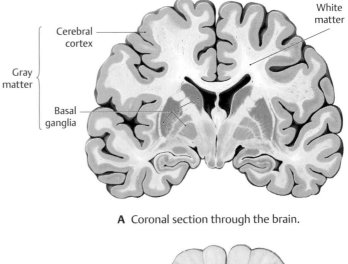

A Coronal section through the brain.

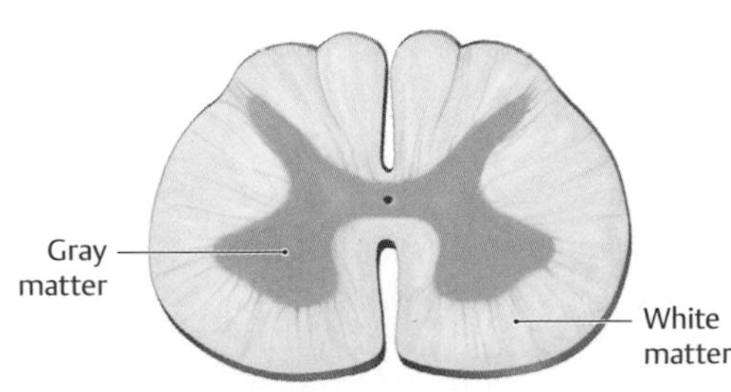

Gray matter
White matter

B Transverse section through the spinal cord.

Table 40.1 Development of the brain

	Primary vesicle	Region		Structure
Neural tube	Prosencephalon (forebrain)	Telencephalon (cerebrum)		Cerebral cortex, white matter, and basal ganglia
		Diencephalon		Epithalamus (pineal), dorsal thalamus, subthalamus, and hypothalamus
	Mesencephalon (midbrain)*			Tectum, tegmentum, and cerebral peduncles
	Rhombencephalon (hindbrain)	Metencephalon	Cerebellum	Cerebellar cortex, nuclei, and peduncles
			Pons*	Nuclei and fiber tracts
		Myelencephalon	Medulla oblongata*	

* The mesencephalon, pons, and medulla oblongata are collectively known as the brainstem.

Fig. 40.5 Embryonic development of the brain

Left lateral view.

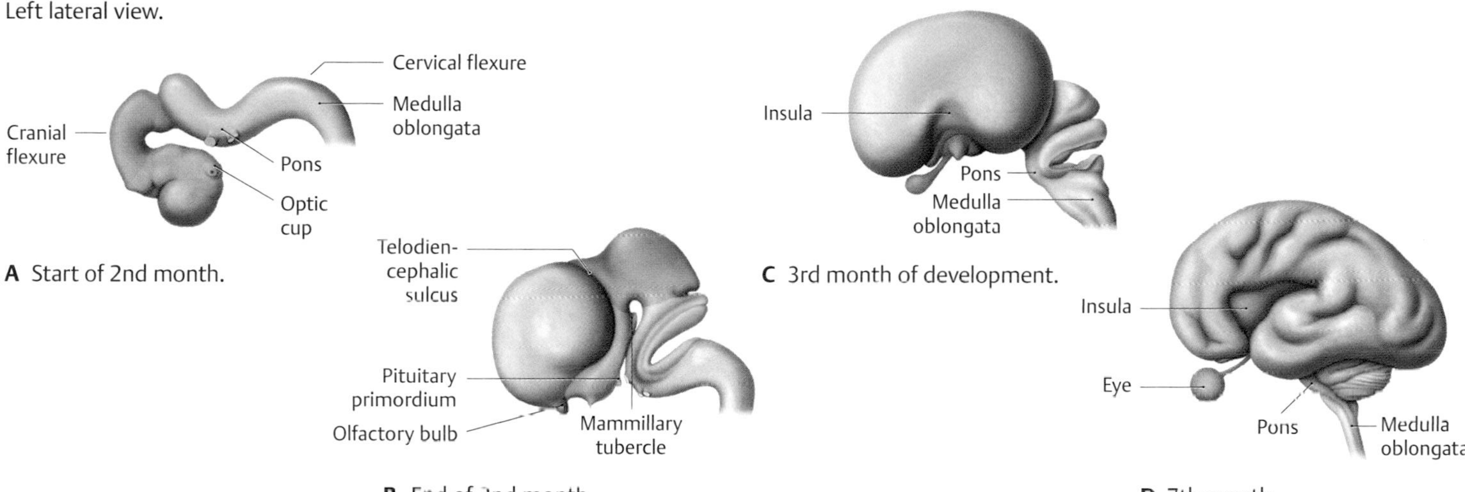

Cervical flexure
Medulla oblongata
Cranial flexure
Pons
Optic cup
Insula
Pons
Medulla oblongata
Telodiencephalic sulcus
Pituitary primordium
Olfactory bulb
Mammillary tubercle
Insula
Eye
Pons
Medulla oblongata

A Start of 2nd month.

B End of 2nd month.

C 3rd month of development.

D 7th month.

Fig. 40.6 Adult brain

See Fig. 40.12 for lobes of the cerebrum. CN, cranial nerve.

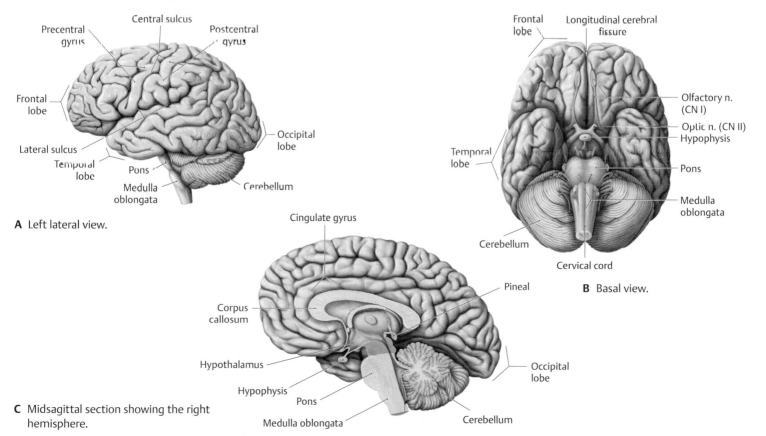

A Left lateral view.

B Basal view.

C Midsagittal section showing the right hemisphere.

Telencephalon

Fig. 40.7 Divisions of the telencephalon

Coronal section, anterior view. The telencephalon is divided into the cerebral cortex, white matter, and basal ganglia. The cerebral cortex is further divided into the allocortex and isocortex (neocortex).

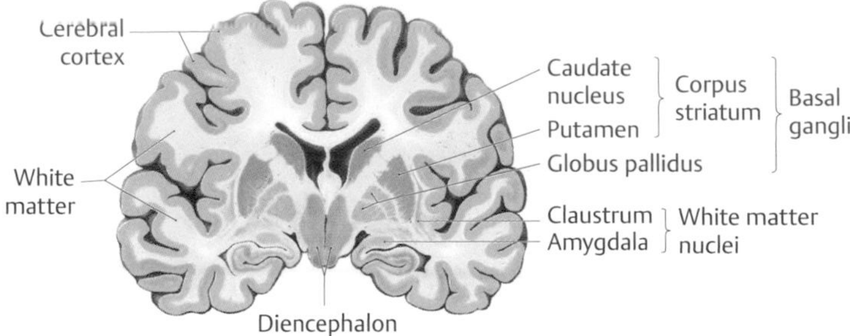
Cerebral cortex
White matter
Caudate nucleus
Putamen
Corpus striatum
Basal ganglia
Globus pallidus
Claustrum
Amygdala
White matter nuclei
Diencephalon

Fig. 40.8 White matter

A special preparation technique was used to show the fiber structure of the superficial layer of white matter.

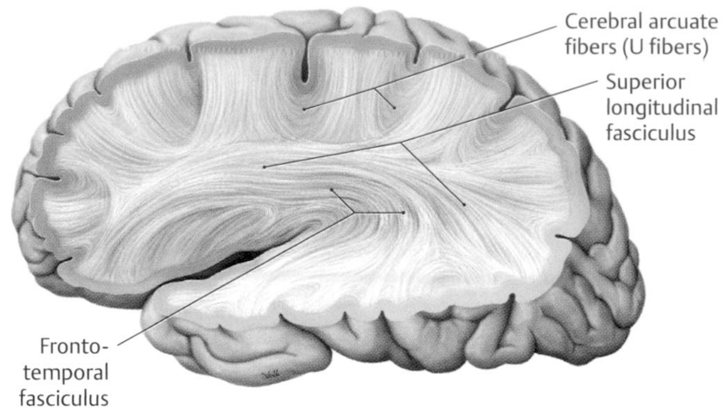
Cerebral arcuate fibers (U fibers)
Superior longitudinal fasciculus
Fronto-temporal fasciculus

A Lateral view of left hemisphere.

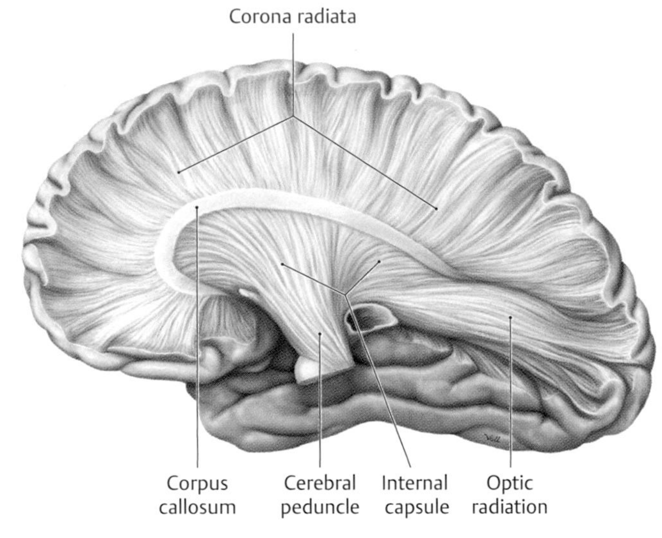
Corona radiata
Corpus callosum
Cerebral peduncle
Internal capsule
Optic radiation

B Medial view of right hemisphere.

Fig. 40.9 Basal ganglia

Transverse section, superior view. The basal ganglia are an essential component of the motor system (see p. 641).

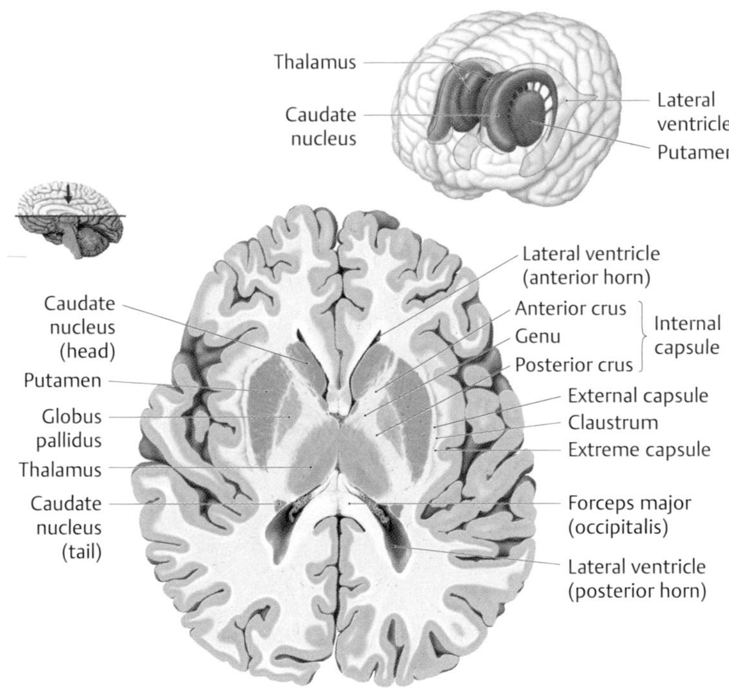
Thalamus
Caudate nucleus
Lateral ventricle
Putamen
Lateral ventricle (anterior horn)
Caudate nucleus (head)
Putamen
Globus pallidus
Thalamus
Caudate nucleus (tail)
Anterior crus
Genu
Posterior crus
Internal capsule
External capsule
Claustrum
Extreme capsule
Forceps major (occipitalis)
Lateral ventricle (posterior horn)

Fig. 40.10 Allocortex

The three-layered allocortex consists of the olfactory cortex (blue) and the hippocampus (pink).

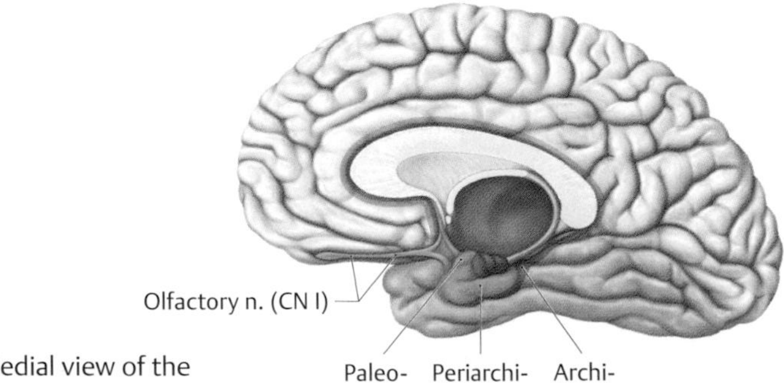
Olfactory n. (CN I)
Paleo-cortex
Periarchi-cortex
Archi-cortex

A Medial view of the right hemisphere.

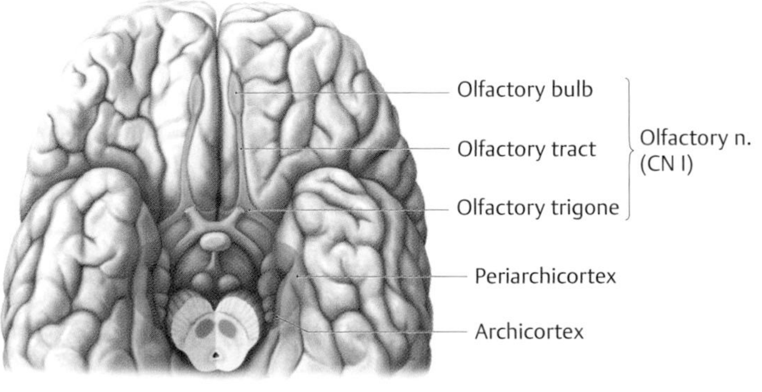
Olfactory bulb
Olfactory tract
Olfactory trigone
Olfactory n. (CN I)
Periarchicortex
Archicortex

B Basal view.

Fig. 40.11 Isocortex: Columnar organization

Morphological considerations divide the isocortex into six horizontal layers; functional considerations divide it into cortical columns.

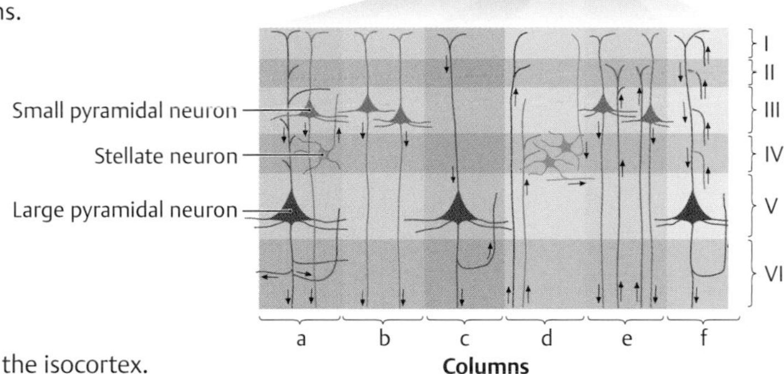
Cortical column
Cerebral cortex (neocortex)
Small pyramidal neuron
Stellate neuron
Large pyramidal neuron
I
II
III
IV
V
VI
a
b
c
d
e
f
Columns
Molecular layer (I)
External granular layer (II)
External pyramidal layer (III)
Internal granular layer (IV)
Internal pyramidal layer (V)
Multiform layer (VI)
Layers

A Histology of the isocortex.

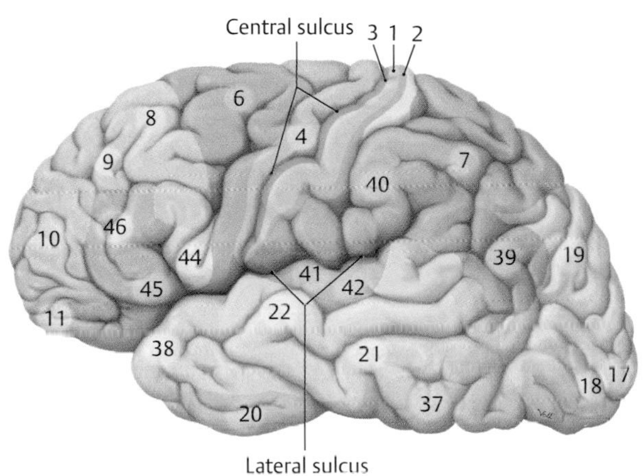
Central sulcus
Lateral sulcus

B Brodmann (cortical) areas, lateral view of the left cerebral hemisphere.

Central sulcus
Parieto-occipital sulcus
Calcarine sulcus

C Brodmann (cortical) areas, medial view of the right cerebral hemisphere.

Fig. 40.12 Lobes in the cerebral hemispheres

The isocortex also may be functionally divided into association areas (lobes).

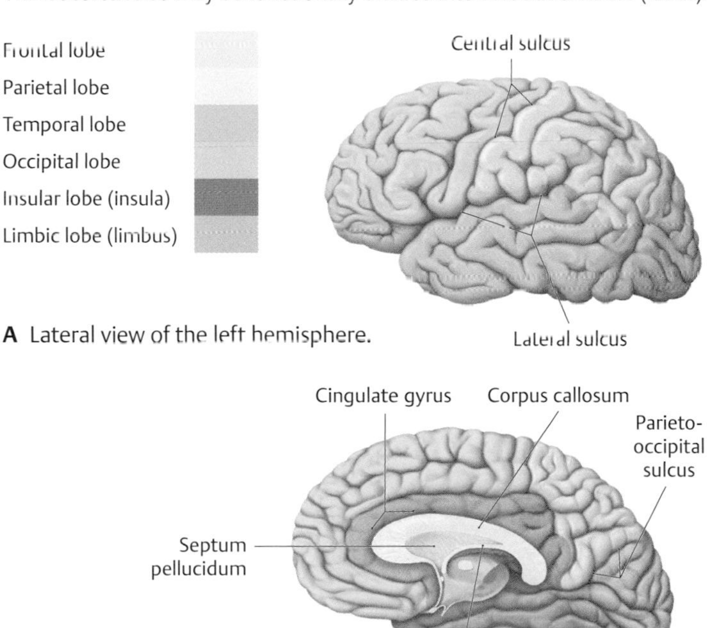
Frontal lobe
Parietal lobe
Temporal lobe
Occipital lobe
Insular lobe (insula)
Limbic lobe (limbus)
Central sulcus
Lateral sulcus
Cingulate gyrus
Corpus callosum
Parieto-occipital sulcus
Septum pellucidum
Fornix

A Lateral view of the left hemisphere.

C Medial view of the right hemisphere.

Insula

B Lateral view of the retracted left cerebral hemisphere.

Frontal pole
Olfactory n. (CN I)
Optic n. (CN II)
Hypophysis
Mammillary body
Mesencephalon
Occipital pole
Longitudinal cerebral fissure

D Basal view with the brainstem removed.

Telencephalon & Diencephalon

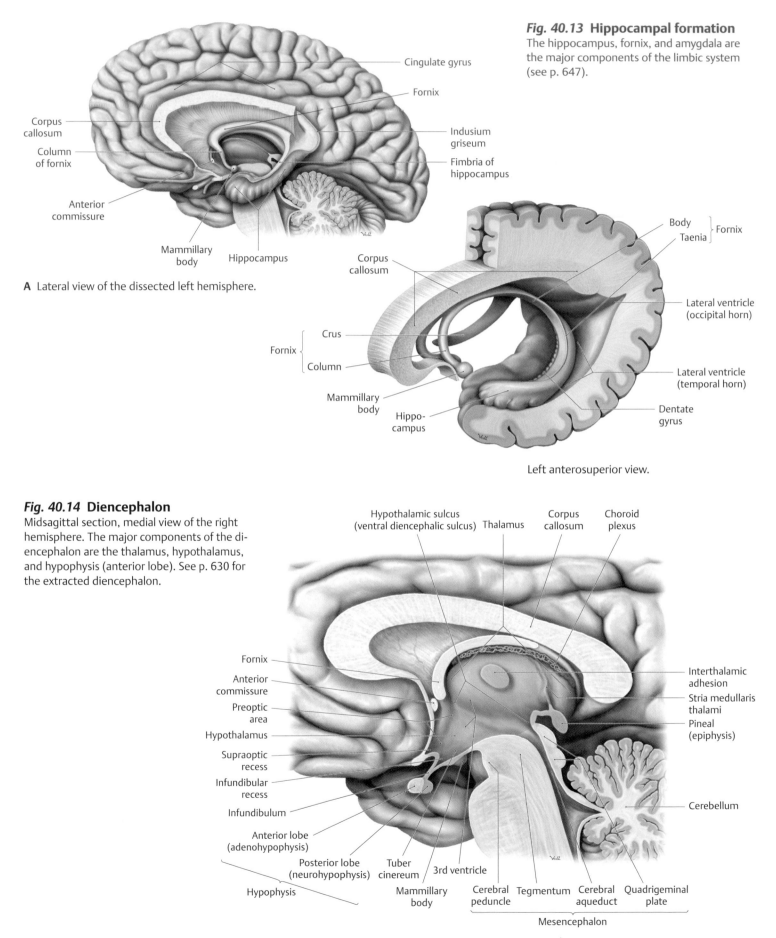

Fig. 40.13 **Hippocampal formation**
The hippocampus, fornix, and amygdala are the major components of the limbic system (see p. 647).

Cingulate gyrus
Fornix
Corpus callosum
Indusium griseum
Column of fornix
Fimbria of hippocampus
Anterior commissure
Mammillary body
Hippocampus

A Lateral view of the dissected left hemisphere.

Body
Taenia
Fornix
Corpus callosum
Lateral ventricle (occipital horn)
Fornix: Crus, Column
Lateral ventricle (temporal horn)
Mammillary body
Hippocampus
Dentate gyrus

Left anterosuperior view.

Fig. 40.14 **Diencephalon**
Midsagittal section, medial view of the right hemisphere. The major components of the diencephalon are the thalamus, hypothalamus, and hypophysis (anterior lobe). See p. 630 for the extracted diencephalon.

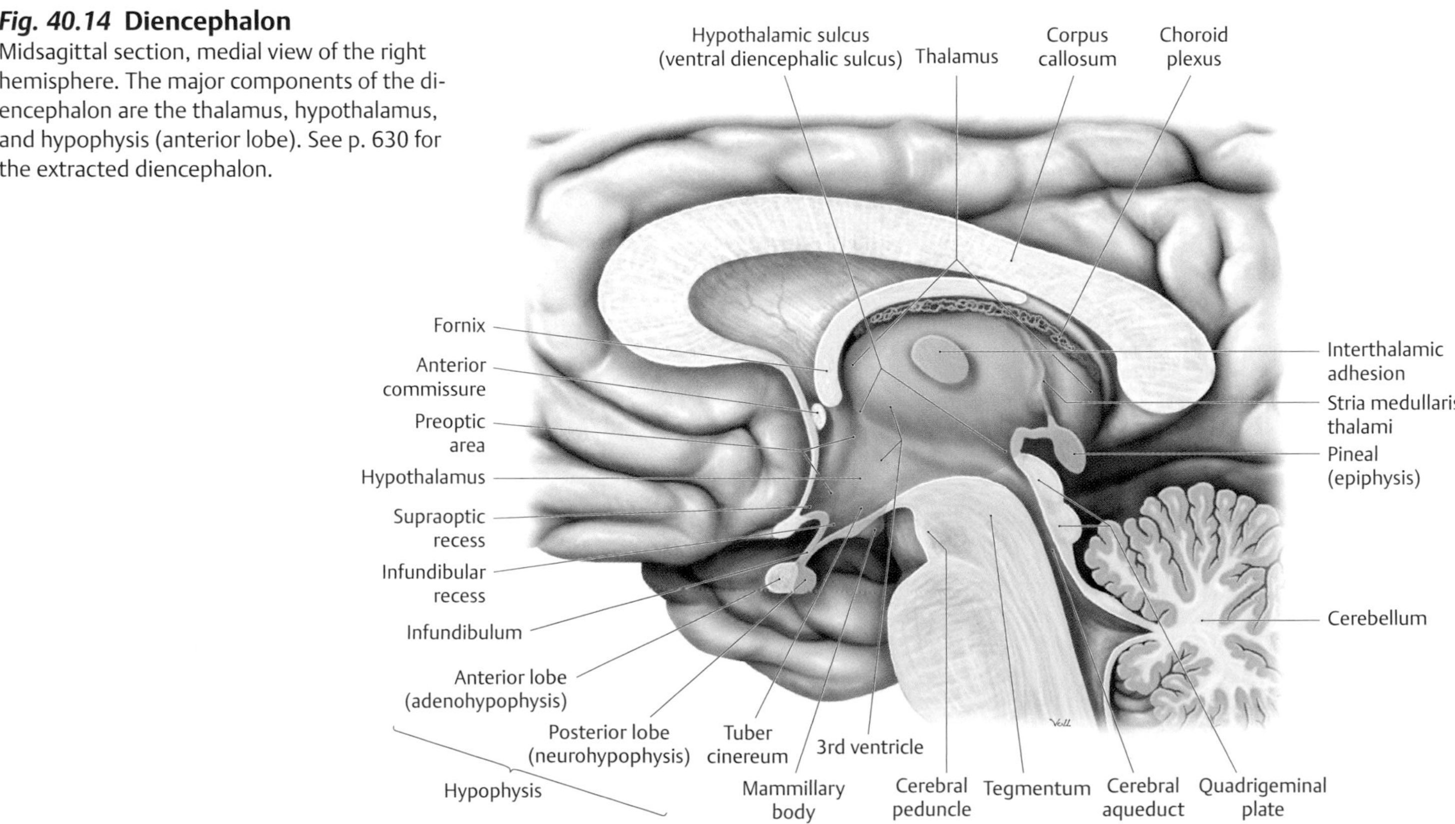
Hypothalamic sulcus (ventral diencephalic sulcus)
Thalamus
Corpus callosum
Choroid plexus
Fornix
Anterior commissure
Preoptic area
Hypothalamus
Supraoptic recess
Infundibular recess
Infundibulum
Anterior lobe (adenohypophysis)
Posterior lobe (neurohypophysis)
Hypophysis
Tuber cinereum
Mammillary body
3rd ventricle
Cerebral peduncle
Tegmentum
Cerebral aqueduct
Quadrigeminal plate
Mesencephalon
Interthalamic adhesion
Stria medullaris thalami
Pineal (epiphysis)
Cerebellum

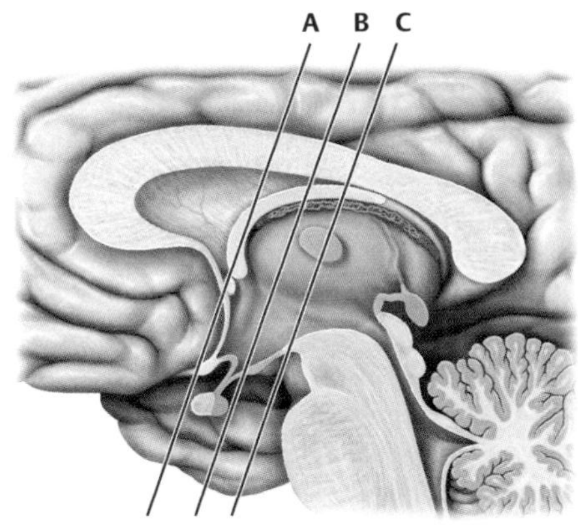
A
B
C

Table 40.2 Structures of the telencephalon

①	Corpus callosum
②	Septum pellucidum
③	Lateral ventricle
④	Fornix
⑤	Caudate nucleus
⑥	Internal capsule
⑦	Putamen
⑧	Globus pallidus
⑨	Cavum septi pellucidi
⑩	Anterior commissure
⑪	Lateral olfactory stria
⑫	Choroid plexus
⑬	Basal ganglia
⑭	Amygdala
⑮	Hippocampus

Table 40.3 Structures of the diencephalon

Ⓟ	Preoptic recess		
OC	Optic chiasm		
3V	3rd ventricle		
OT	Optic tract		
In	Infundibulum		
Ⓣ	Thalamus (with thalamic nuclei):		
		Ⓡ	Reticular nucleus of thalamus
		Ⓔ	External medullary lamina
		Ⓥ	Ventrolateral thalamic nuclei
		Ⓘ	Internal medullary lamina
		Ⓜ	Medial thalamic nuclei
		Ⓐ	Anterior thalamic nuclei
		Ⓟ	Paraventricular nuclei
Ⓢ	Subthalamic nucleus		
SN*	Substantia nigra		
MF	Mammillothalamic fasciculus		
MB	Mammillary body		

*Actually a structure of the mesencephalon.

Fig. 40.15 **Telencephalon and diencephalon: Internal structure**
Coronal section.

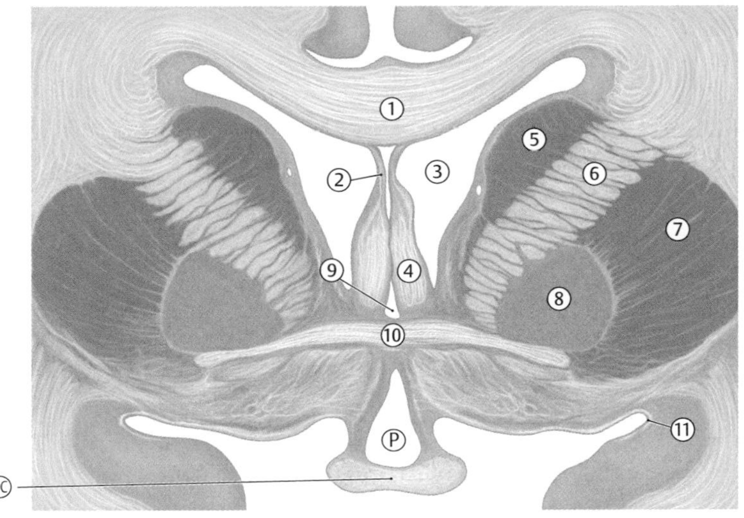
①
②
③
④
⑤
⑥
⑦
⑧
⑨
⑩
⑪
Ⓟ
OC

A Level of the optic chiasm.

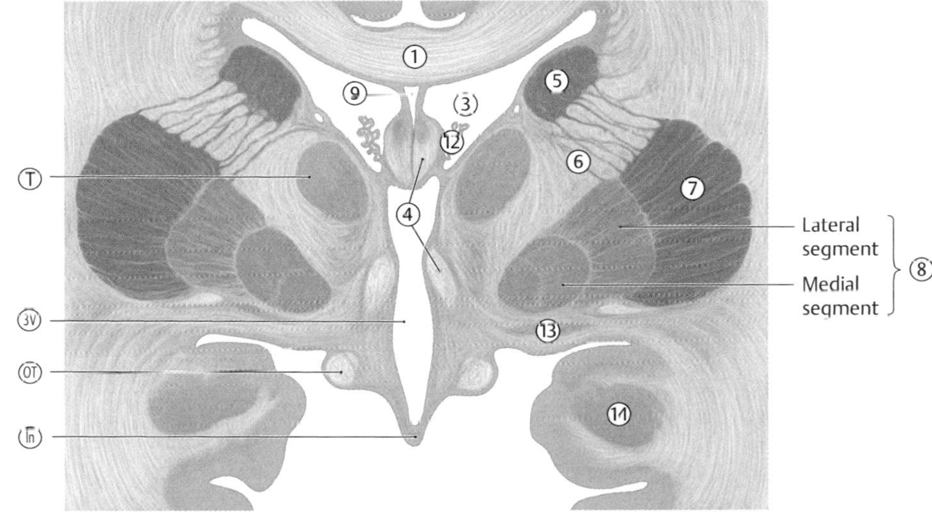
①
⑨
③
⑫
⑤
⑥
⑦
Ⓣ
④
Lateral segment
Medial segment
⑧
3V
⑬
OT
⑭
In

B Level of the tuber cinereum.

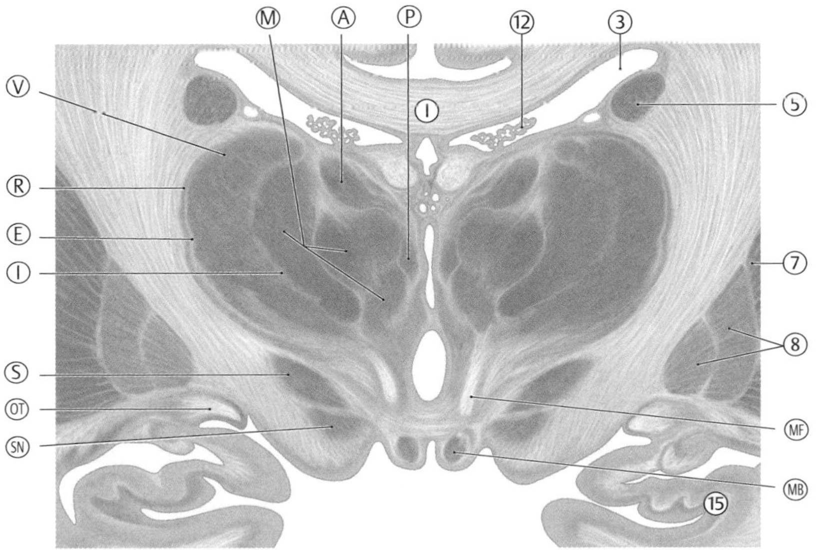
Ⓜ
Ⓐ
Ⓟ
⑫
③
Ⓥ
Ⓘ
⑤
Ⓡ
Ⓔ
Ⓘ
⑦
⑧
Ⓢ
OT
SN
MF
MB
⑮

C Level of the mammillary bodies.

Diencephalon, Brainstem & Cerebellum

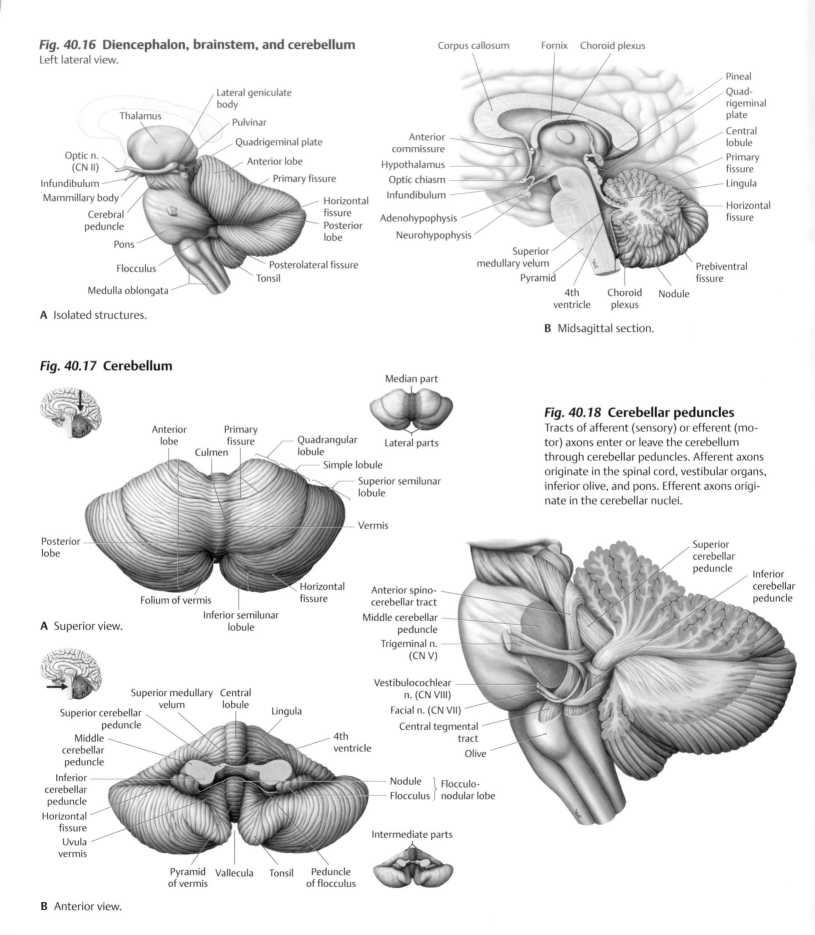

Fig. 40.16 Diencephalon, brainstem, and cerebellum
Left lateral view.

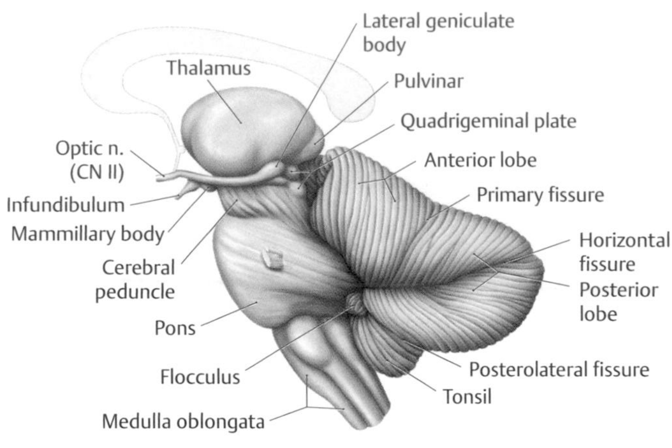
Lateral geniculate body
Thalamus
Pulvinar
Quadrigeminal plate
Optic n. (CN II)
Anterior lobe
Infundibulum
Primary fissure
Mammillary body
Horizontal fissure
Cerebral peduncle
Posterior lobe
Pons
Posterolateral fissure
Flocculus
Tonsil
Medulla oblongata

A Isolated structures.

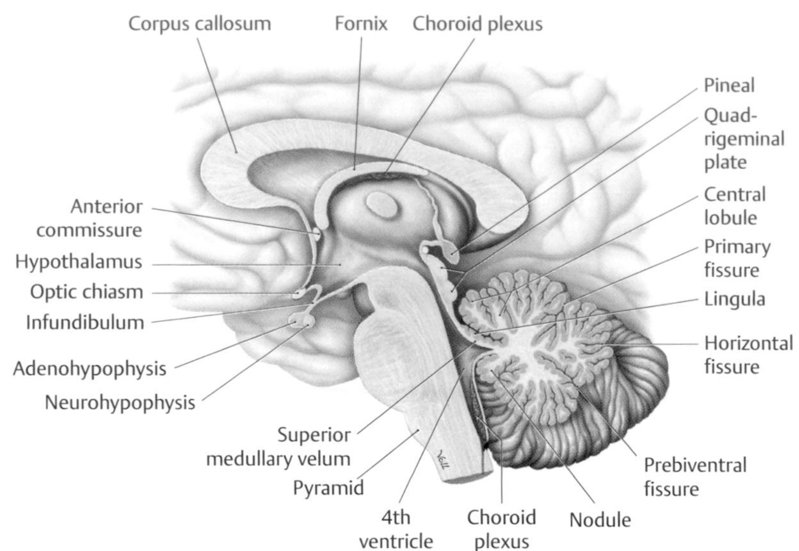
Corpus callosum
Fornix
Choroid plexus
Pineal
Quad-rigeminal plate
Anterior commissure
Central lobule
Hypothalamus
Primary fissure
Optic chiasm
Lingula
Infundibulum
Horizontal fissure
Adenohypophysis
Neurohypophysis
Superior medullary velum
Prebiventral fissure
Pyramid
4th ventricle
Choroid plexus
Nodule

B Midsagittal section.

Fig. 40.17 Cerebellum

Median part
Anterior lobe
Primary fissure
Quadrangular lobule
Lateral parts
Culmen
Simple lobule
Superior semilunar lobule
Vermis
Posterior lobe
Horizontal fissure
Folium of vermis
Inferior semilunar lobule

A Superior view.

Superior medullary velum
Central lobule
Superior cerebellar peduncle
Lingula
Middle cerebellar peduncle
4th ventricle
Inferior cerebellar peduncle
Nodule
Flocculus
Flocculo-nodular lobe
Horizontal fissure
Uvula vermis
Intermediate parts
Pyramid of vermis
Vallecula
Tonsil
Peduncle of flocculus

B Anterior view.

Fig. 40.18 Cerebellar peduncles
Tracts of afferent (sensory) or efferent (motor) axons enter or leave the cerebellum through cerebellar peduncles. Afferent axons originate in the spinal cord, vestibular organs, inferior olive, and pons. Efferent axons originate in the cerebellar nuclei.

Superior cerebellar peduncle
Inferior cerebellar peduncle
Anterior spino-cerebellar tract
Middle cerebellar peduncle
Trigeminal n. (CN V)
Vestibulocochlear n. (CN VIII)
Facial n. (CN VII)
Central tegmental tract
Olive

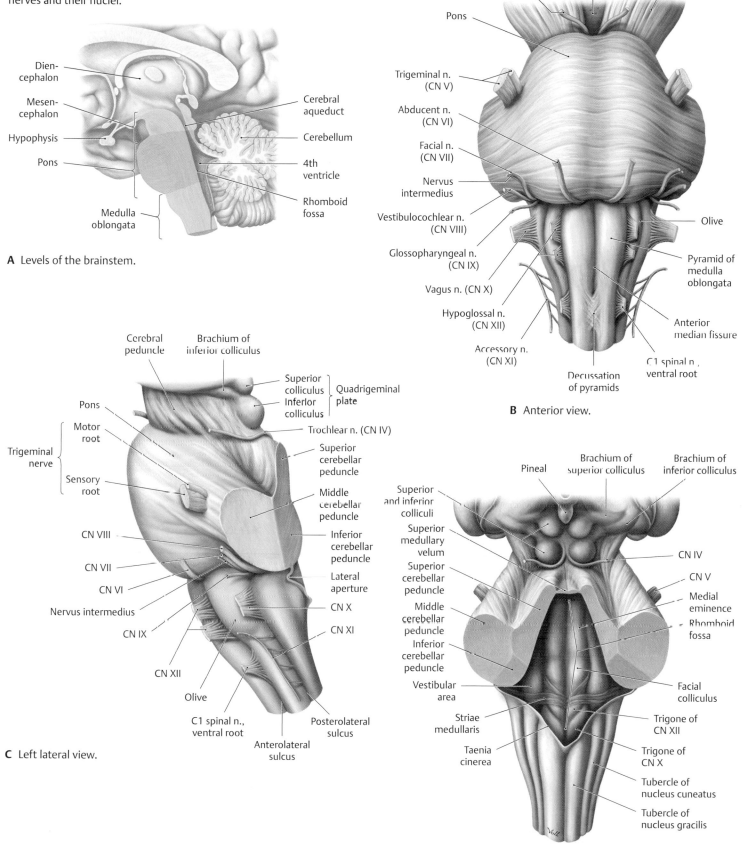

***Fig. 40.19* Brainstem**

The brainstem is the site of emergence and entry of the 10 pairs of true cranial nerves (CN III–XII). See p. 496 for an overview of the cranial nerves and their nuclei.

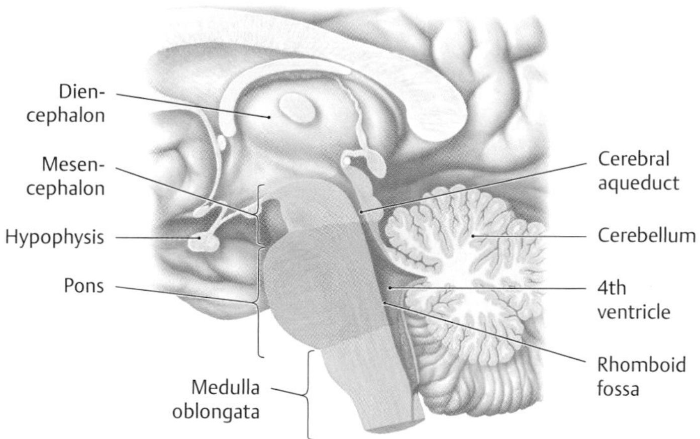

Dien-
cephalon
Mesen-
cephalon
Hypophysis
Pons
Medulla
oblongata
Cerebral
aqueduct
Cerebellum
4th
ventricle
Rhomboid
fossa

A Levels of the brainstem.

Oculomotor n. (CN III)
Interpeduncular fossa
Cerebral peduncle
Pons
Trigeminal n. (CN V)
Abducent n. (CN VI)
Facial n. (CN VII)
Nervus intermedius
Vestibulocochlear n. (CN VIII)
Glossopharyngeal n. (CN IX)
Vagus n. (CN X)
Hypoglossal n. (CN XII)
Accessory n. (CN XI)
Decussation of pyramids
C1 spinal n., ventral root
Anterior median fissure
Pyramid of medulla oblongata
Olive

B Anterior view.

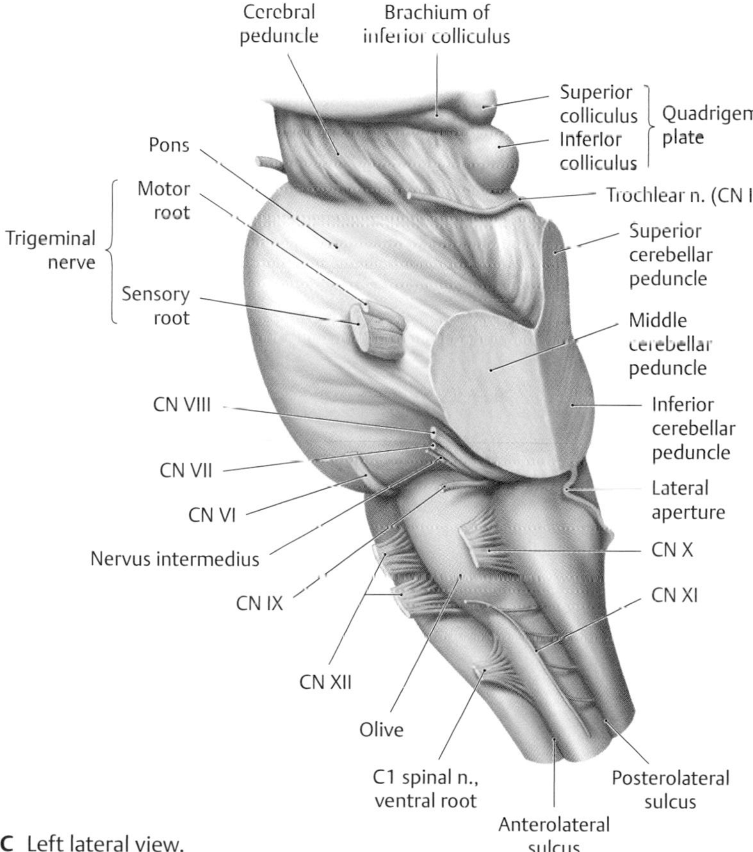

Cerebral
peduncle
Brachium of
inferior colliculus
Superior
colliculus
Inferior
colliculus
Quadrigeminal
plate
Pons
Trigeminal
nerve
Motor
root
Sensory
root
Trochlear n. (CN IV)
Superior
cerebellar
peduncle
Middle
cerebellar
peduncle
Inferior
cerebellar
peduncle
CN VIII
CN VII
CN VI
Nervus intermedius
CN IX
CN XII
Olive
Lateral
aperture
CN X
CN XI
C1 spinal n.,
ventral root
Anterolateral
sulcus
Posterolateral
sulcus

C Left lateral view.

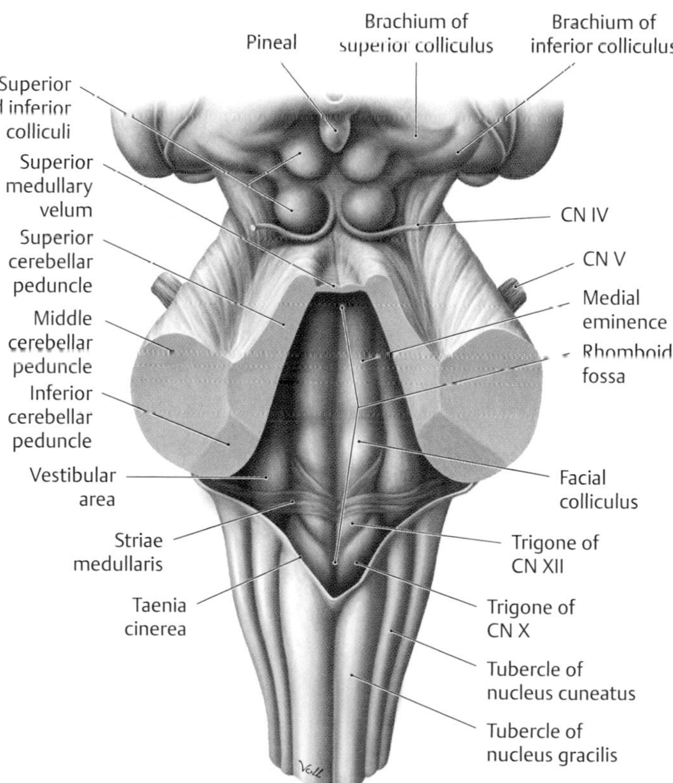

Pineal
Brachium of
superior colliculus
Brachium of
inferior colliculus
Superior
and inferior
colliculi
Superior
medullary
velum
Superior
cerebellar
peduncle
Middle
cerebellar
peduncle
Inferior
cerebellar
peduncle
Vestibular
area
Striae
medullaris
Taenia
cinerea
CN IV
CN V
Medial
eminence
Rhomboid
fossa
Facial
colliculus
Trigone of
CN XII
Trigone of
CN X
Tubercle of
nucleus cuneatus
Tubercle of
nucleus gracilis

D Posterior view.

Fig. 40.20 Circulation of cerebrospinal fluid (CSF)

The brain and spinal cord are suspended in CSF. Produced continually in the choroid plexus, CSF occupies the subarachnoid space and ventricles of the brain and drains through arachnoid granulations into the dural venous sinus system (primarily the superior sagittal sinus) of the cranial cavity. Smaller amounts drain along proximal portions of the spinal nerves into venous plexuses or lymphatic pathways.

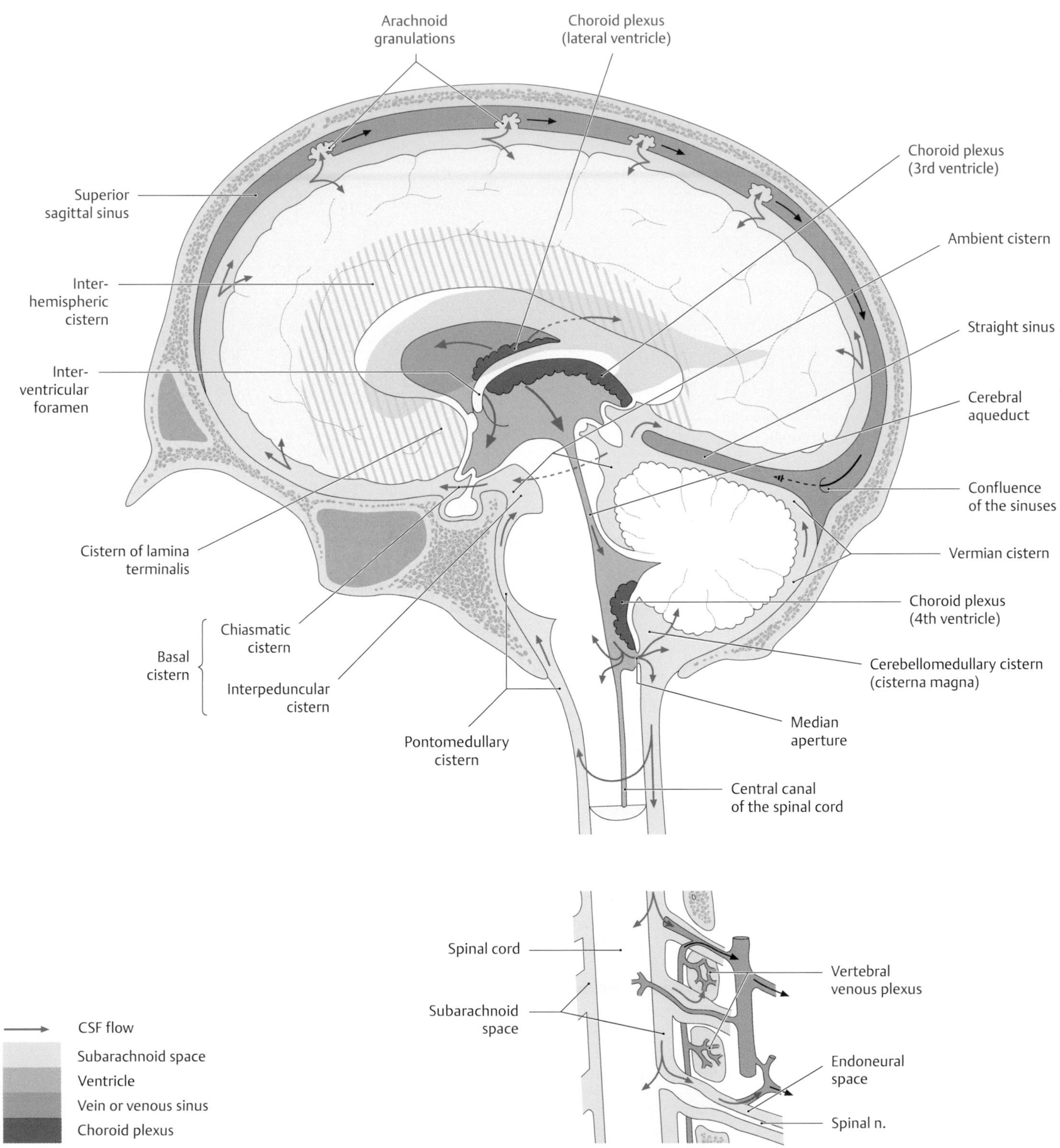

Arachnoid granulations
Choroid plexus (lateral ventricle)
Choroid plexus (3rd ventricle)
Ambient cistern
Straight sinus
Cerebral aqueduct
Confluence of the sinuses
Vermian cistern
Choroid plexus (4th ventricle)
Cerebellomedullary cistern (cisterna magna)
Median aperture
Central canal of the spinal cord
Superior sagittal sinus
Inter-hemispheric cistern
Inter-ventricular foramen
Cistern of lamina terminalis
Basal cistern
Chiasmatic cistern
Interpeduncular cistern
Pontomedullary cistern
Spinal cord
Subarachnoid space
Vertebral venous plexus
Endoneural space
Spinal n.
CSF flow
Subarachnoid space
Ventricle
Vein or venous sinus
Choroid plexus

Fig. 40.21 Ventricular system

The ventricular system is a continuation of the central spinal canal into the brain. Cast specimens are used to demonstrate the connections between the four ventricular cavities.

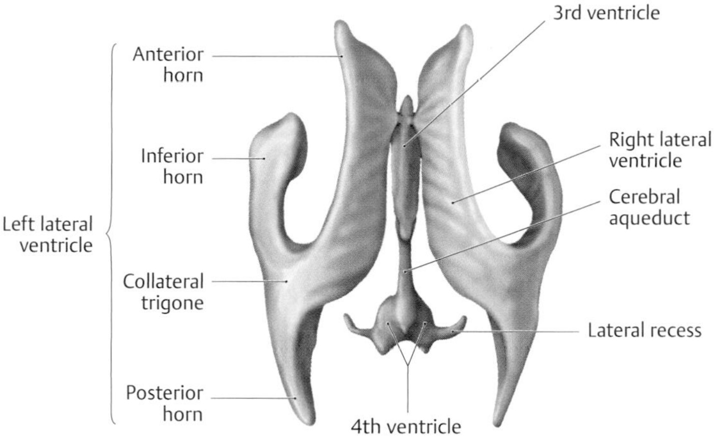

Left lateral ventricle
Anterior horn
Inferior horn
Collateral trigone
Posterior horn
3rd ventricle
Right lateral ventricle
Cerebral aqueduct
Lateral recess
4th ventricle

A Superior view.

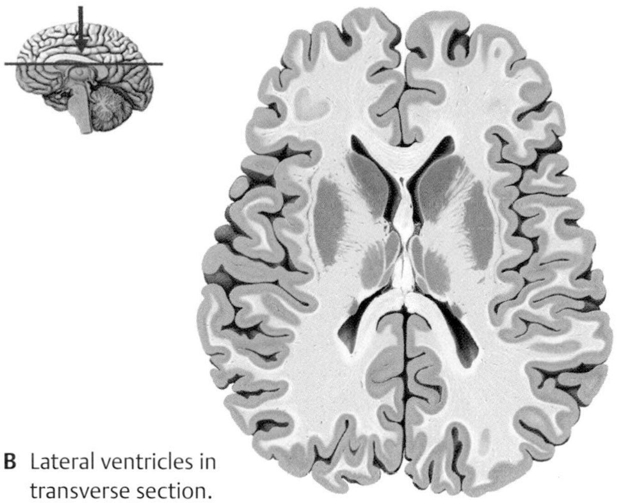

B Lateral ventricles in transverse section.

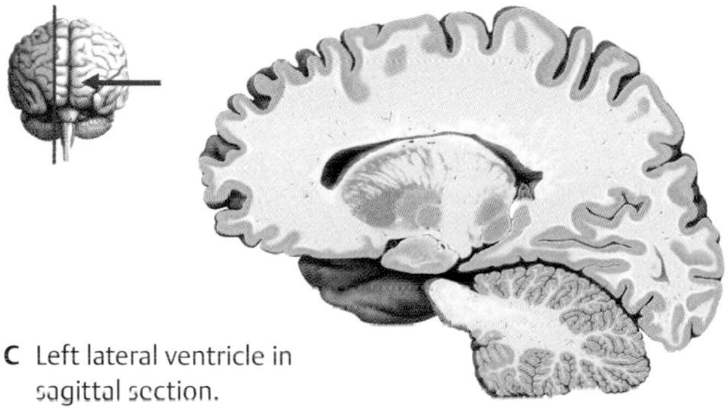

C Left lateral ventricle in sagittal section.

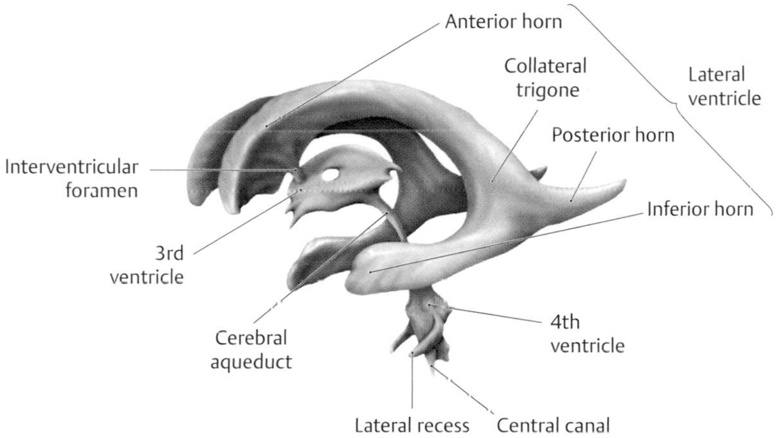

Anterior horn
Collateral trigone
Lateral ventricle
Posterior horn
Inferior horn
Interventricular foramen
3rd ventricle
Cerebral aqueduct
4th ventricle
Lateral recess
Central canal

D Left lateral view.

Fig. 40.22 Ventricular system in situ

Left lateral view.

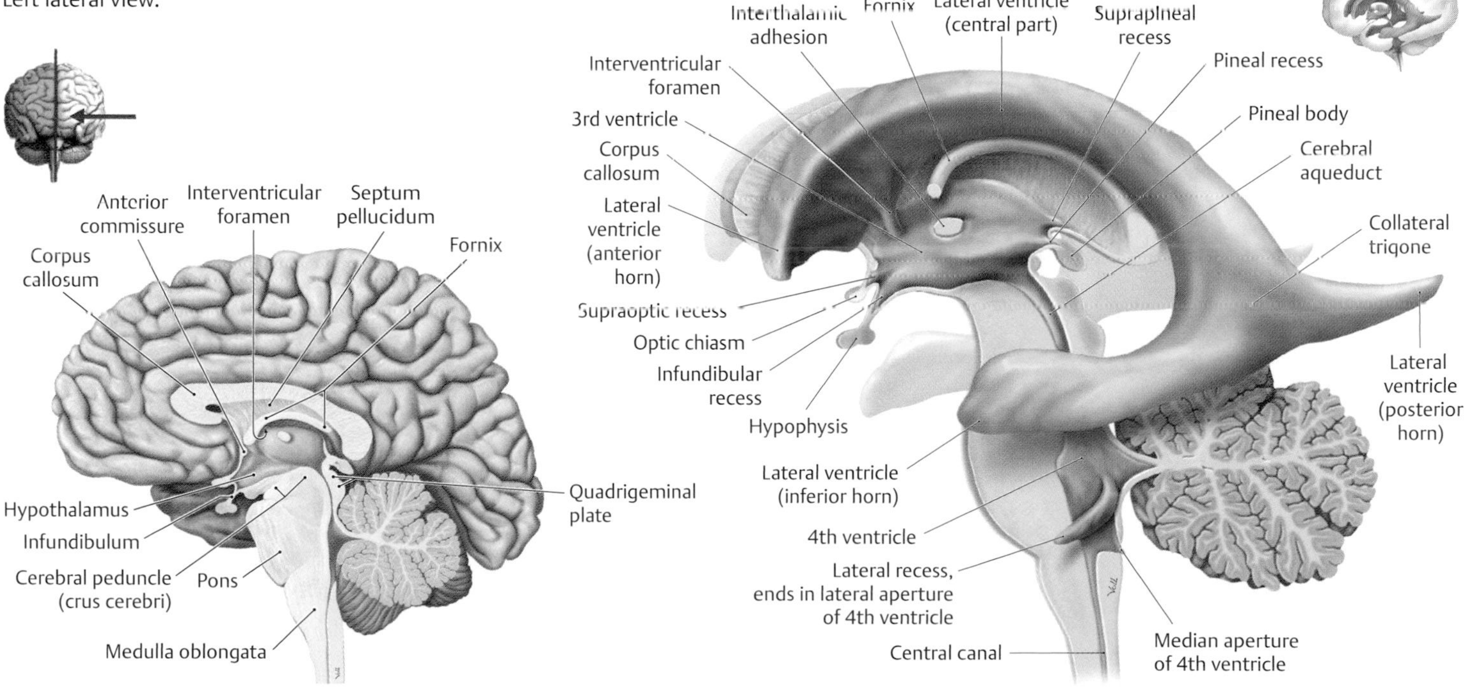
Anterior commissure
Interventricular foramen
Septum pellucidum
Corpus callosum
Fornix
Hypothalamus
Infundibulum
Cerebral peduncle (crus cerebri)
Pons
Medulla oblongata
Quadrigeminal plate
Interthalamic adhesion
Fornix
Lateral ventricle (central part)
Suprapineal recess
Pineal recess
Interventricular foramen
3rd ventricle
Pineal body
Corpus callosum
Cerebral aqueduct
Lateral ventricle (anterior horn)
Collateral trigone
Supraoptic recess
Optic chiasm
Infundibular recess
Hypophysis
Lateral ventricle (posterior horn)
Lateral ventricle (inferior horn)
4th ventricle
Lateral recess, ends in lateral aperture of 4th ventricle
Central canal
Median aperture of 4th ventricle

A 3rd and 4th ventricles in the midsagittal section.

B Ventricular system with neighboring structures.

Veins of the Brain

Fig. 41.1 Superficial cerebral veins

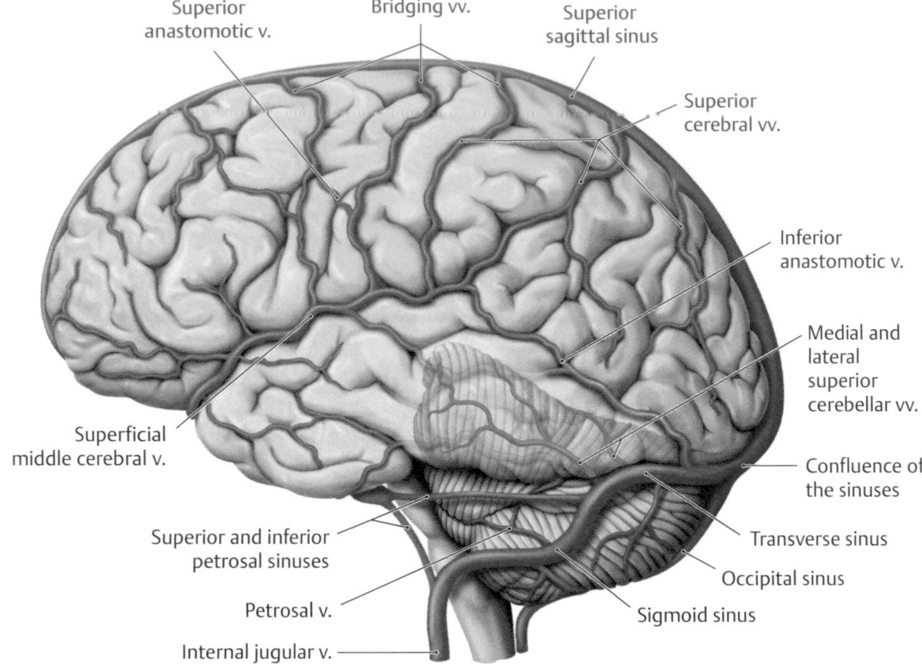
Superior anastomotic v.
Bridging vv.
Superior sagittal sinus
Superior cerebral vv.
Inferior anastomotic v.
Medial and lateral superior cerebellar vv.
Confluence of the sinuses
Transverse sinus
Occipital sinus
Sigmoid sinus
Superficial middle cerebral v.
Superior and inferior petrosal sinuses
Petrosal v.
Internal jugular v.

A Lateral view of the left hemisphere.

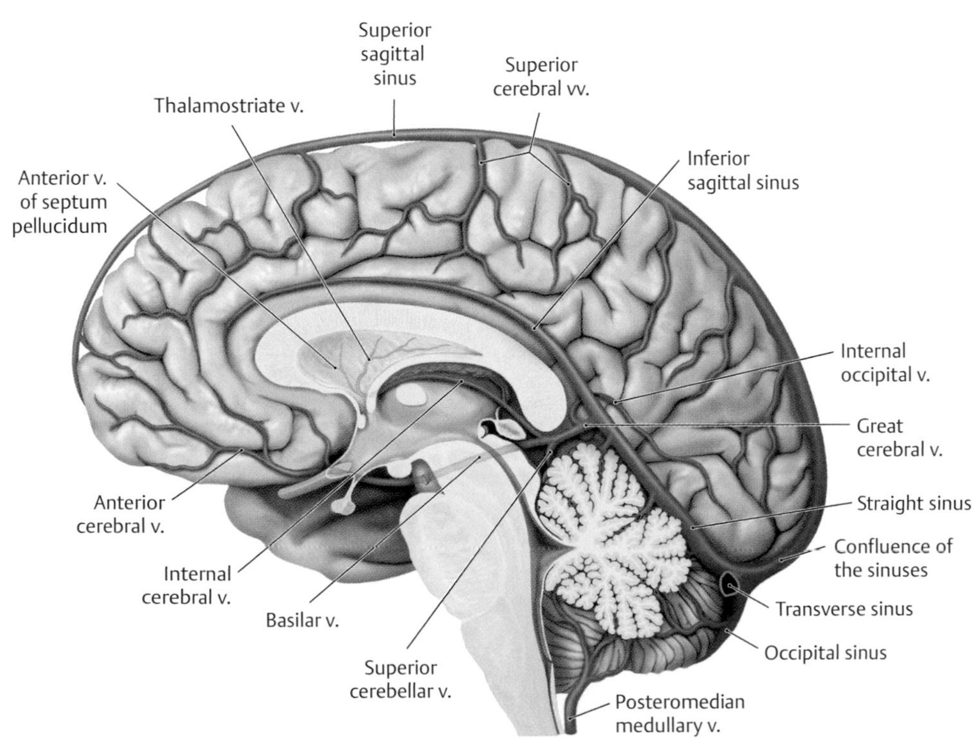
Superior sagittal sinus
Superior cerebral vv.
Thalamostriate v.
Inferior sagittal sinus
Anterior v. of septum pellucidum
Internal occipital v.
Great cerebral v.
Straight sinus
Confluence of the sinuses
Transverse sinus
Occipital sinus
Anterior cerebral v.
Internal cerebral v.
Basilar v.
Superior cerebellar v.
Posteromedian medullary v.

B Medial view of the right hemisphere.

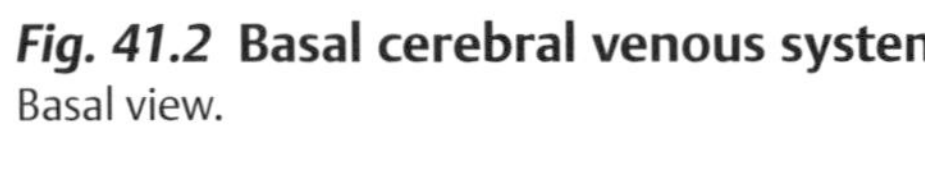

Fig. 41.2 Basal cerebral venous system
Basal view.

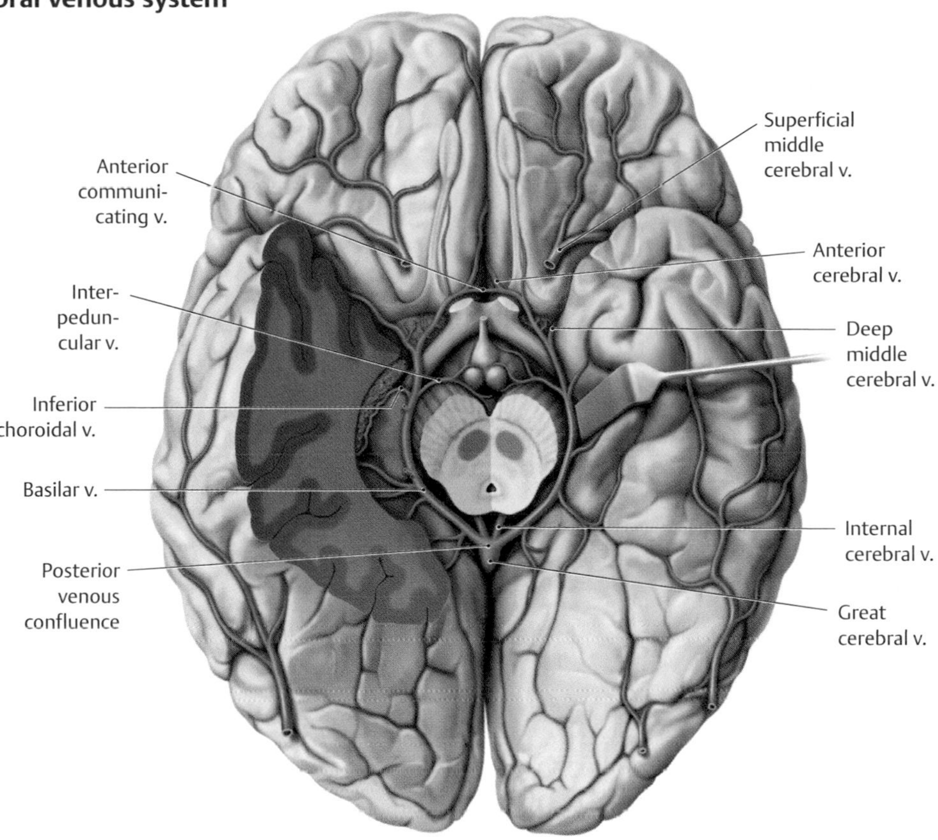
Anterior communicating v.
Inter-peduncular v.
Inferior choroidal v.
Basilar v.
Posterior venous confluence
Superficial middle cerebral v.
Anterior cerebral v.
Deep middle cerebral v.
Internal cerebral v.
Great cerebral v.

Fig. 41.3 Veins of the brainstem
Basal view.

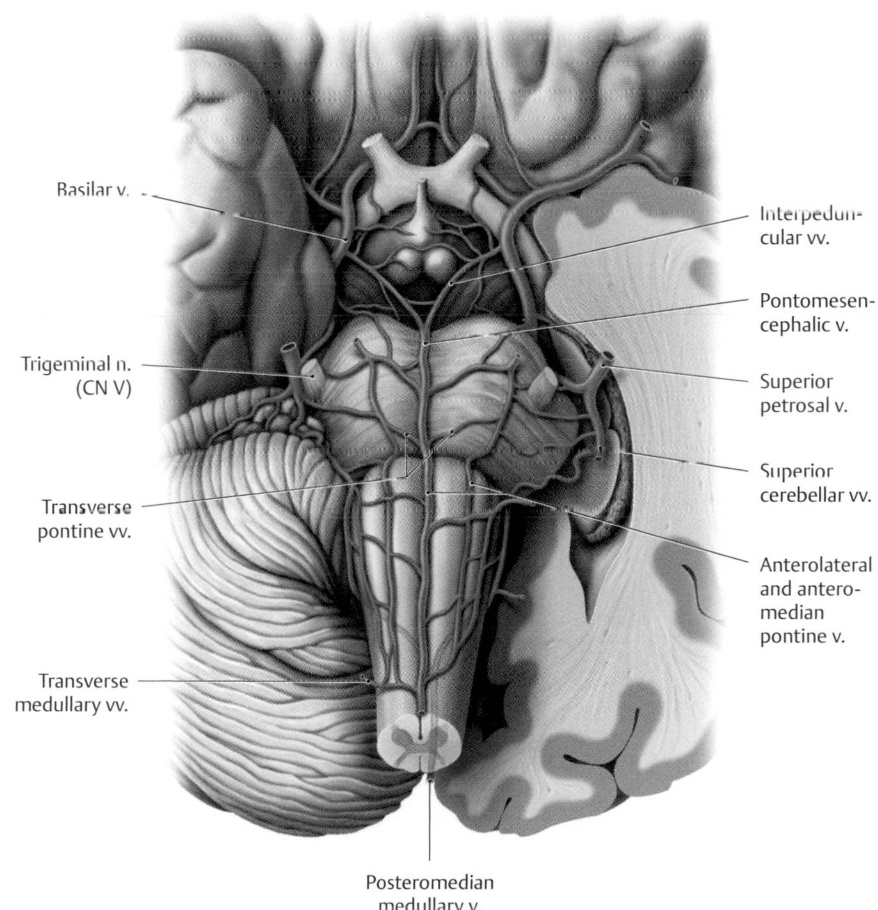
Basilar v.
Trigeminal n. (CN V)
Transverse pontine vv.
Transverse medullary vv.
Interpeduncular vv.
Pontomesen-cephalic v.
Superior petrosal v.
Superior cerebellar vv.
Anterolateral and antero-median pontine v.
Posteromedian medullary v.

Arteries of the Brain

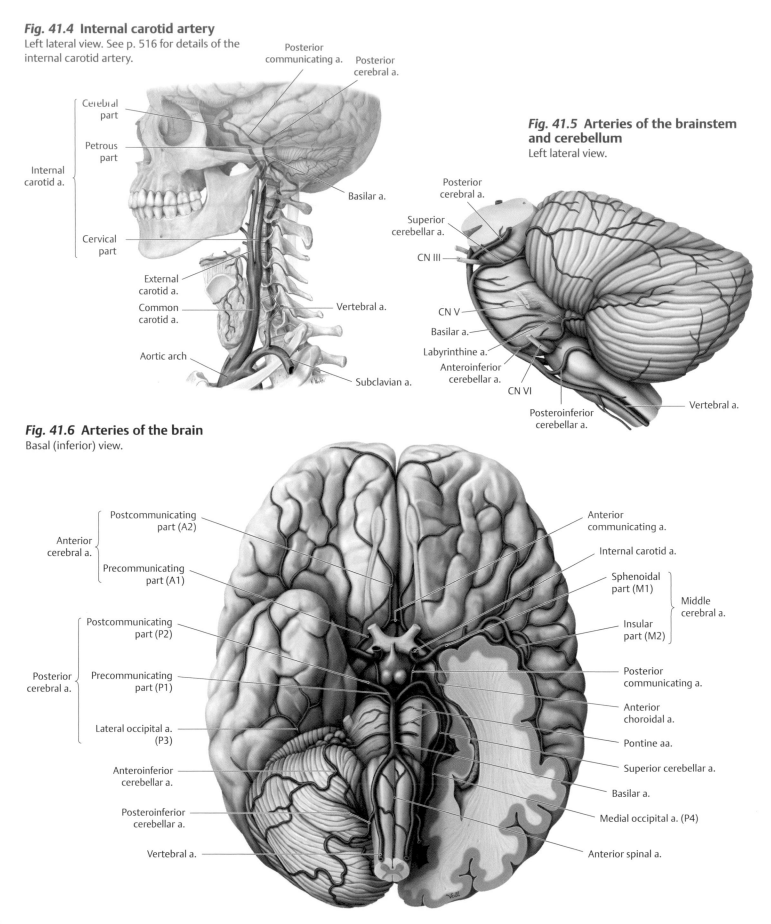

Fig. 41.4 **Internal carotid artery**
Left lateral view. See p. 516 for details of the internal carotid artery.

Posterior communicating a.
Posterior cerebral a.
Internal carotid a.
Cerebral part
Petrous part
Cervical part
Basilar a.
External carotid a.
Common carotid a.
Vertebral a.
Aortic arch
Subclavian a.

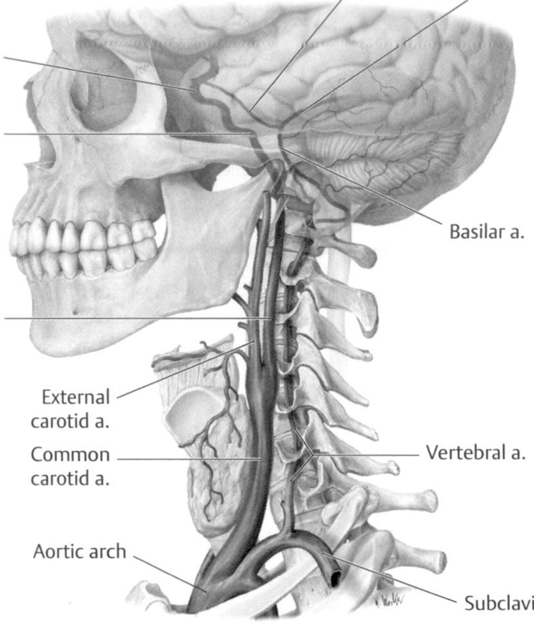

Fig. 41.5 **Arteries of the brainstem and cerebellum**
Left lateral view.

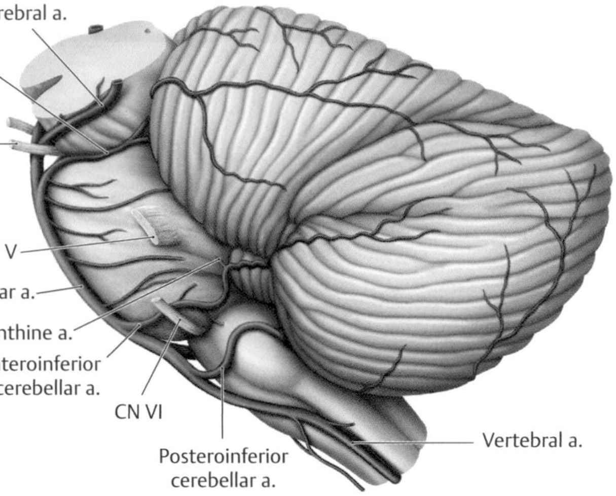

Posterior cerebral a.
Superior cerebellar a.
CN III
CN V
Basilar a.
Labyrinthine a.
Anteroinferior cerebellar a.
CN VI
Posteroinferior cerebellar a.
Vertebral a.

Fig. 41.6 **Arteries of the brain**
Basal (inferior) view.

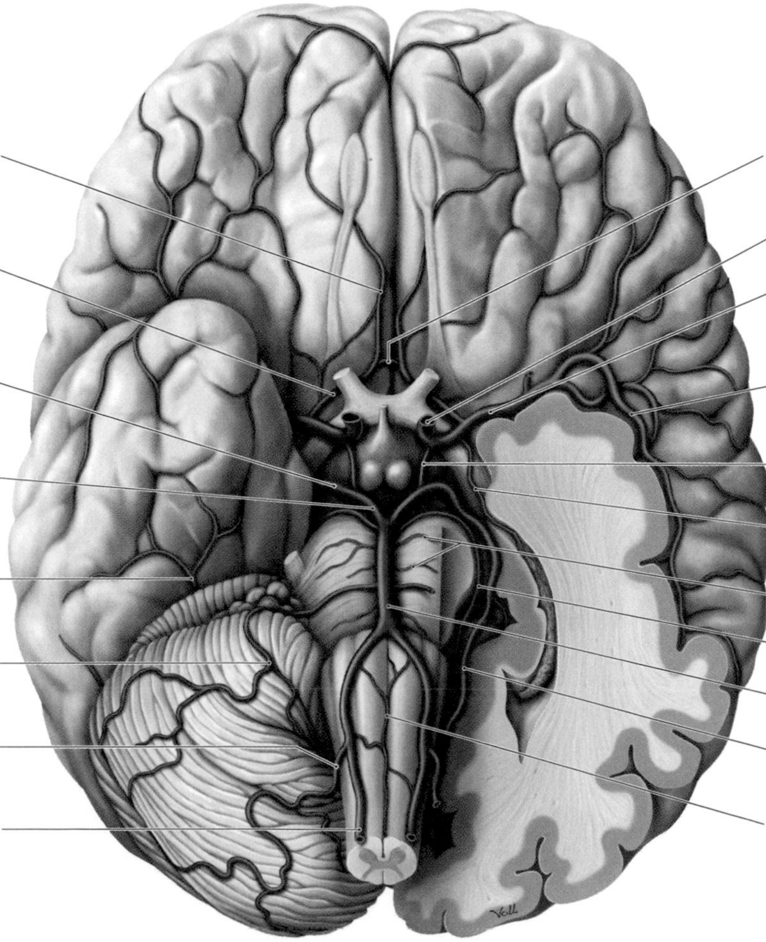

Anterior cerebral a.
Postcommunicating part (A2)
Precommunicating part (A1)
Posterior cerebral a.
Postcommunicating part (P2)
Precommunicating part (P1)
Lateral occipital a. (P3)
Anteroinferior cerebellar a.
Posteroinferior cerebellar a.
Vertebral a.
Anterior communicating a.
Internal carotid a.
Middle cerebral a.
Sphenoidal part (M1)
Insular part (M2)
Posterior communicating a.
Anterior choroidal a.
Pontine aa.
Superior cerebellar a.
Basilar a.
Medial occipital a. (P4)
Anterior spinal a.

Fig. 41.7 Cerebral arteries

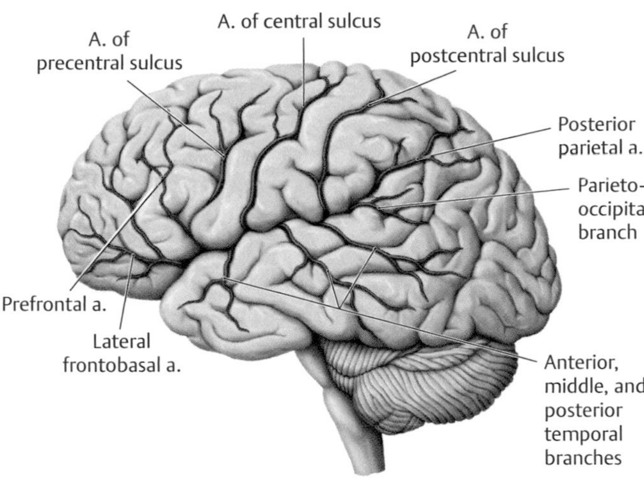
A. of central sulcus
A. of precentral sulcus
A. of postcentral sulcus
Posterior parietal a.
Parieto-occipital branch
Prefrontal a.
Lateral frontobasal a.
Anterior, middle, and posterior temporal branches

A Middle cerebral artery. Lateral view of the left hemisphere.

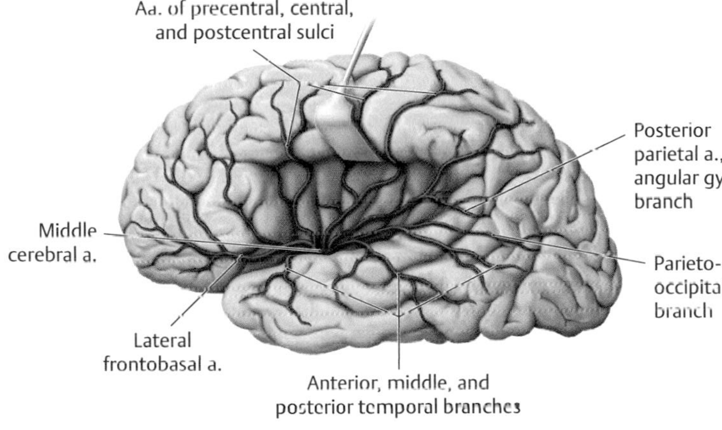
Aa. of precentral, central, and postcentral sulci
Posterior parietal a., angular gyral branch
Middle cerebral a.
Parieto-occipital branch
Lateral frontobasal a.
Anterior, middle, and posterior temporal branches

B Middle cerebral artery. Left lateral view with the lateral sulcus retracted.

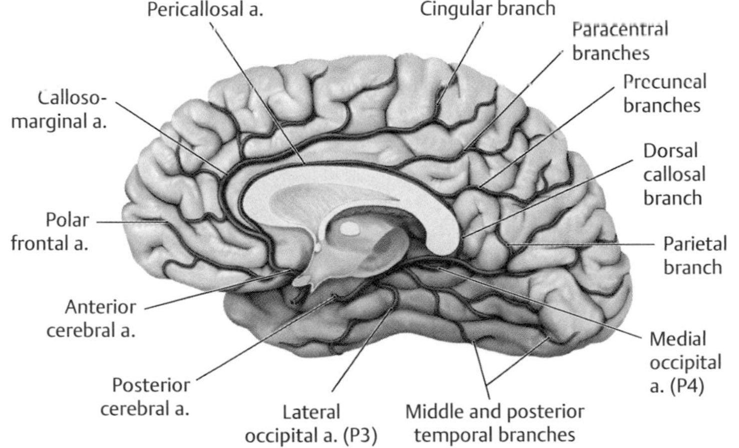
Pericallosal a.
Cingular branch
Paracentral branches
Precuneal branches
Calloso-marginal a.
Dorsal callosal branch
Polar frontal a.
Parietal branch
Anterior cerebral a.
Medial occipital a. (P4)
Posterior cerebral a.
Lateral occipital a. (P3)
Middle and posterior temporal branches

C Anterior and posterior cerebral arteries. Medial view of the right hemisphere.

Fig. 41.8 Cerebral arteries: Distribution areas

The central gray and white matter have a complex blood supply (yellow) that includes the anterior choroidal artery.

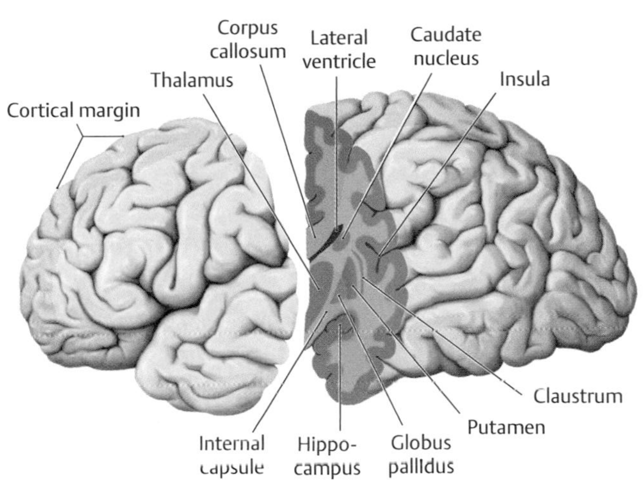
Corpus callosum
Lateral ventricle
Caudate nucleus
Thalamus
Insula
Cortical margin
Claustrum
Putamen
Internal capsule
Hippo-campus
Globus pallidus
Anterior cerebral a.
Middle cerebral a.
Posterior cerebral a.

A Lateral view of the left hemisphere.

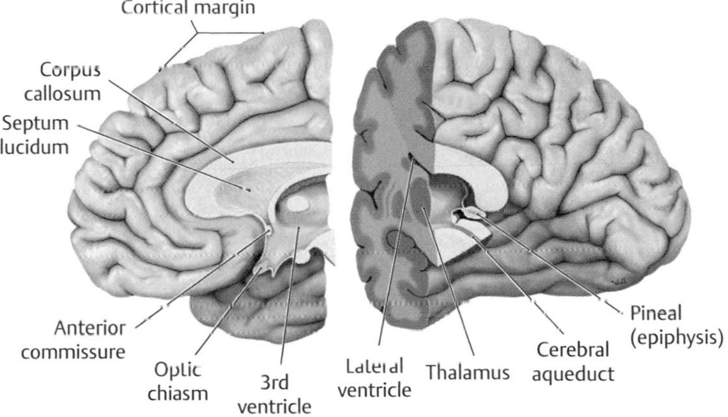
Cortical margin
Corpus callosum
Septum pellucidum
Anterior commissure
Optic chiasm
3rd ventricle
Lateral ventricle
Thalamus
Cerebral aqueduct
Pineal (epiphysis)

B Medial view of the right hemisphere.

Circuitry

Fig. 42.1 Divisions of the nervous system

Direction of information flow divides nerve fibers into two types: afferent (sensory) fibers, which transmit impulses toward the central nervous system (CNS), and efferent (motor) fibers, which transmit impulses away. The nervous system may also be divided into a somatic and an autonomic part. The somatic nervous system mediates interaction with the environment, whereas the autonomic (visceral) nervous system coordinates the function of the internal organs.

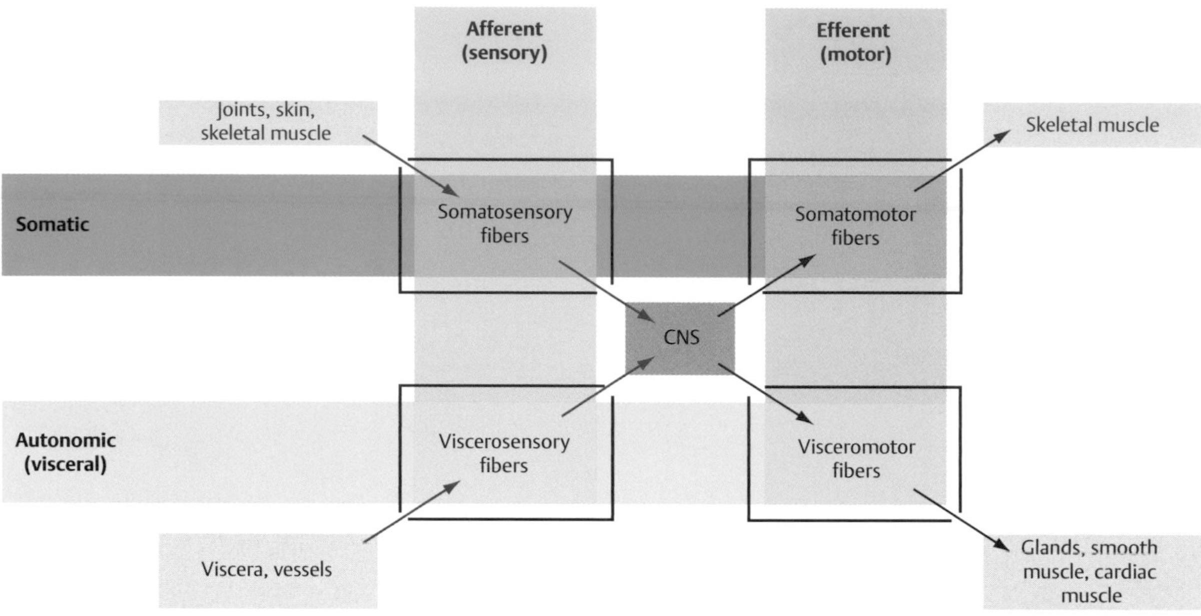
Afferent (sensory)
Efferent (motor)
Joints, skin, skeletal muscle
Skeletal muscle
Somatic
Somatosensory fibers
Somatomotor fibers
CNS
Autonomic (visceral)
Viscerosensory fibers
Visceromotor fibers
Viscera, vessels
Glands, smooth muscle, cardiac muscle

Fig. 42.2 Organization of the gray matter

Left oblique anterosuperior view. The gray matter of the spinal cord is divided into three columns (horns). Afferent (blue) and efferent (red) neurons within these columns are clustered according to function.

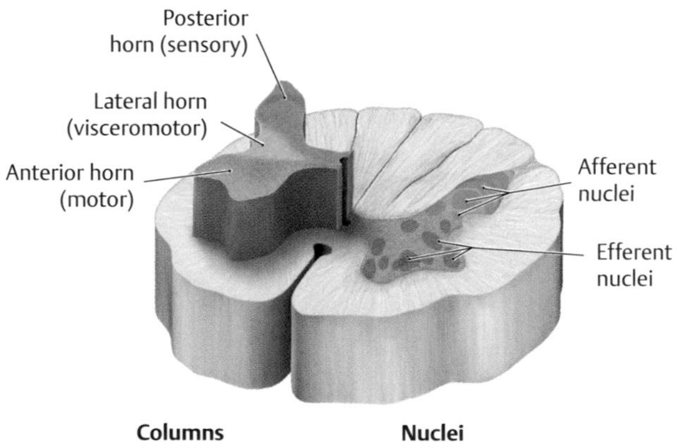
Posterior horn (sensory)
Lateral horn (visceromotor)
Anterior horn (motor)
Afferent nuclei
Efferent nuclei
Columns
Nuclei

Fig. 42.3 Muscle innervation

Indicator muscles are innervated by motor neurons in the anterior horn of one spinal cord segment. Most muscles (multisegmental muscles) receive innervation from a motor column, a vertical arrangement of motor nuclei spanning several segments.

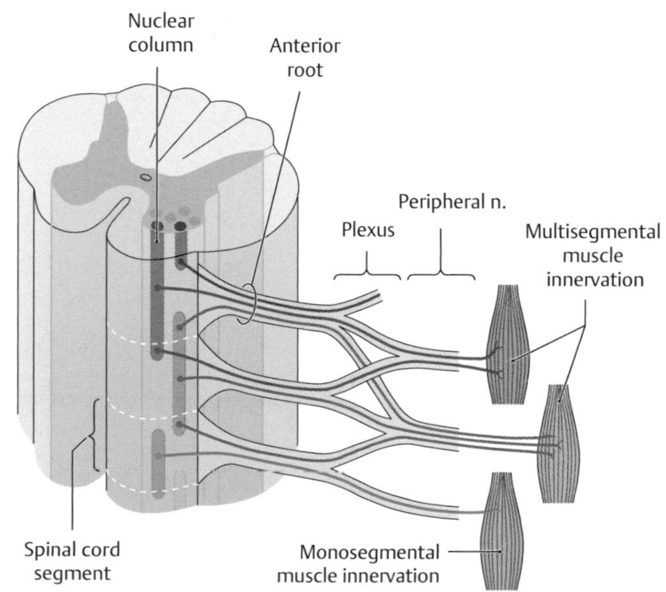
Nuclear column
Anterior root
Peripheral n.
Plexus
Multisegmental muscle innervation
Spinal cord segment
Monosegmental muscle innervation

Fig. 42.4 **Reflexes**
Muscular function at the unconscious (reflex) level is controlled by the gray matter of the spinal cord.

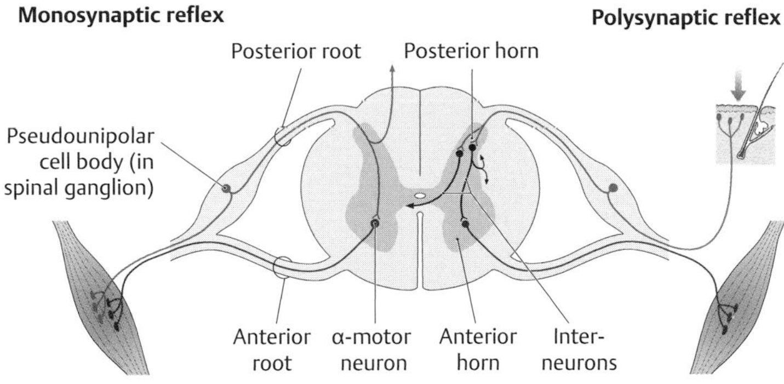

Monosynaptic reflex
Polysynaptic reflex
Posterior root
Posterior horn
Pseudounipolar cell body (in spinal ganglion)
Anterior root
α-motor neuron
Anterior horn
Inter-neurons

A Polysynaptic reflexes may be mediated by receptors inside of or remote from the muscle (i.e., skin); these receptors act via interneurons to stimulate muscle contraction.

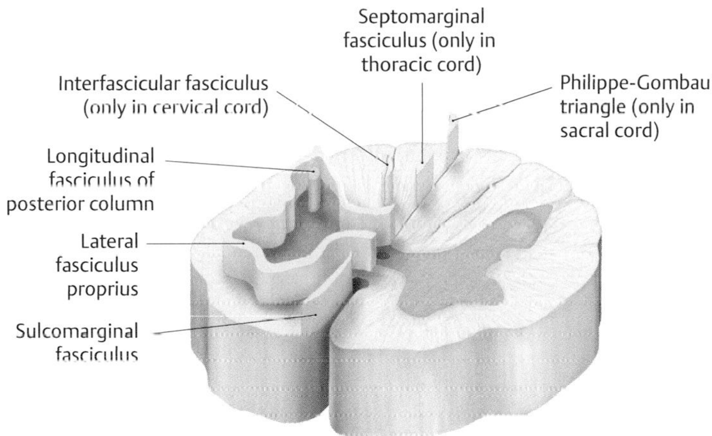

Septomarginal fasciculus (only in thoracic cord)
Interfascicular fasciculus (only in cervical cord)
Philippe-Gombault triangle (only in sacral cord)
Longitudinal fasciculus of posterior column
Lateral fasciculus proprius
Sulcomarginal fasciculus

B Principal intrinsic fascicles of the spinal cord. The intrinsic fascicles are the conduction apparatus of the intrinsic circuits, allowing axons to ascend and descend to coordinate spinal reflexes for multisegmental muscles.

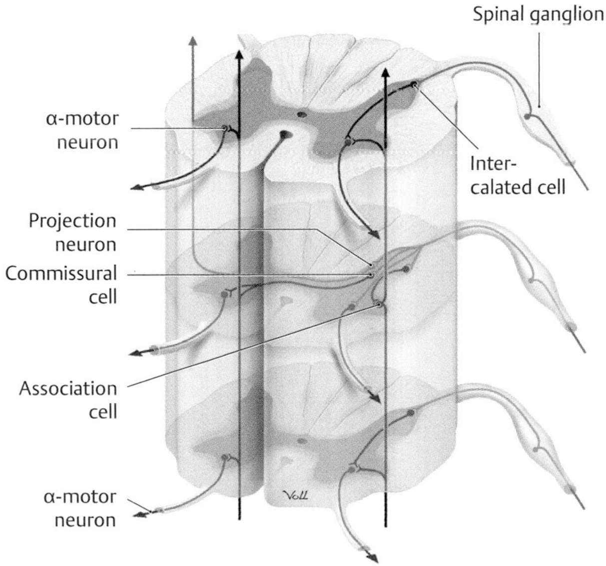

Spinal ganglion
α-motor neuron
Inter-calated cell
Projection neuron
Commissural cell
Association cell
α-motor neuron

C Intrinsic circuits of the spinal cord.

Fig. 42.5 **Sensory and motor systems**
The sensory system (see p. 640) and motor system (see p. 641) are so functionally interrelated they may be described as one (sensorimotor system).

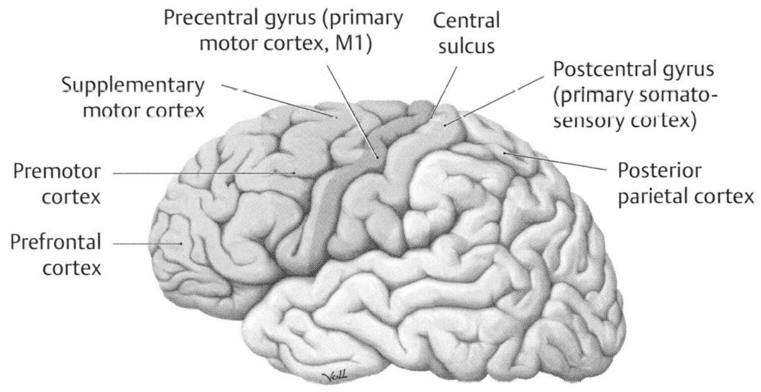

Precentral gyrus (primary motor cortex, M1)
Central sulcus
Supplementary motor cortex
Postcentral gyrus (primary somato-sensory cortex)
Premotor cortex
Posterior parietal cortex
Prefrontal cortex

A Cortical areas of the sensorimotor system. Lateral view of the left hemisphere.

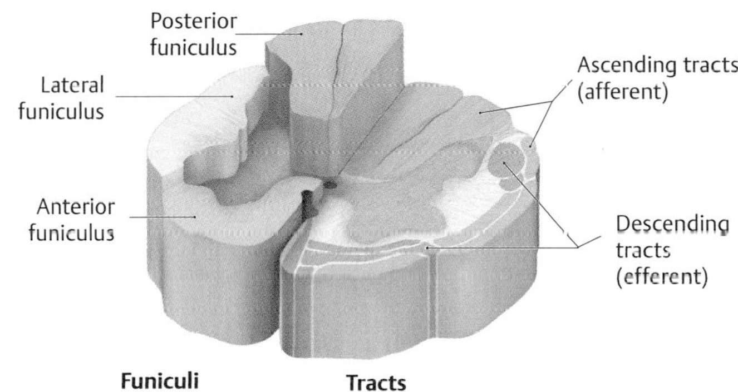

Posterior funiculus
Lateral funiculus
Ascending tracts (afferent)
Anterior funiculus
Descending tracts (efferent)
Funiculi
Tracts

B White matter of the spinal cord. The white matter of the spinal cord contains ascending tracts (afferent, see p. 640) and descending tracts (efferent, see p. 641), which are the CNS equivalent of peripheral nerves.

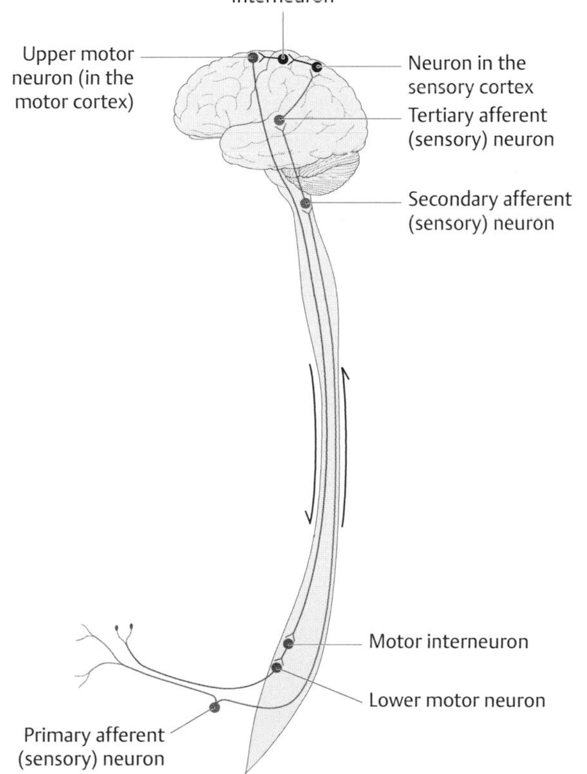

Interneuron
Upper motor neuron (in the motor cortex)
Neuron in the sensory cortex
Tertiary afferent (sensory) neuron
Secondary afferent (sensory) neuron
Motor interneuron
Lower motor neuron
Primary afferent (sensory) neuron

C Overview of sensorimotor integration.

Sensory & Motor Pathways

Fig. 42.6 Sensory pathways (ascending tracts)

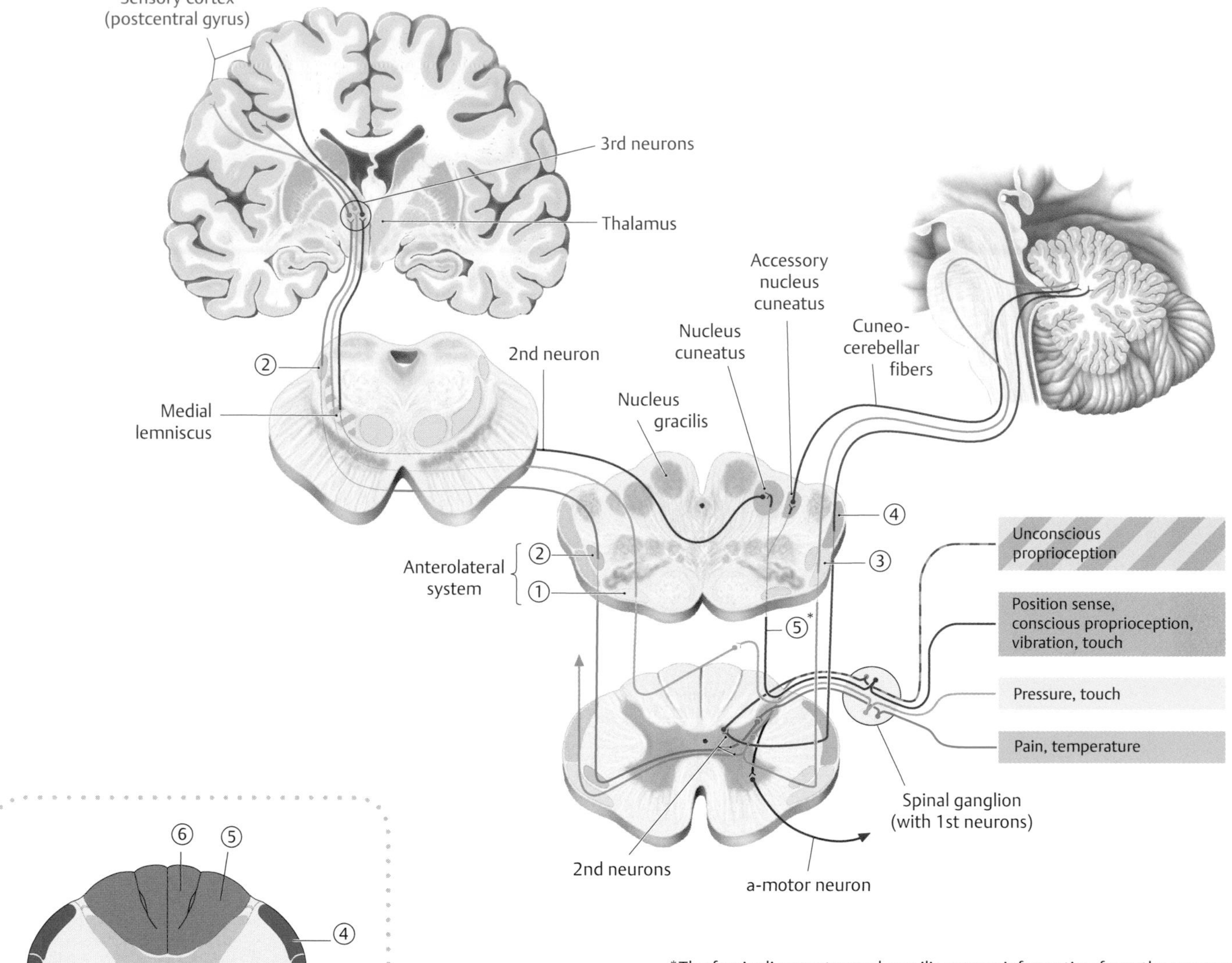
Sensory cortex
(postcentral gyrus)
3rd neurons
Thalamus
Accessory
nucleus
cuneatus
Nucleus
cuneatus
Cuneo-
cerebellar
fibers
2nd neuron
Nucleus
gracilis
②
Medial
lemniscus
④
Unconscious
proprioception
Anterolateral
system
②
①
③
Position sense,
conscious proprioception,
vibration, touch
⑤*
Pressure, touch
Pain, temperature
Spinal ganglion
(with 1st neurons)
2nd neurons
a-motor neuron
⑥
⑤
④
③
②
①

*The fasciculi cuneatus and gracilis convey information from the upper and lower limbs, respectively. At this spinal cord level, only the fasciculus cuneatus is present.

Table 42.1 Ascending tracts of the spinal cord

	Tract	Location	Function		Neurons
①	Anterior spino-thalamic tract	Anterior funiculus	Pathway for crude touch and pressure sensation		1st afferent neurons located in spinal ganglia; contain 2nd neurons and cross in the anterior commissure
②	Lateral spino-thalamic tract	Anterior and lateral funiculi	Pathway for pain, temperature, tickle, itch, and sexual sensation		
③	Anterior spino-cerebellar tract	Lateral funiculus	Pathway for unconscious coordination of motor activities (unconscious proprioception, automatic processes, e.g., jogging, riding a bike) to the cerebellum		Projection (2nd) neurons receive proprioceptive signals from 1st afferent fibers originating at the 1st neurons of spinal ganglia
④	Posterior spino-cerebellar tract				
⑤	Fasciculus cuneatus	Posterior funiculus	Pathway for position sense (conscious proprioception) and fine cutaneous sensation (touch, vibration, fine pressure sense, two-point discrimination)	Conveys information from *upper* limb (not present below T3)	Cell bodies of 1st neuron located in spinal ganglion; pass uncrossed to the dorsal column nuclei
⑥	Fasciculus gracilis*			Conveys information from *lower* limb	

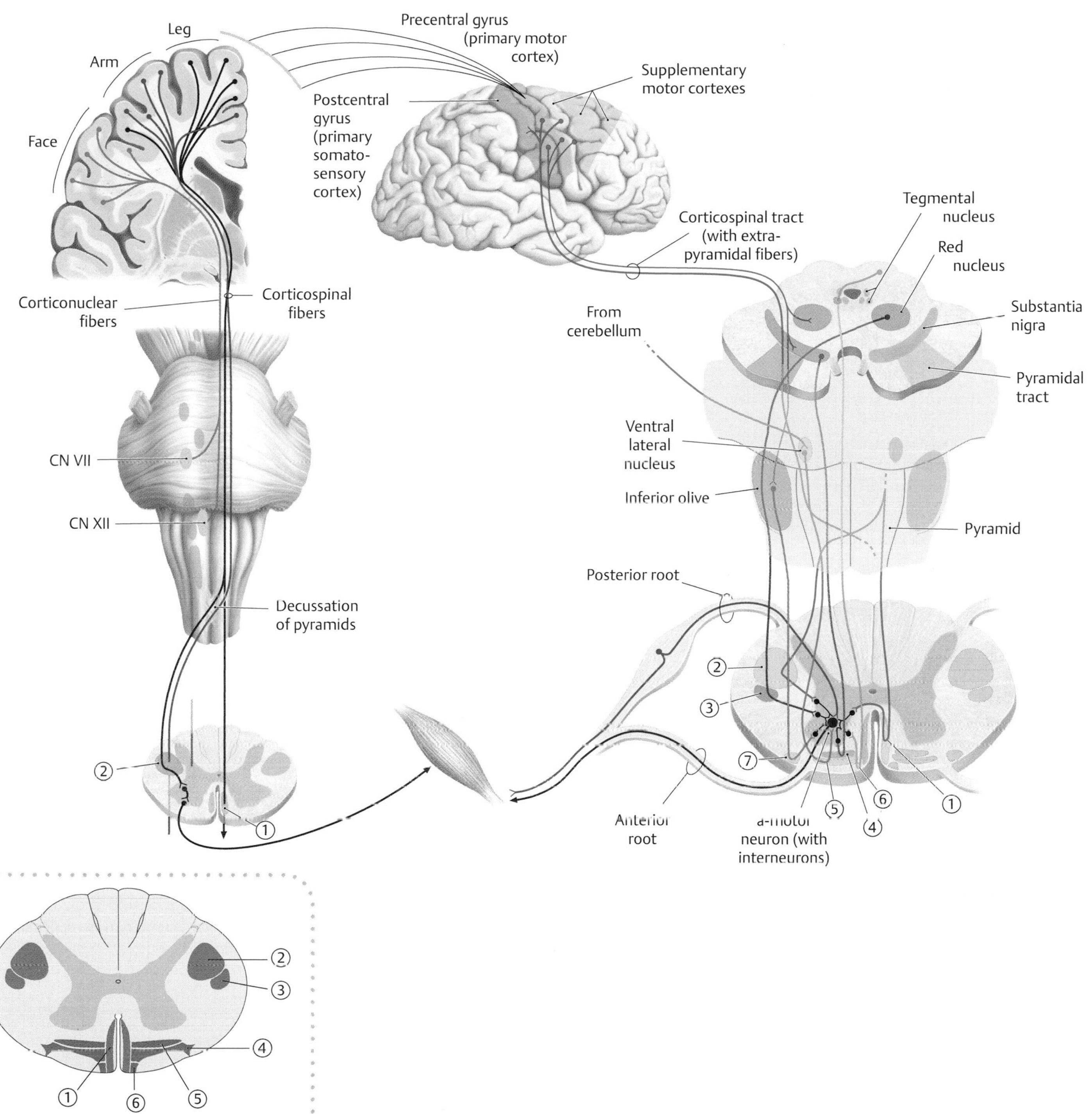
Pyramidal (corticospinal) tract
Extrapyramidal motor system
Leg
Arm
Face
Precentral gyrus (primary motor cortex)
Supplementary motor cortexes
Postcentral gyrus (primary somatosensory cortex)
Corticonuclear fibers
Corticospinal fibers
Corticospinal tract (with extrapyramidal fibers)
Tegmental nucleus
Red nucleus
Substantia nigra
Pyramidal tract
From cerebellum
Ventral lateral nucleus
Inferior olive
Pyramid
CN VII
CN XII
Decussation of pyramids
Posterior root
Anterior root
α-motor neuron (with interneurons)
①
②
③
④
⑤
⑥
⑦

Fig. 42.7 **Motor pathways (descending tracts)**

Table 42.2 Descending tracts of the spinal cord

Tract			Function	
Pyramidal tract	①	Anterior corticospinal tract	Most important pathway for voluntary motor function	Originates in the motor cortex *Corticonuclear* fibers to motor nuclei of cranial nerves *Corticospinal* fibers to motor cells in anterior horn of the spinal cord *Corticoreticular* fibers to nuclei of the reticular formation
	②	Lateral corticospinal tract		
Extrapyramidal motor system	③	Rubrospinal tract	Pathway for automatic and learned motor processes (e.g., walking, running, cycling)	
	④	Reticulospinal tract		
	⑤	Vestibulospinal tract		
	⑥	Tectospinal tract		
	⑦	Olivospinal tract		

Sensory Systems (I)

Table 42.3 Special sensory qualities (senses)

Sense	Cranial nerve		Ref.
Vision	Optic n. (CN II)		See p. 499
Balance	Vestibulocochlear n. (CN VIII)	Vestibular branch	See p. 506
Hearing		Cochlear branch	See p. 506
Taste	Facial n. (CN VII)		See p. 504
	Glossopharyngeal n. (CN IX)		See p. 508
	Vagus n. (CN X)		See p. 510
Smell	Olfactory n. (CN I)		See p. 498

Fig. 42.8 Visual system: Overview

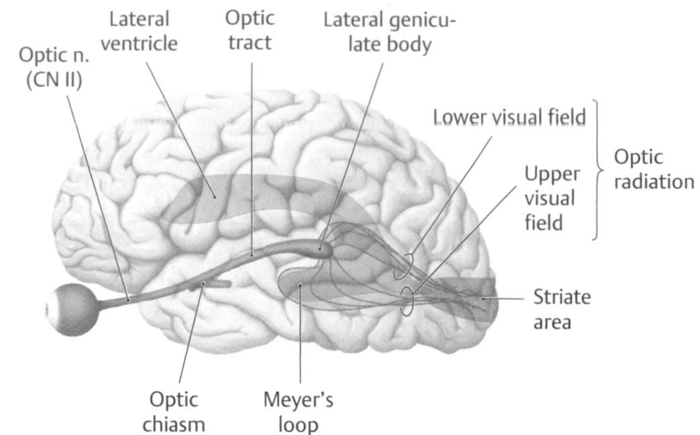
Optic n.
(CN II)
Lateral
ventricle
Optic
tract
Lateral genicu-
late body
Lower visual field
Upper
visual
field
Optic
radiation
Striate
area
Optic
chiasm
Meyer's
loop

A Left lateral view.

B Inferior view.

Fig. 42.9 Visual pathways

90% of optic nerve fibers terminate in the lateral geniculate body on neurons that project to the striate area (visual cortex). This forms the geniculate pathway, responsible for conscious visual perception. The remaining 10% travel along the medial root of the optic tract, forming the non-geniculate pathway. This pathway plays an important role in the unconscious regulation of vision-related processes and reflexes.

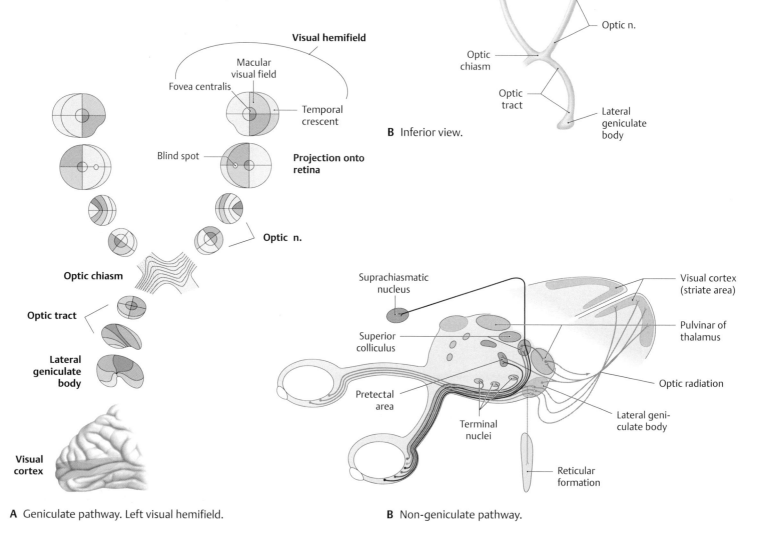

A Geniculate pathway. Left visual hemifield.

B Non-geniculate pathway.

Clinical

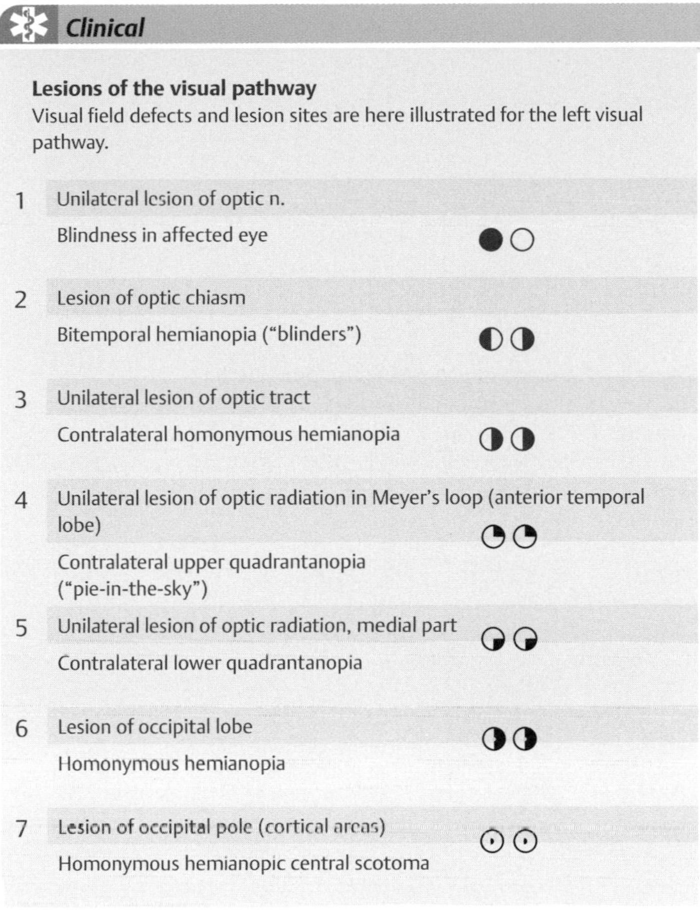

Lesions of the visual pathway

Visual field defects and lesion sites are here illustrated for the left visual pathway.

	Lesion / Defect
1	Unilateral lesion of optic n.
	Blindness in affected eye
2	Lesion of optic chiasm
	Bitemporal hemianopia ("blinders")
3	Unilateral lesion of optic tract
	Contralateral homonymous hemianopia
4	Unilateral lesion of optic radiation in Meyer's loop (anterior temporal lobe)
	Contralateral upper quadrantanopia ("pie-in-the-sky")
5	Unilateral lesion of optic radiation, medial part
	Contralateral lower quadrantanopia
6	Lesion of occipital lobe
	Homonymous hemianopia
7	Lesion of occipital pole (cortical areas)
	Homonymous hemianopic central scotoma

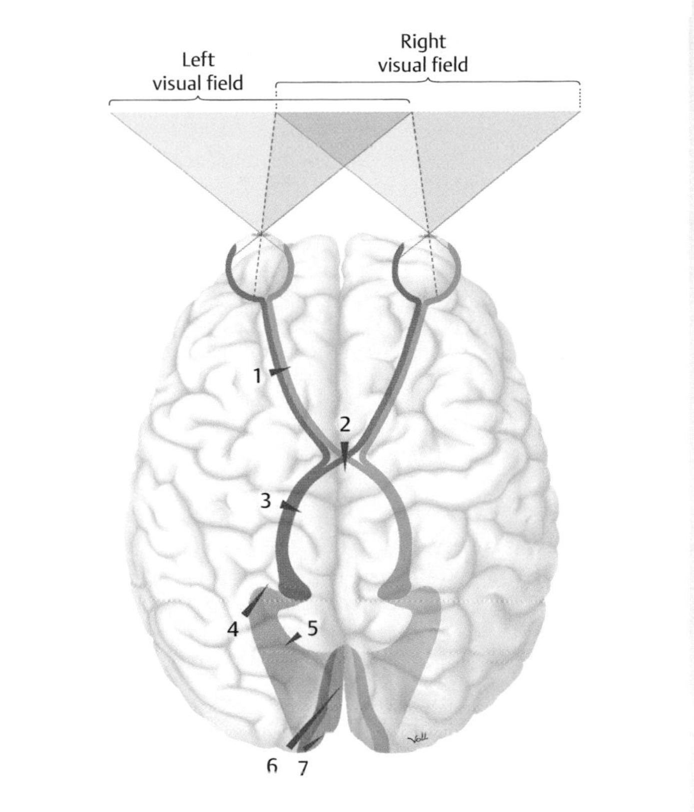
Left
visual field
Right
visual field
1
2
3
4
5
6
7

Fig. 42.10 Reflexes of the visual system

The reflexes of the visual system are mediated by the optic (afferent) and oculomotor (efferent) nerves.

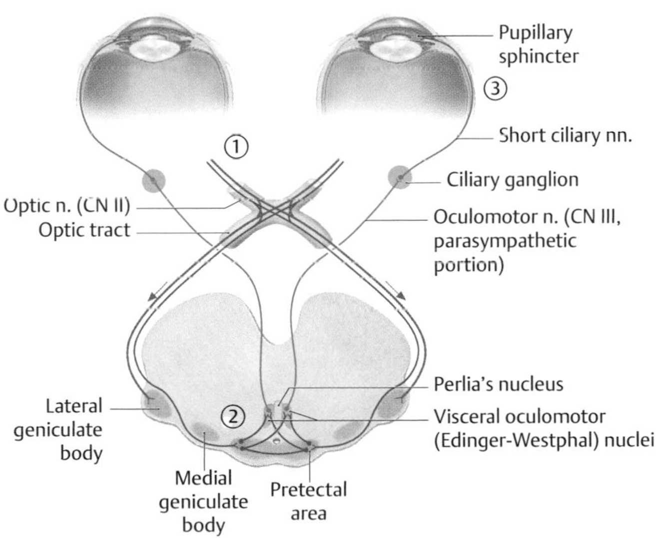
Pupillary
sphincter
③
Short ciliary nn.
①
Ciliary ganglion
Optic n. (CN II)
Optic tract
Oculomotor n. (CN III,
parasympathetic
portion)
Perlia's nucleus
Lateral
geniculate
body
②
Visceral oculomotor
(Edinger-Westphal) nuclei
Medial
geniculate
body
Pretectal
area

A Pupillary light reflex.
① Incoming light is transmitted via the optic nerve.
② Large amounts of light are transmitted to the pretectal area, bypassing the geniculate pathway.
③ The neurons of the visceral oculomotor nucleus synapse on the ciliary ganglion, which induces contraction of the pupillary sphincter.

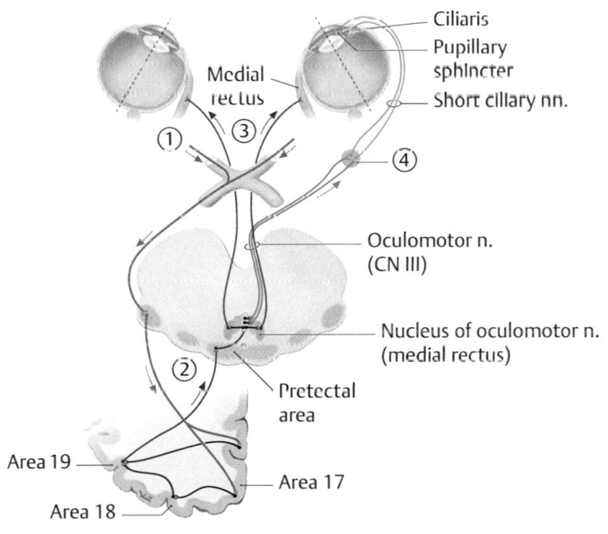
Ciliaris
Pupillary
sphincter
Medial
rectus
Short ciliary nn.
①
③
④
Oculomotor n.
(CN III)
Nucleus of oculomotor n.
(medial rectus)
②
Pretectal
area
Area 19
Area 17
Area 18

B Pathways for convergence and accommodation.
① Light is received from an approaching object.
② Information is relayed via the primary (17) and secondary (19) visual cortexes to the nuclei of the oculomotor nerve.
③ Convergence: Constriction of the medial rectus muscles converges the visual axes of the eyes, keeping the approaching image on the fovea centralis, the point of maximum visual acuity.
④ Accommodation: The curvature of the lens is increased via contraction of the ciliary muscles. The sphincter pupillae also contracts.

Sensory Systems (II)

Fig. 42.11 Balance
Human balance is regulated by the visual, proprioceptive, and vestibular systems. All three systems send afferent fibers to the vestibular nuclei, which then distribute them to the spinal cord (motor support), cerebellum (fine motor function), and brainstem (oculomotor function). Proprioception ("position sense") is the perception of limb position in space. *Note:* Efferents to the thalamus and cortex control spatial sense; efferents to the hypothalamus regulate vomiting in response to vertigo.

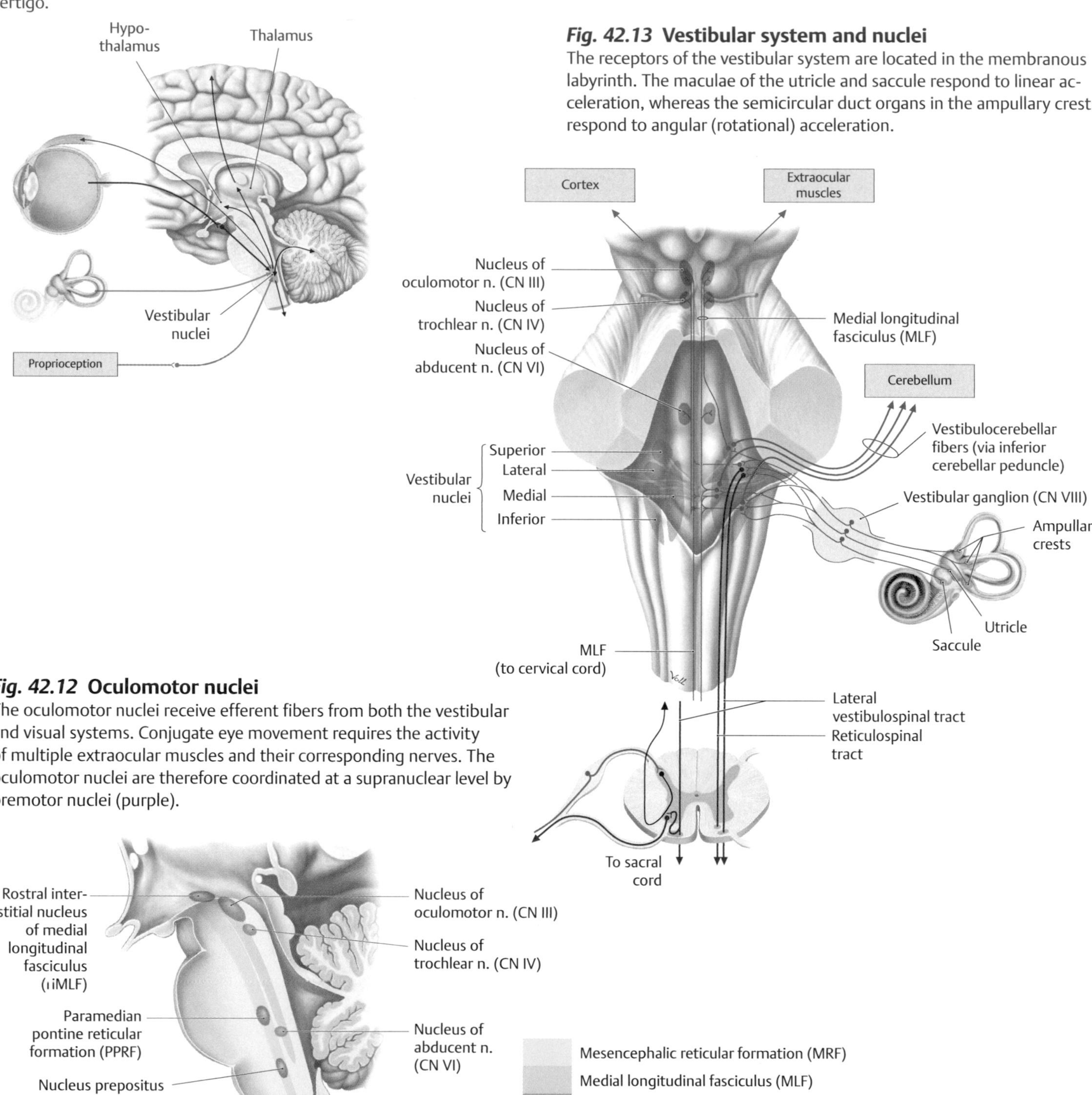

Hypo-thalamus
Thalamus
Vestibular nuclei
Proprioception
Cortex
Extraocular muscles
Nucleus of oculomotor n. (CN III)
Nucleus of trochlear n. (CN IV)
Nucleus of abducent n. (CN VI)
Medial longitudinal fasciculus (MLF)
Cerebellum
Vestibulocerebellar fibers (via inferior cerebellar peduncle)
Vestibular nuclei
Superior
Lateral
Medial
Inferior
Vestibular ganglion (CN VIII)
Ampullary crests
Utricle
Saccule
MLF (to cervical cord)
Lateral vestibulospinal tract
Reticulospinal tract
To sacral cord
Rostral interstitial nucleus of medial longitudinal fasciculus (riMLF)
Paramedian pontine reticular formation (PPRF)
Nucleus prepositus hypoglossi
Nucleus of oculomotor n. (CN III)
Nucleus of trochlear n. (CN IV)
Nucleus of abducent n. (CN VI)
Mesencephalic reticular formation (MRF)
Medial longitudinal fasciculus (MLF)
Oculomotor nuclei
Premotor nuclei

Fig. 42.13 Vestibular system and nuclei
The receptors of the vestibular system are located in the membranous labyrinth. The maculae of the utricle and saccule respond to linear acceleration, whereas the semicircular duct organs in the ampullary crests respond to angular (rotational) acceleration.

Fig. 42.12 Oculomotor nuclei
The oculomotor nuclei receive efferent fibers from both the vestibular and visual systems. Conjugate eye movement requires the activity of multiple extraocular muscles and their corresponding nerves. The oculomotor nuclei are therefore coordinated at a supranuclear level by premotor nuclei (purple).

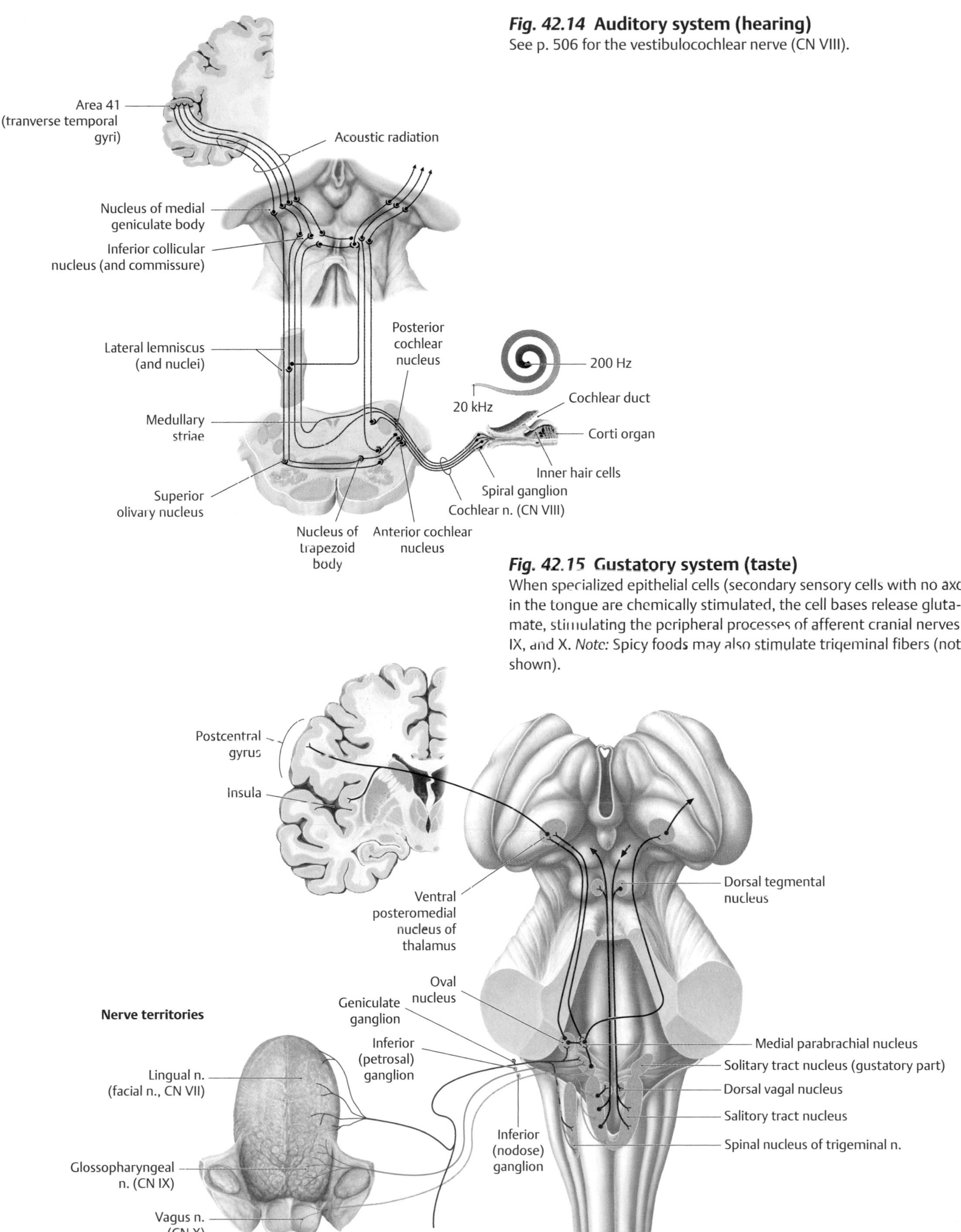
Area 41
(tranverse temporal
gyri)
Acoustic radiation
Nucleus of medial
geniculate body
Inferior collicular
nucleus (and commissure)
Lateral lemniscus
(and nuclei)
Posterior
cochlear
nucleus
200 Hz
20 kHz
Cochlear duct
Corti organ
Medullary
striae
Inner hair cells
Spiral ganglion
Cochlear n. (CN VIII)
Superior
olivary nucleus
Nucleus of
trapezoid
body
Anterior cochlear
nucleus
Postcentral
gyrus
Insula
Ventral
posteromedial
nucleus of
thalamus
Dorsal tegmental
nucleus
Nerve territories
Geniculate
ganglion
Oval
nucleus
Inferior
(petrosal)
ganglion
Medial parabrachial nucleus
Solitary tract nucleus (gustatory part)
Dorsal vagal nucleus
Salitory tract nucleus
Spinal nucleus of trigeminal n.
Lingual n.
(facial n., CN VII)
Inferior
(nodose)
ganglion
Glossopharyngeal
n. (CN IX)
Vagus n.
(CN X)

Fig. 42.14 **Auditory system (hearing)**
See p. 506 for the vestibulocochlear nerve (CN VIII).

Fig. 42.15 **Gustatory system (taste)**
When specialized epithelial cells (secondary sensory cells with no axon) in the tongue are chemically stimulated, the cell bases release glutamate, stimulating the peripheral processes of afferent cranial nerves VII, IX, and X. *Note:* Spicy foods may also stimulate trigeminal fibers (not shown).

Sensory Systems (III)

Fig. 42.16 Olfactory system (smell)

The olfactory system is the only sensory system not relayed in the thalamus before reaching the cortex (the prepiriform area is considered the primary olfactory cortex). The olfactory system is linked to other brain areas and can therefore evoke complex emotional and behavioral responses (mediated by the hypothalamus, thalamus, and limbic system): noxious smells induce nausea; appetizing smells evoke salivation.

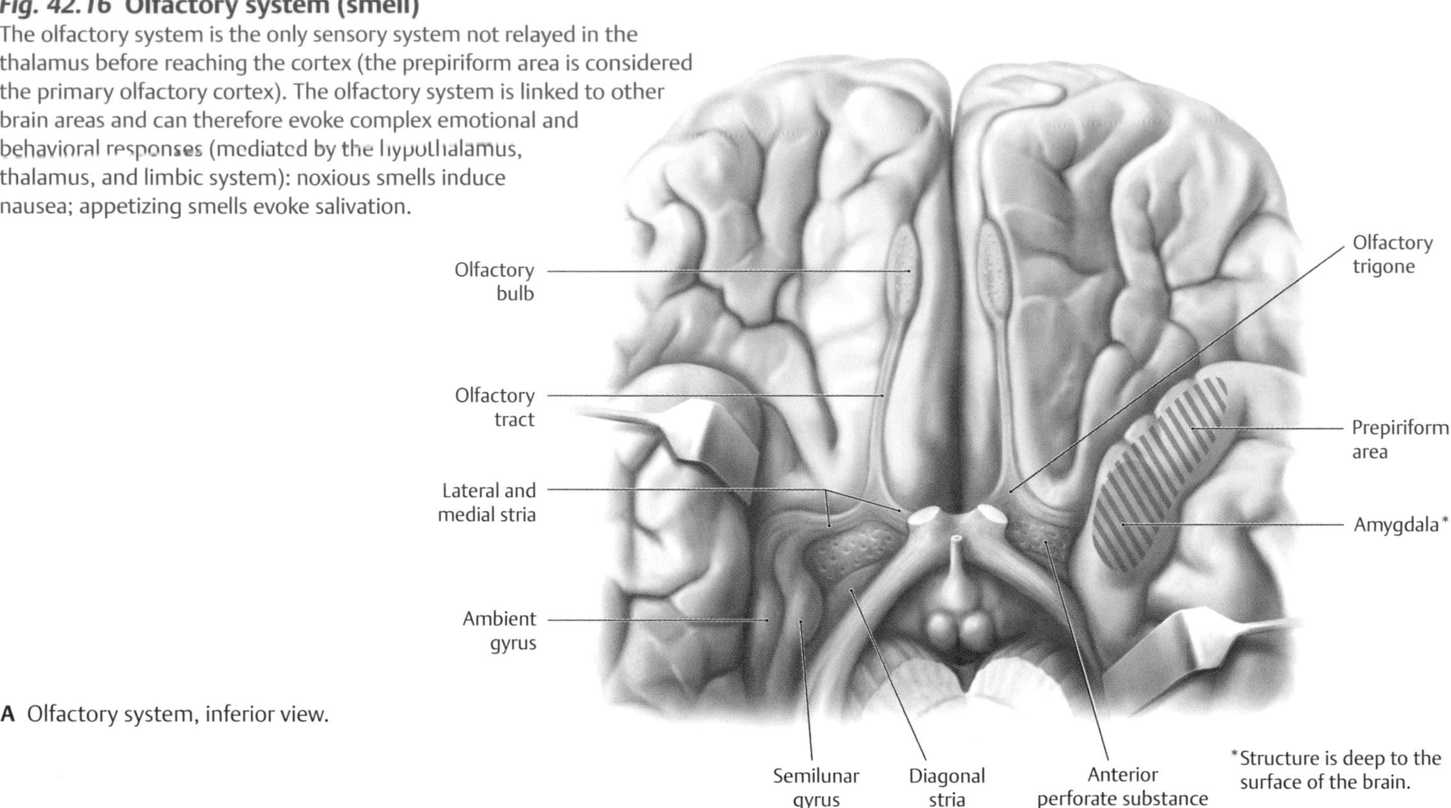
Olfactory bulb
Olfactory tract
Lateral and medial stria
Ambient gyrus
Semilunar gyrus
Diagonal stria
Anterior perforate substance
Olfactory trigone
Prepiriform area
Amygdala*
*Structure is deep to the surface of the brain.

A Olfactory system, inferior view.

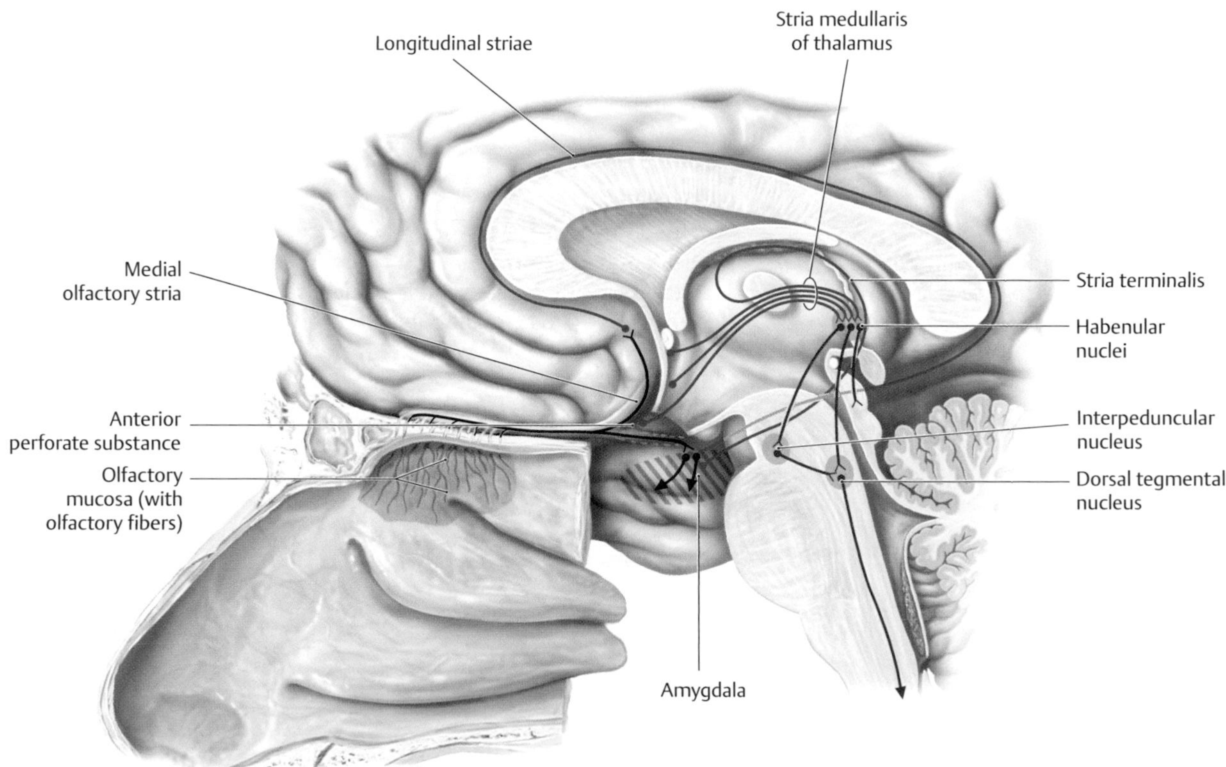
Longitudinal striae
Stria medullaris of thalamus
Medial olfactory stria
Anterior perforate substance
Olfactory mucosa (with olfactory fibers)
Stria terminalis
Habenular nuclei
Interpeduncular nucleus
Dorsal tegmental nucleus
Amygdala

B Olfactory system with nuclei, left lateral view of midsagittal section.

The limbic system, which exchanges and integrates information between the telencephalon, diencephalon, and mesencephalon, regulates drive and affective behavior. It plays a crucial role in memory and learning.

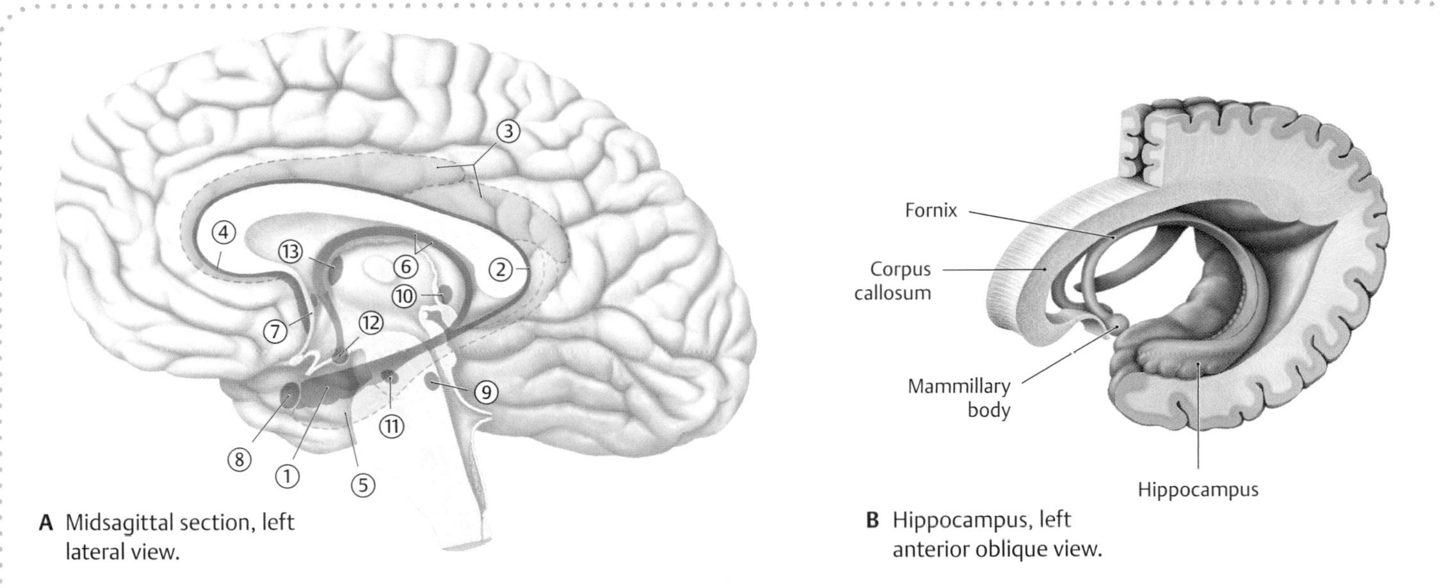
③
④
⑬
⑥
②
⑩
⑦
⑫
⑨
⑪
⑧
①
⑤
Fornix
Corpus callosum
Mammillary body
Hippocampus

A Midsagittal section, left lateral view.

B Hippocampus, left anterior oblique view.

Table 42.4 Structures of the limbic system

Outer arc		Inner arc*		Subcortical nuclei	
①	Parahippocampal gyrus	⑤	Hippocampal formation (hippocampus, entorhinal area of parahippocampal gyrus)	⑧	Amygdala
②	Indusium griseum	⑥	Fornix	⑨	Dorsal tegmental nuclei
③	Subcallosal (paraolfactory) area	⑦	Septal area (septum)	⑩	Habenular nuclei
				⑪	Interpeduncular nuclei
④	Cingulate (limbic) gyrus	Paraterminal gyrus		⑫	Mammillary bodies
				⑬	Anterior thalamic nuclei

* The inner arc also contains the diagonal band of Broca (not shown).

Fig. 42.17 **Limbic system nuclei**
This neuronal circuit (Papez circuit) establishes a connection between information stored at the conscious and unconscious levels.

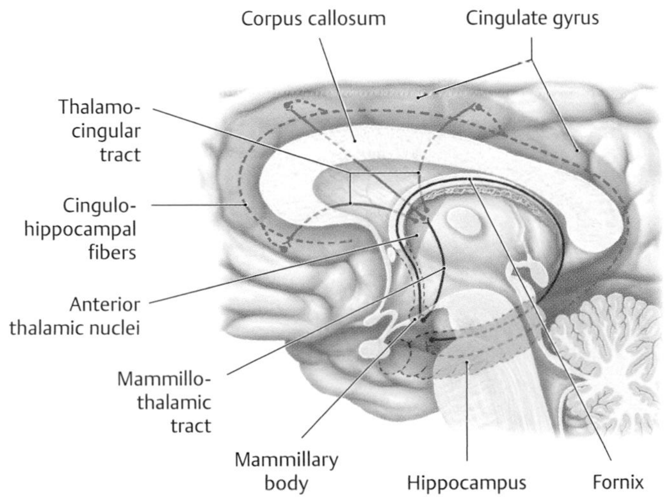
Corpus callosum
Cingulate gyrus
Thalamo-cingular tract
Cingulo-hippocampal fibers
Anterior thalamic nuclei
Mammillo-thalamic tract
Mammillary body
Hippocampus
Fornix

Fig. 42.18 **Limbic regulation of the peripheral autonomic nervous system**
The limbic system receives afferent feedback signals from its target organs. See p. 648 for the autonomic nervous system.

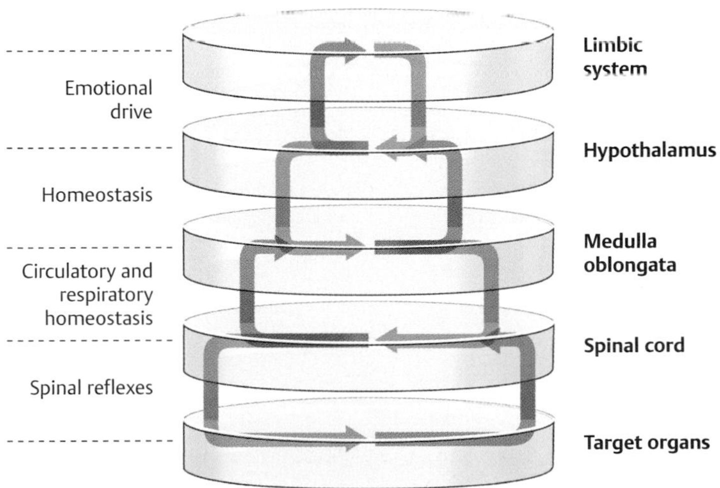
Emotional drive
Homeostasis
Circulatory and respiratory homeostasis
Spinal reflexes
Limbic system
Hypothalamus
Medulla oblongata
Spinal cord
Target organs

Autonomic Nervous System

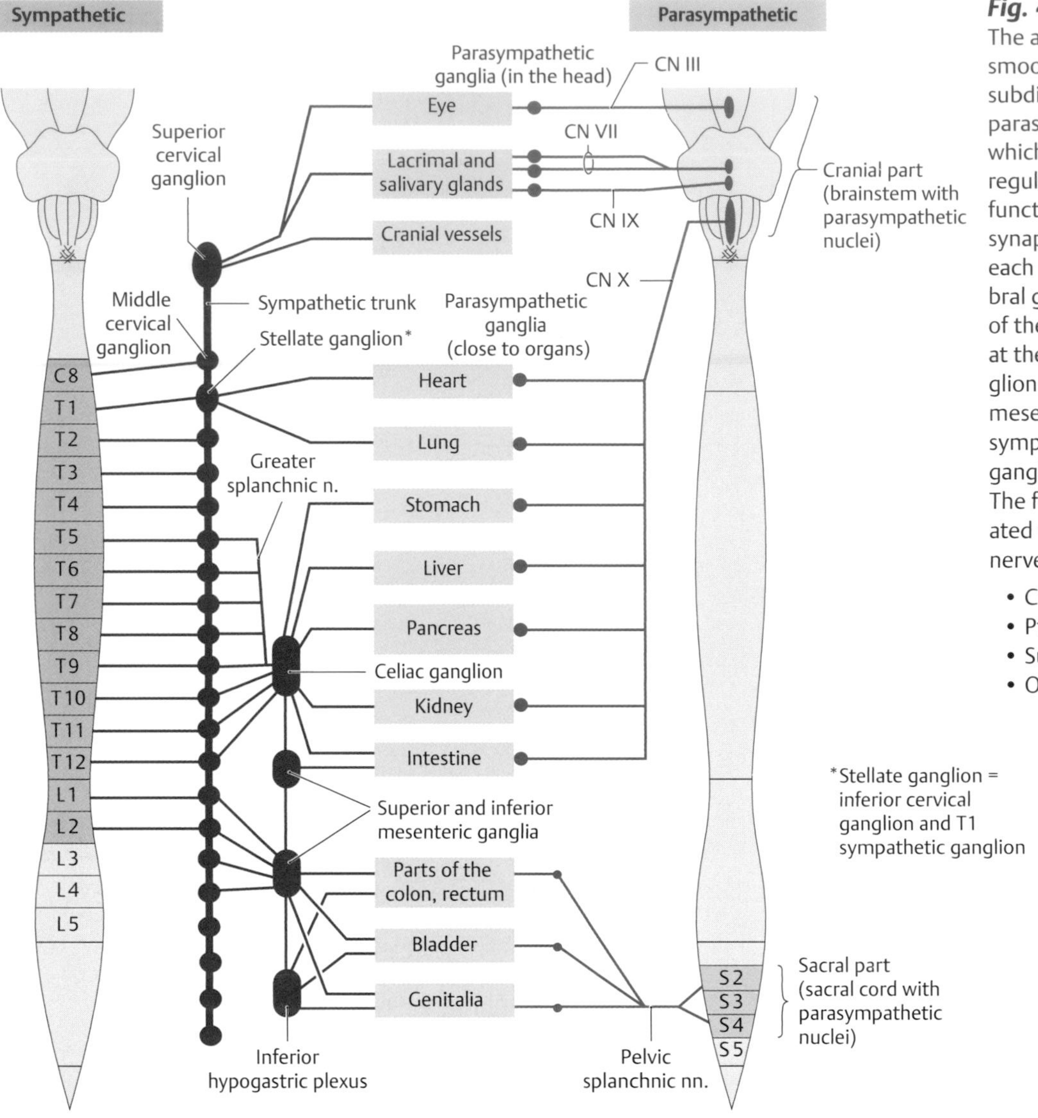
Sympathetic
Parasympathetic
Parasympathetic ganglia (in the head)
CN III
Eye
Superior cervical ganglion
CN VII
Lacrimal and salivary glands
Cranial part (brainstem with parasympathetic nuclei)
Cranial vessels
CN IX
CN X
Middle cervical ganglion
Sympathetic trunk
Stellate ganglion*
Parasympathetic ganglia (close to organs)
C8
T1
T2
T3
T4
T5
T6
T7
T8
T9
T10
T11
T12
L1
L2
L3
L4
L5
Heart
Lung
Greater splanchnic n.
Stomach
Liver
Pancreas
Celiac ganglion
Kidney
Intestine
Superior and inferior mesenteric ganglia
Parts of the colon, rectum
Bladder
Genitalia
Inferior hypogastric plexus
Pelvic splanchnic nn.
S2
S3
S4
S5
Sacral part (sacral cord with parasympathetic nuclei)
*Stellate ganglion = inferior cervical ganglion and T1 sympathetic ganglion

Fig. 43.1 **Autonomic nervous system**
The autonomic nervous system innervates smooth and cardiac muscle and glands. It is subdivided into the sympathetic (red) and parasympathetic (blue) nervous systems, which often act in antagonistic fashion to regulate blood flow, secretions, and organ function (see Table 43.1). The sympathetic synapse occurs within the paired (one on each side of the vertebral column) paravertebral ganglia of the sympathetic trunk or one of the unpaired prevertebral ganglia located at the base of the artery for which the ganglion was named (celiac, superior and inferior mesenteric). Except in the head, the parasympathetic synapse occurs in the terminal ganglion within the wall of the target organ. The four parasympathetic ganglia associated with one of the parasympathetic cranial nerves are as follows:

- Ciliary ganglion, CN III
- Pterygopalatine ganglion, CN VII
- Submandibular ganglion, CN VII
- Otic ganglion, CN IX

Table 43.1 **Effects of the sympathetic and parasympathetic nervous systems**

Organ (organ system)		Sympathetic NS effect	Parasympathetic NS effect
Gastro-intestinal tract	Longitudinal and circular muscle fibers	↓ motility	↑ motility
	Sphincter muscles	Contraction	Relaxation
	Glands	↓ secretions	↑ secretions
Splenic capsule		Contraction	No effect
Liver		↑ glycogenolysis/gluconeogenesis	
Pancreas	Endocrine pancreas	↓ insulin secretion	
	Exocrine pancreas	↓ secretion	↑ secretion
Bladder	Detrusor vesicae	Relaxation	Contraction
	Functional bladder sphincter	Contraction	No effect
Seminal vesicle		Contraction (ejaculation)	
Vas deferens			
Uterus		Contraction or relaxation, depending on hormonal status	
Arteries		Vasoconstriction	Vasodilation of the arteries of the penis and clitoris (erection)

NS, nervous system. See also p. 200.

***Fig. 43.2* Autonomic nervous system circuitry**

The body wall only receives sympathetic postganglionic innervation. Somatic efferent (purple) sympathetic preganglionic fibers exit the spinal cord by the anterior root and synapse in the closest paravertebral (sympathetic) ganglion, accessing it via the white ramus communicans. The postganglionic sympathetic fibers rejoin the anterior and posterior rami via the gray ramus communicans. Visceral efferent fibers pass through the paravertebral ganglion and continue out to a prevertebral ganglion via a splanchnic nerve. They synapse in this distant ganglion, the postganglionic sympathetic fibers passing into the target organ by following its arterial supply. Visceral efferent preganglionic parasympathetic fibers traverse the vagus nerve to the prevertebral ganglion, pass through it, and synapse in an intramural ganglion within the wall of the target organ. The postganglionic parasympathetic fiber is black.

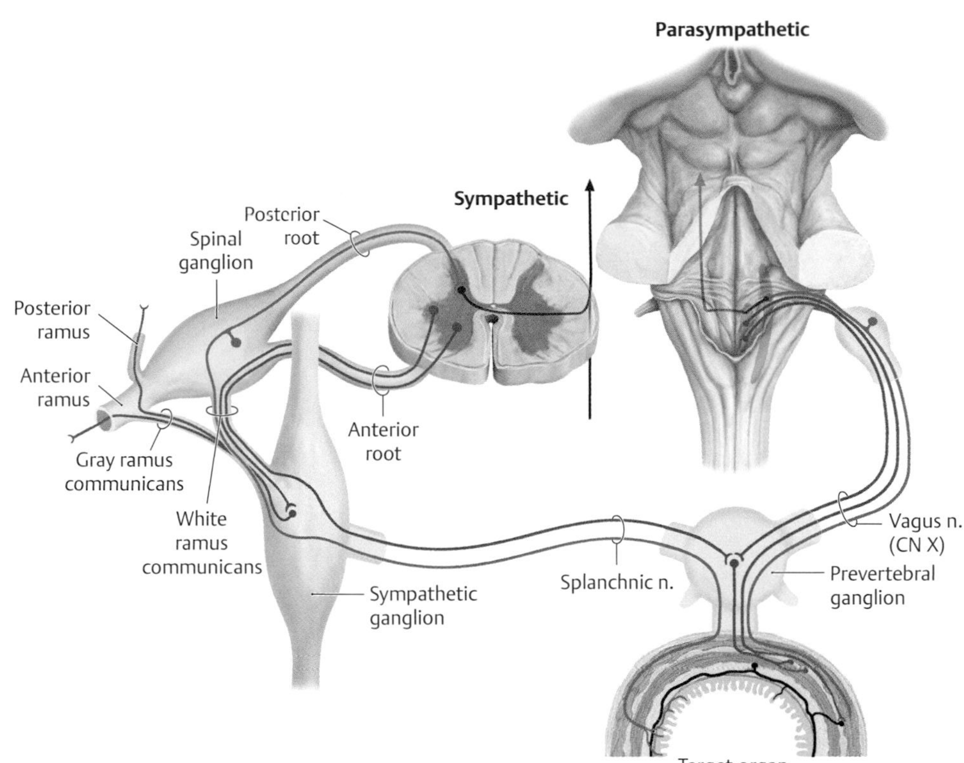

Parasympathetic
Sympathetic
Posterior root
Spinal ganglion
Posterior ramus
Anterior ramus
Gray ramus communicans
White ramus communicans
Anterior root
Sympathetic ganglion
Splanchnic n.
Vagus n. (CN X)
Prevertebral ganglion
Target organ

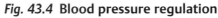

***Fig. 43.3* Modulation of response at target cells by neurotransmitters of the ANS.**

Pre- and postganglionic neurons in the parasympathetic nervous system release acetylcholine(cholinergic neurons), as do preganglionic neurons in the sympathetic division. Postganglionic neurons in the sympathetic nervous system release norepinephrine, except for the suprarenal gland, which releases epinephrine (adrenergic neurons).

Neurotransmitters released by postganglionic neurons of the sympathetic and parasympathetic divisions modulate target cell responses directly by binding to receptors on the target cell or indirectly by binding to receptors on the postganglionic terminals of that or other nearby neurons, thereby modulating further release of neurotransmitters in this figure for the response in cardiac muscle to stimulation by acetylcholine and norepinephrine. This allows for a precise and wide spectrum of responses in the target cell.

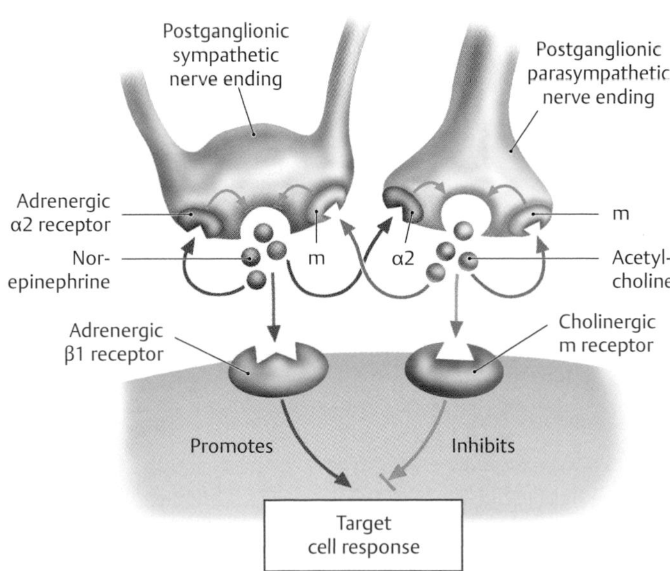

Postganglionic sympathetic nerve ending
Postganglionic parasympathetic nerve ending
Adrenergic α2 receptor
Nor-epinephrine
m
m
α2
Acetyl-choline
Adrenergic β1 receptor
Cholinergic m receptor
Promotes
Inhibits
Target cell response

***Fig. 43.4* Blood pressure regulation**

Not all physiologic responses involve the antagonistic nature of the two divisions of the ANS. Vascular smooth muscle does not receive parasympathetic innervation. Sympathetic fibers may release norepinephrine, inducing the α1 receptor to mediate its contraction (increasing blood pressure). Circulating epinephrine acts on the β2 receptors to induce vasodilation (decreasing blood pressure).

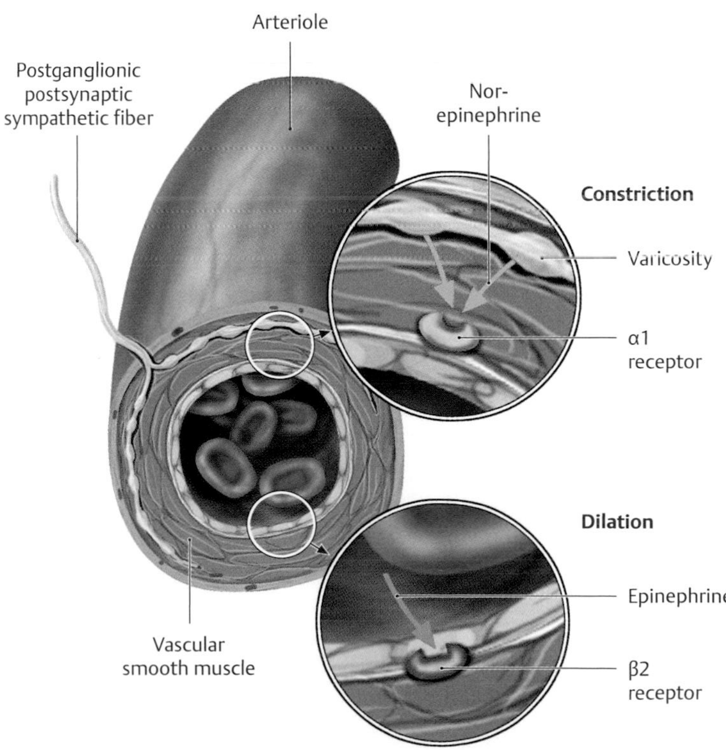

Arteriole
Postganglionic postsynaptic sympathetic fiber
Nor-epinephrine
Constriction
Varicosity
α1 receptor
Dilation
Epinephrine
β2 receptor
Vascular smooth muscle

Index

Index

Note: Clinical applications, imaging, sectional anatomy, and surface anatomy are found under these main headings, broken out by region. Italicized page numbers represent clinical applications. Tabular material is indicated by a “t” following the page number.

A

Abdomen. *See also individual organs*
anastomoses, arterial, 176, 177
arteries of, 176, 176t, 177, 178
autonomic nervous system effects in, 202t, 648t
bones of, 134
divisions of, 148, 148t, 149
greater omental sac, 150–151
lesser omental sac, 152–153. *See also* Bursae, omental
ligaments of, 134
lymphatic drainage of, 192, 192t, 194
mesenteries of, 151, 152, 154, 161, 164
nerves of, 200, 201
neurovasculature of
inguinal region, 142–143, 143t
scrotum,144, 145, 145t
spermatic cord, 144
testis, 145, 145t
organs of by relationship to peritoneum, 148t, 149. *See also individual organs*
planes of, 133t
quadrants of, 132
regions of, 132, 132t
veins of, 184, 184t, 185, 186
walls of
diaphragm, 138–139, 139t
lymphatics of, 194
muscles of, 135, 136–138, 140–141, 140t, 146
nerves of, 200, 201
Acetabulum, 216, 217, 219, 223, 224, 226, 385, 387
labrum of, 385, 387, 388, 445
radiograph of, 217
rim of, 386, 387
roof of, 388, 402, 445
Acoustic radiation, 645
Acromion, 275, 277, 279, 282, 283, 284, 285
relationship to trunk skeleton, 277
Adenohypophysis, 628, 630
Ala
of ilium, 134
nasal, 550
of sacrum
in female, 218
in male, 219
Allocortex, 626
Alveoli, 121
capillary bed on, 126
epithelial lining of, 121
lumen of, 121
pulmonary, 121, 126
respiratory compromise and, *121*
Ampulla
of ductus deferens, 149, 239, 241, 252
hepatopancreatic, sphincter of, 168
rectal, 235
of urethra, 250
of uterine tube, 243
Amygdala, 498, 621, 626, 629t, 646, 647t
Anal canal, 235
blood vessels of, 256
lympathic drainage of, 261, 447
nerves of, 181, 185, 191
regions of, 235t
Anal pecten, 235, 235t
Anastomoses,
arterialof abdomen, 176, 177, 181
of auricle of ear, 559
of superior mesenteric artery, 177
of superior mesenteric artery–inferior pancreatic artery, 181
of celiac trunk, 177
in right and left coronary arteries, *97*
venous
inferior phrenic–suprarenal veins, 173
of head and neck, 523t
Anatomic snuffbox, 374
Anesthesia, lumbar and epidural, *41*
Angina pectoris, *97*
Ankle
ligaments (of region) of, 432–433
mortise of, 382, 404, 428, 429
radiography of, 426, 428
retinacula of, 439
tendon sheaths of, 439
ANS. *See* Autonomic nervous system (ANS)
Ansa cervicalis, 577, 609
superior and inferior roots of, 577, 597, 609
Antihelix, of auricle of ear, 476, 559
Antitragus, of auricle of ear, 476, 559
Antrum
of mastoid bone, 561, 564
pyloric, 156, 157
Anulus fibrosus, 14, 17, 22, 94
disk herniation and, *15*
Anus, 215
Aorta, 61, 104
abdominal, 5, 25, 36, 76, 80, 88, 107, 108, 132, 149, 152, 155, 156, 159, 164, 165, 166, 169, 170, 171, 173, 175, 176, 177, 180, 183, 184, 186, 187, 193, 194, 198, 201, 210, 211, 236, 254, 255, 256, 257, 259, 444
branches of, 176, 176t, 178
distribution of, 178
ascending, 5, 75, 76, 77, *77*, 77t, 80, 84, 88, 89, 90, 91, 92, 93, 95, 96, 97, 99, 100, 101, 116, 124
bifurcation of, 64, 176, 183, 242
descending, 75, 77, *77*, 77t, 101, 114
thoracic, 36, 44, 63, 64, 64t, 69, 76, 80, 82, 85, 87, 88, 101, 104, 106, 107, 107t, 111, 114, 126, 129, 344
branches of, 77t
dissection of, *77*
Aperture
anterior nasal, 479, 551
in brainstem
lateral, 631
median, 632
diaphragmatic, 60, 61
piriform, 479
thoracic
inferior, 52
superior, 52
Apex, 115
of arytenoid cartilage, 598
of heart, 88, 89, 92, 93, 98, 100, 100t, 116, 124
of lung, 114
of tongue, 578, 579
of tooth root, 572
Aponeurosis
bicipital, 290, 312, 318, 366, 367, 376
epicranial. *See* Galea aponeurotica
external oblique, 136, 141, 142, 143, 146, 147, 460, 461, 464
gluteal, 24
internal oblique, 136, 141, 146
latissimus dorsi, 28
lingual, 578
palatine, 575
palmar, 317, 318, 334, 358, 370, 371, 372, 376
atrophy of (Depuytren’s contracture), *334*
plantar, 429, 430, 435, 436, 438, 441, 470, 471
stylopharyngeal, 586
transversus abdominis, 137, 141, 146
Apparatus
auditory
components of, 558
of inner ear, 566
lacrimal, 545
drainage and, *545*
vestibular, of inner ear, 566
Appendix/appendices
of epididymis, 145, 251
of testis, 145, 251
vermiform, 132, 162, 231
Aqueduct
cerebral, 628, 631, 632, 633, 637
cochlear, 560, 566

vestibular, 567
Arachnoid, 40, 41, 524, 526, 632
Arcades, arterial
anastomotic, 559
scapular, 345
Arch
aortic, 36, 74, 76, 77, 82, 85, 87, 88, 89, 92, 93, 100, 103, 104, 107, 108, 109, 114, 116, 124, 125, 126, 603, 636
with thoracic aortic plexus, 99
of atlas (C1)
anterior, 21
posterior, 19, 27
spinous process of, 8
transverse process of, 8
coracoacromial, 283, 285, 286, 287
costal, 133, 138, 289
of cricoid cartilage, 599
of foot
dorsal venous, 446
longitudinal, 435
plantar, 446
deep, 444, 471
transverse, 434
iliopectineal, 142, 147, 461
jugular venous, 595, 606
palatoglossal, 578, 580, 582
palatopharyngeal, 578, 580, 582, 583
palmar venous
deep, 344, 345, 346, 371, 373
superficial, 344, 345, 346, 370, 371, 373
pubic
in female, 218
in male, 219
tendinous
of levator ani, 224
of soleus, 422, 457, 466
vertebral, 7, 9, 11, 14, 19, 20, 21, 22, 25
pedicles of, 15, 23
zygomatic, 477, 478, 482, 531, 532, 617
Archicortex, 626
Area(s)
Brodmann, 627, 643, 645
cortical, of sensorimotor system, 639
Kiesselbach's, 554
preoptic, 628
prepiriform, 498, 646
pretectal, 642, 643
septal, in limbic system, 647t
subcallosal (paraolfactory), 647t
vestibular, in brainstem, 631
of visual cortex, 643
Areola, 70
Arm, 376, 377. *See also* Forearm.
bones of, 276, 280–281, 304–305
lymph vessels of, 347
muscles of, 354–355
anterior, 288–291, 296–299, 302
posterior, 292–295, 300-301, 303
nerves of, 353
topography of
brachial region, 366
cubital region 367
Artery/Arteries (named), 176
alveolar
inferior, 518, 521, 528, 532, 533, 534t, 586, 616, 617
superior
anterior, 521
posterior, 521, 532, 533, 534t
angular, 516, 518, 528, 532, 542
appendicular, 162
arcuate, 174, 179, 444, 469
auditory, internal, 565, 567
auricular
anterior, 559
deep, 521, 534t, 564t, 565
posterior, 517, 517t, 518, 519t, 559
posterior branch, 564t
axillary, 64, 64t, 68, 70, 72, 176, 344, 345, 348, 352, 353, 355t, 357, 363, 364, 365, 366
basilar, 44, 516, 636
brachial, 72, 318, 344, 345, 364, 365, 367, 369, 377
bronchial, 76, 126
buccal, 521, 532, 533, 534t
callosomarginal, 637
caroticotympanic, 564t, 565
carotid
atherosclerosis of, *517*
common, 25, 36, 62, 64, 76, 77, 77t, 80, 82, 85, 88, 92, 107t, 109, 125, 344, 345, 349, 516, 517, 518, 519, 520, 586, 587, 594, 602, 603, 606, 607, 608, 609, 619, 636
external, 36, 516, 517, 519, 520, 530, 531, 554, 559, 564t, 586, 594, 609, 636
branches of, 517t, 518–519, 519t, 520t
internal, 36, 484, 485, 505, 507, 516, 517, 518, 519, 524, 527, 530, 531, 535, 539, 540, 541, 554, 560, 561, 563, 564t, 565, 586, 594, 609, 618, 621, 636
parts and branches of, 516
carpal
dorsal, 345, 375
cecal
anterior, 182, 183, 190, 191
posterior, 182, 190, 191
cerebellar
anteroinferior, 636
posteroinferior, 636
superior, 636
cerebral, 524
anterior, 637
parts of, 636
distribution areas, 637
middle, 524, 526, 637
parts of, 636
posterior, 636, 637
callosal branch, 637
cingular branch, 637
paracentral branch, 637
parietal branch, 637
parts of, 636
precunial branch, 637
temporal branch, 637
cervical
accessory, 45
ascending, 44, 345, 607
deep, 46, 345
superficial, 345, 609, 610, 611
transverse, 47, 345, 607, 608
choroidal
anterior, 636
ciliary
anterior, 547
posterior
long, 540, 547
short, 540, 543, 547
circumflex
humeral, anterior and posterior, 344, 345, 349
scapular, 344, 345, 361, 364, 365
clitoral
deep, 267
dorsal, 247, 267
cochlear
common, 567
proper, 567
colic
left, 155, 159, 171, 173, 177, 183, 191, 209
middle, 149, 150, 153, 160, 177, 182, 183, 190, 191, 209
right, 159, 177, 182, 183, 190, 191, 208, 209
collateral
middle, 344
radial, 344, 369
communicating
anterior, 636
posterior, 516, 636
conjunctival
anterior, 547
coronary
branches of, 96t
disturbed blood flow in, *97*
dominance patterns, 97
left, 94, 96, 96t, 101
anterior interventricular branch, 89
circumflex branch, 96
right, 94, 96, 96t
stenosis of, *97*
cremasteric, 144, 251
crural
anterior, 565
posterior, 565
cystic, 167, 180, 181
branches of, 167
deep, of arm, 345, 361

Artery/Arteries *(continued)*
digital
common palmar, 344, 345, 372, 373
dorsal, 345, 372, 375, 469
palmar, 344, 345, 372, 373
plantar, 444
proper, 444, 470, 471
proper palmar, 345, 372
dorsalis pedis, 444, 469
epigastric
inferior, 143, 146, 147, 150, 154, 160, 175, 176, 178, 186, 236, 254, 257, 444
obturator branch of, 146, 178, 254
superficial, 176, 444, 464
superior, 64, 64t, 68, 176
ethmoidal
anterior, 484, 536t, 540, 543, 554, 555
posterior, 484, 516, 536t, 540, 543, 554
facial, 516, 517, 517t, 518, 519t, 528, 530, 531, 532, 533, 542, 581, 609
transverse, 520, 528, 529
femoral, 142, 143, 144, 146, 147, 176, 178, 186, 257, 268, 270, 271, 444, 445, 458, 460, 461, 464, 473
circumflex
lateral, 444, 445, 464
medial, 444, 445, 463, 464, 465
fibular, 444, 445, 466, 468, 469
foveal, 445
frontal, polar, 637
frontobasal, lateral, 637
gastric
left, 107, 107t, 153, 159, 165, 171, 173, 176, 176t, 177, 180, 181, 182, 188, 189, 190, 191, 207
posterior, 181
right, 176, 176t, 177, 180, 181, 182, 188, 189, 190, 191
short, 181
gastroduodenal, 176, 176t, 177, 180, 181, 182, 188, 189, 190, 191
gastroomental, 207
left, 177, 180, 181, 188, 189
right, 177, 180, 182, 188, 189, 190, 191
genicular
descending, 444, 464
inferior
lateral, 444, 445, 467
medial, 444, 445
middle, 445, 467
superior
lateral, 444, 445, 467
medial, 444, 445, 467
gluteal
inferior, 178, 256, 444, 462, 463, 464, 465
superior, 175, 178, 236, 255, 256, 444, 462, 463, 464, 465
hepatic
common, 63, 107, 153, 159, 169, 171, 173, 176, 176t, 177, 180, 181, 182, 188, 207, 210
proper, 155, 167, 169, 173, 176, 176t, 177, 180, 181, 182, 188, 189, 190, 191
branches of, 166, 167
ileal, 182, 190, 191, 208
ileocolic, 177, 182, 183, 190, 191, 208, 209
colic branch, 182, 183, 190
ileal branch, 182, 183, 190
iliac
circumflex
deep, 146, 176, 178, 186, 257, 444
superficial, 176, 444, 460, 464
common, 149, 155, 175, 176, 176t, 178, 183, 186, 191, 193, 194, 201, 236, 238, 242, 254, 255, 256, 257, 259, 444
ureteral branches of, 187
external, 36, 155, 175, 176, 176t, 230, 233, 236, 237, 238, 242, 247, 256, 257, 260, 444, 464
internal, 36, 175, 176t, 177, 178, 193, 201, 236, 237, 242, 245, 254, 255, 256, 257, 259, 268, 444
anterior trunk of, 175, 236, 255
branches, 254t
iliolumbar, 178, 255
infraorbital, 518, 521, 528, 533, 534t, 535t, 536, 536t, 542
intercostal, 67, 68, 71, 86, 87, 111, 112, 210
anterior, 36, 64, 64t
branches of, 36, 64, 64t
posterior, 36, 44, 47, 64, 64t, 69, 76, 82, 85, 86, 87, 106, 126
branches of, 36, 64, 64t
supreme, 345
interlobar, of kidney, 174, 179
interlobular, of kidney, 179
interosseous
anterior, 318, 344, 345, 369, 373, 377
common, 318, 344, 345
posterior, 318, 344, 345, 369, 377
recurrent, 345, 369
jejunal, 182, 190, 191, 208, 211
labial
inferior, 518
superior, 518
labyrinthine, 484, 636
lacrimal, 540, 543
laryngeal
inferior, 603
superior, 587, 594, 599, 603, 606, 607
lingual, 517, 517t, 518, 519t, 579, 581, 609
deep, 579, 617
lingular, 125t
lumbar, 44, 76, 176t
malleolar
anterior
lateral, 444, 469
medial, 444
marginal, 96, 182
masseteric, 521, 534t
mastoid, 565
maxillary, 517, 517t, 518, 519, 520, 520t, 521, 532, 533, 534, 554, 559, 618
branches of, 521, 534t
divisions of, 520t, 521
ligation of, *521*
terminal branches, 564t
meningeal
middle, 484, 521, 525, 533, 534t, 540, 564t
injury to, *521*
posterior, 484, 621
mesenteric
inferior, 155, 175, 176, 176t, 177, 178, 183, 187, 191, 193, 255, 256, 259
anastomoses of, 177
branches of, 183
superior, 149, 155, 158, 159, 169, 170, 171, 173, 175, 176, 176t, 177, 178, 181, 182, 183, 186, 187, 188, 189, 190, 207, 210, 211, 236
anastomoses of, 177
branches of, 182
metacarpal, 375
dorsal, 345
palmar, 345, 373
metatarsal
dorsal, 444, 469
plantar, 444, 470, 471
musculophrenic, 62, 64
nasal
dorsal, 516, 518, 528, 540, 542
lateral posterior, 534t, 554, 555
nasopalatine, 484
obturator, 146, 178, 245, 255, 256, 257, 445
in female, 237
in male, 270
occipital, 46, 517, 517t, 518, 519t, 525, 529, 586, 587, 612, 613, 618
lateral, 637
medial, 636, 637
ophthalmic, 484, 516, 518, 527, 536, 540, 541, 542, 554
inferior, 542
superior, 542
ovarian, 173, 175, 176t, 178, 186, 187, 189, 236, 237, 238, 242, 243, 245, 255, 257
ureteral branches of, 187
palatine, 534t
descending, 534t, 535t, 554, 555
greater, 484, 534, 534t, 535t, 554, 555, 576, 616
lesser, 484, 534, 534t, 535t, 576
palmar, superficial, 371
palpebral, medial, 540
pancreatic
great, 181
inferior, 181, 189
pancreaticoduodenal, 190, 207
inferior, 177, 188
anterior, 181, 182, 189
posterior, 181, 182, 189

  - superior
    - anterior, 177, 180, 181, 182, 188, 189
    - posterior, 177, 180, 181, 188, 189
- parietal, posterior, 637
  - angular gyral branch, 637
  - parietooccipital branch, 637
  - temporal branch, 637
- penile
  - bulbar, 268
  - deep, 250, 268
    - branches of, 250
  - dorsal, 250, 255, 257, 268, 269
- perforating, 444, 445, 463, 464, 465
- pericallosal, 637
- pericardiacophrenic, 62, 63t, 74, 85, 90
- perineal, 247
  - in female, 267
  - in male, 268
- petrosal
  - greater, 565
  - lesser, 565
  - superficial, 565
- pharyngeal, 594
  - ascending, 517, 517t, 518, 519t, 586
- phrenic
  - inferior, 62, 63, 63t, 76, 107, 173, 175, 176t, 178, 187, 236
  - superior, 62, 63, 63t, 69
- plantar
  - deep, 469
  - lateral, 444, 467, 470, 471
  - medial, 444, 445, 467, 470, 471
- pontine, 636
- popliteal, 407, 444, 445, 465, 466, 467
  - oblique, 467
- posterolateral, right, 96
- prefrontal, 637
- pudendal
  - external, 257, 444, 460, 464
    - in male, 268
  - internal, 232, 234, 256, 463
    - in female, 178, 255, 267
    - in male, 255, 268, 269, 271
- pulmonary, 88, 99, 102, 103
  - branches of, 125t
    - left, 74, 85, 87, 89, 92, 93, 104, 109, 114, 124, 125t
    - right, 84, 85, 91, 92, 93, 95, 104, 114, 124, 125, 125t
- radial, 318, 344, 345, 367, 369, 370, 371, 372, 373, 374, 375
  - dorsal carpal branch, 375
  - recurrent, 344, 367
  - superficial palmar branch, 370, 373
- radicular, anterior, 64
- rectal
  - inferior, 177, 254, 256
    - in female, 255, 267
    - in male, 255, 268
  - middle, 177, 245, 256, 257
    - in female, 178, 237, 255
    - in male, 255, 268
  - superior, 177, 183, 191, 193, 209, 245, 255, 256, 259
- renal, 174, 176, 176t, 179
  - left, 149, 173, 175, 178, 182, 186, 187, 189, 190, 191, 236
    - anterior branch of, 179
    - main trunk, 179
    - posterior branch of, 179
  - renal hypertension and, *179*
  - right, 171, 174, 187, 210
  - stenosis of, *179*
- retinal, central, 540, 546, 547
- sacral
  - lateral, 36, 178
  - medial, 186, 236
  - median, 36, 175, 176t, 178, 245, 254, 255, 256, 257
- scapular, dorsal, 345
- scrotal
  - anterior, 268
  - posterior, 255, 268
- segmental, of lung, 44, 125t, 174, 179
  - segmental medullary
    - anterior, 44
    - posterior, 44
- sigmoid, 177, 183, 191, 209, 256
- sphenopalatine, 533, 534t, 535t, 554
  - bleeding from, *521*
- spinal
  - anterior, 44, 484, 636
  - posterior, 44, 484
- splenic, 63, 149, 153, 155, 159, 169, 170, 171, 173, 176, 176t, 177, 180, 181, 182, 188, 189, 190, 191, 210
  - pancreatic branches of, 181
- sternocleidomastoid, 609
- stylomastoid, 563, 564t, 565
- subarcuate, 565
- subclavian, 36, 44, 62, 64, 64t, 70, 72, 74, 76, 77, 77t, 82, 85, 87, 88, 92, 80, 99, 176, 104, 107, 114, 125, 128, 344, 345, 349, 363, 511, 516, 517, 587, 594, 603, 607, 636
- subcostal, 36
- sublingual, 579
- submental, 518, 579
- subscapular, 344, 363, 365
- sulcal, 44
- supraduodenal, 181
- supraorbital, 516, 536, 540, 542, 543
- suprarenal
  - inferior, 173, 176t, 179
    - left, 175, 176, 176t, 178, 187, 236
  - middle, 173, 174, 176t
    - left, 175, 178, 187, 236
    - right, 174
  - superior, 173
    - left, 63, 175, 176, 176t, 178, 187, 236
    - right, 63, 176, 176t, 187
- suprascapular, 344, 345, 360, 361, 363, 607, 611
- supratrochlear, 516, 518, 536, 540, 543
- sural, 445
- tarsal, 471
  - lateral, 444, 469
  - medial, 467
- temporal
  - deep, 521, 532, 534t
  - middle, 520
  - superficial, 517, 517t, 518, 520t, 528, 529, 532, 533, 559, 581
    - course of, 520
- testicular, 144, 145, 146, 173, 175, 176t, 178, 187, 189, 236, 251, 257
  - ureteral branches of, 187
- thoracic
  - internal, 36, 62, 63, 64, 64t, 68, 69, 70, 74, 76, 107, 112, 113, 176, 210, 344, 345, 607
  - lateral, 64, 64t, 68, 70, 176, 344, 363, 364, 365
  - superior, 64, 64t, 176, 344, 363, 364, 365
- thoracoacromial, 64, 64t, 344, 362, 363, 364, 365
- thoracodorsal, 176, 344, 345, 364, 365
- thyroid
  - inferior, 107t, 345, 587, 594, 602, 603, 607, 609, 619
  - superior, 516, 517, 517t, 518, 519t, 530, 531, 586, 594, 602, 603, 606, 607, 608, 609, 619
- tibial
  - anterior, 444, 445, 469
    - recurrent, 444, 445
  - posterior, 428, 444, 445, 466, 467
  - recurrent
    - posterior, 445, 467
- tubal, 565
- tympanic
  - anterior, 484, 521, 534t, 563, 564t
  - inferior, 564, 564t, 565
  - posterior, 563, 564t
  - superior, 484, 564, 564t, 565
- ulnar, 344, 345, 367, 369, 370, 371, 372, 373, 377
  - recurrent, 344
  - collateral
    - inferior, 318, 344, 366, 367
    - superior, 318, 344, 366, 367
- umbilical, 237, 255, 257
  - obliterated, 103, 237, 254, 257
  - patent part, 257
  - right, 178, 255
  - vaginal branch of, 254
- urethral, 250
  - in male, 268

Artery/Arteries *(continued)*
uterine, 178, 237, 245, 247, 254, 255, 257
tubal branches of, 243, 257
vaginal, 254, 257
branches of, 247
right, 255
vertebral, 17, 36, 40, 44, 46, 64, 107, 344, 345, 484, 516, 517, 519, 525, 586, 594, 613, 618, 619, 620, 621, 636
right, 76
uncinate process proximity to, *17*
vesical
inferior, 245, 257
in female, 178, 237, 255
in male, 255, 270
superior, 245, 254, 257
in female, 237, 255
in male, 255
vestibular, 567
vestibulocochlear, 567
common, 567
zygomaticoorbital, 520, 529
Arteries (of region or organ)
of abdomen, 176
anastomoses of, 176, 177
aorta and major branches, 176
celiac trunk, 177
mesenteric artery
inferior, 177
superior, 177
wall of, anterior, 176
of arm, deep, 344, 361
of auricle, 559
of back, 36
of brain, 636–637
distribution areas, 637
of brainstem, 636
of cerebellum, 636
of diaphragm, 63t
of ductus deferens, 144, 146, 251, 254, 255
of dura mater, 525
of esophagus, 107t
of eyeball, 547
of female external genitalia, 267
of forearm, 345
of hand, 345
of hard palate, 576
of head and neck, 516–517
of heart, 96–97
branches of, 96t
distribution of, 97
of inner ear, 567
of larynx, 603
of lower limb, 444–445
femoral head, 445
thigh and leg, 445
of lungs
arteriogram of, 125
distribution of, 124
of inferior lobe, 125t
of middle lobe, 125t
of superior lobe, 125t
of mediastinum, 84t
of middle ear, 564, 564t
of nasal septum and wall, 554
of neck, 594
of orbit, 540
of pancreatic tail, 181
of pelvis
in female, 254, 255
in male, 254, 255
of penis, 268
of pterygoid canal, 534t
in pterygopalatine fossa, 534t, 535t
of rectum, 256
of retroperitoneum, 155t
of scrotum, 268
of shoulder, posterior, 360–361
of spinal cord, 44
sympathetic and parasympathetic effects on, 648t, 649
of testis, 251
of thigh, 444, 445, 464, 473
of thoracic cavity, 76–77
of thoracic wall, 64t
of tracheobronchial tree, 126
of upper limb, 344–345
lymph vessels and, 347
of vestibular bulb, 247, 267
Asthma, *121*
Atherosclerosis
of carotid artery, *517*
disturbed coronary artery blood flow and, *97*
Atlas (C1), 6, 8–9, 17, 19, 20, 30, 31, 40, 42
arch of, 8, 19, 21, 27
fracture of, *9*
lateral masses of, 9, 18, 19
posterior tubercle of, 18, 21, 30
transverse ligament of, 18, 19, 21, 618
transverse process of, 8, 26, 27, 30, 31, 46
Atrioventricular valves
auscultation sites for, 94t, *95*
Atrium/atria, of heart
left, 84, 88, 91, 92, 93, 96, 98, 100, 101, 102, 103, 108, 116
right, 88, 92, 93, 96, 98, 100, 101, 108, 116, 124
Arteriography. *See* Imaging.
Auditory system, 645
Auricle
of ear, 560
arteries of, 559
innervation of, 559
muscles of, 559
structure of, 559
of heart
left, 92, 93, 101
atrial appendage of, 89, 90, 96
right, 92, 93
atrial appendage of, 89, 96
Auscultation sites, 94t, *95*
Autonomic nervous system (ANS), 638, 648–649
circuits of, 649
effect on abdominal arteries, 202t
parasympathetic, 202, 648
circuitry of, 648t
effect on organs, 202t, 648t
regulatory effects of, 649
peripheral, limbic regulation of, 647
sympathetic, 202, 648
circuits of, 648t
effect on organs, 202t, 648t
regulatory effects of, 648t
Avascular necrosis
humeral fracture and, *281*
scaphoid fractures and, *323*
Axilla, 274
arteries of, 345
lymphatic drainage of, 72, 72t, 347
radial nerve compression in, 353
spaces of, triangular and quadrangular, 361
topography of, 364–365
walls of, 364t
Axis (C2), 6, 8–9, 17, 18, 19, 20, 30, 31, 42, 59, 300
body of, 21
dens of, 5, 6, 55, 383, 554, 580, 582, 586, 618
fracture of, *9*
spinous process of, 18, 26, 27, 30, 46, 593
Axis/axes
of abduction/ adduction, 399
longitudinal
of cervix, 242
of uterus, 242
of vagina, 242
optical, 546
of orbit, 546
of rib cage movement, 56
Axons, 624
myelination of, 624

B

Back. *See also* Vertebral column
arteries of, 36. *See also* Spinal cord, arteries of
bones of. *See* Ribs, Vertebra/vertebrae; Vertebral column
joints of. *See* Vertebral column
ligaments of. *See* Vertebra/vertebrae; Vertebral column
muscles of
craniovertebral joint, 30
extrinsic, 24, 296–301, 296t, 297t, 298t, 299t, 300t, 301t
intrinsic
deep, 29, 34, 34t, 35
intermediate, 28, 29, 32, 32t, 33
prevertebral, 31
short nuchal, 26, 27, 30

superficial, 28, 32, 32t, 33
thoracolumbar fascia and, 24, 25, 28
nerves of, 38, 39
neurovasculature
of nuchal region, 46
of back, 47
veins of, 37. *See also* Spinal cord, veins of.
Balance, cranial nerve associated with, 642t
Bifurcation
aortic, 64, 176, 183, 242
tracheal, 120
Biopsy, percutaneous of liver, *112*
Bladder, urinary, 146, 149, 236
arteries of, 254, 254t, 255
autonomic nervous system effects on, 202t, 648t
in female, 238
lymphatic drainage of, 195, 258, 259, 259t, 261, 447
in male, 239
ligaments of, 345
nerves of, 207, 263, 264, 265
parts of, 237, 238, 239
veins of, 254, 254t, 255
wall structure of, 239
Bleeding. *See also* Hematoma; Hemorrhage.
extracerebral, *525*
nasopharyngeal, *521*
from nose, *555*
Blindness, optic nerve lesion and, *643*
"Blood clots," from lower limb, *125*
Blood flow
disturbed, in coronary arteries, *97*
impeded, in neck, *595*
Blood pressure
optic fundus examination in, *547*
regulation of, 649
renal hypertension and, *179*
Body/bodies
carotid, 586, 609
ciliary, 544, 546, 548, 549
geniculate
lateral, 499, 630, 642, 643
medial, 499, 643
nucleus of, 645
mammillary, 627, 628, 629t, 630, 647t
nerve cell. *See* Gray matter.
pineal, 633
vertebral. *See* Vertebra/Vertebrae.
vitreous, 546, 616, 621
Bones (of region). *See also individual bones*
of abdomen, 134
of back. *See* Vertebra/vertebrae; Vertebral column.
of foot, 424–425
of hand, 322–323
of lower limb, 382–383
of nasal cavity, 550–551
of neck, 588t. *See also* Vertebra/vertebrae; Vertebral column.
of oral cavity, 568–569
of ossicular chain, 562
of paranasal sinuses, 553
of pelvis, 216–217, 218–219
of pterygopalatine fossa, 534t
of skull, 478t
anterior, 479
calvaria, 481
lateral, 478
posterior, 480
of skull base
exterior, 482
interior, 483
of upper limb, 276–281, 304–305, 322–323
of wrist, 322–323
carpal bones, 324–325
Boyd's vein, 447
Brain
in adult, 625
arteries of, 636–637
development of, 625t
in embryo, 625
in nervous system, 624
veins of, 634–635
Brainstem, 630, 631
arteries of, 636
cranial nerves in, 631
levels of, 631
veins of, 635
Breast cancer, *73*
Breast (female), 70
arteries of, 70
cancer of, *73*
cutaneous innervation of, 70
ligaments of, 71
lymph nodes and lymphatics of, 72, 72t
mammary ridges of, 70
mammography of, *73*
nerves of, 70
structures of, 70, 71
veins of, 70
Brim, pelvic, 220
Brodmann areas, 627, 643, 645
Bronchiole, 121, 126
terminal, 121
Bronchus/bronchi
foreign body in, *120*
lobar
inferior, 104, 114, 115, 120, 126, 127
middle, 126, 127
superior, 104, 114, 115, 120, 126, 127
main
left, 76, 77, 87, 88, 105, 107, 109, 111, 120, 124, 126, 127, 129
origin of, 84
right, 76, 77, 85, 105, 109, 111, 120, 124, 126, 127, 129
segmental, 121
subsegmental
large, 121
small, 121
Bulb
carotid, calcified plaque in, *517*
duodenal, 158
olfactory, 498, 554, 555, 626, 646
penile, veins of, 254
vestibular, 233, 238, 240, 247, 248, 249
blood vessels of, 267
Bulbourethral glands, 232, 239, 241, 241t, 250, 252, 253, 269
Bulla, ethmoid, 486, 551
Bundle, atrioventricular (of His), 98
Bursa(e)
acromial
subcutaneous, 287
of calcaneal tendon, 429
gastrocnemio-semimembranosus, *409*
iliopectineal, 461
infrapatellar, 414, 415
of ischium, 385
omental, 149, 152, 153, 156, 170, 171, 210
boundaries of, 152, 153t
location of, 152
recess of
inferior, 152
splenic, 152, 164
superior, 152
vestibule of, 152, 153, 164
wall of, posterior, 152
periarticular, of knee, 409
prepatellar, 407, 415
semimembranosus, 409
subacromial, 285, 286–287
subcoracoid, 285
subdeltoid, 286, 287, 363
subtendinous
of gastrocnemius
lateral, 409
medial, 409, 467
of subscapularis, 285, 286, 287, 363
trochanteric, 387, 463, 465

C

Calcaneus, 382, 405, 417, 418, 420, 422, 423, 424, 425, 426, 427, 428, 429, 430, 431, 432, 433, 434, 443
Calvaria, bones of, 481
Calyx
major , 174, 179
minor, 174
Canal(s)
adductor, 444, 446
anal, 235
blood vessels of, 256
lymphatic drainage of, 261, 447
nerves of, 185, 191
regions of, 235t
auditory
external, 558, *558*, 559, 560, 561
irrigation of, *557*

Canal(s) *(continued)*
carotid, 482, 484, 556
central, of spinal cord, 632, 633
cervical, 243
cochlear, 566
condylar, 482, 484
of dens, apical ligament of, 21
external auditory, 558
facial, 504, 561
hypoglossal, 21, 482, 483, 484, 513
venous plexus of, 484
incisive, 484, 550, 568
infraorbital, 536t, 537, 616
inguinal, 142, 143t, 147, 241, 461t
mandibular, 616, 617
obturator, 224, 270
optic, 483, 484, 487, 499, 536, 536t, 537, 568
palatine
greater, 535t, 568
lesser, 535t
palatovaginal, 482
pelvic, in female, 221
for petrosal nerves, hiatus of, 484
pterygoid, 487, 505, 534t, 535t, 568
pudendal (Alcock's canal), 463
pyloric, 156, 157
sacral, 7, 7t, 12, 13, 218, 219, 223, 454
of Schlemm, 546, 548
glaucoma and, *548*
semicircular, 506, 566
anterior, 507, 558, 560, 561, 565, 566
lateral, 558, 560, 561, 566
orientation and position for caloric testing, *557*
posterior, 507, 558, 560, 561, 566
vertebral, 5, 14, 22, 23, 210
cauda equina in, 41
intervertebral disk relationship to, 14
Canaliculus
lacrimal, inferior and superior, 545
tympanic, 509
Canine teeth, 572
Capitate, 275, 322t, 324, 325, 326, 327, 330, 331, 371
Capitellum, 280, 281, 306, 309
Capsule
acromioclavicular joint, 282
articular, 325
of atlantoaxial joint, lateral, 20
of atlantooccipital joint, 19, 20
lateral, 18
in brain
external, 626
extreme, 626
internal, 626, 629t, 637
of elbow joint, 309, 355t, 357t
of facet joint, 21, 22
of glenohumeral joint, 285, 286, 287
of head
extreme, 621
internal, 620, 621
of hip joint, 388–389
of interphalangeal joint
distal, 329
proximal, 329
of knee joint, 409, 414
attachment of, 414, 415
outpouching in, *409*
of metacarpophalangeal joint, 329, 353t, 357t
of metatarsophalangeal joint, 432, 433, 443
perirenal fat, 171, 172, 175, 210, 236
prostatic, 252
renal fibrous, 172, 174, 179
of shoulder joint, 353t, 361
of temporomandibular joint, 489, 531, 570, 571
innervation of, 571
Tenon's, 544
of wrist, 353t, 357t
of zygapophyseal joint, 19, 20
Carcinoma
of breast, *73*
gastric, *614*
Cardiac cycle, *98*
Cardiac murmur, *95*
Cardiac tamponade, *91*
Cardiac valves
aortic, 84, 91, 94, 94t, 95
auscultation site for, 94t, *95*
atrioventricular
left (bicuspid or mitral), 93, 94t, 95
right (tricuspid), 93, 94t, 95
auscultation of, *95*
sites for, 94t
pulmonary, 94, 94t, 95
auscultation site for, 94t, *95*
semilunar, 95
Carina
at tracheal bifurcation, 120
urethral, 246
Carpal bones, 276, 322t, 324–325
distal row, 325
fractures of, *323*
proximal row, 325
Cartilage
alar, 550
arytenoid, 120, 598, 599, 600, 619
of auricle, 559
corniculate, 598, 599
costal, 52, 53, 53t, 57, 59, 136, 277, 283, 289, 298t
cricoid, 104, 105, 120, 477, 580, 598, 599, 601, 619
epiglottic, 598, 599, 601, 619, 620
laryngeal, 598
nasal
lateral, 550
septal, 550
thyroid, 50, 76, 84, 85, 99, 105, 120, 476, 591, 598, 599, 601, 602, 606, 607, 608, 619, 620, 621
tracheal, 120, 601
triradiate
of hip bone, 217
junction of, 217
radiograph of, 217
Caruncle, lacrimal, 545
Cauda equina, 5, 15, 40, 41, 43, 454, 624
lesion of, 42
Cavity
abdominopelvic
classification of organs of, 148
divisions of, 148–149
layers of, 132
mesenteries of, 148, 151, 154
peritoneum of
parietal, 148, 151
visceral, 148
quadrants of, 132
cranial
dural sinuses in, 526
neurovascular pathways exiting/entering, 484–485
glenohumeral joint, 285
glenoid, *277*, 279, 283, 284, 286, 287, 299, 363
of larynx, 601
nasal, 552, 554–555, 617
bones of, 550–551
neurovasculature of, 554–555
paranasal air sinuses in, 552–553
oral, 550, 560, 616, 620
arteries of, 579
bones of, 568–573
boundaries of, 580, 580t
cavities and spaces of, 568, 570, 580
contents of, 572–573, 578–579
joints of, 570, 571
ligaments of, 570, 580
lymphatic drainage of, 579, 580
muscles of, 571, 574, 575, 577, 578, 580
oral floor (suprahyoid), 574, 575t
soft palate, 575t
nerves of, 571, 576–577, 579
neurovasculature of, 579
organization of, 580
salivary glands in, 581
teeth in, 572–573
veins of, 579
pericardial, 84, 90, 91
cardiac tamponade and, *91*
peritoneal, 148, 150, 172
divisions of, 148
infracolic, 150
mesenteries and mesenteric recesses in, 151
structures of, 150
mesenteries of, 148, 154
organs of, 148, 148t, 154
posterior wall of, 155
of scrotum, 145
supracolic, 150

pleural, 51, 74, 74t, 75, 85, 110–111, 172
boundaries and reference points of, 110t
lymph nodes of, 128
lymphatic dainage of, 128
movement in respiration, 122
in pneumothorax, *123*
positive pressure in, 123
projection onto thorax, 51
synovial, of wrist, 371
thoracic
arteries of, 76–77
divisions of, 74–75
lymphatics of, 80–81
lymph nodes, 108
major structures of, 74t
veins of, 78–79
tympanic, 558, 560–561, 562, 566
anatomic relationships of, 561
arteries of middle ear and, 564
glossopharyngeal nerve (CN IX) in, 509
ossicular chain in, 563
roof of, 507, 561
wall of
anterior, 507, 561
posterior, 507
uterine
extrauterine pregnancies and, *243*
Cavum septi pellucidi, 629t
Cecum, 132, 154, 160, 161, 162–163, 230, 231
arteries of, 176, 176t, 177, 182, 183
lymphatics of, 192, 192t, 193, 198, 199
nerves of, 202, 202t, 203, 204, 205, 209
veins of, 190, 191
Cell(s)
air
of ethmoid, 486, 616, 617, 620
of mastoid, 507, 560, 561, 577
inner hair, 645
Center of gravity, 5, 383
shifted, 455
Central nervous system (CNS)
organization of, 624, 638
Cerebellum, 620, 625, 628, 630, 631
arteries of, 636
in brain development, 625t
flocculus of, 506
frontal lobe of, 616
Cerebrospinal fluid (CSF)
circulation of, 632
cisterns for, 632
in dural sac, 15
extracting sample of, *41*
Cerebrum. *See also* Telencephalon
frontal lobe of, 617
Cervix of uterus, 233, 237, 238, 240, 243, 244, 245, 247, 270
supravaginal part, 243, 246
vaginal part, 243, 246
Chambers
of eyeball
anterior, 546, 548
posterior, 546, 548
pulp, of tooth, 572
Chiasm. *See also* Optic chiasm
crural, 419, 423
plantar, 419, 423
Choanae, 482, 550, 554, 568, 580, 582, 587
Chorda tympani, 484, 504, 505, 507, 533, 561, 563, 564, 566, 577
Chordae tendineae, 93, 95
Choroid, 546, 547, 549
Circle, arterial
of iris
greater, 547
lesser, 547
of Zinn, 547
Circulation
of blood, 88
fetal structures, derivatives of, 103t
portal, 88
postnatal, 103
prenatal, 102
pulmonary, 88
of cerebrospinal fluid, 632
Cistern
ambient, 632
basal, 632
cerebellomedullary, (cisterna magna) 21, 632
chiasmatic, 632
interhemispheric, 632
interpeduncular, 632
of lamina terminalis, 632
pontocerebellar, 620
pontomedullary, 632
vermian, 632
Cisterna chyli, 80, 192, 194, 195, 258, 261
Claustrum, 621, 626, 637
Clavicle, 24, 55, 60, 72, 87, 116, 275, 276–278, 282, 283, 284, 285, 287, 288, 289, 293, 296, 298, 299, 345, 350, 362, 363, 477, 589, 604, 605, 608, 610
head of, 476, 589
relationship to trunk skeleton, 277
Cleft, anal, 225
Clitoris, 238, 240, 246, 248
body of, 249
crus of, 233, 238, 240, 247, 249, 267
glans of, 215, 227, 240, 249, 266
prepuce of, 215, 248, 249
Clivus, 483, 554
CN (cranial nerves), 496–513. *See also individually named nerves under* Nerves (named)
CNS. *See* Central nervous system (CNS)
Coccyx, 4, 5, 6, 12–13, 36, 42, 134, 215, 218, 220, 221, 222, 223, 224, 225, 226, 234, 270
Cochlea, 507, 558, 560, 566
canal, compartments of, 566
spiral ganglia of, 506, 567
Colliculus, 598, 599
facial, 631
inferior, 631
brachium of, 631
seminal, 233, 250, 252
superior, 631, 642
brachium of, 631
Colon, 162–163
arteries of, 176, 176t, 177, 182, 183
ascending, 132, 150, 153, 154, 155, 157, 159, 160, 161, 162, 163, 164, 183, 198, 209
attachment of, 173
descending, 132, 151, 153, 154, 155, 157, 159, 161, 162, 163, 164, 165, 171, 183, 209, 210
attachment of, 173
lymphatic drainage of, 192, 192t, 193, 198, 199
nerves of, 202, 202t, 203, 204, 205, 209
sigmoid, 151, 162, 163, 183, 228, 229, 230, 231, 234, 247
transverse, 132, 149, 150, 151, 152, 153, 154, 159, 161, 162, 163, 164, 171, 172, 183, 198, 209, 210, 211
veins of, 190, 191
Colonoscopy
in colon carcinoma, *163*
in ulcerative colitis, *163*
Column(s)
anal, 235
cortical, in cerebral cortex, 627
of fornix, 628
renal, 174
vaginal
anterior, 246
vertebral. *See* Vertebral column
Commissure
of brain
anterior, 628, 629t, 630, 633, 637
of labia
anterior, 248
posterior, 215, 248, 249
of lips, 476
Computed tomography (CT). *See* Imaging
Concha(e), 486
cymba, 559
of ear, 559
of ethmoid bone. *See* Concha(e), nasal.
nasal, 582
inferior, 478t, 479, 537, 545, 553, 555, 583, 587, 620
middle, 479, 486, 537, 551, 552, 553 555, 568, 583, 587, 616, 620
superior, 486, 498, 537, 551, 552, 553, 555
Conduction system, cardiac, 98
Condyle
femoral
lateral, 382, 384, 385, 404, 406, 407, 410, 412, 413, 414

Condyle, femoral *(continued)*
medial, 382, 384, 385, 404, 406, 407, 410, 412, 413, 414
occipital, 18, 480, 482
tibial
head of, 405
lateral, 380, 382, 406, 417, 420, 421, 468
medial, 382, 403, 406, 422, 423
Confluences, cerebral
of venous sinuses, 632, 634, 635
Conjunctiva, ocular, 544, 546, 548
Contracture, Depuytren's, *334*
Conus arteriosus, 93
Conus elasticus, 599, 600, 601
Conus medullaris, 5, 40, 41
lesion of, 42
Cord
of brachial plexus, 348t, 349, 363
division into terminal branches, 349
lateral, 354, 364, 365, 366
long (terminal) branches of, 354t–357t
short branches of, 354t
medial, 354, 364, 365, 366
long (terminal) branches of, 354t, 355t
short branches of, 354t
posterior, 352–353, 364, 365
long (terminal) branches of, 351t
short branches of, 351t, 352–353
cervical, 625
spermatic, 136, 137, 142, 143, 147, 255, 269, 271, 451, 460, 464
contents of, 144
coverings of, 144
spinal, 40–41, 42, 43, 624
arteries of, 44
ascending (sensory) tracts of, 640t
cauda equina and, 41
cerebrospinal fluid circulation and, 632
cervical, 40
descending (motor) tracts of, 641t
developmental stages of, 41
dural sac in, 41
lesions of, 42
meningeal layers of, 40
nerves of, 43
in nervous system, 624
segments of, and spinal nerves, 42
veins of, 45
white matter of, 639
Cornea, 544, 546, 548
Cornua
coccygeal, 12, 454
sacral, 12, 454
Corona radiata, 626
Corpus callosum, 625, 626, 627, 628, 629t, 630, 633, 637, 647
Corpus cavernosum, of penis, 239, 241, 250, 252, 253, 269, 271
Corpus spongiosum, of penis, 239, 241, 250, 252, 253, 269
Corpus striatum, 626
Cortex
cerebral, 524, 624, 626, 627
margins of, 637
neurons in, 639
motor, supplementary cortexes, 641
primary olfactory, 646
renal, 165, 174
sensory, 640
visual, 642
Corti, organ of, 645
Costal bone
body of, 53t
neck of, 53t
Cranial nerves (CN), 496–513. *See also individually named nerves under* Nerves (named)
Cranium. *See also* Cavity, cranial
bones of, 478t, 524
inner and outer tables, 524, 526
neurocranium, bones of, 478t
viscerocranium, bones of, 478t
Crest
ampullary, 644
external occipital, 482
frontal, 481, 483
iliac, 2, 3, 24, 28, 29, 47, 133, 134, 138, 141, 172, 216, 217, 218, 219, 222, 232t, 292, 301t, 351
intertrochanteric, 384, 386, 389, 399
lacrimal, 536
lateral supracondylar, 319
nasal, 550, 568
of rib head, 57
of rib neck, 55
sacral, 7, 12, 13, 218, 219, 454
sphenoid, 487, 550
supraventricular, 93
transverse, 507
urethral, 250
Crista galli, 483, 486, 524, 537, 550, 551, 553
Crista terminalis, 93
Crohn's disease, *161*
Crus/crura
of brain
anterior, 626
posterior, 626
of clitoris, 233, 238, 240, 247, 249, 267
of diaphragm
left, 61, 138, 139, 158
right, 60, 61, 138, 139, 165
of fornix, 628
of inguinal ring, superficial, 142, 143
of penis, 231, 233, 239, 250
CSF. *See* Cerebrospinal fluid (CSF)
Cuboid, 420, 424, 425, 426, 427, 430, 432, 433, 434
articular surface, 431
tuberosity of, 423, 425, 441
Culmen, 630
Cuneiform, 429, 434
intermediate, 424, 425, 426, 427, 434, 440
lateral, 424, 425, 426, 427, 434
medial, 420, 423, 424, 425, 426, 427, 430, 432, 434, 435, 440, 443, 471
navicular, 427
Curvature
of stomach
greater, 153, 156, 157
lesser, 156, 157
of uterus, 242
Cusp, of cardiac valves, 94, 95
Cyst, synovial popliteal, *409*

D

Degenerative diseases, of lumbar spine, *11*
Dendrites, 624
Dens of axis (C2), 5, 6, 8, 9, 18, 21
in craniovertebral joints, 18
facet for, 9
ligaments of, 18
posterior articular surface of, 19
Dental panoramic tomogram (DPT), 573
Dentition. *See* Teeth
Depuytren's contracture, *334*
Dermatomes, 42
of back, 39
disk herniation and, *15*
of head and neck, 596
of lower limb, 459
of thoracic wall, 67
of upper limb, 359
Diaphragm (thoracic), 5, 51, 60, 62, 67, 69, 74, 75, 76, 79, 80, 82, 84, 85, 86, 87, 88, 89, 107, 108, 109, 111, 112, 122, 128, 138, 139, 139t, 146, 152, 157, 159, 165, 171, 172, 173, 194
blood vessels of, 62, 63, 63t
crus of
left, 138, 139, 158
right, 60, 138, 139, 165
dome of
left, 60, 138
right, 60, 138
during respiration, 56
hepatic surfaces of, 152, 155, 159
hiatus (opening) of, 60, 61
aortic, 60, 138, 139, 178
caval, 60, 61, 63, 138, 139
esophageal, 60, 61,63,138, 139
innervation of, 60t, 62, 63
ligaments of, 60, 60t, 61
muscles of, 138–139, 139t
parts of, 60t
abdominal, 104
costal, 60t, 61, 63
lumbar, 60t, 63
sternal, 60t

Diaphragm (pelvic), 215, 232, 235
fascia of, 235
inferior, 232, 234
superior, 232, 234, 237
innervation of, 226t
Diaphragma sellae, 484, 485, 524
Diastole, ventricular, 94
Diencephalon, 626, 630, 631
in brain development, 625t
components of, 629t
internal structures of, 629t
Diploë, inner and outer tables of, 524, 526
Diplopia, *539*
Disk
articular, 283, 570, 571
ulnocarpal, 325, 327, 331
intervertebral, 4, 5, 6, 14–15, 17, 20, 21, 22, 23, 52, 57, 223, 619
herniation of, *15*
structure of, 14
optic, 546
Dislocation
elbow joint, injury assessment and, *307*
femoral head, necrosis and, *445*
of hip, diagnosing, *387*
of temporomandibular joint, *571*
Diverticulum/diverticula
duodenal, *159*
epiphrenic, 105
esophageal, *105*
hypopharyngeal (pharyngo-esophageal), *105*
parabronchial, 105
Zenker's, 105
Dorsum of foot, 380
muscles of, 440t
neurovasculature of, 469
Dorsum of hand, 338–339. *See also* Hand.
anatomic snuffbox, 374
arteries of, 345
lymphatic drainage of, 347
nerves of, 374
neurovasculature of, 374–375
sensory innervation of, 374
structures of
deep, 375
superficial, 375
veins of, 346, 358
Duct(s)
alveolar, sac of, 121
bile, 167, 168, 169, 173, 180
common, 155, 158, 210
extrahepatic, 168
hepatic, 168
location of, 168
obstruction in (gallstones), *169*
cochlear, 566, 645
cystic, 167, 168, 169
ejaculatory, 241, 252, 253
orifice of, 252
endolymphatic, 566
excretory, 241
hepatic, 167, 173
common, 168, 169
left, 168, 169
right, 167, 168, 169
hepatopancreatic, 169
lactiferous, 71, 73
lymphatic, right, 80, 81, 347, 614
nasolacrimal, 545, 552, 552t
pancreatic, 168, 169, 170
accessory, 158, 168, 170
main, 158
parotid, 528, 529, 530, 531, 581
semicircular, 507
anterior, 566, 567
lateral, 567
posterior, 567
submandibular, 579, 581
terminal, 71, 73
lobular unit (TDLU), 71, 73
thoracic, 80, 81, 87, 108, 129, 192, 198, 258, 607, 614
Ductules
efferent, 145, 251
prostatic, 250
Ductus deferens, 144, 145, 146, 175, 228, 231, 236, 237, 239, 241, 241t, 251, 255, 257, 270
ampulla of, 149, 239, 241, 252
arteries of, 144, 146, 251, 254
autonomic nervous system effects on, 202t, 648t
veins of, 144, 146
Ductus reuniens, 566
Duodenum, 132, 152, 155, 156, 157, 158–159, 164, 166, 173, 180, 183, 198, 210
arteries of, 176, 176t, 177, 181, 182
endoscopy of papillary region of, *159*
lymphatic drainage of, 192, 192t, 193, 197
nerves of, 202, 202t, 203, 204, 205, 206, 208
papillary region, 159
parts of, 158
ascending part, 155, 158, 159, 169, 170, 171, 173
descending part, 153, 155, 158, 159, 165, 168, 169, 170, 171, 172, 211
horizontal part, 149, 154, 155, 158, 159, 161, 164, 168, 170, 171, 173
superior part, 154, 155, 156, 158, 159, 161, 164, 168, 170, 171, 173
veins of, 185, 188, 190
Dura mater, 15, 40, 41, 481, 524, 567
arteries of, 525
folds of, 524
innervation of, 525
layers of, 526
sinuses of. *See* Sinus, dural
Dysplasia, of hip
diagnosing, *387*
ultrasonography of, 387

E

Ear
arteries of, 557, 559, 560, 561, 562, 564, 565, 567
cavities and spaces of, 556, 558, 560, 561, 562–566
external, 558–559
inner, 566–567
auditory apparatus of, 566
blood vessels of, 567
bones of, 556–557
vestibular apparatus of, 566
joints of, 562–564
lymphatic drainage of, 566–567
middle, 558, *563*
arteries of, 564t
mastoid air cells and, *557*
ossicular chain of, 562–563
tympanic cavity of, 560–561
tympanic membrane of, 562–563
muscles of, 492t, 559
nerves of, 559–561, 563–567
neurovasculature of, 557, 560–561, 563–565, 567
regions of, 557, 559
veins of, 567
ECG (electrocardiogram). *See* Electrocardiogram (ECG).
Edema, pulmonary, *117*
Effusion, pleural, 68
Electrocardiogram (ECG), *98*
Embolism, pulmonary, *125*
Eminence
hypothenar, 274, 275, 371
iliopubic, 134, 219, 461
intercondylar, 405, 406
medial, in brainstem, 631
pyramidal, 563
radial carpal, 330
thenar, 274, 275, 356t, 371
ulnar carpal, 330
Emphysema, pulmonary, *117*
Endometrium, 242, 243
Epicondyle
of femur
lateral, 380, 384, 406, 410, 421, 422
medial, 380, 382, 384, 406, 410, 412
of humerus
lateral, 275, 280, 281, 289, 306, 309, 313, 315, 319, 321, 369
medial, 275, 280, 281, 288, 289, 306, 309, 313, 315, 317, 318, 319, 321, 357
Epididymis, 144, 145, 241, 241t, 251, 257, 260
appendix of, 145, 251
blood vessels of, 251
body of, 145, 251
head of, 145, 251
nerves of, 204t
tail of, 145, 251

Epidural anesthesia, *41*
Epigastrium, 50
Epiglottis, 578, 580, 582, 583, 587, 598, 599, 600, 601, 603
Epiphysis, 628, 637
Epitympanum, 561
Erb's point, 610
Esophagus, 61, 63, 69, 75, 76, 77, 82, 84, 86, 87, 88, 91, 104–105, 108, 109, 114, 149, 156, 157, 158, 159, 161, 169, 173, 178, 186, 194, 584, 585, 601, 602, 603, 619
  arteries of, 107, 107t
  autonomic innervation of, 106
  constrictions of, 104, 116
  esophageal diverticula, *105*
  lymphatic drainage of, 108–109
  nerves of, 106
  neurovasculature of, 106
  parts of, 104
    abdominal, 104, 105, 106
    cervical, 84, 85, 104, 106
    thoracic, 75, 82, 84, 85, 104, 105, 106
  structure of, 105
  veins of, 107, 107t
  wall of, 105
Ethmoid bone, 478t, 479, 483, 486, 498, 536, 537, 550, 553, 568
Expiration
  lung contraction in, 123
  in normal respiration *vs.* pneumothorax, *123*
  pleural cavity contraction in, 122
  thoracic cage during, 56
Extension, of knee joint
  cruciate and collateral ligaments in, 413
  menisci in, 411
Eye
  conjugate movements of, 644
  cornea of, 548
  in embryonic brain development, 625
  iris of, 548
  lacrimal apparatus of, 545
  lens of. *See* Lens
  pupil of, 549
Eyeball, 544
  blood vessels of, 547
  fundus of, *547*
  muscles associated with. *See* Muscles (of region or organ), extraocular
  structure of, 546
Eyelid, 544, 545

F

Face. *See also* Facial expression
  innervation of
    motor, 514
    sensory, 515
  neurovasculature of, superficial, 528
Facet(s)
  of laryngeal cartilage
    articular, 598, 600
  of vertebra
    articular, 57
      anterior, 8, 9
      inferior, 8, 9, 10, 11, 16, 17, 22, 23
      posterior, 8
      for rib tubercle, 57
      superior, 7, 8, 9, 10, 11, 12, 14, 16, 17, 18, 22, 23, 57
    costal, 4, 7, 16, 57
      inferior, 7, 10
      superior, 7, 10
    on transverse process, 10
    for dens, 9
Facial expression, muscles of, 488–489, 492t, 493t
  motor innervation of, 514
  origins and insertions of, 490
Falx cerebri, 524, 526, 617
Farsightedness, 549
Fascia
  abdominal, superficial, 142, 143, 460
    deep layer of, 253
  antebrachial, 334, 372
  axillary, 362
  biceps, 365, 367
  brachial, 362
  buccopharyngeal, 602
  bulbar, 544
  Camper's, 146
  cervical, 84
  clavipectoral, 362, 364t
  cremasteric, 142, 144, 145, 145t, 147, 251
  deep cervical, 84, 602, 605t
    investing (superficial) layer, 25, 84, 602, 605t, 606, 609, 610
    pretracheal muscular layer, 25, 84, 602, 605t, 606, 610
    pretracheal visceral layer, 25, 84, 602, 605t, 606, 610
    prevertebral layer, 602, 605t, 610, 611
  of diaphragm (pelvic)
    inferior, 225, 230, 231, 234, 235, 247
    superior, 230, 231, 234, 235, 237, 247
  endothoracic, 61, 67, 68, 69, 111, 112, 139
  gluteal, 462
    of gluteus maximus, 462
    of gluteus medius, 462, 465
  of leg, deep, 466, 468
  nuchal, 25
  obturator, 224, 225, 230, 247
  paravaginal, 233
  paravesicular, 231
  pectoral, 71
  pelvic
    parietal, 239, 245
    visceral, 239, 245
      of bladder, 228, 229
      of rectum, 228, 229
  penile, 239
    deep, 250, 253, 268
    superficial, 250, 268
  perineal (Colles')
    deep, 232, 232t
    superficial, 232, 232t, 247
      in female, 225, 230, 232, 233
      in male, 225, 232, 233, 239
  pharyngobasilar, 585, 586
  plantar, deep layer of, 471
  psoas, 25
  rectoprostatic, 228, 253, 271
  renal
    anterior layer, 25, 172
    posterior layer, 25
    retrorenal layer, 172
  Scarpa's, 146
  spermatic
    external, 142, 144, 145, 145t, 251, 268
    internal, 143, 144, 145, 145t, 147, 251, 257
  of testis, superficial deep layer, 145, 251
  thoracic, superficial, 71, 362
  thoracolumbar, 2, 24, 25, 28, 47, 292, 293, 351, 399, 589
    deep layer, 25, 29
    superficial layer, 24, 25, 28
  transversalis, 25, 137, 143, 146, 147
  visceral, 25
Fasciculus
  dorsal longitudinal, 498
  frontotemporal, 626
  interfascicular, 639
  lateral proprius, 639
  longitudinal
    medial (MLF), 644
      rostral interstitial nucleus of (riMLF), 644
    of posterior column, 639
    superior, 626
  mammillothalamic, 629t
  septomarginal, 639
  sulcomarginal, 639
Fasciculus cuneatus, 640t
Fasciculus gracilis, 640t
Fat capsule, perirenal, 171, 172, 175, 210, 236
Fat pad
  buccal, 617
  in elbow joint injury assessment, *307*
  humeroulnar joint, 307
  infrapatellar, 414, 415
  pararenal, 174
  retrosternal, 84, 86
  tibial, 415
Femur, 382, 384, 387, 388, 400, 401, 406, 408, 409, 410, 414, 415, 416, 420, 421, 422, 423, 472, 473
  epicondyle of. *See* Epicondyle, of femur
  fractures of, *385*
  head of, 233, 270, 385, 386, 387, 445
    arteries of, 445
    in hip joint, MRI of, 385
    necrosis of, *445*
  neck of, 382, 385, 386, 387, 389
    vessels in, 445

shaft of, 387
Fetal circulatory structures, derivatives of, 103t
Fibers. *See also* Cranial nerves
cerebral arcuate (U fibers), 626
corticobulbar, 512, 513
corticonuclear, 641t
corticoreticular, 641t
corticospinal, 641t
cuneocerebellar, 640
intercrural, of superficial inguinal ring, 142, 143
nerve. *See* Axons
in nervous system
afferent (sensory), 638
efferent (motor), 638
olfactory, 498, 554, 555
of optic nerve, 642
parasympathetic, postganglionic, 129, 509, 649
prerectal, 224
Purkinje, 55, 98
somatomotor, 638
somatosensory, 638
sympathetic, postganglionic, 649
vestibulocerebellar, 644
visceromotor, 638
viscerosensory, 638
zonular, 546, 548, 549
Fibula, 382, 399, 400, 401, 402, 404–405, 406, 408, 409, 410, 412, 413, 414, 423, 426, 428, 429, 432, 433, 439, 467, 468, 472, 473
fractures of, *405*
head of, 380, 382, 390, 397, 403, 404, 406, 408, 411, 412, 413, 416, 417, 420, 421, 422, 423, 456, 468, 469
neck of, 404, 406, 456
nerves of, 456, 456t
shaft of, 404
Filia olfactoria, 485
Fimbriae
at abdominal ostium, 243
of hippocampus, 628
Finger
arteries of, 345
bones of. *See* Metacarpel(s); Phalanx/phalanges.
ligaments of, 332–333
lymphatic drainage of, 347
neurovaculature of, 372
veins of, 346
Fissure
anterior median, 631
cerebral
horizontal, 630
longitudinal, 625, 627
primary, 630
of lung, 115, 118
horizontal, 100, 111, 114, 115, 118, 119
oblique, 100, 111, 114, 115, 118, 119
optical, superior, 499
orbital
inferior, 482, 503, 535t, 536t, 537, 539, 568
superior, 484, 487, 503, 536t, 537, 539, 542, 553, 568
palpebral, muscles of, 492t
petrotympanic, 482, 484, 556, 563, 570
pterygopalatine, 504
tympanomastoid, 556
Fistula, ileorectal, *163*
Flexion, of uterus, 242
Flexure
cervical, 625
colic
left (splenic), 150, 151, 154, 159, 161, 162, 163, 164, 165, 169, 171, 183, 210
right (hepatic), 153, 154, 157, 159, 161, 162, 163, 164, 169
cranial, 625
duodenal, 158
inferior, 158
superior, 158
duodenojejunal, 154, 158, 160, 161, 164, 211
perineal, 234
sacral, 234
Flocculus, 630
of cerebellum, 506
peduncle of, 630
Floor
oral
lymphatic drainage of, 579
muscles of, 574, 575t, 590t, 591
innervation of, 577
of orbit, 537, 544
pelvic
muscles of, 224–225, 226, 226t
in female, 230
innervation of, 226t
Fluid accumulation
abnormal pleural, drainage of, *68*
cardiac tamponade and, *91*
radiographic findings in lung, *117*
Fold
alar, 414
aryepiglottic, 583, 600, 601
circular, of intestine,158, 159, 160
in dura mater, 524
malleolar
anterior, 561
posterior, 561
superior, 561
rectal, transverse
inferior, 235
middle, 235
superior, 235
rectouterine, 230, 237
rugal, of stomach, 156
salpingopharyngeal, 555, 580, 582
semilunar, of colon 162
sublingual, 574, 579, 581
umbilical
lateral, 146, 150, 154, 160, 230, 231
medial, 146, 147, 150, 151, 154, 230, 231
median, 146, 150, 151, 154, 160, 230, 231
uterosacral, 234, 237, 243
vesical, transverse, 230, 231
vestibular, 580, 601
vocal, 580, 601
Folium, of vermis, 630
Foot, 382
arches of, 434–435
dorsal venous, 446
longitudinal, 434, 435
plantar, 434, 446
deep, 444, 471
transverse, 434
bones of, 380, 424–425
compartments of
anterior, 429, 430
posterior, 429, 430
dorsum of foot
muscles of, 440t
neurovasculature of, 469
joints of, 426–431
distal articular surfaces, 427
proximal articular surfaces, 427
radiograph of, 425
ligaments of, 432–433
muscles of, 426, 428, 429, 436–443, 440t, 441t, 442t
dorsum of foot, 440t
sole of foot, 436–437, 441t, 442t, 443
neurovasculature of, 466–471
radiograph of, 42
regions of, 381
sole of foot
arteries of, 444
muscles of, 436–437, 441t, 442t, 443
nerves of, 457
neurovasculature of, 470–471
veins of, 446
subdivisions of, 424
Foramen/foramina
ethmoid
anterior, 480, 536t
posterior, 480, 536t
incisive, 480, 482, 568, 576
infraorbital, 477, 478, 479, 503, 536, 545
interventricular, 632, 633
intervertebral, 4, 10, 11, 14, 21, 23, 40
jugular, 482, 483, 484, 508, 510, 512, 526
mandibular, 480, 503, 533, 569, 570
mastoid, 480, 482, 484, 556
mental, 477, 478, 479, 569
obturator, 216, 217, 218, 219, 224
omental (epiploic), 149, 152, 153, 153t, 154, 161, 164
palatine, greater/lesser, 482, 484, 568, 576
parietal, 481
for pterygoid plexus, 568

Foramen/foramina *(continued)*
sacral
anterior, 6, 12, 13, 43, 219, 223, 454
posterior, 6, 12, 13, 43, 219, 454
scapular, *278*
sciatic, greater/lesser, 222, 223, 463t
sphenopalatine, 535t, 551, 555
stylomastoid, 482, 484, 504, 505, 533, 556, 577
for superior laryngeal artery and nerve, 599
supraorbital, 479, 536t
transverse, 7, 8, 16, 20
vertebral artery in, 17
vertebral, 7, 7t, 9, 11, 14, 16, 17, 18, 53
internotch, 10
zygomaticoorbital, 536, 537
Foramen cecum, 578
Foramen lacerum, 482, 483, 484
Foramen magnum, 482, 483, 484, 512, 513, 523
Foramen ovale, 482, 483, 484, 487, 503, 526, 533, 568
Foramen rotundum, 484, 487, 503, 535t, 536
Foramen spinosum, 482, 483, 484, 487
Forearm, 376, 377
arteries of, 345
bones of, 276, 304–305
joints of
elbow (cubital), 306–307
radioulnar, 310–311
muscles of
anterior, 312–313, 316–317
posterior, 314–315, 318–321
nerves of, 356–357
topography of
anterior, 368
cubital region, 367
posterior, 369
Forebrain (prosencephalon), 625t
Forehead, muscles of, 492t
Fornix, 627, 630, 633, 647t
conjunctival, superior, 544
vaginal
anterior, 238, 242, 246
lateral, 243
posterior, 238, 242, 246
Fossa(e)
acetabular, 217, 387, 388, 445, 461
axillary, 274
cerebral, 483
coronoid, 280, 306, 307, 309
cranial, 483
anterior, 485, 527, 537t, 541, 550, 551, 553, 616
middle, 485, 527, 537t, 541, 551
posterior, 483, 485
cubital, 346, 366, 367
venipuncture in, *346*
hyaloid, 546
hypophyseal, 483, 487, 550, 551, 554
iliac, 141
in female, 218
in male, 216, 219
incisive, 568, 572
infraclavicular, 50, 274, 362
infraspinous, 279, 284, 285, 297t, 360
infratemporal
deep neurovascular layer, 533
mandibular nerve (CN V_3) in, 533
superficial neurovascular layer, 532
inguinal
lateral, 146, 147, 231
medial, 146, 147
interpeduncular, 631
ischioanal, 234, 271, 463
in female, 230, 233, 244
in male, 231
jugular, 50
of lacrimal sac, 536
lateral malleolar, 404, 405
mandibular, 482, 556, 570, 571
navicular, 250, 253
olecranon, 280, 281, 307, 308
ovalis, 93
limbus of, 93
paravesical
in female, 230
in male, 233
popliteal, 394, 409, 457
Baker's cyst in, *409*
MRI of, 409
pterygoid, 487, 568
pterygopalatine, 534t, 536, 537t, 621
radial, 280, 306, 309
rhomboid, 631
scaphoid, 559
splenic, 173
subscapular, 279, 297t
supraclavicular, lesser, 604
supraspinous, 55, 279, 297t
supravesical, 146, 147, 230
temporal, neurovasculature of, 531
tonsillar, 582, 586
triangular, 559
trochanteric, 384
Fovea, 384
articular, of radius, 304, 305, 308t, 311
centralis, 546, 549, 642
of femoral head, 385, 388
pterygoid, 569, 570
Foveolae, granular, 481, 526
Fractures
cervical spine, *9*
distal radial, *311*
of elbow joint
injury assessment and, *307*
median nerve injury and, *356*
facial (Le Fort), *479*
femoral, *385*
head of, necrosis and, *445*
fibular, *405*
radiography of, 405
humeral, *281*
axillary nerve injury and, *352*
of scaphoid, *323*
Frenulum
of ileum, 162
of lower lip, 580
of tongue, 579
of upper lip, 580
Frontal bone, 476, 477, 478t, 479, 481, 483, 536, 537, 550, 553
Fundus
of eyeball, *547*
of stomach, 105, 107
Funiculus
anterior, 639
lateral, 639
posterior, 639

G

Galea aponeurotica, 488, 489, 526
Gallbladder, 150, 152, 153, 154, 157, 161, 164, 165, 167, 168–169, 171, 180, 210, 211
arteries of, 176, 176t, 177, 180
body of, 168
fundus of, 167, 168
infundibulum of, 168
lymphatic drainage of, 192, 192t, 193, 196, 197
neck of, 168
nerves of, 202, 203, 204, 205, 206
veins of, 185
Ganglion/ganglia
aorticorenal, 204t, 205, 207, 208, 264
basal, of brain, 624, 626, 629t
celiac, 202, 204t, 205, 207, 208
cervical
inferior, 99
middle, 106, 127, 587, 607
superior, 202, 530, 531, 586, 587, 609
cervicothoracic, 127
ciliary, 501, 503, 541, 543, 643
cochlear, 507
geniculate, 504, 505, 507, 561, 566, 577
hypogastric
superior, 205
impar, 204, 205, 262
inferior
nodose, 645
petrosal, 645
lumbar, sympathetic trunk, 204, 205, 207, 262, 263
mesenteric
inferior, 202, 204t, 205, 207, 209, 262
superior, 202, 204t, 205, 207, 208
otic, 509, 533
pelvic, 203, 204t
prevertebral, 649

pterygopalatine, 503, 504, 505, 515, 535, 555, 576
sacral, 204, 205, 207, 262
of solitary tract, 508, 509, 510
spinal, 40, 41, 43, 67, 639, 640, 649
spiral, of cochlea, 507, 567
stellate, 587, 607
submandibular, 505, 577, 579, 586
sympathetic, 202, 648, 649
cord, 43
thoracic, 82, 106, 127
trigeminal, 503, 504, 514, 515, 527, 541, 555, 577, 621
vestibular, 506, 507, 566, 567, 644
Gastric carcinoma, *614*
Genitalia. *See also* individual genital organs.
in female, 240, 240t, 242, 247, 248-249
arteries of, 254, 254t
blood vessels of, 255, 257, 266, 267
external, 240, 240t, 242, 248–249
episiotomy and, *249*
innervation of, 263, 266
autonomic, 265
internal, 240, 240t
lymphatic drainage of, 259, 259t, 260
mesenteries of, 242
nerves of, 262, 263, 265, 266, 267
neurovasculature of, 266
veins of, 254, 254t
in male, 241, 241t
arteries of, 257
blood vessels of, 255, 257, 268, 269
external, 250–251
innervation of, 263, 268, 269
autonomic, 265
internal, 241, 241t
lymphatic drainage of, 259, 259t, 261
nerves of, 262, 263, 268, 269
neurovasculature of, 268
veins of, 254, 254t, 268
Genu, 626
Girdle
pelvic, 216-217, 382
shoulder, 277–278
relationship to ribs and sternum, 277
Glabella, 478
Gland(s). *See also specific glands*
accessory sex, in male, 241t, 251–252
areolar, 70
bulbourethral, 239, 241, 241t, 250, 251, 252, 253, 269
cerumen, 558
ciliary, 544
lacrimal, 501, 503, 505, 542, 545
lingual, anterior, 579
nasal, 505
parathyroid, 602, 606
parotid, 509, 528, 529, 581, 586, 605, 608, 610, 611, 618
accessory, 581
pineal, 625, 628, 630, 631, 637
salivary, 581
sebaceous
of ear, 558
of eye, 544
seminal, 228, 241, 241t, 251, 252, 253, 271
nerves of, 264, 265
sublingual, 505, 578, 581, 586
submandibular, 505, 531, 581, 609, 621
suprarenal, 172–173, 175
arteries of, 176, 176t, 177, 178, 179
autonomic nervous system effects on, 202t, 648t
left, 172, 173, 175
lymphatic drainage of, 192, 192t, 193, 195
nerves of, 202, 202t, 24, 205, 207, 262, 264
right, 172, 173 175
veins of, 184, 184t, 186, 187
thyroid, 25, 85, 99, 580, 583, 586, 602, 603, 608, 609, 619
urethral, orifices of, 250
of vestibular and vocal folds, 601
vestibular (Bartholin's), 240, 248
Glaucoma
angle-closure, *548*
open-angle, *548*
Globus pallidus, 620, 626, 637
segments of, 629t
Gluteal region
cavities and spaces of, 463, 463t
nerves of, 454
neurovasculature of, 462, 463
muscles of, 393, 398t
veins of, 462
Gray matter
cerebral arteries distribution areas and, 637
in CNS, 624
columns (horns) of, 637
nuclei of, 638
organization of, 638
Groove
arterial, 481, 483
in temporal bone, 556
capitulotrochlear, 281, 306, 309
costal, 67, 68, 69, 111
deltopectoral, 50, 274, 346
for fibularis longus tendon, 425
for flexor hallucis longus tendon, 431
of humerus, 280, 281
for inferior vena cava, in liver, 167
infraorbital, 536
intertubercular, 280, 281, 283, 285, 286, 301t, 355, 364t
malleolar, for tibialis posterior tendon, 404
mylohyoid, 570
radial, 280, 295
radial nerve in, 353
for sigmoid sinus, 556
for subclavian artery, 55, 593
for subclavius muscle, 278
for superior sagittal sinus, 481
for transverse sinus, 483
ulnar, 280, 281, 306, 308, 321, 357
ulnar nerve in, 366
for vertebral artery, 8, 9, 18
Gustatory system, 645
Gutter, paracolic, 155
Gyrus/gyri
ambient, 498, 646
cingulate (limbic), 625, 627, 628, 647t
dentate, 621, 628
parahippocampal, 647t
paraterminal, 647t
postcentral, 625, 640, 641, 645
precentral, 513, 625, 641
semilunar, 498, 646

H

Hamate, 322t, 324, 325, 327, 331, 371
hook of, 275, 317, 323, 325, 330, 371
Hamulus, pterygoid, 482, 487, 575, 585
Hand. *See also* Finger; Thumb
arteries of, 345
deep 373, 375
superficial, 372, 373, 375
bones of, 275, 276, 322–323
"clawing" of, ulnar nerve damage and, *357*
dorsum of. *See* Dorsum of hand
functional position of, *329*
intertendinous connections, 314
dorsal digital extension, 321
joints of, 326–327
ligaments of, 328–329, 334–335
lymphatic drainage of, 347
muscles of, 274, 340–343
deep intrinsic, 336
of dorsum, 338–339
hypothenar, 334, 335, 340–341, 340t
metacarpal, 336–337, 342–343, 342t
middle intrinsic, 335, 336
origns and insertions, 337
superficial intrinsic, 334–335
thenar, 334, 335, 340–341, 340t
nerves of, 356–357, 375
deep, 373, 375
superficial, 372, 373, 375
neurovasculature of, 372
palm of. *See* Palm of hand
surface anatomy of, 275
tendons of, 274, 338–339
Haustra, colonic, 162, 163
Head. *See also* Brain; Cavity, oral; Ear; Eye; Nose; Orbit; Pharynx
arteries of, 484, 485, 505, 507, 508, 511, 516–517, 525, 534
bones of, 477–482, 486–487
cavities and spaces of, 481–483, 485, 524–527
organs of. *See individually named organs.*

Head *(continued)*
muscles of, 485–495
nerves of, 484, 485, 496–515, 525, 533, 535
neurovasculature of, 484, 524, 526–533
superficial, 529
palpable bony prominences of, 477
regions of, 476, 515, 530
surface anatomy of, 476
veins of, 481, 484, 501, 507, 522–523, 523t
Hearing
auditory system for, 645
cranial nerve associated with, 642t
ossicular chain in, *563*
Hearing loss, conductive, *563*
Heart, 5, 89, 101
arteries of, 96–97, 96t
autonomic nerves and plexuses of, 99
ausculation sites of, 94–95, 95t
borders of, 100, 100t
cardiac tamponade and, *91*
chambers of, 93
circulation, 88
pre- and postnatal, 102–103, 103t
conduction system in, 98
disturbed coronary blood flow, *97*
electrocardiogram of, *98*
functions and relations, 88–89, 91
nerves of, 98, 99
lymphatic drainage of, 108
MRI of, 100–101
pericardium, 90–91
portal system collateral pathways to, 185
radiographs of, 100–101
relations of, 88, 91
septal defects in, *103*
skeletal structure of, 94
spaces and cavities, 91
structures of, 100t, 101
surfaces of, 92
valves of, 94–95. *See also* Cardiac valves.
veins of, 96t, 96–97
Heart sounds, auscultation sites for, 94t, *95*
Helicotrema, 566
Helix, of auricle of ear, 476, 559
Hematoma
compartment syndrome and, *469*
epidural, *521*, 524, *525*
subdural, *525*
Hemianopia
bitemporal, *643*
homonymous, *643*
contralateral, *643*
Hemorrhage
extracerebral, *525*
subarachnoid, *525*
subdural, 524
Hernia/herniation
inguinal and femoral hernias, *147*
intervertebral disk, *15*
Hiatus
of adductor magnus, 391, 392, 395, 401, 444, 445, 446, 465
aortic, 60, 61, 76, 78, 80, 138, 139, 178
basilic, 346
of canal for petrosal nerves, 484, 504
esophageal, 60, 61, 63, 78, 85, 105, 138, 139
levator, 224
maxillary, 536, 551
sacral, 12, 40, 41, 223, 454
epidural anesthesia and, *41*
in female, 218
in male, 219
triceps, 361t
of ulnar tunnel
distal, 371
proximal, 371
urogenital, 226
Hilum
of kidney, 172, 174
of lung, 115, 116
of spleen, 170
Hindbrain. *See* Rhombencephalon
Hip, 216, 217, 382
hyperextension of, nerve entrapment and, *450*
muscles of, 381, 390–403
nerves of, 448–459
radiography of, 386–387
regions of, 381
radiograph of, 386–387
Hippocampus, 628, 629t, 637, 647, 647t
fimbria of, 628
His, bundle of, 98
Horn(s)
anterior, 44
of gray matter, 637
of lateral brain venticles, 626, 628, 633
posterior, 44
Humerus, 276, 277, 280–281, 283, 285, 286, 287, 303t, 376, 377
condyle of, 280, 281
epicondyle of. *See* Epicondyle, of humerus
head of, 280, 281, 282, 283, 284, 285, 287, 363, 364
pronator teres and, 313, 317, 318
supinator and, 315
intertubercular groove of, 364t
neck of
anatomical, 280, 281, 284
surgical, 280
shaft of, 280, 281
Hyoid bone, 99, 478t, 569, 574, 578, 579, 580, 581, 591, 599, 601, 603, 604, 608, 609, 620
body of, 569
horns of, 569, 585, 598, 599, 621
muscle origins and insertions, 491
Hyperopia, 549
Hypertension
optic fundus examination in, *547*
renal artery, *179*
Hypophysis, 527, 537t, 625, 627, 628, 631, 633. *See also* Gland(s), parotid
Hypothalamus, 625, 628, 630, 633, 644
Hypotympanum, 561

I

Ileum, 132, 149, 150, 154, 158, 160, 163, 198, 231
arteries of, 176, 176t, 177, 182, 183
Crohn's disease and, *161*
lymphatic drainage of, 192, 192t, 193, 198
nerves of, 202, 202t, 203, 205, 208
terminal, 161, 162
veins of, 185, 190
Ilium, 163, 216, 217, 223, 237, 247, 387, 399
in female, 244
in male, 237
radiograph of, 217
ala (wing) of, 134
Imaging
of abdomen
arteriography
of stenosis of renal artery, anterior view, *179*
computed tomography (CT)
of tranverse section through L1, 211
colonoscopy
of ulcerative colitis, *163*
of colon carcinoma, *163*
endoscopy
of duodenum, papillary region, *159*
of gastic ulcer, *157*
of gastritis, *157*
of large intestine, *163*
of stomach, *157*
MRI
of coronal section of ileum with Crohn's disease, *161*
of transverse section through L2, inferior view, 165
of transverse section through T12, inferior view, 165
radiography
of anterior view of large intestine with colitis, *163*
of anterior view of large intestine with Crohn's disease, *161*
of anterior view of large intestine, 163
ultrasonography
of gallstones, *169*
of back
MRI
of midsagittal section through cervical spine, 21
of midsagittal section of disk herniation in lumbar spine, *15*
radiography
of left lateral view of normal cervical spine, 8
of left lateral view of "whiplash" in cervical spine, *9*

of left lateral view of normal lumbar spine, *11*
of left lateral view of osteoporitic lumbar spine, *11*
of anteroposterior view of sacrum, 13
of head
MRI
of coronal section of paranasal sinuses, 553
opthalmoscopy
of optic fundus, *547*
radiography
of dental panoramic tomogram, 573
ultrasound
of carotid artery atherosclerosis, *517*
of limb (lower)
MRI
of transverse section of Baker's cyst in popliteal fossa *409*
of transverse section femoral head, hip joint, 385
of sagittal section of knee joint, 415
radiography
of anteroposterior view of bones of foot, 425
of anteroposterior view of bones and joints of foot 426
of lateral view of joints of ankle, 428
of posterior view of fibular fracture, *405*
of anteroposterior view of hip joint, 387
of anterioposterior, lateral, and sunrise (60 degrees flexion) views of knee joint, 407
ultrasonography
of normal hip, of infant, 387
of hip dysplasia, of infant, 387
of limb (upper)
MRI
of sagittal section of elbow joint, 307
of coronal section of shoulder, 285
of coronal section of wrist and hand, 327
radiography
of anteroposterior view of shoulder, 284
of anteroposterior view of wrist, *323*
of anterioposterior view of wrist with scaphoid fracture, *323*
of neck
MRI
of midsagittal section through cervical spine, 21
radiography
of left lateral view of normal cervical spine, 8
of left lateral view of "whiplash" in cervical spine, *9*
of pelvis and perineum
MRI
of coronal section of accessory sex glands, 252
of midsagittal section of prostate, prostatic carcinoma, *253*
radiography
of lateral view of acetabulum, of child, 217
of thorax
arteriography, of anterior view of pulmonary arteries and veins, 125
bronchogram, of anterior view of right lung, 118
computed tomography (CT), of transverse section of thorax, 75
mammography, of breast, breast cancer *73*
MRI
of transverse section of thorax through heart, 101
of tranverse section of thorax through heart, aortic dissection, *77*
radiography
of posteroanterior and left lateral views of heart, 100
of posteroanterior and left lateral views of lungs, 116
of posteroanterior view of lungs, lingular pneumonia, *117*
of posteroanterior view of lungs, pulmonary edema, *117*
of posteroanterior view of lungs, pulmonary emphysema, *117*
of anteroposterior view of lungs, tuberculosis, *117*
Impressions
on clavicle, for costclavicular ligament, 278
on liver, for organs, 166
on lung, for organs, 115
Incisors, 572
Incisure
frontal, 479, 536t
intertragic, 559
tympanic, 561
Incus, 558, 560, 561, 562, 563, 564
Indusium griseum, 628, 647t
Infracolic compartment
mesenteries and mesenteric recesses of, 151
structures of, 150
Infundibulum, 243, 628, 629t, 630, 633
of ethmoid bone, 486
of gallbladder, 168
of hypophysis, 628, 629t, 630, 633
of uterine tube, 243
Inguinal region
lymphatic drainage of, 460
muscles of, 142
nerves of, 451
neurovasculature of, 142–143, 143t, 460, 461
structures in, 146, 461
veins of, 460
Inlet
esophageal, 84, 104
obturator, in female, 270
pelvic, 220, 232t
divisions of, 232t
measurements of, 220, 221
thoracic, 75, 84, 122
Innervation, sensory cutaneous
of anterior trunk, 200
of back, 39
of breast (female), 70
of dorsum of hand, 374
of gluteal region, 454
of head, 515
of inguinal region, 451t
of lower limb, 459
of neck, 515, 597
in nuchal region, 596
of palm of hand, 372
of thoracic wall, 66
of upper limb, 359
Inspiration
diaphragm position during, 56
lung expansion in, 123
in normal respiration *vs.* pneumothorax, *123*
pleural cavity expansion in, 122
pleural defect during, 123
thoracic cage during, 56
Insula, 627, 637, 645
in embryonic brain, 625
Interneurons, of spinal cord, 639
Interspinous distance, of pelvis, 220
Intestine, large, 162, 163. *See also* Appendix; Cecum; Colon
carcinoma of, *163*
colitis of, *163*
Innervation of, 209
lymphatic drainage of, 198, 199
Intestine, small, 132, 158, 164. *See also* Duodenum; Ileum; Jejunum
innervation of, 208
lymphatic drainage of, 198
mesenteries of, 161
Iris, 544, 546, 548, 549
arterial circle of
greater, 547, 548
lesser, 547, 548
Ischium, 234
body of, 216, 217
radiograph of, 217
Isocortex
columnar organization of, 627
layers of, 627
Isthmus
of fauces, 580
of prostate, 252
of thyroid gland, 602
of uterine tube, 243

J

Jejunum, 132, 149, 150, 158, 159, 160, 163, 165, 169, 170, 171, 198, 211
arteries of, 176, 176t, 177, 182
lymphatic drainage of, 192, 192t, 193, 198
nerves of, 202, 202t, 203, 205, 208
veins of, 185, 190
Joints (named)
acromioclavicular, 55, 276, 282, 283
injuries to, *283*
atlantoaxial, 16t
lateral, 17, 20
median, 18, 618
atlantooccipital, 16t, 19, 20
lateral, 18
calcaneocuboid, 427
carpometacarpal, 326, 327
dorsal, of thumb, 326, 327, 330
costotransverse, 52
costovertebral, 57
craniovertebral, 16t, 18–19
cricoarytenoid, 599
cricothyroid, 599
cuneonavicular, 427
elbow (cubital), 276, 306–307
arterial network of, 369
injuries to, assessing, *307*
ligaments of, 308–309, 308t
median nerve and, 356t
musculocutaneous nerve and, 355t
topography of, 367
ulnar nerve and, 357t
femoropatellar, 385, 407
glenohumeral, 282, 284–285
bony elements of, 284
capsule and ligaments of, 285
cavity of, 285
MRI of, 285
radiograph of, 284
hip, 386–387
bones of, 382, 383, 384, 385, 386, 387
capsule of, 388–389
dislocation or dysplasia of, diagnosing, *387*
ligaments of, 388–389
muscles of, 390–403
radiography of, 386–387
humeroradial, 306, 308t
humeroulnar, 306, 307, 308t
incudomalleolar, 562, 563
incudostapedial, 562, 563, 564
interphalangeal, 275, 380
distal, 326, 327, 328, 332, 333, 339
promimal, 333
proximal, 326, 327, 328, 332, 339
of thumb, 326, 327
intervertebral, 16t
knee, 406–411, 415
Baker's cyst, *409*
bones of, 406–407
bursae of, 408–409
capsule of, 408–409
cavities and spaces of, 414–415
extension of, 413
fibular fracture and, *405*
flexion of, 413
ligaments of, 408t, 408–409, 410, 412–413
cruciate, rupture of, *413*
menisci of, 410–411
MRI of, 415
radiographs of, 407
rotation of, 413
surfaces of, 384, 385, 406–407
metacarpophalangeal, 275, 326, 327, 328, 332, 339, 372
radial nerve and, 353t
of thumb, 326, 327
ulnar nerve and, 357t
metatarsophalangeal, 427
midcarpal, 326, 327, 331
articular surfaces of, 325
radiocarpal, 326, 327, 331
articular surfaces of, 325
radioulnar, 310–311
distal, 305, 311, 326, 327, 331
pronation, 310
proximal, 305, 306, 308t, 311
rotation, 311
supination, 310
sacrococcygeal, 12
sacroiliac, 13, 216, 218, 223
scapuloclavicular, 282
shoulder, 276
sternoclavicular, 55, 277, 282, 283, 477
sternocostal, 57, 283
subtalar, 428–429
and ligaments of, 430
talocalcaneal, 429
talocalcaneonavicular, 429
talocrural, 428–429
ligaments of, 432t
in plantar flexion, 428, 432
talonavicular, 427
tarsometatarsal, 426, 427
temporomandibular, 569, 570–571
capsule innervation, 571
dislocation of, *571*
ligaments of, 570
mandible and, 569
movement of, 571
uncovertebral, 16t, 17
zygapophyseal, 8, 10, 11, 19, 20
intervertebral facet, 16t
Joints (of region or structure)
of ankle, 383
of coccyx, 454
of foot, 426–431
of hand, 326–327
of hip, 382, 383. *See also* Joint, hip.
of knee, 382, 383. *See also* Joint, knee.
of neck, 588t
of shoulder, 282–285, 284
of thoracic cage, 56–57
of thumb, 326, 327
of upper limb, 275
of wrist, 326–327
Jugum sphenoidale, 483, 487
Junction
anorectal, 235
cervicothoracic, 4
chondro-osseous, 59
craniocervical, 4
esophagogastric, 105
jugulofacial venous, 579, 614
jugulosubclavian, *614*
jugulosubclavian venous, 614
lumbosacral, 4
thoracolumbar, 4
of triradiate cartilage, 217

K

Kidneys, 25, 132, 172–175, 210
arteries of, 176, 176t, 177, 178, 179
autonomic nervous system effects on, 202t, 648t
borders of, 174
fundus of, 238
left, 152, 155, 156, 159, 164, 169, 170, 171, 173, 175, 210, 211, 236
lymphatic drainage of, 192, 192t, 195, 193
nerves of, 202, 202t, 204, 205, 207, 262, 264
pole of
inferior, 174
superior, 174
relations of, 172, 211
renal hypertension and, *179*
right, 153, 155, 157, 159, 164, 165, 166, 171, 172, 173, 175, 188, 236
structure of, 174
veins of, 184, 184t, 186, 187
Kiesselbach's area, nosebleeds and, *555*
Kyphosis, *4*

L

Labium majus/labia majora, 215, 240, 247, 248
Labium minus/labia minora, 215, 238, 240, 246, 247, 248, 266
Labrum
glenoid, 284, 286, 287, 363
ileocecal, 162
ileocolic, 162
Labyrinth
cochlear, 566
innervation of, 567
Lacrimal bone, 478t, 536, 551
Lacrimal drainage, *545*
Lamina
cervical vertebra, 7, 9, 10, 17
of cricoid cartilage, 599

medullary, of thalamus
external, 629t
internal, 629t
thoracic vertebra, 7, 10
thoracolumbar spine, 23
vertebral arch, 20
Lamina cribosa, 546
constricted optic nerve in, *548*
Lamina terminalis
cistern of, 632
Landmarks
lines. *See* Line(s); Reference lines
palpable. *See* Palpable bony prominences
spinous processes. *See* Process, spinous
Laryngopharynx, 580, 620
Larynx, 5, 477, 599, 601t
cartilages of, 598
muscles of, 600, 600t
neurovasculature of, 603
vestibular and vocal folds of, 601
Leg
arteries of, 445, 466–467
bones of, 382, 404–405
fibular fracture, *405*
compartments of, 468t
compartment syndrome in, *469*
lower, 382
muscles of, 381, 416–423, 420t, 421t, 422t, 423t
anterior compartment, 416–417, 421t
lateral compartment, 417, 420t
posterior compartment, 418–419
deep flexors, 423t
superficial flexors, 422t
nerves of, 456, 466–467
neurovasculature of, 466–467
anterior leg, 469
regions of, 381
topography of
lateral and anterior leg, 468–469
posterior and medial leg, 466–467
veins of, 466–467
Lemniscus
lateral, 645
medial, 640
Lens, 544, 546, 548, 549
and ciliary body, 549
light reflection by, 549
Ligaments (named)
acromioclavicular, 282, 283, 285, 287
rupture of, *283*
alar, of dens, 18, 19
annular, 120, 308t, 309, 311, 332, 333, 335, 339, 436
radial head dislocation and, *309*
anococcygeal, 224, 225, 227
apical, of dens, 18, 19, 21
arcuate
lateral, 60, 61, 138, 139, 201
medial, 60, 61, 138, 139, 201
median, 60, 61, 138, 139
pubic, 224
bifurcate, 430, 432, 433
broad, of uterus, 230, 237, 242
mesometrium of, 257
calcaneocuboid, dorsal, 430, 433
calcaneofibular, 432t, 433
calcaneonavicular, plantar, 429, 430, 432, 435, 438, 443
cardinal, of uterus, 244, 245, 247
carpometacarpal
dorsal, 328
palmar, 329
cervical, transverse, 230, 233, 244, 247
collateral, 327, 333, 339, 412–413
accessory, 332
in finger flexion and extension, 332
lateral, of knee, 407, 408, 408t, 409, 410, 411, 412, 413, 414
medial, of knee, 408, 408t, 409, 410, 411, 412, 413
radial, 308t, 309, 327
radiocarpal, 325
ulnar, 308t, 309, 327
ulnar carpal, 325, 328, 331
conoid, 283
coracoacromial, 282, 283, 286, 287, 360
coracoclavicular, 283, 285, 287
injury to, *283*
coracohumeral, 285
coronary, 166, 167
costoclavicular, 283
costotransverse, 57
lateral, 57
superior, 57
costoxiphoid, 57
cricoarytenoid, 599
median, 603
middle, 600
cricothyroid, 599, 602
median, 120, 599, 601
cricotracheal, 599
median, 599
cruciate, 407, 412–413
anterior, 408t, 411, 412, 413, 414, 415
meniscal attachment sites, 411
posterior, 408t, 411, 412, 413, 415
rupture of, *413*
cruciform, 332, 333, 335, 436, 441
deltoid, 432t, 433
denticulate, 40
falciform, 167
of liver, 146, 150, 157, 210
of femoral head, 270, 385, 387, 388, 445
fundiform, of penis, 136
gastrocolic, 152, 153
gastrosplenic, 153, 154, 155, 161, 164, 170
glenohumeral, 285
hepatoduodenal, 152, 154, 155, 157, 159, 161, 164, 166, 171, 173
margin of, 207
hepatoesophageal, 157
hepatogastric, 149, 154, 156, 157, 161, 164, 170
hyoepiglottic, 601
iliofemoral, 388, 389, 391
ilioinguinal, 461
iliolumbar, 134, 222, 389
inguinal, 132, 133, 134, 136, 137, 141, 142, 143, 147, 194, 214, 222, 257, 388, 389, 390, 399, 444, 446, 447, 449, 451, 453, 460, 461, 464
nerve entrapment by, *450*
reflected, 460, 461
intercarpal
dorsal, 328
palmar, 329
interclavicular, 283
interfoveolar, 143, 147
interosseous metacarpal, 327
interspinous, 14, 20t, 21, 22
intertransverse, 18, 20t, 22, 23
intraarticular, 57
ischiofemoral, 388, 389
lacunar, 142, 143, 147, 460, 461
lateral, 489, 570
of bladder, 245
latissimus dorsi, 61, 139
longitudinal
anterior, 20t, 21, 22, 23, 59, 134, 222, 389, 390
posterior, 19, 20t, 21, 22, 23
meniscofemoral, posterior, 408t, 411, 412
metacarpal
deep transverse, 329, 332, 333, 335, 339
dorsal, 328
palmar, 329
superficial transverse, 335, 436
metatarsal, deep transverse, 434
nuchal, 18, 19, 20t, 21, 300, 476, 605
of ovary, 229, 230, 237, 238, 242, 243, 244
palmar, 329, 333, 336, 339
palmar carpal, 330, 370, 371, 373
palpebral
lateral, 542
medial, 545
patellar, 390, 391, 393, 397, 402, 407, 408, 408t, 410, 411, 412, 414, 415, 416, 417, 469. *See also* Retinaculum, patellar
pectineal, 134, 143
perineal, transverse, 247
in male, 269
phalangoglenoid, 332
phrenicocolic, 153
phrenicosplenic, 159
plantar, 434, 438
long, 430, 432, 433, 435, 437, 438, 443
popliteal
arcuate, 408t, 409
oblique, 408t, 409

Ligaments (named) *(continued)*
pterygospinous, 570
pubic, arcuate, 269
pubofemoral, 389
puboprostatic, 237
pubovesical, 244
pulmonary, 115
radiocarpal
dorsal, 328
palmar, 329
radiotriquetral, 331
radioulnar
dorsal, 311, 329, 331
palmar, 311, 329, 331
round
of liver, 146, 150, 151, 154, 157, 160, 161, 164, 167, 168
of uterus, 147, 229, 230, 233, 237, 238, 240, 244, 247, 255, 257
sacrococcygeal, 454
anterior, 223
sacroiliac
anterior, 134, 222, 223, 224, 389
interosseous, 134, 222, 223
posterior, 222, 223, 388, 389
sacrospinous, 134, 138, 222, 223, 224, 227, 270, 388, 389, 399, 463
sacrotuberous, 134, 222, 223, 224, 227, 388, 389, 394, 395, 399, 403, 455, 457, 462, 463, 465
scapular
inferior transverse, 293t
superior transverse, 283, 285, 287, 292, 293t, 350
ossified, *278*
sphenomandibular, 570
splenorenal, 170
stapedial, 562
annular, 563
sternoclavicular
anterior, 282, 283
posterior, 282
sternocostal, radiate, 57, 59
stylomandibular, 570
supraspinous, 20t, 21, 22
suspensory
of breast (Cooper's), 71
of duodenum, 158
of ovary, 230, 233, 238, 240, 242, 243, 247, 255
of penis, 239, 257, 268
syndesmotic, 433
talocalcaneal, interosseous, 426, 429, 430, 433
talofibular
anterior, 432, 432t, 433
posterior, 432t, 433
talonavicular, dorsal, 432, 433
tarsal, dorsal, 432, 433
thyroepiglottic, 599
thyrohyoid, 580, 599, 601
median, 599, 603, 606, 607
tibiofibular
anterior, 432, 432t, 433
posterior, 432, 432t, 433
transverse
of acetabulum, 388
of atlas (C1), 18, 19, 21, 618
of humerus, 285, 286
of knee, 408t, 411, 412
superficial, of metacarpal, 436
transverse carpal. *See* Retinaculum, flexor
transverse perineal. *See* Cardinal ligament of uterus
trapezoid, 283
triangular
left, 166, 167
right, 166, 167
ulnocarpal, palmar, 329
ulnolunate, 331
ulnotriquetral, 331
umbilical, median, 175, 236, 237, 240, 241
uterosacral, 243, 244, 270
vesicouterine, 244
vestibular, 601
median, 599
vocal, 599, 601
Ligaments (of region or structure)
of acetabulum, 388
of ankle and foot, 432–433
subtalar joint and, 430
of craniovertebral joints, 18–19
of elbow, 308t
of fibular head, 410, 412
of fingers, 332–333
of hand, 328–329
of hip joint, 388–389
of incus
posterior, 563
superior, 563
of knee, 408t, 409, 411, 412
of malleus
anterior, 563
lateral of, 561
superior, 563
of neck, 588t
of pelvis, 134–135, 222–223, 245
in female, 244, 245
in male, 134
of sacroiliac joint, 223
of shoulder, 282, 283
acromioclavicular joint, injury to, *283*
glenohumeral joint, 285
posterior, 360–361
of temporomandibular joint, 570
of ulnocarpal, 331
of uterus, 244
of vena cavae, 167, 168
of vertebral arch, 20t
of vertebral body, 20t
of vertebral column, 20, 22
cervical spine, 21
thoracolumbar spine, 22–23
of wrist, 330–331
Ligamentum arteriosum, 87, 89, 90, 92, 104, 125
Ligamentum flavum, 14, 19, 20t, 21, 22, 23
Ligamentum teres femoris. *See* Ligament of femoral head
Ligamentum teres hepatis. *See* Round ligament of liver
Ligamentum venosum, 103, 167
Light reflex, pupillary, 643
Limb (lower). *See also* Ankle; Foot; Leg; Thigh
arteries of, 444–445
bones of, 380, 382–383, 384
of leg, 404–405
of thigh, 406–407
innervation of, 450, 454, 459
joints of, 382, 383, 385, 386, 426–431
hip, 386–389
knee, 406–415
foot, 426–431
ligaments of, 388–389, 408t, 408–409, 410, 412–413, 432–433
lymphatic drainage of, 447, 460, 467
muscles of, 381, 390–403, 416–423, 436–443
of hip, thigh and gluteal region, 390–403
of leg, 416–423
nerves of, 448–456, 459
lumbar plexus, 450–453
lumbosacral plexus, 448t, 448–449
sacral plexus, 454–456
superficial, 458
neurovasculature, 462–471
gluteal, 393, 398t, 454, 462, 463, 463t
inguinal, 460, 461
regions of, 380
veins of, 446–447
deep, 446
perforating, 447
of sole of foot, 446
superficial, 446, 458
Limb (upper), 274–377. *See also* Arm; Axilla; Finger; Forearm; Hand; Joint, elbow; Shoulder; Wrist
arteries of, 344–345
bones of, 276–277
lymphatic drainage of, 346–347
nerves of
brachial plexus, 348–357
superficial, 358–359
regions of, 274
veins of, 346–347
superficial, 358
Limbic system
components of, 628
function of, 647
nuclei of, 647

in peripheral autonomic nervous system regulation, 647
structures of, 647
Limbus, corneoscleral, 546
Limen nasi, 555
Line(s)
anocutaneous, 235
anterior midline, 100
arcuate, 134, 137, 141, 146, 150, 160, 216, 218, 223, 224, 460
axillary
anterior, 51
posterior, 51
dentate, 235
epiphyseal, 387
gluteal
inferior, 217
posterior, 399
intercondylar, 384
intertrochanteric, 384, 386, 389, 399, 402
lateral, 384
midaxillary, 51, 110
midclavicular, 51, 110, 133
of mandible
mylohyoid, 569, 591
oblique, 569
nuchal
inferior, 27, 30, 35, 480, 482, 593
superior, 18, 26, 27, 29, 30, 33, 35, 293, 300, 480, 482, 593
supreme, 480, 482
parasternal, 51
paravertebral, 110
pectineal, 216, 384, 386
of reference. *See* Reference lines
scapular, 110
semilunar, 132, 137
soleal, 404, 406, 423
sternal, 51, 110
supracondylar, 384
transverse, of sacrum, 12
Linea alba, 132, 136, 137, 140, 141, 142, 146, 460
Linea aspera, 384, 386, 403
Linea terminalis, 220, 221, 452
Lingula,
of lung, 115, 118t
of cerebellum, 570, 630
Lingular pneumonia, *117*
Lip
commissure of, 476
frenulum of, upper/lower, 554, 580
Liver, 67, 84, 103, 111, 112, 132, 149, 152, 156, 164, 165, 166–167 170, 172, 180, 211
arteries of, 166, 176, 176t, 177, 180
attachment to diaphragm, 91, 166
autonomic nervous system effects on, 202t, 648t
borders of, 167
lobes of, 167
caudate, 152, 165, 167, 168
left, 150, 152, 154, 157, 161, 164, 165, 167, 168, 210
quadrate, 167, 168
right, 150, 152, 153, 154, 157, 161, 164, 165, 167, 168, 169, 171, 210
lymphatic drainage of, 192, 192t, 193, 196, 197
MRI of, 165
nerves of, 166, 202, 202t, 204, 205, 206
percutaneous biopsy of, *112*
segments of, 166, 166tveins of, 166, 184t. 185, 188
Lobectomy, of lung, *119*
Lobes
of brain
anterior, 628, 630
in cerebral hemispheres, 627
frontal, 616, 617, 625
occipital, 625
lesions of, *643*
posterior, 628, 630
temporal, 527, 625
flocculonodular, 630
of liver
caudate, 152, 165, 167, 168
left, 150, 152, 154, 157, 161, 164, 165, 167, 168, 210
quadrate, 167, 168
right, 150, 152, 153, 154, 157, 161, 164, 165, 167, 168, 169, 171, 210
of lung
arteries and veins of, 125t
bronchopulmonary segments of, 118–119, 118t
inferior, 112, 114, 115, 124
left
Inferior, 115
superior, 115
opacity in lung diseases, 116
removal, *119*
right
inferior, 115
middle, 115
superior, 115
of mammary gland, 71
of prostate, 252
of thyroid gland, 602, 608
Lobule(s)
of cerebellum,
central, 630
quadrangular, 630
semilunar, inferior/superior, 630
simple, 630
mammary, 71, 73
testicular, 145
Lordosis, *4*
nerve entrapment and, *450*
Lower limb. *See* Limb (lower)
Lumbar puncture, *41*
Lunate, 322t, 324, 325, 326, 327, 330, 331, 388
Lung(s), 114
arteries of, 124–125, 125t, 128
borders of, 115
boundaries of, 110
collapsed, 123
diseases of, *117*
lobe opacity in, 116
fissures of, 115, 118
horizontal, 100, 111, 114, 115, 118, 119
oblique, 100, 111, 114, 115, 118, 119
innervation of, 127
left, 51, 74, 75, 88, 101, 123, 124, 128, 129, 165
lobes of. *See* Lobes, of lung
ligaments of, 115
lymphatic drainage of, 128–129
pneumothorax, *123*
pulmonary embolism, *125*
radiographs of
diseased lung, *117, 118*
normal lung, 116
regions of, 115
resection of, *119*
respiratory mechanics of, 110, 122–123
right, 51, 67, 74, 75, 88, 89, 100, 102, 111, 112, 123, 124, 128, 129, 165, 172
segmentation of, 118–119, 118t
arteries and veins of, 124–125, 125t
lymphatics of, 128– 129
neurovasculature of, 126–127
veins of, 124–125, 125t, 127, 128,
Lunule of semilunar valves, 95
Lymph nodes (named),
aortic, 258,258t
lateral, 193, 258t, 259
left, 192, 192t, 193, 193t, 194, 195, 258t, 259, 259t
right, 192, 192t, 193, 193t, 194, 195, 259, 259t
axillary, 72, 347
apical, 72
central, 72
humeral, 72
interpectoral, 72
levels of, 72t
pectoral, 72
subscapular, 72
brachiocephalic, 84, 86, 108
bronchopulmonary, 81, 108, 109, 128, 129
celiac, 108, 192t, 194, 196, 197, 198, 211, 258t
cervical, 72
deep, 579, 615t
superficial, 610, 615t
anterior, 615
lateral, 615
tumor metastasis via, *614*

Lymph nodes (named) *(continued)*
colic
intermediate, 199
left, 199
middle, 199
right, 199
cubital, 72
cystic, 197
epicolic, 199
gastric, left, 196, 197
gastroomental, 196
hepatic, 196, 197
ileocolic, 198, 199
iliac
common, 192, 192t, 193, 193t, 194, 195, 258, 258t, 259, 259t, 260, 261, 447
external, 193, 193t, 194, 259, 259t, 260, 261, 447, 460
internal, 193, 193t, 194, 259, 259t, 261, 447
inguinal
deep, 147, 193, 193t, 194, 259, 259t, 260, 261, 447
inferior, 460
superficial, 193, 193t, 259, 447, 460
horizontal group, 193, 193t, 194, 259, 259t, 260, 261
vertical group, 193, 193t, 194, 259, 259t, 260, 261
superolateral, 447, 460
superomedial, 447, 460
intercostal, 80, 81, 108
intrapulmonary, 81, 128, 129
jugular, 579
lateral group, 615
juxta-intestinal, 198
lacunar, intermediate, 194, 261
lumbar, 192, 192t, 258, 258t, 447
intermediate, 194, 195, 210, 260, 261
left lateral aortic, 192, 194, 195, 260
preaortic.*See* Lymph nodes, preaortic.
retroaortic. *See* Lymph nodes, retroaortic.
right lateral aortic (caval), 192, 194, 195, 260
mastoid, 615
mesenteric
inferior, 192t, 193, 193t, 194, 199, 258t, 259, 259t, 260, 261
intermediate, 198
superior, 192t, 193t, 194, 197, 198, 199, 258t, 259, 259t
obturator, 261
occipital, 612, 615
pancreatic, 196, 197
pancreaticoduodenal, 197
paracolic, 199
paraesophageal, 81, 109
parasternal, 72, 81, 128
tumor spread and, *73*
paratracheal, 81, 108, 109, 128, 129
parotid
deep, 615
superficial, 615
pericardial, lateral, 87
phrenic
inferior, 109, 128, 192t, 194
superior, 84, 87, 91, 108
popliteal
deep, 447, 467
superficial, 447
preaortic, 192, 193t, 195, 258, 258t, 259, 259t
prececal, 199
prevertebral, 108
promontory, 195, 260, 261
rectal, superior, 199
retroaortic, 192, 192t, 194, 258t
retroauricular, 615
retrocaval, 194, 195
retropharyngeal, 586
retropyloric, 197
Rosenmüller's, 460, 461
sacral, 193, 193t, 194, 259, 259t, 260, 261
sigmoid, 199
splenic, 196, 197
submandibular, 579, 615
submental, 579, 615
subpyloric, 196, 197
supraclavicular, 72
gastric carcinoma metastasis to, *614*
suprapyloric, 196, 197
supratrochlear, 72
thoracic, 81
tracheobronchial, 81, 84, 108, 109, 128
inferior, 108, 109, 129
superior, 128, 129
Lymph nodes (of region or organ)
of abdomen, 192, 192t, 258, 258t
parietal, 194
of abdominal wall, posterior, 194
of duodenum, 197
of ileum, 198
of inguinal region, 460
of jejunum, 198
of large intestine, 201
of liver, 196
of lower limb
deep, 447
superficial, 447
of mediastinum, 108, 109
of oral floor, 579
of pancreas, 197
of pelvis, 192, 193, 193t, 258, 259, 259t
parietal, 194
of pleural cavity, 128
of popliteal region, 467
of cervical region of neck , 615
of spleen, 197
of stomach, 196
of thoracic cavity, 108
in thoracic wall, 81
of tongue, 579
of urinary organs, 195
Lymphadenectomy, sentinel, *73*
Lymphatic drainage
of abdomen, 258
of bladder, 193, 259
of duodenum, 197
of female breast, *73*
of genitalia
female, 193, 259
male, 193, 259
of internal organs, 193
of intestines, 198
of liver, 197
of lower limb, 447
of mediastinum, 84t
of oral floor, 579
of pancreas, 197
of pelvic organs, 261
of pelvis, 258–259
of pleural cavity, 128
of rectum, 193, 259
of spleen, 197
of stomach, 197
of thoracic cavity, 80–81
of thoracic wall, 128
of tongue, 579
of upper limb, 347
of urethra, 193, 259
Lymphatic system, tumor metastatis via, *73*
Lymphomas, systemic, *614*

M

Macula lutea, *547*
Male accessory sex glands, 251–252
Malleolus
lateral, 380, 382, 404, 405, 417, 418, 420, 421, 422, 423, 426, 428, 429, 432, 433, 439, 446, 456, 457, 466, 468
articular surface of, 405, 429
medial, 380, 382, 404, 405, 416, 418, 421, 422, 423, 426, 428, 429, 430, 432, 433, 434, 435, 439, 466, 467, 469
articular surface of, 405
Malleus, 558, 560, 561, 562, 563
Mandible, 30, 478t, 479, 480, 569, 574, 578, 579, 586, 605, 606, 608, 620
body of, 569, 617
borders of, 476
head of, 569, 570, 571, 591
muscle origins and insertions, 490
neck of, 570
Manubrium, 133, 138. *See also* Sternum
Mastication
muscles of, 489, 494t–495t
motor innervation of, 514
origins and insertions of, 490–491

Mastoid bone,
antrum of, 564
aditus to, 561
Maxilla, 21, 477, 478t, 479, 480, 482, 536, 537, 550, 551, 554, 616, 618, 620
Meatus
acoustic
external, 478, 556, 570
internal, 483, 507, 556, 566
nasal
inferior, 551, 552t, 553, 555, 616
middle, 551, 552t, 555, 616
superior, 486, 551, 552t, 553, 555, 560
Mediastinum, 84, 86–87, 91
contents of, 84t, 85
divisions of, 75, 84
inferior, 74, 74t, 75, 84t
anterior, 75, 84t, 100
middle, 75, 84t
posterior, 75, 84t, 100
lymphatic drainage of, 108–109
structures of, 86–87
superior, 74t, 75, 84, 84t
testicular, 145, 251
Medulla, renal, 174
Medulla oblongata, 40, 630, 631, 633. *See also* Brainstem
in adult brain, 625
in brain development, 625t
in embryonic brain, 625
glossopharyngeal nerve (CN IX) and, 508
hypoglossal nerve (CN XII) and, 513
olive of, 510
pyramid of, 631
vagus nerve (CN X) and, 510
vestibulocochlear nerve (CN VIII) and, 506
Membrane(s)
atlantooccipital
anterior, 20, 21
posterior, 19, 20, 21, 27
of brain and spinal cord, 40, 524
arachnoid. *See* Arachnoid
dura mater. *See* Dura mater.
pia mater. *See* Pia mater.
external intercostal, 59
fibrous, 385, 389, 407, 445
interosseous, 305, 315, 317, 319, 327, 331, 345, 369, 377, 399, 403, 404, 408, 412, 417, 419, 420, 423, 433, 444, 468, 472
crural, 404
obturator, 134, 222, 223, 271, 388
perineal, 232t, 238
in female, 225, 230, 232, 247
in male, 225, 231, 232, 250
quadrangular, 601
sartorius, 453
stapedial, 563
synovial, 285, 389, 407, 411, 445
tectorial, 18, 19, 20, 21
thyrohyoid, 599, 603
thyroid, 608
tympanic, 504, 558, 560, 561, 562, 564
arteries of middle ear and, 564
mucosal lining of, 562
quadrants of, 562
in otoscopy, *558*
sound waves and, *563*
Meninges, layers of, 40, 524
Meningitis, *557*
Meniscus, of knee joint, 410–411
cruciate ligaments and, 411
injury to, *411*
lateral, 410, 411, 412, 413, 414
medial, 410, 411, 412, 413, 414
Bucket-handle tear, 411
movements of, 411
Mesencephalon, 499, 625t, 627, 628, 631. *See also* Brainstem
Mesentery, 149, 151, 152, 154, 161, 164
root of, 151, 155, 159, 171, 173
Mesoappendix, 155, 162
Mesocolon
sigmoid, 151, 154, 155, 161, 162, 163, 228, 229, 231, 234
transverse, 149, 150, 151, 152, 153, 160, 162, 163, 211
root of, 154, 161, 164, 171, 173, 181
Mesometrium, of broad ligament of uterus, 242, 243, 257
Mesorectum, 245
Mesosalpinx, 237, 242, 243
Mesotympanum, 561
Mesovarium, 242, 243
Metacarpals, 275, 276, 277, 317, 319, 321, 322t, 324, 325, 326, 327, 331, 332, 333, 372, 374
in dorsal digital extension, 339
of thumb, 326
Metatarsals, 382, 420, 422, 423, 424, 425, 426, 427, 428, 429, 430, 432, 433, 434, 436, 437, 439, 440, 441, 467, 471
Metencephalon, in brain development, 625t
Midbrain. *See* Mesencephalon
Modiolus, 566, 567
Mons pubis, 215, 248
Mortise, of ankle, 382, 404, 428, 429
Motor system, 639
Mouth. *See* Cavity, oral.
MRI. *See* Imaging
Mucoperiosteum, of hard palate, 618
Multiple sclerosis, optic fundus examination and, *547*
Muscle edema, compartment syndrome and, *469*
Muscle weakness, small gluteal, *455*
Muscles (named)
abductor digiti minimi, 327, 335, 336, 337, 338, 340t, 341, 357t, 370, 372, 373, 426, 436, 437, 438, 439, 441, 441t, 457, 470, 471
abductor hallucis, 426, 428, 435, 436, 437, 438, 441, 441t, 444, 457, 467, 470, 471
abductor pollicis
brevis, 335, 337, 340t, 341, 353t, 370, 372, 373
longus, 312, 314, 315, 318, 320t, 321, 335, 337, 369, 376, 377
accessory, bundle of, 585
adductor brevis, 391, 392, 396, 400, 400t, 445, 452, 464, 472, 473
adductor hallucis, 434, 435, 437, 438, 442t, 443, 457, 471
oblique head, 434, 438
transverse head, 434, 437, 438
adductor longus, 390, 391, 392, 393, 396, 400, 400t, 445, 452, 464, 472, 473
adductor magnus, 233, 266, 269, 271, 390, 391, 392, 393, 394, 395, 396, 401, 401t, 443, 445, 446, 452, 457, 462, 463, 464, 465, 471, 472, 473
adductor minimus, 391, 392, 401
adductor pollicis, 335, 336, 337, 340t, 341t, 357t, 372, 373
head of, 336
anconeus, 292, 294, 295, 303t, 314, 315, 353t, 369
anococcygeal, 226
articularis genus, 402t
arytenoid
oblique, 585, 587, 600
transverse, 585, 587, 600, 601t
auricular
anterior, 489, 492t, 559
posterior, 489, 492t, 559
superior, 489, 492t, 559
biceps brachii, 72, 274, 286, 287, 288, 289, 290, 291, 302t, 312, 313, 318, 354t, 355t, 362, 364, 365, 366, 367, 369, 376
long and short, head of, 355, 376, 377
biceps femoris, 381, 391, 392, 395, 397, 403t, 418, 419, 466, 467, 473
long head, 394, 395, 396, 403, 417, 456, 457, 463, 465, 472
short head, 395, 396, 403, 417, 456, 457, 465, 467, 472
brachialis, 288, 290, 291, 295, 302t, 318, 353t, 354t, 355t, 366, 367, 369, 376, 377
forearm, 312, 313
brachioradialis, 274, 291, 294, 295, 313, 314, 315, 318, 318t, 319, 353t, 367, 369, 376, 377
forearm, 312
buccinator, 488, 490, 493t, 514, 529, 533, 581, 584, 616, 617, 618
bulbospongiosus, 149, 227, 227t, 238
in female, 225, 232, 233, 247, 248, 249, 266
in male, 225, 232, 233, 239, 250, 253, 269
ciliary, 548, 549, 643
coccygeus, 138, 224, 226, 226t

Muscles (named) *(continued)*
coracobrachialis, 287, 288, 289, 290, 291, 298t, 354t, 355t, 363, 364, 365, 376
corrugator cutis ani, 235
corrugator supercilii, 488, 490
cremaster, 136, 137, 142, 143, 144, 145, 145t, 147, 251
cricoarytenoid
lateral, 601t
posterior, 585, 587, 601t, 603
cricothyroid, 511, 584, 601t, 602, 603, 606, 607, 608
lateral, 603
deltoid, 2, 24, 47, 50, 68, 274, 287, 288, 289, 290, 291, 292, 294, 295, 296t, 352t, 360, 361, 362, 363, 364, 365, 366, 376
depressor anguli oris, 488, 489, 490, 493t, 589
depressor labii inferioris, 488, 489, 490, 493t
depressor septi nasi, 490
digastric, 604, 609
anterior belly, 490, 491, 574, 575t, 577, 584, 590t, 591, 604, 608, 616, 617, 620, 621
posterior belly, 504, 574, 575t, 583, 584, 585, 590t, 591, 604
extensor carpi radialis longus, 274, 291, 292, 294, 295, 312, 313, 314, 315, 318, 318t, 337, 353t, 367, 369, 370, 376, 377
extensor carpi radialis brevis, 291, 292, 294, 295, 312, 313, 314, 315, 318, 318t, 319, 337, 369, 370, 376, 377
extensor carpi ulnaris, 274, 292, 294, 314, 315, 320t, 321, 331, 337, 338, 353t, 369, 377
extensor digiti minimi, 314, 315, 320t, 321, 337, 338, 353t, 377
extensor digitorum, 274, 292, 294, 314, 315, 320t, 321, 337, 338, 353t, 369, 374, 377, 428, 439, 440
extensor digitorum brevis, 416, 417, 439, 440, 440t, 469
extensor digitorum longus, 416, 417, 421, 421t, 439, 456, 468, 469, 471, 473
extensor hallucis brevis, 416, 417, 439, 440, 440t, 469, 471
extensor hallucis longus, 381, 416, 417, 421, 421t, 439, 456, 469, 471
extensor indicis, 314, 315, 320t, 321, 337, 353t, 369, 374
extensor pollicis brevis, 314, 315, 320t, 321, 336, 337, 338, 353t, 377
extensor pollicis longus, 314, 315, 320t, 321, 337, 353t, 369, 377
fibularis brevis, 416, 417, 418, 419, 420, 420t, 428, 437, 438, 439, 456, 466, 469, 473
fibularis longus, 381, 397, 416, 417, 418, 419, 420, 420t, 428, 434, 436, 437, 438, 439, 456, 466, 468, 469, 473
fibularis tertius, 416, 417, 420, 421, 421t, 439
flexor brevis, 418
flexor carpi radialis, 274, 312, 313, 316t, 317, 318, 334, 337, 356t, 370, 373, 376, 377
flexor carpi radialis brevis, 373
flexor carpi radialis longus, 373
flexor carpi ulnaris, 274, 292, 294, 312, 313, 314, 315, 316t, 317, 318, 335, 337, 357t, 370, 371, 373, 376, 377
flexor digiti minimi, 370
flexor digiti minimi brevis, 335, 336, 337, 340t, 341, 372, 373, 436, 437, 438, 442t, 443, 471
flexor digitorum, 437, 473
flexor digitorum brevis, 428, 435, 436, 437, 438, 441, 441t, 443, 457, 470, 471
flexor digitorum longus, 396, 418, 419, 423, 423t, 428, 435, 436, 437, 438, 439, 443, 466, 467
flexor digitorum longus medius, 395
flexor digitorum profundus, 291, 294, 313, 314, 315, 316t, 317, 337, 356t, 357t, 377
flexor digitorum superficialis, 312, 313, 316t, 317, 318, 337, 356t, 369, 370, 373, 376, 377
humeroulnar head of, 369
radial head of, 369
flexor hallucis brevis, 418, 435, 436, 437, 438, 443, 471
flexor hallucis longus, 418, 419, 423, 423t, 428, 435, 436, 437, 438, 439, 466, 467
flexor pollicis brevis, 335, 336, 337, 340t, 341, 356t, 357t, 370, 372, 373
head of, 335
flexor pollicis longus, 312, 313, 316t, 317, 318, 334, 337, 356t, 369, 370, 373, 376, 377
gastrocnemius, 381, 393, 397, 407, 418, 422, 422t, 457, 465, 466, 467, 468, 469, 472
lateral heads, 394, 395, 396, 417, 418, 419, 422, 466, 467
medial heads, 394, 395, 396, 409, 416, 418, 419, 422, 467
gemellus, 398t
inferior, 394, 395, 396, 399, 455, 462, 463, 472
superior, 394, 395, 396, 399, 455, 462, 463, 472
genioglossus, 490, 491, 513, 578, 580, 581, 616, 617, 621
paralysis of, 513
geniohyoid, 490, 491, 574, 575t, 577, 578, 580, 581, 590t, 591, 597, 616, 617
gluteus maximus, 2, 24, 28, 29, 138, 225, 249, 266, 269, 270, 271, 381, 393, 394, 395, 396, 397, 398t, 399, 455, 462, 465, 472
gluteus medius, 2, 381, 391, 394, 395, 396, 397, 398t, 399, 455, 462, 465, 472
gluteus minimus, 233, 391, 392, 394, 395, 396, 398t, 399, 455, 463, 465, 472
gracilis, 266, 269, 390, 391, 392, 393, 394, 395, 400, 400t, 416, 418, 452, 462, 463, 464, 465, 466, 467, 472, 473
helicis major, 559
helicis minor, 559
hyoglossus, 491, 513, 574, 575t, 578, 581, 584, 617
hypothenar, 274, 275, 318,340, 340t, 371
iliacus, 138, 140t, 141, 146, 175, 201, 233, 236, 247, 257, 390, 391, 392, 393, 398t, 399, 451, 453, 461
iliococcygeus, 224, 226, 226t
iliocostalis, 28, 165
iliocostalis cervicis, 29, 32t, 33, 588t
iliocostalis lumborum, 29, 32t, 33
iliocostalis thoracis, 29, 32t, 33
iliopsoas, 138, 141, 142, 147, 270, 390, 391, 392, 396, 398t, 399, 453, 461, 464
infrahyoid, 25, 590t, 591, 597
infraspinatus, 24, 286, 293, 294, 295, 297t, 350t, 363
intercostal, 61, 71, 86, 87, 139
external, 28, 29, 58t, 59, 67, 69, 113, 136
innermost, 58t, 67, 69
internal, 58t, 59, 67, 69, 113, 136, 138
interossei, 339, 374, 405, 416, 426, 439
atrophy of, ulnar nerve damage and, *357*
dorsal, 327, 335, 337, 338, 342t, 343, 357t, 373, 375, 436, 437, 438, 442t, 443, 469
palmar, 336, 337, 342t, 343, 357t
plantar, 435, 436, 437, 438, 442t, 443, 471
slip, in dorsal digital extention, 339
interspinales cervicis, 27, 29, 34t, 35
interspinales lumborum, 29, 34t, 35
intertransversarii cervicis, 27
intertransversarii laterales lumborum, 29, 34t, 35
intertransversarii mediales lumborum, 29, 34t, 35
intertransversarii posteriores cervicis, 34t, 35, 613
ischiocavernosus, 227, 227t, 238
in female, 225, 232, 247, 249, 266, 267
in male, 225, 232, 239, 250, 252, 269
latissimus dorsi, 2, 24, 25, 47, 61, 69, 72, 165, 274, 285, 287, 288, 289, 290, 291, 292, 293, 294, 295, 301t, 351t, 360, 362, 364t, 365, 366
aponeurotic origin of, 24
levator anguli oris, 488, 490, 493t, 618
levator ani, 224, 226, 226t, 227, 234, 235, 238, 256
in female, 225, 229, 230, 233, 244, 247, 249, 266, 267
in male, 225, 228, 231, 232, 233, 239, 269, 271
tendinous arch of, 224
levator labii superioris, 488, 489, 493t
levator labii superioris alaeque nasi, 488, 489, 490, 492t, 493t

levator palpebrae superioris, 501, 538, 539, 542, 543, 544, 545, 616
levator scapulae, 24, 25, 293, 294, 295, 300t, 350t, 589, 611, 619
levator veli palatini, 491, 560, 575t, 584, 585, 618, 621
levatores costarum breves, 29, 34t, 35
levatores costarum longi, 29, 34t, 35
longissimus capitis, 26, 27, 29, 32t, 33, 46, 490, 491, 588t, 613, 619
longissimus cervicis, 32t, 33, 588t, 619
longissimus thoracis, 29, 32t, 33, 165
longitudinal
  inferior, 578
  superior, 578
longus capitis, 31t, 491, 592t, 593, 620
longus colli, 25, 592t, 593, 619
  inferior oblique part, 31t
  superior oblique part, 31t
  vertical part, 31t
lumbricals, 335, 336, 339, 342t, 343, 356, 357t, 373, 435, 436, 437, 438, 442t, 443, 457, 471
  slip, in dorsal digital extention, 339
masseter, 488, 489, 490, 491, 494t, 528, 529, 531, 532, 533, 581, 583, 585, 586, 610, 617, 618
mentalis, 488, 489, 490, 493t
multifidus, 29, 34t, 35
muscularis (detrusor vesicae), 239
musculus uvulae, 575t, 585, 587
mylohyoid, 490, 491, 574, 575t, 577, 578, 581, 584, 590t, 591, 608, 616, 617, 620, 621
nasalis, 488, 490, 492t
oblique
  of auricle, 559
  external, 2, 24, 28, 47, 61, 68, 69, 132, 135, 136, 137, 139, 140t, 141, 142, 146, 151, 154, 155, 157, 160, 165, 173, 288, 292, 293, 451, 460, 461
  inferior, 31, 501, 538t, 539, 544, 616
  internal, 24, 28, 29, 47, 61, 68, 135, 136, 137, 139, 140t, 141, 142, 143, 146, 151, 154, 155, 157, 160, 173, 292, 293
  superior, 501, 538t, 539, 542, 543, 617
obliquus capitis inferior, 26, 27, 29, 30t, 46, 592t, 593, 613, 620, 621
obliquus capitis superior, 26, 27, 29, 30t, 46, 490, 491, 592t, 593, 613
obturator externus, 226t, 233, 391, 392, 396, 401, 401t, 452
obturator internus, 138, 224, 225, 226, 226t, 227, 230, 231, 232, 233, 234, 239, 247, 249, 270, 271, 393, 394, 395, 396, 398t, 399, 455, 462, 463, 465, 472
occipitofrontalis, 492t
  frontal belly, 488, 489
  occipital belly, 489, 490
omohyoid, 360, 363, 491, 590t, 597, 605, 609, 619
  inferior belly, 72, 476, 591, 609, 611
  superior belly, 591, 606
opponens digiti minimi, 335, 336, 337, 340t, 341, 357t, 373, 437, 438, 442t, 443, 471
opponens pollicis, 327, 335, 336, 337, 340t, 341, 356t, 370, 373
ora serrata, 546, 549
orbicularis oculi, 488, 489, 490, 492t, 544, 616
orbicularis oris, 488, 490, 493t, 621
palatoglossus, 575t, 578
palatopharyngeus, 575t, 585, 586, 587, 620, 621
palmaris brevis, 335, 340t, 357t, 370, 371, 372, 376
palmaris longus, 312, 316t, 317, 318, 356t, 371, 373, 376, 377
papillary
  anterior, 93, 95, 98
  posterior, 93, 95
  septal, 93, 95
pectinate, 93
pectineus, 142, 143, 147, 270, 390, 391, 392, 396, 400, 400t, 452, 453, 460, 464
pectoralis major, 50, 68, 71, 72, 274, 288, 289, 290, 291, 298t, 354t, 362, 363, 364t, 365, 366, 376
  abdominal part, 136
  sternocostal part, 136
pectoralis minor, 71, 72, 289, 290, 291, 299t, 347, 354t, 362, 363, 364t, 365, 366
perineal
  deep transverse, 149, 224, 226, 227, 227t, 238, 247, 249, 250
    in female, 232, 233, 246, 266, 267
    in male, 233, 252, 253, 268
  superficial transverse, 226, 227, 227t, 249
    in female, 225, 266, 267
    in male, 225, 269
pharyngeal constrictors
  inferior, 85, 105, 584t, 585, 586, 603, 621
    cricopharyngeal part, 105
    thyropharyngeal part, 105
  middle, 584t, 585, 586
  superior, 584t, 585, 586
piriformis, 138, 224, 226, 226t, 227, 254, 390, 391, 392, 393, 394, 395, 396, 398t, 399, 444, 446, 455, 462, 463, 465, 472
plantaris, 394, 395, 396, 418, 419, 422, 422t, 465, 466, 467, 472
platysma, 488, 490, 493t, 589t, 602, 606, 616, 619
popliteus, 395, 396, 403, 409, 418, 419, 423, 423t, 466, 467
procerus, 488, 492t, 621
pronator quadratus, 312, 313, 316t, 317, 318, 334, 356t, 369, 370, 373
pronator teres, 290, 291, 312, 313, 315, 316t, 317, 318, 356t, 367, 369, 376, 377
psoas major, 25, 60, 61, 138, 139, 140t, 141, 146, 165, 175, 201, 211, 236, 245, 257, 390, 391, 392, 393, 398t, 399, 451, 453, 461
psoas minor, 60, 135, 138, 140t, 201, 393, 399
pterygoid
  lateral, 489, 490, 491, 495t, 514, 532, 533, 571, 618, 621
  medial, 489, 490, 491, 495t, 514, 532, 533, 583, 585, 586, 617, 618, 621
pubococcygeus, 224, 226t, 234
puborectalis, 224, 226t, 234
pupillary dilator, 548
pyramidalis, 137, 140t, 141
quadratus femoris, 233, 392, 394, 395, 396, 398t, 399, 455, 462, 463, 465, 472
quadratus lumborum, 25, 29, 60, 61, 135, 138, 139, 140t, 141, 165, 201, 451
quadratus plantae, 435, 437, 438, 442t, 443, 457, 470, 471
quadriceps femoris, 132, 214, 391, 392, 402, 402t, 415, 453, 464, 473
rectus
  inferior, 501, 538t, 539, 542, 544, 616, 617, 621
  lateral, 501, 538t, 539, 542, 543, 546, 617, 621
  medial, 501, 538t, 539, 542, 543, 546, 616, 617, 643
  superior, 501, 538t, 539, 542, 543, 544, 617, 621
rectus abdominis, 61, 63, 68, 132, 135, 136, 137, 139, 140t, 141, 142, 143, 146, 149, 150, 151, 154, 160, 163, 165, 228, 230, 231, 270, 451, 460
rectus capitis anterior, 31t, 491, 592t, 593
rectus capitis inferior, 593
rectus capitis lateralis, 31t, 491, 592t, 593
rectus capitis posterior major, 26, 27, 29, 30t, 46, 490, 491, 592t, 593, 613, 620, 621
rectus capitis posterior minor, 26, 27, 29, 30, 30t, 46, 490, 491, 592t, 593, 613, 620
rectus femoris, 381, 390, 391, 392, 393, 395, 396, 397, 402, 402t, 416, 417, 453, 464, 472
rhomboid major, 24, 28, 47, 293, 294, 295, 300t, 350t, 363
rhomboid minor, 28, 293, 294, 295, 300t, 350t, 589
risorius, 488, 489, 493t
rotatores breves, 34t, 35
rotatores longi, 34t, 35
rotatores thoracis breves, 29
rotatores thoracis longi, 29
salpingopharyngeus, 560, 585, 587
sartorius, 132, 147, 214, 381, 390, 391, 392, 393, 397, 402, 402t, 416, 453, 464, 472, 473

Muscles (named) *(continued)*
scalene, 25, 82, 355, 356
anterior, 55, 58t, 59, 62, 74, 76, 78, 99, 107, 345, 349, 352, 353, 592t, 593, 597, 607, 608, 609, 611, 619
middle, 58t, 59, 76, 78, 345, 349, 352, 592t, 593, 597, 608, 609, 611, 619
posterior, 58t, 59, 345, 592t, 593, 611, 619
semimembranosus, 381, 391, 392, 393, 394, 395, 396, 403, 403t, 409, 418, 457, 458, 462, 463, 465, 466, 467, 472, 473
semispinalis capitis, 26, 27, 28, 29, 34t, 35, 46, 292, 293, 490, 491, 588t, 612, 613, 618, 620, 621
semispinalis cervicis, 26, 34t, 35, 46, 588t, 619
semispinalis thoracis, 34t, 35
semitendinosus, 381, 390, 391, 392, 393, 394, 395, 396, 403, 403t, 457, 462, 463, 465, 466, 467, 472, 473
serratus anterior, 24, 50, 69, 136, 282, 288, 289, 290, 291, 293, 299t, 350t, 363, 364t, 365, 366
serratus posterior inferior, 24, 25, 28, 32t, 33, 47, 293
serratus posterior superior, 32t, 33
soleus, 395, 396, 416, 417, 418, 419, 422, 422t, 457, 466, 467, 468, 469, 472, 473
spinalis, 28, 29
spinalis cervicis, 29, 32t, 33, 620
spinalis thoracis, 29, 32t, 33
splenius capitis, 26, 27, 28, 29, 32t, 33, 46, 47, 292, 293, 490, 491, 588t, 611, 612, 613, 618, 619, 620, 621
splenius cervicis, 26, 28, 29, 32t, 33, 293, 588t, 619
stapedius, 563
sternocleidomastoid, 24, 25, 26, 27, 46, 50, 288, 289, 292, 293, 362, 476, 490, 491, 529, 581, 586, 587, 588, 589t, 602, 604, 605, 606, 608, 609, 610, 611, 612, 613, 619
paralysis of, 512t
sternohyoid, 491, 584, 590t, 591, 597, 604, 605, 606, 608, 609, 619
sternothyroid, 491, 590t, 591, 597, 606, 609, 619
styloglossus, 491, 513, 578, 583, 584, 586
stylohyoid, 491, 504, 574, 575t, 581, 584, 585, 590t, 591
stylopharyngeus, 491, 508, 584, 585, 586
subclavius, 289, 290, 291, 299t, 350t, 362, 363
subcostal, 58t, 59
subscapularis, 282, 285, 286, 287, 289, 290, 291, 297t, 351t, 363, 364, 364t, 365, 366
subtendinous bursa of, 286, 287
supinator, 291, 294, 312, 313, 314, 315, 320t, 321, 353t, 367, 369
suprahyoid, 490, 574, 575t, 577, 590t, 591
supraspinatus, 24, 285, 286, 289, 290, 291, 293, 294, 295, 297t, 350t, 360, 589
tarsal
inferior, 544
superior, 542, 544
temporalis, 489, 490, 491, 494t, 531, 532, 533, 617
temporoparietal, 489, 559
tensor fasciae latae, 143, 147, 381, 390, 391, 394, 395, 396, 397, 398t, 399, 451, 455, 458, 462, 463, 464, 465, 472
tensor tympani, 558, 561, 563, 564, 565
nerve of, 533
tensor veli palatini, 491, 560, 575t, 584, 585, 618
nerve of, 533
teres major, 2, 24, 274, 287, 288, 289, 290, 291, 292, 293, 294, 295, 301t, 351t, 352t, 360, 361, 364t, 365, 366,376
teres minor, 2, 286, 293, 294, 295, 297t, 361
thyroarytenoid, 601, 601t, 603
thyrohyoid, 513, 584, 591, 597, 603, 606, 608, 609, 619
thyrothyroid, 590t
tibialis anterior, 381, 393, 397, 416, 417, 419, 421, 421t, 428, 438, 439, 456, 468, 469, 471
tibialis posterior, 395, 396, 418, 419, 423, 423t, 434, 436, 437, 438, 439, 466, 467, 473
transverse, of auricle, 559
transversus abdominis, 29, 60, 61, 135, 137, 138, 140t, 141, 142, 143, 146, 147, 151, 154, 155, 157, 160, 173, 201, 451, 460
transversus thoracis, 58t, 59, 138
trapezius, 2, 24, 25, 26, 27, 28, 47, 285, 287, 288, 289, 290, 291, 292, 293, 294, 295, 300t, 360, 362, 363, 476, 490, 491, 588, 589t, 604, 605, 607, 608, 610, 611, 612, 618, 619, 621
paralysis of, 512t
triceps brachii, 2, 24, 274, 292, 294, 295, 303t, 312, 314, 315, 318, 353t, 361, 365, 366, 367, 369, 376, 377
triceps surae, 417, 419, 422t, 439, 467, 472
vastus intermedius, 390, 391, 392, 395, 402, 402t, 453, 464, 472
vastus lateralis, 381, 390, 391, 392, 395, 397, 402, 402t, 408, 416, 417, 453, 464, 472, 473
vastus medialis, 381, 390, 391, 392, 393, 396, 402, 402t, 408, 416, 453, 464, 472
vocalis, 601, 601t
zygomaticus major, 488, 489, 490, 493t, 528
zygomaticus minor, 488, 490, 493t

Muscles (of region or organ)
of abdomen, 132
of abdominal wall
anterior, 140t, 141
anterolateral, 136–137, 140t, 141
lateral, 25
posterior, 138, 140t, 141
of arm, 274, 296t–303t
anterior, 288–291
innervation and actions, 296t–303t
posterior, 292–295
of auricle, 559
of back, 24–35
deep segmental, 33t
intermediate intrinsic, 32t
intrinsic, 25–29, 32t, 61, 69, 139
superficial (extrinsic), 24
transversospinal, 33t
of diaphragm (thoracic), 60–61, 60t, 138–139, 139t
of diaphragm (pelvic), 226t
of ear, 492t
of esophagus, 105
of eye
extraocular, 538-539, 538t
cranial nerves of, 500t, 501
impaired coordination of, *539*
innervation of, 539
extraorbital, testing of, 539
intraocular, innervation of, 549
facial
of expression, 488–489, 492t, 493t
of mastication, 489, 494t, 495t
motor innervation of, 514
of fauces, 585
of foot, 438
of dorsum, 440t
of sole, 436–437, 441t, 442t, 443
of forearm
anterior, 312–313, 316–317
posterior, 314–315, 320–321
radialis group, 318–319
of forehead, 492t
gluteal, 394, 395, 396, 398t
anterior, 394–397
deep muscles, 399
horizontally-oriented muscles, 398
posterior, 394–397
small, weakness in, *455*
superficial muscles, 399
vertically-oriented muscles, 398
of hand, 274, 340–343, 340t, 342t
of dorsum, 338–339
middle and deep layers, 336–337
superficial and middle layers, 334–335
of hip. *See also* Thigh
anterior, 390–393
posterior, 394–397
of inguinal region, 142

of larynx, 601
actions of, 601t
of leg
anterior, 416–417, 421t
lateral, 417, 420t
posterior, 418–419
deep flexors, 423t
superficial flexors, 422t
of lower limb, 381
of mouth, 493t
of neck, 493t
infrahyoid, 588t
lateral (deep), 588t
nuchal (instrinsic back), 588t
prevertebral, 31t, 588t
superficial, 588t, 589, 589t
suprahyoid, 588t
of nose, 492t
in nuchal region, 26–27, 30t
of oral cavity
oral floor (suprahyoid), 574, 575t, 577, 590t, 591
soft palate, 575t, 585
of palpebral fissure, 492t
of pelvic floor, 224–225, 226, 226t, 230
of pelvic wall, 226t
of pelvis, 132
of perineum, 224, 226, 227, 227t
of pharyngotympanic (auditory) tube, 585
of pharynx, 584–585, 584t
of rotator cuff, 297t
of shoulder, 274, 296–303t
anterior, 288–291
posterior, 292–295, 360–361
of skull, 490
of skull base, 491
of thigh
anterior, 390–393, 402t
medial
deep layer, 401t
superficial layer, 400t
posterior, 394–397, 403t
of thorax, 50
of tongue, 578
Mydriasis, 549
Myelencephalon, in brain development, 625t
Myelination, of axons, 624
Myocardial infarction, types of, *97*
Myometrium, 242, 243, 261
Myopia, 549

N

Naris, 550
Nasal bone, 477, 478t, 479, 536, 550
Nasion, 479, 550
Nasopharynx, 580
infection in, *557*
Navicular bone, 422, 424, 425, 426, 427, 428, 429, 430, 432, 433, 434, 435, 440
Nearsightedness, 549
Neck. *See also* Larynx; Pharynx; Vertebra/Vertebrae; Vertebral column
arteries of, 516–517, 594
bones of, 4, 7, 7t, 8–9, 588t
cavities and spaces of, 601
chronic pain in, *17*
joints of, 16–17, 16t, 19–19, 30, 588, 588t, 590, 599, 618
ligaments of, 20–21, 20t, 588, 588t, 599–603, 605–608, 618
lymphatic drainage of, 604, 610, 612, 614, 615
deep, 615t
superficial, 615t
muscles of, 26–27, 30, 30t, 31, 493t, 588–593, 600–602, 604, 605
craniovertebral joint, 30
infrahyoid, 588t, 590t, 591
lateral (scalene), 588t, 592t, 593
nuchal (instrinsic back), 588t
prevertebral, 31, 588t, 592t, 593
short nuchal, 26, 27, 30
suboccipital, 592t, 593
superficial, 588, 589, 589t
suprahyoid, 588t, 590t, 591
nerves of, 39, 519, 596–597
neurovasculature of, 46, 47, 603, 606–613, 616–621
organs of. *See individually named organs*
regions of, 476, 604
surface anatomy of, 476, 477
topography of, 407, 604–605
veins of, 594, 595
anastomoses, 523t
deep, 523
impeded flow in, *595*
superficial, 522t
Necrosis
avascular. *See* Avascular necrosis
femoral head, *445*
Nerve compression
in leg, *469*
of radial nerve, *353*
of spinal nerve, *15, 17*
of suprascapular nerve, *278*
Nerve entrapment, lateral femoral cutaneous nerve, *450*
Nerve injury
abducent nerve (CN Vi), 500t
facial nerve (CN VII), 505t
glossopharyngeal nerve (CN IX), 509t
hypoglossal nerve (CN XII), 513t
oculomotor nerve (CN III), 500t
trigeminal nerve (CN V), 502t
trochlear nerve (CN IV), 500t
vagus (CN X), 510t
vestibulocochlear nerve (CN VIII), 506t
Nerves (named)
abducent (CN VI), 484, 485, 496, 497t, 500t, 501, 527, 536t, 539, 541, 542, 543, 587, 631, 636
course of, 501
nucleus of, 497, 500, 644
origin and functional fiber types of, 497t
accessory (CN XI), 47, 300t, 360, 484, 485, 496, 497t, 512t, 531, 586, 587, 607, 608, 609, 610, 611, 612, 614, 618, 619, 621, 631
lesions of, 512
origin and functional fiber types of, 497t
spinal nucleus of, 497
spinal root of, 484
alveolar
inferior, 503, 514, 515, 532, 533, 576, 577, 586, 616, 617, 618
superior, 576
anterior, 503, 576
middle, 503, 576
posterior, 532, 533, 576
ampullary
anterior, 507
lateral, 507
posterior, 507
anococcygeal, 266, 449
antebrachial
lateral, 355t, 358, 367
medial, 348t, 349, 354t, 358, 359, 366, 367
posterior, 353t, 358, 374
auricular
great, 39, 46, 362, 515, 529, 559, 596t, 597, 606, 610, 611, 612, 613
posterior, 504
auriculotemporal, 503, 509, 514, 515, 528, 529, 530, 532, 533, 559, 571, 576
axillary, 39, 296t, 298t, 348t, 349, 351t, 352, 352t, 359, 361, 365
branches of, 352t
injury to, *352*
sensory distribution, 352, 359
brachial
lateral
inferior, 353t, 358, 360
posterior, 360
superior, 352t, 358, 360
medial, 348t, 349, 354t, 358, 366
posterior, 353t, 358, 365, 366
buccal, 503, 514, 515, 532, 533, 576
caroticotympanic, 509
carotid, common, 99
cavernous, of penis, 263
cervical, 525
cardiac, 99
plexus, branches of, 360
transverse, 515, 596t, 597, 606, 610
deep, 611
ciliary
long, 503, 541, 543
short, 503, 541, 543, 643

Nerves (named) *(continued)*
circumflex humeral, posterior, 361
clitoral, dorsal, 247, 266, 267
clunial, 454, 459
inferior, 47, 266, 448, 454, 454t, 458, 462, 465
middle, 39, 47, 266, 454, 458, 462, 465
superior, 39, 47, 66, 266, 454, 458, 462, 465
coccygeal, 449
cochlear (CN VIII), 507, 560, 561, 566, 567, 645
branches of, 450, 451, 452, 453, 458
cutaneous dorsal
of foot, 466
intermediate, 456, 458, 469
lateral, 457, 458, 468, 469
medial, 456, 458, 469
femoral, 451t, 453
lateral, 201, 448, 448t, 449, 450, 451, 451t, 458, 459, 460, 461, 464
posterior, 266, 269, 448, 448t, 449, 454, 454t, 458, 459, 462, 463, 465
fibular
medial, 456
lateral
of big toe, 456
sural
lateral, 448, 456, 458, 465, 466, 468
medial, 457, 458, 465, 466, 468
digital
common plantar, 457, 470
dorsal, 353t, 372, 374, 469
palmar, 372, 373, 374
common, 356t, 357t, 359
proper, 356t, 357t, 359, 372
proper plantar, 457, 470, 471
ethmoidal
anterior, 503, 525, 536t, 543, 555
posterior, 503, 525, 536t, 543
facial (CN VII), 484, 485, 496, 497t, 504, 505t, 507, 528, 530, 531, 532, 533, 559, 561, 563, 564, 565, 566, 567, 577, 578, 581, 587, 606, 609, 610, 630, 631
branches of, 504, 514, 528, 530, 577, 609
course of, 505t
nuclei of, 497, 504
femoral, 142, 147, 200, 201, 270, 271, 448, 449, 450, 453, 453t, 458, 459, 461, 464
branches of, 201, 449, 450, 451, 452, 453t
lateral, entrapment of, *450*
fibular
branches of, 469
common, 407, 448, 448t, 449, 456, 456t, 459, 465, 466, 467, 468
cutaneous distribution, 456
deep, 448, 456, 456t, 458, 468, 469, 471
superficial, 448, 456, 456t, 458, 468, 469, 473
frontal, 484, 501, 503, 527, 536, 541, 542, 543
genitofemoral, 173, 200, 201, 448, 448t, 449, 450, 451, 451t, 459, 460, 461
femoral branch, 201
genital branch, 142, 143, 144, 201, 266
labial branch, 266
glossopharyngeal (CN IX), 484, 496, 497t, 508t, 577, 578, 579, 586, 587, 618, 621, 630, 631, 645
branches of, 508t
course of, 508
nuclei of, 497, 508
gluteal
inferior, 448t, 449, 454t, 455, 462, 463, 465
superior, 448t, 449, 454t, 455, 462, 463, 465
hypogastric, 205, 207, 209, 245, 262, 263
hypoglossal (CN XII), 484, 485, 496, 497t, 513t, 531, 577, 579, 586, 587, 597, 606, 609, 618, 621, 631
lesions of, 513
nuclei of, 497, 513
unilateral palsy, *579*
iliac, external, 201
iliohypogastric, 39, 172, 173, 200, 201, 448, 448t, 449, 450, 451, 451t, 454, 458, 459, 462, 465
anterior cutaneous branch, 143, 201
lateral cutaneous branch, 201
ilioinguinal, 142, 143, 172, 173, 200, 201, 266, 268, 448, 448t, 449, 450, 451, 451t, 458, 459, 460
infraorbital, 503, 515, 528, 529, 530, 535t, 536t, 542, 544, 576, 616, 617
infratrochlear, 503, 530, 541, 542, 543
intercostal, 39, 47, 62, 63, 66, 67, 68, 69, 71, 82, 86, 87, 106, 111, 112, 200, 210
course of, 67
sensory distribution of, 359
intercostobrachial, 66, 349, 354t, 358
cutaneous distribution of, 354, 359
interosseous
anterior, 348t, 377
anterior antebrachial, 366t
posterior, 353t, 369, 377
labial, posterior, 266, 267
lacrimal, 484, 501, 503, 536, 541, 542, 543
laryngeal
inferior, 511, 587, 603
branches of, 603
recurrent, 106, 127, 607
left, 82, 87, 90, 99, 106, 511t, 587, 603, 608
right, 82, 99, 106, 511t, 587, 603
superior, 99, 127, 510, 511t, 586, 587, 599, 603, 606, 607, 609
branches of, 607
lingual, 503, 504, 505, 514, 515, 532, 533, 576, 577, 578, 579, 586, 617, 618, 620, 645
mandibular (CN V_3), 484, 496, 502t, 504, 505, 514, 515, 525, 533, 541, 555, 571, 576, 577, 597
course of, 503
in infratemporal fossa, 533
meningeal branch of, 484
in sensory innervation of face, 515
masseteric, 503, 514, 515, 533, 571, 576
maxillary (CN V_2), 484, 496, 502t, 504, 505, 514, 515, 525, 527, 541, 555, 576, 597, 621
course of, 503
in orbit, 536t
in pterygopalatine fossa, 535t
in sensory innervation of face, 515
median, 68, 316t, 318, 340t, 342t, 348t, 349, 354t, 363, 364, 365, 366, 367, 369, 370, 371, 373, 374, 377
injury to, *356*
palmar branch, 358, 359
sensory distribution of, 356, 359
mental, 503, 515, 528, 529, 530, 532, 576
musculocutaneous, 298t, 302t, 348t, 349, 354t, 355t, 364, 367, 369, 377
sensory distribution of, 355, 359
mylohyoid, 515, 533, 577
nasociliary, 484, 503, 536, 541, 542, 543
nasopalatine, 484, 535t, 554, 555, 576
obturator, 146, 200, 201, 257, 263, 270, 448, 448t, 449, 451t, 452, 452t, 458, 459, 464
cutaneous distribution of, 452
occipital
3rd., 39, 46, 47, 596t, 611, 613
greater, 39, 46, 515, 529, 596t, 597, 612, 613, 621
lesser, 39, 46, 515, 529, 559, 596t, 597, 610, 611, 612
oculomotor (CN III), 484, 485, 496, 497t, 500t, 527, 536t, 539, 541, 542, 543, 587, 620, 631, 636, 643
course of, 501
nuclei of, 497, 500, 644
olfactory (CN I), 484, 496, 497t, 498, 617
in brain, 625, 626, 627
filia olfactoria of, 485
sense associated with, 630
ophthalmic (CN V_1), 496, 499, 502t, 504, 514, 515, 525, 527, 541, 555, 596, 597
course of, 503
in orbit, 536
in sensory innervation of face, 515
optic (CN II), 484, 485, 496, 499, 501, 524, 527, 536t, 538, 540, 541, 542, 543, 546, 547, 617, 620, 621, 642, 643
in brain, 625, 627, 630
constricted, glaucoma and, *548*

lesion of, *643*
sense associated with, 630
palatine
greater, 484, 534t, 555, 576
lesser, 484, 534t, 555, 576
pectoral
lateral, 298t, 348t, 349, 354t, 362, 363, 364
medial, 298t, 299t, 348t, 349, 354t, 362, 363, 364
penile, dorsal, 263, 268, 269
pericardiacophrenic, 85
perineal, 234
in female, 266, 267
in male, 268, 269
petrosal
deep, 484, 535
greater, 484, 504, 505, 507, 535, 561, 566
lesser, 484, 507, 509, 533, 561, 566
pharyngeal, 535
phrenic, 62, 63, 74, 85, 87, 89, 90, 91, 99, 101, 111, 348, 349, 352, 597, 607, 608, 609, 611, 619
plantar
lateral, 448, 457, 457t, 467, 470, 471
medial, 448, 457, 457t, 467, 470, 471
pterygoid, 576
lateral, 503, 514
medial, 503, 514
pudendal, 227t, 234, 263, 266, 267, 268, 269, 271, 448, 448t, 449, 454t, 462, 463, 465
branches of, 266
labial branches, anterior/posterior, 267
radial, 302t, 303t, 318t, 320t, 348t, 349, 351t, 353t, 365, 367, 372, 374, 377
compression of, *353*
damage to, humeral fracture and, *281*
deep branch of, 353
posterior, 361
sensory distribution of, 353, 359
superficial branches of, 353t, 358
rectal, inferior, 263, 266, 267, 268, 269
saccular, 507, 567
sacculoampullary, 507
sacral, 205, 207, 262
saphenous, 448, 449, 453, 453t, 458, 464, 466, 468, 471
scapular, dorsal, 300t, 348t, 349, 350t
sciatic, 200, 270, 271, 448, 448t, 449, 454t, 455, 456–457, 459, 462, 463, 465, 472, 473
branches of, 456t, 457t
scrotal, posterior, 263, 268, 269
spinal, 17, 39, 40, 42, 47, 349, 350, 351, 352, 515, 577, 619, 620, 632
branches of, 67
in neck, 596, 596t, 619
in nervous system, 624
in posterolateral disk herniation, *15*
splanchnic, 42, 649
greater, 63, 82, 106, 127, 203, 205, 207, 208
lesser, 205, 207, 208
lumbar, 202, 203, 204, 263
pelvic, 202, 205, 207, 245, 262, 263
sacral, 202
thoracic, 202, 203
stapedial, 504
subcostal, 66, 172, 173, 200, 201, 449
suboccipital, 39, 46, 596t, 613
subscapular, 298t, 349, 364
lower, 301t, 348t, 351t, 364, 365
upper, 348t, 351t, 365
supraclavicular, 39, 66, 70, 358, 360, 362, 515, 596t, 597, 606, 610
intermediate, 610, 611
lateral, 610, 611
medial, 610
sensory distribution, 359
supraorbital, 501, 503, 515, 527, 528, 529, 536t, 541, 542, 543
suprascapular, 298t, 348t, 349, 350t, 352t, 360, 361, 607
compression of, *278*
in scapular notch, 350
supratrochlear, 503, 515, 527, 528, 529, 541, 542, 543
sural, 448, 457, 458, 465, 466, 468
temporal, deep, 503, 514, 532, 533, 571
thoracic, long, 299t, 348t, 349, 350t, 363, 364, 365
thoracodorsal, 301t, 348t, 349, 351t, 364, 365
tibial, 407, 448, 448t, 449, 456, 457, 457t, 459, 465, 466, 467
cutaneous distribution, 457
transverse, of neck, 362
trigeminal (CN V), 485, 496, 502t, 505, 533, 541, 555, 576, 587, 631
motor and sensory roots of, 527
nuclei of, 497, 502, 645
in oral cavity, 504
origin and functional fiber types of, 497t
sensory branches of, 515
trochlear (CN IV), 484, 485, 496, 500t, 527, 536t, 539, 541, 542, 543, 631
course of, 501
nucleus of, 497, 500, 644
origin and functional fiber types of, 497t
tympanic, 507, 508, 508t, 509, 561, 565
ulnar, 68, 316t, 318, 340t, 342t, 348t, 349, 354t, 363, 364, 365, 366, 367, 369, 370, 371, 372, 373, 374, 377
branches of
communicating, 353t
dorsal and palmar, 358, 359
injury to, *357*
sensory distribution of, 357, 359
utricular, 507, 567
utriculoampullary, 507
vagus (CN X), 25, 74, 82, 85, 86, 87, 89, 90, 91, 99, 106, 111, 127, 202, 484, 496, 510t, 559, 578, 586, 587, 602, 603, 607, 608, 609, 618, 619, 621, 631, 645, 649
branches in neck, 511t
course of, 511
nuclei of, 497, 510t
origin and functional fiber types of, 497t
sense associated with, 630
vestibular, 507, 560, 561, 566, 567
vestibulocochlear (CN VIII), 484, 485, 507, 558, 567, 587, 631
cochlear part, 496, 506t
membranous labyrinth innervation and, 567
nuclei of, 497
origin and functional fiber types of, 497t
senses associated with, 630
in temporal bone, 507
vestibular part, 506, 506t
zygomatic, 503, 535t, 536t, 576
Nerves (of region or organ)
of abdominal organs, 206, 207
of abdominal walls, 200
of back, 38
cutaneous innervation of, 39
of brachial plexus, 348t, 349
of cranium, 496–513, 624
cavernous sinus and, 527
classification of, 497t
nuclei of, 497, 497t
of diaphragm, 62, 63
of genitalia
female, 266
male, 269
of hard palate, 576
of heart, 99
of larynx, 603
of lower limb, superficial cutaneous, 459–460
of lumbosacral plexus, 448t, 449
lumbar part, 201, 448t, 450t, 450–453, 452t, 453t
sacral part, 448t, 454t, 455, 456t, 457t
of nasal septum and wall, 555
of neck
anterolateral, sensory and motor innervation, 597
nuchal region innervation, 596
spinal nerve branches, 576t
of penis, 268
of perineum
in female, 266
in male, 269
of pterygopalatine fossa, 535t
of retroperitoneum, 155t
of scrotum, 268
senses and, 630, 642t
of shoulder, posterior, 360–361
to the subclavius, 299t, 348t, 349, 350t
of tensor tympani, 533

Nerves (of region or organ) *(continued)*
of tensor veli palatini, 533
of thoracic cavity, 82
parasympathetic nervous system, 83t
sympathetic nervous system, 83t
of thoracic wall, 66–67
Nervous system
autonomic (visceral). *See* Autonomic nervous system (ANS)
central. *See* Central nervous system (CNS)
circuitry of, 638–639
divisions of, 638
fiber types in, 638
overview, 624–625
peripheral, 624
sensorimotor, 639
somatic, 638
Nervus intermedius, 504, 507, 567, 587, 631
Network (vascular)
calcaneal, 466
carpal
dorsal, 345, 375
palmar, 345
dorsal venous, 346, 358
of foot, 446
of elbow and lateral epicondyle, 369
patellar, 464
Neuroanatomy
autonomic nervous system, 648–649
brain and spinal cord, 626–633
arteries of, 636–637
veins of, 634–635
circuitry in, 638–639
of motor pathways, 641
of sensory pathways, 640
of sensory systems, 642–647
Neurocranium, bones of, 478t
Neurohypophysis, 628, 630
Nipple, 70, 71, 73
Node
atrioventricular (AV), 98, 99
sinoatrial (SA), 98, 99
Nodule, of semilunar valve, 95
Nose
arteries of, 554–555
bones of, 550–551
cavities and spaces of, 552, 550–555
muscles of, 492t, 554, 555
nerves of, 554–555
neurovasculature of, 554–555
regions of, 540, 552, 553
septum of, 498, 552, 554, 582, 583
arteries of, 554
deviated, *553*
mucosa of, 554
nerves of, 554, 555
paranasal air sinuses in, 552–553
wall of
arteries of, 554, 555
mucosa of, 555
nerves of, 555
Nosebleeds, *555*
Notch
acetabular, 217
angular, 156
articular, superior, 7
cardiac, 115
clavicular, 52, 54, 57
costal, 54
frontal, 477
intercondylar, 384, 406, 412
jugular, 52, 476
mandibular, 569
mastoid, 482, 556
radial, 304, 305, 308t
scapular, 55, 277, 279, 283, 284, 285, 350, 360, 361t, 365
sciatic
greater, 463
in female, 218
in male, 217
lesser, 463
in female, 218
in male, 217
suprajugular, 50
supraorbital, 477
suprasternal, 476
tentorial, 524
thyroid, superior, 477
trochlear, 304, 305, 307, 308t, 311
ulnar, 311
vertebral
inferior, 10, 11
superior, 7, 10, 11, 14
Nucleus/nuclei
caudate, 620, 626, 629t, 637
cochlear, 506, 645
of cranial nerves, 497, 500
abducent nerve (CN VI), 500t, 644
accessory (CN XI), 512t
facial nerve (CN VII), 504t
glossopharyngeal nerve (CN IX), 508, 509t
hypoglossal nerve (CN XII), 513t
oculomotor nerve (CN III), 500t, 644
trigeminal nerve (CN V), 502t, 508, 645
trochlear nerve (CN IV), 500t, 644
vagus nerve (CN X), 106, 127, 202, 510, 510t
vestibulocochlear nerve (CN VIII), 506t
Edinger-Westphal, 643
geniculate, 645
habenular, 498, 646, 647t
inferior collicular, 645
interpeduncular, 498, 646, 647t
of limbic system, 647
of medial geniculate body, 645
olivary, superior, 645
oval, 645
parabrachial, medial, 645
paraventricular, 629t
Perlia's, 643
premotor, 644
red, 641
salivatory, 497
inferior, 497, 508
superior, 497, 504, 505
of solitary tract, 497t, 504, 505, 508, 510, 645
spinal, of trigeminal nerve (CN V), 508, 645
subthalamic, 629t
suprachiasmatic, 642
tegmental, 498, 641
dorsal, 645, 646, 647t
terminal, 642
thalamic
anterior, 629t, 647, 647t
medial, 629t
posteromedial, ventral, 645
reticular, 629t
superior, 620
ventrolateral, 629t
of trapezoid body, 645
ventral, lateral, 641
vestibular, 644
inferior, 506
lateral, 506
medial, 506
superior, 506
Nucleus ambiguus, 497t, 508, 510, 512t
Nucleus cuneatus, 631, 640, 643
Nucleus gracilis, 631, 640
Nucleus prepositus hypoglossi, 644
Nucleus pulposus, 14, 15, 17, 22
disk herniation and, *15*
"Nursemaid's elbow," *309*

O

Occipital bone, 20, 21, 26, 31, 476, 477, 478t, 480, 481, 618
basilar part, 20, 21, 31
Olecranon, 24, 274, 275, 276, 292, 294, 303t, 304, 305, 369
fossa of, 280, 281, 307, 308
Olfactory system, 646
Olive
inferior, 630, 631, 641
superior, nucleus of, 645
Omentum
greater, 148, 149, 150, 151, 152, 153, 154, 157, 161, 162, 163, 164, 172, 180, 183, 188, 210
lesser, 148, 149, 150, 152, 154, 156, 157, 161, 164, 170, 180
Opacity, in lung radiography, 116
Opening
caval, 60, 61, 63, 85, 138, 139
saphenous, 147, 257, 460
Optic chiasm, 499, 527, 537t, 541, 560, 630, 633, 637, 642
lesion of, *643*
Optic cup, in embryonic brain, 625
Optic radiation, 499, 626, 642
lesion of, *643*

Orbit, 479, 552, 553
arteries of, 539, 540, 546, 547
axis of, 546
oculomotor palsy and, *539*
bones of, 536–537
cavities and spaces of, 536, 537, 542, 545
cranial nerves in, 541
floor of, 537, 544
margins of, 476, 479
muscles of, 538t, 538–539, 544, 545, 546, 548
actions of, 538
cranial nerves of, 500t
course of, 501
impaired coordination of, *539*
innervation of, 539
nerves of, 541, 548
neurovasculature of, 540–543
oculomotor nerve (CN III), 501
optic nerve (CN II) in, 499
organs of, 544–549
periorbita, 527, 541, 544
roof of, 544
structures surrounding, 537t
topography of, 542–543, 544
veins of, 540
Organ of Corti, 645
Orifice
cardiac, 152, 154, 155
of ejaculatory duct, 252
ileocecal, 162
pyloric, 156, 158
ureteral, 233
in female, 238, 240
in male, 239, 241, 270
urethral
external, 215, 227, 238, 246, 248, 266
in male, 250
internal, 233, 239
of urethral glands, 239
vaginal, 215, 246, 247, 248, 266
Oropharynx, 575, 580, 619
Os, uterine, 246, 247
external, 243, 244
internal, 243
Ossicles, auditory. *See* Ossicular chain
Ossicular chain
bones of, 562
in hearing, *563*
in tympanic cavity, 563, 564
Ossification center, 387
Osteophytes, spinal nerve compression and, *17*
Osteoporosis, *11*
femoral fractures and, *385*
Ostium
of maxillary sinus, 553
of sphenoid sinus, 568
uterine, 243
Outlet
pelvic, 220
in female, 221
measurements of, 220, 221
plane of, 221
thoracic, 75
Outpouching, cystic, of knee joint capsule, 409
Oval window, ossicular chain and, *563*
Ovary, 233, 237, 240, 240t, 242–243, 257, 261
arteries of, 176, 176t
ligaments of, 233, 238, 242, 243, 244,
lymphatic drainage of, 258, 259, 259t, 261
nerves of, 263
veins of, 184, 184t

P

Pain
acute abdominal, *149*
chronic neck, *17*
referred, *264*
sense of, 640
Palate
hard, 554, 560, 568, 575, 580
neurovasculature of, 576
soft, 554, 575, 580, 582, 583, 617, 618
muscles of, 575t, 585
Palatine bone, 478t, 480, 482, 534t, 537, 550, 551, 568
Paleocortex, 626
Palm of hand
arteries of, 345
lymphatic drainage of, 347
nerves of, 358, *372–373*
neurovaculature of, *373*
sensory innervation of, 327, 373
surface anatomy of, 275
veins of, 346, 358
Palsy
abducent nerve, *539*
hypoglossal nerve, unilateral, *579*
oculomotor nerve, *539*
trochlear nerve, *539*
ulnar nerve, *357*
Pancreas, 132, 149, 152, 153, 154, 156, 158, 159, 161, 164, 166, 169, 170, 171, 173, 180, 210, 211
arteries of, 176, 176t, 177, 178, 179
autonomic nervous system effects on, 202t, 648t
body of, 155, 164, 170, 171
head of, 155, 170, 171, 211
lymphatic drainage of, 192, 192t, 193, 197
neck of, 173
nerves of, 202, 202t, 203, 204, 205
tail of, 155, 170, 171, 173
uncinate process of, 149, 170, 171
veins of, 185, 188
Papilla
duodenal
endoscopy of, *159*
major, 158, 168
minor, 158, 168
ileal, 162
renal, 174
sublingual, 574, 579, 581
Paracolpium, 244
Paralysis
accessory nerve (CN XI), 512t
hypoglossal nerve (CN XI), 513
hypoglossal nerve (CN XII), 513t
Parietal bone, 476, 477, 478t, 479, 480, 481, 482, 553
Patella, 380, 382, 385, 390, 393, 397, 400, 401, 402, 406, 407, 410, 411, 412, 414, 415, 416, 417, 420, 468, 469
articular surface of, 414
radiography of, 407
Pathway
geniculate, 642
motor (descending tracts), 641
non-geniculate, 642
sensory (ascending tracts), 640
visual, for convergence and accommodation, 643
of visual system, 499, 642
lesions of, *643*
Pecten anus, 235, 235t
Pecten pubis, 218, 219, 223
Pedicle
of cervical vertebra, 7, 9
of thoracic vertebra, 7, 10
of vertebral arch, 20, 23
Peduncle
cerebellar, 630
inferior, 630, 631
middle, 630, 631
superior, 630, 631
cerebral, 626, 628, 630, 631, 633
of flocculus, 630
Pelvic brim, 220
Pelvis, 232. *See also individual organs*
arteries of, 254, 254t.
in female, 254, 254t, 255
in male, 254, 254t, 255
autonomic nerve plexuses in, 205, 262
autonomic nervous system effects in, 202t, 648t
bones of, 216–217, 218–219
pelvic girdle, 216
contents of
in female, 229
in male, 228
divisions of, 232t
false (greater) pelvis, 221, 232, 232t
childbirth and, *218*
fascia of, 245
pelvic inlet, 220
pelvic outlet, 220
perineum, 215, 232
true (lesser) pelvis, 221, 232

Pelvis *(continued)*
gender-specific features of, 220–221, 220t
ligaments of
pelvic girdle, 222–223
deep pelvis and fascia, 244–245
lymphatic drainage of, 192, 193, 193t, 258, 259, 259t, 447
parietal, 194
muscles of
pelvic floor, 224, 225, 226, 226t, 249
perineum, 225, 226, 227, 227t
nerves of. *See individual organs*
of trunk wall, 200, 201
organs of. *See individual organs*
peritoneal relationships in, 148t, 149
female, 230
male, 231
spaces of
in female, 229, 230–233, 232t
in male, 228, 231–233, 232t
veins of, 254, 254t, 255
Penis, 215, 227t, 232, 241, 241t, 250, 257, 260
arteries of, 250, 255, 257, 268, 269
body of, 250
bulb of, 231, 232, 233, 239, 241, 250
corpus cavernosum of, 239, 241, 250, 252, 253, 269, 271
tunica albuginea of, 250, 251, 268
corpus spongiosum of, 239, 241, 250, 252, 253, 269
crus of, 227t, 231, 232 233, 239, 250
dorsum of, 257
glans of, 145, 215, 241, 250, 251, 253, 257, 268
corona of, 204, 250, 268
innervation of, 202, 268
ligament of
fundiform, 136,
suspensory, 239, 257, 268
lymphatic drainage of, 447
MRI of, 252
nerves of, 250, 263, 268, 269
neurovasculature of, 268, 269
root of, 250
septum of, 250
tunica dartos of, 251
veins of, 250, 252, 254, 255, 257, 268, 269
Periarchicortex, 626
Pericardium, 63, 69, 88, 91, 92
fibrous, 74, 85, 87, 89, 90, 91, 99, 108, 109, 111, 112, 113
left atrium, 85
left ventricle, 85
posterior, 90
serous, 91, 111
parietal layer, 89, 90, 91
visceral layer, 89, 91
Perineum, 232, 232t
body of, 225, 226, 227
in female, 229, 230
in male, 228, 231
divisions of, 232t
innervation of
in female, 266
in male, 269
neurovasculature of
in female, 266–267
in male, 268–269
regions of
in female, 215
in male, 215
spaces of
in female, 230–233, 232t
in male, 231–233, 232t
Peritoneum, 148
parietal, 25, 105, 111, 148, 151, 155, 157, 159, 166, 171, 172, 173, 210, 228, 234
of abdominal wall, 146, 147
of abdominopelvic cavity, 148, 150, 151, 239
layers of, 148
of uterus, 247
relationships in, 230
in female, 232, 244
in male, 232
retroperitoneum, 172
visceral, 111, 148, 210, 253
of abdominopelvic cavity, 148, 150, 239
of bladder, 228, 237
layers of, 148
of rectum, 228, 229, 235
of uterus, 237, 242, 246
Pes anserinus, 390, 391, 393, 394, 402, 403, 416, 469
Petit, iliolumbar triangle of, 47
Petrous bone, 560
arteries of middle ear and, 565
Peyer's patches, 160
Phalanx/phalanges, 275, 276, 277, 317, 322t, 326, 382
distal, 317, 321, 326, 327, 333, 421, 424, 425, 426, 432, 440
middle, 326, 327, 333, 424, 425, 426, 440
proximal, 321, 326, 327, 332, 333, 424, 425, 426, 432, 434, 440
Pharyngotympanic (auditory) tube
infection in, *557*
muscles of, 585
Pharynx, 583, 586
arteries of, 581
cavities and spaces of, 586
internal organs of, 581–583
lymphatic drainage of, 582, 586
mucosa of, 583
muscles of, 584–585, 584t
nerves of, 581
neurovasculature of, 587
veins of, 581
Waldeyer's ring in, 582
structures in, 582t
Philippe-Gombault triangle, 639
Philtrum, 476
Pia mater, 524, 526
Pisiform, 275, 317, 322t, 324, 325, 327, 330, 370, 371
Plain film imaging. *See* Imaging
Plate(s)
cribriform, 483, 484, 485, 486, 498, 525, 543, 550, 551, 553, 554, 555, 560
of ethmoid bone
orbital, 616
perpendicular, 486, 537, 553
of palatine bone, 551
of pterygoid process, 487, 551, 568
lateral, 618
quadrigeminal, of mesencephalon, 628, 630, 631, 633
Pleura
cavity of, 51, 74, 74t, 75, 85, 110–111, 172
boundaries and reference points of, 110, 110t
lymph nodes of, 128
lymphatic dainage of
peribronchial network, 128
subpleural network, 128
movement in respiration, 122
projection onto thorax, 51
divisions of, 112
drainage of fluid from, *68*
innervation of, 113
parietal, 51, 67, 68, 85, 111
cervical part, 85, 104, 114
costal part, 63, 67, 69, 86, 87, 111, 112, 114
diaphragmatic part, 63, 67, 74, 85, 111, 112
injury to, pneumothorax and, *123*
mediastinal part, 63, 85, 89, 90, 91, 104, 111, 112, 113, 114
parts of, 111
recesses of, 111, 113
costodiaphragmatic, 111
costomediastinal, 111, 113
regions of, 111
visceral, 67, 68, 111, 112
Plexus
arterial
celiac, 204t
branches of, 203
pial vascular, 547
lymphatic
axillary lymphatic, 72
nerve
autonomic, 204, 204t, 208, 209
of abdomen, 205
of heart, 65, 99
of pelvis, 205, 262

brachial, 25, 82, 87, 99, 104, 348, 348t, 363, 607, 608, 609, 611
cords of. *See* Cord, of brachial plexus
carotid
internal, 484, 507, 509, 535, 541, 561
cervical, 530
branches of, 360, 596, 597
coccygeal, 449
deferential, 263, 265
esophageal, 106
gastric, 99, 207
anterior, 106, 203, 207
posterior, 106, 203
hepatic, 203, 207, 208
hypogastric, 265
inferior, 203, 204t, 207, 209, 262, 263, 270
superior, 204t, 207, 209, 262, 263
iliac plexus, 207, 262, 263
intermesenteric, 200, 204, 205, 207, 209, 262, 263, 265
lumbar, 200, 201, 448t, 449, 450t, 451
lumbosacral, 448t, 449
mesenteric, 202
inferior, 203, 204t, 207, 209, 262, 263
superior, 203, 204t, 208
ovarian, 204t, 205, 208, 262, 263, 265
pancreatic, 203, 207
parotid, 504, 505, 581
pharyngeal, 508
pulmonary, 99, 127
renal, 204t, 205, 207, 208, 264
sacral, 175, 178, 200, 205, 236, 245, 257, 262, 263, 266, 268, 449, 464
nerves of, 448t, 454t, 455, 456t, 457t
splenic, 203, 207, 208
suprarenal, 204t, 205, 207
testicular, 204t, 205, 207, 208, 262, 265
tympanic, 507, 509, 561, 577
ureteral, 205, 207, 262, 263, 264
venous
of anal canal, 235
basilar, 526
of bladder, 238
choroid, 628, 629t, 630, 632
hemorrhoidal, 235
pampiniform, 144, 145, 251, 257
of pharynx, 586
pterygoid, 522, 523t, 595
prostatic, 207, 262, 263, 254, 265, 268
rectal,186
inferior, 203, 263
middle, 203, 207, 262, 263
superior, 203
testicular, 144, 145
of thyroid, 603
uterine, 186, 247, 254, 255
uterovaginal, 270
vaginal, 247, 254, 255
vertebral, 210, 632
external, 37, 40, 41, 45, 65, 523, 523t
internal, 37, 40, 41, 45, 65
uterovaginal, 263, 265
vesical, 186, 207, 262, 264, 265, 268
vesicoprostatic, 270
of vestibular bulb, 267
Pneumatization, of paranasal sinuses, by age, 552
PNS. *See* Peripheral nervous system (PNS)
Poles
of cerebral hemispheres, 627
of kidneys
inferior, 174
superior, 174
occipital, 499
uterine, 242, 243
vascular, 242, 243
Pons, 630, 631, 633. *See also* Brainstem
in adult brain, 625
in brain development, 625t
in embryonic brain, 625
facial nerve (CN VII) and, 504
trigeminal nerve (CN V) and, 502
vestibulocochlear nerve (CN VIII) and, 506
Portal system, collateral pathways to heart of, 185
"Position sense," 644
Pouch
perineal
deep, 232t
superficial, 232t
rectouterine, 229, 230, 237, 242, 246, 270
rectovesical, 149, 228, 231, 239, 253
suprapatellar, 414, 415
vesicouterine, 230, 242, 246
Pregnancy
ectopic, *243*
nerve entrapment in, *450*
tubal, *243*
Premolar teeth, 572
Prepuce, 239, 253
Pressure. *See also* Blood pressure
intracranial, optic fundus examination and, *547*
intraocular, glaucoma and, *548*
in pleural cavity, 123
Pressure, sense of, 640
Process
alveolar, of mandible, 569
anterior, of malleus, 563
articular, of vertebrae, 6, 7, 7t, 8, 9
of calcaneal tuberosity
lateral, 424
medial, 424, 425
ciliary, 549
clinoid
anterior, 483, 487, 568
posterior, 483, 487
condylar, 569
coracoid, 55, 275, 277, 279, 282, 283, 284, 285, 286, 287, 289, 299, 302t, 354, 355, 365, 366
coronoid, 304, 305, 306, 307, 311, 317, 531, 569, 570, 591, 617
costal, of vertebrae 6, 7, 7t, 8, 9
of greater trochanter, 2
mammillary, 11
mastoid, of temporal bone, 18, 26, 27, 30, 33, 476, 477, 478, 480, 482, 556, *557*, 570, 574, 577, 593
of maxilla, 550, 551
muscular, of arytenoid cartilage, 598, 599, 600
palatine, of maxilla, 482, 537, 553, 568, 616, 620
posterior, 550
of posterior talus, 431
pterygoid, of maxilla, 482, 487, 534, 551, 568, 570, 576, 585
pyramidal, 568
of sacral articular tuberosity, 454
spinous, of vertebrae, 6, 7, 7t, 8, 9
styloid, 19, 478, 480, 482, 489, 556, 557, 558, 570, 574, 578, 579, 585
of radius, 275, 304, 305, 311, 319, 322, 323, 324, 325, 326, 331, 374
of temporal bone, 18
of ulna, 275, 304, 305, 311, 322, 323, 324, 325, 326
of vertebrae, 6, 7, 7t, 8
transverse, of vertebrae, 6, 7, 7t, 8
uncinate
of cervical vertebrae, 8, 9, 17, 486, 551, 553
of pancreas, 149, 170, 171
vocal, of arytenoid cartilage, 598, 599, 600
xiphoid, 52, 54, 57, 59, 60, 84, 134, 136, 141, 289
zygomatic, of temporal bone, 482, 556, 570
Processus vaginalis, 144
Promontory, sacral, 4, 5, 7, 12, 13, 134, 218, 219, 222, 223, 389, 390, 393, 399
Proprioception, 640, 644
Prosencephalon, 625t
Prostate, 146, 149, 228, 231, 232, 233, 239, 241, 241t, 245, 251, 252, 253, 255, 271
carcinoma of, *253*
hypertrophy of, *253*
nerves of, 264, 265
Protuberance
mental, 476, 569
occipital
external, 18, 19, 20, 21, 26, 27, 30, 476, 477, 480, 482
internal, 20
Pubic symphysis, 132, 133, 134, 214, 222, 223, 224, 226, 227, 236, 245
in female, 218, 220, 237, 244, 247
in male, 216, 219, 220, 220t, 236, 237, 239, 253, 271

Pubis, 217, 234, 245
in female, 219, 244, 270
in male, 237, 252
radiograph of, 217
Pulvinar, 630, 642
Puncta
inferior, 545
superior, 545
Pupil size, regulation of, 548, 549
Putamen, 621, 626, 629t, 637
Pyramid(s)
cerebellar, 630
decussation of, 631, 641t
of medulla oblongata, 631
medullary, 179
in motor pathway, 641
renal, 165, 174
of vermis, 630

R

Radial tear, *411*
Radiation
acoustic, 645
optic, 626, 642
lesions of, *643*
Radiography. *See* Imaging
Radius, 276, 277, 304–305, 376, 377
"Colles' fracture" of, *311*
fossa of, 280, 306, 309
head of, 275, 304, 305, 306, 309
lunula of, 311
radius fracture of, *311*
subluxation of, *309*
neck of, 304, 306
shaft of, 304, 305
styloid process of, 275, 304, 305
Ramus communicans/rami communicantes, 87
gray, 43, 67, 205, 262, 263, 649
white, 42, 67, 649
Ramus/rami
of bones
ischial, 216, 217, 218
ischiopubic, 238, 239
of mandible, 532, 569, 591, 617, 618
pubic
inferior, 217, 218, 231, 232, 233
superior, 216, 218
of spinal nerves, 40, 42, 43, 43t, 47
anterior
of head, 515, 517
of intercostal nerves, 67, 69
of neck, 596t, 597
of sacral plexus, 205, 454
in autonomic nervous system circuits, 649
meningeal, 43, 67
posterior, 360
of brachial plexus, 349
of head, 515
of intercostal nerves, 66
of neck, 596, 596t, 597
and spinal cord segments, 42
Raphe
anococcygeal, 224
mylohyoid, 574, 591
perineal, 215, 248
pharyngeal, 105, 585, 586
pterygomandibular, 584
Recess. *See also* Mortise
of 4th. ventricle, 633
axillary, 285, 286, 287
costal groove, 67
costodiaphragmatic, 67, 111, 112, 113, 114, 123, 173
costomediastinal, 101, 111, 113
duodenal
inferior, 151, 159
superior, 151, 159
hepatorenal, 172
inferior
ileocecal, 151
of omental bursa, 152
infundibular, 633
intersigmoidal, 151
lateral, 633
mesenteric, in infracolic compartment, 151
pineal, 633
piriform, 583, 601, 619
preoptic, 629t
retrocecal, 151
sacciform, 308, 309
sphenoethmoidal, 552t, 555
splenic, 170
of omental bursa, 152, 164
subpopliteal, 409, 414
superior
of omental bursa, 152
of tympanic membrane, 561
supraoptic, 628, 633
suprapineal, 633
Rectum, 149, 154, 155, 160, 161, 162, 163, 175, 186, 234–235, 235t, 236, 245
arteries of, 176, 176t, 177, 183, 254, 254t, 256
blood vessels of, 255, 256
lymphatic drainage of, 259, 259t, 260, 261, 447
nerves of, 185, 191, 263
regions of, 235t
veins of, 254, 254t, 256
Reference lines
of back
paravertebral, 3t
posterior, 3t
scapular, 3t
of pleural cavity
midaxillary, 110t
midclavicular, 110t
paravertebral, 110t
scapular, 110t
sternal, 110t
of thorax, 51
Referred pain, *264*
Renal medulla, 174
Renal pelvis, 174, 179
Respiration
diaphragm position during, 56
mechanics of, 122–123
thoracic cage during, 56
Respiratory compromise, conditions causing, *121*
Rete testis, 145, 251
Reticular formation, 498, 642
mesencephalic, 644
paramedian pontine (PPRF), 644
Retina, 544, 546, 549
Retinaculum
of ankle, 439
extensor, of foot
inferior, 439, 467, 469
superior, 439, 469
extensor, of hand, 338, 369, 374, 375
fibular
inferior, 439
superior, 439
flexor, of foot, 439, 466, 467
flexor, of hand, 330, 334, 335, 336, 356, 357, 368, 370, 371, 372, 373, 376
patellar
longitudinal, 402
lateral, 408, 408t
medial, 408, 408t
medial, 402
transverse
lateral, 408, 408t
medial, 408, 408t
tibialis anterior, 467
Retroperitoneum
structures of, 155t
Rhombencephalon, in brain development, 625t
Ribs, 2, 29, 31, 33, 52, 54, 55, 57, 59, 60, 61, 62, 67, 68, 74, 76, 78, 82, 87, 88, 111, 112, 122, 134, 141, 172, 277, 283, 287, 288, 299, 301t, 345, 349, 350, 351, 363, 364, 449
head of, 53t, 55
joint of, 57
movement axes of, 56
during respiration, 56
neck of, 55
shaft of, 53, 55
shoulder girdle, relationship to, 277
structural elements of, 53t
types of, 53, 53t
Ridge
mammary, of female breast, 70
marginal (epiphyseal ring), 14
petrous, 483
supracondylar
lateral, 280, 281, 307
medial, 280, 281, 306
Rima glottidis, 601, 601t
Rima vestibuli, 601

Ring
common tendinous, 501, 538, 539, 542
femoral, 147, 461
fibrous, of heart, 94
inguinal
deep, 137, 143t, 146, 147, 230
superficial, 132, 136, 141, 143t, 144, 147, 214, 268, 450, 451, 458, 460, 461
intercrural fibers of, 142, 143
crura of, 142, 143
umbilical, 141
venous, in spinal cord, 45
Root
of ansa cervicalis, superior and inferior, 577, 597, 609
in autonomic nervous system circuitry
anterior, 641, 649
posterior, 641, 649
cochlear, 506, 507, 558
median nerve, 364
lateral and medial, 356
nasociliary
to ciliary ganglion, 503
sensory, 541
of spinal nerve
anterior, 67, 631
posterior, 67
of tongue, 578, 583
of tooth, 572
of trigeminal nerve (CN V)
motor root, 527, 541, 631
sensory root, 527, 541, 631
Rotation, of distal radioulnar joint, 311
Rotator cuff, muscles of, 297t
Rugae
in stomach, 156
in vagina, 246, 247
Rupture, of cruciate ligaments, *413*

S

Sac(s)
dural, 15, 41
endolymphatic, 560, 566, 567
greater, omental, 150, 152
hernial, peritoneum of, *147*
lacrimal, 542, 545
lesser, omental. *See* Bursa(e), omental
Saccule, 507, 566, 644
laryngeal, 601
Sacrum, 2, 6, 13, 15, 35, 134, 163, 216, 223, 224, 234, 244, 351, 380, 388, 393
ala (wing) of, 7, 12, 13, 218, 219
apex of, 12
base of, 7, 13, 215, 218, 219
hiatus of, 218, 219, 223
kyphosis of, *4*
lateral part of, 7, 12, 13
promontory of, 12, 13
surface of
anterior, 13
articular, 12, 13
posterior, 13
wing of. *See* ala
Scala tympani, 566
Scala vestibuli, 566
Scalp, 481, 526
Scaphoid, 322t, 324, 325, 326, 327, 330, 331, 371, 374
fractures of, *323*
Scapula, 276, 277, 278, 279
inferior angle of, 279
neck of, 279
acromion of. *See* Acromion
neurovascular passageways of, 361t
ossified transverse ligament of, *278*
relationship to trunk skeleton, 277
spine of, 279
superior angle of, 279
Sclera, 544, 546, 548, 549
Scotoma, central, *643*
Scrotum, *144, 145*, 215, 241, 241t, 251, 253, 260
neurovasculature of, 268
Sectional anatomy
of abdomen
coronal section
of anterior abdominal wall, 146, 147
of muscles of abdominal wall, 138
midlongitudinal section
of kidney, posterior view, 174
midsagittal section
of abdominopelvic cavity, in male, 148, 149
of muscles of abdominal wall, 138
sagittal section
of inguinal region, 143t
of omental bursa (lesser sac), 152
of right kidney, 172
transverse section
of anterior abdominal wall, 146
of axial CT scan through L1, 211
of left kidney, 156
of liver, 156, 164
of liver through T12, 165
of omental bursa (lesser sac), 152
of pancreas, 156, 171
of spermatic cord, 144
of spleen, 156, 171
of stomach, 156
through L1, inferior view, 210
through L2, inferior view, 211
through T8, inferior and superior views, 139
through T12, inferior view, 210
of back
coronal section
of uncovertebral joints, 17
midsagittal
of cervical spine ligaments, 21
of lumbar spine, disk herniation, *15*
of spine, 5
of thoracolumbar junction, 22
sagittal section
of intervertebral disk, 14
transverse section
of cauda equina in situ, *41*
of cervical spine, 40
of sacral formina, 43
of sacrum, 13
of spinal cord, 38
of thoracolumbar fascia, 25
of vertebral column, 38
of head
coronal section
of cavernous sinus, through middle cranial fossa, 527
of ear, 558
of external auditory canal, 558
of meninges, 524
of orbit, bones of, 537
of paranasal sinuses, 552, 553
through anterior orbital margin, 616
through orbital apex, 617
of tongue, 578
midsagittal section
of cranial fossae, 483
of cranial nerve nuclei, 497
of dura mater, arteries of, 525
of oral cavity, 580
parasagittal section
of nasal cavity, 550, 554
of nasal septum, 554
of olfactory nerve (CN I), 498
sagittal section
of dural sinus, 526
of eyelids and conjunctiva, 544
of facial nerve (CN VII), 504, 577
of head, through inner third of orbit, 621
of head, through medial orbital wall, 620
of nasal cavity, 551, 555
of nasal wall, 555
of orbit, 544
of paranasal sinuses, 552
of pharyngeal tonsils, 582
of temporomandibular joint, 570
of tympanic cavity, 561
of vestibulocochlear nerve (CN VIII), 507
transverse section
of calvarial structure, 481
of cochlear canal, compartments of, 566
of eyeball, 546, 547
of facial nerve (CN VII) nuclei, 504
of glossopharyngeal nerve (CN IX) nuclei, 508
of hypoglossal nerve (CN XII) nuclei, 513
of lens, light reflection by, 549
of oculomotor nerve (CN III) nucleus, 500
through anterior segment of eye, 548
through median atlantoaxial joint, 618

Sectional anatomy
of head
transverse section *(continued)*
tonsillar fossa, 586
of trigeminal nerve (CN V) nuclei, 502
of vagus nerve (CN X) nuclei, 510
of vestibulocochlear nerve (CN VIII) nuclei, 506, 507
of lower limb
coronal section
of femoral head, arteries of, 445
of foot joints, 426
of foot neurovasculature, 471
of hip joint, 387
of subtaler joint, 428
of talocrural joint, 428
midsagittal section
of hip, thigh, gluteal regions, medial muscles, 393
of knee joint, 415
sagittal section
of knee joint, 415
of longitudinal arch stabilization, 435
of subtaler joint, 429
of talocrural joint, 429
transverse section
of femoral head, in hip joint, 385
of femoropatellar joint, 407
of fibula, 405of leg, 468t, 472–473
of sacrum, emerging spinal nerve, 454
of thigh, 472–473
of tibia, 405
of neck
coronal section
of vestibular and vocal folds, 601
midsagittal
of laryngeal cavity, 601
transverse section
at C5 vertebral body, 619
at C7/T1 vertebral junction, 619
of cervical fascia, 605
of thyroid and parathyroid glands, 602, 605
in neuroanatomy
coronal section
of diencephalon, 629
of gray and white matter, 624
of telencephalon, 626, 629
midsagittal section
of brain, 625
of brainstem, 630
of cerebellum, 630
of cerebrospinal fluid spaces, 632
of diencephalon, 628, 630
of limbic system structures, 647
of olfactory system with nuclei, 646
of ventricular system, 632–633
sagittal section
of ventricular system, 633
transverse section
of basal ganglia, 626
of gray and white matter, 624
of ventricular system, 633
of pelvis and perineum
coronal section
of anal canal, 235
of cardinal ligaments of uterus, 244
of diaphragm (pelvic), 138
of genital organs, female, 247
of muscles of pelvic floor, female, 230
of muscles of pelvic floor, male, 231
of pelvis, female, 232–233, 238
of pelvis, male, 232–233
of prostate, 252
of rectum, 235
of urethra, 238–239
of urinary bladder, 238–239
of urogenital triangle, 232
of uterine tube, 243
of uterus, 243
of vagina, 246
longitudinal section
of penis, 250
midsagittal section
of diaphragm (pelvic), 138
of false pelvis, 221
of innervation, female perineum and genitalia, 266
of neurovasculature, male perineum and genitalia, 268
of spaces, peritoneal and subperitoneal, 230–231
of true pelvis, 221
of urethra, 238–239
of urinary bladder, 238–239
of uterus, curvature of, 242
of vagina, 246
parasagittal section
of innervation of pelvis, 263
of pelvis, contents of, 228–229
sagittal section
of blood vessels of pelvis, 255
of epididymis, 145, 251
of prostate, 252–253
of spermatic cord, 144
of testis, 145t, 251
transverse section
of body of penis, 250
of fascia of pelvis, 245
of ligaments of pelvis, 245
of prostate, 252
of root of penis, 250
of spermatic cord, 144
of testis, 145t
through bladder and seminal glands, 270
through bladder and uterine cervix, 270
through prostate and anal canal, 271
of thorax
coronal section
of chest wall, for chest tube insertion, *68*
of costodiaphragmatic recess, 111
of diaphragm, 60
of intercostal nerves, course of, 67
of mediastinum, 75
of percutaneous liver biopsy, *112*
of peribronchial lymphatic network of pleural cavity, 128
of thoracic cavity, 74
midsagittal section
of mediastinum, 75, 84
parasagittal section
of mediastinum, 86–87
sagittal section
of breast, 71
of mediastinum, 91
transverse section
of aortic dissection, *77*
of costovertebral joints, 57
of heart, 101
of intercostal structures, 69
of lung relations, 114
of thoracic lymph nodes at level of tracheal bifurcation, 81
of mediastinum, 74
of parietal pleura, 111
of subpleural lymphatic network of pleural cavity, 128
of upper limb
coronal section
of shoulder joint, 284, 285
of subacromial and subdeltoid bursae, 287
of wrist and hand, 327
longitudinal section
of fingertip, 333
sagittal section
of anterior shoulder, 362
of glenoid cavity, 286
of humeroulnar joint, 307
of subacromial bursa, 286
transverse section
of arm, 376, 377
of carpal tunnel, 330 371
of extensor tendons, dorsal compartments, 338
of extensor tendons, extensor digitorum, 339
of forearm, 376, 377
of metacarpal, third, 333
of radius, 305
of shoulder, 363, 364t
of ulna, 305
of ulnar tunnel, 330, 371
Segmentation of lungs, 118, 118t, 119
arteries and veins of, 125t
bronchopulmonary segments of , 119
Sella(e)
diaphragma, 485
dorsum, 483, 487, 554
tuberculum, 487

Sella turcica, 21, 483
Semilunar valves, of heart, 95
Seminiferous structures, of testis, 241, 241
Senses, cranial nerves associated with, 642t
Sensorimotor system, 639
  cortical areas of, 639
  integration in, 639
Sensory system, 639
  balance, 644
  special qualities of, 642t
  visual, 642–643
Septal defects, *103*
Septum/septa
  dural, 524
  interalveolar, 121
  interatrial, 93, 95
  intermuscular
    of lower limb, 361, 366, 367
    of upper limb, 468, 473
  interventricular, 93, 95, 98, 101
    trabeculae carneae of, 93
  lingual, 578
  nasal, 498, 552, 554, 555, 582, 583, 616, 617
    deviated, *553*
  orbital, 542, 544, 545
  penile, 250
  plantar
    lateral, 436, 471
    medial, 436
  rectovaginal, 230, 246
  rectovesical, 231, 239, 270
  scrotal, 145, 149, 239, 253
  of sphenoid sinus, 568
  testicular, 145, 251
  vesicovaginal, 246
Septum pellucidum, 627, 629t, 633
Sesamoid, 323, 425, 427, 428, 441, 443
Sex glands, accessory, in male, 241t, 252
Sheath
  carotid, 25, 602, 605t, 619
  myelin, 624
  rectus, 137, 142, 146, 288, 298t
    anterior layer of, 135, 136, 141, 146
    posterior layer of, 137, 138, 141, 146, 147
  of tendon. *See* Tendon sheath
Shoulder
  arteries of, 345
  bones of, 278–279
  bursae of
    subacromial, 286–287
    subdeltoid, 287
  joints of, 282
    acromioclavicular, 283
    glenohumeral, 284–285
    scapulothoracic, 282
    shoulder girdle, 282
    sternoclavicular, 283
  girdle, relationship to ribs and sternum, 277
  muscles of
    anterior, 288–291, 296–299, 302
    posterior, 292–295, 300–301, 303
  nerves of. *See* Brachial plexus
  topography of
    anterior, 362–363
    posterior, 360
Sinus (es)
  coronary, 90, 92, 94, 96
  dural (venous), 481, 526, 526t
    carotid, 508
    cavernous, 522, 523, 523t, 526t, 527, 540, 541, 595
      orbit and, 537t
    confluence of, 522, 523, 524, 526, 632, 634
      in cranial cavity, 526
      at skull base, 483
      superior, 632
    intercavernous, anterior and posterior, 526t
    marginal, 526
    occipital, 526t, 634
    petrosal
      inferior, 484, 523, 526t, 634
      superior, 523, 526t, 634
      petrosquamous, 526
    sagittal, 526
      inferior, 485, 526t, 634
      superior, 485, 522, 523, 523t, 524, 526t, 595, 617, 632, 634
    sigmoid, 37, 507, 522, 523, 523t, 526t, 560, 561, 583, 586, 634
    sphenoparietal, 526t
    straight, 632, 634
    transverse, 37, 522, 523, 523t, 526t, 595, 621, 634
  lactiferous, 71, 73
  paranasal, 552, 553, 553t
    ethmoid, 537t, 551, 552, 552t, 553
    frontal, 481, 483, 498, 537t, 550, 551, 552t, 553, 554, 620, 621
    infection of, *553*
    maxillary, 536, 537t, 539, 544, 552t, 553, 568, 616, 617, 621
    sphenoid, 537t, 550, 551, 552t, 554, 555, 560, 620, 621
  pericardial
    oblique, 90
    transverse, 90, 91
  renal, 165, 174
  scleral venous, 547
Sinusitis, *553*
Skull
  bones of, 478–479, 478t, 480–481
  muscles of, origins and insertions, 490
Skull base
  bones of
    exterior, 482
    interior, 483
  muscles of, origins and insertions, 491
Smell
  cranial nerve associated with, 642t
  olfactory system for, 646
Snuffbox, anatomic, 374
Sole of foot, 381
  arteries of, 444
  muscles of, 436–437
    deep instrinsic, 442t, 443
    superior instrinsic, 441t
  nerves of, 457
  neurovasculature of, 470–471
  veins of, 446
Sound waves, ossicular chain and, *563*
Space
  endoneural, 632
  epidural, 15, 40, 41
  episcleral, 544
  intercostal, 112
    chest tube insertion via, *68*
    percutaneous liver biopsy via, *112*
  interscalene, 349, 363, 593
  lateropharyngeal, 586
  mesorectal, 245
  parapharyngeal, 586
  perineal, subcutaneous, 233
  pleural, 68, 123
    chest tube insertion into, *68*
  presacral, 245
  quadrangular, of axilla, 361, 361t
  rectoperitoneal, 231
  rectopubic, in male, 231
  rectorectal (presacral), 230
  rectovaginal, 245
  retro-inguinal, 461t
  retroperitoneal, 245
    pelvic, 238, 247
  retropharyngeal, 586, 602, 621
  retropubic, 245
    in female, 230
    in male, 239, 253
  retrorectal, 245
  subacromial, 282, 286–287
  subarachnoid, 21, 524, 632
  subglottic, 601t
  supraglottic, 601t
  transglottic, 601t
  triangular, of axilla, 361, 361t
  vesicovaginal, 245
Sphenoid bone, 478t, 479, 480, 483, 487, 534t, 537, 551, 553
Sphincter
  anal
    external, 227, 227t, 234, 235, 238
      innervation of, 227t
    internal, 235
  of bile duct, 168
  of hepatopancreatic ampulla, 168
  pupillary, 548, 643
    innervation of, 549
  pyloric, 156, 158

Sphincter *(continued)*
urethral
external, 227t
in female, 230
innervation of, 227t
in male, 231, 239, 252
Spine. *See also* Vertebrae;Vertebral column
cervical, 4, 7, 8–9
injuries in, *9*
lordosis of, *4*
curvatures of, *4*
development of, *4*,41
lumbar, 4, 7, 11
anesthesia adminstration via, *41*
disk herniation in, *15*
lordosis of, *4*
nerve entrapment and, *450*
osteoporotic, radiograph of, *11*
sacral, 4, 7, 12–13
coccyx and, 12–13
thoracic, 4, 7, 10
kyphosis of, *4*
Spine (of structure)
iliac
anterior inferior, 215, 217, 218, 219, 222, 227, 402
anterior superior, 214, 215, 216, 217, 218, 219, 222, 223, 380, 382, 386
posterior inferior, 216, 217, 218, 219, 222, 386
in female, 218
in male, 216, 217, 219
posterior superior, 216, 217, 218, 219, 222, 223, 224, 380, 382, 386, 388, 389, 397, 403, 463
superior inferior, in male, 216, 219
ischial, 216, 217, 218, 219, 222, 223, 224, 270, 386
of nose
anterior, 478, 479, 550, 568
posterior, 568
of scapula, 274, 275
origin and functional fiber types of, 497t
Spleen, 132, 152, 170, 171
autonomic nervous system effects on, 202t, 648t
arteries of, 177, 181
lymphatic drainage of, 192, 193, 197
nerves of, 202, 202t, 203, 204, 205, 206
veins of, 185, 189
Spondylolisthesis, traumatic, *9*
Spondylophyte, 15
Stapes, 558, 561, 562
conductive hearing loss and, *563*
Stenosis, of coronary artery, *97*
Sternum, 52, 53, 53t, 54, 55, 57, 59, 60, 61, 63, 69, 75, 84, 88, 90, 91, 101, 104, 122, 128
body of, 88, 100, 134, 138
manubrium of. *See* Manubrium
shoulder girdle, relationship to, 277
xiphoid process of. *See* Xiphoid process
Stomach, 5, 89, 106, 108, 109, 132, 149, 150, 152, 156, 157,159, 164, 166, 170, 180, 210
arteries of, 176, 176t, 177, 180
body of, 156, 157, 211
cardia of, 156, 157
curvature of
greater, 156, 157
lesser, 156, 157
fundus of, 156, 157
gastritis and, *157*
lymphatic drainage of, 192, 192t, 193, 196, 197
MRI of, 165
muscular layers of, 156
nerves of, 202, 202t, 203, 204, 205, 206
pyloric part, 156
quadrants of, 157
relations of, 156
ulcers of, *157*
veins of, 185, 188
Stria medullaris thalami, 628, 631, 645, 646
lateral olfactory, 629t
Stria terminalis, 646
Stroma
of iris, 548
of spermatic cord, 144
Substantia nigra, 629t, 641
Sulcus/sulci
anterolateral, 631
in brain, 625
calcanei, 431
calcarine, 627
central, 625, 627
artery of, 637
coronary, 92, 93
gluteal, 462
hypothalamic, 628
interventricular
anterior, 92
posterior, 92
lateral, 625, 627
palatine, 620
parietooccipital, 627
plantar
lateral, 470
medial, 470
postcentral, artery of, 637
posterolateral, 631
precentral, artery of, 637
for spinal nerve, 7, 8, 9, 16, 17, 20
telodiencephalic, 625
terminal, 578
Sulcus tali, 431
Surface anatomy
of abdomen, 132–133
of back, 2–3
of hand, 274–275
of head, 476–477
of lower limb, 380–381
of neck, 476 –477
of pelvis, 214–215
of perineum, 215
of thorax, 50–51
of upper limb, 274–275
Sustentaculum tali, 425, 427, 428, 429, 430, 431, 432, 434, 435, 443
Suture
coronal, 478, 481
incisive, 572
lambdoid, 477, 478, 480, 481
palatine
median, 482, 568, 572, 576
transverse, 482, 568, 572
sagittal, 477, 480, 481
sphenofrontal, 478
sphenoparietal, 478
sphenosquamous, 478
squamous, 478
Systole, ventricular, 94

T

Taenia, of fornix, 628
body of, 628
column of, 628
Taenia cinerea, 628
Talonavicular bone, 426
Talus, 405, 422, 423, 424, 425, 426, 427, 428, 429, 430, 431, 432, 433, 434, 435, 440
Tarsals, 382, 424
Tarsus
inferior, 542, 544
superior, 542, 544
Taste
cranial nerve associated with, 642t
gustatory system for, 645
tongue innervation and, 578
Teeth, 479, 480, 572–573
coding of, 572
dental panoramic tomogram of, 573
histology of, 572
principal parts of, 572
Tegmen tympani, 564
Tegmentum, 628
Telencephalon, 626–627
in brain development, 625t
divisions of, 626
internal structures of, 629t
Temperature, sense of, 640
Temporal bone, 477, 478t, 479, 480, 482, 483, 553, 556–557, 558, 561, 566
facial nerve (CN VII) in, 504
parts of, 480, 557
structures of, *557*
vestibulocochlear nerve in, 507
Tendon sheath
of ankle, 439
carpal and digital, 335
communication between, *335*
dorsal carpal, 338

common flexor, 334
of extensor carpi ulnaris muscle, 331
intertubercular, 286
in intertubercular groove, 287
Tendons (named)
Achilles', 381, 417, 418, 422, 429, 435, 439, 466, 467, 472. *See also* Tendon, calcaneal
biceps brachii, 274, 286, 290, 312, 318, 363, 365, 366, 367, 369, 376
biceps femoris, common, 417
brachioradialis, 319, 338
calcaneal, 418
calcaneus brevis, 440
central tendon of diaphragm, 60, 61, 63, 69, 138, 139
conjoint, 135
extensor, of hand, dorsal compartments for, 338, 338t
extensor carpi radialis brevis, 314, 338, 369, 371, 374, 375
extensor carpi radialis longus, 314, 327, 338, 369, 371, 374, 375
extensor carpi ulnaris, 311, 338, 371, 375
extensor digiti minimi, 338, 371, 375
extensor digitorum, of hand, 274, 333, 338, 371, 375, 381
dorsal digital extension, 314, 339
extensor digitorum brevis, 439, 469
extensor digitorum longus, 421, 439, 469
extensor hallucis brevis, 440, 469
extensor hallucis longus, 421, 439, 467, 469
extensor indicis, 338, 371
extensor pollicis brevis, 335, 338, 369, 371, 374, 375
extensor pollicis longus, 338, 369, 371, 374, 375
dorsal, 314
fibularis brevis, 420
fibularis longus, 420, 435, 437, 438, 443
fibularis tertius, 421
flexor carpi radialis, 318, 335, 336, 376
passage for, 330
flexor carpi ulnaris, 329, 335, 336
flexor digitorum brevis, 436, 437, 470, 471
flexor digitorum longus, 423, 437, 442, 443, 457, 470, 471
flexor digitorum profundus, 312, 332, 333, 334, 335, 336, 339, 369, 371, 372
flexor digitorum superficialis, 312, 332, 333, 334, 335, 336, 339, 368, 369, 371, 372
flexor hallucis longus, 436, 437, 457, 470, 471
flexor pollicis longus, 312, 313, 335, 336, 371
gracilis, 400
iliopsoas, 445
intermediate
of digastric muscle, 574
of omohyoid, 591
interossei, dorsal, of foot, 435
palmaris longus, 274, 318, 334, 370, 372, 376
plantaris, 418, 422, 467, 473
quadriceps femoris, 390, 402, 410, 414, 415
rectus femoris, 408
semimembranous, 403
of stapedius, 561
supraspinatus, 287
superior oblique, 538
tensor tympani, 561, 563
tibialis anterior, 438, 469
tibialis posterior, 423, 437, 438, 443
vastus intermedius, 408
Tendons (of region)
of hand, 274, 338–339, 338t
dorsal digital expansion, 321, 339
intertendinous connections, 314, 338
Tenia coli, 150, 154, 160, 161, 162, 228, 229, 234
Tension (valve) pneumothorax, *123*
Tentorium cerebelli, 485, 524, 525, 526, 620
Testis, 241, 241t, 251, 257, 260,
appendix of, 145, 251
arteries of, 176, 176t
blood vessels of, 145, 251
coverings of, 145, 145t, 241t
lobules of, 145
lymphatic drainage of, 258, 259, 259t, 261
mediastinum of, 145, 251
nerves of, 265
veins of, 184, 184t, 251
Test/testing
caloric, for vertigo diagnosis, *557*
of extraorbital muscles, 539
for small gluteal muscle weakness and, *455*
Thalamus, 499, 626, 628, 629t, 630, 637, 640, 644
pulvinar of, 630, 642
Thigh, 382
arteries of, 445, 462–465
bones of, 382, 384
gluteal region and, 465
muscles of, 390–397, 398t, 400t, 400–403, 401t, 402t, 403t
anterior, 390–393, 402t
medial
deep layer, 401t
superficial layer, 400t
posterior, 394–397, 403t
nerves of, 462–465
neurovasculature of, 462–465
topography of
anterior thigh, 464
posterior thigh, 465
veins of, 462–465
Thorax. *See also individual organs*
cavity of
arteries of, 76–77, 77t
lymphatic drainage of, 80–81, 108
mediastinum
divisions and contents, 74, 74t, 75, 84, 84t, 85, 86–87
nerves of, 82–83, 83t
organs of, 74, 74t, 84, 84t. *See also individual organs*
pleural cavities, 51,110, 111. *See also* Pleura
divisions and contents, 74, 74t
veins of, 78–79, 79t
chest tube insertion into, *68*
respiratory changes in, 56, 122
skeletal structure of, 52–53
walls of
arteries of, 64, 64t
bones of, 52–53, 53t, 54–55
joints of, 52, 55, 56–57
muscles of, 50, 58–59
nerves of, 66–67
neurovasculature of, 68–69
veins of, 65
Thromboembolus, from lower limb, *125*
Thumb
digital nerves of, 372
joints of, 326, 327
Thymus, 74, 84, 85, 86
Tibia, 404–405, 406
head of, 404
shaft of, 404
Tongue, 578–579, 580
lymphatic drainage of, 579
muscles of, 578
nerve injury to, 513t
unilateral hypoglossal nerve palsy, *579*
neurovasculature of, 579
structure of, 578
Tonsil, 630
infections of, *583*
lingual, 578, 580, 582t, 586, 601
palatine, 578, 580, 582, 582t, 586, 621
veins of, 523t
pharyngeal, 554, 555, 560, 580, 582, 582t, 583, 585
tubal. *See* Tonsil, pharyngeal.
Torticollis, 512t
Torus tubarius, 554, 580, 582
with lymphatic tissue, 580
Touch, sense of, 640
Trabeculae
arachnoid, 524
cancellous, 487
carneae, 93
septomarginal, 93, 95, 98
Trachea, 5, 25, 74, 75, 76, 77, 84, 85, 86, 88, 99, 100, 104, 105, 107, 108, 109, 119, *120*, 124, 126, 127, 128, 129, 598, 602
bifurcation of, 120
cervical part, 82, 104, 120
foreign body aspiration and, *120*
thoracic part, 104, 120
Tract
cingulohippocampal, 647
corticospinal
anterior, 641t
lateral, 641t

Tract *(continued)*
of extrapyramidal motor system, 641t
iliopubic, 147
iliotibial, 381, 390, 391, 392, 394, 397, 398, 399, 416, 417, 455, 464, 465, 472, 473
mammillothalamic, 647
olfactory, 498, 626, 646
olivospinal, 641t
optic, 629t, 642, 643
lesion of, *643*
termination of, 499
pyramidal, 641t
reticulospinal, 641t, 644
rubrospinal, 641t
semi-iliotibial tendinosus, 418
of sensorimotor system
ascending (afferent), 639
descending (efferent), 639
solitary, nucleus of, 645
spinocerebellar
anterior, 630, 640t
superior, 640t
spinothalamic
anterior, 640t
lateral, 640t
tectospinal, 641t
tegmental, central, 630
thalamocingular, 647
vestibulospinal, 641t
lateral, 644
Tragus, of auricle of ear, 476, 559
Trapezium, 317, 322t, 324, 325, 326, 327, 371, 374
Trapezoid, 322t, 324, 325, 326, 327, 330, 331
Tree, bronchial
conditions associated with, *121*
conducting portion of, 121
divisions of, 121
movement during respiration, 110
neurovasculature of, 126–127
respiratory portion of, 121
Trendelenburg's test, small gluteal muscle weakness and, *455*
Triangle(s)
anal, 215
carotid, 604t, 609
caval, 61
cervical
anterior, 606–607
posterior, lymph node in, 615
clavipectoral, 50, 274
femoral, 464
Hesselbach's, 143, 146, 147
iliolumbar (of Petit), 47
Killian's, 105
lateral cervical, neurovascular structures of, 363
lumbar, 2
fibrous (of Grynfeltt), 47
internal oblique, 24
lumbocostal (Bochdalek's), 60, 61, 139
muscular, 604t
of neck regions and divisions, 604t
occipital, 604t, 612
omoclavicular (subclavian), 604t
Philippe-Gombault, 639
sternocostal, 61, 139
submandibular (digastric), 604t
submental, 604t
suboccipital, 613
urogenital, 215, 232
Trigone
collateral, of left lateral ventricle, 633
femoral, 380
fibrous
left, 94
right, 94
olfactory, 626, 646
urinary, 238, 239
Triquetrum, 275, 322t, 324, 325, 327, 330, 331, 371
Trochanter
greater, 380, 382, 384, 385, 386, 387, 388, 389, 394, 399, 400, 401, 402
lesser, 141, 382, 384, 386, 388, 389, 399, 400, 401, 402, 445
Trochlea
of femur, radiography of, 407
of humerus, 280, 281, 306, 307, 309
Trunk
arterial
brachiocephalic, 74, 76, 77t, 80, 82, 86, 88, 89, 92, 99, 104, 114, 125, 126, 344, 349, 511, 587, 608
costocervical, 36, 345
pulmonary, 88, 89, 90, 91, 92, 93, 99, 100, 102, 103, 104, 114, 124, 125
thyrocervical, 36, 64, 76, 107t, 344, 345, 363, 517, 594, 603, 607, 608, 619
lymphatic
bronchomediastinal
left, 80, 81, 129
right, 81, 129
coronary
left, 108
right, 108
jugular, 80
left, 108
lumbar
left, 80, 258, 261
right, 80, 258, 261
lumbosacral, 263, 449
intestinal, 258
subclavian, 80
left, 80, 81, 129
right, 80, 81, 129
nerve
brachial plexus, 348–357
lower, 349
middle, 349
upper, 349
celiac, 62, 63, 76, 80, 107, 176, 176t, 177, 180, 181, 211, 236
anastomoses of, 177
distribution of, 180
to pancreas, duodenum, and spleen, 181
to stomach, liver, and gallbladder, 180
sympathetic, 63, 82, 86, 87, 99, 106, 111, 201, 202, 205, 262
in anterior cervical region, 607
of deep lateral cervical region, 609
interganglionic, 205, 262
lumbar ganglia of, 207, 262, 263
in pharyngeal space, 586, 587
right, 106
sacral ganglia of, 207, 262
vagal
anterior, 82, 91, 106, 205, 206, 208
hepatic branch, , 206, 208
pyloric branch, 206, 208
posterior, 91, 106, 205, 206, 207, 208
celiac branch, 205, 206, 207, 208
hepatic branch, 206, 207
Trunk (of body), hip bones relation to, 383
Tube
neural, 625t
pharyngotympanic, 507, 558, 560, 561, 564, 565, 585, 620, 621
uterine, 229, 230, 233, 237, 240, 240t, 242, 243, 244, 255, 257, 261
ampulla of, 243
isthmus of, 243
Tuber cinereum, 628
Tubercle
anterior, 7, 8, 9, 16, 17, 20, 31
articular, 556, 570, 571
conoid, 278
corniculate, 583, 587, 600, 601
costal, 52, 53t, 55, 57
cuneiform, 583, 587, 600, 601
dorsal, of radius, 304, 305, 311, 314, 321, 324, 325, 331
genial
inferior, 569
superior, 569
greater, of humerus, 275
iliac, 216, 217, 219, 222
infraglenoid, 279, 284, 303t
lesser, of humerus, 275
mammillary
in embryonic brain, 625
mental, 569
of nucleus cuneatus, 631
of nucleus gracilis, 631
pharyngeal, 482
posterior, 7, 8, 9, 16, 17, 20
of atlas (C1), 18, 21, 30
pubic, 132, 134, 141, 142, 214, 218, 222, 224, 380, 386, 461
scalene, 55, 593
of scaphoid, 275, 323, 325, 330

supraglenoid, 279, 284, 302t
of trapezium, 317, 323, 324, 325, 330
Tuberculosis, *117*
Tuberosity
of 5th metatarsal, 380, 382, 420, 423, 424, 425, 427, 428, 434, 436, 437, 439, 440, 441, 443
calcaneal, 380, 422, 423, 424, 425, 428, 431, 436, 441
lateral process of, 424
medial process of, 424, 425
of cuboid bone, 423, 425, 441
deltoid, 280, 296
of digitorum brevis, 439
of digitorum longus, anterior, 439
of distal phalanx, 323, 326, 333
gluteal, 384, 386, 399, 403
greater, 2, 50, 350
of humerus, 280, 281, 283, 284, 285, 286, 289, 297, 298, 301t
iliac, 134
in female, 218
in male, 215, 216, 219
ischial, 2, 222, 223, 224, 226, 227, 380, 382, 386, 389, 394, 399, 403, 461, 462
in female, 215, 218, 220, 225, 266, 267
in male, 215, 216, 219, 220, 225, 269, 271
lesser, 50
maxillary, 534t
of medial tibial condyle, 380
navicular, 380, 427
radial, 291, 302t, 304, 305, 306, 309, 317
sacral, 12, 13, 223
of sacral articular process, 454
for serratus anterior, 55
tibial, 382, 397, 401, 402, 404, 406, 408, 410, 413, 416, 421
ulnar, 302t, 304, 305, 306, 309, 317
Tumor metastasis
in breast cancer, *73*
to cervical lymph nodes, *614*
Tunica albuginea, 145, 250, 251, 268
Tunica dartos, 144, 145, 145t, 251
Tunica vaginalis, 144, 145, 145t, 251
Tunnel
carpal, 324, 330, 370, 371
ligaments of, 330
structures of, 371
for fibularis longus tendon, 430
radial, 353, 367
tarsal, 467
ulnar, 318, 330, 370, 371, 372
structures of, 371

U

Ulna, 276, 277, 304, 376, 377
head of, 275, 311
in humeroulnar joint, 307
olecranon of, 303t, 304, 305
shaft of, 275, 304, 305
styloid process of, 275, 304, 305, 311, 322, 323, 324, 325, 326
Umbilical cord, 103
Umbo, 561
Uncus, 498, 620
Upper limb. *See* Limb (upper)
Ureter(s), 236–237
in female, 237, 238
in male, 236,237
wall structure of, 239
Urethra, 186
ampulla of, 250
in female, 238
fossa of, navicular, 250, 253
lymphatic drainage of, 195, 258, 259, 259t, 261, 447
in male, 239
membranous part, 233, 250, 252
preprostatic part, 250
prostatic part, 250, 252, 271
spongy part, 232, 239, 241, 250, 252, 253
wall of, 239
Urinary bladder. *See* Bladder, urinary
Urinary tract, autonomic nervous system effects on, 202t, 648t
Urogenital system, in female, 240
Uterus, 229, 230, 232, 237, 240, 240t, 242–243, 244, 261
autonomic nervous system effects on, 202t, 648t
body of, 238, 242, 243, 246
longitudinal axis of, 242
cervix of, 233, 238, 240, 243, 244, 247, 270
supravaginal part, 243, 246
vaginal part, 243, 246
curvature of, 242
flexion of, 242
fundus of, 230, 233, 238, 242, 243, 247, 257
ligaments of, 244, 245
lymphatic drainage of, 258, 259, 259t, 261, 447
nerves of, 263, 265
and uterine tube, 243
version of, 242
Utricle, 507, 566, 644
Uvula, 555, 560, 575, 580, 582, 583
Uvula vermis, 630

V

Vagina, 186, 215, 229, 230, 232, 233, 238, 240, 240t, 243, 244, 246, 247
longitudinal axis of, 242
lymphatic drainage of, 258, 259, 259t, 261
nerves of, 265
posterior commissure of, 215
structure of, 246
vestibule of, 227, 232, 233, 246, 247
wall of
anterior, 243, 246
posterior, 246, 247
Vallecula, 630
Valves
anal, 235
of foramen ovale, 93
of heart. *See* Cardiac valves
of Kerckring, 158
Valvular heart disease, heart sounds and, 94t, *95*
Vasa recta, 182
Vasocorona, spinal cord, 44
Veins (named), 358
alveolar, inferior, 616, 617
anastomotic
inferior, 634
superior, 634
angular, 522, 523t, 528, 529, 532, 540, 542, 595
antebrachial, median, 346, 358, 367
anterior
of right ventricle, 96
of septum pellucidum, 634
appendicular, 185, 190
arcuate, 174
articular, posterior, 595
auditory, internal, 567
auricular, posterior, 522, 523t
axillary, 65, 68, 70, 346, 363, 364, 365, 366
azygos, 37, 45, 62, 63, 65, 69, 75, 78, 79, 80, 84, 85, 86, 101, 107, 107t, 109, 127, 165, 184t, 185
basilar, 634
basilic, 72, 274, 346, 358, 367
median, 346, 367
basivertebral, 45
Boyd's, 447
brachial, 72, 346, 364, 365, 367, 377
brachiocephalic, 79t
left, 37, 45, 62, 74, 78, 79, 80, 84, 86, 89, 104, 107t, 108, 114, 124, 127, 522, 595, 603
right, 37, 65, 74, 78, 79, 80, 88, 89, 104, 107, 108, 124, 127
bridging, 524, 526, 634
ostia of, 524
bronchial, 127
cardiac
anterior, 96t
great, 96, 96t
left posterior, 96t
middle, 96, 96t
oblique, 96
small, 96, 96t
cecal, 190, 191
cephalic, 65, 68, 274, 346, 358, 362, 363, 364, 367
accessory, 346, 358
median, 346
cerebellar
medial and lateral, 634
superior, 634, 635

Veins (named) *(continued)*
cerebral, 524
anterior, 634
great, 526, 634
inferior, 526
internal, 634
middle
deep, 634
superficial, 634
superior, 526, 634
cervical
deep, 45, 595
superficial, 610, 611
choroidal, inferior, 634
clitoral
deep, 267
dorsal, deep, 247, 267
Cockett's, 447
colic, 185
left, 155, 159, 171, 173, 185, 191
middle, 150, 153, 160, 185, 188, 189, 190, 191
right, 185, 190, 191
communicating, anterior, 634
cremasteric, 144, 251
cubital, 346
deep median, 346, 367
median, 274, 346, 358, 367
cystic, 185
digital
dorsal, 358
palmar, 346
diploic, 481, 524
Dodd's, 447
emissary, 481, 484, 526
condylar, 484, 523t, 621
posterior, 618
mastoid, 523t
occipital, 523t
parietal, 523t
epidural
lateral, 45
medial, 45
epigastric, 458
inferior, 143, 146, 147, 150, 154, 160, 175, 185, 186, 236, 257
superficial, 65, 446, 460
superior, 68, 185
esophageal, 107, 185, 188
ethmoidal
anterior, 536t
posterior, 536t
facial, 522, 523, 528, 529, 530, 531, 532, 533, 540, 542, 581, 595, 603, 609
common, 531, 532, 609
deep, 523
femoral, 65, 142, 143, 144, 146, 147, 178, 186, 257, 268, 270, 271, 446, 447, 458, 460, 461, 464, 473
anterior, cutaneous, 446, 460
circumflex
lateral, 446
medial, 446
deep, 446
femoropopliteal, 446
fibular, 446, 468
gastric
left, 107, 107t, 185, 188, 189, 190, 191
right, 185, 188, 189, 190, 191
short, 185, 188, 189
gastroomental
left, 185, 188, 189
right, 185, 188, 189, 190, 191
genicular, 446
gluteal
inferior, 186, 256, 462, 463
superior, 186, 255, 256, 462, 465
hemiazygos, 37, 45, 62, 63, 65, 79, 80, 87, 107, 107t, 111, 127, 184t, 185
accessory, 37, 65, 78, 79, 79t, 80, 87, 107, 107t, 127
hepatic, 79, 88, 103, 155, 159, 166, 167, 168, 169, 171, 173, 184t, 186, 188, 189
ileal, 185, 190, 191
ileocolic, 190, 191
iliac
circumflex
deep, 146, 186, 257
superficial, 65, 446, 458, 460
common, 45, 65, 79, 149, 155, 184, 184t, 185, 186, 191, 228, 238, 254, 255, 256, 257, 447
external, 37, 45, 65, 175, 186, 230, 233, 236, 237, 238, 247, 254, 255, 256, 257, 446, 447, 460, 464
internal, 37, 45, 175, 186, 236, 245, 254, 255, 256, 257, 268, 447
anterior trunk of, 175, 236, 255
infraorbital, 536, 536t, 540
intercapitular, 346, 358
intercostal, 45, 67, 68, 71, 86, 87, 111, 112, 210
anterior, 37, 65, 79t
left superior, 79t, 87
posterior, 37, 47, 62, 65, 69, 79, 79t, 107
right superior, 79t
right supreme, 78
interlobar, of kidney, 174
interosseous, of upper limb,
anterior, 346, 377
posterior, 377
interpeduncular, 634
intervertebral, 37, 45
jejunal, 185, 190, 191
jugular
anterior, 522t, 595, 606
external, 65, 68, 79t, 107, 362, 363, 522t, 529, 587, 595, 606, 607, 609, 610, 611, 619
left, 62, 78
impeded flow in, 595
internal, 25, 37, 45, 65, 72, 74, 79t, 80, 107, 108, 363, 484, 507, 522t, 523, 530, 531, 560, 561, 579, 586, 587, 595, 602, 603, 606, 607, 608, 609, 614, 618, 619, 634
left, 62, 78, 85, 88, 104, 124
right, 79, 124, 129
labial, posterior, 267
labyrinthine, 484
lacrimal, 540
laryngeal
inferior, 587, 603
superior, 603
lingual, 579, 595
deep, 579, 617, 620
lumbar, 37, 45, 63, 78, 79, 184t, 185, 186, 189
marginal
left, 96
right, 96
maxillary, 522, 523, 595
medullary
posteromedian, 635
transverse, 635
meningeal, middle, 526
mesenteric
inferior, 185, 189, 190, 191, 256
superior, 155, 158, 159, 169, 170, 171, 173, 181, 185, 188, 189, 190, 191, 210, 211
metatarsal, plantar, 446
musculophrenic, 63t, 79t
nasal, dorsal, 540, 542
obturator, 146, 186, 255, 256, 257, 270
occipital, 522, 523t, 529, 595, 612
internal, 634
ophthalmic, 540
inferior, 522, 523t, 535t, 536, 540, 543, 595
superior, 484, 501, 522, 523t, 526, 536, 540, 542, 543, 595
ovarian, 184t, 237, 238, 242, 243, 245
left, 173, 175, 184, 186, 187, 189, 236, 257
right, 175, 184, 186, 187, 236, 255
palatine, external, 523
palmar metacarpal, 346
pancreatic, 185
pancreaticoduodenal, 188, 189, 190
inferior, 185
superior posterior, 185
paraumbilical, 146, 185
penile
bulbar, 268
deep, 254, 268
dorsal, 250
deep, 255, 257, 268, 269
superficial, 250, 253, 268
perforator, 346, 367

pericardiacophrenic, 63t, 74, 79t, 85, 90
pericardial, 79t
periumbilical, 65, 185
petrosal, 634
  superior, 635
phrenic
  inferior, 63t, 173, 175, 184, 184t, 186, 187, 236
  superior, 63t, 79t
plantar
  lateral, 446, 470, 471
  medial, 446
pontine
  anterolateral, 635
  anteromedian, 635
  transverse, 635
pontomesencephalic, 635
popliteal, 407, 446, 447, 465, 466, 467
portal, 155, 159, 165, 166, 167, 168, 173, 180, 181, 182, 185, 188, 189, 190, 191, 196, 210, 211, 256
  cancer metastases and, *185*
pudendal
  external, 446, 458, 460
    in male, 257, 268, 460
  internal, 186, 232, 234, 256, 463
    in female, 255, 267
    in male, 255, 268, 269, 271
pulmonary, 88, 99, 125, 125t
  inferior, 125t
    left, 124, 125
    right, 124, 125
  left, 79, 85, 87, 88, 90, 91, 92, 93, 96, 102, 103, 124
  right, 79, 85, 88, 90, 92, 93, 96, 104, 114, 124
  superior, 125t
    left, 93, 124, 125
    right, 124, 125
radial, 346
radicular
  anterior, 45
  posterior, 45
rectal
  inferior, 185, 254, 255, 256, 267
  middle, 185, 186, 255, 256
  superior, 185, *185*, 191, 255, 256
renal, 173, 174, 175, 184, 184t, 185, 186, 187
  segmental, 174
retinal, central, 547
retromandibular, 522, 523, 586
sacral
  lateral, 186, 255
  medial, 186, 236
  median, 175, 184t, 256, 257
saphenous
  accessory, 446, 458
  great, 65, 147, 446, 447, 458, 460, 466
  small, 446, 447, 458, 466, 467
scrotal
  anterior, 268
  posterior, 254, 255, 268
sigmoid, 185, 191, 256
spinal, 45, 484
  anterior, 45
  posterior, 45
splenic, 149, 155, 170, 171, 173, 181, 185, 188, 189, 190, 191, 210
subclavian, 37, 45, 65, 70, 74, 79t, 107, 185, 346, 362, 363, 522, 595, 607
  left, 62, 78, 80, 85, 87, 88, 104, 114, 124
  right, 78, 79, 80, 124, 129, 611
subcostal, 37, 45, 65
submental, 522
sulcal, 45
superficial palmar, 371
superficial thoracoepigastric, 65
suprarenal, 184t
  inferior, 187
  left, 173, 175, 184, 186, 187, 189, 236
  middle, 187
  right, 174, 175, 184, 186, 187, 236
suprascapular, 522
supratrochlear, 540
temporal
  deep, 523
  superficial, 522, 523t, 528, 529, 532, 533, 581, 595
testicular, 144, 145, 146, 184t, 251, 257
  left, 173, 175, 184, 187, 189, 236
  right, 175, 184, 187, 236
thalamostriate, 634
thoracic
  internal, 37, 63, 65, 68, 69, 70, 74, 79t, 112, 113, 185, 210
    right, 78
  lateral, 68, 70, 72
thoracodorsal, 346
thoracoepigastric, 65, 68, 346
  superficial, 65
thymic, 79t
thyroid
  inferior, 62, 78, 79, 79t, 107, 107t, 127, 603, 608
  middle, 603, 608
  superior, 522, 530, 531, 595, 603, 608, 619
tibial
  anterior, 446, 469
  posterior, 428, 446, 447
transverse cervical, 362
ulnar, 346
uterine, 186, 254, 255, 257
vertebral, 40, 595, 619
  right, 45
vesical, 255, 257
  inferior, 186, 255
  superior, 255
vorticose, 547
Veins (of region or organ)
  of abdomen, 184
  of azygos system, 79
    superior vena cava and, 78
  of back, 37
  of brain, 634–635
    basal venous system, 635
  of brainstem, 635
  of cochlear aqueduct, 567
  of diaphragm, 63t
  of ductus deferens, 144, 146, 251
  of duodenum, 188
  of eyeball, 547
  of genitalia
    female, 257, 267
    male, 257
  of head and neck
    anastomotic, 523t
    deep, 523
    principal superficial, 522t
  of heart, 96
    divisions of, 96t
  of inguinal region, 460
  of inner ear, 567
  of larynx, 603
  of lower limb, 459
  of mediastinum, 84t
  of neck, 595
  of occiput, 523
  of orbit, 540
  of palatine tonsil, 523t
  of pancreas, 189
  of pelvis, 254t
    in female, 254, 255
    in male, 254, 255
  of penile bulb, 254
  of penis, 268
  of posterior arch, of foot, 447
  of pterygopalatine fossa, 535t
  pulmonary, 124, 125, 125t
    arteriogram of, 125
    tributaries of, 125t
  of rectum, 256
  of retroperitoneum, 155t
  of round window, 567
  of scalp, 526
  of scrotum, 268
  of spinal cord, 45
  of spleen, 189
  of stomach, 188
  of testis, 251
  of thigh, 473
  of thoracic cavity, 78–79
  of tracheobronchial tree, 127
  of upper limb, 275, 346
    lymph vessels and, 347
  of vestibular aqueduct, 567
  of vestibular bulb, 267
Velum, superior medullary, 630, 631

Vena cavae, 99
inferior, 25, 37, 45, 61, 62, 63, 65, 69, 75, 78, 79, 88, 90, 91, 92, 93, 96, 109, 124, 152, 155, 156, 158, 159, 164, 165, 166, 168, 169, 170, 171, 173, 175, 178, 180, 181, 182, 183, 185, 186, 187, 188, 189, 190, 191, 193, 194, 196, 201, 210, 211, 236, 254, 256, 257, 259, 447
in caval opening, 85
tributaries of, 184, 184t
superior, 37, 45, 51, 62, 65, 74, 75, 78, 79, 80, 85, 88, 89, 90, 91, 92, 93, 96, 98, 99, 100, 104, 107, 108, 109, 114, 116, 124, 127, 185
impeded flow in, *595*
thoracic tributaries of, 79t
Venipuncture, *346*
Ventricles
of brain
3rd., 628, 629t, 633, 637
4th., 630, 631, 633
CSF circulation and, 632
lateral, 499, 620, 626, 629t, 633, 637, 642
of heart
diastole in, 94
left, 88, 89, 92, 93, 96, 98, 100, 101, 102, 103, 108, 116, 124
right, 88, 89, 92, 93, 96, 98, 100, 102, 103, 108, 124
systole in, 94
laryngeal, 601
Ventricular septal defect (VSD), *103*
Vermiform appendix, 132, 162
Vermis, 630
folium of, 630
pyramid of, 630
Vertebra prominens (C7), 2, 3, 6, 8, 17, 20, 21, 31, 35, 40, 42, 277, 288, 300, 301t, 349, 354, 476, 477, 619
spinal nerve and, 17
spinous process of, 5, 8, 27, 33, 619
and T1 vertebral junction, 619
transverse process, 27
Vertebrae, 4, 6, 7, 8, 9, 10, 11, 12, 13
body of, 6, 7, 7t,
cervical, 4, 7, 7t, 8–9
C1. *See* Atlas (C1)
C2. *See* Axis (C2)
C7. *See* Vertebra prominens (C7)
joints of, 16–17, 16t, 18–19
ligaments of, 20–21, 20t
lumbar, 4, 7t, 8–9, 11, 15, 277
processes of, 6, 7, 7t
sacral, 4, 7, 7t, 12–13
structural elements of, 7, 7t
thoracic, 4, 7, 7t, 8–9, 10, 52–53, 277, 289, 354
spinal cord segment and, 127
spinal nerve and, 619
Vertebral column, 4–5, 40. *See also* Spine
bones of, 4, 6–7
intervertebral disk in, 14
herniation of, posterior and posterolateral, *15*
joints of, 16–17
craniovertebral, 16t, 18–19
regions of, 4
vertebrae comprising, 6
Vesica urinaria, 245
Vesicle, seminal. *See* Gland, seminal
Vestibular system, 644
Vestibule, 240, 248
of auditory canal, 558, 560
labial
inferior, 620
superior, 620
laryngeal, 619
nasal, 555
oral, 580, 586, 616
Vincula
brevia, 339, 372
longum, 339, 372
Viscerocranium, bones of, 478t
Vision, cranial nerve associated with, 642t
Visual field, 499, 642, 643
Visual system, 642–643
pathways, lesions of, *643*
pathways of, 642, 643
reflexes of, 643
Vomer, 478t, 479, 482, 537, 550, 553, 568, 576, 616
VSD (ventricular septal defect), *103*
Vulva, 240t

W

“Whiplash” injury, *9*
White matter, 626
cerebral arteries distribution areas and, 637
in CNS, 624
of spinal cord, 639
Window
oval, 507, 561, 562, 566, 567
round, 507, 566, 567
vein of, 567
Wing, iliac. *See* Iliac, ala
Wrist. *See also* Tunnel, carpal
bones of, 322–323, 324–325
carpal region, 370–371
carpal tunnel, 372
joints of, 326–327
ligaments of, 328–331
neurovasculature of, anatomic snuffbox, 374
surface anatomy of, 275
ulnar tunnel of, 370, 371

Z

Zona orbicularis, 445
Zygomatic bone, 476, 478, 479, 482, 536, 553